Clinical Pharmacy and Therapeutics

Commissioning Editor: Pauline Graham
Development Editor: Nicola Lally
Project Manager: Kerrie-Anne McKinlay
Designer/Design Direction: Kirsteen Wright
Illustration Manager: Bruce Hogarth
Illustrators: David Graham/Andrew Bezear

Clinical Pharmacy and Therapeutics

EDITED BY

Roger Walker BPharm, PhD, FRPharmS, FFPH

Professor of Pharmacy Practice,
Welsh School of Pharmacy,
Cardiff University,
Cardiff UK

and

Chief Pharmaceutical Officer,
Welsh Government,
Cardiff, UK

Cate Whittlesea BSc, MSc, PhD, MRPharmS

Senior Lecturer, Institute of Pharmaceutical Science
Kings College London,
London, UK

FIFTH EDITION

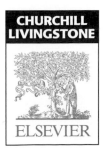

CHURCHILL LIVINGSTONE
ELSEVIER

Edinburgh London New York Oxford Philadelphia St Louis Sydney Toronto 2012

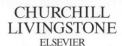

CHURCHILL
LIVINGSTONE
ELSEVIER

First edition 1994
Second edition 1999
Third edition 2003
Fourth edition 2007
Fifth edition 2012

ISBN 978-0-7020-4293-5
  Reprinted 2011, 2012 (twice)
International ISBN 978-0-7020-4294-2
  Reprinted 2012

British Library Cataloguing in Publication Data
A catalogue record for this book is available from the British Library

Library of Congress Cataloging in Publication Data
A catalog record for this book is available from the Library of Congress

Notices
Knowledge and best practice in this field are constantly changing. As new research and experience broaden our understanding, changes in research methods, professional practices, or medical treatment may become necessary.

  Practitioners and researchers must always rely on their own experience and knowledge in evaluating and using any information, methods, compounds, or experiments described herein. In using such information or methods they should be mindful of their own safety and the safety of others, including parties for whom they have a professional responsibility.

  With respect to any drug or pharmaceutical products identified, readers are advised to check the most current information provided (i) on procedures featured or (ii) by the manufacturer of each product to be administered, to verify the recommended dose or formula, the method and duration of administration, and contraindications. It is the responsibility of practitioners, relying on their own experience and knowledge of their patients, to make diagnoses, to determine dosages and the best treatment for each individual patient, and to take all appropriate safety precautions.

  To the fullest extent of the law, neither the Publisher nor the authors, contributors, or editors, assume any liability for any injury and/or damage to persons or property as a matter of products liability, negligence or otherwise, or from any use or operation of any methods, products, instructions, or ideas contained in the material herein.

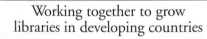

Printed in China

Preface

In both primary and secondary care the use of medicines is the most common intervention in healthcare. Medicines use, however, is not without risk. Drug selection and prescribing is increasingly complex and demanding, and undertaken as part of a multi-disciplinary process that involves pharmacists, some of whom are now prescribers in their own right, along with doctors, nurses and other members of the healthcare team. All must strive to promote safe, appropriate and cost-effective prescribing that respects patient choice and promotes adherence. This book has been written to help the reader understand and address many of these issues. It is unashamedly written from a pharmacy perspective, although we do hope those from other disciplines will also find it of use.

We have made considerable effort to update each chapter and ensure the content is relevant to current practice. Selected website addresses have been included to assist those who want to obtain further information and many references are now available electronically and this has been indicated where appropriate. However, knowledge in therapeutics progresses rapidly, changes to dose regimens and licensed indications are frequent, safety issues emerge with established drugs and new medicines appear at regular intervals. Yesterday another landmark study was published adding to, or perhaps altering, the evidence base for a specific treatment. Together with the ongoing publication of national guidelines and frameworks, the face of therapeutics is ever changing. It is therefore inevitable that some sections of this book will date more quickly than others.

In practice many licensed drugs are used 'off label' or "near label" when prescribed for a certain indication or used in a specific patient group such as children. To omit reference to these agents in the relevant chapter would leave an apparent gap in therapeutic management. As a consequence we have encouraged our authors to present details of all key drugs used along with details of the prescribed regimens even if not licensed for that specific indication. There is, however, a downside to this approach. The reader must always use this text critically and with caution. If this is done the book will serve as a valuable learning resource and help the reader understand some of the principles of therapeutics. We hope that, in some small way, this will also assist in achieving positive patient outcomes.

Roger Walker
Cate Whittlesea

Acknowledgements

In 2011, as in 1994 when the first edition was published, undergraduate and postgraduate students help sustain our enthusiasm and commitment while continuing to be the inspiration and the *raison d'etre* for this book. To all those who have provided feedback in the past, thank you. For those who would like to comment on this edition, we welcome your feedback; please contact us at walkerR@cardiff.ac.uk or cate.whittlesea@kcl.ac.uk.

We remain indebted to all authors who, through their hard work, patience and tolerance, have contributed to the fifth edition of this book. We are particularly grateful to those who have again contributed to another edition of this textbook and who strive, along with us, to produce an ever better book. To our first-time authors, we are very grateful that you agreed to contribute, that you accepted our cryptic editorial comments in good faith and still managed to submit on time. We hope that you will continue to work with us on future editions.

A textbook of this size cannot, of course, be produced without the invaluable help, support and occasional comments of numerous colleagues, particularly those within the Public Health Wales, the Welsh School of Pharmacy, Cardiff University, and the Institute of Pharmaceutical Science, King's College London. It would be invidious to name individuals who have helped us, in part for fear of offending anyone we might miss. We do, however, continue to make one exception to this rule. The administrative support from Marilyn Meecham has been invaluable. She has co-ordinated this new edition from the outset and was often called upon to present the polite face of two chastened editors. Thanks Marilyn.

It was with great sadness that in November 2010 we heard of the untimely death of Professor Steve Hudson. Steve was a friend and colleague who had a broad knowledge of clinical pharmacy and was one of the movers, shakers and thinkers central to the establishment of clinical pharmacy in the UK in the 1980's. He contributed to the first edition of this book in 1994 and his most recent update is included in the current edition. It is our loss that he will be unable to review his latest contribution in print.

Finally, and on a personal note, we would like thank our close families for their support and tolerance with our indulgence in editing this text. At times it may have appeared that everything in our lives took second place to 'the book'. We are eternally grateful for their understanding, particularly when we got our priorities in life wrong. Without the unfailing support of Ann and Alex, this book would never have materialized.

Roger Walker
Cate Whittlesea

Contributors

Alya Abdul-Wahab BSc MB BS MRCP
Dermatology Registrar, St John's Institute of Dermatology, Guys & St Thomas' NHS Trust, London, UK
57. Eczema and psoriasis

Christopher Acomb BSc MPharm MRPharmS
Clinical Pharmacy Manager (Professional Development), Pharmacy Department, St James's University Hospital, Leeds, UK
49. Anaemia

Sharon D. Andrew BSc MPharm MRPharmS
Regional Scientific Services Manager, Allergan Ltd. Marlow, Buckinghamshire, UK
55. Glaucoma

Sotiris Antoniou BPharm MSc DipMgt IPresc MRPharmS
Consultant Pharmacist, Cardiovascular Medicine, Barts and the London NHS Trust, North East London Cardiovascular and Stroke Network, London, UK
22. Arrhythmias

David Baldwin MB BS DM FRCPsych
Professor of Psychiatry, University of Southampton, Southampton, UK
28. Anxiety disorders

Catrin Barker BSc MSc PGDipClinPharm
Acting Deputy Chief Pharmacist, Pharmacy Department, Alder Hey Children's NHS Foundation Trust, Liverpool, UK
10. Paediatrics

Andrew Berrington MRCP FRCPath
Consultant Microbiologist, City Hospitals Sunderland, Sunderland, UK
35. Respiratory infections

Stephen Bleakley BPharm, MSc MCMHP
Locality Lead Pharmacist, Royal Hants Hospital, Southampton, UK
27. Insomnia
28. Anxiety disorders

David Branford PhD MRPharmS
Chief Pharmacist, Derbyshire Mental Health Services, Derby, UK
30. Schizophrenia

Geraldine Brough MB ChB FRCP
Associate Specialist in Rheumatology and Honorary Lecturer, Royal Free Hospital, London, UK
53. Rheumatoid arthritis and osteoarthritis

David J. Burn MD FRCP MA MB BS
Professor of Movement Disorder Neurology and Honorary Consultant Neurologist, Institute for Ageing and Health, Newcastle University, Newcastle upon Tyne, UK
32. Parkinson's disease

Susan Calvert FRCOG
Consultant Obstetrician and Gynaecologist, Bradford Royal Infirmary, Bradford, UK
45. Menstrual cycle disorders
46. Menopause

Laura Cameron BPharm DipPharmPractice MRPharmS
Haematology Pharmacist, Guy's & St Thomas' NHS Foundation Trust, London, UK
51. Lymphomas

Neil J.B. Carbarns BSc MB ChB FRCPath
Consultant Medical Microbiologist, Aneurin Bevan Health Board, Nevill Hall Hospital, Abergavenny, Wales, UK
36. Urinary tract infections

Paul Cockwell MB BCh PhD MRCP FRCP
Consultant Nephrologist, Queen Elizabeth Hospital, Birmingham, UK
17. Acute kidney injury
18. Chronic kidney disease and end-stage renal disease

Jonathan Cooke MPharm PhD MRPharmS
Director of Research and Development, Clinical Director of Pharmacy and Medicines Management, School of Pharmacy and Pharmaceutical Sciences, Faculty of Medical and Human Sciences, University of Manchester, South Manchester University Hospitals NHS Trust, Wythenshawe Hospital, Manchester, UK; Visiting Professor in the Infectious Diseases and Immunity Section, Division of Infectious Diseases, Department of Medicine, Imperial College, London, UK
8. Pharmacoeconomics

Allan Cosslett BPharm, MRPharmS
Lecturer/Disability Officer/Deputy Admissions Officer
& Director of Undergraduate Studies, Welsh School of
Pharmacy, Cardiff University, Cardiff, UK
7. Parenteral nutrition

Anthony Cox Bsc(Hons) DipClinPharm PhD MRPharmS
Lecturer in Clinical Therapeutics, Pharmacy Practice
Group, Aston University, Birmingham, UK
5. Adverse drug reactions

Daniel Creamer BSc MD FRCP
Consultant Dermatologist, Kings College Hospital NHS
Foundation Trust, London, UK
56. Drug-induced skin disorders

Duncan Cripps BPharm PGDipHospPharm MEd
Education and Training Pharmacist, Plymouth Hospitals
NHS Trust, Plymouth, UK
25. Asthma
26. Chronic obstructive pulmonary disease

Sarah Cripps BPharm MSc MRPharmS (IPresc)
Gastroenterology Pharmacist, Oxford Radcliffe Hospitals
NHS Trust, Oxford, UK
13. Inflammatory bowel disease

Amy Cunnington MPharm Dip Pharm Prac
Education & Training Pharmacist, Chapel Allerton
Hospital, Leeds, UK
54. Gout and hyperuricaemia

J. Graham Davies BPharm MSc PhD FRPharmS
Professor of Clinical Pharmacy and Therapeutics, Kings
College London, London, UK
1. Clinical pharmacy process

Nemesha Desai MBBS BSC MRCP PGCHE
Consultant Dermatologist, St John's Institute of
Dermatology, Guys & St Thomas' NHS Trust,
London, UK
57. Eczema and psoriasis

Soraya Dhillon MBE BPharm PhD FRPharmS
Foundation Professor Head, School of Pharmacy,
University of Hertfordshire, Hatfield, UK
31. Epilepsy

Tobias Dreischulte MSc MRPharmS
Research Pharmacist, University of Dundee, Dundee, UK
21. Chronic heart failure

Alexander Dyker MBChB Bsc MSc MD FRCP(Glasgow)
Consultant in Medicine, Clinical Pharmacology
and Stroke Medicine, Newcastle Hospitals, Newcastle
upon Tyne, UK
19. Hypertension

Clive Edwards BPharm PhD MRPharmS FICR(Hon)
Formerly Prescribing Adviser, North Tyneside Primary Care
Trust, Newcastle upon Tyne, UK
6. Laboratory data

Bridget Featherstone BSc DipClinPharm IP
Lead Pharmacist for Transplantation, Addenbrooke's NHS
Trust, Cambridge, UK
15. Adverse effects of drugs on the liver

Martin Fisher MB BS BSc FRCP
Consultant Physician HIV/AIDS, Brighton and Sussex
University Hospitals NHS Trust, Brighton, UK
41. HIV infection

Ray Fitzpatrick BSc PhD FRPharmS
Clinical Director of Pharmacy, Royal Wolverhampton
Hospitals NHS Trust; Professor of Clinical Pharmacy,
Wolverhampton University, Wolverhampton, UK
3. Practical pharmacokinetics

Kevin P. Gibbs BPharm, DipClinPharm Cert Health Econ,
PgC Evidence-based Hth Care PgC Law & Ethics MRPharmS
Clinical Pharmacy Manager, Bristol Royal Infirmary,
Bristol, UK
25. Asthma
26. Chronic obstructive pulmonary disease

Peter Golightly
Director, West Midlands and Trent Regional Medicines
Information Centre, Good Hope Hospital NHS Trust,
West Midlands, UK
47. Drugs in pregnancy and lactation

Elena Grant BPharm MSc MRPharmS
Senior Medicines Information Pharmacist, West Midlands
Medicines Information Centre, Good Hope Hospital, Heart
of England NHS Foundation Trust, West Midlands, UK
47. Drugs in pregnancy and lactation

James W. Gray MRCP FRCPath
Consultant Microbiologist, The Birmingham Children's
Hospital NHS Trust, Diana, Princess of Wales Children's
Hospital, Birmingham, UK
37. Gastro-intestinal infections
38. Infective meningitis

Elizabeth Hackett BSc (hons) MSc
Principal Pharmacist for Diabetes, University Hospitals
Leicester, Leicester, UK
44. Diabetes mellitus

Keith Harding MB ChB FRCGP FRCP FRCS
Sub Dean of Innovation & Engagement / Head of Section
of Wound Healing, Department of Dermatology & Wound
Healing, Cardiff University, Cardiff, UK
58. Wounds

Susanna Harwood BPharm(hons) DipClinPharm IPresc
Pharmacist, University Hospital of Wales, Cardiff, UK
7. Parenteral nutrition

Tina Hawkins Bsc(Hons) ClinDipPharm IPresc
Advanced Clinical Pharmacist, Chapel Allerton
Hospital Leeds Teaching Hospital NHS Trust,
Leeds, UK
54. Gout and hyperuricaemia

Gregory J. Hobbs BMBS FRCA FFPMRCA
Consultant in Pain Medicine, Nottingham University
Hospitals NHS Trust, Nottingham, UK
33. Pain

Samantha Holloway MSc CertEd(FE) RN
Senior Professional Tutor / Course Director, Dept of
Dermatology and Wound Healing, Cardiff University,
Cardiff, UK
58. Wounds

Philip Howard BPharm(Hons) DipClinPharm IPresc MRPharmS
Consultant Antimicrobial Pharmacist, Leeds Teaching
Hospital NHS Trust, Leeds, UK
*39. Surgical site infection and antimicrobial
prophylaxis*

Steve A. Hudson MPharm BPharm FRPharmS
Deceased
Professor of Pharmaceutical Care, Strathclyde
Institute of Biomedical Sciences, Glasgow, UK
21. Chronic heart failure

Graham Jackson MA MB BS FRCP FRCPath MD
Consultant Haematologist, Freeman Hospital,
Newcastle upon Tyne, UK
50. Leukaemia

Stephen Jackson MA, FRCP
Consultant, Leicester General Hospital, Leicester, UK
44. Diabetes mellitus

Gail Jones MD MRCP FRCPath
Consultant Haematologist, Freeman Hospital, Newcastle
upon Tyne, UK
50. Leukaemia

Patrick T.F. Kennedy MB BCh BAO BMedSci MRCP MD
Senior Lecturer & Consultant Hepatologist, Barts and The
London School of Medicine, London, UK
16. Liver disease

Moira Kinnear Bsc MSc ADCPT MRPharmS
Head of NHS Lothian Pharmacy Education, Research
and Development, Western General Hospital, Edinburgh;
Lecturer in Clinical Practice, University of Strathclyde,
Glasgow, UK
12. Peptic ulcer disease

Roger Knaggs BSc BMedSci PhD MRPharmS
Specialist Pharmacist in Anaesthesia and Pain Management,
Queens Medical Centre, Nottingham, UK
33. Pain

Andrzej Kostrzewski MSc MMedEd PhD MRPharmS FHEA
Academic Lead for Clinical Development, University of
Herefordshire, Hatfield, UK
3. Practical pharmacokinetics

Janet Krska BSc PhD MRPharmS
Professor of Pharmacy Practice, School of Pharmacy and
Biomolecular Sciences, Liverpool John Moores University,
Liverpool, UK
5. Adverse drug reactions

Alan Lamont BMedSci(Hons) MBChB FRCR FRCP (Edinburgh)
Consultant Oncologist, Colchester General Hospital,
Essex, UK
52. Solid tumours

Heather Leake Date BSc MSc IPresc MRPharmS
Consultant Pharmacist HIV/Sexual Health, Brighton and
Sussex University Hospitals NHS Trust, Brighton, UK
and Honorary Senior Lecturer, University of Brighton,
Brighton, UK
41. HIV infection

Catherine Loughran BPharm MSc MRPharmS(IPresc)
Lead Pharmacist Haematology, Leicester Royal Infirmary,
Leicester, UK
51. Lymphomas

John J. McAnaw BSc PhD MRPharmS
Head of Pharmacy, NHS 24; Honorary Lecturer in Clinical
Practice, Strathclyde Institute of Pharmacy & Biomedical
Sciences, Glasgow, UK
21. Chronic heart failure

Duncan McRobbie MSc MRPharmS
Associate Chief Pharmacist, Clinical Services and Lead
Cardiac Pharmacist,
Guy's and St Thomas' Hospital NHS Foundation Trust,
London, UK
1. Clinical pharmacy process
20. Coronary Heart disease

John Marriott PhD BSc MRPharmS
Professor of Clinical Pharmacy, School of Clinical and
Experimental Medicine, University of Birmingham,
Birmingham, UK
17. Acute kidney injury
18. Chronic kidney disease and end-stage renal disease

Helen Marlow BPharm(Hons) MRPharmS Dip Clin Pharm
Visiting Lecturer, Non-Medical Prescribing, Kings College
London, London, UK
2. Prescribing

Kay Marshall BPharm PhD FRPharmS MBA
Head of the Bradford School of Pharmacy, University of Bradford, Bradford, UK
45. Menstrual cycle disorders
46. Menopause

Emma Mason BSc MB ChB MRCP
Honorary Senior Lecturer in Palliative Medicine and Pharmacology, University College of Medicine, Cardiff, UK
34. Nausea and vomiting

Maria Martinez MPharm(hons) DipClinPharm MSc MRPharmS
Renal Transplant, Nephrology and Urology Specialist Pharmacist, University Hospitals of Leicester, Leicester, UK
48. Prostate disease

Manjusha Narayanan MBBS, MD, FRCPath
Consultant Microbiologist, Royal Victoria Infirmary, Newcastle upon Tyne, UK
42. Fungal infections

Lika K. Nehaul LRCPI LRCSI MSc FFPH
Consultant in Communicable Disease Control, National Public Health Service for Wales, Mamhilad House, Pontypool, UK
40. Tuberculosis

Anthony J Nunn BPharm, FRPharmS, HonFRCPCH
Associate Director, NIHR Medicines for Children Research Network, University of Liverpool, UK.
10. Paediatrics

John O'Grady MD FRCPI
Consultant Hepatologist, Institute of Liver Studies, King's College Hospital, London, UK
16. Liver disease

Mike Page MD FRCP
Consultant Physician, Royal Glamorgan Hospital, Llantrisant, Wales, UK
43. Thyroid and parathyroid disorders

Dee Pang BPharm
Principal Pharmacist - Medicine, Royal Free Hospital, London, UK
53. Rheumatoid arthritis and osteoarthritis

Peter Pratt BSc MPhil MRPharmS
Chief Pharmacist, Community Health Sheffield, Michael Carlisle Centre, Sheffield, UK
29. Affective disorders

Ali Robb MRCP FRCPath
Consultant Microbiologist, Newcastle upon Tyne Hospitals, Newcastle upon Tyne, UK
35. Respiratory infections

Philip A. Routledge OBE MD FRCP FRCPE FRCGP(Hon) FBTS
Professor, Section of Pharmacology, Therapeutics and Toxicology, Cardiff University, Cardiff, UK
23. Thrombosis
34. Nausea and vomiting

Paula Russell BA Mod (Chem) MApplSc MRPharmS
Principal Pharmacist, Regional Drugs and Therapeutics Centre, Newcastle upon Tyne, UK
47. Drugs in pregnancy and lactation

Paul Rutter BPharm PhD MRPharmS
Principal Lecturer, Department of Pharmacy, University of Wolverhampton, Wolverhampton, UK
14. Constipation and diarrhoea

Josemir W. Sander MD MRCP PhD
Professor of Neurology, Queen Square, London, UK
31. Epilepsy

Robyn Sanderson MPharm(Hons), PG Dip Pharm Practice, MRPharmS
Specialist Pharmacist, St James University Hospital, Leeds, UK
49. Anaemia

Jonathan Sandoe MB ChB, PhD, FRCPath
Consultant Microbiologist, Leeds Teaching Hospitals NHS Trust, Leeds, UK
39. Surgical site infection and antimicrobial prophylaxis

Mini Satheesh MPharm, MSc(Clin.Pharm), MRPharmS(IPresc)
Renal and Urology Specialist Pharmacist, University Hospitals Leicester, Leicester, UK
48. Prostate disease

Hamsaraj G.M. Shetty BSc MB BS FRCP(London), FRCP(Edin)
Consultant Physician & Honorary Senior Lecturer, University Hospital of Wales & Cardiff University, Cardiff, UK
11. Geriatrics
23. Thrombosis

Michele Sie BPharm MSc IPresc MCMHP
Consultant Pharmacist, St Bernards Hospital, West London Mental Health NHS Trust, London, UK
27. Insomnia

Simon Sporton BSc MD FRCP
Consultant Cardiologist, Bart's and The London NHS Trust, London, UK
22. Arrhythmias

Stephanie Stringer MBChB, MRCP
Clinical Fellow in Nephrology, Queen Elizabeth Hospital, Birmingham, UK
17. Acute kidney injury
18. Chronic kidney disease and end-stage renal disease

Lucy C. Titcomb BSc MRPharmS MCPP
Lead Ophthalmic Pharmacist, Birmingham and Midland
Eye Centre, Birmingham, UK
55. Glaucoma

Ruben Thanacoody MD FRCP(Edin)
Consultant Physician, Royal Victoria Infirmary; Honorary
Clinical Senior Lecturer, Institute of Cellular Medicine,
Newcastle University, Newcastle-upon-Tyne, UK
4. Drug interactions

Sean Turner BPharm MSc DipClinPharm
Director of Pharmacy, Children, Youth and Women's
Health Service, Adelaide, South Australia, Australia
10. Paediatrics

Roger Walker BPharm PhD FRPharmS FFPH
Professor of Pharmacy Practice, Welsh School of Pharmacy,
Cardiff University; Consultant in Pharmaceutical Public
Health, Public Health Wales, Cardiff, UK
24. Dyslipidaemia

Sarah Walsh MB BCh BAO BMedSci MRCP
Consultant Dermatologist, King's College Hospital,
London, UK
56. Drug-induced skin disorders

Martin P. Ward Platt MB ChB MD FRCP FRCPCH
Consultant Paediatrician and Honorary Clinical Reader in
Neonatal and Paediatric Medicine, Royal Victoria Infirmary,
Newcastle upon Tyne, UK
9. Neonates

David Webb BPharm MSc MRPharmS HonFCPP
Director, East & South East England Specialist Pharmacy
Services; Visiting Professor, School of Pharmacy, University
of London, London, UK
1. Clinical pharmacy process

Cate Whittlesea BSc (Pharmacy) MSc Econ PhD MRPharmS
Senior Lecturer Pharmacy Practice, Kings College London,
London, UK
2. Prescribing

Helen Williams BPharm(Hons) PGDip(Cardiol) MRPharmS IPresc
Consultant Pharmacist for Cardiovascular Disease,
Southwark Health and Social Care, London, UK
24. Dyslipidaemia

Netty Wood DipPharmPract, MRPharmS (IPresc)
Lead Pharmacist, Essex Cancer Network, Essex, UK
52. Solid tumours

Ken Woodhouse MD FRCP FHEA
Professor of Medicine and Geriatric Medicine, School
of Medicine, Cardiff University, Cardiff, UK
11. Geriatrics

Hilary Wynne MA MD FRCP
Consultant Physician, Freeman Hospital, Newcastle upon
Tyne, UK
6. Laboratory data

Laura Yates MBChB DRCOG MRCPCH PhD
Head of Teratology, UK Teratology Information Service,
Newcastle upon Tyne, UK
47. Drugs in pregnancy and lactation

Contents

Section 1 General 1

1. **Clinical pharmacy process** 2
    D.G. Webb, J.G. Davies, D. McRobbie

2. **Prescribing** 14
    H. Marlow, C. Whittlesea

3. **Practical pharmacokinetics** 32
    R. Fitzpatrick, A. Kostrzewski

4. **Drug interactions** 50
    H.K.R. Thanacoody

5. **Adverse drug reactions** 62
    J. Krska, A.R. Cox

6. **Laboratory data** 76
    H.A. Wynne, C. Edwards

7. **Parenteral nutrition** 96
    S.J. Harwood, A.G. Cosslett

8. **Pharmacoeconomics** 116
    J. Cooke

Section 2 Life stages 123

9. **Neonates** 124
    M.P. Ward Platt

10. **Paediatrics** 132
    C. Barker, A.J. Nunn, S. Turner

11. **Geriatrics** 149
    H.G.M. Shetty, K. Woodhouse

Section 3 Therapeutics 161

12. **Peptic ulcer disease** 162
    M. Kinnear

13. **Inflammatory bowel disease** 185
    S.E. Cripps

14. **Constipation and diarrhoea** 209
    P. Rutter

15. **Adverse effects of drugs on the liver** 222
    B.E. Featherstone

16. **Liver disease** 238
    P. Kennedy, J.G. O'Grady

17. **Acute kidney injury** 255
    P. Cockwell, S. Stringer, J. Marriott

18. **Chronic kidney disease and end-stage renal disease** 272
    J. Marriott, P. Cockwell, S. Stringer

19. **Hypertension** 295
    A.G. Dyker

20. **Coronary heart disease** 312
    D. McRobbie

21. **Chronic heart failure** 333
    S.A. Hudson, J. McAnaw, T. Dreischulte

22. **Arrhythmias** 354
    S. Sporton, S. Antoniou

23. **Thrombosis** 376
    P.A. Routledge, H.G.M. Shetty

24. **Dyslipidaemia** 389
    R. Walker, H. Williams

25. **Asthma** 412
    K.P. Gibbs, D. Cripps

26. **Chronic obstructive pulmonary disease** 431
    D. Cripps, K.P. Gibbs

27. **Insomnia** 446
    S. Bleakley, M. Sie

28. **Anxiety disorders** 454
    S. Bleakley, D. Baldwin

29. **Affective disorders** 465
    J.P. Pratt

30. **Schizophrenia** 479
    D. Branford

31. **Epilepsy** 489
    J.W. Sander, S. Dhillon

32. **Parkinson's disease** 507
    D.J. Burn

33. **Pain** 519
    R.D. Knaggs, G.J. Hobbs

34. **Nausea and vomiting** 535
    E. Mason, P.A. Routledge

35. **Respiratory infections** 545
    A. Robb, A.W. Berrington

36. **Urinary tract infections** 561
    N.J.B. Carbarns

37. **Gastro-intestinal infections** 573
    J.W. Gray

38. **Infective meningitis** 584
    J.W. Gray

39. **Surgical site infection and antimicrobial prophylaxis** 596
    P. Howard, J.A.T. Sandoe

40. **Tuberculosis** 608
    L.K. Nehaul

41. **HIV infection** 621
    H. Leake Date, M. Fisher

42. **Fungal infections** 654
    M. Narayanan

43. **Thyroid and parathyroid disorders** 669
    M.D. Page

44. **Diabetes mellitus** 685
    Elizabeth A. Hackett, Stephen N.J. Jackson

45. **Menstrual cycle disorders** 711
    K. Marshall, S. Calvert

46. **Menopause** 725
    K. Marshall, S. Calvert

47. **Drugs in pregnancy and lactation** 739
    P. Russell, L. Yates, E. Grant, P. Golightly

48. **Prostate disease** 753
    M. Martinez, M. Satheesh

49. **Anaemia** 769
    C. Acomb, R. Sanderson

50. **Leukaemia** 786
    G. Jackson, G. Jones

51. **Lymphomas** 803
    L. Cameron, C. Loughran

52. **Solid tumours** 818
    N. Wood, A. Lamont

53. **Rheumatoid arthritis and osteoarthritis** 832
    D.J. Pang, G.M. Brough

54. **Gout and hyperuricaemia** 848
    T. Hawkins, A. Cunnington

55. **Glaucoma** 861
    L.C. Titcomb, S.D. Andrew

56. **Drug-induced skin disorders** 880
    S. Walsh, D. Creamer

57. **Eczema and psoriasis** 893
    A. Abdul-Wahab, N. Desai

58. **Wounds** 910
    S. Holloway, K. Harding

Section 4 Appendices 927

Appendix 1 **Medical abbreviations** 928

Appendix 2 **Glossary** 938

Index 944

SECTION 1

GENERAL

1 Clinical pharmacy process

D. G. Webb, J. G. Davies and D. McRobbie

Key points

- Clinical pharmacy comprises a set of functions that promote the safe, effective and economic use of medicines for individual patients.
- The emergence of clinical pharmacy has allowed pharmacists to shift from a product-oriented role towards direct engagement with patients and the problems they encounter with medicines.
- The practice of clinical pharmacy is generally an essential component of pharmaceutical care.
- Pharmaceutical care is a co-operative, patient-centred system for achieving specific and positive patient outcomes from the responsible provision of medicines.
- The three key elements of the care process are patient assessment, determining the care plan and evaluating the outcome.
- The ability to consult with patients is a key process in the delivery of pharmaceutical care and requires regular review and development regardless of experience.
- The clinical pharmacy process has been incorporated into a professional development framework that can be used to enhance skills and knowledge.

Clinical pharmacy, unlike the discipline of pharmacy, is a comparatively recent and variably implemented form of practice. It encourages pharmacists and support staff to shift their focus from a solely product-oriented role towards more direct engagement with patients and the problems they encounter with medicines. Over the past 20 years there has been an emerging consensus that the practice of clinical pharmacy itself should grow from a collection of patient-related functions to a process in which all actions are undertaken with the intention of achieving explicit outcomes for the patient. In doing so, clinical pharmacy moves to embrace the philosophy of pharmaceutical care (Hepler and Strand, 1990).

This chapter provides a practical framework within which a knowledge and understanding of therapeutics and practice can be best utilised. It describes a pragmatic approach to applying both the principles of pharmaceutical care and the specific skills of clinical pharmacy in a manner that does not depend on the setting of the practitioner or patient.

Development of clinical practice in pharmacy

The emergence of clinical pharmacy as a form of practice has been attributed to the poor medicines control systems that existed in hospitals during the early 1960s (Cousins and Luscombe, 1995). Although provoked by similar hospital-centred problems, the nature of the professional response differed between the USA and the UK.

In the USA, the approach was to adopt unit dose dispensing and pursue decentralisation of pharmacy services. In the UK, the unification of the prescription and the administration record meant this document needed to remain on the hospital ward and required the pharmacist to visit the ward to order medicines. Clinical pharmacy thereby emerged from the presence of pharmacists in these patient areas and their interest in promoting safer medicines use. This was initially termed 'ward pharmacy' but participation in medical ward rounds in the late 1970s signalled the transition to clinical pharmacy.

Medication safety may have been the spur but clinical pharmacy in the 1980s grew because of its ability to promote cost-effective medicines used in hospitals. This role was recognised by the UK government, which, in 1988, endorsed the implementation of clinical pharmacy services to secure value for money from medicines. Awareness that support depended, to an extent, on the quantification of actions and cost savings led several groups to develop ways of measuring pharmacists' clinical interventions. Coding systems were necessary to aggregate large amounts of data in a reliable manner and many of these drew upon the eight steps (Table 1.1) of the drug use process (DUP) indicators (Hutchinson et al., 1986).

The data collected from these early studies revealed that interventions had very high physician acceptance rates, were made most commonly at the 'select regimen' and 'need for drug' stages of the DUP, and were influenced by hospital ward type (intensive care and paediatrics having the highest rates), pharmacist grade (rates increasing with grade) and time spent on wards (Barber et al., 1997).

Despite the level of activity that intervention monitoring revealed, together with evidence of cost containment and a broadly supportive health care system, frustrations began to appear. These, in part, stemmed from a lack of certainty about the fundamental purpose of clinical pharmacy and

Table 1.1 Drug use process (DUP) indicators

DUP stage	Action
Need for a drug	Ensure there is an appropriate indication for each drug and that all medical problems are addressed therapeutically
Select drug	Select and recommend the most appropriate drug based upon the ability to reach therapeutic goals, with consideration of patient variables, formulary status and cost of therapy
Select regimen	Select the most appropriate drug regimen for accomplishing the desired therapeutic goals at the least cost without diminishing effectiveness or causing toxicity
Provide drug	Facilitate the dispensing and supply process so that drugs are accurately prepared, dispensed in ready-to-administer form and delivered to the patient on a timely basis
Drug administration	Ensure that appropriate devices and techniques are used for drug administration
Monitor drug therapy	Monitor drug therapy for effectiveness or adverse effects in order to determine whether to maintain, modify or discontinue
Counsel patient	Counsel and educate the patient or caregiver about the patient's therapy to ensure proper use of medicines
Evaluate effectiveness	Evaluate the effectiveness of the patient's drug therapy by reviewing all the previous steps of the drug use process and taking appropriate steps to ensure that the therapeutic goals are achieved

Table 1.2 Definitions of clinical pharmacy, pharmaceutical care and medicines management

Term	Definition
Clinical pharmacy	Clinical pharmacy comprises a set of functions that promote the safe, effective and economic use of medicines for individual patients. Clinical pharmacy process requires the application of specific knowledge of pharmacology, pharmacokinetics, pharmaceutics and therapeutics to patient care
Pharmaceutical care	Pharmaceutical care is a co-operative, patient-centred system for achieving specific and positive patient outcomes from the responsible provision of medicines. The practice of clinical pharmacy is an essential component in the delivery of pharmaceutical care
Medicines management	Medicines management encompasses the way in which medicines are selected, procured, delivered, prescribed, administered and reviewed to optimise the contribution that medicines make to producing informed and desired outcomes of patient care

from tensions between the drive towards specialisation in clinical pharmacy and the need to improve services of a more general level in hospitals and other care settings.

Pharmaceutical care

The need to focus on outcomes of medicines use rather than dwelling only on the functions of clinical pharmacy became apparent (Hepler and Strand, 1990). The launch of pharmaceutical care as the 'responsible provision of drug therapy for the purpose of achieving definite outcomes that improve a patient's quality of life' was a landmark in the topography of pharmacy practice. In reality, this was an incremental step forward, rather than a revolutionary leap, since the foundations of pharmaceutical care as 'the determination of drug needs for a given individual and the provision not only of the drug required but also the necessary services to assure optimally safe and effective therapy' had been established previously (Brodie et al., 1980).

The delivery of pharmaceutical care is dependent on the practice of clinical pharmacy but the key feature of care is that the practitioner takes responsibility for a patient's drug-related needs and is held accountable for that commitment. None of the definitions of pharmaceutical care is limited by reference to a specific professional group. Although pharmacists and pharmacy support staff would expect to, and clearly can, play a central role in pharmaceutical care, it is essentially a co-operative system that embraces the contribution of other professionals and patients (Table 1.2). The avoidance of factionalism has enabled pharmaceutical care to permeate community pharmacy, particularly in Europe, in a way that clinical pharmacy and its bedside connotations did not. It also anticipated health care policy in which certain functions, such as the prescribing of medicines, have been extended beyond their traditional professional origins to be undertaken by those trained and identified to be competent to do so.

Medication-related problems

When the outcome of medicines use is not optimal, a classification (Box 1.1) for identifying the underlying medication-related problem (MRP) has been proposed (Hepler and

Box 1.1 Categories of medication-related problems

Untreated indication
Treatment without indication
Improper drug selection
Too little drug
Too much drug
Non-compliance
Adverse drug reaction
Drug interaction

Strand, 1990). Some MRPs are associated with significant morbidity and mortality. Preventable medication-related hospital admissions in the USA have a prevalence of 4.3%, indicating that gains in public health from improved medicines management would be sizeable (Winterstein et al., 2002). In the UK too, preventable medication-related morbidity has been associated with 4.3% of admissions to a medical unit. In nearly all cases, the underlying MRP was linked to prescribing, monitoring or adherence (Howard et al., 2003).

In prospective studies, up to 28% of accident and emergency department visits have been identified as medication related, of which 70% are deemed preventable (Zed, 2005). Again, the most frequently cited causes were non-adherence and inappropriate prescribing and monitoring. The cost of drug-related morbidity and mortality in the US ambulatory care (outpatient) population was estimated in 2000 to be $177 billion. Hospital admission accounted for 70% of total costs (Ernst and Grizzle, 2001). In England, adverse drug reactions (ADRs) have been identified as the cause of 6.5% of hospital admissions for patients over 16 years of age. The median bed stay with patients admitted with an ADR was 8 days representing 4% of bed capacity. The projected annual cost to the NHS was £466 million, the equivalent of seven 800-bed hospitals occupied by patients admitted with an ADR (Pirmohamed et al., 2004).

The rate for adverse drug events among hospital inpatients in the USA has been quantified as 6.5 per 100 admissions. Overall, 28% of events were judged preventable, rising to 42% of those classified as life-threatening or serious (Bates et al., 1995). The direct cost of medication errors, defined as preventable events that may cause or lead to inappropriate medicines use or harm, in NHS hospitals has been estimated to lie between £200 and £400 million per year. To this should be added the costs arising from litigation (DH, 2004).

The scale of the misadventure that these findings reveal, coupled with increasing concerns about the costs of drug therapy, creates an opportunity for a renaissance in clinical pharmacy practice, providing that it realigns strongly with patient safety, cost-effectiveness and prevention of ill health. In practice, community pharmacists may be uniquely placed to help reduce the level of medication-related morbidity in primary care by virtue of their accessibility and existing relationships.

Benefits of pharmaceutical care

The ability to demonstrate that clinical pharmacy practice improves patient outcomes is of great importance to the pharmaceutical care model. In the USA, for example, pharmacists'

participation in physician ward rounds has been shown to reduce adverse drug events by 78% and 66% in general medical (Kucukarslan et al., 2003) and intensive care settings (Leape et al., 1999), respectively. A study covering 1029 US hospitals was the first to indicate that both centrally based and patient-specific clinical pharmacy services are associated with reduced mortality rates (Bond et al., 1999). The services involved were medicines information, clinical research performed by pharmacists, active pharmacist participation in resuscitation teams and pharmacists undertaking admission medication histories.

In the UK, the focus has been also on prevention and management of medicine-related problems. Recognition that many patients either fail to benefit or experience unwanted effects from their medicines has elicited two types of response from the pharmacy profession. The first response has been to put in place, and make use of, a range of postgraduate initiatives and programmes to meet the developmental needs of pharmacists working in clinical settings. The second has been the re-engineering of pharmaceutical services to introduce schemes for medicines management at an organisational level. These have ranged from specific initiatives to target identified areas of medication risk, such as pharmacist involvement in anticoagulation services, to more general approaches where the intention is to ensure consistency of medicines use, particularly across care interfaces. Medicines reconciliation on hospital admission ensures that medicines prescribed to in-patients correspond to those that the patient was taking prior to admission. Guidance in the UK recommends that medicines reconciliation should be part of standard care and that pharmacists should be involved as soon as possible after the patient has been admitted (NICE and NPSA, 2007). Medicines reconciliation has been defined as:

• Collecting information on medication history using the most recent and accurate sources of information to create a full, and current, list of medicines;
• Verifying this list against the hospital drug chart and ensuring that any discrepancies are identified and acted upon;
• Documenting and communicating any changes, omissions or discrepancies.

This process requires the name of medicines, dosage, frequency and route of administration to be established for all medicines taken prior to admission. The information collected as part of medicines reconciliation is a pre-requisite for medication review, which is a process which considers the appropriateness of treatment and the patient's medication-taking behaviour.

Pharmaceutical consultation

Structured postgraduate education has served to improve the knowledge of clinical pharmacists but fully achieving the goals of pharmaceutical care has proved more challenging. Part of the difficulty has been the requirement to place the patient at the heart of the system, rather than being a relatively passive recipient of drug therapy and associated information. To deliver pharmaceutical care requires more than scientific expertise. It mandates a system that describes the role and responsibilities of the pharmacist and provides the necessary infrastructure to support them in this role and, secondly, a clear process by which the pharmacist can deliver their contribution to patient care.

Pharmaceutical care is predicated on a patient-centred approach to identifying, preventing or resolving medicine-related problems. Central to this aim is the need to establish a therapeutic relationship. This relationship must be a partnership in which the pharmacist works with the patient to resolve medication-related issues in line with the patient's wishes, expectations and priorities. Table 1.3 summarises the three key elements of the care process (Cipolle et al., 1998). Research in chronic diseases has shown that self-management is promoted when patients more fully participate in the goal-setting and planning aspects of their care (Sevick et al., 2007). These are important aspects to consider when pharmacists consult with patients. In community pharmacy, one approach to help patients used their medicines more effectively is medicines use review (MUR). This uses the skills of pharmacists to help patients understand how their medicines should be used, why they take them and to identify any problems patients have in relation to their medicines, providing feedback to the prescriber if necessary. Two goals of MUR are to improve the adherence of patients to prescribed medicines and to reduce medicines wastage.

Clinical guidance on medicines adherence emphasises the importance of patient involvement in decisions about medicines (NICE, 2009).

Recommendations include that health care professionals should:

- adapt their consultation style to the needs of individual patients
- consider any factors which may affect patients' involvement in the consultation
- establish the most effective way of communicating with each patient
- encourage patients to ask about their condition and treatment
- be aware that consultation skills can be improved to enhance patient involvement.

Medicines-taking behaviour

The need for a care process which ensures that the patient is involved at all stages has become clearer as the extent of non-adherence has been revealed. Significant proportions (between 30% and 50%) of patients with chronic conditions do not take their prescribed medicines as directed. Many factors are thought to influence a patient's decision to adhere to a pre-scribed regimen. These include the characteristics of the disease and the treatment used to manage it, the patient's beliefs about their illness and their medicines, as well as the quality of the interaction between the patient and health care practitioner. Non-adherence can be categorised broadly into two types: intentional and unintentional. Unintentional non-adherence may be associated with physical or sensory barriers to taking medicines, for example, not being able to swallow or unable to read the labels, forgetfulness or poor comprehension. Traditionally, pharmacists have played a key role in helping patients overcome these types of problems, but have been less active in identifying and resolving intentional non-adherence.

Intentional (or deliberate) non-adherence may be due to a number of factors. Recent work in health psychology has shaped our understanding of how patients perceive health and illness and why they often decide not to take their medicines. When people receive information about illness and its treatment, it is processed in accordance with their own belief systems. Often patients' perceptions are not in tune with the medical reality and when this occurs, taking medicines may not make sense to the individual. For example, a patient diagnosed with hypertension may view the condition as one that is caused by stress and, during periods of lower stress, may not take their prescribed medicines (Baumann and Leventhal, 1985). Consequently, a patient holding this view of hypertension may be at increased risk of experiencing an adverse outcome such as a stroke.

More recent research has shown that patient beliefs about the necessity of the prescribed medication and concerns about the potential long-term effects have a strong influence on medicines-taking behaviour (Horne, 2001). However, a patient's beliefs about the benefits and risks of medicines are rarely explored during consultation, despite evidence of an association between non-adherence and the patient's satisfaction with the consultation process adopted by practitioners (Ley, 1988).

Consultation process

There are several comprehensive accounts of the functions required to satisfy each stage of the DUP, but few go on to explore how the pharmacist might create a therapeutic relationship with their patient. The ability of a pharmacist to consult effectively is fundamental to pharmaceutical care and this includes establishing a platform for achieving adherence/concordance. Nurturing a relationship with the patient is essential to understanding their medication-related needs.

Descriptions of pharmaceutical consultation have been confined largely to the use of mnemonics such as WWHAM, AS METTHOD and ENCORE (Box 1.2). These approaches

Table 1.3	Key elements of the care process
Element	Purpose
Assessment	The main goal is to establish a full medication history and highlight actual and potential drug-related problems
Care plan	This should clearly state the goals to optimise care and the responsibilities of both the pharmacist and the patient in attaining the stated goals
Evaluation	This reviews progress against the stated patient outcomes

provide the pharmacist with a rigid structure to use when questioning patients about their symptoms but, although useful, serve to make the symptom or disease the focus of the consultation rather than the patient. A common misconception is that health care professionals who possess good communication skills are also able to consult effectively with patients; this relationship will not hold if there is a failure to grasp the essential components of consultation technique. Research into patients' perceptions of their illness and treatment has demonstrated that they are more likely to adhere to their medication regimen, and be more satisfied with the consultation, if their views about illness and treatment have been taken into account and the risks and benefits of treatment discussed. The mnemonic approach to consultation does not address adequately the complex interaction that may take place between a patient and a health care practitioner.

Undertaking a pharmaceutical consultation can be considered as a series of four interlinked phases, each with a goal and set of competencies (Table 1.4). These phases follow a problem-solving pattern, embrace relevant aspects of adherence research and attempt to involve the patient at each stage in the process. For effective consultation, the practitioner also needs to draw upon a range of communication behaviours (Box 1.3). This approach serves to integrate the agendas of both patient and pharmacist. It provides the vehicle for agreeing on the issues to be addressed and the responsibilities accepted by each party in achieving the desired outcomes.

The ability to consult with patients is a key process in the delivery of pharmaceutical care and consequently requires regular review and development, regardless of experience. To ensure these core skills are developed, individuals should use trigger questions to prompt reflection on their approach to consulting (Box 1.4).

Box 1.2 Mnemonics used in the pharmacy consultation process

WWHAM
Who is it for?
What are the symptoms?
How long has it been going on?
Action taken?
Medicines taken?

AS METTHOD
Age of the patient?
Self or for someone else?
Medicines being taken?
Exactly what do you mean (by the symptom)?
Time and duration of the symptom
Taken any action (medicine or seen the doctor)?
History of any disease?
Other symptoms?
Doing anything to alleviate or worsen the symptom?

ENCORE
Evaluate the symptom, its onset, recurrence and duration.
No medication is always an option.
Care when dealing with specific patient groups, notably the elderly, the young, nursing mothers, pregnant women, those receiving specific medication such as methotrexate and anticoagulants, and those with particular disease, for example, renal impairment.
Observe the patient for signs of systemic disturbance and ask about presence of fever, loss of weight and any accompanying physiological disturbance.
Refer when in doubt.
Explain any course of action recommended.

Box 1.3 Consultation behaviours

Active listening
Appropriate use of open and closed questions
Respect patient
Avoid jargon
Demonstrate empathy
Deal sensitively with potentially embarrassing or sensitive issues

---

Table 1.4 Pharmaceutical consultation process

Element	Goal	Examples of associated competencies
Introduction	Building a therapeutic relationship	Invites patient to discuss medication or health-related issue Discusses structure and purpose of consultation Negotiates shared agenda
Data collection and problem identification	Identifying the patient's medication-related needs	Takes a full medication history Establishes patient's understanding of their illness Establishes patient's understanding of the prescribed treatment Identifies and prioritises patient's pharmaceutical problems
Actions and solutions	Establishing an acceptable management plan with the patient	Involves patient in designing management plan Tailors information to address patient's perception of illness and treatment Checks patient's understanding Refers appropriately
Closure	Negotiating safety netting strategies with the patient	Provides information to guide action when patient experiences problems with management plan Provides further appointment or contact point

Box 1.4 Key postconsultation questions

Do I know more now about the patient?
Was I curious?
Did I really listen?
Did I find out what really mattered to them?
Did I explore their beliefs and expectations?
Did I identify the patient's main medication-related problems?
Did I use their thoughts when I started explaining?
Did I share the treatment options with them?
Did I help my patient to reach a decision?
Did I check that they understood what I said?
Did we agree?
Was I friendly?

Clinical pharmacy functions and knowledge

The following practical steps in the delivery of pharmaceutical care are based largely on the DUP. The 'select regimen' and 'drug administration' indicators have been amalgamated at step 3.

Step 1. Establishing the need for drug therapy

For independent prescribers this step includes establishing a diagnosis and then balancing the risks and benefits of treatment against the risks posed by the disease. Current practice for most pharmacists means that another professional, most frequently a doctor, will have diagnosed the patient's presenting condition and any co-existing disease. The pharmacist's role, therefore, is often one of providing information to the independent prescriber on the expected benefits and risks of drug therapy by evaluating both the evidence base and individual patient factors. Pharmacists also draw on these concepts as they become more involved in prescribing and adjusting therapy for patients under their care.

The evidence for one specific mode of therapy may not be conclusive. In this circumstance, the pharmacist will need to call on their understanding of the principles of pharmaceutical science and on clinical experience to provide the best advice possible.

Step 1.1. Relevant patient details

Without background information on the patient's health and social circumstances (Table 1.5) it is difficult to establish the existence of, or potential for, MRPs. When this information is

Table 1.5 Relevant patient details

Factor	Implications
Age	The very young and the very old are most at risk of medication-related problems. A patient's age may indicate their likely ability to metabolise and excrete medicines and have implications for step 2 of the drug use process
Gender	This may alter the choice of the therapy for certain indications. It may also prompt consideration of the potential for pregnancy or breast feeding
Ethnic or religious background	Racially determined predispositions to intolerance or ineffectiveness should be considered with certain classes of medicines, for example, ACE inhibitors in Afro-Caribbean people. Formulations may be problematic for other groups, for example, those based on blood products for Jehovah's Witnesses or porcine-derived products for Jewish patients
Social history	This may impact on ability to manage medicines and influence pharmaceutical care needs, for example, living alone or in a care home or availability of nursing, social or informal carers
Presenting complaint	Symptoms the patient describes and the signs identified by the doctor on examination. Pharmacists should consider whether these might be attributable to the adverse effects of prescribed or purchased medicines
Working diagnosis	This should enable the pharmacist to identify the classes of medicines that would be anticipated on the prescription based on current evidence
Previous medical history	Understanding the patient's other medical conditions and their history helps ensure that management of the current problem does not compromise a prior condition and guides the selection of appropriate therapy by identifying potential contraindications
Laboratory or physical findings	The focus should be on findings that may affect therapy, such as • renal function • liver function • full blood count • blood pressure • cardiac rhythm Results may convey a need for dosage adjustment or presence of an adverse reaction

lacking a review solely of prescribed medicines will probably be of limited value and risks making a flawed judgement on the appropriateness of therapy for that individual.

Current and co-existing conditions with which the patient presents can be established from various sources. In medical notes, the current diagnosis (Δ) or differential diagnoses (ΔΔ) will be documented, as well as any previous medical history (PMH). Other opportunities to gather information come from discussion with the patient and participation in medical rounds. In primary care, general medical practitioners' computer systems carry information on the patient's diagnosis.

Once the diagnosis and PMH are established it is then possible to identify the medicines that would be expected to be prescribed for each indication, based on contemporary evidence. This list of medicines may be compiled from appropriate national or international guidelines, local formularies and knowledge of current practice.

Step 1.2. Medication history

A medication history is the part of a pharmaceutical consultation that identifies and documents allergies or other serious adverse medication events, as well as information about how medicines are taken currently and have been taken in the past. It is the starting point for medicines reconciliation and medication review.

Obtaining accurate and complete medication histories has been shown to have a positive effect on patient care and pharmacists have demonstrated that they can compile such histories with a high degree of precision and reliability as part of medicines reconciliation. The benefit to the patient is that prescribing errors of omission or transcription are identified and corrected early, reducing the risk of harm and improving care.

Discrepancies between the history recorded by the medical team and that which the pharmacist elicits fall into two categories: intentional (where the medical team has made a decision to alter the regimen) or unintentional (where a complete record was not obtained). Discrepancies should be clarified with the prescriber or referred to a more senior pharmacist. Box 1.5 lists the key components of a medication history.

Step 2. Selecting the medicine

The issues to be tackled at this stage include clinical and cost-effective selection of a medicine in the context of individual patient care. The list of expected treatments generated at step 1 is now scrutinised for its appropriateness for the patient. This requires three separate types of interaction to be identified: drug–patient, drug–disease and drug–drug. The interactions should be prioritised in terms of likelihood of occurrence and the potential severity of outcome should they occur.

Step 2.1. Identify drug–patient interactions

Many medicines have contraindications or cautions to their use that relate to age groups or gender. Potential drug–patient interactions should be identified that may arise with any of the medicines that could be used to treat the current and pre-existing

---

Box 1.5   Key components of a medication history

1. Introduce yourself to the patient and explain the purpose of the consultation.
2. Identify any allergies or serious adverse reactions and record these on the prescription chart, care notes or patient medication record.
3. Ascertain information about prescribed and non-prescribed treatments from:
   - the patient's recall
   - medicines in the patient's possession
   - referral letter (usually from the patient's primary care doctor)
   - copy of prescriptions issued or a repeat prescription list
   - medical notes
   - contact with the appropriate community pharmacist or primary care doctor.
4. Ensure the following are recorded:
   - generic name of medicine (unless specific brand is required)
   - dose
   - frequency
   - duration of therapy.
5. Ensure items such as inhalers, eye drops, topical medicines, herbal and homeopathic remedies are included, as patients often do not consider these as medicines.
6. Ascertain the patient's medication-taking behaviour.
7. Consider practical issues such as swallowing difficulties, ability to read labels and written information, container preferences, ordering or supply problems.
8. Document the history in an appropriate format.
9. Note any discrepancies between this history and that recorded by other health care professionals.
10. Ascertain if these discrepancies are intentional (from patient, nursing staff, medical staff or medical notes).
11. Communicate non-intentional discrepancies to the prescriber.
12. Document any other important medication-related information in an appropriate manner, for example, implications of chronic renal failure, dialysis, long-term steroid treatment.

---

conditions. Types of drug–patient interactions may include allergy or previous ADR, the impact of abnormal renal or hepatic function or chronic heart failure on the systemic availability of some medicines, and patients' preferences for certain treatment options, formulations or routes of administration.

Step 2.2. Identify drug–disease interactions

A drug–disease interaction may occur when a medicine has the potential to make a pre-existing condition worse. Older people are particularly vulnerable due to the co-existence of several chronic diseases and exposure to polypharmacy. Prevention of drug–disease interactions requires an understanding of the pharmacodynamic properties of medicines and an appreciation of their contraindications.

Step 2.3. Drug–drug interactions

Medicines may affect the action of other medicines in a number of ways. Those with similar mechanisms of action may show an enhanced effect if used together whilst those with opposing actions may reduce each other's effectiveness.

Metabolism of one medicine can be affected by a second that acts as an inducer or inhibitor of the cytochrome P450 enzyme system.

The practitioner should be able to identify common drug interactions and recognise those medicines with increased risk of potential interaction, such as those with narrow therapeutic indices or involving hepatic P450 metabolic pathways. It is important to assess the clinical significance of drug interactions and consider the options for effective management.

The list of potential, evidence-based treatments should be reviewed for possible drug–patient, drug–disease and drug–drug interactions. The refined list can then be compared with the medicines that have been prescribed for the patient. The practitioner should explore any discrepancies to ensure the patient does not experience an MRP. This may necessitate consultation with medical staff or other health care professionals, or referral to a more senior pharmacist.

Step 3. Administering the medicine

Many factors influence the effect that a medicine has at its locus of action. These include the rate and extent of absorption, degree of plasma protein binding and volume of distribution, and the routes of metabolism or excretion. Factors affecting bioavailability may include the extent of absorption of the drug from the gastro-intestinal tract in relation to food and other medicines, or the amount adsorped onto intravenous infusion bags and giving sets when used to administer medicines parenterally.

The liver has extensive capacity for drug metabolism, even when damaged. Nevertheless, the degree of hepatic impairment should be assessed from liver function tests and related to potential changes in drug metabolism. This is particularly important for medicines that require activation by the liver (pro-drugs) or those whose main route of elimination is transformation into water-soluble metabolites.

Table 1.6 summarises the main pharmaceutical considerations for step 3. At this point, the practitioner needs to ensure the following tasks have been completed accurately.

Step 3.1. Calculating the appropriate dose

Where doses of oral medicines require calculation, this is usually a straightforward process based on the weight of the patient. However, medicines to be administered parenterally may require more complex calculations, including knowledge of displacement values (particularly for paediatric doses) and determination of appropriate concentrations in compatible fluids and rates of infusion.

Step 3.2. Selecting an appropriate regimen

Giving medicines via the oral route is the preferred method of administration. Parenteral routes carry significantly more risks, including infection associated with vascular access. This route, however, may be necessary when no oral formulation exists or when the oral access is either impossible or inappropriate because of the patient's condition.

Table 1.6 Pharmaceutical considerations in the administration of medicines

Dose	Is the dose appropriate, including adjustments for particular routes or formulations? Examples: differences in dose between intravenous and oral metronidazole, intramuscular and oral chlorpromazine, and digoxin tablets compared with the elixir
Route	Is the prescribed route available (is the patient nil by mouth?) and appropriate for the patient? Examples: unnecessary prescription of an intravenous medicine when the patient can swallow, or the use of a solid dosage form when the patient has dysphagia
Dosage form	Is the medicine available in a suitable form for administration via the prescribed route?
Documentation	Is documentation complete? Do nurses or carers require specific information to administer the medicine safely? Examples: appropriateness of crushing tablets for administration via nasogastric tubes, dilution requirements for medicines given parenterally, rates of administration and compatibilities in parenteral solutions (including syringe drivers)
Devices	Are devices required, such as spacers for inhalers?

Although simple regimens (once- or twice-daily administration) may facilitate adherence, some medicines possess short half-lives and may need to be given more frequently. The practitioner should be familiar with the duration of action of regularly encountered medicines to ensure dosage regimens are designed optimally.

Step 4. Providing the medicine

Ensuring that a prescription is legal, legible, accurate and unambiguous contributes in large measure to the right patient receiving the right medicine at the right time. For the majority of pharmacists this involves screening prescriptions written by other professionals, but those acting as supplementary and independent prescribers need to be cognisant of guidance on prescribing, such as that contained within the British National Formulary, when generating their prescriptions.

In providing a medicine for an individual, due account must be taken of the factors that influence the continued availability and supply of the medicine within the hospital or community setting, for example, formulary and drug tariff status, primary/secondary shared care arrangements, and whether the prescribed indication is within the product licence. This is particularly important with unlicensed or non-formulary medicines when information and agreement on continuation of prescribing, recommended monitoring and availability of supply are transferred from a hospital to primary care setting.

Risks in the dispensing process are reduced by attention to products with similar names or packaging, patients with similar names, and when supplying several family members at the same time. Medicines should be labelled accurately, with clear dosage instructions and advisory labels, and presented appropriately for patients with specific needs, for example, the visually impaired, those unable to read English or with limited dexterity.

Step 5. Monitoring therapy

Monitoring criteria for the effectiveness of treatment and its potential adverse effects can be drawn from the characteristics of the prescribed medicines used or related to specific patient needs. Close monitoring is required for medicines with narrow therapeutic indices and for the subset of drugs where therapeutic drug monitoring may be beneficial, for example, digoxin, phenytoin, theophylline and aminoglycosides. Anticoagulant therapy, including warfarin and unfractionated heparin, is associated with much preventable medication-related morbidity and always warrants close scrutiny.

Throughout this textbook, details are presented on the monitoring criteria that may be used for a wide range of medicines. Patients with renal or hepatic impairment or an unstable clinical condition need particular attention because of the likely requirement for dosage adjustment or change in therapy.

Step 6. Patient advice and education

There is a vast quantity of information on drug therapy available to patients. The practitioner's contribution in this context is to provide accurate and reliable information in a manner that the patient can understand. This may require the pharmacist to convey the benefits and risks of therapy, as well as the consequences of not taking medicines.

Information about medicines is best provided at the time of, or as soon as possible after, the prescribing decision. In the hospital setting, this means enabling patients to access information throughout their stay, rather than waiting until discharge. With many pharmacy departments providing medicines in patient packs, the patient can be alerted to the presence of information leaflets, encouraged to read them and ask any questions they may have. This approach enables the patient to identify their own information needs and ensures the pharmacist does not create a mismatch between their own agenda and that of the patient. However, there will be a need to explain clearly the limitations of leaflets, particularly when medicines are prescribed for unlicensed indications.

Although the research on adherence indicates the primacy of information that has been tailored to the individual's needs, resources produced by national organisations, such as Diabetes UK (www.diabetes.org.uk) and British Heart Foundation (www.bhf.org.uk), may also be of help to the patient and their family or carers. In addition, patients often require specific information to support their daily routine of taking medicines. All written information, including medicines reminder charts, should be dated and include contact details of the pharmacist to encourage patients to raise further queries or seek clarification.

Step 7. Evaluating effectiveness

The provision of drug therapy for the purpose of achieving definite outcomes is a fundamental objective of pharmaceutical care. These outcomes need to be identified at the outset and form the basis for evaluating the response to treatment. Practitioners delivering pharmaceutical care have a responsibility to evaluate the effectiveness of therapy by reviewing steps 1–6 above and taking appropriate action to ensure the desired outcomes are achieved. Depending on the duration of direct engagement with a patient's care, this may be a responsibility the pharmacist can discharge in person or it may necessitate transfer of care to a colleague in a different setting where outcomes can be assessed more appropriately.

Case study

The following case is provided to illustrate the application of several steps in the delivery of pharmaceutical care. It is not intended to be a yardstick against which patient care should be judged.

Case 1.1

Mr JB, a 67-year-old retired plumber, has recently moved to your area and has come to the pharmacy to collect his first prescription. He has a PMH of coronary heart disease (CHD) and has recently had a coronary artery stent inserted. He has a long history of asthma which is well controlled with inhaled medicines.

Step 1. Establishing the need for drug therapy

What classes of medicines would you expect to be prescribed for these indications?

Mr JB gives a complete medication history that indicates he takes his medicines as prescribed, he has no medication-related allergies, but does suffer from dyspepsia associated with acute use of non-steroidal anti-inflammatory agents. He has a summary of his stent procedure from the hospital that indicates normal blood chemistry and liver function tests.

Step 2. Selecting the medicine

What drug–patient, drug–disease and drug–drug interactions can be anticipated (Table 1.7).

Steps 3 and 4. Administering and providing the medicines

What regimen and individualised doses would you recommend for Mr JB (Table 1.8).

Table 1.7 The case of Mr JB: potential drug interactions with the patient, the disease or other drugs

	Drug–patient interactions	Drug–disease interactions	Drug–drug interactions
Medicines that should be prescribed for CHD			
Aspirin	Previous history of dyspepsia	Aspirin should be used with caution in asthma	Combination of antiplatelet agents increases risk of bleeding
Clopidogrel	Previous history of dyspepsia		
Statins			Possible increased risk of myopathy if simvastatin given with diltiazem
β-Blockers		β-Blocker contraindicated in asthma	Combination of different agents to control angina may lead to hypotension
Diltiazem			Reduces metabolism of simvastatin thereby increasing the risk of side effects
Nitrates (GTN spray)	Previous history of side effects (e.g. headache, flushing) may result in patient not using spray when required		
Medicines that may be prescribed for asthma			
β2-Agonist inhalers	Patient's ability to use inhaler devices effectively	β2-Agonists can cause tachycardia	
Steroid inhalers			
Antimuscarinic inhalers		Antimuscarinic agents can cause tachycardia and atrial fibrillation	Antimuscarinics may reduce effect of sublingual nitrate tablets (failure to dissolve under tongue owing to dry mouth)

CHD, coronary heart disease.

Table 1.8 The case of Mr JB: possible therapeutic regimen

	Recommendation	Rationale
Medicines that should be prescribed for CHD		
Aspirin	75 mg daily orally after food	Benefit outweighs risk if used with PPI
Clopidogrel	75 mg daily orally after food	Benefit outweighs risk if used with PPI. Length of course should be established in relation to previous stent
Lansoprazole	15 mg daily orally	Decreases risk of GI bleeds with combination antiplatelets. Concerns about some PPIs reducing the effectiveness of clopidogrel makes selection of specific PPI important
Simvastatin	20 mg daily orally	Low dose selected due to diltiazem reducing the metabolism of simvastatin and increasing the risk of side effect
Nitrates	2 puffs sprayed under the tongue when required for chest pain	

Continued

This predicted regimen can be compared with the prescribed therapy and any discrepancies resolved with the prescriber. Step 4 (provision) in Mr JB's case would be relatively straightforward.

Steps 5, 6 and 7. Monitoring therapy, patient education and evaluation

What criteria would you select to monitor Mr JB's therapy and what information would you share with the patient? What indicators would convey effective management of his condition (Table 1.9).

Quality assurance of clinical practice

Quality assurance of clinical pharmacy has tended to focus on the review of performance indicators, such as intervention rates, or rely upon experienced pharmacists to observe and comment on the practice of others using local measures. The lack of generally agreed or national criteria raises questions about the consistency of these assessments, where they take place, and the overall standard of care provided to patients. Following the Bristol Royal Infirmary Inquiry (2001) into

Table 1.8 The case of Mr JB: possible therapeutic regimen—cont'd

	Recommendation	Rationale
Diltiazem	90 mg m/r twice a day	Used for rate control as β-blockers contraindicated in asthma
Ramipril	10 mg daily	To reduce the progression of CHD and heart failure
Medicines that may have been prescribed		
Salbutamol inhaler	2 puffs (200 μcg) to be inhaled when required	Patient should follow asthma treatment plan if peak flow decreases
Beclometasone inhalers	2 puffs (400 μcg) twice a day	Asthma treatment plan which may include increasing the dose of inhaled steroids if peak flow decreases

CHD, coronary heart disease; PPI, proton pump inhibitor; GI, gastro-intestinal; m/r, modified release.

Table 1.9 The case of Mr JB: monitoring criteria and patient advice

	Recommendation
Drugs that should be prescribed for CHD	
Aspirin	Ask patient about any symptoms of dyspepsia or worsening asthma
Clopidogrel	Ask patient about any symptoms of dyspepsia
Lansoprazole	If PPIs don't resolve symptoms, primary care doctor should be consulted
Simvastatin	Liver function tests 3 months after any change in dose, or annually. Creatine kinase only if presenting with symptoms of unexplained muscle pain. Cholesterol levels 3 months after any change in dose, or annually if at target
Nitrates (GTN spray)	Frequency of use to be noted. Increasing frequency that results in a resolution of chest pain should be reported to primary care doctor and anti-anginal therapy may be increased. ANY use that does not result in resolution of chest pain requires urgent medical attention
Diltiazem	Blood pressure and pulse monitored regularly
Ramipril	Renal function and blood pressure monitored within 2 weeks of any dose change, or annually
Drugs that may have been prescribed for asthma	
Salbutamol inhaler	Salbutamol use should be monitored as any increase in requirements may require increase in steroid dose
Beclometasone inhalers	Monitor for oral candidiasis

paediatric cardiac surgery, there has been much greater emphasis on the need for regulation to maintain the competence of health care professionals, the importance of periodic performance appraisal coupled with continuing professional development, and the introduction of revalidation.

The challenges for pharmacists are twofold: first, to demonstrate their capabilities in a range of clinical pharmacy functions and second, to engage with continuing professional development in a meaningful way to satisfy the expectations of pharmaceutical care and maintain registration with, for example, the General Pharmaceutical Council in the UK. The pragmatic approach to practice and the clinical pharmacy process outlined throughout this chapter has been incorporated into a professional development framework, called the General Level Framework (GLF) available at: www.codeg. org, that can be used to develop skills, knowledge and other attributes irrespective of the setting of the pharmacist and their patients.

References

Barber, N.D., Batty, R., Ridout, D.A., 1997. Predicting the rate of physician-accepted interventions by hospital pharmacists in the United Kingdom. Am. J. Health Syst. Pharm. 54, 397–405.

Bates, D.W., Cullen, D.J., Laird, N., et al., 1995. Incidence of adverse drug events and potential adverse drug events in hospitalized patients. J. Am. Med. Assoc. 274, 29–34.

Baumann, L.J., Leventhal, H., 1985. I can tell when my blood pressure is up, can't I? Health Psychol. 4, 203–218.

Bond, C.A., Raehl, C.L., Franke, T., 1999. Clinical pharmacy services and hospital mortality rates. Pharmacotherapy 19, 556–564.

Bristol Royal Infirmary Inquiry, 2001. The Report of the Public Inquiry into Children's Heart Surgery at the Bristol Royal Infirmary 1984–1995. Learning from Bristol. Stationery Office, London. Available at: http://www.bristol-inquiry.org.uk/final_report/rpt_print.htm.

Brodie, D.C., Parish, P.A., Poston, J.W., 1980. Societal needs for drugs and drug related services. Am. J. Pharm. Educ. 44, 276–278.

Cipolle, R.J., Strand, L.M., Morley, P.C. (Eds.), 1998. Pharmaceutical Care Practice. McGraw-Hill, New York.

Cousins, D.H., Luscombe, D.K., 1995. Forces for change and the evolution of clinical pharmacy practice. Pharm. J. 255, 771–776.

Department of Health, 2004. Building a Safer NHS for Patients: Improving Medication Safety. Department of Health, London. Available at: http://www.dh.gov.uk/en/Publicationsandstatistics/Publications/PublicationsPolicyAndGuidance/DH_4071443.

Ernst, F.R., Grizzle, A.J., 2001. Drug-related morbidity and mortality: updating the cost of illness model. J. Am. Pharm. Assoc. 41, 192–199.

Hepler, C.D., Strand, L.M., 1990. Opportunities and responsibilities in pharmaceutical care. Am. J. Hosp. Pharm. 47, 533–543.

Horne, R., 2001. Compliance, adherence and concordance. In: Taylor, K., Harding, G. (Eds.), Pharmacy Practice. Taylor and Francis, London.

Howard, R.L., Avery, A.J., Howard, P.D., et al., 2003. Investigation into the reasons for preventable drug related admissions to a medical admissions unit: observational study. Qual. Saf. Health Care 12, 280–285.

Hutchinson, R.A., Vogel, D.P., Witte, K.W., 1986. A model for inpatient clinical pharmacy practice and reimbursement. Drug Intell. Clin. Pharm. 20, 989–992.

Kucukarslan, S.N., Peters, M., Mlynarek, M., et al., 2003. Pharmacists on rounding teams reduce preventable adverse drug events in hospital general medicine units. Arch. Intern. Med. 163, 2014–2018.

Leape, L.L., Cullen, D.J., Clapp, M.D., et al., 1999. Pharmacist participation on physician rounds and adverse drug events in the intensive care unit. J. Am. Med. Assoc. 282, 267–270.

Ley, P., 1988. Communicating with Patients. Improving Communication, Satisfaction and Compliance. Croom Helm, London.

National Institute for Health and Clinical Excellence and National Patient Safety Agency, 2007. Technical Patient Safety Solutions for Medicines Reconciliation on Admission of Adults to Hospital. NICE, London. Available at http://www.nice.org.uk/nicemedia/pdf/PSG001GuidanceWord.doc.

National Institute for Health and Clinical Excellence, 2009. Medicines adherence: involving patients in decisions about prescribed medicines and supporting adherence. Clinical Guideline 76. NICE, London. Available at http://www.nice.org.uk/nicemedia/pdf/CG76NICEGuideline.pdf.

Pirmohamed, M., James, S., Meakin, S., et al., 2004. Adverse drug reactions as cause of admission to hospital: prospective analysis of 18 820 patients. Br. Med. J. 329, 15–19.

Sevick, M.A., Trauth, J.M., Ling, B.S., et al., 2007. Patients with complex chronic diseases: perspectives on supporting self management. J. Gen. Intern. Med. 22, 438–444.

Winterstein, A.G., Sauer, B.C., Helper, C.D., et al., 2002. Preventable drug-related hospital admissions. Ann. Pharmacother. 36, 1238–1248.

Zed, P.J., 2005. Drug-related visits to the emergency department. J. Pharm. Pract. 18, 329–335.

2 Prescribing

H. Marlow and C. Whittlesea

Key points

- Prescribers need to assess and manage the potential benefits and harms of treatment.
- Patients should receive cost-effective medication appropriate to their clinical needs, in doses that meet their requirements and for an adequate period of time.
- Respect for patient autonomy, obtaining consent and sharing decision making is a fundamental part of the prescribing process.
- The consultation is a fundamental part of clinical practice and requires effective interpersonal reasoning and practical skills.
- Using a consultation framework is recommended to ensure relevant issues are covered.
- Prescribing is a complex mix of factors - evidence, external influences and cognitive biases - and these should be recognised.

To prescribe is to authorise by means of a written prescription the supply of a medicine. Prescribing incorporates the processes involved in decision making undertaken by the prescriber before the act of writing a prescription. Historically, prescribing has been the preserve of those professionals with a medical, dental or veterinary training. As the role of other health care professionals such as pharmacists and nurses has expanded, prescribing rights have in turn been extended to them. The premise for this development has been that it better utilises the training of these professional groups, is clinically appropriate and improves patient access.

Regardless of the professional background of the individual prescriber, the factors that motivate them to prescribe a particular medicine are a complex mix of evidence of effectiveness and harm, external influences and cognitive biases. A rational approach to prescribing uses evidence and has outcome goals and evaluates alternatives in partnership with the patient. With the advent of new professional groups of prescribers (non-medical prescribers), it is increasingly important to understand the components of rational and effective prescribing, and the influences on this process. There is a need for a systematic approach to prescribing, and an understanding of the factors that influence the decision to prescribe a medicine. These issues will be covered in the following sections. Initially, the fundamentals of rational and effective prescribing will be discussed, followed by a brief outline of the acquisition of prescribing rights by pharmacists and the associated legal framework. The final section will cover the prescribing process and the factors that influence this.

Rational and effective prescribing

Prescribing a medicine is one of the most common interventions in health care used to treat patients. Medicines have the potential to save lives and improve the quality of life, but they also have the potential to cause harm, which can sometimes be catastrophic. Therefore, prescribing of medicines needs to be rational and effective in order to maximise benefit and minimise harm. This is best done using a systematic process that puts the patient at the heart of the process (Fig. 2.1).

What is meant by rational and effective prescribing?

There is no universally agreed definition of good prescribing. The WHO promotes the rational use of medicines, which requires that patients receive medications appropriate to their clinical needs, in doses that meet their own individual requirements, for an adequate period of time, and at the lowest cost to them and their community. However, a more widely used framework for good prescribing has been described (Barber, 1995) and identifies what the prescriber should be trying to achieve, both at the time of prescribing and in monitoring treatment thereafter. The prescriber should have the following four aims:

- Maximise effectiveness
- Minimise risks
- Minimise costs
- Respect the patient's choices.

This model links to the four key principles of biomedical ethics: beneficence, non-maleficence, justice and veracity, and respect for autonomy, and can be applied to decision making at both an individual patient level and when making decisions about medicines for a wider population, for example in a Drug and Therapeutics Committee. One of the strengths of this model is the consideration of the patient's perspective and the recognition of the inherent tensions between the four key aims.

Another popular framework to support rational prescribing decisions is known as STEPS (Preskorn, 1994). The STEPS

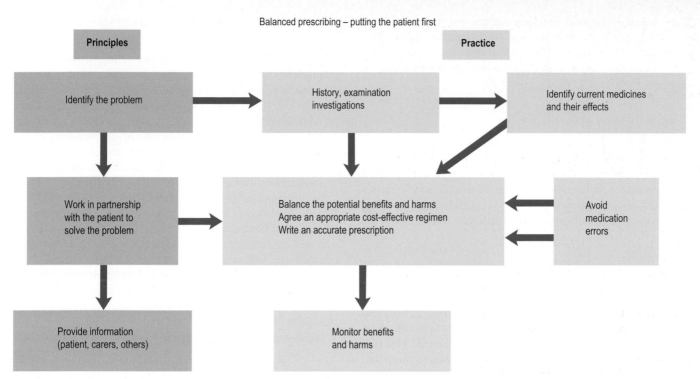

Balanced prescribing – putting the patient first

Fig. 2.1 A framework for good prescribing (from Background Briefing. A blueprint for safer prescribing 2009 © Reproduced by permission of the British Pharmacological Society.)

model includes five criteria to consider when deciding on the choice of treatment:

- Safety
- Tolerability
- Effectiveness
- Price
- Simplicity.

Inappropriate or irrational prescribing

Good prescribing is sometimes defined as the lack of irrational prescribing. Prescribing can be described as irrational for many reasons:

- Poor choice of a medicine
- Polypharmacy or co-prescribing of interacting medicine
- Prescribing for a self-limiting condition
- Continuing to prescribe for a longer period than necessary
- Prescribing too low a dose of a medicine
- Prescribing without taking account of the patient's wishes.

Inappropriate or irrational prescribing can result in serious morbidity and mortality, particularly when childhood infections or chronic diseases such as hypertension, diabetes, epilepsy and mental disorders are being treated. Inappropriate prescribing also represents a waste of resources and, as in the case of antimicrobials, may harm the health of the public by contributing to increased antimicrobial resistance. Finally, an over-willingness to prescribe stimulates inappropriate patient demand and fails to help the patient understand when they should seek out support from a health care professional.

Pharmacists as prescribers and the legal framework

Evolution of non-medical prescribing

Independent prescribing is defined as 'prescribing by a practitioner (doctor, dentist, nurse, pharmacist) who is responsible and accountable for the assessment of patients with undiagnosed or diagnosed conditions and for decisions about the clinic management required including prescribing' (DH, 2006).

In 1986, a report was published in the UK ('Cumberlage report') which recommended that community nurses should be given authority to prescribe a limited number of medicines as part of their role in patient care (Department of Health and Social Security, 1986). Up to this point, prescribing in the UK had been the sole domain of doctors, dentists and veterinarians. This was followed in 1989 by a further report (the first Crown report) which recommended that community nurses should prescribe from a limited formulary (DH, 1989). The legislation to permit this was passed in 1992.

At the end of the 1990s, in line with the then UK government's desire to widen access to medicines by giving patients quicker access to medicines, improving access to service and making better use of the skills of health care professionals, the role of prescriber was proposed for other health care professionals. This change in prescribing to include non-medical prescribers (pharmacists, nurses and optometrists) was developed following a further review (Crown, 1999).

This report suggested the introduction of supplementary prescribers, that is, non-medical health professionals who could prescribe after a diagnosis had been made and a clinical management plan drawn up for the patient by a doctor (Crown, 1999).

Supplementary prescribing

The Health and Social Care Act 2001 allowed pharmacists and other health care professionals to prescribe. Following this legislation, in 2003, the Department of Health outlined the implementation guide allowing pharmacists and nurses to qualify as supplementary prescribers (DH, 2003). In 2005, supplementary prescribing was extended to physiotherapists, chiropodists/podiatrists, radiographers and optometrists (DH, 2005).

Supplementary prescribing is defined as a voluntary prescribing partnership between an independent prescriber (doctor or dentist) and a supplementary prescriber (nurse, pharmacist, chiropodists/podiatrists, physiotherapists, radiographers and optometrists) to implement an agreed patient-specific clinical management plan with the patient's agreement. This prescribing arrangement also requires information to be shared and recorded in a common patient file. In this form of prescribing the independent prescriber, that is the doctor or if appropriate the dentist, undertakes the initial assessment of the patient, determines the diagnosis and the initial treatment plan. The elements of this patient-specific plan, which are the responsibility of the supplementary prescriber, are then documented in the patient-specific clinical management plan. The legal requirements for which are detailed in Box 2.1. Supplementary prescribers can prescribe Controlled Drugs and also both off-label and unlicensed medicines.

Box 2.1 Overview of the requirements for a clinical management plan for supplementary prescribing

Legal requirements
Patient details
- Name of the patient to whom the plan relates
- Patient allergies
- Difficulties patient has with medicines

Disease and treatment
- Condition
- Class or name of medicines
- Limitations on doses, strength or time of treatment
- When to seek advice from, or refer back to independent prescriber
- Arrangements for notification of adverse drug reactions or incidents

Prescriber information
- Name of independent prescriber (doctor or dentist)
- Name of supplementary prescriber (pharmacist, nurse, physiotherapists, chiropodists/podiatrists, radiographers and optometrists)
- Start date
- Review date

Non-medical independent prescribing

Following publication of a report on the implementation of nurse and pharmacist independent prescribing within the NHS in England (DH, 2006), pharmacists were enabled to become independent prescribers as defined under the Medicines and Human Use (Prescribing; Miscellaneous Amendments) Order of May 2006. Pharmacist independent prescribers were able to prescribe any licensed medicine for any medical condition within their competence except Controlled Drugs and unlicensed medicines. The restriction on Controlled Drugs included those in Schedule 5 (CD Inv.POM and CD Inv.P) such as co-codamol. At the same time, nurses could also become qualified as independent prescribers (formerly known as Extended Formulary Nurse Prescribers) and prescribe any licensed medicine for any medical condition within their competence, including some Controlled Drugs. Since 2008, optometrists can also qualify as independent prescribers to prescribe for eye conditions and the surrounding tissue. They cannot prescribe for parenteral administration and they are unable to prescribe Controlled Drugs.

Following a change in legislation in 2010, pharmacist and nurse, non-medical prescribers, were allowed to prescribe unlicensed medicines (DH, 2010).

From the above it should be evident that in the UK suitably qualified pharmacists can prescribe as either supplementary or independent prescribers.

Accountability

Prescribers have the authority to make prescribing decisions for which they are accountable both legally and professionally. Accountability when prescribing covers three aspects – the law, the statutory professional body and the employer.

The law of Tort, the concept of a 'civil wrong', includes clinical negligence. In such a claim, the patient needs to demonstrate that the prescriber caused them injury or damage. For this allegation to be substantiated the patient needs to prove that the prescriber owed them a duty of care, that this duty of care was breached and that this caused the injury identified, and also that the injury was foreseeable. The law of Tort also permits actions for breach of confidentiality and also for battery, should a patient be treated without consent. Therefore, prescribers (independent and supplementary) are legally and professionally accountable for their decisions. This includes decisions not to prescribe and also ensuring that the prescription is administered as directed. The legal responsibility for prescribing always lies with the individual who signed the prescription. In addition, prescribers also have a responsibility to ensure the instructions are clear and not open to misinterpretation.

If a prescriber is an employee then the employer expects the prescriber to work within the terms of his/her contract, competency and within the rules/policies, standard operating procedure and guidelines, etc. laid down by the organisation. Therefore, working as a prescriber, under these conditions, ensures that the employer has vicarious liability. So should any patient be harmed through the action of the prescriber and he/she is found in a civil court to be negligent, then under these circumstances the employer is responsible for any compensation to the patient. Therefore, it is important to always work within these frameworks, as working outside these requirements makes the prescriber personally liable for such compensation. To reinforce this message it has been stated that the job descriptions of non-medical prescribers should incorporate a clear statement that prescribing forms part of the duties of their post (DH, 2006).

Ethical framework

Four main ethical principles of biomedical ethics have been set out for use by health care staff in patient–practitioner relationships (Beauchamp and Childress, 2001). These principles are respect for autonomy, non-maleficence, beneficence, justice and veracity and need to be considered at all points in the prescribing process.

Autonomy

Autonomy recognises an individual patient's right to self-determination in making judgements and decisions for themselves and encompasses informed patient consent. Respect for autonomy is therefore a form of personal liberty which freely permits patients to choose whether they wish to have treatment in accordance with their own plans.

Confidentiality. Confidentiality is a fundamental right with respect to patient autonomy. Therefore, patients have the right to confidentiality, and consent is required to disclose information regarding their health and treatment.

Consent. Obtaining consent from a patient for treatment can be divided into three components: voluntariness, information and competency. Consent is invalid when it is given under pressure or coercion. Therefore, it is important that consent is obtained for each act and not assumed because this is a routine assessment or procedure and therefore can be carried out automatically. It is essential the patient understands their diagnosis, the benefit and rationale of the proposed treatment and the likelihood of its success together with the associated risks and consequences, for example side effects. Therefore, a prescriber needs to discuss these aspects with the patient. In addition, potential alternative treatments should also be discussed to allow the patient to make a comparison with the proposed plan. The prognosis if no treatment is prescribed should also be discussed. Such a wide-ranging discussion may require more than one appointment and reinforces the necessity for an ongoing patient–professional relationship focused on the needs of the patient. Associated with this is the need to determine if the patient has the competency to make decisions for themselves with respect to vulnerable groups such as those who have learning disabilities, children and the elderly. Young people aged 16 and 17 are normally presumed to be able to consent to their own treatment.

Gillick competence is used to determine if children have the capacity to make health care decisions for themselves. Children under 16 years of age can give consent as long as they can satisfy the prescriber that they have capacity to make this decision.

However, with the child's consent, it is a good practice to involve the parents in the decision-making process. In addition, children under 16 may have the capacity to make some decisions relating to their treatment, but not others. So it is important that an assessment of capacity is made related to each decision. There is some confusion regarding the naming of the test used to objectively assess legal capacity to consent to treatment in children under 16, with some organisations and individuals referring to Fraser guidance and others Gillick competence. Gillick competence is the principle used to assess the capacity of children under 16, while the Fraser guidance refers specifically to contraception (Wheeler, 2006).

The Mental Capacity Act (2005) protects the rights of adults who are unable to make decisions for themselves. The fundamental concepts within this act are the presumption that every adult has capability and should be supported to make their own individual decision. The five key principles are listed in Box 2.2. Therefore, any decision made on their behalf should be as unrestrictive as possible and must be in the patient's own interest, not biased by any other individual or organisation's benefit. Advice regarding patient consent is listed in Box 2.3.

Non-maleficence

At the heart of the principle of non-maleficence is the concept of not knowingly causing harm to the patient. The principle is expressed in the Hippocratic Oath. This obligation not to harm is distinct from the obligation to help others. While

---

Box 2.2 Overview of the five principles of the Mental Capacity Act

- A person is assumed to have capacity unless it is established that he/she lacks capacity.
- A person should not be treated as unable to make a decision unless all practical steps to enable him/her to do this have been taken without success.
- A person cannot be treated as unable to make a decision because he/she makes an unwise decision.
- Acts or decisions made for or on behalf of a person who lacks capacity must be in that person's best interests.
- Before an act or decision is made, the purpose has to be reviewed to assess if it can be achieved as effectively in a way that is less restrictive of the person's rights/freedom of action.

Box 2.3 Advice on patient consent

- Take care when obtaining consent.
- Give the patient understandable information about all significant possible adverse outcomes.
- Ensure the patient has the opportunity to ask questions/consider his/her options.
- Document the advice/warnings provided in the patient's notes.
- Invite the patient to sign to say that he/she understands, and accepts the risks explained.
- Record in the patient's notes if they decline to undergo a treatment/procedure.

codes of all health care professionals outline obligations not to harm clients, many interventions result in some harm, however transitory. Sometimes one act can be described as having a 'double effect', that is, two possible effects: one good effect (intended) and one harmful effect (unintended). The harmful effect is allowed if proportionally it is less than the good effect. Therefore, it is important for prescribers to review both the potential positive effects of treatment, for example symptom control, and the negative effects, for example side effects. It is also important to consider both acts of commission and omission, as a failure to prescribe can also cause harm to the patient.

Beneficence

This is the principle of doing good and refers to the obligation to act for the benefit of others that is set out in codes of professional conduct, for example, pharmacists' code of ethics and professional standards and guidance (Royal Pharmaceutical Society of Great Britain, 2009). Beneficence is referred to both physical and psychological benefits of actions and also related to acts of both commission and omission. Standards set for professionals by their regulatory bodies such as the General Pharmaceutical Council can be higher than those required by law. Therefore, in cases of negligence the standard applied is often that set by the relevant statutory body for its members.

Justice and veracity

This last principle is related to the distribution of resources to ensure that such division or allocation is governed by equity and fairness. This is often linked to cost-effectiveness of treatment and potential inequalities if treatment options are not offered to a group of patients or an individual. However, as a prescriber it is important to consider the evidence base for the prescribed medicine and also to review the patient as an individual to ensure the treatment offered adheres to this principle. This principle of fairness and freedom from discrimination therefore encompasses Human Rights including the need for assessment of medication as part of the Disability Discrimination Act. Health care professionals have a duty under this act to make reasonable adjustments to ensure that all patients have the same opportunity for good health. Therefore, a prescriber should also assess with the patient that the medication prescribed can be accessed by them. Veracity or 'truth telling' underpins both effective communication and patient consent.

Professional frameworks for prescribing

Each professional regulatory body has standards to which their members must adhere. Members are accountable to such bodies for their practice and can be sanctioned by these bodies if their actions do not adhere to these standards. Therefore, individuals will be held accountable by their respective statutory body for their prescribing decisions.

The professional standards for pharmacists are defined within 'Medicines, Ethics and Practice' and contain additional requirements for pharmacists who are qualified as non-medical prescribers and also good practice guidance (Royal Pharmaceutical Society of Great Britain, 2009). This guidance provides advice on a wide range of areas including self-audit, promotions, gifts from drug companies, written agreement with the employing organisation describing the prescriber's scope of practice, liability and indemnity arrangements, competency to prescribe and not just prescribing and dispensing a medicine.

Off-label and unlicensed prescribing

For a medicine to be licensed for use in a specific country, the manufacturer must obtain a marketing authorisation, formerly called the product license. This details the patients, conditions and purpose under which the medicine is licensed for use. Any medicine which does not have a marketing authorisation for the specific country where it is prescribed is termed 'unlicensed'. Unlicensed medicines prescribed include new medicines undergoing clinical trial, those licensed and imported from another country but not licensed in the country where they are to be used. It also includes 'specials' manufactured to meet a specific patient's needs or produced when two licensed medicines are mixed for administration.

However, if a licensed medicine is prescribed outside that specified in the marketing authorisation then this is described as 'off-label'. This happens in practice, for example many medicines are not licensed for use in children but are prescribed for them. In addition, some established medicines are prescribed for conditions outside their marketing authorisation, for example amitriptyline for neuropathic pain and azathioprine in Crohn's disease. The British National Formulary includes information on off-label use as an annotation of 'unlicensed indication' to inform health care professionals. The details of a medicine's marketing authorisation are provided in the Summary of Product Characteristics.

The company which holds the marketing authorisation has the responsibility to compensate patients who are proven to have suffered unexpected harm caused by the medicine when prescribed and used in accordance with the marketing authorisation. Therefore, if a medicine is prescribed which is either unlicensed or off-label, the prescriber carries professional, clinical and legal responsibility and is therefore liable for any harm caused. Best practice on the use of unlicensed and off-label medicines is described in Box 2.4. In addition, all health care professionals have a responsibility to monitor the safety of medicines. Suspected adverse drug reactions should therefore be reported in accordance with the relevant reporting criteria.

Prescribing across the interface between primary and secondary care

When a patient moves between care settings, there is a risk that a 'gap' in care will take place. These 'gaps' in care are almost always as a result of poor communication and frequently involve medicines, particularly when the patient is

Box 2.4 Advice for prescribing unlicensed and off-label medicines (from Drug Safety Update, 2009; 2: 7, with kind permission from MHRA)

Consider

- Before prescribing an unlicensed medicine be satisfied that an alternative licensed medicine would not meet the patient's needs.
- Before prescribing an off-label medicine be satisfied that such use would better serve the patient's needs than an appropriately licensed alternative.
- Before prescribing an unlicensed medicine or using an off-label medicine:
  - be satisfied that there is a sufficient evidence base and/ or experience of using the medicine to show its safety and efficacy;
  - take responsibility for prescribing the medicine and for overseeing the patient's care, including monitoring and follow up;
  - record the medicine prescribed and, where common practice is not being followed, the reason for prescribing the medicine; you may wish to record that you have discussed this with the patient.

Communicate

- You give patients, or those authorising treatment on their behalf, sufficient information about the proposed treatment, including known serious or common adverse drug reactions, to enable them to make an informed decision.
- Where current practice supports the use of a medicine outside the terms of its license, it may not be necessary to draw attention to the license when seeking consent. However, it is a good practice to give as much information as patients or carers require or which they see as relevant.
- You explain the reasons for prescribing an off-label medicine or prescribing an unlicensed medicine where there is little evidence to support its use, or where the use of the medicine is innovative.

discharged from hospital into a community setting. So far, there is no evidence-based solution to these problems. The primary care prescriber with the responsibility for the continuing management of the patient in the community may be required to prescribe medicines with which they are not familiar. The prescriber should be fully informed and competent to prescribe a particular medicine for his/her patient. Supporting information from the hospital, in the form of shared care guidelines, can help inform the prescriber about medicines with which they may not be very familiar. Overall, the decision about who should take responsibility for continuing care or prescribing treatment after the initial diagnosis or assessment should be based on the patient's best interests rather than on the health care professional's convenience or the cost of the medicine. However, it is legitimate for a prescriber to refuse to prescribe where they consider they have insufficient expertise to accept responsibility for the prescription or where the product is of a very specialised nature and/or requires complex ongoing monitoring. Professional bodies are developing principles for communication between health care professionals in primary and secondary care to improve patient safety.

Clinical governance

Clinical governance is defined as 'the system through which NHS organisations are accountable for continuously improving the quality of their services and safeguarding high standards of care, by creating an environment in which clinical excellence will flourish' (DH, 1998). It is a process embraced by the NHS to ensure that the quality of health care embedded within organisations is continuously monitored and improved. Clinical governance parallels corporate governance within commercial organisations and as such provides a systematic set of mechanisms such as duties, accountabilities and rules of conduct to deliver quality health care.

Clinical governance is described as having seven pillars:

- Patient, service user, carer and public involvement
- Risk management
- Clinical audit
- Staffing and management
- Education, training and continuing professional development (CPD)
- Research and clinical effectiveness
- Use of information.

Within the NHS, standards of practice have been developed and monitored to ensure risks are managed and controlled. As part of this framework the performance of staff is also assessed and remedial action taken, if required. NHS organisations have clinical governance requirements for their staff which include requirements for non-medical prescribing.

Professional bodies have also incorporated clinical governance into their codes of practice. The four tenants of clinical governance are to ensure clear lines of responsibility and accountability; a comprehensive strategy for continuous quality improvement; policies and procedures for assessing and managing risks; procedures to identify and rectify poor performance in staff. Therefore, the professional bodies such as those of pharmacists, nurses and optometrists have also identified clinical governance frameworks for independent prescribing as part of their professional codes of conduct. The General Pharmaceutical Council, the UK pharmacy regulator, code of practice provided a framework not only for the individual pharmacist, non-medical prescriber, but also for their employing organisation. Suggested indicators for good practice are detailed in Box 2.5.

Competence and competency frameworks

Competence can be described as the knowledge, skills and attributes required to undertake an activity to a specific minimum standard within a defined environment. A competency framework is a group of competencies identified as essential to effectively perform a specific task. It can be used by an individual or an organisation to assess performance in this defined area. For example, it can be used for staff selection/ recruitment, training and performance review.

The National Prescribing Centre has published a competency framework for pharmacist prescribers

Box 2.5 Overview of clinical governance practice recommendations for prescribers

- Ensure effective communication with patients and carers to meet the patient's needs, so that the patient can make informed choices about their treatment.
- Prescribe within competence (scope of practice).
- Obtain patient consent for investigations and management.
- Document in the patient's medical record, a comprehensive record of the consultation and the agreed treatment plan.
- Undertake full assessment of patients competently and with consent.
- Prescribe safely, legally, appropriately, clinically and cost-effectively with reference to national and local guidelines.
- Assess and manage risk of treatment and associated investigations.
- Prescribe and refer in accordance with the clinical management plan if relevant.
- Ensure the secure storage of prescriptions and follow the relevant organisational procedures if they are lost or stolen.
- Ensure wherever possible separation of prescribing and dispensing; prescribing and administration.
- Audit prescribing practice.
- Identify and report incidents and adverse drug reactions.
- Participate in and record continuing professional development relating to prescribing.
- Follow organisational procedures for dealing with the pharmaceutical industry regarding gifts and hospitality.

(Granby and Picton, 2006) which is described in Table 2.1. This framework is composed of three areas: the consultation, prescribing effectively and prescribing in context. These three areas are further subdivided to provide nine competencies each with an overarching statement. The nine competencies are:

- Clinical and pharmaceutical knowledge
- Establishing options
- Communicating with patients
- Prescribing safety
- Prescribing professionally
- Improving prescribing practice
- Information in context
- The NHS in context (the principles apply to all health care organisations)
- The team and individual context.

Each of these competencies is supported by a series of statements/behavioural indicators, all of which an individual needs to demonstrate they have achieved the overall competency (Table 2.1). Prescribers can review their prescribing performance using the nine competencies and the associated 77 behavioural indicators using this framework as a self-assessment tool. The framework is particularly useful when structuring ongoing CPD.

Table 2.1 Overview of the National Prescribing Centre competency framework for pharmacists (Granby and Picton, 2006)

Competency area	Competency	Behaviour indicator
Consultation	Clinical and pharmaceutical knowledge	10 statements For example, understands the conditions being treated, their natural progress and how to assess their severity
	Establishing options	14 statements For example, assesses the clinical condition using appropriate techniques and equipment
	Communicating with patients	11 statements For example, explains the nature of the patient's condition, the rationale behind and potential risks and benefits of management options
Prescribing effectively	Prescribing safely	9 statements For example, only prescribes a medicine with adequate, up-to-date knowledge of its actions, indications, contraindications, interactions, cautions, dose and side effects
	Prescribing professionally	8 statements For example, accepts personal responsibility for own prescribing and understands the legal and ethical implications of doing so
	Improving prescribing practice	7 statements For example, reports prescribing errors and near misses, reviews practice to prevent recurrences
Prescribing in context	Information in context	6 statements For example, critically appraises the validity of information sources (e.g. promotional literature, research)
	The NHS in context	5 statements For example, follows relevant local and national guidance for medicines use (e.g. local formularies, care pathways, NICE guidance)
	The team and individual context	7 statements For example, establishes relationships with colleagues based on understanding, trust and respect for each other's roles

The prescribing process

Consultation

The consultation is a fundamental part of the prescribing process and the prescriber needs to understand and utilise this in order to help them practise effectively. The medical model of disease, diagnosis and prescribing is often central to practice, but an understanding of the patient's background together with their medical beliefs and anxieties is equally important in helping the prescribers understand their own role and behaviours alongside those of their patients. A broad range of practical skills are needed in the consultation:

- *Interpersonal skills:* the ability to communicate and make relationships with patients.
- *Reasoning skills:* the ability to gather appropriate information, interpret the information and then apply it both in diagnosis and management.
- *Practical skills:* the ability to perform physical examinations and use clinical instruments.

The style in which the consultation is undertaken is also important. The paternalistic prescriber–patient relationship is no longer appropriate. This has been replaced in modern health care by a more patient-centred focus that ensures patient autonomy and consent. This uses a task-orientated approach to keep consultation times to a reasonable duration and set parameters to ensure a realistic expectation from the consultation.

An example of this is the Calgary Cambridge framework which can be used to structure and guide patient consultations (Silverman et al., 2005). The framework is represented in Fig. 2.2. The five key stages of the consultation are:

- Initiating the session
- Gathering information
- Physical examination
- Explanation and planning
- Closing the session.

In addition to these stages there are two key tasks performed throughout the consultation. These are 'providing structure' and 'building the patient–prescriber relationship'. These two tasks are vital in ensuring an effective consultation. For a patient–prescriber communication to be effective, it is important that this focuses on interaction between the patient and the prescriber and is not just passive transmission of information. Feedback from the patient about the information received is essential for effective communication and will be covered in more detail below.

Building relationships

Non-verbal communication is important and can be used by the prescriber to gain information from the patient. Facial expressions and body posture can give clues about how the patient is feeling, for example anxious or tired. Proximity and

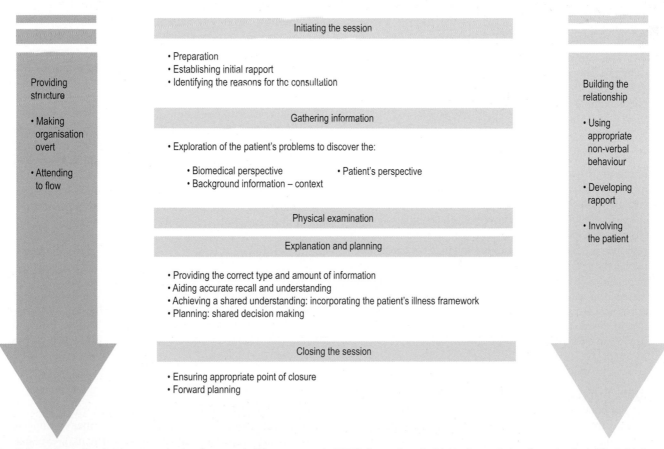

Fig. 2.2 Calgary Cambridge consultation framework (Silverman et al., 2005). Reproduced with kind permission from the Radcliffe Publishing Ltd, Oxford.

eye contact are also important to determine if the patient is activity engaged in the conversation or are they distracted. Such non-verbal clues, for example anxiety, tiredness and pain, can then be explored verbally with the patient.

The prescribers also need to review their own non-verbal communication to ensure this reinforces the verbal message they are giving to the patient. For example, doctors who face the patient, make eye contact and maintain an open posture were regarded by their patients to be more interested and empathic (Harrigan et al., 1985). Also health care professionals in primary care who demonstrated non-verbal intimacy (close distance, leaning forward, appropriate body orientation and touch) had increased patient satisfaction (Larsen and Smith, 1981).

As eye contact is an important non-verbal form of communication, obtaining information from patient records and documenting the consultation could undermine these skills. Therefore, it is important to read notes in advance of the consultation and avoid writing up the outcome while the patient is speaking. Indicating to the patient that references need to be made to their record or information documented ensures the patient is informed about the break in the consultation. This strategy should be adopted for both paper and computer-based records.

Developing rapport is also essential to building an effective patient–prescriber relationship. This can be achieved by providing an accepting response to the patient's concerns and expectations. This is achieved by acknowledging the patient's views and valuing their contribution and accepting this information in a non-judgemental way. This does not necessarily mean that the prescriber agrees with information but that they accept that this is a legitimate view from the patient's perspective. This can be reinforced by summarising the patient's view. The prescriber should acknowledge the patient's coping efforts and self-care. Avoiding jargon and explaining complex concepts in simple terms, to enable patients to understand the diagnosis and management, is also important.

Providing structure

This is important in the patient–prescriber consultation to enable the five key stages to be effectively completed. The prescriber needs to establish the boundaries for the consultation, that is, the time available and the topics covered and termination of the consultation. Therefore, as the power in the consultation is with the prescriber, it is his/her responsibility to guide the consultation and involve the patient. This is to ensure a patient-centred collaborative partnership is established. This can be achieved by using problem identification, screening and agenda-setting skills. The use of a logical sequence, signposting from one part of the consultation to the next and including an initial and end summary, will provide an effective structure to the consultation.

Initiating the session

During the first stage of the consultation the prescriber needs to greet the patient and confirm his/her identity. They should also ensure the environment for the consultation is appropriate for maintaining eye contact and ensuring confidentiality. The prescriber should also introduce him/herself, his/her role and gain relevant consent. During this stage the prescriber must demonstrate respect for the patient and establish a patient-centred focus. Using initially open and then closed questions the prescriber needs to identify the patient's problem/issues. By adopting this approach and actively listening, the prescriber is able to confirm the reason for the consultation and identify other issues. This allows the prescriber to negotiate an agenda for the next stages of the consultation through agreement with the patient and taking into account both the patient and prescriber's needs. This initial stage is vital for the success of the consultation as many patients have hidden agendas which, if not identified at this stage, can lead to these concerns not being addressed. Beckman and Frankel (1984) studied doctors' listening skills and identified that even minimal interruptions by doctors to initial patients' statements at the beginning of the consultation prevented patients' concerns from being expressed. This resulted in either these issues not being identified at all or they were raised by patient's late in the consultation

Gathering information

The aim of this stage is to explore the problem identified from both the patient and prescriber's perspective to gain background information which is both accurate and complete. Britten et al. (2000) identified that lack of patient participation in the consultation led to 14 categories of misunderstanding between the prescriber and patient. These included patient information unknown to the prescriber, conflicting information from the patient and communication failure with regard to the prescriber's decision. During this stage the illness framework, identified by exploring the patient's ideas, concerns, expectations and experience of his/her condition and effect on his/her life, is combined with the information gained by the prescriber through his/her biomedical perspective. This encompasses signs, symptoms, investigations and underlying pathology. Assimilation of this information leads the prescriber to a differential diagnosis. By incorporating information from both viewpoints, a comprehensive history detailing the sequence of events can be obtained using questioning, listening and clarification. This ends with an initial summary where the prescriber invites the patient to comment and contribute to the information gathered.

Physical examination

At the start of this stage it is important to again obtain the patient's consent for any examination by explaining the process and rationale for the assessment. The environment, for example room temperature and screening for the examination, is important and the prescriber should review this to ensure the patient's comfort.

Explanation and planning

This stage of the consultation incorporates three aspects: the differential diagnosis/hypothesis, the prescriber's management plan (investigations and alternative treatments), explanation and negotiating the plan of action with the patient.

In one UK study, doctors were found to overestimate the extent to which they completed the tasks of discussing the risk of medication, checking the ability of the patient to follow the treatment plan and obtaining the patient's input and view on the medication prescribed (Makoul et al., 1995).

In order to successfully accomplish this stage of the consultation, the prescriber needs to use a number of skills and also to involve the patient. The prescriber should ensure he/she gives the correct type and amount of information. This is done by assessing the patient's prior knowledge by employing both open and closed questions. By organising the information given into chunks which can be easily assimilated the prescriber can then check the patient understands the information given. Questioning the patient regarding additional information they require also helps to ensure the patient's involvement and maintains rapport. The prescriber must determine the appropriate time to give explanations and also allow the patient time to consider the information provided. Signposting can also be a useful technique to employ during this stage. Once again the language used should be concise, easy to understand and avoid jargon. Using diagrams, models and written information can enhance and reinforce patient understanding. The explanation should be organised into discreet sections with a logical sequence so that important information can be repeated and summarised. Box 2.6 summarises the issues the prescriber should consider before prescribing a medicine.

Box 2.6 Issues the prescriber should reflect upon before prescribing a medicine (National Prescribing Centre, 1998)

- What is the drug?
  - Is it novel?
  - Is it a line extension?
- What is the drug used for?
  - Licensed indications
  - Any restrictions on initiation
  - Does first line mean first choice?
- How effective is the drug?
  - Is there good evidence for efficacy?
  - How does it compare with existing drugs?
- How safe is the drug?
  - Are there published comparative safety data?
  - Has it been widely used in other countries?
  - Are the details contained in the Summary of Product Characteristics understood?
  - Are there clinically important drug interactions?
  - Are there monitoring requirements?
  - Can it be used long term?
- Who should not receive this drug?
  - Are there patients in whom it is contraindicated?
- Does the drug provide value for money?
  - Is there good evidence of cost-effectiveness compared to other available interventions?
  - What impact will this drug have on the health care budget?
- What is its place in therapy?
  - What advantages are there?
  - Are the benefits worth the cost?
  - Are there some patients that would particularly benefit?

To achieve shared understanding and shared decision making, it is important to incorporate the patient's perspective by relating the information given to the patient's illness framework. The patients also need to have the opportunity to ask questions, raise doubts and obtain clarification. This can be undertaken effectively by taking the patient's beliefs, culture, abilities and lifestyle into account when discussing treatment options, for example fasting during Ramadan, or use of memory aids to support adherence. The prescriber should also explain his/her rationale for the management plan identified and also discuss possible alternatives. By involving and negotiating with the patient in this way, a mutually acceptable treatment plan can be identified which allows the patient to take responsibility for his/her own health.

Closing the session

The effectiveness of the end of a consultation is as important as the preceding stages. A number of steps are undertaken during the closing stage. These include agreeing a contract with the patient as to the next steps to be taken by both patient and prescriber, for example additional investigations and/or referral. Safety net strategies are also employed and discussed, so the patient can identify unexpected outcomes or treatment failure and also understand who and how to contact the prescriber or another health care professional if appropriate. The end summary is an essential component of this stage and is used to briefly and accurately identify the management plan established during the previous stage in the consultation. This is followed by final checking that the patient has understood and consented to this management plan. At the end of the consultation the patient is given another opportunity to ask any final questions.

Communicating risks and benefits of treatment

Explaining the risks and benefits of treatment in an effective manner is an essential skill for health care professionals. This ensures patient's consent to treatment is informed and that the patient has an opportunity to participate in shared decision making about their treatment. Before this stage of the consultation is reached, the health care professional has to know the evidence about treatment, be able to apply it to the individual patient in front of them and then be able to communicate risks and benefits in terms the patient can understand.

It is important to communicate the risks and benefits of treatment in relation to medicines. This is because many medicines are used long term to treat or prevent chronic diseases, but we know they are often not taken as intended. Sometimes these medicines do not appear to have any appreciable beneficial effect on patients' symptoms, for example medicines to treat hypertension. Most patients want to be involved in decisions about their treatment, and would like to be able to understand the risks of side effects versus the likely benefits of treatment, before they commit to the inconvenience of taking regular medication. An informed patient is more likely to be concordant with treatment, reducing waste of health care resources including professional time and the waste of medicines which are dispensed but not taken.

Communicating risk is not simple (Paling, 2003). Many different dimensions and inherent uncertainties need to be taken into account, and patients' assessment of risk is primarily determined by emotions, beliefs and values, not facts. This is important, because patients and health care professionals may ascribe different values to the same level of risk. Health care professionals need to be able to discuss risks and benefits with patients in a context that would enable the patient to have the best chance of understanding those risks. It is also prudent to inform the patient that virtually all treatments are associated with some harm and that there is almost always a trade-off between benefit and harm. How health care professionals present risk and benefit can affect the patient's perception of risk.

Some important principles to follow when describing risks and benefit to patients:

- Remember patients' assessments of risk are primarily determined by emotions, not by facts
- Communicate the trade-off between benefits and harms
- Avoid purely descriptive terms of risk, for example 'low risk'
- Use a consistent denominator, for example 1 in 100, 5 in 100; not 1 in 100, 1 in 20
- Use absolute numbers (not relative, or percentages)
- Describe outcomes in both a negative and positive perspective
- Use visual aids and probabilities.

Visual patient decision aids are becoming increasingly popular as a tool that health care professionals can use to support discussions with patients by increasing their knowledge about expected outcomes and helping them to relate these to their personal values (National Prescribing Centre, 2008). Further information about using patient decision aids can be found at http://www.npci.org.uk/therapeutics/mastery/mast4/patient_decision_aids/patient_decision_aid1.php

Adherence

Adherence has been defined as the extent to which a patient's behaviour matches the agreed recommendation from the prescriber. When a patient is non-adherent this can be classified as intentional or unintentional non-adherence (National Institute for Health and Clinical Excellence, 2009).

Unintentional non-adherence occurs when the patient wishes to follow the treatment plan agreed with the prescriber, but is unable to do so because of circumstances beyond their control. Examples of this include forgetting to take the medicine at the defined time or an inability to use the device prescribed. Strategies to overcome such obstacles include medication reminder charts, use of multi-compartment medication dose systems, large print for those with poor eyesight, aids to improve medication delivery, for example inhaler-aids, tube squeezers for ointments and creams, and eye drop administration devices. A selection of these devices is detailed in a guide to the design of dispensed medicines (National Patient Safety Agency, 2007).

Intentional non-adherence occurs when the patient decides he/she does not wish to follow the agreed treatment plan. This may occur because of the patient's beliefs, his/her perceptions or motivation. Therefore, it is important that all of these aspects are included in the discussion between the patient and prescriber when the treatment plan is developed. The patient needs to fully appreciate his/her medical condition and its prognosis in order to understand the rationale for the treatment options discussed. Also the effect of not taking the treatment needs to be explicitly explored with the patient. The benefits of the treatment plan as well as side effects also need to be explored with the patient. The patient information leaflet (PIL) can be used to support this discussion. The patient's previous experience of medicines and associated side effects should be explored as this gives the prescriber vital information about perceptions and motivation. Adherence to existing prescribed medication should be explored non-judgementally. For example, asking the patient how often he/she has missed taking doses at the prescribed time over the previous 7 days would enable the prescriber to assess adherence but also explore lifestyle factors or side effects which may impact on the patient. These can then be discussed and strategies developed to optimise adherence.

Studies have demonstrated that between 35% and 50% of medicines prescribed for chronic conditions are not taken as recommended (National Institute for Health and Clinical Excellence, 2009). Therefore, it is the prescriber's responsibility to explore with the patient their perceptions of medicines to determine if there are any reasons why they may not want to or are unable to use the medicine. In addition, any barriers which might prevent the patient from using the treatment as agreed, for example manual dexterity, eyesight, memory, should be discussed and assessed. Such a frank discussion should enable the patient and prescriber to jointly identify the optimum treatment regimen to treat the condition. In addition, information from the patient's medical records can be used to assess adherence. For example, does the frequency of requests for repeat medication equate to the anticipated duration of use?

Review of unused medicines can be undertaken and it is also important to assess the patient's administration technique on an ongoing basis for devices, for example asthma inhalers to optimise correct technique. This can be achieved, for example, on carrying out a medicine's reconciliation on hospital admission when the patient's prescribed medicines are compared to what they were taking before admission through discussion with patients/carers and review of primary care records.

As it is likely that at some point all patients will forget to take their medicine, it is important to give all patients information on what to do should a dose be missed. For individuals taking medication for treatment of a chronic condition, adherence should not be assumed and therefore assessment of adherence should form an ongoing discussion at each consultation.

Medication review

Medication review has been defined as 'a structured, critical examination of a patient's medicines with the objective of reaching an agreement with the patient about treatment, optimising the impact of medicines, minimising the number of medication-related problems and reducing waste' (Medicines Partnership, 2002).

It is important that medicines are prescribed appropriately and that patients continue to achieve benefits from their medicines. The regular review of medicines is a key part of a good prescribing process and has many potential benefits for patients including:

- Improves the current and future management of the patient's medical condition;
- Provides an opportunity to develop a shared understanding between the patient and the health care professional about medicines and their role in the patient's treatment;
- Improves health outcomes through optimal medicines use;
- Reduces adverse events related to medicines;
- Provides an opportunity to empower the patient and carers to be actively involved in their care and treatment;
- Reduces unwanted or unused medicines.

Many medicines prescribed for patients are used to treat chronic long-term conditions and are consequently prescribed regularly on a long-term basis. Frequently, patients obtain these medicines using a repeat prescribing system. This enables the patients to obtain further supplies of their medicine without routinely having to see their primary care doctor or prescriber, thereby reducing unnecessary consultations. In the UK, repeat prescribing accounts for about 60–75% of all prescriptions and 80% of cost. Robust systems and processes are essential in primary care to ensure repeat prescribing is safe and not wasteful. Reviewing a patient's medication forms an essential element of a robust repeat prescribing process.

Medication reviews can be carried out in many different care settings, by a variety of health care professionals and in many different ways. Different types of medication review are required to meet the needs of patients for different purposes. A medication review can be from a simple review of the prescription to an in-depth clinical medication review. However, the aim of all types of medication review is to achieve the following:

- Give patients the chance to raise questions and highlight problems they are having with their medicines.
- Seek to improve or optimise the benefit of treatment for an individual patient.
- Review should be carried out in a systematic way by a competent health care professional.
- Have any proposed changes from the review agreed with the patient.
- Review should be clearly documented in the patient's medical notes.
- Monitor and record the outcome of any change in medication.

The benefits of medication review are now being recognised by health policy makers, and in the UK, community pharmacists are required to carry out different levels of medication review as part of their normal clinical activities. Medication reviews are often targeted towards patient groups who are more likely to have problems with their medicines, for example the elderly, patients taking more than four medicines regularly, patients in care homes, those on medicines with special monitoring requirements. Characteristics of different types of medication review are described in Table 2.2.

The key elements of an advanced clinical medication review are:

- Pre-planning and advance warning for the patient
- Identifying ALL medicines being taken
- Patient's understanding of treatment

Table 2.2 Characteristics of types of medication review (adapted from Clyne et al., 2008)

	Purpose of the review	Requires patient to be present	Access to patient's notes
Prescription review	Address technical issues relating to the prescription, for example anomalies, changed items, cost-effectiveness	No (any resulting changes to prescribed medicines must involve the patient/carer)	Possibly (community pharmacist may not have access to patient's clinical notes)
Concordance and compliance medication review	Address issues relating to the patient's medicine-taking behaviour and use of medicines	Usually (any resulting changes to prescribed medicines must involve the patient/carer)	Possibly (community pharmacist may not have access to patient's clinical notes)
Clinical medication review	Address issues relating to the patient's use of medicines in the context of their clinical condition	Yes	Yes

Medication reviews include all medicines, including prescription, complementary and over the counter medicines. Prescription review may relate to one therapeutic area only.

- Appropriateness of treatment
- Review of physiological tests and measurements
- Review of efficacy
- Side effects and interactions
- Practicalities of medicines usage
- Future treatment plans
- Opportunities for questions and concerns.

The NO TEARS approach (Lewis, 2004) is also a useful prompt to assist such a review (Table 2.3).

Factors that influence prescribers

A prescriber is subject to various influences which may impact upon their decision making when deciding whether to prescribe a medicine and which medicine to prescribe. Some of these influences may result in poor decision making; therefore, it is important to have an understanding of these influences and how they may impact on prescribing decisions.

A range of influences that affect the prescribing decisions made by primary care doctors have been identified (Fig. 2.3).

Patients and prescribing decisions

The prescribing and use of medicines is strongly influenced by cultural factors that affects patients and prescribers alike. Issues such as whether the patient expects a prescription or whether the prescriber thinks the patient expects a prescription both influence the decision to prescribe. Patients may want a prescription for a whole variety of reasons, some of which are more valid than others. Beyond wanting a medicine for its therapeutic effect, a prescription for a medicine may demonstrate to the patient that their illness is recognised, be seen as a symbol of care, offer legitimacy for time off work because of illness, or fit with their health beliefs. Patients who frequently consult and receive a prescription are more likely to repeat the experience, and expect a prescription at their next consultation.

A number of studies have found that doctors sometimes feel under pressure from patients to prescribe, although patients may not always expect a prescription from the doctor. However, while patients often expect to receive a medicine, they may also have more complex agendas that need to be explored in the consultation. Patients may have mixed attitudes towards medicines and reluctance to take medicines is quite common. Whilst a medicine may be prescribed for its pharmacological effect, there may be other associated reasons

Table 2.3 The NO TEARS approach to medication review

NO TEARS	Questions to think about
Need and indication	Why is the patient taking the medicine, and is the indication clearly documented in the notes? Do they still need the medicine? Is the dose appropriate? Has the diagnosis been confirmed or refuted? Would a non-drug treatment be better? Does the patient know what their medicines are for?
Open questions	Use open questions to find out what the patient understands about their medicines, and what problems they may be having with them.
Tests and monitoring	Is the illness under control? Does treatment need to be adjusted to improve control? What special monitoring requirements are there for this patient's medicines? Who is responsible for checking test results?
Evidence and guidelines	Is there new evidence or guidelines that mean I need to review the patient's medicines? Is the dose still appropriate? Do I need to do any other investigations or tests?
Adverse effects	Does the patient have any side effects? Are any of the patient's symptoms likely to be caused by side effects of medicines, including OTC and complementary medicines? Are any of the patients' medicines being used to treat side effects of other medicines? Is there any new advice or warnings on side effects or interactions?
Risk reduction and prevention	If there is time, ask about alcohol use, smoking, obesity, falls risk or family history, for opportunistic screening. Is treatment optimised to reduce risks?
Simplification and switches	Can the patient's medicines regimen be simplified? Are repeat medicines synchronised for prescribing at the same time? Explain any changes in medicines to the patient.

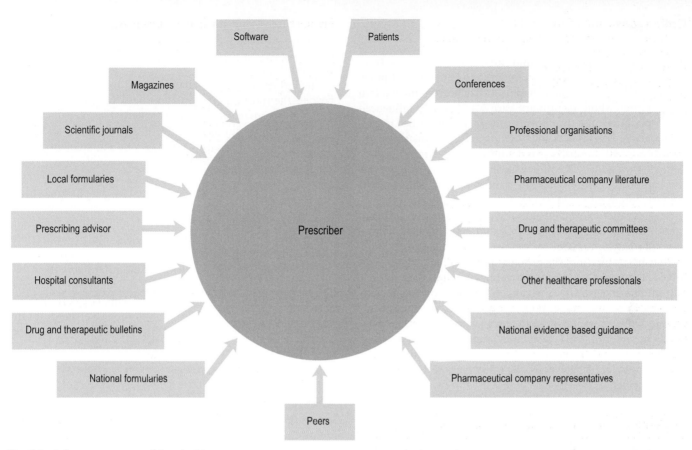

Fig. 2.3 Influences on prescribing decisions

to prescribe for a patient, for example to end the consultation, to avoid doing anything else or having to say 'no', to maintain contact with the patient, as a response to carer anxiety, or to fulfil the patient's expectation.

The informed patient

Health care is moving to a position of greater shared decision making with patients and development of the concept of patient autonomy. This is being supported through the better provision of information for patients about their prescribed medicines. The EU directive 2001/83 (European Commission, 2001) requires that all pharmaceutical products are packaged with an approved PIL, which provides information on how to take the medicine and possible adverse effects. Other important developments that have increased patients' access to information, albeit of variable quality, include the role of the media in general and the amount of attention they give to health and health-related matters, the emergence of the Internet, and the development of patient support groups. The reporting in the media of concerns regarding the safety of MMR vaccine and the subsequent rapid drop in MMR vaccinations rates in children is a good example of the importance of these developments in influencing patients and prescribing.

Direct advertising of medicines to patients is allowed in the USA and New Zealand, but not in Europe. Advertising medicines in this way is clearly effective in increasing sales of medicines, as evidenced by the increased spending and prescriptions for advertised drugs, compared to non-advertised drugs in these countries. This has led to concern that direct to consumer advertising encourages unnecessary and inappropriate use of medication. In the UK, education for patients may be provided by the manufacturer through sponsored disease awareness campaigns but there is concern that these encourage individuals to seek advice or treatment from their doctor for conditions that have been incorrectly self diagnosed. These campaigns may also help to raise awareness of conditions that have not been well managed in the past. However, they can also act as covert advertisements for prescription. Such campaigns, which may be established by a drug company with or without the endorsement of a patient group, often take place at the same time as a drug's launch and may involve aggressive promotion. As a consequence there have been calls to control the influence of companies on the production of disease awareness campaigns that impact on the individual patient, who then exerts pressure on the prescriber for a specific medicine.

Health care policy

National policy and guidelines, for example National Service Frameworks and guidance from NICE in the UK, have a significant influence on prescribing, although the influence may not be as great as expected for some medicines (Prescribing Support Unit, 2009).

Colleagues

Several studies have found that health care professionals in primary care (both doctors and nurses) rely on advice from trusted colleagues and opinion leaders as a key source of information on how to manage patients. It has been estimated that 40% of prescribing in primary care was strongly influenced by hospitals because the choice of medicine prescribed in general practice was often guided by hospital specialists through their precedent prescribing and educational advice (National Audit Office, 2007). The Pharmaceutical Industry recognise the value of identifying 'key opinion' leaders amongst the medical community and will try to cultivate them to influence their peers and fellow clinicians, by paying them for a consultancy, lecture fees, travel, research and articles favourable to that company's products.

Pharmacists, in both the primary and secondary care, themselves have an influence on prescribing through their roles as clinical pharmacists, or as part of their work advising on prescribing in primary care. Pharmacists are often regarded as trusted colleagues, and as such can have an important influence on prescribing. In whichever sector they are working, pharmacists need to be aware that their advice and decisions may be influenced by exactly the same factors that influence the prescriber.

Pharmaceutical industry

The pharmaceutical industry has a very wide and important influence on prescribing decisions affecting every level of health care provision, from the medicines that are initially discovered and developed through clinical trials, to the promotion of medicines to the prescriber and patient groups, the prescription of medicines and the compilation of clinical guidelines. There are over 8000 pharmaceutical company representatives in the UK trying to persuade prescribers to prescribe their company's product. This represents a ratio of about 1 representative for every 7.5 doctors (House of Commons Health Committee, 2005) with 1 representative for every 4 primary care doctors (National Audit Office, 2007). Whilst representatives from the pharmaceutical industry can provide useful and important new information to prescribers about medicines, the information presented is not without bias and rarely provides any objective discussion of available competitor products.

The influence of the pharmaceutical industry extends well beyond the traditional selling approach of using representatives, and is increasingly sophisticated. The pharmaceutical industry spends millions on advertising, company sponsored information from medical journals and supplements, sponsorship to attend conferences and meetings, and medical education. Over half of postgraduate education and training for doctors in the UK is sponsored by the pharmaceutical industry. The wide variety, volume and intensity of marketing activities the industry engage in are an important influence on prescribing by health care professionals. But on asking prescribers if they are influenced by the pharmaceutical industry, they usually deny that drug promotion affects their own prescribing practices, although they do believe that it affects other prescribers' prescribing habits. This is clearly not the case, as research has shown that even the use of modest samples, gifts and food exerts a significant influence on prescriber behaviour.

Cognitive factors

Most prescribing decisions are made using the processes our brains develop to handle large volumes of complex information quickly. This rapid decision making is aided by heuristics, strategies that provide shortcuts that allow us to make quick decisions. This type of decision making largely relies on a small number of variables that we believe are important based on information collected by brief reading in summary journals (e.g. Bandolier, Drug and Therapeutics Bulletin and articles in popular doctors' and nurses' magazines mailed free of charge) and talking to colleagues. However, it is important to recognise that cognitive biases affect these heuristics (or shortcuts) involved in rapid decision making, and that experts as well as generalists are just as fallible to cognitive biases in decision making. At least 43 cognitive biases in decision making have been described. Some examples of cognitive biases that may affect prescribing decisions are shown in Table 2.4.

Table 2.4   Examples of types of cognitive biases that influence prescribing

Type of cognitive bias	Description
Novelty preference	The belief that the progress of science always results in improvements and that newer treatments are generally better than older treatments
Over optimism bias	Tendency of people to over-estimate the outcome of actions, events or personal attributes to a positive skew
Confirmation bias	Information that confirms one's already firmly held belief is given higher weight than refuting evidence
Mere exposure effect	More familiar ideas or objects are preferred or given greater weight in decision making
Loss aversion	To weigh the avoidance of loss more greatly than the pursuit of an equivalent gain
Illusory correlation	The tendency to perceive two events as causally related, when in fact the connection between them is coincidental or even non-existent

Strategies to influence prescribing

Health care organisations at local and national levels have been seeking to influence prescribing behaviour over many years, both to control expenditure on medicines and to improve quality of care. Medicines are one of the most well-researched interventions in health care, with a relative wealth of evidence to support their use. Despite this, there is still a wide variation in prescribing practice between clinicians and between health care organisations. This may reflect variation in clinical practice arising from the inconsistent implementation of evidence-based medicine and the impact of the many factors that influence prescribing. Strategies to improve prescribing can be managerial and process orientated, or more supportive and educationally orientated. Strategies that use a combination of different interventions on a repeat basis are more likely to be successful at influencing prescribing.

Managerial approaches to influence prescribing

Formularies are restricted lists of medicines, to which prescribers are encouraged or required to adhere. This helps consistency of prescribing, ensures that prescribers are familiar with a range of medicines, and can help contain costs. In secondary care, prescribers can usually only prescribe those medicines included within the formulary, as these are the medicines stocked in the pharmacy. In primary care a formulary is generally advisory in nature and less restrictive as community pharmacies can supply any reimbursable medicine. Medicines are included in a formulary if they are deemed to have met rational criteria based on clinical and cost-effectiveness. Health care organisations usually have a process for deciding which medicines are included within their local formulary, keeping the formulary updated, and monitoring the implementation of local formulary decisions. Some formularies are developed to cover prescribing in both primary and secondary care, which mean they can have a significant influence on prescribing patterns in the whole of a local health economy. Over recent years, formularies have developed beyond just being a list of medicines and often include useful advice for prescribers, for example about disease management.

Local and national guidelines

Guidelines for the use of a medicine, a group of medicines or the management of a clinical condition may be produced for local or national use. They can be useful tools to guide and support prescribers in choosing which medicines they should prescribe. Ideally, guidelines should make evidence-based standards of care explicit and accessible, and aid clinical decision making. The best-quality guidelines are usually those produced using systematically developed evidence-based statements to assist clinicians in making decisions about appropriate health care for specific clinical circumstances. In the UK, there is an accreditation scheme to recognise organisations who achieve high standards in producing health or social care guidance. Examples of accredited guidelines are those produced by NICE (National Institute for Health and Clinical Excellence, www.nice.org.uk) and SIGN (Scottish Intercollegiate Guideline Network, www.sign.ac.uk). Local guidelines are often developed to provide a local context and interpretation of national guidance, and offer guidance on managing patients between primary and secondary care. However, despite the availability of good quality accessible clinical guidelines, implementation in practice remains variable.

Clinical decision support systems are increasingly popular as a way of improving clinical practice, and influence prescribing. These often utilise interactive computer programs that help clinicians with decision-making tasks at the point of care, and also help them keep up-to-date, and support implementation of clinical guidelines. Clinical knowledge summaries (www.cks.nhs.uk) is a decision support system developed for use in primary care that includes PILs, helps with differential diagnosis, suggests investigations and referral criteria, and gives screens that can be shared between the patient and the prescriber in the surgery.

Incentives

In an effort to contain prescribing costs, some health care systems use direct incentives to influence clinical behaviour and, in particular, prescribing. The incentives, which are usually financial, may be direct to the prescriber or offer some benefits to the prescriber's patients. They can have a significant impact on prescribing practice. Typically, primary care doctors are given indicative prescribing budgets and are expected to meet the prescribing needs of their patients from within this budget. Financial incentive schemes to reward good fiscal management of prescribing budgets and improve the quality of prescribing are used to encourage prescribers to change their practice. Incentive schemes usually influence what is prescribed, rather than whether a prescription is written. The most effective schemes are simple to understand, have achievable targets, and require information about prescribing patterns to be readily available. However, incentives schemes for prescribing need to be managed carefully in order not to create perverse incentives, such as increasing the referral of patients to another part of the health care system, or causing an increase in overall health care costs.

Provision of comparative (benchmarking) information

The provision of benchmarked information on comparative prescribing patterns to primary care doctors is an important influence on prescribing behaviour. Using appropriate benchmarking data brings the behaviour of practices into a local and national context. Benchmarking can provide the basis for making clinicians aware of the potential for change and allows them to understand the potential outcome of any actions. Various prescribing indicators have been developed both locally and nationally to measure and compare quality and cost-effectiveness of prescribing. Ideally, indicators used should be evidence based, utilise available data sources and be validated.

Support and education

One of the challenges for modern health care organisations is to ensure consistent implementation of evidence-based interventions and influence clinical practice. Simply providing prescribers with information or education about an evidence-based intervention rarely produces a change in practice. There is a need to understand the concerns that the adopting clinician may have about the change, recognise that these concerns are often legitimate but may change over time and that the concerns must be addressed and overcome before successful adoption can occur. Interpersonal influence, particularly through the use of trusted colleagues or opinion leaders, is a powerful way to change practice. This is the basis for using pharmacists as prescribing advisers or 'academic detailers' to influence prescribing practice particularly in primary care. Prescribing advisers present evidence-based tailored messages, allow the exchange of information and try to negotiate and persuade clinicians to change practice. Clinicians see pharmacists as a trusted and credible source of prescribing information, who can be moderately successful in changing practice, particularly if linked with an incentive.

In order to change prescribing practice, pharmacists need to be aware of how to use an adoption model-based approach to convey key messages to the prescriber to help them change practice. One such model is known as AIDA (see Table 2.5)

More sophisticated multifaceted educational interventions can also be effective at changing prescribing behaviour but need to be flexible to meet the needs of individual clinicians. This sort of combination approach includes small group learning, audit and feedback, practical support to make changes in practice, and involvement and education of patients.

Table 2.5 AIDA adoption model for influencing prescribers

Awareness	Make the prescriber aware of the issues, prescribing data and evidence for the need to change
Interest	Let the prescriber ask questions and find out more about the proposed change: what the benefits are, what the prescriber's concerns are
Decision	Help the prescriber come to a decision to make a change. How can the change be applied to their patients, what support is there to overcome the barriers to change, provide further information and training to support the change
Action	Action of making a change by the prescriber. Support this with simple reminders, patient decision support, feedback data and audit

Conclusion

While medicines have the capacity to improve health, they also have the potential to cause harm. Prescribing of medicines needs to be rational and effective in order to maximise benefit and minimise harm. Good prescribing should ensure the patient's ideas, concerns and expectations are taken into account. This can be effectively managed by adopting a consultation framework and using patient decision aids to support shared decision making with the patient. Prescribers need to be aware of their responsibilities and accountability particularly when prescribing off-label or unlicensed medicines. They also need to work within their organisation's clinical governance framework. The influences and biases that affect prescribing need to be recognised and minimised by utilising trusted independent sources of information to inform prescribing decisions.

References

Audit Commission, 2003. Primary Care Prescribing – A Bulletin for Primary Care Trusts. Audit Commission, London.

Barber, N., 1995. What constitutes good prescribing? Br. Med. J. 310, 923–925.

Beauchamp, T.L., Childress, J.F., 2001. Principles of Biomedical Ethics, fifth ed. Oxford University Press, Oxford.

Beckman, H.B., Frankel, R.M., 1984. The use of videotape in internal medicine training. J. Gen. Intern. Med. 9, 517–521.

Britten, N., Stevenson, F.A., Barry, C.A., Barber, N., Bradley, C.P., 2000. Misunderstandings in prescribing decision in general practice: qualitative study. Br. Med. J. 320, 484–488.

Clyne, W., Blenkinsopp, A., Seal, R., 2008. A Guide to Medication Review. National Prescribing Centre, Liverpool.

Crown, J., 1999. Review of Prescribing, Supply and Administration of Medicines. Department of Health, London. Available at: http://www.dh.gov.uk/prod_consum_dh/groups/dh_digitalassets/@dh/@en/documents/digitalasset/dh_4077153.pdf.

Department of Health and Social Security, 1986. Neighbourhood Nursing. A Focus for Care, Report of the community nursing review. HMSO, London.

De Vries, T.P.G.M., Henning, R.H., Hogerzeil, H.G., et al., 1994. Guide to Good Prescribing – A Practical Manual. WHO, Geneva.

DH, 1989. Review of Prescribing, Supply and Administration of Medicines (The Crown Report). Department of Health, London.

DH, 2003. Supplementary Prescribing by Nurses and Pharmacists with the NHS in England: A Guide for Implementation. Department of Health, London. Available at: http://www.dh.gov.uk/prod_consum_dh/groups/dh_digitalassets/@dh/@en/documents/digitalasset/dh_4068431.pdf.

DH, 2005. Supplementary Prescribing by Nurses, Pharmacists, Chiropodists/Podiatrists, Physiotherapists and Radiographers Within the NHS in England: A Guide for Implementation. Department of Health, London. Available at: http://www.dh.gov.uk/en/Publicationsandstatistics/Publications/PublicationsPolicyAndGuidance/DH_4110032.

DH, 2006. Improving Patients' Access to Medicines. A Guide to Implementing Nurse and Pharmacist Independent Prescribing Within the NHS in England. Department of Health, London. Available online at: http://www.dh.gov.uk/prod_consum_dh/groups/dh_digitalassets/@dh/@en/documents/digitalasset/dh_4133747.pdf.

DH, 2009. Reference Guide to Consent for Examination or Treatment, second ed. Department of Health, London. Available at: http://www.dh.gov.uk/prod_consum_dh/groups/dh_digitalassets/documents/digitalasset/dh_103653.pdf.

DH, 2010. Changes to Medicines Legislation to Enable Mixing of Medicines Prior to Administration in Clinical Practice. Department of Health, London. Available at: http://webarchive. nationalarchives.gov.uk/+/www.dh.gov.uk/en/Healthcare/ Medicinespharmacyandindustry/Prescriptions/ TheNon-MedicalPrescribingProgramme/DH_110765.

European Commission, 2001. Proposal for a Directive of the European Parliament and of the Council Amending Directive 2001/83/EC on the Community Code Relating to Medicinal Products for Human Use. Available at: http://pharmacos.eudra.org/F2/review/doc/ finaltext/011126-COM_2001_404-EN.pdf.

Granby, T., Picton, C., 2006. Maintaining Competency in Prescribing. An Outline Framework to Help Pharmacists Prescribers. Available at: http://www.npc.co.uk/prescribers/resources/competency_framework_ oct_2006.pdf.

Greenhalgh, T., Macfarlane, F., Maskrey, N., 2010. Getting a better grip on research: the organisational dimension. InnovAiT 3, 102–107.

Harrigan, J.A., Oxman, T.E., Rosenthal, R., 1985. Rapport expressed through non-verbal behavior. J. Nonverbal. Behav. 9, 95–110.

House of Commons Health Committee, 2005. The Influence of the Pharmaceutical Industry HC 42-I. The Stationery Office, London.

Larsen, K.M., Smith, C.K., 1981. Assessment of non-verbal communication in patient-physician interview. J. Fam. Pract. 12, 481–488.

Lewis, T., 2004. Using the NO TEARS tool for medication review. Br. Med. J. 329, 434.

Makhinson, M., 2010. Biases in medication prescribing: the case of second-generation antipsychotics. J. Psychiatr. Pract. 16, 15–21.

Makoul, G., Arnston, P., Scofield, T., 1995. Health promotion in primary care physician-patient communication and decision about prescription medicines. Soc. Sci. Med. 41, 1241–1254.

Medicines Partnership, 2002. Room for Review. A Guide to Medication Review: The Agenda for Patients, Practitioners and Managers. Medicines Partnership, London.

Medicines and Healthcare products Regulatory Agency, 2009. Off-label use or unlicensed medicines: prescribers' responsibilities. Drug Safety Update 2, 7.

Mossialos, E., Mrazek, M., Walley, T., 2004. Regulating Pharmaceuticals in Europe: Striving for Efficiency, Equity and Quality. Open University Press, Maidenhead.

National Audit Office, 2007. Prescribing Costs in Primary Care. The Stationery Office, London.

National Institute for Health and Clinical Excellence, 2009. Medicines Adherence Involving Patients Indecisions About Prescribed Medicines and Supporting Adherence. Clinical Guideline 76. NICE, London. Available at: http://www.nice.org.uk/nicemedia/ live/11766/43042/43042.pdf.

National Patient Safety Agency, 2007. Design for Patient Safety: A Guide to the Design of Dispensed Medicines. NPSA, London.

National Prescribing Centre, 1998. Prescribing New Drugs in General Practice. MeReC Bulletin 9, 21–24.

National Prescribing Centre, 2008. Using Patient Decision Aids. MeReC Extra No. 36. Available at http://www.npc.co.uk/ebt/merec/ other_non_clinical/resources/merec_extra_no36.pdf.

Paling, J., 2003. Strategies to help patients understand risks. Br. Med. J. 327, 745–748.

Prescribing Support Unit, 2009. Use of NICE Appraised Medicines in the NHS in England – Experimental Statistics. The Health and Social Care Information Centre, Prescribing Support and Primary Care. Available at: http://www.ic.nhs.uk/webfiles/publications/niceappmed/ Use%20of%20NICE%20appraised%20medicines%20in%20the%20 NHS%20in%20England.pdf.

Preskorn, S.H., 1994. Antidepressant drug selection: criteria and options. J. Clin. Psychiatr. 55 (Suppl A), 6–22; discussion 23–4, 98–100.

Royal Pharmaceutical Society of Great Britain, 2007. Clinical Governance Framework for Pharmacist Prescribers and Organisations Commissioning or Participating in Pharmacy Prescribing. RPSGB, London.

Royal Pharmaceutical Society of Great Britain, 2009. Medicines Ethics and Practice: A Guide for Pharmacists and Pharmacy Technicians. RPSGB, London.

Silverman, J., Kurtz, S., Draper, J., 2005. Skills for Communicating with Patients, second ed. Radcliffe Publishing, Oxford.

Wheeler, R., 2006. Gillick or Fraser? A plea for consistency over competence in children. Br. Med. J. 332, 807.

Further reading

Appelbe, G.E., Wingfield, J., 2009. Dale and Appelbe's Pharmacy Law and Ethics, ninth ed. Pharmaceutical Press, London.

Horne, R., Weinman, J., Barber, N., et al., 2005. Concordance, adherence and compliance in medicine taking. Report for the National Co-ordinating Centre for NHS Service Delivery and Organisation R&D, London. Available at: http://www.sdo.nihr.ac.uk/ files/project/76-final-report.pdf.

NHS Litigation Authority, 2003. Clinical Negligence. A Very Brief Guide for Clinicians. NHS Litigation Authority, London.

3 Practical pharmacokinetics

R. Fitzpatrick and A. Kostrzewski

Key points

- Pharmacokinetics can be applied to a range of clinical situations with or without therapeutic drug monitoring (TDM).
- TDM can improve patient outcomes but is only necessary for drugs with a low therapeutic index, where there is a good concentration response relationship, and where there is no easily measurable physiological parameter.
- Sampling before steady state is reached or before distribution is complete, leads to erroneous results.
- The volume of distribution can be used to determine the loading dose.
- The elimination half-life determines the time to steady state and the dosing interval.
- Kinetic constants determine the rate of absorption and elimination.
- Clearance determines the maintenance dose.
- Creatinine clearance can be reliably estimated from population values.
- Use of actual blood level data wherever possible to assist dose adjustment is advisable. However, population pharmacokinetic values can be used for digoxin, theophylline and gentamicin.
- Once daily dosing of gentamicin is a realistic alternative to multiple dosing.
- TDM is essential in the dose titration of lithium and phenytoin, but of little value for valproate, or the newer anticonvulsants.

Clinical pharmacokinetics may be defined as the study of the time course of the absorption, distribution, metabolism and excretion of drugs and their corresponding pharmacological response. In practice, pharmacokinetics makes it possible to model what may happen to a drug after it has been administered to a patient. Clearly, this science may be applied to a wide range of clinical situations, hence the term 'clinical pharmacokinetics'. However, no matter how elegant or precise the mathematical modelling, the relationship between concentration and effect must be established before pharmacokinetics will be of benefit to the patient.

General applications

Clinical pharmacokinetics can be applied in daily practice to drugs with a low therapeutic index, even if drug level monitoring is not required.

Time to maximal response

By knowing the half-life of a drug, the time to reach a steady state may be estimated (Fig. 3.1), and also when the maximal therapeutic response is likely to occur, irrespective of whether drug level monitoring is needed.

Need for a loading dose

The same type of information can be used to determine whether the loading dose of a drug is necessary, since drugs with longer half-lives are more likely to require loading doses for acute treatment.

Dosage alterations

Clinical pharmacokinetics can be useful in determining dosage alteration if the route of elimination is impaired through end organ failure (e.g. renal failure) or drug interaction. Using limited pharmacokinetic information such as the fraction that should be excreted unchanged (f_e value), which can be found in most pharmacology textbooks, quantitative dosage changes can be estimated.

Choosing a formulation

An understanding of the pharmacokinetics of absorption may also be useful in evaluating the appropriateness of particular formulations of a drug in a patient.

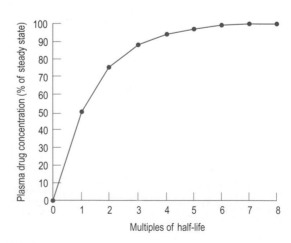

Fig. 3.1 Time to steady state.

Application to therapeutic drug monitoring

Clinical pharmacokinetics is usually associated with therapeutic drug monitoring (TDM), and its subsequent utilisation. When TDM is used appropriately, it has been demonstrated that patients suffer fewer side effects than those who are not monitored (Reid et al., 1990). Although TDM is a proxy outcome measure, a study with aminoglycosides (Crist et al., 1987) demonstrated shorter hospital stays for patients where TDM was used. Furthermore, a study on the use of anticonvulsants (McFadyen et al., 1990) showed better epilepsy control in those patients where TDM was used. A literature review of the cost-effectiveness of TDM concluded that emphasis on just cost is inappropriate and clinical relevance should be sought (Touw et al., 2007). There are various levels of sophistication for the application of pharmacokinetics to TDM. Knowledge of the distribution time and an understanding of the concept of steady state can facilitate determination of appropriate sampling times.

For most drugs that undergo first-order elimination, a linear relationship exists between dose and concentration, which can be used for dose adjustment purposes. However, if the clearance of the drug changes as the concentration changes (e.g. phenytoin), then an understanding of the drug's pharmacokinetics will assist in making correct dose adjustments.

More sophisticated application of pharmacokinetics involves the use of population pharmacokinetic data to produce initial dosage guidelines, for example nomograms for digoxin and gentamicin, and to predict drug levels. Pharmacokinetics can also assist in complex dosage individualisation using actual patient specific drug level data.

Given the wide range of clinical situations in which pharmacokinetics can be applied, pharmacists must have a good understanding of the subject and of how to apply it to maximise their contribution to patient care.

Basic concepts

Volume of distribution

The apparent volume of distribution (V_d) may be defined as the size of a compartment which will account for the total amount of drug in the body (A) if it were present in the same concentration as in plasma. This means that it is the apparent volume of fluid in the body which results in the measured concentration of drug in plasma (C) for a known amount of drug given, that is:

$$C = \frac{A}{V_d}$$

This relationship assumes that the drug is evenly distributed throughout the body in the same concentration as in the plasma. However, this is not the case in practice, since many drugs are present in different concentrations in various parts of the body. Thus, some drugs which concentrate in muscle tissue have a very large apparent volume of distribution, for example digoxin. This concept is better explained in Fig. 3.2.

The apparent volume of distribution may be used to determine the plasma concentration after an intravenous loading dose:

$$C = \frac{\text{loading dose}}{V_d} \quad (1)$$

Conversely, if the desired concentration is known, the loading dose may be determined:

$$\text{loading dose} = \text{desired } C \times V_d \quad (2)$$

In the previous discussion, it has been assumed that after a given dose a drug is instantaneously distributed between the various tissues and plasma. In practice this is seldom the case. For practical purposes it is reasonable to generalise by referring to plasma as one compartment and tissue as if it were another single separate compartment. However, in reality there will be many tissue subcompartments. Thus, in pharmacokinetic terms the body may be described as if it were divided into two compartments: the plasma and the tissues.

Figure 3.3 depicts the disposition of a drug immediately after administration and relates this to the plasma concentration–time graph.

Initially, the plasma concentration falls rapidly, due to distribution and elimination (α phase). However, when an equilibrium is reached between the plasma and tissue (i.e. the distribution is complete), the change in plasma concentration is only due to elimination from the plasma (β phase), and the plasma concentration falls at a slower rate. The drug is said to follow a two-compartment model. However, if distribution

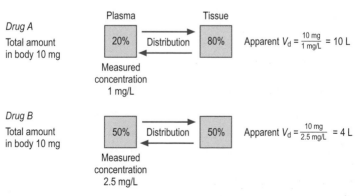

Fig. 3.2 Distribution: more of drug A is distributed in the tissue compartment resulting in a higher apparent volume of distribution than drug B, where more remains in the plasma.

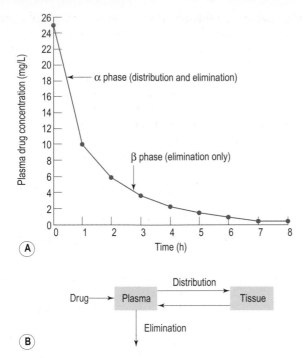

(A)

(B)

Fig. 3.3 (A) Two-compartment model showing two phases in the plasma concentration–time profile. (B) Representation of a two-compartment model showing distribution of drug between plasma and tissue compartments.

is completed quickly (within minutes), then the α phase is not seen, and the drug is said to follow a one-compartment model.

The practical implications of a two-compartment model are that any sampling for monitoring purposes should be carried out after distribution is complete. In addition, intravenous bolus doses are given slowly to avoid transient side effects caused by high peak concentrations.

Elimination

Drugs may be eliminated from the body by a number of routes. The primary routes are excretion of the unchanged drug in the kidneys, or metabolism (usually in the liver) into a more water soluble compound for subsequent excretion in the kidneys, or a combination of both.

The main pharmacokinetic parameter describing elimination is clearance (CL). This is defined as the volume of plasma completely emptied of drug per unit time. For example, if the concentration of a drug in a patient is 1 g/L and the clearance is 1 L/h, then the rate of elimination will be 1 g/h. Thus, a relationship exists:

$$\text{rate of elimination} = CL \times C \qquad (3)$$

Total body elimination is the sum of the metabolic rate of elimination and the renal rate of elimination. Therefore:

$$\text{total body clearance} = CL\ (\text{metabolic}) + CL\ (\text{renal})$$

Thus, if the fraction eliminated by the renal route is known (f_e), then the effect of renal impairment on total body clearance can be estimated.

The clearance of most drugs remains constant for each individual. However, it may alter in cases of drug interactions, changing end-organ function or autoinduction. Therefore, it is clear from equation (Eq.) (3) that as the plasma concentration changes so will the rate of elimination. However, when the rate of administration is equal to the rate of elimination, the plasma concentration is constant (C^{ss}) and the drug is said to be at a steady state.

At steady state:

$$\text{rate in} = \text{rate out}$$

At the beginning of a dosage regimen the plasma concentration is low. Therefore, the rate of elimination from Eq. (3) is less than the rate of administration, and accumulation occurs until a steady state is reached (see Fig. 3.1).

$$\text{rate of administration} = \text{rate of elimination} = CL \times C^{ss} \qquad (4)$$

It is clear from Eq. (3) that as the plasma concentration falls (e.g. on stopping treatment or after a single dose), the rate of elimination also falls. Therefore, the plasma concentration–time graph follows a non-linear curve characteristic of this type of first-order elimination (Fig. 3.4). This is profoundly different from a constant rate of elimination irrespective of plasma concentration, which is typical of zero-order elimination.

For drugs undergoing first-order elimination, there are two other useful pharmacokinetic parameters in addition to the volume of distribution and clearance. These are the elimination rate constant and elimination half-life.

The elimination rate constant (k_e) is the fraction of the amount of drug in the body (A) eliminated per unit time. For example, if the body contains 100 mg of a drug and 10% is eliminated per unit time, then $k_e = 0.1$. In the first unit of time, 0.1×100 mg or 10 mg is eliminated, leaving 90 mg. In the second unit of time, 0.1×90 mg or 9 mg is eliminated, leaving 81 mg. Elimination continues in this manner. Therefore:

$$\text{rate of elimination} = k_e \times A \qquad (5)$$

Combining Eqs. (3) and (5) gives

$$CL \times C = k_e \times A$$

and since

$$C = \frac{A}{V_d}$$

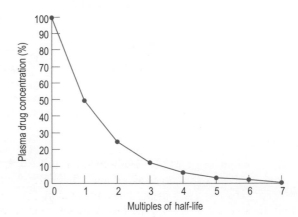

Fig. 3.4 First-order elimination.

then

$$CL \times \frac{A}{V_d} = k_e \times A$$

Therefore,

$$CL = k_e \times V_d \qquad (6)$$

Elimination half-life ($t_{1/2}$) is the time it takes for the plasma concentration to decay by half. In five half-lives the plasma concentration will fall to approximately zero (see Fig. 3.4).

The equation which is described in Fig. 3.4 is

$$C_2 = C_1 \times e^{-k_e \times t} \qquad (7)$$

where C_1 and C_2 are plasma concentrations and t is time.

If half-life is substituted for time in Eq. (7), C_2 must be half of C_1.

Therefore,

$$0.5 \times C_1 = C_1 \times e^{-k_e \times t_{1/2}}$$

$$0.5 = e^{-k_e \times t_{1/2}}$$

$$\ln 0.5 = -k_e \times t_{1/2}$$

$$0.693 = -k_e \times t_{1/2}$$

$$t_{1/2} = \frac{0.693}{k_e} \qquad (8)$$

There are two ways of determining k_e, either by estimating the half-life and applying Eq. (8) or by substituting two plasma concentrations in Eq. (7) and applying natural logarithms:

$$\ln C_2 = \ln C_1 - (k_e \times t)$$

$$k_e \times t = \ln C_1 - \ln C_2$$

$$k_e = \frac{\ln C_1 - \ln C_2}{t}$$

In the same way as it takes approximately five half-lives for the plasma concentration to decay to zero after a single dose, it takes approximately five half-lives for a drug to accumulate to the steady state on repeated dosing or during constant infusion (see Fig. 3.1).

This graph may be described by the equation

$$C = C^{ss}[1 - e^{-k_e \times t}] \qquad (9)$$

where C is the plasma concentration at time t after the start of the infusion and C^{ss} is the steady state plasma concentration. Thus (if the appropriate pharmacokinetic parameters are known), it is possible to estimate the plasma concentration any time after a single dose or the start of a dosage regimen.

Absorption

In the preceding sections, the intravenous route has been discussed, and with this route all of the administered drug is absorbed. However, if a drug is administered by any other route it must be absorbed into the bloodstream. This process may or may not be 100% efficient.

The fraction of the administered dose which is absorbed into the bloodstream is the bioavailability (F). Therefore, when applying pharmacokinetics for oral administration, the dose or rate of administration must be multiplied by F. Bioavailability F is determined by calculating the area under the concentration time curve (AUC). The rationale for this is described below.

The rate of elimination of a drug after a single dose is given by Eq. (3). By definition the rate of elimination is amount of drug eliminated per unit time.

The amount eliminated in any one unit of time $dt = CL \times C \times dt$

The total amount of drug eliminated $= \sum_0^\infty CL \times C \times dt$

As previously explained, CL is constant. Therefore,

Total amount eliminated $= CL \times \sum C \times dt$ from start until C is zero.

$\sum C \times dt$ from start until zero is actually the area under the plasma concentration–time curve (Fig. 3.5).

After a single i.v. dose the total amount eliminated is equal to the amount administered D i.v.

Therefore, D i.v. $= CL \times$ AUC i.v. or $CL = $ D i.v. /AUC.

However, for an oral dose the amount administered is $F \times$ D p.o.

As CL is constant in the same individual,

$$CL = F \times \text{D p.o.}/\text{AUC p.o.} = \text{D i.v.}/\text{AUC i.v.}$$

Rearranging gives

$$F = (\text{D i.v.} \times \text{AUC p.o.}) / (\text{D p.o.} \times \text{AUC i.v.})$$

In this way, F can be calculated from plasma concentration–time curves.

Dosing regimens

From the preceding sections, it is possible to derive equations which can be applied in clinical practice.

From Eq. (1) we can determine the change in plasma concentration ΔC immediately after a single dose:

$$\Delta C = \frac{S \times F \times \text{dose}}{V_d} \qquad (10)$$

where F is bioavailability and S is the salt factor, which is the fraction of active drug when the dose is administered as a salt (e.g. aminophylline is 80% theophylline, therefore $S = 0.8$).

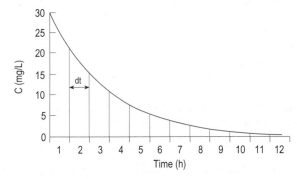

Fig. 3.5 The area under the concentration time curve (AUC) is the sum of C × dt.

Conversely, to determine a loading dose:

$$\text{loading dose} = \frac{\text{desired change in } C \times V_d}{S \times F} \quad (11)$$

At the steady state it is possible to determine maintenance dose or steady state plasma concentrations from a modified Eq. (4):

$$\text{rate in} = \frac{S \times F \times \text{dose}}{T} = CL \times \text{average } C^{ss} \quad (12)$$

where T is the dosing interval.

Peak and trough levels

For oral dosing and constant intravenous infusions, it is usually adequate to use the term 'average steady state plasma concentration' (average C^{ss}). However, for some intravenous bolus injections it is sometimes necessary to determine peak and trough levels (e.g. gentamicin).

At the steady state, the change in concentration due to the administration of an intravenous dose will be equal to the change in concentration due to elimination over one dose interval:

$$\Delta C = \frac{S \times F \times \text{dose}}{V_d} = C_{max} - C_{min}$$

Within one dosing interval the maximum plasma concentration (C_{max}^{ss}) will decay to the minimum plasma concentration (C_{min}^{ss}) as in any first-order process.

Substituting C_{max}^{ss} for C_1 and C_{min}^{ss} for C_2 in Eq. (7):

$$C_{max}^{ss} = C_{max}^{ss} \times e^{-k_e \times t}$$

where t is the dosing interval.

If this is substituted into the preceding equation:

$$\frac{S \times F \times \text{dose}}{V_d} = C_{max}^{ss} - (C_{max}^{ss} \times e^{-k_e \times t})$$

Therefore,

$$C_{max}^{ss} = \frac{S \times F \times \text{dose}}{V_d[1 - e^{-k_e \times t}]} \quad (13)$$

$$C_{min}^{ss} = \frac{S \times F \times \text{dose}}{V_d(1 - e^{-k_e \times t})} \times e^{-k_e \times t} \quad (14)$$

Interpretation of drug concentration data

The availability of the technology to measure the concentration of a drug in plasma should not be the reason for monitoring. There are a number of criteria that should be fulfilled before therapeutic drug monitoring is undertaken. These are:

• the drug should have a low therapeutic index;
• there should be a good concentration–response relationship;
• there are no easily measurable physiological parameters.

In the absence of these criteria being fulfilled, the only other justification for undertaking TDM is to monitor adherence or to confirm toxicity. When interpreting TDM data, a number of factors need to be considered.

Sampling times

In the preceding sections, the time to reach the steady state has been discussed. When TDM is carried out as an aid to dose adjustment, the concentration should be at steady state. Therefore, approximately five half-lives should elapse after initiation or after changing a maintenance regimen, before sampling. The only exception to this rule is when toxicity is suspected. When the steady state has been reached, it is important to sample at the correct time. It is clear from the discussion above that this should be done when distribution is complete (see Fig. 3.3).

Dosage adjustment

Under most circumstances, provided the preceding criteria are observed, adjusting the dose of a drug is relatively simple, since a linear relationship exists between the dose and concentration if a drug follows first-order elimination (Fig. 3.6A). This is the case for most drugs.

Capacity limited clearance

If a drug is eliminated by the liver, it is possible for the metabolic pathway to become saturated, since it is an enzymatic system. Initially the elimination is first-order, but once saturation of the system occurs, elimination becomes zero-order. This results in the characteristic dose–concentration graph seen in Fig. 3.6B. For the majority of drugs eliminated by the liver, this effect is not seen at normal therapeutic doses and only occurs at very high supratherapeutic levels, which is why the kinetics of some drugs in overdose is different from normal. However, one important exception is phenytoin, where saturation of the enzymatic pathway occurs at therapeutic doses. This will be dealt with in the section on phenytoin.

Increasing clearance

The only other situation where first-order elimination is not seen is where clearance increases as the plasma concentration increases (Fig. 3.6C). Under normal circumstances, the plasma protein binding sites available to a drug far outnumber

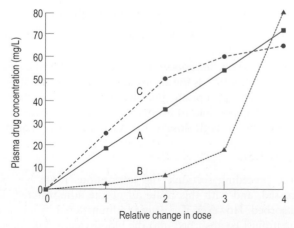

Fig. 3.6 Dose–concentration relationships: (A) first-order elimination, (B) capacity-limited clearance, (C) increasing clearance.

the capacity of the drug to fill those binding sites, and the proportion of the total concentration of drug which is protein bound is constant. However, this situation is not seen in one or two instances (e.g. valproate and disopyramide). For these particular drugs, as the concentration increases the plasma protein binding sites become saturated and the ratio of unbound drug to bound drug increases. The elimination of these drugs increases disproportionate to the total concentration, since elimination is dependent on the unbound concentration.

Therapeutic range

Wherever TDM is carried out, a therapeutic range is usually used as a guide to the optimum concentration. The limits of these ranges should not be taken as absolute. Some patients may respond to levels above or below these ranges, whereas others may experience toxic effects within the so-called therapeutic range. These ranges are only adjuncts to dose determination, which should always be done in the light of clinical response.

Clinical applications

Estimation of creatinine clearance

Since many drugs are renally excreted, and the most practical marker of renal function is creatinine clearance, it is often necessary to estimate this in order to undertake dosage adjustment in renal impairment. The usual method is to undertake a 24-h urine collection coupled with a plasma creatinine measurement. The laboratory then estimates the patient's creatinine clearance. The formula used to determine creatinine clearance is based upon the pharmacokinetic principles in Eq. (3).

The rate of elimination is calculated from the measurement of the total amount of creatinine contained in the 24-h urine sample divided by 24, that is,

$$\frac{\text{amount of creatinine}}{24} = \text{rate of excretion (mg/h)}$$

Using this rate of excretion and substituting the measured plasma creatinine for C^{ss} in Eq. (4), the creatinine clearance can be calculated.

However, there are practical difficulties with this method. The whole process is cumbersome and there is an inevitable delay in obtaining a result. The biggest problem is the inaccuracy of the 24-h urine collection.

An alternative approach is to estimate the rate of production of creatinine (i.e. rate in) instead of the rate of elimination (rate out). Clearly this has advantages, since it does not involve 24-h urine collections and requires only a single measure of plasma creatinine. There are data in the literature relating creatinine production to age, weight and sex since the primary source of creatinine is the breakdown of muscle.

Therefore, equations have been produced which are rearrangements of Eq. (4), that is,

$$\text{creatinine clearance} = \frac{\text{rate of production}}{C^{ss}}$$

Rate of production is replaced by a formula which estimates this from physiological parameters of age, weight and sex.

It has been shown that the equation produced by Cockcroft and Gault (1976) appears to be the most satisfactory. A modified version using SI units is shown as

$$\underset{\text{(mL/min)}}{\text{creatinine clearance}} = \frac{F \times [(140 - \text{age in years}) \times \text{weight (kg)}]}{\text{plasma creatinine (μmol/L)}}$$

where $F = 1.04$ (females) or 1.23 (males).

There are limitations using only plasma creatinine to estimate renal function. The modification of diet in renal disease (MDRD) formula can be used to estimate glomerular filtration rate (eGFR). This formula uses plasma creatinine, age, sex and ethnicity (Department of Health, 2006).

$$\begin{aligned} \text{eGFR} = {} & 175 \times [\text{plasma creatinine (μmol/L)} \times 0.011312]^{-1.154} \\ & \times [\text{age in year}]^{-0.203} \times [1.212 \text{ if patient is black}] \\ & \times [0.742 \text{ if female}] \end{aligned}$$

eGFR = glomerular filtration rate (mL/min per 1.73 m²).

The MDRD should be used with care when calculating doses of drugs, as most of the published dosing information is based on Cockcroft and Gault formula. In patients with moderate to severe renal failure, it is best to use the Cockcroft and Gault formula to determine drug dosing.

Digoxin

Action and uses

Digoxin is the most widely used of the digitalis glycosides. Its primary actions on the heart are those of increasing the force of contraction and decreasing conduction through the atrioventricular node. Currently, its main role is in the treatment of atrial fibrillation by slowing down the ventricular response, although it is also used in the treatment of heart failure in the presence of sinus rhythm. The primary method of monitoring its clinical effect in atrial fibrillation is by measurement of heart rate but knowledge of its pharmacokinetics can be helpful in predicting a patient's dosage requirements.

Plasma concentration–response relationship

- <0.5 μcg/L: no clinical effect
- 0.7 μcg/L: some positive inotropic and conduction blocking effects
- 0.8–2 μcg/L: optimum therapeutic range (0.5–0.9 μcg/L in patients >65)
- 2–2.5 μcg/L: increased risk of toxicity, although tolerated in some patients
- >2.5 μcg/L: gastro-intestinal, cardiovascular system and central nervous system toxicity.

Distribution

Digoxin is widely distributed and extensively bound in varying degrees to tissues throughout the body. This results in a high apparent volume of distribution. Digoxin volume of distribution can be estimated using the equation 7.3 L/kg (ideal body weight (BWt)) which is derived from population data. However, distribution is altered in patients with renal impairment, and a more accurate estimate in these patients is given by:

$$V_d = 3.8 \times \text{ideal BWt} + (3.1 \times \text{creatinine clearance (mL/min)})$$

A two-compartment model best describes digoxin disposition (see Fig. 3.3), with a distribution time of 6–8 h. Clinical effects are seen earlier after intravenous doses, since the myocardium has a high blood perfusion and affinity for digoxin. Sampling for TDM must be done no sooner than 6 h postdose, otherwise an erroneous result will be obtained.

Elimination

Digoxin is eliminated primarily by renal excretion of unchanged drug (60–80%), but some hepatic metabolism occurs (20–40%). The population average value for digoxin clearance is:

$$\text{digoxin clearance (mL/min)} = 0.8 \times \text{BWt}$$
$$+ (\text{creatinine clearance (mL/min)})$$

However, patients with severe congestive heart failure have a reduced hepatic metabolism and a slight reduction in renal excretion of digoxin:

$$\text{digoxin clearance (mL/min)} = 0.33 \times \text{BWt}$$
$$+ (0.9 \times \text{creatinine clearance (mL/min)})$$

Ideal body weight should be used in these equations.

Absorption

Digoxin is poorly absorbed from the gastro-intestinal tract, and dissolution time affects the overall bioavailability. The two oral formulations of digoxin have different bioavailabilities:

$$F(\text{tablets}) = 0.65$$
$$F(\text{liquid}) = 0.8$$

Practical implications

Using population averages it is possible to predict plasma concentrations from specific dosages, particularly since the time to reach the steady state is long. Population values are only averages, and individual values may vary. In addition, a number of diseases and drugs affect digoxin disposition.

As can be seen from the preceding discussion, congestive heart failure, hepatic and renal diseases all decrease the elimination of digoxin. In addition, hypothyroidism increases the plasma concentration (decreased metabolism and renal excretion) and increases the sensitivity of the heart to digoxin. Hyperthyroidism has the opposite effect. Hypokalaemia, hypercalcaemia, hypomagnesaemia and hypoxia all increase the sensitivity of the heart to digoxin. There are numerous drug interactions reported of varying clinical significance. The usual cause is either altered absorption or clearance.

Theophylline

Theophylline is an alkaloid related to caffeine. It has a variety of clinical effects including mild diuresis, central nervous system stimulation, cerebrovascular vasodilatation, increased cardiac output and bronchodilatation. It is the last which is the major therapeutic effect of theophylline. Theophylline does have some serious toxic effects. However, there is a good plasma concentration–response relationship.

Plasma concentration–response relationship

- <5 mg/L: no bronchodilatation[1]
- 5–10 mg/L: some bronchodilatation and possible anti-inflammatory action
- 10–20 mg/L: optimum bronchodilatation, minimum side effects
- 20–30 mg/L: increased incidence of nausea, vomiting[2] and cardiac arrhythmias
- >30 mg/L: cardiac arrhythmias, seizures.

Distribution

Theophylline is extensively distributed throughout the body, with an average volume of distribution based on population data of 0.48 L/kg.

Theophylline does not distribute very well into fat, and estimations should be based on ideal body weight. A two-compartment model best describes theophylline disposition, with a distribution time of approximately 40 min.

Elimination

Elimination is a first-order process primarily by hepatic metabolism to relatively inactive metabolites.

The population average for theophylline clearance is 0.04 L/h/kg, but this is affected by a number of diseases/drugs/pollutants. Therefore, this value should be multiplied by:

- 0.5 where there is cirrhosis, or when cimetidine, erythromycin or ciprofloxacin are being taken concurrently due to enzyme inhibition in the liver;
- 0.4 where there is congestive heart failure with hepatomegaly due to reduced hepatic clearance;
- 0.8 where there is severe respiratory obstruction (FEV1 < 1 L);
- 1.6 for patients who smoke (defined as more than 10 cigarettes per day), since smoking stimulates hepatic metabolism of theophylline.

Neonates metabolise theophylline differently, with 50% being converted to caffeine. Therefore, when it is used to treat neonatal apnoea of prematurity, a lower therapeutic range is used (usually 5–10 mg/L), since caffeine contributes to the therapeutic response.

---

[1] Some patients exhibit a clinical effect at these levels which has been attributed to possible anti-inflammatory effects.
[2] Nausea and vomiting can occur within the therapeutic range.

Product formulation

Aminophylline (the ethylenediamine salt of theophylline) is only 80% theophylline. Therefore, the salt factor (S) is 0.8. Most sustained-release (SR) preparations show good bioavailability but not all SR preparations are the same, which is why advice in the BNF recommends patients are maintained on the same brand.

Practical implications

Intravenous bolus doses of aminophylline need to be given slowly (preferably by short infusion) to avoid side effects due to transiently high blood levels during the distribution phase. Oral doses with sustained release preparations can be estimated using population average pharmacokinetic values and titrated proportionately according to blood levels and clinical response. In most circumstances, sustained release preparations may be assumed to provide 12h cover. However, more marked peaks and troughs are seen with fast metabolisers (smokers and children). In these cases, the sustained release preparation with the lowest k_a value may be used twice daily (e.g. Uniphyllin ($k_a = 0.22$)). Alternatively, thrice daily dosage is required if a standard ($k_a = 0.3$–0.4) sustained release product is used (e.g. Phyllocontin ($k_a = 0.37$) or Nuelin SA ($k_a = 0.33$)).

Gentamicin

Clinical use

The spectrum of activity of gentamicin is similar to other aminoglycosides but its most significant activity is against *Psuedomonas aeruginosa*. It is still regarded by many as first choice for this type of infection.

Therapeutic range

Gentamicin has a low therapeutic index, producing dose-related side effects of nephro- and ototoxicity. The use of TDM to aid dose adjustment is essential if these toxic effects which appear to be related to peak and trough plasma levels are to be avoided. It is generally accepted that the peak level (drawn 1h post-dose after an intravenous bolus or intramuscular injection) should not exceed 12 mg/L and the trough level (drawn immediately pre-dose) should not exceed 2 mg/L.

The above recommendations relate to multiple daily dosing of gentamicin. If once daily dosing is used, then different monitoring and interpretation parameters apply as described at the end of this section.

Distribution

Gentamicin is relatively polar and distributes primarily into extracellular fluid. Thus, the apparent volume of distribution is only 0.3 L/kg. Gentamicin follows a two-compartment model with distribution being complete within 1h.

Elimination

Elimination is by renal excretion of the unchanged drug. Gentamicin clearance is approximately equal to creatinine clearance.

Practical implications

Since the therapeutic range is based on peak (1h post-dose to allow for distribution) and trough (pre-dose) concentrations, it is necessary to be able to predict these from any given dosage regimen.

Initial dosage. This may be based on the patient's physiological parameters. Gentamicin clearance may be determined directly from creatinine clearance. The volume of distribution may be determined from ideal body weight. The elimination constant k_e may then be estimated using these parameters in Eq. (6). By substituting k_e and the desired peak and trough levels into Eq. (7), the optimum dosage interval can be determined (add on 1h to this value to account for sampling time). Using this value (or the nearest practical value) and the desired peak or trough value substituted into Eq. (13) or Eq. (14), it is possible to determine the appropriate dose.

Changing dosage. This is not as straightforward as for theophylline or digoxin, since increasing the dose will increase the peak and trough levels proportionately. If this is not desired, then use of pharmacokinetic equations is necessary. By substituting the measured peak and trough levels and the time between them into Eq. (7), it is possible to determine k_e (and the half-life from Eq. (8) if required). To estimate the patient's volume of distribution from actual blood level data, it is necessary to know the C_{max}^{ss} immediately after the dose (time zero), not the 1h value which is measured. To obtain this, Eq. (7) may be used, this time substituting the trough level for C_2 and solving for C_1. Subtracting the trough level from this C_{max}^{ss} at time zero, the volume of distribution may be determined from Eq. (10). Using these values for k_e and V_d, derived from actual blood level data, a new dose and dose interval can be determined as before.

Once daily dosing. There are theoretical arguments for once daily dosing of gentamicin, since aminoglycosides display concentration-dependent bacterial killing, and a high enough concentration to minimum inhibitory concentration (MIC) ratio may not be achieved with multiple dosing. Furthermore, aminoglycosides have a long post-antibiotic effect. Aminoglycosides also accumulate in the kidneys, and once daily dosing could reduce renal tissue accumulation. There have been a number of clinical trials comparing once daily administration of aminoglycosides with conventional administration. A small number of these trials have shown less nephrotoxicity, no difference in ototoxicity, and similar efficacy with once daily administration.

Initial dosage for a once daily regimen is 5–7 mg/kg/day for patients with a creatinine clearance of >60 mL/min. This is subsequently adjusted on the basis of blood levels. However, monitoring of once daily dosing of gentamicin is different to multiple dosing. One approach is to take a blood sample 6–14h after the first dose and plot the time and result on a standard concentration-time plot (the Hartford nomogram, Nicolau et al., 1995; Fig. 3.7). The position of the individual patient's point in relation to standard lines on the nomogram indicates what the most appropriate dose interval should be (either 24, 36 or 48h). Once daily dosing of gentamicin has not been well studied in pregnant or breastfeeding women, patients with major burns, renal failure, endocarditis or cystic

If result available within 24 h

- Use graph below to select dose interval. Use serum concentration and time interval between start of infusion and sample to plot intercept (see example given on graph).
- Give next dose (7 mg/kg by infusion as above) after interval indicated by graph.
  If result falls above upper limit for Q48 h, abandon once daily regimen. Measure gentamicin concentration after another 24 h and adopt multiple daily dose regimen if result <2 mg/L
  If result falls on Q24 h sector it is not necessary to recheck gentamicin concentration within 5 days unless patient's condition suggests renal function may be compromised.

- **Graph:**   Use values of plasma concentration and time interval to find intercept
                  (Example given of 6 mg/L after 10 h yields dose interval of 36 h)

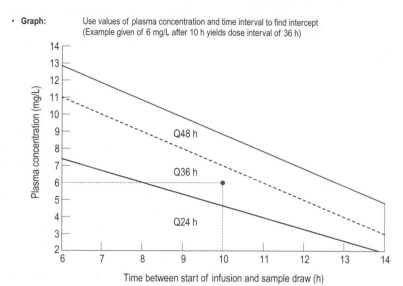

MONITORING

- Repeat U&E daily. Calculate creatinine clearance from serum creatinine to check dose interval has not changed.
- If dose interval has to be changed, check gentamicin concentration 6 – 14 h after start of next infusion note time of start of infusion and time of sampling and use graph to verify correct dose interval.

Fig. 3.7   Nomogram for adjustment of once daily gentamicin dosage (Nicolau et al., 1995).

fibrosis. Therefore, it cannot be recommended in these groups and multiple daily dosing should be used.

Lithium

Lithium is effective in the treatment of acute mania and in the prophylaxis of manic depression. The mechanism of action is not fully understood, but it is thought that it may substitute for sodium or potassium in the central nervous system. Lithium is toxic, producing dose-dependent and dose-independent side effects. Therefore, TDM is essential in assisting in the management of the dosage.

Dose-dependent effects

The plasma concentration–response relationship derived on the basis of the 12-h standardised lithium level (measured 12 h after the evening dose of lithium) is shown below:

- <0.4 mmol/L: little therapeutic effect
- 0.4–1.0 mmol/L: optimum range for prophylaxis
- 0.8–1.2 mmol/l: optimum range for acute mania
- 1.2–1.5 mmol/L: causes possible renal impairment
- 1.5–3.0 mmol/L: causes renal impairment, ataxia, weakness, drowsiness, thirst, diarrhoea

- 3.0–5.0 mmol/L: causes confusion, spasticity, dehydration, convulsions, coma, death. (Levels above 3.5 mmol/L are regarded as a medical emergency.)

Dose-independent effects

These include tremor, hypothyroidism (approximately 10% of patients on chronic therapy), nephrogenic diabetes insipidus, gastro-intestinal upset, loss in bone density, weight gain (approximately 20% of patients gain more than 10 kg) and lethargy.

Distribution

Lithium is unevenly distributed throughout the body, with a volume of distribution of approximately 0.7 L/kg. Lithium follows a two-compartment model (see Fig. 3.3) with a distribution time of 8 h (hence, the 12-h sampling criterion).

Elimination

Lithium is excreted unchanged by the kidneys. Lithium clearance is approximately 25% of creatinine clearance, since there is extensive reabsorption in the renal tubules.

In addition to changes in renal function, dehydration, diuretics (particularly thiazides), angiotensin-converting enzyme inhibitors (ACE inhibitors) and non-steroidal anti-inflammatory drugs (NSAIDs) (except aspirin and sulindac) all decrease lithium clearance. Conversely, aminophylline and sodium loading increase lithium clearance.

Notwithstanding the above factors, there is a wide inter-individual variation in clearance, and the lithium half-life in the population varies between 8 and 35 h with an average of approximately 18 h. Lithium clearance shows a diurnal variation, being slower at night than during the day.

Practical implications

In view of the narrow therapeutic index, lithium should not be prescribed unless facilities for monitoring plasma lithium concentrations are available. Since lithium excretion is a first-order process, changes in dosage result in a proportional change in blood levels. Blood samples should be drawn 12 h after the evening dose, since this will allow for distribution and represent the slowest excretion rate. Population pharmacokinetic data (particularly the volume of distribution) cannot be relied upon to make initial dosage predictions, although renal function may give an approximate guide to clearance. Blood level measurements are reported in SI units and therefore it is useful to know the conversion factors for the various salts.

- 100 mg of lithium carbonate is equivalent to 2.7 mmol of lithium ions
- 100 mg of lithium citrate is equivalent to 1.1 mmol of lithium ions.

Phenytoin

Phenytoin is used in the treatment of epilepsy (see Chapter 31). Use is associated with dose-independent side effects which include hirsutism, acne, coarsening of facial features, gingival hyperplasia, hypocalcaemia and folic acid deficiency. However, phenytoin has a narrow therapeutic index and has serious concentration-related side effects.

Plasma concentration–response relationship

- <5 mg/L: generally no therapeutic effect
- 5–10 mg/L: some anticonvulsant action with approximately 50% of patients obtaining a therapeutic effect with concentrations of 8–10 mg/L
- 10–20 mg/L: optimum concentration for anticonvulsant effect
- 20–30 mg/L: nystagmus, blurred vision
- >30 mg/L: ataxia, dysarthria, drowsiness, coma.

Distribution

Phenytoin follows a two-compartment model with a distribution time of 30–60 min. The apparent volume of distribution is 1 L/kg.

Elimination

The main route of elimination is via hepatic metabolism. However, this metabolic route can be saturated at normal therapeutic doses. This results in the characteristic non-linear dose/concentration curve seen in Fig. 3.6B. Therefore, instead of the usual first-order pharmacokinetic model, a Michaelis–Menten model, used to describe enzyme activity, is more appropriate.

Using this model, the daily dosage of phenytoin can be described by

$$\frac{S \times F \times \text{dose}}{T} = \frac{V_{\max} \times C^{ss}}{K_m + C^{ss}} \qquad (15)$$

K_m is the plasma concentration at which metabolism proceeds at half the maximal rate. The population average for this is 5.7 mg/L, although this value varies greatly with age and race.

$V_{\max}$ is the maximum rate of metabolism of phenytoin and is more predictable at approximately 7 mg/kg/day.

Since clearance changes with blood concentration, the half-life also changes. The usual reported value is 22 h, but this increases as concentration increases. Therefore, it is difficult to predict when the steady state will be reached. However, as a rule of thumb, 1–2 weeks should be allowed to elapse before sampling after a dosage change.

In overdose, it can be assumed that metabolism of the drug is occurring at the maximum rate of $V_{\max}$. Therefore, the decline in plasma concentration is linear (zero-order) at approximately 7 mg/L/day.

Practical implications

Since the dose/concentration relationship is non-linear, changes in dose do not result in proportional changes in plasma concentration (see Fig. 3.6B). Using the Michaelis–Menten model, if the plasma concentration is known at one dosage, then $V_{\max}$ may be assumed to be the population average (7 mg/kg/day), since this is the more predictable parameter, and K_m calculated using Eq. (15). The revised values of K_m can then be used in Eq. (15) to estimate the new dosage required to produce a desired concentration. Alternatively, a nomogram may be used to assist in dose adjustments (Fig. 3.8).

Care is needed when interpreting TDM data and making dosage adjustments when phenytoin is given concurrently with other anticonvulsants, since these affect distribution and metabolism of phenytoin. Since phenytoin is approximately 90% protein bound, in patients with a low plasma albumin and or uraemia, the free fraction increases and therefore an adjusted total phenytoin should be calculated or a free salivary level taken. To adjust the observed concentration in hypoalbuminaemia the following equation can be applied:

$$C_{\text{adjusted}} = \frac{C_{\text{observed}}}{0.9 \times (C_{\text{albumin}} / 44) + 0.1}$$

Albumin concentration is in g/L.

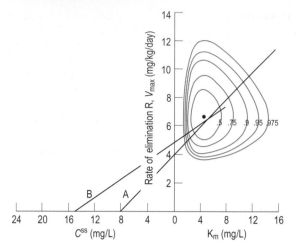

Fig. 3.8 Orbit graph. The most probable values of V_{max} and k_m for a patient may be estimated using a single steady-state phenytoin concentration and a known dosing regimen. The eccentric circles or 'orbits' represent the fraction of the sample patient population whose k_m and V_{max} values are within that orbit. (1) Plot the daily dose of phenytoin (mg/kg/day) on the vertical line (rate of elimination). (2) Plot the steady-state concentration (C^{ss}) on the horizontal line. (3) Draw a straight line connecting C^{ss} and daily dose through the orbits (line A). (4) The coordinates of the mid point of the line crossing the innermost orbit through which the line passes are the most probable values for the patient's V_{max} and k_m. (5) To calculate a new maintenance dose, draw a line from the point determined in Step 4 to the new desired C^{ss} (line B). The point at which line B crosses the vertical line (rate of elimination) is the new maintenance dose (mg/kg/day). The line A represents a C^{ss} of 8 mg/l on 276 mg/day of phenytoin acid (300 mg/day of sodium phenytoin) for a 70 kg patient. Line B has been drawn assuming the new desired steady-state concentration was 15 mg/L (μg/mL). The original figure is modified so that R and V_{max} are in mg/kg/day of phenytoin acid (modified from Evans et al., 1992).

In ureamic patients with severe renal failure, the unbound fraction is approximately doubled, so the target concentration needs to be half the normal concentration or apply the adjusted concentration equation if albumin level is known.

The oral formulations of phenytoin show good bioavailability. However, tablets and capsules contain the sodium salt ($S = 0.9$), whereas the suspension and infatabs are phenytoin base ($S = 1$). Intramuscular phenytoin is slowly and unpredictably absorbed, due to crystallisation in the muscle tissue, and is therefore not recommended. Fosphenytoin, a prodrug of phenytoin, is better absorbed from the intramuscular site. Doses should be expressed as phenytoin equivalent. Fosphenytoin sodium 1.5 mg is equivalent to phenytoin sodium 1 mg.

Carbamazepine

Carbamazepine is indicated for the treatment of partial and secondary generalised tonic-clonic seizures, primary generalised tonic-clonic seizures, trigeminal neuralgia, and prophylaxis of bipolar disorder unresponsive to lithium. There are a number of dose-independent side effects, including various dermatological reactions and, more rarely, aplastic anaemia

and Stevens–Johnson syndrome. However, the more common side effects are concentration related.

Plasma concentration–response relationship when used in the treatment of epilepsy

- <4 mg/L: little therapeutic benefit
- 4–12 mg/L: optimum therapeutic range for monotherapy
- >9 mg/L: possible side effects of nystagmus, diplopia, drowsiness and ataxia, particularly if patients are on other anticonvulsant therapy
- >12 mg/L: side effects common, even on monotherapy.

Distribution

Carbamazepine is distributed widely in various organs, with the highest concentration found in liver and kidneys. Carbamazepine is 70–80% protein bound and shows a wide variation in the population average apparent volume of distribution (0.8–1.9 L/kg). This wide variation is thought to be due to variations in absorption (since there is no parenteral form) and protein binding.

Elimination

Carbamazepine is eliminated almost exclusively by metabolism, with less than 2% being excreted unchanged in the urine. Elimination is a first-order process, but carbamazepine induces its own metabolism (auto-induction). Therefore, at the beginning of therapy, clearance is 0.01–0.03 L/h/kg, rising to 0.05–0.1 L/h/kg on chronic therapy. Auto-induction begins in the first few days of commencing therapy and is maximal at 2–4 weeks.

Since clearance changes with time, so does half-life, with reported values as long as 35 h after a single dose, decreasing to 5–7 h on regular dosing.

Absorption

Absorption after oral administration is slow, with peak concentrations being reached 2–24 h post-dose (average 6 h). Absorption is incomplete, with bioavailability estimated at approximately 80% ($F = 0.8$).

Practical implications

Use of pharmacokinetic equations is limited, due to the auto-induction effect. However, there are a number of important practical points:

- Blood samples should not be drawn before the steady state, which will not be achieved until 2–4 weeks after starting therapy to allow for auto-induction, or 3–4 days after subsequent dose adjustments.
- When sampling, the trough level should be measured because of the variable absorption pattern.
- Complex calculations are not helpful, but as a rule of thumb each 100 mg dose will increase the plasma concentration at the steady state by approximately 1 mg/L in adults.

- A number of other drugs (including phenytoin) when given concurrently will affect carbamazepine metabolism and subsequent blood levels.

Phenobarbital

Phenobarbital is indicated in all forms of epilepsy except absence seizures. Although there is a clear concentration–response relationship, routine plasma concentration monitoring is less useful than for other drugs, since tolerance occurs.

Plasma concentration–response relationship

- <15 mg/L: little therapeutic effect
- 15–40 mg/L: optimum range
- 40–50 mg/L: sedation, confusion (elderly), although may be tolerated by some patients
- >60 mg/L: serious toxic effect of ataxia, lethargy, stupor, coma.

The sedation which commonly manifests early on in therapy becomes less with continued therapy.

Distribution

Phenobarbital readily distributes into most body tissues and is 50% protein bound. The population-average volume of distribution is 0.7–1 L/kg.

Elimination

Phenobarbital is primarily (80%) metabolised by the liver, with approximately 20% being excreted unchanged in the urine. Elimination is a first-order process, but is relatively slow with a population average clearance of approximately 0.004 L/h/kg. However, as with theophylline, clearance in children is increased and is approximately twice the adult clearance. Applying Eqs. (6) and (8) to these population values gives an estimate of the half-life of the order of 5 days. This is much shorter in children and longer in the elderly.

Practical application

In view of the long half-life, single daily dosage is possible with phenobarbital. Samples for therapeutic monitoring may be drawn any time during a dose interval, since concentration fluctuation between doses is minimal. However, the patient should be at the steady state, which takes 2–4 weeks (1–2 weeks in children). The pharmacokinetics of phenobarbital may be altered by liver and (less markedly) renal disease, but are not affected by the concurrent administration of other anticonvulsants.

Primidone

Like phenobarbital, primidone is effective in the treatment of tonic–clonic and partial seizures. Much of the anticonvulsant activity of primidone is due to the metabolites phenobarbital and phenylethylmalonamide. Therefore, primidone plasma concentrations are only useful to confirm transient toxicity.

Toxic manifestations such as sedation, nausea and ataxia are seen at concentrations greater than 15 mg/L. The plasma concentration should be drawn approximately 3 h post dose, which corresponds to the peak concentration.

Phenylethylmalonamide assays are not routinely available, although this metabolite probably contributes to anticonvulsant activity. Measurement of phenobarbital levels is of limited value, since conversion of primidone to phenobarbital is variable between individuals. However, phenobarbital levels may be helpful in dosage selection, where seizures are not adequately controlled despite regular dosage, or where there is suspected toxicity.

Valproate

Sodium valproate as valproic acid in the bloodstream has a broad spectrum of anticonvulsant activity, being useful in generalised absence, generalised tonic–colonic and partial seizures.

Plasma concentration–response relationship

There is no clear concentration–response relationship for valproate, although a range of 50–100 mg/L is often quoted as being optimal, with 50% of patients showing a response at levels above 80 mg/L. Levels above 100 mg/L do not confer any additional therapeutic benefits. Although there is no clear relationship between plasma levels and toxic effects, the rare hepatotoxicity associated with valproate appears to be related to very high levels of over 150 mg/L.

Distribution

Valproate is extensively bound to plasma protein (90–95%), and unlike other drugs, it can saturate protein binding sites at concentrations greater than 50 mg/L, altering the free fraction of drug. Therefore, the apparent volume of distribution of valproate varies from 0.1 to 0.5 L/kg.

Elimination

Elimination of valproate is almost entirely by hepatic metabolism, with less than 5% being eliminated by the kidneys.

As a result of the saturation of protein binding sites and the subsequent increase in the free fraction of the drug, clearance of the drug increases at higher concentrations. Therefore, there is a non-linear change in plasma concentration with dose (illustrated in Fig. 3.6C).

Practical implications

In view of the lack of a clear concentration–response relationship and the variable pharmacokinetics, there are limited indications for the measurement of valproate levels. In most cases, dosage should be based on clinical response. Valproic acid can take several weeks to become fully active, so adjustment of doses must not be made quickly.

In a few cases where seizures are not controlled at high dosage, a plasma level may be helpful in confirming treatment failure. If monitoring is to be undertaken, levels should be drawn at steady state (2–3 days). A trough sample will be the most useful, since wide fluctuations of blood levels may occur during a dose interval.

Lamotrigine, vigabatrin, gabapentin, tiagabine, topiramate, pregabalin, lacosamide and levetiracetam

These newer medicines are indicated for the treatment of a range of types of epilepsy and some with additional indications. All are used as adjunctive treatment with other anticonvulsants, and some indicated for monotherapy.

Plasma concentration–response relationship

There is no clear relationship between plasma concentration and response for these newer anticonvulsants. The situation is further complicated by the fact that these preparations are usually used as add-on therapy with other anticonvulsants.

Practical implications

While these newer anticonvulsants have narrow therapeutic indices and inter- and intra-individual variation in pharmacokinetics, there is not enough evidence to support routine TDM, and dosage should be titrated to clinical response.

Ciclosporin

Ciclosporin is a neutral lipophilic cyclic endecapeptide extracted from the fungus *Tolypocladium inflatum gams*. It is a potent immunosuppressive agent, used principally to reduce graft rejection after organ and tissue transplantation. The drug has a low therapeutic index, with a number of toxic effects including nephrotoxicity, hepatotoxicity, gastro-intestinal intolerance, hypertrichosis and neurological problems. Efficacy in reducing graft rejection as well as the main toxic effect of nephro- and hepatotoxicity appear to be concentration related.

Plasma concentration–response relationship

With all drugs that are monitored the therapeutic range is a window with limits, which are not absolute. It is even more difficult to define a therapeutic range for ciclosporin, since there are a number of influencing factors. First, the measured concentration varies depending on sampling matrix (i.e. whole blood or plasma). Second, it depends on whether the assay is specific for ciclosporin alone or non-specific to include metabolites. A target concentration varies between centres, but is commonly around 100–200 ng/mL in the first 6 months after transplantation and 80–150 ng/mL from 6 months onwards. Levels below the lower limit

of this window are associated with an increased incidence of graft rejection. Levels above the upper limit are associated with an increased incidence of nephrotoxicity and hepatotoxicity.

Distribution

Ciclosporin is highly lipophilic and is distributed widely throughout the body with a volume of distribution of 4–8 L/kg. There is variable distribution of ciclosporin within blood, since the whole blood concentration is approximately twice the plasma concentration. Within plasma, ciclosporin is 98% protein bound.

Elimination

Ciclosporin is eliminated primarily by hepatic metabolism, with wide inter-individual variation in clearance (0.1–2 L/h/kg). In children these values are approximately 40% higher, with a resulting increased dosage requirement on a milligram per kilogram basis. In elderly patients or patients with hepatic impairment a lower clearance rate has been observed.

Practical implications

In addition to the wide inter-patient variability in distribution and elimination pharmacokinetic parameters, absorption of standard formulations of ciclosporin is variable and incomplete ($F = 0.2$–0.5 in normal subjects). In transplant patients this variation in bioavailability is even greater, and increases during the first few months after transplant. Furthermore, a number of drugs are known to interact with ciclosporin. All these factors suggest that therapeutic drug monitoring will assist in optimum dose selection, but the use of population averages in dose prediction is of little benefit, due to wide inter-patient variation. When using TDM with ciclosporin a number of practical points need to be considered:

- The sampling matrix should be whole blood, since there is a variable distribution of ciclosporin between blood and plasma.
- Samples should represent trough levels and be drawn at the steady state, which is achieved 2–3 days after initiating or changing the dosage (average half-life is 9 h).
- Ciclosporin concentration monitoring should be undertaken every 2–3 days in the immediate postoperative phase until the patient's clinical condition is stable. Thereafter, monitoring can be undertaken every 1–2 months.
- TDM should be performed when changing brands of ciclosporin, since there are marked differences in the bioavailability of different brands.

Summary pharmacokinetic data for drugs with therapeutic plasma concentrations are listed in Table 3.1.

Table 3.1 Summary of pharmacokinetic data

Drug	Therapeutic range of plasma concentrations	V_d (L/kg)	CL (L/h/kg)	Half-life (h)
Digoxin	0.8–2.0 μcg/L (0.5–0.9 μcg/L in patients >65) 1–2.6 nmol/L (0.625 nmol/L – 1.1 nmol/L in patients >65)	7.3	See text	36
Theophylline	10–20 mg/L 55–110 μmol/L	0.48	0.04	8
Gentamicin	Peak 5–12 mg/L, trough <2 mg/L	0.3	1 × CL (creatinine)	2
Lithium	0.4–0.8 mmol/L	0.5–1	0.2 × CL (creatinine)	18
Phenytoin	10–20 mg/L 40–80 μmol/L	1	K_m = 5.7 mg/L V_{max} = 7 mg/kg/day	
Carbamazepine	4–12 mg/L 17–50 μmol/L	0.8–1.9	0.05–1	
Phenobarbital	15–40 mg/L 65–172 μmol/L	0.7–1	0.004	120
Primidone	<15 mg/L <69 μmol/L	0.6		
Valproate	<100 mg/L <693 μmol/L			
Ciclosporin	Varies between centres 100–200 ng/mL (first 6 months after transplantation) 80–150 ng/mL (from 6 months onwards)			9

Population pharmacokinetic parameters are based on averages. The degree of variability around the average is different for each drug. See text for variability.

Case studies

Case 3.1

You are reviewing a formulary submission for a new formulation of a product, which has reportedly an improved side effect profile due to better absorption characteristics. However, there is conflicting evidence in the literature over the absorption of the new preparation. One paper, which is available to you, shows a concentration-time profile for the oral formulation after a single oral dose of 250 mg as in Table 3.2.

The paper also quotes an area under the curve (AUC) after a single i.v. dose of 200 mg as 87 mg/L/h.

Table 3.2 Concentration-time profile for the oral formulation after a single oral dose of 250 mg

Time after administration	1h	2h	3h	4h	5h	6h	7h	8h	9h	10h	11h	12h
Concentration (mg/L)	10	18	12.7	9	6.4	4.5	3.2	2.25	1.6	1.1	0.78	0.55

Questions

1. What is the AUC after the single oral dose of 250 mg?
2. What is the bioavailability of the new formulation?

Answers

1. Draw the concentration-time profile on a piece of paper; try to do it reasonably accurately but it does not have to be exact. Draw down vertical lines from the curve at each 1-h time interval to create a series of trapeziums (the first one is actually a triangle). Calculate the area of each trapezium from the formula

   Area of trapezium = (sum of the height of each side/2) × width (1h)

   Then add all the areas together (assume a value of 0 after 12h)

   AUC p.o. = 69.99 mg/L/h

2. From the equation $F = \dfrac{D\,\text{i.v.} \times \text{AUC p.o.}}{D\,\text{p.o.} \times \text{AUC i.v.}}$

   $F = 200 \times 69.99 / 250 \times 87$
   $F = 0.64$

Case 3.2

An 86-year-old lady is admitted to hospital by her primary care doctor, with increasing shortness of breath. She lives alone, is independent and has a flat on the 5th floor of a block of flats. She has a stable plasma creatinine of 150 µmol/L

She is 55 kg, 4′ 11″ tall.

She is known to have recently diagnosed atrial fibrillation, osteoporosis and ischaemic heart disease.

Her current medication is:

Aspirin	300 mg daily
Adcal D3	Two tablets daily
Imdur	60 mg daily
Simvastatin	40 mg daily
Senna	7.5 mg daily
Digoxin	62.5 µcg daily

She has been taking digoxin in a dose of 62.5 µcg daily for the last 3 weeks.

Questions

1. Calculate the predicted digoxin level for this lady.
2. A digoxin blood level is reported to be 1.0 µcg/L. List the reasons for the difference between the measured and predicted digoxin levels.
3. The hospital doctor queries if he should increase the dose of digoxin as the blood level is on the low side. Use an evidence-based approach to reply to the clinician.

Answers

1. Her predicted glomerular filtration rate is calculated from Cockcroft-Gault equation:

$$\text{Creatinine clearance (mL/min)} = \frac{F \times [(140 - \text{age in years}) \times \text{weight (kg)}]}{\text{plasma creatinine (µmol/L)}}$$

$$\text{Creatinine clearance (CL}_{cr}) = \frac{1.04(140 - 86)55}{150} = 20.6 \text{ mL/min}$$

On the assumption that the patient has severe congestive heart failure, the predicted digoxin level is calculated using the equation:

$$CL_{dig} = 0.33 \times IBW + 0.9 \times CL_{cr}$$
$$= (0.33 \times 55) + (0.9 \times 20.6) = 36.69 \text{ mL/min} = 2.2 \text{ L/h}$$

Ideal body weight (IBW (kg)):

$$\text{Male} = 50 + (2.3 \times \text{height in inches over 5 feet})$$

$$\text{Female} = 45.5 + (2.3 \times \text{height in inches over 5 feet})$$

Equation (4) rate of administration = rate of elimination = $CL \times C^{ss}$

Rearranging Eq. (4):

$$C_{ssave} = \frac{\text{Dose} \times S \times F}{CL_{dig} \times \tau} = \frac{62.5 \times 1 \times 0.63}{2.2 \times 2.4} = 0.75 \,\mu\text{cg/L}$$

2. The predicted level is less than the measured level, this may be because:
   - The level has been taken less than 6 h after the oral dose
   - Suspected non-adherence
   - Congestive heart failure has affected the renal function
3. A subgroup analysis of the Digitalis Investigation Group suggested that participants >65 years who had low blood levels (0.5–0.9 µcg/L) had reductions in all – cause mortality. It has also been suggested that digoxin may be associated with an increased risk of problems in patients with atrial fibrillation (Gjesdal et al., 2008).
   Therefore, the dose of digoxin should not be increased.

Case 3.3

A 68-year-old man (72 kg, 5′ 2″ tall) is admitted to the medical ward from intensive care as he is in a stable condition. He was admitted 2 days ago with Gram negative sepsis identified from a blood culture. He was commenced on gentamicin 5 mg/kg once daily as per the hospital protocol.

Current laboratory results are:

Urea	31.6 mmol/L (3.2–7.5 mmol/L)
Creatinine	168 µmol/L (71–133 µmol/L)

Gentamicin levels were taken 1 and 8 h after the first dose and reported as 19 and 10 mg/L, respectively.

Questions

1. Calculate the patient's elimination constant k_e.
2. Calculate the plasma concentration at C° immediately after the injection.
3. Using the plasma concentration at C° calculate the level you would expect the patient to achieve immediately prior to his next dose.
4. Calculate the dosage interval you would recommend aiming for a trough of 1 mg/L.

Answers

1. As the two plasma levels are known the elimination constant k_e is calculated from the following equation.

$$k_e = \frac{\ln C_1 - \ln C_2}{t}$$

Using the plasma levels reported:

$$k_e = \frac{\ln 19 - \ln 10}{7}$$

$$k_e = 0.092 \text{ h}^{-1}$$

2. The plasma concentration at C° immediately after the injection is calculated as:

$$C^t = C^\circ \times e^{-k_e \times t}$$

$$19 = C^\circ \times e^{-0.092 \times 1}$$

$$C^\circ = 20.8 \text{ mg/L}$$

3. The plasma concentration at C° is then used to calculate the expected level to be achieved immediately prior to his next dose.

$$C^t = C^\circ \times e^{-k_e \times t}$$

$$C^t = 20.8 \times e^{-0.092 \times 24}$$

$$= 2.2 \text{ mg/L}$$

4. The dosage interval can then be calculated for a trough of 0.5 mg/L

$$Cp^t = Cp^\circ \times e^{-k_e \times t}$$

$$\ln 0.5 = \ln 20.8 \times (-0.092 \times t)$$

$$-0.693 = 3.03 \times (-0.092 \times t)$$

$$t = 40.52 \text{ h}$$

As this time interval is more than 24 h and could potentially become nephrotoxic/ototoxic, an alternative antibiotic should be prescribed.

Case 3.4

A 68-year-old Argentinean man (69 kg) was found wandering in the street. A neighbour alerted the police. He was described as being confused and agitated. The patient could not speak English and on admission to hospital could not give a history. The neighbour told the ambulance staff the patient was normally well, but known to be taking medicines for a mental disorder. The ambulance staff found lithium and amisulpride in the man's pockets.

A sample of lithium was taken and reported as 2.5 mmol/L (0.6–1 mmol/L). His plasma creatinine was 160 µmol/L so the lithium was stopped.

Questions

1. Calculate the patient's pharmacokinetic parameters clearance (CL), volume of distribution (V_d), elimination constant (k_e) using population data.
2. Estimate the time for the lithium level to decrease to the middle of the normal range.
3. Briefly describe the symptoms of lithium toxicity.

Answers

1. Population data suggests that the clearance of lithium can be calculated using the following equation:

$$\text{Clearance} = 0.25 \times \text{CrCL (L/h)}$$

The patient's creatinine clearance (CrCL) is calculated using the Cockcroft and Gault equation:

$$\text{Creatinine clearance (CrCL)} = \frac{1.23 \times (140 - \text{age}) \times \text{weight in kg}}{\text{Plasma creatinine (µmol/L)}}$$

$$\text{Creatinine clearance (CrCL)} = \frac{1.23 \times (140 - 68) \times 69}{160} = 38.2 \text{ mL/min}$$

Convert 38.2 mL/min to L/h

$$\frac{38.2 \times 60}{1000} = 2.29 \text{ L/h}$$

Lithium clearance = $0.25 \times 2.29 = 0.573$ L/h

Population data suggests that the volume of distribution (V_d) for lithium is 0.7 L/Kg.

Therefore, for this patient the volume of distribution:

$$V_d = 0.7 \times 69$$
$$V_d = 48.3 \text{ L}$$

The elimination rate constant k_e is calculated:

$$CL = k_e \times V_d \quad \text{to give } k_e = \frac{CL}{V_d}$$

$$k_e = \frac{0.573}{48.3}$$

$$k_e = 0.01186 \text{ h}^{-1}$$

2. The time it will take for this man's lithium level to return to the middle of the normal range (0.6-1 mmol/L), that is, 0.7 mmol/L is calculated using:

$$\text{Time to decay} = \frac{\ln Cp^1 - \ln Cp^2}{k_e}$$

$$\text{Time to decay} = \frac{\ln 2.5 - \ln 0.7}{0.01186}$$

$$\text{Time to decay} = 107.3 \text{ h} = 4.5 \text{ days}$$

3. Acute lithium toxicity tends to present with gastro-intestinal symptoms. If the toxicity is due to an increase in dose, symptoms will include neuromuscular signs, for example, ataxia and tremor. This is sometimes referred to as acute on chronic toxicity. Chronic toxicity is harder to treat due to tissue deposition and involves neurological problems.

Case 3.5

Mr B is a 38-year old, 63 kg man who suffers from asthma. He has been admitted to hospital and Nuelin S.A. 500 mg 12 hourly (6 am and 6 pm) has been added to his regimen. He responds well to this treatment but unfortunately after 2 days of treatment two doses are missed (evening dose and following morning dose). The clinical team is anxious to discharge him, so it is decided to give him a loading dose of aminophylline at 10 am before restarting him on maintainence therapy.

Questions

1. Was the patient at steady state before the medication was omitted?
2. What is the estimated theophylline level at 10 am?
3. The levels were then checked and the theophylline level was reported as 4 mg/L. What loading dose of i.v. aminophylline would you recommend?

Answers

1. His pharmacokinetic parameters can be calculated from population data

$$\text{Clearance} = 63 \text{ kg} \times 0.04 \text{ L/h/kg} = 2.52 \text{ L/h}$$

$$V_d = 63 \text{ kg} \times 0.45 \text{ L/kg} = 28.3 \text{ L}$$

$$k_e = \frac{CL}{V_d}$$

$$k_e = 0.089 \text{ h}^{-1}$$

Using Eq. (8), $t_{\frac{1}{2}} = 0.693/k_e$

The patient's half-life ($t_{1/2}$) = 7.8 h.

It can therefore be assumed he was at steady state after 48 h of treatment (more than 5 × half-life).

2. To calculate his levels at 10 am it is assumed that S.R. theophylline behaves like an i.v. infusion ($F = 1.0$). Although this is not strictly true, Nuelin S.A. has a good slow release profile.

From Eq. (12)

$$\frac{S \times F \times \text{dose}}{T} = \text{Average } C^{ss} \times \text{CL}$$

$$\text{Average} C^{ss} = \frac{S \times F \times \text{dose}}{T \times \text{CL}}$$

$$\text{Average} C^{ss} = \frac{500 \times 1}{12 \times 2.52}$$

$$\text{Average} C^{ss} = 16.5 \text{mg} / \text{L}$$

To calculate theophylline concentration at 10 am, $C^{10\,am}$ need to delay this for 16 h as the morning dose from the previous day will have provided a steady dose of theophylline until the evening (first missed dose), so starting dose is C^{ss}.

Using Eq. (7)

$$C_2 = C_1 \times e^{-k_e \times t}$$

$$C^{10\,am} = 16.5 \times e^{-k_e \times 16}$$

$$C^{10\,am} = 16.5 \times e^{-0.089 \times 16}$$

$$C^{10\,am} = 3.97 \text{mg/L}$$

3. To calculate a loading dose the change in theophylline concentration (C) to be achieved needs to be calculated:

$$C = \text{desired } C \ (15 \text{ mg}/\text{L}) - \text{actual} \ (4 \text{ mg}/\text{L})$$

From Eq. (1):

$$\text{Loading dose} = C \times V_d$$

$$\text{Loading dose} = 11 \times 28.3 \text{ L}$$

$$\text{Loading dose} = 311 \text{ mg of theophylline}$$

Aminophylline is only 80% theophylline, therefore

$$\text{Loading dose} = \frac{311}{0.8}$$

Aminophylline loading dose = 390 mg aminophylline to be administered by slow i.v. bolus.

Case 3.6

A 29-year-old man (70 kg) was diagnosed with TB meningitis 2 months ago. He is currently in hospital because of social issues. His liver function and other biochemical results are within the normal range. He was started on phenytoin capsules 350 mg daily at the time of diagnosis.

His current medication is:

Pyridoxine	12.5 mg daily
Rifater	four tablets daily
Phenytoin capsules	350 mg daily

One month after being started on this medication his phenytoin plasma level is measured as 7 mg/L

Questions

1. Using population data, calculate this man's predicted phenytoin plasma level.
2. Explain the difference between the predicted and actual phenytoin level
3. Using the phenytoin plasma level reported, assume steady state. Calculate this patient's V_{max}.
4. Calculate the dose required to obtain a plasma level of 10 mg/L at steady state.
5. Compare your answer using the orbit plot.

Answers

1. Using population data, calculate this man's predicted plasma level.
   F, bioavailabilty; S, salt factor; V_{max}, maximum rate of metabolism; K_m, Michaelis-Menten constant.
   $V_{max} = 7$ mg/kg/day, $K_m = 5.7$ mg/L, $D = 350$ mg, $F = 1$, $S = 0.92$.
   Rearranging Eq. (15):

$$\frac{S \times F \times \text{dose}}{T} = \frac{V_{max} \times C^{ss}}{K_m + C^{ss}}$$

$$C^{ss} = \frac{K_m \times (S \times F \times \text{dose})}{(V_{max} \times T) - (S \times F \times \text{dose})}$$

$$C^{ss} = \frac{5.7 \times 0.92 \times 350}{70 \times 7 \times 1 - (0.92 \times 350)}$$

$$C^{ss} = \frac{1835.4}{490 - 322}$$

$$C^{ss} = 10.93 \text{ mg/L}$$

2. There are a number of potential reasons for the difference between the predicted and actual level:
   - The patient is not at steady state. This is unlikely as he has been on this medication from diagnosis 2 months ago.
   - The patient is not taking the phenytoin prescribed. This is also unlikely because as a hospital inpatient the nursing staff have been giving him his medication.
   - There is an interaction between the rifampacin and phenytoin. This is the most likely reason.

3. Using the plasma level reported, assume steady state. Calculate this patient's actual V_{max}.
   Using $K_m = 5.7$ mg/L

$$\text{Current phenytoin plasma level } 7 = \frac{5.7 \times (350 \times 1 \times 0.92)}{V_{max} - (350 \times 1 \times 0.92)}$$

$$7 = \frac{1834.4}{V_{max} - 322}$$

$$V_{max} - 322 = \frac{1834.4}{7}$$

$$V_{max} = 262.2 + 322$$

$$V_{max} = 584 \text{ mg/day}$$

4. Calculate the dose required to obtain a plasma level of 10 mg/L at steady state:

$$\frac{S \times F \times \text{dose}}{T} = \frac{V_{max} \times C^{ss}}{K_m + C^{ss}}$$

$$\frac{S \times F \times \text{dose}}{1} = \frac{584 \times 10}{5.7 + 10}$$

$$\text{Dose} = \frac{371.97}{0.92}$$

$$\text{Dose} = 404 \text{ mg/day}$$

The nearest practical dose would be 400 mg per day and a level checked again in 2 weeks.

References

Cockcroft, D.W., Gault, M.H., 1976. Prediction of creatinine clearance from plasma creatinine. Nephron 16, 31–41.

Crist, K.D., Nahata, M.C., Ety, J., 1987. Positive impact of a therapeutic drug monitoring program on total aminoglycoside dose and hospitalisation. Ther. Drug Monit. 9, 306–310.

Department of Health, 2006. Estimated Glomerular Filtration Rate (eGFR). Department of Health Publications, London. Available from: //www.dh.gov.uk/en/Publicationsandstatistics/Publications/PublicationsPolicyAndGuidance/DH_4133020.

Evans, W.E., Shentag, J.J., Jusko, W.J. (Eds.), 1992. Applied Pharmacokinetics, 3rd edn. Applied Therapeutics. Lippincott Williams & Wilkins, Baltimore, pp. 586–617.

Gjesdal, K., Feyzi, J., Olssen, S.B., 2008. Digitalis: a dangerous drug in atrial fibrillation? Analysis of the SPORTIF III and V data. Heart 94, 191–196.

McFadyen, M.L., Miller, R., Juta, M., et al., 1990. The relevance of a first world therapeutic drug monitoring service to the treatment of epilepsy in third world conditions. S. Afr. Med. J. 78, 587–590.

Nicolau, D.P., Freeman, C.D., Belliveau, P.P., et al., 1995. Experience with a once daily aminoglycoside program administered to 2,184 adult patients. Antimicrob. Agents Chemother. 39, 650–655.

Reid, L.D., Horn, J.R., McKenna, D.A., 1990. Therapeutic drug monitoring reduces toxic drug reactions: a meta-analysis. Ther. Drug Monit. 12, 72–78.

Touw, D.J., Neef, C., Thomson, A.H., et al., 2007. Cost-effectiveness of therapeutic drug monitoring: an update. Eur. J. Hosp. Pharm. Sci. 13, 83–91.

Further reading

Begg, E.J., Barclay, M.L., Duffull, S.B., 1995. A suggested approach to once daily aminoglycoside dosing. Br. J. Clin. Pharmacol. 39, 605–609.

Burton, M.E., Shaw, L.M., Schentag, J.J., 2006. Applied Pharmacokinetics and Pharmacodynamics: Principles of Therapeutic Drug Monitoring, fourth ed. Lippincott Williams & Wilkins, Baltimore.

Dhillon, S., Kostrzewski, A., 2006. Clinical Pharmacokinetics. Pharmaceutical Press, London.

Elwes, R.D.C., Binnie, C.D., 1996. Clinical pharmacokinetics of newer antiepileptic drugs. Clin. Pharmacokinet. 30, 403–415.

Jermain, D.M., Crismon, M.L., Martin, E.S., 1991. Population pharmacokinetics of lithium. Clin. Pharmacokinet. 10, 376–381.

Lemmer, B., Bruguerolle, B., 1994. Chronopharmacokinetics: are they clinically relevant? Clin. Pharmacokinet. 26, 419–427.

Luke, D.R., Halstenson, C.E., Opsahl, J.A., et al., 1990. Validity of creatinine clearance estimates in the assessment of renal function. Clin. Pharmacol. Ther. 48, 503–508.

Rambeck, B., Boenigk, H.E., Dunlop, A., et al., 1980. Predicting phenytoin dose: a revised nomogram. Ther. Drug Monit. 1, 325–354.

Tserng, K., King, K.C., Takieddine, F.N., 1981. Theophylline metabolism in premature infants. Clin. Pharmacol. Ther. 29, 594–600.

Winter, M.E., 2003. Basic Clinical Pharmacokinetics. Lippincott Williams & Wilkins, Baltimore.

Yukawa, E., 1996. Optimisation of antiepileptic drug therapy: the importance of plasma drug concentration monitoring. Clin. Pharmacokinet. 31, 120–130.

4   Drug interactions

H. K. R. Thanacoody

Key points

- Drug interactions can cause significant patient harm and are an important cause of morbidity.
- Most clinically important drug interactions occur as a result of either decreased drug activity with diminished efficacy or increased drug activity with exaggerated or unusual effects. Drugs with a narrow therapeutic range, such as theophylline, lithium and digoxin, or a steep dose–response curve, such as anticoagulants, oral contraceptives and anti-epileptics, are often implicated.
- The most important pharmacokinetic interactions involve drugs that can induce or inhibit enzymes in the hepatic cytochrome P450 system.
- Pharmacodynamic interactions are difficult to classify but their effects can often be predicted when the pharmacology of co-administered drugs is known.
- In many cases, potentially interacting drugs can be given concurrently provided the possibility of interaction is kept in mind and any necessary changes to dose or therapy are initiated promptly. In some situations, however, concurrent use of potentially interacting drugs should be avoided altogether.
- Suspected adverse drug interactions should be reported to the appropriate regulatory authority as for other adverse drug reactions.

Drug interactions have been recognised for over 100 years. Today, with the increasing availability of complex therapeutic agents and widespread polypharmacy, the potential for drug interactions is enormous and they have become an increasingly important cause of adverse drug reactions (ADR).

Despite regulatory requirements to define the safety profile of new medicines including their potential for drug–drug interactions before marketing, the potential for adverse interactions is not always evident. This was illustrated by the worldwide withdrawal of the calcium channel blocker mibefradil, within months of launch, following reports of serious drug interactions (Li Wan Po and Zhang, 1998). In the past decade, a number of medicines have been either withdrawn from the market, for example, terfenadine, grepafloxacin and cisapride, or had their use restricted because of prolongation of the QT interval on the electrocardiogram, for example, thioridazine. Drug interactions are an important cause of QT prolongation which increases the risk of developing a life-threatening ventricular arrhythmia known as torsade de pointes (Roden, 2004).

The increasing availability and non-prescription use of herbal and complementary medicines has also led to greater awareness of their potential for adverse interactions. St John's wort, a herbal extract used for treatment of depression, can cause serious interactions as a result of its enzyme-inducing effects. Drug interactions with food and drink are also known to occur, exemplified by the well-known interaction between monoamine oxidase inhibitor antidepressants (MAOIs) and tyramine-containing foodstuffs. Grapefruit juice is a potent inhibitor of cytochrome P450 3A4 and causes clinically relevant interactions with a number of drugs including simvastatin and atorvastatin, thereby increasing the risk of statin-induced adverse reactions such as myopathy and myositis.

Although medical literature is awash with drug interaction studies and case reports of adverse drug interactions, only a relatively small number of these are likely to cause clinically significant consequences for patients. The recognition of clinically significant interactions requires knowledge of the pharmacological mechanisms of drug interactions and a thorough understanding of high-risk drugs and vulnerable patient groups.

Definition

An interaction is said to occur when the effects of one drug are altered by the co-administration of another drug, herbal medicine, food, drink or other environmental chemical agents (Baxter, 2010). The net effect of the combination may manifest as an additive or enhanced effect of one or more drugs, antagonism of the effect of one or more drugs, or any other alteration in the effect of one or more drugs.

Clinically significant interactions refer to a combination of therapeutic agents which have direct consequences on the patient's condition. Therapeutic benefit can be obtained from certain drug interactions, for example, a combination of different antihypertensive drugs may be used to improve blood pressure control or an opioid antagonist may be use to reverse the effect of an overdose of morphine. In this chapter, we will concentrate on clinically significant interactions which have the potential for undesirable effects on patient care.

Epidemiology

Accurate estimates of the incidence of drug interactions are difficult to obtain as published studies frequently use different criteria for defining a drug interaction, and for distinguishing between clinically significant and non-significant interactions. Some of the early studies uncritically compared prescribed drugs with lists of possible drug interactions without taking into account their potential clinical significance.

The reported incidence of drug–drug interactions in hospital admissions ranged from 0% to 2.8% in a review which included nine studies, all of which had some design flaws (Jankel and Fitterman, 1993). In the Harvard Medical Practice Study of adverse events, 20% of events in acute hospital inpatients were drug related. Of these, 8% were considered to be due to a drug interaction, suggesting that interactions are responsible for less than 2% of adverse events in this patient group (Leape et al., 1992).

In a 1-year prospective study of patients attending an Emergency Department, 3.8% resulted from a drug–drug interaction and most of these led to hospital admissions (Raschetti et al., 1999). In a prospective UK study carried out on hospital inpatients, ADR were responsible for hospital admission in 6.5% of cases. Drug interactions were involved in 16.6% of adverse reactions, therefore being directly responsible for leading to hospital admission in approximately 1% of cases (Pirmohamed et al., 2004).

Few studies have attempted to quantify the incidence of drug–drug interactions in the outpatient hospital setting and in the community. In the early 1990s, a community pharmacy study in the USA revealed a 4.1% incidence of interactions, while a Swedish study reported an incidence of 1.9%. In the outpatient setting, the availability of newer drugs for a variety of chronic conditions has increased the risk of drug–drug interactions in this patient group.

Although the overall incidence of serious adverse drug interactions is low, it remains a potentially preventable cause of morbidity and mortality.

Susceptible patients

The risk of drug interactions increases with the number of drugs used. In a hospital study, the rate of ADR in patients taking 6–10 drugs was 7%, rising to 40% in those taking 16–20 drugs, with the exponential rise being largely attributable to drug interactions (Smith et al., 1969). In a high-risk group of emergency department patients, the risk of potential adverse drug interaction was 13% in patients taking 2 drugs and 82% in those taking 7 or more drugs (Goldberg et al., 1996).

Although polypharmacy is common and often unavoidable, it places certain patient groups at increased risk of drug interactions. Patients at particular risk include those with hepatic or renal disease, those on long-term therapy for chronic disease, for example, HIV infection, epilepsy, diabetes, patients in intensive care, transplant recipients, patients undergoing complicated surgical procedures and those with more than one prescriber. Critically ill and elderly patients are

---

Box 4.1 Examples of drugs with high risk of interaction

Concentration-dependent toxicity
Digoxin
Lithium
Aminoglycosides
Cytotoxic agents
Warfarin

Steep dose–response curve
Verapamil
Sulphonylureas
Levodopa

Patient dependent on therapeutic effect
Immunosuppressives, e.g., ciclosporin, tacrolimus
Glucocorticoids
Oral contraceptives
Antiepileptics
Antiarrhythmics
Antipsychotics
Antiretrovirals

Saturable hepatic metabolism
Phenytoin
Theophylline

---

at increased risk not only because they take more medicines but also because of impaired homeostatic mechanisms that might otherwise counteract some of the unwanted effects. Interactions may occur in some individuals but not in others. The effects of interactions involving drug metabolism may vary greatly in individual patients because of differences in the rates of drug metabolism and in susceptibility to microsomal enzyme induction. Certain drugs are frequently implicated in drug interactions and require careful attention (Box 4.1).

Mechanisms of drug interactions

Drug interactions are conventionally discussed according to the mechanisms involved. These mechanisms can be conveniently divided into those with a pharmacokinetic basis and those with a pharmacodynamic basis. Drug interactions often involve more than one mechanism. There are some situations where drugs interact by unique mechanisms, but the most common mechanisms are discussed in this section.

Pharmacokinetic interactions

Pharmacokinetic interactions are those that affect the processes by which drugs are absorbed, distributed, metabolised or excreted. Due to marked interindividual variability in these processes, these interactions may be expected but their extent cannot be easily predicted. Such interactions may result in a change in the drug concentration at the site of action with subsequent toxicity or decreased efficacy.

Absorption

Following oral administration, drugs are absorbed through the mucous membranes of the gastro-intestinal tract. A number of factors can affect the rate of absorption or the extent of absorption (i.e. the total amount of drug absorbed).

Changes in gastro-intestinal pH. The absorption of a drug across mucous membranes depends on the extent to which it exists in the non-ionised, lipid-soluble form. The ionisation state depends on the pH of its milieu, the pK_a of the drug and formulation factors. Weakly acidic drugs, such as the salicylates, are better absorbed at low pH because the non-ionised form predominates.

An alteration in gastric pH due to antacids, histamine H_2 antagonists or proton pump inhibitors therefore has the potential to affect the absorption of other drugs. The clinical significance of antacid-induced changes in gastric pH is not certain, particularly since relatively little drug absorption occurs in the stomach. Changes in gastric pH tend to affect the rate of absorption rather than the extent of absorption, provided that the drug is acid labile. Although antacids could theoretically be expected to markedly influence the absorption of other drugs via this mechanism, in practice, there are very few clinically significant examples. Antacids, histamine H_2 antagonists and omeprazole can significantly decrease the bioavailability of ketoconazole and itraconazole, which require gastric acidity for optimal absorption, but the absorption of fluconazole and voriconazole is not significantly altered by changes in gastric pH.

The alkalinising effects of antacids on the gastro-intestinal tract are transient and the potential for interaction may be minimised by leaving an interval of 2–3 h between the antacid and the potentially interacting drug.

Adsorption, chelation and other complexing mechanisms. Certain drugs react directly within the gastro-intestinal tract to form chelates and complexes which are not absorbed. The drugs most commonly implicated in this type of interaction include tetracyclines and the quinolone antibiotics that can complex with iron, and antacids containing calcium, magnesium and aluminium. Tetracyclines can chelate with divalent or trivalent metal cations such as calcium, aluminium, bismuth and iron to form insoluble complexes, resulting in greatly reduced plasma tetracycline concentrations.

Bisphosphonates are often co-prescribed with calcium supplements in the treatment of osteoporosis. If these are taken concomitantly, however, the bioavailability of both is significantly reduced, with the possibility of therapeutic failure.

The absorption of some drugs may be reduced if they are given with adsorbents such as charcoal or kaolin, or anionic exchange resins such as colestyramine or colestipol. The absorption of propranolol, digoxin, warfarin, tricyclic antidepressants, ciclosporin and levothyroxine is reduced by colestyramine.

Most chelation and adsorption interactions can be avoided if an interval of 2–3 h is allowed between doses of the interacting drugs.

Effects on gastro-intestinal motility. Since most drugs are largely absorbed in the upper part of the small intestine, drugs that alter the rate at which the stomach empties its contents can affect absorption. Drugs with anticholinergic effects, such as tricyclic antidepressants, phenothiazines and some antihistamines, decrease gut motility and delay gastric emptying. The outcome of the reduced gut motility can either be an increase or a decrease in drugs given concomitantly. For example, tricyclic antidepressants can increase dicoumarol absorption, probably as a result of increasing the time available for its dissolution and absorption. Anticholinergic agents used in the management of movement disorders have been shown to reduce the bioavailability of levodopa by as much as 50%, possibly as a result of increased metabolism in the intestinal mucosa.

Opioids such as diamorphine and pethidine strongly inhibit gastric emptying and greatly reduce the absorption rate of paracetamol, without affecting the extent of absorption. Codeine, however, has no significant effect on paracetamol absorption. Metoclopramide increases gastric emptying and increases the absorption rate of paracetamol, an effect which is used to therapeutic advantage in the treatment of migraine to ensure rapid analgesic effect. It also accelerates the absorption of propranolol, mefloquine, lithium and ciclosporin. This type of interaction is rarely clinically significant.

Induction or inhibition of drug transport proteins. The oral bioavailability of some drugs is limited by the action of drug transporter proteins, which eject drugs that have diffused across the gut lining back into the gut. At present, the most well-characterised drug transporter is P-glycoprotein. Digoxin is a substrate of P-glycoprotein and drugs that inhibit P-glycoprotein, such as verapamil, may increase digoxin bioavailability with the potential for digoxin toxicity (DuBuske, 2005).

Malabsorption. Drugs such as neomycin may cause a malabsorption syndrome leading to reduced absorption of drugs such as digoxin. Orlistat is a specific long-acting inhibitor of gastric and pancreatic lipases, thereby preventing the hydrolysis of dietary fat to free fatty acids and triglycerides. This can theoretically lead to reduced absorption of fat-soluble drugs co-administered with orlistat. There has been recent concern about potential decreased absorption of levothyroxine and anti-epileptic drugs such as valproate sodium and lamotrigine, although the exact mechanism for the postulated interactions is presently unclear.

Most of the interactions that occur within the gut result in reduced rather than increased absorption. It is important to recognise that the majority result in changes in absorption rate, although in some instances the total amount (i.e. extent) of drug absorbed is affected. For drugs that are given chronically on a multiple dose regimen, the rate of absorption is usually unimportant provided the total amount of drug absorbed is not markedly altered. On the other hand, delayed absorption can be clinically significant where the drug affected has a short half-life or where it is important to achieve high plasma concentrations rapidly, as may be the case with analgesics or hypnotics. Absorption interactions can often be avoided by allowing an interval of 2–3 h between administration of the interacting drugs.

Drug distribution

Following absorption, a drug undergoes distribution to various tissues including to its site of action. Many drugs and their metabolites are highly bound to plasma proteins. Albumin is the main plasma protein to which acidic drugs such as warfarin are bound, while basic drugs such as tricyclic antidepressants, lidocaine, disopyramide and propranolol are generally bound to α_1-acid glycoprotein. During the process of distribution, drug interactions may occur, principally as a result of displacement from protein-binding sites. A drug displacement interaction is defined as a reduction in the extent of plasma protein binding of one drug caused by the presence of another drug, resulting in an increased free or unbound fraction of the displaced drug. Displacement from plasma proteins can be demonstrated in vitro for many drugs and has been thought to be an important mechanism underlying many interactions in the past. However, clinical pharmacokinetic studies suggest that, for most drugs, once displacement from plasma proteins occurs, the concentration of free drug rises temporarily, but falls rapidly back to its previous steady-state concentration due to metabolism and distribution. The time this takes will depend on the half-life of the displaced drug. The short-term rise in the free drug concentration is generally of little clinical significance but may need to be taken into account in therapeutic drug monitoring. For example, if a patient taking phenytoin is given a drug which displaces phenytoin from its binding sites, the total (i.e. free plus bound) plasma phenytoin concentration will fall even though the free (active) concentration remains the same.

There are few examples of clinically important interactions which are entirely due to protein-binding displacement. It has been postulated that a sustained change in steady-state free plasma concentration could arise with the parenteral administration of some drugs which are extensively bound to plasma proteins and non-restrictively cleared, that is, the efficiency of the eliminating organ is high. Lidocaine has been given as an example of a drug fitting these criteria.

Drug metabolism

Most clinically important interactions involve the effect of one drug on the metabolism of another. Metabolism refers to the process by which drugs and other compounds are biochemically modified to facilitate their degradation and subsequent removal from the body. The liver is the principal site of drug metabolism, although other organs such as the gut, kidneys, lung, skin and placenta are involved. Drug metabolism consists of phase I reactions such as oxidation, hydrolysis and reduction, and phase II reactions, which primarily involve conjugation of the drug with substances such as glucuronic acid and sulphuric acid. Phase I metabolism generally involves the cytochrome P450 (CYP450) mixed function oxidase system. The liver is the major site of cytochrome 450-mediated metabolism, but the enterocytes in the small intestinal epithelium are also potentially important.

CYP450 isoenzymes. The CYP450 system comprises 57 isoenzymes, each derived from the expression of an individual gene. As there are many different isoforms of these enzymes, a classification for nomenclature has been developed, comprising a family number, a subfamily letter and a number for an individual enzyme within the subfamily (Wilkinson, 2005). Four main subfamilies of P450 isoenzymes are thought to be responsible for most (about 90%) of the metabolism of commonly used drugs in humans: CYP1, CYP2, CYP3 and CYP4. The most extensively studied isoenzyme is CYP2D6, also known as debrisoquine hydroxylase. Although there is overlap, each cytochrome 450 isoenzyme tends to metabolise a discrete range of substrates. Of the many isoenzymes, a few (CYP1A2, CYP2C9, CYP2C19, CYP2D6, CYP2E1 and CYP3A4) appear to be responsible for the human metabolism of most commonly used drugs.

The genes that encode specific cytochrome 450 isoenzymes can vary between individuals and, sometimes, ethnic groups. These variations (polymorphisms) may affect metabolism of substrate drugs. Interindividual variability in CYP2D6 activity is well recognised (see Chapter 5). It shows a polymodal distribution and people may be described according to their ability to metabolise debrisoquine. Poor metabolisers tend to have reduced first-pass metabolism, increased plasma levels and exaggerated pharmacological response to this drug, resulting in postural hypotension. By contrast, ultra-rapid metabolisers may require considerably higher doses for a standard effect. About 5–10% of white Caucasians and up to 2% of Asians and black people are poor metabolisers.

The CYP3A family of P450 enzymes comprises two isoenzymes, CYP3A4 and CYP3A5, so similar that they cannot be easily distinguished. CYP3A is probably the most important of all drug-metabolising enzymes because it is abundant in both the intestinal epithelium and the liver and it has the ability to metabolise a multitude of chemically unrelated drugs from almost every drug class. It is likely that CYP3A is involved in the metabolism of more than half the therapeutic agents that undergo alteration by oxidation. In contrast to other cytochrome 450 enzymes, CYP3A shows continuous unimodal distribution, suggesting that genetic factors play a minor role in its regulation. Nevertheless, the activity of the enzyme can vary markedly among members of a given population.

The effect of a cytochrome 450 isoenzyme on a particular substrate can be altered by interaction with other drugs. Drugs may be themselves substrates for a cytochrome 450 isoenzyme and/or may inhibit or induce the isoenzyme. In most instances, oxidation of a particular drug is brought about by several CYP isoenzymes and results in the production of several metabolites. So, inhibition or induction of a single isoenzyme would have little effect on plasma levels of the drug. However, if a drug is metabolised primarily by a single cytochrome 450 isoenzyme, inhibition or induction of this enzyme would have a major effect on the plasma concentrations of the drug. For example, if erythromycin (an inhibitor of CYP3A4) is taken by a patient being given carbamazepine (which is extensively metabolised by CYP3A4), this may lead to toxicity due to higher concentrations of carbamazepine. Table 4.1 gives examples of some drug substrates, inducers and inhibitors of the major cytochrome 450 isoenzymes.

Table 4.1 Examples of drug substrates, inducers and inhibitors of the major cytochrome P450 enzymes

P450 isoform	Substrate	Inducer	Inhibitor
CYP1A2	Caffeine Clozapine Imipramine Olanzapine Theophylline Tricyclic antidepressants R-warfarin	Omeprazole Lansoprazole Phenytoin Tobacco smoke	Amiodarone Cimetidine Fluoroquinolones Fluvoxamine
CYP2C9	Diazepam Diclofenac Losartan Statins SSRIs S-warfarin	Barbiturates Rifampicin	Amiodarone Azole antifungals Isoniazid
CYP2C19	Cilostazol Diazepam Lansoprazole	Carbamazepine Rifampicin Omeprazole	Cimetidine Fluoxetine Tranylcypromine
CYP2D6	Amitriptyline Codeine Dihydrocodeine Flecainide Fluoxetine Haloperidol Imipramine Nortriptyline Olanzapine Ondansetron Opioids Paroxetine Propranolol Risperidone Thioridazine Tramadol Venlafaxine	Dexamethasone Rifampicin	Amiodarone Bupropion Celecoxib Duloxetine Fluoxetine Paroxetine Ritonavir Sertraline
CYP2E1	Enflurane Halothane	Alcohol (chronic) Isoniazid	Disulfiram
CYP3A4	Amiodarone Terfenadine Ciclosporin Corticosteroids Oral contraceptives Tacrolimus R-warfarin Calcium channel blockers Donepezil Benzodiazepines Cilostazol	Carbamazepine Phenytoin Barbiturates Dexamethasone Primidone Rifampicin St John's wort Bosentan Efavirenz Nevirapine	Cimetidine Clarithromycin Erythromycin Itraconazole Ketoconazole Grapefruit juice Aprepitant Diltiazem Protease inhibitors Imatinib Verapamil

Enzyme induction. The most powerful enzyme inducers in clinical use are the antibiotic rifampicin and antiepileptic agents such as barbiturates, phenytoin and carbamazepine. Some enzyme inducers, notably barbiturates and carbamazepine, can induce their own metabolism (autoinduction). Cigarette smoking, chronic alcohol use and the herbal preparation St John's wort can also induce drug-metabolising enzymes. Since the process of enzyme induction requires new protein synthesis, the effect usually develops over several days or weeks after starting an enzyme-inducing agent. Similarly, the effect generally persists for a similar period following drug withdrawal. Enzyme-inducing drugs with short half-lives such as rifampicin will induce metabolism more rapidly than inducers with longer half-lives, for example, phenytoin, because they reach steady-state concentrations more rapidly. There is evidence that the enzyme induction process is dose dependent, although some drugs may induce enzymes at any dose.

Enzyme induction usually results in a decreased pharmacological effect of the affected drug. St John's wort is now known to be a potent inducer of CYP3A (Mannel, 2004). Thus, when a patient receiving ciclosporin, tacrolimus, HIV-protease inhibitors, irinotecan or imatinib takes St John's wort, there is a risk of therapeutic failure with the affected drug. However, if the affected drug has active metabolites, this may lead to an increased pharmacological effect. The effects of enzyme induction vary considerably between patients and are dependent upon age, genetic factors, concurrent drug treatment and disease state. Some examples of interactions due to enzyme induction are shown in Table 4.2.

Enzyme inhibition. Enzyme inhibition is responsible for many clinically significant interactions. Many drugs act as inhibitors of cytochrome 450 enzymes (see Box 4.2). A strong inhibitor is one that can cause ≥5-fold increase in the plasma area-under-the-curve (AUC) value or more than 80% decrease in clearance of CYP3A substrates. A moderate inhibitor is one that can cause ≥2- but <5-fold increase in the AUC value or

Table 4.2 Examples of interactions due to enzyme induction

Drug affected	Inducing agent	Clinical outcome
Oral contraceptives	Rifampicin	Therapeutic failure of contraceptives
	Rifabutin	Additional contraceptive precautions required
	Modafinil	Increased oestrogen dose required
Ciclosporin	Phenytoin Carbamazepine St John's wort	Decreased ciclosporin levels with possibility of transplant rejection
Paracetamol	Alcohol (chronic)	In overdose, hepatotoxicity may occur at lower doses
Corticosteroids	Phenytoin Rifampicin	Increased metabolism with possibility of therapeutic failure

Box 4.2 Examples of enzyme inhibitors frequently implicated in interactions

Antibacterials	**Cardiovascular drugs**
Ciprofloxacin	Amiodarone
Clarithromycin	Diltiazem
Erythromycin	Quinidine
Isoniazid	Verapamil
Metronidazole	**Gastro-intestinal drugs**
Antidepressants	Cimetidine
Duloxetine	Esomeprazole
Fluoxetine	Omeprazole
Fluvoxamine	**Antirheumatic drugs**
Nefazodone	Allopurinol
Paroxetine	Azapropazone
Sertraline	Phenylbutazone
Antifungals	**Other**
Fluconazole	Aprepitant
Itraconazole	Bupropion
Ketoconazole	Disulfiram
Miconazole	Grapefruit juice
Voriconazole	Imatinib
Antivirals	Propoxyphene
Amprenavir	Sodium valproate
Indinavir	
Nelfinavir	
Ritonavir	
Saquinavir	

Table 4.3 Examples of interactions due to enzyme inhibition

Drug affected	Inhibiting agent	Clinical outcome
Anticoagulants (oral)	Ciprofloxacin Clarithromycin	Anticoagulant effect increased and risk of bleeding
Azathioprine	Allopurinol	Enhancement of effect with increased toxicity
Clopidogrel	Lansoprazole	Reduced anti-platelet effect
Carbamazepine Phenytoin Sodium valproate	Cimetidine	Antiepileptic levels increased with risk of toxicity
Sildenafil	Ritonavir	Enhancement of sildenafil effect with risk of hypotension

50–80% decrease in clearance of sensitive CYP3A substrates when the inhibitor is given at the highest approved dose and the shortest dosing interval. A weak inhibitor is one that can cause ≥1.25- but <2-fold increase in the AUC values or 20–50% decrease in clearance of sensitive CYP3A substrates when the inhibitor is given at the highest approved dose and the shortest dosing interval.

Concurrent administration of an enzyme inhibitor leads to reduced metabolism of the drug and hence an increase in the steady-state drug concentration. Enzyme inhibition appears to be dose related. Inhibition of hepatic metabolism of the affected drug occurs when sufficient concentrations of the inhibitor are achieved in the liver, and the effects are usually maximal when the new steady-state plasma concentration is achieved. Thus, for drugs with a short half-life, the effects may be seen within a few days of administration of the inhibitor. Maximal effects may be delayed for drugs with a long half-life.

The clinical significance of this type of interaction depends on various factors, including dosage (of both drugs), alterations in pharmacokinetic properties of the affected drug such as half-life and patient characteristics such as disease state. Interactions of this type are again most likely to affect drugs with a narrow therapeutic range such as theophylline, ciclosporin, oral anticoagulants and phenytoin. For example, starting treatment with an enzyme inhibitor such as ritonavir in a patient taking sildenafil could result in a marked increase in sildenafil plasma concentrations. Some examples of interactions due to enzyme inhibition are shown in Table 4.3.

The isoenzyme CYP3A4, in particular, is present in the enterocytes. Thus, after oral administration of a drug, cytochrome 450 enzymes in the intestine and the liver may reduce the portion of a dose that reaches the systemic circulation, that is, the bioavailability of the drug. Drug interactions resulting in inhibition or induction of enzymes in the intestinal epithelium can have significant consequences. For example, by selectively inhibiting CYP3A4 in the enterocyte, grapefruit juice can markedly increase the bioavailability of some oral calcium channel blockers, including felodipine (Wilkinson, 2005). Such an interaction is usually considered to be a drug metabolism interaction, even though the mechanism involves an alteration in drug absorption. A single glass of grapefruit juice can cause CYP3A inhibition for 24–48 h and regular consumption may continuously inhibit enzyme activity. Consumption of grapefruit juice is therefore not recommended in patients receiving drugs that are extensively metabolised by CYP3A such as simvastatin, tacrolimus and vardenafil.

Enzyme inhibition usually results in an increased pharmacological effect of the affected drug, but in cases where the affected drug is a pro-drug which requires enzymatic metabolism to active metabolites, a reduced pharmacological effect may result. For example, clopidogrel is metabolised via CYP2C19 to an active metabolite which is responsible for its anti-platelet effect. Proton pump inhibitors such as lansoprazole are inhibitors of CYP2C19 and may lead to reduced effectiveness of clopidogrel when used in combination

Predicting interactions involving metabolism. Predicting drug interactions is not easy for many reasons. First, individual drugs within a therapeutic class may have different effects on an isoenzyme. For example, the quinolone antibiotics ciprofloxacin and norfloxacin inhibit CYP1A2 and have been reported to increase plasma theophylline levels, whereas moxifloxacin is a much weaker inhibitor and appears not to interact in this way. While atorvastatin and simvastatin are metabolised predominantly by the CYP3A4 enzyme, fluvastatin is metabolised by CYP2C9 and pravastatin is not metabolised by the CYP450 system to any significant extent.

Identification of cytochrome P450 isoenzymes involved in drug metabolism using in vitro techniques are now an important step in the drug development process. However, findings of in vitro studies are not always replicated in vivo and more detailed drug interaction studies may be required to allow early identification of potential interactions. Nevertheless, some interactions affect only a small proportion of individuals and may not be identified unless large numbers of volunteers or patients are studied.

Suspected drug interactions are often described initially in published case reports and are then subsequently evaluated in formal studies. For example, published case reports indicate that some antibiotics reduce the effect of oral contraceptives, although this interaction has not been demonstrated in formal studies. Another factor complicating the understanding of metabolic drug interactions is the finding that there is a large overlap between the inhibitors/inducers and substrates of the drug transporter protein P-glycoprotein and those of CYP3A4. Therefore, both mechanisms may be involved in many of the drug interactions previously thought to be due to effects on CYP3A4.

Elimination interactions

Most drugs are excreted in either the bile or urine. Blood entering the kidneys is delivered to the glomeruli of the tubules where molecules small enough to pass across the pores of the glomerular membrane are filtered through into the lumen of the tubules. Larger molecules, such as plasma proteins and blood cells, are retained. The blood then flows to other parts of the kidney tubules where drugs and their metabolites are removed, secreted or reabsorbed into the tubular filtrate by active and passive transport systems. Interactions can occur when drugs interfere with kidney tubule fluid pH, active transport systems or blood flow to the kidney, thereby altering the excretion of other drugs.

Changes in urinary pH. As with drug absorption in the gut, passive reabsorption of drugs depends on the extent to which the drug exists in the non-ionised lipid-soluble form. Only the non-ionised form is lipid soluble and able to diffuse back through the tubular cell membrane. Thus, at alkaline pH, weakly acidic drugs (pK_a 3.0–7.5) largely exist as ionised lipid-insoluble molecules which are unable to diffuse into the tubule cells and will therefore be lost in the urine. The renal clearance of these drugs is increased if the urine is made more alkaline. Conversely, the clearance of weak bases (pK_a 7.5–10) is higher in acid urine. Strong acids and bases are virtually completely ionised over the physiological range of urinary pH and their clearance is unaffected by pH changes.

This mechanism of interaction is of very minor clinical significance because most weak acids and bases are inactivated by hepatic metabolism rather than renal excretion. Furthermore, drugs that produce large changes in urine pH are rarely used clinically. Urine alkalinisation or acidification has been used as a means of increasing drug elimination in poisoning with salicylates and amphetamines, respectively.

Changes in active renal tubule excretion. Drugs that use the same active transport system in the kidney tubules can compete with one another for excretion. Such competition between drugs can be used to therapeutic advantage. For example, probenecid may be given to increase the plasma concentration of penicillins by delaying renal excretion. With the increasing understanding of drug transporter proteins in the kidneys, it is now known that probenecid inhibits the renal secretion of many other anionic drugs via organic anion transporters (OATs; Lee and Kim, 2004). Increased methotrexate toxicity, sometimes life-threatening, has been seen in some patients concurrently treated with salicylates and some other non-steroidal anti-inflammatory drugs (NSAIDs). The development of toxicity is more likely in patients treated with high-dose methotrexate and those with impaired renal function. The mechanism of this interaction may be multifactorial but competitive inhibition of methotrexate's renal tubular secretion is likely to be involved. If patients taking methotrexate are given salicylates or NSAIDs concomitantly, the dose of methotrexate should be closely monitored.

Changes in renal blood flow. Blood flow through the kidney is partially controlled by the production of renal vasodilatory prostaglandins. If the synthesis of these prostaglandins is inhibited by drugs such as indometacin, the renal excretion of lithium is reduced with a subsequent rise in plasma levels. The mechanism underlying this interaction is not entirely clear, as plasma lithium levels are unaffected by other potent prostaglandin synthetase inhibitors, for example, aspirin. If an NSAID is prescribed for a patient taking lithium, the plasma levels should be closely monitored.

Biliary excretion and the enterohepatic shunt. A number of drugs are excreted in the bile, either unchanged or conjugated, for example, as the glucuronide, to make them more water soluble. Some of the conjugates are metabolised to the parent compound by the gut flora and are then reabsorbed. This recycling process prolongs the stay of the drug within the body but if the gut flora are diminished by the presence of an antibacterial, the drug is not recycled and is lost more quickly. This mechanism has been postulated as the basis of an interaction between broad-spectrum antibiotics and oral contraceptives. Antibiotics may reduce the enterohepatic circulation of ethinyloestradiol conjugates, leading to reduced circulating oestrogen levels with the potential for therapeutic failure. There is considerable debate about the nature of this interaction as the evidence from pharmacokinetic studies is not convincing. However, due to the potential adverse consequences of pill failure, most authorities recommend a conservative approach, including the use of additional contraceptive precautions to cover the short-term use of broad-spectrum antibiotics.

Drug transporter proteins. Drugs and endogenous substances are now known to cross biological membranes not just by passive diffusion but by carrier-mediated processes, often known as transporters. Significant advances in the identification of various transporters have been made and although their contribution to drug interactions is not yet clear, they are now thought to play a role in many interactions formerly attributed to cytochrome 450 enzymes (DuBuske, 2005).

P-glycoprotein (P-gp) is a large cell membrane protein that is responsible for the transport of many substrates, including drugs. It is a product of the ABCB1 gene (previously known as the multidrug resistance gene, MDR1) and a member of the adenosine triphosphate (ATP)-binding cassette family of transport proteins (ABC transporters). P-glycoprotein is found in high levels in various tissues including the renal proximal tubule, hepatocytes, intestinal mucosa, the pancreas and the blood–brain barrier. P-glycoprotein acts as an efflux pump, exporting substances into urine, bile and the intestinal lumen. Its activity in the blood–brain barrier limits drug accumulation in the central nervous system (CNS). Examples of some possible inhibitors and inducers of P-glycoprotein are shown in Table 4.4. The pumping actions of P-glycoprotein can be induced or inhibited by some drugs. For example, concomitant administration of digoxin and verapamil, a P-glycoprotein inhibitor, is associated with increased digoxin levels with the potential for digoxin toxicity. There is an overlap between CYP3A4 and P-glycoprotein inhibitors, inducers and substrates. Many drugs that are substrates for CYP3A4 are also substrates for P-glycoprotein. Therefore, both mechanisms may be involved in many of the drug interactions initially thought to be due to changes in CYP3A4. Digoxin is an example of the few drugs that are substrates for P-glycoprotein but not CYP3A4.

Pharmacodynamic interactions

Pharmacodynamic interactions are those where the effects of one drug are changed by the presence of another drug at its site of action. Sometimes these interactions involve competition for specific receptor sites but often they are indirect and involve interference with physiological systems. They are much less easy to classify than interactions with a pharmacokinetic basis.

Antagonistic interactions

It is to be expected that a drug with an agonist action at a particular receptor type will interact with antagonists at that receptor. For example, the bronchodilator action of a selective β_2-adrenoreceptor agonist such as salbutamol will be antagonised by β-adrenoreceptor antagonists. There are numerous examples of interactions occurring at receptor sites, many of which are used to therapeutic advantage. Specific antagonists may be used to reverse the effect of another drug at receptor sites; examples include the opioid antagonist naloxone and the benzodiazepine antagonist flumazenil. α-Adrenergic agonists such as metaraminol may be used in the management of priapism induced by α-adrenergic antagonists such as phentolamine. There are many other examples of drug classes that have opposing pharmacological actions, such as anticoagulants and vitamin K and levodopa and dopamine antagonist antipsychotics.

Additive or synergistic interactions

If two drugs with similar pharmacological effects are given together, the effects can be additive (see Table 4.5). Although not strictly drug interactions, the mechanism frequently contributes to ADR. For example, the concurrent use of drugs with CNS-depressant effects such as antidepressants, hypnotics, antiepileptics and antihistamines may lead to excessive drowsiness, yet such combinations are frequently encountered. Combinations of drugs with arrhythmogenic potential such as antiarrhythmics, neuroleptics, tricyclic antidepressants and those producing electrolyte imbalance (e.g. diuretics) may lead to ventricular arrhythmias and should be avoided. Another example which has assumed greater importance of late is the risk of ventricular tachycardia and torsade de pointes associated with the concurrent use of more than one drug with the potential to prolong the QT interval on the electrocardiogram (Roden, 2004).

Serotonin syndrome

Serotonin syndrome (SS) is associated with an excess of serotonin that results from therapeutic drug use, overdose or inadvertent interactions between drugs. Although severe cases are uncommon, it is becoming increasingly well recognised in patients receiving combinations of serotonergic drugs (Boyer and Shannon, 2005). It can occur when two or more drugs affecting serotonin are given at the same time or after one serotonergic drug is stopped and another started. The

Table 4.4 Examples of inhibitors and inducers of P-glycoprotein

Inhibitors	Atorvastatin
	Ciclosporin
	Clarithromycin
	Dipyridamole
	Erythromycin
	Itraconazole
	Ketoconazole
	Propafenone
	Quinidine
	Ritonavir
	Valspodar
	Verapamil
Inducers	Rifampicin
	St John's wort

Table 4.5 Examples of additive or synergistic interactions

Interacting drugs	Pharmacological effect
NSAID, warfarin, clopidogrel	Increased risk of bleeding
ACE inhibitors and K-sparing diuretic	Increased risk of hyperkalaemia
Verapamil and β-adrenergic antagonists	Bradycardia and asystole
Neuromuscular blockers and aminoglycosides	Increased neuromuscular blockade
Alcohol and benzodiazepines	Increased sedation
Pimozide and sotalol	Increased risk of QT interval prolongation
Clozapine and co-trimoxazole	Increased risk of bone marrow suppression

syndrome is characterised by symptoms including confusion, disorientation, abnormal movements, exaggerated reflexes, fever, sweating, diarrhoea and hypotension or hypertension. Diagnosis is made when three or more of these symptoms are present and no other cause can be found. Symptoms usually develop within hours of starting the second drug but occasionally they can occur later. Drug-induced SS is generally mild and resolves when the offending drugs are stopped. Severe cases occur infrequently and fatalities have been reported.

SS is best prevented by avoiding the use of combinations of several serotonergic drugs. Special care is needed when changing from a selective serotonin reuptake inhibitor (SSRI) to an MAOI and vice versa. The SSRIs, particularly fluoxetine, have long half-lives and SS may occur if a sufficient wash-out period is not allowed before switching from one to the other. When patients are being switched between these two groups of drugs, the guidance in manufacturers' Summaries of Product Characteristics should be followed. Many drugs have serotonergic activity as their secondary pharmacology and their potential for causing the SS may not be readily recognised, for example linezolid, an antibacterial with monoamine oxidase inhibitory activity has been implicated in several case reports of SS.

Many recreational drugs such as amfetamines and their derivatives have serotonin agonist activity and the SS may ensue following the use of other serotonergic drugs.

Drug or neurotransmitter uptake interactions

Although seldom prescribed nowadays, the MAOIs have significant potential for interactions with other drugs and foods. MAOIs reduce the breakdown of noradrenaline in the adrenergic nerve ending. Large stores of noradrenaline can then be released into the synaptic cleft in response to either a neuronal discharge or an indirectly acting amine. The action of the directly acting amines adrenaline, isoprenaline and noradrenaline appears to be only moderately increased in patients taking MAOIs. In contrast, the concurrent use of MAOIs and indirectly acting sympathomimetic amines such as amphetamines, tyramine, MDMA (ecstasy), phenylpropanolamine and pseudoephedrine can result in a potentially fatal hypertensive crisis. Some of these compounds are contained in proprietary cough and cold remedies. Tyramine, contained in some foods, for example cheese and red wine, is normally metabolised in the gut wall by monoamine oxidase to inactive metabolites. In patients taking MAOI, however, tyramine will be absorbed intact. If patients taking MAOIs also take these amines, there may be a massive release of noradrenaline from adrenergic nerve endings, causing a sympathetic overactivity syndrome, characterised by hypertension, headache, excitement, hyperpyrexia and cardiac arrhythmias. Fatal intracranial haemorrhage and cardiac arrest may result. The risk of interactions continues for several weeks after the MAOI is stopped as new monoamine oxidase enzyme must be synthesised. Patients taking irreversible MAOIs should not take any indirectly acting sympathomimetic amines. All patients must be strongly warned about the risks of cough and cold remedies, illicit drug use and the necessary dietary restrictions.

Drug–food interactions

It is well established that food can cause clinically important changes in drug absorption through effects on gastro-intestinal absorption or motility, hence the advice that certain drugs should not be taken with food, for example, iron tablets and antibiotics. Two other common examples already outlined include the interaction between tyramine in some foods and MAOIs, and the interaction between grapefruit juice and the calcium channel blocker felodipine. With improved understanding of drug metabolism mechanisms, there is greater recognition of the effects of some foods on drug metabolism. The interaction between grapefruit juice and felodipine was discovered serendipitously when grapefruit juice was chosen to mask the taste of ethanol in a study of the effect of ethanol on felodipine. Grapefruit juice mainly inhibits intestinal CYP3A4, with only minimal effects on hepatic CYP3A4. This is demonstrated by the fact that intravenous preparations of drugs metabolised by CYP3A4 are not much affected whereas oral preparations of the same drugs are. Some drugs that are not metabolised by CYP3A4 show decreased levels with grapefruit juice, such as fexofenadine. The probable reason for this is that grapefruit juice inhibits some drug transporter proteins and possibly affects organic anion-transporting polypeptides, although inhibition of P-glycoprotein has also been suggested. The active constituent of grapefruit juice is uncertain. Grapefruit contains naringin, which degrades during processing to naringenin, a substance known to inhibit CYP3A4. Although this led to the assumption that whole grapefruit will not interact, but that processed grapefruit juice will, some reports have implicated the whole fruit. Other possible active constituents in the whole fruit include bergamottin and dihydroxybergamottin.

Initial reports of an interaction between cranberry juice and warfarin, prompting regulatory advice that the international normalised ratio (INR) should be closely monitored in patients taking this combination, have not been confirmed by subsequent controlled studies.

Cruciferous vegetables, such as brussels sprouts, cabbage and broccoli, contain substances that are inducers of the CYP450 isoenzyme CYP1A2. Chemicals formed by burning (e.g. barbecuing) meats additionally have these properties. These foods do not appear to cause any clinically important drug interactions in their own right, but their consumption may add another variable to drug interaction studies, so complicating interpretation.

Drug–herb interactions

There has been a marked increase in the availability and use of herbal products in the UK over the past decade, which include Chinese herbal medicines and Ayurvedic medicines. Up to 24% of hospital patients report using herbal remedies (Constable et al., 2007). Such products often contain pharmacologically active ingredients which can give rise to clinically significant interactions when used inadvertently with other conventional drugs.

Extracts of *Glycyrrhizin glabra* (liquorice) used for treating digestive disorders may cause significant interactions in patients using digoxin or diuretics. It may exacerbate hypokalaemia induced by diuretic drugs and precipitate digoxin toxicity. Herbal products such as Chinese ginseng (*Panax ginseng*), Chan Su (containing bufalin) and Danshen may also contain digoxin-like compounds which can interfere with digoxin assays, leading to falsely elevated levels being detected.

A number of herbal products have anti-platelet and anti-coagulant properties and may increase the risk of bleeding when used with aspirin or warfarin. Herbal extracts containing coumarin-like constituents include Alfalfa (*Medicago sativa*), Angelica (*Angelica archangelica*), Dong Quai (*Angelica polymorpha, A. dahurica, A. atropurpurea*), chamomile, horse chestnut and red clover (*Trifolium pratense*) which can potentially lead to interactions with warfarin. Herbal products with anti-platelet properties include Borage (*Borago officinalis*), Bromelain (*Ananas comosus*), capsicum, feverfew, garlic, Ginkgo (*Ginkgo biloba*) and turmeric amongst others.

Other examples of drug–herb interactions include enhancement of hypoglycaemic (for example Asian ginseng) and hypotensive (for example hawthorn) effects, and lowering of seizure threshold (for example evening primrose oil and *Shankapushpi*). The most widely discussed drug–herb interactions are those involving St John's wort (*Hypericum* extract) used for depression but these only represent a minority of the potential interactions. It is therefore imperative that patients are specifically asked about their use of herbal medicines as they may not volunteer this information.

Conclusion

Whilst one should acknowledge the impossibility of memorising all potential drug interactions, health care workers need to be alert to the possibility of drug interactions and take appropriate steps to minimise their occurrence. Drug formularies and the Summary of Product Characteristics provide useful information about interactions. Other resources that may also be of use to prescribers include drug safety updates from regulators such as the Medicines and Health care products Regulatory Agency (available at http://www.mhra.gov.uk/index.htm), interaction alerts in prescribing software and the availability of websites which highlight interactions for specific drug classes, for example, HIV drugs (http://www.hiv-druginteractions.org/).

Possible interventions to avoid or minimise the risk of a drug interaction include:

(1) Switching one of the potential interacting drugs.
(2) Allowing an interval of 2–3 h between administration of the interacting drugs.

(3) Altering the dose of one of the interacting drugs, for example, reducing the dose of the drug which is likely to have an enhanced effect as a result of the interaction. In this case, the dose is generally reduced by one-third or half with subsequent monitoring for toxic effects either clinically or by therapeutic drug monitoring. Conversely, if the drug is likely to have reduced effects as a result of the interaction, the patient should be monitored similarly for therapeutic failure and the dose increased if necessary.
(4) Advising patients to seek guidance about their medication if they plan to stop smoking, or start a herbal remedy, as they may need close monitoring during the transition.

Overall, it is important to anticipate when a potential drug interaction might have clinically significant consequences for the patient. In these situations, advice should be given on how to minimise the risk of harm, for example, by recommending an alternative treatment to avoid the combination of risk, by making a dose adjustment or by monitoring the patient closely.

Case studies

Case 4.1

Mrs C is a 62-year-old woman with a history of hypertension, atrial fibrillation and type 2 diabetes. She is a non-smoker and obese. Her current medication comprises flecainide 100 mg twice a day, aspirin 75 mg daily, simvastatin 40 mg and diltiazem 180 mg daily. Mrs C is suffering from a respiratory tract infection and her primary care doctor has prescribed a 5-day course of clarithromycin.

Questions

1. Are there likely to be any clinically significant drug interactions?
2. What advice do you give?

Answers

1. There is potential for interaction between simvastatin and diltiazem and between simvastatin and clarithromycin. Some statins, particularly simvastatin and atorvastatin, are metabolised by cytochrome P450 (CYP3A4) and co-administration of potent inhibitors of this enzyme may particularly increase plasma levels of these statins and so increase the risk of dose-related side effects, including rhabdomyolysis. Clarithromycin is a potent inhibitor of CYP3A4 and diltiazem is a less potent inhibitor.
2. Current advice is that diltiazem and simvastatin may be given together provided the simvastatin dose does not exceed 40 mg daily, so it is reasonable for this therapy to be continued. However, clarithromycin should not be given together with simvastatin. Myopathy and rhabdomyolysis have been reported in patients taking the combination. Mrs C should be advised not to take her simvastatin while she is taking clarithromycin and to start taking it again after she has completed the course of antibiotic.

Case 4.2

A 19-year-old woman is on long-term treatment with minocycline 100 mg daily for acne. She wishes to start using the combined oral contraceptive and her doctor has prescribed a low-strength pill (containing ethinyloestradiol 20 μcg with norethisterone 1 mg). The doctor contacts the pharmacist for advice on whether the tetracycline will interfere with the efficacy of the oral contraceptive.

Question

Is there a clinically significant interaction in this situation?

Answer

Contraceptive failure has been attributed to doxycycline, lymecycline, oxytetracycline, minocycline and tetracycline in about 40 reported cases, seven of which specified long-term antibacterial use. There is controversy about whether or not a drug interaction occurs but if there is one it appears to be very rare. Controlled trials have not shown any effect of tetracycline or doxycycline on contraceptive steroid levels. The postulated mechanism is suppression of intestinal bacteria resulting in a fall in enterohepatic recirculation of ethinyloestradiol. Overall, there is no evidence that this is clinically important.

In the case of long-term use of tetracyclines for acne, a small number of cases of contraceptive failure have been reported. Nevertheless, the only well-designed, case–control study in dermatological practice indicated that the incidence of contraceptive failure due to this interaction could not be distinguished from the general and recognised failure rate of oral contraceptives. The UK Family Planning Association advises that women on long-term antibiotic therapy need only take extra precautions for the first 3 weeks of oral contraceptive use because, after about 2 weeks, the gut flora becomes resistant to the antibiotic. In addition, there is some evidence that ethinyloestradiol may accentuate the facial pigmentation that can be caused by minocycline.

Case 4.3

A 48-year-old man with a history of epilepsy is admitted to hospital with tremor, ataxia, headache, abnormal thinking and increased partial seizure activity. His prescribed medicines are phenytoin 300 mg daily, clonazepam 6 mg daily and fluoxetine 20 mg daily. It transpires that fluoxetine therapy had been initiated 2 weeks previously. The patient's phenytoin level is found to be 35 mg/L; at the last outpatient clinic visit 4 months ago, it was 18 mg/L.

Question

What is the proposed mechanism of interaction between fluoxetine and phenytoin and how should it be managed?

Answer

Fluoxetine is believed to inhibit the metabolism of phenytoin by the cytochrome P450 isoenzyme CYP2C9, potentially leading to increased plasma phenytoin levels. There are a number of published case reports and anecdotal observations of phenytoin toxicity occurring with the combination, but the available evidence is conflicting. A review by the U.S. Food and Drug Administration suggested that a marked increase in plasma phenytoin levels, with accompanying toxicity, can occur within 1–42 days (mean onset time of 2 weeks) after starting fluoxetine. If fluoxetine is added to treatment with phenytoin, the patient should be closely monitored. Ideally the phenytoin plasma levels should be monitored and there may be a need to reduce the phenytoin dosage.

Case 4.4

A 79-year-old man presented to hospital with a 3-day history of increasing confusion and collapse. He had a history of chronic lumbosacral pain, treated with oxycodone 10 mg twice daily and amitriptyline 75 mg daily. Five days before hospital admission he had been prescribed tramadol 100 mg four times daily for worsening sciatica. On admission the patient had a Glasgow Coma Scale of 11 and he was delirious and hallucinating. There were no focal neurological signs. Over the next 2 days he became increasingly unwell, confused and sweaty with pyrexia and muscular rigidity. Biochemical tests showed a metabolic acidosis (base deficit of 10.7) and an elevated creatine kinase level of 380 IU/L. There was no evidence of infection. At this stage a diagnosis of probable serotonin syndrome was made.

Questions

1. What is serotonin syndrome and what drugs are most commonly associated with it?
2. How is serotonin syndrome managed?

Answers

1. Serotonin syndrome is often described as a clinical triad of mental status changes, autonomic hyperactivity and neuromuscular abnormalities. However, not all these features are consistently present in all patients with the disorder. Symptoms arising from a serotonin excess range from diarrhoea and tremor in mild cases to delirium, neuromuscular rigidity, rhabdomyolysis and hyperthermia in life-threatening cases. Disturbance of electrolytes, transaminases and creatine kinase may occur. Clonus is the most important finding in establishing the diagnosis of the serotonin syndrome. The differential diagnosis includes neuroleptic malignant syndrome, sepsis, hepatic encephalopathy, heat stroke, delirium tremens and anticholinergic reactions. Serotonin syndrome may not be recognised in some cases because of its protean manifestations. A wide range of drugs and drug combinations has been associated with the serotonin syndrome, including MAOIs, tricyclic antidepressants, SSRIs, opioids, linezolid and $5HT_1$-agonists. Tramadol is an atypical opioid analgesic with partial μ antagonism and central reuptake inhibition of serotonin (5HT) and noradrenaline. At high doses it may also induce serotonin release. Tramadol is reported as causing serotonin syndrome alone (in a few case reports) and in combination with SSRIs, venlafaxine and atypical antipsychotics.
2. Management of the serotonin syndrome involves removal of the precipitating drugs and supportive care. Many cases typically resolve within 24 h after serotonergic drugs are stopped but symptoms may persist in patients taking medicines with long half-lives or active metabolites. The $5HT_{2A}$-antagonist cyproheptadine and atypical antipsychotic agents with $5HT_{2A}$-antagonist activity, such as olanzapine, have been used to treat serotonin syndrome, although their efficacy has not been conclusively established.

Case 4.5

A 42-year-old woman is on long-term treatment with azathioprine 100 mg daily and bendroflumethiazide 2.5 mg daily. The latter was discontinued after an episode of gout but she had three further episodes over the following year. Her doctor considers prescribing allopurinol as prophylaxis.

Question

Is this likely to cause a clinically significant interaction?

Answer

Azathioprine is metabolised in the liver to mercaptopurine and then converted to an inactive metabolite by the enzyme xanthine oxidase. Allopurinol is an inhibitor of xanthine oxidase and will lead to the accumulation of mercaptopurine which can cause bone marrow suppression and haematological abnormalities such as neutropenia and thrombocytopenia.

The dose of azathioprine should be reduced by at least 50% and close haematological monitoring is required if allopurinol is used concomitantly.

Case 4.6

A 68-year-old woman is on long-term treatment with lansoprazole for gastro-oesophageal reflux disease and warfarin for atrial fibrillation. She is admitted with haematemesis. On direct questioning, she also revealed that she takes various herbal medicines which contain chamomile, horse chestnut, garlic, feverfew, ginseng and St John's wort.

Question

What drug–herb interactions may have contributed to her presentation to hospital?

Answer

Garlic, feverfew and ginseng all inhibit platelet aggregation by inhibiting the production or release of prostaglandins and thromboxanes. In addition, chamomile and horse chestnut contain coumarin-like constituents which can potentiate the anticoagulant effect of warfarin. St John's wort is a potent enzyme inducer and may induce the metabolism of lansoprazole via CYP2C19, thereby reducing the effectiveness of lansoprazole.

Although the effects of herbs individually may be small, their combined effects may lead to serious complications.

References

Baxter, K. (Ed.), 2010. Stockley's Drug Interactions, ninth ed. Pharmaceutical Press, London.

Boyer, E.W., Shannon, M., 2005. Current concepts: the serotonin syndrome. N. Engl. J. Med. 352, 1112–1120.

Constable, S., Ham, A., Pirmohamed, M., 2007. Herbal medicines and acute medical emergency admissions to hospital. Br. J. Clin. Pharmacol. 63, 247–248.

DuBuske, L.M., 2005. The role of P-glycoprotein and organic anion-transporting polypeptides in drug interactions. Drug Saf. 28, 789–801.

Goldberg, R.M., Mabee, J., Chan, L., et al., 1996. Drug–drug and drug–disease interactions in the ED: analysis of a high-risk population. Am. J. Emerg. Med. 14, 447–450.

Jankel, C.A., Fitterman, L.K., 1993. Epidemiology of drug–drug interactions as a cause of hospital admissions. Drug Saf. 9, 55–59.

Leape, L.L., Brennan, T.A., Laird, N., et al., 1992. The nature of adverse events in hospitalised patients: results of the Harvard Medical Practice Study II. N. Engl. J. Med. 324, 377–384.

Lee, W., Kim, R.B., 2004. Transporters and renal drug elimination. Ann. Rev. Pharmacol. Toxicol. 44, 137–166.

Li Wan Po, A., Zhang, W.Y., 1998. What lessons can be learnt from withdrawal of mibefradil from the market? Lancet 351, 1829–1830.

Mannel, M., 2004. Drug interactions with St John's wort: mechanisms and clinical implications. Drug Saf. 27, 773–797.

Pirmohamed, M., James, S., Meakin, S., et al., 2004. Adverse drug reactions as cause of admission to hospital: prospective analysis of 18820 patients. Br. Med. J. 329, 15–19.

Raschett, R., Morgutti, M., Menniti-Ippolito, F., et al., 1999. Suspected adverse drug events requiring emergency department visits or hospital admissions. Eur. J. Clin. Pharmacol. 54, 959–963.

Roden, D.M., 2004. Drug-induced prolongation of the QT interval. N. Engl. J. Med. 350, 1013–1022.

Smith, J.W., Seidl, L.G., Cluff, L.E., 1969. Studies on the epidemiology of adverse drug reactions v. clinical factors influencing susceptibility. Ann. Intern. Med. 65, 629.

Wilkinson, G.R., 2005. Drug therapy: drug metabolism and variability among patients in drug response. N. Engl. J. Med. 352, 2211–2221.

5 Adverse drug reactions

J. Krska and A. R. Cox

Key points

- An adverse drug reaction is an unintended noxious response occurring after the normal use of a drug, which is suspected to be associated with the drug.
- Adverse drug reactions can be classified as type A, which are most common and related to the drug's pharmacological effect, or type B, which are rare and unpredictable, although other classes of reaction can be identified.
- Few adverse reactions are identified during pre-marketing studies; therefore, pharmacovigilance systems to detect new adverse drug reactions are essential.
- Spontaneous reporting schemes are a common method of pharmacovigilance which depend primarily on health professionals.
- Patients are encouraged to contribute to post-marketing surveillance schemes in some countries.
- Adverse drug reactions are a significant cause of morbidity and mortality, are responsible for approximately 1 in 20 hospital admissions and are a considerable financial burden on health systems.
- Predisposing factors for adverse drug reactions include age, female gender, ethnicity, genetic factors, co-morbidities and concomitant medication.
- Many adverse drug reactions may be preventable through rational prescribing and careful monitoring of drug therapy.
- Health professionals need to be able to identify and assess adverse drug reactions and play a major role in preventing their occurrence.
- Patients want to receive information about adverse drug reactions; therefore, communicating the risks of using medicines is an important skill for health professionals.

Introduction

All medicines with the ability to produce a desired therapeutic effect also have the potential to cause unwanted adverse effects. Health professionals should have an awareness of the burden that adverse drug reactions (ADRs) place on health services and the public, the identification and avoidance of ADRs and their important role in post-marketing surveillance of medicines to ensure their continued safety.

Risks associated with medicinal substances are documented throughout history; for example, William Withering's 1785 account provides a meticulous description of the adverse effects of digitalis. However, it was the thalidomide disaster that captured public attention and brought about major regulatory changes in drug safety. Thalidomide was first marketed by Chemie Grünenthal in 1957 and distributed in the UK by Distillers Ltd, whose chief medical advisor stated, 'If all the details of this are true, then it is a most remarkable drug. In short, it is impossible to give a toxic dose.' In 1958, thalidomide was recommended for use in pregnant and nursing mothers without supporting evidence. An Australian doctor, Jim McBride, and a German doctor, Widukund Lenz, independently associated thalidomide exposure with serious birth defects and thalidomide was withdrawn in December 1961. Thalidomide left behind between 8000 and 12,000 deformed children and an unknown number of deaths *in utero*.

The 1970s saw another unexpected and serious adverse reaction. The cardioselective beta-adrenergic receptor blocker practolol, launched in June 1970, was initially associated with rashes, some of which were severe. A case series of psoriasis-like rashes linked to dry eyes, including irreversible scarring of the cornea, led other doctors to report eye damage, including corneal ulceration and blindness, to regulators. Cases of sclerosing peritonitis, a bowel condition associated with significant mortality, were also reported. Practolol had remained on the market for 4 years; over 100,000 people had been treated and hundreds were seriously affected.

Some adverse effects can be more difficult to differentiate from background events occurring commonly in the population. The COX-II selective non-steroidal anti-inflammatory drugs (NSAIDs), celecoxib (introduced 1998) and rofecoxib (introduced 1999), were marketed on the basis of reduced gastro-intestinal ADRs in comparison to other non-selective NSAIDs. Apparent excesses of cardiovascular events, which were noted during clinical trials and in elderly patient groups, were ascribed to the supposed cardio-protective effects of comparator drugs. However, in September 2004, a randomised controlled trial of rofecoxib in the prevention of colorectal cancer showed the drug to be associated with a significantly increased risk of cardiovascular events. Celecoxib was also associated with a dose-related increased risk of cardiovascular events in clinical trials. Rofecoxib was voluntarily withdrawn from the market. Further research has provided evidence of thrombotic risk with non-selective NSAIDs, in particular diclofenac. This risk appears to extend to all NSAID users, irrespective of baseline cardiovascular risk.

Not all drug safety issues are related to real effects. In 1998, a widely-publicised paper by Andrew Wakefield and co-authors, later retracted, alleged a link between MMR vaccine and autism, and led to a crisis in parental confidence in the vaccine. This had a detrimental effect on vaccination rates, resulting in frequent outbreaks of measles and mumps, despite epidemiological and virological studies showing no link between MMR vaccine and autism. The MMR vaccine controversy illustrates how media reporting of drug safety information can influence patients' views of medicines and can cause significant harm. Poor presentation of drug safety issues in the media often creates anxiety in patients about medicines which they may be using, regardless of their benefits.

Assessing the safety of drugs

When drugs are newly introduced to the market, their safety profile will be provisional. While efficacy and evidence of safety must be demonstrated for regulatory authorities to permit marketing, it is not possible to discover the complete safety profile of a new drug prior to its launch. Pre-marketing clinical trials involve on average 2500 patients, with perhaps a hundred patients using the drug for longer than a year. Therefore, pre-marketing trials do not have the power to detect important reactions that occur at rates of 1 in 10,000, or fewer, drug exposures. Often, only pharmacologically predictable ADRs with short onset times may be identified in clinical trials, nor can pre-marketing trials detect ADRs which are separated in time from drug exposure. Additionally, patients within trials are often carefully selected, without the multiple disease states or complex drug histories of patients in whom the drug will eventually become used. Furthermore, the patient's perspective is also frequently excluded from clinical trial safety assessments, with ADRs being assessed only by the clinicians who run them (Basch, 2010). For these reasons, rare and potentially serious adverse effects often remain undetected until a wider population is exposed to the drug. The vigilance of health professionals is an essential factor in discovering these new risks, together with regulatory authorities who continuously monitor reports of adverse effects throughout the lifetime of a marketed medicinal product.

As a result of this monitoring, the safety profile of established drugs is often well known, although new risks are occasionally identified. However, an important part of the therapeutic management of medical conditions is the minimisation of these well-known risks through rational prescribing and careful monitoring of drug therapy. Current evidence suggests that this could be improved.

Definitions

Having clear definitions of what constitutes an ADR is important. The World Health Organization (WHO) defines an ADR as 'a response to a drug that is noxious and unintended and occurs at doses normally used in man for the prophylaxis, diagnosis or therapy of disease, or for modification of physiological function' (WHO, 1972). The use of the phrase 'at doses normally used in man' distinguishes the noxious effects of drugs during normal medical use from toxic effects caused by poisoning. Whether an effect is considered noxious depends on both the drug's beneficial effects and the severity of the disease for which it is being used. There is no need to prove a pharmacological mechanism for any noxious response to be termed an ADR.

The terms ADR and adverse drug effect can be used interchangeably; adverse reaction applies to the patient's point of view, while adverse effect applies to the drug. The terms suspected ADR or reportable ADR are commonly used in the context of reporting ADRs to regulatory authorities, for example, through the UK's Yellow Card Scheme, operated by the Medicines and Healthcare Regulatory Authority (MHRA). Although the term 'side effect' and ADR are often used synonymously, the term 'side effect' is distinct from ADR. A side effect is an unintended effect of a drug related to its pharmacological properties and can include unexpected benefits of treatment.

The WHO definition has been criticised for excluding the potential for contamination of a product, ADRs that include an element of error, and ADRs associated with pharmacologically inactive excipients in a product. The use of the term 'drug' also excluded the use of complementary and alternative treatments, such as herbal products. In an attempt to overcome these points, the following definition of an ADR was proposed, 'An appreciably harmful or unpleasant reaction, resulting from an intervention related to the use of a medicinal product, which predicts hazard from future administration and warrants prevention or specific treatment, or alteration of the dosage regime, or withdrawal of the product' (Edwards and Aronson, 2000).

It is important also to avoid confusion with the term adverse drug event (ADE). An ADR in a patient is an adverse outcome that is attributed to a suspected action of a drug, whereas an ADE is an adverse outcome that occurs after the use of a drug, but which may or may not be linked to use of the drug. It therefore follows that all ADRs are ADEs, but that not all ADEs will be ADRs. This distinction is important in the assessment of the drug safety literature, since the term ADE can be used when it is not possible to suggest a causal link between a drug treatment and an adverse outcome. The suspicion of a causal relationship between the drug and the adverse effect is central to the definition of an ADR.

Classification of ADRs

Classification systems for ADRs are useful for educational purposes, for those working within a regulatory environment and for clarifying thinking on the avoidance and management of ADRs.

Rawlins–Thompson classification

The Rawlins–Thompson system of classification divides ADRs into two main groups: Type A and Type B (Rawlins, 1981). Type A reactions are the normal, but quantitatively exaggerated, pharmacological effects of a drug. They include the primary pharmacological effect of the drug, as well as any secondary pharmacological effects of the drug, for example, ADRs caused by the antimuscarinic activity of tricyclic antidepressants. Type A reactions are most common, accounting for 80% of reactions.

Type B reactions are qualitatively abnormal effects, which appear unrelated to the drug's normal pharmacology, such as hepatoxicity from isoniazid. They are more serious in nature, more likely to cause deaths, and are often not discovered until after a drug has been marketed. The Rawlins–Thompson classification has undergone further elaboration over the years (Table 5.1) to take account of ADRs that do not fit within the existing classifications (Edwards and Aronson, 2000).

The DoTS system

The DoTS classification is based on *Do*se relatedness, *T*iming and patient *S*usceptibility (Aronson and Ferner, 2003). In contrast to the Rawlins–Thompson classification, which is defined only by the properties of the drug and the reaction, the DoTS classification provides a useful template to examine the various factors that both describe a reaction and influence an individual patient's susceptibility.

DoTS first considers the dose of the drug, as many adverse effects are clearly related to the dose of the drug used. For example, increasing the dose of a cardiac glycoside will increase the risk of digitalis toxicity. In DoTS, reactions are divided into toxic effects (effects related to the use of drugs outside of their usual therapeutic dosage), collateral effects (effects occurring within the normal therapeutic use of the drug) and hyper-susceptibility reactions (reactions occurring in sub-therapeutic doses in susceptible patients). Collateral effects include reactions not related to the expected pharmacological effect of the drug or off-target reactions of the expected therapeutic effect in other body systems. It is worth noting that approximately 20% of newly marketed drugs have their dosage recommendations reduced after marketing, often due to drug toxicity.

The time course of a drug's presence at the site of action can influence the likelihood of an ADR occurring. For example, rapid infusion of furosemide is associated with transient hearing loss and tinnitus, and a constant low dose of methotrexate is more toxic than equivalent intermittent bolus doses. DoTS categorises ADRs as either time-independent reactions or time-dependent reactions. Time-independent reactions occur at any time within the treatment period, regardless of the length of course. Time-dependent reactions range from rapid and immediate reactions, to those reactions which can be delayed.

The final aspect of the DoTS classification system is susceptibility, which includes factors such as genetic predisposition, age, sex, altered physiology, disease and exogenous factors such as drug interactions (Table 5.2)

Factors affecting susceptibility to ADRs

Awareness of the factors which increase the risk of ADRs is key to reducing the burden on individual patients by informing prescribing decisions. The risk that drugs pose to patients

Table 5.1 Extended Rawlins–Thompson classification of adverse drug reactions

Type of reaction	Features	Examples
Type A: Augmented pharmacological effect	Common Predictable effect Dose-dependent Low morbidity Low mortality	Bradycardia associated with a beta-adrenergic receptor antagonist
Type B: Bizarre effects not related to pharmacological effect	Uncommon Unpredictable Not dose-dependent High morbidity High mortality	Anaphylaxis associated with a penicillin antibiotic
Type C: Dose-related and time-related	Uncommon Related to the cumulative dose	Hypothalamic pituitary–adrenal axis suppression by corticosteroids
Type D: Time-related	Uncommon Usually dose-related Occurs or becomes apparent some time after use of the drug	Carcinogenesis
Type E: Withdrawal	Uncommon Occurs soon after withdrawal of the drug	Opiate withdrawal syndrome
Type F: Unexpected failure of therapy	Common Dose-related Often cause by drug interactions	Failure of oral contraceptive in presence of enzyme inducer

Table 5.2 DoTS system of ADR classification

Dose relatedness	Time relatedness	Susceptibility
Toxic effects: ADRs that occur at doses higher than the usual therapeutic dose	*Time-independent reactions*: ADRs that occur at any time during treatment.	Raised susceptibility may be present in some individuals, but not others. Alternatively, susceptibility may follow a continuous distribution – increasing susceptibility with impaired renal function.
Collateral effects: ADRs that occur at standard therapeutic doses	*Time-dependent reactions*: *Rapid reactions* occur when a drug is administered too rapidly. *Early reactions* occur early in treatment then abate with continuing treatment (tolerance). *Intermediate reactions* occur after some delay, but if reaction does not occur after a certain time, little or no risk exists.	*Factors include*: genetic variation, age, sex, altered physiology, exogenous factors (interactions) and disease.
Hypersusceptability reactions: ADRs that occur at sub-therapeutic doses in susceptible patients	*Late reactions* risk of ADR increases with continued-to-repeated exposure, including withdrawal reactions. *Delayed reactions* occur some time after exposure, even if the drug is withdrawn before the ADR occurs.	

varies dependent on the population exposed and the individual characteristics of patients. Some reactions may be unseen in some populations, outside of susceptible subjects. Other reactions may follow a continuous distribution in the exposed population. Although many susceptibilities may not be known, a number of general factors which affect susceptibility to ADRs and others which affect the propensity of specific drugs to cause ADRs have been elucidated.

Age

Elderly patients may be more prone to ADRs, with age-related decline in both the metabolism and elimination of drugs from the body. They also have multiple co-morbidities and are, therefore, exposed to more prescribed drugs. Chronological age is, therefore, arguably a marker for altered physiological responses to drugs and for the presence of co-morbidities and associated drug use rather than a risk *per se*. As the population ages, the mitigation of preventable ADRs in the elderly will become increasingly important.

Children differ from adults in their response to drugs. Neonatal differences in body composition, metabolism and other physiological parameters can increase the risk of specific adverse reactions. Higher body water content can increase the volume of distribution for water-soluble drugs, reduced albumin and total protein may result in higher concentrations of highly protein bound drugs, while an immature blood–brain barrier can increase sensitivity to drugs such as morphine. Differences in drug metabolism and elimination and end-organ responses can also increase the risk. Chloramphenicol, digoxin, and ototoxic antibiotics such as streptomycin are examples of drugs that have a higher risk of toxicity in the first weeks of life.

Older children and young adults may also be more susceptible to ADRs, a classic example being the increased risk of extrapyramidal effects associated with metoclopramide. The use of aspirin was restricted in those under the age of 12, after an association with Reye's syndrome was found in epidemiological studies. Additionally, children can be exposed to more adverse effects due to the heightened probability of dosing errors and the relative lack of evidence for both safety and efficacy.

Gender

Women may be more susceptible to ADRs. In addition, there are particular adverse reactions that appear to be more common in women than men. For example, impairment of concentration and psychiatric adverse events associated with the anti-malarial mefloquine are more common in females.

Females are more susceptible to drug-induced torsade de pointes, a ventricular arrhythmia linked to ventricular fibrillation and death. Women are also over-represented in reports of torsades de pointes associated with cardiovascular drugs (such as sotalol) and erythromycin. This increased susceptibility in women is thought to be due to their longer QTc interval compared to men.

Co-morbidities and concomitant medicines use

Reductions in hepatic and renal function substantially increase the risk of ADRs. A recent study examining factors that predicted repeat admissions to hospital with ADRs in older patients showed that co-morbidities such as congestive cardiac failure, diabetes, and peripheral vascular, chronic pulmonary, rheumatological, hepatic, renal, and malignant diseases were strong predictors of readmissions for ADRs, while advancing age was not. Reasons for this could be pharmacokinetic and pharmacodynamic changes associated with pulmonary, cardiovascular, renal and hepatic insufficiency, or drug interactions because of multiple drug therapy (Zhang et al., 2009).

Ethnicity

Ethnicity has also been linked to susceptibility to ADRs, due to inherited traits of metabolism. It is known, for example, that the cytochrome P450 genotype, involved in drug metabolism, has varied distribution among people of differing ethnicity. For example, CYP2C9 alleles associated with poor metabolism can affect warfarin metabolism and increase the risk of toxicity. This occurs more frequently in white individuals compared to black individuals.

Examples of ADRs linked to ethnicity include the increased risk of angioedema with the use of ACE inhibitors in black patients (McDowell et al., 2006), the increased propensity of white and black patients to experience central nervous system ADRs associated with mefloquine compared to patients of Chinese or Japanese origin, and differences in the pharmacokinetics of rosuvastatin in Asian patients which may expose them to an increased risk of myopathy. However, susceptibility based on ethnicity could be associated with genetic or cultural factors and ethnicity can be argued to be a poor marker for a patient's genotype.

Pharmacogenetics

Pharmacogenetics is the study of genetic variations that influence an individual's response to drugs, and examines polymorphisms that code for drug transporters, drug-metabolising enzymes and drug receptors. A greater understanding of the genetic basis of variations that affect an individual's response to drug therapy has promised to lead to a new era of personalised medicine. Arguably, pharmacogenetics has yet to deliver on an appreciable scale, the reduction in ADRs that was predicted. However, there are some important examples of severe ADRs that may be avoided with knowledge of a patient's genetic susceptibility.

As already noted, major genetic variation is found in the cytochrome CYP450 group of isoenzymes. This can result in either inadequate responses to drugs, or increased risk of ADRs. Clinically relevant genetic variation has been seen in CYP2D6, CYP2C9, CYP2C19 and CYP3A5. A large effect on the metabolism of drugs can occur with CYP2C9, which accounts for 20% of total hepatic CYP450 content.

The narrow therapeutic index of warfarin, its high inter-individual variability in dosing and the serious consequences of toxicity have made it a major target of pharmacogenomic research. Studies of genetic polymorphisms influencing the toxicity of warfarin have focused on CYP2C9, which metabolises warfarin and vitamin K epoxide reductase (VKOR), the target of warfarin anticoagulant activity. Genetic variation in the VKORC1 gene, which encodes VKOR, influences warfarin dosing by a threefold greater extent than CYP2C9 variants. In 2007, the U.S. Food and Drug Administration (FDA) changed the labelling requirement for warfarin, advising that a lower initial dose should be considered in people with certain genetic variations. However, concerns remain because genetic variation only accounts for a proportion of the variability in drug response and clinicians may obtain a false sense of reassurance from genetic testing leading to complacency in monitoring of therapy. In addition, there appears to be little evidence of additional benefit (Laurence, 2009), in terms of preventing major bleeding events, compared to careful monitoring of the INR (see chapter 23)

A success story for pharmacogenetics is the story of the nucleoside analogue reverse transcriptase inhibitor (NRTI) abacavir. Hypersensitivity skin reactions to abacavir are a particular problem in the treatment of human immunodeficiency virus (HIV) infection. Approximately 5–8% of patients taking abacavir develop a severe hypersensitivity reaction, including symptoms such as fever, rash, arthralgia, headache, vomiting and other gastro-intestinal and respiratory disturbances. Early reports that only a subset of patients was affected, a suspected familial predisposition, the short onset time (within 6 weeks of starting therapy), and an apparent lower incidence in African patients led to suspicion of a genetic cause. Subsequent research revealed a strong predictive association with the human leukocyte antigen HLA-B*5701 allele in Caucasian and Hispanic patients. The presence of the allele can be used to stratify the predicted risk of hypersensitivity as high risk (>70%) for carriers of HLA-B*5701 and low risk (<1%) for non-carriers of HLA-B*5701. Evidence from the practical use of HLA-B*5701 screening has shown substantial falls in the incidence of hypersensitivity reactions, as well as a more general improved compliance with the medication (Lucas et al., 2007).

Another example of a success story for pharmacogenetics involves the cutaneous ADRs Stevens–Johnson syndrome (SJS) and toxic epidermal necrolysis (TEN). Both are serious reactions associated with substantial morbidity and mortality in which up to 40% of patients with TEN may die. SJS and TEN have been associated with numerous drugs, although the incidence of these reactions is extremely rare. Anti-epileptic drugs, such as carbamazepine and phenytoin, are known causes of SJS and TEN. The reactions are more common in South East Asian populations, including those from China, Thailand, Malaysia, Indonesia, the Philippines and Taiwan and, to a lesser extent, India and Japan. The presence of HLA allele, HLA-B*1502, for which genetic testing is available, indicates an increased risk of skin reactions for carbamazepine, phenytoin, oxcarbamazepine and lamotrigine. The FDA has recommended HLA-B*1502 screening before using carbamazepine and phenytoin in South East Asian individuals.

Erythrocyte glucose-6-phophatase dehydrogenase (G6PD) deficiency

G6PD deficiency is present in over 400 million people worldwide. It is a sex-linked inherited enzyme deficiency, leading to susceptibility to haemolytic anaemia. Patients with low levels of G6PD are predisposed to haemolysis with oxidant drugs such as primaquine, sulphonamides and nitrofurantoin. There are many variants of the genotype, leading to varied susceptibilities in individuals.

Porphyrias

The porphyrias are a heterogeneous group of inherited disorders of haem biosynthesis. The disorders are transmitted as autosomal dominants, with the exception of the rare congenital porphyria, which is recessive. The effects of drugs are of most importance in patients with acute porphyrias, in which certain commonly prescribed agents may precipitate life-threatening attacks. Other trigger factors include alcohol and changes in sex hormone balance. In the acute porphyrias, patients develop abdominal and neuropsychiatric disturbances, and they excrete in their urine excessive amounts of the porphyrin precursors 5-aminolaevulinic acid (ALA) and porphobilinogen.

A number of drugs may induce excess porphyrin synthesis. However, it is extremely difficult to predict whether or not a drug may cause problems in patients with porphyria and the only factors shown to be clearly linked with porphyrinogenicity are lipid solubility and membrane fluidisation, that is, the ability to disrupt the phospholipid bilayer of the cell membrane. A number of commonly used drugs induce ALA synthase in the liver, but there is wide variation between porphyric patients in their sensitivity to drugs which may trigger attacks. Thus, whereas a single dose of a drug may be sufficient to trigger an acute attack in one patient, another may require a number of relatively large doses of the same drug to produce any clinically significant effect. Lists of drugs which are known to be unsafe and drugs which are thought to be safe for use in acute porphyria are available in the British National Formulary.

Immunological reactions

The immune system is able to recognise drugs as foreign substances, leading to allergic reactions. Smaller drug molecules (<600 Da) can bind with proteins to trigger an immune response, or larger molecules can trigger an immune response directly. The immune response is not related to the pharmacological action of the drug and prior exposure to the drug is required. Immunological reactions are often distinct recognisable responses.

Allergic reactions range from rashes, serum sickness and angioedema to the life-threatening bronchospasm and hypotension associated with anaphylaxis. Patients with a history of atopic or allergic disorders are at higher risk. Immunological (hypersensitivity) reactions are split into four main types (Table 5.3).

Formulation issues contributing to ADRs

Although ADRs caused by product formulation issues are rare, because of stringent regulatory control, examples have occurred and regulatory authorities remain vigilant for such problems. In 1937, the S.E. Massengill Company in the USA developed a liquid preparation of an early antibiotic sulphanilamide which contained 72% diethylene glycol. Over a 2-week period, 353 patients received the elixir, 30% of whom died, including 34 children. Sadly, episodes of diethylene glycol poisoning have been reported in contemporary times, in countries which include Nigeria, India, Argentina and Haiti. In 2006, cough medicines made using glycerin contaminated with diethylene glycol, sourced from China, were responsible for the suspected deaths of over 300 people in Panama.

Osmosin was a slow-release preparation of indometacin which used a novel osmotic pump to deliver the drug through a laser-drilled hole in an impervious tablet. Osmosin was withdrawn in 1983 after 36 fatal gastro-intestinal haemorrhages, suspected to be caused by the tablet becoming lodged against the mucosa of the gastro-intestinal tract and exposing the mucosa to high localised concentrations of indometacin.

Adverse reactions have also been associated with excipient changes. In Australia and New Zealand, a decision to change

Table 5.3 Classification of immunological (hypersensitivity) reactions

Classification	Mechanism	Symptoms/signs and examples
Type I (immediate)	Drug/IgE complex to mast cells release of histamine and leukotrienes.	Pruritis, urticaria, bronchoconstriction, angioedema, hypotension, shock, for example, penicillin anaphylaxis.
Type II (cytotoxic)	IgG and complement binding to (usually) red blood cell. Cytotoxic T-cells lyse the cell.	Haemolytic anaemia and thrombocytopaenia, for example, associated with cephalosporins, penicillins and rifampicin.
Type III (immune complex)	Drug antigen and IgG or IgM form immune complex, attracting macrophages and complement activation.	Cutaneous vasculitis, serum sickness, for example, associated with chlorpromazine and sulphonamides.
Type IV (delayed type)	Antigen presentation with major histocompatibility complex protein to T-cells and cytokine and inflammatory mediator release.	Usually occur after 7–20 days. Macular rashes and organ failure, including Stevens–Johnson syndrome and toxic epidermal necrolysis, for example, associated with neomycin and sulphonamides.

the formulation of phenytoin to one used in the USA led to previously stable patients developing severe adverse reactions, including coma. In the US formulation calcium sulphate dihydrate was replaced with lactose. Unfortunately, it was subsequently found that the calcium salt slowed absorption of phenytoin, while the lactose in the new formulation increased its absorption.

Although excipients are often referred to as inert substances, serious adverse reactions such as anaphylaxis and angioedema have been reported to these substances. Sweeteners, flavourings, colouring agents/dyes and preservatives have all been associated with adverse reactions (Kumar, 2003).

Epidemiology of ADRs

ADRs are widespread, as shown by both systematic reviews and large-scale studies. A review of 69 studies from many countries in 2002 found that ADRs were responsible for an estimated 2.6% of admissions to hospitals and that between 3.5% and 7.3% of in-patients may suffer an ADR. More recent data, however, shows these to be under-estimates. A prospective study (Pirmohamed et al., 2004) found that 6.5% out of 18,820 admissions to medical units were caused by ADRs, with 2.3% of patients dying as a result. A similar prospective study of 3695 in-patient episodes found that 14.7% of those admitted to medical or surgical wards experienced an ADR during their stay. These were more common in women, older patients and in those admitted to surgical wards (Davies et al., 2009).

In primary care, estimates for the incidence of ADRs are more difficult to obtain. Some studies have relied on patients' reports of ADRs, either to postal questionnaires or telephone surveys. These provide varying estimates in ADR incidence and prevalence, but are hampered by the lack of information about non-responders. Nonetheless, estimates are of the order of 25% in the USA (Ghandi et al., 2003) and 30% in the UK (Jarernsiripornkul et al., 2002). A systematic review in 2007 found an incidence of overall ADEs, including ADRs, of 14.9 per 1000 person-months in primary care settings.

A widely quoted figure is that ADRs are between the fourth and sixth leading cause of death in the USA. This is based on an extrapolation of a meta-analysis of studies carried out in the USA, which showed that the incidence of serious ADRs causing hospital admission or occurring during admissions was 6.7% and resulted in an incidence of fatal ADRs of 0.32% (Lazarou et al., 1998). The study has been criticised for its methodology; however, more recent work from Sweden has identified that ADRs were responsible for 3% of deaths there (Wester et al., 2008), while in England ADRs were shown to occur in 0.4% of all patients admitted to hospital. This latter study showed that mortality was higher in those experiencing an ADR than in those who did not. Furthermore, the median length of stay in patients who experienced an ADR was 20 days compared to 8 days and costs associated with in-patient ADRs were calculated to be £171 million annually for the NHS in England (Davies et al., 2009). Costs to the NHS associated with admissions

due to ADRs have been estimated as £466 million annually (Pirmohamed et al., 2004).

Pharmacovigilance and epidemiological methods in ADR detection

As already noted, the inherent weaknesses of pre-marketing studies mean that post-marketing surveillance of medicines is essential to detect previously unnoticed adverse effects of treatment. The science of this process is called pharmacovigilance and has been defined as 'the study of the safety of marketed drugs under the practical conditions of clinical use in large communities'. Pharmacovigilance is concerned with the detection, assessment and prevention of adverse effects or any other possible drug-related problems, with the ultimate goal of achieving rational and safe therapeutic decisions in clinical practice.

Spontaneous reporting

Pharmacovigilance uses multiple methods, but the following will focus on spontaneous reporting systems. Spontaneous reporting systems collect data about suspected ADRs in a central database. Cases are not collected in a systematic manner, but accumulate through reports submitted spontaneously by people who make a connection between a drug and a suspected drug-induced event. In the UK, the spontaneous reporting scheme is the Yellow Card scheme. In some countries reporting is a voluntary activity, in others reporting is a legal requirement. There is no evidence that such a requirement increases reporting rates.

Spontaneous reporting has a number of advantages. It is relatively cheap to administer, can follow a product throughout its life and can also accept reports to over-the-counter medication and herbal treatments. Such schemes are, however, passive surveillance systems, which rely on the ability of health professionals to recognise possible ADRs and to distinguish these from symptoms related to underlying disease. It is important to emphasise that only a suspicion of a causal link between a drug and an adverse event is required, not confirmation of the association. One disadvantage of spontaneous reporting systems is their inability to quantify the risk. Such systems supply a numerator (the number of reports), but estimates of the incidence of reactions cannot be made because the population exposed to the drug cannot be ascertained accurately. Furthermore, only a minority of reactions are reported. Spontaneous reports are, however, an important form of evidence leading to drug withdrawals and are crucial for hypothesis generation.

Signal detection

A signal can be described as a possible causal relationship between an adverse event and a drug, which was previously unknown. One useful analogy for signal detection in a spontaneous reporting database is to think of a radio signal, which is disguised by the background radio 'noise'. Statistical methods of signal generation can be thought of as methods of tuning in to capture the radio signal from the background noise.

Statistical approaches scan the data accumulated through spontaneous reports for 'drug–adverse event pairs' that are disproportionately present within the database as a whole. Such calculations can be run automatically by modern computer systems, providing the opportunity to scan large databases for potential signals of new ADRs. Only rarely will a signal provide such strong evidence that a restriction on use of the drug or its withdrawal is immediately required.

However, while these mathematical approaches do develop hypotheses and give the illusion of an objective estimate of risk, they are not conclusive in themselves. A signal could be due to causes other than the drug. Confounding factors such as particular groups of patients being 'channelled' into receiving a drug can influence reporting. Similarly, reports may be received and analysed by a varied set of people with differing levels of understanding, competence, training, experience and awareness. There is also a tendency for reporting rates to be higher with newly introduced drugs, while articles in the media, regulatory action and even legal cases can provoke reporting of particular reactions. For that reason, the strength of the signal also depends on the quality of the individual spontaneous reports.

Causality assessment

The assessment of whether a drug is responsible for a suspected ADR is of great importance in both the regulatory environment and within the pharmaceutical industry. Reporters to spontaneous reporting schemes are requested to submit suspected ADRs and such reports contain variable levels of information. For example, since re-challenge with the suspected drug is often ethically unacceptable, very few reports contain such information.

As already noted, while a safety signal can arise from the accumulation of reported cases of the event in a database, causality assessment of individual cases may influence the subsequent decision-making process. However, often causality is difficult to prove in pharmacovigilance and a high degree of suspicion may be all that is necessary for regulatory action.

One of the most common methods of causality assessment in use is unstructured clinical assessment, also known as global introspection. Expert review of clinical information is undertaken and a judgement is made about the likelihood of the reaction being due to drug exposure. The assessment of complex situations, often with missing information, is open to variation between different assessors and studies have shown marked disagreement between experts. The WHO international monitoring centre uses global introspection for case assessment, assigning standardised causality categories to suspected ADRs (Table 5.4).

A number of alternative methods of assessing causality have been developed using standardised decision algorithms in an attempt to increase objectivity and reduce assessor bias.

Table 5.4 WHO causality categories for ADRs

Category	Description
Certain	Pharmacologically definitive, with re-challenge if necessary
Probably/likely	Reasonable temporal relationship, unlikely to be attributed to disease processes or other drugs, with reasonable dechallenge response
Possible	Reasonable temporal relationship, but could be explained by concurrent disease or drugs. No information on withdrawal
Unlikely	Temporal relationship improbable, concurrent disease or drugs provide plausible explanation
Conditional/unclassified	An event which requires more data for assessment
Unassessable/ unclassifiable	An event that cannot be judged because of insufficient/contradictory information which cannot be supplemented or verified

One of those most commonly used to assess causality is the Naranjo algorithm. This uses a questionnaire and points are added or taken away based on the responses to each question, such as *'Did the adverse reaction reappear when the drug was re-administered?'* The total score is then used to place the assessed reaction on the following scale: definite, probable, possible or doubtful. Algorithms may be less open to the effects of confounding variables, such as underlying disease states or concomitant drugs, but variation in assessor judgements still occur.

Yellow Card Scheme

The UK's Yellow Card Scheme was established in 1964 following the thalidomide tragedy. The Scheme is operated by the Medicines and Health care Products Regulatory Authority (MHRA). Health care professionals and coroners can submit reports of suspected ADRs using a Yellow Card (found in the British National Formulary) or using an on-line form (http://www.yellowcard.gov.uk). An association between the medicine and the event does not have to be confirmed. A suspicion is sufficient for a report to be submitted. The MHRA request that all serious suspected ADRs are reported by health care professionals concerning established medicines (drugs and vaccines). For newer drugs and vaccines, all suspected ADRs should be reported, even if minor events. Newer medicines under intensive surveillance are identified with an inverted black triangle symbol in product information and standard prescribing texts. Black triangle status is generally maintained for at least 2 years, but the period varies, depending on how much information is obtained about a product's continued safety. All suspected ADRs occurring in children should be reported even if the medicine has been used off-label.

Information from Yellow Card reports is entered into a database, suspected reactions are categorised using the internationally accepted Medical Dictionary for Regulatory Affairs (MedDRA) and the resultant signals generated by the combined reports are then assessed for causality. Where there is a valid signal which may be an ADR, further work may be required to assess the association further. This could involve requesting further details from reporters, contacting manufacturers, reviewing the literature or conducting pharmacoepidemiological studies. The MHRA estimates that about 40% of the safety signals investigated by the Agency are generated from spontaneous reports.

When new ADRs are identified and an association confirmed, the MHRA may take action in the form of changes to the Summary of Product Characteristics (SmPC) and/ or the patient information leaflet (PIL), restricting usage or withdrawing marketing authorisation for the medicine. Withdrawal of marketing authorisation or change in use requires that prescribers and suppliers be informed immediately, but such information is also usually publicised in the media; hence, patients are often aware of these actions and may present with requests for information and advice.

Unfortunately, spontaneous reporting systems, including the Yellow Card Scheme, suffer from severe under-reporting. A systematic review estimated this to be between 82% and 98% (Hazell and Shakir, 2006). There are a variety of reasons for this, including lack of certainty that the medicine caused the symptom, but it is important to emphasise that such certainty is not required. There is also no requirement to provide the patient name or contact details, only those of the actual reporter; hence, confidentiality, also cited as a reason for under-reporting, is no longer an issue. Furthermore, the MHRA have systems in place to check for duplicate reports covering the same incident, thereby eliminating concern about two people submitting reports about the same event in a given patient.

Direct patient reporting

Patients have been permitted to report directly to MHRA since October 2005, with the number of reports increasing steadily since then. Respondents to a survey of UK patient reporters indicated that the facility to report was important and most had an understanding of the purpose of reporting. Many considered it provided an opportunity to influence the content of PILs so that other patients may be better informed. However, there remains a need to further increase awareness of direct patient reporting among both the public and health professionals.

Despite the limited awareness of direct patient reporting, in the main people find it relatively easy to report suspected ADRs (McLernon et al., 2011). The majority of people who reported a suspected ADR identified it as such through issues relating to timing, as outlined in the causality methods used by pharmacovigilance experts, or by accessing information about the medicine from the PIL (Krska et al., 2011). There

are a number of countries world-wide which accept patient reports. It has been suggested that these advantages include faster signal generation, avoiding the filtering effect of interpretation of events by health professionals and not least, maintaining the number of reports at a time when reporting by health professionals may be reducing.

A comparison of the content of patient reports submitted to MHRA in the first 2 years of the scheme indicated they were more likely to describe the impact of the ADR than in reports submitted by health professionals. Comparisons of the ADR reports submitted indicated a wider range of ADRs were reported by patients to more medicines. However, the proportion of reactions judged serious by MHRA was similar between both patients and health professionals. Overall, patient reports make a useful contribution to pharmacovigilance.

Published case reports

The first suspicions of a less common or unpredictable reaction may often be seen in a case report from a practitioner. As seen by the cases of thalidomide and practolol, astute and vigilant clinicians submitting case reports to the medical press has been of importance in drug safety. Case reports have been described as a form of non-systematic voluntary reporting. However, reports are not solicited and their appearance in the medical literature is in the gift of medical editors. Editors may demand a causal link, or a case series, requiring higher standards of investigation than regulatory agencies demand from a spontaneous report. These high standards can prevent case histories from reaching publication and deter many clinicians. Furthermore, the time it takes for a case report about a suspected ADR to be published could be several months, during which time more patients may be exposed to the potential risk.

Cohort studies

Cohort studies are prospective pharmacoepidemiological studies that monitor a large group of patients taking a particular drug over a period of time. Ideally such studies compare the incidence of a particular adverse event in two groups of patients, those taking the drug of interest and, another group, matched for all important characteristics except the use of the drug. These studies can indicate the relative risks associated with the adverse event in people exposed to the drug being studied.

Case–control studies

Case–control studies compare the extent of drug usage in a group of patients who have experienced the adverse event with the extent of usage among a matched control group who are similar in potentially confounding factors, but have not experienced the event. By comparing the prevalence of drug taking between the groups, it may be possible to identify whether significantly more people who experienced the event also took a particular drug. Examples of associations which have been established by case–control studies are Reye's syndrome and aspirin and the relationship between maternal diethylstilboestrol ingestion and vaginal adenocarcinoma in female offspring. Case–control studies are an effective method of confirming whether or not a drug causes a given reaction once a suspicion has been raised. Being retrospective, they rely on good record-keeping about drug use and are not capable of detecting previously unsuspected adverse reactions.

Roles of health professionals

Ensuring medicines are used safely is fundamental to the role of all health professionals who prescribe, supply, administer, monitor or advise on their use. When selecting a medicine for an individual patient, whether this is to be prescribed or sold, the health professional should take account of all relevant patient factors, which may predispose to an ADR. As outlined above, this includes co-morbidities, concomitant drugs, renal and liver function and genetic predisposition. Importantly, it is invaluable to have information about the patient's ADR history. Studies have repeatedly shown that this is poorly documented, leading to inappropriate re-use of medicines which have previously caused problems. Hence, another important role of all health professionals is the documentation of identified ADRs. The patient may have information about this if documentation is insufficient; therefore, questioning the patient about his/her ability to tolerate specific medicines or extracting a full ADR history should be considered at every opportunity.

Identifying and assessing ADRs in clinical practice

Outside the pharmacovigilance environment of companies and regulatory agencies, the identification of potential ADRs is an essential component of clinical practice. Although assessments in practice may lack the formality of expert or algorithmic assessment, they are likely to take into account similar factors, such as whether the clinical event is commonly drug related, the temporal relationship with drug use, a dose relationship and exclusion of other possible causes. A list of such factors is set out in Box 5.1.

There are many triggers which can lead to the suspicion of an ADR. For example, changes in medicines, dose reduction, prescription of medicines used to treat allergic reactions or those frequently used to counteract the effects of other drugs. Simple questioning of patients could easily be incorporated into many aspects of routine care to increase the chances of detecting potential ADRs.

The process of identifying an ADR then involves making a judgement about whether or not a particular event such as a symptom, condition or abnormal test result could be related to a drug used in the patient experiencing the event. The prior experiences of the patient with other medicines should also be taken into consideration.

Every opportunity should be taken to question patients about their experience, to determine whether they perceive any adverse events which could be due to medicines. While

---

> **Box 5.1** Factors that may raise or suppress suspicion of a drug-induced event (Shakir, 2004)
>
> The *temporal relationship* between the exposure to the drug and the subsequent event
>
> The *clinical and pathological characteristics of the event* – events which are known to be related to drug use, rather than disease processes
>
> The *pharmacological plausibility* – based on the observer's knowledge of pharmacology
>
> *Existing information* in published drug information sources – whether or not the event has been noted by others
>
> *Concomitant medication* – which may be considered the cause of an event
>
> *Underlying and concurrent illnesses* – may alter the event or be considered the cause of the event
>
> *De-challenge* – disappearance of symptoms after dose reduction or cessation of therapy
>
> *Re-challenge* – reappearance of symptoms after dose increases or recommencement of therapy
>
> *Patient characteristics* and previous medical history – past history of the patient may colour the view of the event
>
> The potential for *drug interactions*

---

routinely asking simple questions is important, it is of equal value to develop a positive attitude towards the patients' perception of suspected ADRs. There is some evidence that health professionals may dismiss patients who report that they have experienced an ADR, but many patients identify such problems appropriately, using factors such as onset, effect of dose change, effect of de-challenge or even re-challenge, as well as the information sources freely accessible to them (Krska et al., 2011). To ascertain whether a symptom reported by a patient can be reasonably suspected of being an ADR requires careful questioning.

As stated above, the MHRA encourage reporting of all serious suspected ADRs to established drugs and all suspected ADRs to new drugs or vaccines. If not reporting themselves, health professionals should consider encouraging others to report. For example, a community pharmacist may have insufficient information to complete a Yellow Card as fully as possible, so may encourage a general practitioner to report. Alternatively, a hospital pharmacist may report on behalf of a consultant clinician. Encouraging others to report also extends to providing information about reporting and educating others, including patients, to report. Community pharmacies and general medical practices should all have a supply of Yellow Cards for patients, but patients may require advice and support in completing these. Pharmacists in particular, because of their role in dispensing prescriptions, may also be involved in educating and supporting others in preventing ADRs and in developing methods to detect ADRs through prescription monitoring.

Preventing ADRs

The majority of ADRs are thought to be preventable; hence, there is potential to dramatically reduce the costs associated with ADRs and possibly also deaths. Assessing preventability is a difficult area, since it involves judgements and many different methods have been developed for making these judgements. The approach of Hallas et al. (1990) is widely used, providing definitions of avoidability which range from definite (due to a procedure inconsistent with present-day knowledge or good medical practice) to unevaluable (poor data or conflicting evidence). Recent estimates suggest that between 53% and 72% of hospital admissions due to ADEs are preventable, while a meta-analysis (Beijer and de Blaey, 2002) showed that 88% of ADRs causing hospital admission in the elderly were preventable. However, not all ADRs are absolutely preventable and assessments using hindsight are unlikely to replicate clinical decision making at the point of prescribing. Preventability also varies from those with clear solutions, such as the prescribing of a teratogenic drug to a female of child bearing age, to those where the drug increases the risk of an event that occurs within the population.

ADRs can be prevented by checking previous ADR history, minimising the use of drugs known to carry a high risk of ADRs and tailoring drug selection to individuals based on the factors which predispose them to ADRs. Strategies are still required to minimise the burden of ADRs, but many recent initiatives have the potential to do so. For example, electronic decision support, increasing regular review of medicines, improved sharing of information about patients between health care providers and the increasing availability of guidance on drug selection and appropriate use should all increase rational prescribing, which may have an effect on the incidence of ADRs.

Monitoring therapy

Monitoring the effects of drugs either by direct measurement of serum concentration or by measurement of physiological markers is another potential mechanism to reduce the risk of ADRs. For example, it has been estimated that one in four of preventable drug-related hospital admissions are caused by failure to monitor renal function and electrolytes (Howard et al., 2003).

Clozapine, used for the management of treatment resistant schizophrenia and psychosis, is associated with significant risk of agranulocytosis. Mandatory monitoring of white blood cell counts has effectively eliminated the risk of fatal agranulocytosis.

Ideally, advice on monitoring should be clear, provide an evidence-based frequency of monitoring and acceptable values. However, robust evidence for the optimal monitoring frequency is limited, hampering specific guidance on monitoring. Guidelines vary between various expert bodies and drug information sources. An examination of the adequacy of manufacturers' advice on monitoring for haematological ADRs found that advice was too vague to be useful to prescribers (Ferner et al., 2005).

Currently, monitoring is often neglected, although practitioners may take greater care when treating the elderly and those with more co-morbidities (McDowell., 2010). Warfarin remains one of the top 10 drugs involved in drug-induced admissions, despite a clearly defined monitoring requirement.

Explaining risks to patients

Numerous studies have shown that patients want to receive information about side effects, although one study comparing patients' views to those of health professionals found that the latter viewed providing side effect information as of much less importance than patients did in receiving it. One of the main sources of information about ADRs is the PIL, which must be provided every time a medicine is prescribed or supplied. Ultimately, patients then have to make a decision about whether or not to use the medicine. Therefore, they have a right to receive understandable information about the potential for harm that a medicine may cause, to enable them to make an informed decision. While there may still be debate about whether the provision of information on side effects encourages reduced adherence to taking medicines or spurious reporting of adverse effects, it is clear that this information is useful to patients and its availability will increase. Patients do use the PIL when suspected adverse events are experienced, to assist in ascribing the cause of the problem; therefore, as outlined above, side effect information should be understandable and there is now a requirement to test information leaflets with patients prior to granting a marketing authorisation for a medicine.

Patients increasingly access a wide range of information sources about medicines and ADRs themselves; indeed, they are actively encouraged to do so. Hence, they may question judgements about the selection of individual products they have been prescribed or sold. In this situation, the health professional must be able to interpret the information accessed by the patient to ensure it is unbiased and accurate.

The EU recommends using verbal terms to describe the risk of experiencing an ADR, ranging from '*very common*' (for rates of more than 1 in 10) to '*very rare*' (for rates of less than 1 in 10,000). The MHRA advocates combining words with frequencies, for example, '*Common (affects more than 1 in 100 persons)*'. Studies show that patients tend to over-estimate the risk when these are described using words only and that patients differ in their understanding of what the terms mean. Percentages, particularly those below 1%, are also not understood by everybody. This lack of understanding of the risks of experiencing an ADR can potentially reduce willingness to use the medicine.

Another approach is the use of pictures, such as faces, graphs or charts. One example is the 'Paling palette', which is a grid of 1000 stick figures to convey information on the chances of experiencing a particular outcome. A similar method is a 'Cates plot' which is a grid of 100 faces or 1000 faces for rarer events, coloured differently and either smiling or downcast depending on the outcome. An example of a Cates plot is provided in Fig. 5.1. These types of icon grids are mainly used to convey the potential benefits and risks of a particular action, but can also be used to explain the risks of getting a side effect. Cates plots have been used to good effect by the UK's National Prescribing Centre. However, there are people who do not find these easy to understand (Ancker et al., 2006).

Much work has been undertaken on risk communication. It is important to appreciate that, when communicating information

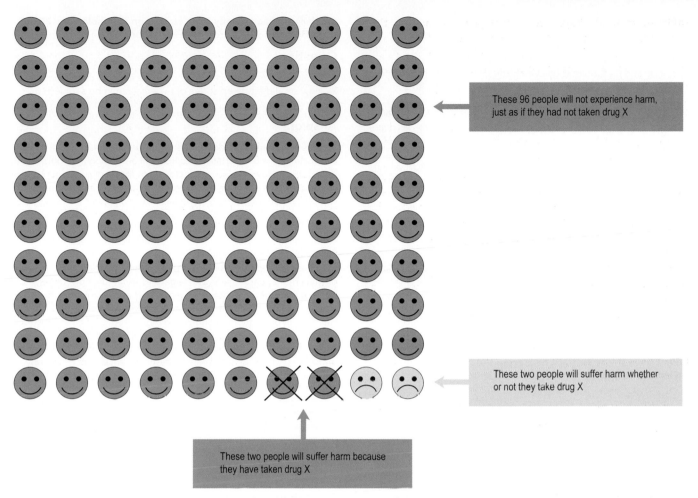

These 96 people will not experience harm, just as if they had not taken drug X

These two people will suffer harm whether or not they take drug X

These two people will suffer harm because they have taken drug X

Fig. 5.1 Acute coronary syndrome (ACS) patient decision aid: aspirin plus clopidogrel versus aspirin alone. Copyright National Prescribing Centre, reproduced by permission.

about potential ADRs, how risks are perceived will be affected by the relationship between the health professional and the patient, the patient's prior experience and beliefs, how information is framed and the context in which it is given. Patients may also have views on the acceptability of ADRs, which should be taken into account when selecting a product for an individual. An ADR which is viewed as minor by health professionals may be considered to reduce quality of life by one patient, while another patient may be happy to accept this for the potential benefit the medicine offers. Even when drugs are withdrawn from the market for safety reasons, significant numbers of patients will feel they were willing to accept the harm–benefit of the drug. Communicating the harms and benefits of medicines is, therefore, an important role of health professionals.

Case studies

Case 5.1

Mr KM is a fairly active 69-year-old. He has regularly presented his repeat prescription for atenolol 50 mg daily, aspirin 75 mg daily and simvastatin 40 mg daily to the same community pharmacy for several years. Last month diltiazem SR 60 mg twice daily was added, as he had been getting increasing angina symptoms. He asks for a topical product to treat neck pain, which has developed in the last few days which he puts down to a 'frozen shoulder'.

Questions

1. Could this be an ADR and why did it develop now?
2. Is it appropriate to change to another statin?
3. What actions should the pharmacist take?

Answers

1. Neck pain, 'frozen shoulder' and such descriptions are typical of the muscular pain which is induced by statins. The incidence of mild muscle pain with statins is between 2% and 7% in clinical trials. The onset varies from a few weeks to over 2 years after starting treatment, the incidence is dose-related and the severity ranges from mild aches to severe pain, causing reduced mobility. Older people, who may have reduced renal function or liver function, are at greater risk of statin-induced myopathy.

Diltiazem can inhibit the metabolism of simvastatin due to its actions on cytochrome P450 isoenzyme CYP3A4, thereby increasing the risk of myopathy.

Statin-induced myopathy ranges from mild myopathies and myalgias, to myositis, to rare cases of potentially life-threatening rhabdomyolysis, in which muscle cell walls are disrupted and the contents leak into the systemic circulation. Muscle pain in patients taking statins should, therefore, always be taken seriously.

2. The problem is associated with all drugs in the class. Although simvastatin and atorvastatin, the most widely prescribed, are both lipophilic and metabolised by cytochrome P450 3A4 and, therefore, may be most likely to cause muscle pain, there is no reliable comparative data on different statins.

3. Creatinine kinase (CK) levels should have been measured before initiating statin therapy, but regardless of whether or not this was done, a CK level should be measured now, plus liver function tests. Mr KM's primary care doctor should be contacted to inform him about the suspected ADR and the patient encouraged to report the ADR via the Yellow Card Scheme. It may be appropriate to discontinue or reduce the dose of the simvastatin, depending on the result of the CK level and the severity of the symptoms. The problem may not resolve immediately on discontinuation. Grapefruit juice can increase blood levels of simvastatin and high alcohol intake increases the risk of myopathy, so the pharmacist should also warn Mr KL about avoiding these.

Case 5.2

A 39-year-old male taking varenicline for smoking cessation reports that he has been suffering from vivid dreams and has become increasingly aggressive towards his family. Last night he had a major argument with his wife. His wife mentioned he hadn't been the same since he started the varenicline and he would like to know if this was a possible cause.

Questions

1. Is varenicline a possible cause of his vivid dreams and aggression?
2. Is this a reportable adverse drug reaction?

Answers

1. Varenicline has been associated with neuropsychiatric ADRs, including depression, suicidal thoughts, suicidal behaviour and aggression. Vivid dreams and other sleep disorders have also been reported. Prescribers have been warned that such reactions have been reported. Assessing the cause of this reaction is difficult, since smoking cessation itself is associated with exacerbations of underlying psychiatric illness and the risk of symptoms of depression. As varenicline dosing starts 1–2 weeks before stopping smoking, a key question is how long the patient has been taking the drug, and if the symptoms appeared before the smoking cessation date.

2. If a health professional considers that a patient's symptoms are a possible ADR to a newer drug, then they should be reported to regulatory authorities (in the UK, this would be through the MHRA's Yellow Card Scheme). Only a suspicion is necessary to report a reaction, not proven causality. In the case of intensively monitored medicines (identified by an inverted black triangle in the BNF), any reaction, no matter how trivial should be reported. Patients can also report directly to regulatory authorities in some countries, including the UK. Neuropsychiatric reactions such as this are commonly reported by patients.

Case 5.3

A 65-year-old man with heart failure is admitted to hospital with a potassium level of 7.1 mmol/L. Already stabilised on lisinopril 20 mg daily, he had recently been started on spironolactone 25 mg daily. He had a serum creatinine of 160 μmol/L.

Questions

1. What is the mechanism of any possible adverse drug reaction?
2. How should future episodes of hyperkalaemia be avoided?

Answers

1. Spironolactone, an aldosterone receptor antagonist, has a beneficial effect on mortality and hospital admission in patients with heart failure. However, spironolactone can increase potassium serum levels due to its effect on aldosterone. When used in combination with ACE inhibitors, serious hyperkalaemia can occur.

Although clinical trials of spironolactone showed no risk, cases have been reported in the literature and other epidemiological studies have indicated that in real-world clinical situations, the incidence of hyperkalaemia is increased.

2. Care should be taken when prescribing spironolactone outside of trial criteria, particularly with regard to renal function. Other susceptibilities for the development of hyperkalaemia include diabetes and the elderly due to reduced aldosterone production. Changes in other therapy should be monitored, as well as episodes of acute illness. Those with mildly increased serum potassium should have a reduced dose of spironolactone. More intensive monitoring of potassium levels at the commencement of therapy might be useful, although the hyperkalaemia can occur months after initiation.

Case 5.4

A 55-year-old woman attending a warfarin out-patient clinic has a raised INR. On questioning it is discovered that she has recently started taking glucosamine for muscle aches for the last 2 weeks.

Questions

1. What is the likelihood that glucosamine was responsible for the rise in the INR?
2. Should this reaction be reported to regulatory authorities?

Answers

1. Glucosamine is a popular supplement purchased for 'joint health'. It is commonly used by older patients. Spontaneous reports of interactions between warfarin and glucosamine have been submitted to UK, Australian and US regulators. Additional cases have been reported in the literature. While there is no known mechanism and no formal interaction studies, the published cases and spontaneous reports are sufficient evidence to suggest a potential interaction. Given the wide use of glucosamine, the interaction may be rare, although under-reporting is common.

Assessment of this individual case requires further questioning to eliminate other confounding factors such as changes in diet or adherence issues.

2. Interactions with, or adverse reactions to, complementary and alternative remedies can be reported to spontaneous reporting schemes, such as the Yellow Card Scheme. Collation of such reports allows regulators to gather further information on the suspected reaction, and any susceptibilities that may in time provide useful information to other users.

References

Ancker, J., Senathirajah, Y., Kukafka, R., et al., 2006. Design features of graphs in health risk communication: a systematic review. J. Am. Med. Inform. Assoc. 13, 608–618.

Aronson, J.K., Ferner, R.E., 2003. Joining the DoTS: new approach to classifying adverse drug reactions. Br. Med. J. 327, 1222–1225.

Basch, E., 2010. The missing voice of patients in drug-safety reporting. N. Engl. J. Med. 362, 865–869.

Beijer, H.J., de Blaey, C.J., 2002. Hospitalisations caused by adverse drug reactions (ADR): a meta-analysis of observational studies. Pharm. World Sci. 24, 46–54.

Davies, E.C., Green, C.F., Taylor, S., et al., 2009. Adverse drug reactions in hospital in-patients: a prospective analysis of 3965 patient-episodes. PLoS ONE 4, e4439 doi:10.1371/journal.pone.0004439.

Edwards, I.R., Aronson, J.K., 2000. Adverse drug reactions: definitions, diagnosis, and management. Lancet 356, 1255–1259.

Ferner, R.E., Coleman, J., Pirmohammed, M., et al., 2005. The quality of information on monitoring for haemotological adverse drug reactions. Br. J. Pharmacol. 60, 448–451.

Ghandi, T.K., Weingart, S.N., Borus, J., et al., 2003. Adverse drug events in ambulatory care. N. Engl. J. Med. 348, 1556–1564.

Hallas, J., Harvald, B., Gran, L.F., et al., 1990. Drug-related hospital admissions: the role of definitions and intensity of data collection and the possibility of prevention. J. Intern. Med. 228, 83–90.

Hazell, L., Shakir, S.A., 2006. Under-reporting of adverse drug reactions: a systematic review. Drug Saf. 29, 385–396.

Howard, R., Avery, A.J., Howard, P.D., et al., 2003. Investigations into the reasons for preventable admissions to a medical admissions unit. Qual. Saf. Health Care 12, 280–285.

Jarernsiripornkul, N., Krska, J., Capps, P.A.G., et al., 2002. Patient reporting of potential adverse drug reactions: A methodological study. Br. J. Clin. Pharmacol. 53, 318–325.

Kumar, A., 2003. Adverse effects of pharmaceutical excipients. Adverse Drug React. Bull. 222, 851–854.

Krska, J., Anderson, C.A., Murphy, E., Avery, A.J., on behalf of the Yellow Card Study Collaboration. How do patient reporters identify adverse drug reactions? A qualitative study of reporting via the UK Yellow Card Scheme. Drug Saf. 2011. In press.

Laurence, J., 2009. Getting personal: the promises and pitfalls of personalized medicine. Transl. Med. 154, 269–271.

Lazarou, J., Pomeranz, B.H., Corey, P.N., 1998. Incidence of adverse drug reactions in hospitalized patients. J. Am. Med. Assoc. 279, 1200–1205.

Lucas, A., Nolan, D., Mallal, S., 2007. HLA-B*5701 screening for susceptibility to a bacavir hypersensitivity. J. Antimicrob. Chemother. 59, 591–595.

McDowell, S.E., 2010. Monitoring of patients treated with antihypertensive therapy for adverse drug reactions. Adverse Drug React. Bull. 261, 1003–1006.

McDowell, S.E., Coleman, J.J., Ferner, R.E., 2006. Systematic review and meta-analysis of ethnic differences in risks of adverse reactions to drugs used in cardiovascular medicine. Br. Med. J. 332, 1177–1181.

McLernon D.J., Bond C.M., Fortnum H., Hannaford P.C., Krska J., Lee A.J., Watson M.C., Avery A.J., on behalf of the Yellow Card Study Collaboration. Patient experience of reporting adverse drug reactions via the Yellow Card Scheme in the UK. Pharmacoepidemiol. Drug Saf. 2011. Published early on-line: doi: 10.1002/pds.2117.

Pirmohamed, M., James, S., Meakin, S., et al., 2004. Adverse drug reactions as cause of admission to hospital: prospective analysis of 18 820 patients. Br. Med. J. 329, 15–19.

Rawlins, M.D., 1981. Clinical pharmacology: adverse reactions to drugs. Br. Med. J. 282, 974–976.

Shakir, S.A.W., 2004. Causality and correlation in pharmacovigilance. In: Talbot, T., Waller, P. (Eds.), Stephens' Detection of New Adverse Drug Reactions, fifth ed. John Wiley and Sons Ltd, Chichester, pp. 329–343.

Wester, K., Jonnson, A.K., Sigset, O., et al., 2008. Incidence of fatal adverse drug reactions: a population based study. Br. J. Clin. Pharmacol. 65, 573–579.

WHO, 1972. International drug monitoring: the role of national centres. Tech. Rep. Ser. 498, 1–25.

Zhang, M., Holman, C.D.J., Price, S.D., et al., 2009. Co-morbidity and repeat admission to hospital for adverse drug reactions in older adults: retrospective cohort study. Br. Med. J. 338, a2752.

Further reading

Aronson, J.K., Ferner, R.E., 2005. Clarification of terminology in drug safety. Drug Saf. 28, 851–870.

Cates Plot. Dr. Chris Cates' EBM Website. http://www.nntonline.net/visualrx/cates_plot/ (Accessed 16th March 2011).

Drug Safety Update. MHRA, London. Available at: http://www.mhra.gov.uk/Publications/Safetyguidance/DrugSafetyUpdate.

Lee, A., 2006. Adverse Drug Reactions, second ed. Pharmaceutical Press, London.

Talbot, J., Waller, P., 2004. Stephens' Detection of New Adverse Drug Reactions, fifth ed. John Wiley & Sons Ltd, Chichester.

Waller, P., 2010. An Introduction to Pharmacovigilance. Wiley-Blackwell, Oxford.

6 Laboratory data

H. A. Wynne and C. Edwards

Key points

- Biochemical and haematological tests provide useful information for the diagnosis, screening, management, prognosis and monitoring of disease and its response to treatment.
- Reference ranges are important guides which generally represent the test values from 95% of the healthy population (mean ± 2 standard deviations).
- A series of values, rather than a single test value, is often required to ensure clinical relevance and eliminate erroneous values due to patient variation and analytical or sampling errors.
- A wide variety of intracellular enzymes may be released into the blood following damage to tissues such as hepatocytes and skeletal muscle. These can be measured in serum to provide useful diagnostic information.
- Commonly requested biochemical test profiles include the so-called 'Us and Es' (urea and electrolytes), liver function tests, troponins and C-reactive protein.
- Commonly requested haematological test profiles include full blood count, differential white cell count, erythrocyte sedimentation rate (ESR), serum folate and vitamin B_{12} and iron status, and clotting screen.
- Drug therapy can cause abnormal test results.
- Drugs can have an important role in preventing or treating abnormalities.

This chapter will consider the common biochemical and haematological tests that are of clinical and diagnostic importance. For convenience, each individual test will be dealt with under a separate heading and a brief review of the physiology and pathophysiology will be given where appropriate to explain the basis of biochemical and haematological disorders.

It is usual for a reference range to be quoted for each individual test (see Tables 6.1 and 6.4). This range is based on data obtained from a sample of the general population which is assumed to be disease-free. Many test values have a normal distribution and the reference values are taken as the mean ± 2 standard deviations (SD). This includes 95% of the population. The 'normal' range must always be used with caution since it takes little account of an individual's age, sex, weight, height, muscle mass or disease state, many of which variables can influence the value obtained. Although reference ranges are valuable guides, they must not be used as sole indicators of health and disease. A series of values rather than a simple test value may be required in order to ensure clinical relevance and to eliminate erroneous values caused, for example, by spoiled specimens or interference from diagnostic or therapeutic procedures. Furthermore, a disturbance of one parameter often cannot be considered in isolation without looking at the pattern of other tests within the group.

Further specific information on the clinical and therapeutic relevance of each test may be obtained by referral to the relevant chapter in this book.

Biochemical data

The homeostasis of various elements, water and acid–base balance are closely linked, both physiologically and clinically. Standard biochemical screening includes several measurements which provide a picture of fluid and electrolyte balance and renal function. These are commonly referred to colloquially as 'Us and Es' (urea and electrolytes) and the major tests are described below.

Sodium and water balance

Sodium and water metabolism are closely interrelated both physiologically and clinically, and play a major role in determining the osmolality of serum.

Water constitutes approximately 60% of body weight in men and 55% in women (women have a greater proportion of fat tissue which contains little water). Approximately two-thirds of body water is found in the intracellular fluid (ICF) and one-third in the extracellular fluid (ECF). Of the ECF 75% is found within interstitial fluid and 25% within serum (Fig. 6.1). Total body water is regulated by the renal action of antidiuretic hormone (ADH), the renin angiotensin–aldosterone system, noradrenaline/norepinephrine and by thirst which is stimulated by rising plasma osmolality.

In general, water permeates freely between the ICF and ECF. Cell walls function as semipermeable membranes, with water movement from one compartment to the other being controlled by osmotic pressure: water moves into the compartment with the higher osmotic concentration. The osmotic content of the two compartments is generally the same, that is, they are isotonic, which ensures normal cell membrane integrity and cellular processes. However, the kidneys are an exception to the rule.

Table 6.1 Biochemical data: typical normal adult reference values measured in serum

Laboratory test	Reference range
Urea and electrolytes	
Sodium	135–145 mmol/L
Potassium	3.4–5.0 mmol/L
Calcium (total)	2.12–2.60 mmol/L
Calcium (ionised)	1.19–1.37 mmol/L
Phosphate	0.80–1.44 mmol/L
Magnesium	0.7–1.00 mmol/L
Creatinine	75–155 µmol/L
Urea	3.1–7.9 mmol/L
Estimated glomerular filtration rate (eGFR)	≥ 90 ml/min/1.73m²
Glucose	
Fasting	3.3–6.0 mmol/L
Non-fasting	<11.1 mmol/L
Glycated haemoglobin	Non-diabetic subjects <43 mmol/mol
	Inadequate control >58 mmol/mol
Liver function tests	
Albumin	34–50 g/L
Bilirubin (total)	<19 µmol/L
Enzymes	
Alanine transaminase	<45 U/L
Aspartate transaminase	<35 U/L
Alkaline phosphatase	35–120 U/L
γ-Glutamyl transpeptidase	<70 U/L
Ammonia	
Men	15–50 µmol/L
Female	10–40 µmol/L
Amylase	<100 U/L
Cardiac markers	
Troponin I	(99th percentile of upper reference limit) 0.04 µcg/L
Other tests	
C-reactive protein (CRP)	0–5 mg/L
Osmolality	282–295 mOsmol/kg
Uric acid	0.15–0.47 mmol/L
Parathyroid hormone (adult with normal calcium)	10–65 ng/L
25-Hydroxyvitamin D	>75 nmol/L (optimal)
	>50 nmol/L (sufficient)
	30–50 nmol/L (insufficient)
	12–30 nmol/L (deficient)
	<12 nmol/L (severely deficient)

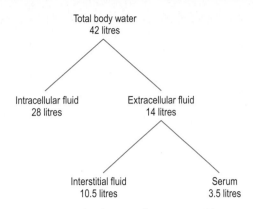

Fig. 6.1 Approximate distribution of water in a 70 kg man.

The amount of water taken in and lost by the body depends on intake, diet, activity and the environment. Over time the intake of water is normally equal to that lost (Table 6.2). The minimum daily intake necessary to maintain this balance is approximately 1100 mL. Of this, 500 mL is required for normal excretion of waste products in urine, whilst the remaining volume is lost via the skin in sweat, via the lungs in expired air, and in faeces. The kidneys regulate water balance, water being filtered, then reabsorbed in variable amounts depending primarily on the level of ADH.

Water depletion

Water depletion will occur if intake is inadequate or loss excessive. Excessive loss of water through the kidney is unusual except in diabetes insipidus or following the overuse of diuretics.

Patients with fever will lose water through the skin and ventilated patients will lose it through the lungs. Diarrhoea causes water depletion. Water loss is usually compensated for if the thirst mechanism is intact or can be responded to, but this may not occur in patients who are unconscious, have swallowing difficulties or are disabled. Severe water depletion may induce cerebral dehydration causing confusion, fits, coma and circulatory failure.

The underlying cause for the water depletion should be identified and treated. Replacement water should be given orally, where possible, or by nasogastric tube, intravenously

The osmolality of the ECF is largely determined by sodium and its associated anions, chloride and bicarbonate. Glucose and urea have a lesser, but nevertheless important, role in determining ECF osmolality. Protein, especially albumin, makes only a small (0.5%) contribution to the osmolality of the ECF but is a major factor in determining water distribution between the two compartments. The contribution of proteins to the osmotic pressure of serum is known as the colloid osmotic pressure or oncotic pressure.

The major contributor to the osmolality of the ICF is potassium.

Table 6.2 Typical daily water balance for a healthy 70 kg adult

	Input (mL)		Output (mL)
Oral fluids	1400	Urine	1500
Food	700	Lung	400
Metabolic oxidation	400	Skin	400
		Faeces	200
Total	2500		2500

or subcutaneously as necessary with 5% dextrose in water or, in patients with associated sodium deficits, isotonic saline. Hypotonic saline is sometimes used, but with great caution, where neurologic effects of hypertonicity predominate. Hypernatraemia should be corrected slowly: not more than half of the water deficit should be corrected in the first 12–24 h.

Water excess

Water excess is usually associated with an impairment of water excretion such as that caused by renal failure or the syndrome of inappropriate secretion of the antidiuretic hormone arginine vasopressin (SIADH). This syndrome has several causes including chest infections and some tumours, particularly small cell carcinoma of the lung. Excess intake is rarely a cause of water excess since the healthy adult kidney can excrete water at a rate of up to 2 mL/min. Patients affected usually present with signs consistent with cerebral overhydration, although if it is of gradual onset, over several days, they may be asymptomatic. Hyponatraemia is usually present.

Water and ECF osmolality

If the body water content changes independent of the amount of solute, osmolality will be altered (the normal range is 282–295 mmol/kg of water). A loss of water from the ECF will increase its osmolality and result in the movement of water from the ICF to ECF. This increase in ECF osmolality will stimulate the hypothalamic thirst centres to promote a desire to drink while also stimulating the release of vasopressin or ADH. ADH increases the permeability of the renal collecting ducts to water and promotes water reabsorption with consequent concentration of urine.

If the osmolality of the ECF falls, there is no desire to drink and no secretion of ADH. Consequently, a dilute urine is produced which helps restore ECF osmolality to normal.

The secretion of ADH is also stimulated by angiotensin II, arterial and venous baroreceptors, volume receptors, stress (including pain), exercise and drugs such as morphine, nicotine, tolbutamide, carbamazepine and vincristine. If blood volume decreases by more than 10%, the hypovolaemia stimulates ADH release and overrides control based on osmolality.

Sodium distribution

The body of an average 70 kg man contains approximately 3000 mmol of sodium. Most of this sodium is freely exchangeable and is extracellular. The normal serum range is 135–145 mmol/L. In contrast, the ICF concentration of sodium is only about 10 mmol/L.

Each day approximately 1000 mmol of sodium is secreted into the gut and 25,000 mmol filtered by the kidney. The bulk of this is recovered by reabsorption from the gut and renal tubules. It should be clear, therefore, that partial failure of homeostatic control can potentially have major consequences.

Sodium and ECF volume

The ECF volume is dependent upon total body sodium since sodium is almost entirely restricted to the ECF, and water intake and loss are regulated to maintain a constant concentration of sodium in the ECF compartment.

Sodium balance is maintained by renal excretion. Normally, 70% of filtered sodium is actively reabsorbed in the proximal tubule, with further reabsorption in the loop of Henle. Less than 5% of the filtered sodium load reaches the distal tubule where aldosterone can stimulate further sodium reabsorption.

Other factors such as natriuretic peptide hormone can also affect sodium reabsorption. This hormone is secreted by the cardiac atria in response to atrial stretch following a rise in atrial pressure associated with, say, volume expansion. It is natriuretic (increases sodium excretion in urine) and, amongst other actions, reduces aldosterone concentration.

Sodium depletion

Inadequate oral intake of sodium is rarely the cause of sodium depletion, although inappropriate parenteral treatment may occasionally be implicated. Sodium depletion commonly occurs with water depletion, resulting in dehydration or volume depletion. The normal response of the body to the hypovolaemia includes an increase in aldosterone secretion (which stimulates renal sodium reabsorption) and an increase in ADH secretion if ECF volume depletion is severe.

The serum sodium level can give an indication of depletion, but it must be borne in mind that the serum sodium may be:

- increased, for example, where there is sodium and water loss but with predominant water loss, as occurs in excessive sweating;
- normal, for example, where there is isotonic sodium and water loss, as occurs from burns or a haemorrhage;
- decreased, for example, sodium loss with water retention as would occur if an isotonic sodium depletion were treated with a hypotonic sodium solution.

Sodium excess

Sodium excess can be due to either increased intake or decreased excretion. Excessive intake is not a common cause, although hypernatraemia can be associated with excessive intravenous saline infusion or unreplaced hypotonic water depletion, due to impaired access to free water or impaired thirst.

Sodium excess is usually due to impaired excretion. It may also be caused by a primary mineralocorticoid excess, for example, Cushing's syndrome or Conn's syndrome. However, it is often due to a secondary hyperaldosteronism associated with, for example, congestive cardiac failure, nephrotic syndrome, hepatic cirrhosis with ascites, or renal artery stenosis. Sodium and water retention causes oedema.

Hypernatraemia

The signs and symptoms of hypernatraemia include muscle weakness and confusion.

Drug-induced hypernatraemia is often the result of a nephrogenic diabetes insipidus-like syndrome whereby the renal tubules are unresponsive to ADH. The affected patient presents with polyuria, polydipsia or dehydration.

- Lithium and phenytoin are the most commonly implicated drugs. The diabetes insipidus-like syndrome with lithium has been reported after only 2 weeks of therapy. The syndrome is usually reversible on discontinuation. Whilst affected, however, many patients are unresponsive to exogenous ADH.
- Demeclocycline can also cause diabetes insipidus and can be used in the management of patients with the syndrome of inappropriate ADH secretion (SIADH).
- Phenytoin generally has a less pronounced effect on urinary volume than lithium or demeclocycline, and does not cause nephrogenic diabetes insipidus. It inhibits ADH secretion at the level of the central nervous system.

Hypernatraemia can be caused by a number of other drugs (Box 6.1) and by a variety of mechanisms; for example, hypernatraemia secondary to sodium retention is known to occur with corticosteroids whilst the administration of sodium-containing drugs parenterally in high doses also has the potential to cause hypernatraemia.

Hyponatraemia

A fall in the serum sodium level can be the result of sodium loss, water retention in excess of sodium usually resulting from defects in free water excretion due to low ECF volume or inappropriate secretion of ADH. Increased water intake may also contribute, or a combination of both factors. A number of drugs have also been implicated as causing hyponatraemia (Box 6.2).

The inappropriate secretion of ADH is the mechanism underlying many drug-induced hyponatraemias. In this syndrome, the drug may augment the action of endogenous ADH (e.g. chlorpropamide), increase the release of ADH (e.g. carbamazepine), or have a direct ADH-like action on the kidney (e.g. oxytocin or, more obviously, desmopressin). Hyponatraemia can also be induced by mechanisms different from those described above. Lithium may cause renal damage and a failure to conserve sodium. Likewise the natriuretic action of diuretics can predispose to hyponatraemia.

Box 6.1 Examples of drugs known to cause hypernatraemia

Adrenocorticotrophic hormone
Anabolic steroids
Androgens
Corticosteroids
Lactulose
Oestrogens
Oral contraceptives
Sodium bicarbonate

Box 6.2 Examples of drugs known to cause hyponatraemia

Amitriptyline and other tricyclic antidepressants
Amphotericin
Angiotensin converting enzyme inhibitors
Carbamazepine
Cisplatin
Clofibrate
Cyclophosphamide
Diuretics
Heparin
Lithium
Miconazole
NSAIDs
Opiates
Tolbutamide
Vasopressin
Vincristine

Potassium

The total amount of potassium in the body, like sodium, is 3000 mmol. About 10% of the body potassium is bound in red blood cells (RBCs), bone and brain tissue and is not exchangeable. The remaining 90% of total body potassium is free and exchangeable with the vast majority having an intracellular location, being pumped in and out by Na/K-ATPase pumps. This is controlled by mechanisms aimed at ensuring stable intracellular to extracellular ratios, and hence correct muscular and neuronal excitability. Only 2% of the exchangeable total body potassium is in the ECF, the compartment from where the serum concentration is sampled and measured. Consequently, the measurement of serum potassium is not an accurate index of total body potassium, but together with the clinical status of a patient it permits a sound practical assessment of potassium homeostasis.

The serum potassium concentration is controlled mainly by the kidney with the gastro-intestinal tract normally having a minor role. The potassium filtered in the kidney is almost completely reabsorbed in the proximal tubule. Potassium secretion is largely a passive process in response to the need to maintain membrane potential neutrality associated with active reabsorption of sodium in the distal convoluted tubule and collecting duct. The extent of potassium secretion is determined by a number of factors including:

- the amount of sodium available for exchange in the distal convoluted tubule and collecting duct;
- the availability of hydrogen and potassium ions for exchange in the distal convoluted tubule or collecting duct;
- the ability of the distal convoluted tubule or collecting duct to secrete hydrogen ions;
- the concentration of aldosterone;
- tubular fluid flow rate.

As described above, both potassium and hydrogen can neutralise the membrane potential generated by active sodium reabsorption and consequently there is a close relationship between potassium and hydrogen ion homeostasis. In acidosis, hydrogen ions are normally secreted in preference to potassium and potassium moves out of cells, that is, hyperkalaemia is often associated with acidosis, except in renal tubular acidosis. In alkalosis, fewer hydrogen ions will be present and potassium moves into cells and potassium is excreted, that is, hypokalaemia is often associated with alkalosis.

The normal daily dietary intake of potassium is of the order of 60–200 mmol, which is more than adequate to replace that lost from the body. It is unusual for a deficiency in intake to account for hypokalaemia. A transcellular movement of potassium into cells, loss from the gut or excretion in the urine are the main causes of hypokalaemia.

Hypokalaemia

Transcellular movement into cells. The shift of potassium from the serum compartment of the ECF into cells accounts for the hypokalaemia reported following intravenous or, less frequently, nebulised administration of β-adrenoreceptor agonists such as salbutamol. Parenteral insulin also causes a shift of potassium into cells, and is used for this purpose in the acute management of patients with hyperkalaemia. Catecholamines, for example, adrenaline/epinephrine and theophylline also have this effect.

Loss from the gastro-intestinal tract. Although potassium is secreted in gastric juice, much of this, together with potassium ingested in the diet, is reabsorbed in the small intestine. Stools do contain some potassium, but in a patient with chronic diarrhoea or a fistula, considerable amounts of potassium may be lost and precipitate hypokalaemia. Likewise, the abuse of laxatives increases gastro-intestinal potassium loss and may precipitate hypokalaemia. Analogous to the situation with diarrhoea, the potassium secreted in gastric juice may be lost following persistent vomiting and can also contribute to hypokalaemia.

Loss from the kidneys. Mineralocorticoid excess, whether it be due to primary or secondary hyperaldosteronism or Cushing's syndrome, can increase urinary potassium loss and cause hypokalaemia. Likewise, increased excretion of potassium can result from renal tubular damage. Nephrotoxic antibiotics such as gentamicin have been implicated in this.

Many drugs which can induce hypokalaemia do so by affecting the regulatory role of aldosterone upon potassium–sodium exchange in the distal tubule and collecting duct. Administered corticosteroids mimic aldosterone and can, therefore, increase potassium loss.

The most commonly used groups of drugs that can cause hypokalaemia are thiazide and loop diuretics. Both groups of drugs increase the amount of sodium delivered and available for reabsorption at the distal convoluted tubule and collecting duct. Consequently, this will increase the amount of potassium excreted from the kidneys. Some of the drugs known to cause hypokalaemia are shown in Box 6.3.

Clinical features. The patient with moderate hypokalaemia may be asymptomatic, but the symptoms of more severe hypokalaemia include muscle weakness, hypotonia, paralytic ileus, depression and confusion. Arrhythmias may occur. Typical changes on the electrocardiogram (ECG) are of ST depression, T wave depression/inversion and prolonged

Box 6.3   Examples of drugs known to cause hypokalaemia
Amphotericin
Aspirin
Corticosteroids
Diuretics
Gentamicin
Glucose
Insulin
Laxatives
Penicillin G (sodium salt)
Piperacillin + tazobactam
Salicylates
Sodium bicarbonate
Sodium chloride
Terbutaline
Ticarcillin + clavulanic acid

P–R interval. Although hypokalaemia tends to make anti-arrhythmic drugs less effective, the action of digoxin, in contrast, is potentiated leading to increased signs of toxicity. Insulin secretion in response to a rising blood glucose concentration requires potassium and this mechanism may be impaired in hypokalaemia. Rarely there may be impaired renal concentrating ability with polyuria and polydipsia.

Hypokalaemia is managed by giving either oral potassium or intravenous suitability dilute potassium solutions, depending on its severity and the clinical state of the patient.

Hyperkalaemia

Hyperkalaemia may arise from excessive intake, decreased elimination or shift of potassium from cells to the ECF. It is rare for excessive oral intake to be the sole cause of hyperkalaemia. The inappropriate use of parenteral infusions containing potassium is probably the most common iatrogenic cause of excessive intake. Hyperkalaemia is a common problem in patients with renal failure due to their inability to excrete a potassium load.

The combined use of potassium-sparing diuretics such as amiloride, triamterene or spironolactone with an angiotensin converting enzyme (ACE) inhibitor, which will lower aldosterone, is a recognised cause of hyperkalaemia, particularly in the elderly. Mineralocorticoid deficiency states such as Addison's disease where there is a deficiency of aldosterone also decrease renal potassium loss and contribute to hyperkalaemia. Those at risk of hyperkalaemia should be warned not to take dietary salt (NaCl) substitutes in the form of KCl.

The majority of body potassium is intracellular. Severe tissue damage, catabolic states or impairment of the energy-dependent sodium pump, caused by hypoxia or diabetic ketoacidosis, may result in apparent hyperkalaemia due to potassium moving out of and sodium moving into cells. If serum potassium rises, insulin release is stimulated which, through increasing activity in Na/K-ATPase pumps, causes potassium to move into cells. Box 6.4 gives examples of some drugs known to cause hyperkalaemia.

Angiotensin converting enzyme inhibitors
Antineoplastic agents (cyclophosphamide, vincristine)
Non-steroidal anti-inflammatory drugs
β-Adrenoreceptor blocking agents
Ciclosporin
Digoxin (in acute overdose)
Diuretics, potassium sparing (amiloride, triamterene, spironolactone)
Heparin
Isoniazid
Lithium
Penicillins (potassium salt)
Potassium supplements
Tetracycline

Haemolysis during sampling or a delay in separating cells from serum will result in potassium escaping from blood cells into serum and causing an artefactual hyperkalaemia.

Clinical features. Hyperkalaemia can be asymptomatic but fatal. An elevated potassium level has many effects on the heart: notably the resting membrane potential is lowered and the action potential shortened. Characteristic changes of the ECG precede ventricular fibrillation and cardiac arrest.

In emergency management of a patient with hyperkalaemia (>6.5 mmol/L ± ECG changes), calcium gluconate (or chloride) at a dose of 10 mL of 10% solution is given intravenously over 5 min. This does not reduce the potassium concentration but antagonises the effect of potassium on cardiac tissue. Immediately thereafter, glucose 50 g with 20 units soluble insulin, for example, by intravenous infusion will lower serum potassium levels within 30 min by increasing the shift of potassium into cells.

If acidosis is present, bicarbonate administration may be considered.

The long-term management of hyperkalaemia may involve the use of oral or rectal polystyrene cation-exchange resins which remove potassium from the body. Chronic hyperkalaemia, in renal failure, is managed by a low potassium diet.

Calcium

The body of an average man contains about 1 kg of calcium and 99% of this is bound within bone. Calcium is present in serum bound mainly to the albumin component of protein (46%), complexed with citrate and phosphate (7%), and as free ions (47%). Only the free ions of calcium are physiologically active. Calcium metabolism is regulated by 1,25-dihydroxycholecalciferol (vitamin D) which, when serum calcium is low, is secreted to promote gastro-intestinal absorption of calcium, and by parathyroid hormone (PTH) which is inhibited by increased serum concentrations of calcium ions. PTH is secreted in response to low calcium concentrations and increases serum calcium by actions on osteoclasts, kidney and gut.

The serum calcium level is often determined by measuring total calcium, that is, that which is free and bound but the measurement of free or ionised calcium offers advantages in some situations.

In alkalosis, hydrogen ions dissociate from albumin, and calcium binding to albumin increases, together with an increase in complex formation. If the concentration of ionised calcium falls sufficiently, clinical symptoms of hypocalcaemia may occur despite the total serum calcium concentration being unchanged. The reverse effect, that is, increased ionised calcium, occurs in acidosis.

Changes in serum albumin also affect the total serum calcium concentration independently of the ionised concentration. A variety of equations are available to estimate the calcium concentration and many laboratories report total and adjusted calcium routinely. A commonly used formula is shown in Fig. 6.2. Caution must be taken when using such a formula in the presence of disturbed blood hydrogen ion concentrations.

Hypercalcaemia

Hypercalcaemia may be caused by a variety of disorders, the most common being primary hyperparathyroidism in which there is autonomous growth of PTH-producing cells and malignancy. Hypercalcaemia of malignancy is seen in multiple myeloma and carcinomas which metastasise in bone. It is also seen in squamous carcinoma of the bronchus, as a result of a peptide with PTH-like activity, produced by the tumour. Hypercalcaemia also occurs in thyrotoxicosis, vitamins A and D intoxication, acute renal failure, renal transplantation and acromegaly. PTH measurement can be pivotal in the establishment of the cause of hypercalcaemia.

Thiazide diuretics, lithium, tamoxifen and calcium supplements used in the management of osteoporosis are examples of some of the drugs which can cause hypercalcaemia.

An artifactual increase in total serum calcium may sometimes be seen as a result of a tourniquet being applied during venous sampling. The resulting venous stasis may cause redistribution of fluid from the vein into the extravascular space, and the temporary haemoconcentration will affect albumin levels.

Management of hypercalcaemia involves correction of any dehydration with normal saline followed by furosemide which inhibits tubular reabsorption of calcium. Bisphosphonates are used to inhibit bone turnover.

For albumin < 40 g/L:

Corrected calcium = [Ca] + 0.02 × (40 − [alb]) mmol/L

For albumin > 45 g/L:

Corrected calcium = [Ca] − 0.02 ([alb] − 45) mmol/L

Fig. 6.2 Formula for correction of total serum calcium concentration for changes in albumin concentration; albumin concentration = [alb] (albumin units = g/L); calcium concentration = [Ca] (total calcium units = mmol/L).

Hypocalcaemia

Hypocalcaemia can be caused by a variety of disorders including severe malnutrition, hypoalbuminaemia, hypoparathyroidism, pancreatitis and those that cause vitamin D deficiency, for example, malabsorption, reduced exposure to sunlight, liver disease and renal disease. In alkalaemia, which may occur when a patient is hyperventilating, there is an increase in protein binding of calcium, which can result in a fall in serum levels of ionised calcium, manifesting itself as paraesthesiae or tetany.

Drugs that have been implicated as causing hypocalcaemia include bisphosphonates which suppress formation and function of osteoclasts, phenytoin, phenobarbital, aminoglycosides, phosphate enemas, calcitonin, cisplatin, mithramycin and furosemide.

Biochemical measurements of serum calcium, phosphate and alkaline phosphatase can be normal in some patients with vitamin D deficiency and osteomalacia. The recent development of non-radioactive automated assays for serum PTH and 25-hydroxy vitamin D (25-OHD) has made measurement of these two hormones possible in many laboratories. There is a lack of consensus regarding a specific level of 25-OHD that is indicative of vitamin D deficiency, but this has usually been established by assessing the point at which serum PTH starts to rise. This, together with methodological and technical issues, prevents direct comparison of values across laboratories. Clinical decision limits for PTH and 25-OHD are laboratory specific and must be interpreted within the clinical context of each patient.

Phosphate

About 85% of body phosphate is in bone, 15% in ICF and only 0.1% in ECF. Its major function is in energy metabolism. Serum levels are regulated by absorption from the diet, which is partly under the control of vitamin D, and PTH which controls its excretion by the kidney and resorption from bone. The recent identification of genes encoding for renal phosphate transporters or associated proteins, and the discovery of a new hormone, fibroblast growth factor 23 and its emerging role in the bone–kidney axis which regulates systemic phosphate, has improved knowledge of homeostasis.

Hypophosphataemia

Clinical features. Severe hypophosphataemia can cause general debility, anorexia, anaemia, muscle weakness and wasting and some bone pain and skeletal wasting. As phosphorus is ubiquitous in various foods, inadequate dietary phosphorus intake requires near starvation. Refeeding of those recovering from energy depletion as a result, for example, of alcoholic bouts or diabetic ketoacidosis, without adequate provision of phophorus, can precipitate hypophosphataemia.

Hyperphosphataemia

Hyperphosphataemia occurs in chronic renal failure. Less common causes are secondary to rhabdomyolysis, tumour lysis or severe haemolysis. Hyperphosphataemia can cause hypocalcaemia. Treatment of hyperphosphataemia requires identification and correction of the underlying cause.

Magnesium

Magnesium is an essential cation, found primarily in bone, muscle and soft tissue. About 1% of the total body content is in the ECF. As an important cofactor for numerous enzymes and ATP, it is critical in energy requiring metabolic processes, protein synthesis, membrane integrity, nervous tissue conduction, neuromuscular excitability, muscle contraction, hormone secretion and in intermediary metabolism. Serum magnesium levels are usually maintained within a tight range (0.7–1.0 mmol/L). Although a serum concentration of less than this usually indicates some level of magnesium depletion, serum levels may be normal in spite of low intracellular magnesium due to magnesium depletion. Hypocalcaemia is a prominent manifestation of moderate to severe magnesium deficiency in humans.

Hypomagnesaemia is frequently seen in critically ill patients. Causes include excessive gastro-intestinal losses, renal losses, surgery, trauma, infection, malnutrition and sepsis. The drugs most likely to induce significant hypomagnesaemia are cisplatin, amphotericin B and ciclosporin, but it is also a potential complication of treatment with amikacin, gentamicin, laxatives, pentamidine, tobramycin, tacrolimus and carboplatin. A hypomagnesaemic effect of furosemide and hydrochlorothiazide is questionable and routine monitoring and treatment are not required. Use of digoxin has been associated with hypomagnesaemia, possibly by enhancing magnesium excretion, which may predispose to digoxin toxicity, for example, dysrhythmias.

Where treatment is indicated, oral supplements are available but because of their slow onset of action and gastro-intestinal intolerance the intravenous route is often preferred and especially in critically ill patients with severe symptomatic hypomagnesaemia.

Hypermagnesaemia is most commonly caused by renal insufficiency and excess iatrogenic magnesium administration.

Creatinine

Serum creatinine concentration is largely determined by its rate of production, rate of renal excretion and volume of distribution. It is frequently used to evaluate renal function.

Creatinine is produced at a fairly constant rate from creatine and creatine phosphate in muscle. Daily production is a function of muscle mass and declines with age from 24 mg/kg/day in a healthy 25-year-old to 9 mg/kg/day in a 95-year-old. Creatinine undergoes complete glomerular filtration with little reabsorption by the renal tubules. Its clearance is, therefore, usually a good indicator of the glomerular filtration rate (GFR). As a general rule, and only at the steady state, if the serum creatinine doubles this equates to a 50% reduction in the GFR and consequently renal function. The serum creatinine level can be transiently elevated following meat ingestion, but less so than urea, or strenuous exercise. Individuals with a high muscle bulk produce more creatinine and, therefore, have a higher serum creatinine level compared to an otherwise identical but less muscular individual.

The value for creatinine clearance is higher than the true GFR due to the active tubular secretion of creatinine. In a patient with a normal GFR, this is of little significance. However, in an individual in whom the GFR is low (<10 mL/min), the tubular secretion may make a significant contribution to creatinine elimination and overestimate the GFR. In this type of patient, the breakdown of creatinine in the gut can also become a significant source of elimination. Some drugs including trimethoprim and cimetidine inhibit creatinine secretion, reducing creatinine clearance and elevating serum creatinine without affecting the GFR.

Measured and estimated GFR

GFR measured as the urinary or plasma clearance of an ideal filtration marker such as inulin is the best overall measure of kidney function but techniques are complex and expensive. Urinary clearance of creatinine allows estimation of GFR, but blood sampling and timed urine collection have practical difficulty and are subject to error.

In the steady state, the serum level of creatinine is related to the reciprocal of the GFR and estimating equations based on this, as well as age, sex, race and body size are in use to facilitate the detection, evaluation and management of chronic kidney disease. The Cockcroft Gault formula is not adjusted for body-surface area whereas the Modification of Diet in Renal Disease (MDRD) study equation is, and is more accurate in older and obese people. Estimates of GFR using these equations fall within the same interval for guiding dose adjustment of renally excreted drugs. Accuracy of estimates of GFR cannot be relied upon in patients with rapidly changing kidney function, those with unusual body habitus or diet, without chronic kidney disease and in patients with estimates of GFR of 60 mL/1.73 m^2 or greater.

Urea

The catabolism of dietary and endogenous amino acids in the body produces large amounts of ammonia. Ammonia is toxic and its concentration is kept very low by conversion in the liver to urea. Urea is eliminated in urine and represents the major route of nitrogen excretion. The urea is filtered from the blood at the renal glomerulus and undergoes significant tubular reabsorption of 40–50%. This tubular reabsorption is pronounced at low rates of urine flow but is reduced in advanced renal failure. Serum urea is a less reliable marker of GFR than creatinine. Urea levels vary widely with diet, rate of protein metabolism, liver production and the GFR. A high protein intake from the diet, tissue breakdown, major haemorrhage in the gut, and consequent absorption of the protein from the blood, and corticosteroid therapy may produce elevated serum urea levels (up to 10 mmol/L). Urea concentrations of more than 10 mmol/L are usually due to renal disease or decreased renal blood flow following shock or dehydration. As with serum creatinine levels, serum urea levels do not begin to increase until the GFR has fallen by 50% or more.

Production is decreased in situations where there is a low protein intake and in some patients with liver disease. Thus, non-renal as well as renal influences should be considered when evaluating changes in serum urea concentrations.

Arterial blood gases

Arterial blood gas analysis provides a rapid and accurate assessment of oxygenation, alveolar ventilation and acid–base status, the three processes which maintain pH homeostasis. The maintenance of arterial CO_2 tension (PaCO$_2$) depends on the quantity of CO_2 produced in the body and its removal through alveolar ventilation. High PaCO$_2$ (>6.1 kPa) indicates alveolar hypoventilation and low PaCO$_2$ (<4.5 kPa) implies alveolar hyperventilation.

The adequate delivery of oxygen to the tissues depends upon the cardiopulmonary system, arterial oxygen tension (PaO$_2$), oxygen concentration in inspired air and haemoglobin content and its affinity for oxygen. Oxygen saturation is measured by pulse oximetry or by arterial blood gas analysis. Hypoxaemia is defined as a PaO$_2$ of less than 12 kPa at sea level in an adult patient breathing room air.

Bicarbonate and acid–base

Bicarbonate acts as part of the carbonic acid–bicarbonate buffer system, which is important to maintain acid–base balance and thus the pH of the blood. pH homeostasis is accomplished through the interaction of lungs, kidneys and blood buffers. This interaction is best represented by the Henderson–Hasselbalch equation, an equation by which the pH of a buffer solution, blood plasma being one, can be determined (Fig. 6.3).

Plasma bicarbonate is controlled mainly by kidney and blood buffers. The lungs control the PaCO$_2$.

In metabolic acidosis such as that which occurs in renal failure, diabetic ketoacidosis or salicylate poisoning, bicarbonate levels fall. In metabolic alkalosis, the plasma bicarbonate concentration is high. This can occur, for instance, when there is a loss of hydrogen ions from the stomach, as in severe vomiting, or loss through the kidneys, as in mineralocorticoid excess or severe potassium depletion. In the latter situation, an increase in sodium reabsorption in the kidney results in bicarbonate retention and a loss of hydrogen ions. The blood buffer system of carbonic acid/bicarbonate base can act immediately to prevent excessive change in pH. The respiratory system takes a few minutes but the kidneys up to several days to readjust H$^+$ ions concentration.

$$pH = pKa + Log_{10} \frac{[HCO_3^-]}{\alpha\, pCO_2}$$

Fig. 6.3 The Henderson–Hasselbalch equation. pH, plasma pH; pK$_a$, negative log to base 10 of the apparent overall dissociation constant of carbonic acid; [HCO$_3^-$], plasma bicarbonate concentration; α, solubility of carbon dioxide in blood at 37 °C; pCO$_2$, partial pressure of carbon dioxide in blood.

Glucose

The serum glucose concentration is largely determined by the balance of glucose moving into, and leaving, the extracellular compartment. In a healthy adult, this movement is capable of maintaining serum levels below 10 mmol/L, regardless of the intake of meals of varying carbohydrate content.

The renal tubules have the capacity to reabsorb glucose from the glomerular filtrate, and little unchanged glucose is normally lost from the body. Glucose in the urine (glycosuria) is normally only present when the concentration in serum exceeds 10 mmol/L, the renal threshold for total reabsorption.

Normal ranges for serum glucose concentrations are often quoted as non-fasting (<11.1 mmol/L) or fasting (3.3–6.0 mmol/L) concentration ranges. Fasting serum glucose levels between 6.1 and 7.0 mmol/L indicate impaired glucose tolerance. When symptoms are typical of diabetes, a fasting level above 7.0 mmol/L or a 2 h post-glucose or random serum glucose level ≥11.1 mmol/L is consistent with a diagnosis of diabetes. Other signs and symptoms, if present, are notably those attributable to an osmotic diuresis, and will suggest clinically the diagnosis of diabetes mellitus.

Glycated haemoglobin

Glucose binds to a part of the haemoglobin molecule to form a small glycated fraction. Normally, about 5% of haemoglobin is glycated, but this amount is dependent on the average blood glucose concentration over the lifespan of the red cells (about 120 days) and where red cell lifespan is reduced this leads to low glycated haemoglobin levels. The major component of the glycated fraction is referred to as HbA_{1C}.

Measurement of HbA_{1C} is well established as an indicator of chronic glycaemic control in patients with diabetes. Several methods exist for its determination, but the International Federation of Clinical Chemistry and Laboratory Medicine has recently approved a reference measurement procedure which is analytically specific. As a consequence, laboratories are moving over to measure the substance fraction of the valyl-I-fructosylated haemoglobin β-chains with the unit millimole per mole, and away from the non-specific HbA_{1C} as measured by various non-standardised laboratory procedures.

Uric acid

The production of uric acid, the end product of purine metabolism, is catalysed by xanthine oxidase, an enzyme linked to oxidative stress, endothelial dysfunction and heart failure. The purines, which are used for nucleic acid synthesis, are produced by the breakdown of nucleic acid from ingested meat or synthesised within the body.

Monosodium urate is the form in which uric acid usually exists at the normal pH of body fluids. The term urate is used to represent any salt of uric acid.

Two main factors contribute to elevated serum uric acid levels: an increased rate of formation and reduced excretion. Uric acid is poorly soluble and an elevation in serum concentration can readily result in deposition, as monosodium urate, in tissues or joints. Deposition usually precipitates an acute attack of gouty arthritis. The aim of treatment is to reduce the concentration of uric acid and prevent further attacks of gout. It has been hypothesised that measurement of urate could serve as a marker of cardiovascular risk because the serum uric acid level is an independent predictor of all causes of mortality in patients at high risk of cardiovascular disease, independent of diuretic use.

Liver function tests (LFTs)

Routine LFTs give information mainly about the activity or concentrations of enzymes and compounds in serum rather than quantifying specific hepatic functions and must be interpreted in the context of the patient's characteristic and the pattern of the abnormalities. Results are useful in confirming or excluding a diagnosis of clinically suspected liver disease, and monitoring its course.

Serum albumin levels and prothrombin time (PT) indicate hepatic protein synthesis; bilirubin is a marker of overall liver function.

Transaminase levels indicate hepatocellular injury and death, while alkaline phosphatase levels estimate the amount of impedance of bile flow.

Albumin

Albumin is quantitatively the most important protein synthesised in the liver, with 10–15 g/day being produced in a healthy man. About 60% is located in the interstitial compartment of the ECF, the remainder in the smaller, but relatively impermeable, serum compartment where it is present at a higher concentration. The concentration in the serum is important in maintaining its volume since it accounts for approximately 80% of serum colloid osmotic pressure. A reduction in serum albumin concentration often results in oedema.

Albumin has an important role in binding, among others, calcium, bilirubin and many drugs. A reduction in serum albumin will increase free levels of agents which are normally bound and adverse effects can result if the 'free' entity is not rapidly cleared from the body.

The serum concentration of albumin depends on its rate of synthesis, volume of distribution and rate of catabolism. Synthesis falls in parallel with increasing severity of liver disease or in malnutrition states where there is an inadequate supply of amino acids to maintain albumin production. Synthesis also decreases in response to inflammatory mediators such as interleukin. A low serum albumin concentration will occur when the volume of distribution of albumin increases, as happens, for example, in cirrhosis with ascites, in fluid retention states such as pregnancy or where a shift of albumin from serum to interstitial fluid causes dilutional hypoalbuminaemia after parenteral infusion of excess protein-free fluid. The movement of albumin from serum into interstitial fluid is often associated with increased capillary permeability in postoperative patients or those with septicaemia.

Other causes of hypoalbuminaemia include catabolic states associated with a variety of illnesses and increased loss of albumin, either in urine from damaged kidneys, as occurs in the nephrotic syndrome, or via the skin following burns or a skin disorder such as psoriasis, or from the intestinal wall in a protein-losing enteropathy. The finding of hypoalbuminaemia and no other alteration in liver tests virtually rules out hepatic origin of this abnormality.

Albumin's serum half-life of approximately 20 days precludes its use as an indicator of acute change in liver function but levels are of prognostic value in chronic disease.

An increase in serum albumin is rare and can be iatrogenic, for example, inappropriate infusion of albumin, or the result of dehydration or shock.

A shift of protein is known to occur physiologically when moving from lying down to the upright position. This can account for an increase in the serum albumin level of up to 10 g/L and can contribute to the variation in serum concentration of highly bound drugs which are therapeutically monitored.

Bilirubin

At the end of their life, RBCs are broken down by the reticuloendothelial system, mainly in the spleen. The haemoglobin molecules, which are subsequently liberated, are split into globin and haem. The globin enters the general protein pool, the iron in haem is reutilised, and the remaining tetrapyrrole ring of haem is degraded to bilirubin. Unconjugated bilirubin, which is water insoluble and fat soluble, is transported to the liver tightly bound to albumin. Unconjugated hyperbilirubinaemia in adults is most commonly the result of haemolysis, or Gilbert's syndrome due to genetic defects in UDP-glucronyltransferase. It is actively taken up by hepatocytes, conjugated with glucuronic acid and excreted into bile. The conjugated bilirubin is water soluble and secreted rapidly into the gut where it is broken down by bacteria into urobilinogen, a colourless compound, which is subsequently oxidised in the colon to urobilin, a brown pigment excreted in faeces. Some of the urobilinogen is absorbed and most is subsequently re-excreted in bile (enterohepatic circulation). A small amount is absorbed into the systemic circulation and excreted in urine, where it too may be oxidised to urobilin. The presence of increased conjugated bilirubin is usually a sign of liver disease.

The liver produces 300 mg of bilirubin each day. However, because the mature liver can metabolise and excrete up to 3 g daily, serum bilirubin concentrations are not a sensitive test of liver function. As a screening test they rarely do other than confirm the presence or absence of jaundice. In chronic liver disease, however, changes in bilirubin concentrations over time do convey prognostic information.

An elevation of serum bilirubin concentration above 50 μmol/L (i.e. approximately 2.5 times the normal upper limit) will reveal itself as jaundice, seen best in the skin and sclerae. Elevated bilirubin levels can be caused by increased production of bilirubin (e.g. haemolysis, ineffective erythropoiesis), impaired transport into hepatocytes (e.g. interference with bilirubin uptake by

drugs such as rifampicin or due to hepatitis), decreased excretion (e.g. with drugs such as rifampicin and methyltestosterone, intrahepatic obstruction due to cirrhosis, tumours, etc.) or a combination of the above factors.

The bilirubin in serum is normally unconjugated, bound to protein, not filtered by the glomeruli and does not normally appear in the urine. Bilirubin in the urine (bilirubinuria) is usually the result of an increase in serum concentration of conjugated bilirubin and indicates an underlying pathological disorder.

Enzymes

The enzymes measured in routine LFTs are listed in Table 6.1. Enzyme concentrations in the serum of healthy individuals are normally low. When cells are damaged, increased amounts of enzymes are detected as the intracellular contents are released into the blood.

It is important to remember that the assay of 'serum enzymes' is a measurement of catalytic activity and not actual enzyme concentration and that activity can vary depending on assay conditions. Consequently, the reference range may vary widely between laboratories.

While the measurement of enzymes may be very specific, the enzymes themselves may not be specific to a particular tissue or cell. Many enzymes arise in more than one tissue and an increase in the serum activity of one enzyme can represent damage to any one of the tissues which contain the enzymes. In practice, this problem may be clarified because some tissues contain two or more enzymes in different proportions which are released on damage. For example, alanine and aspartate transaminase both occur in cardiac muscle and liver cells, but their site of origin can often be differentiated, because there is more alanine transaminase in the liver than in the heart. In those situations where it is not possible to look at the relative ratio of enzymes, it is sometimes possible to differentiate the same enzyme from different tissues. Such enzymes have the same catalytic activity but differ in some other measurable property, and are referred to as isoenzymes.

The measured activity of an enzyme will be dependent upon the time it is sampled relative to its time of release from the cell. If a sample is drawn too early after a particular insult to a tissue there may be no detectable increase in enzyme activity. If it is drawn too late, the enzyme may have been cleared from the blood.

Alkaline phosphatase

Alkaline phosphatase is an enzyme which transports metabolites across cell membranes. Alkaline phosphatases are found in the canalicular plasma membrane of hepatocytes, in bone where they reflect bone building or osteoblastic activity, and in the intestinal wall and placenta, kidneys and leucocytes. Each site of origin produces a specific isoenzyme of alkaline phosphatase, which can be electrophoretically separated if concentrations are sufficiently high. Hepatic alkaline phosphatase is present on the surface of bile duct epithelia.

Disorders of the liver which can elevate alkaline phosphatase include intra- or extra-hepatic cholestasis, space-occupying lesions, for example, tumour or abscess, and hepatitis. Drug-induced liver injury, for example, by ACE inhibitors or oestrogens, may present with a cholestatic pattern, that is, a preferential increase in alkaline phosphatase.

Physiological increases in serum alkaline phosphatase activity also occur in pregnancy due to release of the placental isoenzyme and during periods of growth in children and adolescents when the bone isoenzyme is released.

Pathological increases in serum alkaline phosphatase of bone origin may arise in disorders such as osteomalacia and rickets, Paget's disease of bone, bone tumours, renal bone disease, osteomyelitis and healing fractures. Alkaline phosphatase is also raised as part of the acute-phase response, for example, intestinal alkaline phosphatase may be raised in active inflammatory bowel disease. If in doubt, the origin of the enzyme can be indicated by assessment of γ-glutamyl transpeptidase (see next section) or electrophoresis to separate alkaline phosphatase isoenzymes.

Transaminases

The two transaminases of diagnostic use are aspartate transaminase (AST; also known as aspartate aminotransferase) and alanine transaminase (ALT; also known as alanine aminotransferase). These enzymes catalyse the transfer of α-amino groups from aspartate and alanine to the α-keto group of ketoglutaricacid to generate oxalacetic and pyruvic acid. They are found in many body tissues, with the highest concentration in hepatocytes and muscle cells. In the liver, ALT is localised solely in cytoplasm whereas AST is cytosolic and mitrochondrial.

Serum AST levels are increased in a variety of disorders including liver disease, crush injuries, severe tissue hypoxia, myocardial infarction, surgery, trauma, muscle disease and pancreatitis. ALT is elevated to a similar extent in the disorders listed which involve the liver, though to a lesser extent, if at all, in the other disorders. In the context of liver disease, increased transaminase activity indicates deranged integrity of hepatocyte plasma membranes and/or hepatocyte necrosis. They may be raised in all forms of viral and non-viral, acute and chronic liver disease, most markedly in acute viral, drug induced (e.g. paracetamol poisoning), alcohol related and ischaemic liver damage. Non-alcoholic fatty liver disease is now the most common cause of mild alteration of aminotransferase levels in the developed world.

γ-Glutamyl transpeptidase

γ-Glutamyl transpeptidase (Gamma GT; also known as γ-glutamyl transferase) is present in high concentrations in the liver, kidney and pancreas, where it is found within the endoplasmic reticulum of cells. It is a sensitive indicator of hepatobiliary disease but does not differentiate a cholestatic disorder from hepatocellular disease. It can also be elevated in alcoholic liver disease, hepatitis, cirrhosis and non-hepatic disease such as pancreatitis, congestive cardiac failure, chronic obstructive pulmonary disease and renal failure.

Serum levels of γ-glutamyl transpeptidase activity can be raised by enzyme induction by certain drugs such as phenytoin, phenobarbital, rifampicin and oral contraceptives.

Serum γ-glutamyl transpeptidase activity is usually raised in an individual with alcoholic liver disease. However, it can also be raised in heavy drinkers of alcohol who do not have liver damage, due to enzyme induction. Its activity can remain elevated for up to 4 weeks after stopping alcohol intake.

Although it lacks specificity, it has a high sensitivity for liver disease, and is thus useful for identifying the cause of a raised alkaline phosphatase level.

Ammonia

The concentration of free ammonia in the blood is very tightly regulated and is exceeded by two orders of magnitude by its derivative, urea. The normal capacity for urea production far exceeds the rate of free ammonia production by protein catabolism under normal circumstances, such that any increase in free blood ammonia concentration is a reflection of either biochemical or pharmacological impairment of urea cycle function or fairly extensive hepatic damage. Clinical signs of hyperammonaemia occur at concentrations >60 mmol/L and include anorexia, irritability, lethargy, vomiting, somnolence, disorientation, asterixis, cerebral oedema, coma and death; appearance of these findings is generally proportional to free ammonia concentration. Causes of hyperammonaemia include genetic defects in the urea cycle and disorders resulting in significant hepatic dysfunction. Ammonia plays an important role in the increase in brain water which occurs in acute liver failure. Measurement of the blood ammonia concentration in the evaluation of patients with known or suspected hepatic encephalopathy can help in diagnosis and assessing the effect of treatment. Valproic acid can induce hyperammonaemic encephalopathy as one of its adverse neurological effects.

Amylase

The pancreas and salivary glands are the main producers of serum amylase. The serum amylase concentration rises within the first 24 h of an attack of pancreatitis and then declines to normal over the following week. Although a number of abdominal and extra-abdominal conditions including loss of bowel integrity through infarction or perforation, chronic alcoholism, post-operative states and renal failure can result in a high amylase activity, in patients with the clinical picture of severe upper abdominal symptoms the specificity and sensitivity of an amylase level over 1000 IU/L in the diagnosis of pancreatitis is over 90%. There is a lack of prognostic significance of absolute values of amylase as values are directly related to the degree of pancreatic duct obstruction and inversely related to severity of pancreatic disease.

Cardiac markers

Troponins

Cardiac troponin I (cTnI) and cardiac troponin T (cTnT) are regulatory proteins that control the calcium-mediated interaction between actin and myosin in cardiac muscle. They are the preferred biomarker for myocardial necrosis as they have near absolute myocardial tissue specificity as well as high clinical sensitivity. The major international cardiac societies have introduced an international definition and classification for myocardial infarction which depends on the detection of a rise and/or fall (≥20%) of troponin with at least one value above the 99th percentile of the upper reference limit (URL) plus at least one of the following: (i) symptoms of ischaemia, or (ii) ECG evidence or imaging evidence of ischaemia. Sampling of cTn at two time points, usually admission and 12h from worst pain, is usually needed, although if it is entirely clear that there has been a myocardial infarction, particularly in a late presentation, a second sample may not be needed. They contribute significantly to stratification of individuals with acute coronary syndromes, either alone or in combination with admission ECG or a predischarge exercise stress test. The decision as to whether to monitor cTnI or cTnT in a given laboratory is a balance between cost, availability of automated instrumentation and assay performance in which there is not yet standardisation between laboratories. Cardiac troponins offer extremely high tissue specificity and sensitivity but do not discriminate between ischaemic and non-ischaemic mechanisms of myocardial injury, such as myocarditis, cardiac surgery and sepsis. New, more sensitive assays are being developed, although studies will be required to define the clinical significance of minor releases of cTn and its relation to cardiac tissue viability.

Creatine kinase (CK)

CK is an enzyme which is present in relatively high concentrations in heart muscle, skeletal muscle and in brain in addition to being present in smooth muscle and other tissues. Levels are markedly increased following shock and circulatory failure, myocardial infarction and muscular dystrophies. Less marked increases have been reported following muscle injury, surgery, physical exercise, muscle cramp, an epileptic fit, intramuscular injection and hypothyroidism. The most important adverse effects associated with statins are myopathy and an increase in hepatic transaminases, both of which occur infrequently. Statin-associated myopathy represents a broad clinical spectrum of disorders, from mild muscle aches to severe pain and restriction in mobility, with grossly elevated CK levels. In rhabdomyolysis, a potentially life-threatening syndrome resulting from the breakdown of skeletal muscle fibres as a result of ischaemic crush injury, for example, large quantities of CK are measurable in the blood with the level of CK in the blood predicting the developments of acute renal failure. Medications and toxic substances that increase the risk of rhabdomyolysis are shown in Table 6.3.

Table 6.3 Medications and toxic substances that increase the risk of rhabdomyolysis

Direct myotoxicity	Indirect muscle damage
HMG-CoA reductase inhibitors, especially in combination with fibrate-derived lipid-lowering agents such as niacin (nicotinic acid) Ciclosporin Itraconazole Erythromycin Colchicine Zidovudine Corticosteroids	Alcohol Central nervous system depressants Cocaine Amphetamine Ecstasy (MDMA) LSD Neuromuscular blocking agents

HMG-CoA, 3-hydroxy-3-methylglutaryl coenzyme A; LSD, lysergic acid diethylamide; MDMA, methylene dioxymethamphetamine.

CK has two protein subunits, M and B, which combine to form three isoenzymes, BB, MM and MB. BB is found in high concentrations in the brain, thyroid and some smooth muscle tissue. Little of this enzyme is present in the serum, even following damage to the brain. The enzyme found in serum of normal subjects is the MM isoenzyme which originates from skeletal muscle.

Cardiac tissue contains more of the MB isoenzyme than skeletal muscle. Following a myocardial infarction there is a characteristic increase in serum CK activity. Although measurement of activity of the MB isoenzyme was used in the past to detect myocardial damage, cardiac troponin measurement is now the preferred biomarker.

Lactate dehydrogenase (LD)

Lactate dehydrogenase has five isoenzymes (LD1–LD5). Total LD activity is rarely measured because of the lack of tissue specificity. Levels of activity are elevated following damage to the liver, skeletal muscle and kidneys, in both megaloblastic and immune haemolytic anaemias, and in intravascular haemolysis such as occurs in thrombotic thrombocytopenic purpura and paroxysmal nocturnal haemoglobinuria. In lymphoma, a high LD activity indicates a poor prognosis. Elevation of LD1 and LD2 occurs after myocardial infarction, renal infarction or megaloblastic anaemia; LD2 and LD3 are elevated in acute leukaemia; LD3 is often elevated in some malignancies; and LD5 is elevated after damage to liver or skeletal muscle.

Tumour markers

Tumour markers are defined as a qualitative or quantitative alteration or deviation from normal of a molecule, substance or process that can be detected by some type of assay above and beyond routine clinical and pathological evaluation. They may be detected within malignant cells, surrounding stroma or metastases, or as soluble products in blood, secretions or excretions. In order to be useful clinically, the precise use of the marker in altering clinical management should have been defined by data based on a reliable assay, and a validated clinical outcome trial.

Whilst only a few markers contribute to the diagnosis of cancer, serial measurements can be useful in assessing the presence of residual disease and response to treatment. A detailed discussion of each marker, which include prostatic-specific antigen, human chorionic gonadotropin, α-fetoprotein, carcinoembryonic antigen, cancer antigen (CA125 and CA19) is outside the scope of this chapter. Updated National Academy of Clinical Biochemistry Laboratory Medicine Practice Guidelines for the use of tumour markers in the clinic were published in 2008 to encourage their optimal use. Use in predicting response to therapy and, therefore, targeting therapy is increasingly used: for breast cancer, oestrogen and progesterone receptors are mandatory for predicting response to hormone therapy, and human epidermal growth factor receptor-2 (HER2) measurement is mandatory for predicting response to trastuzumab.

Prostatic specific antigen (PSA) is a serine protease produced by normal and malignant prostatic epithelium and secreted into seminal fluid. Only minor amounts leak into the circulation from the normal prostate, but the release is increased in prostatic disease. It is not recommended for prostate cancer screening but is useful for the detection of recurrence and response to therapy. Free PSA measurement can improve distinguishing of malignant from benign prostatic disease when total PSA is <10 μcg/L, although results for free PSA differ between commercially available assay methods and require harmonisation.

Immunoglobulins

Immunoglobulins are antibodies which are produced by B lymphocytes. They are detected on elctrophoresis as bands in three regions: α, β and γ, with most occurring in the γ region. Hypergammaglobulinaemia may result from stimulation of B cells and produces an increased staining of bands in the γ region on electrophoresis. This occurs in infections, chronic liver disease and autoimmune disease.

In some diseases such as chronic lymphatic leukaemia, lymphoma and multiple myeloma, a discrete, densely staining band (paraprotein) can be seen in the γ region. In multiple myeloma, abnormal fragments of immunoglobulins are produced (Bence-Jones protein) which clear the glomerulus and are found in the urine.

Haematology data

The haematology profile is an important part of the investigation of many patients and not just those with primary haematological disease.

Typical measurements reported in a haematology screen, with their normal values, are shown in Table 6.4, whilst a list of the common descriptive terms used in haematology is presented in Table 6.5.

Table 6.4 Haematology data: typical normal adult reference values

Haemoglobin	11.5–16.5 g/dL
Red blood cell (RBC) count	$3.8–4.8 \times 10^{12}$/L
Reticulocyte count	$50–100 \times 10^{9}$/L
Packed cell volume (PCV)	0.36–0.46 L/L
Mean cell volume (MCV)	83–101 fL
Mean cell haemoglobin (MCH)	27–34 pg
Mean cell haemoglobin concentration (MCHC)	31.5–34.5 g/dL
White cell count (WBC)	$4.0–11.0 \times 10^{9}$/L

Differential white cell count:
  Neutrophils (30–75%)
  Lymphocytes (5–15%)
  Monocytes (2–10%)
  Basophils (<1%)
  Eosinophils (1–6%)
	
	$2.0–7.0 \times 10^{9}$/L
	$1.5–4.0 \times 10^{9}$/L
	$0.2–0.8 \times 10^{9}$/L
	$<0.1 \times 10^{9}$/L
	$0.04–0.4 \times 10^{9}$/L

Platelets	$150–450 \times 10^{9}$/L
Erythrocyte sedimentation rate (ESR)	1–35 mm/h
D-dimers	0–230 ng/mL
Ferritin	15–300 μcg/L
Total iron binding capacity (TIBC)	47–70 μmol/L
Serum B_{12}	170–700 ng/L
Red cell folate	160–600 μcg/l
Iron	11–29 μmol/L
Transferrin	1.7–3.4 g/L

RBC count

RBCs are produced in the bone marrow by the process of erythropoiesis. One of the major stimulants of this process is erythropoietin, produced mainly in the kidney. Immature erythroblasts develop into mature erythrocytes which are then released into the circulation:

erythroblasts

↓

normoblasts (nucleated)

↓

reticulocytes (non-nucleated)

↓

erythrocytes

Normally, only reticulocytes and non-nucleated mature erythrocytes are seen in the peripheral blood.

Table 6.5 Descriptive terms in common use in haematology

Anisocytosis	Abnormal variation in cell size (usually refers to RBCs), for example, red cells in iron deficiency anaemia
Agranulocytosis	Lack of granulocytes (principally neutrophils)
Aplastic	Depression of synthesis of all cell types in bone marrow (as in aplastic anaemia)
Basophilia	Increased number of basophils
Hypochromic	MCHC low, red cells appear pale microscopically
Leucocytosis	Increased white cell count
Leucopenia	Reduced white cell count
Macrocytic	Large cells
Microcytic	Small cells
Neutropenia	Reduced neutrophil count
Neutrophilia	Increased neutrophil count
Normochromic	MCHC normal; red cells appear normally pigmented
Pancytopenia	Decreased number of all cell types: it is synonymous with aplastic anaemia
Poikilocytosis	Abnormal variation in cell shape, for example, some red cells appear pear shaped in macrocytic anaemias
Thrombocytopenia	Lack of platelets

The lifespan of a mature red cell is usually about 120 days. If this is shortened, as for instance in haemolysis, the circulating mass of red cells is reduced and with it the supply of oxygen to tissues is decreased. In these circumstances, red cell production is enhanced in healthy bone marrow by an increased output of erythropoietin by the kidneys. Under normal circumstances red cells are destroyed by lodging in the spleen due to decreasing flexibility of the cells. They are removed by the reticuloendothelial system.

A high RBC (erythrocytosis or polycythaemia) indicates increased production by the bone marrow and may occur as a physiological response to hypoxia, as in chronic airways disease, or as a malignant condition of red cells such as in polycythaemia rubra vera.

Reticulocytes

Reticulocytes are the earliest non-nucleated red cells. They owe their name to the fine net-like appearance of their cytoplasm which can be seen, after appropriate staining, under the microscope and contains fine threads of ribonucleic acid (RNA) in a reticular network. Reticulocytes normally represent between 0.5% and 1.0% of the total RBC and do not feature significantly in a normal blood profile. However, increased production (reticulocytosis) can be detected in times of rapid red cell regeneration as occurs in response to haemorrhage or haemolysis. At such times the reticulocyte count may reach 40% of the RBC. The reticulocyte count may be useful in assessing the response of the marrow to iron, folate or vitamin B_{12} therapy. The count peaks at about 7–10 days after starting such therapy and then subsides.

Mean cell volume (MCV)

The MCV is the average volume of a single red cell. It is measured in femtolitres (10^{-15} L). Terms such as 'microcytic' and 'macrocytic' are descriptive of a low and high MCV, respectively. They are useful in the process of identification of various types of anaemias such as caused by iron deficiency (microcytic) or vitamin B_{12} or folic acid deficiency (megaloblastic or macrocytic).

Packed cell volume (PCV)

The PCV or haematocrit is the ratio of the volume occupied by red cells to the total volume of blood. It can be measured by centrifugation of a capillary tube of blood and then expressing the volume of red cells packed in the bottom as a percentage of the total volume. It is reported as a fraction of unity or as a percentage (e.g. 0.45% or 45%). The PCV is calculated nowadays as the product of the MCV and RBC. The PCV often reflects the RBC and will, therefore, be decreased in any sort of anaemia. It will be raised in polycythaemia. It may, however, be altered irrespective of the RBC, when the size of the red cell is abnormal, as in macrocytosis and microcytosis.

Mean cell haemoglobin (MCH)

The MCH is the average weight of haemoglobin contained in a red cell. It is measured in picograms (10^{-12} g) and is calculated from the relationship:

$$MCH = \frac{Haemoglobin}{RBC}$$

The MCH is dependent on the size of the red cells as well as the concentration of haemoglobin in the cells. Thus, it is usually low in iron-deficiency anaemia when there is microcytosis and there is less haemoglobin in each cell, but it may be raised in macrocytic anaemia.

Mean cell haemoglobin concentration (MCHC)

The MCHC is a measure of the average concentration of haemoglobin in 100 mL of red cells. It is usually expressed as grams per litre but may be reported as a percentage. The MCHC will be reported as low in conditions of reduced haemoglobin synthesis, such as in iron-deficiency anaemia. In contrast, in macrocytic anaemias the MCHC may be normal or only slightly reduced because the large red cells may contain more haemoglobin, thus giving a concentration approximating that of normal cells. The MCHC can be raised in severe prolonged dehydration. If the MCHC is low, the descriptive term 'hypochromic' may be used (e.g. a hypochromic anaemia) whereas the term 'normochromic' describes a normal MCHC.

Haemoglobin

The haemoglobin concentration in men is normally greater than in women, reflecting in part the higher RBC in men. Lower concentrations in women are due, at least in part, to menstrual loss.

Haemoglobin is most commonly measured to detect anaemia. In some relatively rare genetic diseases, the haemoglobinopathies, alterations in the structure of the haemoglobin molecule can be detected by electrophoresis. Abnormal haemoglobins which can be detected in this manner include HbS (sickle haemoglobin in sickle cell disease) and HbA_2 found in β-thalassaemia carriers.

Platelets (thrombocytes)

Platelets are formed in the bone marrow. A marked reduction in platelet number (thrombocytopenia) may reflect either a depressed synthesis in the marrow or destruction of formed platelets.

Platelets are normally present in the circulation for 8–12 days. This is useful information when evaluating a possible drug-induced thrombocytopenia, since recovery should be fairly swift when the offending agent is withdrawn.

A small fall in the platelet count may be seen in pregnancy and following viral infections. Severe thrombocytopenia may result in spontaneous bleeding. A reduced platelet count is also found in disseminated intravascular coagulation, which manifests clinically as severe haemorrhages, particularly in the skin and results in rapid consumption of clotting factors and platelets.

An increased platelet count (thrombocytosis) occurs in malignancy, inflammatory disease and in response to blood loss.

White blood cell (WBC) count

White cells (leucocytes) are of two types: the granulocytes and the agranular cells. They are made up of various types of cells (Fig. 6.4) with different functions and it is logical to consider them separately. A haematology profile often reports a total white cell count and a differential count, the latter separating the composition of white cells into the various types.

Neutrophils

Neutrophils or polymorphonucleocytes (PMNs) are the most abundant type of white cell. They have a phagocytic function, with many enzymes contained in the lysosomal granules. They are formed in the bone marrow from the stem cells which form myoblasts and these develop through a number of

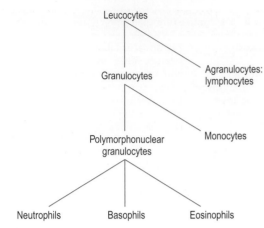

Fig. 6.4   Types of white cells.

stages into the neutrophil with a multiple-segmented nucleus. Neutrophils constitute approximately 40–70% of circulating white cells in normal healthy blood. Their lifespan is 10–20 days. The neutrophil count increases in the presence of infection, tissue damage (e.g. infarction) and inflammation (e.g. rheumatoid arthritis, acute gout). Neutropenia, also described as agranulocytosis in its severest forms, is associated with malignancy and drug toxicity, but may also occur in viral infections such as influenza, infectious mononucleosis and hepatitis.

Basophils

Basophils normally constitute a small proportion of the white cell count. Their function is poorly understood but basophilia occurs in various malignant and premalignant disorders such as leukaemia and myelofibrosis.

Eosinophils

Eosinophils constitute normally less than 6% of white cells. Their function appears to be concerned with inactivation of mediators released from mast cells, and eosinophilia is, therefore, apparent in many allergic conditions such as asthma, hay fever and drug sensitivity reactions as well as some malignant diseases.

Lymphocytes

Lymphocytes are the second most abundant white cells in the circulating blood, but the majority of them are found in the spleen and other lymphatic tissue. They are formed in the bone marrow. An increase in lymphocyte numbers occurs particularly in viral infections such as rubella, mumps, infectious hepatitis and infectious mononucleosis.

Monocytes

Monocytes are macrophages. Their numbers increase in some infections such as typhoid, subacute bacterial endocarditis, infectious mononucleosis and tuberculosis.

Other blood tests

Erythrocyte sedimentation rate (ESR)

The ESR is a measure of the settling rate of red cells in a sample of anticoagulated blood, over a period of 1 h, in a cylindrical tube.

In youth, the normal value is less than 10 mmol/h, but normal values do rise with age. The Westergren method, performed under standardised conditions, is commonly used in haematology laboratories. The ESR is strongly correlated with the ability of red cells to aggregate into orderly stacks or rouleaux. In disease, the most common cause of a high ESR is an increased protein level in the blood, such as the increase in acute-phase proteins seen in inflammatory disease. Proteins are thought to affect the repellent surface charges on red cells and cause them to aggregate into rouleaux and hence the sedimentation rate increases. Although some conditions may cause a low ESR, the test is principally used to monitor inflammatory disease. The ESR may be raised in the active phase of rheumatoid arthritis, inflammatory bowel disease, malignant disease and infection. The ESR is non-specific and, therefore, of little diagnostic value, but serial tests can be helpful in following the progress of disease, and its response to treatment.

C-reactive protein (CRP)

CRP, named for its capacity to precipitate the somatic C-polysaccharide of streptococcus pneumoniae, was the first acute-phase protein to be described. This non-specific acute-phase response occurs in animals in response to tissue damage, infection, inflammation and malignancy. Production of CRP is rapidly and sensitively upregulated, in hepatocytes, under the control of cytokine (IL-6) originating at the site of pathology. It recognises altered self and foreign molecules, as a result of which it activates complement and generates pro-inflammatory cytokines and activation of the adaptive immune system.

Serum concentrations rise by about 6 h, peaking around 48 h. The serum half-life is constant at about 19 h, so serum level is determined by synthesis rate, which therefore reflects the intensity of the pathological process stimulating this, and falls rapidly when this ceases. CRP values are not diagnostic, however, but can only be interpreted in knowledge of all other clinical and pathological results. In most diseases, the circulating value of CRP reflects ongoing inflammation or tissue damage more accurately than do other acute-phase parameters such as serum viscosity or the ESR. Drugs reduce CRP values by affecting the underlying pathology providing the acute-phase stimulus.

Coagulation

Coagulation is the process by which a platelet and fibrin plug is formed to seal a site of injury or rupture in a blood vessel. The current model of a 'coagulation network' differs from the previous popular cascade scheme. It proposes that blood coagulation is localised on the surfaces of activated cells in three overlapping steps: initiation, amplification and propagation. Coagulation is initiated when a tissue factor (TF) bearing cell is exposed to blood flow, following either damage of endothelium such as by perforation of a vessel wall or activation by chemicals, cytokines or the inflammatory process. The formation of a clot then involves a complex interaction between platelets and factor VIII bound to von Willebrand factor which leave the vascular space and adhere to collagen and other matrix components at the site of injury. The coagulation process is amplified when enough thrombin is generated on or near the TF bearing cells to trigger full activation of platelets and coagulation co-factors on the platelet surface. It ends with the generation of sufficient thrombin, to clot fibrinogen. To prevent inappropriate propagation of the thrombus, the process is controlled by naturally occurring anticoagulants and the fibrinolytic system, the final effector of which is plasmin which cleaves fibrin into soluble degradation products. The interaction between TF and factor VII is the most important in the initiation of coagulation and many of the coagulation reactions occur on the surface of cells (particularly platelets). The cellular model of normal haemostasis is shown in Fig. 6.5. Despite the complexity of this model, the basic coagulation tests can still be interpreted in relation to the 'intrinsic', 'extrinsic', and 'final common pathway' components of the traditional and previously held cascade (Fig. 6.6). The extrinsic pathway can be considered to consist of the factor VIIa/TF complex working with the factor Xa/Va complex and the intrinsic pathway to consist of factor XIa working with the complexes of factors VIIIa/IXa and factors Xa/Va. The extrinsic pathway operates on the TF bearing cell to initiate and amplify coagulation with the intrinsic pathway operating on the activated platelet surface to produce the burst of thrombin to form and stabilise the fibrin clot.

Monitoring anticoagulant therapy

The blood tests for the adequacy of the extrinsic pathway, prothombin time (PT) and the intrinsic pathway, activated partial thromboplastin time (aPTT) do not reflect the complexity of haemostasis in vivo, or the risk of bleeding. This requires interpretation of the result in the clinical context of surgical or accidental trauma or medical illness.

One stage PT

Measuring the PT is the most commonly used method for monitoring oral anticoagulation therapy. The PT is responsive to depression of three of the four vitamin K dependent factors (factors II, VII and X). The PT is measured by adding calcium and thromboplastin (a phospholipid-protein extract of tissue that promotes the activation of factor X by factor VIII) to citrated plasma.

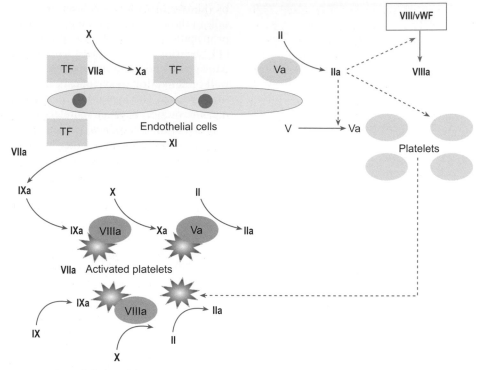

Fig. 6.5 Normal haemostasis; the cellular model.

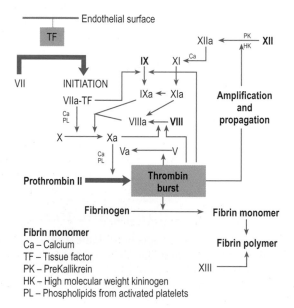

Fibrin monomer
Ca – Calcium
TF – Tissue factor
PK – PreKallikrein
HK – High molecular weight kininogen
PL – Phospholipids from activated platelets

Fig. 6.6 Coagulation network.

International Normalised Ratio (INR)

The results of the test are commonly expressed as a ratio of the PT time of the patient compared with that of the normal control. This is known as the INR, a system used to standardise reporting worldwide.

$$INR = \left\{ \frac{\text{Patient's PT}}{\text{Control PT}} \right\}^{ISI}.$$

The ISI is the international sensitivity index and represents the responsiveness of a given thromboplastin to the reduction of vitamin K dependent clotting factors and is allocated to commercial preparations of thromboplastin to standardise them. More responsive thromboplastins have lower ISI values.

The target value varies according to the indication for the anticoagulant, but for most, including for thrombo-embolic prophylaxis in atrial fibrillation, is 2.5. For some indications including recurrent deep vein thrombosis and pulmonary embolism whilst on warfarin, the target is higher at 3.5.

The most common use of the PT and INR is to monitor oral anticoagulant therapy, but the PT is also useful in assessing liver function because of its dependence on the activity of clotting factors I, II, V, VII and X which are produced in the liver. It may be prolonged also by deficiency in vitamin K, and consumptive coagulopathy. Obstructive jaundice may decrease the absorption of vitamin K and thereby increase PT. PT will respond to parenteral administration of vitamin K, which is ineffective when jaundice is caused by decreased functioning liver mass.

Activated partial thromboplastin time (APTT)

The APTT is the most common method for monitoring unfractionated heparin therapy.

A thromboplastic reagent is added to an activator such as activated silicone or kaolin. If the activator is kaolin, the test may be referred to as the PTTK (partial thromboplastin time kaolin) or the KCCT (kaolin–cephalin clotting time). Cephalin is a brain extract supplying the thromboplastin.

The mixture of thromboplastin and activator is mixed with citrated plasma to which calcium is added, and the time for the mixture to clot is recorded. The desirable APTT for optimal heparin therapy is between 1.5 and 2.5 times the normal control.

Low molecular weight heparins are effective and safe for the prevention and treatment of venous thromboembolism, and because they provide more predictable anticoagulant activity than unfractionated heparin it is usually not necessary to monitor the APTT during treatment. Laboratory monitoring using an anti-factor Xa assay may be of value in certain clinical settings, including patients with renal insufficiency, and use of fractionated heparin for prolonged periods in pregnancy or in newborns and children.

D-dimers

D-dimers are degradation products of fibrin clots, formed by the sequential action of three enzymes, thrombin, factor VIIIa and plasmin which degrades cross-linked fibrin to release fibrin degradation products and expose the D-dimer antigen. D-dimer assays measure an epitope on fibrin degradation products using monoclonal antibodies. As each has its own unique specificity, there is no standard unit of measurement or performance and clinicians need to be aware of that of their institution. Levels of D-dimers in the blood are raised in conditions associated with coagulation and are used to detect venous thromboembolism, although they are influenced by the presence of co-morbid conditions such as cancer, surgery and infectious diseases. D-dimer measurement has been most comprehensively validated in the exclusion of venous thromboembolism in certain patient populations and in the diagnosis and monitoring of coagulation activation in disseminated intravascular coagulation. More recently, assays are being used in the prediction of the risk of VTE recurrence. Diagnosis of DVT or PE should include a clinical probability assessment as well as D-dimer measurements. In patients with a low clinical probability of pulmonary embolism, a negative quantitative D-dimer test result effectively excludes PE. In suspected DVTs, D-dimer measurements combined with a clinical prediction score and compression ultrasonography study have a high predictive value.

Xanthochromia

Xanthochromia is a yellow discolouration of cerebrospinal fluid caused by haemoglobin catabolism. It is thought to arise within several hours of subarachnoid haemorrhage (SAH) and can help to distinguish the elevated red cell count observed after traumatic lumbar puncture from that observed following SAH, particularly if few red cells are present. Spectrophotometry to detect the presence of both oxyhaemoglobin and bilirubin, which both contribute to xanthochromia following SAH, is used, although some hospitals rely on visual inspection.

Iron, transferrin and iron binding

Iron is necessary for the functioning of all mammalian cells, but is particularly important in cells producing haemoglobin and myoglobin. Iron circulating in the serum is bound to transferrin. It leaves the serum pool and enters the bone marrow where it becomes incorporated into haemoglobin in developing red cells. Serum iron levels are extremely labile and fluctuate throughout the day and, therefore, provide little useful information about iron status.

Transferrin, a simple polypeptide chain with two iron binding sites, is the plasma iron binding protein which facilitates its delivery to cells bearing transferrin receptors. Measurement of total iron binding capacity (TIBC), from which the percentage of transferrin saturation with iron may be calculated, gives more information. Saturation of 16% or lower is usually taken to indicate an iron deficiency, as is a raised TIBC of greater than 70 μmol/L.

Ferritin is an iron storage protein found in cell cytosol. It acts as a depot, accepting excess iron and allowing for mobilisation of iron when needed. Serum ferritin measurement is the test of choice in patients suspected of having iron deficiency anaemia.

In normal individuals, the serum ferritin concentration is directly related to the available storage iron in the body. The serum ferritin level falls below the normal range in iron deficiency anaemia, and its measurement can provide a useful monitor for repletion of iron stores after iron therapy. Ferritin is an acute-phase protein and levels may be normal or high in the anaemia of chronic disease, such as occurs in rheumatoid arthritis or chronic renal disease.

Iron balance is regulated by hepcidin, a circulating peptide hormone, which aims to provide iron as needed, whilst avoiding excess iron promoting formation of toxic oxygen radicals.

Iron overload causes high concentrations of serum ferritin, as can liver disease and some forms of cancer. Genetic iron overload results from mutations in molecules which regulate hepcidin production or activity.

Vitamin B$_{12}$ and folate

In the haematology literature, B$_{12}$ refers not only to cyanocobalamin but also to several other cobalamins with identical nutritional properties. Folic acid, which can designate a specific compound, pteroylglutamic acid, is also more commonly used as a general term for the folates. Deficiency of cobalamin can result both in anaemia, usually macrocytic, and neurological disease, including neuropathies, dementia and psychosis. Folate deficiency produces anaemia, macrocytosis, depression, dementia and neural tube defects.

Liver disease tends to increase B$_{12}$ levels, and they may be reduced in folate deficient patients: malabsorption of B$_{12}$ may result from long-term ingestion of antacids such as proton-pump inhibitors or H$_2$-receptor antagonists or biguanides (metformin). Serum folate levels tend to increase in B$_{12}$ deficiency, and alcohol can reduce levels. RBC folate is a better measure of folate tissue stores.

Current assays analyse total B$_{12}$ concentration, only a small percentage of which is metabolically active. Varying test sensitivities and specificities result from the lack of a precise 'gold standard' for the diagnosis of cobalamin deficiency. In the future, new assays for the active component which is carried on holotranscobalamin may be of greater relevance if their clinical usefulness can be established.

Case studies

Case 6.1

Mr F is a 70-year-old man who presents with diffuse pains in his arms and legs. He is Asian, from Pakistan, and has been in England for 50 years.
He has the following biochemical test results:

Alkaline phosphatase	436 U/L
Total calcium	2.27 mmol/L
Ionised calcium	1.10 mmol/L
Phosphate	0.97 mmol/L
Vitamin D	6 nmol/L
Parathyroid hormone	434 ng/L
Urea	4.6 mmol/L
Creatinine	63 µmol/L

Questions

1. With respect to Mr F's blood results, what is the diagnosis?
2. How should he be treated?
3. How should he be monitored?

Answers

1. The diagnosis is osteomalacia due to vitamin D deficiency.
2. Vitamin D deficiency is caused by dietary deficiency of vitamin D and deficient endogenous production due to poor sunlight exposure. A deficit in activation can result from liver or kidney disease. People at high or low latitude, especially housebound, and people with dark coloured skin are at particular risk.
   Vitamin D_2 (cholecalciferol) or vitamin D_3 (ergocalciferol) is given orally in doses of 2000–4000 IU (0.05–0.1 mg) daily for 6–12 weeks, followed by daily supplements of 200–400 IU. The dose needed to achieve levels in the sufficient range sometimes requires daily doses over 800 IU. Where osteomalacia is due to intestinal malabsorption, higher doses of vitamin D and large doses of calcium may be required. In some instances, oral vitamin D is ineffective and the parenteral (intramuscular) route is required. In renal impairment, 1α hydroxylated vitamin D is usually prescribed.
3. Serum calcium should be monitored frequently during the first 1–2 months of therapy and less frequently once a stable dose has been established which has ensured return to normal of calcium, alkaline phosphatase and parathyroid hormone levels.

Case 6.2

A 70-year-old man on a hospital medical ward has a fast pulse rate and falling blood pressure. His recent drug history is warfarin as thrombo-embolic prophylaxis for chronic atrial fibrillation and erythromycin for a recent chest infection. He has vomited a moderate quantity of blood.

Haematology results:	Hb 8.8 g/dL
	RBC 4.7 × 10¹²/L
Platelets	570 × 10⁹/L
INR	6.0

MCV, MCH and the rest of the blood profile are normal

Clinical biochemistry:	Urea 11.6 mmol/L

Creatinine is normal and sodium and potassium concentrations are normal.

Questions

1. What is the cause of this patient's low haemoglobin?
2. What is the likely cause of his raised urea level?
3. What might have contributed to his over-anticoagulation as evidenced by his INR?

Answers

1. The cause of his low haemoglobin is a gastro-intestinal bleed. The picture is one of blood loss, manifested by a loss of red cells and haemoglobin. The red cells are of normal size and colour. As haemoglobin is normal immediately after a bleed, this man's bleed must have begun sufficiently long ago for haemodilution, through ingestion of fluid, to have occurred.
2. A raised urea in the presence of a normal creatinine may signify dehydration or gastro-intestinal bleeding. In this case, given the blood picture, the latter is more likely. Blood in the gastro-intestinal tract is a source of protein which will be absorbed into the hepatic portal system and converted to urea in the liver.
3. Erythromycin inhibits the cytochrome P450 system, particularly the CYP3A4 isoenzyme. CYP1A2 and CYP3A4 are the main enzymes for the inactivation of (R)-warfarin. Erythromycin, therefore, potentiates warfarin's action. The patient has been ill and in hospital and, therefore, his recent intake of vitamin K containing foods, for example, green leafy vegetables may well have been lower than is usual for him. Antibiotics can reduce synthesis of vitamin K by gut bacteria but this has little, if any, effect upon anticoagulation, and interactions with warfarin previously attributed to this mechanism have since been attributed to other modes of interaction.

Case 6.3

An 80-year-old patient with a history of Type II diabetes mellitus is admitted to hospital after an episode of vomiting and diarrhoea, followed by increasing confusion and drowsiness. His medication includes bendroflumethiazide and gliclazide. On examination he has a reduced level of consciousness, is dehydrated, and has a low blood pressure.
Biochemistry results show:

Sodium	158 mmol/L
Potassium	4.6 mmol/L
Urea	44 mmol/L
Creatinine	250 µmol/L
Random blood glucose	38 mmol/L

Arterial blood gases on air:

pH	7.39
pCO_2	5.0 kPa
Actual bicarbonate	24 mmol/L
pO_2	12.7 kPa

Questions

1. What is the diagnosis?
2. Why is the sodium raised?
3. What do his blood gases indicate?

Answers

1. The patient has hyperglycaemic hyperosmolar non-ketotic coma, evidenced by his clinical signs, raised blood glucose, sodium, urea and creatinine.

2. This is evidence of water depletion. This patient is dehydrated because of vomiting and diarrhoea, bendroflumethiazide and the osmotic diuresis caused by hyperglycaemia.
3. Normal serum pH and bicarbonate concentration show that he does not have metabolic ketoacidosis, the condition which only occurs in patients with Type I diabetes and which may be precipitated by infection.

Case 6.4

An 83-year-old man presents with a few weeks history of tiredness, unsteadiness and an abnormal sensation in both hands and feet. On examination he is ataxic with poor co-ordination due to absent joint position and vibration sense. Clinical diagnosis is of sensory ataxia due to dorsal column pathology. His drug treatment includes long-term metformin for Type 2 diabetes mellitus and lansoprazole.
Haematology results show:

Haemoglobin	8.9 g/dL
MCV	110 fL
B_{12}	128 ng/L
Red cell folate	300 μcg/L

Questions

1. What is the likely cause of this patient's symptoms and signs?
2. How should his neurological features be investigated?
3. What term describes this type of anaemia?
4. What drug treatment should he receive?

Answers

1. Subacute combined degeneration of the spinal cord and anaemia due to vitamin B_{12} deficiency.
2. Magnetic Resonance Imaging (MRI) of the spine. This is likely to show signal abnormality in the posterior columns of the spinal cord.
3. Macrocytic anaemia.
4. Parenteral administration, usually by intramuscular injection of vitamin B_{12}. In the UK, several loading doses are given followed by maintenance injections (e.g. 1000 μcg every 3 months) for the patient's lifetime. Treatment with pharmacological doses of oral cyanocobalamin is occasionally given, for example, if the patient has needle phobia or is allergic to the IM B_{12} preparation.

Further reading

Hoffbrand A.V., Moss P.A.H., Pettit, J.E. (Eds.), 2006. Essential Haematology, fifth ed. Blackwell, Oxford.

Gaw A. (Ed), 2008. Clinical Biochemistry: An Illustrated Colour Text, fourth ed. Churchill Livingstone, London.

7 Parenteral nutrition

S.J. Harwood and A.G. Cosslett

Key points

- Parenteral nutrition is indicated in people who are malnourished or at risk of malnutrition due to a non-functional, inaccessible or perforated gastro-intestinal tract or who have inadequate or unsafe enteral nutritional intake.

- Combinations of oral diet, enteral feeding and parenteral nutrition, either peripherally or centrally, may be appropriate.

- Parenteral nutrition regimens should be tailored to the nutritional needs of the patient and should contain a balance of seven essential components: water, L-amino acids, glucose, lipid with essential fatty acids, vitamins, trace elements and electrolytes.

- Advances in technology alongside expertise in pharmaceutical stability often permit the required nutrients to be administered from a single container. Increasingly, standard formulations are used, including licensed preparations.

- Parenteral nutrition must be compounded under validated aseptic conditions by trained specialists.

- Prescriptions are guided by baseline nutritional assessment, calculation of requirements using a range of algorithms, knowledge of the patient's disease status and ongoing monitoring.

- The incidence of complications with parenteral nutrition is reducing; knowledge of management is improving.

Introduction

Malnutrition

Malnutrition can be described as a deficiency, excess, or imbalance of energy, protein, and other nutrients that causes measurable adverse effects on body tissue, size, shape, composition, function and clinical outcome.

In UK hospitals, most malnutrition appears to be a general undernutrition of all nutrients (protein, energy and micronutrients) rather than marasmus (insufficient energy provision) or kwashiorkor (insufficient protein provision). Alternatively, there may be a specific deficiency, such as thiamine in severe hepatic disease.

Multiple causes may contribute to malnutrition. They may include inadequate or unbalanced food intake, increased demand due to clinical disease status, defects in food digestion or absorption, or a compromise in nutritional metabolic pathways. Onset may be acute or insidious.

Even mild malnutrition can result in problems with normal body form and function with adverse effects on clinical, physical and psychosocial status. Symptoms may include impaired immune response, reduced skeletal muscle strength and fatigue, reduced respiratory muscle strength, impaired thermoregulation, impaired skin barrier and wound healing. In turn, these predispose the patient to a wide range of problems including infection, delayed clinical recovery, increased clinical complications, inactivity, psychological decline and reduced quality of life. As symptoms may be non-specific, the underlying malnutrition may be left undiagnosed. Early nutrition intervention is associated with reduced average length of hospital stay and linked cost savings.

Nutrition screening

Routine screening is recommended by the Malnutrition Advisory Group of the British Association of Parenteral and Enteral Nutrition (BAPEN). This group has worked to promote awareness of the clinical significance of malnutrition and has produced guidelines to monitor and manage malnutrition. A range of screening criteria and tools have been developed and refined to assess nutritional status. Examples include the relatively simple and reproducible body mass index tool with consideration of other key factors (Table 7.1), and the BAPEN 'MUST' tool (Malnutrition Universal Screening Tool; BAPEN, 2003). Body weight should not be used in isolation; significant weight fluctuations may reflect fluid disturbances, and muscle wasting may be due to immobility rather than undernutrition. More complex anthropometry measurements are sometimes indicated to track changes.

Incidence of undernutrition

The incidence of undernutrition in hospitalised patients is not accurately known, although it is estimated as being between 20% and 40%.

Indications for parenteral nutrition (PN)

PN is a nutritionally balanced aseptically prepared or sterile physicochemically stable solution or emulsion for intravenous administration. It is indicated whenever the gastro-intestinal tract is inaccessible, perforated or non-functional or when enteral nutrition is inadequate or unsafe. PN should be considered if the enteral route is not likely to be possible for more

Table 7.1	Body mass index as a screening tool
BMI (kg/m²)	BMI category
<18.5	Underweight
18.5–25	Ideal BMI
25–29.9	Overweight
>30	Obese
Body mass index (BMI) = weight (kg)/height (m)²	

than 5 days. PN may fulfill the total nutritional requirements or may be supplemental to an enteral feed or diet.

The simplest way to correct or prevent undernutrition is through conventional balanced food; however, this is not always possible. Nutritional support may then require oral supplements or enteral tube feeding. Assuming the gut is functioning normally, the patient will be able to digest and absorb their required nutrients. These include water, protein, carbohydrate, fat, vitamins, minerals and electrolytes; however, if the gut is not accessible or functioning adequately to meet the patient's needs, or gut rest is indicated, then PN may be used. While the enteral route is the first choice, this may still fail to provide sufficient nutrient intake in a number of patients. Complications and limitations of enteral nutrition need to be recognised.

A decision pathway can be followed to guide initial and ongoing nutritional support. While many are published, a locally tailored and regularly updated pathway is favoured. A useful starting point may be found at Fig. 7.1.

Close monitoring should ensure the patient's needs are met; a combination of nutrition routes is sometimes the best course. Where possible, patients receiving PN should also receive enteral intake, even minor gut stimulation has been linked with a reduction in the incidence of bacterial translocation through maintaining gut integrity and preventing overgrowth and cholestatic complications. PN should not be stopped abruptly but should be gradually reduced in line with the increasing enteral diet.

Nutrition support teams

A report published by the Kings Fund Report (1992) highlighted the issue of malnutrition both in the hospital and home setting. The findings led to the development of the British Association of Enteral and Parenteral Nutrition (BAPEN) and nutrition support teams throughout the UK. These multidisciplinary nutrition support teams comprise a doctor, nurse, pharmacist and dietitian. They function in a variety of ways, depending on the patient populations and resources. In general, they adopt either a consultative or an authoritative role in nutrition management. Many studies have shown their positive contribution to the total nutritional care of the patient through efficient and appropriate selection and monitoring of feed and route.

Components of a PN regimen

In addition to water, six main groups of nutrients need to be incorporated in a PN regimen (Table 7.2). The aim is to provide appropriate sources and amounts of all the equivalent building blocks in a single daily admixture.

Water volume

Water is the principal component of the body and accounts for approximately 60% and 55% of total body weight in men and women, respectively. Usually, homeostasis maintains appropriate fluid levels and electrolyte balance, and thirst drives the

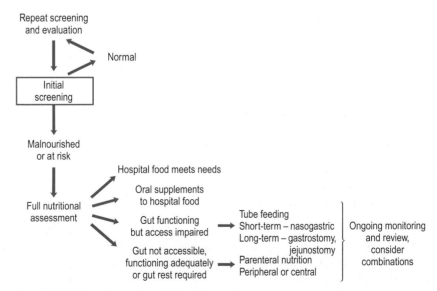

Fig. 7.1 Decision pathway to guide initial and ongoing nutritional support.

Table 7.2 Oral and equivalent parenteral nutrition source

Oral diet	Parenteral nutrition source
Water	Water
Protein	L-amino acids mixture
Carbohydrate	Glucose
Fat with essential fatty acids	Lipid emulsions with essential fatty acids
Vitamins	Vitamins
Minerals	Trace elements
Electrolytes	Electrolytes

healthy person to drink; however, some patients are not able physically to respond by drinking and so this homeostasis is ineffective. There is risk of over- or underhydration if the range of factors affecting fluid and electrolyte balance is not fully understood and monitored. In general, an adult patient will require 20–40 ml/kg/day fluid; however, Table 7.3 describes other factors that should be considered in tailoring input to needs.

Amino acids

Twenty L-amino acids are required for protein synthesis and metabolism, and the majority of these can be synthesised endogenously. Eight are called 'essential' amino acids because they cannot be synthesised (isoleucine, leucine, lysine, methionine, phenylalanine, threonine, tryptophan and valine). A further group of 'conditionally essential' amino acids (arginine, choline, glutamine, taurine and S-adenosyl-L-methionine) are defined as the patient's needs exceed synthesis in clinically stressed conditions. Also, due to the immature metabolic pathways of neonates, infants and children, some other amino acids are essential in the young patient, and these include histidine, proline, cysteine, tyrosine and taurine. Immature neonatal metabolism does not fully metabolise glycine, methionine, phenylalanine and threonine and so requirements are reduced.

To balance the patient's amino acid requirements and the chemical characteristics of the amino acids (solubility, stability and compatibility), a range of commercially available licensed solutions has been formulated containing a range of amino acid profiles (Table 7.4). Aminoplasmal®, Aminoven, Synthamin® and Vamin® are designed for adult patients. The amino acid profiles of Primene® and Vaminolact® are specifically tailored to neonates, infants and children (reflecting the amino acid profile of maternal cord blood and breast milk, respectively).

L-glutamine was initially excluded from formulations due to its low solubility and relatively poor stability in the aqueous environment; however, it is recognised that there is a clinical need for this amino acid in catabolic stress, and it is now available as an additive (Dipeptiven®) and as an amino acid solution containing a dipeptide form of glutamine (Glamin®) in which the peptide bond cleaves in the blood, releasing free L-glutamine. Research is also considering the rationale and merits of supplementing arginine, glutathione and ornithine α-ketoglutarate.

Table 7.3 Factors affecting fluid requirements

Consider increasing fluid input	Consider reducing fluid input
Signs/symptoms of dehydration	Signs/symptoms of fluid overload
Fever: increased insensible losses from lungs in hyperventilation and from skin in sweating. Allow 10–15% extra water per 10°C above normal	High humidity: reduced rate of evaporation
Acute anabolic state: increased water required for increased cell generation	Blood transfusion: volume input
High environmental temperature or low humidity: increased rate of evaporation	Cardiac failure: may limit tolerated blood volume
	Drug therapy: assess volume and electrolyte content of infused drug
Abnormal GI loss (vomiting, wounds, ostomies, diarrhoea): consider both volume loss and electrolyte content	
Burns or open wound(s): increased water evaporation	
	Renal failure: fluid may accumulate so reduce input accordingly or provide artificial renal support
Blood loss: assess volume lost and whether replaced by transfusion, colloid, crystalloid	

Table 7.4 Examples of amino acid and consequential nitrogen content of licensed amino acid solutions available in the UK

Name	Nitrogen content (g/L)	Electrolytes present
Aminoplasmal® 5% E	8	Potassium, magnesium, sodium and dihydrogen phosphate
Aminoplasmal® 10%	16	
Aminoven® 25	25.7	
Glamin®	22.4	
Hyperamine® 30	30	Sodium
Primene® 10%	15	
Synthamin® 9	9.1	Potassium, magnesium, sodium and acid phosphate
Synthamin® 9 EF	9.1	
Synthamin® 14	14	Potassium, magnesium, sodium and acid phosphate
Synthamin® 14 EF	14	
Synthamin® 17	17	Potassium, magnesium, sodium and acid phosphate
Synthamin® 17 EF	17	
Vamin® 9 Glucose	9.4	Potassium, magnesium, sodium and calcium
Vamin® 14	13.5	Potassium, magnesium, sodium and calcium
Vamin® 14EF	13.5	
Vamin® 18EF	18	
Vaminolact®	9.3	

For adults, PN solutions are generally prescribed in terms of the amount of nitrogen they provide, rounding to the nearest gram; for example, 9, 11, 14 or 18 g nitrogen regimens may be prescribed. Assuming adequate energy is supplied, most adult patients achieve nitrogen balance with approximately 0.2 g nitrogen/kg/day, although care should be taken with overweight patients.

A 24-h urine collection can be used as an indicator of nitrogen loss, assuming all urine is collected and urea or volume output is not compromised by renal failure; however, a true nitrogen output determination requires measurement of nitrogen output from all body fluids, including urine, sweat, faeces, skin and wounds. Nitrogen balance studies can indicate the metabolic state of the patient (positive balance in net protein synthesis, negative balance in protein catabolism).

Urinary urea constitutes approximately 80% of the urinary nitrogen. The universally accepted conversion factor for nitrogen to protein is 1 g nitrogen per 6.25 g of protein.

Amino acid solutions are hypertonic to blood and should not be administered alone into the peripheral circulation.

Energy

Many factors affect the energy requirement of individual patients and these include age, activity and illness (both severity and stage). Predictive formulae can be applied to estimate the energy requirement, for example, the Harris Benedict equation or the more commonly used Schofield equation, which is shown below in Table 7.5.

Alternatively, calorimetry techniques can be used; however, no single method is ideal or suits all scenarios. Often it is found that two methods result in different recommendations. The majority of adults can be appropriately maintained on 25–35 non-protein kcal/kg/day. There is debate over whether to include amino acids as a source of calories since it is simplistic to assume they are either all spared for protein synthesis or fed into the metabolic pathways (Krebs cycle) and contribute to the release of energy-rich molecules. In general, we refer to 'non-protein energy' and sufficient lipid and glucose energy is supplied to spare the amino acids. As a rough guide, the non-protein energy-to-nitrogen ratio is approximately 150:1, although an ideal ratio for all patients has not been absolutely defined. A lower ratio is considered for critically ill patients, while higher ratios are considered for less catabolic patients.

Dual energy

In general, energy should be sourced from a balanced combination of lipid and glucose; this is termed 'dual energy' and is more physiological than an exclusive glucose source. Typically, the fat-to-glucose ratio remains close to the 60:40–40:60 ranges.

Dual energy can minimise the risk of giving too much lipid or glucose since complications increase if the metabolic capacity of either is exceeded. A higher incidence of acute adverse

Table 7.5 Schofield equation

Age (years)	Male	Female
15–18	BMR = 17.6 × weight (kg) + 656	BMR = 13.3 × weight (kg) + 690
18–30	BMR = 15.0 × weight (kg) + 690	BMR = 14.8 × weight (kg) + 485
30–60	BMR = 11.4 × weight (kg) + 870	BMR = 8.1 × weight (kg) + 842
>60	BMR = 11.7 × weight (kg) + 585	BMR = 9.0 × weight (kg) + 656

BMR, basal metabolic rate.

effects is noted with faster infusion rates and higher total daily doses, especially in patients with existing metabolic stress. It is, therefore, essential that the administered dose complements the energy requirements and the infusion rate does not exceed the metabolic capacity.

While effectively maintaining nitrogen balance, lipid inclusion is seen to confer a number of advantages (Box 7.1). Some patients, notably long-term home patients, do not tolerate daily lipid infusions and need to be managed on an individual basis. Depending on the enteral intake and nutritional needs, lipids are prescribed for a proportion of the days. A trial with the newer generation lipid emulsions may be appropriate.

Glucose

Glucose is the recommended source of carbohydrate (1 g anhydrous glucose provides 4 kcal). Table 7.6 indicates the energy provision and tonicity for a range of concentrations. Glucose 5% is regarded as isotonic with blood. The higher concentrations cause phlebitis if administered directly to peripheral veins and should, therefore, be given by a central vein or in combination with compatible solutions to reduce the tonicity.

The glucose infusion rate should generally be between 2 and 4 mg/kg/min. An infusion of 2 mg/kg/min (equating to approximately 200 g (800 kcal) per day for a 70 kg adult) represents the basal glucose requirement, whereas 4 mg/kg/day is regarded as the physiological optimal rate. Higher levels are

tolerated by some patients especially those at home on PN, but monitoring of blood glucose is required at least initially. Care needs to be taken as glucose oxidation occurs, but there is an increased conversion to glycogen and fat. If excess glucose is infused and the glycogen storage capacity exceeded, the circulating glucose level rises, *de novo* lipogenesis occurs (production of fat from glucose) and there is an increased incidence of metabolic complications.

Lipid emulsions

Lipid emulsions are used as a source of energy and for the provision of the essential fatty acids, linoleic and alpha-linolenic acid. Supplying 10 kcal energy per gram of lipid, they are energy rich and can be infused directly into the peripheral veins since they are relatively isotonic with blood.

Typically, patients receive up to 2.5 g lipid/kg/day. For practical compounding reasons, and assuming clinical acceptance, this tends to be rounded to 100 g or 50 g. Details of lipid emulsions available within the UK can be found in Table 7.7.

Lipid emulsions are oil-in-water formulations. Figure 7.2 shows the structure of triglycerides (three fatty acids on a glycerol backbone) and a lipid globule, stabilised at the interface by phospholipids. Ionisation of the polar phosphate group of the phospholipid results in a net negative charge of the lipid globule and an electromechanically stable formulation. The lipid globule size distribution is similar to that of the naturally occurring chylomicrons (80–500 nm), as indicated in Fig. 7.3.

The first-generation lipid emulsions have been in use since the 1970s and utilise soybean oil as the source of long chain fatty acids. More recent research on lipid metabolic pathways and clinical outcomes has indicated that the fatty acid profile of soybean oil alone is not ideal. For example, it is now recognised that these lipid emulsions contain

---

Box 7.1 Examples of the advantages of dual energy systems over glucose-only energy systems

Minimise risk of hyperglycaemia and related complications
Prevent and reverse fatty liver (steatosis)
Reduce carbon dioxide production and respiratory distress
Meet higher calorie requirements of septic and trauma patients when glucose oxidation reduced and lipid oxidation increased
Reduce metabolic stress
Support immune function
Improve lean body mass and reduce water retention
Permit peripheral administration, through reduced tonicity
Facilitate fluid restriction, as lipid is a concentrated source of energy
Are a source of essential fatty acids, preventing and correcting deficiency

---

Table 7.6 Energy provision and tonicity of glucose solutions

Concentration (w/v)	Energy content (kcal/L)	Osmolarity (mOsmol/L)
5%	200	278
10%	400	555
20%	800	1110
50%	2000	2775
70%	2800	3885

Table 7.7 Examples of licensed lipid emulsions available in the UK

Lipid emulsion type	Details of products with kJ per litre
Soybean oil	Intralipid® 10% (4600), 20% (8400), 30% (12600)
Purified olive oil/soybean oil	ClinOleic® 20% (8360)
Medium chain triglycerides/soybean oil	Lipofundin® MCT/LCT 10% (4430), 20% (8000)
Purified structured triglycerides	Structolipid® 20% (8200)
Omega-3-acid triglycerides/soybean oil/medium chain triglycerides	Lipidem® (7900)
Highly refined fish oil	Omegaven® (4700)
Fish oil/olive oil/soybean oil/medium chain triglycerides	SMOFLipid® (8400)

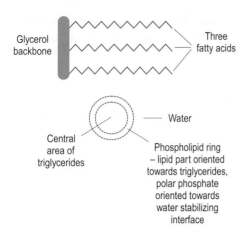

Fig. 7.2 Triglyceride structure and composition of lipid emulsion globule.

excess essential polyunsaturated fatty acids, resulting in a qualitative and quantitative compromise to the eicosanoid metabolites that have important roles in cell structure, haemodynamics, platelet function, inflammatory response and immune response.

The molecular structure of the fatty acids has an important impact on the patient's oxidative stress. Two strategies have been applied to overcome this: a reduction in the polyunsaturated fatty acid content through an improved balance of fatty acids or the inclusion of medium chain fatty acids. This has resulted in the development of lipid emulsions that include olive oil (rich in monounsaturated oleic acid and antioxidant α-tocopherol with an appropriate level of essential polyunsaturated fatty acids), fish oil (rich in omega 3 fatty acids) and medium chain triglycerides or structured triglycerides (reduced long chain fatty acid content). Clinical application of these newer lipid emulsions depends upon good clinical studies within the relevant patient population. Such studies should evaluate the efficacy of energy provision and clinical tolerance and report improvements in the eicosanoid-dependent functions or oxidative stress.

Both egg and soybean phospholipids include a phosphate moiety. There is a debate as to whether this is bioavailable.

Therefore, some manufacturers include the phosphate content in their stability calculations, while others do not.

The 20% lipid emulsions are favoured, especially in paediatrics, as they contain less phospholipid than the 10% emulsions in relation to triglyceride provision. If there is incomplete clearance of the infused phospholipids, lipoprotein X, an abnormal phospholipid-rich low-density lipoprotein, is generated and a raised blood cholesterol observed. The incidence of raised lipoprotein X levels is greater with the 10% emulsions as they present proportionally more phospholipid.

Lipid clearance monitoring is particularly important in patients who are at risk of impaired clearance, including those who are hyperlipidaemic, diabetic, septic, have impaired renal or hepatic function or are critically ill (Crook, 2000).

Micronutrients

Micronutrients have a key role in intermediary metabolism, as both co-factors and co-enzymes. For example, zinc is required by over 200 enzyme systems and affects many diverse body functions including acid–base balance, immune function and nucleic acid synthesis. It is evident, therefore, that the availability of micronutrients can affect enzyme activity and total metabolism. When disease increases the metabolism of the major substrates, the requirement for micronutrients is increased. Some of the micronutrients also play an essential role in the free radical scavenging system. These include the following:

- copper, zinc and manganese, in the form of superoxide dismutase, dispose of superoxide radicals
- selenium, in the form of glutathione peroxidase, removes hydroperoxyl compounds
- vitamin C is a strong reducing agent
- vitamins A, E and ß-carotene react directly with free radicals

By the time a patient starts PN, they may have already developed a deficiency of one or more essential nutrients. By the time a specific clinical deficiency is observed, for example,

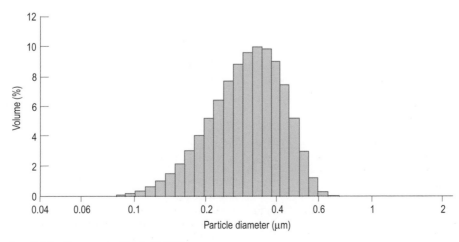

Fig. 7.3 Lipid globule size distribution curve of Ivelip® 20%.

Box 7.2   Factors affecting micronutrient requirements

Baseline nutritional state on starting parenteral nutrition
- Acute or chronic onset of illness
- Dietary history
- Duration and severity of inadequate nutritional intake

Increased loss
- Small bowel fistulae/aspirate: rich in zinc
- Biliary fluid loss: rich in copper
- Burn fluid loss: rich in zinc, copper, selenium

Increased requirement
- Increased metabolism: acute in anabolic phase following catabolic phase of critically ill
- Active growth

Organ function
- Liver failure: copper and manganese clearance reduced
- Renal failure: aluminium, chromium, zinc and nickel clearance reduced

---

depigmentation of hair in copper deficiency or skin lesions in zinc deficiency, the patient will already have tried to compensate to maintain levels, compromised intracellular enzyme activity and antioxidant systems and expressed non-specific symptoms such as fatigue and impaired immune response. A summary of factors that affect micronutrient needs is presented in Box 7.2.

Measuring blood levels of vitamins and trace elements in acutely ill patients is of limited value. It is recommended that these are measured every 1–6 months depending on levels, and in patients at home on PN (NICE, 2006). Deficiency states are clinically significant but, with non-specific symptoms, they are often difficult to diagnose.

Micronutrient experts prefer to prevent a deficit developing and compromising the clinical state, rather than perform regular monitoring of blood results.

Micronutrients should be included daily from the start of the PN. The requirements are increased during critical illness and in chronically depleted patients. Patients with major burns and trauma or with artificial renal support can quickly become depleted. Their supplementation may influence the outcome of the disease. Even if the patient has reasonable levels and reserves initially, they can quickly become depleted if they are not supported by daily administration. Additional oral or enteral supplements may be considered if there is some intestinal absorption. However, copper deficiency can increase iron absorption and zinc intake can decrease copper absorption.

The micronutrients naturally fall into two groups: the trace elements and vitamins. Micronutrients should be added to all PN infusions under appropriate, controlled, environmental conditions prior to administration (NICE, 2006).

Trace elements

Trace elements are generally maintained at a relatively constant tissue concentration and are present to a level of less than 1 mg/kg body weight. They are essential; deficiency results in structural and physiological disorders which, if identified early enough, can be resolved by re-administration. Ten essential trace elements are known: iron, copper, zinc, fluorine, manganese, iodine, cobalt (or as hydroxycobolamin), selenium, molybdenum and chromium. Adult reference ranges for daily requirements of trace metals can be found in Table 7.8. Currently two preparations are commercially available for adults (Decan®, Additrace®) together with a single paediatric preparation (Peditrace®).

Various recommended baseline doses have been published but no single licensed preparation provides all trace elements at the dose required. Concern over neurotoxicity with accumulated manganese, especially in liver failure, led to a reduction in the advised daily dose and recommendations for plasma monitoring. Recognising the benefits of zinc and selenium on the free radical scavenging system, some specialists advise an increase in the administered dose. Some patients, notably those with burns, renal replacement therapy and/or multiple trauma, as well as long-term patients, may require extra trace elements (Fleming, 1989).

Vitamins

There are two groups of vitamins: the water-soluble vitamins and the fat-soluble vitamins. Fat-soluble vitamins are stored in the body fat, whereas excess water-soluble vitamins are renally cleared; therefore, if there is inadequate provision, deficiency states for the water-soluble vitamins reveal themselves first. The adult reference range for daily requirements of vitamins can be found in Table 7.9. Commercially available preparations are Solivito® N (water soluble), Vitlipid® N Adult/Infant (fat soluble), Cernevit® (water and fat soluble).

In an attempt to reduce the risk of osteoporosis, especially in home PN patients, there have been recent changes to recommended biochemical vitamin D levels (Holick, 2007). Patients on long-term PN should have vitamin D levels measured

Table 7.8   Adult daily reference range for trace elements

Sex	Age	Iron (µmol/day)	Zinc (µmol/day)	Copper (µmol/day)	Selenium (µmol/day)
Male	19–50+	160	145	19	0.9
Female	19–50	260	110	19	0.8
Female	50+	160	110	19	0.8

Table 7.9 Adult daily reference ranges for vitamins (adapted from Department of Health, 1991)

Sex	Age	Thiamin (mg/day)	Riboflavin (mg/day)	Niacin (mg/day)	Vit B6 (mg/day)	Vit B12 (µcg/day)	Folate (µcg/day)	Vit C (mg/day)	Vit A (µcg/day)	Vit D (µcg/day)
Male	19–50	1.0	1.3	17	1.4	1.5	200	40	700	–
Male	50+	0.9	1.3	16	1.4	1.5	200	40	700	–[a]
Female	19–50	0.8	1.1	13	1.2	1.5	200	40	600	–
Female	50+	0.8	1.1	12	1.2	1.5	200	40	600	–[a]

[a] After age 65, the recommended normal daily intake is 10 µcg/day for male and females.

every 6 months. If low, this should be supplemented in order to help protect against osteoporosis which is a well recognised complication of home PN.

Electrolytes

Electrolytes are included to meet the patient's needs. Typical daily parenteral requirements are

- sodium (1–1.5 mmol/kg)
- potassium (1–1.5 mmol/kg)
- calcium (0.1–0.15 mmol/kg)
- magnesium (0.1–0.2 mmol/kg)
- phosphate (0.5–0.7 mmol/kg).

Depending upon the stability of the patient's clinical state, they are kept relatively constant or adjusted on a near daily basis, reflecting changes in blood biochemistry. Tables, for example, British National Formulary can be used to guide electrolyte replacement if there is excessive gastro-intestinal waste or high losses through burns. Hypophosphataemia should be corrected before starting parenteral or enteral nutrition to avoid the refeeding syndrome. Varying amounts of electrolytes are lost from the different gastro-intestinal secretions. Table 7.10 gives an indication of the content of various gastro-intestinal secretions. This should be taken into account when formulating PN for a patient who may have such losses.

Administration of PN

Routes of administration

PN can be administered peripherally or centrally.

Peripheral route

Administration of PN via a peripheral venous catheter should be considered for patients who are likely to need short-term feeding (less than 14 days) and who have no other need for central venous access. Peripheral lines are less costly than central lines and they may be inserted at the bedside providing the patient has good venous access. Ultrasound machines may be used to aid placement. There is no need for a chest X-ray

to confirm placement as the line does not reach the central circulation. Mid-lines should be considered which are usually about 20 cm long.

Care should be taken when formulating PN to be administered via a peripheral catheter with regard to the tonicity of the solution.

Some indications and contraindications to the use of the peripheral route are summarised in Box 7.3.

Peripheral administration is sometimes complicated or delayed by phlebitis, where an insult to the endothelial vessel wall causes inflammation, redness, pain and possible extravasation. Hot and cold compresses have been used to treat this. A 5 mg glyceryl trinitrate patch placed where the line tip is estimated to be may cause some local vasodilation which is believed to prevent thrombophlebitis (Khawaja and Williams, 1991). Peripheral tolerance can be influenced by a range of factors (Box 7.4).

Many consider that the tonicity of the infused solution or emulsion is a key factor defining peripheral infusion tolerance. The total number of osmotically active particles in the intracellular and extracellular fluids is essentially the same, approximately 290–310 mOsmol/L. When a lipid emulsion is included, infusions of approximately three times this osmolarity are generally well tolerated via the peripheral route and there are reports of success with higher levels. However, other factors should also be considered. Patient factors, such as vein

Box 7.3 Indications and contraindications to the use of peripheral parenteral nutrition

Indications
- Duration of feed likely to be short term
- Supplemental feeding
- Compromised access to central circulation, for example, local trauma, surgery or thrombosis
- No immediate facilities or trained staff to insert central catheter
- High risk of fungal or bacterial sepsis, for example, patients with purulent tracheostomy secretions, immune deficiency state, history of repeated sepsis
- Contraindication to central venous catheterisation

Contraindications
- Inadequate or inaccessible peripheral veins
- Large volumes of administration
- High calorie/nitrogen requirements alongside fluid restrictions (admixture osmolarity too high)

Box 7.4 Factors that improve tolerance to peripheral lines

- Aseptic insertion and line care
- Selection of large vessel with good blood flow and direct path, for example, cephalic vein
- Fine-bore catheter (22G) for minimal trauma on insertion and disturbance of blood flow
- Fine polyurethane catheter
- Secure catheter to minimise physical trauma
- Glyceryl trinitrate patch distal to insertion site, over tip to vasodilate vein
- Flushing of lines not in use
- Low-tonicity infusions
- Inclusion of lipid emulsion; venoprotective and isotonic with blood

fragility and blood flow, may mean that some infusion episodes are better tolerated than others. The osmolarity of a PN formulation can be estimated by applying the following equation:

$$= \frac{\sum [osmolarity_n (mOsmol/L) \times volume_n (L)]}{Total\ volume(L)},$$

where n indicates the component.

By considering the macronutrients included in the regimen, that is, the amino acids, glucose and lipid, an estimation of the osmolarity can be made. The value will be increased by electrolyte or micronutrient additions; however, since the peripheral tolerance is affected by so many factors, including tonicity, and because the limit is only an estimate, the effect of these additions is relatively low unless high levels of monovalent ions are included.

Central route

The central venous route is indicated when longer-term feeding is anticipated, high tonicity or large volume formulations are required, or the peripheral route is inaccessible. The rapid and turbulent blood flow in the central circulation and the constant movement of the heart ensure rapid mixing and reduce the risk of osmotically induced injury to the endothelium.

A range of single-, double-, triple- and quadruple-lumen central lines are available and one lumen must be dedicated for the intravenous nutrition. These lines require skilful insertion, usually into the jugular or subclavian vein, and confirmation of their position by X-ray. This relatively invasive and costly procedure is performed by trained medical staff. Tunnelling of the line to an appropriate exit site facilitates line care and may reduce the incidence of significant line sepsis. The femoral route is not favoured due to a higher incidence of sepsis. If cared for well, a tunnelled central line placed in a patient receiving home PN may last for many years.

Peripherally Inserted Central Catheters (PICCs)

PICCs are typically inserted into a peripheral vein, usually the cephalic or basilic in the upper arm, with the exit tip in the superior vena cava just above the right atrium. As the name suggests, they are used for the central administration of infusions. Single- and double-lumen versions are available; some also have a one-way valve to prevent backflow. Insertion is less invasive than for conventional central lines and can be undertaken by trained nurse practitioners at the bedside. A chest X-ray is necessary to confirm placement.

Infusion control

Pumps

PN must always be administered under the control of an infusion pump. Acute overload of fluid, nutrition and electrolytes can have morbid consequences.

Infusion pumps should be used with an appropriate infusion or giving set which is compatible with both the infusion pump and the PN admixture. For home patients, small, simple battery-powered ambulatory pumps are favoured.

Temperature

PN should be at room temperature when it is infused. It must, therefore, be removed from the refrigerator in which it is stored approximately 2 h before connection. No external heat should be applied, although intermittent inversion of the bag may help.

If a cold admixture is infused, the patient may experience infusion discomfort, and the acute release of gas from where it was dissolved in the admixture may cause the pump to alarm 'air in line'.

Compounded formulations

Historically, PN was administered from a series of separate bottles, where health care staff had to accurately and safely manage a combination of giving sets, infusion rates and total infusion times. Most patients now receive their complete nutrition from a single daily bag of a pharmaceutically stable PN formulation.

Various terms are used to describe the PN formulation, depending on whether lipid is included. If it contains lipid, it is called a 3-in-1, ternary or all-in-one admixture, if no lipid is present, the terms 2-in-1, binary or aqueous admixture are used. Various methods now exist for compounding PN, these range from high-tech, computer run compounding machines through to basic principle techniques such as gravity filling.

Standardised formulations

Depending on the type (size and specialty) of the hospital, a range of standard formulations are maintained and supported with prescribing guidelines. These may be compounded from scratch, compounded from 'base-bags' locally or by a licensed unit, or purchased as licensed ready-to-use presentations.

The range is specifically selected to meet the needs of the patients managed by the hospital and will typically include a low-tonicity regimen suitable for peripheral administration, a higher calorie and nitrogen regimen for central administration to catabolic patients and a high-tonicity regimen for fluid-restricted patients. Baseline electrolytes will generally be included, although the flexibility for reduced levels is usually offered.

Licensed ready-to-use products

A range of licensed ready-to-use preparations are available and should have micronutrients added prior to infusing. For convenience, baseline electrolyte levels are included in many formulations and meet the needs of most patients and additional electrolytes may be added up to the limits set by the manufacturer. Electrolyte-free options are also available. Some are licensed for use in paediatrics and/or for peripheral use. Manufacturers advise on stability and shelf-life for electrolyte and micronutrient additions. The range of ready-to-use products includes:

- triple chamber bags (OliClinomel®, Kabiven®, StructoKabiven® and Nutriflex® Lipid ranges): chambers separately pre-filled with lipid, amino acid and glucose and terminally sterilised, these are activated by applying external pressure so weak seal peels open, mixing the contents to form a 3-in-1 formulation.
- dual chamber bags (Clinimix® and Nutriflex® ranges): chambers separately pre-filled with amino acid and glucose and terminally sterilised, these are activated to form a 2-in-1 formulation. They provide the flexibility to allow staff to omit or add a compatible lipid.

The range of commercially available PN formulations is continually expanding. For hospital pharmacies who do not have compounding facilities, this offers an opportunity to ensure the correct formulation is given to meet individual patients needs. PN formulations are now available with micronutrients added and with extended shelf-lives when stored in a refrigerator.

Cyclic infusions

Cyclic PN is when the daily requirements are administered over a short period. A classic example is the stable home patient who administers their feed overnight, freeing themselves from the constraints of an infusion during the day. This enables them to have more physical freedom and improves their quality of life. Some patients, however, prefer to administer their PN during the day time. This is made possible by use of a small ambulatory pump and a back pack in which they may carry their PN.

Since cyclic feeding more closely simulates the human feeding pattern and is a closer match to normal hormonal and metabolic cycles, it also offers a range of metabolic and clinical advantages. Steatosis, fatty infiltration of the liver, is less common and may be corrected by employing cyclic feeding because the feed-free period facilitates lipolysis and fat mobilisation. Peripheral tolerance may be improved as the endothelia recover between infusion periods.

Initially, the patient should receive the PN infusion slowly over the full 24 h, as tolerated, the rate of infusion can be increased slowly to decrease the infusion time. This should be done over a series of days. During this period, the patient must be monitored closely for any signs of fluid, electrolyte or acid-base imbalance and hyper/hypoglycaemia. For example, on stopping the infusion, rebound hypoglycaemia may occur.

Pharmaceutical issues

Having identified the balance of nutrients required for a patient in a single day, it is necessary to formulate a physically and chemically stable aseptically prepared admixture. PN admixtures contain over 50 chemical entities and, as such, are extremely complex and have many chemical interactions taking place which could lead to instability in the final formulation. Professional advice or appropriate reference material should

Table 7.10 Electrolyte content of gastro-intestinal secretions

Intestinal tract locality	Volume (ml)	Sodium (mmol/L)	Potassium (mmol/L)	Chloride (mmol/L)	Bicarbonate (mmol/L)
Saliva	1500	10	25	10	30
Gastric juice (fasting)	1500	60	15	90	15
Pancreatic fistula	700	140	5	75	120
Biliary fistula	500	145	5	100	40
Jejunostomy	2000–3000	110	5	100	30
Ileostomy	500	115	8	45	30
Proximal colostomy	300	80	20	45	30
Diarrhoea	500–1500	120	25	90	45

be sought and used before compounding and administering of PN takes place. Manufacturers and third party experts can advise on stability issues.

Physical stability

Physical instability takes a number of forms including precipitation of crystalline material and breakdown of the lipid emulsion.

Precipitation

Precipitation carries two key risks. First, the potential to infuse solid particles to the narrow pulmonary capillaries may result in fatal emboli. Second, the prescribed nutrients may not be infused to the patient. Clinically dangerous precipitates may not always be visible to the naked eye, especially if lipid emulsion is present. They may also develop over time, and an apparently 'safe' admixture may develop fatal precipitates when in use.

Precipitation of solid is epitomised by the formation of calcium phosphate; this is of special concern in neonatal admixtures where the requirements to prevent hypophosphataemic rickets and severe osteopenia may exceed the safe concentrations. Such concentrations are rarely seen in adult regimens. It is known that calcium and phosphate can form a number of different salt forms each with different solubility profiles, for example, $Ca(H_2PO_4)_2$ which is highly soluble in comparison to $CaHPO_4$ and $Ca_3(PO_4)_2$. $Ca_3(PO_4)_2$ precipitation occurs relatively immediate and has a white, fluffy amorphous appearance; however, $CaHPO_4.2H_2O$ precipitation is time mediated and has a more crystalline appearance.

Factors affecting calcium phosphate precipitation are shown in Table 7.11. Practical measures can be taken to minimise the risks; these include accurate calculation of the proposed formulation, comparison against professionally defined comprehensive matrices and thorough mixing. Solubility curves and algorithms should be used with extreme caution, even if they are quoted for a specific amino acid source, this is because they do not consider all the factors and do not consistently identify risk. Assuming the sodium content can be tolerated, use of an organic phosphate salt form may be beneficial due to the higher solubility of the sodium glycerophosphate salt form.

Trace elements have also been associated with clinically significant precipitation; these include iron phosphate and copper sulphide (hydrogen sulphide from the minor degradation of cysteine/cystine). These very fine precipitate forms are less likely to cause occlusion of catheters or lung capillaries, but have been associated with significant clinical delivery losses when they are taken up by inline filtration devices.

Lipid destabilisation

The oil-in-water lipid emulsions are sensitive to destabilisation by a range of factors including the presence of positively charged ions, pH changes and changes in environmental

Table 7.11 Factors affecting calcium phosphate precipitation

Factor	Mechanism and effect
pH	Low pH supports solubility, whereas a higher pH supports precipitation. Depending on the amount and buffering capacity of the amino acids, this can be affected by different concentrations and sources of glucose solution and acetate salt forms.
Temperature	Higher temperatures associated with greater precipitation, increased availability of free calcium to interact and a shift to the more insoluble salt forms.
Amino acids	Buffer pH changes. Complex with calcium so less available to react with phosphate. Both the source of amino acid and the relative content are important.
Magnesium	Complex with phosphate forming soluble salts rather than less soluble calcium salts.
Calcium salt form	Calcium chloride dissociates more readily than calcium gluconate, releasing it to react with the phosphate.
Phosphate salt form	Monobasic salts, for example, dipotassium phosphate, dissociate more readily than dibasic salts, for example, potassium acid phosphate, releasing phosphate to react with the calcium. Organic salts, such as sodium glycerophosphate and glucose-1-phosphate, are more stable.
Mixing order	Optimum stability achieved by only permitting calcium and phosphate to come together in a large volume admixture. Agitate between additions to avoid pockets of concentration.

temperature. The lipid globules may come together and coalesce to form larger globules and release free oil; this could occlude the lung microvasculature and cause respiratory and circulatory compromise and lead to death.

Positively charged ions destabilise the admixture by drawing the negatively charged lipid globules together, overwhelming the electromechanical repulsion of the charged phospholipids and increasing their tendency to join or coalesce. Divalent and trivalent ions have a more significant effect; therefore, there are tightly defined limits for the amount of Ca^{2+}, Mg^{2+} and Fe^{3+} that can be added to a 3-in-1 admixture. Although the limits for the other polyvalent ions (such as zinc and selenium) are also controlled, because they are given in micromolar or nanomolar quantities, they are less of a problem. Low concentrations of amino acids and extremes of glucose concentration (high and low) also reduce the stability of the emulsion and increase the tendency for creaming and cracking of the lipid emulsion.

The naked eye can identify large-scale destabilisation, as shown in Table 7.12; however, the limitations of this method need to be recognised; clinically significant destabilisation might not be visible to the naked eye. In practice, stability laboratories use specialised technical equipment to determine defined criteria so as to establish the physical stability of a formulation. These tests include assessing changes in lipid globule size distribution with optical microscopes, and variety of particle size analysis instruments against the defined limits of pharmaceutical acceptance. A wide safety margin is applied.

Chemical stability

Chemical stability takes many forms, notably chemical degradation of the vitamins and amino acids.

Vitamin stability

Many vitamins readily undergo chemical degradation, and vitamin stability often defines the shelf-life of a given formulation.

Vitamin C (ascorbic acid), the least stable component, is generally regarded as the marker for vitamin degradation. Vitamin C oxidation is accelerated by heat, oxygen and certain trace elements, including copper. Other examples include vitamin A photolysis and vitamin E photo-oxidation. Measures that minimise oxygen presence, such as minimal aeration during compounding, evacuation of air at the end of compounding and use of multi-laminated oxygen barrier bags, and light protection of admixture containers and delivery sets are recommended.

Amino acid stability

The amino acid profile should be maintained for the shelf-life of the formulation and manufacturers perform assays to confirm this prior to issuing stability reports.

Maillard reaction

The Maillard reaction is a complex pathway of chemical reactions that starts with a condensation of the carbonyl group of the glucose and the amino group of the amino acid. At present, relatively little is known about the clinical effects of these Maillard reaction products; however, it is prudent to minimise their presence by protecting from light and avoiding high temperatures.

Microbial contamination

PN is a highly nutritious medium whose hypertonicity will partially limit microbial growth potential. Growth in the presence of lipid emulsion is greater. Pharmaceutical developments have enabled terminal sterilisation of many of the components, including the multi-chamber bag presentations; however, additional manipulations should only be performed using validated aseptic techniques in appropriate pharmaceutically clean environments by suitably trained staff. Nurses, patients and carers must be trained to apply aseptic methods when connecting and disconnecting infusions, for this reason, many centres have documented line care and PN protocols.

Shelf-life and temperature control

The manufacturer may be able to provide physical and chemical stability data to support a formulation for a shelf-life of up to 90 days at 2–8°C followed by 24h at room temperature for infusion; this assumes that a strict aseptic technique is used during compounding. Units holding a manufacturing license covering aseptic compounding of PN are potentially able to assign this full shelf-life (if stability data is available), whilst unlicensed units are limited to a maximum shelf-life of 7 days.

PN must be stored and transported within the defined temperature limits and should not be exposed to temperature cycling (e.g. the formulations must not freeze); for this reason, a validated cold-chain must be employed especially when delivering formulations to home care patients. Pharmaceutical-grade fridges should be used and monitored

Table 7.12 Lipid instability

	Description	Visual observation
Stable, normal emulsion	Lipid globules equally dispersed. Suitable for administration	Normal emulsion
Light creaming	Lipid globules rising to the top of the bag. Slight layering visible. Readily redisperses on inverting the bag. Suitable for administration	Light creaming
Heavy creaming, flocculation	Lipid globules coming together but not joining. Rising to the top of the bag. More obvious layering visible. Readily redisperses on inverting the bag. Acceptable for administration	Heavy creaming
Coalescence	Lipid globules come together, coalesce to form larger globules and rise to the surface. Larger globules join, releasing free oil. Irreversible destabilisation of the lipid emulsion. Not suitable for administration	Cracked. Oil layer viewed close up

to ensure appropriate air cycling and temperature mainte-nance. The temperature during the infusion period should be known with neonatal units and their patient incubators classically maintained at higher temperatures; therefore, for-mulations used for this environment must have been stability-validated at these temperatures.

Drug stability

The addition of drugs to PN admixtures, or Y-site co-administration, is actively discouraged unless the compatibil-ity has been formally confirmed. Wherever possible, the PN should be administered through a dedicated line. Multilumen catheters can be used to infuse PN separately from other infusion(s); however, extreme competition for intravenous access may prompt consideration of drug and PN combina-tions. Many factors need to be considered: the physical and chemical stability of the PN, the physical and chemical stabil-ity of the drug, the bioavailability of the drug (especially when a lipid emulsion is present) and the effect of stopping and starting Y-site infusions on the actual administration rates. It is not possible to reliably extrapolate data from a specific PN com-position, between brands of solutions and salt forms or between brands or doses of drugs. A range of studies has been performed and published; however, these should be used with caution.

In practice, drugs should only be infused with PN when all other possibilities have been exhausted. These may include gaining further intravenous access and changing the drug(s) to clinically acceptable non-intravenous alternatives. The relative risks of stopping and starting the PN infusion and repeatedly breaking the infusion circuit should be fully con-sidered before sharing a line for separate infusions of PN and drug. In most cases, the risks outweigh the benefits; however, if this option is adopted, the line must be flushed before and after with an appropriate volume of solution known to be sta-ble with both the PN and the drug. Strict aseptic technique should be adopted to minimise the risk of contaminating the line and infusions.

Filtration

All intravenous fluids pass through the delicate lung microvas-culature with its capillary diameter of 8–12 µm. The presence of particulate matter has been demonstrated to cause direct embolisation, direct damage to the endothelia, formation of granulomata and formation of foreign body giant cells, and to have a thrombogenic effect. In addition, the presence of microbial and fungal matter can cause a serious infection or inflammatory response.

Precautions taken to minimise the particulate load of the compounded admixture must include:

- use of filter needles or straws (5 µm) during compounding to catch larger particles such as cored rubber from bottles and glass shards from ampoules
- air particle levels kept within defined limits in aseptic rooms by the use of air filters and non-shedding clothing and wipes

- use of quality raw materials with minimal particulate presence, including empty bags and leads
- confirmation of physical and chemical stability of the formulation prior to aseptic compounding applying approved mixing order (stability for the required shelf-life time and conditions)

Guidelines have been published that endorse the use of fil-ters, especially for patients requiring intensive or prolonged parenteral therapy, including home patients, the immuno-compromised, neonates and children (Bethune et al., 2001). The filter should be placed as close to the patient as possible and validated for the PN to be used. For 2-in-1 formulations, 0.2 µm filters may be used, for 3-in-1 formulations, validated 1.2 µm filters may be used.

Light protection

It is widely recognised that exposure to light, notably photo-therapy light and intense sunlight, may increase the degrada-tion rate of certain constituents such as vitamins A and E. It is recommended that all regimens should be protected from light both during storage and during infusion, since

- the presence of a lipid emulsion does not totally protect against vitamin photodegradation
- the Maillard reaction is influenced by light exposure
- ongoing research suggests lipid peroxidation is accelerated by a range of factors, including exposure to certain wavelengths of light
- validated bag and delivery set covers should only be used

Nutritional assessment and monitoring

Initial assessment

Once screening has identified that a patient is in need of nutri-tional intervention, a more detailed assessment is performed; this will include an evaluation of nutritional requirements, the expected course of the underlying disease, consideration of the enteral route and, where appropriate, identification of access routes for PN. This will be supported by a clinical assessment that will include:

- clinical history
- dietary history
- physical examination
- anthropometry including muscle function tests
- biochemical, haematological and immunological review.

Monitoring

PN monitoring has a number of objectives. It should

- evaluate ongoing nutritional requirements, including fluid and electrolytes
- determine the effectiveness of the nutritional intervention

- facilitate early recognition of complications
- identify any deficiency, overload or toxicity to individual nutrients
- determine discrepancies between prescribed, delivered and received dose.

Regular monitoring contributes to the success of the PN and a monitoring protocol should be in place for each individual patient. Baseline data should be recorded so deviations can be recognised and interpreted. In the early stages, while the patient is in the acute stage of their illness and the nutritional requirements are being established, the frequency of monitoring will be greatest. Some tests may be defined by the underlying disease state, rather than by the presence of PN *per se*. As the patient's status stabilises, the frequency of monitoring will reduce, although the range of parameters monitored is likely to increase. Examples of parameters monitored include the following:

- *Clinical symptoms or presentation:* may be specific, for example, thrombophlebitis, or non-specific, for example, confusion.
- *Temperature, blood pressure and pulse:* vigilance for the risk of sepsis.
- *Fluid balance and weight:* acute weight changes reflect fluid gain or loss and prompt review of the volume of the PN. Slow, progressive changes are more likely to reflect nutritional status.
- *Nitrogen balance:* an assessment of urine urea and insensible loss and their relation to nitrogen input. It is difficult to obtain accurate figures.
- *Visceral proteins*: albumin levels may indicate malnutrition but its long half-life limits sensitivity to detect acute changes in nutritional status. Other markers with a shorter half-life may be more useful, for example, transferrin.
- *Haematology:* platelet counts and clotting studies for thrombocytopenia.
- *C-reactive protein:* monitor the inflammatory process.
- *Blood glucose:* hyperglycaemia is a relatively frequent complication. Management includes either a reduction in the infused dose or lengthening of the infusion period. If these measures fail, insulin may be used. Hyperglycaemia may also indicate sepsis. Rebound hypoglycaemia can occur when an infusion is stopped. If this is a problem, the infusion should be tapered off during the last hour or two of the infusion. Some infusion pumps are programmed to do this automatically.
- *Lipid tolerance:* turbidity, cholesterol and triglyceride profiles required.
- *Electrolyte profile:* indicates appropriate provision or complicating clinical disorder. In the first few days, low potassium, magnesium and/or phosphate with or without clinical symptoms may reflect the refeeding syndrome (see below).
- *Liver function tests:* an abnormal liver profile may be observed and it is often difficult to identify a single cause. PN and other factors such as sepsis, drug therapy and underlying disease may all interplay. In adults,

PN-induced abnormalities tend to be mild, reversible and self-limiting. In the early stages, fatty liver (steatosis) is seen. In longer-term patients, a cholestatic picture tends to present. Varying the type of lipid used and removing lipid from some formulations may be of benefit.

- *Anthropometry:* assesses longer-term status.
- *Acid–base profile:* indicative of respiratory or metabolic compromise and may require review of PN formulation.
- *Vitamin and trace element screen:* a range of single compounds or markers to consider tolerance and identify deficiencies, although of limited value as some tests are non-specific and inaccurate.
- *Catheter entry site:* vigilance for phlebitis, erythema, extravasation, infection, misplacement.

Complications

Complications of PN fall into two main categories: catheter-related and metabolic (Box 7.5). Overall, the incidence of such complications has reduced because of increased knowledge and skills together with more successful management (Maroulis and Kalfarentzos, 2000).

Line sepsis

This is a serious and potentially life-threatening condition. Monitoring protocols should ensure that signs of infection are identified early and a local decision pathway should be in place to guide efficient diagnosis and management. Management will depend upon the type of line and the source of infection. Alternative sources of sepsis should be considered. Initially, the PN is usually stopped.

Box 7.5 Examples of complications during parenteral nutrition

Catheter-related
- Thrombophlebitis (peripheral)
- Catheter-related infection, local or systemic
- Venous thrombosis
- Line occlusion (lipid, thrombus, particulate, mechanical)
- Pneumothorax, catheter malposition, vessel laceration, embolism, hydrothorax, dysrhythmias, incorrect placement (central)

Metabolic
- Hyperglycaemia or hypoglycaemia
- Electrolyte imbalance
- Lipid intolerance
- Refeeding syndrome
- Dehydration or fluid overload
- Specific nutritional deficiency or overload
- Liver disease or biliary disease
- Gastro-intestinal atrophy
- Metabolic bone dysfunction (in long term)
- Thrombocytopenia
- Adverse events with parenteral nutrition components
- Essential fatty acid deficiency

Line occlusion

Line occlusion may be caused by a number of factors, including:

- fibrin sheath forming around the line, or a thrombosis blocking the tip
- internal blockage of lipid, blood clot or salt and drug precipitates
- line kinking
- particulate blockage of a protective line filter.

Management will depend on the cause of the occlusion; in general, the aim is to save the line and resume feeding with minimum risk for the patient. The use of locks and flushes with alteplase (for fibrin and thrombosis), ethanol (for lipid deposits) and dilute hydrochloric acid (for salt and drug precipitates) may be considered. In some cases, the lines may need to be replaced.

These complications can be minimised by having a dedicated line for PN, flushing the line well with sodium chloride 0.9% before and after use and a regular slow flush of ethanol 20% may be used to prevent lipid deposition.

Refeeding syndrome

Patients should be assessed as to their risk of developing refeeding syndrome (see Table 7.13). Refeeding syndrome can be defined as 'the potentially fatal shifts in fluids and electrolytes that may occur in malnourished patients receiving nutrition'. Undernourished patients are catabolic and their major sources of energy are fat and muscle. As the PN infusion (which contains glucose) starts, this catabolic state is pushed to anabolic which in turn causes a surge of insulin. As the insulin levels increase, there is an intracellular shift of magnesium, potassium and phosphate, and acute hypomanganesaemia, hypokalaemia and hypophosphataemia result. This can cause cardiac and neurological dysfunction and may be fatal. PN should be gradually increased over a period of 2–7 days depending on the patient's body mass index and risk of developing refeeding syndrome. Oral thiamine and vitamin B compound strong or full dose intravenous vitamin B preparation may be administered before PN is started and for the first few days of infusion.

Table 7.13 Risk factors for developing refeeding syndrome (NICE, 2006)

One or more of the following:	Two or more of the following:
BMI <16 kg/m²	BMI <18.5 kg/m²
Unintentional weight loss greater than 15% within the last 3–6 months	Unintentional weight loss greater than 10% within the last 3–6 months
Little or no nutritional intake for more than 10 days	Little or no nutritional intake for more than 5 days
Low levels of potassium, phosphate or magnesium prior to feeding	A history of alcohol abuse or drugs including insulin, chemotherapy, antacids or diuretics

Specific disease states

Liver

Although abnormal liver function tests associated with short-term PN are usually benign and transient, liver dysfunction in long-term PN patients is one of the most prevalent and severe complications. Its underlying pathophysiology, however, largely remains to be elucidated. The content of PN should be examined and care should be taken not to overfeed with glucose and/or lipid. Supplementation with taurine in the formulation has been reported to ameliorate PN associated cholestasis through promoted bile flow. Various lipid preparations are now available, including preparations containing fish oils which have been reported to be beneficial in reversing liver disease (De Meijer et al., 2009). Lipid emulsions containing a mix of medium and long chain triglycerides are also available and have an improved liver tolerability. Due to the complexity of liver function, the range of potential disorders and its role in metabolism, the use of PN in liver disease is not without problems. Consensus guidelines for the use of PN in liver disease have been published (Plauth et al., 2009). Nutritional intervention may be essential for recovery, although care must be exercised with amino acid input and the risk of encephalopathy, calorie input and metabolic capacity, and the reduced clearance of trace elements such as copper and manganese (Maroulis and Kalfarentzos, 2000). Low-sodium, low-volume feeds are indicated if there is ascites. Cyclic feeding appears useful, especially in steatosis.

Renal failure

Fluid and electrolyte balance demand close attention, and guidelines for nutrition in adult renal failure are available (Cano et al., 2009). A low volume and poor quality urine output may necessitate a concentrated PN formulation with a reduction in electrolyte content, particularly a reduction in potassium and phosphate. In the polyuric phase or the nephrotic syndrome, a higher volume formulation may be required. If there is fluid retention, ideal body weight should be used for calculating requirements rather than the actual body weight.

The metabolic stress of acute renal failure and the malnutrition of chronic renal failure may initially demand relatively high nutritional requirements; however, nitrogen restriction may be necessary to control uraemia in the absence of dialysis or filtration and to avoid uraemia-related impaired glucose tolerance, because of peripheral insulin resistance, and lipid clearance.

Micronutrient requirements may also change in renal disease. For example, renal clearance of zinc, selenium, fluoride and chromium is reduced and there is less renal 1α-hydroxylation of vitamin D.

Intradialytic PN (IDPN) may be administered at the same time as dialysis; however, this is not without complications. High blood sugars and fluid overload can be a problem and there is uncertainty as to how much of the PN is retained by the body and how much is removed by dialysis. Administration requires local guidelines and monitoring to be in place (Foulks, 1999; Lazarus, 1999).

Pancreatitis

Acute pancreatitis is a metabolic stress that requires high-level nutritional support and pancreatic rest to recover. Guidelines for nutrition in acute pancreatitis are available (Gianotti et al., 2009). While enteral nutrition stimulates the pancreas, PN does not appear to. Hyperglycaemia may occur and require exogenous insulin.

Sepsis and injury

Significant fluctuations in macronutrient metabolism are seen during sepsis and injury. There are two metabolic phases: the 'ebb' phase of 24–48 h and the following 'flow' phase. The initial hyperglycaemia, reflecting a reduced utilisation of glucose, is followed by a longer catabolic state with increased utilisation of lipid and amino acids. The effect of the different lipid emulsions on immune function is the subject of much research. It is important not to overfeed and also to consider the reduced glucose tolerance during the critical days. This is due to increased insulin resistance and incomplete glucose oxidation. Exogenous insulin may be required.

Respiratory

While underfeeding and malnutrition can compromise respiratory effort and muscle function, overfeeding can equally compromise respiratory function due to increased carbon dioxide and lipid effects on the circulation. While chronic respiratory disease may be linked with a long-standing malnutrition, the patient with acute disease will generally be hypermetabolic.

Cardiac failure

Cardiac failure and multiple drug therapy may limit the volume of PN that can be infused. Concentrated formulations are used and, as a consequence of the high tonicity, administered via the central route. Close electrolyte monitoring and adjustment is required. Cardiac drugs may affect electrolyte clearance. Although central lines may already be in use for other drugs or cardiac monitoring, it is essential to maintain a dedicated lumen or line for the feed.

Diabetes mellitus

Diabetic patients can generally be maintained with standard dual-energy regimens. It is important to use insulin to manage blood glucose rather than reduce the nutritional provision of the feed. Close glucose monitoring will guide exogenous insulin administration. This should be given as a separate infusion (sliding scale) or, if the patient is stable, in bolus doses. Insulin should not be included within the PN formulation due to stability problems and variable adsorption to the equipment. Y-site infusion with the PN should be avoided as changes in insulin rates will be delayed and changes in feed rates will result in significant fluctuations in insulin administration. Extra potassium and phosphate may be required due to the impact of the glucose and insulin. Long-term PN patients may need differing insulin regimes depending on the glucose load (aqueous/lipid) in the formulation. Although using oral antihypoglycaemic agents with PN may be considered, care should be taken as to the potentially erratic absorption and so varying blood glucose levels.

Cancer and palliative care

Nutritional support in cancer and palliative care is guided by the potential risks and benefits of the intervention, alongside the wishes of the patient and their carers. Further research is required to evaluate the effects of PN on length and quality of life.

Standard PN may be useful during prolonged periods of gastro-intestinal toxicity, as in bone marrow transplant patients. The use of PN is not thought to stimulate tumour growth (Nitenberg and Raynard, 2000).

Short bowel syndrome

The small intestine is defined as 'short' if it is less than 100 cm. Treatment options depend upon which part of the gut has been removed and the functional state of the remaining organ. The surface area for absorption of nutrition and reabsorption of fluid and electrolytes is significantly compromised. Fluid and electrolyte balance needs to be managed closely due to the high-volume losses. High-volume PN formulations with raised electrolyte content (notably sodium and magnesium) may be required. Vitamin and trace element provision is very important.

Long-term PN

Home care is well established in the UK, with some patients successfully supported for over 20 years. Total or supplemental PN may be appropriate. Trace elements, notably selenium, should be managed closely as requirements may be increased.

Most patients are extremely well informed about their underlying disease and their PN; many also benefit from support group PINNT (Patients on Intravenous and Nasogastric Nutrition Therapy) and LITRE (Looking into the Requirements for Equipment), a standing committee of BAPEN which looks at equipment issues.

There are an increasing number of patients at home on PN. Scotland and Wales now have designated networks to care for these patients. Many patients are trained to connect and disconnect their PN and to care for their central lines. Patients are encouraged to lead as active and normal life as possible. Foreign travel is now possible for patients on home PN, as are most other normal daily activities and sports (Staun et al., 2009).

Paediatric PN

Nutritional requirements

Early nutritional intervention is required in paediatric patients due to their low reserve, especially in neonates. Where possible, premature neonates should commence feeding from day 1. In addition to requirements for the maintenance of body tissue, function and repair, it is also important to support growth and development, especially in the infant and adolescent.

Typical guidelines for average daily requirements of fluid, energy and nitrogen are shown in Table 7.14. The dual-energy approach is favoured in paediatrics. Approximately 30% of the non-protein calories are provided as lipid using a 20% emulsion. Most centres gradually increase the lipid provision from day 1 from 1 g/kg/day to 2 g/kg/day and then 3 g/kg/day, monitoring lipid clearance through the serum triglyceride level. This ensures the essential fatty acid requirements of premature neonates are met.

Formulation and stability issues

Many centres use standard PN formulations including the specific paediatric amino acid solutions (Primene® or Vaminolact®). Prescriptions and formulations are tailored to reflect clinical status, biochemistry and nutritional requirements.

Micronutrients are included daily. Paediatric licensed preparations are available and are included on a ml/kg basis up to a maximum total volume (Peditrace®, Solivito® N and Vitlipid® N Infant). Electrolytes are also monitored and included in all formulations on a mmol/kg basis. Acid–base balance should be considered. Potassium and sodium acetate salt forms are used in balance with the chloride salt forms in neonatal formulae to avoid excessive chloride

Table 7.14 Suggested paediatric daily PN requirements (adapted from Koletzko et al., 2005)

		Day 1	Day 2	Day 3	Day 4	Na+	K+	Ca²⁺	Mg²⁺
		>1 month but <10 kg				mmol/kg/day			
Fluid requirement	100 ml/kg								
						3	2.5	0.6	0.1
Nitrogen	g/kg	0.15	0.2	0.3	0.4				
Glucose	g/kg	10	12	14	16				
Lipid	g/kg	1	2	2	3				
Phosphate[a]	mmol/kg/day	0.5	0.58	0.58	0.6				
		10–15 kg							
Fluid requirement	1000 ml + 50 ml/kg for each kg above 10 kg								
						3	2.5	0.2	0.07
Nitrogen	g/kg	0.15	0.2	0.3	0.3				
Glucose	g/kg	6	8	10	12				
Lipid	g/kg	1.5	2	2.5	2.5				
Phosphate[a]	mmol/kg/day	0.23	0.27	0.3	0.3				
		16–20 kg							
Fluid requirement	1000 ml + 50 ml/kg for each kg above 10 kg								
						3	2	0.2	0.07
Nitrogen	g/kg	0.15	0.2	0.3	0.3				
Glucose	g/kg	4	6	8	10				
Lipid	g/kg	1.5	2	2	2				
Phosphate[a]	mmol/kg/day	0.22	0.26	0.26	0.26				

Continued

Table 7.14 Suggested paediatric daily PN requirements (adapted from Koletzko et al., 2005)—Cont'd

21–30 kg							
Fluid requirement	1500 ml + 20 ml/kg for each kg above 20 kg						
					3	2	0.2	0.07
Nitrogen	g/kg	0.2	0.3	0.3			
Glucose	g/kg	4	6	8			
Lipid	g/kg	1	2	2			
Phosphate[a]	mmol/kg/day	0.18	0.26	0.26			
>30 kg							
Fluid requirement	1500 ml + 20 ml/kg for each kg above 20 kg						
					3	2	0.2	0.07
Nitrogen	g/kg	0.15	0.2				
Glucose	g/kg	3	5				
Lipid	g/kg	1	2				
Phosphate[a]	mmol/kg/day	0.18	0.25				

[a] includes phosphate from lipid emulsion and Vitlipid® preparations.

input contributing to acidosis (acetate is metabolised to bicarbonate, an alkali). In the initial stages, neonates tend to hypernatraemia due to relatively poor renal clearance; this should be reflected in the standard formulae used.

Due to the balance of nutritional requirements, a relatively high glucose requirement with high calcium and phosphate provision, the neonatal and paediatric prescription may be supplied by a separate 2-in-1 bag of amino acids, glucose, trace elements and electrolytes and a lipid syringe with vitamins. These are generally given concurrently, joining at a Y-site. Older children can sometimes be managed with 3-in-1 formulations. A single infusion is particularly useful in the home care environment. Some ready-to-use formulations are licensed for use in paediatrics and include the Kabiven® and OliClinomel® range.

Improved stability profiles with the new lipid emulsions, and increasing stability data, may support 3-in-1 formulations that meet the nutritional requirements of younger children.

Concerns over the contamination of calcium gluconate with aluminium and the association between aluminium contamination of neonatal PN and impaired neurological development have favoured the use of calcium chloride over gluconate; however, chloride load should be considered if the former is used. If calcium gluconate is to be used it must be from plastic containers.

Heparin

Historically, low concentrations of heparin were included in 2-in-1 formulations in an attempt to improve fat clearance through enhanced triglyceride hydrolysis, prevent the formation of fibrin around the infusion line, reduce thrombo-sis and reduce thrombophlebitis during peripheral infusion; however, this is no longer recommended. It is recognised that when the 2-in-1 formulation comes into contact with the lipid phase, calcium-heparin bridges form between these lipid globules, destabilising the formulation. Also, there is limited evidence of clinical benefit of the heparin inclusion.

Route of administration

Peripheral administration is less common in neonates and children due to the risk of thrombophlebitis; however, it is useful when low-concentration, short-term PN is required and there is good peripheral access. The maximum glucose concentration for peripheral administration in paediatrics is generally regarded to be 12%. However, considering all the other factors that can affect the tonicity of a regimen and peripheral tolerance, it is clear that this is a relatively simplistic perspective. Many centres favour a limit of 10% with close clinical observation.

Central administration is via a PICC, a long-term tunnelled central line, a jugular or subclavian line. Femoral lines are a less preferred option owing to their location and, therefore, high risk of becoming infected.

Case study

Case 7.1

Mrs B, aged 47, was admitted for investigation of chronic diarrhoea and 6 kg weight loss over the past 3 months.
See Table 7.15.

Table 7.15 Clinical details for Case 7.1

Day	Clinical observation/event	PN changes
1	Admitted to gastroenterology ward from clinic for investigation of chronic diarrhoea and weight loss. Current weight 49 kg, height 1.65 m. Usual weight 55 kg, 1.65 m. Estimated current energy requirement 1500 kcal.	
2	Contrast study revealed intestinal fistula between small bowel and transverse colon. Diarrhoea approx. 1.5 L/day.	
3	Case discussed with surgeons. For PN for 2–3 weeks prior to surgery to improve nutritional status. Patient made 'nil by mouth'. Central line inserted for PN use only.	PN prescribed (considering both fluid and electrolytes from other therapies, and potassium loss from diarrhoea of approx. 30–70 mmol/L): Volume 2 L, nitrogen 9 g, carbohydrate 400 kcal, lipid 550 kcal, Na^+ 230 mmol, K^+ 80 mmol, Ca^{2+} 5 mmol, Mg^{2+} 11 mmol, phosphate 35 mmol and micronutrients added (daily).
4	Biochemistry results: Na^+ 129 mmol/L (135–145 mmol/L), K^+ 3.2 mmol/L (3.4–5.0 mmol/L), urea 6.9 mmol/L (3.1–7.9 mmol/L), Cr 86 µmol/L (75–1550 µmol/L), corr Ca^{2+} 2.3 mmol/L (2.12–2.60 mmol/L), Mg^{2+} 0.75 mmol/L (0.7–1.0 mmol/L), phosphate 0.85 mmol/L (0.80–1.44 mmol/L). Temperature/pulse/respiration normal, diarrhoea losses reduced to 800 mL/day.	Regimen unchanged.
5	Biochemistry results: Na^+ 132 mmol/L, K^+ 3.1 mmol/L, urea 4.3 mmol/L, Cr 85 µmol/L, corr Ca^{2+} 2.2 mmol/L, Mg^{2+} 0.50 mmol/L, phosphate 0.60 mmol/L	PN regimen unchanged. Additional 20 mmol Mg^{2+} prescribed in 500 mL of saline infused over 6 h.
6	Biochemistry results: Na^+ 138 mmol/L, K^+ 3.5 mmol/L, urea 3.0 mmol/L, Cr 86 µmol/L, corr Ca 2.2 mmol/L, Mg^{2+} 0.78 mmol/L, phosphate 0.9 mmol/L. Diarrhoea reduced to 500 mL/day.	PN regimen changed to: Volume 2 L, nitrogen 11 g, carbohydrate 800 kcal, lipid 800 kcal, Na^+ 100 mmol, K^+ 80 mmol, Ca^{2+} 5 mmol, Mg^{2+} 15 mmol, phosphate 40 mmol.
7	Biochemistry results: Na^+ 139 mmol/L, K^+ 4.1 mmol/L, urea 2.8 mmol/L, Cr 78 µmol/L, Mg^{2+} 0.95 mmol/L, phosphate 1.3 mmol/L.	K^+ reduced to 60 mmol, Mg^{2+} reduced to 10 mmol, phosphate reduced to 30 mmol.

Questions

1. Calculate Mrs B's current body mass index (BMI)
2. Why were the calories provided in the initial bags less than Mrs B's requirements?
3. Why should potassium, magnesium and phosphate levels be monitored closely and explain a possible reason for the slight drop in these biochemical values on day 5?
4. Explain why the amounts of sodium and potassium were chosen in the initial formulation.
5. What additional vitamin should have been prescribed prior to PN starting?
6. Why was no extra magnesium given in the PN on day 5?
7. How much nutrition can be provided to promote weight gain and how could this be provided?

Answers

1. 18 kg/m².
2. Mrs B's significant weight loss, low BMI and likely malabsorption place her at risk of refeeding syndrome. An initial maximum rate of 10–20 kcal/kg is recommended. In practice, this is often achieved by administering half the patient's nutritional requirements over 24 h; however, the provision of adequate quantities of magnesium, potassium and phosphate can be problematic. It is also essential that sufficient micronutrients are provided, especially thiamine, to ensure effective metabolism of the macronutrients provided.
3. Potassium, magnesium and phosphate are all driven intracellularly during the refeeding response.
4. In 1500 mL of diarrhoea, Mrs B will lose approximately 180 mmol sodium and 38 mmol potassium; this should be added

to her basic requirements of 50 mmol sodium and 50 mmol potassium.

5. Oral thiamine or full dose intravenous vitamin B should have been prescribed to minimise the risk of refeeding syndrome.
6. Extra magnesium could not be added to the regimen on day 5 due to the stability limits for the regimen prescribed. The lipid content of the regimen places tight limits on the divalent ion content. This can be overcome by using lipid-free regimens, but this must be considered in the context of the patient's long-term nutritional plan.
7. Mrs B's predicted basic metabolic rate is only 1250 kcal. Allowing for activity, energy expenditure can be expected to increase to 1500 kcal. The provision of additional calories to promote weight gain is only appropriate if the patient is in an anabolic state and able to utilise the additional energy and nitrogen effectively to gain functional tissue. Excessive calorie intake in the face of ongoing catabolism is most likely to increase metabolic stress and increase the risk of complications such as abnormal LFTs. An additional 400–1000 kcal/day is considered sufficient to promote weight gain. The increased calories can be provided within a 3-in-1 regimen but care should be taken not to exceed the predicted glucose oxidation rate or lipid intake of 1.5 g/kg/day.

Acknowledgement

This chapter is based on the contribution which first appeared in the fourth edition of this textbook edited by S.J. Dunnett.

References

Bethune, K., Allwood, M., Grainger, C., et al., 2001. Use of filters during the preparation and administration of parenteral nutrition: position paper and guidelines prepared by a British Pharmaceutical Nutrition Group Working Party. Nutrition 17, 403–408.

British Association of Parenteral and Enteral Nutrition, 2003. Malnutrition Universal Screening Tool. Available at: www.bapen.org.uk/musttoolkit.html.

Cano, N.J.M., Aparicio, M., Brunori, G., et al., 2009. ESPEN guidelines on parenteral nutrition: acute renal failure. Clin. Nutr. 28, 401–414.

Crook, M.A., 2000. Lipid clearance and total parenteral nutrition: the importance of monitoring of plasma lipids. Nutrition 16, 774–775.

De Meijer, V.E., Gura, K.M., Le, H.D., 2009. Fish oil-based emulsions prevent and reverse parenteral nutrition associated liver disease: the Boston experience. J. Parent. Ent. Nutr. 33, 541–547.

Department of Health, 1991. Dietary Reference Values for Food Energy and Nutrients for the United Kingdom. Report of the panel on dietary reference values of the committee on medical aspects of food policy. DH, London.

Fleming, C.R., 1989. Trace element metabolism in adult patients requiring total parenteral nutrition. Am. J. Clin. Nutr. 49, 573–579.

Foulks, C.J., 1999. An evidence-based evaluation of intradialytic parenteral nutrition. Am. J. Kidney Dis. 33, 186–192.

Gianotti, L., Meier, R., Lobo, D., et al., 2009. ESPEN guidelines on nutrition in pancreatitis. Clin. Nutr. 28, 428–435.

Holick, M., 2007. Vitamin D deficiency. N. Engl. J. Med. 357, 266–281.

Khawaja, H.T., Williams, J.D., 1991. Transdermal glyceryl trinitrate to allow peripheral total parenteral nutrition: a double blind placebo controlled feasibility study. J. R. Soc. Med. 84, 69–72.

Kings Fund Report, 1992. A Positive Approach to Nutrition as Treatment. Kings Fund, London.

Koletzko, B., Goulet, O., Hunt, J., 2005. Guidelines on paediatric parenteral nutrition of the European Society of Paediatric Gastroenterology, Hepatology and Nutrition (ESPGHAN) and the European Society for Clinical Nutrition and Metabolism (ESPEN), supported by the European Society of Paediatric Research (ESPR). J. Pediatr. Gastroenterol. Nutr. 41, S1–S4 Available at: http://espghan.med.up.pt/joomla/position_papers/con_22.pdf.

Lazarus, J.M., 1999. Recommended criteria for initiating and discontinuing intradialytic parenteral nutrition. Am. J. Kidney Dis. 33, 211–216.

Maroulis, J., Kalfarentzos, F., 2000. Complications of parenteral nutrition at the end of the century. Clin. Nutr. 19, 299–304.

National Institute for Health and Clinical Excellence, 2006. Nutrition Support in Adults CG32. NICE, London. Available at: http://www.nice.org.uk/guidance/CG32.

Nitenberg, G., Raynard, B., 2000. Nutritional support of the cancer patient: issues and dilemmas. Crit. Rev. Oncol./Haematology 34, 137–168.

Plauth, M., Cabre, E., Canpillo, B., et al., 2009. ESPEN guidelines on parenteral nutrition: hepatology. Clin. Nutr. 28, 436–444.

Staun, M., Pironi, L., Bozzetti, F., et al., 2009. ESPEN guidelines on parenteral nutrition: home parenteral nutrition (HPN) in adult patients. Clin. Nutr. 28, 467–479.

Further reading

Austin, P., Stroud, M. (Eds.), 2007. Prescribing Adult Intravenous Nutrition. Pharmaceutical Press, London.

Ainsworth, S.B., Clerihew, L., McGuire, W., 2007. Percutaneous central venous catheters versus peripheral cannulae for delivery of parenteral nutrition in neonates. Cochrane Database Syst. Rev. 3. Art. No.: CD004219. doi:10.1002/14651858.CD004219.pub3.

Baskin, J.L., Pui, C.H., Reiss, U., et al., 2009. Management of occlusion and thrombosis with long-term indwelling central venous catheters. Lancet 374, 159–169.

Goulet, O., 2009. Some new insights in intestinal failure-associated liver disease. Curr. Opin. Org. Transplant. 14, 256–261.

Lloyd, D.A., Gabe, S.M., 2007. Managing liver dysfunction in parenteral nutrition. Proc. Nutr. Soc. 66, 530–538.

Misra, S., Kirby, D.F., 2000. Micronutrient and trace element monitoring in adult nutrition support. Nutr. Clin. Pract. 15, 120–126.

Schofield, 1985. Equations for estimating basal metabolic rate (BMR). Clin. Nutr. 39C, 5–41.

Shenkin, A., 1995. Trace elements and inflammatory response: implications for nutritional support. Nutrition 11, 100–105.

Useful websites

British Pharmaceutical Nutrition Group. Available at: http://. www.bpng.co.uk.

American Society for Parenteral and Enteral Nutrition. Available at: http://www.nutritioncare.org/

8 Pharmacoeconomics

J. Cooke

Key points

- Expenditure on medicines is increasing at a greater rate than other health care costs.
- Increasingly governments are employing health economics to help prioritise between different medicines and other health technologies.
- In health economics, consequences of a treatment can be expressed in monetary terms (cost–benefit), natural units of effectiveness (cost-effectiveness) and in terms of patient preference or utility (cost–utility).
- Head-to-head studies offer the best way of determining overall effectiveness and cost-effectiveness.
- Sensitivity analysis can be used to address areas of uncertainty.
- Medication non-adherence, medication errors and unwanted drug effects place a considerable burden on societal health care costs.
- Decision analysis techniques offer a powerful tool for comparing alternative treatment options.

The demand for and the cost of health care are growing in all countries. Many governments are focusing their activities on promoting the effective and economic use of resources allocated to health care. The increased use of evidence-based programmes not only concentrates on optimizing health outcomes but also utilises health economic evaluations.

While there have been marked gains in life expectancy in those countries which make up the Organization for Economic Co-operation and Development (OECD), health costs have also risen in all of them. The USA spent 16% of its national income (gross domestic product, GDP) on health in 2007, a value considerably greater than many other OECD countries (Fig. 8.1).

Medicines form a small but significant proportion of total health care costs; this has been increasing consistently as new medicines are marketed. For example, the overall NHS expenditure on medicines in England in 2008 was £11.6 billion. Primary care expenditure was £8.1 million and hospital use accounted for 28.7% of the total cost at £3.3 million, up from 25.8% in 2007. The cost of medicines has increased by 3.4% overall and by 15.2% in hospitals.

Most OECD countries have seen growth in spending on medicines outstrip growth in total health spending over this period. In the USA and Australia, pharmaceutical spending has increased at more than double the rate of growth in total health spending (OECD, 2009).

There are a number of reasons why prescribing costs are increasing:

- Demographic changes have resulted in an ageing population which is living longer and has greater needs for therapeutic interventions. This patient group is more susceptible to unwanted effects of medicines which in turn consume more resources.
- More patients have complex clinical problems and co-morbidities that have higher dependency on medicines.
- Health screening programmes and improved diagnostic techniques are uncovering previously non-identified diseases, which subsequently require treatment.
- The marketing of new medicines that offer more effective and less toxic alternatives to existing agents. Invariably these are more expensive, especially biotechnology medicines, such as monoclonal antibodies which can cost in excess of £30,000 per patient per year.
- The use of existing agents becoming more widespread as additional indications for their use are found.
- Increasing numbers of standards in guidelines of care are being set by national bodies such as the National Institute for Health and Clinical Excellence (NICE).
- Public and patients have a higher expectation of their rights to access high-cost health care.
- Higher acquisition costs are also due to inflation and currency fluctuations.

In the UK, health reforms over the past decade have addressed the quality of care through promotion of quality and safety standards. The formation of NICE in 1998

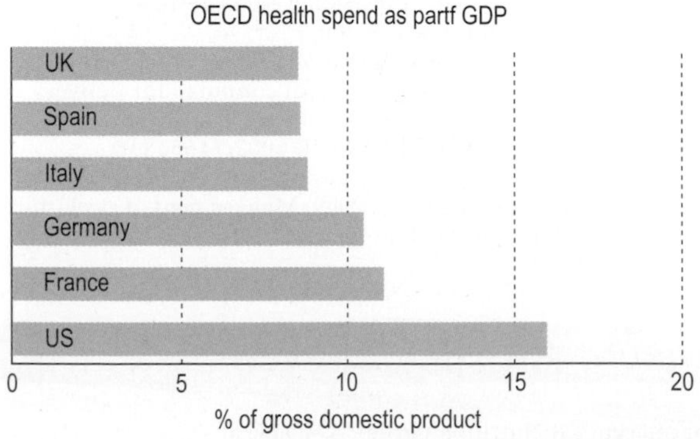

Fig. 8.1 Comparison of health spend as a percentage of gross domestic product in different countries in 2007 (OECD, 2009).

'to improve standards of patient care and to reduce inequities in access to innovative treatment' has formalised this process. NICE undertakes appraisals of medicines and other treatments (health technologies) and addresses the clinical and cost-effectiveness of therapies and compares outcomes with alternative use of NHS funds. The increased use of evidence-based programmes not only concentrates on optimizing health outcomes but also utilises health economic evaluations. Formalised health technology assessments provide an in-depth and evidence-based approach to this process.

Terms used in health economics

Pharmacoeconomics can be defined as the measurement of both the costs and consequences of therapeutic decision making. Pharmacoeconomics provides a guide for decision makers on resource allocation but does not offer a basis on which decisions should be made. Pharmacoeconomics can assist in the planning process and help assign priorities where, for example, medicines with a worse outcome may be available at a lower cost and medicines with better outcome and higher cost can be compared.

When economic evaluations are conducted it is important to categorise various costs. Costs can be direct to the organisation, that is physicians' salaries, the acquisition costs of medicines, consumables associated with drug administration, staff time in preparation and administration of medicines, laboratory charges for monitoring effectiveness and adverse drug reactions. Indirect costs include lost productivity from a disease which can manifest itself as a cost to the economy or taxation system as well as economic costs to the patient and the patient's family. All aspects of the use of medicines may be allocated costs, both direct, such as acquisition and administration costs, and indirect, such as the cost of a given patient's time off work because of illness, in terms of lost output and social security payments. The consequences of drug therapy include benefits for both the individual patient and society at large and may be quantified in terms of health outcome and quality of life, in addition to the purely economic impact.

It is worthwhile here to describe a number of definitions that further qualify costs in a health care setting. The concept of *opportunity cost* is at the centre of economics and identifies the value of opportunities which have been lost by utilizing resources in a particular service or health technology. This can be valued as the benefits that have been forsaken by investing the resources in the best alternative fashion. Opportunity cost recognises that there are limited resources available for utilising every treatment, and therefore the rationing of health care is implicit in such a system.

Average costs are the simplest way of valuing the consumption of health care resources. Quite simply, they represent the total costs (i.e. all the costs incurred in the delivery of a service) of a health care system divided by the units of production. For example, a hospital might treat 75,000 patients a year (defined as finished consultant episodes, FCEs) and have a total annual revenue cost of £150 million. The average cost per FCE is, therefore, £2000.

Fixed costs are those which are independent of the number of units of production and include heating, lighting and fixed staffing costs. *Variable costs*, on the other hand, are dependent on the numbers of units of productivity. The cost of the consumption of medicines is a good example of variable costs.

The inevitable increases in the medicines budget in a particular institute which is treating more patients, or treating those with a more complex pathology, have often been erroneously interpreted by financial managers as a failure to effectively manage the budget. To better describe the costs associated with a health care intervention, economists employ the term '*marginal costs*' to describe the costs of producing an extra unit of a particular service. The term '*incremental cost*' is employed to define the difference between the costs of alternative interventions.

Choice of comparator

Sometimes a claim is made that a treatment is cost effective. But cost effective against what? As in any good clinical trial, a treatment has to be compared against a reasonable comparator. The choice of comparator is crucial to this process. A comparator that is no longer in common use or in a dose that is not optimal will result in the evaluated treatment being seen as more effective than it actually is. Sadly many evaluations of medicines fall into this trap as sponsors seldom wish to undertake head-to-head studies against competitors. Again, the reader has to be careful when interpreting economic evaluations from settings which are different from those in local practice. A common error can be made when viewing international studies that have different health care costs and ways of treating patients and translating them directly into 'one's own practice'.

In addition, hospital charges, including those for hotel services such as heating and lighting overheads, meals and accommodation, which may constitute a major cost, should be considered. These are frequently included in an average cost per patient day.

Types of health economic evaluations

Cost–benefit analysis (CBA)

In CBA, consequences are measured in terms of the total cost associated with a programme where both costs and consequences are measured in monetary terms. While this type of analysis is preferred by economists, its use in health care is problematical as it is frequently difficult to ascribe monetary values to clinical outcomes such as pain relief, avoidance of stroke or improvements in quality of life.

Methods are available for determining cost–benefit for individual groups of patients that centre around a concept known as *contingent valuation*. Specific techniques include *willingness to pay*, where patients are asked to state how much they would be prepared to pay to avoid a particular event or symptom, for example pain or nausea following day-care surgery. Willingness to pay can be fraught with difficulties of interpretation in countries with socialised health care systems which are invariably funded out of general taxation. *Willingness to accept* is a similar concept but is based on the minimum amount an individual person or population would receive in order to be prepared to lose or reduce a service.

CBA can be usefully employed at a macro level for strategic decisions on health care programmes. For example, a countrywide immunisation programme can be fully costed in terms of resource utilisation consumed in running the programme. This can then be valued against the reduced mortality and morbidity that occur as a result of the programme.

CBA can be useful in examining the value of services, for example centralised intravenous additive services where a comparison between a pharmacy-based intravenous additive service and ward-based preparation by doctors and nurses may demonstrate the value of the centralised pharmacy service, or a clinical pharmacokinetics service where the staffing and equipment costs can be offset against the benefits of reduced morbidity and mortality.

Cost-effectiveness analysis (CEA)

CEA can be described as an examination of the costs of two or more programmes which have the same clinical outcome as measured in physical units, for example lives saved or reduced morbidity. Treatments with dissimilar outcomes can also be analysed by this technique. Where two or more interventions have been shown to be or are assumed to be similar, then if all other factors are equal, for example convenience, side effects, availability, etc., selection can be made on the basis of cost. This type of analysis is called cost-minimisation analysis (CMA). CMA is frequently employed in formulary decision making where often the available evidence for a new product appears to be no better than for existing products. This is invariably what happens in practice as clinical trials on new medicines are statistically powered for equivalence as a requirement for licensing submission.

As previously described, CEA examines the costs associated with achieving a defined health outcome. While these outcomes can be relief of symptoms such as nausea and vomiting avoided, pain relieved, etc., CEA frequently employs years of life gained as a measure of the success of a particular programme. This can then offer a method of incrementally comparing the costs associated with two or more interventions. For example, consider a hypothetical case of the comparison of two drug treatments for the management of malignant disease.

Treatment 1 represents a 1-year course of treatment for a particular malignant disease. Assume that this is the current standard form of treatment and that the average total direct costs associated with this programme are £A per year. This will include the costs of the medicines, antiemetics, inpatient stay, radiology and pathology. Treatment 2 is a new drug treatment for the malignancy which as a result of comparative controlled clinical trials has demonstrated an improvement in the average life expectancy for this group of patients from 3.5 years for treatment 1 to 4.5 years for treatment 2. The average annual total costs for treatment 2 are £B. A comparative table can now be constructed.

Strategy	Treatment costs	Effectiveness
Treatment 1	£A	3.5 years
Treatment 2	£B	4.5 years

Incremental cost-effectiveness ratio:

$$= £B - £A / (4.5 - 3.5) \text{ per life year gained.}$$

Cost–utility analysis (CUA)

An alternative measurement for the consequences of a health care intervention is the concept of utility. Utility provides a method for estimating patient preference for a particular intervention in terms of the patient's state of well-being. Utility is described by an index which ranges between 0 (representing death) and 1 (perfect health). The product of utility and life years gained provides the term quality-adjusted life-year (QALY).

There are a number of methods for the calculation of utilities.

- The *Rosser–Kind matrix* relies on preferences from population samples from certain disease groups.
- The *visual analogue scale* method seeks to obtain patient preferences for their perceived disease state by scoring themselves on a line scaled between 0 and 1 as above.
- The *standard gamble* method requires individuals to choose between living the rest of their lives in their current state of health or making a gamble of an intervention which will restore them to perfect health. Failure of the gamble will result in instant death. The probabilities of the gamble are varied until there is indifference between the two events.
- The *time trade-off* method requires individuals to decide how many of their remaining years of life expectancy they would be prepared to exchange for complete health.

Using the previous model, if treatment 1 provides on average an increase of 3.5 years life expectancy but that this is valued at a utility of 0.9, then the health gain for this intervention is 0.9 × 3.5 = 3.15 QALYs. Similarly, if the increase in life expectancy with treatment 2 only has a utility of 0.8 (perhaps because it produces more nausea) then the health gain for this option becomes 0.8 × 4.5 = 3.6 QALYS. An incremental CUA can be undertaken as follows:

Strategy	Treatment costs	Effectiveness	Utility
Treatment 1	£A	3.5 years	0.9
Treatment 2	£B	4.5 years	0.8

Incremental cost–utility ratio:

$$= (£B - £A) / [(4.5 × 0.8) - (3.5 × 0.9)] \text{ per QALY gained.}$$

The calculation of QALYs provides a method which enables decision makers to compare different health interventions and assign priorities for decisions on resource allocation. However, the use of QALY league tables has provided much debate amongst stakeholders of health care as to their value and use.

According to NICE, there is no empirical basis for assigning a particular value (or values) to the cut-off between cost-effectiveness and cost-ineffectiveness. The general view is that those interventions with an incremental cost-effectiveness ratio of less than £20,000 per QALY should be supported and that there should be increasingly strong reasons for accepting as cost-effective interventions with an incremental cost-effectiveness ratio of over £30,000 per QALY.

Costs and consequences

Discounting

Discounting is an economic term which is based mainly on a time preference that assumes individuals prefer to forego a part of the benefits of a programme if they can have those benefits now rather than fully in an uncertain future. The value of this preference is expressed by the discount rate. There is intense debate amongst health economists regarding the value for this annual discount level and whether both costs and consequences should be subjected to discounting. If a programme does not exceed 1 year then discounting is felt to be unnecessary.

Decision analysis

Decision analysis offers a method of pictorial representation of treatment decisions. If the results from clinical trials are available, probabilities can be placed within the arms of a decision tree and outcomes can be assessed in either monetary or quality units. An example of this can be found in the assessment of glycoprotein IIb/IIIa inhibitors in acute coronary syndrome (National Institute for Health and Clinical Excellence, 2002). The evidence of clinical and economic outcomes compares percutaneous coronary intervention and coronary artery bypass grafting. To populate a decision tree, it is necessary to obtain information from the literature on the probabilities for the clinical benefits and risks of each procedure (Table 8.1). The costs of the various procedures, consumables and bed stay are then calculated (Table 8.2). From these a decision tree can be constructed that determines the cost-effectiveness of one intervention over another (Fig. 8.2).

Table 8.1 Baseline probabilities used in the short-term model of percutaneous coronary intervention (PCI) versus coronary artery bypass graph (CABG; National Institute for Health and Clinical Excellence, 2002)

Node	Description	Probability	Parameters of the beta distribution	
			α	β
A	Acute PCI	0.05	53	980
B	Repeat revasc.	0.048	8	157
C	Repeat revasc. PCI	1.00	–	–
D	Death (revasc. PCI)	0.00	0.01	7.99
E	MI (revasc. PCI)	0.13	1	7
F	Death (revasc. CABG)	0.00	–	–
G	MI (revasc. CABG)	0.00	–	–
H	Death (no repeat revasc.)	0.03	5	152
I	MI (no repeat revasc.)	0.03	5	147
J	CABG	0.05	47	933
K	Death (CABG)	0.11	5	42
L	MI (CABG)	0.07	3	39
M	6-month revasc.	0.05	48	885
N	6-month revasc. PCI	0.48	23	25
O	Death (6-month revasc. PCI)	0.09	2	21
P	MI (6-month revasc. PCI)	0.10	2	19
Q	Death (6-month revasc. CABG)	0.00	0.01	24.99
R	MI (6-month revasc. CABG)	0.16	4	21

Table 8.1 Baseline probabilities used in the short-term model of percutaneous coronary intervention (PCI) versus coronary artery bypass graph (CABG; National Institute for Health and Clinical Excellence, 2002)—cont'd

Node	Description	Probability	Parameters of the beta distribution	
			α	β
S	Death (no revasc.)	0.08	68	817
T	MI (no revasc.)	0.05	40	777
	Baseline risk of gastro-intestinal bleeding:			
	(i) Undergoing PCI in acute period	0.00	0.01	52.99
	(ii) Undergoing CABG in acute period	0.02	1	46
	(iii) No initial revasc.	0.01	12	921

CABG, coronary artery bypass graft; MI, myocardial infarction; PCI, percutaneous coronary intervention; revasc., revascularisation intervention; MI, myocardial infarction.

Table 8.2 Unit costs used in the analysis of percutaneous coronary intervention (PCI) versus coronary artery bypass graph (CABG; National Institute for Health and Clinical Excellence, 2002)

Unit cost	Unit	Base-case value
PCI	Procedure	£1410.04
CABG	Procedure	£4902.22
Repeat PCI	Per diem	£2976
Angiogram	Procedure	£748.25
Cardiac ward	Day	£157.47
Non-cardiac ward	Day	£244.00
CCU	Day	£459.04
Outpatient	Visit	£59.70
Cardiac day case	Visit	£108.58
Non-cardiac day case	Visit	£182.00
Guidewire	Item	£61.75
Stent	Item	£599.01
Guiding catheter	Item	£37.05
Blood	Unit	£85.00
Full blood count	Item	£4.00
Endoscopy	Item	£246.00
Tirofiban	12.5 mg vial	£146.11 (+VAT)
Eptifibatide	20 mg vial	£15.54 (+VAT)
Eptifibatide	75 mg vial	£48.84 (+VAT)

Table 8.2 Unit costs used in the analysis of percutaneous coronary intervention (PCI) versus coronary artery bypass graph (CABG; National Institute for Health and Clinical Excellence, 2002)—cont'd

Unit cost	Unit	Base-case value
Abciximab	10 mg vial	£280.00 (+VAT)
Omeprazole	28 tab pack 10 mg	£18.91
Clopidogrel	28 tab pack 75 mg	£35.31

CABG, coronary artery bypass graft; CCU, coronary care unit; PCI, percutaneous coronary intervention.

If there is uncertainty about the robustness of the values of the variables within the tree, they can be varied within defined ranges to see if the overall direction of the tree changes. This is referred to as *sensitivity analysis* and is one of the most powerful tools available in an economic evaluation.

Economic evaluation of medicines

A number of countries have introduced explicit guidelines for the conduct of economic evaluations of medicines. Others require economic evaluations before allowing a medicine onto an approved list or formulary. Guidelines have been published which aim to provide researchers and peer reviewers with background guidance on how to conduct an economic evaluation and how to check its quality (Drummond et al., 2005), whilst others (National Institute for Health and Clinical Excellence, 2009a,b) have set out how they incorporate health economics in the evaluation of medicines.

Risk management of unwanted drug effects

Avoiding the adverse effects of medicines has become a desirable goal of therapeutic decision makers as well as those who promote quality assurance and risk management. Not only can there be

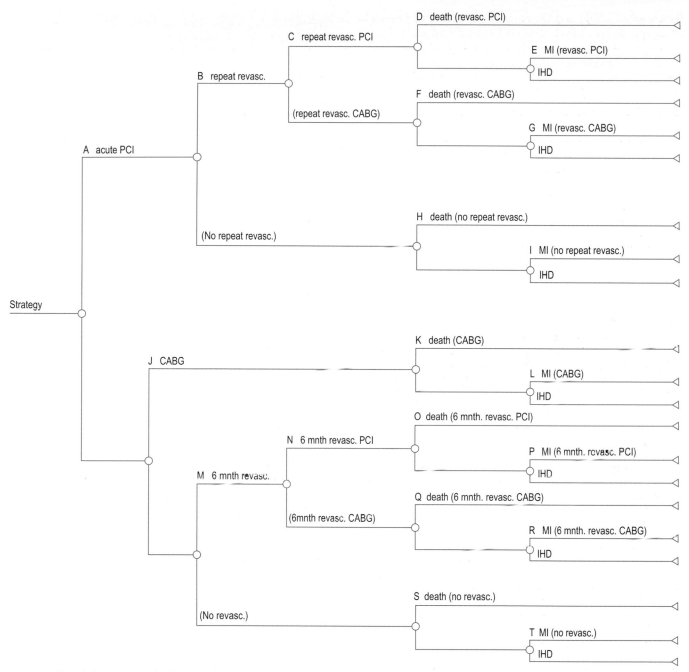

Fig. 8.2 Clinical decision tree for choices of percutaneous coronary intervention (PCI) versus coronary artery bypass graph (CABG; National Institute for Health and Clinical Excellence, 2002). MI, myocardial infarction; IHD, ischaemic heart disease; revasc., revascularisation intervention.

significant sequelae in terms of increased morbidity associated with adverse drug effects but the economic consequences can be considerable. For example, gentamicin is often regarded as a relatively inexpensive antibiotic but in the USA each case of nephrotoxicity has been reported to cost several thousands of pounds in terms of additional resources consumed even without any assessment of the reduction in a patient's quality of life. The increasingly litigious nature of society has resulted in economic valuation of perceived negligence, for example, with irreversible vestibular toxicity associated with prolonged unmonitored aminoglycoside therapy. As a result, many health care systems have targeted a significant reduction in the number of serious errors in the use of prescribed medicines.

Medication non-adherence

The costs of non-adherence with medicines are considerable. In the USA, it has been calculated that 11% of all admissions to hospital are directly associated with some form of non-adherence. This equates to two million hospital admissions a year in the USA resulting from medication non-adherence at a total cost of over £5 billion. In addition, lost work productivity through non-adherence has been estimated to cost in excess of a further £3 billion per year. The scale of the problem in the UK is probably similar.

In the UK, between a half and one-third of all medicines prescribed for long-term conditions are not taken as recommended

(Horne et al., 2005) and the estimated drug cost of unused or unwanted medicines in the NHS in England is around £100 million a year (Department of Health, 2008) annually. National guidance on medicines adherence has been issued (National Institute for Health and Clinical Excellence, 2009a,b).

Incentives and disincentives

There are good examples of both incentives and disincentives being used in the NHS to save money. In England, the contract for hospitals penalises those organisations that fail to achieve their targets for reducing *Clostridium difficile* infections. Good antimicrobial stewardship is essential for addressing this as each case of *Clostridium difficile* infection can cost at least £4000. Reduction in prescribing of both fluoroquinolones and second and third generation cephalosporins is associated with a reduction in *Clostridium difficile* infection (Department of Health and Health Protection Agency, 2008). It follows from this that reducing the use of these agents can reduce acquisition costs of the medicines.

Examples of incentives to reduce expenditure can be seen within the NHS commissioning processes in England. A typical example involves a scheme where commissioners must make 1.5% of contract value (or equivalent non-contract activity value) available for each provider's quality and innovation scheme and these include prescribing targets (Department of Health, 2010).

Conclusion

A fundamental element of the use of pharmacoeconomics in practice is the viewpoint from which the analysis is conducted. Ideally this should be from a societal perspective but frequently it is from a government or Department of Health

---

Box 8.1   Ten examples of the application of pharmacoeconomics in practice

- The value of one treatment over another in terms of the cost for each unit of health gained
- Avoidance of costs associated with the failure to use an appropriate medicine, for example antimicrobial surgical prophylaxis
- Avoidance of the costs of the side effects or adverse effects of a medicine
- Financial planning and horizon scanning for new medicines
- Prioritisation of health care resources
- Health gain, quality of life issues and patient preferences
- Duration of care and balance between inpatient, day care and outpatient care
- Changes in legislative controls, for example reclassification of medicines from prescription only to pharmacy status
- Costs of concordance and non-concordance
- Economics of health service delivery

---

viewpoint. Purchasers of health care may also have a different perspective from provider units, and the viewpoint of clinicians may differ from that of the patient. The pharmaceutical industry will probably have another viewpoint that will be focused on their particular products. As a consequence, with all economic evaluations the perspective from which they have been analysed should be clear.

The effect of having budgets that are rigorously defended in every section of the health service, as occurs with the medicines budget, is to deny the application of economic decision making in the most efficient way for the population served. It is clear that pharmacoeconomics has an important part to play in the practice of therapeutics (Box 8.1) and needs to be an integral part of all planned therapeutic developments.

References

Department of Health, 2008. Pharmacy in England, Building on Strengths – Delivering the Future. DH, London. pp. 1–141.

Department of Health, 2010. Using the Commissioning for Quality and Innovation (CQUIN) Payment Framework – An Addendum to the 2008 Policy Guidance for 2010/11. Department of Health, London.

Department of Health and Health Protection Agency, 2008. Clostridium difficile: How to Deal with the Problem. DH, London.

Drummond, M.F., Sculpher, M.J., Torrance, G.W., et al. (Eds.), 2005 Methods for the Economic Evaluation of Health Care Programmes, third ed. Oxford University Press, Oxford.

Horne, R., Weinman, J., Barber, N., et al., 2005. Concordance, Adherence and Compliance in Medicine-Taking. Report for the National Co-ordinating Centre for NHS Service Delivery and Organisation R & D.

National Institute for Health and Clinical Excellence, 2002. Guidance on the Use of Glycoprotein IIb/IIIa Inhibitors in the Treatment of Acute Coronary Syndromes. NICE, London. Available at: http://guidance.nice.org.uk/TA47/Guidance/pdf/English.

National Institute for Health and Clinical Excellence, 2009a. The Guidelines Manual 2009. NICE, London. pp. 81–91. Available at: http://www.nice.org.uk/media/68D/29/The_guidelines_manual_2009_Chapter_7_Assessing_cost_effectiveness.pdf.

National Institute for Health and Clinical Excellence, 2009b. Medicines Adherence: Involving Patients in Decisions About Prescribed Medicines CG 76. NICE, London. Available at: http://guidance.nice.org.uk/CG76/Guidance/pdf/English.

OECD, 2009. Health Data. Available at: http://www.ecosante.org/index2.php?base=OCDE&langh=ENG&langs=ENG&sessionid=.

Further reading

Audit Commission, 2005. Managing the Financial Implications of NICE Guidance. Audit Commission Publications, Wetherby.

Bootman, J.L. (Ed.), 2004. Principles of Pharmacoeconomics. Harvey Whitney Books Co., Cincinnati.

Drummond, M.F. (Ed.), 2005. Methods for the Economic Evaluation of Health Care Programmes. Oxford University Press, Oxford.

Øvretveit, J., 2009. Does Improving Quality Save Money? A Review of Evidence of Which Improvements to Quality Reduce Costs to Health Service Providers. The Health Foundation, London.

Rascati, K.L. (Ed.), 2009. Essentials of Pharmacoeconomics. Lippincott Williams & Wilkins, Philadelphia.

Walley, T., Haycox, A., Boland, A. (Eds.), 2003. Pharmacoeconomics. Elsevier, London.

LIFE STAGES

9 Neonates

M. P. Ward Platt

Key points

- The survival of very premature babies has been greatly increased through the use of antenatal betamethasone and neonatal surfactant treatment to prevent and treat surfactant deficiency.
- The feto-placental unit creates a unique route for drug delivery.
- Drug disposition and metabolism in the neonate are very different from those at any other time of life.
- Preterm babies grow very fast, so doses have to be re-calculated at regular intervals.
- Drug elimination in the neonate can be much slower than in children, especially in the first week, so dose intervals have to be longer.

The earliest in pregnancy at which newborn babies can sometimes survive is around 23 weeks' gestation, when survival is about 10% for liveborn babies. Conventionally, any baby born at less than 32 weeks is regarded as being at relatively high risk of death or disability. About 7.5% of all births are technically 'premature' (<37 weeks) but only 1.4% of births take place before 32 weeks of gestation. Likewise, 7% of all babies are low birth weight (LBW), for example, <2500 g, and 1.4% are very low birth weight (VLBW). However, it is the gestation at birth rather than the birth weight which is of more practical and prognostic value. The definitions of selected terms used for babies are given in Table 9.1.

Because mothers with high-risk pregnancies will often be transferred for delivery to a hospital capable of providing neonatal intensive care, the proportion of preterm and LBW babies cared for in such units is greater than in smaller maternity units in peripheral hospitals. In the population as a whole, between 1% and 2% of all babies will receive intensive care, and the most common reason for this among preterm babies is the need for respiratory support of some kind. Over three-quarters of babies born at 25 weeks' gestation now survive to discharge home.

Babies of less than 32 weeks' gestation invariably need some degree of special or intensive care, and generally go home when they are feeding adequately, somewhere between 35 and 40 weeks of postmenstrual age. So although in epidemiological terms the neonatal period is up to the first 28 postnatal days, babies may be 'neonatal' inpatients for as long as 3 or 4 months; during this time their weight may triple and their physiology and metabolism will change dramatically.

Drug disposition

Absorption

An important and unique source of drug absorption, available until birth, is the placenta. Maternal drugs pass to the fetus and back again during pregnancy, but from delivery, any drugs present in the neonatal circulation can no longer be eliminated by that route and must be dealt with by the baby's own systems. Important examples of maternal drugs which may adversely affect the newborn baby include opiates given for pain relief during labour, β-blockers given for pregnancy-induced hypertension and benzodiazepines for eclamptic seizures. In addition, a mother may be given a drug with the intention of treating not her but her fetus. An example of this is the use of corticosteroids to promote fetal lung maturation when preterm delivery is planned or expected. In this situation, betamethasone is normally the drug of choice as prednisolone is metabolised in the placenta and does not reach the fetus.

Enteral drug absorption is erratic in any newborn baby and unavailable in the ill baby because the stomach does not always empty effectively. Therefore, most drugs are given intravenously to ensure maximum bioavailability. Some drugs, such as paraldehyde and diazepam (for neonatal seizures) and paracetamol (for simple analgesia), can be given rectally. The trachea may be used as the preferred route of administration when surfactant administration is required or where adrenaline (epinephrine) is given for resuscitation. The buccal route may be used to administer glucose gel in the treatment of hypoglycaemia. In the very preterm baby of 28 weeks' gestation or less, the skin is extremely thin and a poor barrier to water loss; consequently it is also permeable to substances in contact with it. This is harmful to the baby if there is prolonged skin contact with alcohol, as in chlorhexidine in 70% methylated spirit, which causes severe chemical burn and has resulted in systemic methyl alcohol poisoning. The intramuscular route is normally avoided in premature babies because of their small muscle bulk, although the notable exceptions to this are the administration of vitamin K and naloxone.

Distribution

Drugs are distributed within a baby's body as a function of their lipid and aqueous solubility, as at any other time of life. The main difference in the neonate is that the size of the body water pool under renal control is related not to the baby's

Table 9.1 Definitions of terms

Normal length of human pregnancy (term)	37 up to 42 completed weeks of gestation
Preterm	<37 weeks of gestation at birth
Post-term	42 completed weeks onwards
Neonatal period	Up to the 28th postnatal day
Low birth weight (LBW)	<2500 g
Very low birth weight (VLBW)	<1500 g
Extremely low birth weight (ELBW)	<1000 g

surface area but to body weight. Furthermore, the absolute glomerular filtration rate increases logarithmically with post-conceptional age irrespective of the length of a baby's gestation. This has implications for predicting the behaviour of water-soluble drugs such as gentamicin. The amount of adipose tissue can vary substantially between different babies. Any baby born more than 10 weeks early, and babies of any gestation who have suffered intrauterine growth restriction, may have little body fat. Conversely, the infant of a diabetic mother may have a particularly large fat layer and this affects the retention of predominantly lipid-soluble drugs. Protein binding in the plasma is influenced by the amount of albumin available and this in turn is related to gestation, with albumin values found 12 weeks prior to term being only two-thirds of adult concentrations.

Metabolism

The metabolic fate of drugs in the newborn is not qualitatively different to that in the older child, for example, hydroxylation, oxidation and conjugation to sulphate or glucuronide. It is the efficiency with which these processes are carried out that distinguishes the baby from the older person. In addition to the immaturity of the metabolic pathways for drug disposal, drug metabolism is also affected by the physiological hyperbilirubinaemia of the newborn. The bilirubin can compete both for enzyme-binding sites and for glucuronate, and may thus affect drug metabolism for as long as unconjugated hyperbilirubinaemia persists.

Elimination

The relative immaturity of hepatic and renal function results in correspondingly slow elimination of most drugs from the neonate. This is not necessarily a problem, so long as due account is taken of the slow elimination and dose intervals are modified accordingly. It may even be a useful property, as with phenobarbital, which when given as a loading dose (usually 20 mg/kg) will remain in circulation for days in useful therapeutic quantities, often avoiding the need for further

doses. On the other hand, drugs such as gentamicin and vancomycin, which have a relatively narrow therapeutic index, must be given far less frequently than in children or adults and serum drug levels must be assayed to avoid toxicity.

There has been little study of pharmacodynamics in the term or preterm neonate. Most clinicians work on the assumption that the kinetics of drug behaviour are so different in this group of patients that the pharmacodynamic properties must follow the same pattern. In practice, the most important pharmacodynamic effect is probably that of the behaviour of opiates derived from the mother in labour. Pethidine and diamorphine are the opiates most likely to cause significant respiratory depression in the neonate. Such respiratory depression can be treated with naloxone, and a special neonatal preparation (20 μcg/mL) is available. However, after birth the opiates and their metabolites have a long serum half-life in the baby whereas the naloxone is rapidly eliminated. The initial dramatic effect of naloxone can give a false sense of security, as the baby may become narcosed after a few hours following transfer to the postnatal ward. To try to prevent this late-onset narcosis, adult naloxone (400 μcg/mL) may be given intramuscularly to ensure it remains active over several hours. Even when the respiratory effects have disappeared, opiates may have prolonged behavioural effects on both mother and baby.

Major clinical disorders

Respiratory distress syndrome (RDS)

Among preterm babies the most commonly encountered disorder is RDS (also sometimes called hyaline membrane disease from its appearance on lung histology, or surfactant deficiency lung disease in recognition of the aetiology). The root cause of this disease is the lack of sufficient pulmonary surfactant at the time of birth. The condition is rare in babies born at or near term and becomes increasingly likely the more preterm a birth takes place. It is now quite unusual to see classical RDS because it is prevented both by the use of antenatal betamethasone in the mother and the postnatal administration of surfactant to babies at highest risk (see below).

Clinically, RDS is manifested by obvious difficulty with breathing, with nasal flaring, rib recession, tachypnoea and a requirement for oxygen therapy. The natural history is that RDS becomes worse over the first 2 days, reaches a plateau and then gradually improves. The use of antenatal steroid therapy to the mother, and surfactant therapy for the infant, has not only transformed the clinical course of this condition but also greatly reduced mortality.

A relatively big baby born around 32–34 weeks of gestation with mild RDS may need no more treatment than extra oxygen. In contrast, smaller, more premature or more severely affected babies need some degree of mechanical assistance: either continuous positive airway pressure by nasal prongs or full artificial ventilation through an endotracheal tube. A few babies require high inspired concentrations of oxygen (up to 100%) for several days. Fortunately, pulmonary oxygen toxicity is not as much a problem to the neonate as it is to the adult, though it may have a causal role in the development of bronchopulmonary dysplasia. The major concern is the damage that prolonged arterial hyperoxia can do to the retina, resulting in retinopathy of prematurity. The goal is to give enough inspired oxygen to keep the arterial partial pressure within a range of about 6–12 kPa.

Mechanical ventilation is not a comfortable experience, for adults or children, but it has taken a long time to appreciate that this may also be true for premature babies. Paralysing agents such as pancuronium are sometimes given to ventilated neonates but these only prevent the baby from moving and are not sedative. Pancuronium is widely used, partly because it wears off slowly so that the baby is not suddenly destabilised. Shorter acting agents such as atracurium are often used for temporary paralysis for intubation. Whether or not the baby is paralysed, morphine is commonly given either as intermittent doses or as an infusion, to provide narcosis and analgesia to reduce the distress of neonatal intensive care.

Antenatal steroids given to the mother reduce the incidence, severity and mortality of RDS caused by surfactant deficiency. Unfortunately, it is not possible to identify and treat all mothers whose babies could benefit. Babies of less than 32 weeks' gestation gain most benefit because they are at greatest risk of death and disability from RDS. Optimum treatment is four oral doses of 6 mg betamethasone, each given 12-hourly, or two doses of 12 mg intramuscularly 24 h apart.

Similarly, the introduction of exogenous surfactant, derived from the pig or calf, has revolutionised the management of RDS. Natural surfactants derived from animals are currently more effective than artificial synthetic ones. The first dose should be given as soon as possible after birth since the earlier it is given, the greater the benefit (Soll, 1999).

There are several other important ways of treating babies in respiratory failure. Inhaled nitric oxide dilates pulmonary arterioles and lowers the excessive pulmonary blood pressure which often complicates respiratory failure. Persistent pulmonary hypertension may also complicate early onset septicaemia and meconium aspiration syndrome; in term and near-term babies, nitric oxide is both more effective than the previous drug therapies and much less likely to lead to systemic hypotension. However, it does not reduce mortality or major complications when used in babies with birth weights less than 1500 g (Van Meurs et al., 2005).

For some babies of at least 34 weeks of gestation and at least 2 kg birth weight, extracorporeal membrane oxygenation (ECMO), in which a baby is in effect put on partial heart–lung bypass for a few days, may be life-saving when ventilation and nitric oxide fails (ECMO Collaborative Trial Group., 1996).

Patent ductus arteriosus (PDA)

PDA can be a problem in the recovery phase of RDS, and usually shows itself as a secondary increase in respiratory distress and/or ventilatory requirement, an increasing oxygen requirement, wide pulse pressure and a characteristic heart murmur. Physiologically, as pressure in the pulmonary artery falls, an open duct allows blood from the aorta to flow into the pulmonary artery, which engorges the lungs and reduces their compliance, while putting strain on the heart. Echocardiography is used to confirm the clinical suspicion. About one-third of all babies with birth weights less than 1000 g will develop signs of PDA, for example, the characteristic heart murmur, but treatment is only needed when the baby is haemodynamically compromised. When treatment is needed the options are either medical treatment (with indometacin or ibuprofen) or surgical ligation.

Indometacin is usually given intravenously in the UK, because when given enterally its absorption is unpredictable and it may need to be given before the baby has started enteral feeds. The alternative is intravenous ibuprofen. Potential serious side effects of both drugs include renal impairment, gastric haemorrhage and gut perforation. Surgery is considered when one or more courses of medical treatment fail to close the PDA or if drugs are contraindicated for any reason. There are no good randomised controlled trials to guide clinicians on the best approach to managing PDA.

Bronchopulmonary dysplasia (BPD)

BPD, also sometimes generically known as chronic lung disease of prematurity, most frequently occurs in very immature babies who have undergone prolonged respiratory support. The factors predisposing to BPD are the degree of prematurity, the severity of RDS, infection, the occurrence of PDA, oxygen toxicity and probably intrinsic genetic factors. BPD can be defined as oxygen dependency lasting more than 28 days from birth, but this definition is not very useful in that many babies born at less than 28 weeks of gestation require oxygen for 28 days or more, but few still need it after 8 weeks. A more useful functional and epidemiological definition of established BPD is oxygen dependency at 36 weeks of postmenstrual age, in a baby born before 32 weeks.

Established BPD not severe enough to need continuing mechanical ventilation is either treated with nasal continuous positive airway pressure with or without oxygen supplementation, or if less severe again is treated with oxygen through nasal cannulae. Enough oxygen must be used to maintain an oxygen saturation high enough to control pulmonary artery pressure, while avoiding chronic low-grade hyperoxia which could contribute to retinopathy of prematurity. Optimum oxygen saturations in these babies have not been rigorously defined but the outcome of several large trials is awaited.

A chronic inflammatory process is part of the pathology of BPD, and for this reason much attention has been given to the role of corticosteroids in treating it. Steroid use generally results in a rapid fall in oxygen requirements, but does not improve mortality. Indeed, there is evidence that when dexamethasone is used within the first 1 or 2 weeks there may even be an increased rate of cerebral palsy, so one of the principal indications for steroid use is when a baby remains ventilator dependent at the age of 4 weeks or more. A wide variety of treatment regimens has been tested in trials and there is no standard approach; both the initial dose (usually between 50 and 250 μcg/kg) and the rate of reduction of dose are generally individualised to the baby. Side effects such as hypertension and glucose intolerance are common, although mostly reversible, but the effects on growth can be more serious if steroids are given for a long time.

BPD leads to increases in both pulmonary artery pressures and lung water content. The consequent strain on the heart can lead to heart failure, with excessive weight gain, increasing oxygen requirements and clinical signs such as oedema and a cardiac 'gallop' rhythm. The first-line treatment for heart failure, as in any age group, is with diuretics. Thiazides improve pulmonary mechanics as well as treating heart failure (Brion et al., 2002). Sometimes furosemide is used but its side effects are significant urinary loss of potassium and calcium, and renal calcification. An alternative is to combine a thiazide with spironolactone which causes less calcium and potassium loss. By reducing lung water content, diuretics can also improve lung compliance and reduce the work of breathing. However, BPD is not routinely treated with diuretics, since many babies do well without them. Systemic hypertension sometimes occurs among babies with BPD and may need treatment with antihypertensive drugs such as nifedipine.

For some babies with severe BPD, in whom echocardiography demonstrates pulmonary arterial pressures close to, or greater than, systemic pressure, many neonatologists try sildenafil, as there has been considerable experience using this drug off-label to prevent pulmonary hypertensive crises in babies after cardiac surgery. However, sildenafil has very variable pharmacokinetics in babies, so the dose is difficult to define, and the commonly recommended upper limit of 2 mg/kg four times a day may not be sufficient for some babies (Ahsman et al., 2010).

Significantly preterm babies still in oxygen at 36 weeks' postmenstrual age are almost certain to need oxygen at home after discharge, and home oxygen programmes for ex-premature babies with BPD are now widespread. Most babies manage to wean off supplementary oxygen in a few months but a very few may need it for up to 2 years.

Infection

Important pathogens in the first 2 or 3 days after birth are group B β-haemolytic streptococci and a variety of Gram-negative organisms, especially *Escherichia coli*. Coagulase-negative staphylococci and *Staphylococcus aureus* are more important subsequently. In general, it is wise to use narrow-spectrum agents and short courses of antibiotics whenever possible, and to discontinue blind treatment quickly, for example, after 48 h if confirmatory evidence of bacterial infection, such as blood culture, is negative. The most serious neonatal infections are listed in Table 9.2.

Superficial candida infection is common in all babies, but systemic candida infection is a particular risk in very preterm babies receiving prolonged courses of broad-spectrum antibiotics, with central venous access, and receiving intravenous feeding. Increasingly, units are adopting policies of prophylaxis with either enteral nystatin or systemic fluconazole in the highest risk preterm babies.

It is usual to start antibiotics prophylactically whenever preterm labour is unexplained, where there has been prolonged

Table 9.2 Serious neonatal infections and pathogens

Septicaemia	*Staphylococcus epidermidis*, group B streptococci, *Escherichia coli*
Systemic candidiasis	*Candida* spp.
Necrotizing enterocolitis	No single causal pathogen
Osteomyelitis	*Staphylococcus aureus*
Meningitis	Group B streptococci, *E. coli*

rupture of the fetal membranes prior to delivery, and when a baby is ventilated from birth. A standard combination for such early treatment is penicillin G and an aminoglycoside, to cover group B streptococci and Gram-negative pathogens. Treatment can be stopped after 48 h if cultures prove negative. Blind treatment starting when a baby is more than 48 h old has to take account of the expected local pathogens, but will always include cover for *S. aureus*. Cephalosporins such as cefotaxime and ceftazidime have been heavily promoted for use in the blind treatment of neonatal infection on the grounds of their lower toxicity when compared to aminoglycosides, their wide therapeutic index and the absence of any need to monitor serum concentrations. Their main disadvantage is the breadth of their spectrum which may result in fungal overgrowth or the spread of resistance, although they compare favourably with ampicillin in this regard. Since courses of blind treatment are often only for 48 h, and the antibiotics can be stopped when cultures are negative, there is often no need to measure levels in babies receiving aminoglycosides, thereby negating much of the apparent advantage of cephalosporins. Moreover, there is now good evidence for giving gentamicin 24 hourly rather than more frequently, as it has similar efficacy and less potential for toxicity.

Methicillin-resistant *S. aureus* (MRSA) has emerged as a real problem in hospitals in recent years, but there is little evidence that neonatal units are a particularly hazardous environment.

The most important active viral infection in neonates is cytomegalovirus (CMV), and the most important one from which to protect babies in the UK is vertically transmitted human immuno-deficiency virus (HIV). For CMV, which is now thought to be a major factor in non-hereditary sensorineural hearing loss, treatment is with intravenous ganciclovir and oral valganciclovir.

For HIV, the goal of management is to prevent 'vertical' transmission from mother to baby. The main strategy to combat this is to use aggressive maternal treatment throughout pregnancy to suppress the maternal viral load. Current practice is to give the baby zidovudine, as a single agent, for 4 weeks when the maternal viral load is low, or triple therapy if the load is high.

Necrotizing enterocolitis (NEC)

NEC is an important complication of neonatal intensive care, and can arise in any baby. However, it most commonly occurs in premature babies and those already ill. It is especially associated with being small for gestational age, birth asphyxia and the presence of a PDA. Since many sick babies have multiple problems, it has been difficult to disentangle causal associations from spurious links to conditions that occur anyway in ill infants, such as the need for blood transfusion. There is general agreement that the pathophysiology is related to damage of the gut mucosa, which may occur because of hypotension or hypoxia, coupled with the presence of certain organisms in the gastro-intestinal tract that invade the gut wall to give rise to the clinical condition. It almost never arises in a baby who has never been fed, whilst early 'minimal' feeding, and initiating feeding with human breast milk, appears to be protective. Probably the most important protection that can be given exogenously is enteral probiotics (AlFaleh & Bassler, 2008).

A baby who becomes ill with NEC is often septicaemic and may present acutely with a major collapse, respiratory failure and shock, or more slowly with abdominal distension, intolerance of feeds with discoloured gastric aspirates and blood in the stool. The medical treatment is respiratory and circulatory support if necessary, antibiotics, and switching to intravenous feeding for a period of time, usually 7–10 days. One of the most difficult surgical judgements is deciding if and when to operate to remove necrotic areas of gut or deal with a perforation.

The antibiotic strategy for NEC is to cover Gram-positive, Gram-negative and anaerobic bacteria. Metronidazole is used to cover anaerobes in the UK but clindamycin is preferred in some other countries. As with other drugs, metronidazole behaves very differently in neonates compared with older children and adults, having an elimination half-life of over 20 h in term babies. The elimination half-life is up to 109 h in preterm babies, partly due to poor hepatic hydroxylation in infants born before 35 weeks' gestation. There is probably a case to be made for monitoring serum levels of this drug, but in practice this is seldom done.

Haemorrhagic disease of the newborn

Haemorrhagic disease of the newborn, better described as vitamin K-dependent bleeding, is very rare but it may cause death or disability if it presents with an intracranial bleed. Except in the case of malabsorption, it affects only breast-fed babies because they get very little vitamin K in maternal milk, and their gut bacteria do not synthesise it. Formula fed infants get sufficient vitamin K in their diet.

There are several possible strategies for giving vitamin K with a view to preventing haemorrhagic disease. An intramuscular injection of phytomenadione 1 mg (0.5 mL) can be given either to every newborn baby or selectively to babies who have certain risk factors such as instrumental delivery, preterm birth, etc. Vitamin K can be given orally, so long as an adequate number of doses is given, and this has been shown to be effective in preventing disease (Wariyar et al., 2000). Intramuscular injections are an invasive and unpleasant intervention for the baby since muscle bulk is small in the newborn, and particularly the preterm, and other structures such as the sciatic nerve can be damaged even if the intention is to give the injection into the lateral thigh. Intramuscular injections can be reserved for those babies with doubtful oral absorption, for example, all those admitted for special care, or at high risk because of enzyme-inducing maternal drugs such as anticonvulsants.

Apnoea

Apnoea is the absence of breathing. Babies (and adults) normally have respiratory pauses, but preterm babies in particular are prone to prolonged pauses in respiration of over 20 s which can be associated with significant falls in arterial oxygenation. Apnoea usually has both central and obstructive components, is often accompanied by bradycardia, and requires treatment to prevent life-threatening episodes of arterial desaturation.

Episodes of apnoea and bradycardia can be treated in three ways: intubating and mechanically ventilating the baby, giving nasal continuous positive airway pressure (nCPAP) or giving respiratory stimulants such as caffeine or doxapram. The main goal of medical treatment is to reduce the number and severity of the episodes without having to resort to artificial ventilation. Caffeine both reduces apnoea in the short term, and improves long-term outcome (Schmidt et al., 2006). Doxapram is occasionally given as an adjunct to both caffeine and nCPAP, to avoid resorting to mechanical ventilation. Most clinicians stop giving respiratory stimulants when the baby is around 34 weeks of postmenstrual age, by which time most babies will have achieved an adequate degree of cardiorespiratory stability and no longer need even the most basic forms of monitoring device.

Seizures

Seizures may arise as part of an encephalopathy, when they are accompanied by altered consciousness, or as isolated events when the baby is neurologically normal between seizure episodes. Investigations are directed to finding an underlying cause but in about half of all term babies having fits without an encephalopathy, no underlying cause can be found.

Just as with children and adults, treatment may be needed to control an acute seizure which does not terminate quickly, or given long term to prevent the occurrence of fits. In the neonate, the first-choice anticonvulsant for the acute treatment of seizures is phenobarbital because it is effective, seldom causes respiratory depression, and is active for many hours or days because of its long elimination half-life. Diazepam is sometimes used intravenously or rectally but it upsets temperature control, causes unpredictable respiratory depression, and is very sedating compared to phenobarbital. Paraldehyde is occasionally used because it is easy to give rectally, is relatively non-sedating and short acting. It is excreted by exhalation and the smell can make the working environment quite unpleasant for staff. Phenytoin is often used when fits remain uncontrolled after two loading doses of phenobarbital (total 40 mg/kg) but is not usually given long term because of its narrow therapeutic index. When seizures are intractable, options include clonazepam, midazolam or lidocaine; the last two are given as infusions. There is little experience with intravenous sodium valproate in the neonate. Longer term treatment is commonly with phenobarbital but after the first few postnatal months, carbamazepine or sodium valproate is more suitable.

Hypoxic–ischaemic encephalopathy (HIE), which usually results either from intrapartum asphyxia or from an antepartum insult such as placental abruption, is an important cause of seizures. Convulsions are a marker of a more severe insult; they usually occur within 24 h of birth and may last for several days, after which they spontaneously resolve. The less severely affected babies quickly return to neurological normality. No drug has been shown to improve outcome when given after the insult has occurred, but cooling a baby to between 33 and 34 °C for 72 h has been shown to improve the degree of neurodisability among survivors and has rapidly become standard therapy (Edwards et al., 2010).

The therapeutic dilemma lies in the degree of aggression with which convulsions should be treated, since no conventional anticonvulsant is very effective in reducing electrocerebral seizure activity, even when the clinical manifestations of seizures are abolished, and as stated before, convulsions tend naturally to cease after a few days. However, seizures which compromise respiratory function need to be treated to prevent serious falls in arterial oxygen tension and possible secondary neurological damage. Also, babies with frequent or continuous seizure activity are difficult to nurse and cause great distress to their parents. Therefore, in practice it is usual to try to suppress the clinical manifestation of seizure activity, and phenobarbital remains the most commonly used first-line treatment. Where a decision is taken to keep a baby on anticonvulsant medication, therapeutic drug monitoring can provide helpful information and may need to be repeated from time to time during follow-up.

Principles and Goals of Therapy

The ultimate aim of neonatal care at all levels is to maximise disability-free survival and identify treatable conditions which would otherwise compromise growth or development. It follows that potential problems should be anticipated and the complexities of intensive care should be avoided if at all possible.

Many of the drugs used in neonatal care are not licensed for such use, or are used off-label. There is a high potential for errors because of the small doses used, which sometimes calls for unusual levels of dilution when drawing up drugs. Constant vigilance, electronic prescribing and the use of specialised neonatal formularies are all important in preventing harm.

Rapid growth

Once the need for intensive care has passed, the growth of a premature baby can be very rapid indeed if the child is being fed with a high-calorie formula modified for use with preterm infants. Indeed, most babies born at 27 weeks, and weighing around 1 kg, can be expected to double their birth weight by the time they are 8 weeks old. Since the dose of all medications

is calculated on the basis of body weight, constant review of dose is necessary to maintain efficacy, particularly for drugs that may be given for several weeks such as respiratory stimulants, diuretics and anticonvulsants. Conversely, all that is necessary to gradually wean a baby from a medication is to hold the dose constant so that the baby gradually 'grows out' of the drug. This practice is frequently used with diuretic medication in BPD, the need for which becomes less as the baby's somatic growth reduces the proportion of damaged lung in favour of healthy tissue.

Therapeutic drug monitoring

The assay of serum concentrations of various drugs has a place in neonatal medicine, particularly where the therapeutic index of a drug is narrow. It is routine to assay levels of antibiotics such as aminoglycosides and vancomycin, of which the trough measurement is of most value since it is accumulation of the drug which must be avoided. More rarely, it may be necessary to assay minimal inhibitory or bactericidal concentrations of antibiotics in blood or cerebrospinal fluid if serious infections are being treated, but constraints on sampling limit the frequency with which this may be undertaken.

Where phenobarbital or other anticonvulsants are given long term, intermittent measurement of serum levels can be a useful guide to increasing the dose. All these drugs have a long half-life, so it is most important that drug concentrations are not measured too early, or too frequently, to prevent inappropriate changes in dose being made before a steady state is reached.

Avoiding harm

Intramuscular injections are considered potentially harmful because of the small muscle bulk of babies. However, it is not always easy to establish venous access and occasionally it may be necessary to use the intramuscular route instead. For vaccines the intramuscular route is unavoidable.

For sick preterm infants ventilated for respiratory failure, handling of any kind is a destabilising influence, so the minimal necessary intervention should be the rule. Merely opening the doors of an incubator can destabilise a fragile baby. It is, therefore, a good practice to minimise the frequency of drug administration and to try to coordinate the doses of different medications.

Time-scale of clinical changes

In babies, the time-scale for starting drug treatments is very short because the clinical condition of any baby can change with great rapidity. For example, where a surfactant is required it should be given as soon as possible after birth to premature babies who are intubated and ventilated. Similarly, infection can be rapidly progressive, so starting antibiotics is a priority when the index of suspicion is high or where congenital bacterial infection is likely. The same applies for antiretroviral drugs when a baby is born to a mother positive for HIV, especially if the maternal viral load is high.

For the sick preterm infant, this model applies to a wide range of interventions. It is seldom possible to wait a few hours for a given drug, and this has obvious implications for the level of support required by a neonatal service.

Early urgent immunisation with hepatitis B vaccine and the administration of anti-hepatitis B immunoglobulin are very important in preventing vertical transmission of hepatitis B when the mother is e-antigen positive. Of less urgency, but considerable importance, is making sure that premature babies who are still on the neonatal unit 8 weeks after birth get their routine immunisations, since these should be given according to chronological age irrespective of prematurity.

Patient and parent care

It is all too easy to take a mechanistic approach to neonatal medicine, on the grounds that premature infants cannot communicate their needs. Such an approach to therapy is inappropriate. Even when receiving intensive care, any infant who is not either paralysed or very heavily sedated does in fact respond with a wealth of cues and non-verbal communication in relation to their needs. Monitors, therefore, do not replace clinical skills, but provide supplementary information and advance warning of problems. Even the most premature babies show individual characteristics, which emphasises that individualised care is as important in this age group as in any other. In particular, neonatal pain and distress have effects on nociception and behaviour well into the childhood years.

Involvement of parents in every aspect of care is a necessary goal in neonatal clinical practice, and care is increasingly regarded as a partnership between professionals and parents rather than the province of professionals alone. Routine administration of oral medication is thus an act in which parents may be expected to participate, and for those whose baby has to be discharged home still requiring continuous oxygen, the parent will rapidly obtain complete control, with support from the hospital and the primary health care team. The growing number of babies who survive very premature birth but whose respiratory state requires continued support after discharge presents an increasing therapeutic challenge for the future.

Case studies

Case 9.1

Ms A went into labour as a result of an antepartum haemorrhage at 28 weeks of gestation. There was no time to give her steroids when she arrived at the maternity unit and her son, J, was born by vaginal delivery in good condition. However, he required intubation and ventilation at the age of 10 min to sustain his breathing; surfactant was immediately given down the endotracheal tube. He was not weighed at the time but was given intramuscular vitamin K and then taken to the special care unit. On arrival in the unit, baby J was weighed (1270 g) and placed in an incubator for warmth. He was connected to a ventilator. Blood was taken for culture and basic haematology, and he was prescribed antibiotics. A radiograph confirmed the diagnosis of respiratory distress syndrome.

Questions

1. Which antibiotic(s) would be appropriate initially for baby J?
   Over the next 2 days, baby J required modest ventilation and remained on antibiotics. A second dose of surfactant was given 12 h after the first. Parenteral feeding was commenced on day 2 as per unit policy, and on day 3 very slow continuous milk feeding into his stomach was started. Blood cultures were negative at 48 h and the antibiotics were stopped. On day 4 he was extubated into 30% oxygen.

   On day 5, baby J looked unwell with a rising oxygen requirement, increased work of breathing and poor peripheral perfusion. Examination revealed little else except that his liver was enlarged and a little firm, his pulses rather full and easy to feel and there was a moderate systolic heart murmur. One possibility was infection.
2. Which antibiotics would be appropriate for baby J on day 5? Another possibility was a patent arterial duct leading to heart failure.
3. How could his heart failure and patent ductus arteriosus be treated?
   After appropriate treatment he looked progressively better and when the blood culture was negative after 2 days, the antibiotics were stopped. By the age of 2 weeks, baby J was on full milk feeds and the duct had closed. He was in air. However, he began to have increasingly frequent episodes of spontaneous bradycardia, sometimes following apnoeic spells in excess of 20 s duration. Examination between episodes showed a healthy, stable baby. Investigations such as haematocrit, serum sodium and an infection screen were normal.
4. At 2 weeks, which drug of choice could be used to treat his apnoea and bradycardia? What would be the expected duration of treatment with this drug?

Answers

1. Blind antibiotic cover is usually started until negative blood cultures are received. Penicillin and gentamicin would provide good cover for streptococci and Gram-negative organisms, which are the most likely potential pathogens at this stage. A suitable dose would be 30 mg/kg of penicillin every 12 h and 2.5 mg/kg of gentamicin every 12 h. Alternatively, a third-generation cephalosporin such as cefotaxime could be used for initial blind treatment. If cultures were negative at 48 h, antibiotics could be stopped provided that there were no clinical indications to continue.
2. At day 5, antibiotic treatment should take account of the likely pathogens such as S. aureus and others causing nosocomial infections. A suitable choice for the former would be flucloxacillin, if there was no concern about MRSA, or vancomycin if there was. The vancomycin starting dose would be 15 mg/kg every 12 h. The addition of another agent with good Gram-negative activity such as gentamicin or a third-generation cephalosporin would provide good cover.
3. Intravenous indometacin or ibuprofen would be suitable for the treatment of patent ductus arteriosus. Furosemide (1 mg/kg as a single dose) is the drug of choice for acute heart failure.
4. Caffeine is now the drug of choice. A suitable dose of caffeine for baby J would be a loading dose of 20 mg/kg with maintenance dose of 5 mg/kg/day, increasing to 10 mg/kg/day if necessary. The frequency of episodes of apnoea and bradycardia should decline immediately. The treatment is likely to continue until he is about 34 weeks of postmenstrual age, when his control of breathing should be mature enough to maintain good respiratory function.

Case 9.2

Baby B was born at 25 weeks' gestation and was ventilated for 5 days before being extubated onto continuous positive airways pressure. On extubation she was initially in air, but now at the age of 4 weeks she is mostly in about 30% oxygen, fully fed on milk, and growing well. Her chest X-ray shows the pattern typical of chronic lung disease. One morning she is noticed to be in 45% oxygen, she has had a large weight gain and she looks quite oedematous all over.

Questions

1. What do these symptoms suggest?
   After careful evaluation, baby B is given an oral dose of furosemide 1 mg/kg, following which the oedema goes down, her weight falls and her oxygen requirement returns to 30%.
2. What are the disadvantages of giving regular furosemide in this situation?
   A thiazide diuretic and spironolactone are prescribed. Four days later, routine biochemistry tests show a sodium of 125 mmol/L.
3. What is the choice the attending team has to make?

Answers

1. The symptoms suggest heart failure. Medical examination would probably have revealed an enlarged liver, and the heart might have had a 'gallop' rhythm as well. In babies, the symptoms and signs commonly suggest both left and right ventricular failure.
2. Regular treatment with furosemide causes hypercalcuria, as well as excessive loss of sodium and potassium. Chronic hypercalcuria can lead to nephrocalcinosis. For this reason, a combination of thiazides and spironolactone is commonly used.
3. The sodium is low (but the normal range in preterm babies is 130–140 mmol/L, lower than in children and adults). That it is low is probably an effect of the diuretics. The choice lies between carrying on with the diuretics and supplementing the sodium intake, or stopping the diuretics and observing the baby for any recurrence of heart failure.

References

Ahsman, M.J., Witjes, B.C., Wildschut, E.D., et al., 2010. Sildenafil exposure in neonates with pulmonary hypertension after administration via a nasogastric tube. Arch. Dis. Childhood. Fetal Neonatal Ed. 95, F109–F114.

AlFaleh, K.M., Bassler, D., 2008. Probiotics for prevention of necrotizing enterocolitis in preterm infants. Cochrane Database of Systematic Reviews Issue 1, Art No. CD005496. doi: 10.1002/14651858.CD005496, Available at: pub2 clinical/pdf/CD005496_standard.pdf.

Brion, L.P., Primhak, R.A., Ambrosio-Perez, I., 2002. Diuretics acting on the distal renal tubule for preterm infants with (or developing) chronic lung disease. Cochrane Database of Systematic Reviews Issue 1, Art No. CD001817. doi: 10.1002/14651858.CD001817, Available at: http://onlinelibrary.wiley.com/o/cochrane/clsysrev/articles/CD001817/frame.html.

ECMO Collaborative Trial Group, 1996. UK collaborative randomised trial of neonatal extracorporeal membrane oxygenation. UK Collaborative ECMO Trial Group. Lancet 348, 75–82.

Edwards, A.D., Brocklehurst, P., Gunn, A.J., et al., 2010. Neurological outcomes at 18 months of age after moderate hypothermia for perinatal hypoxic ischaemic encephalopathy: synthesis and meta-analysis of trial data. Br. Med. J. c363, 340.

Schmidt, B., Roberts, R.S., Davis, P., et al., 2006. Caffeine therapy for apnea of prematurity. N. Engl. J. Med. 354, 2112–2121.

Soll, R., 1999. Early versus delayed selective surfactant treatment for neonatal respiratory distress syndrome. Cochrane Database of Systematic Reviews Issue 4, Art No. CD001456.

Van Meurs, K.P., Wright, L.L., Ehrenkranz, R.A., et al., 2005. Inhaled nitric oxide for premature infants with severe respiratory failure. N. Engl. J. Med. 353, 13–22.

Wariyar, U., Hilton, S., Pagan, J., et al., 2000. Six years' experience of prophylactic oral vitamin K. Arch. Dis. Childhood. Fetal Neonatal Ed. 82, F64–68.

Further reading

Lissauer T, Fanaroff A.A. (Eds.), 2006. Neonatology at a Glance. Wiley-Blackwell, Oxford.

Northern Neonatal Network, 2006. Neonatal Formulary: Drug Use in Pregnancy and the First Year of Life, fifth ed. Wiley-Blackwell, Oxford.

Rennie, J.M., Robertson, N.R.C., 2002. A Manual of Neonatal Intensive Care, fourth ed. Arnold, London.

Young, T.E., Magnum, B., 2009. NeoFax: A Manual of Drugs Used in Neonatal Care, 22nd ed. Thomson Reuters, Montvale.

10 Paediatrics

C. Barker, A. J. Nunn and S. Turner

Key points

- Children are not small adults.
- Patient details such as age, weight and surface area need to be accurate to ensure appropriate dosing.
- Weight and surface area may change in a relatively short time period and necessitate dose adjustment
- Pharmacokinetic changes in childhood are important and have a significant influence on drug handling and need to be considered when choosing an appropriate dosing regimen for a child.
- The ability of the child to use different dosage forms changes with age, so a range should be available, for example, oral liquid, dispersible tablets, capsules.
- The availability of a medicinal product does not mean it is appropriate for use in children.
- The use of an unlicensed medicine in children is not illegal, although it must be ensured that the choice of drug and dose is appropriate.

Paediatrics is the branch of medicine dealing with the development, diseases and disorders of children. Infancy and childhood is a period of rapid growth and development. The various organs, body systems and enzymes that handle drugs develop at different rates; hence, drug dosage, formulation, response to drugs and adverse reactions vary throughout childhood. Compared with adult medicine, drug use in children is not extensively researched and the range of licensed drugs in appropriate dosage forms is limited.

For many purposes it has been common to subdivide childhood into the following periods:

- neonate: the first 4 weeks of life
- infant: from 4 weeks to 1 year
- child: from 1 year to 12 years

For the purpose of drug dosing, children over 12 years of age are often classified as adults. This is inappropriate because many 12 year olds have not been through puberty and have not reached adult height and weight. The International Committee on Harmonization (2001) has suggested that childhood be divided into the following age ranges for the purposes of clinical trials and licensing of medicines:

- preterm newborn infant
- term newborn infants (0–27 days)
- infants and toddlers (28 days to 23 months)
- children (2–11 years)
- adolescents (12–16/18 years)

These age ranges are intended to reflect biological changes: the newborn (birth to 4 weeks) covers the climacteric changes after birth, 4 weeks to 2 years the early growth spurt, 2–11 years the gradual growth phase and 12–18 years puberty and the adolescent growth spurt to final adult height. Manufacturers of medicines and regulatory authorities are working towards standardising the age groups quoted in each product's Summary of Product Characteristics.

Demography

The 2001 census revealed that dependent children still make up a substantial number of people, at 11.7 million, but figures published by the Office for National Statistics in 2009 indicate that over the last 25 years the percentage of the population aged 16 years and under has decreased from 21% to 19%. This trend is predicted to continue and by 2033 the percentage of the population under 16 years old is predicted to be 18%. The UK census in 2011 will be the next opportunity to confirm this trend.

Children make substantial use of hospital-based services. It has been estimated that of the 14 million attendances at hospital emergency departments reported each year in England, 2.9 million were for children. At the same time there were 4.5 million outpatient attendances and 700,000 in-patient admissions. The 10 most common admission diagnoses in a specialist children's hospital over an 18-month period are shown in Table 10.1.

Congenital anomalies

Congenital anomalies remain an important cause of infant and child mortality in England and Wales, and account for an increasing proportion of infant deaths. The National Congenital Anomaly System (NCAS), established in 1964 in the wake of the thalidomide tragedy, has monitored congenital anomalies nationally in England and Wales. Registers such as NCAS are important in planning service delivery and alerting specialists to conditions where research is required. However, it relies on voluntary notifications and collaborates with local registers to improve the quality and quantity of data (see Useful Paediatric Websites at end of chapter).

Table 10.1 Top 10 diagnoses on admission to a specialist children's hospital

Ranking	Diagnosis
1	Respiratory tract infections
2	Chronic diseases of tonsils and adenoids
3	Asthma
4	Abdominal and pelvic pain
5	Viral infection (unspecified site)
6	Non-suppurative otitis media
7	Inguinal hernia
8	Unspecified head injury
9	Gastroenteritis/colitis
10	Undescended testicle

Data for 2008 are available but there is ongoing discussion about the future direction of the recording service, given the wide variability in reporting between areas with and without regional congenital anomaly registers. In 2007, a new classification of congenital anomalies was introduced to include tighter rules for deciding which congenital anomalies should be included in the Office for National Statistics report making year on year comparisons more difficult.

In 2008, there were 175 central nervous system (CNS) anomalies, for example, hydrocephalus, 282 cleft lip/palate, 932 heart and circulatory, 258 hypospadias and 225 Down's syndrome reported to NCAS.

Neural tube defects (spina bifida) are one example of devastating congenital malformations that have been influenced by public health intervention programmes. The results of a long-term study (MRC Vitamin Study Research Group, 1991) showed that folate supplementation prevented 72% of neural tube defects when given to women at high risk of having a child with a neural tube defect. Hence, folate supplementation is now part of the routine advice given in antenatal clinics.

Cancer

Cancer is very rare in childhood; around 1700 new cases are diagnosed in children less than 15 years old in the UK each year. About one-third of all childhood cancers are leukaemias and of these, about 80% are of the acute lymphoblastic type (ALL). Although rare, childhood cancer is the most common cause of death from illness in children aged between 1 and 15 years of age.

As a consequence of the technical advances in treatment and the centralisation of services in specialist centres, a much greater number of childhood cancer sufferers are surviving to adulthood.

Asthma, eczema and hay fever

Asthma, eczema and hay fever (allergic rhinitis) are among the most common chronic diseases of childhood and most of the affected children are managed in primary care. During the 1970s and 1980s there was considerable expansion of epidemiological research into these disorders, prompted mainly by concern about the increase in hospital admissions for childhood asthma despite the availability of effective anti-asthma medication. These studies failed to identify any demographic, perinatal or environmental factor which could explain more than a small proportion of the large changes in prevalence of asthma, hay fever or eczema. Incidence rates of acute asthma in children under 5 years old were reported to be 1.5 per 1000 per week in 1991; the rates for children aged 5–14 years old were 0.9 per 1000 per week. Between 1993 and 2000 the incidence rates for both groups declined, but asthma continues to be an important childhood illness placing a burden on the health service.

Infections

Despite a dramatic decline in the incidence of childhood infectious diseases during the twentieth century, they remain an important cause of ill health in childhood. Major advances in the prevention of infections have been achieved through the national childhood vaccination programme.

The importance of maintaining high vaccine uptake has been demonstrated by the resurgence of vaccine-preventable diseases where children have not been vaccinated. Adverse publicity surrounding the MMR (measles, mumps and rubella) vaccine, involving a possible association with Crohn's disease and autism, resulted in a loss of public confidence in the vaccine and a decrease in MMR coverage. This occurred in spite of rigorous scientific investigation and evidence refuting the claims. The annual coverage for MMR for 2-year olds declined from 92% in 1992 to 87% in 2000 and data for 2004 show that it dropped to 81.5%. Although this decline is far less than that seen for pertussis in the 1970s, if MMR coverage remains at this level or declines further, resurgences of MMR in primary schoolchildren will become more common. NHS information centre data revealed 85% of children in England had received the MMR vaccine in 2007/8. However, to achieve herd immunity, 95% of children need to be immunised; unless this figure is improved a measles epidemic still remains a possibility.

An important gastro-intestinal infection that appears to be increasing is infection with verotoxin-producing *Escherichia coli* (VTEC). This is important because it is the main cause of haemolytic uraemic syndrome, a severe condition which can lead to acute renal failure in children. VTEC is an example of an emerging infection. Before the 1980s it was unknown and during the 1990s reports of infection with VTEC in children in the UK tripled from 172 in 1991 to 531 in 1999. In 2009 the rates of VTEC 0157 decreased as age increased, with significantly higher rates in the 0–4 year age group (8 per 100,000) than in 5–9 year olds (4 per 100,000) and a further decrease (2 per 100,000) in the 10–19 year age group. It is a public health priority to improve VTEC 0157 surveillance and improve diagnostic testing.

Respiratory syncytial virus (RSV) is the most important cause of lower respiratory tract infection in infants and young children in the UK, in whom it causes bronchiolitis, tracheobronchitis and pneumonia. It is responsible for seasonal outbreaks of respiratory tract infection most commonly between October and April. The main burden of disease is borne by children under 2 years and there are around 7000–10000 confirmed laboratory reports of RSV in children in England and Wales each year. During the winter months, RSV is the single greatest cause of admission to hospital in children.

Mental health disorders

Mental health disorders are another emerging concern in the child health arena. In 2004, 1 in 10 children and young people aged 5–16 years old had a clinically diagnosed mental health disorder. These included 4% with an emotional disorder such as depression or anxiety, 6% with a conduct disorder, 2% with a hyperkinetic disorder and 1% with less common disorders, for example, autism, tics.

Groups at particular high risk of psychiatric disorder include children in the care system, young people who are homeless and young offenders. Longitudinal evidence has confirmed that many child psychiatric disorders persist well into adult life. Biological, psychological and social factors all seem likely to contribute to the risk of psychiatric disorders, and may act in combination.

Drugs, smoking and alcohol

The harm that drugs, smoking and drinking can do to the health of children and young people is recognised and a number of targets have been set in an attempt to reduce prevalence. Recent figures on smoking, alcohol and drug use among young people have been provided by the NHS Information Centre in their 2008 report.

In 2008, 6% of schoolchildren smoked regularly (at least once a week). Girls are more likely to smoke than boys and the prevalence increases with age. Around 14% of 15-year olds smoke regularly compared to 0.5% of 11-year olds. However, the prevalence of smoking amongst children has halved since its peak in the mid-1990s (13% in 1996), suggesting a decline in prevalence to below government targets. In 2007, the minimum age for buying tobacco was increased from 16 years old to 18 years old.

More than half of pupils (52%) aged 11–15 years have drunk alcohol in their lifetime. In 2008, a national survey identified that the mean amount of alcohol consumed by pupils who had drunk in the last week was 14.6 units. Boys drink more than girls and older pupils drink more than younger pupils. In one large survey, 17% of pupils aged 11–15 years old admitted to being drunk in the last 4 weeks.

The prevalence of drug use has declined since 2001. In 2008, 22% of pupils said that they had ever used drugs with 33% reporting that they had ever been offered drugs. Pupils were most likely to have taken cannabis (9%). Five percent of pupils had sniffed glue or other volatile substances in the last year and 2.9% had sniffed poppers. Overall, 3.6% of pupils had taken class A drugs in the last year.

Nutrition and exercise

Health during childhood can impact upon well-being in later life. Good nutrition and physical exercise are vital both for growth and development and for preventing health complications in later life. In addition, dietary patterns in childhood and adolescence have an influence on dietary preferences and eating patterns in adulthood.

In 2000, an international definition of overweight and obesity in childhood and adolescence was proposed to help calculate internationally comparable prevalence rates of overweight and obesity in children and adolescents. The definition interprets overweight and obesity in terms of reference points for body mass index (BMI, in kg/m^2) by age and sex, and is linked to the widely used adult overweight cut-off point of 25 and adult obesity cut-off point of 30.

In 2004, it was estimated that 14% of boys and 17% of girls aged 2–15 years of age were obese. Probable reasons for a rise in overweight and obesity in children are changes in diets and an inactive lifestyle. There is evidence that obesity at an early age tends to continue to adulthood.

Being overweight is linked to the development of type 2 diabetes, high blood pressure, heart disease, stroke, certain cancers and other types of illnesses. Therefore, healthy eating is not only important in relation to weight but also contributes to reducing the risk of heart disease, stroke and some cancers in later life. It is recommended that a well-balanced diet providing all the nutrients required should include at least five portions of fruit and vegetables a day. It is now practice in many areas for infant children (aged 4–7 years) each day to be provided with a piece of free fruit during school break time.

The normal child

Growth and development are important indicators of a child's general well-being and paediatric practitioners should be aware of the normal development milestones in childhood. In the UK, development surveillance and screening of babies and children is well established through child health clinics.

Weight is one of the most widely used and obvious indicators of growth, and progress is assessed by recording weights on a percentile chart (Fig. 10.1). A weight curve for a child which deviates from the usual pattern requires further investigation. Separate recording charts are used for boys and girls and since percentile charts are usually based on observations of the white British population, adjustments may be necessary for some ethnic groups. The World Health Organization (WHO) has challenged the widely used growth charts, based on growth rates of infants fed on formula milk. In 2006, it published new growth standards based on a study of more than 8000 breast-fed babies from six countries around the world. The optimum size is now that of a breast-fed baby. Recently, new growth charts have been introduced for children

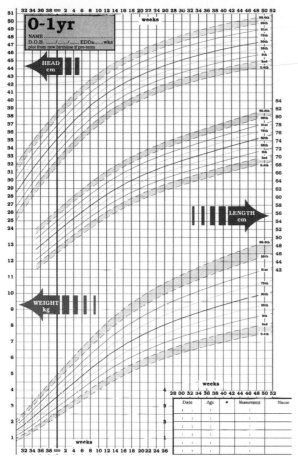

Fig. 10.1 Example of a centile chart (Child Growth Foundation).

from birth to 4 years of age. These combine the UK and WHO data. Copies can be accessed at http://www.rcpch. ac.uk/Research/UK-WHO-Growth-Charts.

Height (or length in children less than 2 years of age) is another important tool in developmental assessment. In a similar way to weight, height or length should follow a percentile line. If this is not the case or if growth stops completely, then further investigation is required. The normal rate of growth is taken to be 5 cm or more per year and any alteration in this growth velocity should be investigated.

For infants up to 2 years of age, head circumference is also a useful parameter to monitor. In addition to the above, assessments of hearing, vision, motor development and speech are undertaken at the child health clinics. A summary of age-related development is shown in Fig. 10.2.

Child health clinics play a vital role in the national childhood immunisation programme, which commences at 2 months of age. Immunisation is a major success story for preventive medicine, preventing diseases that have the potential to cause serious damage to a child's health, or even death. An example of the impact that immunisation can have on the profile of infectious diseases is demonstrated by the meningitis C immunisation campaign, which began in November 1999. The UK was the first country to introduce the meningitis C conjugate (MenC) vaccine and uptake levels have been close to 90%. The programme was targeted at under-20 year olds and has been a

huge success, with a 90% reduction in cases in that age group. Authorities were hoping to mirror the success of the meningitis C campaign with the introduction of the seven valent pneumococcal vaccine into the routine UK childhood immunisation schedule in April 2006. Post-licensing surveillance has shown a large reduction in both invasive and non-invasive disease incidence due to vaccine serotypes in vaccinated individuals. However, during the same period, the UK has seen an increase in invasive disease due to the non-vaccine serotypes, caused for a large part by the six serotypes not covered by the seven valent vaccine, but present in a new 13 valent vaccine. In April 2010, the 13 valent pneumoccocal vaccine replaced the seven valent vaccine in the standard immunisation schedule. Human papilloma virus vaccine has also recently been introduced to the immunisation programme in the UK for females aged 12–13 years of age, to reduce the risk of cervical cancer.

Advice on the current immunisation schedule can be found in the current edition of the British National Formulary for Children.

Drug disposition

Pharmacokinetic factors

An understanding of the variability in drug disposition is essential if children are to receive rational and appropriate drug therapy (Anderson and Holford, 2008, 2009). For convenience, the factors that affect drug disposition will be dealt with separately. However, when treating a patient all the factors have a dynamic relationship and none should be considered in isolation.

Absorption

Oral absorption. The absorption process of oral preparations may be influenced by factors such as gastric and intestinal transit time, gastric and intestinal pH and gastrointestinal contents. Posture, disease state and therapeutic interventions such as nasogastric aspiration or drug therapy can also affect the absorption process. It is not until the second year of life that gastric acid output increases and is comparable on a per kilogram basis with that observed in adults. In addition, gastric emptying time only approaches adult values at about 6 months of age.

The bioavailability of sulphonamides, digoxin and phenobarbital has been studied in infants and children of a wide age distribution. Despite the different physicochemical properties of the drugs, a similar bioavailability pattern was observed in each case. The rate of absorption was correlated with age, being much slower in neonates than in older infants and children. However, few studies have specifically reported on the absorption process in older infants or children. The available data suggest that in older infants and children orally administered drugs will be absorbed at a rate and extent similar to those in healthy adults. Changes in the absorption rate would appear to be of minor importance when compared to the age-related differences of drug distribution and excretion.

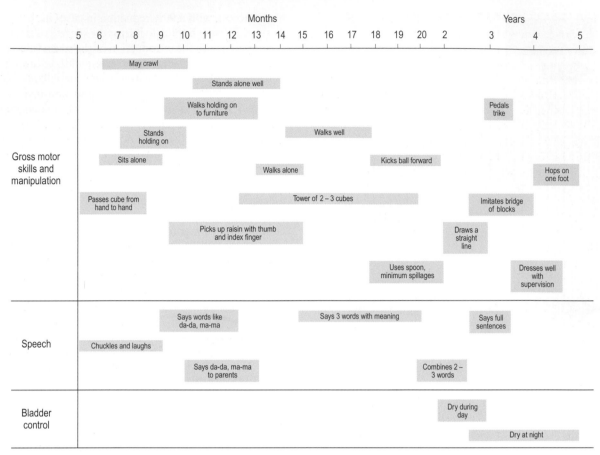

Fig. 10.2 A summary of the various stages of development.

Intramuscular absorption. Absorption in infants and children after intramuscular (i.m.) injection is noticeably faster than in the neonatal period, since muscle blood flow is increased. On a practical note, intramuscular administration is very painful and should, where possible, be avoided. The route should not be used for the convenience of staff if alternative routes of administration are available.

Intraosseous absorption. This is a useful route of administration in patients in whom intravenous access cannot be obtained. It is especially useful in paediatric cardiorespiratory arrests where rapid access is required. A specially designed needle is usually inserted into the flat tibial shaft until the marrow space is reached. This route is considered equivalent to the intravenous route for rate of drug absorption, and most drugs can be given by this route.

Topical absorption. Advances in transdermal drug delivery systems have led to an increased use of this route of administration. For example, patch formulations of hyoscine hydrobromide have been found to be very useful to dry up secretions in children with excess drooling; likewise fentanyl patches can be useful in pain management. Percutaneous absorption, which is inversely related to the thickness of the stratum corneum and directly related to skin hydration, is generally much greater in the newborn and young infant than in the adult. This can lead to adverse drug reactions (ADRs). For example, the topical application of a preparation containing prilocaine and lidocaine (EMLA) should not be used in preterm infants because of concerns about significant absorption of prilocaine in this age group, which may lead to methaemoglobinaemia. The development of needle-free subcutaneous jet injection systems appears to bring many benefits as a method of drug administration. They have been shown to give comparable levels to standard subcutaneous injections and overcome the problems of needle phobia, with less pain on administration. This system has been used with growth hormone, insulin, sedation prior to procedures and vaccination in children.

Another route of topical absorption is ophthalmically. Significant amounts of drugs may be absorbed from ophthalmic preparations through ophthalmic or nasolacrimal duct absorption; for example, administration of phenylephrine eye drops can lead to hypertensive episodes in children.

Rectal absorption. The rectal route of administration is generally less favoured in the UK than in other European countries. It can be useful in patients who are vomiting or in infants or children reluctant or unable to take oral medication. The mechanism of rectal absorption is probably similar to that of the upper part of the gastro-intestinal tract, despite differences in pH, surface area and fluid content. Although some products are erratically absorbed from the rectum, the rapid onset of action can be invaluable; for example, rectal diazepam solution produces a rapid cessation of seizures in epilepsy and can be easily administered by parents in an emergency.

Buccal absorption. The buccal cavity is a potentially useful route of administration in patients who cannot tolerate medications via the oral route; for example, postoperative patients or those with severe nausea. Highly lipophilic drugs can rapidly cross the buccal mucosa. Fentanyl is available as a lozenge formulation (Actiq®). This has been used to relax children before painful procedures and as a treatment for breakthrough pain in palliative care patients, although it remains unlicensed for use in children. Midazolam has also been administered via this route for the acute treatment of seizures and is favoured over rectal diazepam for this purpose.

There are a number of 'melt' and 'wafer' formulations available, for example, piroxicam and ondansetron. These preparations have the advantage of palatability; however, they are not absorbed via the buccal muscosa but require swallowing and enteral absorption of the active constituent. Desmopressin for buccal absorption has been introduced as an alternative to the tablet formulation 120 µcg is given buccally compared to 200 µcg orally.

Intranasal absorption. The intranasal route is another useful route of administration. Medicines can be administered intranasally for their local action, for example, sympathomimetics, or for their systemic effects, for example, desmopressin in the treatment of diabetes insipidus. Midazolam has been widely used intranasally in children for the treatment of anxiety prior to procedures and also for the treatment of childhood seizures. Highly lipophilic analgesics such as fentanyl are used via this route for the treatment of acute pain, particularly in situations where intravenous access is difficult, for example, reduction of fractures in the emergency department. Diamorphine may be administered by nasal instillation and is preferred to intramuscular or oral morphine.

Significant systemic absorption of medicines given intranasally for their local effect can also occur; for example, corticosteroids used in the treatment of allergic rhinitis have led to cushingoid symptoms and growth suppression.

Inhalation absorption. Direct delivery of drug therapies to the lungs has been the mainstay of treatment for asthma for many years. However, systemic absorption of corticosteroids used in the treatment of asthma may produce adrenal suppression.

The administration of insulin by inhalation for the treatment of both type 1 and type 2 diabetes mellitus in adults was anticipated to be of benefit in children. The first licensed product (for adults) was launched in 2006 but was withdrawn in 2007 due to disappointing worldwide sales. No similar product has replaced it.

Distribution

A number of factors that determine drug distribution within the body are subject to change with age. These include vascular perfusion, body composition, tissue-binding characteristics and the extent of plasma protein binding.

As a percentage of total body weight, the total body water and extracellular fluid volume decrease with age (Table 10.2). Thus, for water-soluble drugs such as aminoglycosides, larger doses on a milligram per kilogram of body weight basis are required in the neonate than in the older child to achieve similar plasma concentrations.

Table 10.2 Extracellular fluid volume and total body water as a percentage of body weight at different life stages

Age	Total body water (%)	Extracellular fluid (%)
Preterm neonate	85	50
Term neonate	75	45
3 months	75	30
1 year	60	25
Adult	60	20

Protein binding. Despite normal blood pH, free fatty acid and bilirubin levels in infants, binding to plasma proteins is reduced as a result of low concentrations of both globulins and albumin. It has been suggested that binding values comparable with those seen in adults are reached within the third year of life for acidic drugs, whereas for basic drugs adult values are not reached until between 7 and 12 years of life. The clinical significance of this reduction in infants and older children is minimal. The influence of disease states, such as renal impairment, on plasma protein binding is more important.

Drug metabolism

At birth the majority of the enzyme systems responsible for drug metabolism are either absent or present in considerably reduced amounts compared with adult values, and evidence indicates that the various systems do not mature at the same time. This reduced capacity for metabolic degradation at birth is followed by a dramatic increase in the metabolic rate in the older infant and young child. In the 1–9 year age group in particular, metabolic clearance of drugs is shown to be greater than in adults, as exemplified by theophylline, phenytoin and carbamazepine. Thus, to achieve plasma concentrations similar to those observed in adults, children in this age group may require a higher dosage than adults on a milligram per kilogram basis (Table 10.3).

Metabolic pathways that play only a minor role in adults may play a more significant role in children and compensate for any deficiencies in the normal adult metabolic pathway. For example, glucuronidation accounts for up to 70% of the metabolic pathway of paracetamol in adulthood; however,

Table 10.3 Theophylline dosage in children older than 1 year

Age	Dosage (mg/kg/day)
1–9 years	24
9–12 years	20
12–16 years	18
Adult	13

Table 10.4 Renal clearance of gentamicin

	Plasma half-life
Small premature infants weighing less than 1.5 kg	11.5 h
Small premature infants weighing 1.5–2 kg	8 h
Term infants and large premature infants less than 1 week of age	5.5 h
Infants 1 week to 6 months	3–3.5 h
Infants more than 6 months to adulthood	2–3 h

in the early newborn period glucuronidation is deficient, accounting for less than 20% of paracetamol metabolism. This is compensated for by a more pronounced sulphate conjugation and this leads to an apparently normal half-life in newborns. Paracetamol appears to be less toxic in children than in adults and this may be in part explained by the compensatory routes of metabolism.

Renal excretion

The anatomical and functional immaturity of the kidneys at birth limits renal excretory capacity. Below 3–6 months of age the glomerular filtration rate is lower than that of adults, but may be partially compensated for by a relatively greater reduction in tubular reabsorption. Tubular function matures later than the filtration process. Generally, the complete maturation of glomerular and tubular function is reached only towards 6–8 months of age. After 8 months the renal excretion of drugs is comparable with that observed in older children and adults. Changes in renal clearance of gentamicin provide a good example of the maturation of renal function (Table 10.4).

Other factors

In addition to age-related changes in drug disposition, nutritional status and disease states can influence drug handling. High plasma clearance of antibiotics such as penicillins and aminoglycosides has been demonstrated in children with cystic fibrosis; increased elimination of furosemide has been reported in children with nephrotic syndrome, while prolonged elimination of furosemide has been reported in infants with congestive cardiac failure. Altered protein binding has been demonstrated in hepatic disease, nephrotic syndrome, malnutrition and cardiac failure.

Drug therapy in children

Dosage

Doses of medicines in children should be obtained from a paediatric dosage handbook and should not be extrapolated from the adult dose. There are a number of such texts available

internationally. The information within them may be based on evidence from clinical studies in children or reflect the clinical experience of the contributors. In the UK, the BNF-C (see Further reading section) is a national formulary which includes prescribing guidelines and drug monographs. It contains information on licensed, unlicensed and off-label use of medicines. When consulting any dosage reference resource, care should be taken to identify the dosage convention being used. Most formularies use a single dose convention and indicate the number of times the dose should be repeated in a 24-h period. Other formularies indicate the total daily dose and the number of doses this is divided into. Some formularies combine both conventions. Confusing the total daily dose with the single dose to be repeated may have catastrophic consequences and the single dose convention has become the preferred convention.

While age, weight and height are the easiest parameters to measure, the changing requirement for drug dosage during childhood corresponds most closely with changes in body surface area (BSA). Nomograms which allow the surface area to be easily derived are available. There are practical problems in using the surface area method for prescribing; accurate height and weight may be difficult to obtain in a sick child, and manufacturers rarely provide dosage information on a surface area basis. The surface area formula for children has been used to produce the percentage method, giving the percentage of adult dose required at various ages and weights, although use should be reserved for exceptional circumstances (Table 10.5).

In selecting a method of dosage calculation, the therapeutic index of the drug should be considered. For agents with

Table 10.5 Percentage of adult dose required at various ages and body weights

	Mean weight for age (lb)	Mean weight for age (kg)	Percent of adult dose
Newborn (full term)	7.7	3.5	12.5
2 months	10	4.5	15
4 months	14	6.5	20
1 year	22	10	25
3 years	33	15	33.3
7 years	50	23	50
10 years	66	30	60
12 years	86	39	75
14 years	110	50	80
16 years	128	58	90
Adult	150	68	100

a narrow therapeutic index, such as cytotoxic agents, where recommendations are quoted per square metre, dosing must be based on the calculated surface area. However, there may be exceptions, for example, in children less than 1 year of age who have a proportionally larger surface area than other age groups. In children less than 1 year, dosages of chemotherapeutic agents are often based on weight rather than surface area to prevent overestimation of the dose in this age group.

For drugs with a wide therapeutic index, such as penicillin, single doses may be quoted for a wide age range. Between these two extremes, doses are quoted in milligrams per kilogram and this is the most widely used method of calculation. Whichever method is used, the resulting dosage should be rounded sensibly to facilitate dose measurement and administration and subsequently modified according to response or adverse effects.

It is important to note that none of the available methods of dosage calculation account for the change in dosage interval that may be required because of age-related changes in drug clearance. Where possible, the use of therapeutic drug monitoring to confirm the appropriateness of a dose is recommended.

Choice of preparation

The choice of preparation and its formulation will be influenced by the intended route of administration, the age of the child, availability of preparations, other concomitant therapy and, possibly, underlying disease states. The problems of administering medicines to children were reviewed by the European Medicines Evaluation Agency (EMEA, 2005).

Buccal route

Drugs may be absorbed rapidly from the buccal cavity (the cheek pouch) or they may dissolve when administered and be swallowed and absorbed from the stomach. 'Melt®' technology, for example, desmopressin, piroxicam, ondansetron, in which the drug and flavourings are freeze-dried into a rapidly dissolving pellet, can be very useful. The 'melt' dissolves instantly into a very small volume which is difficult for the child to reject. Gels, sprays and liquids can also be administered into the buccal cavity, using drugs such as midazolam to treat seizures.

Oral route

The oral route is usually the most convenient but in an uncooperative child it can be the least reliable. Safe and effective drug therapy requires accurate administration, yet the 5-mL spoon is a difficult means of administering liquid medicines. Use of an oral syringe can provide controlled administration, ensure accurate measurement of the calculated dose and avoids the need for dilution of preparations with syrup. Use of oral syringes (which will not fit an intravenous Luer connector) are mandatory in UK practice. Concentrated formulations may be administered as oral drops in a very small volume. Although convenient, there could be significant dosage errors if drops are not delivered accurately.

In general, liquid preparations are more suitable for children under 7 years of age; there is a wide variability in the age at which children can swallow tablets and capsules but some quite young children can cope with solid dose formulations, especially mini-tablets. Some commercially available products contain excipients such as alcohol, propylene glycol and dyes that may cause adverse effects or be inappropriate for use in children with particular disease states. The osmolality and tonicity of preparations may be important; necrotizing enterocolitis (a disorder seen in the neonatal period) has been associated with many different factors including high-osmolality infant feeding formulae and pharmaceutical preparations, although a causal relationship has not been established. Oral liquids with high-osmolality or extremes of pH may irritate the stomach and should be diluted for administration. Sugar-free preparations may be necessary in the diabetic child or be desirable in other children for the prevention of dental caries. It is, however, important to be aware of the potential problems associated with substitutes for sucrose. The artificial sweetening agent aspartame, used in some preparations, should be used with caution in children with phenylketonuria because of its phenylalanine content. Other substitutes such as sorbitol and glycerol may not contribute to dental caries but produce diarrhoea if large doses are given. In these instances, a specially formulated preparation containing a higher amount of the active drug in small volume may be preferable.

Injection solutions can sometimes be administered orally, although their concentration and pH must be considered together with the presence of unsuitable excipients. Powders or small capsules may be prepared and used as an alternative. However, lactose is a common diluent in powders and caution must be exercised in children with lactose intolerance as a result of an inborn error of metabolism, or temporarily following gastro-intestinal diseases or gut surgery.

Parents are often discouraged from adding the dose of medicine to an infant's feed. Quite apart from potential interactions which may arise with milk feeds, if the entire feed is not taken a proportion of the dose will be lost. It is also important to advise parents when it is not appropriate to crush solid dosage forms (e.g. sustained-release preparations). However, it should be recognised that addition of a medicine to a food or liquid may be the only way of rendering an unpalatable medicine acceptable. Whenever possible, evidence that this is pharmaceutically acceptable should be sought.

Manufacturers are increasingly recognising the difficulties associated with administration of medicines to children and are responding with novel formulations.

Mini tablets of just a few millimetres diameter may be useful to ease administration and allow flexibility of dosage. They may be presented in capsules or counted from bulk and can be individually coated for positioned or sustained release. Increased surface area may present larger quantities of excipients to the child and requires careful control.

If an age-appropriate formulation is not available, for example, for a medicine used off-label, a liquid oral preparation may be prepared extemporaneously, often by crushing the 'adult' tablets and suspending the powder in commercial or locally produced suspending agents. Alternatively the 'adult' dosage form may be manipulated, for example, by splitting tablets. Due consideration must be given to safety, accuracy and stability, when modifying dosage forms.

Nasogastric and gastrostomy administration

Medicines may be administered into the stomach via a nasogastric tube in the unconscious child or when swallowing is difficult. A gastrostomy tube may be placed into the stomach transcutaneously if the problem is long term, for example, in some children with cerebral palsy. Enteral nutrition may also be administered through such tubes. Drugs such as phenytoin may adsorb to the plastic of the tubes and interact with enteral feeds, requiring special administration techniques to ensure bioavailability. Suitability of drugs for nasogastric or gastrostomy tube administration should always be checked.

Intranasal route

Several drugs, such as desmopressin, diamorphine, fentanyl and midazolam, have been shown to be absorbed from the nasal mucosa. This route may avoid the need for injections but administration may be difficult in the uncooperative child and drugs administered may irritate the mucosa or be painful.

Rectal route

Although the rectal route can be useful, it is limited by the range of products available and the dosage inflexibility associated with rectal preparations. Some oral liquid preparations such as chloral hydrate and carbamazepine can be administered rectally. The route is useful in the unconscious child in the operating theatre or intensive care unit and it is not uncommon to administer perioperative analgesics such as diclofenac and paracetamol and the antiemetic ondansetron using suppository formulations. Parents and teachers may express concerns about using this route, fearing accusations of child abuse, but it is an important route of administration for diazepam or paraldehyde in the fitting child. Increasingly, buccal administration of midazolam may be preferred.

When oral and rectal routes are inappropriate, the parenteral route may be necessary.

Parenteral route

The problems associated with the administration of intramuscular injections in infants and children have been described earlier in this chapter. The route has a limited role in paediatric drug therapy and should not be used routinely. The intravenous route of administration is more widely used, but it is still associated with a number of potential problems that are outlined below.

Intravenous access. The practical difficulties of accessing small veins in the paediatric patient do not require explanation. However, these difficulties can often explain the sites of access that are chosen. Scalp veins, commonly used in newborn infants, are often very prominent in this age group, allowing easy access. It is also more difficult for the infant to dislodge a cannula from this site than from a site on the arm or foot. Likewise the umbilical artery offers a useful route for monitoring the patient but can also be used for drug administration in some circumstances. Vasoconstrictive drugs, such as adrenaline (epinephrine), dopamine and isoprenaline, should not be given by this route.

Fluid overload. In infants and children, the direct administration of intravenous fluids from the main infusion container is associated with the risk of inadvertent fluid overload. This problem can be avoided by the use of a paediatric administration set and/or a volumetric infusion device to control the flow rate. A paediatric administration set incorporates a graduated volumetric chamber with a maximum capacity of 150 mL. Although this system is intended primarily as a safety device, the volume within the burette chamber can be readily adjusted, allowing its use for intermittent drug administration and avoiding the need for the 'piggyback system' commonly used in adult intravenous administration.

Dilution of parenteral preparations for infusion may also cause inadvertent fluid overload in children. In fluid-restricted or very young infants, it is possible that the volume of diluted drug can exceed the daily fluid requirement. In order to appreciate this problem, the paediatric practitioner should become familiar with the fluid volumes that children can tolerate. As a guide these volumes can be calculated using the following formula: 100 mL/kg for the first 10 kg, plus 50 mL/kg for the next 10 kg, plus 20 mL/kg thereafter. Worked examples are given in Table 10.6. It is important to remember that these volumes do not account for losses such as those caused by dehydration, diarrhoea or artificial ventilation. While the use of more concentrated infusion solutions may overcome the problem of fluid overload, stability data on concentrated solutions are often lacking. It may, therefore, be necessary to manipulate other therapy to accommodate the treatment or even to consider alternative treatment options. Fluid overload may also result from excessive volumes of flushing solutions and is described later. Guidance on selecting appropriate intravenous fluids for administration to children to avoid fluid induced hyponatraemia are available (National Patient Safety Agency, 2007).

Lack of suitable paediatric formulations. A large number of parenteral products are only available in adult dose sizes.

Table 10.6 Calculation of standard daily fluid requirements in paediatric patients

15 kg patient	35 kg patient
100 mL/kg × 10 kg = 1000 mL	100 mL/kg × 10 kg = 1000 mL
Plus 50 mL/kg × 5 kg = 250 mL	Plus 50 mL/kg × 10 kg = 500 mL
Total = 1250 mL/day	Plus 20 mL/kg × 15 kg = 300 mL
	Total = 1800 mL/day

The concentrations of these products can make it difficult to measure the small doses required in paediatrics. Dilution to achieve measurable concentrations, miscalculations and misinterpretation of decimal points may lead to errors. 'Ten times' errors are common particularly when drawing the dose from a single ampoule or vial that contains sufficient for an adult patient.

Displacement volume. Reconstitution of powder injections in accordance with manufacturers' directions usually makes no allowance for the displacement volume of the powder itself. Hence, the final volume may be greater than expected and the concentration will, therefore, be less than expected. This can result in the paediatric patient receiving an underdose, which becomes even more significant in younger patients receiving smaller doses or more concentrated preparations. Paediatric units usually make available modified reconstitution directions which take account of displacement volumes.

Rates of infusion. The slow infusion rates often necessary in paediatrics may influence drug therapy. The greater the distance between the administration port and the distal end of the delivery system, and the slower the flow rate, the longer the time required for the drug to be delivered to the patient. In very young infants and children, it may take several hours for the drug to reach the patient, depending on the point of injection. This is an important consideration if dosage adjustments are being made in response to plasma level monitoring. Bolus injections should always be given as close to the patient as possible.

Dead space. Following administration via an injection port, a residual amount of drug solution can remain trapped at the port. If dose volumes are small the trapped fluid may represent a considerable proportion of the intended dose. Similarly, the volume of solution required to prime the intravenous lines or the in-line filters (i.e. the dead space) can be a significant proportion of the intended dose. This problem can be minimised by ensuring that drugs are flushed at an appropriate rate into the main infusion line after administration via an injection port or through a filter, and by priming the lines initially with a compatible solution. The small volumes required to prime filters and tubing specifically designed for infants and children can be used to minimise the dead space. Modern filter materials can produce less adsorption of drugs so that more of the drug is delivered to the patient.

It is important to remember that flushing volumes can add a significant amount to the daily fluid and sodium intake, and it may be important to record the volume of flushing solutions used in patients susceptible to fluid overload.

Excipients. Analogous to oral preparations, excipients may be present in parenteral formulations and can be associated with adverse effects. Benzyl alcohol, polysorbates and propylene glycol are commonly used agents which may induce a range of adverse effects in children including metabolic acidosis, altered plasma osmolality, central nervous system depression, respiratory depression, cardiac arrhythmias and seizures. Knowledge of the products that contain these ingredients may influence drug selection.

Many hospitals have established centralised intravenous additive services (CIVAS) that prepare single intravenous doses under aseptic conditions, thus avoiding the need for preparation at ward level. Such services have not only significantly decreased the risks associated with intravenous therapy, particularly in the paediatric population, but can also produce considerable cost savings.

Pulmonary route

The use of aerosol inhalers for the prevention and treatment of asthma presents particular problems for children because of the coordination required. The availability of breath-activated devices and spacer devices and large-volume holding chambers has greatly improved the situation. Guidance has been published on the use of inhaler devices in children less than 5 years of age (National Institute for Health and Clinical Excellence, 2000) and older children (National Institute for Health and Clinical Excellence, 2002) and updated in 2008 (British Thoracic Society and Scottish Intercollegiate Guidelines Network, 2008). Recent experience has shown that different types of large-volume holding chambers alter drug delivery and absorption and should not be considered as interchangeable.

It must be remembered that drugs can be absorbed into the systemic circulation after pulmonary administration or may be absorbed by the enteral route when excess drug is swallowed. High-dose corticosteroid inhalation may suppress the adrenal cortical axis and growth by this mechanism.

Dose regimen selection

A summary of the factors to be considered when selecting a drug dosage regimen or route of administration for a paediatric patient is shown in Table 10.7.

Counselling, adherence and concordance

Parents or carers are often responsible for the administration of medicines to their children and, therefore, the concordance and adherence of both parties must be considered. Literature about non-adherence and concordance in children is limited, but the problem is considered to be widespread and similar to that reported in adults.

Non-adherence may be caused by several factors such as patient resistance to taking the medicine, complicated dosage regimens, misunderstanding of instructions and apparent ineffectiveness or side effects of treatment. In older children and adolescents who may be responsible for their own medication, different factors may be responsible for non-adherence; for example, they may be unwilling to use their medication because of peer pressure.

Several general principles should be considered in an attempt to improve adherence. Adherence is usually better when fewer medicines are prescribed. Attention should be given to the formulation, taste, appearance and ease of

Table 10.7 Factors to be considered when selecting a drug dosage regimen or route of administration for a paediatric patient

Factor	Comment
1. Age/weight/surface area	Is the weight appropriate for the stated age? If it is not, confirm the difference. Can the discrepancy be explained by the patient's underlying disease, for example, patients with neurological disorders such as cerebral palsy may be significantly underweight for their age? Is there a need to calculate dosage based on surface area, for example, cytotoxic therapy? Remember heights and weights may change significantly in children in a very short space of time. It is essential to recheck the surface area at each treatment cycle using recent heights and weights
2. Assess the appropriate dose	The age/weight of the child may have a significant influence on the pharmacokinetic profile of the drug and the manner in which it is handled. In addition, the underlying disease state may influence the dosage or dosage interval
3. Assess the most appropriate interval	In addition to the influence of disease states and organ maturity on dosage interval, the significance of the child's waking day is often overlooked. A child's waking day is generally much shorter than that of an adult and may be as little as 12 h. Instructions given to parents particularly should take account of this, for example, the instruction 'three times a day' will bear no resemblance to 'every 8 hours' in a child's normal waking day. If a preparation must be administered at regular intervals, then the need to wake the child should be discussed with the parents or preferably an alternative formulation, such as a sustained-release preparation, should be considered
4. Assess the route of administration in the light of the disease state and the preparations and formulations available	Some preparations may require manipulation to ensure their suitability for administration by a specific route. Even preparations which appear to be available in a particular form may contain undesirable excipients that require alternatives to be found, for example, patients with the inherited metabolic disorder phenylketonuria should avoid oral preparations containing the artificial sweetener aspartame because of its phenylalanine content
5. Consider the expected response and monitoring parameters	Is the normal pharmacokinetic profile altered in children? Are there any age-specific or long-term adverse effects, such as on growth, that should be monitored?
6. Interactions	Drug interactions remain as important in reviewing paediatric prescriptions as they are in adult practice. However, drug–food interactions may be more significant; particularly drug–milk interactions in babies having 5–6 milk feeds per day
7. Legal considerations	Is the drug licensed? If an unlicensed drug is to be used, the pharmacist should have sufficient information to support its use

administration of treatment. The regimen should be simple and tailored to the child's waking day. If possible the child should be involved in choosing a suitable preparation when choice is available.

Many health professionals often counsel the parents/carer only, rather than involving the child in the counselling process. Where possible, treatment goals should be set in collaboration with the child. Studies have shown that parents consider the 8–10 year age group the most appropriate at which to start including the child in the counselling process. As well as verbal instruction, parents often want written information. However, current patient information leaflets (PILs) must reflect the Summary of Product Characteristics (SmPC) and so are often inappropriate. If a drug is used in an 'off-label' manner, statements such as 'not recommended for use in children' may cause confusion and distress. Care needs to be taken, therefore, to ensure that the information provided, whether written or spoken, is appropriate for both the parent and the child.

Information provided with medicines is often complex and may not always be relevant to children. The Royal College of

Paediatrics and Child Health in conjunction with other bodies have launched a range of information leaflets on medicines for parents and carers. The leaflets cover off-label use of specific drugs and aim to provide appropriate and accurate and easily understandable information on dosage and side effects to those administering medicines to children. The leaflets can be downloaded from the website: www.medicinesforchildren.org.uk

Medicines in schools

Children who are acutely ill will be treated with medicines at home or in hospital, although during their recovery phase it may be possible to return to school. Children with chronic illness such as asthma or epilepsy, and children recovering from acute illnesses, may require medicines to be administered whilst at school. In addition, there are some medical emergencies which may occur at school or on school trips that require prompt drug administration before the arrival of the emergency services. These emergencies include anaphylaxis (associated with food allergy or insect stings), severe asthma attacks and seizures.

Policies and guidance

There is considerable controversy over the administration of medicines in schools. There is no legal or contractual duty on school staff to administer medicine or supervise a pupil taking it. This is a voluntary role. Some support staff may have specific duties to provide medical assistance as part of their contract. Policies and procedures are required to ensure that prescribed medicines are labelled, stored and administered safely and appropriately, and that teachers and care assistants are adequately trained and understand their responsibilities.

Advice has been provided for schools and their employers on how to manage medicines in schools (Department for Education and Skills, 2005). The roles and responsibilities of employers, parents and carers, governing bodies, head teachers, teachers and other staff and of local health services are all explained. The advice considers staffing issues such as employment of staff, insurance and training. Other issues covered include drawing up a health care plan for a pupil, confidentiality, record keeping, the storage, access and disposal of medicines, home-to-school transport, and on-site and off-site activities. It also provides general information on four common conditions that may require management at school: asthma, diabetes, epilepsy and anaphylaxis.

Responsibility for common medicines

Responsible pupils should be allowed to administer their own medication. Asthmatics should carry their 'reliever' inhaler (e.g. salbutamol or terbutaline), a spare should be available in school, and easy access before and during sports assured. There should be no need to have 'preventer' inhalers at school since two or three times daily administration schedules are appropriate and can avoid school hours. Medicines with a two or three times daily administration schedule should be supplied wherever possible so that dosing during school hours is avoided. Sustained-release preparations or drugs with intrinsically long half-lives may be more expensive but avoid the difficulties of administration at school. Sustained-release methylphenidate and atomoxetine, both used in the management of attention deficit hyperactivity disorder or ADHD, are examples. When administration at school is unavoidable, the school time doses can be provided in a separate, labelled container.

Special schools

Some children with severe, chronic illness will go to special rather than mainstream schools where their condition can receive attention from teachers and carers who have undergone appropriate training. Some special schools will be residential. Pupils may also attend another institution for respite care. Particular attention to communication of changes to drug

treatment between parents, primary care doctors, hospital doctors and school staff is required if medication errors are to be avoided.

Monitoring parameters

Paediatric vital signs (Table 10.8) and haematological and biochemical parameters (Table 10.9) change throughout childhood and differ from those in adults. The figures presented in the tables are given as examples and may vary from hospital to hospital.

Table 10.8 Paediatric vital signs

	Age		
	<1 year	2–5 years	5–12 years
Heart rate (beats/min)	120–140	100–120	80–100
Blood pressure (systolic) (mmHg)	70–90	80–90	90–110
Respiratory rate (breaths/min)	25–45	25–30	16–25

Table 10.9 Biochemical and haematology reference ranges

	Neonate	Child	Adult
Albumin (g/L)	24–48	30–50	35–55
Bilirubin (µmol/L)	<200	<15	<17
Calcium (mmol/L)	1.8–2.8	2.15–2.7	2.20–2.55
Chloride (mmol/L)	95–110	95–110	95–105
Creatinine (µmol/L)	28–60	30–80	50–120
Haemoglobin (g/dL)	18–19	11–14	13.5–18.0 (males) 12–16 (females)
Haematocrit	0.55–0.65	0.36–0.42	0.4–0.45 (males) 0.36–0.44 (females)
Magnesium (mmol/L)	0.6–1.0	0.6–1.0	0.7–1.0
Phosphate (mmol/L)	1.3–3.0	1.0–1.8	0.85–1.4
Potassium (mmol/L)	4.0–7.0	3.5–5.5	3.5–5.0
Sodium (mmol/L)	130–145	132–145	135–145
Urea (mmol/L)	1.0–5.0	2.5–6.5	3.0–6.5
White cell count (×10⁹/L)	6–15	5–14	3.5–11

Assessment of renal function

There are a number of methods of measuring renal function in children. These include the use of ^{51}Cr-EDTA, ^{99m}Tc-DTPA and using serum and urine creatinine concentrations over a timed period. However, despite some limitations, serum creatinine and estimated creatinine clearance are the most frequently used and most practical methods for day-to-day assessment of renal function.

In adults, several formulae and nomograms are available for calculating and estimating renal function. However, these cannot be extrapolated to the paediatric population; the Cockcroft and Gault equation and the estimated GFR (eGFR) equation are validated only for patients aged 18 years and over.

A number of validated models are available for use in children. These equations use combinations of serum creatinine, height, weight, BSA, age and sex to provide a simple estimate of creatinine clearance. A number of these equations have been further modified to better predict creatinine clearance; however, the advantage of simplicity is thereby lost. Several examples with their validated age ranges are shown below:

- Traub and Johnson (age 1–18 years)

$$\text{Creatinine clearance} \atop (\text{mL/min/1.73}\,\text{m}^2) = \frac{42 \times \text{height (cm)}}{\text{Serum creatinine (mmol/L)}}$$

- Counahan-Barratt (age 2 months to 14 years)

$$\text{Creatinine clearance} \atop (\text{mL/min/1.73}\,\text{m}^2) = \frac{38 \times \text{height (cm)}}{\text{Serum creatinine (mmol/L)}}$$

- Schwartz

$$\text{Creatinine clearance} \atop (\text{mL/min/1.73}\,\text{m}^2) = \frac{k \times \text{height (cm)}}{\text{Serum creatinine (mmol/L)}}$$

where k varies dependent on the age of the patient:

> low birth weight infants = 30
> normal infants 0–18 months = 40
> girls 2–16 years = 49
> boys 2–13 years = 49
> boys 13–16 years = 60

Whichever equation is chosen, it should be borne in mind that there are limitations to their use; for example, they should not be used in rapidly changing renal function, anorexic or obese patients, and they should not be taken as an accurate measure but as a guide to glomerular filtration rate.

Adverse drug reactions

The incidence of ADRs in children outside the neonatal period is thought to be less than at all other ages; however, the nature and severity of the ADRs that children experience may differ from those experienced by adults.

Studies have shown an incidence of ADRs in paediatric patients of between 0.2% and 22% of patients. The wide range reflects the limited number of formal prospective and retrospective studies examining the incidence and characteristics of ADRs in the paediatric age group and the variations in study setting, patient group and definition of ADR used. Data can also be skewed by vaccination campaigns since adverse effects are common and reporting encouraged. One consistent finding is that the greater the number of medications the child is exposed to, the greater the risk of ADRs.

ADRs in infants and older children typically occur at lower doses than in adults, and symptoms may be atypical. Examples include:

- enamel hypoplasia and permanent discolouration of the teeth with tetracyclines
- growth suppression with long-term corticosteroids in prepubertal children
- paradoxical hyperactivity in children treated with phenobarbital
- hepatotoxicity associated with the use of sodium valproate. There are three major risk factors:
  - age under 3 years
  - child receiving other anticonvulsants
  - developmental delay
- increased risk of Reye's syndrome with the use of salicylates in children with mild viral infection. Reye's syndrome is a life-threatening illness associated with drowsiness, coma, hypoglycaemia, seizures and liver failure. The mechanism of this toxicity remains unknown but aspirin should generally be avoided in children under 16 years of age.

Many ADRs occur less frequently in the paediatric population, for example, gastro-intestinal bleeds with NSAIDs, hepatotoxicity with flucloxacillin and severe skin reactions with trimethoprim/sulfamethoxazole.

The reporting of ADRs is particularly important because the current system of drug development and authorisation not only deprives children of useful drugs because of the lack of clinical trials in children but may also exclude them from epidemiological studies of ADRs to prescribed drugs. The Commission on Human Medicines strongly encourages the reporting of all suspected ADRs in children, including those relating to unlicensed or off-label use of medicines, even if the intensive monitoring symbol (an inverted black triangle) has been removed. This reporting scheme has been extended in recent years to allow pharmacists, nurses and patients/carers to report suspected ADRs.

Medication errors

In contrast to ADRs, medication errors occur as a result of human mistakes or system flaws. Medication errors are now recognised as an important cause of adverse drug events in paediatric practice and should always be considered as a possible causative factor in any unexplained situation. They can produce a variety of problems ranging from minor discomfort to death. In the USA, it is estimated that

100–150 deaths occur annually in children in hospitals due to medication errors. The actual reported incidence of errors varies considerably between studies, ranging from 0.15% to 17% of admissions. However, different reporting systems and criteria for errors make direct comparisons between studies difficult.

The incidence of medication errors and the risk of serious errors occurring in children are significantly greater than in adults. The causes are many and include:

- Heterogeneous nature of the paediatric population and the corresponding lack of standard dosage.
- Calculation errors by the prescriber, pharmacist, nurse or caregiver.
- Lack of available dosage forms and concentrations appropriate for administration to children, necessitating additional calculations and manipulations of commercially available products or preparation of extemporaneous formulations from raw materials.
- Lack of familiarity with paediatric dosing guidelines.
- Confusion between adult and paediatric preparations.
- Limited published information.
- Need for precise dose measurement and appropriate drug delivery systems; absence leads to administration errors and use of inappropriate measuring devices.
- Ten-fold dosing errors are particularly important and potentially catastrophic; but reports still appear regularly in the published literature.

The reporting and prevention of medication errors is important. The causes of medication errors are usually multifactorial and it is essential that when investigating medication errors, particular focus should be placed on system changes.

Licensing medicines for children

Medicines licensing process

All medicines marketed in the UK must have been granted a product licence (PL) under the terms of the Medicines Act 1968, or a marketing authorisation (MA) following more recent European legislation on the authorisation of medicines. The aim of licensing is to ensure that medicines have been assessed for safety, quality and efficacy. In the UK, evidence submitted by a pharmaceutical company is assessed by the Medicines and Healthcare products Regulatory Agency (MHRA) with independent advice from the Commission on Human Medicines (CHM) and its paediatric medicines expert group.

The licensed indications for a drug are published in the SmPC. Many medicines granted a product license or MA for adult use have not been scrutinised by the licensing authorities for use in children. This is reflected by contraindications or cautionary wording in the SmPC. There has been a lack of commercial incentive to develop medicines for the relatively small paediatric market and perceived difficulties in carrying out clinical trials in this group. It is not illegal to use medicines for indications or ages not specified in the data sheet but to ensure safe and effective treatment, health professionals should have adequate supporting information about the intended use before proceeding. Failure to ensure that the use of a medicine is reasonable could result in a suit for negligence if the patient comes to harm.

Unlicensed and 'off-label' medicines

It has been reported that up to 35% of drugs used in a children's hospital and 10% of drugs used in general practice may be used outside the terms of the approved, licensed indications (McIntyre et al., 2000, Turner et al., 1998). The term 'off-label' is often used to describe this. Because many of these medicines will have been produced in 'adult' dose forms, such as tablets, it is often necessary to prepare extemporaneously a suitable liquid preparation for the child. This may be made from the licensed dose form, for example, by crushing tablets and adding suitable excipients, or from chemical ingredients. An appropriate formula with a validated expiry period and ingredients to approved standards should be used. Care must be taken to ensure accurate preparation, particularly when using formulae or ingredients which are unfamiliar.

On some occasions the drug to be used has no product license or MA, perhaps because it is only just undergoing clinical trials in adults, has been imported from another country, has been prepared under a 'specials' manufacturing licence or is being used for a rare condition for which it has not previously been employed. As with 'off-label' use, there must always be information to support the quality, efficacy and safety of the medicine as well as information on the intended use. There is always a risk in using such a medicine, which must be balanced against the seriousness of the child's illness and discussed with the parents if practicable.

Many authorities require that the patient should always be informed if the medicine prescribed is unlicensed or 'off-label' and even that written informed consent be obtained before treatment begins. In many situations, in paediatrics, this would be impractical but if parents are not informed the PIL included with many medicines may cause confusion since it may state that it is 'not for use in children'. Patient or parent information specific to the situation should be prepared and provided.

Recent legislation on medicines for children

The worldwide legislation on medicines for children is changing. This is in recognition of the limited research and small number of licensed medicines brought about by a lack of incentive for commercial development. Both Europe and the USA have orphan drugs regulations designed to offer incentives for the development of medicines for rare diseases. Although not exclusively for paediatric conditions, the regulations have assisted the development of important drugs such as antiretrovirals (HIV/AIDS), alendronate (osteogenesis imperfecta), α-galactosidase (Fabry's disease), sodium phenylbutyrate (hyperammonaemia) and ibuprofen injection (closure of patent ductus arteriosus).

The USA has had regulations designed to promote the development of paediatric preparations for more than 10 years (Best Pharmaceuticals for Children Act 2002 and Pediatric Research Equity Act 2003). However, these regulations have resulted in few significant developments in medicines for children in other countries. In the European Union, the 'European Parliament and Council Regulation (EC) on medicinal products for paediatric use' became law in January 2007. Thereafter, pharmaceutical companies wishing to market medicines for adults must agree to a Paediatric Investigation Plan with the EMEA. In return for such development, the company will receive an additional 6 months market exclusivity for its product. There are also expected to be incentives for developing paediatric formulations and indications for off-patent medicines.

Several European governments have funded paediatric clinical trials networks to stimulate research and help undertake studies resulting from the paediatric medicines regulations. In the UK, the Medicines for Children Research Network (MCRN) is part of the UK National Institute for Health Research and has six local research networks in England with equivalent provision in the other UK countries. Research and development of paediatric formulations is part of the MCRN programme.

The WHO has a 'Make medicines child size' programme to stimulate the development of age-appropriate formulations of medicines for children, particularly for those which appear in the List of Essential Medicines for Children. In June 2010, the first ever WHO model formulary for children was released to provide information on how to use over 240 essential medicines for treating illness and disease in children from 0 to 12 years of age. A number of individual countries have developed their own formularies over the years, but until now there was no single comprehensive guide for all countries (available at: http://www.who.int/childmedicines/en/).

Service frameworks

National service frameworks (NSFs) are long-term strategies for improving specific areas of care. Two paediatric service frameworks have been published; one for paediatric intensive care (Department of Health, 2002) and another for children, young people and maternity services (Department of Health, 2004) and continue to influence practice.

The service framework for paediatric intensive care defines the nature of paediatric intensive care, the elements of a high-quality paediatric intensive care service and a policy framework for the future organisation of services. Standards for district general hospitals, lead centres, major acute general hospitals and specialist hospitals are set out and cover medical and nurse staffing, facilities, and clinical effectiveness and management. Other aspects considered include retrieval services, education and training needs, and the implications for audit and research.

The framework for children, young people and maternity services sets standards for children's health and social services, and the interface of those services with education. It establishes clear standards for promoting the health and well-being of children and young people and for providing high-quality services which meet their needs.

The recommendations that relate to the use of medicines for children and young people include:

- All children and young people should receive medicines that are safe and effective, in formulations that can be easily administered and are appropriate to their age, having minimum impact on their education and lifestyle.
- Medicines should be prescribed, dispensed and administered by professionals who are well trained, informed and competent to work with children to improve health outcomes and minimise harm and any side effects of medicines.
- Children and young people and their parents or carers should be well informed and supported to make choices about their medicines and competent in the administration of medicines.

Markers of good practice are defined as:

- The use of medicines in children is based on the best available evidence of clinical use and cost-effectiveness and safety, ideally derived from clinical trials but also including, where appropriate, medicines that are not licensed for their age group or for their particular health problem ('off-label') or those that do not have a licence at all ('unlicensed') in order to achieve the best possible health outcomes and minimise harm and side effects.
- In all settings and whatever the circumstances, children and young people have equitable access to clinically safe and cost-effective medicines in age-appropriate formulations.
- Appropriate information and decision support are available for professionals who prescribe, dispense and administer medicines for children and young people.
- Children, young people and their parents/carers receive consistent, up-to-date, comprehensive, timely information on the safe and effective use of medicines.
- In all settings, professionals enable parents, young people and, where appropriate, children to be active partners in the decisions about the medicines prescribed for them.
- Primary and secondary care providers should ensure that the use of medicines in children is incorporated in their clinical governance and audit arrangements.
- The contribution of pharmacists to the effective and safe use of medicines in children is maximised.

Case studies

Case 10.1

Name: PT
Age: 7 years old
Sex: Male
Weight: 16 kg

Presenting condition:	Presented in the emergency department with a 2-day history of worsening groin and hip pain. Could not bear weight. Patient was febrile with a temperature of 39.2°C, vomiting and dehydrated. There was no history of injury.
Previous medical history:	Nil of note
Allergies:	No known drug allergies
Drug history:	Nil of note

Differential diagnosis:	Septic arthritis, osteomyelitis
Tests:	Urea and electrolytes
	Full blood count
	CRP, ESR
	Blood culture and sensitivities
	X-ray (hips and abdomen)
	Bone scan
Results:	Bone scan revealed right pubic osteomyelitis
	CRP = 56 mg/L (normal range 0–10 mg/L)
	ESR = 34 mm/h (normal range 1–10 mm/h)
	Blood culture revealed *Staphylococcus aureus* sensitive to flucloxacillin
Prescribed:	Flucloxacillin i.v. 800 mg four times a day for 2 weeks. To be followed by oral flucloxacillin 800 mg four times a day for 4 weeks
Progress:	Temperature settled and ESR/CRP decreased following initiation of antibiotic therapy

On the third day of treatment the patient developed a raised red rash which was suspected of being an allergic reaction to flucloxacillin. Treatment was changed to i.v. clindamycin 160 mg three times a day (10 mg/kg/dose) for 2 weeks followed by oral clindamycin 160 mg three times a day for a further 4 weeks.

Question

Comment on the drug therapy and any monitoring required.

Answer

There are a number of points to consider in this patient.
- Body weight appears low for age; therefore, need to check if the weight is correct (expected weight for a 7-year old to be approx. 23 kg). If incorrect, doses of medication will need to be recalculated.
- Recommended i.v. dose of flucloxacillin of 50 mg/kg/dose is correct. However, usual maximum oral dose of flucloxacillin is 25 mg/kg/dose. This is because of the increased risk of gastric side effects with high oral doses of flucloxacillin.
- There is a need to consider compliance with oral flucloxacillin therapy due to poor palatability of the suspension formulation (if the child would not take capsules) and the frequent dosing regimen.
- Whilst the risk of flucloxacillin-induced hepatotoxicity is low in children, there is a need to consider measuring baseline and repeat liver function tests because of the prolonged course (more than 2 weeks) of flucloxacillin therapy.
- Clindamycin has good oral bioavailability, so i.v. therapy may be unnecessary.
- The recommended dose of clindamycin by i.v. infusion is up to 10 mg/kg dose 6 hourly in severe infection. The infusion should be diluted to 6 mg/mL with sodium chloride 0.9% or dextrose 5% (or a combination) and administered over 30–60 min at a maximum rate of 20 mg/kg/h. Consider 160 mg in 27 mL sodium chloride 0.9% over 30 min.
- The recommended standard oral dose of clindamycin is 3–6 mg/kg/dose four times a day. This may contribute to problems with adherence to long-term therapy. A three times daily dosing regimen is to be preferred, particularly as this child may return to school, and four times daily dosing would require a dose to be administered at school which may be problematic.
- Consideration should be given to how to administer clindamycin. Clindamycin palmitate suspension, which was palatable, is no longer available as a licensed preparation in the UK. Whilst

extemporaneous formulations are available that use clindamycin hydrochloride capsules, the palatability of the resultant suspension is a major concern, particularly given the prolonged course of therapy. A 75 mg/5 mL suspension, licensed in Belgium, can be imported. From a safety and efficacy perspective it is preferable to use such a product, which has been through a regulatory process similar to that of the UK, than to compound an extemporaneous preparation, which has not undergone appropriate pharmaceutical/pharmacokinetic evaluation.
- Consideration could be given to decreasing the dose of clindamycin to 150 mg three times a day to accommodate capsules, although the child may have difficulty taking these.
- The most serious adverse effect of clindamycin is antibiotic-associated colitis. Therefore, it is important to monitor for diarrhoea. If this arises treatment should be discontinued.

Case 10.2

Name: CS
Age: 18 months old
Sex: Female
Weight: 10 kg

Presenting condition:	Severe right-sided abdominal pain
	Vomiting and loss of appetite
	Increased temperature 38.2°C
Previous medical history:	Nil of note
Allergies:	No known allergies
Drug history:	Nil of note
Tests:	Ultrasound
Provisional diagnosis:	Appendicitis

CS went to theatre where an appendicectomy was performed. The appendix was noted to be perforated.

Prescribed:	Morphine 50 mg in 50 mL to run at 1–4 mL/h (10–40 µcg/kg/h)
	Paracetamol 200 mg four times a day as required orally or per rectum
	Diclofenac 12.5 mg twice a day as required per rectum.
	or
	Ibuprofen 100 mg four times a day as required orally when tolerating milk
	Five days of i.v. antibiotic therapy with:
	Gentamicin 70 mg daily
	Ampicillin 250 mg four times a day
	Metronidazole 75 mg three times a day

Question

Comment on the patient's drug therapy.

Answer

- The morphine dose is incorrect. If the infusion is prepared as directed, 1 mL/h will actually provide 100 µcg/kg/h. This is a 10-fold overdose which is a medication error frequently seen in children.
- There is a need to consider how to administer the appropriate rectal dose of paracetamol to this child. Often post appendicectomy patients will need to be nil by mouth for several days. Rectal bioavailability is lower than oral bioavailability and there may be a need to consider giving a larger rather than smaller paracetamol dose, that is, possibly 250 mg/rectum 8 hourly rather than 125 mg 6 hourly, for up to 48 h, but not exceeding 90 mg/kg/day.
- Suggest that paracetamol and NSAID are administered regularly in addition to the morphine for at least the first few days post-surgery. Multimodal analgesic therapy is recommended.

- There will be a need to monitor CS for side effects. Nausea, vomiting and pruritus all occur frequently with morphine but can be treated/prevented.
- Young children are particularly susceptible to developing myoclonic jerks with morphine. These are often worrying for parents but resolve on withdrawal of the morphine.
- NSAIDs are well tolerated by children and the risk of adverse events is much lower in children than the adult population. However, it is important to ensure adequate hydration status postoperatively, particularly when using NSAIDs. Acute renal failure has been reported in children who have been treated with NSAIDs and not adequately hydrated.
- The choice of antibiotics for CS is appropriate. High-dose (7 mg/kg) once-daily aminoglycoside (gentamicin/tobramycin) therapy is now routinely used in children. It is administered by short infusion over 20 min. Plasma drug levels should be monitored to achieve a 18–24 h trough level of <1 mg/L. Monitor urea and electrolytes and serum creatinine. Ampicillin can be given as a bolus injection over 3–5 min. Metronidazole should be given as a short infusion over 20 min.

References

Anderson, B.J., Holford, N.H.G., 2008. Mechanism-based concepts of size and maturity in pharmacokinetics. Annu. Rev. Pharmacol. Toxicol. 48, 303–332.

Anderson, B.J., Holford, N.H., 2009. Mechanistic basis of using body size and maturation to predict clearance in humans. Drug. Metab. Pharmacokinet. 24, 25–36.

British National Formulary for Children, 2010. Pharmaceutical Press, London. Available at: www.bnfc.nhs.uk/bnfc/

British Thoracic Society and Scottish Intercollegiate Guidelines Network, 2008. British Guideline on the Management of Asthma. SIGN, Edinburgh. Available at: http://www.sign.ac.uk/guidelines/fulltext/101/index.html

Department for Education and Skills, 2005. Managing Medicines in Schools and Early Years Settings. Department for Education and Skills, London. Available at: http://publications.education.gov.uk/eOrderingDownload/1448–2005PDF-EN-02.pdf

Department of Health, 2002. National Service Framework for Paediatric Intensive Care. Stationery Office, London.

Department of Health, 2004. The National Service Framework for Children, Young People and Maternity Services. Stationery Office, London. Available at: http://www.dh.gov.uk/en/Publicationsandstatistics/Publications/PublicationsPolicyAndGuidance/DH_4089100

European Medicines Evaluation Agency, 2005. Reflection Paper: Formulations of Choice for the Paediatric Population. EMEA, London. Available at: http://www.ema.europa.eu/docs/en_GB/document_library/Scientific_guideline/2009/09/WC500003782.pdf

International Committee on Harmonization, 2001. Note for Guidance on Clinical Investigation of Medicinal Products in the Paediatric Population. European Medicines Agency, London. Available at: http://www.ema.europa.eu/docs/en_GB/document_library/Scientific_guideline/2009/09/WC500002926.pdf

McIntyre, J., Conroy, S., Avery, A., et al., 2000. Unlicensed and off label prescribing of drugs in general practice. Arch. Dis. Child. 83, 498–501.

MRC Vitamin Study Research Group, 1991. Prevention of neural tube defects: results of the Medical Research Council vitamin study. Lancet 338, 131–137.

National Institute for Health and Clinical Excellence, 2000. Guidance on the Use of Inhaler Systems (Devices) in Children Under the Age of 5 Years with Chronic Asthma. Technology Appraisal 10. NICE, London. Available at http://www.nice.org.uk/nicemedia/pdf/NiceINHALERguidance.pdf

National Institute for Health and Clinical Excellence, 2002. Inhaler Devices for Routine Treatment of Chronic Asthma in Older Children (aged 5–15 years). Technology Appraisal No. 38. NICE, London. Available at http://www.nice.org.uk/nicemedia/live/11450/32338/32338.pdf

National Patient Safety Agency, 2007. Reducing the Risk of Hyponatraemia When Administering Intravenous Solutions to Children. NPSA, London. Available at: http://www.nrls.npsa.nhs.uk/resources/?EntryId45=59809

Turner, S., Longworth, A., Nunn, A.J., et al., 1998. Unlicensed and off-label drug use in paediatric wards: prospective study. Br. Med. J. 316, 343–345.

Further reading

Advanced Life Support Group, 2005. Advanced Paediatric Life Support: The Practical Approach, fourth ed. Blackwell, London.

Advanced Life Support Group, 2005. Prehospital Paediatric Life Support: The Practical Approach. BMJ Books, London.

Behrman, R.E., Kliegman, R.M., Jenson, H.B., et al. (Eds.), 2007. Nelson Textbook of Pediatrics, eighteenth ed. W. B. Saunders, Philadelphia.

Lewisham and North Southwark Health Authority, 2005. Guy's, St Thomas's and Lewisham Hospitals Paediatric Formulary, seventh ed. Lewisham and North Southwark Health Authority, London.

NHS Education for Scotland (NES), 2009. An Introduction to Paediatric Pharmaceutical Care. Available online at: www.nes.scot.nhs.uk/pharmacy.

Phelps, S.J., Hak, E.B., 2007. Teddy Bear Book: Pediatric Injectable Drugs, eighth ed. American Society of Health System Pharmacists, Bethesda.

Taketomo, C., Hodding, J.H., Kraus, D.M., 2009. Pediatric Dosage Handbook, sixteenth ed. Lexi-Comp, Hudson.

Useful websites

Child Growth Standards: www.who.int/childgrowth/en/

Contact a Family (for families with disabled children): www.cafamily.org.uk/

Immunization against infectious diseases: www.dh.gov.uk/PolicyAndGuidance/HealthAndSocialCareTopics/GreenBook/

Neonatal and Paediatric Pharmacists Group (NPPG): www.nppg.org.uk/

Royal College of Paediatrics and Child Health: www.rcpch.ac.uk/

The National Congenital Anomalies System: www.statistics.gov.uk/CCI/SearchRes.asp?term=congenital+anomalies

Geriatrics 11

H. G. M. Shetty and K. Woodhouse

Key points

- The elderly form about 18% of the population and receive about one-third of health service prescriptions in the UK.
- Ageing results in physiological changes that affect the absorption, metabolism, distribution and elimination of drugs.
- Alzheimer's disease and vascular dementia are the most important diseases of cognitive dysfunction in the elderly. Donepezil, rivastigmine and galantamine are inhibitors of acetylcholinesterase and improve cognitive function in Alzheimer's disease.
- The elderly patient with Parkinson's disease is more susceptible to the adverse effects of levodopa such as postural hypotension, ventricular dysrhythmias and psychiatric effects.
- Aspirin, dipyridamole and clopidogrel reduce the reoccurrence of non-fatal strokes in the elderly.
- Treatment of elevated systolic and diastolic blood pressure in the elderly with a low dose thiazide diuretic, β-blocker, calcium antagonist or angiotensin-converting enzyme (ACE) inhibitor have all been shown to be beneficial.
- Urinary incontinence can be classified as stress incontinence, overflow incontinence or due to detrusor instability. Stress incontinence is not amenable to drug therapy. The most common drugs used in detrusor instability are oxybutynin and tolterodine.
- Non-steroidal anti-inflammatory drugs (NSAIDs) are more likely to cause gastroduodenal ulceration and bleeding in the elderly.

The elderly have multiple and often chronic diseases. It is not surprising, therefore, that they are the major consumers of drugs. Elderly people receive about one-third of National Health Service (NHS) prescriptions in the UK. In most developed countries, the elderly now account for 25–40% of drug expenditure.

A survey of drug usage in 778 elderly people in the UK showed that 70% had been on prescribed medication and 40% had taken one or more prescribed drugs within the previous 24 h; 32% were taking cardiovascular drugs, and the other therapeutic categories used in decreasing order of frequency were for disorders of the central nervous system (24%), musculoskeletal system (10%), gastro-intestinal system (8%) and respiratory system (7%). The most commonly used drugs were diuretics; analgesics; hypnotics, sedatives and anxiolytics; antirheumatic drugs; and β-blockers.

Institutionalised patients tend to be on larger numbers of drugs compared with patients in the community. One study has shown that patients in long-term care facilities are likely to be receiving, on average, eight drugs. Psychotropic drugs are used widely in nursing or residential homes.

For optimal drug therapy in the elderly, a knowledge of age-related physiological and pathological changes that might affect handling of and response to drugs is essential. This chapter discusses the age-related pharmacokinetic and pharmacodynamic changes which might affect drug therapy and the general principles of drug use in the elderly.

There has been a steady increase in the number of elderly people, defined as those over 65 years of age, since the beginning of the twentieth century. They formed only 4.8% of the population in 1901, increasing to 15.2% in 1981 and about 18% in 2001. In 2008, there were 4.8 million people over the age of 75 years in the UK. Their number is projected to increase to 5.8 million by 2018 and to 8.7 million by 2033 – a rise of 81% over 25 years. In addition, the number of people over 85 years of age is also projected to increase from 1.3 million in 2008 to 3.3 million in 2033. The number of centenarians is projected to increase from 11,000 in 2008 to 80,000 in 2033 (Office for National Statistics, 2010). The significant increase in the number of very elderly people will have important social, financial and health care planning implications.

Pharmacokinetics

Ageing results in many physiological changes that could theoretically affect absorption, first-pass metabolism, protein binding, distribution and elimination of drugs. Age-related changes in the gastro-intestinal tract, liver and kidneys are

- reduced gastric acid secretion
- decreased gastro-intestinal motility
- reduced total surface area of absorption
- reduced splanchnic blood flow
- reduced liver size
- reduced liver blood flow
- reduced glomerular filtration
- reduced renal tubular filtration.

149

Absorption

There is a delay in gastric emptying, reduction in gastric acid output and splanchnic blood flow with ageing. These changes do not significantly affect the absorption of the majority of drugs. Although the absorption of some drugs such as digoxin may be slower, the overall absorption is similar to that in the young.

First-pass metabolism

After absorption, drugs are transported via the portal circulation to the liver, where many lipid-soluble agents are metabolised extensively (more than 90–95%). This results in a marked reduction in systemic bioavailability. Obviously, even minor reductions in first-pass metabolism can result in a significant increase in the bioavailability of such drugs.

Impaired first-pass metabolism has been demonstrated in the elderly for several drugs, including clomethiazole, labetalol, nifedipine, nitrates, propranolol and verapamil. The clinical effects of some of these, such as the hypotensive effect of nifedipine, may be significantly enhanced in the elderly. In frail hospitalised elderly patients, that is, those with chronic debilitating disease, the reduction in pre-systemic elimination is even more marked.

Distribution

The age-related physiological changes which may affect drug distribution are

- reduced lean body mass
- reduced total body water
- increased total body fat
- lower serum albumin level
- α_1-acid glycoprotein level unchanged or slightly raised.

Increased body fat in the elderly results in an increased volume of distribution for fat-soluble compounds such as clomethiazole, diazepam, desmethyl-diazepam and thiopental. On the other hand, reduction in body water results in a decrease in the distribution volume of water-soluble drugs such as cimetidine, digoxin and ethanol.

Acidic drugs tend to bind to plasma albumin, while basic drugs bind to α_1-acid glycoprotein. Plasma albumin levels decrease with age and therefore the free fraction of acidic drugs such as cimetidine, furosemide and warfarin will increase. Plasma α_1-acid glycoprotein levels may remain unchanged or may rise slightly with ageing, and this may result in minimal reductions in free fractions of basic drugs such as lidocaine. Disease-related changes in the level of this glycoprotein are probably more important than age *per se*.

The age-related changes in distribution and protein binding are probably of significance only in the acute administration of drugs because, at steady state, the plasma concentration of a drug is determined primarily by free drug clearance by the liver and kidneys rather than by distribution volume or protein binding.

Renal clearance

Although there is a considerable interindividual variability in renal function in the elderly, in general the glomerular filtration rate declines, as do the effective renal plasma flow and renal tubular function. Because of the marked variability in renal function in the elderly, the dosages of predominantly renally excreted drugs should be individualised. Reduction in dosages of drugs with a low therapeutic index, such as digoxin and aminoglycosides, may be necessary. Dosage adjustments may not be necessary for drugs with a wide therapeutic index, for example, penicillins.

Hepatic clearance

Hepatic clearance (Cl_H) of a drug is dependent on hepatic blood flow (Q) and the steady state extraction ratio (E), as can be seen in the following formula:

$$Cl_H = Q \times \frac{C_a - C_v}{C_a} = Q \times E$$

where C_a and C_v are arterial and venous concentrations of the drug, respectively. It is obvious from the above formula that when E approaches unity, Cl_H will be proportional to and limited by Q. Drugs which are cleared by this mechanism have a rapid rate of metabolism, and the rate of extraction by the liver is very high. The rate-limiting step, as mentioned earlier, is hepatic blood flow, and therefore drugs cleared by this mechanism are called 'flow limited'. On the other hand, when E is small, Cl_H will vary according to the hepatic uptake and enzyme activity, and will be relatively independent of hepatic blood flow. The drugs which are cleared by this mechanism are termed 'capacity limited'.

Hepatic extraction is dependent upon liver size, liver blood flow, uptake into hepatocytes, and the affinity and activity of hepatic enzymes. Liver size falls with ageing and there is a decrease in hepatic mass of 20% and 40% between the third and tenth decade. Hepatic blood flow falls equally with declining liver size. Although it is recognised that the microsomal mono-oxygenase enzyme systems are significantly reduced in ageing male rodents, evidence suggests that this is not the case in ageing humans. Conjugation reactions have been reported to be unaffected in the elderly by some investigators, but a small decline with increasing age has been described by others.

Impaired clearance of many hepatically eliminated drugs has been demonstrated in the elderly. Morphological changes rather than impaired enzymatic activity appear to be the main cause of impaired elimination of these drugs. In frail debilitated elderly patients, however, the activities of drug-metabolising enzymes such as plasma esterases and hepatic glucuronyltransferases may well be impaired.

Pharmacodynamics

Molecular and cellular changes that occur with ageing may alter the response to drugs in the elderly. There is, however, limited information about these alterations because of the technical difficulties and ethical problems involved in measuring them. It is not surprising, therefore, that there is relatively little information about the effect of age on pharmacodynamics.

Changes in pharmacodynamics in the elderly may be considered under two headings:

- those due to a reduction in homeostatic reserve and
- those that are secondary to changes in specific receptor and target sites.

Reduced homeostatic reserve

Orthostatic circulatory responses

In normal elderly subjects, there is blunting of the reflex tachycardia that occurs in young subjects on standing or in response to vasodilatation. Structural changes in the vascular tree that occur with ageing are believed to contribute to this observation, although the exact mechanism is unclear. Antihypertensive drugs, drugs with α receptor blocking effects (e.g. tricyclic antidepressants, phenothiazines and some butyrophenones), drugs which decrease sympathetic outflow from the central nervous system (e.g. barbiturates, benzodiazepines, antihistamines and morphine) and antiparkinsonian drugs (e.g. levodopa and bromocriptine) are, therefore, more likely to produce hypotension in the elderly.

Postural control

Postural stability is normally achieved by static reflexes, which involve sustained contraction of the musculature, and phasic reflexes, which are dynamic, short term and involve transient corrective movements. With ageing, the frequency and amplitude of corrective movements increase and an age-related reduction in dopamine (D_2) receptors in the striatum has been suggested as the probable cause. Drugs which increase postural sway, for example hypnotics and tranquillisers, have been shown to be associated with the occurrence of falls in the elderly.

Thermoregulation

There is an increased prevalence of impaired thermoregulatory mechanisms in the elderly, although it is not universal. Accidental hypothermia can occur in the elderly with drugs that produce sedation, impaired subjective awareness of temperature, decreased mobility and muscular activity, and vasodilatation. Commonly implicated drugs include phenothiazines, benzodiazepines, tricyclic antidepressants, opioids and alcohol, either on its own or with other drugs.

Cognitive function

Ageing is associated with marked structural and neurochemical changes in the central nervous system. Cholinergic transmission is linked with normal cognitive function, and in the elderly the activity of choline acetyltransferase, a marker enzyme for acetylcholine, is reduced in some areas of the cortex and limbic system. Several drugs cause confusion in the elderly. Anticholinergics, hypnotics, H_2 antagonists and β-blockers are common examples.

Visceral muscle function

Constipation is a common problem in the elderly as there is a decline in gastro-intestinal motility with ageing. Anticholinergic drugs, opiates, tricyclic antidepressants and antihistamines are more likely to cause constipation or ileus in the elderly. Anticholinergic drugs may cause urinary retention in elderly men, especially those who have prostatic hypertrophy. Bladder instability is common in the elderly, and urethral dysfunction more prevalent in elderly women. Loop diuretics may cause incontinence in such patients.

Age-related changes in specific receptors and target sites

Many drugs exert their effect via specific receptors. Response to such drugs may be altered by the number (density) of receptors, the affinity of the receptor, postreceptor events within cells resulting in impaired enzyme activation and signal amplification, or altered response of the target tissue itself. Ageing is associated with some of these changes.

α-Adrenoceptors

α_2-Adrenoceptor responsiveness appears to be reduced with ageing while α_1-adrenoceptor responsiveness appears to be unaffected.

β-Adrenoceptors

β-Adrenoceptor function declines with age. It is recognised that the chronotropic response to isoprenaline infusion is less marked in the elderly. Propranolol therapy in the elderly produces less β-adrenoceptor blocking effect than in the young. In isolated lymphocytes, studies of cyclic adenosine monophosphate (AMP) production have shown that on β-adrenoceptor stimulation the dose–response curve is shifted to the right, and the maximal response is blunted.

An age-related reduction in β-adrenoceptor density has been shown in animal adipocytes, erythrocytes and brain, and also in human lymphocytes in one study, although this has not been confirmed by other investigators. As maximal response occurs on stimulation of only 0.2% of β-adrenoceptors, a reduction in the number by itself is unlikely to account for age-related changes. Some studies have shown a reduction in high-affinity binding sites with ageing, in the absence of change in total receptor numbers, and others have suggested that there may be impairment of postreceptor transduction mechanisms with ageing that may account for reduced β-adrenoceptor function.

Cholinergic system

The effect of ageing on cholinergic mechanisms is less well known. Atropine produces less tachycardia in elderly humans than in the young. It has been shown in ageing rats that the hippocampal pyramidal cell sensitivity to acetylcholine is reduced. The clinical significance of this observation is unclear.

Benzodiazepines

The elderly are more sensitive to benzodiazepines than the young, and the mechanism of this increased sensitivity is not known. No difference in the affinity or number of benzodiazepine-binding sites has been observed in animal studies. Habituation to benzodiazepines occurs to the same extent in the elderly as in the young.

Warfarin

The elderly are more sensitive to warfarin. This phenomenon may be due to age-related changes in pharmacodynamic factors. The exact mechanism is unknown.

Digoxin

The elderly appear to be more sensitive to the adverse effects of digoxin, but not to the cardiac effects.

Common clinical disorders

This section deals in detail only with the most important diseases affecting older people. Other conditions are mentioned primarily to highlight areas where the elderly differ from the young or where modifications of drug therapy are necessary.

Dementia

Dementia is characterised by a gradual deterioration of intellectual capacity. Alzheimer's disease (AD), vascular dementia (VaD), dementia with Lewy bodies and frontotemporal dementia are the most important diseases of cognitive dysfunction in the elderly. AD has a gradual onset, and it progresses slowly. Forgetfulness is the major initial symptom. The patient has difficulty in dressing and other activities of daily living. He or she tends to get lost in his or her own environment. Eventually, the social graces are lost. VaD is the second most important cause of dementia. It usually occurs in patients in their 60s and 70s, and is more common in those with a previous history of hypertension or stroke. It is commonly associated with mood changes and emotional lability. Physical examination may reveal focal neurological deficits. A number of drugs and other conditions cause confusion in the elderly, and their effects may be mistaken for dementia. These are listed in Box 11.1.

In patients with AD, damage to the cholinergic neurones connecting subcortical nuclei to the cerebral cortex has been

---

Box 11.1 Drugs causing confusion in the elderly

Antiparkinsonian drugs
Barbiturates
Benzodiazepines
Diuretics
Hypoglycaemic agents
Monoamine oxidase inhibitors
Opioids
Steroids
Tricyclic antidepressants

---

consistently observed. Postsynaptic muscarinic cholinergic receptors are usually not affected, but ascending noradrenergic and serotonergic pathways are damaged, especially in younger patients. Based on those abnormalities, several drugs have been investigated for the treatment of AD. Lecithin, which increases acetylcholine concentrations in the brain, 4-aminopyridine, piracetam, oxitacetam and pramiracetam, all of which stimulate acetylcholine release, have been tried, but have produced no, or unimpressive, improvements in cognitive function. Anticholinesterases block the breakdown of acetylcholine and enhance cholinergic transmission. Donepezil, galantamine and rivastigmine are recommended for treatment of patients with AD of moderate severity only (those with a Mini Mental State Examination (MMSE) score of between 10 and 20 points; NICE, 2009). Donepezil is a piperidine-based acetylcholinesterase inhibitor. It has been shown to improve cognitive function in patients with mild to moderately severe AD. However, it does not improve day-to-day functioning, quality-of-life measures or rating scores of overall dementia. Rivastigmine is a non-competitive cholinesterase inhibitor. It has been shown to slow the rate of decline in cognitive and global functioning in AD. Galantamine, a reversible and competitive inhibitor of acetylcholinesterase, has also been shown to improve cognitive function significantly and is well tolerated. Adverse effects of cholinesterase inhibitors include nausea, vomiting, diarrhoea, weight loss, agitation, confusion, insomnia, abnormal dreams, muscle cramps, bradycardia, syncope and fatigue. Treatment with these drugs should only be continued in people with dementia who show an improvement or no deterioration in their minimental score, together with evidence of global (functional and behavioural) improvement after first few months of treatment. The treatment effect should then be reviewed critically every 6 months, before a decision to continue drug therapy is made.

Memantine, an N-methyl-D-aspartate (NMDA) antagonist, has also been used for the treatment of moderate to severe AD. It acts mainly on subtypes of glutamate receptors related to memory (i.e. NMDA), resulting in improvements in cognition. It has also been shown to have some beneficial effects on behaviour and its use is recommended in patients with moderate to severe AD as part of well-designed clinical studies (NICE, 2009).

Deposition of amyloid (in particular the peptide β/A4) derived from the Alzheimer amyloid precursor protein (APP) is an important pathological feature of the familial form of

AD that accounts for about 20% of patients. Point mutation of the gene coding for APP (located in the long arm of chromosome 21) is thought to be associated with familial AD. Future treatment strategies, therefore, might involve development of drugs which inhibit amyloidogenesis.

In some studies, donepezil and galantamine have been shown to improve cognition, behaviour and activities of daily living in patients with VaD, and in those with AD and coexistent cerebrovascular disease. Memantine has been reported to stabilise progression of VaD compared with placebo. However, acetylcholinesterase inhibitors and memantine should not be prescribed for the treatment of cognitive decline in patients with VaD, except as part of properly constructed clinical studies (National Collaborating Centre for Mental Health, 2007). Aspirin therapy has also been reported to slow the progression of VaD. The incidence of VaD is likely to decrease with other stroke prevention strategies such as smoking cessation, anticoagulation for atrial fibrillation, control of hypertension and hyperlipidemia.

Parkinsonism

Parkinsonism is a relatively common disease of the elderly with a prevalence between 50 and 150 per 100,000. It is characterised by resting tremors, muscular rigidity and bradykinesia (slowness of initiating and carrying out voluntary movements). The patient has a mask-like face, monotonous voice and walks with a stoop and a slow shuffling gait.

The elderly are more susceptible than younger patients to some of the adverse effects of antiparkinsonian drugs. Age-related decline in orthostatic circulatory responses, means that postural hypotension is more likely to occur in elderly patients with levodopa therapy. The elderly are more likely to have severe cardiac disease, and levodopa preparations should be used with caution in such patients because of the risk of serious ventricular dysrhythmias. Psychiatric adverse effects such as confusion, depression, hallucinations and paranoia occur with dopamine agonists and levodopa preparations. These adverse effects may persist for several months after discontinuation of the offending drug and may result in misdiagnosis (e.g. of AD) in the elderly. Bromocriptine and other ergot derivatives should be avoided in elderly patients with severe peripheral arterial disease as they may cause peripheral ischaemia. 'Drug holidays', which involve discontinuation of drugs, for example, for 2 days per week, may reduce the incidence of adverse effects of antiparkinsonian drugs, but their role is questionable.

Stroke

Stroke is the third most common cause of death and the most common cause of adult disability in the UK. About 110,000 people in England and Wales have their first stroke each year and about 30,000 people go on to have further strokes (National Collaborating Centre for Chronic Conditions, 2008). The incidence of stroke increases by 100-fold from the fourth to the ninth decade. About 85% of strokes are ischaemic and 15% are due to haemorrhages.

Treatment of acute stroke

Thrombolytic agents. The National Institute of Neurological Disorders and Stroke (1995) in the United States showed that, compared with placebo, thrombolysis with tissue plasminogen activator (rt-PA) within 3 h of onset of ischaemic stroke improved clinical outcome at 3 months despite increased incidence (6%) of symptomatic intracranial bleeding. Several studies have since confirmed the efficacy of intravenous rt-PA, administered within 3 h and up to 4.5 h, in acute ischaemic stroke. The odds ratio for improved outcome at 3 months, however, decreases from 2.5, if treatment is given between 0 and 90 min, to 1.3 between 181 and 270 min. A pooled analysis of the major randomised placebo-controlled trials of rt-PA (alteplase) for acute stroke showed large parenchymal haemorrhage in 5.2% of 1850 patients assigned to alteplase and 1.0% of 1820 controls, with no clear relation to onset of stroke to time of treatment (OTT). Adjusted odds of mortality increased with OTT (from 0.78 for 0–90 min to 1.22 for 181–270 min; Lees et al., 2010). Most of the clinical trials with rt-PA have excluded patients over 80 years of age. However, analysis of data from studies which have included patients over the age of 80 years, indicates that thrombolysis is effective in this age group but may be associated with a higher risk of bleeding. The currently ongoing International Stroke Trial 3 is specifically investigating the safety and efficacy of rt-PA in patients aged 80 years or more.

Antiplatelet therapy. Aspirin in doses of 150–300 mg commenced within 48 h of onset of ischaemic stroke has been shown to reduce the relative risk of death or dependency by 2.7% up to 6 months after the event in two large studies (Chen et al., 2000).

Anticoagulation. Use of intravenous unfractionated heparin and low molecular weight heparin have not been shown to be beneficial and are associated with increased risk of intracranial haemorrhage.

Neuroprotective agents. A large number of neuroprotective agents have been used for treatment of acute ischaemic stroke but none have been shown to have long-term beneficial effects.

Secondary prevention

Aspirin in doses of 75–1500 mg/day reduces the risk of stroke recurrence by about 23% as compared with placebo. This is likely to be due to its antiplatelet effect. Clopidogrel has been shown to reduce the relative risk for stroke recurrence by 8% compared with aspirin. When compared with aspirin alone, the combination of aspirin (75 mg daily) plus extended-release dipyridamole (200 mg twice daily) has been reported to reduce the relative risk by 20–23%. Aspirin plus extended-release dipyridamole has not been shown to be superior to clopidogrel alone in preventing recurrent stroke (Sacco et al., 2008). Clopidogrel plus aspirin (75 mg each daily) compared with aspirin alone is associated with an absolute increase in the risk for life-threatening bleeding by 1.3%, and therefore this combination is not recommended for secondary stroke prevention (Diener et al., 2004).

In patients with atrial fibrillation who have had a previous stroke or transient ischaemic attack, anticoagulation with warfarin (INR 1.5–2.7) has been shown to be significantly better than aspirin for secondary prevention (Hart et al., 2007). Anticoagulation has not been shown to be effective for secondary prevention in patients with sinus rhythm. Dabigatran, an oral direct thrombin inhibitor, at a dose of 110 mg twice daily is associated with similar rates of stroke and systemic embolism but lower rates of major haemorrhage. At a dose of 150 mg twice daily, it is associated with lower rates of stroke and systemic embolism but similar rates of major haemorrhage compared with warfarin (Connolly et al., 2009). Unlike warfarin, this drug does not require routine monitoring of anticoagulation. Two orally administered Factor Xa inhibitors, apixaban and rivaroxaban, are currently under investigation for stroke prevention in atrial fibrillation.

Adequate control of hypertension, diabetes, hyperlipidaemia, stopping smoking and reducing alcohol consumption are also important in secondary stroke prevention.

Primary prevention

A number of randomised controlled trials have shown that anticoagulation with warfarin compared with placebo reduces the risk of stroke in patients with atrial fibrillation (Hart et al., 2007). Control of risk factors such as hypertension, hyperlipidaemia, diabetes, and smoking is likely to play an important role in primary prevention.

Osteoporosis

Osteoporosis is a progressive disease characterised by low bone mass and micro-architectural deterioration of bone tissue resulting in increased bone fragility and susceptibility to fracture. It is an important cause of morbidity in postmenopausal women. The most important complication of osteoporosis is fracture of the hip. Fractures of wrist, vertebrae and humerus also occur. Increasing age is associated with higher risk of fractures, which occur mostly in those aged over 75 years. In the UK, over 200,000 fractures occur each year, costing the NHS £1.8 billion per year, of which 87% is spent on hip fractures (Poole and Compston, 2006).

Prevention

As complications of osteoporosis have enormous economic implications, preventive measures are extremely important. Regular exercise has been shown to halve the risk of hip fractures. Stopping smoking before the menopause reduces the risk of hip fractures by 25%.

Treatment

Vitamin D and calcium. Vitamin D deficiency is common in elderly people. Treatment for 12–18 months with 800 IU of vitamin D plus 1.2 g of calcium given daily has been shown to reduce hip and non-vertebral fractures in elderly women (mean age 84 years) living in sheltered accommodation. It is not known whether vitamin D supplementation alone reduces hip fractures. Calcium supplementation on its own does not reduce fracture incidence and is no longer recommended for treatment of osteoporosis.

Calcitriol and alfacalcidol. Calcitriol (1,25-dihydroxyvitamin D), the active metabolite of vitamin D, and alfacalcidol, a synthetic analogue of calcitriol, reduce bone loss and have been shown to reduce vertebral fractures, but not consistently. Serum calcium should be monitored regularly in patients receiving these drugs.

Bisphosphonates. Bisphosphonates, synthetic analogues of pyrophosphate, bind strongly to the bone surface and inhibit bone resorption. Currently, three oral bisphosphonates are available for the treatment of osteoporosis: alendronate, etidronate and risedronate. Alendronate can be given either daily (10 mg) or weekly (70 mg) with equal efficacy. It is effective in reducing vertebral, wrist and hip fractures by about 50%. Etidronate is given cyclically with calcium supplements to reduce the risk of bone mineralisation defects. It reduces the risk of vertebral fractures by 50% in postmenopausal women. There is no evidence to support its effectiveness in preventing hip fractures. Risedronate reduces vertebral fractures by 41% and non-vertebral fractures by 39%. It has been shown to significantly reduce the risk of hip fractures in postmenopausal women. Alendronate and risedronate are currently used as first-line drugs in older women with osteoporosis.

Intravenous ibandronate, given at a dose of 3 mg once every 3 months, can be used for treatment of postmenopausal osteoporosis. It can also be given orally at a dose of 150 mg once monthly.

All bisphosphonates cause gastro-intestinal side effects. Alendronate and risedronate are associated with severe oesophageal reactions including oesophageal stricture. Patients should not take these tablets at bed-time and should be advised to stay upright for at least 30 min after taking them. They should avoid food for at least 2 h before and after taking etidronate. Alendronate and risedronate should be taken 30 min before the first food or drink of the day. Bisphosphonates should be avoided in patients with renal impairment.

Strontium ranelate, which both increases bone formation and reduces bone resorption, reduces vertebral and non-vertebral (including hip) fractures in postmenopausal women with osteoporosis. It is well tolerated. It can be used in those who are unable to tolerate alendronate or risedronate. It should be avoided in patients with severe renal disease (creatinine clearance below 30 mL/min). It can be used with caution in patients at increased risk of venous thromboembolism and those with phenylketonuria.

Hormone replacement therapy (HRT). Oestrogens increase bone formation and reduce bone resorption. They also increase calcium absorption and decrease renal calcium loss. HRT, if started soon after the menopause, is effective in preventing vertebral fractures but has to be continued lifelong if protection against fractures is to be maintained. It is associated with increased risk of endometrial cancer, breast cancer and venous thromboembolism. One study has shown that HRT may increase the risk of deaths due to myocardial disease in elderly women with pre-existing ischaemic heart disease. It should be avoided in older patients.

Raloxifene. Raloxifene, an oral selective oestrogen receptor modulator (SERM) that has oestrogenic actions on bone and anti-oestrogenic actions on the uterus and breast. It reduces the risk of vertebral fractures, but not those at other sites. Adverse effects include hot flushes, leg cramps, and risk of venous thromboembolism. It also protects against breast cancer. Its use is restricted, as a second-line drug, to younger postmenopausal women with vertebral osteoporosis.

Parathyroid hormone peptides. Teriparatide is the recombinant portion of human parathyroid hormone, amino acid sequence 1–34, of the complete molecule (which has 84 amino acids). It reduces vertebral and non-vertebral fractures in postmenopausal women. It does not reduce hip fractures. It is given subcutaneously at a dose of 20 μcg daily. The recombinant (full 1–84 amino acid sequence) parathyroid hormone peptide (Preotact®) can also be used at a dose of 100 μcg daily. It has similar efficacy as teriparatide. Both these drugs are expensive and teriparatide is associated with an increased risk of osteosarcoma in animal studies.

Calcitonin. Calcitonin inhibits osteoclasts and decreases the rate of bone resorption, reduces bone blood flow and may have central analgesic actions. It is effective in all age groups in preventing vertebral bone loss. It is costly and has to be given parenterally or intranasally. It should not be given for more than 3–6 months at a time to avoid its inhibitory effects on bone resorption and formation, which usually disappear after 2–4 weeks. Antibodies do develop against calcitonin, but they do not affect its efficacy. Calcitonin is useful in treating acute pain associated with osteoporotic vertebral fractures.

Arthritis

Osteoarthrosis, gout, pseudogout, rheumatoid arthritis and septic arthritis are the important joint diseases in the elderly. Treatment of these conditions is similar to that in the young. If possible, NSAIDs should be avoided in patients with osteoarthrosis. Total hip and knee replacements should be considered in patients with severe arthritis affecting these joints.

Hypertension

Hypertension is an important risk factor for cardiovascular and cerebrovascular disease in the elderly. The incidence of myocardial infarction is 2.5 times higher, and that of cerebrovascular accidents twice as high in elderly hypertensive patients compared with non-hypertensive subjects. Elevated systolic blood pressure is the single most important risk factor for cardiovascular disease and more predictive of stroke than diastolic blood pressure.

Blood pressure lowering has been shown to be beneficial in those patients below and above the age of 65 years with no substantial variation in reduction in major vascular events with different drug classes (Blood Pressure Lowering Treatment Trialists' Collaboration, 2008). There is evidence that treatment of both systolic and diastolic blood pressure in the elderly is beneficial. One large study has shown reductions in cardiovascular events, and mortality associated with cerebrovascular accidents in treated elderly patients with hypertension (Amery et al., 1986). The treatment did not reduce the total mortality significantly. Another study (SHEP, 1991), which used low-dose chlortalidone to treat isolated systolic hypertension (systolic blood pressure 160 mmHg or more with diastolic blood pressure less than 95 mmHg), showed a 36% reduction in the incidence of stroke, with a 5-year benefit of 30 events per 1000 patients. It also showed a reduction in the incidence of major cardiovascular events with a 5-year absolute benefit of 55 events per 1000 patients. In addition, this study reported that antihypertensive therapy was beneficial even in patients over the age of 80 years. There is increasing evidence that antihypertensive therapy in patients over 80 years of age is beneficial. Subgroup meta-analysis of seven randomised controlled trials, which included 1670 patients over 80 years, showed that antihypertensive therapy for about 3.5 years reduces the risk of heart failure by 39%, strokes by 34% and major cardiovascular events by 22% (Gueyffier, 1999). In one placebo-controlled study which included 3845 patients who were 80 years of age or older and had a sustained systolic blood pressure of 160 mmHg or more, treatment with the diuretic indapamide (sustained release, 1.5 mg) plus perindopril (2 or 4 mg) to achieve the target blood pressure of 150/80 mmHg resulted in a 30% reduction in the rate of fatal or non-fatal stroke, a 39% reduction in the rate of death from stroke, a 21% reduction in the rate of death from any cause, a 23% reduction in the rate of death from cardiovascular causes and a 64% reduction in the rate of heart failure (Beckett et al., 2008).

Treatment of hypertension

Non-pharmacological. In patients with asymptomatic mild hypertension, non-pharmacological treatment is the method of choice. Weight reduction to within 15% of desirable weight, restriction of salt intake to 4–6 g/day, regular aerobic exercise such as walking, restriction of ethanol consumption and stopping smoking are the recommended modes of therapy.

Pharmacological

Thiazide diuretics. Thiazides lower peripheral resistance and do not significantly affect cardiac output or renal blood flow. They are effective, cheap, well tolerated and have also been shown to reduce the risk of hip fracture in elderly women by 30%. They can be used in combination with other antihypertensive drugs. Adverse effects include mild elevation of creatinine, glucose, uric acid and serum cholesterol levels as well as hypokalaemia. They should be used in low doses, as higher doses only increase the incidence of adverse effects without increasing their efficacy.

β-Adrenoceptor blockers. Although theoretically the β-blockers are expected to be less effective in the elderly, they have been shown to be as effective as diuretics in clinical studies. Water-soluble β-blockers such as atenolol may cause fewer adverse effects in the elderly.

Calcium antagonists. Calcium antagonists act as vasodilators. Verapamil and, to some extent, diltiazem decrease cardiac output. These drugs do not have a significant effect on lipids or the central nervous system. They may be more effective in the elderly, particularly in the treatment of isolated systolic hypertension. Adverse effects include headache, oedema and postural hypotension. Verapamil may cause conduction disturbances and decrease cardiac output. The use of short-acting dihydropyridine calcium antagonists, for example nifedipine, is controversial. Some studies indicate adverse outcomes with these agents, particularly in those patients with angina or myocardial infarction.

ACE inhibitors and angiotensin receptor blockers (ARBs): ACE inhibitors and ARBs used for treatment of hypertension are discussed elsewhere (see chapter 19). These drugs should be used with care in the elderly, who are more likely to have underlying atherosclerotic renovascular disease that could result in renal failure. Excessive hypotension is also more likely to occur in the elderly.

Myocardial infarction

The diagnosis of myocardial infarction in the elderly may be difficult in some patients because of an atypical presentation (Bayer et al., 1986). In the majority of patients, chest pain and dyspnoea are the common presenting symptoms. Confusion may be a presenting factor in up to 20% of patients over 85 years of age. The diagnosis is made on the basis of history, serial electrocardiograms and cardiac enzyme estimations.

The principles of management of myocardial infarction in the elderly are similar to those in the young. Thrombolytic therapy has been shown to be safe and effective in elderly patients.

Cardiac failure

In addition to the typical features of cardiac failure, that is, exertional dyspnoea, oedema, orthopnoea and paroxysmal nocturnal dyspnoea (PND), elderly patients may present with atypical symptoms. These include confusion due to poor cerebral circulation, vomiting and abdominal pain due to gastro-intestinal and hepatic congestion, or insomnia due to PND. Dyspnoea may not be a predominant symptom in an elderly patient with arthritis and immobility. Treatment of cardiac failure depends on the underlying cause and is similar to that in the young. Diuretics, ACE inhibitors, β-blockers and digoxin are the important drugs used in the treatment of cardiac failure in the elderly.

Leg ulcers

Leg ulcers are common in the elderly. They are mainly of two types: venous or ischaemic. Other causes of leg ulcers are blood diseases, trauma, malignancy and infections (Cornwall et al., 1986), but these are less common in the elderly. Venous ulcers occur in patients with varicose veins who have valvular incompetence in deep veins due to venous hypertension. They are usually located near the medial malleolus and are associated with varicose eczema and oedema. These ulcers are painless unless there is gross oedema or infection. Ischaemic ulcers, on the other hand, are due to poor peripheral circulation, and occur on the toes, heels, foot and lateral aspect of the leg. They are painful and are associated with signs of lower limb ischaemia, such as absent pulse or cold lower limb. There may be a history of smoking, diabetes or hypertension.

Venous ulcers respond well to treatment, and over 75% heal within 3 months. Elevation of the lower limbs, exercise, compression bandage, local antiseptic creams when there is evidence of infection, with or without steroid cream, are usually effective. There is no evidence of benefit from the use of oral zinc sulphate in patients with chronic leg ulcers. Dressings impregnated with silver have not been shown to be better than simple low-adherent dressings for the healing of venous leg ulcers. Use of 5% Eutectic Mixture of Local Anaesthetics (EMLA): lidocaine–prilocaine cream results in statistically significant reduction in debridement pain scores but it appears to have no impact on wound healing. Ibuprofen dressings have not been shown to offer pain relief (Briggs et al., 2010). Antiseptics should not be used when there is granulation tissue. Topical streptokinase may be useful to remove the slough on ulcers. Gel colloid occlusive dressings may also be useful in treating chronic ulcers. Skin grafting may be necessary for large ulcers. Ischaemic ulcers do not respond well to medical treatment, and the patients should be assessed by vascular surgeons.

Urinary incontinence

Urinary incontinence in the elderly may be of three main types:

Stress incontinence: due to urethral sphincter incompetence. It occurs almost exclusively in women and is associated with weakening of pelvic musculature. Involuntary loss of small amounts of urine occurs on performing activities which increase intra-abdominal pressure, for example, coughing, sneezing, bending, lifting, etc. It does not cause significant nocturnal symptoms.

Overflow incontinence: constant involuntary loss of urine in small amounts. Prostatic hypertrophy is a common cause and is often associated with symptoms of poor stream and incomplete emptying. Increased frequency of micturition at night is often a feature. Use of anticholinergic drugs and diabetic autonomic neuropathy are other causes.

Detrusor instability: causes urge incontinence where a strong desire to pass urine is followed by involuntary loss of large amounts of urine either during the day or night. It is often associated with neurological lesions or urinary outflow obstruction, for example, prostatic hypertrophy, but in many cases the cause is unknown.

Stress incontinence is not amenable to drug therapy. In patients with prostatic hypertrophy α_1-blockers such as prazosin, indoramin, alfuzosin, terazosin, and tamsulosin have all been shown to increase peak urine flow rate and improve symptoms in about 60% of patients. They reduce outflow obstruction by blocking α_1-receptors and thereby relaxing prostate smooth muscle. Postural hypotension is an important adverse effect and occurs in between 2% and 5% of patients.

5α-Reductase converts testerone to dihydrotesterone (DHT) which plays an important role in the growth of prostate. The 5α-reductase inhibitor finasteride reduces the prostate volume by 20% and improves peak urine flow rate. The clinical effects, however, might not become apparent until after 3–6 months of treatment. Main adverse effects are reductions in libido and erectile dysfunction in 3–5% of patients.

Several antimuscarinic drugs including darifenacin, oral and transdermal oxybutynin, modified-release propiverine, solifenacin, and modified-release tolterodine have been licensed for overactive bladder syndrome. All these drugs are similar in efficacy and cause antimuscarinic side effects such as dry mouth, blurred vision and constipation. Immediate-release oxybutynin is the least expensive drug and is more likely to cause adverse effects. Transdermal and modified release preparations are better tolerated, but are more expensive (Anon, 2007).

Constipation

The age-related decline in gastro-intestinal motility and treatment with drugs which decrease gastro-intestinal motility predispose the elderly to constipation. Decreased mobility, wasting of pelvic muscles and a low intake of solids and liquids are other contributory factors. Faecal impaction may occur with severe constipation, which in turn may cause subacute intestinal obstruction, abdominal pain, spurious diarrhoea and faecal incontinence. Adequate intake of dietary fibre, regular bowel habit and use of bulking agents such as bran or ispaghula husk may help to prevent constipation. When constipation is associated with a loaded rectum, a stimulant laxative such as senna or bisacodyl may be given. Frail, ill elderly patients with a full rectum may have atonic bowels that will not respond to bulking agents or softening agents, and in such cases a stimulant is more effective. A stool-softening agent such as docusate sodium is effective when stools are hard and dry. For severe faecal impaction a phosphate enema may be needed. Long-term use of stimulant laxatives may lead to abuse and atonic bowel musculature.

Gastro-intestinal ulceration and bleeding

Gastro-intestinal bleeding associated with peptic ulcer is less well tolerated by the elderly. The clinical presentation may sometimes be atypical with, for example, patients presenting with confusion. *Helicobacter pylori* infection is common and its treatment is similar to that in younger patients. NSAIDs are more likely to cause gastroduodenal ulceration and bleeding in the elderly (Griffin et al., 1988).

Principles and goals of drug therapy in the elderly

A thorough knowledge of the pharmacokinetic and pharmacodynamic factors discussed is essential for optimal drug therapy in the elderly. In addition, some general principles based on common sense, if followed, may result in even better use of drugs in the elderly.

Avoid unnecessary drug therapy

Before commencing drug therapy it is important to ask the following questions:

- Is it really necessary?
- Is there an alternative method of treatment?

In patients with mild hypertension, non-drug therapies which are of proven efficacy should be considered in the first instance. Similarly, unnecessary use of hypnotics should be avoided. Simple measures such as emptying the bladder before going to bed to avoid having to get up, avoidance of stimulant drugs in the evenings or night, or moving the patient to a dark, quiet room may be all that is needed.

Effect of treatment on quality of life

The aim of treatment in elderly patients is not just to prolong life but also to improve the quality of life. To achieve this, the correct choice of treatment is essential. In a 70-year-old lady with severe osteoarthrosis of the hip, for example, total hip replacement is the treatment of choice rather than prescribing NSAIDs with all their attendant adverse effects.

Treat the cause rather than the symptom

Symptomatic treatment without specific diagnosis is not only bad practice but can also be potentially dangerous. A patient presenting with 'indigestion' may in fact be suffering from angina, and therefore treatment with proton pump inhibitors or antacids is clearly inappropriate. When a patient presents with a symptom every attempt should be made to establish the cause of the symptom and specific treatment, if available, should then be given.

Drug history

A drug history should be obtained in all elderly patients. This will ensure the patient is not prescribed a drug or drugs to which they may be allergic, or the same drug or group of drugs to which they have previously not responded. It will help to avoid potentially serious drug interactions.

Concomitant medical illness

Concurrent medical disorders must always be taken into account. Cardiac failure, renal impairment and hepatic dysfunction are particularly common in the elderly, and may increase the risk of adverse effects of drugs.

Choosing the drug

Once it is decided that a patient requires drug therapy, it is important to choose the drug likely to be the most efficacious and least likely to produce adverse effects. It is also necessary to take into consideration coexisting medical conditions. For example, it is inappropriate to commence diuretic therapy to treat mild hypertension in an elderly male with prostatic hypertrophy.

Dose titration

In general, elderly patients require relatively smaller doses of all drugs compared with young adults. It is recognised that the majority of adverse drug reactions in the elderly are dose related and potentially preventable. It is, therefore, rational to start with the smallest possible dose of a given drug in the least number of doses and then gradually increase both, if necessary. Dose titration should obviously take into consideration age-related pharmacokinetic and pharmacodynamic alterations that may affect the response to the chosen drug.

Choosing the right dosage form

Most elderly patients find it easy to swallow syrups or suspensions or effervescent tablets rather than large tablets or capsules.

Packaging and labelling

Many elderly patients with arthritis find it difficult to open child-resistant containers and blister packs. Medicines should be dispensed in easy-to-open containers that are clearly labelled using large print.

Good record keeping

Information about a patient's current and previous drug therapy, alcohol consumption, smoking and driving habits may help in choosing appropriate drug therapy and when the treatment needs to be altered. It will help to reduce costly duplications and will also identify and help to avoid dangerous drug interactions.

Regular supervision and review of treatment

A UK survey showed that 59% of prescriptions to the elderly had been given for more than 2 years, 32% for more than 5 years and 16% for more than 10 years. Of all prescriptions given to the elderly, 88% were repeat prescriptions; 40% had not been discussed with the doctor for at least 6 months, especially prescriptions for hypnotics and anxiolytics. It also showed that 31% of prescriptions were considered pharmacologically questionable, and 4% showed duplication of drugs. It is obvious that there is a need for regular and critical review of all prescriptions, especially when long-term therapy is required.

Adverse drug reactions (ADRs)

It is recognised that ADRs occur more frequently in the elderly. A multicentre study in the UK in 1980 showed that ADRs were the only cause of admission in 2.8% of 1998 admissions to 42 units of geriatric medicine. It also showed that ADRs were contributory to a further 7.7% of admissions. On the basis of this study it can be estimated that up to 15,000 geriatric admissions per annum in the UK are at least partly due to an ADR. Obviously, this has enormous economic implications.

The elderly are more susceptible to ADRs for a number of reasons. They are usually on multiple drugs, which in itself can account for the increased incidence of ADRs. It is, however, recognised that ADRs tend to be more severe in the elderly, and gastro-intestinal and haematological ADRs are more common than would be expected from prescribing figures alone. Age-related pharmacokinetic and pharmacodynamic alterations and impaired homeostatic mechanisms are the other factors which predispose the elderly to ADRs, by making them more sensitive to the pharmacological effects of the drugs. Not surprisingly, up to 80% of ADRs in the elderly are dose-dependent and therefore predictable.

Adherence

Although it is commonly believed that the elderly are poor compliers with their drug therapy, there is no clear evidence to support this. Studies in Northern Ireland and continental Europe have shown that the elderly are as adherent with their drug therapy as the young, provided that they do not have confounding disease. Cognitive impairment, which is common in old age, multiple drug therapy and complicated drug regimens may impair adherence in the elderly. Poor adherence may result in treatment failure. The degree of adherence required varies depending on the disease being treated. For treatment of a simple urinary tract infection, a single dose of an antibiotic may be all that is required, and therefore compliance is not important. On the other hand, adherence of 90% or more is required for successful treatment of epilepsy or difficult hypertension. Various methods have been used to improve adherence. These include prescription diaries, special packaging, training by pharmacists and counselling.

Conclusion

The number of elderly patients, especially those aged over 75 years, is steadily increasing, and they are accounting for an ever-increasing proportion of health care expenditure in the West. Understanding age-related changes in pharmacodynamic factors, avoiding polypharmacy and regular and critical review of all drug treatment will help in the rationalisation of drug prescribing, reduction in drug-related morbidity and also the cost of drug therapy for this important subgroup of patients.

Case studies

Case 11.1

An 80-year-old woman presented to an out-patient clinic with a history of severe giddiness and a few episodes of blackouts. She was being treated for angina and hypertension. She had been on bendroflumethiazide 2.5 mg once daily, and slow-release isosorbide mononitrate 60 mg once daily for a few years. Her general practitioner had recently commenced nifedipine SR 20 mg twice daily for poorly controlled hypertension. On examination her blood pressure was 120/70 mmHg while supine and 90/60 mmHg on standing up.

Question

What is the underlying problem in this patient, and could it be caused by any of the medications that the patient is taking?

Answer

This patient obviously has significant postural hypotension. All her drugs have the potential to produce postural hypotension, and when used together they may produce symptomatic postural hypotension.

It is important to recognise that some drugs such as nifedipine and nitrates have impaired first-pass metabolism in the elderly and that their clinical effects are enhanced. In addition, orthostatic circulatory responses are also impaired in the elderly. The need for antihypertensive drugs should be carefully assessed in all elderly patients, and, if therapy is indicated, the smallest dose of drug should be commenced and increased gradually. Patients should also be told to avoid sudden changes of posture.

Case 11.2

An 85-year-old man was admitted to hospital with anorexia, nausea and vomiting. He was known to have atrial fibrillation, congestive cardiac failure and chronic renal impairment. He was on digoxin 250 μcg once daily and furosemide 80 mg twice daily.

His serum biochemistry revealed the following (normal range in parentheses):

Potassium	4.5 mmol/L	(3.5–5)
Urea	40 mmol/L	(3.0–6.5)
Creatinine	600 μmol/L	(50–120)
Digoxin	3.5 μcg/L	(1–2)

Question

What are the likely causes of medical problems in this patient and how should the drug therapy be altered?

Answer

The patient's biochemical results confirm the presence of renal impairment and digoxin toxicity. The renal impairment could be related to the relatively high dose of furosemide which needs to be reduced. As digoxin is predominantly excreted through the kidneys, the dose should be reduced in severe renal impairment. In such

situations, digitoxin, which is predominantly metabolised in the liver, can be used instead of digoxin.

Case 11.3

An 80-year-old woman with a previous history of hypothyroidism presented with a history of abdominal pain and vomiting. She had not moved her bowels for the previous 7 days. Two weeks earlier her general practitioner had prescribed a combination of paracetamol and codeine to control pain in her osteoarthritic hips.

Question

What are the likely underlying causes of this patient's bowel dysfunction?

Answer

This patient developed severe constipation after taking a codeine-containing analgesic. Ageing is associated with decreased gastro-intestinal motility. Hypothyroidism, which is common in the elderly, is also associated with reduced gastro-intestinal motility. Whenever possible, drugs that are known to reduce gastro-intestinal motility should be avoided in the elderly.

Case 11.4

A 75-year-old lady who suffered from osteoarthritis of hip and knee joints presented with a history of passing black stools. Her drug therapy included diclofenac 50 mg three times daily and paracetamol 1 g as required.

Question

What is the likely cause of this patient's symptoms?

Answer

The likely cause is upper gastro-intestinal bleeding due to diclofenac, which is an NSAID. Elderly people are more prone to develop ulceration in stomach and duodenum with NSAIDs compared with young patients.

Case 11.5

A 70-year-old man was found by his general practitioner to have hypertension and was commenced on lisinopril 5 mg once a day. He had a previous history of peripheral vascular disease for which he had required angioplasty. Two weeks after commencing antihypertensive treatment, he presented with lack of appetite, nausea and decreased urine output.

Question

What do you think has happened and is the most likely underlying problem?

Answer

The patient is probably developing renal failure. With a previous history of peripheral vascular disease, he is likely to have bilateral renal artery stenosis. ACE inhibitors can cause renal failure in the presence of bilateral renal stenosis by reducing blood supply to the kidneys.

References

Amery, A., Birkenhager, W., Brixko, P., et al., 1986. Efficacy of antihypertensive drug treatment according to age, sex, blood pressure, and previous cardiovascular disease in patients over the age of 60. Lancet 2, 589–592.

Anon, 2007. Update on drugs for overactive bladder syndrome. Drug Ther. Bull. 45, 44–48.

Bayer, A.J., Chadha, J.S., Farag, R.R., et al., 1986. Changing presentation of myocardial infarction with increasing old age. J. Am. Geriatr. Soc. 34, 263–266.

Beckett, N.S., Peters, R., Fletcher, A.E., et al., for the HYVET Study Group, 2008. Treatment of hypertension in patients 80 years of age or older. N. Engl. J. Med. 358, 1887–1898.

Blood Pressure Lowering Treatment Trialists' Collaboration, 2008. Effects of different regimens to lower blood pressure on major cardiovascular events in older and younger adults: meta-analysis of randomised trials. Br. Med. J. 336, 1121–1123.

Briggs, M., Nelson, E.A., 2010. Topical agents or dressings for pain in venous leg ulcers. Cochrane Database Syst. Rev. 4, CD001177. Doi: 10.1002/14651858.CD001177.

Chen, Z.M., Sandercock, P., Pan, H.C., et al., 2000. Indications for early aspirin use in acute ischaemic stroke: a combined analysis of 40,000 randomised patients from the Chinese acute stroke trial and the international stroke trial. On behalf of the CAST and IST collaborative groups. Stroke 31, 1240–1249.

Connolly, S.J., Ezekowitz, M.D., Yusuf, S., et al., RE-LY Steering Committee and Investigators, 2009. Dabigatran versus warfarin in patients with atrial fibrillation. N. Engl. J. Med. 36, 1139–1151.

Cornwall, J.V., Dore, C.J., Lewis, J.D., 1986. Leg ulcers: epidemiology and aetiology. Br. J. Surg. 73, 693–696.

Diener, H.C., Bogousslavsky, J., Brass, L.M., et al., 2004. Aspirin and clopidogrel compared with clopidogrel alone after recent ischaemic stroke or transient ischaemic attack in high-risk patients (MATCH): randomised, double-blind, placebo-controlled trial. Lancet 364, 331–337.

Griffin, M.R., Ray, W.A., Schaffner, W., 1988. Non-steroidal anti-inflammatory drug use and death from peptic ulcer in elderly persons. Ann. Intern. Med. 109, 359–363.

Gueyffier, F., Bulpitt, C., Boissel, J.P., et al., 1999. Antihypertensive drugs in very old people:a subgroup meta-analysis of randomised controlled trials. Lancet 353, 793–796.

Hart, R.G., Pearce, L.A., Aguilar, M.I., 2007. Meta-analysis antithrombotic therapy to prevent stroke in patients who have nonvalvular atrial fibrillation. Ann. Intern. Med. 146, 857–867.

Lees, K.R., Bluhmki, E., von Kummer, R., et al., 2010. Time to treatment with intravenous alteplase and outcome in stroke: an updated pooled analysis of ECASS, ATLANTIS, NINDS, and EPITHET trials. Lancet 375, 1695–1703.

National Collaborating Centre for Mental Health, 2007. Dementia. A NICE–SCIE guideline on supporting people with dementia and their carers in health and social care. National Clinical Practice Guideline Number 42. The British Psychological Society & The Royal College of Psychiatrists, London.

National Collaborating Centre for Chronic Conditions 2008. Stroke. National Clinical Guideline for Diagnosis and Initial Management of Acute Stroke and Transient Ischaemic Attack (TIA). Royal College of Physicians, London.

National Institute for Health and Clinical Excellence, 2009. Donepezil, galantamine, rivastigmine (review) and memantine for the treatment of Alzheimer's disease. Technology Appraisal 111, (amended). NICE, London.

National Institute of Neurological Disorders on Stroke rt-PA Stroke Study Group, 1995. Tissue plasminogen activator for acute ischaemic stroke. N. Engl. J. Med. 333, 1581–1587.

Office for National Statistics, 2010. Population trends 139 office for national statistics. Newport . Available at http://www.statistics.gov.uk/statbase/product.asp?vlnk=6303.

Poole, K.E.S., Compston, J.E., 2006. Osteoporosis and its management. Br. Med. J. 333, 1251–1256.

Sacco, R.L., Diener, H.C., Yusuf, S., et al., for the PRoFESS Study Group, 2008. Aspirin and extended-release dipyridamole versus clopidogrel for recurrent stroke. N. Engl. J. Med. 359, 1238–1251.

SHEP Cooperative Research Group, 1991. Prevention of stroke by antihypertensive drug treatment in older persons with isolated systolic hypertension: final results of the systolic hypertension in the elderly programme (SHEP). J. Am. Med. Assoc. 265, 3255–3264.

Further reading

Adams, R.J., Albers, G., Alberts, M.J., 2008. Update to the AHA/ASA recommendations for the prevention of stroke in patients with stroke and transient ischemic attack. Stroke 39, 1647–1652.

Iqbal, P., Castleden, C.M., 1997. Management of urinary incontinence in the elderly. Gerontology 43, 151–157.

Prisant, L.M., Moser, M., 2000. Hypertension in the elderly: can we improve results of therapy. Arch. Intern. Med. 160, 283–289.

Scottish Intercollegiate Guidelines Network, 2008. Management of patients with stroke or TIA: assessment, investigation, immediate management and secondary prevention. A National Clinical Guideline. SIGN, Edinburgh. Available at http://www.sign.ac.uk/pdf/sign108.pdfv.

THERAPEUTICS

12 Peptic ulcer disease

M. Kinnear

Key points

- The two main types of peptic ulcer disease are those associated with *Helicobacter pylori* and those associated with non-steroidal anti-inflammatory drugs (NSAIDs) and aspirin.
- Ulcer-like dyspepsia does not correlate with diagnosis of peptic ulcer.
- Uninvestigated dyspepsia without alarm symptoms may be treated empirically without an endoscopic diagnosis.
- An *H. pylori* test and treat strategy means it is unknown if the patient has an ulcer.
- Triple therapy with a proton pump inhibitor (PPI), clarithromycin and amoxicillin twice daily for 7 days is currently the recommended first-line *H. pylori* eradication regimen.
- Patient adherence influences the success of *H. pylori* eradication therapy.
- *H. pylori* eradication therapy does not have a role in the management of gastro-oesophageal reflux disease (GORD). Its benefit in the management of functional dyspepsia is small.
- Associated risks of *Clostridium difficile* infection, pneumonia and osteoporosis have led to judicious use of PPIs.
- Patients who need to continue NSAID therapy are the only patients with peptic ulcer disease in whom continued ulcer-healing therapy is necessary after the ulcer has healed and *H. pylori* has been eradicated.
- Upper gastro-intestinal symptoms in NSAID users do not correlate well with presence or absence of peptic ulcers.
- The risk of ulcers associated with NSAID use is common to all non-specific NSAIDs and is dose dependent. The risk is maintained during treatment and decreases once treatment is stopped.
- Risk factors for NSAID-induced gastro-intestinal complications include previous history of peptic ulcer or gastro-intestinal bleeding, age >65, concomitant use of aspirin, anticoagulants or corticosteroids.
- Adding a PPI to non-specific NSAIDs provides a similar reduction in risk of gastro-intestinal toxicity to that offered by cyclo-oxygenase-2 (COX-2) inhibitors alone.
- Enteric coating or taking them with food does not reduce the risk of upper gastro-intestinal bleeding associated with NSAIDs and low-dose aspirin.
- Adding a PPI to aspirin is associated with lower risk of recurrent gastro-intestinal bleeding than clopidogrel alone.
- Concomitant PPI therapy may decrease clopidogrel activity through competitive hepatic metabolism; the combination is not recommended unless dual antiplatelet therapy is indicated.

- *H. pylori* eradication has a greater effect on decreasing recurrent peptic ulcer bleeding rate than PPIs alone in patients who continue low-dose aspirin; an additive effect is seen if both strategies are used.
- Cardiovascular risks must be weighed against gastro-intestinal risks in deciding whether or not to discontinue aspirin and for how long in patients who present with gastro-intestinal bleeding.
- Approximately one-third of deaths from gastro-intestinal bleeding are due to NSAIDs, and up to one-third of NSAID/aspirin deaths are attributed to low-dose aspirin.
- High dose intravenous PPI therapy is indicated to prevent re-bleeding in patients at high risk (active bleeding or non-bleeding visible vessel) following endoscopic haemostatic treatment for bleeding peptic ulcer. It is not recommended in those at low risk or pre-endoscopy.
- *H. pylori* eradication reduces re-bleeding rate in patients with gastro-intestinal bleeding but eradication treatment can be delayed until normal oral intake is resumed.
- Adding a PPI to a COX-2 inhibitor (in those not at cardiovascular risk) decreases the re-bleeding rate in those patients at high risk of re-bleeding in comparison to COX-2 inhibitors alone. No comparison has been made with non-selective NSAID in combination with PPI.

The term 'peptic ulcer' describes a condition in which there is a discontinuity in the entire thickness of the gastric or duodenal mucosa that persists as a result of acid and pepsin in the gastric juice (Fig. 12.1). Oesophageal ulceration due to acid reflux is generally classified under GORD. This definition excludes carcinoma and lymphoma, which may also cause gastric ulceration, and also excludes other rare causes of gastric and duodenal ulceration such as Crohn's disease, viral infections and amyloidosis. About 10% of the population in developed countries is likely to be affected at some time by peptic ulcer, with the prevalence for active ulcer disease being about 1% at any particular point in time.

Peptic ulcer disease often presents to clinicians as dyspepsia. However, not all patients with dyspepsia have peptic ulcer disease. Dyspepsia is defined as persistent or recurrent pain or discomfort centred in the upper abdomen. The most common causes of dyspepsia are non-ulcer or functional dyspepsia, GORD and peptic ulcer. Other causes include gastric cancer, pancreatic or biliary disease. Peptic ulcer accounts for 10–15% of dyspepsia, and oesophagitis for about 20%. However, 60–70% of patients have no obvious abnormality and have functional dyspepsia or endoscopy-negative GORD. Dyspepsia is a common symptom and affects about 40% of

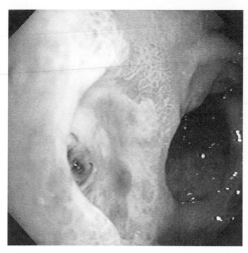

Fig. 12.1 Duodenal ulcer seen at endoscopy. Note also a visible blood vessel that is a stigma of recent haemorrhage.

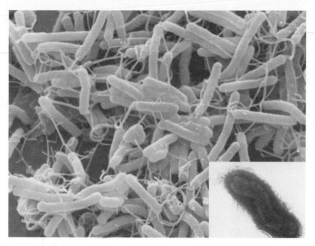

Fig. 12.2 *Helicobacter pylori*. The Gram-negative spiral bacterium *H. pylori*, formerly known as *Campylobacter pylori*, was isolated serendipitously from patients with gastritis by Barry Marshall and Robin Warren in 1982. Seven years later, it was conceded that *H. pylori* is responsible for most cases of gastric and duodenal ulcer.

people annually. It is the reason for 5–10% of consultations with primary care physicians, and up to 70% of referrals to gastro-intestinal units are patients with dyspepsia. However, the widely adopted test and treat recommendation for uninvestigated dyspepsia has reduced endoscopy referrals.

Epidemiology

The incidence of duodenal ulcer is now declining, which follows the decline in *H. pylori* infection. However, hospital admission rates for gastro-intestinal bleeding associated with gastric and duodenal ulcers are rising, especially in older patients. This is probably a consequence of increased prescriptions for low-dose aspirin, NSAIDs, antiplatelets, anticoagulants and selective serotonin reuptake inhibitors (SSRI). Over the previous decade there has been an increase in idiopathic peptic ulcer disease in patients who test negative for *H. pylori* and who do not take NSAIDs or aspirin. In some countries, up to one-quarter of peptic ulcers are idiopathic and there is a decrease in prevalence of *H. pylori* infection. Idiopathic ulcers should be investigated to attempt to identify the underlying cause following careful reassessment of *H. pylori* status and medication history.

Infection by *H. pylori*, a spiral bacterium of the stomach, remains an important epidemiological factor in causing peptic ulcer (Fig. 12.2). Most *H. pylori* infections are acquired by oral–oral and oral–faecal transmission. The most important risk factors for *H. pylori* infection are low social class, overcrowding and home environment during childhood, for example, bed sharing. Transmission may occur within a family, a fact demonstrated by the finding that family members, especially spouses, may have the same strain of *H. pylori*. *H. pylori* seropositivity increases with age as colonisation persists for the lifetime of the host. Subjects who become infected with *H. pylori* when young are more likely to develop chronic or atrophic gastritis with reduced acid secretion that may protect them from developing duodenal ulcer. However, it may promote development of gastric ulcer as well as gastric cancer.

Duodenal ulcer seems to develop in those who are infected with *H. pylori* at the end of childhood or later. Historically, developing countries have a higher ratio of duodenal ulcer to gastric ulcer but as rates of *H. pylori* infection decline with improvements in hygiene and rates of gastric ulcer increase with the use of ulcerogenic drugs, this ratio of duodenal to gastric ulcer is declining. The prevalence of *H. pylori* still tends to be higher in the Asian adult population in whom a lower parietal cell mass has been found. These factors together with slower metabolism may explain the greater efficacy of PPIs in Asian populations. There may be other genetic, environmental or cultural factors influencing peptic ulcer disease.

Pathogenesis

There are two common forms of peptic ulcer disease: those associated with the organism *H. pylori* and those associated with the use of aspirin and NSAIDs. Less common is ulcer disease associated with massive hypersecretion of acid which occurs in the rare gastrinoma (Zollinger–Ellison) syndrome.

Helicobacter pylori

This organism is a Gram-negative microaerophilic bacterium found primarily in the gastric antrum of the human stomach (see Fig. 12.2). Ninety-five percent or more of duodenal ulcers and 80–85% of gastric ulcers are associated with *H. pylori*. The bacterium is located in the antrum and the acid-secreting microenvironment of the corpus of the stomach is less hospitable to the bacterium. In the developed world, reinfection rates are low, about 0.3–1.0% per year, whereas in the developing world reinfection rates are higher, approximately 20–30%. Ulcerogenic strains of *H. pylori*, ulcer-prone hosts, age of infection and interaction with other ulcerogenic factors such as NSAIDs determine peptic ulcer development

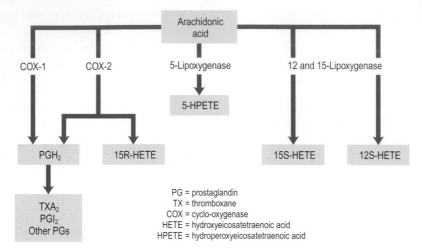

Fig. 12.3 Arachidonic acid pathway.

following *H. pylori* infection. The contribution of *H. pylori* infection to the risk of ulcers in NSAID users is not clear but there appears to be an additive effect. The risk of peptic ulcer in long-term NSAID users is greater in those who test positive for *H. pylori* and eradication of *H. pylori* in these patients prior to commencing NSAID treatment has been shown to reduce the risk of *H. pylori* NSAID-associated peptic ulcer.

Although the majority of species in the *H. pylori* genus have been associated with pathology, some are more virulent than others which probably explains why, in combination with host-related factors, only 5–10% of those infected go on to develop peptic ulcer disease.

The underlying pathophysiology associated with *H. pylori* infection involves the production of cytotoxin-associated gene A (*CagA*) proteins and vacuolating cytotoxins, such as vac A, which activate the inflammatory cascade. *CagA* status and one genotype of the vac A gene are also predictors of ulcerogenic capacity of a strain. In addition, a number of enzymes produced by *H. pylori* may be involved in causing tissue damage and include urease, haemolysins, neuraminidase and fucosidase.

Gastrin is the main hormone involved in stimulating gastric acid secretion, and gastrin homeostasis is also altered in *H. pylori* infection. The hyperacidity in duodenal ulcer may result from *H. pylori*-induced hypergastrinaemia. The elevation of gastrin may be a consequence of bacterially mediated decrease of antral D cells that secrete somatostatin, thus losing the inhibitory modulation of somatostatin on gastrin, or direct stimulation of gastrin cells by cytokines liberated during the inflammatory process. Long-standing hypergastrinaemia leads to an increased parietal cell mass. High acid content in the proximal duodenum leads to metaplastic gastric-type mucosa, which provides a niche for *H. pylori* infection followed by inflammation and ulcer formation.

Non-steroidal anti-inflammatory drugs

Three patterns of mucosal damage are caused by NSAIDs. These include superficial erosions and haemorrhages, silent ulcers detected at endoscopy and ulcers causing clinical symptoms and complications. Weak acid NSAIDs, such as acetylsalicylic acid, are concentrated from the acidic gastric juice into mucosal cells, and may produce acute superficial erosions via inhibition of COX and by mediating the adherence of leucocytes to mucosal endothelial cells. Enteric coating may prevent this superficial damage but does not demonstrate any clinical benefit in terms of reduction of gastro-intestinal bleeding or ulceration (Bhatt et al., 2008). The major systemic action of NSAIDs that contributes to the formation of ulcers is the reduction of mucosal prostaglandin production. All NSAIDs share the ability to inhibit COX (Fig. 12.3). The presence of NSAID-induced ulcers does not correlate with abdominal pain and NSAIDs themselves often mask ulcer pain. Approximately 20% of patients taking NSAIDs experience symptoms of dyspepsia but symptoms correlate poorly with the presence of mucosal damage. Ulcers and ulcer complications occur in approximately 4% of NSAID users every year. Patients taking NSAIDs have a four-fold increase in risk of ulcer complications compared with non-users. The risk of ulcer bleeding in low-dose aspirin users is two- to three-fold and there may be differences in risk factors. For example, the risk with aspirin is less influenced by age than the risk associated with NSAIDs (McQuaid and Laine, 2006) and *H. pylori* may have greater influence on the risk of bleeding with low-dose aspirin than with NSAIDs (Lanza et al., 2009).

Each year, in the UK population over the age of 60 years, there are ~3500 hospitalisations and over 400 deaths associated with NSAIDs. The risk of ulcer complications (Box 12.1) is progressive depending upon the number of risk factors present (Lanza et al., 2009). The most important risk factors

---

Box 12.1 Risk factors for NSAID ulcers

Age greater than 65 years
Previous peptic ulceration/bleeding
High dose of NSAID or more than one NSAID (including aspirin)
Short-term history of NSAID use (<1 month)
Concomitant corticosteroid or anticoagulant use
Cardiovascular disease

are a history of ulcer complications and advancing age, particularly over 75 years. Ulcers have been found to be more common in patients who have taken NSAIDs for less than 3 months, with the highest risk observed during the first month of treatment. The risk increases with higher doses of NSAID but mucosal damage occurs with even very low doses of NSAIDs, particularly aspirin. Corticosteroids alone are an insignificant ulcer risk, but potentiate the ulcer risk when added to NSAIDs, particularly in daily doses of at least 10 mg prednisolone (Lanza et al., 2009).

Low-dose aspirin (75 mg/day) alone increases the risk of ulcer bleeding and this effect may be due to the antiplatelet action, independent of other risk factors. Concomitant use of aspirin with NSAIDs further increases the risk. There is no evidence that anticoagulants increase the risk of NSAID ulcers but they are associated with an increase in the risk of haemorrhage. The presence of cardiovascular disease is also considered as an independent risk factor.

Selective cyclo-oxygenase-2 inhibitors

The gastro-intestinal side effects of conventional NSAIDs are mediated through the inhibition of COX-1 (see Fig. 12.3). COX-1 stimulates synthesis of homeostatic prostaglandins while COX-2 is predominantly induced in response to inflammation. Selective COX-2 inhibitors tend not to reduce the mucosal production of protective prostaglandins to the same extent as NSAIDs. COX-2 inhibitors are, therefore, considered to be safer than non-selective NSAIDs in patients at high risk of developing gastro-intestinal mucosal damage. Although studies have confirmed the reduction of endoscopic and symptomatic ulcers (Hooper et al., 2004), an increase in cardiovascular risk, including heart attack and stroke, has resulted in the withdrawal of some COX-2 inhibitors from the market. Additional contraindications are now in place for those COX-2 inhibitors that remain on the market. Amongst the new contraindications is the recommendation that they should not be taken by patients with established heart or cerebrovascular disease, or taken in combination with low-dose aspirin as this negates any beneficial gastro-intestinal protective effects. The need for and choice of anti-inflammatory agent should therefore take into account gastro-intestinal, cardiovascular and other risks such as potential cardio-renal effects. For all agents, the lowest effective dose should be used for the shortest duration.

Candidates for COX-2 inhibitors are patients at high risk of NSAID-related gastro-intestinal events but who do not require low-dose aspirin therapy. The lowering of risk of gastro-intestinal events is similar for COX-2 inhibitors and non-selective NSAIDs combined with a gastroprotective agent.

Nitric oxide-releasing NSAIDs

Nitric oxide (NO)-releasing NSAIDs are being investigated to see if the gastric mucosa protection associated with nitric oxide prevents ulceration when prostaglandins are inhibited by NSAIDs (Fiorucci et al., 2007). Nitric oxide is coupled to the NSAID via an ester, resulting in prolonged release of nitric oxide. Nitric oxide itself has anti-inflammatory effects adding to the potency of the NSAID. Animal studies suggest NO-releasing agents, such as naproxcinod, have minimum cardiovascular and gastro-intestinal toxicity.

Clinical manifestations

Upper abdominal pain occurring 1–3 h after meals and relieved by food or antacids is the classic symptom of peptic ulcer disease. The relationship to meals is more marked in duodenal ulcer than in gastric ulcer. However, the symptoms of peptic ulcer disease lack specificity; they do not distinguish between duodenal ulcer, gastric ulcer or functional dyspepsia. Anorexia, weight loss, nausea and vomiting, heartburn and eructation can all occur with peptic ulcer disease. Patients with predominant symptoms of heartburn are likely to have GORD. Complications of peptic ulcer disease may occur with or without previous dyspeptic symptoms. These are haemorrhage, chronic iron-deficiency anaemia, pyloric stenosis and perforation. In the elderly, the presentation is more likely to be silent and gastro-intestinal bleeding may be the first clinical sign of disease. Peptic ulcer bleeding is the most frequent and severe complication of peptic ulcer disease. Physical examination may be negative or reveal epigastric tenderness. Peptic ulcers in the past tended to relapse and remit, and 70–80% of ulcers relapse within 1–2 years after being healed by antisecretory therapy. This tendency to relapse is dramatically reduced by eradication of *H. pylori*.

Patient assessment

Presenting symptoms of dyspepsia require careful assessment to judge the risk of serious disease or to provide appropriate symptomatic treatment. Symptom subgroups such as ulcer, reflux and dysmotility type may be useful in identifying the predominant symptom subgroup to which a patient belongs. Many patients have symptoms which fit more than one subgroup (Box 12.2). Many patients seek reassurance, lifestyle advice and symptomatic treatment with a single consultation, others have chronic symptoms. In some cases, medications may be the cause of dyspepsia and should be reviewed (Box 12.3).

Patients at any age who present with alarm features (Box 12.4) should be referred for endoscopic investigation. These groups of patients are at a higher risk of underlying serious disease such as cancer, ulcers or severe oesophagitis. Referral is also recommended for patients over the age of 55 if symptoms are unexplained or persistent despite initial management (NICE, 2004; SIGN, 2003). Malignant disease is rare in young people and in those without alarm features.

Patients with predominant reflux-like symptoms are likely to respond to acid-suppressing therapy and one month's treatment of standard dose of PPI should be given in patients whose symptoms persist despite antacid and lifestyle adjustment. Eradication of *H. pylori* is not beneficial in GORD.

In those patients who do not have reflux-like dyspepsia, testing for the presence of *H. pylori* is recommended. Eradication treatment should be prescribed for those who test positive and empirical acid suppression for those who test negative. The small proportion of patients with symptoms due to ulcers should be cured. Overall, in functional dyspepsia, symptom control is poor but a small and significant benefit of eradication treatment has been shown. Acid suppression is only of benefit in a small proportion of patients with functional dyspepsia. There is no evidence to support other pharmacological therapies and non-pharmacological strategies may have a future role in functional dyspepsia. Patients should be reassured that the condition is common and not serious. National guidelines (NICE, 2004) provide algorithms to guide practitioners through the management of patients presenting with dyspepsia (Fig. 12.4A and B).

Investigations

Endoscopy

Endoscopy is generally the investigation of choice for diagnosing peptic ulcer, and the procedure is sensitive, specific and safe. However, it is also invasive and expensive. Routine endoscopy in patients presenting with dyspepsia without alarm features (see Box 12.4) is not necessary. Endoscopic investigation should be undertaken in patients with alarm features and in those patients over 55 years who present with unexplained or persistent symptoms of dyspepsia. Biopsies may be taken to exclude malignancy and uncommon lesions such as Crohn's disease.

Patients with upper gastro-intestinal bleeding have traditionally undergone endoscopy whether as an emergency or on the next available list. Most patients do not require endoscopy and in those at low risk, endoscopy and admission to hospital can be avoided by application of a scoring system. The most widely used is the Rockall risk scoring system which includes endoscopic findings to predict poor outcome. Pre-endoscopic scoring systems are available (Stanley et al., 2009) such as the abbreviated Rockall score or the Glasgow–Blatchford score (GBS) which identify low-risk patients who can be managed safely without endoscopy or admission to hospital.

Wireless capsule endoscopy is also available to investigate NSAID-induced ulceration of the small intestine causing gastro-intestinal haemorrhage and is preferable to radiological imaging.

Radiology

Double-contrast barium radiography should detect 80% of peptic ulcers. However, endoscopy is more accurate and almost always preferred. A Gastrograffin® meal is used to diagnose peptic perforation in patients presenting with an acute abdomen, if a plain abdominal X-ray is not diagnostic.

H. pylori detection

There are several methods of detecting *H. pylori* infection. They include non-invasive tests such as serological tests to detect antibodies, [^{13}C] urea breath tests and stool antigen tests. Urea breath tests have a sensitivity and specificity over 90% and are accurate for both initial diagnosis and confirmation of eradication. The breath test is based on the principle that urease activity in the stomach of infected individuals hydrolyses urea to form ammonia and carbon dioxide. The test contains carbon-labelled urea which, when hydrolysed, results in production of labelled carbon dioxide which appears in the patient's breath. The stool antigen test uses an enzyme immunoassay to detect *H. pylori* antigen in stool. This test also has a sensitivity and specificity over 90% and can be used in the initial diagnosis and also to confirm eradication. However, the breath test is preferable and more convenient. Serological tests are based on the detection of anti-*H. pylori* IgG antibodies but are not able to distinguish between active or previous exposure to infection. Near patient serology tests are not recommended (Malfertheiner et al., 2007) as they are inaccurate.

Invasive tests requiring gastric antral biopsies include urease tests, histology and culture. Of these, the biopsy urease test is widely used. Agar-based biopsy urease tests are designed to be read at 24h, whereas the strip-based biopsy urease tests can be read at 2h following incubation with the biopsy material.

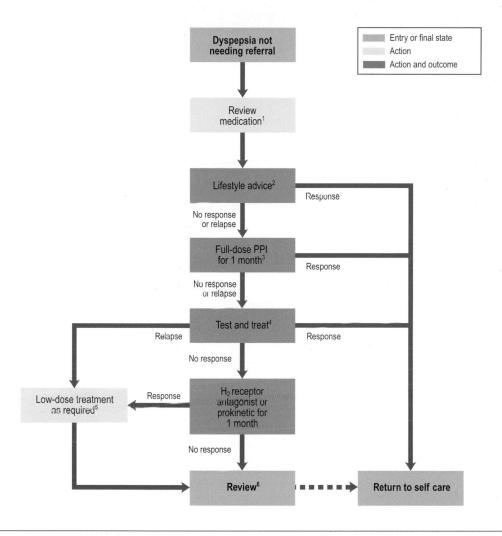

(A)

	Entry or final state
	Action
	Action and outcome

1 Review medications for possible causes of dyspepsia, for example, calcium antagonists, nitrates, theophyllines, bisphosphonates, steroids and NSAIDs.

2 Offer lifestyle advice, including advice on healthy eating, weight reduction and smoking cessation, promoting continued use of antacid/alginates.

3 There is currently inadequate evidence to guide whether full dose PPI (proton pump inhibitor) for 1 month or *H. pylori* test and treat should be offered first. Either treatment may be tried first with the other offered if symptoms persist or return.

4 Detection: use carbon-13 urea breath test, stool antigen test or, when performance has been validated, laboratory based serology.
Eradication: use PPI, amoxicillin, clarithromycin 500 mg (PAC$_{500}$) regimen or a PPI, metronidazole, clarithromycin 250 mg (PAC$_{250}$) regimen.
Do not retest even if dyspepsia remains unless there is a strong clinical need.

5 Offer low-dose treatment with a limited number of repeat prescriptions. Discuss the use of treatment on an as-required basis to help patients manage their own symptoms.

6 In some patients with an inadequate response to therapy it may become appropriate to refer to a specialist for a second opinion. Emphasise the benign nature of dyspepsia. Review long-term patient care at least annually to discuss medication and symptoms.

Fig. 12.4 (A) Decision algorithm for management of uninvestigated dyspepsia.

Continued

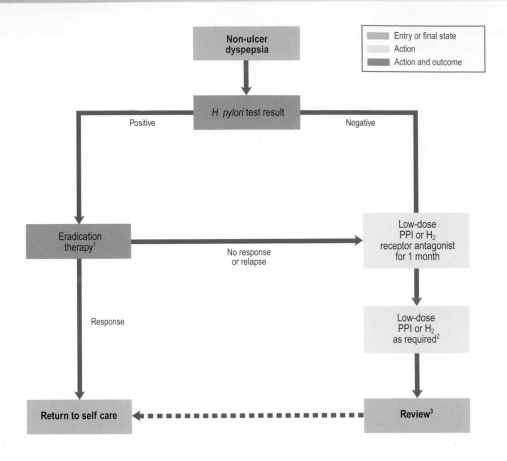

Fig. 12.4, cont'd   (B) Decision algorithm for management of non-ulcer dyspepsia.

1   Use a proton pump inhibitor (PPI), amoxicillin, clarithromycin 500 mg (PAC$_{500}$) regimen or a PPI, metronidazole, clarithromycin 250 mg (PAC$_{250}$) regimen. Do not retest unless there is a strong clinical need.

2   Offer low-dose treatment, possibly on an as-required basis, with a limited number of repeat prescriptions.

3   In some patients with an inadequate response to therapy or new emergent symptoms it may become appropriate to refer to a specialist for a second option. Emphasise the benign nature of dyspepsia. Review long-term patient care at least annually to discuss medication and symptoms.

Increasing the number of biopsy samples increases the sensitivity of the test as infection can be patchy. The accuracy of the urea breath test or biopsy urease test can be reduced by drug therapy; therefore, it is recommended to discontinue PPIs at least 2 weeks before testing and discontinue antibiotics at least 4 weeks before testing to reduce the risk of false-negative results.

The faecal occult blood test is not specific for or sensitive to detection of NSAID-induced gastric damage. A full blood count may provide evidence of blood loss from peptic ulcer.

Treatment

Complications of peptic ulcer disease

Bleeding peptic ulcer

Peptic ulcer is the most common cause of non-variceal upper gastro-intestinal bleeding. Most patients with bleeding peptic ulcer are clinically stable and stop bleeding without any

intervention, whereas other outcomes include re-bleeding and mortality. Endoscopy allows identification of the severity of disease as well as endoscopic haemostatic therapy which is successful in reducing mortality. Endoscopic therapy is necessary only in patients who exhibit high-risk stigmata (active bleeding, non-bleeding visible vessel, adherent clot) on endoscopy.

A number of pharmacological agents have been used for endoscopic injection therapy such as 1:10,000 adrenaline (epinephrine), human thrombin and fibrin glue. Mechanical endoscopic treatment options include thermocoagulation using a heater probe or endoscopic clipping. Combination therapies are superior to monotherapy and a combination of adrenaline 1:10,000 with either thermal or mechanical treatment is recommended (SIGN, 2008; Barkun et al., 2010). Need for surgery, re-bleeding rates and mortality are reduced but bleeding recurs in about 10% of patients and can cause death. Patients with uncontrolled bleeding should receive repeat endoscopic treatment, arterial embolisation or surgery. The risk of recurrent bleeding following endoscopic therapy is reduced by increasing intragastric pH during the first 3 days after the initial bleed and eradication of *H. pylori*. Biopsies taken at the time of endoscopy are used to detect *H. pylori*, or the urea breath test can be used once oral intake is established and *H. pylori* eradication therapy is indicated in those who test positive. Successful eradication of *H. pylori* reduces the rate of re-bleeding to a greater extent than antisecretory non-eradicating therapy (Gisbert et al., 2004). Following successful *H. pylori* eradication and healing of the ulcer, there is no need to continue maintenance antisecretory therapy beyond 4 weeks unless required for prophylaxis of ulcer complications in those continuing to take aspirin or NSAIDs (SIGN, 2008).

Acid suppression reduces the re-bleeding rate and should be given to those patients at high risk of re-bleeding following endoscopic haemostatic therapy. The rationale for this is based on the fact that gastric acid inhibits clot formation and if intragastric pH is maintained above 6 during the first 3 days after the initial bleed, there is opportunity for clot stabilisation and haemostasis. Meta-analysis suggests PPIs significantly reduce re-bleeding rates compared with H_2-receptor antagonists and are the preferred choice of treatment (Leontiadis et al., 2006). In similar dosage regimens, there is no data to suggest any PPI is more efficacious than another. The optimal dose and route of PPI is unknown in this indication, although reduction in mortality is observed in high-risk patients when high dose PPI therapy is given (e.g. 80 mg bolus omeprazole, pantoprazole or esomeprazole followed by 8 mg/h for 72 h) following endoscopic haemostasis (Leontiadis et al., 2007; SIGN, 2008; Barkun et al., 2010).

The use of intravenous PPI therapy before endoscopy in patients with upper gastro-intestinal bleeding does not affect clinical outcome such as re-bleeding, need for surgery or mortality (Dorward et al., 2006). However, this may reduce the need for endoscopic therapy (Lau et al., 2007) as demonstrated in Asian patients in whom PPIs are more effective. Its benefits are not clear and it is not possible to identify patients with a greater likelihood of being at high risk. Therefore, the use of PPIs is not recommended prior to diagnosis by endoscopy (SIGN, 2008) but may be beneficial if early endoscopy is delayed (Barkun et al., 2010).

In those patients at low risk for re-bleeding and in whom endoscopic therapy is not indicated, usual therapeutic doses of oral PPI are given for 4 weeks to heal the ulcer. Aspirin or NSAIDs should be avoided but if strongly indicated, these patients are given concomitant PPI therapy following successful eradication of *H. pylori*. The effect of *H. pylori* eradication on the risk of recurrent ulcer bleeding is greater in patients taking low-dose aspirin than in those taking NSAIDs (Chan et al., 2001). A possible explanation (Lanza et al., 2009) for this might be that aspirin provokes bleeding in *H. pylori* ulcers and after healing, aspirin is less likely to cause ulceration.

In patients for whom there is a clear indication to continue aspirin therapy, addition of a PPI is of benefit in the prevention of recurrent bleeding in aspirin users (Lai et al., 2002). Clopidogrel alone is not a safer alternative than this combination in terms of prevention of recurrent ulcer bleeding. Cardiovascular and gastro-intestinal risks must be taken into consideration when deciding how long aspirin should be discontinued after a gastro-intestinal bleed. In some cases, low-dose aspirin can be restarted with concurrent PPI treatment within 7 days (Barkun et al., 2010). When the combination of aspirin and clopidogrel is indicated, concomitant PPI therapy is recommended in patients at high risk of gastro-intestinal complications despite the potential drug interaction between PPIs and clopidogrel. An increased risk of myocardial infarction has been observed with the combination of clopidogrel and PPIs (MHRA, 2009). Causality is unclear but it is suggested that through competitive enzyme inhibition, PPIs metabolised by CYP2C19 reduce the conversion of clopidogrel to its active metabolite. Concomitant use is discouraged but if necessary, separation of dosage timing is recommended (Laine and Hennekens, 2010).

Pyloric stenosis

Malignancy is the most common cause of gastric outlet obstruction. Peptic ulcer disease is the underlying cause in about 10% of cases. There is limited anecdotal evidence that incomplete gastric outlet obstruction may improve within several months of successful *H. pylori* eradication. Conventional treatment with acid-suppressive therapy may also help. If medical therapy fails to relieve the obstruction, endoscopic balloon dilation or surgery may be required.

Zollinger–Ellison syndrome

This rare syndrome consists of a triad of non-β islet cell tumours of the pancreas that contain and release gastrin, gastric acid hypersecretion and severe ulcer disease. Extrapancreatic gastrinomas are also common and may be found frequently in the duodenal wall. A proportion of these patients have tumours of the pituitary gland and parathyroid gland (multiple endocrine neoplasia type I). Surgical resection of the gastrinoma may be curative. Medical management consists of greater than standard doses of PPIs. The somatostatin analogue octreotide is also effective but has no clear advantage over PPIs. Patients with idiopathic peptic ulcer disease should be investigated for Zollinger–Ellison syndrome and gastrinoma.

Stress ulcers

Severe physiological stress such as head injury, spinal cord injury, burns, multiple trauma or sepsis may induce superficial mucosal erosions or gastroduodenal ulcerations. These may lead to haemorrhage or perforation. Mechanical ventilation and the presence of coagulopathies place patients at particular risk of stress-related mucosal bleeding and may warrant prophylactic treatment (Quenot et al., 2009). Diminished blood flow to the gastric mucosa, decreased cell renewal, diminished prostaglandin production and, occasionally, acid hypersecretion are involved in causing stress ulceration. Intravenous acid-suppression therapy, histamine H_2-receptor antagonists and PPIs, and nasogastric tube administration of sucralfate (4–6 g daily in divided doses) have been used to prevent stress ulceration in the intensive care unit until the patient tolerates enteral feeding. The most commonly used regimen is intravenous ranitidine 50 mg every 8 h reducing to 25 mg in severe renal impairment. Current evidence does not support routine use of prophylaxis and reports of complications associated with bacterial overgrowth in the gastro-intestinal tract in patients receiving acid suppressants should limit use only to those at high risk. Complications include association with hospital acquired *Clostridium difficile* diarrhoea (Dial et al., 2004) and pneumonia (Herzig et al., 2009).

Uncomplicated peptic ulcer disease

Treatment of endoscopically proven uncomplicated peptic ulcer disease has changed dramatically in recent years (Fig. 12.5A and B). Curing of *H. pylori* infection and discontinuation of NSAIDs are key elements for the successful management of peptic ulcer disease.

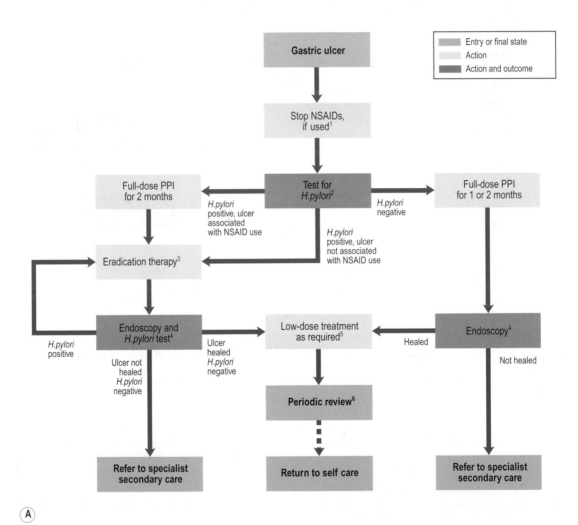

1 If NSAID continuation is necessary, after ulcer healing offer long-term gastric protection or consider substitution to a newer COX-2-selective NSAID.

2 Use a carbon-13 urea breath test, stool antigen test or, when performance has been validated, laboratory-based serology.

3 Use a proton pump inhibitor (PPI), amoxicillin, clarithromycin 500 mg (PAC$_{500}$) regimen or a PPI, metronidazole, clarithromycin 250 mg (PMC$_{250}$) regimen.
   Follow guidance found in the *British National Formulary* for selecting second-line therapies.
   After two attempts at eradication manage as *H. pylori* negative.

4 Perform endoscopy 6 to 8 weeks after treatment. If re-testing for *H.pylori* use a carbon-13 urea breath test.

5 Offer low-dose treatment, possibly used on an as-required basis, with a limited number of repeat prescriptions.

6 Review care annually, to discuss symptoms, promote stepwise withdrawal of therapy when appropriate and provide lifestyle advice. In some patients with an inadequate response to therapy it may become appropriate to refer to a specialist.

Fig. 12.5 (A) Management algorithm for gastric ulcer.

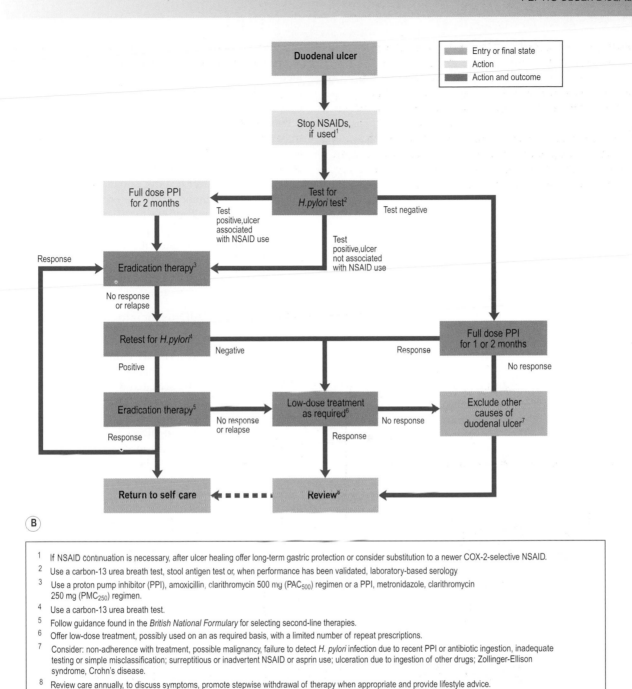

Fig. 12.5, cont'd (B) Management algorithm for duodenal ulcer.

1. If NSAID continuation is necessary, after ulcer healing offer long-term gastric protection or consider substitution to a newer COX-2-selective NSAID.

2. Use a carbon-13 urea breath test, stool antigen test or, when performance has been validated, laboratory-based serology

3. Use a proton pump inhibitor (PPI), amoxicillin, clarithromycin 500 mg (PAC_{500}) regimen or a PPI, metronidazole, clarithromycin 250 mg (PMC_{250}) regimen.

4. Use a carbon-13 urea breath test.

5. Follow guidance found in the *British National Formulary* for selecting second-line therapies.

6. Offer low-dose treatment, possibly used on an as required basis, with a limited number of repeat prescriptions.

7. Consider: non-adherence with treatment, possible malignancy, failure to detect *H. pylori* infection due to recent PPI or antibiotic ingestion, inadequate testing or simple misclassification; surreptitious or inadvertent NSAID or asprin use; ulceration due to ingestion of other drugs; Zollinger-Ellison syndrome, Crohn's disease.

8. Review care annually, to discuss symptoms, promote stepwise withdrawal of therapy when appropriate and provide lifestyle advice.

H. pylori eradication

It is known that *H. pylori* infection is associated with over 90% of duodenal ulcers and 80% of gastric ulcers. Cure of this infection with antibiotic therapy and simultaneous treatment with conventional ulcer-healing drugs facilitates symptom relief and healing of the ulcer and reduces the ulcer relapse rate. Antibiotics alone, or acid-suppressing agents alone, do not eradicate *H. pylori*. Both therapies act synergistically as growth of the organism occurs at elevated pH and antibiotic efficacy is enhanced during growth. Additionally, increasing intragastric pH may enhance antibiotic absorption. Recent studies limited to one country (Italy) suggest that sequential antibiotic treatment may be advantageous in overcoming emerging antibiotic resistance but the complexity of sequential regimens has the potential to affect adherence (Jafri et al., 2008)

High eradication rates are achieved by a short course of triple therapy consisting of a PPI, clarithromycin and amoxicillin or metronidazole in a twice-daily simultaneous regimen. European guidelines recommend 1 week of therapy, whereas the US guidelines recommend 10–14 days of therapy and achieve 7–9% better eradication rates (Malfertheiner et al., 2007).

Triple therapy consists of:

- OCA: omeprazole 20 mg, clarithromycin 500 mg and amoxicillin 1 g or
- OCM: omeprazole 20 mg, clarithromycin 250 mg and metronidazole 400 mg.

A lower dose of clarithromycin (250 mg twice daily) is effective and recommended when combined with metronidazole (NICE, 2004). However, some prescribers prefer to recommend 500 mg twice daily to achieve consistency and avoid prescribing errors.

Omeprazole may be replaced with any of the other PPI drugs. Local resistance rates determine the most appropriate first-line regimen, with OCA preferred in areas of high metronidazole resistance. In the UK, resistance to metronidazole has been reported in about 50% of *H. pylori* isolates, and resistance to clarithromycin in about 10%, although this is rising. Resistance to amoxicillin is rare. Sensitivity testing is of little value as *in vitro* resistance to either drug does not preclude eradication when those drugs are used as part of a triple therapy regimen. In patients with hypersensitivity to penicillin, the OCM regimen or substitution of amoxicillin from the OCA regimen with tetracycline 500 mg twice daily is used. If patients have recently received antibiotic treatment for any indication, a regimen avoiding that antibiotic is preferred.

Failure of a first-line regimen to achieve eradication will necessitate treatment with another triple therapy regimen or with a bismuth-based quadruple regimen. Recommended second-line triple therapy regimens include a PPI, amoxicillin or tetracycline and metronidazole. Most four-drug regimens contain bismuth subsalicylate, metronidazole, tetracycline or amoxicillin and a PPI and are generally not as well tolerated by patients as triple therapy regimens. Quadruple therapy may be used first-line where there is high prevalence of clarithromycin resistance. The indication should be reviewed in patients who are refractory to conventional as well as quadruple eradication therapies, to determine the importance of eradication before proceeding to endoscopic biopsies and determination of antibiotic sensitivity after culture. This strategy is rarely justified in dyspepsia.

Successful eradication relies upon patients adhering to their medication regimen. It is, therefore, important to educate patients about the principles of eradication therapy and also about coping with common adverse effects associated with their regimen. Diarrhoea is the most common adverse effect and should subside after treatment is complete. In rare cases, this can be severe and continue after treatment. If this happens, patients should be advised to return to their doctor as rare cases of antibiotic-associated colitis have been reported. If drugs are not taken as intended, then non-adherence may result in antibiotic resistance, should the antibiotic concentration at the site of infection decrease to a level where resistance may emerge.

If eradication is successful, uncomplicated active peptic ulcers heal without the need to continue ulcer-healing drugs beyond the duration of eradication therapy (Gisbert et al., 2004). Patients with persistent symptoms after eradication therapy should have their *H. pylori* status rechecked. This should be carried out no sooner than 4 weeks after discontinuation of therapy to avoid false-negative results due to suppression rather than eradication of the organism. If the patient is *H. pylori* positive, an alternative eradication regimen should be given. If eradication was successful but symptoms persist, gastro-oesophageal reflux or other causes of dyspepsia should be considered.

Patients who have had a previous gastro-intestinal bleed from a gastric ulcer should continue ulcer-healing therapy for a further 3 weeks in addition to eradication therapy. *H. pylori* eradication should be confirmed. The need for routine endoscopy to confirm ulcer healing is unclear but should be undertaken where malignancy is suspected.

Other accepted indications for *H. pylori* eradication include mucosal-associated lymphoid tissue (MALT) lymphoma of the stomach, severe gastritis, and in patients with a high risk of gastric cancer such as those with family history of the disease.

Treatment of NSAID-associated ulcers

NSAID-associated ulcers may be *H. pylori* positive. Although the presence of *H. pylori* may enhance the efficacy of acid suppression, eradication is generally recommended in infected patients with NSAID-associated ulcers as it is difficult to differentiate between *H. Pylori* or NSAID as the cause of the ulcer (Malfertheiner et al., 2009). If NSAIDs are discontinued, most uncomplicated ulcers heal using standard doses of a PPI, H_2-receptor antagonist, misoprostol or sucralfate. Healing is impaired if NSAID use is continued. Studies have demonstrated conflicting results, in terms of the comparative healing rates between PPIs and H_2-receptor antagonists, in this situation (Yeomans et al., 2006; Goldstein et al., 2007). PPIs demonstrate higher healing rates at 4 weeks but similar healing rates to H_2-receptor antagonists at 8 weeks. There is no evidence that high-dose PPI is better than treatment with the standard dose. Although effective, misoprostol use is limited by treatment-related adverse events.

Prophylaxis of NSAID ulceration

NSAIDs should be avoided in patients who are at risk of gastro-intestinal toxicity (see Box 12.1). However, some patients with chronic rheumatological conditions may require long-term NSAID treatment, in which case the lowest effective dose should be used. Dyspepsia is not a risk factor for ulcer complications but in those patients at high risk of ulcer complication, the NSAID should be stopped and investigation undertaken if dyspepsia develops.

Data suggests that *H. pylori* increases, has no effect on or decreases ulcer risk in NSAID users (Malfertheiner et al., 2007, 2009). The value of eradication of *H. pylori* in chronic NSAID users is, therefore, unclear but there may be some benefit in screening and eradicating *H. pylori* in patients about to start NSAIDs. The benefit is less apparent in those patients at low risk of peptic ulcer. In patients with a history of bleeding or non-bleeding ulcer, guidelines recommend screening for and eradicating *H. pylori* before starting low-dose aspirin (Bhatt et al., 2008). When using NSAIDs in patients with a previous bleeding ulcer, PPI maintenance therapy is more effective secondary prophylaxis than *H. pylori* eradication alone, but a combination of both treatments is additive.

Treatment options for ulcer prophylaxis in patients at risk of peptic ulcer but who require NSAIDs, include co-therapy with acid-suppressing agents or a synthetic prostaglandin analogue, or substitution of a selective COX-2 inhibitor for a non-selective NSAID (Hooper et al., 2004). Comparison of study outcomes requires interpretation of whether ulcers are detected symptomatically or by endoscopy. The prostaglandin analogue, misoprostol at a dose of 800 μcg daily is effective at reducing NSAID-associated ulcer complications and symptomatic ulcers. Adverse effects, primarily diarrhoea, abdominal pain and nausea, limit its use as lower doses are less effective. PPIs are effective at reducing endoscopically diagnosed ulcers and dyspepsia symptoms but the effect on symptomatic ulcers is unclear. Studies have not demonstrated any advantage in using higher than standard doses of PPIs to reduce risk of ulcers. Standard doses of H_2-receptor antagonists are effective at reducing the risk of endoscopic duodenal ulcers. However, reduction in the risk of gastric ulcers requires double this dose. Gastroprotective agents licensed for prophylaxis of NSAID ulceration are listed in Table 12.1.

In low-dose aspirin users, standard-dose PPIs are more effective than high dose H_2-receptor antagonists in preventing recurrent ulcer bleeding following ulcer healing and eradication of *H. pylori* (Ng et al., 2010). However, in those patients who do not have a history of peptic ulcer bleeding, high-dose H_2-receptor antagonists might be an alternative to PPIs (Taha et al., 2009).

Given the contraindications to selective COX-2 inhibitors, their use is limited and further studies are required to clarify their place in minimising risk of ulcers in both primary and secondary prophylaxis. In patients with no history of peptic

ulcer bleeding but with risk factors, a combination of COX-2 inhibitor with a PPI was similar in efficacy to a combination of non-selective NSAID with a PPI (Scheiman et al., 2006). In patients with a history of ulcer bleeding, a combination of selective COX-2 inhibitor with a PPI reduced recurrent ulcer bleeding compared to COX-2 inhibitor alone (Chan et al., 2007). This was not compared to a combination of a non-selective NSAID and a PPI. Although an earlier study suggested COX-2 inhibitors alone offered similar protection to that offered by a combination of non-selective NSAID with PPI (Lai et al., 2005), results suggest that in high-risk patients with a history of gastro-intestinal bleeding in whom an NSAID is indicated where alternative analgesic therapies have failed and in whom there are no contraindications to selective COX-2 inhibitors, a combination of PPI with a selective COX-2 inhibitor may be the safest strategy.

H. pylori-negative, NSAID-negative ulcers

Ulceration in the absence of *H. pylori* infection or NSAID or aspirin use is rare and validation of negative medication history and *H. pylori* status should be confirmed using biopsy samples and a careful medication history including over the counter preparations. Many analgesics contain aspirin or NSAIDs and some patients purchase low-dose aspirin.

Gastro-oesophageal reflux disease

GORD is the term used to describe any symptomatic clinical condition or histopathological alteration resulting from episodes of reflux of acid, pepsin and, occasionally, bile into the oesophagus from the stomach (Moayyedi and Talley, 2006). Heartburn is the characteristic symptom, and the patient may also complain of acid regurgitation and dysphagia. Complications include oesophageal stricture, oesophageal ulceration and formation of specialised columnar-lined oesophagus at the gastro-oesophageal junction known as Barrett's oesophagus (Shaheen and Richter, 2009). The mechanism of acid reflux is multifactorial and involves transient lower oesophageal sphincter relaxations, reduced tone of the lower oesophageal sphincter, hiatus hernia and abnormal oesophageal acid clearance. The severity of inflammation of the oesophageal mucosa is described as categories of oesophagitis (Los Angeles A–D). However, approximately two-thirds of patients with GORD have normal mucosa on endoscopy. Hypersensitivity to normal acid exposure may be the cause of symptoms in this group of patients. Progression from non-erosive reflux disease to erosive oesophagitis and Barrett's oesophagus is rare.

Management of GORD focuses on symptom control rather than endoscopic findings, and therefore careful symptom evaluation is required (Box 12.5). Patients with alarm features or those who fail to respond to medical treatment should be referred for endoscopic investigation. *H. pylori* eradication is not recommended in the management of GORD (Malfertheiner et al., 2007).

Strategies for initial treatment include lifestyle measures such as weight loss and smoking cessation in combination

Table 12.1	Drugs for prophylaxis for NSAID-induced ulceration	
Drug	**Licensed indication**	**Prophylaxis dose**
Omeprazole	Prophylaxis of further DU or GU	20 mg every day
Esomeprazole	Prophylaxis of DU or GU	20 mg every day
Lansoprazole	Prophylaxis of DU or GU	15–30 mg every day
Pantoprazole	Prophylaxis of DU or GU	20 mg daily
Misoprostol	Prophylaxis of DU or GU	200 μcg 2–4 times a day
Ranitidine	Prophylaxis of DU	150 mg twice a day
Ranitidine	Prophylaxis of DU (unlicensed)	300 mg twice day

DU, duodenal ulcer; GU, gastric ulcer.

Box 12.5 Symptoms associated with gastro-oesophageal reflux disease

Heartburn and regurgitation
Belching
Upper abdominal discomfort
Bloating and postprandial fullness
Chest pain
Hoarseness
Cough

with antacids. These measures may be effective in patients with no significant impairment of quality of life. When quality of life is impaired, acid-suppression therapy is the basis of effective treatment. A course of standard-dose PPI therapy is most effective for symptom relief, healing of oesophagitis and maintenance of remission in patients with GORD (Fig. 12.6).

Compared with erosive oesophagitis, there is a diminished response to acid suppression in non-erosive reflux disease but PPIs remain the most effective agents. Most patients respond after 4 weeks' treatment and after initial control of symptoms, therapy can be withdrawn. If symptoms return, intermittent courses can be given or, alternatively, on-demand single doses can be taken immediately as symptoms occur. Patients who relapse frequently may require continuous maintenance therapy using the lowest dose of acid suppression which provides effective symptom relief.

Escalating doses can be used in the small number of patients who do not respond to initial treatment. These patients should be investigated to confirm diagnosis. Those with a normal upper endoscopy may require pH monitoring or motility tests. Twice-daily dosing may be required in patients with persistent symptoms. A selected group of patients may benefit from anti-reflux surgery rather than the escalation of acid-suppressing

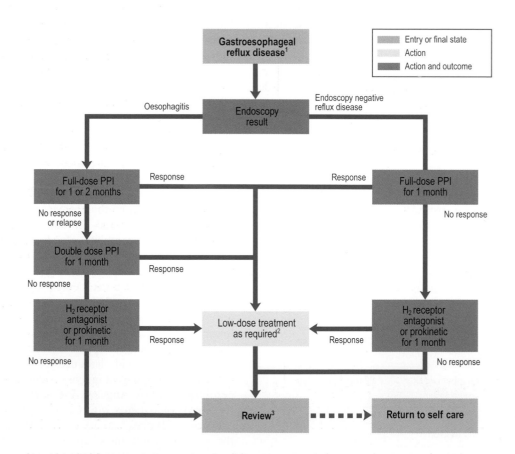

[1] GORD refers to endoscopically determined oesophagitis or endoscopy-negative reflux disease. Patients with uninvestigated 'reflux-like' symptoms should be managed as patients with uninvestigated dyspepsia.
There is currently no evidence that *H. pylori* should be investigated in patients with GORD.

[2] Offer low-dose treatment, possibly used on an as-required basis, with a limited number of repeat prescriptions.

[3] Review long-term patient care at least annually to discuss medication and symptoms.
In some patients with an inadequate response to therapy or new emergent symptoms it may become appropriate to refer to a specialist for a second opinion.

A minority of patients have persistent symptoms despite proton pump inhibitor (PPI) therapy and this group remains a challenge to treat.
Therapeutic options include doubling the dose of PPI therapy, adding an H_2 receptor antagonist at bedtime and extending the length of treatment.

Fig. 12.6 Management algorithm for gastro-oesophageal reflux disease.

treatment. Patients with endoscopically severe oesophagitis (Los Angeles class C or D) should be kept on standard-dose PPIs long-term to maintain symptom relief and prevent the development of complications such as Barrett's oesophagus or oesophageal adenocarcinoma.

Ulcer-healing drugs

Proton pump inhibitors

The PPIs are all benzimidazole derivatives that control gastric acid secretion by inhibition of gastric H^+, K^+-ATPase, the enzyme responsible for the final step in gastric acid secretion from the parietal cell (Fig. 12.7).

The PPIs are inactive prodrugs that are carried in the bloodstream to the parietal cells in the gastric mucosa. The prodrugs readily cross the parietal cell membrane into the cytosol. These drugs are weak bases and therefore have a high affinity for acidic environments. They diffuse across the secretory membrane of the parietal cell into the extracellular secretory canaliculus, the site of the active proton pump (see Fig. 12.7). Under these acidic conditions the prodrugs are converted to their active form, which irreversibly binds the proton pump, inhibiting acid secretion. Since the 'active principle' forms at a low pH it concentrates selectively in the acidic environment of the proton pump and results in extremely effective inhibition of acid secretion. The different PPIs (omeprazole, esomeprazole, lansoprazole, pantoprazole and rabeprazole) bind to different sites on the proton pump, which may explain their differences in potency on a milligram per milligram basis.

PPIs require an enteric coating to protect them from degradation in the acidic environment of the stomach. This delays absorption and a maximum plasma concentration is reached after 2–3h. Different formulations have been developed for patients with swallowing difficulties but these still rely upon some form of enteric coating (Table 12.2). New immediate-release formulations are under development which may overcome problems with enteric-coated granules blocking enteral feeding tubes.

Since these drugs irreversibly bind to the proton pump they have a sustained duration of acid inhibition which does not correlate with the plasma elimination half-life of 1–2h. The apparent half-life is approximately 48h. This prolonged duration of action allows once-daily dosing of PPIs, although twice-daily dosing is recommended in some cases of erosive oesophagitis or Barrett's oesophagus when a sustained gastric pH of greater than 4.0 is required. All PPIs are most effective if taken about 30min before a meal as they inhibit only actively secreting proton pumps. Meals are the main stimulus to proton pump activity. The optimal dosing time is 30–60min before the first meal of the day.

Intravenous PPIs are most frequently used to prevent recurrent ulcer bleeding in high-risk patients. Intravenous preparations are therapeutically equivalent to oral preparations. In the UK, omeprazole, pantoprazole and esomeprazole can be given intravenously.

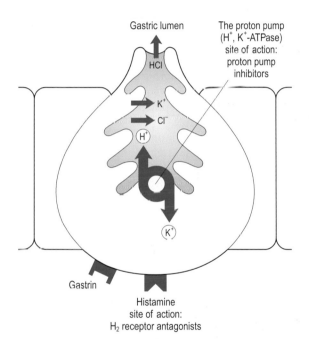

Fig. 12.7 Receptor stimulation of acid secretion.

Table 12.2 Available formulations of proton pump inhibitors

	Omeprazole	Lansoprazole	Pantoprazole	Rabeprazole	Esomeprazole
Capsule or tablet	√	√ (sucked)	√	√	√
Capsule granules can be dispersed in uncarbonated water or juice (pH < 5) or yoghurt	√				
Dispersible tablet	√	√			√
Granules for oral suspension					√
Intravenous	√		√		√
Available over the counter	√				

PPIs are metabolised in the liver to various sulphate conjugates that are extensively eliminated by the kidneys (80%). With the exception of severe hepatic dysfunction, no dose adjustments are necessary in liver disease or in renal disease. Apart from minor differences in bioavailability in the first few days of oral dosing, pharmacokinetics are similar among all PPIs. The antisecretory effect is also similar among all agents when administered chronically in equivalent standard doses.

Adverse drug reactions

Experience suggests that PPIs are a remarkably safe group of drugs. The most commonly reported side effects are diarrhoea, headaches, abdominal pain, nausea, fatigue and dizziness which resolve on drug discontinuation (Table 12.3). Possible mechanisms for diarrhoea include bacterial overgrowth, changes in intestinal pH and bile salt abnormalities. Diarrhoea is most commonly associated with lansoprazole, particularly in the elderly. Some cases of persistent chronic watery diarrhoea associated with lansoprazole have been diagnosed as microscopic colitis. This may be explained by the unique ability of lansoprazole to inhibit colonic proton pumps which may have an effect on colonic secretion and pH. Apart from the association between lansoprazole and diarrhoea, the incidence of adverse reactions is similar among the drugs in this group.

Loss of gastric acidity has been associated with colonisation of the normally sterile upper gastro-intestinal tract. Associations with increased risk of respiratory tract infections and *C. difficile*-associated disease have prompted more judicious use of PPIs. Long-term use may also decrease bone density and increase risk of hip fractures.

Drug interactions

The cytochrome P450 enzyme system is classified into a number of subgroups, several of which are involved in drug metabolism. All PPIs are metabolised to varying degrees by the same cytochrome P450 isoenzymes, CYP2C19 and CYP3A. All except rabeprazole are metabolised primarily via the CYP2C19 isoenzyme. This suggests rabeprazole may be less influenced by other drugs metabolised through this system or by genetic changes in hepatic metabolism. The affinity of individual PPIs for these enzymes influences the incidence of clinically relevant drug interactions.

- Pantoprazole has lower affinity for the enzyme system than the other PPIs and is also metabolised by a sulphotransferase which is non-saturable and not part of the cytochrome P450 system. Rabeprazole is also metabolised through a non-enzymatic pathway.
- Omeprazole inhibits CYP2C9 and 2C19, the isoenzymes involved in the metabolism of, for example, phenytoin (2C9), *S*-warfarin (2C9), diazepam (2C19) and *R*-warfarin (2C19). Omeprazole 40 mg daily can decrease the clearance of phenytoin, but phenytoin levels were unchanged after a dose of 20 mg of omeprazole daily. Therefore, phenytoin plasma concentrations should be monitored when omeprazole is taken concomitantly. Omeprazole may increase the coagulation time in patients receiving warfarin therapy, especially if doses higher than 20 mg daily are given. Changes in the plasma concentration of the less potent (*R*) enantiomer of warfarin have been observed; therefore, monitoring of the international normalised ratio (INR) is recommended during concomitant therapy. The metabolism of benzodiazepines, particularly diazepam, may be decreased by omeprazole. Similar interactions are likely with esomeprazole.
- Lansoprazole is a weak inducer of CYP1A2 and concurrent administration results in increased theophylline clearance.

Other isolated interactions have been reported:

- Omeprazole can increase the concentration of ciclosporin.
- Clarithromycin increases esomeprazole concentrations; however, omeprazole has also increased clarithromycin concentration.
- Lansoprazole has reduced the efficacy of the oral contraceptive pill.
- Clarithromycin has increased plasma lansoprazole concentration.
- Lansoprazole has increased plasma concentration of tacrolimus.
- Omeprazole has increased the concentration of escitalopram.
- Omeprazole has decreased renal elimination of methotrexate.

Approximately 3% of the Caucasian and 20% of the Asian population are poor metabolisers of PPIs due to genetic polymorphism associated with CYP2C19. High plasma concentrations are achieved and the relative capacity for metabolism by other isoenzymes may alter and result in drug interactions. In practice, the genotype of a patient is unknown. The relative contribution of CYP2C19 to PPI metabolism is greatest with omeprazole and least with rabeprazole. The observation of decreased clopidogrel activity and increased cardiovascular events has been linked to competitive inhibition of CYP2C19 possibly caused by concomitant treatment with PPIs.

Table 12.3 Common adverse reactions to ulcer-healing drugs

Proton pump inhibitors	H₂-receptor antagonists	Sucralfate
Diarrhoea	Diarrhoea	Constipation
Headache	Headache	
Abdominal pain	Abdominal pain	
Nausea	Confusion	
Fatigue		
Dizziness		

The use of symptom-driven, on-demand PPI therapy may prove problematic if used concomitantly with warfarin or phenytoin. Careful monitoring should be undertaken. All acid-suppressing drugs potentially decrease the absorption of some drugs by increasing gastric pH. Reduction in absorption of ketoconazole and increased absorption of digoxin have been reported with PPIs. The absorption of drugs formulated as pH-dependent, controlled-release products may also be altered. Very few clinically important drug interactions have been reported despite the widespread use of these agents.

Clinical use

PPIs relieve symptoms and heal peptic ulcers faster than H_2-receptor antagonists. They also heal ulcers that are refractory to H_2-receptor antagonists. All PPIs provide similar *H. pylori* eradication rates and ulcer healing when used at their recommended doses. Standard doses of PPIs are used concomitantly with non-selective NSAIDs and with low-dose aspirin in patients at risk of peptic ulcers or ulcer bleeding. High dose intravenous PPIs are used to prevent recurrent bleeding in high-risk patients (active bleeding or non-bleeding visible vessel) during the initial 72 h after a bleed. In GORD, PPIs heal oesophagitis and control symptoms more rapidly than H_2-receptor antagonists. Differences between PPIs in terms of speed of symptom relief are observed only in the first few days of treatment. Patients with severe oesophagitis should continue long-term PPI therapy, whereas those with milder GORD should be stepped down in terms of acid suppression and therapy withdrawn if symptoms are controlled. On-demand therapy is used to maintain symptom control. Patients with functional dyspepsia should not routinely receive long-term treatment with PPIs. PPIs can be purchased over the counter for short-term relief of heartburn.

H_2-receptor antagonists

The H_2-antagonists are all structural analogues of histamine. They competitively block the histamine receptors in gastric parietal cells, thereby preventing acid secretion. Pepsinogen requires acid for conversion to pepsin and so when acid output is reduced, pepsin generation is, in turn, also reduced.

All the available drugs (cimetidine, ranitidine, famotidine, nizatidine) have similar properties. Maximum plasma concentration is reached within 1–3 h after administration. First-pass hepatic metabolism varies, ranitidine being most extensively metabolised which explains the difference between the intravenous and oral dose. All H_2-antagonists are eliminated to a variable and significant extent via the kidneys, and all require dosage reduction in moderate-to-severe renal impairment. They are equally effective at suppressing daytime and nocturnal acid secretion while they do not cause total achlorhydria. The evening dose of a H_2-antagonist is particularly important because during the daytime, gastric acid is buffered for long periods by food; however, during the night this does not occur and the intragastric pH may fall below 2.0 for several hours. For healing oesophagitis, intragastric pH must remain above 4.0 for 18 h or more per day. H_2-receptor antagonists

are, therefore, not effective in healing oesophagitis. Adding a bedtime dose of H_2-receptor antagonist to PPI therapy may enhance nocturnal gastric pH control in patients in whom nocturnal gastric acid breakthrough is problematic.

The role of H_2-receptor antagonists in the management of peptic ulcer disease has diminished. H_2-receptor antagonists are less effective than PPIs in eradication regimens, in treating ulcers when NSAIDs are continued, and in prophylaxis of NSAID-induced ulcers. H_2-receptor antagonists do effectively heal ulcers in patients who discontinue their NSAID and they also have a role in continuing acid suppression for symptomatic treatment following eradication therapy. Their main role is in the empirical management of dyspepsia symptoms. If patients with mild symptoms gain adequate relief, it is not necessary to use a PPI. H_2-receptor antagonists are preferred over PPIs in the second-line treatment of heartburn in pregnancy, although there is growing evidence to support safe use of PPIs in those not controlled by H_2-receptor antagonists. H_2-receptor antagonists can be purchased in doses lower than those prescribed for the management of heartburn and indigestion.

Adverse drug reactions

H_2-receptor antagonists are a remarkably safe group of drugs with a lower risk of side effects than PPIs. The risk of any adverse reaction is below 3% and serious adverse reactions account for less than 1%. Diarrhoea and headache are the most common and occasionally mental confusion and rashes have been reported (see Table 12.3). Hepatotoxicity is a rare adverse effect. Cimetidine, due to its antiandrogenic effects, has been associated with gynaecomastia and impotence when used in high doses.

Drug interactions

Although many drug interactions have been suggested with cimetidine, many have only been demonstrated *in vitro* and are of doubtful clinical significance. Cimetidine inhibits the activity of cytochrome P450 and consequently retards oxidative metabolism of some drugs. This interaction is potentially important for drugs with a narrow therapeutic index. The clearance of theophylline is reduced to about 40% of normal, and raised plasma levels occur as a result. Phenytoin metabolism is reduced, and toxicity is theoretically possible. The metabolism of a number of benzodiazepines, including diazepam, flurazepam and triazolam, is impaired and levels are raised.

The interaction with warfarin has frequently been cited as justification to change to an alternative H_2-antagonist which binds less intensively to the CYP 450 system; however, careful investigation has shown that this interaction is complex. The metabolism of (*R*)-warfarin is affected to a greater degree than that of (*S*)-warfarin. As the (*S*) enantiomer is the more potent, the pharmacodynamic effects of the interaction may be modest, although the plasma warfarin concentrations may be increased. Current opinion suggests that warfarin may safely be added with appropriate monitoring when patients are already taking cimetidine in regular daily doses. Other H_2-antagonists should be used in patients who are difficult to stabilise on warfarin or for whom frequent monitoring is not feasible.

All acid-suppressing drugs potentially decrease the absorption of drugs such as ketoconazole and other pH-dependent controlled-release products by increasing gastric pH.

Bismuth chelate

Bismuth has been included in antacid mixtures for many decades but fell from favour because of its neurotoxicity. Bismuth chelate is a relatively safe form of bismuth that has ulcer-healing properties comparable to those of H_2-antagonists. Its mode of action is not clearly understood but it is thought to have cytoprotective properties. Bismuth is toxic to *H. pylori* and was one of the first agents to be used to eradicate the organism and reduce ulcer recurrence. Tripotassium dicitratobismuthate in combination with tetracycline, metronidazole and a PPI is used in quadruple therapy regimens in patients resistant to triple therapy.

Adverse drug reactions

Small amounts of bismuth are absorbed from bismuth chelate, and urinary bismuth excretion may be raised for several weeks after a course of treatment. The risks of bismuth intoxication are small if these products are used at the recommended dose and for short courses of treatment. Bismuth may accumulate in patients with impaired renal function. The most commonly reported events are nausea, vomiting, blackened tongue and dark faeces.

Sucralfate

Sucralfate is the aluminium salt of sucrose octasulphate. Although it is a weak antacid, this is not its principal mode of action in peptic ulcer disease. It has mucosal protective effects including stimulation of bicarbonate and mucus secretion and stimulation of mucosal prostanoids. At pH less than 4.0 it forms a sticky viscid gel that adheres to the ulcer surface and may afford some physical protection. It is capable of adsorbing bile salts. These activities appear to reside in the entire molecular complex and are not due to the aluminium ions alone. Sucralfate has no acid-suppressing activity. At a dose of 2 g twice daily, sucralfate is effective in the treatment of NSAID-induced duodenal ulcers, if the NSAID is stopped. However, it is not effective in the treatment and prevention of NSAID-related gastric ulcers. It has also been used in the prophylaxis of stress ulceration. The liquid formulation is often used as the tablets are large and difficult to swallow.

Adverse drug reactions

Constipation appears to be the most common problem with sucralfate, and this is thought to be related to the aluminium content (see Table 12.3). About 3–5% of a dose is absorbed, and therefore there is a risk of aluminium toxicity with long-term treatment. This risk is correspondingly greater in patients with renal impairment. Caution is required to avoid oesophageal bezoar formation around a nasogastric tube in patients managed in the intensive care unit.

Drug interactions

Sucralfate may bind to other agents in the gastro-intestinal tract and reduce the absorption of other drugs. Therefore, it should be taken at least 2 h following other medicines.

Antacids

Antacids have a place in symptomatic relief of dyspepsia, in particular symptoms associated with GORD. They have a role in the management of symptoms which sometimes remain for a short time after *H. pylori* eradication of uncomplicated duodenal ulcer.

The choice of antacid lies between aluminium-based and magnesium-based products, although many proprietary products combine both. Calcium-based products are unsuitable as calcium stimulates acid secretion. Antacids containing sodium bicarbonate are unsuitable for regular use because they deliver a high sodium load and generate large quantities of carbon dioxide. It should be noted that magnesium trisilicate mixtures contain a large amount of sodium bicarbonate. Some products contain other agents such as dimeticone or alginates. Products containing sodium alginate with a mixture of antacids are effective in relief of symptoms in GORD but are not particularly effectual antacids.

Aluminium-based antacids cause constipation, and magnesium-based products cause diarrhoea. When combination products are used, diarrhoea tends to predominate as a side effect. Although these are termed 'non-absorbable', a proportion of aluminium and magnesium is absorbed and the potential for toxicity exists, particularly with coexistent renal failure.

Antacids provide immediate symptom relief and a more rapid response is achieved with liquid preparations. They have a limited duration of action and need to be taken several times a day, usually after meals and at bedtime. Administration should be separate from drugs with potential for chelation, such as tetracycline and ciprofloxacin, and also pH-dependent controlled-release products.

Patient care

Patient education

Patients who present with symptoms of dyspepsia should be assessed in terms of risk of serious disease. Referral for investigation is indicated if they exhibit alarm features. Patients with predominant reflux-like symptoms are likely to respond to antacid/alginate medicines. In those with reflux-like symptoms, lifestyle should be assessed as weight loss is known to improve reflux symptoms in obese patients and raising the head of the bed may improve nocturnal symptoms of heartburn. A medication history, including purchased medicines, should be undertaken to identify likely or possible drug-induced causes of symptoms. Symptoms of dyspepsia are associated with many medicines including aspirin, NSAIDs and corticosteroids. Other agents are associated with gastro-oesophageal reflux and include those with antimuscarinic effects, for example, tricyclic antidepressants, or those which relax muscle tone, for example, calcium channel blockers and nitrates, or those which cause oesophageal mucosal damage, for example, biphosphonates. Clinical medication review allows assessment of the benefits and risks associated with medicines and referral to the prescriber may be necessary. Patients who do not respond to 2 weeks of symptomatic relief medication should be referred to the primary care doctor.

Patients should be advised to seek the pharmacist's advice when purchasing over-the-counter analgesic preparations. Patients with risk factors for peptic ulcer disease should be advised to avoid over-the-counter aspirin and NSAIDs and to use paracetamol-based products. Taking aspirin or NSAIDs with or after food may decrease the risk of dyspepsia symptoms but does not decrease the risk of ulcer complications. Before prescribing NSAID or aspirin therapy, patients should be assessed in terms of both cardiovascular and gastro-intestinal risk. Benefits must outweigh risks in NSAID users and if NSAIDs are necessary in those at risk of ulcer complications, prophylaxis should be prescribed. Consideration should be given to screening for *H. pylori*. Patients should be aware of the optimum time of administration of PPIs, the dose and duration of therapy. Misoprostol should not be used in pregnant women, and women of child-bearing age should be warned appropriately.

Patients with diagnosed peptic ulcer disease need to be educated about the current principles of therapeutic management determined by the diagnosis and, if appropriate, the balanced risks associated with continued aspirin or NSAID therapy. Uncomplicated disease requires a short course of treatment which may or may not include eradication of *H. pylori*. Patients need to know the importance of adherence to eradication therapy for successful treatment and to avoid development of resistance to antibiotics. Previous adverse reactions should be established; for example, patients who are sensitive to penicillin need an eradication regimen which does not include amoxicillin. Patients should be warned of the specific side effects to be expected from the regimen chosen for them and advised what to do should they experience any of these effects. Patients taking metronidazole must avoid alcohol as they might have a disulfiram-like reaction with sickness and headache. Patients also need to know how their therapy will be followed up. In most patients, a single treatment course is required and there is no need for maintenance therapy unless they require prophylaxis treatment to reduce risks associated with continued NSAID or low-dose aspirin therapy.

Patient monitoring

Treatment success in uncomplicated peptic ulcer disease is measured by review of the patient in terms of symptom control. Patients with complicated ulcers or those who continue to have symptoms will receive a urea breath test and/or an endoscopy to confirm successful eradication of *H. pylori*. Very few patients require follow-up endoscopy. Patients should be aware of what their review will entail and when their review will take place. If patients comply with their medication the review process may be kept to a minimum.

Following eradication therapy, some patients continue to experience symptoms of abdominal pain. Patients should be reassured that these symptoms will resolve spontaneously, but if necessary an antacid preparation can be recommended to relieve symptoms until review. Patients receiving treatment for NSAID-induced ulceration should continue their ulcer-healing therapy for 4 weeks. If the NSAID or aspirin has been discontinued there is no need to continue ulcer treatment therapy once the ulcer has healed unless the NSAID or aspirin must also be continued.

Patients with iron-deficiency anaemia following a bleeding ulcer may be prescribed oral iron therapy. If patients suffer side effects such as constipation or diarrhoea, the dose of iron should be reduced. Treatment with iron should be for at least 3 months. Iron preparations are best absorbed from an empty stomach but if gastric discomfort is felt, the preparation should be taken with food.

Some common therapeutic problems in the treatment of peptic ulcer disease are summarised in Table 12.4.

Table 12.4 Common therapeutic problems in peptic ulcer disease

	Comments
Ulcer-like symptoms of dyspepsia are not specific for peptic ulcer disease and are often present in functional (non-ulcer) dyspepsia	Predominant heartburn differentiates GORD from dyspepsia. Patients with GORD are likely to respond to antisecretory therapy
In uncomplicated patients with ulcer-like symptoms of dyspepsia, there is controversy about whether a 1-month course of acid suppression or test and for *H. pylori* should be carried out initially	Identification and eradication of *H. pylori* will benefit those with ulcers and a small proportion of *H. pylori*-positive patients with functional dyspepsia. A course of acid suppression will have similar outcomes but ulcers may relapse. Eradication of *H. pylori* plays no role in management of GORD
A test and treat policy is cost-effective compared with initial endoscopy in patients with uncomplicated dyspepsia	There is no evidence to support widespread eradication of *H. pylori* in primary care
Patients on proton pump inhibitors (PPIs) can have false-negative results for *H. pylori*	PPIs should be withdrawn at least 2 weeks before urea breath test or biopsy urease testing (endoscopy)

Continued

Table 12.4 Common therapeutic problems in peptic ulcer disease—cont'd

	Comments
Following a 7-day eradication therapy regimen, antisecretory therapy can normally be stopped	Longer courses of acid-suppressive therapy should be reserved for patients with active ulcers complicated by bleeding and/or NSAID use
First-line eradication therapy comprises twice-daily PPI, amoxicillin 1 g and clarithromycin 500 mg	Metronidazole can be substituted in those patients allergic to amoxicillin and for second-line therapy. When combined with metronidazole, the dose of clarithromycin can be reduced to 250 mg
Use of high dose intravenous PPIs	Intravenous PPI use is not recommended before endoscopic diagnosis in gastro-intestinal bleeding. High dose intravenous PPI is recommended for 72 h after endoscopic haemostatic therapy in patients at high risk of re-bleeding from peptic ulcer
In patients with NSAID-associated active peptic ulcer disease who test positive for *H. pylori*, the cause of the ulcer may not be confirmed	The ulcer should be healed with a PPI for 4 weeks and *H. pylori* eradicated. Eradication of *H. pylori* reduces the risk of recurrent bleeding
The treatment of NSAID-associated ulcers may differ depending upon whether or not the NSAID must be continued	If NSAIDs are withdrawn, healing rates at 4 weeks are best with PPIs and are similar between H_2-receptor antagonists and PPIs after 8 weeks. PPIs are continued only if NSAIDs are continued
Patients in whom low-dose aspirin is indicated but have risk factors for peptic ulcer disease	Use of aspirin should be considered carefully, especially for primary prophylaxis of cardiovascular disease. Enteric coating does not reduce this risk. Clopidogrel is not a safer alternative than aspirin in combination with a PPI
There is an increased risk of bleeding with dual antiplatelet therapy	PPIs are thought to decrease conversion of clopidogrel to active metabolite, thus decreasing efficacy of clopidogrel. If dual antiplatelet therapy is indicated after PCI, use H_2 receptor antagonist unless high risk (previous gastro-intestinal bleed), when PPI indicated
NSAID use in elderly patients	Patients over 65 years of age are at increased risk of peptic ulcer disease associated with NSAIDs and often present with 'silent ulcers'. NSAIDs (prescription and non-prescription) should be avoided in the elderly
Patients who are candidates for COX-2 inhibitors	COX-2 inhibitors are associated with less gastro-intestinal toxicity than non-selective NSAIDs. COX-2 inhibitors are contraindicated in cardiovascular disease. The reduction in gastro-intestinal risk associated with COX-2 inhibitors is similar to reduction in risk associated with non-selective NSAIDs in combination with gastroprotective agents
Criteria and regimens to administer for stress ulcer prophylaxis are unclear	Intravenous H_2-receptor antagonist therapy is given to patients at risk until enteral feeding is tolerated. Definite risk factors include mechanical ventilation, presence of coagulopathy and spinal cord injury. Controversial risks include head injury, sepsis, burns, multiple trauma, steroid therapy
Patients who require long-term PPI therapy	Those in whom long-term NSAIDs or low-dose aspirin are indicated and who have risk factors for associated upper gastro-intestinal complications. Patients with endoscopically diagnosed GORD who either have severe erosive oesophagitis or severe symptoms which can only be controlled with maintenance therapy

PCI, percutaneous coronary intervention.

Case studies

Case 12.1

A 62-year-old man (Mr BD) presented to A&E following haematemesis and melaena. He suffered no pain. His past medical history included non-ST-elevated myocardial infarction (NSTEMI) for which he had undergone percutaneous coronary intervention (PCI)

and bare metal stent insertion 4 months previously. Mr BD stopped smoking 2 years previously, drinks alcohol in moderation and is not obese. He was taking the following prescribed medicines:

Aspirin (dispersible) 75 mg
Clopidogrel 75 mg
Ramipril 2.5 mg twice daily
Simvastatin 40 mg daily
Atenolol 100 mg
GTN spray prn

On investigation Mr BD's haemoglobin concentration was 8 g/dL (11.5–16.5 g/dL) with an MCV of 90 fL (83–101 fL). His blood pressure was 98/60 mmHg with a heart rate of 120 beats per minute and respiratory rate of 20 beats per minute. There was no jaundice or stigmata of liver disease. Plasma urea was 18 mmol/L (3.1–7.9 mmol/L) with a creatinine of 87 μmol/L (75–155 μmol/L). INR was 1.0. Serum sodium was 142 mmol/L (135–145 mmol/L) and serum potassium was 4.3 mmol/L (3.4–5.0 mmol/L). Endoscopy revealed an actively bleeding gastric ulcer.

Questions

1. What immediate treatment should Mr BD receive?
2. What treatment should he receive at the time of endoscopy?
3. Why should biopsies be taken at the time of endoscopy?
4. What pharmacological treatment should be given to reduce the risk of re-bleeding following endoscopic haemostatic therapy?
5. What was the likely cause of the bleeding ulcer?
6. When should antiplatelet therapy be restarted and with which agent(s)?
7. Is gastroprotection indicated following ulcer healing?
8. Summarise Mr BD's educational needs in terms of his medicines.

Answers

1. Mr BD's age, comorbidity and clinical signs of shock place him at risk of death and in need of emergency hospital admission for aggressive resuscitation with intravenous fluids and red cell transfusion. Either colloid or crystalloid solutions can be used for volume restoration prior to administering blood products. Sodium chloride 0.9% is appropriate fluid replacement. Following resuscitation, early endoscopic examination should be undertaken, within 24 h of presentation. There is no evidence to support the use of intravenous PPIs prior to diagnosis by endoscopy. The most frequent cause of upper gastro-intestinal bleeding is peptic ulcer disease. If Mr BD is nauseated, an antiemetic should be prescribed.
2. The clinical markers suggest urgent endoscopy is indicated. Patients who are shocked and have active peptic ulcer bleeding are at high risk of continuing to bleed and should receive haemostatic endoscopic therapy. Endoscopic treatment is indicated only for those with high-risk lesions (active bleeding, non-bleeding visible vessels or adherent blood clot). Endoscopic injection of large volume (at least 13 mL) 1:10,000 adrenaline achieves haemostasis through vasoconstriction and haemostasis is sustained if this is combined with thermal coagulation or mechanical endoscopic clipping. The patient should receive combination endoscopic therapy.
3. The presence of H. pylori should be sought at the time of endoscopy. Biopsies should be taken from the antrum and the body of the stomach. Samples are sent for testing for the presence of malignant cells and samples are used for the rapid urease test for H. pylori. The presence of bleeding may reduce the sensitivity of the rapid urease test and if negative results are obtained, a urea breath test can be undertaken once oral intake is established.
4. In high-risk patients who have received endoscopic haemostatic therapy, high dose intravenous PPI therapy reduces the risk of re-bleeding. The optimum dose and route is unclear but improved mortality is observed in high-risk patients when a dose of 80 mg bolus followed by 8 mg/h infusion for 72 h is given. Maintaining intragastric pH above 6 is considered to stabilise clot formation and prevent re-bleeding

   If a positive test for H. pylori was obtained, oral eradication therapy should be given, although there is no evidence to suggest this must be given in the acute phase so should wait until oral intake is established. H. pylori eradication therapy is effective in prevention of re-bleeding from peptic ulcer. Ulcer healing can be achieved with an additional 3 weeks treatment with standard-dose PPI.

5. Mr BD was taking dual antiplatelet therapy to reduce the risk of myocardial infarction and cardiovascular death. These agents act synergistically through different pathways. Aspirin is a thromboxane A_2 inhibitor and clopidogrel is an adenosine diphosphate (ADP) inhibitor. Both these agents carry an increased risk of bleeding events, the risk being additive with dual therapy. Mr BD did not have any additional risk factors for peptic ulcer disease but it is important to take a careful medication history to identify if he had been taking NSAID analgesics and ensure he avoids such medicines in the future. The bleeding peptic ulcer was likely caused by the combination of aspirin and clopidogrel.

6. In patients with NSTEMI, most benefit is gained from the addition of clopidogrel to aspirin therapy in the first 3 months. Prolonged treatment for 12 months is indicated if a drug-eluting stent is inserted but as this patient had a bare metal stent inserted 4 months previously, the benefit from the addition of clopidogrel does not outweigh the gastro-intestinal bleeding risk and consideration should be given to discontinuation of clopidogrel. Aspirin should be continued at a dose of 75 mg daily. There is no evidence to suggest enteric coating is of any benefit, so the dispersible formulation should be continued. It is suggested that aspirin should be restarted within 7 days of discontinuation to maintain cardiovascular secondary prevention.

7. Standard dose of PPI should be continued as maintenance therapy in this patient to reduce the risk of further aspirin induced gastro-intestinal bleeding.

8. Mr BD needs to be aware of both his cardiovascular and gastro-intestinal risks. He does need to continue aspirin but he should be aware of the need to discontinue clopidogrel now as it is 4 months following his NSTEMI and the benefit does not outweigh the risk. He should not to take any other aspirin or NSAID containing medicines.

   Mr BD should be prescribed 7 days treatment with twice-daily omeprazole 20 mg, amoxicillin 1 g and clarithromycin 500 mg after ascertaining he is not penicillin sensitive. The importance of this treatment in prevention of re-bleeding should be emphasised to encourage adherence to the prescribed course which he may complete after discharge from hospital. Aspirin will be restarted and the dose of omeprazole will be reduced to 20 mg daily. A repeat endoscopy will be undertaken only if malignancy was suspected. Mr BD will return for a breath test to confirm eradication of H. pylori, although there is a risk of a false-negative result with concomitant omeprazole therapy.

   The anaemia associated with the acute bleed was treated with a blood transfusion and should not require additional oral iron therapy which is indicated in the case of microcytic anaemia more commonly caused by chronic bleeding

Case 12.2

A 57-year-old woman (Mrs MG) presents with symptoms of epigastric pain which has interfered with her normal activities over the previous few weeks. Medication history reveals that Mrs MG takes no prescribed medicines and occasional paracetamol as an analgesic for minor ailments. Although she has occasional heartburn, this is not the predominant symptom. Mrs MG has not vomited and does not have difficulty or pain on swallowing. She has not lost weight recently and has normal stools with no evidence of bleeding. The pain is not precipitated by exercise and does not radiate to the arms and neck. Mrs MG is a non-smoker and only takes a small quantity of alcohol on social occasions. She has an allergy to penicillin.

Questions

1. How should Mrs MG be treated?
2. Which *H. pylori* test should be used in primary care?

Answers

1. It is important to ascertain if Mrs MG has alarm features which should be investigated particularly as her age places her at higher risk of gastro-intestinal cancer. However, cancer is very rare in the absence of alarm features, and therefore initial management strategies are suggested prior to referral for investigation. Symptom assessment also suggests the pain is not cardiac in nature. Most patients with ulcer-like epigastric pain have functional dyspepsia but a small proportion have peptic ulcer disease. Her symptoms are affecting her quality of life, so an initial strategy of testing for *H. pylori* would be appropriate and if positive a 7-day course of twice-daily eradication therapy of omeprazole 20 mg, metronidazole 400 mg and clarithromycin 250 or 500 mg can be prescribed. Mrs MG should be advised to complete the course of therapy to avoid eradication failure and/or resistance to antibiotics. The potential interaction between metronidazole and alcohol should be explained to the patient in terms of the risk of nausea, vomiting, flushing and breathlessness which may occur during and for a few days after discontinuing metronidazole. Patients should also be alerted to the common adverse effect of diarrhoea associated with triple therapy. Patients should be encouraged to cope with the inconvenience but report symptoms to their doctor if they continue after the course of treatment is finished. If Mrs MG has an uncomplicated ulcer, it should heal with this treatment and if she has functional dyspepsia, a small proportion of patients obtain symptom relief. If Mrs MG tests negative for *H. pylori*, a 4-week course of standard-dose PPI can be given for symptomatic relief. If symptoms persist despite eradication therapy, successful eradication should be confirmed 4 weeks after treatment and eradication repeated if necessary. If patients over 55 years of age do not respond to either of these initial management strategies, referral for further investigation should be undertaken.
2. The most accurate non-invasive *H. pylori* test is the carbon-13 urea breath test. Alternative tests are the stool antigen test and a laboratory-based serology test. Local facilities and costs determine the choice of tests. Serology tests based on measurement of serum antibody are commonly used for initial detection of *H. pylori* but cannot be used to confirm eradication since circulating antibody remains for several weeks after removal of antigen.

Case 12.3

A 68-year-old woman (Ms WR) presents for review of her medication. Her medical history includes hypertension and osteoarthritis of the knees. Ms WR receives a regular prescription for:

Bendroflumethiazide 2.5 mg
Naproxen 500 mg twice daily

Ms WR stopped smoking 4 years previously and drinks no more than 10 units of alcohol per week. She is overweight with a BMI of 30 kg/m². Ms WR occasionally purchases an antacid to treat symptoms of heartburn if she's eaten a large meal at night. Her blood pressure was 148/92 mmHg with a pulse of 82 beats per minute.

Routine blood tests revealed:

		Reference range
Sodium	138 mmol/L	135–145 mmol/L
Potassium	3.9 mmol/L	3.4–5.0 mmol/L
Creatinine	110 μmol/L	75–155 μmol/L
Blood glucose	6.8 mmol/L	<11.1 mmol/L
Total cholesterol	4.5 mmol/L	<4.0 mmol/L
Haemoglobin	12.0 g/dL	11.5–16.5 g/dL

Questions

1. What is the mechanism for NSAID-induced peptic ulcer disease?
2. What are the risks associated with NSAID use in this patient?
3. What are the options for treating her pain and minimising the risk of peptic ulceration?

Answers

1. NSAIDs cause superficial erosions, but the main mechanism for causing ulcers in through their systemic inhibition of mucosal prostaglandin production. COX-1 is the enzyme responsible for synthesis of prostaglandins responsible for gastro-intestinal mucosal protection through maintenance of blood flow and production of mucus and bicarbonate. Another isoform of COX, COX-2 is involved in the inflammatory response and the prostaglandins produced are associated with pain and inflammation. The anti-inflammatory action of NSAIDs is thought to be as a result of inhibition of COX-2. Inhibition of COX-1 is thought to be responsible for the gastro-intestinal and renal adverse effects of NSAIDs.
2. Age-related reduction in the synthesis of prostaglandins and secretion of bicarbonate from the gastro-intestinal mucosa is the probable reason for the age-related increase in incidence of peptic ulcer bleeding. Patients over 60 years of age are at higher risk of peptic ulcer complications than their younger counterparts and the risk is much higher in those above 75 years of age. Other risk factors include a previous history of peptic ulcer disease, in particular peptic ulcer bleeding. Dyspepsia symptoms do not correlate with those who develop peptic ulcer disease and are, therefore, not a risk factor and can be treated symptomatically. Concomitant drug therapy such as aspirin, corticosteroids and anticoagulants increase the risk of peptic ulcer complications. In this case, the patient's age places her at risk, and therefore the benefits of the NSAID should be weighed against the risks and potential options for risk management considered.

   Age is also a risk factor for NSAID-induced decrease in renal perfusion caused by inhibition of prostaglandin-stimulated renal blood flow, a compensatory mechanism which is activated when renal perfusion is impaired. Withdrawal of NSAID therapy can improve renal perfusion and associated haemodynamic effects such as hypertension
3. The safest option for Ms WR is to manage the pain with regular use of a paracetamol-based product and to withdraw the NSAID thus removing the risk of peptic ulcer disease but also removing the potential detrimental effect the NSAID may have on blood pressure since the patient is just above the target for blood pressure control. Weight loss may also help to reduce the burden on her knees and may also have some positive effect on her blood pressure.

   The relative risk of ulcer complications has been compared among groups of NSAIDs with naproxen being of intermediate risk. Different NSAIDs vary in their selectivity for COX isoenzymes and may account for the relative toxicities observed. Selective COX-2 inhibitors are associated with low risk but are contraindicated in patients with cardiovascular disease as they have been associated with an increased incidence of myocardial infarction. However, some other non-selective NSAIDs have also been associated with thrombotic risk, although naproxen seems to have the lowest risk and so is an appropriate choice of NSAID if indicated in this patient. There is no clear evidence to test for and eradicate *H. pylori* in chronic NSAID users.

An assessment of Ms WR's pain should be undertaken and the risks associated with naproxen use should be explained to the patient who may be willing to change to regular paracetamol with the addition of codeine if necessary. Otherwise adding a standard dose of PPI to naproxen reduces the gastro-intestinal risks but not the renal risks.

References

Barkun, A.N., Bardou, M., Kuipers, E.J., et al., 2010. International consesus recommendations on the management of patients with nonvariceal upper gastro-intestinal bleeding. Ann. Intern. Med. 152, 101–113.

Bhatt, D.L., Scheiman, J., Abraham, N.S., et al., 2008. Expert consensus document on reducing the gastro-intestinal risks of antiplatelet therapy and NSAID use: a report of the American College of Cardiology Foundation Task Force on Clinical Expert Consensus Documents. J. Am. Coll. Cardiol. 52, 1502–1517.

Chan, F.K., Chung, S.C., Suen, B.Y., et al., 2001. Preventing recurrent upper gastro-intestinal bleeding in patients with *Helicobacter pylori* infection who are taking low dose aspirin or naproxen. N. Engl. J. Med. 344, 967–973.

Chan, F.K.L., Wong, V.W.S., Suen, B.Y., et al., 2007. Combination of a cyclo-oxygenase-2 inhibitor and a proton-pump inhibitor for prevention of recurrent ulcer bleeding in patients at very high risk: a double-blind, randomised trial. Lancet 369, 1621–1626.

Dial, S., Alrasadi, K., Manoukian, C., et al., 2004. Risk of Clostridium difficile diarrhea among hospital inpatients prescribed proton pump inhibitors: cohort and case–control studies. Can. Med. Assoc. J. 171, 33–38.

Dorward, S., Sreedharan, A., Leontiadis, G.I., et al., 2006. Proton pump inhibitor treatment initiated prior to endoscopic diagnosis in upper gastro-intestinal bleeding. Cochrane Database Syst. Rev. 4, No. CD005415.

Fiorucci, S., Santucci L Distrutti, E., 2007. NSAIDs, Coxibs CINOD and H2S-releasing NSAIDs, what lies beyond the horizon? Dig. Liver Dis. 39, 1043–1051.

Gisbert, J.P., Khorrami, S., Carballo, F., et al., 2004. *H. pylori* eradication therapy vs. antisecretory non-eradication therapy (with or without long-term maintenance antisecretory therapy) for the prevention of recurrent bleeding from peptic ulcer. Cochrane Database Syst. Rev. 2, No. CD004062.

Goldstein, J.L., Johanson, J.F., Hawkey, C.J., et al., 2007. Clinical trial: healing of NSAID-associated gastric ulcers in patients continuing NSAID therapy – a randomised study comparing rantidine with esomeprazole. Aliment. Pharmacol. Ther. 26, 1101–1111.

Herzig, S.J., Howell, M.D., Ngo, L.H., et al., 2009. Acid-suppressive medication use and the risk for hospital-acquired pneumonia. J. Am. Med. Assoc. 301, 2120–2128.

Hooper, L., Brown, T.J., Elliott, R.A., et al., 2004. The effectiveness of five strategies for the prevention of gastro-intestinal toxicity induced by non-steroidal anti-inflammatory drugs: systematic review. Br. Med. J. 329, 948–952.

Jafri, N.S., Hornung, C.A., Howden, C.W., 2008. Meta-analysis: sequential therapy appears superior to standard therapy for Helicobacter pylori infection in patients naïve to treatment. Ann. Intern. Med. 148, 923–931.

Lai, K.C., Lam, S.K., Chu, K.M., et al., 2002. Lansoprazole for the prevention of recurrences of ulcer complications from long-term low dose aspirin use. N. Engl. J. Med. 346, 2033–2038.

Lai, K.C., Chu, K.M., Hui, W.M., et al., 2005. Celecoxib compared with lansoprazole and naproxen to prevent gastro-intestinal ulcer complications. Am. J. Med. 118, 1271–1278.

Laine, L., Hennekens, C., 2010. Proton pump inhibitor and clopidogrel interaction: fact or fiction? Am. J. Gastroenterol. 105, 34–41.

Lanza, F.L., Chan, F.K., Quigley, E.M.Practice Parameters Committeee of the American College of Gastroenterology, 2009. Guidelines for prevention of NSAID-related ulcer complications. Am. J. Gastroenterol. 104, 728–738.

Lau, J.Y., Leung, W.K., Wu, J.C., et al., 2007. Omeprazole before endoscopy in patients with gastro-intestinal bleeding. N. Engl. J. Med. 356, 1631–1640.

Leontiadis, G.I., Sharma, V.K., Howden, C.W., 2006. Proton pump inhibitor treatment for acute peptic ulcer bleeding. Cochrane Database Syst. Rev. 1, No. CD002094.

Leontiadis, G.I., Sharma, V.K., Howden, C.W., 2007. Proton pump inhibitor therapy for peptic ulcer bleeding: cochrane collaboration meta-analysis of randomised controlled trials. Mayo Clin. Proc. 82, 286–296.

Malfertheiner, P., Megraud, F., O'Morain, C., et al., 2007. Current concepts in the management of Helicobacter pylori infection: the Maastricht III Consensus Report. Gut 56, 772–781.

Malfertheiner, P., Chan, F.K.L., McColl, E.L., 2009. Peptic ulcer disease. Lancet 374, 1449–1461.

McQuaid, K.R., Laine, L., 2006. Systematic review and meta-analysis of adverse events of low-dose aspirin and clopidogrel in randomised controlled trials. Am. J. Med. 119, 624–638.

MHRA, 2009. Clopidogrel and proton pump inhibitors: interaction. Drug Safety Update 2, 2–3.

Moayyedi, P., Talley, N.J., 2006. Gastro-oesophageal reflux disease. Lancet 367, 2086–2100.

National Institute for Health and Clinical Excellence, North of England Dyspepsia Guideline Development Group, 2004. Dyspepsia – management of dyspepsia in adults in primary care. Clinical Guideline 17. NICE, London.

Ng, F.H., Wong, S.Y., Lam, K.F., et al., 2010. Famotidine is inferior to pantoprazole in preventing recurrence of aspirin-related peptic ulcers or erosions. Gastroenterology 138, 82–88.

Quenot, J.P., Theiry, N., Barbar, S., 2009. When should stress ulcer prophylaxis be used in the ICU? Curr. Opin. Crit. Care 15, 139–143.

Scheiman, J.M., Yeomans, N.D., Talley, N.J., et al., 2006. Prevention of ulcers by esomeprazole in at-risk patients using non-selective NSAIDs and COX-2 inhibitors. Am. J. Gastroenterol. 101, 701–710.

Scottish Intercollegiate Guidelines Network, 2003. Dyspepsia. Guideline No. 68. Scottish Intercollegiate Guidelines Network, Edinburgh.

Scottish Intercollegiate Guidelines Network, 2008. Management of Acute Upper and Lower Gastro-intestinal Bleeding Guideline 105. Scottish Intercollegiate Guideline Network, Edinburgh.

Shaheen, N.J., Richter, J.E., 2009. Barrett's oesophagus. Lancet 373, 850–861.

Stanley, A.J., Ashley, D., Dalton, H.R., et al., 2009. Outpatient management of patients with low risk upper gastro-intestinal haemorrhage: multicentre validation and prospective evaluation. Lancet 373, 42–47.

Taha, A.S., McCloskey, C., Prasad, R., et al., 2009. Famotidine for the prevention of peptic ulcers and oesophagitis in patients taking low dose aspirin (FAMOUS): a phase III, randomised, double-blind, placebo-controlled trial. Lancet 374, 119–125.

Yeomans, N.D., Svedberg, L.E., Naesdal, J., 2006. Is ranitidine therapy sufficient for healing peptic ulcers associated with non-steroidal anti-inflammatory drug use? Int. J. Clin. Pract. 60, 1401–1407.

Further reading

Boparai, V., Rajagopalan, J., Triadafilopoulos, G., 2008. Guide to the use of proton pump inhibitors in adult patients. Drugs 68, 925–947.

Latimer, N., Lord, J., Grant, R.L., et al., 2009. Cost effectiveness of COX-2 selective inhibitors and traditional NSAIDs alone or in combination with a proton pump inhibitor for people with arthritis. Br. Med. J. 339, b2538.

Lazzaroni, M., Bianchi Porro, G., 2009. Management of NSAID-induced gastro-intestinal toxicity. Drugs 69, 51–69.

Van Pinxteren, B., Numans, M.E., Bonis, P.A., et al., 2004. Short-term treatment with proton pump inhibitors, H_2 receptor antagonists and prokinetics for gastro-oesophageal reflux disease-like symptoms and endoscopy negative reflux disease. Cochrane Database Syst. Rev. 3, No. CD002095.

Inflammatory bowel disease 13

S. E. Cripps

Key points

- Ulcerative colitis and Crohn's disease are the two most common inflammatory bowel diseases (IBD) of the gut. Both are chronic relapsing conditions with a high morbidity and remain largely incurable.

- Ulcerative colitis and Crohn's disease are similar but there are contrasting features which relate to the site of involvement and extent of inflammation across the bowel wall. Ulcerative colitis is limited to the large bowel and the mucosa, whereas Crohn's disease frequently involves the small intestine with inflammation extending through the bowel wall to the serosal surface.

- The aims of treatment are to control acute attacks promptly and effectively, induce remission, maintain remission and identify patients who will benefit from surgery.

- Choice and route of therapy will depend on site, extent and severity of the disease together with knowledge of current or previous treatment.

- A reduction in inflammation with corticosteroids and aminosalicylates is the mainstay of treatment, with immunosuppressants (e.g. azathioprine, methotrexate, ciclosporin) and biologic agents (e.g. infliximab and adalimumab), reserved for more severe and refractory cases.

- The management of IBD poses a challenge to the multidisciplinary team both clinically and economically.

- National standards for IBD aim to ensure patients receive consistent, high-quality care and IBD services throughout the UK are evidence based, engaged in local and national networking, based on modern IT and meet specific minimum standards.

Introduction

Inflammatory bowel disease (IBD) can be divided into two chronic inflammatory disorders of the gastro-intestinal tract, namely Crohn's disease (CD) and ulcerative colitis (UC). Crohn's disease affects any part of the gastro-intestinal tract whereas ulcerative colitis affects the colon and rectum only. Current available treatment for IBD is not curative. IBD follows a relapsing and remitting course that is unpredictable and causes disruption to a patient's lifestyle and places a burden on the workplace and healthcare setting. The management of IBD patients poses a challenge to the multidisciplinary team both clinically and economically.

Epidemiology

The incidence of IBD is greater in North America, Europe, Australia and New Zealand, although the incidence in Africa, Asia and South America is rising steadily. This increase in developing countries may be due to improved sanitation and vaccination programmes along with a decreased exposure to enteric infections. Jewish and Asian people living in USA and UK are more commonly affected by IBD than those living in Israel and Asia. There appears to be no association between IBD and social class. The peak incidence of IBD occurs between 10 and 40 years, although it can occur at any age, with 15% of cases diagnosed in individuals over the age of 60 years. The incidence appears equal between males and females, although some studies in Crohn's disease show a slight female predominance. Up to 240,000 people are affected by IBD in the UK.

The incidence of new cases of ulcerative colitis in Europe and USA is 2–8 per 100,000 per year with a prevalence of 40–80 per 100,000 per year. The incidence has remained fairly static over the last 40 years. In the UK, Crohn's disease occurs with a similar frequency to ulcerative colitis with around 4 per 100,000 per year and a prevalence of 50 per 100,000. The rates in central and southern Europe are lower. In South America, Asia and Africa, Crohn's disease is uncommon but appears to be on the rise (Mpofu and Ireland, 2006).

Aetiology

The causative agents of IBD are largely unknown, although a number of factors are thought to play a role.

Environmental

Diet

Evidence that dietary intake is involved in the aetiology of IBD is inconclusive, although several dietary factors have been associated with IBD, including fat intake, fast food ingestion, milk and fibre consumption, and total protein and energy intake. A large number of case-control studies have reported a causal link between the intake of refined carbohydrates and Crohn's disease (Gibson and Shepherd, 2005). The mechanism for diet as a trigger is very poorly understood.

185

During the course of the disease, patients are able to identify foods which aggravate or exacerbate their symptoms, for example, milk or spicy foods. Up to 5% of patients with ulcerative colitis improve by avoiding cow's milk, whilst patients with Crohn's disease improve if they start to take elemental (amino acid based), oligomeric (peptides) and polymeric (whole protein) feeds, although symptoms may return when their normal diet is reintroduced.

Those that are breastfed as infants have a reduced risk of developing IBD (Mpofu and Ireland, 2006).

Smoking

There is a higher rate of smoking amongst patients with Crohn's disease than in the general population, with up to 40% of patients with the disease being smokers. Smoking worsens the clinical course of the disease and increases the risk of relapse and the need for surgery. Fewer patients with ulcerative colitis smoke (approximately 10%). Former smokers are at the highest risk of developing ulcerative colitis, while current smokers have the least risk. Stopping smoking can provoke the emergence of ulcerative colitis. This indicates that smoking may help to prevent the onset of the disease. The explanation for this is unclear. However, it is thought that in addition to its effect on the inflammatory response, the chemicals absorbed from cigarette smoke affect the smooth muscle inside the colon, potentially altering gut motility and transit time. In some studies, nicotine has been shown to be an effective treatment for ulcerative colitis (Guslandi, 1999).

Infection

Exposure to *Mycobacterium paratuberculosis* has been considered a causative agent of Crohn's disease, although current evidence indicates it is not an aetiological factor.

Ulcerative colitis may present after an episode of infective diarrhoea, but overall there is little evidence to support the role of a single infective agent.

Enteric microflora

Enteric microflora plays an important role in the pathogenesis of IBD because the gut acts as a sensitising organ that contributes to the systemic immune response. Patients with IBD show a loss of immunological tolerance to intestinal microflora and consequently antibiotics often play a role in the treatment of IBD. More recently, manipulating the intestinal flora using probiotics, prebiotics and symbiotic has proven to be an effective therapeutic strategy. Probiotics such as *Bifidobacteria* and *Lactobacilli* alter the intestinal microflora balance favourably. Prebiotics stimulate the growth of specific, beneficial microorganisms in the colon whilst synbiotics, a combination of both prebiotics and probiotics, have been successfully used.

Drugs

Non-steroidal anti-inflammatory drugs (NSAIDs) such as diclofenac have been reported to exacerbate IBD (Felder et al., 2000). It is thought this may result from direct inhibition of the synthesis of cytoprotective prostaglandins. Antibiotics may also precipitate a relapse in disease due to a change in the enteric microflora. The risk of developing Crohn's disease is thought to be increased in women taking the oral contraceptive pill, possibly caused by vascular changes.

MMR vaccine. There has been much debate about the link between bowel disease and measles, measles vaccine or combined measles, mumps and rubella (MMR) immunisation. However, current evidence has indicated no proven correlation.

Appendicectomy

Appendicectomy has a protective effect in both Crohn's disease and ulcerative colitis (Radford-Smith et al., 2002). It is unclear whether this protective effect is immunologically based or whether individuals who develop appendicitis and consequently have an appendicectomy are physiologically, genetically or immunologically distinct from the population that is predisposed to IBD.

Stress

Some patients find that stress triggers a relapse in their IBD and this has been reproduced in animal models. It is thought that stress activates inflammatory mediators at enteric nerve endings in the gut wall. In addition to stress as a trigger factor, living with IBD can also be stressful. Its chronic nature, lack of curative treatment, distressing symptoms and impact on lifestyle make it difficult for patients to cope.

Genetic

Fifteen percent of first degree relatives have IBD. There is mounting evidence that Crohn's disease and ulcerative colitis result from an inappropriate response of the immune system in the mucosa of the gastro-intestinal tract to normal enteric flora (Ahmad et al., 2004). Since the mid-1990s there has been considerable progress in understanding the contribution of genetics to IBD susceptibility and phenotype.

Mutations of the gene CARD15/NOD2 located on chromosome 16 have been associated with small intestinal Crohn's disease in white but not oriental populations. Two other genes have been recently linked with Crohn's disease (OCTN1 on chromosome 5 and DLG5 on chromosome 10).

Genetic studies in ulcerative colitis have shown human lymphocyte antibody (HLA) is more strongly linked. Genotype related to pattern of disease (HLA-DRI*103) is 5–11 times more common in patients who have undergone colectomy.

Ethnic and familial

Jews are more prone to IBD than non-Jews, with Ashkenazi Jews having a higher risk than Sephardic Jews. In North America, IBD is more common in whites than blacks. First-degree relatives of those with IBD have a 10-fold increase in risk of developing the disease. A familial link is supported from research showing a 15-fold greater concordance for IBD in monozygotic (identical) than dizygotic (non-identical) twins (Jess et al., 2005).

cytokines, such as interleukin-10 and transforming growth factor-β, to control inflammation and effector pathways. In Crohn's disease, it is also thought that T-cells are resistant to apoptosis after inactivation. Non-pathogenic bowel flora appears to be an essential factor.

Pathophysiology

In individuals with IBD, trigger factors typically cause a severe, prolonged and inappropriate inflammatory response in the gastro-intestinal tract and the ongoing inflammatory reaction leads to an alteration in the normal architecture of the digestive tract. Genetically susceptible individuals seem unable to downregulate immune or antigen non-specific inflammatory responses. It is thought that chronic inflammation is characterised by increased activity of effector lymphocytes and pro-inflammatory cytokines that override normal control mechanisms. Others, however, have suggested that IBD may result from a primary failure of regulatory lymphocytes and

Disease location

The character and distribution, both macroscopic and microscopic, of chronic inflammation define and distinguish ulcerative colitis and Crohn's disease. Table 13.1 shows the differences in location and distribution of ulcerative colitis and Crohn's disease. Figure 13.1 details the histological differences.

Crohn's disease

Crohn's disease can affect any part of the gut from the mouth to the anus. Approximately 45% of patients have ileocaecal disease, 25% colitis only, 20% terminal ileal disease, 5% small

Table 13.1 Location and distribution of ulcerative colitis and Crohn's disease

	Ulcerative colitis	Crohn's disease
Location	Colon and rectum 40% proctitis 20% pancolitis 10–15% backwash ileitis	Entire gut (mouth to anus, rectal sparing) 45% ileocaecal disease 25% colitis only 20% terminal ileal disease 5% small bowel disease 5% anorectal, gastroduodenal, oral disease
Distribution	Continuous, diffuse No granulomas Inflammation of mucosa Ulceration if fine and superficial	Often discontinuous and segmental 'skip lesions' Full thickness (transmural) Granulomatous inflammation Deep ulceration with mucosal extension
Fissures, fistulae and stricture	Absent	Common
Perianal disease	Absent	Present

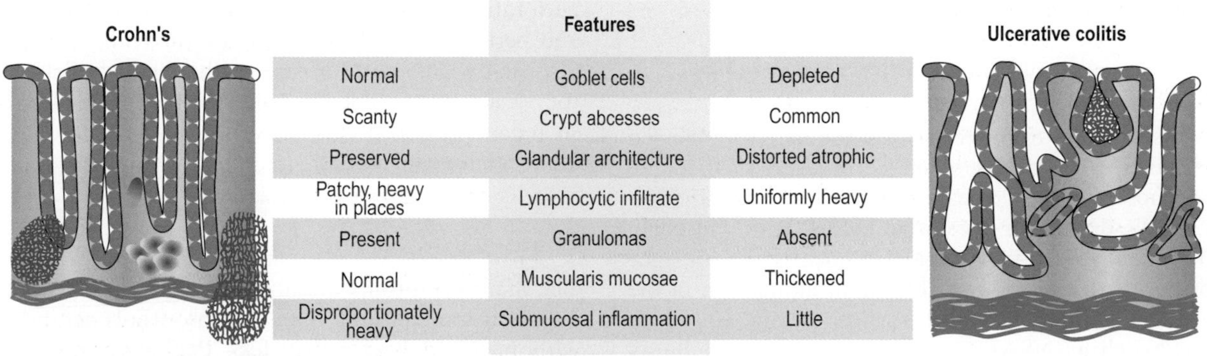

Crohn's	Features	Ulcerative colitis
Normal	Goblet cells	Depleted
Scanty	Crypt abcesses	Common
Preserved	Glandular architecture	Distorted atrophic
Patchy, heavy in places	Lymphocytic infiltrate	Uniformly heavy
Present	Granulomas	Absent
Normal	Muscularis mucosae	Thickened
Disproportionately heavy	Submucosal inflammation	Little

Fig. 13.1 Histological features in the rectal biopsy that help to distinguish between ulcerative colitis and Crohn's disease (from Misiewicz et al., 1994, with kind permission from Blackwell Scientific Publications, Oxford).

bowel disease and 5% anorectal, gastroduodenal or oral disease. Crohn's disease can involve one area of the gut or multiple areas, with unaffected areas in between being known as 'skip lesions'. The areas of the small bowel affected are typically thickened and narrow. A 'red ring' is often the first visible abnormality seen on colonoscopy. This is a lymphoid follicular enlargement with a surrounding ring of erythema, which develops into aphthoid ulceration and may progress to deep fissuring ulcers with a cobblestone appearance, fibrosis and strictures. Intestinal strictures arise from chronic and extensive inflammation and fibrosis and bowel obstruction may arise. Local gut perforation may cause abscesses which may also lead to fistulae.

Microscopically, inflammation extends through all layers of the bowel. Inflammatory cells are seen throughout, resulting in ulceration and microabscess formation. Non-caseating epithelioid cells, sometimes with Langhans' giant cells, are seen in about 25% of colonic biopsies and in 60% of surgically resected bowel. Chronic inflammation in the small intestine, colon, rectum and anus leads to an increased risk of carcinoma.

Ulcerative colitis

At first presentation, ulcerative colitis is confined to the rectum (proctitis) in 40% of cases, the sigmoid and descending colon (left-sided colitis) in 40% and the whole colon (total ulcerative colitis or pancolitis) in 20% of cases. Proctitis extends to involve more of the colon in a minority, with 15–30% of patients developing more extensive disease over 10 years. The reason why some patients have extensive disease and some have limited disease is unknown. In severe total ulcerative colitis, there may also be inflammation of the terminal ileum. This is known as 'backwash ileitis' but is not clinically significant. The colon appears mucopurulent, erythematous and granular with superficial ulceration that in severe cases leads to ulceration. As the colon heals by granulation, post-inflammatory polyps may form.

Microscopically, superficial inflammation is seen with inflammatory cells infiltrating the lamina propria and crypts. Crypt abscesses occur, the crypt structure is lost and goblet cell depletion arises as mucin is lost. Dysplasia, which can potentially progress to carcinoma, may be seen in biopsies taken from patients with long-standing total colitis.

Other types of colitis

Crohn's disease yet to be classified (sometimes referred to indeterminate colitis) is when chronic colitis persists, yet the pathology of the disease has not been identified as either Crohn's disease or ulcerative colitis. In microscopic colitis, the main feature is watery diarrhoea in the presence of a normal colonoscopy and chronic inflammation in the absence of crypt architectural distortion on mucosal biopsies. Drugs such as NSAIDs and proton pump inhibitors (PPIs) are implicated as the cause in up to 50% of cases of microscopic colitis. Diversion colitis is when inflammation occurs in the defunctioned loop of a colostomy causing a mucous discharge. Pseudomembranous colitis is caused by *Clostridium difficile*, usually after prolonged or multiple antibiotics. The use of PPIs predisposes patients to infection. It is diagnosed by sigmoidoscopy and detection of *C. difficile* toxin in the stool.

Clinical manifestation

The clinical differences between Crohn's disease and ulcerative colitis are described in Table 13.2.

Crohn's disease

The clinical features of Crohn's disease depend largely on the site of the bowel affected, the extent, severity and the pathological process in each patient. Crohn's disease tends to be more disabling than ulcerative colitis with 25% of patients unable to work 1 year after diagnosis. The predominant symptoms in Crohn's disease are diarrhoea, abdominal pain and weight loss. Weight loss occurs in most patients, irrespective of disease location. Ten to twenty percent of patients will have weight loss greater than 20%. The main cause is decreased oral intake, although malnutrition is also common. There is a slight increase in mortality in patients with extensive Crohn's disease.

Small bowel, ileocaecal and terminal ileal disease

Patients present with pain and/or a tender palpable mass in the right iliac fossa with weight loss and diarrhoea, which usually contains no blood. Diarrhoea is caused by mucosal inflammation, bile salt malabsorption that causes steatorrhoea or bacterial growth proximal to a stricture. Small bowel obstruction may also occur as a consequence of inflammation, fibrosis and stricture formation. Patients often describe a more generalised intermittent pain which is colicky with loud gurgling bowel sounds (borborygmi), abdominal distension, vomiting and constipation. When inflammation or abscesses are the predominant pathology, many patients present with constant pain and fever. Enteric fistulae occur and may involve the skin, bladder or vagina. Although rare, perforation of the gut may present with an acute abdomen and peritonitis. Vitamin B_{12} and folic acid deficiencies predispose patients with disease of the terminal ileum to macrocytic anaemia, while bile acid malabsorption also occurs in such patients and predisposes them to cholesterol gallstones and oxalate renal stones.

Colitis

The main symptoms are abdominal pain, profuse and frequent diarrhoea (more than six loose stools per day) with or without blood, and weight loss. Patients also complain of lassitude, anorexia and nausea and appear thin, tachycardic, anaemic, malnourished and febrile. Colitis may present

Table 13.2 Clinical differences between ulcerative colitis and Crohn's disease

Symptom	Ulcerative colitis	Crohn's disease
Prominent symptom	Bloody diarrhoea	Diarrhoea, abdominal pain, weight loss 30%, no gross bleeding
Fever	++	++
Abdominal pain	Variable	++
Diarrhoea	+++	+++
Rectal bleeding	+++	++
Weight loss	+	++
Sign of malnutrition	+	++
Abdominal mass	–	++
Dehydration	+++	++
Iron-deficiency anaemia, raised CPR/ESR, hypoalbuminaemia	++	++

CPR, C-reactive protein; ESR, erythrocyte sedimentation rate; +, the likelihood this symptom will be present; –, symptom absent in patient.

insidiously with minimal discomfort. Patients with severe involvement of the colon or the terminal ileum often have electrolyte abnormalities, hypoalbuminaemia and iron-deficiency anaemia. Extra-intestinal complications are more common in those patients with large bowel disease.

Perianal disease

Patients may present with an anal fissure, fistula or a perirectal abscess. These symptoms can have a significant impact on the patient's lifestyle.

Gastroduodenal and oral disease

These are both rare conditions. Gastroduodenal Crohn's disease presents as dyspepsia, pain, weight loss, anorexia, nausea and vomiting. Oral disease is very painful and may cause chronic ulceration resulting in anorexia.

Stricturing Crohn's disease

Patients presenting with pain, vomiting and constipation and a diagnosis of stricturing disease can lead to perforation if not surgically treated, although this is rare (see Fig. 13.2)

Ulcerative colitis

Typical symptoms of ulcerative colitis include bloody diarrhoea (the most predominant symptom) with mucus, abdominal pain with fever, and weight loss in severe cases. The typical

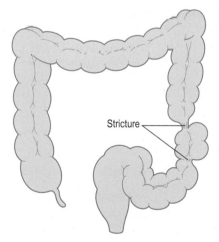

Fig. 13.2 Stricture formation in Crohn's disease.

appearance of a patient diagnosed with Crohn's disease is low BMI, malabsorption, weight loss and growth retardation. Frank blood loss is more common in ulcerative colitis than Crohn's disease. The symptoms of ulcerative colitis are similar to Crohn's colitis with patients being tachycardic, anaemic, febrile, fatigued, dehydrated and thin. Approximately 50% of patients with ulcerative colitis have some form of relapse each year, and severe attacks can be life-threatening. Up until the 1960s, one-third of ulcerative colitis patients died from the condition; with advances in medical and surgical treatment death is now extremely rare.

Acute severe disease

In addition to the typical symptoms of ulcerative colitis, patients with acute severe disease may present with more than six bloody stools per day (10–20 liquid stools per day is not unusual), with a fever (>37.8 °C), tachycardia (>90 bpm), anaemia (Hb < 10.5 g/dL) or elevated inflammatory markers (ESR > 30 mm/h; CRP > 8). Severity is commonly assessed using the Truelove and Witts criteria (see investigations).

Moderately active disease

Stool frequency is less than six motions each day with diarrhoea, mucus and rectal bleeding. Moderatively active disease is more common in 'left-sided' disease. Toxic megacolon is rare in patients with rectosigmoidal involvement, and the incidence of colon cancer is much lower in these patients than those with total colitis.

Proctitis

The manifestations of active proctitis are less severe. These are tenesmus, pruritus ani, rectal bleeding and mucous discharge. Patients are often constipated.

Toxic dilatation

This can occur in untreated severe ulcerative colitis. There is a high risk of perforation with a mortality of 50%.

Extra-intestinal complications of IBD

Around 20–30% of patients with IBD will present with extra-intestinal manifestations. They are more commonly seen in patients where IBD affects the colon. Complications affect the joints, skin, bone, eyes, liver and biliary tree and are more common in active disease. Figure 13.3 highlights some of the extra-intestinal features of IBD.

Joints and bones

Arthropathies occur in 10% of patients with IBD, are more common in women and are a well-recognised complication of IBD. Patients with pauciarticular disease, characterised by arthritis limited to five or fewer joints, often experience a flare in the arthropathy when there is an exacerbation of the IBD symptoms. When the IBD relapse is treated, the arthropathy improves. In contrast, in polyarticular arthropathy, a chronic condition which affects more than five joints, a flare of the IBD appears not to be temporally related to the activity of the arthropathy. About 5% of patients with IBD also have ankylosing spondylitis. This is thought to be immunologically mediated and not associated with IBD activity. Osteopenia, potentially leading to osteoporosis, is often seen in patients with IBD because of chronic steroid use (particularly when the cumulative dose of prednisolone exceeds 10 g) and/or malabsorption.

Skin

Both erythema nodosum and pyoderma gangrenosum are associated with IBD. Erythema nodosum appears as tender, hot, red nodules that subside over a few days to leave a brown

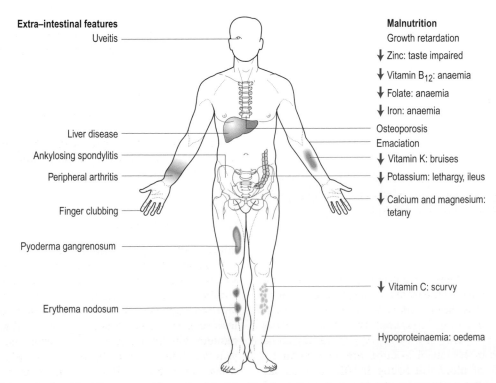

Extra–intestinal features
- Uveitis
- Liver disease
- Ankylosing spondylitis
- Peripheral arthritis
- Finger clubbing
- Pyoderma gangrenosum
- Erythema nodosum

Malnutrition
Growth retardation
↓ Zinc: taste impaired
↓ Vitamin B₁₂: anaemia
↓ Folate: anaemia
↓ Iron: anaemia
Osteoporosis
Emaciation
↓ Vitamin K: bruises
↓ Potassium: lethargy, ileus
↓ Calcium and magnesium: tetany
↓ Vitamin C: scurvy
Hypoproteinaemia: oedema

Fig. 13.3 Some of the extra-intestinal illnesses and features of malnutrition found in patients with inflammatory bowel disease (from Misiewicz et al., 1994, with kind permission from Blackwell Scientific Publications, Oxford).

skin discolouration. Disease flares are normally directly related to IBD activity in the 8% of patients affected.

Pyoderma gangrenosum presents as a discrete pustule that develops into an ulcer. In the 2% of patients affected, IBD activity does not appear to be directly related to the pyoderma gangrenosum, which may begin or worsen when the IBD is quiescent.

Sweet's syndrome (an acute febrile neutrophillic dermatosis) which has some similarity to erythema nodosum may also be associated with IBD.

Eye

Ocular complications are infrequent, occurring in less than 10% of cases. Episcleritis (intense burning and itching with localised area of blood vessels) is the most common complication of IBD. Scleritis, which involves more of the eye, may impair vision. Uveitis (headache, burning red eye, blurred vision) is often associated with joint and skin manifestations of IBD. Conjunctivitis is frequently seen in IBD patients but is not specific and no true association has been demonstrated.

Hepatobiliary

Biliary complications of IBD are gallstones and sclerosing cholangitis which occurs in 5% of patients with ulcerative colitis but less frequently in those with Crohn's disease. Conversely the prevalence of IBD (mostly ulcerativ colitis) in patients with sclerosing cholangitis is 70–80%. Sclerosing cholangitis, found predominantly in males, is a chronic cholestatic condition characterised by inflammation and fibrosis of the intrahepatic and extrahepatic bile ducts. Patients present with obstructive jaundice, cholangitis and raised liver enzymes (alkaline phosphatase and γ-glutamyltranspeptidase). Endoscopic retrograde cholangiopancreatography (ERCP) is useful in diagnosing and aiding the stenting of strictures. There is an increased risk of cholangiocarcinoma, with a liver transplant the only cure. Hepatic complications of IBD include fatty liver, pericholangitis, chronic active hepatitis and cirrhosis.

Thromboembolic

Thromboembolic complications occur in around 1–2% of IBD patients. The most common cause of death in hospitalised IBD patients is pulmonary embolism (Solem et al., 2004).

Anaemia

Around one-third of patients have haemoglobin levels below 12 g/dL. The main causes are chronic intestinal bleeding with iron loss (bowel inflammation) which causes a microcytic anaemia whereas the chronic inflammatory disease can cause normocytic anaemia giving rise to mixed features anaemia. Folate, iron, vitamin B_{12} malabsorption are also common. The side effects of commonly used drugs in IBD, for example, methotrexate and azathioprine can give rise to symptoms of anaemia.

Investigations

Radiological, pathological and clinical investigations help to confirm diagnosis, disease recurrence and response to treatment. Differential diagnoses of IBD include carcinoma, infection, drug-induced colitis, ischaemia, radiation damage, irritable bowel syndrome and diverticulitis.

Endoscopy

The key diagnostic investigation in IBD is lower gastrointestinal tract endoscopy (sigmoidoscopy and colonoscopy), which allows direct visualisation of the large bowel and histopathological assessment from biopsies. The risk of developing colorectal cancer is 7–10% after 20 years in patients with colonic disease. Therefore, routine surveillance colonoscopy is essential in the early detection of colorectal cancer. Treatment response to biologics, for example infliximab, can be assessed via mucosal healing seen at colonoscopy.

In patients with severe symptoms, it is sometimes necessary to delay a full colonoscopy because of the increased risk of perforation. Wireless capsule endoscopy is a relatively new procedure where the small bowel can be viewed and can be useful in patients with non-stricturing Crohn's disease.

Radiology

Radiological imaging is complementary to clinical and endoscopic assessment. It is used in the initial evaluation or diagnosis, preoperative review, to highlight the presence of complications during exacerbations and to evaluate extraintestinal manifestations. Radiological examination still plays a key role in IBD affecting the small bowel, although endoscopy has generally replaced conventional X-ray examinations of the colon.

Computed tomography (CT scan) and magnetic resonance imagery (MRI) are the best radiological methods for locating and defining fistulae and abscesses in active Crohn's disease.

Radiolabelled leucocyte scans that utilise autologous leucocytes labelled with [99]technetium-hexamethylenamine oxime may provide further information of disease site and severity.

Laboratory findings

Although not diagnostic, active disease is suggested in patients with raised inflammatory markers that include erythrocyte sedimentation rate (ESR) and C-reactive protein (CRP) in addition to a low haemoglobin and raised platelet count. Vitamin B_{12} may be low in patients with chronic terminal ileal disease. Low red cell folate and serum albumin, magnesium, calcium, zinc and essential fatty acids also indicate chronic inflammation and malabsorption. Anti-*Saccharomyces cerevisiae* antibodies (ASCA) are more likely to be present in Crohn's disease. Serology can be used to exclude infection as a cause of diarrhoea.

Malabsorption, indicated by low serum trace elements, for example, magnesium and zinc, is not seen in ulcerative colitis. Low albumin may indicate relapse in active disease. Patients with sclerosing cholangitis often present with altered liver function tests.

Stool tests

Red and white blood cells can be seen on microscopic examination of fresh stools. Microscopic identification of infective cells such as amoeba may also be visualised. *C. difficile* toxin can be assessed through culture and toxin assay. Stool tests do not diagnose IBD but contribute to excluding alternative diagnoses.

Clinical assessment tools

The Crohn's Disease Activity Index (CDAI) or the Harvey–Bradshaw Index (HBI) is used in most clinical trials to define remission in Crohn's disease. However, in clinical practice the CDAI is rarely used as it needs to be measured prospectively and is complex. The HBI is a simple measure of stool frequency, pain and other clinical features that is increasingly used to document selection for and response to biologic therapy. A CDAI of <150 or an HBI ≤3 suggests patient is in remission (NICE, 2010).

The Truelove and Witts criteria is a useful tool in defining the severity of ulcerative colitis (see Table 13.3). A severe attack is defined as more than six bloody stools a day plus one or more of the following: pulse >90 beats/min, temperature >37.8 °C, haemoglobin <10.5 g/dL or ESR >30 mm/h. In this case, the patient should be admitted to hospital.

Remission in ulcerative colitis is defined as complete resolution of symptoms with a normal bowel pattern (<3 stools/day), no urgency and no visible bleeding. Mucosal healing is confirmed by endoscopy. Steroid-free remission is the goal of therapy.

Table 13.3 Truelove and Witts criteria for assessing severity of ulcerative colitis (Travis et al., 2008)

Feature	Mild	Moderate	Severe
Motions per day	<4	4–6	>6
Rectal bleeding	Little	Moderate	Large amounts
Temperature	Apyrexial	Intermediate	>37.8 °C on 2 of 4 days
Pulse rate	Normal	Intermediate	>90 bpm
Haemoglobin	Normal	Intermediate	<10.5 g/dL
ESR	Normal	Intermediate	>30 mm/h

ESR, erythrocyte sedimentation rate.

Treatment of inflammatory bowel disease

At present there is no cure for IBD since the exact cause of the condition is unknown. A wide range of drugs and nutritional supplements are available to maintain the patient in long periods of remission in both Crohn's disease and ulcerative colitis. However, surgical intervention will eventually become necessary when the patient relapses and fails to respond to drug therapy. Since the majority of people with IBD are diagnosed under the age of 30, effective treatment and avoidance of relapses is of paramount importance in this chronic long-term condition.

Nutritional therapy

Nutritional therapy can be considered as an adjunctive or primary treatment. Although a potential problem for all patients with IBD, patients with Crohn's disease are at particular risk of becoming malnourished and developing a variety of nutritional deficiencies (Fig. 13.3). It is, therefore, important for patients to receive optimal nutrition and dietary manipulation as needed. Low-fibre diets help to reduce clinical symptoms of intestinal obstruction in Crohn's disease (Fernandes-Banares et al., 1999). Functional and structural damage to the small bowel can cause malabsorption problems and occasionally patients may require a low-lactose diet. Patients with poor oral intake and loss of appetite often respond to supplemental enteral feeds. Enteral nutrition in the form of an elemental or polymeric diet can be used as primary therapy and is widely employed in paediatrics (Heuschkel and Walker-Smith, 1999).

Patients who have extensive small bowel resection may experience many nutritional deficiencies because of malabsorption. Iron depletion, hypoproteinaemia, deficiencies in water- and fat-soluble vitamins, trace elements and electrolytes may all occur and must be corrected using a suitable replacement regimen.

Where appropriate, and when enteral nutrition is not indicated or adequate, a total parenteral nutrition (TPN) regimen may be prescribed. Some patients receive concurrent enteral and parenteral feeding.

Drug treatment

The main goals of drug treatment are to treat acute attacks promptly and effectively, induce and maintain remission, limit drug toxicity, modify the pattern of disease, avoid and/or manage complications and select patients who will benefit from surgery. Morbidity and mortality can also be reduced by the prompt use of effective and appropriate drug therapy. The choice of drug and route of administration depends on the site, extent and severity of the disease together with the individual's treatment history. Drug therapy is often required for many years and patient preference, acceptability and possible side effects not only affect choice but will impact on medication adherence. There is a need for therapeutic strategy and consistency in the management of patients with IBD.

Corticosteroids, aminosalicylates and immunosuppressive agents (immunomodulators) such as azathioprine are the mainstays of treatment. Immunomodulators are not licensed for use in IBD but are routinely used.

Modern advances in treatment, such as the use of humanised monoclonal antibody preparations and other biologic agents which modify the affected biochemical inflammatory pathways, now have a significant role in treatment of the disease. These are likely to be the main area of future development.

Other drugs such as antibiotics, for example, metronidazole, are helpful in some cases, while colestyramine, thalidomide, sodium cromoglicate, bismuth and arsenical salts, nicotine, lidocaine, sucralfate, new steroid entities, cytoprotective agents, aloe vera, probiotics and fish oils are rarely used. However, for some patients they provide alternative or supplemental therapy.

The choice of drug treatment is dependent on whether it is prescribed to induce remission or as maintenance therapy. The majority of patients are managed successfully as hospital outpatients or by their primary care doctor. Only severe extensive or fulminant disease requires hospitalisation and the use of parenteral therapy and/or surgical intervention. Oral medication can be given to most patients for maintenance of moderate disease.

The route of administration is a particularly important factor in IBD. In contrast to most other conditions, minimal systemic absorption and maximal intestinal wall drug levels are required with oral therapy. Several delivery strategies have been used to achieve this including the chemical modification of drug molecules, delayed and controlled-release formulations and the use of bioadhesive particles.

Disease confined to the anus, rectum or left side of the colon is more appropriately treated with rectally administered topical preparations where the drug is applied directly to the site of inflammation (Table 13.4).

These topical preparations have reduced systemic absorption and fewer side effects. Choice of formulation depends on the site of inflammation and also consideration of presentation, acceptability, patient preference and cost. Adherence to topical therapy is generally poor and good patient education is required for effective benefit.

Proctitis is best treated with suppositories. Where inflammation affects the rectum and sigmoid colon (up to 15–20 cm), foam enemas are preferred. In more extensive disease extending to the splenic flexure (30–60 cm), liquid enemas are the agents of choice. However, patients often require a combination of different rectal preparations because, for example, over 90% of liquid enemas bypass the rectum and thereby exert no therapeutic benefit at that site. As a consequence, a suppository may also be required to treat rectal inflammation. The propellant action of foam applicators also results in some preparations by-passing the rectal mucosa. Enemas or suppositories should be administered just before bedtime in a supine position as this allows a much longer retention time. Liquid enemas can be warmed and should be inserted while lying in the left lateral position.

An algorithm for drug treatment in IBD is shown in Fig. 13.4.

Table 13.4 Comparison of commercially available preparations for rectal administration in inflammatory bowel disease

Generic name (proprietary name)	Formulation	Site of release
Sulfasalazine (Salazopyrin®)	Suppositories	Rectum
	Retention enema	Transverse, descending colon and rectum
Mesalazine (Pentasa®, Salofalk®)	Retention enema	Transverse, descending colon and rectum
Mesalazine (Asacol®, Salofalk®)	Foam enema	Rectum and rectosigmoid colon
Mesalazine (Asacol®®, Pentasa®, Salofalk®)	Suppositories	Rectum
Prednisolone sodium phosphate (Predsol®)	Retention enema	Transverse, descending colon and rectum
	Suppositories	Rectum
Prednisolone sodium metasulphobenzoate (Predenema®)	Retention enema	Transverse and descending colon
Prednisolone sodium metasulphobenzoate (Predfoam®)	Foam enema	Rectum and rectosigmoid colon
Prednisolone sodium phosphate (Predsol®)	Retention enema	Transverse and descending colon
Hydrocortisone acetate (Colifoam®)	Foam enema	Rectum and rectosigmoid colon
Budesonide (Entocort®®)	Retention enema	Rectum and rectosigmoid colon

Corticosteroids

The glucocorticoid properties of hydrocortisone and prednisolone are the mainstay of treatment in active ulcerative colitis and Crohn's disease. Prednisolone administered orally or rectally is the steroid of choice, although in emergency situations hydrocortisone or methylprednisolone is used when the parenteral route is required. Corticosteroids have direct anti-inflammatory and immunosuppressive actions which rapidly control symptoms. They can be used either alone or in combination, with a suitable mesalazine (5-aminosalicylic acid, 5-ASA) formulation or immunosuppressant, to induce remission.

Oral corticosteroids should not be used for maintenance treatment because of serious long-term side effects, and abrupt withdrawal should be avoided. Patients should be maintained on aminosalicylates or immunosuppressants, as appropriate, or referred for surgery.

Formulations. Oral prednisolone will control mild and moderate IBD and 70% of patients improve after 2–4 weeks of 40 mg/day. This is gradually reduced over the next 4–6 weeks

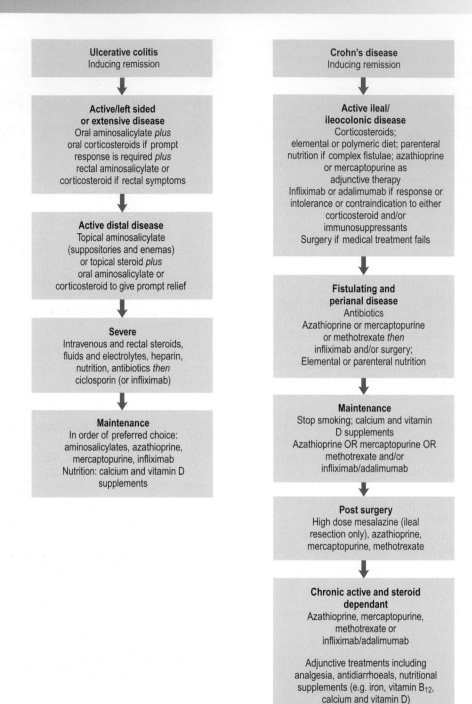

Fig. 13.4 Drug treatment algorithm for inflammatory bowel disease.

to prevent acute adrenal insufficiency and early relapse. An example of a reducing oral prednisolone regime is detailed in Box 13.1.

Oral corticosteroids should be taken in the morning to mimic the diurnal rhythm of the body's cortisol secretion and prevent sleep disturbance. Uncoated steroid tablets are suitable for most patients while enteric-coated preparations do not offer any proven advantage and should be avoided in patients with short bowel or strictures because of poor absorption and bolus release at stricture sites.

Box 13.1 An example of a reducing regimen for oral steroids

40 mg/day for 1 week
30 mg/day for 1 week
20 mg/day for 4 weeks
15 mg/day for 1 week
10 mg/day for 1 week
5 mg/day for 1 week then stop

Local regimen used at the Oxford Radcliffe Hospitals NHS Trust

Severe extensive or fulminant disease requires hospitalisation. Patients are given either hydrocortisone sodium succinate, administered intramuscularly or intravenously at doses of 100 mg three or four times a day, or methylprednisolone 15–20 mg three or four times a day, for 5 days. No additional benefit is gained after 7–10 days. Additional therapy used in severe disease may include intravenous fluid and electrolyte replacement, blood transfusion, topical therapy for rectal and/or colonic involvement, prophylactic heparin (IBD is associated with increased coagulopathy), antibiotics and nutritional support, including possible parenteral nutrition. Oral prednisolone therapy is normally introduced as soon as possible and withdrawn over the following 6–8 weeks. Too rapid reduction is associated with relapse.

Prednisolone at doses higher than 40 mg/day increases the incidence of adverse effects and has little therapeutic advantage. Short-term side effects include moon face, acne, sleep and mood disturbance, dyspepsia, hypokalamia, hypernatraemia and glucose intolerance. Prolonged use can cause cataracts, osteoporosis and increased risk of infection. Doses below 20 mg are not generally effective in active disease (St Clair Jones, 2006). A typical treatment algorithm for the management of an acute attack of IBD is presented in Fig. 13.5.

Rectal corticosteroid preparations are available as suppositories, foam and liquid enemas. In the acute setting, some hospitals make up their own liquid enemas using 100 mg hydrocortisone sodium succinate injection in 100 mL sodium chloride 0.9%. This unlicensed preparation is administered via a burette and soft catheter over 30 min. It is often well tolerated and gives better therapeutic results compared with commercial preparations.

The distribution and absorption characteristics of rectally administered steroids vary greatly. Hydrocortisone (e.g. Colifoam®) is readily absorbed from the rectal mucosa with high peak concentrations compared to prednisolone sodium metasulphobenzoate (e.g. Predenema®) and, to a lesser extent, Predfoam®. Topical preparations may play a role either alone or in combination with oral steroids.

Other steroids

Budesonide, available orally and rectally, is currently licensed for Crohn's disease affecting the ileum and descending colon. It is less effective than conventional corticosteroids in inducing remission in active Crohn's disease, but has fewer side effects than prednisolone because of its rapid and extensive first-pass metabolism. However, the absorbed drug has a higher affinity for glucocorticoid receptors 50–100 times that of prednisolone and so long-term treatment is not advocated. Budesonide has shown to be of benefit in microscopic colitis (Travis et al., 2005). Budesonide enemas are effective in inducing remission in distal ulcerative colitis and are comparable to conventional steroids but probably less effective than mesalazine enemas (Marshall and Irvine, 1997).

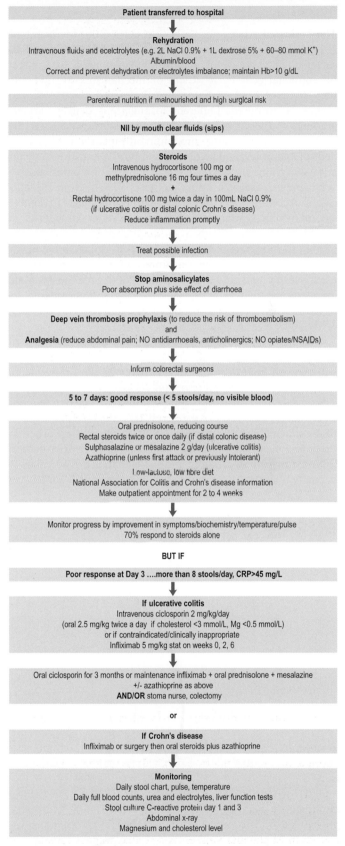

Fig. 13.5 Treatment algorithm for a severe attack of inflammatory bowel disease.

Aminosalicylates

The aminosalicylates currently licensed for the treatment of IBD include sulphasalazine, mesalazine, olsalazine and balsalazide. Their mode of action is unclear but a local effect on epithelial cells by a variety of mechanisms to moderate the release of lipid mediators, cytokines and reactive oxygen species is proposed. Different formulations deliver variable amounts of the active component, mesalazine (5-ASA), to the gut lumen where it exerts a predominantly local action independent of blood levels. The dissolution profile and site of ulceration determine the effectiveness of different preparations.

Diagnosis, disease location, activity, side effect profile, efficacy and cost all affect the choice of aminosalicylate. Available as oral or rectal preparations, aminosalicylates can be used in combination with steroids to induce and maintain remission, in mild to moderate ulcerative colitis. Sulfasalazine is considerably cheaper but the newer aminosalicylates are generally used (Sutherland and MacDonald, 2006). Aminosalicylate maintenance therapy with doses of 1.2 g and above appears to reduce the risk of colorectal cancer by up to 75% (Van Staa et al., 2005).

The use of aminosalicylates in Crohn's disease is less well established (Dignass et al., 2010). There is evidence of patient benefit with high-dose mesalazine (over 2 g/day) in reducing relapse post-small bowel resection.

Sulfasalazine consists of sulfapyridine diazotised to mesalazine. It is broken down by bacterial azoreductase in the colon to mesalazine and sulfapyridine. Sulfapyridine is absorbed in the colon, metabolised by hepatic acetylation or hydroxylation followed by glucuronidation and excreted in urine. Mesalazine is partly absorbed, metabolised by the liver and excreted via the kidneys as n-acetyl 5-ASA. However, the majority is acetylated as it passes through the intestinal mucosa. Sulfasalazine itself is poorly absorbed and that which is absorbed is recycled back into the gut, via the bile, either unchanged or as the n-acetyl metabolite.

Elimination of sulfapyridine depends on the patient's acetylator phenotype. Those who inherit the 'slow' acetylator phenotype experience more side effects. The dissolution profile of the drug and the site of ulceration determine effectiveness (Fig. 13.6). The optimal dose of sulfasalazine to achieve and maintain remission is usually in the range of 2–4 g per day in 2–4 divided doses. Acute attacks require 4–8 g per day in divided doses until remission occurs, but at these doses associated side effects are often observed.

About 30% of patients taking sulfasalazine experience adverse effects which are either dose related and dependent on acetylate phenotype or idiosyncratic and not dose related. Dose-related side effects include nausea, vomiting, abdominal pain, diarrhoea, headache, metallic taste, haemolytic anaemia, reticulocytosis and methaemoglobinaemia. Side effects which are not dose related include rashes, aplastic anaemia, agranulocytosis, pancreatitis, hepatic and pulmonary dysfunction, renal impairment, peripheral neuropathy and oligospermia. In 3% of patients, acute intolerance may be seen. This often resembles colitis and includes bloody diarrhoea. Adverse effects usually occur during the first 2 weeks of therapy, the majority being related to plasma sulfapyridine levels. Sulfasalazine metabolites are responsible for the yellow colouration of bodily fluids and staining of soft contact lenses.

Mesalazine is tolerated by 80% of patients who are intolerant of sulphasalazine. Many of the sulphonamide-related adverse

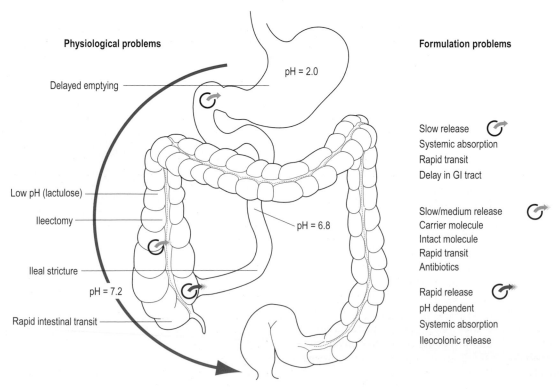

Fig. 13.6 Physiological and formulation problems encountered with mesalazine and delivery systems.

effects of sulfasalazine are avoided by using one of the newer aminosalicylate formulations. However, mesalazine alone can still cause side effects, including blood disorders, pancreatitis, renal dysfunction and lupoid phenomenon. Patients should be counselled on how to recognise and report blood dyscrasias and if they occur, treatment should be stopped.

Formulations. Mesalazine is unstable in acid medium and rapidly absorbed from the gastro-intestinal tract. To increase stability and/or alter the site of release, 5-ASA is modified by different delivery systems (see Fig. 13.6). Mesalazine dose is more important than the delivery system and the lowest systemic absorption preparation should be used. The different delivery systems developed are:

- acrylic resin-coated mesalazine tablet that releases drug pH-dependently;
- ethyl cellulose-coated mesalazine granules that release drug in a time controlled manner;
- diazotisation of mesalazine to itself or to an inert carrier.

All mesalazine preparations are licensed for UC, however only Mesren® MR and Asacol® MR are licensed for Crohn's disease. There are six modified release oral preparations currently licensed in the UK. Asacol® MR, Ipacol®, Mesren® MR and Mezavant® XL contain mesalazine coated with an acrylic resin, Eudragit-S. Mesren® MR and Ipacol® are generic versions of Asacol® MR. Mezavant® XL, recently licensed, is a modified release mesalazine formulation with a patented multi-matrix release system allowing less frequent dosing which may be beneficial in patients experiencing difficulty with a high tablet burden. Salofalk® contains mesalazine coated with

Eudragit-L. All these preparations provide pH-dependant release of mesalazine at the mid to terminal ileum and the colon, at pH 7 (Asacol® MR, Mesren® MR, Mezavant® XL) and pH 6 (Ipacol®, Salofalk®). As dissolution occurs at a lower pH with Ipacol® and Salofalk®, this results in a lower ileocolonic mucosal concentration of mesalazine compared with the other pH-dependant release products. There is little clinical difference between the available pH-dependant products Asacol® MR, Mesren® MR and Mezavant® XL. However, cost may contribute to initiating new patients with the cheaper generic. Pentasa® tablets and granules comprise ethyl cellulose-coated granules of mesalazine which are released in the stomach. Mesalazine is leached slowly and continuously from the granules throughout the gastro-intestinal tract at all physiological pH.

It is very important to maintain patients on the same brand of mesalazine as some may relapse because of the different release profiles of the active drug. Therefore, mesalazine should always be prescribed by brand.

Evidence suggests that there is no difference in splitting the dose of mesalazine products as licensed, compared to taking the total dose once daily.

Dipentum® 250mg capsules and 500mg tablets contain olsalazine sodium, a dimer of mesalazine. Like sulfasalazine, it remains intact until it reaches the colon where it undergoes bacterial cleavage, releasing two molecules of mesalazine. Olsalazine-induced diarrhoea may help patients with distal disease and proximal constipation. Colazide® 750mg capsules contain balsalazide sodium, a pro-drug of mesalazine, which relies on bacterial cleavage in the colon, releasing mesalazine from 4-aminobenzoyl β-alanine, the inert carrier molecule.

Table 13.5 Comparison of available oral aminosalicylate preparations for patients with IBD

Generic (proprietary) name	Formulation	Release profile	Site of release
Sulfasalazine (Salazopyrin®)	Compressed tablet, plain and film coated	Azo-linked, independent of pH	Terminal ileum and colon
Mesalazine (Asacol®)	Compressed tablet, acrylic coating	Acrylic coating dissolving at pH 7	Terminal ileum and colon
Mesalazine (Mesren®)	Compressed tablet, acrylic coating	Acrylic coating dissolving at pH 7	Terminal ileum and colon
Mesalazine (Salofalk®)	Compressed tablet and/or capsule, acrylic coating	Acrylic coating dissolving at pH 6	Terminal ileum and colon
Mesalazine (Mezavant® XL)	Compressed tablet, acrylic coating	Multi-matrix release system	Terminal ileum and colon
Mesalazine (Ipacol®)	Compressed tablet and/or capsule, acrylic coating	Acrylic coating dissolving at pH 6	Mid-jejunum ileum and colon
Mesalazine (Pentasa®)	Microgranules coated with ethyl cellulose and compressed into tablets. Granules also available	Disintegration not dependent on pH. Slow dissolution rate	Stomach, duodenum, jejunum, ileum and colon
Olsalazine (Dipentum®)	Hard gelatin capsules and tablets, uncoated	Azo-linked disintegration independent of pH	Terminal ileum and colon
Balsalazide (Colazide)	Hard gelatin capsules	Azo-linked disintegration independent of pH	Terminal ileum and colon

Table 13.5 compares the oral aminosalicylate preparations currently available.

Mesalazine enemas (1 g in 100 mL), foam enemas (1 g per application) or suppositories (250 mg, 500 mg and 1 g) are effective alternatives for treating distal ulcerative colitis and proctitis. The optimum rectal dose is 1 g. Rectal administrations of 5-ASA formulations are significantly better than rectal corticosteroids in inducing remission in ulcerative colitis but steroids are considerably cheaper (Travis et al., 2008). In severe ulcerative colitis, oral and topical formulations should be combined to give prompt symptom relief. Topical and oral 5-ASA is better than either alone (Marteau et al., 2005).

Immunosuppressants

Azathioprine, 6-mercaptopurine, methotrexate, ciclosporin and mycophenolate are immunosuppressants used in patients unresponsive to steroids and aminosalicylates or who relapse when steroids are withdrawn. They are used to induce and maintain remission. All are unlicensed for use in IBD but are routinely used. Treatment may be for up to 5 years because earlier withdrawal increases the rate of relapse. They can take several weeks to work and require regular monitoring.

Thioguanines (azathioprine, mercaptopurine). Azathioprine is metabolised to 6-mercaptopurine by the liver. Both azathioprine and 6-mercaptopurine have steroid-sparing properties. Although the action in IBD is unclear, their active metabolites inhibit purine ribonucleotide synthesis which may in turn inhibit lymphocyte function, primarily T-cells. Mercaptopurine is further metabolised to 6-thioguanine nucleotides.

The main indications for thioguanines are when patients

- require two or more steroid courses in 1 year;
- have chronic active disease unresponsive to steroids or 5-ASAs;
- relapse when steroids are withdrawn (within 3 months) or when the dose is reduced below 15 mg;
- require post-operative prophylaxis of complex Crohn's disease (fistulising or extensive disease).

Oral maintenance doses for azathioprine are usually 2–2.5 mg/kg/day and for mercaptopurine, 1–1.5 mg/kg/day. Doses are adjusted to patient response, tolerance, white cell and platelet counts. Patients are usually prescribed a reducing dose of corticosteroid in addition because mercaptopurine and azathioprine can take several weeks to show a therapeutic benefit.

Seventy percent of patients will tolerate azathioprine. Of the remaining 30%, most will tolerate mercaptopurine. The most common side effects occur within 2–3 weeks of starting treatment and rapidly stop on withdrawal. These include flu-like symptoms (myalgia, headache), nausea and diarrhoea. Nausea is reduced by taking the medicine with food. Although rare (<3%), leucopenia can develop suddenly and unpredictably. Hepatotoxicity and pancreatitis have also been reported in less than 5% of patients. Thioguanine has been used but is associated with a greater risk of hepatotoxicity. There is no evidence that the incidence of lymphoma increases with the use of these agents (St Clair Jones, 2006).

The value of assessing thiopurine methyl transferase (TPMT) activity and genotype, especially prior to initiating treatment, is debatable. Patients who develop leucopenia and are TPMT deficient have a greater risk of myelotoxicity. However, this may not apply in IBD. Some gastroenterologists measure TPMT if a patient has relapsed on doses greater than 2 mg/kg/day to identify fast metabolisers who may respond to higher doses. Measuring TPMT activity to identify the 0.3% of non-metabolisers who are at high risk of rapid leucopenia has also been recommended (Carter et al., 2004).

One of the most significant drug interactions is with allopurinol which inhibits the principal pathway for detoxification of azathioprine and mercaptopurine. Patients receiving these drugs concomitantly should have their dose of azathioprine reduced to approximately one-third to a quarter of the usual dose.

Methotrexate. A low-dose regimen of methotrexate is effective in inducing and maintaining remission in patients with chronically active Crohn's disease. Patients receive once-weekly doses of methotrexate ranging from 15 to 25 mg on the same day each week. These can be given orally or by subcutaneous or intramuscular injection. Oral medication is more practical, although parenteral administration may be more effective and better tolerated. Methotrexate is reserved for patients intolerant or unresponsive to thioguanines.

Methotrexate metabolites inhibit dihydrofolate reductase, although this cytotoxic action does not explain the drug's anti-inflammatory effect. Inhibition of cytokine and eicosanoid synthesis and modification of adenosine levels probably contribute.

Adverse effects associated with methotrexate are essentially gastro-intestinal (nausea, vomiting, diarrhoea and stomatitis). These may also be reduced by prescribing weekly doses of folic acid 5 mg. Folic acid should not be taken on the same day as the methotrexate. Monitoring is undertaken because of the serious side effects of hepatotoxicity, bone marrow suppression and pneumonitis.

Methotrexate is teratogenic and all male and female patients should be counselled about using contraception while taking the medication and also for 3 months after therapy is withdrawn. Guidance to improve the safety of methotrexate use and minimise the potential risk of overdose has been issued (NPSA, 2006). Measures include the issue of patient hand-held monitoring cards detailing dose and blood test results, comprehensive written and verbal medicines information, dispensing one strength of tablet (2.5 mg) and ensuring inpatient medication charts clearly state once-weekly dosing and the number and strength of tablets routinely used. An aide memoire commonly recommended to patients to remember dose frequency is to take methotrexate on Mondays and folic acid on Fridays.

Ciclosporin. Ciclosporin is a calcineurin inhibitor that acts at an early stage on precursors of helper T-cells by interfering with the release of interleukin-2. This inhibits the formation of the cytotoxic lymphocytes which cause tissue damage. Both controlled and uncontrolled studies suggest that ciclosporin is effective rescue therapy for severe ulcerative colitis failing to respond to intravenous steroids (Campbell et al., 2005). Its use in Crohn's disease is unproven.

The effectiveness of ciclosporin at doses of 2–5 mg/kg/day in treating IBD has been studied in patients refractory to conventional drug therapy (Van Assche et al., 2003). A dose of 2 mg/kg has been shown to be as effective as 4 mg/kg. Patient response to this treatment has varied, with adverse effects causing withdrawal of treatment in some cases. However, some patients have stopped concurrent steroid therapy and have remained in remission for some time.

When patients with severe colitis fail to show a response to treatment with parenteral steroids, then ciclosporin at an intravenous dose of 2 mg/kg/day should be considered. If patients respond to parenteral ciclosporin they can subsequently be maintained on an oral dose for 3–6 months. If the patient has a low plasma magnesium (<0.5 mmol/L) or low cholesterol (<3 mmol/L), they are at an increased risk of ciclosporin-induced seizures when given intravenously. In these circumstances, treatment with an oral ciclosporin preparation, for example, Neoral®, at a dose of 5 mg/kg/day is preferred. Ciclosporin therapy is used for many patients, but normally as a bridge to colectomy or starting maintenance treatment with azathioprine or mercaptopurine. Infliximab is an alternative 'rescue therapy' for acute severe colitis (NICE, 2008a) if ciclosporin is contraindicated or clinically inappropriate. A multi-centre randomised controlled trial (CONSTRUCT) is underway comparing the clinical and cost-effectiveness of infliximab and ciclosporin in the treatment of steroid resistant acute severe colitis.

Forty percent of patients who receive ciclosporin develop minor side effects such as tremor, paraesthesia, headache, gum hyperplasia, burning sensations of the hands and feet and hirsutism. Major complications include nephrotoxicity, neurotoxicity, hepatotoxicity and hypertension. There has been 1–2% mortality reported in some case series. Ciclosporin blood levels should be monitored and maintained within the range of 100–200 ng/mL. Grapefruit juice, macrolide antibiotics (mainly erythromycin and clarithromycin), ketoconazole, fluconazole, itraconazole, diltiazem, verapamil, oral contraceptives and protease inhibitors are just some of the drugs that increase ciclosporin levels and toxicity.

In severe proctitis, refractory to standard treatments, ciclosporin enemas have been used with some success at a dose of 250 mg at night for 1 month. No commercial preparation is available.

Tacrolimus. Tacrolimus is an alternative calcineurin inhibitor to ciclosporin that has shown some benefit in inducing remission in ulcerative colitis. It is of limited value in Crohn's disease.

Mycophenolate. It has been suggested that mycophenolate mofetil is effective and well tolerated in IBD. Although used if other treatments have failed, there is little evidence regarding its use in clinical practice.

Monitoring of immunosuppressants. Major concerns about the use of immunosuppressive agents are related to bone marrow suppression and hepatotoxicity. Therefore, patients should be monitored regularly and have routine blood counts and liver function tests including plasma bilirubin and alkaline phosphatase. These should be undertaken every 2–3 weeks for the first 2–3 months and then bimonthly. Although often advised, there is no evidence that more frequent monitoring is more effective. Patients should be taught to recognise the signs of bone marrow suppression and educated about the need for earlier blood tests and the increased risk of infection due to immunosuppression. It is recommended that all patients initiated or maintained on immunosuppressants are provided with a record card detailing current dose and blood test results. This should be shown to their doctor and pharmacist at each visit. There should be good shared care policies in place between primary and secondary care in the management of patients on immunomodulators.

The incidence of lymphomas in patients receiving immunosuppressants when compared with other treatments is of concern. Patients should be advised to avoid live vaccines while taking immunosuppressants, including corticosteroids. Guidance on appropriate action following abnormal blood results is provided in Box 13.2.

Biologic agents

Since their introduction over a decade ago, biological therapy targeting tumour necrosis factor alpha (TNF-α) has revolutionised the management of IBD. These agents are efficacious in treating signs and symptoms of Crohn's disease and ulcerative colitis, reducing corticosteroid requirements and draining fistulae, achieving mucosal healing and reducing the need for major abdominal surgery or hospitilisation. They are indicated for patients who have failed or are intolerant or who have contraindications to conventional therapy including corticosteroids and immunomodulators. Not all patients will require biological therapy which is expensive and is a significant cost to the Health Service. Some patients may derive greater benefit from early use of these agents such as patients who are steroid dependant or who have complex fistulising disease.

Biologic agents that are licensed for use in IBD are infliximab (Remicade®) and adalimumab (Humira®). At present there are no direct comparative studies of the two agents. Certolizumab pegol (Cimzia®) has also shown benefit and is an alternative in some cases; however, it is currently not licensed for use in IBD. All these monoclonal antibodies inhibit the functional activity of the pro-inflammatory cytokine TNF-α which damages cells lining the gut, causing pain, cramping and diarrhoea. Colonic biopsies post-treatment with these agents show a substantial reduction in TNF-α and a reduction in the commonly elevated plasma inflammatory marker C-reactive protein. Table 13.6 summarises the anti-TNF agents used. All appear to have similar efficacy, although there are more data on infliximab than adalimumab or certolizumab. Natalizumab, another monoclonal antibody, has also shown promise in treating active Crohn's disease. It works by inhibiting the migration of leucocytes into the CNS thereby reducing inflammation. It is unlicensed in IBD.

Box 13.2 Guidance on dealing with abnormal blood results for patients on immunosuppressant therapy

Baseline U&Es, LFTs and FBC should be carried out prior to initiation of therapy. These should be repeated at 2 weeks, 4 weeks then every 2–3 months.

Methotrexate should be *stopped* and the relevant expert advice obtained if any of the following occur:

WBC	$<4 \times 10^9$ L^{-1}
Neutrophils	$<2 \times 10^9$ L^{-1}
Platelets	$<150 \times 10^9$ L^{-1}
AST/ALT	$>3 \times$ normal range

- Unexplained respiratory symptoms, for example, dyspnea, dry cough, especially if accompanied by fever and sweats
- Renal impairment
- Mouth or throat ulceration/rash/unexplained bleeding/fever/ alopecia/recurrent sore throats, infections, fever or chills/ nausea/vomiting/diarrhoea

Azathioprine or mercaptopurine should be *stopped* and the relevant expert advice obtained if any of the following occur:

WBC	$<4 \times 10^9$ L^{-1}
Neutrophils	$<2 \times 10^9$ L^{-1}
Platelets	$<150 \times 10^9$ L^{-1}
AST/ALT	$>3 \times$ normal range

- Significant reduction in renal function
- Mouth or throat ulceration/rash/unexplained bleeding/fever/ upper abdominal or back pain/alopecia/recurrent sore throats, infections, fever or chills/nausea/vomiting/diarrhoea
- Nausea may be relieved by taking the dose with/after food or in divided doses

Ciclosporin should be *stopped* and the relevant expert advice obtained if any of the following occur:
- High blood levels (will require dose adjustment)
- Significant reduction in renal function
- Uncontrolled hypertension

Drug blood levels should be done at similar intervals to FBC. A 12-h trough level should be taken, that is, before a dose. Target level within the range of 100–200 ng/mL. It takes 2–3 days to reach steady state after dose change

U&Es, urea and electrolytes; LFTs, liver function tests; FBC, full blood count; WBC, white blood cells; ALT, alanine transaminase; AST, aspartate transaminase.

Table 13.6 Summary of anti-TNF agents used in IBD

Agent	Licensed/(unlicensed) indication	Dose
Infliximab	*Crohn's disease*	
	Induction of remission in severe active disease	5 mg/kg intravenously at weeks 0 and 2
	Maintenance treatment	5 mg/kg intravenously 6 weeks after initial dose then every 8 weeks or further dose of 5 mg/kg if signs and symptoms recur
	Fistulising	5 mg/kg intravenously at weeks 0, 2 and 6 (consult product literature)
Infliximab	*Ulcerative colitis*	
	Induction of remission in moderate to severe active disease	5 mg/kg intravenously at weeks 0, 2 and 6
	Maintenance of remission in severe active disease	5 mg/kg intravenously every 8 weeks; discontinue if no response 14 weeks after initial dose
	Extra-intestinal manifestations (unlicensed)	5 mg/kg intravenously
Adalimumab	*Crohn's disease*	
	Induction of remission in severe active disease	80 mg subcutaneously at week 0, 40 mg at week 2 and or accelerated regime of 160 mg at week 0, 80 mg at week 2
	Maintenance treatment	40 mg subcutaneously on alternate weeks, increasing to weekly if loss of response
Certolizumab pegol	*Crohn's disease (unlicensed)*	
	Used in moderate to severe disease when patients who have lost response to or are intolerant of infliximab or adalimumab	
	Induction	400 mg subcutaneously at weeks 0, 2 and 4
	Maintenance treatment	400 mg subcutaneously every 4 weeks

National guidance has been issued on the use of infliximab in ulcerative colitis (NICE, 2008a,b) and infliximab and adalimumab in the treatment of Crohn's disease (NICE, 2010). The latter guidance indicates treatment should be started with the less expensive drug, taking into account drug administration costs, required dose and product price per dose. This may need to be varied for individual patients due to differences in the method of administration and treatment schedules.

A combination of infliximab with azathioprine has been shown to be superior to monotherapy in inducing remission and mucosal healing in Crohn's patients naïve to both agents. The rate of infliximab-related infusion reactions was also less with combination treatment and there was no significant difference seen with the rate of serious infection (Colombel et al., 2010). For scheduled treatment, the concomitant immunomodulator should be reviewed and stopped after 6–12 months. It remains unclear whether the same applies to other anti-TNF agents. In practice, the same principles apply with other immunomodulators such as methotrexate.

Natalizumab should not be combined with an immunosuppressant or prolonged steroids as this may increase the risks of progressive multifocal leucoencephalopathy (D'Haens et al., 2010).

There is currently no specific guidance on how long anti-TNF agents should be continued for. Preliminary evidence suggests that many patients in clinical remission for greater than 1 year, with a normal C-reactive protein and complete mucosal healing on endoscopy will remain in remission during the following year after stopping treatment. Whether remission is then sustained or whether the behaviour of disease is altered in the long term is currently unknown (D'Haens et al., 2010). NICE guidance on the treatment of Crohn's disease recommends that infliximab or adalimumab treatment should be given until treatment failure (including the need for surgery) or until 12 months after initiation of treatment, whichever is shorter. Patients should then have their disease reassessed and continue treatment if there is clear evidence of ongoing active disease and treatment is still clinically appropriate. Treatment can be restarted if patients subsequently relapse.

Loss of response or intolerance to anti-TNF agents can be managed by optimising dosing regimes, switching to agents or switching class, for example, to natalizumab. Reasons for a loss of response should be assessed.

Monoclonal antibodies are contraindicated in patients with tuberculosis (TB) and, therefore, all patients should have a chest X-ray prior to administration to exclude latent TB. Infliximab increases the risk of TB five-fold. Other contraindications include moderate to severe cardiac failure, history of malignancy (excluding non-melanoma skin cancer), sepsis (including pelvic or perianal), optic neuritis. Intestinal stricturing is a relative contraindication (obstruction may be exacerbated through rapid healing at the stricture site) along with chronic hepatitis B/C carriers, primary failure or absence of inflammatory activity (normal C-reactive protein). Patients who receive live vaccines should not receive biological therapy for 3 months. Patients on biologics should be vaccinated against tetanus, pneumococcus species, influenza and hepatitis B. Young females should also be vaccinated for the human papilloma virus.

Anti-TNF agents should only be prescribed by a gastroenterologist with experience of IBD, and in the case of infliximab, administered in a setting where there are adequate resuscitation facilities available and patients are closely monitored. Patients self-administering adalimumab at home should be counselled on how to recognise signs of infection, for example, fever, productive cough, toothache, stinging on passing urine or if neurological symptoms develop.

Infliximab. Infliximab is a chimeric human murine monoclonal antibody, licensed for treating severe active Crohn's disease (with or without fistulae) which is refractory or intolerant to corticosteroids or conventional immunosuppressants alone or if surgery is inappropriate. Treatment may be repeated if the condition responded to the initial course but subsequently relapsed. Infliximab is also licensed for moderate to severe active ulcerative colitis (acute exacerbation) requiring hospitilisation and/or possible surgical intervention and if unresponsive to conventional treatments. Infliximab may half the need for colectomy in steroid refractory patients with acute ulcerative colitis. It remains to be determined whether infliximab is superior to ciclosporin (D'Haens et al., 2010).

In severe active Crohn's disease, infliximab is administered by intravenous infusion, at a dose of 5 mg/kg over a 2-h period, repeated after 2 weeks. If a clinical response is seen, then a maintenance dose of 5 mg/kg every 8 weeks should be given. Alternatively, a dose could be given when signs and symptoms recur. Fixed interval dosing may be superior to intermittent dosing because of the reduced risk of immunogenicity (NICE, 2010).

In active fistulising Crohn's disease where disease has not responded to conventional therapy (including antibiotics, drainage and immunosuppressive therapy) or who are intolerant or have contraindications to conventional therapy, an initial dose of 5 mg/kg is given, repeated at 2 and 6 weeks after the first infusion is given. If no response is seen after three doses, no further treatment should be given (NICE, 2010).

Trials in inflammatory Crohn's disease have shown an 81% response rate at 4 weeks. After 12 weeks, 48% of patients still had a response. In fistulising disease, 68% of patients experienced a 50% reduction in the number of draining fistulas at two or more consecutive visits. If a loss of response is seen the dose can be increased to 10 mg/kg (unlicensed) or the dosing interval shortened. An alternative is to switch treatment to adalimumab.

In treatment-refractory, moderate to severe acute exacerbation of ulcerative colitis, the licensed dose regimen is 5 mg/kg at weeks 0, 2 and 6. The optimal maintenance strategy after induction therapy is currently unknown. Treatment should be discontinued if no response is seen after 14 weeks. In azathioprine naïve patients responding to infliximab induction, azathioprine is an option instead of infliximab for maintenance (Travis et al., 2008). Although unlicensed, infliximab has shown to be of benefit in extra-intestinal manifestations such as pyoderma gangrenosum and peripheral and axial naturopathies

All doses should be preceded with intravenous corticosteroid (hydrocortisone 200 mg) unless the patient has been taking an immunosuppressant for more than 3 months.

In some patients, infliximab has been associated with either infusion (during or shortly after infusion) or delayed hypersensitivity reactions. It may also affect the normal body immune responses in a significant number of patients. Other side effects include headache, dizziness, nausea, rash, raised liver function tests, abdominal pain, fatigue, etc.

Adalimumab. Adalimumab is a fully humanised anti-TNF monoclonal antibody which is licensed for the treatment of severe active Crohn's disease in patients who are refractory or intolerant to corticosteroids and conventional immunomodulators. It may also be used in those patients who have primary or secondary non-response to infliximab or developed a hypersensitivity reaction. Unlike infliximab it is not licensed for acute ulcerative colitis.

As adalimumab is fully humanised it is less immunogenic than infliximab. It also has the advantage of being given as a subcutaneous injection which enables patients to self-administer at home, therefore reducing nursing time and hospital bed occupancy. This also lends itself to supply by home delivery services. The licensed dose is an initial induction of 80 mg followed by 40 mg at week 2 and then 40 mg on alternate weeks thereafter as maintenance. An accelerated dose of 160 mg followed by 80 mg and then 40 mg on alternate weeks maintenance is more commonly used, particularly in those patients who have previously been on infliximab. The maintenance dose can be increased to 40 mg weekly if a diminished or suboptimal response is seen but treatment should be stopped if no response is seen within 12 weeks of the initial dose.

Infliximab may be of benefit in patients initiated on adalimumab as the first-line anti-TNF agent but who lose response to, or develop adverse effects. The efficacy of infliximab in patients with no initial response to adalimumab needs to be evaluated.

Certolizumab. Certolizumab is a pegylated monoclonal antibody fragment TNF-α antibody. It is currently used for those patients who have lost response to or have become intolerant to infliximab or adalimumab. It is given at an induction dose of 400 mg subcutaneously at weeks 0, 2 and 4 and then if a response is seen, once every 4 weeks as maintenance.

Antibiotics

Metronidazole has been used in Crohn's disease associated with perianal disease, sepsis associated with fistulae, perforation and bacterial overgrowth in the small bowel. Doses of 0.6–1.5 g/day are typically used and well tolerated. Metronidazole appears to be ineffective in ulcerative colitis. The associated paraesthesia appears to be dose related, occurring frequently with treatment of greater than 3 months duration. In such patients, doses should be gradually reduced or the drug alternated with another antibiotic, for example, ciprofloxacin, tetracycline or rifabutin, which have shown some limited benefit. The metabolite of metronidazole has a free nitro group and this is probably responsible for the drug's local activity. It also inhibits phospholipase A, contributing to a reduction in damage induced by polymorphonuclear leucocytes.

Other antibacterials are used if specifically indicated, especially when the causative bacterial agents have been identified.

Pseudomembranous colitis caused by *C. difficile* usually occurs after prolonged or multiple antibiotics. This can be distinguished from other causes of colitis by biopsy and stool culture. If it is unclear whether a patient has pseudomembranous or acute colitis, treatment with metronidazole or vancomycin and steroids is advised. A colonoscopy can be performed once symptoms resolve.

Other treatments

Thalidomide. The use of thalidomide, under specialist supervision, is restricted to refractory cases of Crohn's disease. Thalidomide acts as a TNF-α inhibitor and probably stabilises lysosomal membranes. At therapeutic doses it also inhibits the formation of superoxide and hydroxyl radicals, both potent oxidants capable of causing tissue damage. Daily doses in the range of 50–400 mg have proved beneficial when used for periods of 1 week to several months. Side effects during treatment include sedation, dry skin and reduced libido. Thalidomide is teratogenic and should never be used in women of child-bearing age.

Antidiarrhoeals. Codeine diphenoxylate and loperamide should be used with caution to treat diarrhoea and abdominal cramping in IBD. Their use may mask inflammation, infection, obstruction or colonic dilation, thereby delaying correct diagnosis.

Colestyramine. Colestyramine has been used in Crohn's disease following ileal resection to reduce diarrhoea associated with bile acid malabsorption caused by the decrease in small bowel absorptive surface area and the cathartic effect of bile salts on the colon. Doses of up to 4 g three times a day inhibit the secretion of water and electrolytes stimulated by bile acids.

Fish oils (omega-3 fatty acids). Fish liver oils containing eicosapentaenoic and docosahexaenoic acids have been used with some success in the treatment of both ulcerative colitis and Crohn's disease. These products cause unpleasant regurgitation which renders them unpalatable in long-time use. Enteric-coated preparations have reduced this problem. It is thought that fish oils work by diverting fatty acid metabolism from leukotriene B4 to the formation of the less inflammatory leukotriene B5.

Miscellaneous treatments. There are many limited trials, studies and case series in the literature evaluating other therapies for ulcerative colitis and Crohn's disease. These include probiotics, sodium cromoglicate, bismuth and arsenic salts, sucralfate, nicotine, oxygen-derived free radical scavengers, somatostatin analogues, lidocaine, chloroquine, d-penicillamine, carbomers, antituberculous agents, heparin, aloe vera, probiotics and worm therapy (helminths). In general, these treatments are not recommended, although the variety illustrates the limitations of current therapy. When a patient is not responding to conventional agents, consideration should be given to referral to a specialist centre for a review of current therapy and a plan of future management. Alternative and complementary treatments, for example, acupuncture, aromatherapy may have a role.

Leukapheresis has been shown to have some benefit in patients with IBD. It involves removal of leucocytes from the blood, either through an adsorptive system or by centrifugation. In each system, venous blood is removed in a continuous flow, anticoagulated, processed to deplete the leukocytes and returned to the circulation (see NICE, 2005). Table 13.7 summarises the pharmacological profile of drugs used in adults with IBD.

Future treatments

Future therapy is focusing on the ability of drugs to target a specific point in the inflammatory process, such as TNF, interleukins (IL-10, 11, 12), T-cell surface antigens and stem cell transplantation.

Table 13.7 Pharmacological profile of drugs used in adults with inflammatory bowel disease

Pharmacological group	Daily dose	$t^{1/2}$ (h)	Metabolism
Steroids			
Hydrocortisone	125–250 mg as foam enema 100–400 mg in 0.9% w/v in sodium chloride intravenously	1.5	Hepatic metabolism 70% and 30% unchanged
Prednisolone	20–60 mg orally 20 mg as foam or liquid enema 5–10 mg as suppositories	3	Hepatic metabolism 70% and 30% unchanged
Budesonide	3–9 mg orally 20 mg as enema	2.8	90% hepatic metabolism
Aminosalicylates			
Mesalazine	500 mg–1.5 g as suppositories 1 g as enema 1.2–2.4 g orally	0.7–2.4	Local and systemic Hepatic acetylation, glucuronidation
Olsalazine	1–3 g orally	1.0	Local and systemic Hepatic acetylation, glucuronidation
Sulfasalazine	3 g as enema 1–2 g as suppositories 4–8 g orally	5–8	Colonic azo-reduction Local and systemic acetylation Hepatic glucuronidation
Balsalazide	3–6.75 g orally	1.0	Local and systemic hepatic acetylation
Antibiotics			
Metronidazole	600 mg–1.2 g orally 1.5 g intravenously	6–24	Hepatic metabolism
Immunosuppressants			
Azathioprine	2–2.5 mg/kg orally	3	Hepatic metabolism to 6-mercaptopurine
6-Mercaptopurine	1–1.5 mg/kg orally	1.5	Hepatic metabolism to inactive metabolite
Methotrexate	15–25 mg by intramuscular or subcutaneous injection weekly 15–25 mg orally weekly	3–10	Insignificant metabolism at low doses
Ciclosporin	2 mg/kg intravenously 5 mg/kg orally	19–27	Mainly hepatic metabolism
Monoclonal antibody			
Infliximab	5 mg/kg intravenous infusion every 8 weeks (maintenance)	8–9 days	Unknown
Adalimumab	40 mg subcutaneous injection every 2 weeks	10–19 days	Unknown
Certolizumab	400 mg subcutaneous injection every 4 weeks	14 days	Unknown
Miscellaneous			
Arsenic salts	250 mg–1 g rectally	72	Tissue deposition excreted unchanged
Bismuth salts	200 mg–1.2 g rectally	60–80	Tissue deposition excreted unchanged
Fish oils	3–4 g	None	Used in the arachidonic acid cycle
Sodium cromoglicate	200–800 mg orally 100–400 mg rectally	Unknown	Poorly absorbed, excreted unchanged in urine and bile
Nicotine	5–15 mg transdermally	0.5–2.0	Hepatic oxidation to cotinine 5% excreted unchanged
Lidocaine	200–800 mg rectally	1–2	Hepatic de-ethylation and hydrolysis 3% excreted unchanged Largely excreted unchanged
Human growth hormone	1.5–5 mg daily by subcutaneous injection	0.5–4	Unknown
Thalidomide	100–400 mg orally	7–16	Hydrolysis
Colestyramine	4–12 g orally		Not absorbed
Probiotics, for example, VSL#3	1–2 sachets daily orally		Poorly absorbed

Surgical treatment

Fifty to eighty percent of Crohn's disease patients will require surgery within 5–10 years of diagnosis. In contrast, 20–30% of ulcerative colitis patients will usually undergo colectomy with 5 years.

In ulcerative colitis, surgical colectomy, temporary ileostomy and ileoanal pouch construction are all curative. These are the surgical interventions of choice, although proctocolectomy and permanent ileostomy also have a role. Curative surgery is not possible in Crohn's disease as recurrence elsewhere in the gut is inevitable. Complications in the course of their illness result in about 70% of patients with Crohn's disease requiring at least one surgical procedure. If a significant length of gut is removed this can result in short gut syndrome which may require long-term parenteral nutrition and medication to control a high-output stoma if present, for example, PPIs, loperamide, codeine phosphate, isotonic fluids.

Patient care

The impact of a diagnosis of IBD should not be underestimated. In general, most patients are diagnosed when they are relatively young and the disease can have a significant effect on the rest of their life. In addition to managing symptoms, the condition can result in loss of education and difficulty in gaining employment or insurance. In young patients, it can cause psychological problems and growth failure or retarded sexual development. Anxiety and loss of self-esteem are commonly described. In addition to pharmacological treatments, psychological support is also important. Medical treatment with corticosteroids and immunosuppressants causes secondary health problems such as infection and surgery may result in complications such as intestinal failure. The care of patients with IBD is, therefore, a challenge for the multidisciplinary team.

All patients should be educated about their illness and medication and reminded that even in periods of remission it is important to continue taking prescribed therapy. This should take the form of verbal and written information. Drug use is invariably lifelong and patients are likely to receive several different treatments during the course of their illness due to intolerance or lack of response. Certain patients such as female or those newly diagnosed patients may require more tailored information about the condition or treatment. Patients with poor dexterity may find the use of rectal preparations difficult and these preparations may, therefore, be poorly tolerated. Leaflets about IBD and insurance or employment for patients with IBD have been prepared by the National Association for Colitis and Crohn's Disease (www.nacc.org.uk). Patients should also be warned about unreliable information sources.

Patients and primary care doctors may require additional reassurance as several of the treatments used, for example, azathioprine, are unlicensed for IBD. Regular blood monitoring of aminosalicylates and immunosuppressants is essential to ensure patients avoid toxicity associated with these drugs.

All patients taking steroids must be issued with a steroid card. Shared care policies between primary care doctors, gastroenterologists and patients may also be appropriate.

If relapse occurs in some patients, they are advised to increase the dose of their current oral therapy and/or commence rectal administration of a corticosteroid before contacting their doctor. If symptoms do not improve within 48 h they should arrange a review with their specialist.

Effective home treatment of proctitis is important because tenesmus and occasional faecal incontinence, apart from being distressing, limit further treatment. Good counselling on the administration of topical therapy is important to ensure effectiveness and adherence.

IBD affects young adults, so pregnancy is not uncommon. Poorly controlled IBD can affect fertility and pregnancy. Good nutrition, stopping smoking and adherence to medication is important. Active disease is a risk factor for pre-term delivery and low birth weight. Infertility associated with sulfasalazine therapy would indicate the use of alternative aminosalicylate therapy. With the exception of methotrexate, which is contraindicated in pregnancy, most drugs used in the treatment of IBD do not present a significant hazard. However, patients are strongly advised to first discuss any plans for pregnancy with their gastroenterologist. Care of pregnant women should be done jointly by a gastroenterologist and obstetrician.

Encouraging patients to stop smoking, especially those with Crohn's disease, can have a significant impact on the course of the disease.

Long-term steroid use and underlying IBD both contribute to a higher risk of developing osteoporosis. This is prevalent in up to 50% of the patient population with IBD. Patients with Crohn's disease appear more susceptible to osteoporosis than those with ulcerative colitis. Regular DEXA-scanning should be considered and preventive treatment with bisphosphonate and/or calcium and vitamin D supplements may be necessary. Guidance for the treatment of osteoporosis in IBD has been published by the British Society of Gastroenterology.

IBD patients often develop microcytic anaemia because of malabsorption and chronic blood loss. Assessment of the blood film and serum ferritin can differentiate between iron deficiency and anaemia of chronic disease. Oral iron supplements are generally poorly tolerated and parenteral iron may be required. Guidance of the treatment of iron-deficiency anaemia in IBD has been published (Gasche et al., 2007). Megaloblastic anaemias are uncommon, although vitamin B_{12} and folate deficiencies occur and may benefit from appropriate supplementation.

The European Crohn's and Colitis Organisation have published evidence-based consensus guidelines on the prevention, diagnosis and management of opportunistic infections in IBD (Rahier et al., 2009). These highlight which vaccinations should be offered on diagnosis of IBD. UK practice currently recommends influenza, and pneumococcal vaccine in immunosupressed patients only, along with HPV vaccines for females aged 12–18 years in line with other national guidelines. IBD patients in the UK are also advised to receive the swine flu vaccine if immunocompromised.

In 2009, National IBD Standards were published by key stakeholders involved in the care of patients with IBD to improve the service provided for people with a diagnosis of IBD across the UK. The aim of the standards is to ensure patients receive consistent, high-quality care and that IBD services throughout the UK are evidence based, engaged in local and national networking, based on modern IT and audit, meet specific minimum standards. The delivery of patient-focused care requires a multidisciplinary approach which should comprise medical gastroenterologist, nurse specialist, pharmacist, dietician, psychologist, colorectal surgeon, primary care doctor, radiologist and histopathologist.

Case studies

Case 13.1

Miss A has been receiving maintenance treatment with infliximab for Crohn's disease for the last 6 months but is now losing response and the decision is made to switch her to adalimumab. She weighs 65 kg and is currently taking azathioprine 100 mg daily and Adcal D$_3$ two tablets daily. She is hoping to start a family within the next year.

Questions

1. What dose of adalimumab (Humira®) should be prescribed?
2. For how long should combination treatment with azathioprine and adalimumab (Humira®) continue?
3. What advice would you give regarding immunisation for patients on biologic agents?
4. Is adalimumab (Humira®) safe in pregnancy and breastfeeding?

Answers

1. The licensed dosing schedule for severe active Crohn's disease is 80 mg, then 40 mg 2 weeks after initial dose or an accelerated regimen (more commonly used in practice) of 160 mg followed by 80 mg 2 weeks after initial dose; the maintenance dose is 40 mg on alternate weeks, increased if necessary to 40 mg weekly. Treatment should be reviewed if no response is seen within 12 weeks of the initial dose. Adalimumab is administered by subcutaneous injection.
2. The risk of developing immunogenicity and loss of response to adalimumab must be balanced against potential toxicities of combining biologic agents with immunosuppressants such as azathioprine. There is no definitive duration of overlap but a period of 6 months is common and then the immunomodulator can be stopped.
3. Patients should have annual vaccination against influenza (seasonal flu) and swine flu. Pneumococcal polysaccharide vaccine (doses at 0 and 3 years) is also recommended as anyone who gets a viral pneumonia when they are immunocompromised is at high risk of pneumococcal co-infection.
4. As adalimumab is a relatively new drug, little is known about its effect in pregnancy. The manufacturer advises to avoid and take adequate contraception during and for at least 5 months after the last dose. Patients should be advised that if they are planning a pregnancy or are already pregnant and are receiving adalimumab then they must inform their specialist. Adalimumab has been assigned to pregnancy category B by the FDA. Animal studies have revealed no teratogenic, embryotoxic or fetotoxic effects.

There are no controlled data in human pregnancy. Adalimumab is only recommended for use during pregnancy when benefit outweighs risk. To monitor outcomes of pregnant women exposed to adalimumab, a pregnancy registry has been established.

The priority is to keep the mother well and in remission. Although very low amounts of adalimumab may be transferred into breast milk, there is no risk to the baby, because adalimumab is a protein that is digested, so cannot be absorbed. The benefits of breastfeeding generally outweigh any theoretical risk while using adalimumab. Information changes rapidly, so it is important to discuss this with a specialist gastroenterologist.

Case 13.2

Miss B, a 30-year-old woman has a known history of ulcerative colitis and presents with bloody diarrhoea (12 motions/day), pyrexia, CRP 84 mg/L, platelets 545 × 10^9 L^{-1}, haemoglobin 10.5 g/dL. She is admitted to hospital for intensive medical management with intravenous and rectal steroids, fluid and electrolyte replacement and subcutaneous heparin.

Questions

1. What is the rationale for prescribing Miss B intravenous steroids and what biochemical monitoring should be undertaken?
2. Miss B is complaining of abdominal pain and the doctor is considering starting codeine phosphate or diclofenac. What advice would you give them?

   By day 3 of intensive therapy, Miss B is still passing more than six stools a day and her C-reactive protein remains greater than 45 mg/L. The decision is made to start infliximab. The patient weighs 65 kg.
3. What assessments should be made prior to administering infliximab?
4. What dose would you recommend and what advice would you give the nursing staff about administration?

Answers

1. Intravenous administration is appropriate as absorption of oral steroids could be erratic and unpredictable in severe inflammation or in patients who are systemically unwell. A parenteral steroid also ensures rapid attainment of drug levels. The mineralocorticoid properties of hydrocortisone may cause sodium and water retention, and hypokalaemia and glucocorticoid property may produce a rise in blood sugar levels. In case the patient requires second-line treatment with ciclosporin, a magnesium level and cholesterol level should be done.
2. Regular use of opiates such as codeine phosphate should be avoided as the resulting reduction in gastro-intestinal motility may precipitate a toxic megacolon and perforation. For this reason, antidiarrhoeal agents such as loperamide should also be avoided. NSAIDs, by reducing cyclo-oxygenase enzyme activity, may potentially increase production of proinflammatory leukotrienes and increase bleeding. Paracetamol is safe and may be prescribed. The anti-inflammatory action of the intravenous steroids should also reduce pain. However, pain is uncommon in ulcerative colitis because the inflammation is mucosal. The patient should be reviewed to ensure perforation is not overlooked.
3. Definite contraindications to anti-TNF therapy are sepsis, including pelvic or perianal sepsis, TB, optic neuritis or other demyelinating disorders, infusion reactions (previous sensitivity to either agent or murine products), cancer (past or present) or cardiac failure (moderate to severe NYHA III or IV – marked limitation of physical activity). Relative contraindications are pregnancy or breastfeeding, obstructive structuring disease

or surgery potentially inappropriate, chronic hepatitis B or C carriers, primary failure or loss of response, absence of inflammatory activity, that is, normal C-reactive protein.

A chest X-ray should be carried out +/− Mantoux test to rule out latent TB as infliximab increases the risk of TB five-fold. Indian or African ethnicity escalates the risk.

4. A 5 mg/kg dose should be prescribed (5 × 65 kg = 300 mg to the nearest whole vial) and infused over 2 h.

Rare infusion-related side effects are hypotension, shortness of breath and flushing. Blood pressure and pulse should be monitored every 30 min. Stopping the infusion temporarily often resolves the symptoms or they can be treated with antihistamines and paracetamol. Anaphylactic reactions are very rare but have been reported. If anaphylaxis occurs then future infusions are not advised. The patient is already receiving IV steroids to minimise the risk of hypersensitivity. Other side effects include lower respiratory tract infection and fatigue.

Case 13.3

Mr C was diagnosed with ulcerative colitis 12 months ago. His past medical history includes surgical resection and radiotherapy for squamous cell carcinoma of the mouth. As a result of this the patient has a Peg-J tube inserted for administration of enteral feed and medication. He is currently prescribed Pentasa® 2 g/day and a reducing course of prednisolone.

Question

1. Is Pentasa® suitable for administration via a Peg-J tube?

Answer

1. Pentasa® MR tablets disperse in water to give M/R granules which are slightly smaller than those in the sachets. However, the tablet contents can only be drawn into a catheter-tipped syringe owing to their size and will only flush down a 16 fr tube without blockage. The granules must not be crushed as this will destroy the modified release mechanism. As Peg-J tubes are typically smaller than 16 fr this preparation is unsuitable for Mr C as are all other oral modified release 5-ASA preparations. An alternative would be topical preparations if clinically appropriate or to consider changing to sulfasalazine liquid preparation.

Case 13.4

Mrs D is admitted to hospital for colectomy and formation of an ileostomy, following unsuccessful medical management of her ulcerative colitis. Her regular drug therapy on admission includes:
Pentasa® 1 g three times a day
Azathioprine 100 mg daily
Prednisolone 5–15 mg/day
Digoxin 125 μcg daily
Aspirin 75 mg daily

Questions

1. Following her operation, Mrs D's ileostomy output is high. What treatment approaches are available for managing high-output stomas?
2. What changes, if any, would you recommend to her current prescription?

Answers

1. High-output stomas lead to dehydration and metabolic disturbance, for example, hypokalaemia, hypernatraemia.

Drinking more can make the situation worse since this flushes the small intestinal contents through and exacerbates dehydration. Food and drink can promote secretion and increase volume.

The causes of high-output stomas need to be considered and may include high lactose intake, partial obstruction, gastric hypersecretion, inappropriate diet, laxatives and diuretics. Treatment options should include high-dose PPI to reduce gastric acid hypersecretion and codeine phosphate (180–240 mg/day) and/or loperamide to reduce gut motility. In the absence of a colon, a dose of loperamide that exceeds 16 mg/day can be used without adverse effect. Octreotide has been used as an alternative to the antimotility drugs but would appear to offer limited benefit and is best reserved for when other measures have been tried. Intake of isotonic fluids with a sodium concentration >90 mmol/L, to allow the jejunum to absorb water, may also be of benefit.

2. As ulcerative colitis is confined to the colon, following colectomy, the patient will no longer require medical treatment for maintenance of her ulcerative colitis, that is, Pentasa® and azathioprine and these can be stopped. Depending on how long the patient has been taking prednisolone, this should be reduced slowly to prevent withdrawal. If the stoma output remains high, careful monitoring of potassium levels should be taken to prevent digoxin toxicity. If potassium supplementation is given, oral modified release preparations should be avoided.

Case 13.5

Mr E was diagnosed with Crohn's disease 4 years ago and also suffers from gout. Although relatively well, during the last year he has required two courses of prednisolone. However, when the dose has been reduced, his symptoms have flared. The decision has been made to start Mr F on azathioprine. He weighs 70 kg.

Questions

1. What dose of azathioprine would you recommend for this patient to re-establish remission?
2. Are there any drugs Mr F should avoid while taking azathioprine?

Answers

1. A dose of 2–2.5 mg/kg should be recommended (150–175 mg). As azathioprine is a steroid-sparing agent this should enable prednisolone to be withdrawn.
2. One of the most significant drug interactions is with allopurinol which inhibits the principal pathway for detoxification of azathioprine and mercaptopurine. Patients receiving allopurinol concomitantly should have their dose of azathioprine reduced to approximately one-third to a quarter of the usual dose. NSAIDs which are often used to treat an acute flare of gout should be avoided in Crohn's disease.

Case 13.6

Mrs F, a 36-year-old woman, is unable to tolerate azathioprine or mercaptopurine for her Crohn's disease and has been started on oral methotrexate 25 mg once weekly.

Questions

1. What counselling points would you discuss with the patient regarding her methotrexate treatment?

2. What is the rationale for also prescribing folic acid?
3. Mrs F asks you if it is safe to become pregnant while taking methotrexate. What advice would you give her?

Answers

1. Methotrexate is effective in maintaining remission in Crohn's disease in patients who do not respond to or tolerate azathioprine or mercaptopurine. Like the thioguanines it has inflammatory and immunosuppressive properties which help to reduce the damage to the bowel wall which is responsible for the symptoms of Crohn's disease. It can take several weeks before patients start to feel the effects.

   Methotrexate should be taken once a week, on the same day of the week. Methotrexate is never taken every day. Methotrexate comes in tablet form in two different strengths: 2.5 and 10 mg. The two strengths are different shapes but are a similar colour. It is important that patients keep an up to date record of the dose they are taking and always check the strength of the tablet they have been given each time they get a prescription. To reduce the risk of confusion and possible overdose, many pharmacies only stock 2.5 mg strength tablets. If patients have problems swallowing large numbers of tablets (in this case 10 × 2.5 mg), they can be dispersed in water. As recommended by the NPSA (2006) in their 'Improving compliance with oral methotrexate' guidelines, patients should be given a monitoring card which details the dose, strength and quantity of tablets to be taken each week and blood test results.

   The most frequent side effects are nausea and vomiting (especially at start of treatment) which can be reduced by taking the dose with food; inflammation and soreness of the mouth, diarrhoea and rash or generalised itchiness. Hair loss can also occur but is reversible on stopping treatment.

   Mrs F should also be advised about the need for regular blood tests as methotrexate suppresses the bone marrow and can affect liver function. If they feel generally unwell or develop unexplained bruising, bleeding, sore throat, fever or malaise, they should contact their doctor. Methotrexate can cause inflammation in the lung tissue leading to a feeling of breathlessness or persistent cough. Although very rare, it should be reported to a doctor as soon as possible.

   Immunisation with live vaccines should also be avoided. Patient should receive vaccination for influenza, pneumococcal and swine flu.
2. Methotrexate is a folate antagonist. In patients who experience gastro-intestinal side effects, folic acid helps to reduce their frequency. It should be taken once weekly, 4 days after the methotrexate. As an aide memoire patients are often advised to take it on a Friday if they take methotrexate on a Monday.
3. It is not safe to take methotrexate during pregnancy. It is essential that men and women of child-bearing potential use a reliable form of contraception during treatment and for at least 3 months after treatment is stopped as methotrexate can damage the developing fetus. If patients are planning a family it is essential they discuss it with their doctor first.

Case 13.7

Mr G is newly diagnosed with mild ulcerative colitis. His abdominal X-ray suggests predominantly disease of the rectum and sigmoid colon. His past medical history includes joint stiffness due to rheumatoid arthritis. He presents at the pharmacy with a prescription for sulphasalazine tablets and Predfoam® one at night.

Questions

1. What advice would you give Mr G about the administration of Predfoam® enemas?
2. What are the side effects associated with the use of topical steroids?

   Mr G expresses concerns to the primary care doctor about the possibility of sulphasalazine impairing fertility as he and his wife hope to start a family. The primary care doctor decides to switch Mr G to mesalazine tablets, 800 mg taken three times a day.
3. Mesalazine 400 mg tablets are available in several different brands. Does it matter which brand is supplied?
4. Does mesalazine cause problems with fertility?

Answers

1. Rectal therapy is appropriate for mild left-sided disease. Enemas are best administered just before bedtime when the supine position allows longer retention times. Predfoam® comes in an aerosol can and the drug is delivered by attaching some plastic rectal tubes to the canister. A new tube is used for each dose. Patients with rheumatoid arthritis may have difficulty in using enemas and this may affect adherence and treatment success. The aerosol canister is flammable and care should be taken.
2. Prednisolone sodium metasulphobenzoate (Predfoam®) is poorly absorbed and the systemic side effects are minimal.
3. Once initiated, patients should remain on the same brand of mesalazine as different brands have different release profiles. Relapse of disease can occur if patients are inadvertently switched to another brand. Prescribers are encouraged to prescribe by brand and not by generic name.
4. Mesalazine does not cause problems with fertility, only sulfasalazine is associated with infertility and this only affects men. Sulfasalazine affects sperm but is reversible on stopping treatment.

Acknowledgements

The author would like to thank Dr Rebecca Palmer (Specialist Registrar, John Radcliffe Hospital, Oxford) and June Beharry (Dietitian, John Radcliffe Hospital, Oxford) for their comments on the chapter.

References

Ahmad, T., Tamboli, C.P., Jewell, D., et al., 2004. Clinical relevance of advances in genetics and pharmacogenetics of IBD. Gastroenterology 126, 1533–1549.

Campbell, S., Travis, S., Jewell, D., 2005. Ciclosporin use in acute ulcerative colitis: a long-term experience. Eur. J. Gastroenterol. Hepatol. 17, 79–84.

Carter, M.J., Lobo, A.J., Travis, S.P.L., et al., 2004. Guidelines for the management of inflammatory bowel disease in adults. Gut 53, (Suppl. V), v1–v16.

Colombel, J.F., Sandborn, W.J., Reinisch, W., et al., 2010. Infliximab, azathiorprine, or combination therapy for Crohn's disease. N. Engl. J. Med. 362, 1383–1385.

D'Haens, G.R., Panaccione, R., Higgins, P.D.R., et al., 2010. The London position statement of the World Congress of Gastroenterology on biological therapy for IBD with the European Crohn's and Colitis Organization: when to start, when to stop, which drug to choose, and how to predict response? Am. J. Gastroenterol. Advance online publication 2 November 2010. doi: 10.1038/ajg.2010.392. Available at: http://www.nature.com/ajg/journal/vaop/ncurrent/full/ajg2010392a.html.

Dignass, A., Van Assche, G., Lindsay, J.O., et al., 2010. The second European evidence based consensus on the diagnosis and management of Crohn's disease: current management 2010. J. Crohns Colitis 4, 28–62.

Felder, J.B., Burton, I.K., Rajapakse, R., 2000. Effects of nonsteroidal anti-inflammatory drugs on inflammatory bowel disease: a case–control study. Am. J. Gastroenterol. 95, 1949–1954.

Fernandes-Banares, F., Honojoso, J., Sanchez-Lombrana, J.L., et al., 1999. Randomised clinical trial of *Plantago ovata* seeds (dietary fiber) as compared with mesalazine in maintaining remission in ulcerative colitis. Am. J. Gastroenterol. 2, 427–433.

Gasche, C., Berstad, A., Befritis, R., et al., 2007. Guidelines on the diagnosis and management of iron deficiency and anaemia in inflammatory bowel diseases. Inflamm. Bowel Dis. 13, 1545–1553.

Gibson, P.R., Shepherd, S.J., 2005. Personal view: food for thought – western lifestyle and susceptibility to Crohn's disease. The FODMAP hypothesis. Aliment. Pharmacol. Ther. 21, 1399–1409.

Guslandi, M., 1999. Nicotine treatment for ulcerative colitis. Br. J. Clin. Pharmacol. 48, 481–484.

Heuschkel, R.B., Walker-Smith, J.A., 1999. Enteral nutrition in inflammatory bowel disease of childhood. J. Parenter. Enteral. Nutr. 23, S29–S32.

Jess, T., Riis, L., Jespersgaard, C., et al., 2005. Disease concordance, zygosity, and NOD2/CARD15 status: follow-up of a population-based cohort of Danish twins with inflammatory bowel disease. Am. J. Gastroenterol. 100, 2486–2492.

Marshall, J.K., Irvine, E.J., 1997. Rectal corticosteroids versus alternative treatments in ulcerative colitis: a meta-analysis. Gut 40, 775–781.

Marteau, P., Probert, C.S., Undgren, S., et al., 2005. Combined oral and enema treatment with Pentasa (mesalazine) is superior to oral therapy alone in patients with mild/moderate active ulcerative colitis: a randomised, double blind, placebo controlled study. Gut 54, 960–965.

Misiewicz, J., Pounder, R.E., Venables, C.W. (Eds.), 1994. Diseases of the Gut and Pancreas, second ed. Blackwell Scientific Publications, Oxford.

Mpofu, C., Ireland, A., 2006. Inflammatory bowel disease – the disease and its diagnosis. Hosp. Pharm. 13, 153–158.

National Institute for Health and Clinical Excellence, 2005. Leukapheresis for Inflammatory Bowel Disease. NICE, London. Available at: http://www.nice.org.uk/nicemedia/live/11178/31403/31403.pdf.

National Institute for Health and Clinical Excellence, 2008a. Infliximab for acute exacerbations of ulcerative colitis. Technology Appraisal No. 163. NICE, London. Available at: http://www.nice.org.uk/nicemedia/pdf/TA163Guidance.pdf.

National Institute for Health and Clinical Excellence, 2008b. Infliximab for subacute manifestations of ulcerative colitis. Technology Appraisal No. 140. NICE, London. Available at: http://www.nice.org.uk/nicemedia/live/11959/40412/40412.pdf.

National Institute for Health and Clinical Excellence, 2010. Infliximab (review) and adalimumab for the treatment of Crohn's disease (includes a review of technology appraisal guidance 40). Technology Appraisal No. 187. NICE, London. Available at: http://www.nice.org.uk/nicemedia/live/12985/48552/48552.pdf.

National Patient Safety Agency, 2006. Patient safety alert 13. Improving Compliance with Oral Methotrexate Guidelines. NPSA, London. Available at: http://www.nrls.npsa.nhs.uk/resources/?entryid45=59800.

Radford-Smith, G.L., Edwards, J.E., Purdie, D.M., 2002. Protective role of appendicectomy on onset and severity of ulcerative colitis and Crohn's disease. Gut 51, 808–813.

Rahier, J.F., Ben-Horin, S., Chowers, Y., et al., 2009. European evidence based consensus on the prevention, diagnosis and management of opportunistic infections in inflammatory bowel disease. J. Crohns Colitis 3, 47–91. Available at: https://www.ecco-ibd.eu/.

Solem, C.A., Loftus, E.V., Tremaine, W.J., et al., 2004. Venous thromboembolism in inflammatory bowel disease. Am. J. Gastroenterol. 99, 97–101.

St Clair Jones, A., 2006. Inflammatory bowel disease – drug treatment and its implications. Hosp. Pharm. 13, 161–166.

Sutherland, L., MacDonald, J.K., 2006. Oral 5-aminosalicylic acid for induction of remission in ulcerative colitis. Cochrane Database Syst. Rev. 2, CD000543. doi:10.1002/14651858.CD000543.pub2.

Travis, S.P.L., Ahmad, T., Collier, J., et al., 2005. Pocket Consultant Gastroenterology, third ed. Blackwell Publishing, Oxford.

Travis, S.P.L., Stange, E.F., Lemann, M., et al., 2008. European evidence-based consensus on the management of ulcerative colitis: current management. J. Crohns Colitis 2, 24–62.

Van Assche, G., D'Haens, G., Noman, M., et al., 2003. Randomised double blind comparison of 4 mg/kg v 2 mg/kg intravenous cyclosporin in severe ulcerative colitis. Gastroenterology 25, 1025–1031.

Van Staa, T.P., Card, T., Logan, R.F., et al., 2005. 5-Aminosalicylate use and colorectal cancer risk in inflammatory bowel disease: a large epidemiological study. Gut 54, 1573–1578.

Further reading

Grosso, A., Bodalia, P., Shah, M., 2009. A review of mesalazine MR formulations in ulcerative colitis. Br. J. Clin. Pharm. 1, 333–336. Available at: http://www.clinicalpharmacy.org.uk/December/review.pdf.

Lewis, N.R., Scott, B.B., 2007. Guidelines for osteoporosis in inflammatory bowel disease and coeliac disease. Available at: http://www.bsg.org.uk.

Quality care: service standards for the healthcare of people who have inflammatory bowel disease (IBD). Available online at: http://www.ibdstandards.org.uk.

Van Assche, G., Dignass, A., Panes, J., et al., 2010. The second European evidence based consensus on the diagnosis and management of Crohn's disease: definitions and diagnosis 2010. J. Crohns Colitis 4, 7–27.

Van Assche, G., Dignass, A., Reinisch, W., et al., 2010. The second European evidence based consensus on the diagnosis and management of Crohn's disease: special situations 2010. J. Crohns Colitis 4, 63–101.

Useful websites

British Society of Gastroenterology,
www.bsg.org.uk/

IBD standards,
www.ibdstandards.org.uk/

Constipation and diarrhoea 14

P. Rutter

Key points

Constipation

- About 90% of people defaecate between three times a day and once every 3 days.
- Constipation is considered infrequent bowel action when it happens twice a week or less that involves straining to pass hard stools accompanied by a sensation of pain or incomplete evacuation.
- Constipation is usually not caused by a serious disease and is corrected by non-drug treatment.
- Non-drug treatment involves increasing fibre intake, increasing fluid intake and encouraging exercise.
- The four main groups of drugs used to treat constipation (bulk forming, stimulant, osmotic and faecal softener) all have proven efficacy compared to placebo.

Diarrhoea

- Diarrhoea is the passage of loose or watery stools, at least three times in a 24-h period, which may be accompanied by anorexia, nausea, vomiting, abdominal cramps or bloating.
- Gastroenteritis is the most common cause of diarrhoea in all age groups.
- In the UK, rotavirus and small round structured virus (SRSV) are the most common causes of gastroenteritis in children.
- In adults, Campylobacter followed by rotavirus are the most common causes.
- Blood in diarrhoea is classed as dysentery and indicates the presence of an invasive organism such as Campylobacter, Salmonella, Shigella or Escherichia coli O157.
- Dehydration is the main complication of acute diarrhoea. Oral rehydration solution is the mainstay of treatment, particularly in children and the elderly.
- Antimotility agents, for example, loperamide, diphenoxylate, codeine, may be given to adults with mild-to-moderate diarrhoea but are not recommended for use in children.

Constipation and diarrhoea are two of the most common disorders of the gastro-intestinal tract. Most adults will suffer from these disorders at some time in their life and while they are often self-limiting, they can cause significant morbidity or occur as a secondary feature to a more serious disorder. For example, constipation may be secondary to hypothyroidism, hypokalaemia, diabetes, multiple sclerosis or gastro-intestinal obstruction. Likewise, diarrhoea may be secondary to ulcerative colitis, Crohn's disease, malabsorption or bowel carcinoma.

Both constipation and diarrhoea can also be drug induced and this should be considered when trying to identify a likely cause and determine effective management.

Constipation

In Western populations, 90% of people defaecate between three times a day and once every 3 days. It is clear, therefore, that to base a definition of constipation on frequency alone is problematic. What is perceived to be constipation by one individual may be normal to another. Most definitions of constipation include infrequent bowel action of twice a week or less that involves straining to pass hard faeces and which may be accompanied by a sensation of pain or incomplete evacuation. A pragmatic definition would simply be the passage of hard stools less frequently than the patient's own normal pattern. Standard criteria for the diagnosis of diarrhoea are available (Longstreth et al., 2006), although they are seldom used in practice.

Incidence

Constipation affects all age groups but is more common in the elderly: up to 20% of elderly people, compared to 8% of middle-aged and 3% of young people, seek medical advice for constipation. In the elderly, poor diet, insufficient intake of fluids, lack of exercise, concurrent disease states and use of drugs that predispose to constipation have all been identified as contributory factors.

Constipation is reported to be twice as common in women than men, although this probably reflects the greater likelihood that they seek medical advice. Constipation is, however, common in late pregnancy (up to 40% of women) due to increased circulating oestrogens, reduced gastro-intestinal motility and delayed bowel emptying caused by displacement of the uterus against the colon. It has also been reported that between 5% and 10% of children have constipation and it is more common in formula-fed babies.

Aetiology

The digestive system can be divided into the upper and lower gastro-intestinal tract. The upper gastro-intestinal tract starts at the mouth and includes the oesophagus and stomach and is

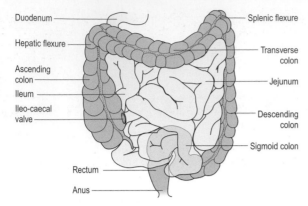

Fig. 14.1 The lower gastro-intestinal tract.

responsible for the ingestion and digestion of food. The lower gastro-intestinal tract consists of the small intestine, large intestine (colon), rectum and anus (Fig. 14.1) and is responsible for the absorption of nutrients, conserving body water and electrolytes, drying the faeces and elimination.

The remains of undigested food are swept along the gastro-intestinal tract by waves of muscular contractions called peristalsis. These peristaltic waves eventually move the faeces from the colon to the rectum and induce the urge to defaecate. By the time the stool reaches the rectum it generally has a solid consistency because most of the water has been absorbed.

Normally there is a net uptake of fluid in the intestine in response to osmotic gradients involving the absorption and secretion of ions, and the absorption of sugars and amino acids. This process is under the influence of the autonomic nervous system (sympathetic and parasympathetic). In those situations where absorption increases, this will generally lead to constipation, whereas a net secretion will result in diarrhoea.

Agents that alter intestinal motility, either directly or by acting on the autonomic nervous system, affect the transit time of food along the gastro-intestinal tract. Since the extent of absorption and secretion of fluid from the gastro-intestinal tract generally parallels transit time, a slower transit time will lead to the formation of hard stools and constipation. Motility is largely under parasympathetic (cholinergic) control, with stimulation bringing about an increase in motility while antagonists such as anticholinergics, or drugs with anticholinergic side effects, decrease motility and induce constipation. This mechanism is distinct from that of the other major group of drugs that induce constipation, the opioids. Opioids cause constipation by maintaining or increasing the tone of smooth muscle, suppressing forward peristalsis, raising sphincter tone at the ileocaecal valve and anal sphincter, and reducing sensitivity to rectal distension. This delays passage of faeces through the gut, with a resultant increase in absorption of electrolytes and water in the small intestine and colon.

It is normally the lower section of the gastro-intestinal tract that becomes dysfunctional during constipation. For convenience, many classify constipation as originating from within the colon and rectum, or externally. Causes directly attributable to the colon or rectum include obstruction from neoplasm, Hirschsprung's disease (absence of neurons in the diseased segment of the internal anal sphincter), outlet obstruction due to rectal prolapse or damage to the pudendal nerve, typically during childbirth. Causes of constipation outside the colon include poor diet, inadequate fibre intake, inadequate water intake, excessive intake of caffeine, use of medicines with constipating side effects or systemic disorders such as hypothyroidism, diabetic autonomic neuropathy, spinal cord injury, cerebrovascular accident, multiple sclerosis or Parkinson's disease.

Differential diagnosis

Constipation is a symptom and not a disease and can be caused by many different factors (Table 14.1) but the overwhelming majority of cases in non-elderly patients will be due to lack of dietary fibre. To aid diagnosis, questions need to be asked about the frequency and consistency of stools, nausea, vomiting, abdominal pain, distension, discomfort, mobility, diet and other concurrent symptoms or disorders the patient may be experiencing. It may also be necessary to ask about access to a toilet or commode. The individual with limited mobility may suppress the urge to defaecate because of difficulty in getting to the toilet. Likewise, lack of privacy or dependency on a nurse or carer for toileting may result in urge suppression that precipitates constipation or exacerbates an underlying predisposition. Patients with unexplained constipation of recent onset or a sudden aggravation of existing constipation associated with abdominal pain and the passage of blood or mucus, and long-standing constipation unresponsive to treatment require further investigation. Investigations include sigmoidoscopy/colonoscopy, barium enema, full blood count and biochemical monitoring including thyroid function tests (Fig. 14.2).

General management

In uncomplicated constipation, education and advice on diet and exercise are the mainstays of management and may adequately control symptoms in many individuals. Typically this advice will include reassurance that the individual does not have cancer, that the normal frequency of defaecation varies widely between individuals, and that mild constipation is not in itself harmful.

If the patient is taking medication for a concurrent disorder this must be assessed for its propensity to cause constipation. In the UK, over 700 medicinal products, including ophthalmic preparations, have constipation listed as a possible side effect. Common examples of medicines involved are presented in Table 14.2.

Non-drug treatment

Non-drug treatment is advocated as first-line therapy for all patient groups, except those who are terminally ill. This often includes advising an increase in fluid intake at the same time as reducing strong or excessive intake of tea or coffee, since these act as a diuretic and serve to make constipation worse.

Table 14.1 Causes of constipation

Cause	Comment
Poor diet	Diets high in animal fats, for example, meats, dairy products, eggs, and refined sugar, for example, sweets, but low in fibre predispose to constipation
Irritable bowel syndrome	Spasm of colon delays transit of intestinal contents. Patients have a history of alternating constipation and diarrhoea
Poor bowel habit	Ignoring and suppressing the urge to have a bowel movement will contribute to constipation
Laxative abuse	Habitual consumption of laxatives necessitates increase in dose over time until intestine becomes atonic and unable to function without laxative stimulation
Travel	Changes in lifestyle, daily routine, diet and drinking water may all contribute to constipation
Hormone disturbances	For example, hypothyroidism, diabetes. Other clinical signs should be more prominent, for example, lethargy and cold intolerance in hypothyroidism and increased urination and thirst in diabetes
Pregnancy	Mechanical pressure of womb on intestine and hormonal changes, for example, high levels of progesterone
Fissures and haemorrhoids	Painful disorders of the anus often lead patients to suppress defaecation, leading to constipation
Diseases	Many disease states may have constipation as a symptom, for example, scleroderma, lupus, multiple sclerosis, depression, Parkinson's disease, stroke
Mechanical compression	Scarring, inflammation around diverticula and tumours can produce mechanical compression of intestine
Nerve damage	Spinal cord injuries and tumours pressing on the spinal cord affect nerves that lead to intestine
Colonic motility disorders	Peristaltic activity of intestine may be ineffective, resulting in colonic inertia
Medication	See Table 14.2
Dehydration	Insufficient fluid intake or excessive fluid loss. Water and other fluids add bulk to stools, making bowel movements soft and easier to pass
Immobility	Prolonged bedrest after an accident, during an illness or general lack of exercise
Electrolyte abnormalities	Hypercalcaemia, hypokalaemia

It is generally recommended that fibre intake in the form of fruit, vegetables, cereals, grain foods, wholemeal bread, etc. be increased to about 30 g/day. The amounts of fibre in commonly eaten foods have been published (MeReC, 2004). Such a diet should be tried for at least 1 month to determine if it has an effect. Most will notice an effect within 3–5 days. Unfortunately, a high-fibre diet is not without problems, with patients complaining of flatulence, bloating and distension, although these effects should diminish over a period of several months. Patients who increase their fibre intake must also be advised to drink 2 L of water a day. Where an intake of this volume cannot be ingested it will be necessary to avoid increasing dietary fibre. An increased level of exercise should also accompany the raised fibre intake as this is thought to help relax and contract the abdominal muscles and help food move more efficiently through the gut.

A high-fibre diet is not recommended in those with megacolon or hypotonic colon/rectum because they do not respond to bulk in the colon. Similarly, a high-fibre diet may not be appropriate in those with opioid-induced constipation.

Drug treatment

Drug treatment is indicated where there is faecal impaction, constipation associated with illness, surgery, pregnancy, poor diet, where the constipation is drug induced, where bowel strain is undesirable, and as part of bowel preparation for surgery. The various laxatives available can be classified as bulk forming, stimulant, osmotic and faecal softeners. A systematic review (Tramonte et al., 1997) identified 36 trials involving 1815 participants that met their inclusion criteria. Twenty of the trials compared laxative against placebo or regular diet, 13 of which demonstrated statistically significant increases in bowel movement. The remaining 16 trials compared different types of laxatives with each other. The review concluded that laxative use was superior to placebo but due to a lack of comparative data could not conclude which laxative group was most efficacious. Further, more recent reviews have found good evidence that macrogols are effective, as are ispaghula husk and bisacodyl, although data is still lacking on which laxative is best (Frizelle and Barclay, 2007).

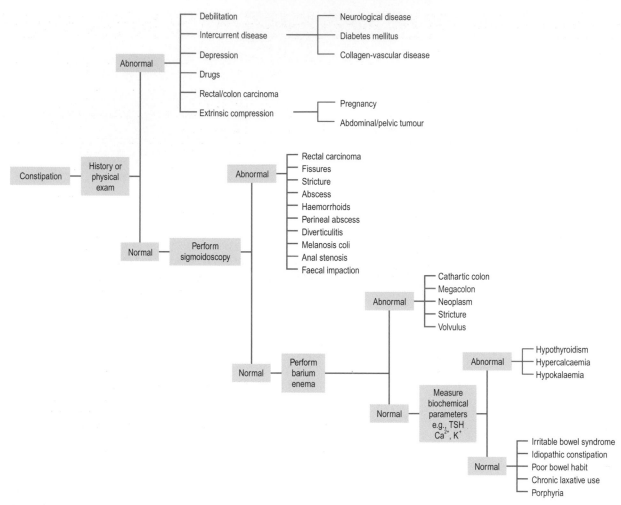

Fig. 14.2 A diagnostic algorithm for constipation.

In general, the fit, active, elderly person should be treated as a younger adult. In contrast, management of constipation in children is often complex. Early treatment is required in children to avoid developing a megarectum, faecal impaction and overflow incontinence. Encouraging the child to use the toilet after meals and increasing dietary fibre have a role alongside oral drug treatment. Depending on circumstances, behavioural therapy may be indicated. In pregnancy, if drug treatment is required, bulk-forming laxatives are first choice, but if stools remain hard then either changing to or adding in lactulose or a macrogol is advocated. Conversely, if stools are soft but the woman still finds difficulty in passing stools then a stimulant laxative should be considered.

Bulk-forming agents. Ispaghula, methylcellulose, sterculia and bran are typical bulk-forming agents and are usually taken as granules, powders or tablets. Their use is most appropriate in situations where dietary intake of fibre cannot be increased and the patient has small hard stools, haemorrhoids or an anal fissure.

The mechanism of action for bulk-forming agents involves polysaccharide and cellulose components that are not digested and which retain fluid, increase faecal bulk and stimulate peristalsis. They may also encourage the proliferation of colonic bacteria and this helps further increase faecal bulk and stool softness. Following ingestion it usually takes 12–36 h before any effect is seen but it may take longer. An adequate volume of fluid should also be ingested to avoid intestinal obstruction. Bulk-forming agents can be used safely long term, during pregnancy or breast feeding but many users will experience problems with flatulence and distension. The use of bulk-forming agents is not recommended in patients with colonic atony, intestinal obstruction or faecal impaction and they are less effective, or may even exacerbate constipation, in those who lack mobility.

Stimulant laxatives. Drugs in this group include bisacodyl, senna and dantron. They directly stimulate colonic nerves that cause movement of the faecal mass, reduce transit time and result in the passage of stool within 8–12 h. As a consequence of their time to onset, oral dosing at bedtime is generally recommended. For a rapid action (within 20–60 min), suppositories can be used. Abdominal cramps are common as an immediate side effect of stimulant laxatives, while electrolyte disturbances and an atonic colon may result from chronic use.

In the elderly, atonic colon is of less concern and prolonged use may be appropriate in a few cases. Stimulant laxatives should be avoided in patients with intestinal obstruction, and

Table 14.2 Examples of medicines known to cause constipation (frequency defined as very common [>10%] or common [1–10%])

α-Blocker	Prazosin
Antacid	Aluminium and calcium salts
Anticholinergic	Trihexyphenidyl, hyoscine, oxybutynin, procyclidine, tolterodine
Antidepressant	Tricyclics, SSRIs, reboxetine, venlafaxine, duloxetine, mirtazepine
Antiemetic	Palonosetron, dolasetron, aprepitant
Antiepileptic	Carbamazepine, oxcarbazepine
Antipsychotic	Phenothiazines, haloperidol, pimozide and atypical antipsychotics such as amisulpride, aripiprazole, olanzapine, quetiapine, risperidone, zotepine, clozapine
Antiviral	Foscarnet
β-Blocker	Oxprenolol, bisoprolol, nebivolol; other β-blockers cause constipation more rarely
Bisphosphonate	Alendronic acid
CNS stimulant	Atomoxetine
Calcium channel blocker	Diltiazem, verapamil
Cytotoxic	Bortezomib, buserelin, cladribine, docetaxel, doxorubicin, exemestane, gemcitabine, irinotecan, mitozantrone, pentostatin, temozolomide, topotecan, vinblastine, vincristine, vindesine, vinorelbine
Dopaminergic	Amantadine, bromocriptine, carbegolide, entacapone, tolcapone, levodopa, pergolide, pramipexole, quinagolide
Growth hormone antagonist	Pegvisomant
Immunosuppressant	Basiliximab, mycophenolate, tacrolimus
Lipid-lowering agent	Colestyramine, colestipol, rosuvastatin, atorvastatin (other statins uncommon) gemfibrozil
Iron	Ferrous sulphate
Metabolic disorder	Miglustat
Muscle relaxant	Baclofen
NSAID	Meloxicam; other NSAIDs, for example, aceclofenac, and COX-2 inhibitors reported as uncommon
Smoking cessation	Bupropion
Opioid analgesic	All opioid analgesics and derivatives
Ulcer healing	All proton pump inhibitors, sucralfate

dantron alone, or in combination with a faecal softener, is restricted for use in constipation in terminally ill patients of all ages, because animal studies have demonstrated that it has carcinogenic and genotoxic properties.

Osmotic laxatives. Osmotic laxatives include magnesium salts, phosphate enemas, sodium citrate enemas, lactulose and macrogols. These agents retain fluid in the bowel by osmosis or change the water distribution in faeces to produce a softer, bulkier stool. Their ingestion should be accompanied by an appropriate fluid intake.

Rectal preparations of phosphates and sodium citrate are useful for quick relief, within 30 min, and bowel evacuation before abdominal radiological procedures, sigmoidoscopy and surgery. Oral magnesium salts such as the sulphate are also indicated for rapid bowel evacuation and have an effect within 2–5 h.

Lactulose is a semisynthetic disaccharide, which is not absorbed from the gut. It increases faecal weight, volume and bowel movement and must be taken regularly. It may take 48 h or longer to work. It is also useful in the treatment of hepatic encephalopathy since it produces an osmotic diarrhoea of low faecal pH that discourages the growth of ammonia-producing organisms. Macrogols are inert polymers of ethylene oxide which induce a laxative effect by sequestering fluid in the bowel and like lactulose may take 48 h or more to exert an effect.

Faecal softeners/emollient laxatives. Docusate sodium is a non-ionic surfactant that has stool-softening properties. It reduces surface tension, increases the penetration of intestinal fluids into the faecal mass and has weak stimulant properties. Rectal docusate has a rapid onset of action but should not be used in individuals with haemorrhoids or anal fissure.

The classic lubricant, liquid paraffin, has no place in modern therapy. It seeps from the anus and is associated with granulomatous reactions following absorption of small quantities, lipoid pneumonia following aspiration and malabsorption of fat-soluble vitamins.

Diarrhoea

Diarrhoea is defined as the increased passage of loose or watery stools relative to the person's usual bowel habit. It may be accompanied by anorexia, nausea, vomiting, abdominal cramps or bloating. It is not a disease but a sign of an underlying problem such as an infection or gastro-intestinal disorder. The most likely cause of diarrhoea in all age groups is viral or bacterial infection; therefore, the following section primarily focuses on acute infective gastroenteritis but also includes reference to drug-induced diarrhoea. Diarrhoea can be associated with other conditions, for example, irritable bowel syndrome, inflammatory bowel disease, colorectal cancer and malabsorption syndromes, but these will not be covered here.

Acute gastroenteritis is most common in children but the precise incidence is not known because many cases are self-limiting and not reported. Nevertheless, diarrhoeal illness in children leads to high consultation rates with primary care doctors and accounts for one in five consultations in the 0–4 age group. It has been estimated that children under the age of 5 years have between one and three bouts of diarrhoea per year. Children in the same age range account for over 5% of consultations to primary care doctors, with 18,000 children a year in England and Wales being admitted to hospital with rotavirus infection.

The incidence of diarrhoea in adults is, on average, just under one episode per person each year. Many of these cases are thought to be food related, with 22% of those consulting a doctor claiming to have 'food poisoning'. Traveller's diarrhoea is another common cause of diarrhoea. For high-risk travel to areas such as Africa, Asia and South America, the reported incidence is more than 20%. Over recent years, *Escherichia coli* O157 has gained prominence because of a number of outbreaks in different communities associated with severe disease and even death. It is, however, an uncommon cause of diarrhoea, accounting for only 0.1% of all cases.

Aetiology

In the UK, rotavirus and small round structured virus (SRSV) are the most common identified causes of gastro-enteritis in children. In adults, Campylobacter followed by rotavirus are the most common causes, although rates of norovirus have reported to be on the increase. Other identified causes include: the bacteria *E. coli*, Salmonella, Shigella, *Clostridium perfringens* enterotoxin; viruses such as adenovirus and astrovirus; and the protozoa Cryptosporidium, Giardia and Entamoeba. These pathogens produce diarrhoea via a number of methods: for example, enterotoxigenic *E. coli* produce enterotoxins that affect gut function with secretion and loss of fluids; by interfering with normal mucosal function, for example, adherent enteropathogenic *E. coli*; or by causing injury to the mucosa and deeper tissues, for example, enteroinvasive *E. coli* or enterohaemorrhagic *E. coli* such as *E. coli* O157. Other organisms, for example, *Staphylococcus aureus* and *Bacillus cereus*, produce preformed enterotoxins which on ingestion induce rapid-onset diarrhoea and vomiting that usually last less than 12 h.

So-called traveller's diarrhoea frequently affects people travelling from an area of more developed standards of hygiene to a less developed area. In many instances, the cause remains unknown, even after stool culture, but where a pathogen is identified, bacterial infection is responsible in over 80% of cases, and associated with ingestion of contaminated food or water and occurs during or shortly after travel. Bacterial pathogens commonly isolated include *E. coli*, Shigella, Salmonella, Campylobacter, Vibrio and Yersinia species. Viruses (10–15% of cases) and parasites (2–10% of cases), such as norovirus, Giardia, Cryptosporidium and Entamoeba, account for the remainder.

Many medicines, particularly broad-spectrum antibiotics such as ampicillin, erythromycin and neomycin, induce diarrhoea secondary to therapy (Table 14.3). With these antibiotics the mechanism involves the overgrowth of antibiotic-resistant bacteria and fungi in the large bowel after several days of therapy. The diarrhoea is generally self-limiting. However, when the overgrowth involves *Clostridium difficile* and the associated production of its bacterial toxin, life-threatening pseudomembranous colitis may be the outcome.

Signs and symptoms

Acute-onset diarrhoea is associated with loose or watery stools that may be accompanied by anorexia, nausea, vomiting, abdominal cramps, flatulence or bloating. When there is blood in the diarrhoea this is classed as dysentery and indicates the presence of an invasive organism such as Campylobacter, Salmonella, Shigella or *E. coli* O157.

The history of symptom onset is important. The duration of diarrhoea, whether other members of the family and contacts are ill, recent travel abroad, food eaten, antibiotic use and weight loss are all important factors to elucidate. The possibility of underlying diseases such as AIDS or infective proctitis in homosexual men must also be considered.

Dehydration is a common problem in the very young and frail elderly and the signs and symptoms must be recognised.

Table 14.3   Examples of medicines known to cause diarrhoea (defined as very common [>10%] or common [1–10%])

α-Blocker	Prazosin
ACE inhibitor	Lisinopril, perindopril
Angiotensin receptor blocker	Telmisartan
Acetylcholinesterase inhibitor	Donepezil, galantamine, rivastigmine
Antacid	Magnesium salts
Antibacterial	All
Antidiabetic	Metformin, acarbose
Antidepressant	SSRIs, clomipramine, venlafaxine
Antiemetic	Aprepitant, dolasetron
Antiepileptic	Carbamazepine, oxcarbazepine, tiagabine, zonisamide, pregabalin, levtiracetam
Antifungal	Caspofungin, fluconazole, flucytosine, nystatin (in large doses), terbinafine, voriconazole
Antimalarial	Mefloquine
Antiprotozoal	Metronidazole, sodium stibogluconate
Antipsychotic	Aripiprazole
Antiviral	Abacavir, emtricitabine, stavudine, tenofovir, zalcitabine, zidovudine, amprenavir, atazanavir, indinavir, lopinavir, nelfinavir, saquinavir, efavirinez, ganciclovir, valganciclovir, adefovir, oseltamivir, ribavrin, fosamprenavir
β-Blocker	Bisoprolol, carvedilol, nebivolol
Bisphosphonate	Alendronic acid, disodium etidronate, ibandronic acid, risedronate, sodium clodronate, disodium pamidronate, tiludronic acid
Cytokine inhibitor	Adalimumab, infliximab
Cytotoxic	All classes of cytotoxics
Dopaminergic	Levodopa, entacapone
Growth hormone antagonist	Pegvisomant
Immunosuppressant	Ciclosporin, mycophenolate, leflunomide
NSAID	All
Ulcer healing	All proton pump inhibitors
Vaccine	Pediacel (5 vaccines in 1), haemophilus, meningococcal
Miscellaneous	Calcitonin, strontium ranelate, colchicine, dantrolene, olsalazine, anagrelide, nicotinic acid, pancreatin, eplerenone, acamprosate

In children, the severity of dehydration is most accurately determined in terms of weight loss as a percentage of body weight prior to the dehydrating episode. Unfortunately, in the clinical situation pre-illness weight is rarely known; therefore, clinical signs of dehydration must be assessed. National Institute for Health and Clinical Excellence (2009) has issued guidance on assessing the level of dehydration in children under 5 years of age and appropriate fluid management depending on the level of dehydration. Symptoms that could indicate mild dehydration are vague and include tiredness, anorexia, nausea and light-headedness.

Symptoms become more prominent in moderate dehydration and include dry mucous membranes, sunken eyes, decreased skin turgor (pinch test of 1–2 s or longer), tachycardia, apathy, dizziness and postural hypotension. In severe dehydration, the above symptoms are more marked and may also include hypovolaemic shock, oliguria or anuria, cold extremities, a rapid and weak pulse and low or undetectable blood pressure.

Investigations

Before any investigations are undertaken a medication history is required to eliminate antibiotic- and other drug-induced diarrhoeas, or the possibility of a laxative overuse-induced diarrhoea. Testing for *C. difficile*-induced pseudomembranous colitis is indicated in those with severe symptoms or where hospitalisation or antibiotic therapy with lincomycins, broad-spectrum β-lactams or cephalosporins has occurred within the preceding 6 weeks.

In general, stool culture is required in patients who are immunocompromised, with bloody diarrhoea, severe symptoms, where there is no improvement within 48 h. Stool culture is also required when there is a history of recent overseas travel to non-Western countries.

Where the diarrhoea persists for more than 10 days, further investigation should be undertaken to exclude parasites such as Giardia, Entamoeba and Cryptosporidium. Acute, severe or persistent diarrhoea in a homosexual male or patient with AIDS warrants referral for specialist advice.

Treatment

Acute infective diarrhoea, including traveller's diarrhoea, is usually a self-limiting disorder. However, depending on the causative agent, a number of complications may have to be dealt with. Dehydration and electrolyte disturbance can be readily treated but may, if severe, progress to acidosis and circulatory failure with hypoperfusion of vital organs, renal failure and death. Toxic megacolon due to infective colitis has been documented; associated arthritis or Reiter's syndrome may complicate the invasive diarrhoeas of Campylobacter and Yersinia; Salmonella species may infiltrate bones, joints, meninges and the gallbladder; and *E. coli* infection may, for example, be complicated by haemolytic uraemic syndrome.

General measures

Patients should be advised on handwashing and other hygiene-related issues to prevent transmission to other family members. Promotion of handwashing has been shown to decrease diarrhoeal episodes by approximately one-third (Ejemot et al., 2008). Exclusion from work or school until the patient is free of diarrhoea is advised. In acute, self-limiting diarrhoea, children, healthcare workers and food handlers should be symptom free for 48 h before returning to school or work. More exacting criteria for return to work, such as testing for negative stool samples, are rarely required.

In both children and adults, normal feeding should be restarted as soon as possible. In weaned and non-weaned children with gastroenteritis, early feeding after rehydration has been shown to result in higher weight gain, no deterioration or prolongation of the diarrhoea and no increase in vomiting or lactose intolerance (Conway and Ireson, 1989, Sandhu et al., 1997). Similarly, breast-feeding infants should continue to feed throughout the rehydration and maintenance phases of therapy. Avoidance of milk or other lactose-containing food is seldom justified.

Dehydration treatment

Since diarrhoea results in fluid and electrolyte loss, it is important to ensure the affected individual maintains adequate fluid intake. Most patients can be advised to increase their intake of fluids, particularly fruit juices with their glucose and potassium content, and soups because of their sodium chloride content. High-carbohydrate foods such as bread and pasta can also be recommended because they promote glucose and sodium co-transport.

Young children and the frail elderly are prone to diarrhoea-induced dehydration and use of an oral rehydration solution (ORS) is recommended. The formula recommended by the World Health Organization (WHO) contains glucose, sodium, potassium, chloride and bicarbonate in an almost isotonic fluid. A number of similar preparations are available commercially in the form of sachets that require reconstitution in clean water before use (Table 14.4). Glucose concentrations between 80 and 120 mmol/L are needed to optimise sodium absorption in the small intestine. Glucose concentrations in excess of 160 mmol/L will cause an osmotic gradient that will result in increased fluid and electrolyte loss. High sodium solutions, in excess of 90 mmol/L, may lead to hypernatraemia, especially in children, and should be avoided. Until recently, the WHO ORS contained 90 mmol/L sodium, as cholera is more common in developing countries and associated with rapid loss of sodium and potassium. However, a systematic review of trials using a reduced osmolarity ORS (Hahn et al., 2002) concluded that solutions with a reduced

Table 14.4 Composition of oral rehydration solutions						
	Osmolarity (mOsm/L)	Glucose (mmol/L)	Sodium (mmol/L)	Chloride (mmol/L)	Potassium (mmol/L)	Base (mmol/L)
Dioralyte®	240	90	60	60	20	Citrate 10
Electrolade®	251	111	50	40	20	Bicarbonate 30
WHO ORS	245	75	75	65	20	Citrate 10

osmolarity compared to the standard WHO formula were associated with fewer unscheduled intravenous infusions, a trend towards reduced stool output and less vomiting in children with mild-to-moderate diarrhoea. Based on this and other findings, the WHO ORS now has a reduced osmolarity of 245 mOsm/L and contains 75 mmol of sodium.

Commercially available solutions in the UK contain lower sodium concentrations as diarrhoea tends to be isotonic, and therefore replacement of large quantities of sodium is less important and indeed may be harmful. The presence of potassium prevents hypokalaemia occurring in the elderly, especially in those taking diuretics. ORS should be routinely used in both primary and secondary care settings. There appears to be no significant difference between intravenous and oral rehydration (Gavin et al., 1996).

For healthy adults, an appropriate substitute for a rehydration sachet is 1 level teaspoonful of table salt plus 1 tablespoon of sugar in 1 L of drinking water. The volume of ORS to be taken in treating mild-to-moderate diarrhoea is dependent on age. In adults, 2 L of oral rehydration fluid should be given in the first 24 h, followed by unrestricted normal fluids with 200 mL of rehydration solution per loose stool or vomit. For children, 30–50 mL/kg of an ORS should be given over 3–4 h. This can be followed with unrestricted fluids, either with normal fluids alternating with ORS or normal fluids with 10 mL/kg rehydration solution after each loose stool or vomit (Murphy, 1998). The solution is best sipped every 5–10 min rather than drunk in large quantities less frequently.

Care is required in diabetic patients who may need to monitor blood glucose levels more carefully.

Drug treatment

Antimotility agents. In acute diarrhoea, antimotility agents such as loperamide, diphenoxylate and codeine are occasionally useful for symptomatic control in adults who have mild-to-moderate diarrhoea and require relief from associated abdominal cramps. Antimotility agents are not recommended for use in children as trial results appear contradictory and any benefits are small with unacceptable levels of side effects observed. Management should initially focus on prevention or treatment of fluid and electrolyte depletion before antimotility agents are considered.

Antimotility agents should be avoided in severe gastroenteritis or dysentery because of the possibility of precipitating ileus or toxic megacolon. All appear to have comparable efficacy but loperamide is the drug of choice given its low incidence of CNS effects.

Diphenoxylate. Diphenoxylate is a synthetic opioid available as co-phenotrope in combination with a subtherapeutic dose of atropine. The atropine is present to discourage abuse but may cause atropinic effects in susceptible individuals. Administration of co-phenotrope at the recommended dosage carries minimal risk of dependence. However, prolonged use or administration of high doses may produce a morphine-type dependence. Its adverse effect profile resembles that of morphine.

In cases of suspected overdose, signs may be delayed for up to 48 h. Young children are particularly susceptible to diphenoxylate overdose where as few as 10 tablets of co-phenotrope may be fatal.

Concurrent use of diphenoxylate with monoamine oxidase inhibitors can precipitate a hypertensive crisis, while the action of CNS depressants such as barbiturates, tranquillisers and alcohol is enhanced.

Loperamide. Loperamide is a synthetic opioid analogue that exerts its action by binding to opiate receptors in the gut wall, reducing propulsive peristalsis, increasing intestinal transit time, enhancing the resorption of water and electrolytes, reducing gut secretions and increasing anal sphincter tone. In uncomplicated diarrhoea, it may have an effect within 1 h of oral administration. It is relatively free of CNS effects at therapeutic doses, although CNS depression may be seen in overdose, particularly in children. As it undergoes hepatic metabolism it should be used with caution in patients with hepatic dysfunction.

Codeine and morphine. The constipating side effect of the opioid analgesics codeine and morphine may be used to treat diarrhoea. Both are susceptible to misuse and, given in large doses, may induce tolerance and psychological and physical dependence. Morphine may still be obtained in combination with agents such as the adsorbent kaolin, for example, kaolin and morphine. However, it has no evidence of efficacy in the treatment of diarrhoea and should not be recommended.

Bismuth subsalicylate. Bismuth subsalicylate is an insoluble complex of trivalent bismuth and salicylate that has been shown to be effective in reducing stool frequency. It possesses antimicrobial activity on the basis of its bismuth content while the salicylate is considered to confer antisecretory properties. At therapeutic doses it is relatively free from side effects, although it may cause blackening of the tongue and stool. The relatively large quantity of the liquid preparation that has to be consumed is seen as a disadvantage.

Antimicrobials. Antibiotics are generally not recommended in diarrhoea associated with acute infective gastroenteritis. Inappropriate use will only contribute further to the problem of resistant organisms. There is, however, a place for antibiotics in patients with positive stool culture where the symptoms are not receding or for travellers' diarrhoea (De Bruyn et al., 2000). In patients presenting with dysentery or suspected exposure to bacterial infection, treatment with a quinolone, for example, ciprofloxacin, may be appropriate. However, quinolones are not without their problems: they may cause tendon damage or induce convulsions in epileptics, in situations that predispose to seizures, and in patients taking NSAIDs. Their use in adolescents is also not recommended because of an association with arthropathy.

Where Campylobacter is the suspect causative organism, patients with severe symptoms or dysentery should receive early treatment with erythromycin or ciprofloxacin. Severe symptoms or dysentery associated with Shigella can also be treated with ciprofloxacin. Nalidixic acid can be used in children and trimethoprim may be appropriate in pregnant women where resistance is not a problem.

The use of antibiotics in patients with Salmonella is not generally recommended because of the likelihood that excretion is prolonged. Antibiotics may, however, be indicated in the very young and the immunocompromised. The benefit of antibiotic use in enterohaemorrhagic infection, for example, *E. coli* O157, is less clear. In this situation, there is evidence that antibiotics cause toxins to be released which may lead to haemolytic uraemic syndrome.

In both amoebic dysentery and giardiasis, metronidazole is the drug of choice. Diloxanide is also used in amoebic dysentery to ensure eradication of the intestinal disease. Antibiotics are not indicated in the treatment of cryptosporidiosis in immunocompromised individuals.

Probiotics. Probiotics have been defined as components of microbial cells or microbial cell preparations that have a beneficial effect on health. Well-known probiotics include lactic acid bacteria and the yeast Saccharomyces. The rationale for their use in infectious diarrhoea is that they act against enteric pathogens by competing for available nutrients and binding sites, making gut contents acid and increasing immune responses. A Cochrane review (Allen et al., 2003) concluded that whilst probiotics in individual studies appeared moderately effective as adjunctive therapy, there were insufficient studies of specific probiotic regimens to inform the development of evidence-based treatment guidelines.

Zinc. The use of zinc has been reviewed in the treatment of diarrhoea in children in developing countries (Lazzerini et al., 2008). In this context, zinc has been shown to be of value in children older than 6 months, probably because they have some prior, underlying deficiency of zinc.

Rotavirus vaccine. Rotavirus vaccine has been shown to protect against the most common strains of rotavirus (G1 and G3), although the benefits of the vaccine are dependant on the type of vaccine used, with rhesus and human rotavirus the most efficacious (Soares-Weiser, 2004).

Some of the common therapeutic problems in the management of individuals with constipation and diarrhoea are outlined in Table 14.5.

Table 14.5 Common therapeutic problems in constipation and diarrhoea

Problem	Comment
Constipation	
Bulk laxative, for example ispaghula, taken at bedtime	Drugs such as ispaghula should not be taken before going to bed because of risk of oesophageal blockage
Urine changes colour	Anthraquinone glycosides, for example senna, are excreted by the kidney and may colour urine yellowish-brown to red colour, depending on pH
Patient claims dietary and fluid advice ineffective in resolving constipation	May find high-fibre diet difficult to adhere to, socially unacceptable, and expect result in less than 4 weeks
Patient taking docusate complains of unpleasant aftertaste or burning sensation	Advise to take with plenty of fluid after ingestion
Sterculia as Normacol® and Normacol Plus® granules or sachets	The granules should be placed dry on the tongue and swallowed immediately with plenty of water or a cool drink. They can also be sprinkled onto and taken with soft food such as yoghurt
Methylcellulose (Celevac®)	Each tablet should be taken with at least 300 mL of liquid
Diarrhoea	
Antimotility agent requested for a young child	Antimotility agents must be avoided in young children or patients with severe gastroenteritis or dysentery
Antimotility agent requested by patient with persistent diarrhoea (>10 days)	Antimotility agent inappropriate. Stool culture required to exclude parasitic infection such as Giardia, Entamoeba and Cryptosporidium
Adult with diarrhoea stops eating and drinking to allow diarrhoea to settle	Patient should eat and drink as normally as possible. Plenty of fluids required to prevent dehydration. Fruit juice (glucose and potassium), soup (salt), bread and pasta (carbohydrate) are of particular benefit
Reconstitution of oral rehydration solution	Each sachet of Diorolyte® and Electrolade® requires 200 mL of water. They should be discarded after 1 h after preparation unless stored in a fridge when they may be kept for 24 h

Case studies

Case 14.1

Mr J, a man in his 30s, asks to speak to the pharmacist. He has constipation and has taken some medicine, lactulose, but he is still finding it difficult to go to the toilet. He asks for a stronger laxative.

Question

What further information do you need to obtain to be in a position to help Mr J?

Answer

Constipation is rarely a symptom of sinister pathology in someone of Mr J's age. The most likely cause is a diet low in fibre and inadequate fluid intake. Establish the duration and nature of the problem and discuss with Mr J his usual diet. Determine if there has been any change to his diet recently, which may have precipitated the constipation. Social factors also play a role in constipation, so it is prudent to ask if there have been any life changes such as a loss of job or difficulties with family life. If his replies to the questions raise no suspicion of underlying medical problems then dietary advice only may be needed. However, since he has already taken lactulose it is likely he will persist in his request for a suitable laxative. Question Mr J on how he took the lactulose and for how long. Patients often have misconceptions on how quickly a medicine will work. A stimulant laxative may be a suitable alternative for Mr J as it has a quicker onset of action.

Case 14.2

Mr A's mother has recently moved in with his family following the death of his father 4 months ago. Although she was formerly a sprightly 78 year old, she is now withdrawn, eats little of the meals prepared for her and no longer goes for her daily walks. Mr A knows she is taking medicine for a long-standing heart complaint and has recently started taking antidepressants. She is complaining of constipation.

Question

Mr A would like to know if there is any medicine suitable to help his mother.

Answer

Constipation is a common problem in the elderly. Activity levels often diminish and many also suffer from medicine-induced constipation exacerbated by reduced muscle tone. Pain on defaecation associated with haemorrhoids is also a common contributory factor. The elderly often have poor dental status or false teeth and consequently avoid high-fibre foods because they are more difficult to chew.

In the case of Mr A's mother, the history provides little insight into the duration of the problem, although there are a number of factors that warrant further investigation. Clearly, a reduction in physical activity has occurred and her diet and fluid intake may have changed. The death of her husband and loss of independence are significant lifestyle issues for Mr A's mother that cannot readily be addressed and probably account for the recent introduction of antidepressants. The identity of her 'heart medicine' may reveal a drug-induced factor that could have been enhanced by the recent prescription for antidepressants. It is also unclear whether she has been constipated previously.

Appropriate exercise, proper diet and sufficient fluid may be the only key actions that need to be taken.

Case 14.3

Mr B is a busy 45-year-old executive who works for a large multinational company. He has noted blood in his stools over the past 2 weeks and for 3 days has had continuous abdominal discomfort. He has discussed his symptoms with his wife and they suspect haemorrhoids are the cause. Mr B is going away on business in 6 days and seeks your advice on a suitable treatment.

Question

What advice should be given to Mr B?

Answer

Blood in the stool is not necessarily serious. If the blood appears fresh and can only be seen on the surface of the stool it is likely the source is the anus or distal colon. It is probably caused by straining and bleeding from haemorrhoids or an anal fissure. Similarly, if the blood appears as specks or as a smear on the toilet paper after defaecation, this is also likely to indicate haemorrhoids, particularly if such a diagnosis has been made previously following clinical examination.

If the blood is mixed with the faeces and has a dark or 'tarry' appearance then a more serious underlying cause is possible. The darker the faeces, the more suggestive they are that there has been an upper GI bleed or a substantial loss of blood from the large bowel. If this is the case the patient should have a proper clinical examination.

Iron or bismuth tablets can cause darkened stools, so it is important to take a medication history from the patient.

However, given Mr B's age, recent onset of symptoms and the presence of continuous abdominal pain accompanying the constipation, a thorough clinical examination is required to eliminate sinister pathology such as bowel obstruction caused by a tumour or diverticular disease.

Case 14.4

A 7-year-old boy in previous good health was admitted to hospital with bloody diarrhoea and dehydration 4 days after attending a children's birthday party. He was treated with intravenous fluids and given nothing by mouth. The day after admission to hospital a colonoscopy revealed haemorrhagic colitis. His diarrhoea seemed to be improving up to day 5 when he experienced a generalised convulsion following which he was transferred to a children's intensive care bed. He was irritable, pale and hypertensive, and an emergency laboratory report revealed thrombocytopenia, hyponatraemia and hyperkalaemia.

Questions

1. What is the likely diagnosis in this child?
2. What specific therapy is required?

Answers

1. This patient probably has haemolytic uraemic syndrome caused by *E. coli* O157. Haemolytic uraemic syndrome is the most common form of acquired renal insufficiency in young children. It is characterised by nephropathy, thrombocytopenia and microangiopathic haemolytic anaemia. Although there are a number of potential causative factors, the most common is the toxin-producing O157 strain of *E. coli*. In 1996, 21 people died from *E. coli* O157 after eating contaminated meat from a butcher's shop in Scotland. In 2001, 13 Girl Guides and their leader contracted *E. coli* O157 after camping in a field in Inverclyde, Scotland, previously grazed by sheep and in 2005 more than 158 children from 42 schools in South Wales were affected by eating contaminated meat, one of whom died.

   The syndrome typically has a pro-drome of bloody diarrhoea occurring 5–7 days before onset of renal insufficiency. Colonoscopy is usually non-specific and shows haemorrhagic colitis. At diagnosis most children are pale and very irritable. Hypertension and hyponatraemia may be associated with convulsions and are generally a consequence of a disorder of fluid and salt balance. Laboratory findings may include anaemia and thrombocytopenia, hyponatraemia, hyperkalaemia, hypocalcaemia and metabolic acidosis. The kidney typically shows signs of glomerular endothelial injury. Capillary thrombosis is quite prominent but with no evidence of immune complex deposition. Similar findings can usually be seen in all other organs including the brain, liver and intestine.

2. Treatment is usually supportive. Fluid and electrolyte balance need to be corrected and the hypertension controlled. In cases with prolonged oliguria or anuria, peritoneal dialysis may be used. Approximately 85% of patients recover normal renal function.

Case 14.5

Mr G is planning to travel to Mexico on business. He was last there 6 months ago but was incapacitated with diarrhoea for 3 of 6 days in a busy work schedule. He does not want a repeat experience on his forthcoming visit and seeks advice about taking a course of antibiotics with him to use as empirical treatment should the need arise.

Questions

1. Is there any evidence that antibiotics are of benefit in traveller's diarrhoea?
2. Are there any problems associated with empirical use of antibiotics in traveller's diarrhoea?

Answers

1. The empirical use of antibiotics has been shown to increase the cure rate in individuals suffering from traveller's diarrhoea. Studies in travellers including students, package tourists, military personnel and volunteers have compared antibiotic use against placebo (De Bruyn et al., 2000). The antibiotics studied have included aztreonam, ciprofloxacin, co-trimoxazole, norfloxacin, ofloxacin and trimethoprim given for durations varying from a single dose to a 5-day treatment course. Overall, antibiotics increased the cure rate at 72 h (defined as cessation of unformed stools or less than one unformed stool/24 h) without additional symptoms.

2. The use of antibiotics in the treatment of traveller's diarrhoea does have problems. Adverse effects in up to 18% of recipients have been reported with gastro-intestinal (cramp, nausea, anorexia), dermatological (rash) and respiratory (cough, sore throat) symptoms the most frequently reported. Antibiotic-resistant isolates have also been reported following the use of ciprofloxacin, co-trimoxazole and norfloxacin. In the USA but not the UK, rifaximin, a semi-synthetic rifamycin derivative that is little absorbed from the gastro-intestinal tract, is licensed for the treatment of traveller's diarrhoea.

References

Allen, S.J., Okoko, B., Martinez, E., et al., 2003. Probiotics for treating infectious diarrhoea. Cochrane Database Syst. Rev. 4, Art No. CD003048. doi: 10.1002/14651858.CD003048.pub2.

Conway, S.P., Ireson, A., 1989. Acute gastroenteritis in well nourished infants: comparison of four feeding regimens. Arch. Dis. Child 64, 87–91.

De Bruyn, G., Hahn, S., Borwick, A., 2000. Antibiotic treatment for travellers' diarrhoea. Cochrane Database Syst. Rev. 3, Art. No. CD002242. doi: 10.1002/14651858.CD002242.

Ejemot, R.I., Ehiri, J.E., Meremikwu, M.M., et al., 2008. Hand washing for preventing diarrhoea. Cochrane Database Syst. Rev. 1, Art. No. CD004265. doi: 10.1002/14651858.CD004265.pub2.

Frizelle, F., Barclay, M., 2007. Constipation in Adults. Clinical Evidence. BMJ Publishing Group Ltd, London, Available at: http://clinicalevidence.bmj.com/ceweb/index.jsp.

Gavin, N., Merrick, N., Davidson, B., 1996. Efficacy of glucose-based oral rehydration therapy. Pediatrics 98, 45–51.

Hahn, S., Kim, Y., Garner, P., 2002. Reduced osmolarity oral rehydration solution for treating dehydration due to diarrhoea in children. Cochrane Database Syst. Rev. 1, Art No. CD002847. doi: 10.1002/14651858.CD002847.

Lazzerini, M., Ronfani, L., 2008. Oral zinc for treating diarrhoea in children. Cochrane Database Syst. Rev. 3, Art No. CD005436. doi: 10.1002/14651858.CD005436.pub2.

Longstreth, G.F., Thompson, W.G., Chey, W.D., et al., 2006. Functional bowel disorders. Gastroenterology 130, 1480–1491.

MeReC, 2004. Approximate dietary fibre content of selected foods. MeReC Bull. 14 (Suppl. 6), 1.

Murphy, M.S., 1998. Guidelines for managing acute gastroenteritis based on a systematic review of published research. Arch. Dis. Child 79, 279–284.

National Institute for Health and Clinical Excellence, 2009. Diarrhoea and Vomiting in Children: Diarrhoea and Vomiting Caused by Gastroenteritis: Diagnosis, Assessment and Management in Children Younger than 5 Years. Clinical Guideline 84. NICE, London, Available at: http://guidance.nice.org.uk/nicemedia/live/11846/43815/43815.doc.

Sandhu, B.K., Isolauri, E., Walker-Smith, J.A., et al., 1997. A multicentre study on behalf of the European Society of Paediatric Gastroenterology and Nutrition Working Group on Acute Diarrhoea: early feeding in childhood gastroenteritis. J. Pediatr. Gastroenterol. Nutr. 24, 522–527.

Soares-Weiser, K., Goldberg, E., Tamimi, G., et al., 2004. Rotavirus vaccine for preventing diarrhoea. Cochrane Database Syst. Rev. 1, Art No. CD002848. doi: 10.1002/14651858.CD002848.pub2.

Tramonte, S.M., Brand, M.B., Mulrow, C.D., et al., 1997. The treatment of chronic constipation in adults. A systematic review. J. Gen. Int. Med. 12, 15–24.

Further reading

Alonso-Coello, P., Guyatt, G., Heels-Ansdell, D., et al., 2005. Laxatives for the treatment of hemorrhoids. Cochrane Database Syst. Rev. 4, Art No. CD004649. doi: 10.1002/14651858.CD004649.pub2.

Bartlett, J.G., 2002. Antibiotic-associated diarrhoea. N. Engl. J. Med. 346, 334–339.

Borum, M.L., 2001. Constipation: evaluation and management. Prim. Care 28, 577–590.

Dupont, H.L., 2009. Systematic review: the epidemiology and clinical features of travellers' diarrhoea. Aliment. Pharmacol. Ther. 30, 187–196.

Khin, M.U., Nyunt-Nyunt, W., Khin, M., et al., 1985. Effect on clinical outcome of breast feeding during acute diarrhoea. Br. Med. J. 290, 587–589.

Pappagallo, M., 2001. Incidence, prevalence and management of opioid bowel dysfunction. Am. J. Surg. 182 (Suppl. 5A), 115–185.

Sellin, J.H., 2001. The pathophysiology of diarrhoea. Clin. Transplant. 15 (Suppl. 4), 2–10.

Xing, J.H., Soffer, E.E., 2001. Adverse effects of laxatives. Dis. Colon. Rectum. 44, 1201–1209.

15 Adverse effects of drugs on the liver

B. E. Featherstone

Key points

- Approximately 20–30% of acute liver failure cases are attributed to drugs.
- Risk of drug-induced liver disorders increases with age and is generally more common in women.
- Generally, drug-induced liver damage is either dose-related or idiosyncratic.
- Drugs can cause all types of liver disorder and should always be considered in patients presenting with liver-related problems.
- The clinical features of drug-induced hepatotoxicity vary widely, depending upon the type of liver damage caused.
- Treatment of drug-induced hepatotoxicity relies on correct diagnosis, prompt withdrawal of the causative agent and supportive therapy.
- Patients given potentially hepatotoxic drugs should be monitored regularly and taught how to recognise signs of liver dysfunction and advised to report symptoms immediately.
- Drugs causing dose-related hepatic toxicity may do so at lower doses in patients with liver disease than in patients with normal liver function and idiosyncratic reactions may occur more frequently in patients with existing liver disease.
- Any new drug has the potential to cause hepatotoxicity. Post-marketing surveillance is important to highlight new potential hepatotoxic effects.

An adverse drug reaction (ADR) is an effect that is unintentional, noxious and occurs at doses used for diagnosis, prophylaxis and treatment. A hepatic drug reaction is an ADR which predominantly affects the liver.

Drugs can induce almost all forms of acute or chronic liver disease, with some drugs producing more than one type of hepatic reaction. Although not a particularly common form of ADR, drugs should always be considered as a possible cause of liver disease.

Epidemiology

The incidence of drug-induced liver disease (DILD) has continued to rise steadily since the late 1960s, although the incidence of idiosyncratic reactions for most drugs remains low, occurring at therapeutic doses from 1 in every 1000 patients to 1 in every 100,000 patients. DILD is not usually life-threatening; however, for the small number of patients who develop drug-induced acute liver failure (ALF) the prognosis is poor, with a 60–80% mortality rate, unless they receive a liver transplant. The incidence and severity of DILD is shown in Fig. 15.1. It is estimated that 15–40% of ALF cases may be attributable to drugs. Classification of ALF suggests three classes: hyperacute, acute and subacute (Table 15.1).

In the early 1990s, acute overdose with paracetamol accounted for 30,000–40,000 hospital admissions and over half the cases of ALF referred to liver units. It is the definite cause of approximately 100 deaths a year in the UK. ALF induced by paracetamol has become an important indication for liver transplantation. Hepatotoxicity induced by such drugs as halothane, the antituberculous agents (isoniazid and rifampicin), psychotropics, antibiotics and cytotoxic drugs still continue to cause concern.

Many drugs cause elevated liver enzymes with apparently no clinically significant adverse effect, although in a few patients there may be significant hepatotoxicity. For example, isoniazid

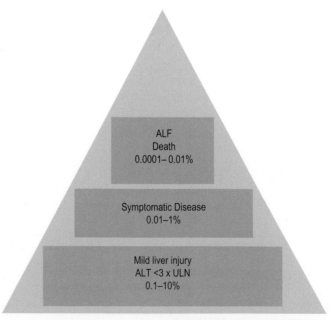

Fig. 15.1 The spectrum of drug-induced liver disease. ALF, acute liver failure; ALT, alanine transferase; ULN, upper limit of normal; % incidence of population taking medication.

Table 15.1 Characteristics of the different types of acute liver failure (Richardson and O'Grady, 2002)

Characteristic	Hyperacute	Acute	Subacute
Transition time from jaundice to encephalopathy	0–7 days	8–28 days	29–84 days
Cerebral oedema	Common	Common	Rare
Renal failure	Early	Late	Late
Ascites	Rare	Rare	Common
Coagulation disorder	Marked	Marked	Modest
Prognosis	Moderate	Poor	Poor

Table 15.2 Examples of drugs that elevate liver enzymes

Drug	Percentage of patients with increase in transaminases
Cefaclor	11%
Cefixime	0.7%
Ciprofloxacin	5%
Chlorpromazine	50%
Diclofenac	15%
Donepezil	MHRA reports[a]
Efavirenz	4%
Heparin/LWMH	5%
Isoniazid	10–36%
Naproxen	4%
Norfloxacin	0.1%
Nevirapine	12%
Niacin	50%
Rifampicin	15–30%
Sodium valproate	11%
SSRIs	MHRA reports[a]
Statins	1–2%
Sulphonamides	10%

[a]Available at: http://www.mhra.gov.uk

causes elevated liver enzymes in 10–36% of patients taking the drug as a single agent. However, only 1% suffer significant hepatotoxicity, with the liver function tests (LFTs) of the majority returning to normal if therapy is discontinued. Other examples of drugs that elevate liver enzymes are shown in Table 15.2.

Although it is not possible to identify patients who will suffer ADRs manifesting in hepatic toxicity, a number of risk factors have been identified.

Risk factors

Pre-existing liver disease

Pre-existing liver disease may increase the risk of developing drug-induced hepatic injury with agents such as methotrexate, cytotoxic agents, aspirin and sodium valproate. In general, patients with liver disease are more likely to suffer ADRs. A past medical history of DILD from any medication has been shown to be a predictor of future DILD from other drugs.

Age

It is generally accepted that the elderly are at an increased risk of ADRs. There are multiple reasons for this, including higher exposure rates and decreased metabolism. Drug-induced hepatic injury is more likely to occur in elderly patients than in those under 35 years of age. Similarly, halothane hepatitis and isoniazid or chlorpromazine hepatotoxicity are more likely in patients over 40 years of age. The severity of the reactions also appears to increase with age, especially in those over 60 years. Sodium valproate toxicity, on the other hand, demonstrates an increased risk of developing serious or fatal hepatotoxicity in those under 3 years, with risk decreasing as age advances. Aspirin is an example of another drug causing hepatotoxicity, specifically in children. Reye's syndrome in children has been linked to the use of aspirin following a viral illness; it is life-threatening and associated with coma, seizures and liver failure. A cholestatic presentation of DILD is more common in older patients and hepatocellular damage is generally more common in younger patients.

Gender

The frequency of drug-induced hepatotoxicity is thought to be more common in females than males, particularly with halothane, isoniazid, flucloxacillin, chlorpromazine, erythromycin and nitrofurantoin. However, evidence from a recent series of more than 600 cases of DILD found that female gender was not a risk factor. There is weak evidence of a gender difference in toxicity of sodium valproate, being more common in boys before puberty and in females after puberty. Cholestatic jaundice associated with co-amoxiclav has been reported to be more common in males than females.

Genetics

Genetic differences that affect an individual's ability to metabolise certain drugs may predispose to DILD. For example, both fast and slow acetylators may be more susceptible to isoniazid-induced liver damage. The conventional view is that rapid acetylators are at risk of increased toxic reactions due to transformation of acetylhydrazine by cytochrome P450 into a reactive metabolite; other studies suggest slow acetylation may result in toxicity due to formation of hydrazine, which is toxic in itself. When starting, isoniazid monitoring of LFTs is recommended monthly for the first 3 months, as toxicity is most likely to occur early in therapy.

Halothane-induced injury has been reported for multiple family members.

It is thought that a genetic predisposition to allergic forms of drug hypersensitivity could be a factor in some types of liver disease. Flucloxacillin liver injury has been associated with the human leukocyte antigen B*5701. Having this HLA haptotype confers an 80-fold increase in susceptibility to liver injury with flucloxacillin.

Enzyme induction

Alcohol, rifampicin and other drugs that induce cytochrome P450 isoenzyme 2El potentiate the risk of hepatotoxicity with other drugs such as paracetamol, isoniazid and halothane. The role of alcohol as a risk factor for DILD is, however, not clear-cut and acute and chronic alcohol consumption may have different effects.

Concomitant therapy with other anticonvulsants, particularly phenytoin and phenobarbital, is a risk factor for toxicity with sodium valproate, where 90% of cases of liver injury are associated with combination therapy.

Polypharmacy

A typical example of this is seen with NSAIDs. The risk of liver disease with NSAIDs is normally extremely low but is increased when NSAIDs are used with other hepatotoxic drugs.

Concurrent diseases and pregnancy

Pre-existing renal disease, diabetes, pregnancy and poor nutrition may all affect the ability of the liver to metabolise drugs effectively and may put the patient at risk of developing liver damage. Table 15.3 summarises the host factors that may predispose a patient to drug hepatotoxicity.

Aetiology

Drug-induced hepatotoxicity may present as an acute insult that may or may not progress to chronic disease, or it can present as an insidious development of chronic disease. The type of lesion may be cytotoxic (cellular destruction) or cholestatic (impaired bile flow). Cytotoxic damage may be further classified as necrotic (cell death) or steatic (fatty degeneration). The liver damage resulting from drug toxicity often presents as a mixed picture of cytotoxic and cholestatic injury.

Table 15.3 Examples of host factors that predispose to drug hepatotoxicity

Host factor	Drug example
Pre-existing liver disease	Methotrexate, aspirin, sodium valproate

Age
  Older
  Younger
	
	Halothane, isoniazid, chlorpromazine, co-amoxiclav, nitrofuratoin
	Aspirin, sodium valproate

Gender
  Female
  Male
	
	Halothane, isoniazid, nitrofurantoin, flucloxacillin, chlorpromazine, erythromycin
	Sodium valproate (in prepubescent boys), co-amoxiclav

Genetics	Halothane, chlorpromazine, phenytoin, carbamazepine, phenobarbital, paracetamol, flucloxacillin
Enzyme induction	Paracetamol, halothane, isoniazid, sodium valproate
Polypharmacy	NSAIDs if used with other hepatotoxic drugs Isoniazid with rifampicin or pyrazinamide Sodium valproate with phenytoin Paracetamol with zidovudine

Concurrent diseases
  Diabetes mellitus
  Renal failure
  Malnutrition
	
	Methotrexate
	Allopurinol, i.v. tetracycline
	Paracetamol

HIV positive with hepatitis C or B co-infection	Antiretroviral agents

Table 15.4 Characteristics of intrinsic and idiosyncratic hepatotoxic reactions

	Intrinsic toxicity		Idiosyncratic toxicity
Mechanism	Direct toxicity	Metabolic abnormality	Hypersensitivity reaction
dose-dependent	Yes	No	No
Predictable	Yes	No	No
Latency	Hours	Weeks to months	1–5 weeks
Type of injury	Usually necrosis	Any	Any
Clinical features	Acute liver failure	Increased liver enzymes, hepatitis, jaundice	Fever, rash, eosinophilia, arthralgias, hepatitis

The mechanisms of drug-induced hepatic damage can be divided into intrinsic (type A) and idiosyncratic (type B) hepatotoxicity (Table 15.4). Intrinsic hepatotoxicity is predictable, dose-dependent and usually has a short latency period ranging from hours to weeks. The majority of individuals who take a toxic dose are affected and exhibit the same type of injury. Examples are paracetamol, salicylates, methotrexate and tetracycline. Other examples are presented in Table 15.5. Toxicity may be avoided by ensuring the doses listed are not exceeded.

Idiosyncratic reactions occur at a low frequency, typically less than 1 in 100 individuals who are exposed to the drug. The latency period is variable, ranging from 5 to 90 days from the initial ingestion of the drug. The type of injury is less predictable and not dose-related. This type of reaction may be due to either drug hypersensitivity or a metabolic abnormality. Examples of drugs that induce idiosyncratic reactions are chlorpromazine, halothane and isoniazid.

The precise mechanisms resulting in DILD are often not completely understood, although injury to the hepatocytes may result directly from interference with intracellular function, membrane integrity or indirectly by immune-mediated damage to cells.

Necrosis

Necrosis is characterised by cytotoxic cellular breakdown (hepatocellular destruction) and is generally associated with a poor prognosis. Drugs commonly associated with DILD have a variable propensity to cause hepatic necrosis. For example, hepatic necrosis has been reported in 3% of cases with co-amoxiclav DILD compared to 89% in individuals with halothane-induced liver injury cases.

Paracetamol causes hepatic necrosis when its normal metabolic pathway is saturated. Subsequent metabolism occurs by an alternative pathway that produces a toxic metabolite which covalently binds to liver cell proteins and causes necrosis.

Steatosis

In steatosis, hepatocytes become filled with small droplets of lipid (microvesicular fatty liver) or occasionally with lipid droplets that are much larger (macrovesicular fatty liver).

Table 15.5 Examples of dose-related drug-induced hepatotoxicity

Drug	Toxic dose
Paracetamol	Single dose >10 g
Tetracycline	>2 g daily (oral), increased risk of toxicity in pregnancy and renal failure
Methotrexate	Weekly dose >15 mg Cumulative dose >2 g in 3 years, increased risk of toxicity in pre-existing liver disease, alcohol abuse, diabetes
6-Mercaptopurine	>2.5 mg/kg
Vitamin A	Chronic use of 40,000 units daily
Cyclophosphamide	Daily dose >400 mg/m²
Salicylates	Chronic use >2 g daily
Anabolic steroids	High dose >1 month
Oral contraceptive	Increased risk with higher oestrogen content, older preparations Duration of treatment
Iron	Single dose >1 g

Tetracyclines are thought to cause steatosis by interfering with synthesis of lipoproteins that normally remove triglycerides from the liver.

Cholestasis

Some drugs injure bile ducts and cause partial or complete obstruction of the common bile duct, resulting in retention of bile acids and the condition known as cholestasis. Cholestasis caused by anabolic and contraceptive steroids is due to inhibition of bilirubin excretion from the hepatocyte into the bile.

The penicillins, although commonly associated with allergic drug reactions, are a very rare cause of liver disease. The isoxazoyl group present in the synthetic β-lactamase resistant oxypenicillins has been implicated as a cause of liver injury. Acute cholestatic hepatitis has increasingly been reported during treatment with flucloxacillin, and in some countries this has become the most important cause of drug-induced cholestatic hepatitis. The incidence appears to be about twice that of the related isoxazoyl penicillins cloxacillin and dicloxacillin. Moreover, there is likely to be underreporting due to a delay in onset of up to 42 days after stopping treatment. Female sex, age over 55 years, longer courses and high daily doses also seem to be associated with a higher risk of liver reaction to flucloxacillin.

Rifampicin causes hyperbilirubinaemia by inhibiting uptake of bilirubin by the hepatocyte as well as inhibiting bilirubin excretion into bile. This is generally not an indication for interrupting rifampicin therapy, although liver function will need to be closely monitored. Other therapeutic agents affect sinusoidal or endothelial cells, which may result in veno-occlusive disease or fibrosis. Vitamin A affects the fat storing cells, causing toxicity that leads to fibrosis.

Pathophysiology

The range of DILDs is illustrated in Table 15.6. Increased serum level of hepatobiliary enzymes without clinical liver disease occurs with variable frequency between drugs but for some agents it may occur in up to half the patients who receive a drug. This may reflect subclinical liver injury.

Hepatocellular necrosis

In severe cases, acute hepatocellular necrosis presents with jaundice and LFT abnormalities, including a modestly raised alkaline phosphatase and a markedly elevated alanine aminotransferase level of up to 200 times the upper limit of the reference range. Prolongation of the prothrombin time occurs but depends on the severity of the injury, increasing dramatically in severe cases. Microscopy reveals necrosis of the hepatocytes in a characteristic pattern.

Steatosis

Steatosis (fatty liver) is the accumulation of fat droplets within liver cells and is associated with abnormal LFTs, although the elevation of alanine aminotransferase is not as high as that seen in acute hepatocellular necrosis. Hyperammonia, hypoglycaemia, acidosis and clotting factor deficiency may also be present. Histologically, the liver damage resembles the acute fatty liver of pregnancy. Fat distribution within the hepatocyte is either microvesicular, as occurs with tetracycline, aspirin and sodium valproate, or macrovesicular where the hepatocyte cell nucleus is displaced to the periphery by a single large fat droplet. This type of damage occurs typically with steroids, methotrexate, alcohol and amiodarone.

A less severe, more chronic form of fatty liver, steatohepatitis, also occurs. Steatohepatitis differs from diffuse fatty

Table 15.6 Examples of adverse drug reactions on the liver

Adverse reaction	Drugs associated with reaction
Hepatocellular necrosis	Paracetamol Propylthiouracil Salicylates Iron salts Allopurinol Dantrolene Halothane Ketoconazole Isoniazid Mithramycin Cocaine 'Ecstasy' (methylenedioxymethamphetamine, MDMA)
Fatty liver	Amiodarone Tetracyclines Steroids Sodium valproate L-Asparaginase
Cholestasis	Oral contraceptives Carbimazole Anabolic steroids Ciclosporin
Cholestasis with hepatitis	Chlorpromazine Tricyclic antidepressants Erythromycin Flucloxacillin Co-amoxiclav ACE inhibitors Sulphonamides Sulphonylureas Phenytoin NSAIDs Cimetidine Ranitidine Trazodone
Granulomatous hepatitis	Phenytoin Allopurinol Carbamazepine Clofibrate Hydralazine Sulphonamides Sulphonylureas
Acute hepatitis	Dantrolene Isoniazid Phenytoin
Chronic active hepatitis	Methyldopa Nitrofurantoin Isoniazid
Fibrosis and cirrhosis	Methotrexate Methyldopa Vitamin A (dose-related)
Vascular disorders	Azathioprine Dactinomycin Dacarbazine

change. Notably, the clinical symptoms and biochemistry resemble chronic parenchymal disease and the histology is similar to that seen in alcoholic hepatitis. Amiodarone is an example of a drug that can cause chronic steatohepatitis associated with phospholipidosis.

Cholestasis

Cholestasis without hepatitis is associated with a raised bilirubin and a normal or minimally raised alanine aminotransferase level. No inflammation or hepatocellular necrosis is seen. In contrast, cholestasis associated with hepatitis presents with raised bilirubin, alanine aminotransferase and alkaline phosphatase levels and a certain amount of liver damage.

Granulomatous hepatitis

Granulomatous hepatitis occurs with modestly elevated LFTs and, usually, normal synthetic liver function. Histology reveals granulomas and tissue eosinophilia.

Acute hepatitis

Acute hepatitis resembles viral hepatitis with LFTs raised in proportion to the severity of the hepatocellular damage. The best indicator of severity is the prothrombin time. Histologically, necrosis and cellular degeneration are seen in combination with an inflammatory infiltrate.

Chronic active hepatitis

Chronic active hepatitis may present as an acute injury or progress to cirrhosis. Serum transaminases are usually raised and albumin is low. The histology resembles that of autoimmune chronic active hepatitis and is associated with circulating autoantibodies. Methyldopa is an example of a drug that can cause chronic active hepatitis.

Fibrosis

In patients with fibrosis, the serum transaminase levels may be only slightly raised, and are not good predictors of hepatic damage. Microscopy shows deposition of fibrous tissues. Fibrosis may proceed to cirrhosis. Such damage may be seen with long-term methotrexate use.

Vascular disorders

A variety of drugs can cause veno-occlusive disease, which is characterised by non-thrombotic narrowing of small centrilobular veins, and is typically caused by cytotoxic agents and some herbal remedies. Use of oral contraceptives or cytotoxic agents may exacerbate an underlying thrombotic disorder and increase the risk of the Budd–Chiari syndrome (obstruction of the large veins) developing

Tumours

Drugs have been associated with a variety of hepatic tumours. The drugs most commonly linked to malignancy are the oral contraceptives, anabolic steroids and danazol.

Clinical manifestations

The clinical features of drug-induced hepatotoxicity vary widely, depending on the type of liver damage caused.

Acute hepatocellular necrosis

In acute hepatocellular necrosis caused by paracetamol, early symptoms include anorexia, nausea and vomiting, malaise and lethargy. Abdominal pain may be the first indication of liver damage but is not usually apparent for 24–48 h. A period of apparent recovery precedes the development of jaundice and production of dark urine. If the liver injury is severe, deterioration follows, with repeated vomiting, hypoglycaemia, metabolic acidosis, bruising and bleeding, drowsiness and hepatic encephalopathy. Oliguria (diminished urine output) and anuria (complete cessation of urine production) may result from acute tubular necrosis. Renal failure may occur even in the absence of severe liver disease. In addition to acute renal failure, myocardial injury and pancreatitis have also been reported. In fatal cases, death from acute hepatic failure occurs between 4 and 18 days after ingestion.

Steatosis

A patient presenting with steatosis generally shows fatigue, nausea, vomiting, hypoglycaemia and confusion. Jaundice is present in severe cases.

Acute hepatitis

Acute hepatitis may present with a prodromal illness with non-specific symptoms or include features of drug allergy followed by anorexia, nausea and vomiting, dark urine, pale stools and jaundice. Jaundice tends to be present in severe cases. Weight loss may also be a feature of acute hepatitis. Fatalities occur in 5–30% of jaundiced patients. Acute hepatitis is second only to paracetamol self-poisoning as a cause of DILD.

Chronic active hepatitis

Drug-induced chronic active hepatitis may present with tiredness, lethargy and malaise, in a manner similar to other types of chronic liver disease. The symptoms may evolve over many months. Gastro-intestinal symptoms are usually present, and patients may show one or more complications of severe liver disease, including ascites, bleeding oesophageal varices or hepatic encephalopathy. If the ADR has an allergic component, a skin rash and other extrahepatic features of a drug allergy such as lymphadenopathy, evidence of bone marrow suppression (particularly petechial haemorrhages) may be present.

Cholestasis

The main clinical feature of pure cholestasis is severe pruritus, with or without other features, according to the severity, such as dark urine, pale stools and jaundice.

Drug-induced cholestatic hepatitis usually presents with gastro-intestinal symptoms following an influenza-like illness. Abdominal pain with typical features of cholestasis then occurs. The pruritus is generally less severe than with pure cholestasis.

Veno-occlusive disease

Veno-occlusive disease may present with painful hepatomegaly, ascites and jaundice along with other features of liver insufficiency. It has been reported following chemotherapy with drugs such as cyclophosphamide, doxorubicin and dacarbazine. It has also been reported as a common complication of bone marrow transplantation.

Hepatic tumours

In general, patients with hepatic tumours present in a similar manner. Abdominal pain may or may not be reported, together with a feeling of fullness after eating. Weight loss, fatigue, anorexia, nausea and, occasionally, vomiting can occur, especially in advanced cases.

Investigations

Various types of investigation are used in the diagnosis of drug-induced hepatotoxicity, with the number and type of tests depending on the clinical presentation. Unfortunately, available laboratory tests do not provide ideal markers for DILD and the diagnosis is generally one of exclusion.

Biochemical tests

Routine LFTs are measured, which generally include total bilirubin, alanine transaminase and alkaline phosphatase. Impairment of the synthetic function of the liver is detected by total protein, albumin and the prothrombin time. Other biochemical tests may include measurement of γ-glutamyl transpeptidase which may be elevated in all forms of liver disease, including drug-induced disease. α-Fetoprotein may be measured to exclude malignancy. Conjugated bilirubin may be measured to establish if there is biliary obstruction.

Serological markers

Serological markers for hepatitis A, B and C and other viruses such as the Epstein–Barr virus should be determined in patients with symptoms of hepatitis with appropriate risk factors to exclude an infective cause.

Radiological investigations

Radiological investigations, such as ultrasound, computed tomography, percutaneous cholangiograms and endoscopic retrograde cholangiopancreatography (ERCP), are used to look for physical obstruction of bile ducts by gallstones, masses or strictures.

Liver biopsy

Liver biopsy is seldom helpful for diagnosis but certain drugs can cause characteristic lesions, such as the distribution of microvesicular fat droplets seen with tetracyclines. Specific diagnostic tests for drug-induced disease exist for few drugs, with halothane being a notable exception.

Other causes of liver dysfunction such as autoimmune chronic active hepatitis, acute severe cholestasis, ischaemic hepatic necrosis, pregnancy-related liver disease, the Budd–Chiari syndrome, rare metabolic disorders or liver disease related to alcohol abuse must also be excluded.

Treatment

The aim of treatment for drug-induced hepatotoxicity is complete recovery. This relies on correct diagnosis, withdrawal of any and all suspected drugs, and supportive therapy, which may include liver transplantation where appropriate.

Diagnosis

Drug-induced hepatic injury should be suspected in every patient with jaundice while ruling out other causes of liver disease by the clinical history and the results of investigations. The typical process in screening patients presenting with jaundice is outlined in Fig. 15.2 and the general approach to the differential diagnosis of acute hepatitis is set out in Fig. 15.3.

Drugs that are commonly prescribed, such as NSAIDs, antimicrobials and antihypertensive agents, are more likely to be implicated in DILD, although the frequency for the individual agents is low. Identifying the causative agent and stopping it is important in reducing the morbidity and mortality associated with DILD. Recovery normally follows discontinuation of a hepatotoxic drug. Serious toxicity or ALF may result if the drug is continued after symptoms appear or the serum transaminases rise significantly. Failure to discontinue the drug may give grounds for claims of negligence.

A detailed and thorough drug history, including use of oral contraceptives, over-the-counter medicines, vitamins, herbal preparations and illicit drug use, should be obtained. Examples of herbal and dietary preparations implicated in causing liver damage are listed in Box 15.1. Attention to the duration of treatment with a specific drug and the relationship to the onset of symptoms is important. The likelihood of a drug-related disease is greatest when the abnormality begins between 5 and 90 days after taking the first dose and within 15 days of taking the last dose. The latent period, that is, the time between starting therapy and the appearance of

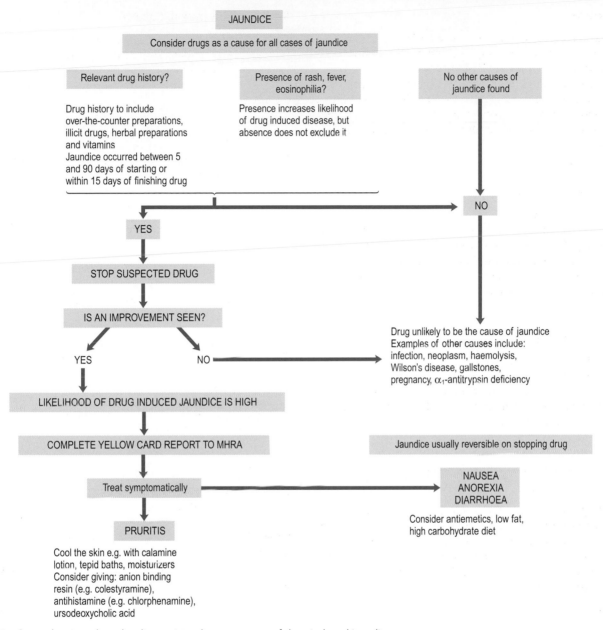

Fig. 15.2 General approach to the diagnosis and management of drug-induced jaundice.

symptoms, may vary but for many drugs is sufficiently reproducible to be of some diagnostic value.

Predisposing factors for liver toxicity should also be noted. If the liver injury is accompanied by fever, rash and eosinophilia, the likelihood of drug-induced disease increases, although lack of these features does not exclude it. Unequivocal diagnosis cannot be made in most circumstances, and improvement on withdrawal of the implicated drug may provide the strongest evidence for drug-induced disease. Time for resolution of the abnormalities is dependent on the individual drug and type of liver disease. In some cases, several months may elapse.

Idiosyncratic reactions may also need to be considered and the literature consulted for previous reports. A key component of secondary prevention is the reporting of all suspected hepatic drug reactions to the appropriate monitoring agency, particularly for newer agents with fewer published cases. Many drugs are approved and licensed before the idiosyncratic reactions are identified as there is little chance of detecting the reaction in the phase III studies which typically involve 300 patients. To detect a single case of clinically significant hepatic injury due to a drug with 95% confidence, the number of patients included in the trial must be about three times the incidence of the reaction. Idiosyncratic reactions occur in about 1 in 10,000 patients so to detect the reaction, the clinical trial would have to study 30,000 patients. Practice points for diagnosing DILD are shown in Box 15.2.

Withdrawal

Once drug-induced hepatotoxicity has been recognised as a possibility, therapy should be stopped. If the patient is receiving more than one potentially hepatotoxic drug, all drugs

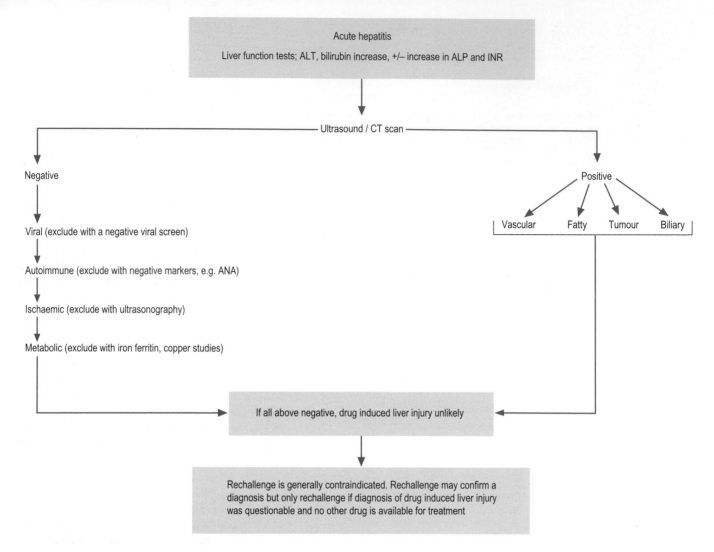

Fig. 15.3 General approach to the differential diagnosis of acute hepatitis. ALT, alanine transferase; ALP, alkaline phosphatase; INR, international normalised ratio; ANA, antinuclear antibodies.

Box 15.1 Examples of herbal remedies and food supplements implicated in hepatotoxicity

Black cohosh
Borage oil
Camellia sinensis
Chapparal (*Larrea tridentata*)
Chinese herbal preparations for skin disorders
Comfrey
Fortorol (food supplement which may contain nimesulide)
Garcinia (*Garcinia camboge*)
Germander (*Teucrium chamaedrys*)
Hydroxycut
Kava kava (*Piper methysticum*)
Khat (*Catha edulis*)
Miradin (food supplement which may contain nimesulide)
Mistletoe (skullcap)
Noni juice (*Morina citrofolia*)
Passion flower (*Passiflora incarnata*)
Ubiquinone
Valerian (*Valeriana officinalis*)

Box 15.2 Practice points for the diagnosis of drug-induced liver disease

- Consider drugs as a cause for all cases of liver damage in patients presenting with liver disease.
- Take a careful drug history include prescription, over the counter, herbal and alternative medicines
- Has the drug implicated been previously reported to cause drug-induced liver disease?
- Does the patient have risk factors for drug-induced liver disease?
- Consider the temporal relation (onset of symptoms between 5 and 90 days after initial exposure?)
- Is there improvement on discontinuation of the suspected agent?
- Rechallenge with the suspected drug is not recommended; however, a positive rechallenge is the most definite evidence of drug-induced disease.

Box 15.3 Examples of drugs associated with the development of chronic liver disease

Amiodarone
Chlorpromazine
Diclofenac
Isoniazid
Methotrexate
Nitrofurantoin

should be stopped. Withdrawal of the agent usually results in recovery that begins within a few days. However, LFTs may take many months or even years to return to normal. Co-amoxiclav and phenytoin are examples of drugs that have been associated with a worsening of the patient's condition for several weeks after withdrawal, and a protracted recovery period of several months. Examples of drugs associated with chronic liver injury are shown in Box 15.3.

Rechallenge

When drug-induced hepatotoxicity has been confirmed by improvement on drug withdrawal, subsequent use in the patient is generally contraindicated. Rechallenge is not normally justified as this is potentially dangerous for the patient, although a positive rechallenge is the most definitive confirmation of drug-induced disease. Inadvertent rechallenge may occur. If the rechallenge is negative, this is usually taken to indicate that the patient may resume using the drug. Another adverse reaction on re-exposure to the drug precludes any further use.

Management

If clinical or laboratory signs of hepatic failure appear, hospitalisation is mandatory.

After withdrawal of the drug, attempts to remove it from the body are only relevant for acute hepatotoxins such as paracetamol, metals or toxic mushrooms such as *Amanita phalloides* (death cap).

If patients present a few hours post-ingestion, any unabsorbed drug may best be removed by gastric lavage, rather than by use of emetics.

Antidotes

Specific antidotes are acetylcysteine and methionine for paracetamol, and desferrioxamine for iron overdose. Desferrioxamine 5–10 g in 50–100 mL of water is administered orally as soon as possible after ingestion for acute iron poisoning. Parenteral desferrioxamine is indicated in addition to oral administration, to chelate absorbed iron where the plasma levels exceed 89.5 μmol/L, where the plasma levels exceed 62.6 μmol/L and there is evidence of free iron, and in patients with signs and symptoms of acute iron poisoning.

Corticosteroids

Immunosuppression with corticosteroids has been used in the management of drug-induced hepatotoxicity, but evidence indicates their use does not affect survival of patients with ALF. However, there have been anecdotal reports of impressive responses to corticosteroids that are persuasive, and it may be appropriate to conduct a short trial in rare types of drug-induced disease.

Supportive treatment

For most patients there is no specific treatment available. General supportive treatment is necessary in liver failure, with appropriate attention to fluid and electrolyte balance.

Nutritional support should be along conventional medical lines. Some patients find that a low-fat, high-carbohydrate diet provides relief from the anorexia, nausea and diarrhoea that may accompany cholestasis.

Pruritus

The main symptom of drug-induced cholestasis is pruritus due to high systemic concentrations of bile acids deposited in tissues. General measures include light clothing (avoid wool) and cooling the skin with tepid baths or calamine lotion, and a general moisturising agent such as aqueous cream. The management of liver-induced pruritus is discussed in more detail in Chapter 16.

Coagulation disorders

Coagulation disorders should be treated by correcting vitamin K deficiency with intravenous phytomenadione injection. This should correct the prothrombin time within 3–5 days. Oral phytomenadione is ineffective in cholestasis. Menadiol sodium phosphate, the water-soluble vitamin K analogue, may be effective in an oral dose of 10 mg daily. If bleeding occurs, infusion of fresh frozen plasma or clotting factor concentrates will be indicated. The administration of other fat-soluble vitamins may also be necessary. Liver transplantation is often considered the treatment of choice for patients with acute hepatic failure induced by drugs.

Long-term treatment

When the DILD is under control, consideration will have to be given to the treatment of the original condition for which the implicated drug was prescribed. In many cases, drug therapy will still be required and caution must, therefore, be exercised, as drugs with similar chemical structures may cause similar hepatotoxicity (Table 15.7).

Hepatotoxicity may occur with different derivatives of a drug. Erythromycin-induced cholestatic hepatitis has been more frequently reported with the estolate preparation than with other erythromycin esters (ethylsuccinate, stearate, propionate and lactobionate). It is not clear which part of the drug is responsible for hypersensitivity.

Table 15.7 Examples of cross-sensitivity within drug groups

	Problem	Action
Phenothiazines	Cross-sensitivity	Avoid
Tricyclics	Cross-sensitivity	Avoid
NSAIDs	Cross-sensitivity	Avoid
Isoniazid, pyrazinamide	Chemically-related	Avoid
Halothane	Avoid enflurane	Isoflurane appears safe

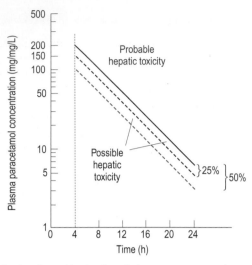

Fig. 15.4 Semilogarithmic plot of plasma paracetamol concentration versus time in hours after ingestion.

Paracetamol-induced hepatotoxicity

Paracetamol causes a dose-related toxicity resulting in centrilobular necrosis. It normally undergoes the phase II reactions of glucuronidation and sulphation. However, paracetamol is metabolised by cytochrome P450 2E1 to *N*-acetyl-*p*-benzoquinoneimine (NABQI) if the capacity of the phase II reactions is exceeded or if cytochrome P450 2E1 is induced. After normal doses of paracetamol, NABQI is detoxified by conjugation with glutathione to produce mercaptopurine and cysteine conjugates. Following overdose, tissue stores of glutathione are depleted, allowing NABQI to accumulate and cause cell damage. Illness, starvation and alcohol deplete glutathione stores and increase the predisposition to paracetamol toxicity, while acetylcysteine and methionine provide a specific antidote by replenishing glutathione stores.

Ingestion of doses as low as 10–15 g of paracetamol have been reported to cause severe hepatocellular necrosis. Removal of unabsorbed paracetamol by gastric lavage may be worthwhile if more than 150 mg/kg body weight has been taken and the patient presents within 4 h of ingestion. Activated charcoal may also be administered to reduce further absorption of paracetamol and facilitate removal of unmetabolised paracetamol from extracellular fluids. This may lessen the effect of any methionine given. A plasma paracetamol concentration should be taken as soon as possible but not within 4 h of ingestion due to the fact that a misleading and low level may be obtained because of continuing absorption and distribution of the drug. The plasma concentration measured should be compared with a standard nomogram reference line of a plot of plasma paracetamol concentration against time in hours after ingestion. This may be a semilogarithmic (Fig. 15.4) or linear (Fig. 15.5) plot. Generally, administration of intravenous acetylcysteine is the treatment of choice for paracetamol overdose when the blood paracetamol level is in the range predictive of possible or probable liver injury (see Fig. 15.4). Patients allergic to acetylcysteine may receive oral methionine.

Acetylcysteine is most effective within 8 h of overdose. However, late administration in patients who present more than 16–24 h post-ingestion may be appropriate. Acetylcysteine administered at this stage will not counteract the oxidative effects of paracetamol but it may have a

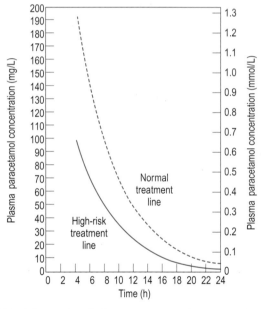

Fig. 15.5 A linear plot of plasma paracetamol concentration versus time in hours after ingestion.

cytoprotective role in hepatic failure, and has been shown to reduce morbidity and mortality in patients who have already developed ALF.

Patient care

Patients may be at risk of drug-induced hepatotoxicity from prescribed drugs or from purchased drugs. Additionally, children may be at risk from medicines that are not stored properly. Parents should be reminded to store all medicines in child resistant containers and out of reach. Deaths from liver failure have occurred in children following overdose with drugs commonly available, such as iron tablets.

Patient counselling

Patients who purchase preparations containing paracetamol should be made aware of the danger of overdosing, which may occur if other preparations containing paracetamol are taken simultaneously. Since 1994 the European guidelines on package labelling have required products containing paracetamol to warn patients of the need to avoid other products containing paracetamol. The pack size of paracetamol sold from general sales outlets has been limited to 16 tablets or capsules (32 where paracetamol is sold under the supervision of a pharmacist) with the aim of limiting availability and reducing residual stocks in the home. This appears to have reduced the incidence of ALF secondary to paracetamol overdose.

All patients should be advised of potential side effects. This information needs to be reinforced with the use of patient information leaflets.

Patients and their carers should be helped to recognise signs of liver disorder and know to report immediately symptoms such as malaise, nausea, fever and abdominal discomfort that may be significant, although non-specific during the first few weeks of any change of therapy. If these are accompanied by elevated LFTs, the drug should be discontinued.

Patients who recover from drug-induced hepatotoxicity should be informed of the causative agent, warned to avoid it in the future, and advised to inform their doctor, dentist, nurse and pharmacist about the occurrence of such an event.

Parents of children commenced on sodium valproate should be warned to report side effects that may be suggestive of liver injury such as the onset of anorexia, abdominal discomfort, nausea and vomiting. Early features include drowsiness and disturbed consciousness. Fever may also be present. The time to onset is between 1 and 4 months in the majority of cases.

The challenge for all members of the health care team is to alert patients to the potentially toxic effects of drugs without creating so much concern that they fail to comply with vital medication. For the limited number of drugs presented in Table 15.8, careful monitoring of LFTs during the first 6 months of treatment is advisable, although not always practical. Thereafter, regular monitoring of LFTs is appropriate in patients who are at greater risk of hepatotoxicity. Such patients would include those with known liver disease, those taking other hepatotoxic drugs, those aged over 40 years, and heavy alcohol consumers. Surveillance should be particularly frequent in the first 2 months of treatment. In patients with no risk factors and normal pretreatment liver function, LFTs

Table 15.8 Examples of drugs where regular monitoring of liver function is recommended

Drug	Baseline measurement[a]	Frequency of monitoring
Anti-TB therapy (isoniazid, rifampicin, pyrazinamide)	Yes	Patients with pre-existing chronic liver disease: check LFTs regularly, every week for the first 2 weeks, then twice a week for the first 2 months. Patients with normal liver function tests and no evidence of pre-existing liver disease: regular monitoring is not necessary but LFTs repeated if signs of liver dysfunction develop, for example, fever, malaise, vomiting or jaundice. Patients with raised pretreatment hepatic transaminases: Two or more times normal: check LFTs weekly for 2 weeks, then twice a week until normal. Under two times normal: check LFTs at 2 weeks. If these transaminases have fallen, further tests are only needed if symptoms occur
Amiodarone	Yes	LFTs checked every 6 months
Cyproterone	Yes	Recheck if any symptoms
Dantrolene	Yes	Repeat LFTs after first 6 weeks of therapy
Itraconazole	Yes	Monitor LFTs if therapy continues for more than 1 month. Recheck if any symptoms
Ketoconazole	Yes	LFTs checked on weeks 2 and 4 of therapy and then every month
Methotrexate	Yes	LFTs checked every 2 weeks for the first 2 months, then monthly for 4 months, then every 3 months
Methyldopa	Yes	Check LFTs at intervals during the first 6–12 weeks of treatment
Micafungin	Yes	Periodic monitoring of LFTs recommended. Recheck if any symptoms
Nevirapine	Yes	Check LFTs every 2 weeks for the first 2 months, then at month 3 and then regularly
Pioglitazone	Yes	Periodic monitoring of LFTs recommended. Recheck if any symptoms

Table 15.8 Examples of drugs where regular monitoring of liver function is recommended—cont'd

Drug	Baseline measurement[a]	Frequency of monitoring
Rosiglitazone	Yes	Periodic monitoring of LFTs recommended. Recheck if any symptoms.
Sodium valproate	Yes	Check LFTs regularly during the first 6 months of therapy
Statins	Yes	LFTs checked 12 weeks after initiation or after a dose increase and periodically thereafter
Sulfasalazine	Yes	LFTs checked every 2 weeks for the first 2 months, then monthly for 4 months then every 3 months
Tipranavir	Yes	Check LFTs on weeks 2, 4 and 8 of treatment and then every 2–3 months
Vildagliptin	Yes	LFTs checked every 3 months for the first year and then periodically

[a]Baseline and subsequent liver function tests (LFTs) difficult to interpret in critically ill patients as LFTs will be affected by multiple factors

need only be repeated if fever, malaise, vomiting, jaundice or unexplained deterioration during treatment occurs.

Since many drugs cause elevation of LFTs there may be difficulty in assessing when to stop a drug, particularly when treating an individual for tuberculosis or epilepsy. An empirical guideline is that the drug should be stopped if the levels of alanine transaminase exceed three times the upper limit of the reference range. Any clinical features of liver disease or drug allergy would require immediate discontinuation of the drug. Conversely, a raised γ-glutamyl transpeptidase level and elevated alanine transaminase level in the absence of symptoms often reflect microsomal induction and would not indicate drug-induced injury.

It should be noted that monitoring of LFTs is not a complete safeguard against hepatotoxicity, as some drug reactions develop very quickly, and the liver enzymes are an unreliable indicator of fibrosis.

Minimising the risk of DILD

Cholestatic jaundice has been reported to occur in about 1 in 6000 patients treated with co-amoxiclav. The risk of acute liver injury with co-amoxiclav is approximately six times that of amoxicillin and increases with treatment courses above 14 days. Hence, the indications for co-amoxiclav have been restricted to cover infections caused by amoxicillin-resistant β-lactam-producing infections.

Patients admitted for procedures requiring a general anaesthetic should be questioned about past exposure and any previous reactions to halothane. Halothane is well known to be associated with hepatotoxicity, particularly if patients are re-exposed. Repeated exposure to halothane within a period of less than 3 months should be avoided, while some increase in risk persists regardless of the time interval since last exposure. Unexplained jaundice or delayed-onset post-operative fever in a patient who has received halothane is an absolute contraindication to future use in that individual. Patients with a family history of halothane-related liver injury should also be treated with caution.

The individuals at greatest risk of halothane hepatitis are obese, post-menopausal women. Halothane may be present in detectable amounts even in theatres equipped with scavenging devices, and it is possible for these small concentrations to provoke a reaction in a highly sensitised individual. If electing to avoid halothane, a halothane-free circuit and operating theatre should be used. Cross-hepatotoxicity with other haloalkanes is a possibility, and enflurane should also be avoided. Isoflurane appears to be safe, as no reports of cross-sensitivity have been published. Some anaesthetists would prefer to use total intravenous anaesthesia in patients who have had a reaction to halothane.

Although hepatic ADRs are rare for most drugs, when they do occur they can cause significant morbidity and mortality. Over 600 drugs have been associated with hepatotoxicity and any new drug released on to the market may have the potential to cause hepatotoxicity. Pemoline, troglitazone and tolcapone are examples of drugs withdrawn from the market due to reports of serious hepatic reactions. These examples help to highlight the importance of post-marketing surveillance and yellow card reporting.

Appropriate selection of drugs, an awareness of predisposing factors and avoidance of toxic dose thresholds and potentially hepatotoxic drug–drug interactions will minimise the risk to patients.

Practice points for patient care and minimising the risk of DILD are outlined in Box 15.4.

Box 15.4 Practice points for minimising the risk of drug-induced liver disease (DILD)

- Minimise DILD by ensuring appropriate monitoring of drugs associated with hepatotoxicity.
- Minimise DILD by following recommendations, for example, use co-amoxiclav for penicillin β-lactam resistant infections only, counsel all patients on paracetamol not to exceed 4 g/day and to be alert to other preparations containing paracetamol.
- Counsel all patients (or carers of patients) on potentially hepatotoxic medicines to recognise and report signs of liver damage.
- Inform all patients who have DILD of the causative agent, and the importance of avoiding this in future.

Case studies

Case 15.1

Mr V, a 39-year-old male, presented to his local hospital following a paracetamol overdose. He had recently separated from his wife, had not been eating properly, went on an alcohol binge and then on impulse had taken approximately 70 paracetamol tablets. He self-referred himself to his local hospital 28 h after the overdose. At presentation he was feeling nauseous and had right subcostal pain. His results at this time were:

	Actual value (normal range)
Paracetamol	18 mg/mL
Albumin	26 g/dL (30–50 g/L)
Alanine transaminase	5435 units/L (0–50 units/L)
Bilirubin	50 µmol/L (<17 µmol/L)
Alakline phosphatase	66 units/L (30–135 units/L)
Prothrombin time	57 s (9.8–12.6 s)
Creatinine	133 (35–125 µmol/L)
Urea	5.6 (0–7.5 mmol/L)

Other test results:
  Hepatitis screen negative
  Autoantibody screen negative

At this stage, supportive treatment was given. However, he deteriorated, with worsening test results and the development of encephalopathy. He was then transferred to a tertiary intensive care unit, with a diagnosis of ALF secondary to paracetamol overdose. His test results on admission to the intensive care unit were:

	Actual value (normal range)
Albumin	22 g/dL (30–50 g/L)
Alanine transaminase	12,477 units/L (0–50 units/L)
Bilirubin	71 µmol/L (<17 µmol/L)
Alakline phosphatase	73 units/L (30–135 units/L)
Prothrombin time	90.8 s (9.8–12.6 s)
Arterial pH	7.226 (7.350–7.450)
Lactate	6.9 (0.4–2.2 mmol/L)
Creatinine	336 (35–125 µmol/L)
Urea	7.4 (0–7.5 mmol/L)

He was put on the liver transplant urgent list and received an orthotopic liver transplant (OLT) the following day.

Questions

1. What risk factors does Mr V have which suggest a worse prognosis?
2. On initial presentation what treatment should be initiated?
3. What is the significance of the high creatinine result?
4. Can Mr V be prescribed paracetamol for pain relief?

Answers

1. The progression of paracetamol toxicity can be categorised into four stages: preclinical, hepatic injury, hepatic failure, and recovery. The prognosis varies depending upon the stage at presentation. Mr V's late presentation to hospital also increases his risk of a worse prognosis. He presented to hospital 28 h after the overdose, with raised ALT and some symptoms of liver injury, indicating that he was in the hepatic injury stage and progressed onto the liver failure stage with the development of encephalopathy. Patients presenting with liver injury have a variable prognosis but patients who present with hepatic failure have a mortality rate of 20–40%. Had he presented in the preclinical stage he would have been expected to make a full recovery with treatment.

   Although Mr V had acutely ingested alcohol at the time of paracetamol overdose, this is not a risk factor for a worse prognosis. Theoretically, acute alcohol ingestion competes with paracetamol for CYP2E1 metabolism resulting in lower formation of NAPQI and thus less toxicity. Chronic alcohol consumption induces the CYP2E1 enzyme resulting in increased NAPQI production and increased risk of hepatotoxicity.

   The fact that Mr V had not been eating properly may have resulted in depleted glutathione stores and a worse prognosis.

   Mr V developed hepatorenal syndrome, this is a poor prognostic indicator and has an associated mortality of 50–100%. A poor prognosis is also associated with the following:

Prothrombin time	>36 s
Creatinine	>200 µmol/L
pH	<7.3
Encephalopathy	Present
Cerebral oedema	Present
Time from onset of jaundice to encephalopathy	0–7 days

2. A plasma paracetamol level needs to be taken as soon as possible, although not within the first 4 h following paracetamol overdose. A toxic screen should be performed to exclude other drug overdoses. Supportive therapy with intravenous fluids and oxygen, if necessary, should be given. This patient should also be treated with N-acetylcysteine. Treatment with N-acetylcysteine is particularly beneficial when administered within 8 h of paracetamol overdose when the blood paracetamol level is in the range predictive of possible or probable liver injury (see Fig. 15.4). However, late administration in patients who present more than 16–24 h post-ingestion is also appropriate. Acetylcysteine administered at this stage will not counteract the oxidative effects of paracetamol but it may have a cytoprotective role in hepatic failure, improving haemodynamics and oxygen use. Late administration of N-acetylcysteine has been shown to reduce morbidity and mortality in patients who have already developed hepatic failure. Available data for use of N-acetylcysteine following paracetamol overdose suggests that, although the evidence for benefit is limited, it should be given to patients with overdose (Brok et al., 2006).

3. Mr V developed renal impairment secondary to the liver damage which is known as the hepatorenal syndrome (HRS). Other causes of renal impairment should be excluded. Where necessary drug doses should be adjusted for renal impairment. Once the liver recovers, or transplantation of the liver occurs, the kidneys are likely to recover.

4. Paracetamol should be avoided in the acute phase following an overdose. However, if following the acute phase, the patient needs either an analgesic or antipyretic, then paracetamol in small doses may be used. Following a liver transplant, standard paracetamol doses can be used as long as the patient is adequately nourished and does not have any psychological issues with the use of paracetamol.

Case 15.2

Ms B is a 43-year-old lady with type 2 diabetes who was commenced on simvastatin 10 mg at night 4 months ago. She has no other relevant past medical history. She does not drink alcohol and does not consume grapefruit. Drug history includes gliclazide MR 60 mg twice a day and aspirin 75 mg daily. A routine blood test revealed an increase in ALT from baseline (pre-simvastatin) of 21 to 197 units/L (0–50 units/L) at 4 months.

Questions

1. What are the likely causes of the increase in ALT?
2. Should liver function tests be routinely monitored in patients on a statin?
3. What action, if any, should be taken in this case?
4. Can statins be used in patients with pre-existing liver disease?

Answers

1. The most likely cause of the increase in ALT is the introduction of simvastatin 4 months previously. All statins are reported to cause elevations in transaminases, which may be transient or persistent. The incidence of transaminitis with statins is low, being reported to occur between 1 in 1000 and 1 in 10,000 patients. Other causes of liver disease should also be considered in this case, for example, non-alcoholic steatohepatitis (NASH) associated with diabetes.

2. Monitoring of liver function tests in patients taking a statin is recommended in the Summary of Product Characteristics, and hence should be monitored for medico legal reasons (McKenney et al., 2006). It is recommended to monitor liver function tests at baseline and then at 12 weeks or after a dose increase. However, the true value for monitoring liver function test is not clear as it does not identify those at risk of liver damage, is expensive and may lead to patient anxiety and unnecessary cessation of statin therapy. Moreover, hepatic function does not appear to be compromised by statin use and there is no apparent link between an elevation in liver function tests and the development of toxicity (McKenney et al., 2006).

3. Ms B had a single high ALT result. The general recommendation is that if the patient is asymptomatic and the transaminase levels are greater than three times the upper limit of normal the test should be repeated. If transaminases are still more than three times upper limit of normal the patient should have a full liver investigation.

   In this case, the simvastatin was switched to pravastatin before a repeat liver function test. Follow-up liver function tests showed that the ALT had returned to within the normal range. It is highly probable that this rise in ALT on simvastatin would have been transient and had the patient continued with simvastatin the ALT would have normalised. However, the patient was anxious, did not want to risk any progression of liver toxicity and was keen to switch to an alternative statin.

4. Statins are contraindicated in ALF and decompensated chronic liver disease. However, they can probably be used safely in liver disease where there is no, or mild, synthetic dysfunction. Statin use may actually improve elevations in transaminases in patients with fatty liver disease (Gomez-Dominguez et al., 2006)

Case 15.3

Mr K, a 28-year-old HIV-infected male, was found to have elevated liver function tests on a routine monitoring sample following initiation of antiretroviral therapy. He had previously been diagnosed with HIV 6 months ago, with a CD count of 330 cells/mm³ and a viral load of 83,000 copies/mL. Relevant past medical history included psychiatric illness. He had been initiated on Kivexa® (abacavir and lamivudine) and nevirapine 5 months ago. He is not on any other medications. Mr K was recalled to the hospital clinic for urgent medication review. In the clinic, Mr K reported a 3-day history of general malaise, abdominal discomfort and nausea. Examination in clinic showed to have a normal blood pressure, a temperature of 37.1 °C and slight visible jaundice. There were no signs of a hypersensitivity reaction. His routine liver function tests were:

	Actual value (normal range)
Albumin	30 g/dL (30–50 g/L)
Alanine transaminase	350 units/L (0–50 units/L)
Bilirubin	90 μmol/L (<17 μmol/L)
Alkaline phosphatase	180 units/L (30–135 units/L)

Questions

1. For which drug would Mr K be having routine liver function tests?
2. What is the significance of looking for signs of hypersensitivity?
3. Does Mr K have any risk factors for developing drug associated hepatotoxicity?
4. What actions should be taken in relation to this patient's antiretroviral therapy?

Answers

1. Hepatotoxicity among HIV-infected persons taking nevirapine is a well recognised adverse effect. The incidence of an asymptomatic increase in hepatic aminotransferase levels is reported as approximately 5–15%, with the incidence of clinically symptomatic hepatitis among persons taking nevirapine of approximately 4% (Martínez et al., 2001). It is recommended that all patients commencing on nevirapine undergo close monitoring during the first 18 weeks of treatment, with liver function tests performed at baseline, then every 2 weeks for the first 2 months again after a further 1 month and regularly thereafter.

2. Signs of hypersensitivity help to diagnose the type of nevirapine induced hepatotoxicty. Two distinct mechanisms and time courses of nevirapine-associated hepatotoxicity have been recognised. The first type is an immune-mediated hypersensitivity reaction, developing within 18 weeks of the start of nevirapine. Most patients with this type of early nevirapine associated hepatotoxicity will have concomitant flu-like symptoms (fever, myalgia, fatigue, malaise, nausea, and vomiting) with or without skin rash. The second, and much less frequent type, typically occurs after 18 weeks of nevirapine therapy and most likely represents an intrinsic toxic drug effect (Soriano et al., 2008).

3. Mr K does not have any risk factors. Risk factors for developing hepatotoxicity with nevirapine include female gender, higher CD4 cell count prior to starting nevirapine (greater than 250 cells/mm³ in females and greater than 400 cells/mm³ in males), chronic hepatitis B or C virus infection, alcoholic liver disease and abnormal baseline hepatic aminotransferase levels (Soriano et al., 2008).

4. In general, nevirapine should be discontinued when increases in hepatic aminotransferase levels occur associated with a rash. Mr K shows signs of clinical hepatitis with symptoms of general malaise, abdominal discomfort and nausea, in conjunction with a raised ALT. He does not show signs of hypersensitivity or rash. His nevirapine therapy should be suspended and his liver function monitored closely. Once his liver function has settled, nevirapine could be cautiously reintroduced with close monitoring. For patients who develop nevirapine-associated hepatitis, the risk of developing hepatitis from subsequent treatment with efavirenz or delavirdine remains unknown. As a consequence, efavirenz or delavirdine should be used with caution if initiated in a patient with prior nevirapine-associated hepatotoxicity.

Acknowledgement

The content of this chapter is based on that which appeared in the fourth edition of this textbook and was written in collaboration with B.E. Cadman.

References

Brok, J., Buckley, N., Gluud, C., 2006. Interventions for paracetamol (acctaminophen) overdose. Cochrane Database Syst. Rev. 2 Art No. CD003328. doi:10.1002/14651858.CD003328.pub2.

Gomez-Dominguez, E., Gisbert, J., Moreno-Monteagudo, J., et al., 2006. A pilot study of atorvastatin treatment in dyslipemid, non alcoholic fatty liver patients. Aliment. Pharmacol. Ther. 23, 1643–1647.

Martínez, E., Blanco, J.L., Arnaiz, J.A., et al., 2001. Hepatotoxicity in HIV-1-infected patients receiving nevirapine-containing antiretroviral therapy. AIDS 15, 1261–1268.

McKenney, J., Davidson, M.H., Jacobson, T.A., et al., 2006. Final conclusions and recommendations of the National Lipid Association Statin Safety Assessment Task Force. Am. J. Cardiol. 97, 89C–94C.

Richardson, P., O'Grady, J., 2002. Acute liver disease. Hosp. Pharm. 9, 131–136.

Soriano, V., Puoti, M., Garcia-Gasco, P., et al., 2008. Antiretroviral drugs and liver injury. AIDS 22, 1–13.

Further reading

Bell, L.N., Chalasani, N., 2009. Epidemiology of idiosyncratic drug-induced liver injury. Semin. Liver Dis. 29, 337–347.

Bjornsson, E., 2007. Long term follow up of patients with mild to moderate drug induced liver injury. Aliment. Pharmacol. Ther. 26, 79–85. Available at: http://www.medscape.com/viewarticle/558756.

Bjornsson, E., 2009. The natural history of drug-induced liver injury. Semin. Liver Dis. 24, 357–363. Available at: http://www.medscape.com/viewarticle/711396.

Heard, K.J., 2008. Acetylcysteine for acetaminophen poisoning. N. Engl. J. Med. 359, 285–292.

Lee, W.L., 2003. Drug induced hepatotoxicity. N. Engl. J. Med. 349, 474–485.

North-Lewis, P. (Ed.), 2008. Drugs and the Liver. Pharmaceutical Press, London.

Suzuki, A., Andrade, R.J., Bjornsson, E., et al., 2010. Drugs associated with hepatotoxicity and their reporting frequency of liver adverse events in VigiBase: unified list based on international collaborative work. Drug Saf. 33, 503–522.

Watkins, P., 2009. Biomarkers for the diagnosis and management of drug induced liver injury. Semin. Liver Dis. 24, 393–399. Available at: http://www.medscape.com/viewarticle/711398.

16 Liver disease

P. Kennedy and J. G. O'Grady

Key points

- The liver is a complex organ central to the maintenance of homeostasis.
- The liver is notable for its capacity to regenerate unless cirrhosis has developed. There are now some data to suggest that cirrhosis is reversible in selected cases, for example treated hepatitis B virus.
- The spectrum of liver disease extends from mild, self-limiting conditions to serious illnesses which may carry significant morbidity and mortality.
- Liver disease is defined as acute or chronic on the basis of whether the history of disease is less than or greater than 6 months, respectively.
- Viral infections and paracetamol overdose are the leading causes of acute liver disease, but a significant number of patients have no defined aetiology (seronegative hepatitis).
- Alcohol abuse and chronic viral hepatitis (B and C) are the major causes of chronic liver disease.
- Cirrhosis may be asymptomatic for considerable periods of time.
- Ascites, encephalopathy, varices and hepatorenal failure are the main serious complications of cirrhosis.
- A careful assessment is required prior to the use of any drug in a patient with liver disease due to unpredictable effects on drug handling.

The liver weighs up to 1500 g in adults and as such is one of the largest organs in the body. The main functions of the liver include protein synthesis, storage and metabolism of fats and carbohydrates, detoxification of drugs and other toxins, excretion of bilirubin and metabolism of hormones, as summarised in Fig. 16.1. The liver has considerable reserve capacity reflected in its ability to function normally despite surgical removal of 70–80% of the organ or the presence of significant disease. It is noted for its capacity to regenerate rapidly. However, once it has been critically damaged multiple complications develop involving many body systems. The distinction between acute and chronic liver disease is conventionally based on whether the history is less or greater than 6 months, respectively.

The hepatocyte is the functioning unit of the liver. Heptocytes are arranged in lobules and within a lobule hepatocytes perform different functions depending on how close they are to the portal tract. The portal tract is the 'service network' of the liver and contains an artery and a portal vein delivering blood to the liver and bile duct which forms part of the biliary drainage system (Fig. 16.2). The blood supply to the liver is 30% arterial and the remainder is from the portal system which drains most of the abdominal viscera. Blood passes from the portal tract through sinusoids that facilitate exposure to the hepatocytes before the blood is drained away by the hepatic venules and veins. There are a number of other cell populations in the liver, but two of the most important are Kuppfer cells, fixed monocytes that phagocytose bacteria and particulate matter, and stellate cells responsible for the fibrotic reaction that ultimately leads to cirrhosis.

Acute liver disease

Acute liver disease is a self-limiting episode of hepatocyte damage which in most cases resolves spontaneously without clinical sequelae. This is a rare condition in which there is a rapid deterioration in liver function with associated encephalopathy (altered mentation) and coagulopathy. Acute liver failure (ALF) carries a significant morbidity and mortality and may require emergency liver transplantation.

Chronic liver disease

Chronic liver disease occurs when permanent structural changes within the liver develop secondary to long-standing cell damage, with the consequent loss of normal liver architecture. In many cases, this progresses to cirrhosis, where fibrous scars divide the liver cells into areas of regenerative tissue called nodules (Fig. 16.3). Conventional wisdom is that this

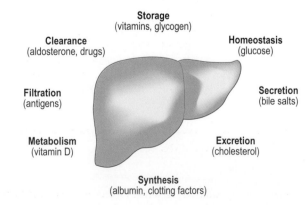

Fig. 16.1 Normal physiological functions of the liver, with examples of each.

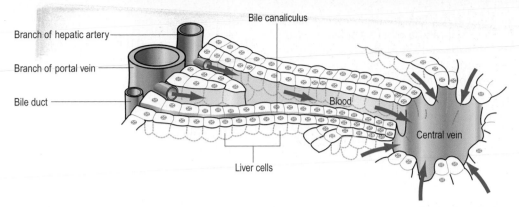

Fig. 16.2 Illustration of the relationship between the three structures that comprise the portal tract, with blood from both the hepatic artery and portal vein perfusing the hepatocytes before draining away towards the hepatic veins (central veins). Each hepatocyte is also able to secrete bile via the network of bile ducts. (Reproduced with permission of McGraw-Hill from Vander, 1980.)

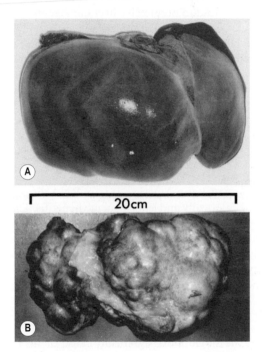

Fig. 16.3 The gross post-mortem appearance of (A) a normal and (B) a cirrhotic liver demonstrating scarring and nodule formation in part B.

process is irreversible, but therapeutic intervention in hepatitis B and haemochromatosis has now repeatedly documented cases of reversal of cirrhosis. Once chronic liver disease progresses, patients are at risk of developing liver failure, portal hypertension or hepatocellular carcinoma. Cirrhosis is a sequel of chronic liver disease of any aetiology and it develops over very variable time periods from 5 to 20 or more years.

Causes of liver disease

Viral infections

Viruses commonly affect the liver, resulting in a transient and innocuous hepatitis. Viruses which target the liver are primarily described as hepatotropic viruses, and each of these can lead to clinically significant hepatitis and in some cases to the development of chronic viral hepatitis with viral persistence. Five human viruses have been well described to date, including hepatitis A (HAV), B (HBV), C (HCV), D (HDV) and E (HEV). Each type of viral hepatitis causes a similar pathology with acute inflammation of the liver. Types A and E are classically associated with an acute and sometimes severe hepatitis which is invariably self-limited, but occasionally fatal. Hepatitis B causes acute hepatitis in adults and 5% of patients become chronic carriers, while 95% of patients infected in the neonatal period are chronically infected. Hepatitis C rarely causes an acute hepatitis but up to 85% of patients become chronic carriers. Both viruses cause chronic liver inflammation or hepatitis, cirrhosis and hepatocellular carcinoma.

Hepatitis A

Hepatitis A virus (HAV) is a non-enveloped RNA virus and a major cause of acute hepatitis worldwide, accounting for up to 25% of clinical hepatitis in the developed world. HAV is an enteric virus and the faecal oral route is the main mechanism of transmission. The virus is particularly contagious and constitutes a public health problem throughout the world. The virus may go unnoticed by the patient in the absence of an icteric episode, particularly in children. However, HAV can cause ALF in less than 1% of patients who are typically older adults. The virus is particularly prevalent in areas of poor sanitation, and often associated with water- and food-borne epidemics. Hepatitis A has a relatively short incubation period (2–7 weeks), during which time the virus replicates and abnormalities in liver function tests can be detected.

Hepatitis B

Up to 500 million people worldwide are chronically infected with the hepatitis B virus (HBV). Chronic HBV is defined as the presence of hepatitis B surface antigens (HBsAg) for a period of more than 6 months. In endemic areas of Africa and the Far East, up to 15–20% of the population are chronic carriers of HBV and exposure to HBV at birth (vertical transmission) is the single most important risk factor for the development of chronic HBV infection. Acquisition of HBV in adulthood is often via sexual transmission and is usually associated with a discrete episode of hepatitis. HBV can also be transmitted parenterally, by the transfusion of blood or blood products from contaminated stocks and by intravenous drug use or needle sharing.

There are many factors that determine the outcome of HBV infection, ranging from age and genetic factors of the host to virus characteristics. Acute HBV infection has a peculiarly long incubation period of 3–6 months, which is generally self-limiting and does not require antiviral therapy. Most patients recover within 1–2 months of the onset of jaundice. The protracted incubation period and the ability of the virus to escape the host immune response contribute to the development of chronic HBV. Chronic HBV is associated with varying levels of viraemia and hepatic inflammation. The level of viraemia, and thus infectivity, was conventionally determined by the presence of the hepatitis Be antigen (HBeAg); and HBeAg loss resulted in a reduction in HBV viraemia and a more favourable outcome. However, HBeAg negative chronic hepatitis with significantly elevated levels of HBV DNA is now recognised as a growing health care problem and is associated with a poorer prognosis. HBeAg negative chronic HBV results as a consequence of the emergence of escape mutants from the core promoter or pre-core regions of the virus. It is estimated that 15–40% of HBV carriers will develop serious sequelae during their lifetime, namely liver cirrhosis and/or hepatocellular carcinoma, which can develop in chronic HBV in the absence of cirrhosis. Childhood infection is associated with a different disease outcome with a higher percentage of patients developing chronic HBV infection, and owing to the protracted exposure to the virus a higher proportion develop cirrhosis and hepatocellular carcinoma.

Hepatitis C

Over 170 million people worldwide are chronically infected with hepatitis C virus (HCV). HCV is a hepatotropic, non-cytopathic, predominantly blood borne virus with greater infectivity than the human immunodeficiency virus (HIV). It is estimated that more than 2.7 million people in the USA are chronically infected with HCV, where it is the leading cause of death from liver disease. The equivalent estimate for the UK is between 200,000 and 500,000, although a considerable proportion of these have not yet been diagnosed. HCV is transmitted parenterally, most commonly through intravenous drug use and the sharing of contaminated needles. Prior to its identification in 1990, HCV (previously known as Non-A, Non-B viral hepatitis) was also contracted through contaminated blood and blood products. The introduction of widespread screening of blood donors and pooled blood products has largely consigned blood transfusion as a mode of transmission to history. There remains a small risk of HCV infection associated with tattooing, electrolysis, ear piercing, acupuncture and sexual contact. The vertical transmission rate from HCV infected mother to child is less than 3%.

Hepatitis D

Hepatitis D virus (HDV) is an incomplete virus that can establish infection only in patients simultaneously infected by HBV. It is estimated that 5% of HBV carriers worldwide are infected with HDV. It is endemic in the Mediterranean basin and is transmitted permucosally, percutaneously or sexually. In other geographical areas, it is confined to intravenous drug users.

HCV infection is associated with the development of a recognised episode of acute hepatitis in only a small percentage of individuals. The majority of patients remain asymptomatic and so are often unaware of the infection or the timing of when they contracted the virus. Symptoms associated with HCV infection tend to be mild constitutional upset with malaise, weakness and anorexia being most commonly reported. Up to 85% of subjects exposed to HCV develop chronic disease, which can lead to progressive liver damage, cirrhosis and hepatocellular carcinoma. Unlike HBV, the risk of developing hepatocellular carcinoma is almost totally linked to the presence of cirrhosis. Approximately 20–30% of patients with chronic HCV infection progress to end-stage liver disease within 20–30 years and alcohol consumption is a recognised co-factor that accelerates disease progression. HCV infection is now the leading worldwide indication for liver transplantation.

Hepatitis E

Hepatitis E virus (HEV) is endemic in India, Asia, the Middle East and parts of Latin America. It is an RNA virus which is transmitted enterically and leads to acute hepatitis. The symptoms of HEV are no different from other causes of viral hepatitis, with an average incubation period of 42 days. It was previously thought that the risk of death was increased in pregnancy, especially in the final trimester, but more recent data do not support this belief.

Alcohol

Alcohol is the single most significant cause of liver disease throughout the Western world accounting for between 40% and 60% of cases of cirrhosis in different countries. In general, deaths from alcoholic liver disease in each country correlate with the consumption of alcohol per head of population, although additional factors can influence this trend. Liver disease related to recent alcohol consumption presents a broad spectrum, ranging from the relatively benign fatty liver disease to the development of alcoholic hepatitis, a condition with an immediate mortality of between 30% and 60%. An estimated 20% of alcohol abusers develop progressive liver fibrosis, which can eventually lead to alcoholic cirrhosis, typically after a period of 10–20 years of heavy indulgence.

The central event in the development of hepatic fibrosis is the transformation of hepatic stellate cells into matrix secreting cells producing pericellular fibrosis. This network of collagen fibres develops around the liver cells and gradually leads to hepatocyte cell death. The extent of fibrosis progresses and micronodular fibrotic bands develop characterising alcoholic cirrhosis. The anatomical changes within the liver increase resistance to blood flow from the portal system, causing an increase in pressure within this system resulting in portal hypertension. As the number of normally functioning liver cells reduces further, because of continued liver cell failure and death, the clinical condition deteriorates progressively with the development of liver failure. The rate of disease progression, and indeed regression, is very strongly linked to whether or not patients continue to consume alcohol.

Non-alcohol related fatty liver disease

Liver pathology that is very similar to alcohol-induced disease is now well recognised in a number of settings including obesity, diabetes mellitus and the metabolic syndrome. As a result, the entities of non-alcoholic fatty liver disease (NAFLD) and non-alcoholic steatohepatitis (NASH) have been introduced. It has been suggested that up to 25% of the U.S. population have NAFLD. The majority of cases of cryptogenic cirrhosis probably reflect the end stage of the NAFLD/NASH disease process even though by that stage the characteristic fatty infiltrate has disappeared.

Immune disorders

Autoimmune disease can affect the hepatocyte or bile duct and is characterised by the presence of auto-antibodies and raised immunoglobulin levels.

Autoimmune hepatitis (AIH)

AIH is an unresolving inflammation of the liver characterised by the presence of auto-antibodies (anti-smooth muscle [type 1] or anti-kidney, liver microsomal [type 2]), hypergammaglobulinemia and an interface hepatitis on liver histology. It is usually a chronic, progressive disease which can occasionally present acutely with a severe hepatitis. AIH typically occurs in young women, between 20 and 40 years, and often with a history or family history of autoimmune disorders.

Primary biliary cirrhosis (PBC)

PBC is an autoimmune disease of the liver which predominantly affects middle aged women (95% of cases are female). It is characterised by the presence of antimitochondrial antibodies and a granulomatous destruction of the interlobular bile ducts leading to progressive ductopenia, fibrosis and cirrhosis. The disease is progressive, albeit over a period of 20 years or longer if diagnosed at an early stage, and liver transplantation is the only effective treatment.

Primary sclerosing cholangitis (PSC)

PSC is an idiopathic chronic inflammatory disease resulting in intra- and extra-hepatic biliary strictures, cholestasis and eventually cirrhosis. There is a strong association with inflammatory bowel disease, particularly ulcerative colitis; 75% of PSC patients have ulcerative colitis and 5–8% of patients with ulcerative colitis develop PSC. It has a predilection for young Caucasian males (mean age at presentation 39 years), but it can occur in infancy or childhood and can affect any race. Cholangiocarcinoma develops in up to 10% of patients with PSC.

Vascular abnormalities

The Budd–Chiari syndrome (BCS) is a rare, heterogeneous and potentially fatal condition related to the obstruction of the hepatic venous outflow tract. The prevalence of underlying thrombophilia is markedly increased in patients with BCS. Affected patients are commonly women with an average age at presentation of 35. Early recognition and immediate use of anticoagulation has vastly improved outcome. More advanced disease can be treated in a number of ways including venoplasty, transjugular intrahepatic portosystemic shunt (TIPS), surgical shunts or liver transplantation.

Metabolic and genetic disorders

There are various inherited metabolic disorders that can affect the functioning of the liver.

Haemochromatosis

Hereditary haemachromatosis (HH) is the most commonly identified genetic disorder in the Caucasian population. It is associated with increased absorption of dietary iron resulting in deposition within the liver, heart, pancreas, joints, pituitary gland and other organs. This can lead to cirrhosis and hepatocellular carcinoma.

Wilson's disease

Wilson's disease is an autosomal recessive disorder of copper metabolism. The disorder leads to excessive absorption and deposition of dietary copper within the liver, brain, kidneys and other tissues. Presentation can vary widely from chronic hepatitis, asymptomatic cirrhosis, ALF to neuropsychiatric symptoms with cognitive impairment.

α_1-Antitrypsin deficiency

This is an autosomal recessively inherited disease and is the most common genetic metabolic liver disease. The disease results in a reduction in α_1-antitrypsin which is protective against a variety of proteases including trypsin, chymotrypsin, elastase and proteases present in neutrophils. The homozygous form of the disease (ZZ phenotype) is associated with the development of liver disease and cirrhosis in 15–30% of both adult and paediatric patients.

Glycogen storage disease

Glycogen storage disease is a rare disease occurring in 1 in 100,000 births. Enzymatic deficiencies at specific steps in the pathway of glycogen metabolism cause impaired glucose production and accumulation of abnormal glycogen in the liver.

Gilbert's syndrome

Gilbert's syndrome is characterised by persistent mild unconjugated hyperbilirubinaemia. It is most frequently recognised in adolescents and young adults with an incidence of between 2% and 7% in the general population. Serum bilirubin levels fluctuate but can increase to 80–100 µmol/L during periods of stress, sleep deprivation, prolonged fasting, menstruation and intercurrent infections. Gilbert's syndrome is an asymptomatic condition requiring no therapy, although patients may inappropriately associate being jaundiced with the symptoms of the condition that triggered the increase in the bilirubin levels.

Drugs

Drugs are an important cause of abnormal liver function tests and acute liver injury, including ALF (DILI drug-induced liver injury). Drugs can also be relevant to a number of chronic liver diseases including steatosis, fibrosis/cirrhosis, autoimmune and vascular disease. In most situations, the drug is implicated because of an appropriate temporal relationship between the disease and drug exposure.

Clinical manifestations

Symptoms of liver disease

In patients who have liver disease, weakness, increased fatigue and general malaise are common but non-specific symptoms. Weight loss and anorexia are more commonly seen in chronic liver disease and loss of muscle bulk is a characteristic of very advanced disease. Abdominal discomfort may be described by patients with an enlarged liver or spleen while distension with ascites is usually the cause in more advanced disease. Abdominal pain is common in hepatobiliary disease, frequently localised to the right upper quadrant. This is often a feature of rapid or gross enlargement of the liver when the pain is thought to be a consequence of capsular stretching. Tenderness over the liver is a symptom of acute hepatitis, hepatic abscess or hepatic malignancy.

Jaundice is the most striking symptom of liver disease and can present with or without pain, depending on the underlying aetiology of disease. Pruritus can be a distressing symptom in cholestatic liver disease and patients usually complain that it is worse at night. Patients with acute and chronic liver disease can develop bleeding complications because of defective hepatic synthesis of coagulation factors and low platelet counts

Signs of liver disease

Cutaneous signs

Hyperpigmentation is common in chronic liver disease and results from increased deposition of melanin. It is particularly associated with PBC and haemachromatosis. Scratch marks on the skin suggest pruritus which is a common feature of cholestatic liver disease. Vascular 'spiders' referred to as spider naevi are small vascular malformations in the skin and are found in the drainage area of the superior vena cava, commonly seen on the face, neck, hands and arms. Examination of the limbs can reveal several signs, none of which are specific to liver disease. Palmar erythema, a mottled reddening of the palms of the hands, can be associated with both acute and chronic liver disease. Dupuytren's contracture, thickening and shortening of the palmar fascia of the hands causing flexion deformities of the fingers, was traditionally associated with alcoholic cirrhosis. It is now considered to be multifactorial in origin and not to reflect primary liver disease. Nail changes, highly polished nails or white nails (leukonychia) can be seen in up to 80% of patients with chronic liver disease. Leukonychia is a consequence of low serum albumin. Finger clubbing is most commonly seen in hypoxaemia related to hepato-pulmonary syndrome, but is also a feature of chronic liver disease (Table 16.1)

Abdominal signs

Abdominal distension, notably of the flanks, is suggestive of ascites which can develop in both acute (less commonly) and chronic liver disease. An enlarged liver (hepatomegaly) is a common finding in acute liver disease. In cirrhotic patients the liver may be large, but alternatively it may be small and shrunken reflecting end-stage chronic disease. An enlarged spleen (splenomegaly) in the presence of chronic liver disease is the most important sign of portal hypertension. Dilated abdominal wall veins are a notable finding in chronic liver disease with the detection of umbilical and para-umbilical veins, a feature of portal hypertension.

Jaundice

Jaundice is the physical sign regarded as synonymous with liver disease and is most easily detected in the sclerae. It reflects impaired liver cell function (hepatocellular pathology)

Table 16.1 Physical signs of chronic liver disease

Common findings	End-stage findings
Jaundice	Ascites
Gynaecomastia & loss of body hair	Dilated abdominal blood vessels
Hand changes:	Fetor hepaticus
Palmar erythema	Hepatic flap
Clubbing	Neurological changes:
Dupuytren's contracture	Hepatic encephalopathy
Leuconychia	Disorientation
Liver mass reduced or increased	Changes in consciousness
Parotid enlargement	Peripheral oedema
Scratch marks on skin	Pigmented skin
Purpura	Muscle wasting
Spider naevi	
Splenomegaly	
Testicular atrophy	
Xanthelasma	
Hair loss	

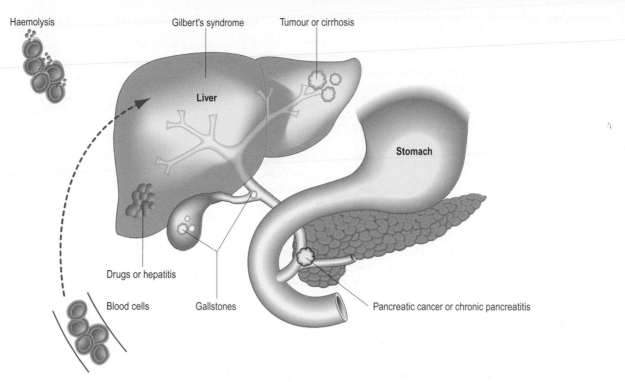

Fig. 16.4 Common causes of jaundice. Obstructive: due to blockage of the bile ducts; Hepatocellular: due to drugs, hepatitis, chronic liver disease or tumour formation; Prehepatic: due to increased blood breakdown such as occurs in haemolysis.

or it can be cholestatic (biliary) in origin. Hepatocellular jaundice is commonly seen in acute liver disease, but may be absent in chronic disease until the terminal stages of cirrhosis are reached. The causes of jaundice are shown in Fig. 16.4.

Portal hypertension

The increased pressure in the portal venous system leads to collateral vein formation and shunting of blood to the systemic circulation. Portal hypertension is an important contributory factor to the formation of ascites and the development of encephalopathy due to bypassing of blood from the liver to the systemic circulation. The major, potentially life-threatening complication of portal hypertension is torrential venous haemorrhage (variceal bleed) from the thin walled veins in the oesophagus and upper stomach. Patients with portal hypertension are often asymptomatic, while others may present with bleeding varices, ascites and/or encephalopathy.

Ascites

Ascites is the accumulation of fluid within the abdominal cavity. The precise mechanism by which ascites develops in chronic liver disease is unclear, but the following are all thought to contribute:

- Activation of the renin–angiotensin–aldosterone axis as a consequence of central hypovolaemia, leading to a reduction in sodium excretion by the kidney and fluid retention. Reduced aldosterone metabolism due to reduced liver function may also contribute to increased fluid retention.
- A reduction in serum albumin and reduced oncotic pressure is thought to contribute to the collection of fluid in the third space. Peripheral oedema (swollen lower limbs) occurs through this mechanism in a manner similar to the development of ascites.
- Portal hypertension and splanchnic arterial vasodilation alters intestinal capillary pressure and permeability and so facilitates the accumulation of retained fluid in the abdominal cavity.

Sexual characteristics

Endocrine changes are well documented in chronic liver disease and tend to be more common in alcoholic liver disease. Hypogonadism is common in patients with cirrhosis and in males results in testicular atrophy, female body hair distribution and gynaecomastia. This is thought, in part, to occur because the cirrhotic liver cannot metabolise oestrogen, leading to feminisation in males. Gynaecomastia is particularly found in alcoholics but is also seen in those taking spironolactone, when there is usually associated tenderness of the nipples. In women with chronic liver disease menstrual irregularity, amenorrhoea and reduced fertility are encountered in those of reproductive age, but few detectable physical signs are seen as a result of gonadal atrophy.

Investigations

All patients with liver disease must undergo a comprehensive and thorough assessment to ascertain the underlying aetiology. Although causes of acute and chronic liver disease may differ, a similar approach is used to investigate both patient groups to ensure no primary cause or co-factor is overlooked.

Biochemical tests

Biochemical liver function tests (LFTs) are simple, inexpensive and easy to perform but usually cannot be used in isolation to make a diagnosis. Biochemical parameters provide very useful information in monitoring disease progression or response to therapy. The liver enzymes usually measured are the aminotransferases which reflect hepatocellular pathology and the cholestatic liver enzymes, alkaline phosphatase and γ-glutamyl transpeptidase. Aspartate transaminase (AST) and alanine transaminase (ALT) are two intracellular enzymes present in hepatocytes which are released into the blood of patients as a consequence of hepatocyte damage. Extremely high values, where transaminases are recorded in the thousands, occur in acute liver disease, for example, viral hepatitis or paracetamol overdose. In chronic hepatitis, serum transaminases are rarely more than five to eight times the normal upper limit. Alkaline phosphatase is present in the canalicular and sinusoidal membranes of the liver but is also present in other sites, especially bone. Concomitant elevation of the enzyme γ-glutamyl transpeptidase confirms the hepatic origin of an elevated alkaline phosphatase. The serum alkaline phosphatase activity may be raised by up to four to six times the normal limit in intrahepatic or extra-hepatic cholestasis. It can also be raised in conditions associated with liver infiltration, such as metastases.

Bilirubin is commonly elevated in hepatocellular pathology and especially in acute hepatitis and end-stage chronic disease. An increase in bilirubin concentration results in jaundice and is usually clinically apparent when the serum bilirubin level exceeds 50 µmol/L. In acute liver disease, the serum bilirubin reflects severity of disease but is of little prognostic value. In chronic liver disease, a gradual increase for no apparent reason usually reflects serious disease progression. Hepatocellular damage, cholestasis and haemolysis can all cause elevations in the serum bilirubin concentration.

Synthetic function capacity is very important in assessing liver disease. Prothrombin time (PT), international normalised ratio (INR) and other coagulation studies are useful short-term markers of the synthetic function, especially in acute liver insults where they reflect the severity of the liver injury. PT or INR are also important indicators of chronic liver disease when combined with albumin levels. Albumin is synthesised in the liver and serum albumin levels reflect liver function over the preceeding months rather than days as with coagulation studies. Alternative causes of hypoalbuminaemia need to be considered, especially proteinuria.

Laboratory investigation of aetiology

All individuals presenting with derangement of liver function should be tested for hepatitis A, B, and C as part of a routine liver disease screen. Auto-antibodies and immunoglobulins to screen for autoimmune disease are also relevant to both acute and chronic liver disease. Serum ferritin, caeruloplasmin (in patients under 40 years), α_1-antitrypsin phenotype and lipid profile are standard investigations in patients with evidence of chronic liver disease.

Imaging techniques

Ultrasound is a non-invasive, low-risk procedure that is pivotal in the preliminary assessment of liver disease as it assesses the size, shape and texture of the liver and screens for dilatation of the biliary tract. In patients with chronic liver disease, it assesses patency of the portal vein and may detect signs of portal hypertension (increased spleen size, ascites). It is also routinely used to screen for hepatocellular carcinoma and other hepatobiliary malignancies. Computed tomography (CT) and magnetic resonance (MR) scans are regularly used for more precise definition of any abnormalities identified on ultrasound.

Liver biopsy

Liver biopsy is an invasive procedure with an associated morbidity and mortality, albeit extremely low. Nevertheless, it remains the gold standard in establishing a diagnosis and assessing the severity of chronic liver disease. Progress has been made in developing techniques to assess liver fibrosis non-invasively and a technique called Fibroscan appears to be effective in patients with HCV. In some instances, liver histology will contribute to the decision-making process with regard to therapy, for example, whether to initiate antiviral therapy for HBV or HCV. In acute hepatic dysfunction, a liver biopsy is usually unnecessary, especially if the condition is self-limiting.

Patient care

Pruritus

Pruritus is a prominent and sometimes distressing symptom of chronic liver disease and tends to be most debilitating in the context of cholestatic conditions. The pathogenesis of pruritus in liver disease is poorly understood but the deposition of bile salts within the skin is considered to be central to its development. However, the concentration of bile salts in the skin does not appear to correlate with the intensity of pruritus. Management of pruritus is variable. Relief of biliary obstruction by endoscopic, radiological or surgical means is indicated in patients with obstructed biliary systems. In other cases, pharmacological agents are used initially but in some cases plasmapheresis, molecular absorbants recirculating system (MARS) or even liver transplantation may be needed.

Anion exchange resins

Colestyramine and colestipol act by binding bile acids and preventing their reabsorption. These anion exchange resins are the first line of therapy in the treatment of pruritus. Colestyramine is usually initiated at a dosage of 4 g once or twice daily, and the dose is then titrated to optimise relief without causing side effects (predominantly gastro-intestinal). Such adverse effects are common and include constipation, diarrhoea, fat and vitamin malabsorption. Palatability is variable and consequently adherence is often a problem. In order to enhance compliance, patients should be advised that the benefits of therapy may take time to become apparent and often up to a week. Anion exchange resins can reduce the absorption of concomitant therapy and such drugs should be taken 1 h prior to or 4 h after colestyramine or colestipol ingestion. Drugs which are susceptible to this interaction include digoxin, thyroxine, ursodeoxycholic acid (UDCA), chlorothiazide, propranolol and the antibiotics tetracycline and penicillin.

Antihistamines

Although frequently used, antihistamines are usually ineffective in the management of the pruritus caused by cholestasis and should not be considered first-line therapy. A non-sedating antihistamine such as cetirizine (10 mg once daily) or loratidine (10 mg once daily) is preferred as these avoid precipitating or masking encephalopathy. Antihistamines such as chlorphenamine or hydroxyzine provide little more than sedative properties, although they may be useful at night if the severity of pruritus is sufficient to prevent a patient from sleeping.

Ursodeoxycholic acid

The bile acid UDCA (10 mg/kg daily in two divided doses) has been used frequently in cholestatic liver disease and long-term use has been shown to be effective in the treatment of pruritus. However, in about 5% of cases it worsens the pruritus.

Rifampicin

Rifampicin induces hepatic microsomal enzymes, which may benefit some patients, possibly by improving bile flow. Rifampicin, administered at a dose of 600 mg/day may be effective in the treatment of pruritus, albeit over a more prolonged period of time (1–3 weeks). It is most commonly used in patients with PBC. Its use is restricted by its potential hepatotoxicity and drug interactions with other agents.

Opioid antagonists

A growing spectrum of opioid antagonists have been used to treat pruritus because it is believed that endogenous opioids in the central nervous system are potent mediators of itch. As a consequence the centrally acting opioid antagonists naloxone, naltrexone and nalmefene are thought to reverse the actions of these endogenous opioids. The use of such agents is limited by their route of administration. Naloxone is given by subcutaneous injection, while naltrexone and nalmefene are reported to be more substantially bioavailable after oral administration. A summary of drugs used in the management of pruritus is shown in Table 16.2.

Table 16.2 Drugs commonly used in the management of pruritus

Drug	Indication	Daily dose	Advantage	Disadvantage
Colestyramine	Cholestatic jaundice Itching (first line)	4–16 g (in two or three divided doses)	Reduce systemic bile salt levels	Poor patient adherence due to unpalatability Diarrhoea/constipation Increased flatulence Abdominal discomfort
Ursodeoxycholic acid	Cholestatic jaundice Itching	10–15 mg/kg (in two divided doses)		Variable response
Menthol 2% in aqueous cream	Itching	As required	Local cooling effect	Variable response
Chlorphenamine	Itching	4–16 mg (in three or four divided doses)	Sedative effects may be useful for night-time itching	May precipitate/aggravate encephalopathy
Hydroxyzine	Itching	25–100 mg (in three or four divided doses)	Sedative effects may be useful for night-time itching	May precipitate/aggravate encephalopathy
Cetirizine	Itching	10 mg (once daily)	Antihistamine with low incidence of sedation	Variable response
Naltrexone	Itching	50 mg/day	Shown to be beneficial in primary biliary cirrhosis	Opiate withdrawal symptoms, usually transient

Topical preparations

Topical therapy may benefit some patients. Calamine lotion or menthol 2% in aqueous cream are standard preparations, but improvement of pruritus with such agents is variable.

Clotting abnormalities

The relationship of liver disease to clotting abnormalities is shown diagrammatically in Fig. 16.5. Haemostatic abnormalities develop in approximately 75% of patients with chronic liver disease and 100% of patients with ALF. The majority of clotting factors (with the exception of factor V) are dependent on vitamin K. Patients with liver disease who develop deranged blood clotting should receive intravenous doses of phytomenadione (vitamin K), usually 10 mg daily for 3 days. Administration of vitamin K to patients with significant liver disease does not usually improve the prothrombin time because the liver is unable to utilise the vitamin to synthesis clotting factors. Oral vitamin K is less effective than the parenteral form and so, has little or no place in the management of clotting abnormalities and bleeding secondary to liver disease.

Aspirin, non-steroidal anti-inflammatory drugs (NSAIDs) and anticoagulants should be avoided in all patients with liver disease because of the risk of altering platelet function, causing gastric ulceration and bleeding. NSAIDs have also been implicated in precipitating renal dysfunction and variceal bleeding in patients with end-stage liver disease. Although COX-2 inhibitors may cause a lower incidence of bleeding complications, currently they are avoided in patients with liver disease as their use still poses a risk.

Ascites

The aim in the treatment of ascites is to mobilise the abnormal collection of third space fluid (intra-abdominal fluid) and this can be achieved by simple measures such as reduced sodium intake. A low-salt diet (60–90 mEq/day) may be enough to facilitate the elimination of ascites and delay reaccumulation of fluid. Salt reduction combined with fluid restriction (approximately 1–1.5 L/day) are practical measures taken to mobilise fluid and provide weight reduction and symptomatic relief.

Aggressive weight reduction in the absence of peripheral oedema should be avoided as it is likely to lead to intravascular fluid depletion and renal failure. Weight loss should not exceed 300–500 g/day in the absence of peripheral oedema and 800–1000 g/day in those with peripheral oedema to prevent renal failure. However, diuretics and/or paracentesis are the cornerstone in the management of moderate to large volume ascites. A sequential approach to the management of ascites is outlined in Box 16.1.

Diuretics

The aldosterone antagonist, spironolactone is usually used as a first-line agent in the treatment of ascites. In most instances, a negative sodium balance and loss of ascitic fluid can be achieved with low doses of diuretics. Spironolactone can be used alone or in combination with a more potent loop diuretic. The specific agents and dosages used are outlined in Table 16.3. Spironolactone acts by blocking sodium reabsorption in the collecting tubules of the kidney. It is usually commenced at 50–100 mg/day, but this varies, depending on the patient's clinical status, electrolyte levels and concomitant drug therapies. It can take many days to have a therapeutic effect, so dose augmentation should be conducted with caution and strict observation of renal parameters. The addition of a loop diuretic, furosemide 40 mg/day enhances the natriuretic activity of spironolactone, and should be used when ascites is severe or when spironolactone alone fails to produce acceptable diuresis.

The use of more potent diuretic combinations may result in excessive diuresis which can lead to renal failure of pre-renal origin. The initiation and augmentation of diuretic therapy should ideally be carried out in hospital. This allows strict urea and electrolyte monitoring to detect impending hyperkalaemia and/or hyponatraemia, which commonly occur with diuretic therapy. It also allows the

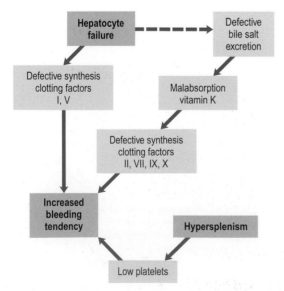

Fig. 16.5 Mechanisms of deranged clotting in chronic liver disease.

Box 16.1 The sequential approach to the management of cirrhotic ascites

Bedrest and sodium restriction (60–90 mEq/day, equivalent to 1500–2000 mg of salt/day)
▼
Spironolactone (or other potassium-sparing diuretic)
▼
Spironolactone and loop diuretic
▼
Large-volume paracentesis and colloid replacement

Other measures
Transjugular intrahepatic portosystemic shunt (TIPS)
Peritonovenous shunt
Consider orthotopic liver transplantation

Table 16.3 Diuretics used in the management of ascites

Drug	Indication	Daily dose	Advantage	Disadvantage
Spironolactone	Fluid retention	50–400 mg	Aldosterone antagonist Slow diuresis	Painful gynaecomastia Variable bioavailability Hyperkalaemia
Furosemide	Fluid retention	40–160 mg	Rapid diuresis Sodium excretion	Nephrotoxic Hypovolaemia Hypokalaemia Hyponatraemia Caution in pre-renal uraemia
Amiloride	Mild fluid retention	5–10 mg	As K⁺-sparing agent or weak diuretic if spironolactone contraindicated	Lacks potency

baseline measurement of urinary sodium excretion, subsequent changes in the diuretic dose should be titrated against urinary sodium excretion. Aggressive and unchecked diuresis will precipitate the hepatorenal syndrome, which has a very poor prognosis. Generally, if the serum sodium level decreases to less than 130 mmol/L or if creatinine levels rise to greater than 130 µmol/L then dose escalation of diuretics should be stopped. Diuretic therapy can be complicated by encephalopathy, hypokalaemia, hyponatraemia and azotaemia. Gynaecomastia and muscle cramps are side effects of diuretic therapy.

Refractory ascites, which occurs in 5–10% of patients with ascites, is associated with a 1-year survival rate of 25–50%. Therapeutic strategies include repeated large volume paracentesis combined with the administration of plasma expanders or alternatively, TIPS. In some patients, liver transplantation may be indicated. Ascites is considered to be refractory or diuretic resistant if there is no response with once daily doses of 400 mg spironolactone and 160 mg furosemide. Again, urinary sodium excretion provides important information in terms of the response to or viability of dose augmentation with diuretic therapy. Patients on lower doses of diuretics are also considered to have refractory ascites if side effects are a problem, for example, hepatic encephalopathy, hyperkalaemia, hyponatraemia or azotemia.

Paracentesis

Repeated large volume paracentesis in combination with albumin administration is the most widely accepted therapy for refractory ascites. Patients generally require paracentesis every 2–4 weeks and the procedure is often performed in the outpatient setting. Paracentesis, however, does not affect the mechanism responsible for ascitic fluid accumulation and so early recurrence is common. Intravenous colloid replacement or plasma expanders are used to prevent adverse effects on the renal and systemic circulation. Colloid replacement in the form of 6–8 g albumin/L of ascites removed (equivalent to 100 mL of 20% human albumin solution [1 unit] for every 2.5 L of ascitic fluid removed) is a standard regimen.

Transjugular intrahepatic portosystemic shunting (TIPS)

TIPS is an invasive procedure, used to manage refractory ascites or control refractory variceal bleeding. It is carried out under radiological guidance. An expandable intrahepatic stent is placed between one hepatic vein and the portal vein by a transjugular approach (Fig. 16.6). In contrast to paracentesis, the use of TIPS is effective in preventing recurrence in patients with refractory ascites. It reduces the activity of sodium retaining mechanisms and improves the renal response to diuretics. However, a disadvantage of this procedure is the high rate of shunt stenosis (up to 30% after 6–12 months) which leads to recurrence of ascites. TIPS can also induce or exacerbate hepatic encephalopathy.

Spontaneous bacterial peritonitis (SBP)

Patients with ascites should be closely observed for SBP as it develops in 10–30% of patients and has a high mortality. Hepatorenal syndrome can complicate SBP in up to 30% of

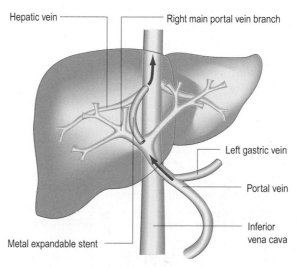

Fig. 16.6 Intrahepatic stent shunt links the hepatic vein with the intraheptic portal vein.

patients and also carries a high mortality. Conventional signs and symptoms of peritonitis are rarely present in such patients and if suspected, treatment with appropriate antibiotics should be started immediately after a diagnostic ascitic tap has been taken. A polymorphonuclear leucocyte count of greater than 250 cells/mm³ is diagnostic of this condition. The causative organism is of enteric origin in approximately three-quarters of infections, and originates from the skin in the remaining one-quarter. Cefotaxime (2 g, 8 hourly) is effective in 85% of patients with SBP and is commonly used as first-line antimicrobial therapy. Other antibiotic regimens have been used including co-amoxiclav, but third-generation cephalosporins are the treatment of choice. The quinolone, norfloxacin (400 mg/day), has a role in the prevention of recurrence of SBP, estimated as 70% at 1-year, and is recommended for long-term antibiotic prophylaxis. However, the emergence of quinolone-resistant bacteria is a growing problem in the management of SBP.

Hepatic encephalopathy

Hepatic encephalopathy is a reversible neuropsychiatric complication that occurs with significant liver dysfunction. The precise cause of encephalopathy remains unclear, but three factors are known to be implicated, namely portosystemic shunting, metabolic dysfunction and an alteration of the blood–brain barrier. It is thought that intestinally derived neuroactive and neurotoxic substances such as ammonia pass through the diseased liver or bypass the liver through shunts and go directly to the brain. This results in cerebral dysfunction. Ammonia is thought to increase the permeability of the blood–brain barrier, enabling other neurotoxins to enter the brain, and indirectly alter neurotransmission. Other substances implicated in causing hepatic encephalopathy include free fatty acids, γ-aminobutyric acid (GABA) and glutamate.

Clinical features of hepatic encephalopathy range from trivial lack of awareness, altered mental state to asterixis (liver flap) through to gross disorientation and coma. During low-grade encephalopathy, the altered mental state may present as impaired judgement, altered personality, euphoria or anxiety. Reversal of day/night sleep patterns is very typical of encephalopathy. Somnolence, semistupor, confusion and, finally, coma can ensue (Table 16.4).

Encephalopathy associated with cirrhosis and/or portalsystemic shunts may develop as a result of specific precipitating factors (Box 16.2) or spontaneously. Common precipitating factors include gastro-intestinal bleeding, SBP, constipation, dehydration, electrolyte abnormalities and certain drugs including narcotics and sedatives. Identification and removal of such precipitating factors is mandatory. Therapeutic management is then aimed at reducing the amount of ammonia or nitrogenous products in the circulatory system. Treatment with laxatives increases the throughput of bowel contents, by reducing transit time and also increases soluble nitrogen output in the faeces. Drug therapies for encephalopathy are summarised in Table 16.5.

Lactulose, a non-absorbable disaccharide, decreases ammonia production in the gut. It is widely used as it is broken down by gastro-intestinal bacteria to form lactic, acetic and formic acids. The effect of lactulose is to acidify the colonic contents which leads to the ionisation of nitrogenous products within the bowel, with a consequent reduction in their absorption from the gastro-intestinal tract. Lactulose is commenced in doses of 30–40 mL/day and titrated to result in two to three bowel motions each day. Patients unable to take oral medication or those with worsening encephalopathy are treated with phosphate enemas.

Antibiotics such as metronidazole or neomycin may also be used to reduce ammonia production from gastro-intestinal bacteria. Metronidazole has been the preferred option in the past, while the use of neomycin has largely been abandoned because of associated toxicity. Recent data has supported the use of the rifaximin, a minimally absorbed antibiotic, for the treatment of acute encephalopathy and the remission of chronic encephalopathy (Bass et al., 2010). Other therapies investigated for the treatment of encephalopathy include L-ornithine-L-aspartate (LOLA), sodium benzoate, L-dopa, bromocriptine and the benzodiazepine receptor antagonist, flumazenil.

Oesophageal varices

Variceal bleeding is the most feared complication of portal hypertension in patients with cirrhosis and there is a 30% lifetime risk of at least one bleeding episode among patients with cirrhosis and varices. Treatment of variceal bleeding includes

Table 16.4 Grading of hepatic encephalopathy

Grade 0	Normal
Subclinical	Abnormal psychometric tests for encephalopathy (e.g. number correction test)
Grade 1	Mood disturbance, abnormal sleep pattern, impaired handwriting +/− asterixis
Grade 2	Drowsiness, grossly impaired calculation ability, asterixis
Grade 3	Confusion, disorientation, somnolent but arousable, asterixis
Grade 4	Stupor to deep coma, unresponsive to painful stimuli

Box 16.2 Precipitating causes of hepatic encephalopathy

- Gastro-intestinal bleeding
- Infection (spontaneous bacterial peritonitis, other sites of sepsis)
- Hypokalaemia, metabolic alkalosis
- High protein diet
- Constipation
- Drugs, opioids and benzodiazepines
- Deterioration of liver function
- Post-surgical TIPS

Table 16.5 Drugs commonly used in the management of encephalopathy

Drug	Dose	Comment	Side effects
Lactulose	15–30 mL orally 2–4 times daily	Aim for 2–3 soft stools daily	Bloating, diarrhoea
Metronidazole	400–800 mg orally daily in divided doses	Metabolism impaired in liver disease	Gastro-intestinal disturbance
Neomycin Used less frequently now	2–4 g orally daily in divided doses	Maximum duration of 48 h	Potential for nephro- and ototoxicity
Rifaxamin	550 mg twice daily	Benefit demonstrated over 6 months use	Allergic reactions, gastro-intestinal disturbance May permit overgrowth *Clostridium difficile*

endoscopic banding, or rarely sclerotherapy, of oesophageal varices in parallel with splanchnic vasoconsrictors and intensive medical care. Patients with variceal bleeding refractory to endoscopic intervention or patients bleeding from ectopic or uncontrolled gastric varices will need TIPS or surgical decompressive shunts. Refractory variceal bleeding should, therefore, be managed in centres with the appropriate expertise.

Initial treatment is aimed at stopping or reducing the immediate blood loss, treating hypovolaemic shock, if present, and subsequent prevention of recurrent bleeding. Immediate and prompt resuscitation is an essential part of treatment. Only when medical treatment has been initiated and optimised should endoscopy be performed. Endoscopy confirms the diagnosis and allows therapeutic intervention. Fluid replace-

ment is invariably required, and should be in the form of colloid or packed red cells and administered centrally. Saline should generally be avoided in all patients with cirrhosis. Fluid replacement must be administered with caution, as overzealous expansion of the circulating volume may precipitate further bleeding by raising portal pressure, thereby exacerbating the clinical situation. A flow chart for the management of bleeding oesophageal varices is shown in Fig. 16.7.

Endoscopic management

Variceal band ligation uses prestretched rubber bands applied to the base of a varix which has been sucked into the banding chamber attached to the front of an endoscope. Variceal

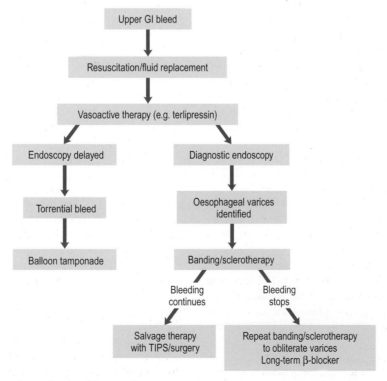

Fig. 16.7 Management of oesophageal variceal haemorrhage.

band ligation (VBL) controls bleeding in approximately 90% of cases. It is at least as effective as sclerotherapy, which it has largely superceded, and is associated with fewer side effects. Balloon tamponade with a Sengstaken–Blakemore balloon or Linton balloon may be used to stabilise a patient with actively bleeding varices by directly compressing the bleeding varices, until more definitive therapy can be undertaken. Balloon tamponade can control bleeding in up to 90% of cases but 50% rebleed when the balloon is deflated. Gastric varices develop in approximately 20% of patients with portal hypertension. The risk of gastric variceal bleeding is lower than that of oesophageal variceal bleeding, but bleeding from fundal varices is more difficult to manage and is associated with a higher mortality. The most effective treatment strategy for fundal varices is now considered to be variceal obturation with tissue adhesives or 'glue injection'. The use of cyanoacrylate injection in the treatment of fundal varices is associated with less rebleeding and is emerging as the treatment of choice in the hands of experienced endoscopists.

Drug treatment

Several pharmacological agents are available for the emergency control of variceal bleeding (Table 16.6). Most act by lowering portal venous pressure. They are generally used to control bleeding in addition to balloon tamponade and emergency endoscopic techniques. Vasopressin was the first vasoconstrictor used to reduce portal pressure in patients with actively bleeding varices. However, its associated systemic vasoconstrictive adverse effects limited its use. The synthetic vasopressin analogue, terlipressin, is highly effective in controlling bleeding and in reducing mortality. It can be administered in bolus doses every 4–6 h and has a longer biological activity and a more favourable side effect profile. Once a diagnosis of variceal bleeding has been established, a vasoactive drug infusion (usually terlipressin) should be started without further delay and continued for 2–5 days. Somatostatin and the somatostatin analogue, octreotide, are reported to cause selective splanchnic vasoconstriction and reduce portal pressure. Although they are reported to cause less adverse effects on the systemic circulation, terlipressin remains the agent of choice.

Transjugular intrahepatic portosystemic shunt (TIPS)

TIPS is now established as the preferred rescue therapy in cases where endoscopic intervention has failed to control bleeding (Fig. 16.7). Recent data suggests the use of early

TIPS, within the first 48 h, may be life saving in patients with advanced liver failure.

Prevention of rebleeding

Endoscopic band ligation (EBL) is performed at regular intervals (1–2 weeks) as part of an eradication programme to obliterate the varices. Once varices have been eradicated, endoscopic follow-up can be performed less frequently (3 monthly) for the first year, then twice yearly thereafter. If varices reappear they should be banded regularly until eradicated again. Non-selective β-blockers, such as propranolol, are the medication of choice to prevent rebleeding and can also be used as primary prophlaxis against variceal bleeding in patients with known varices. The mechanism of action is complex, but they reduce portal hypertension by causing splanchnic vasoconstriction and reduced portal blood flow. At higher doses they can have a more marked negative effect on cardiac output and so must be titrated accordingly.

Acute liver failure

ALF occurs when there is a rapid deterioration in liver function in previously healthy individuals resulting in encephalopathy and a coagulopathy. ALF is a multisystem disorder with cerebral oedema and renal impairment being particularly important complications. In the past, viral hepatitis was a major consideration in the aetiology of ALF. However, the development of a commercial vaccine for hepatitis B has seen a dramatic decline in the contribution of HBV to ALF in Western countries. The most common cause of ALF in the UK and USA is paracetamol (acetaminophen) toxicity. Seronegative hepatitis is the other common aetiological group. Management of ALF is complicated, involving supporting the central nervous system, cardiovascular and renal systems. All patients with ALF are at risk of infection, and prophylactic administration of broad spectrum antibiotics and antifungal agents is standard practice. Coagulopathy and bleeding resulting from liver failure are well-recognised life-threatening complications which require specialised monitoring and early correction.

Liver transplantation

Liver transplantation is the established treatment for selected patients with ALF, decompensated chronic liver disease, inherited metabolic disorders and primary liver cancer. HCV and alcohol-induced end-stage liver disease are the commonest indications for liver transplantation in Europe and the USA. Typical 1 year survival rates are around 90% for elective transplants. Remarkably few transplants fail because of rejection and, nowadays, technical problems, infection and multisystem failure account for most deaths in the first year. Recurrence of the primary disease, malignancy and death with a functioning graft account for most late deaths.

An increasing number of immunosuppressive agents are now available and this has enabled clinicians to tailor immunosuppression to achieve a balance of good graft function

Table 16.6 Drugs used in the treatment of acute bleeding varices

Drug	Dosage and administration
Terlipressin	1–2 mg bolus 4–6 hourly for 48 h
Octreotide	50 μcg/h i.v. infusion for 48 h or longer if patient rebleeds

and an acceptable side effect profile. The calcineurin inhibitors (CNIs), tacrolimus and ciclosporin remain the mainstay of immunosuppressive therapy. Corticosteroids are still commonly used, at least during the first 3 months after transplantation. The other drugs used regularly for long-term immunosuppression include azathioprine, mycophenolate, sirolimus and everolimus. Therapy is monitored closely and increasingly tailored to individual patients, with a particular emphasis on preserving renal function and reducing the risk of cardiovascular disease.

Disease specific therapies

Hepatitis B

The primary goal in the management of chronic HBV infection is to prevent cirrhosis, hepatic failure and hepatocellular carcinoma. The ideal outcome is eradication of HBV with HBsAg loss and the prevention of irreversible liver damage. However, the eradication of HBV is near impossible because of the presence of extra-hepatic reservoirs of HBV and the integration of HBV into the host genome and the presence of an intracellular conversion pathway which replenishes the pool of transcriptional templates in the hepatocyte nucleus without the need for reinfection. For this reason, the main treatment goal is continuous viral suppression and current therapies, specifically with oral antiviral agents, are judged by their ability to provide continuous viral suppression.

It is the persistence of covalently closed circular DNA (cccDNA) which is considered to preclude a 'cure' for HBV. Thus, therapies currently available for the treatment of chronic HBV are measured in terms of HBeAg seroconversion (in eAg positive disease), viral suppression, ALT normalisation and improvement in liver histopathology. More recently, there has been specific focus on HBsAg quantification, with loss of HBsAg considered a surrogate marker of cccDNA levels (Sung et al., 2005). Thus, all therapies in the treatment of HBV should be benchmarked against HBsAg loss, as a marker of drug utility and efficacy.

There is now concensus amongst the major liver disease authorities in terms of their clinical practice guidelines and the recommended agents available for the treatment of chronic HBV infection. Treatment strategies have broadened and include the potent oral antiviral agents tenofovir (Marcellin et al., 2008; National Institute for Health and Clinical Excellence, 2009) and entecavir (National Institute for Health and Clinical Excellence, 2008) as first-line monotherapies. While these two agents have emerged as the leading oral antivirals, the weaker and more outdated agents such as telbivudine, lamivudine and adefovir are still widely used. The use of lamivudine or adefovir as monotherapy is no longer recommended and should be avoided if at all possible, owing to the high rates of resistance reported with these drugs. Pegylated interferon (peginterferon) alfa-2a has re-emerged as a viable alternative to oral antiviral agents in the treatment of chronic HBV. This is due primarily to its potent immunomodulatory effects which gives it a clear advantage over oral antivirals. Significant rates of surface antigen (sAg) loss have been reported in both HBeAg positive and negative disease and the inclusion of surface antigen quantification has provided an objective tool to assess response to pegylated interferon. The advantages of interferon therapy, such as a finite treatment course, good rates of surface antigen loss in selected patients, must be weighed against the disadvantages associated with an injection-based therapy and the inherent side effect profile associated with interferons. Therefore, a careful and rational approach must be followed when considering treatment of chronic HBV. While reported rates of resistance is extremely low with entecavir, and none reported with tenofovir, the treatment landscape for chronic HBV has changed dramatically from the high rates of resistance previously seen with lamivudine and adefovir. However, when commencing oral antiviral agents, the patient must be aware they are potentially embarking on a lifelong course of treatment.

An issue which must be given further consideration is the potential side effect profile of these relatively new drugs, notwithstanding their potency and documented efficacy. The potential for unforeseen side effects must be considered unresolved, as safety data to date are limited by the relatively short period of time that these drugs have been used in clinical practice. Likewise, physicians will need to remain vigilant for the emergence of resistant virus, even with these potent agents with well-described high-genetic barriers to resistance.

Hepatitis C

The primary aim of treating patients with chronic HCV is viral clearance with sustained virologic response (SVR) defined as the absence of viraemia 6 months after antiviral therapy has been discontinued. Viral clearance improves the patient's quality of life and reduces the risk of progression to cirrhosis and hepatocellular carcinoma.

Pegylated interferon and ribavirin combination therapy are now the standard care of chronic HCV (National Institute for Health and Clinical Excellence, 2010). The SVR for treatment of naïve patients is of the order of 55% for genotypes 1 and 4 (48 weeks of therapy) and 80–85% for genotypes 2 and 3 (24 weeks of therapy). The treatment duration, however, can be individualised based on the baseline viral load and the speed of virological response during treatment. Patients failing to achieve a significant reduction in viral load after 12 weeks will normally have therapy discontinued. The current standard of care combination therapy is limited by the side effect profile, complications of therapy and poor patient tolerability. Side effects of therapy include influenza-like symptoms, decrease in haematological parameters (haemoglobin, neutrophils, white blood cell count and platelets), gastrointestinal complaints, psychiatric disturbances (anxiety and depression) and hypo- or hyperthyrodism. It is accepted that these side effects are a major obstacle preventing completion of therapy by hindering compliance or enforcing significant dose reductions. While growth factors (erythropoietin, GCSF) and antidepressants may alleviate some side effects, there remains a clear need for better treatment strategies in chronic HCV infection.

Significant progress has been made in the development of new HCV-specific inhibitors. Data from recent trials have shown a marked improvement in SVR when these new protease inhibitors, telaprevir and boceprevir are given in combination with current standard of care, increasing response rates to 61–75% in genotype 1 HCV infection. It is anticipated that these agents will be available for clinical practice from 2011. Several new HCV-specific inhibitors are currently in clinical evaluation including protease inhibitors, nucleoside and non-nucleoside polymerase inhibitors as well as non-HCV compounds with anti-HCV activity. It is envisaged, as a result of this evolution of HCV therapies, that the treatment options for HCV will become more robust.

Autoimmune hepatitis

Corticosteroids and/or azathioprine are the standard therapy for AIH. Prednisone or prednisolone are administered at doses of 40–60 mg/day alone or at lower doses when combined with azathioprine. The steroid dose is reduced over a 6-week to 3-month period to a target maintenance dose of 7.5 mg/day or lower. The disturbance in aminotransferases usually normalises within 6–12 weeks, but histological remission tends to lag by 6–12 months. Azathioprine at a dose of 1–1.5 mg/kg/day is used as an adjunct to corticosteroid therapy. Azathioprine, used alone, is ineffective in treating the acute phase of AIH. In patients intolerant of azathioprine, or in cases of proven treatment failure, other immunosuppressants have been used, for example, tacrolimus and mycophenolate. Newer corticosteroids such as budesonide, with fewer systemic side effects, have also been used effectively and may have a greater role in the future treatment of AIH.

Primary biliary cirrhosis. Several therapies have been associated with short-term symptomatic improvements in liver function tests. UDCA, the only medication widely used to treat PBC, reduces the retention of bile acids and increases their hepatic excretion. Therefore, it is effective in protecting against the cytotoxic effects of dihydroxy bile acids which accumulate in PBC. However, UDCA does not appear to prevent ongoing bile duct injury and disease progression. Therefore, liver transplantation remains the only effective option in patients with end-stage disease. Immunosuppressive agents such as ciclosporin, azathioprine and methotrexate have also been assessed for the treatment of PBC but clinically significant adverse events outweigh the potential benefits.

Primary sclerosing cholangitis

There is no effective treatment for this condition. UDCA can be used to manage associated cholestasis, and doses as high as 15 mg/kg/day have been advocated despite the limited evidence that it alters the natural history of the disease. Studies with various immunosuppressive agents have been disappointing and transplantation remains the only effective treatment option in patients with advanced disease.

Wilson's disease

This rare autosomal recessive condition is usually managed with chelation therapy. Penicillamine is the agent of choice in Wilson's disease as it promotes urinary copper excretion in affected patients and prevents copper accumulation in presymptomatic individuals. Initial treatment of 1.5–2 g/day is given in divided doses. Initially, neurological symptoms may worsen because of deposition of mobilised copper in the basal ganglia, but symptomatic patients tend to improve over a period of several weeks. Other therapy-related adverse effects include renal dysfunction, haematological abnormalities and disseminated lupus erythematosis. Therefore, regular monitoring of full blood count and electrolytes is required as well as small doses of pyridoxine (25 mg) to counteract the antipyridoxine effect of penicillamine and the associated neurological toxicity. Patients unable to tolerate penicillamine may respond to trientine. This chelating agent is less potent than penicillamine but has fewer adverse effects. Oral zinc is also used but it too is less potent than penicillamine.

Case studies

Case 16.1

A 56-year-old man is admitted to hospital following haematemesis and melaena. He has a known history of alcoholic liver disease (stopped drinking alcohol 1 year ago) with marked ascites.
A provisional diagnosis of bleeding oesophageal varices is made.

A Sengstaken–Blakemore tube is inserted and the balloon inflated as a temporary measure to arrest bleeding. The patient is transferred 8 h later to a specialist regional centre for further management.

Laboratory data on admission are:

Na	124 (133–143 mmol/L)
K	3.0 (3.5–5.0 mmol/L)
Creatinine	131 (80–124 µmol/L)
Urea	14.3 (2.7–7.7 mmol/L)
Bilirubin	167 (3.15 µmol/L)
ALT	24 (0–35 IU/L)
PT	18.9 (13 s)
Albumin	24 (35–50 g/dL)
Hb	8.9 (13.5–18 g/dL)

Drugs on admission:

Spironolactone 200 mg one each morning.

....

Questions

1. What other action would you have recommended before the patient was transferred to the regional centre?
2. What options (drug and/or non-drug) are likely to be available at the regional centre for managing the patient's bleeding varices?
3. What further long-term measures would you recommend for this patient?

....

Answers

1. Initial restoration of circulating blood volume with colloid, followed by cross-matched blood. Fluid replacement is necessary to protect renal perfusion. In view of the patient's ascites, saline should be avoided. Dextrose 5% with added

potassium (hypokalaemia present) would be a reasonable choice. A pharmacological agent to reduce portal pressure, such as terlipressin 1–2 mg every 4–6 h or octreotide 50 μcg/h, should be started. Current evidence supports terlipressin over octreotide. Broad spectrum antibiotics such as cefuroxime and metronidazole should be started intravenously if there is suspicion of abdominal infection or sepsis. There is no evidence that gastric acid suppression is beneficial, but if the bleeding is caused by a gastric mucosal lesion, a proton pump inhibitor such as lansoprazole or omeprazole, or a histamine type-2 receptor antagonist such as ranitidine can be administered.

Spironolactone is likely to be either causing or exacerbating the low sodium and should be discontinued.

Vitamin K, 10 mg intravenously once daily for 3 days, should be administered to try to correct the raised prothrombin time. As the patient has severe liver disease with varices and ascites there is a possibility he may develop encephalopathy. It would be advisable to start lactulose or, if the patient is unable to take medicines orally, administer an enema such as a phosphate enema.

2. *Banding/ligation*: this has a similar efficacy to sclerotherapy but fewer complications. It involves mechanical strangulation of variceal channels by small elastic plastic rings mounted on the tip of the endoscope.

Transjugular intrahepatic portosystemic shunt (TIPS): this can be used to reduce portal pressure, but there is a risk of precipitating encephalopathy.

Banding is the first-line option for managing bleeding oesophageal varices. Patients who continue to bleed after two endoscopic treatments should be considered for TIPS. Surgery involving portal-systemic shunts or devascularisation are possible options if the above alternatives repeatedly fail. Extra-hepatic portal-systemic shunts are situated outside the liver and divert portal blood flow into the systemic circulation bypassing the liver. Devascularisation involves obliteration of the collateral vessels supplying blood to the varices.

3. Banding/ligation can be performed at regular intervals of 1–2 weeks to obliterate the varices. Once varices have been eradicated, endoscopic follow-up should be undertaken every 3 months for the first year then every 6–12 months thereafter. If varices reappear they should be banded regularly until eradicated again. Non-selective β-blockers such as propranolol are used in the prophylaxis of further bleeds, with the dose adjusted until the heart rate is reduced by 25%, but to not less than 55 beats/min.

Case 16.2

A 68-year-old woman with a long-standing history of alcoholic liver disease is admitted to hospital with a 2-week history of vomiting, confusion, increased abdominal distension and worsening jaundice.
On admission laboratory data are as follows:

Na	116 (133–143 mmol/L)
K	3.8 (3.5–5 mmol/L)
Urea	8.5 (3.3–7.7 mmol/L)
Cr	119 (80–124 μmol/L)
Bilirubin	459 (3–17 μmol/L)
Albumin	23 (35–50 g/L)
ALT	23 (0–35 iu/L)
Alk P	524 (70–300 iu/L)
PT	18.6 (13 s)

Drugs on admission are as follows:

Spironolactone: 300 mg each morning.
Temazepam: 10 mg at night.
Lactulose: 10 mL twice daily.

Questions

Discuss the initial treatment plan for the management of:
1. Ascites
2. Nausea and vomiting
3. Confusion

Answers

From the presenting features and LFTs on admission it is apparent that the patient's liver disease is getting progressively worse, probably as a result of continued alcohol intake. She is confused on admission and this suggests encephalopathy, a common complication of chronic liver disease.

1. *Ascites management*. The patient has increased abdominal distension on admission suggestive of worsening ascites. This might be due to poor adherence with spironolactone, or alternatively, her ascites may have become diuretic resistant.

The patient should be sodium restricted and confined to bed. Spironolactone therapy should be stopped in view of the low sodium and confusion, as overuse of diuretics can precipitate encephalopathy. Fluid restriction is necessary to reduce the ascites, but sufficient fluid is required to rehydrate the patient following vomiting.

Paracentesis should be used to manage the ascites. Every litre of ascitic fluid removed should be replaced with 6–8 g of albumin. A diagnostic ascitic tap should be taken to ensure there is no infection in the ascites.

2. *Nausea/vomiting management*. Urea is slightly raised, indicating possible dehydration as a result of vomiting. The patient should be rehydrated with dextrose 5%, not saline, as this will worsen the ascites. Additional potassium should be given to correct the low serum potassium. Note that if the patient has been taking the spironolactone there would normally be an increase in potassium, but in this case the vomiting has probably reduced this. The patient's nausea can be managed with a suitable antiemetic such as domperidone 10 mg four times a day initially and then titrated according to the response.

3. *Confusion*. Confusion may be an early sign of encephalopathy in this patient. Temazepam should be stopped. The patient is on an inadequate dose of lactulose for the management of encephalopathy, so this should be increased to produce 2–3 loose motions per day. A typical dose would be 20 mL three or four times daily. In view of the patient's confusion, it may be worth considering other agents in the management of the encephalopathy, such as metronidazole 400 mg twice daily.

Case 16.3

A 54-year-old woman with primary biliary cirrhosis has been complaining of increasing backache over the last 3 months. Her general condition has deteriorated over the past year during which she has suffered from ascites and encephalopathy. Her main complaint is of continuous back pain, which disturbs her sleep.

Question

How would you manage this patient's back pain?

Answer

Back pain secondary to osteoporosis-related vertebral fractures is common in patients with chronic liver disease, such as primary biliary cirrhosis. This is due to the fact that most patients with primary biliary cirrhosis are postmenopausal women in their late 50s where bone thinning is likely, secondary to both menopausal and liver changes. Once the diagnosis has been confirmed, the patient should be counselled that the bone pain is chronic, tends to be intermittent, and takes several months to settle after each new fracture. Bed rest is useful in the acute situation, but prolonged bed rest can accelerate bone loss.

Although there have been rapid advances in recent years in the treatment of postmenopausal osteoporosis, very few studies have addressed the problems of treating osteoporosis in patients with chronic liver disease. Hormone replacement therapy has not been evaluated in patients with chronic liver disease, and oestrogen therapy is widely believed to be contraindicated in such patients, although there is little evidence to support this. Transdermal oestrogen preparations that avoid the first-pass metabolic effect may be a possible future option.

The patient should be advised to take adequate calcium supplementation of 1–1.5 g/day in addition to her normal diet. Vitamin D deficiencies are common in chronic liver disease and it would be advisable to administer 300,000 units intramuscularly every 3 months.

For symptomatic management of the pain a variety of analgesics are available. The choice of drug is influenced by both the severity of the pain and the degree of liver impairment.

For mild pain, paracetamol is the mainstay of treatment, and may be used in standard doses in the majority of patients with liver dysfunction. Patients pretreated with cytochrome P450 inducing drugs or patients with a history of alcohol abuse are at increased risk of paracetamol-induced liver injury and should receive only short courses at low doses (maximum of 2 g/day for an adult).

Opioid analgesics should usually be avoided in liver disease because of their sedative properties and the risks of precipitating or masking encephalopathy. If a patient has stable mild to moderate liver disease then short-term use of opioids can be considered. Moderate potency opioids, such as dihydrocodeine and codeine, are eliminated almost entirely by hepatic metabolism. Therapy should be initiated at a low dose, and the dosage interval titrated according to the response of the patient. Despite their low potency, these preparations may still precipitate encephalopathy.

In severe pain, the use of potent opioids is usually unavoidable. They undergo hepatic metabolism, and are therefore likely to accumulate in liver disease. To compensate for this it is important to increase the dosage interval when using these drugs. Morphine, pethidine or diamorphine should be administered at doses at the lower end of the dosage range at intervals of 6–8 h. The patient should be regularly observed and the dose titrated according to patient response. In any patient with liver disease receiving an opioid, it is advisable to coprescribe a laxative as constipation can increase the possibility of developing encephalopathy.

NSAIDs should be avoided in patients with liver disease. All NSAIDs can prolong bleeding time via their effects on platelet function. Impaired liver function itself can lead to a reduced synthesis of clotting factors and an increased bleeding tendency. NSAIDs may also be dangerous due to the increased risk of gastro-intestinal haemorrhage and potential to precipitate renal dysfunction.

References

Bass, N.M., Mullen, K.D., Sanyal, A., et al., 2010. Rifaximin treatment in hepatic encephalopathy. N. Engl. J. Med. 362, 1071–1081.

Marcellin, P., Heathcote, E.J., Buti, M., et al., 2008. Tenofovir disoproxil fumarate versus adefovir dipivoxil for chronic hepatitis B. N. Engl. J. Med. 359, 2442–2455.

National Institute for Health and Clinical Excellence, 2008. Entecavir for the Treatment of Chronic Hepatitis B. Technology Appraisal 153. NICE, London, Available at: http://www.nice.org.uk/TA153.

National Institute for Health and Clinical Excellence, 2009. Tenofovir Disoproxil for the Treatment of Chronic Hepatitis B. Technology Appraisal 173. NICE, London, Available at: http://www.nice.org.uk/TA173.

National Institute for Health and Clinical Excellence, 2010. Peginterferon Alfa and Ribavirin for the Treatment of Chronic Hepatitis C. Technology Appraisal 200. NICE, London, Available at: http://www.nice.org.uk/guidance/TA200.

Sung, J.J., Wong, M.L., Bowden, S., et al., 2005. Intrahepatic hepatitis B virus covalently closed circular DNA can be a predictor of sustained response to therapy. Gastroenterology 128, 1890–1897.

Further reading

Foster, G., Reddy, K.R. (Eds.), 2010. Clinical Dilemmas in Viral Liver Disease. John Wiley & Sons, Chichester.

Friedman, L.S., Keeffe, E.B. (Eds.), 2004. Handbook of Liver Disease, second ed. Elsevier Health, London.

Lindor, K.D., Talwalkar, J.A., 2008. Cholestatic Liver Disease. Humana Press, New Jersey.

Mahl, T.E., O'Grady, J., 2006. Fast Facts: Liver Disorders (Fast Facts series). Health Press Limited, Oxford.

Acute kidney injury 17

P. Cockwell, S. Stringer and J. Marriott

Key points

- Acute renal failure (ARF), or acute kidney injury (AKI), is diagnosed when the excretory function of the kidney declines rapidly over a period of hours or days and is usually associated with the accumulation of metabolic waste products and water.
- A wide range of factors can precipitate AKI, including trauma, obstruction of urine flow or any event that causes a reduction in renal blood flow, including surgery and medical conditions, for example, sepsis, diabetes, acute liver disease, rapidly progressive glomerulonephritis.
- Drug involvement in the development of AKI is common.
- There are no specific signs and symptoms of AKI. The condition is typically indicated by raised blood levels of creatinine and/or a low urine output.
- The clinical priorities in AKI are to manage life-threatening complications, correct intravascular fluid balance and establish the cause of the renal failure, reversing factors causing damage where possible.
- The aim of medical treatment is to remove causative factors and maintain patient well-being so that the kidneys have a chance to recover.
- Most measures of renal function are inaccurate when renal function deteriorates or improves rapidly as is usually the case in AKI.
- Treatment of AKI is essentially supportive, though there are conditions that cause AKI that are reversible with specific treatment.
- AKI is a serious condition with mortality rates up to 70%, varying according to cause and at its highest with concurrent failure of other organs.

The diagnostic criteria for AKI is based on an increase in serum creatinine or the presence of oliguria (see Table 17.1). Criteria have recently been introduced for the definition and staging of the condition; the acronym RIFLE is used (Risk, Injury, Failure, Loss and End-stage renal disease (ESRD)), which is now becoming established in clinical practice (see Fig. 17.1).

The large majority of cases of AKI occur in patients who are already hospitalised for other medical conditions; up to 7% of these sustain AKI and this increases to 30% or more in those who are critically ill. Most cases are caused by pre-renal AKI and are reversed with appropriate intervention. However, severe AKI, as defined by the requirement for dialysis treatment, is often associated with failure of one or more non-renal organs (this is called multi-organ failure); in this setting there is a mortality rate of 70% in patients with sepsis and AKI and 45% in patients without sepsis. AKI that occurs in the community is responsible for around 1% of all hospital admissions.

Classification and causes

AKI is not a single disease state with a uniform aetiology, but a consequence of a range of different diseases and conditions. The most useful practical classification comprises three main groupings: (i) pre-renal, (ii) renal, or (iii) post-renal. More than one category may be present in an individual patient. Common causes of each type of AKI are outlined in Table 17.1.

Definition and incidence

Acute renal failure (ARF) is a common and serious problem in clinical medicine. It is characterised by an abrupt reduction (usually within a 48-h period) in kidney function. This results in an accumulation of nitrogenous waste products and other toxins. Many patients become oliguric (low urine output) with subsequent salt and water retention. In patients with pre-existing renal impairment, a rapid decline in renal function is termed 'acute on chronic renal failure'. The nomenclature of ARF is evolving and the term acute kidney injury (AKI) is being increasingly used in clinical practice.

Table 17.1 Classification of acute kidney injury

Acute kidney injury type	Typical % cases	Common aetiology
Pre-renal	40–80	Reversible ↓ renal perfusion through hypoperfusion
Intra-renal (including ATN)	10–50	Renal parenchymal injury
Post-renal	<10	Urinary tract obstruction
ATN, acute tubular necrosis.		

255

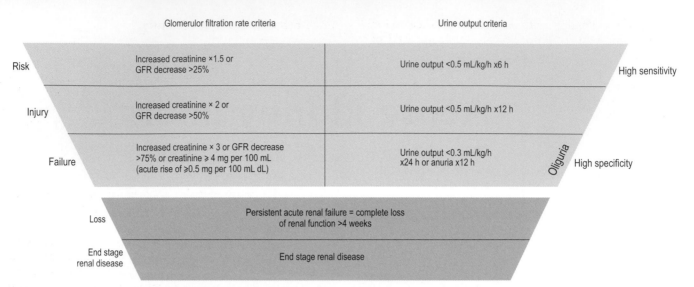

Glomerulor filtration rate criteria	Urine output criteria	
Risk	Increased creatinine ×1.5 or GFR decrease >25%	Urine output <0.5 mL/kg/h x6 h	High sensitivity
Injury	Increased creatinine × 2 or GFR decrease >50%	Urine output <0.5 mL/kg/h x12 h	
Failure	Increased creatinine × 3 or GFR decrease >75% or creatinine ≥ 4 mg per 100 mL (acute rise of ≥0.5 mg per 100 mL dL)	Urine output <0.3 mL/kg/h x24 h or anuria x12 h	High specificity
Loss	Persistent acute renal failure = complete loss of renal function >4 weeks		
End stage renal disease	End stage renal disease		

Fig. 17.1   The RIFLE criteria for the definition and staging of acute renal disease.

The kidneys are pre-disposed to haemodynamic injury owing to hypovolaemia or hypoperfusion. This relates to the high blood flow through the kidneys in normal function; the organs represent 5% of total body weight but receive 25% of blood flow. Furthermore, the renal microvascular bed is unique; firstly, the glomerular capillary bed is on the arterial side of the circulation; secondly, the peri-tubular capillaries are down-stream from the glomerular capillary bed. Finally, renal cells are highly specialised and are, therefore, pre-disposed to ischaemic and inflammatory injury.

Pre-renal acute kidney injury

This is caused by impaired perfusion of the kidneys with blood, and is usually a consequence of decreased intravascular volumes (hypovolaemia) and/or decreased intravascular pressures. Some of the commonest causes of pre-renal AKI are summarised in Fig. 17.2. Perfusion of the kidneys at the level of the microvascular beds (glomerular and tubulo-interstitial) is usually maintained through wide variations in pressure and flow through highly efficient auto-regulatory pathways, such as the renin–angiotensin–aldosterone system (RAAS) and

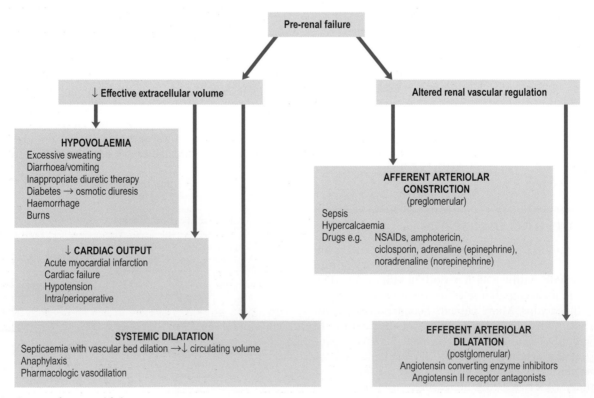

Fig. 17.2   Causes of pre-renal failure.

regulated prostaglandin synthesis. However, when the systolic blood pressure (BP) drops below 80 mmHg, AKI may develop. In individuals with chronic kidney disease (CKD) or in the elderly, this may occur at higher levels of systolic BP. Drugs that inhibit the RAAS, such as angiotension converting enzyme inhibitors (ACE inhibitors) and angiotensin receptor blockers (ARBs), or block the production of prostaglandins, such as non-steroidal anti-inflammatory drugs (NSAIDs), can pre-dispose to the development of pre-renal AKI. These are discussed in more detail below.

Hypovolaemia

This results from any condition that causes intravascular fluid depletion, either directly by haemorrhage or indirectly to compensate for extravascular loss. Examples of this include diarrhoea and vomiting, burns and excessive use of diuretics. Hypotension is a secondary effect of significant hypovolaemia.

Hypotension

In addition to hypovolaemia, hypotension can result from pump (cardiac) failure, of which there are a number of causes, the most common of which is ischaemic heart disease. Another important cause is septic shock, where there is peripheral vasodilatation and low peripheral resistance which leads to profound hypotension despite a high cardiac output.

Intra-renal acute kidney injury

This is caused by a variety of causes (see Tables 17.1 and 17.2), most commonly (in >80% of cases) acute tubular necrosis (ATN). ATN occurs usually as a consequence of a combination of factors, including hypotension, often in the setting of sepsis and nephrotoxic agents including drugs or chemical poisons, or endogenous sources such as myoglobin or haemoglobin.

Acute tubular necrosis

ATN is a diagnosis made by renal biopsy; the findings can include damage to the proximal tubule and the ascending limb of the loop of Henle, interstitial oedema and sparse infiltrating inflammatory cells. Whilst severe and sustained hypoperfusion can lead to ATN, it usually develops when there is a combination of factors including the presence of one or more of a range of nephrotoxins. These may arise exogenously from drugs or chemical poisons, or from endogenous sources such as haemoglobin, myoglobin, crystals (uric acid, phosphate) and toxic products from sepsis or tumours (see Table 17.2). Some endogenous toxins may be released as a direct consequence of drug exposure. For example, myoglobin may be released (rhabdomyolosis) following muscle injury or necrosis, hypoxia, infection or following drug treatment, for example, with fibrates and statins, particularly when both are used in combination. The mechanism of the subsequent damage to renal tissue is not

Table 17.2 Common clinical factors known to cause acute tubular necrosis

Clinical factor	Mechanism
Hypoperfusion	Reduced oxygen/nutrient supply
Radiocontrast media	Medullary ischaemia may result from contrast media induced renal vasoconstriction. The high ionic load of contrast media may produce ischaemia particularly in diabetics and those with myeloma (who produce large quantities of light chain immunoglogulins)
Sepsis	Infection produces endotoxaemia and systemic inflammation in combination with a pre-renal state and nephrotoxins. The immunological response to sepsis involves release of vasoconstrictors and vasodilators (e.g. eicosanoids, nitric oxide) and damage to vascular endothelium with resultant thrombosis
Rhabdomyolysis	Damaged muscles release myoglobin, which can cause ATN through direct nephrotoxicity and by a reduction in blood flow in the outer medulla
Renal transplantation	The procedures and conditions encountered during renal transplantation can induce ischaemic ATN which can be difficult to distinguish from the nephrotoxic effects of immunosuppressive drug therapy used in these circumstances and rejection
Hepatorenal syndrome	Renal vasoconstriction is frequently seen in patients with end-stage liver disease. Progression to ATN is common
Nephrotoxins Aminoglycosides	Aminoglycosides are transported into tubular cells where they exert a direct nephrotoxic effect. Current dosage regimens recommend once daily doses, with frequent monitoring of drug levels, to minimise total uptake of aminoglycoside
Amphotericin	Amphotericin appears to cause direct nephrotoxicity by disturbing the permeability of tubular cells. The nephrotoxic effect is dose dependent and minimised by limiting total dose used, rate of infusion and by volume loading. These precautions also apply to newer liposomal formulations

Continued

Table 17.2 Common clinical factors known to cause acute tubular necrosis—cont'd

Clinical factor	Mechanism
Immunosuppressants	Ciclosporin and tacrolimus cause intra-renal vasoconstriction that may result in ischaemic ATN. The mechanism is unclear but enhanced by hypovolaemia and other nephrotoxic drugs
NSAIDs	Vasodilator prostaglandins, mainly E_2, D_2 and I_2 (prostacyclin), produce an increase in blood flow to the glomerulus and medulla. In normal circumstances, they play no part in the maintenance of the renal circulation. However, increased amounts of vasoconstrictor substances arise in a variety of clinical conditions such as volume depletion, congestive cardiac failure or hepatic cirrhosis associated with ascites. Maintenance of renal blood flow then becomes more reliant on the release of vasodilatory prostaglandins. Inhibition of prostaglandin synthesis by NSAIDs may cause unopposed arteriolar vasoconstriction, leading to renal hypoperfusion
Cytotoxic chemotherapy	For example, cisplatin
Anaesthetic agents	Methoxyflurane, enflurane
Chemical poisons/naturally occurring poisons	Insecticides, herbicides, alkaloids from plants and fungi, reptile venoms

understood fully but probably results from a combination of factors including hypoperfusion, haem-catalysed free radical tubular cytotoxicity and haem cast formation and precipitation leading to tubular injury.

The vascular bed and development of acute tubular necrosis. Regional blood flow within the kidney varies, resulting in relatively hypoxic regions such as the outer medulla. This area is also the site of highly metabolically active parts of the nephron. Owing to the relatively poor oxygen supply and high metabolic demands, the outer medulla is at risk of ischaemia, even under normal conditions. The regulation of regional blood flow in the kidney, and therefore the oxygen supply to these areas, relies upon vasomotor mechanisms mediated in part by adenosine. Adenosine appears to exert either vasoconstrictor or vasodilator effects within the kidney depending upon the relative distribution of A_1 and A_2 receptors.

Clearly, any circumstance that interferes with the delicate balance of blood flow and, therefore, oxygen supply within the kidney can result in ATN because of ischaemia and a greater vulnerability to nephrotoxins. The likelihood of ATN is increased by underlying conditions that pre-dispose to ischaemia such as pre-existing CKD of any cause, atheromatous renovascular disease and cholesterol embolisation from upstream atheromatous plaque rupture.

Common causes of acute tubular necrosis. Table 17.2 shows a summary of some of the common factors encountered clinically that may cause ATN.

Immune and inflammatory renal disease

The kidney is vulnerable to a range of immunological processes that can cause AKI. These are divided into glomerular causes (glomerulonephritis) and interstitial causes (interstitial nephritis). Rarely, acute pyelonephritis, which is an infection of renal parenchyma, usually as a consequence of ascending infection, can cause AKI.

Rapidly progressive glomerulonephritis

Glomerulonephritis refers to an inflammatory process within the glomerulus. If that process causes AKI it is called rapidly progressive glomerulonephritis (RPGN). This is an important cause of AKI occurring without a precipitating other illness. Most cases of RPGN are caused by a small vessel vasculitis; this gives a pattern of injury in the glomerulus that is called a focal segmental necrotising glomerulonephritis (FSNGN) with crescent proliferation; crescents are the presence of cells and extra-cellular matrix in Bowman's space. Most cases of FSNGN are caused by anti-neutrophil cytoplasmic antibody-associated small-vessel vasculitis (SVV). Anti-neutrophil cytoplasmic antibodies (ANCA) refer to the presence of circulating antibodies that are targeted against primary neutrophil cytoplasmic antigens (proteins including proteinase 3 and myeloperoxidase).

The two main types of anti-neutrophil cytoplasmic antibody-associated SVV are Wegener's granulomatosis and microscopic polyangiitis. Other important causes of RPGN include Goodpasture's disease, which is caused by antibodies against glomerular basement membrane (anti-GBM antibodies), Systemic lupus erythematosis (SLE) which usually affects young women and is more common with black ethnicity, and secondary vasculitis are triggered by drugs, infection and tumours. There are many drug triggers for secondary vasculitis; the commonest clinical presentation is a cutaneous vasculitis, secondary to immune complex deposition. Kidney involvement can occur and has been reported with a range of drugs.

Interstitial nephritis

Interstitial nephritis is thought to be a nephrotoxin-induced hypersensitivity reaction associated with infiltration of inflammatory cells into the interstitium with secondary involvement of the tubules. The nephrotoxins involved are usually drugs and/or the toxic products of infection. Drugs that have been most commonly shown to be responsible include NSAIDs, antibiotics (especially penicillins, cephalosporins and quinolones), proton pump inhibitors such as omeprazole, furosemide, allopurinol and azathioprine, although many other drugs have been implicated.

Differentiating pre-renal from renal acute kidney injury

It is sometimes possible to distinguish between cases of pre-renal and renal AKI through examination of biochemical markers (see Table 17.3). In renal AKI, the kidneys are generally unable to retain Na^+ owing to tubular damage. This can be demonstrated by calculating the fractional excretion of sodium (FENa); in practice this is not often done because it lacks sensitivity and specificity and may be difficult to interpret in the elderly who may have pre-existing concentrating defects.

$$FENa = sodium\ clearance/creatinine\ clearance$$

$$FENa = \frac{urine\ sodium \times serum\ creatinine}{serum\ sodium \times urine\ creatinine}$$

If FENa <1%, this indicates pre-renal AKI with preserved tubular function; if FENa >1% this is indicative of ATN. This relationship is less robust if a patient with renal AKI has glycosuria, pre-existing renal disease, has been treated with diuretics, or has other drug-related alterations in renal haemodynamics, for example, through use of ACE inhibitors or NSAIDs. One potential use of urinary electrolytes is in the patient with liver disease and AKI; where the diagnosis of hepato-renal syndrome is being considered, one of the diagnostic criteria is a urinary sodium <10 mmol/L

Post-renal acute kidney injury

Post-renal AKI results from obstruction of the urinary tract by a variety of mechanisms. Any mechanical obstruction from the renal pelvis to the urethral orifice can cause post-renal AKI; these can be divided into causes within the ureters (e.g. calculi or clots), a problem within the wall of ureter (malignancies, benign strictures) and external compression (e.g. retroperitoneal tumours). It is extremely unusual for drugs to be responsible for post-renal AKI. Practolol-induced retroperitoneal fibrosis resulting in bilateral ureteric obstruction is a rare example.

Clinical manifestations

The signs and symptoms of AKI are often non-specific and the diagnosis can be confounded by coexisting clinical conditions. The patient may exhibit signs and symptoms of volume depletion or overload, depending upon the precipitating conditions, course of the disease and prior treatment.

Acute kidney injury with volume depletion

In those patients with volume depletion, a classic pathophysiological picture is likely to be present, with tachycardia, postural hypotension, reduced skin turgor and cold extremities (see Table 17.4). The most common sign in AKI is oliguria, where urine production falls to less than 0.5 mL/kg/h for several hours. This is below the volume of urine required to effectively excrete products of metabolism to maintain a physiological steady state. Therefore, the serum concentration of those substances normally excreted by the kidney will rise and differentially applies to all molecules up to a molecular weight of around 50 kDa. This includes serum creatinine, which at a molecular weight of 113 Da is normally freely filtered by the kidneys but with loss of kidney function the serum level climbs. Whilst the term uraemia is still in widespread use, it merely describes a surrogate for the overall metabolic disturbances that accompany AKI; these include excess potassium, hydrogen ions (acidosis) and phosphate in blood. Most cases of AKI are first identified by an abnormal blood test, though some patients may have symptoms that are specifically attributable to AKI; these include nausea, vomiting, diarrhoea, gastro-intestinal haemorrhage, muscle cramps and a declining level of consciousness.

Table 17.3 Differentiating pre-renal from renal acute kidney injury

Laboratory test	Pre-renal	Renal
Urine osmolality (mOsm/kg)	>500	<400
Urine sodium (mEq/L)	<20	>40
Urine/serum creatinine (µmol/L)	>40	<20
Urine/serum urea (µmol/L)	>8	<3
Fractional excretion of sodium (%)	<1	>2

Table 17.4 Factors associated with acute kidney injury

	Volume depletion	Volume overload
History	Thirst Excessive fluid loss (vomiting or diarrhoea) Oliguria	Weight increase Orthopnoea/nocturnal dyspnoea
Physical examination	Dry mucosae ↓ Skin elasticity Tachycardia	Ankle swelling Oedema Jugular venous distension
	↓ Blood pressure ↓ Jugular venous pressure	Pulmonary crackles Pleural effusion

Acute kidney injury with volume overload

In those patients with AKI who have maintained a normal or increased fluid intake as a result of oral or intravenous administration, there may be clinical signs and symptoms of fluid overload (see Table 17.4).

Diagnosis and clinical evaluation

In hospitalised patients, AKI is usually diagnosed incidentally by the detection of increasing serum creatinine and/or a reduction in urine output.

The assessment of renal function is described in detail in Chapter 18. However, unless a patient is at steady state, measurement of serum creatinine does not provide a reliable guide to renal function. For example, serum creatinine levels will usually rise by only 50–100 μmol/L per day following complete loss of renal function in a previously normal patient. These changes in serum creatinine are not sufficiently responsive to serve as a practical indicator of glomerular filtration rate, particularly in AKI in critical care scenarios.

In the hospital situation, when AKI is detected incidentally, the cause(s) of the condition, such as fluid depletion (hypovolaemia), infection or the use of nephrotoxic drugs, are often apparent on close examination of the clinical history. The development of AKI in this setting is more likely to occur in people with pre-existing CKD. People with normal baseline kidney function usually need to sustain at least two separate triggers for the development of AKI; for example, hypovolaemia will rarely cause AKI in this setting, but when hypovolaemia occurs in the presence of nephrotoxic drugs then AKI may occur. In patients with pre-existing CKD, AKI (i.e. acute on chronic renal failure) can occur in patients with one trigger. By definition, the worse the baseline kidney function, the smaller the trigger required for the development of AKI. Irrespective of the presentation of AKI, it is wise to consider the complete differential diagnosis in all people; active exclusion of post-renal AKI and immune and inflammatory AKI should be considered in all cases. In AKI without an obvious precipitating pre-or post-renal cause, there is a greater need to consider these causes. Although the majority of patients have ATN, other causes such as rapidly progressive glomerulonephritis, interstitial nephritis, multiple myeloma or urinary tract obstruction must be screened for and systematically excluded. In addition to supportive care that is generic for all causes of AKI, disease-specific treatment may also be required. The investigation of AKI is outlined in Fig. 17.3.

Various other parameters should be monitored through the course of AKI. Fluid balance charts that are frequently used may be inaccurate and should not be relied upon exclusively. Records of daily weight are more reliable but are dependent on the mobility of the patient.

Monitoring fluid balance in acute kidney disease

Maintaining appropriate fluid balance in AKI is a critical component of the clinical management of the patient. Detailed clinical assessment includes:

1. Measurement of BP which needs to be interpreted in respect of the baseline for the affected patient together with the patient's heart rate.
2. Auscultation of the heart for the presence of 3rd (and 4th) heart sounds; the presence of these indicate cardiac strain associated with fluid overload.
3. Presence of added sounds in the chest, in particular fine inspiratory crackles that are found in some patients with pulmonary oedema.
4. A chest X-ray for the presence of pulmonary oedema.
5. Pulse oximetry to assess arterial oxygen saturation.
6. Whilst the presence of pitting oedema of the legs or sacrum indicates longer term fluid overload, it may be a useful marker of overall endothelial function and the potential for extravascular fluid accumulation.
7. Decreased skin turgor is a sign of fluid loss.

Intravascular monitoring

Central venous pressure (CVP) can be measured following insertion of a central venous catheter, and is a measure of the pressure in the large systemic veins and the right atrium produced by venous return. CVP assesses circulating volume and, therefore, the degree of fluid deficit, and reduces the risk of pulmonary oedema following over-rapid transfusion. CVP should usually be maintained within the normal range of 5–12 cmH$_2$O.

Most patients with AKI do not require invasive monitoring to the extent described above and recover with supportive care based on careful clinical observations.

Monitoring key parameters in acute kidney disease

Serum electrolytes including potassium, bicarbonate, calcium, phosphate and acid–base balance should be measured on a daily basis. In patients with severe AKI, acid–base balance may need assessing every few hours as this may direct fluid replacement, respiratory support and dialysis treatment.

Course and prognosis

Pre-renal acute kidney injury

The majority of cases will recover within days of onset following prompt correction of the underlying causes. The urine output improves and waste products of metabolism are cleared by the kidneys. Whilst the kidney function usually stabilises to the pre-event baseline, in some patients long-term kidney function resets to lower than previous values.

ATN may be divided into three phases. The first is the oliguric phase where patients have sustained pre-renal AKI and move from the potential for early reversibility to a situation where uraemia and hyperkalaemia develop and the patient may die unless renal replacement therapy (RRT) with dialysis

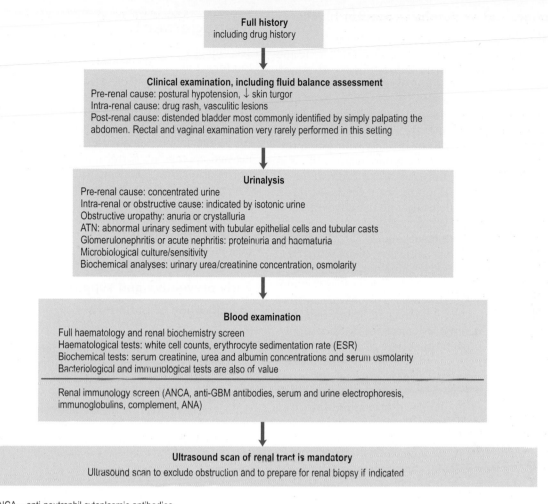

Full history
including drug history

Clinical examination, including fluid balance assessment
Pre-renal cause: postural hypotension, ↓ skin turgor
Intra-renal cause: drug rash, vasculitic lesions
Post-renal cause: distended bladder most commonly identified by simply palpating the abdomen. Rectal and vaginal examination very rarely performed in this setting

Urinalysis
Pre-renal cause: concentrated urine
Intra-renal or obstructive cause: indicated by isotonic urine
Obstructive uropathy: anuria or crystalluria
ATN: abnormal urinary sediment with tubular epithelial cells and tubular casts
Glomerulonephritis or acute nephritis: proteinuria and haematuria
Microbiological culture/sensitivity
Biochemical analyses: urinary urea/creatinine concentration, osmolarity

Blood examination
Full haematology and renal biochemistry screen
Haematological tests: white cell counts, erythrocyte sedimentation rate (ESR)
Biochemical tests: serum creatinine, urea and albumin concentrations and serum osmolarity
Bacteriological and immunological tests are also of value

Renal immunology screen (ANCA, anti-GBM antibodies, serum and urine electrophoresis, immunoglobulins, complement, ANA)

Ultrasound scan of renal tract is mandatory
Ultrasound scan to exclude obstruction and to prepare for renal biopsy if indicated

ANCA – anti-neutrophil cytoplasmic antibodies
GBM – glomelular basement membrane
ANA – anti nuclear antibody

Fig. 17.3 The investigations of acute kidney injury.

is started. The oliguric phase is usually no longer than 7–14 days but may last for 6 weeks. This is followed by a diuretic phase, which is characterised by a urine output that rises over a few days to several litres per day. This phase lasts for up to 7 days and corresponds to the recommencement of tubular function. The onset of this phase is associated with an improving prognosis unless the patient sustains an intercurrent infection or a vascular event. Finally, the patient enters a recovery phase where tubular cells regenerate slowly over several months, although the glomerular filtration rate often does not return to initial levels. The elderly recover renal function more slowly and less completely.

The mortality rate of AKI varies according to the cause but increases when AKI occurs in patients with multi-organ failure, where mortality rates of up to 70% are seen. Higher mortality rates are seen in patients aged over 60 years.

Death resulting from uraemia and hyperkalaemia are very uncommon. Consequently, the major causes of death associated with AKI are septicaemia and intercurrent acute vascular events such as myocardial infarction and stroke. High circulating levels of uraemic toxins that occur in AKI result in general debility. These, together with the significant number of invasive procedures such as bladder catheterisation and intravascular cannulation which are necessary in the management of AKI, leave such patients prone to infection and septicaemia. Uraemic gastro-intestinal haemorrhage is a recognised consequence of AKI, probably as a result of reduced mucosal cell turnover.

Post-renal acute kidney injury

Prompt identification and relief of the obstruction is important. The prognosis is then dependent on the underlying cause of the obstruction of the renal tract and the baseline to which the kidney function returns after the obstruction has been relieved. If the underlying problem is benign then there may be no long-term adverse consequences. However, if the cause of the obstruction is due to an underlying malignancy then long-term survival is dependent on whether this can be cured.

ACE inhibitors and angiotensin receptor blockers in acute kidney injury

ACE inhibitors and ARBs are not directly nephrotoxic and can be used in most patients with kidney disease. However, profound hypotension can occur if they are initiated in susceptible patients such as those who are receiving high dose diuretics as treatment for fluid overload. This might result in the development of pre-renal AKI. It is, therefore, wise to monitor BP and carefully titrate dosages whilst monitoring renal function in such patients. Nonetheless, it is common to see increases in serum creatinine levels of up to 20% on initiation of an ACE inhibitor or ARB and this is not necessarily a cause for discontinuing therapy with these agents.

ACE inhibitor use is, however, absolutely contraindicated when a patient has bilateral renal artery stenosis, or renal artery stenosis in a patient with a single functioning kidney. If an ACE inhibitor or ARB is initiated under these circumstances then pre-renal AKI may ensue. This may occur since the renin–angiotensin system is stimulated by low renal perfusion resulting from stenotic lesions in the arteries supplying the kidneys, most often at the origin of the renal artery from the abdominal aorta. Angiotensin II is produced which causes renal vasoconstriction, in part, through increased efferent arteriolar tone. This creates a 'back pressure' which paradoxically maintains glomerular filtration pressure in an otherwise poorly perfused kidney. If angiotensin II production is inhibited by an ACE inhibitor, or the effect is blocked by an ARB, then efferent arteriole dilatation will result. Since increased efferent vascular tone maintains filtration in such patients, then the overall result of ACE inhibitor or ARB therapy will be to reduce or shut down filtration at the glomerulus and put the patient at risk of pre-renal AKI (see Fig. 17.4).

Management

The aim of the medical management of a patient with AKI is to prolong life in order to allow recovery of kidney function. Effective management of AKI depends upon a rapid diagnosis. If the underlying acute deterioration in renal function is detected early enough, it is often possible to prevent progression. If the condition is advanced, however, management consists mainly of supportive strategies, with close monitoring and appropriate correction of metabolic, fluid and electrolyte disturbances. Patients with severe AKI usually require renal replacement therapy with dialysis. Specific therapies that promote recovery of ischaemic renal damage remain under investigation. Patients with immune-mediated causes of AKI should be treated with appropriate immunosuppressant regimens to treat the underlying cause of the AKI.

Early preventive and supportive strategies

Identification of patients at risk

Any patient who has concurrent or pre-existing conditions that increase the risk of development and progression of AKI must be identified and this includes those with pre-existing CKD, diabetes, jaundice, myeloma and the elderly. These patients either have baseline impaired renal function or are sensitised to the development of AKI by the co-morbid condition. Meticulous attention to fluid balance, assessment of infection and the use of drugs is crucial to minimise the risk of development of AKI.

Withdrawal and avoidance of nephrotoxic agents

Irrespective of whether the aetiology of the AKI directly involves nephrotoxic drugs, the drug and treatment regimens should be examined so that potential nephrotoxins are

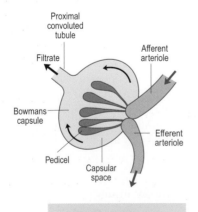
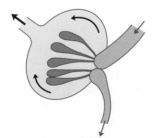
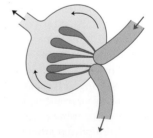

A. Normal glomerulus with efferent arteriolar tone (narrowed outflow of blood) causing a 'back pressure' producing filtration with water and solutes progressing through the capsular space to the proximal convoluted tubule

B. Glomerulus in an untreated patient with renal artery stenosis. There is increased efferent arteriolar tone caused by the vasoconstrictive actions of angiotensin II. The efferent arteriole is narrowed more than normal promoting filtration

C. Glomerulus in a patient with renal artery stenosis but treated with an ACE inhibitor or angiotensin receptor blocker. Blockade of the vasoconstrictive effects of angiotensin II has produced dilation of the efferent arteriole resulting in failure of the back pressure promoting filtration

Fig. 17.4 The actions of ACE inhibition and angiotensin receptor blockade in patients with renal artery stenosis.

withdrawn and avoided in the future in order to avoid exacerbating the condition. Particular care should be taken with ACE inhibitors, NSAIDs, radiological contrast media, and aminoglycosides. The doses should be adjusted of any drugs that are renally excreted or have active metabolites that are excreted renally.

Optimisation of renal perfusion

Initial treatment should include rapid correction of fluid and electrolyte balance to maximise renal perfusion. A central line may be considered to facilitate ease of fluid infusion and monitoring of intravascular volumes. In patients where it is difficult to assess fluid balance by use of clinical examination a urinary catheter may be placed in order that fluid losses may be measured easily. However, with the recent focus on the prevention of catheter-related bacteraemia, central lines are seldom used outside specialist renal and intensive care units.

A diagnosis of acute deterioration of renal function caused by renal underperfusion implies that restoration of renal perfusion would reverse impairment by improving renal blood flow, reducing renal vasoconstriction and flushing nephrotoxins from the kidney. The use of crystalloids in the form of 0.9% sodium chloride is an appropriate choice of intravenous fluid since it replaces both water and sodium ions in a concentration approximately equal to serum. The effect of fluid replacement on urine flow and intravascular pressures should be carefully monitored. However, fluid loading with 1–1.5 L saline at <0.5 L/h is unlikely to cause harm in most patients who do not show signs of fluid overload. There is no evidence that colloids such as gelofusin or albumin provide any additional benefit for volume expansion and renal recovery over the use of 0.9% sodium chloride.

The use of inotropes such as noradrenaline and cardiac doses of dopamine should be restricted to non-renal indications.

Establishing and maintaining an adequate diuresis

Whilst loop diuretics (most commonly furosemide) may facilitate the management of fluid overload and hyperkalaemia in early or established AKI, there is no evidence that these agents are effective for the prevention of, or early recovery from, AKI. It is reasonable to use these agents whilst the urine output is maintained as this provides space for intravenous drugs and parenteral feeding including oral supplements. In experimental settings, loop diuretics decrease renal tubular cell metabolic demands and increase renal blood flow by stimulating the release of renal prostaglandins, a haemodynamic effect inhibited by NSAIDs. However, there is no demonstrable impact on clinical outcomes. Indeed, diuretic therapy should only be initiated in the context of fluid overload. If not, any diuresis might produce a negative fluid balance and precipitate or exacerbate a pre-renal state.

Doses of up to 100 mg/h of furosemide can be given by continuous intravenous infusion. Higher infusion rates may cause transient deafness. The use of continuous infusions of loop diuretics has been shown to produce a more effective diuresis with a lower incidence of side effects than seen with bolus administration. Bolus doses of loop diuretics may induce renal vasoconstriction and be theoretically detrimental to function.

The addition of small oral doses of metolazone may also be considered. Metolazone is a weak thiazide diuretic alone but produces a synergistic action with loop diuretics. In this setting, it should be used with great care as it may initiate a profound diuresis and the patient can rapidly develop intravascular depletion and worsen renal failure

Mannitol. Mannitol has historically been recommended for the treatment of AKI. The rationale for using mannitol in AKI arises from the concept that tubular debris may contribute to oliguria. There is no evidence for mannitol producing benefit in AKI over and above aggressive hydration. Indeed, mannitol can cause volume overload. Consequently, mannitol is now not recommended for patients with AKI.

Dopamine. Historically, dopamine has been recommended at low dose to improve renal blood flow and urine output. Dopamine at low dose acts as a renal vasodilator in normal kidneys, but in renal failure it is a renal vasoconstrictor even at a low dose. This translates into no demonstrable clinical benefit and it should no longer be used. Dopamine has alpha and beta adrenergic effects. Recently, fenoldapam, a pure dopaminergic D_1 agonist has been investigated in small scale clinical trials; the results have shown a trend towards benefit in recovery of renal function from AKI. However, larger trials are needed to identify if fenoldapam has a role in routine clinical practice (Kellum et al., 2008).

Drug therapy and renal auto-regulation

Intra-renal blood flow is controlled by an auto-regulatory mechanism unique to the kidney called tubuloglomerular feedback (TGF). This mechanism produces arteriolar constriction in response to an increased solute load to the distal nephrons. Glomerular filtration rate and kidney workload are thus reduced. It has been proposed that oliguria is an adaptive response to renal ischaemia and therapy designed to improve glomerular filtration rate would increase solute load to the nephrons and might increase kidney workload and worsen AKI. Clearly, reversal of a pre-renal state with fluids is a logical therapeutic aim.

Non-dialysis treatment of established acute kidney injury
Uraemia and intravascular volume overload

In renal failure, the symptoms of uraemia include nausea, vomiting and anorexia, and result principally from accumulation of toxic products of protein metabolism including urea.

Unfortunately, since uraemia causes anorexia, nausea and vomiting, many severely ill patients are unable to tolerate any kind of diet. In these patients and those who are catabolic, the use of enteral or parenteral nutrition should be considered at an early stage.

Intravascular fluid overload must be managed by restricting NaCl intake to about 1–2 g/day if the patient is not hyponatraemic and total fluid intake to less than 1 L/day plus the volume of urine and/or loss from dialysis. Care should be taken with the so-called 'low salt' products, as these usually contain KCl, which will exacerbate hyperkalaemia.

Hyperkalaemia

This is a particular problem in AKI, not only because urinary excretion is reduced but also because intracellular potassium may be released. Rapid rises in extracellular potassium are to be expected when there is tissue damage, as in burns, crush injuries and sepsis. Acidosis also aggravates hyperkalaemia by provoking potassium leakage from healthy cells. The condition may be life-threatening causing cardiac arrhythmias and, if untreated, can result in asystolic cardiac arrest.

Dietary potassium should be restricted to less than 40 mmol/day and potassium supplements and potassium-sparing diuretics removed from the treatment schedule. Emergency treatment is necessary if the serum potassium level reaches 7.0 mmol/L (normal range 3.5–5.5 mmol/L) or if there are the progressive changes in the electrocardiogram (ECG) associated with hyperkalaemia. These include tall, peaked T waves, reduced P waves with increased QRS complexes or the 'sine wave' appearance that often presages cardiac arrest (see Chapter 18, Fig. 18.10).

Emergency treatment of hyperkalaemia consists of the following:

1. 10–30 mL (2.25–6.75 mmol) of calcium gluconate 10% intravenously over 5–10 min; this improves myocardial stability but has no effect on the serum potassium levels. The protective effect begins in minutes but is short lived (<1 h), although the dose can be repeated.
2. 50 mL of 50% glucose together with 8–12 units of soluble insulin over 10 min. Endogenous insulin, stimulated by a glucose load or administered intravenously, stimulates intracellular potassium uptake, thus removing it from the serum. The effect becomes apparent after 15–30 min, peaks after about 1 h and lasts for 2–3 h and will decrease serum potassium levels by around 1 mmol/L.
3. Nebulised salbutamol has also been used to lower potassium; however, this is not effective for all patients and does not permanently lower potassium. If used it is seen as a temporary emergency measure.

Acidosis

The inability of the kidney to excrete hydrogen ions may result in a metabolic acidosis. This may contribute to hyperkalaemia. It may be treated orally with sodium bicarbonate 1–6 g/day in divided doses (though this is not appropriate for acute metabolic acidosis seen in AKI), or 50–100 mmol of bicarbonate ions (preferably as isotonic sodium bicarbonate 1.4% or 1.26%, 250–500 mL over 15–60 min) intravenously may be used. The administration of bicarbonate in acidotic patients will also tend to reduce serum potassium concentrations. Bicarbonate will cause an increase in intracellular Na^+ through activation of the cell membrane Na^+/H^+ exchanger, which promotes increased activity of Na-K ATPase producing increased intracellular sequestration of K^+.

If calcium gluconate is used to treat hyperkalaemia, care should be taken not to mix it with the sodium bicarbonate (by giving this through the same intravenous access site) as the resulting calcium bicarbonate forms an insoluble precipitate. If elevation of serum sodium or fluid overload precludes the use of sodium bicarbonate, extreme acidosis (serum bicarbonate of less than 10 mmol/L) is best treated by dialysis.

Hypocalcaemia

Calcium malabsorption, probably secondary to disordered vitamin D metabolism, can occur in AKI. Hypocalcaemia usually remains asymptomatic, as tetany of skeletal muscles or convulsions does not normally occur until serum concentrations are as low as 1.6–1.7 mmol/L (normal 2.20–2.55 mmol/L). Should it become necessary, oral calcium supplementation with calcium carbonate is usually adequate, and although vitamin D may be used to treat the hypocalcaemia of AKI, it rarely has to be added. Effervescent calcium tablets should be avoided as they contain a high sodium or potassium load.

Hyperphosphataemia

As phosphate is normally excreted by the kidney, hyperphosphataemia can occur in AKI but rarely requires treatment. Should it become necessary to treat, phosphate-binding agents may be used to retain phosphate ions in the gut. The most commonly used agents are calcium containing such as calcium carbonate or calcium acetate and are given with food. For further information see Chapter 18.

Infection

Patients with AKI are prone to infection and septicaemia, which can ultimately cause death. Bladder catheters, central catheters and even peripheral intravenous lines should be used with care to reduce the chance of bacterial invasion. Leucocytosis is sometimes seen in AKI and does not necessarily imply infection. However, pyrexia must be immediately investigated and treated with appropriate antibiotic therapy if accompanied by toxic symptoms such as disorientation or hypotensive episodes. Samples from blood, urine and any other material such as catheter tips should be sent for culture before antibiotics are started. Antibiotic therapy should be broad spectrum until a causative organism is identified.

Other problems

Uraemic gastro-intestinal erosions

These are a recognised consequence of AKI, probably as a result of reduced mucosal cell turnover owing to high circulating levels of uraemic toxins. Proton pump inhibitors are effective and it is unlikely that any one is more advantageous than another. However, proton pump inhibitors should be used with caution in hospitals where there are significant rates of *Clostridium difficile* diarrhoea, as they may pre-dispose to the development of this organism. H_2 antagonists are an appropriate alternative.

Nutrition

There are two major constraints concerning the nutrition of patients with AKI:

- patients may be anorexic, vomiting and too ill to eat;
- oliguria associated with renal failure limits the volume of enteral or parenteral nutrition that can be given safely.

The introduction of dialysis or haemofiltration allows fluid to be removed easily and, therefore, makes parenteral nutrition possible. Large volumes of fluid may be administered without producing fluid overload. The use of parenteral nutrition is rare but where appropriate factors to be considered include fluid balance, calorie/protein requirements, electrolyte balance/requirements, and vitamin and mineral requirements.

The basic calorie requirements are similar to those in a non-dialysed patient, although the need for protein may occasionally be increased in haemodialysis and haemofiltration because of amino acid loss. In all situations, protein is usually supplied as 12–20 g/day of an essential amino acid formulation, although individual requirements may vary.

Electrolyte-free amino acid solutions should be used in parenteral nutrition formulations for patients with AKI as they allow the addition of electrolytes as appropriate. Potassium and sodium requirements can be calculated on an individual basis depending on serum levels. There is usually no need to try to normalise serum calcium and phosphate levels as they will stabilise with the appropriate therapy, or, if necessary, with haemofiltration or dialysis. Water-soluble vitamins are removed by dialysis and haemofiltration but the standard daily doses normally included in parenteral nutrition fluids more than compensate for this loss. Magnesium and zinc supplementation may be required, not only because tissue repair often increases requirements but also because they may be lost during dialysis or haemofiltration.

It is necessary to monitor the serum urea, creatinine and electrolyte levels daily to make the appropriate alterations in the required nutritional support. The glucose concentration should also be checked daily as patients in renal failure sometimes develop insulin resistance. The plasma pH should be checked initially to determine if addition of amino acid solutions is causing or aggravating metabolic acidosis. It is also valuable to check calcium, phosphate and albumin levels regularly, and when practical, daily weighing gives a useful guide to fluid balance.

Renal replacement therapy

Renal replacement therapy is indicated in a patient with AKI when kidney function is so poor that life is at risk. However, it is desirable to introduce renal replacement therapy early in AKI, as complications and mortality are reduced if the serum urea level is kept below 35 mmol/L. Generally, replacement therapy is urgently indicated in AKI to:

1. remove uraemic toxins when severe symptoms are apparent, for example, impaired consciousness, seizures, pericarditis, rapidly developing peripheral neuropathy
2. remove fluid resistant to diuretics, for example, pulmonary oedema
3. correct electrolyte and acid–base imbalances, for example, hyperkalaemia >6.5 mmol/L or 5.5–6.5 where there are ECG changes, increasing acidosis (pH < 7.1 or serum bicarbonate <10 mmol/L) despite bicarbonate therapy, or where bicarbonate is not tolerated because of fluid overload.

Forms of renal replacement therapy

The common types of renal replacement therapy used in clinical practice are:

- haemodialysis
- haemofiltration
- haemodiafiltration
- peritoneal dialysis

Although the basic principles of these replacement therapies are similar, clearance rates, that is, the extent of solute removal, vary.

In all types of renal replacement therapy, blood is presented to a dialysis solution across some form of semi-permeable membrane that allows free movement of low molecular weight compounds. The processes by which movement of substances occur are:

- *Diffusion.* Diffusion depends upon concentration differences between blood and dialysate and molecule size. Water and low molecular weight solutes (up to a molecular weight of about 5000) move through pores in the semi-permeable membrane to establish equilibrium. Smaller molecules can be cleared from blood more effectively as they move more easily through pores in the membrane.
- *Ultrafiltration.* A pressure gradient (either +ve or −ve) across a semi-permeable membrane will produce a net directional movement of fluid from relative high to low pressure regions. The quantity of fluid dialysed is the ultrafiltration volume.
- *Convection.* Any molecule carried by ultrafiltrate may move passively with the flow by convection. Larger molecules are cleared more effectively by convection.

Haemodialysis

In haemodialysis, the form of access used in AKI is a dialysis line. This is placed in a vein (the jugular, femoral or subclavian), which has an arterial lumen through which the blood is removed from the patient and a venous lumen by which it is returned to the patient after passing through a dialyser. The terms arterial and venous lumen can be misleading as both lumens are situated in the same vein. They are part of the same line which bifurcates and has two lumens, the longer lumen is the 'arterial' lumen and the shorter the 'venous' lumen. Heparin is added to the blood as it leaves the body to prevent the dialyser clotting. Blood is then actively pumped through the artificial kidney before being returned to the patient (Fig. 17.5). In those patients at high risk of haemorrhage, the amount of heparin used can be reduced or even avoided altogether. The dialyser consists of a cartridge comprising either a bundle of hollow tubes (hollow fibre dialyser) or a series of parallel flat plates (flat-plate dialyser) made of a synthetic semi-permeable membrane. Flat-plate dialysers are now rarely used. Dialysis fluid flows around the membrane countercurrent (opposite) to the flow of blood in order to maximise diffusion gradients. The dialysis solution is essentially a mixture of electrolytes in water with a composition approximating to extracellular fluid into which solutes diffuse. The ionic concentration of the dialysis fluid can be manipulated to control the rate and extent of electrolyte transfer. Calcium and bicarbonate concentrations can also be increased in dialysis fluid to promote diffusion into blood as replacement therapy. By manipulating the hydrostatic pressure of the dialysate and blood circuits, the extent and rate of water removal by ultrafiltration can be controlled.

Haemodialysis can be performed in either intermittent or continuous schedules. The latter regimen is preferable in the critical care situation, providing 24-h control, and minimising swings in blood volume and electrolyte composition that are found using intermittent regimens. The haemodialysis described in this section is indistinguishable from that used as maintenance therapy for many patients with end stage renal failure, the method of access in this group is often via an arterio-venous fistula (see Chapter 18).

The capital cost of haemodialysis is considerable, requires specially trained staff, and is seldom undertaken outside a renal unit. It does, however, treat renal failure rapidly and is, therefore, essential in hypercatabolic renal failure where urea is produced faster than, for example, it could be removed by peritoneal dialysis. Haemodialysis can also be used in patients who have recently undergone abdominal surgery in whom peritoneal dialysis would be ill advised.

Haemofiltration

Haemofiltration is an alternative technique to dialysis where simplicity of use, fine fluid balance control and low cost have ensured its widespread use in the treatment of AKI.

A similar arrangement to haemodialysis is employed but dialysis fluid is not used. The hydrostatic pressure of the blood drives a filtrate, similar to interstitial fluid, across a high permeability dialyser (passes substances of molecular weight up to 30,000) by ultrafiltration. Solute clearance occurs by convection. Commercially prepared haemofiltration fluid may then be introduced into the filtered blood in quantities sufficient to maintain optimal fluid balance. As with haemodialysis, haemofiltration can be intermittent or continuous. In continuous arterio-venous haemofiltration (CAVH), blood is diverted, usually from the femoral artery, and returned to the femoral vein; this is now very seldom used. In continuous venovenous haemofiltration (CVVH), a dual lumen vascular catheter is inserted into a vein (as described above). Blood is removed from the body via the distal lumen (the one furthest from the right side of the heart) in a process assisted by a blood pump, passed through a haemofilter and returned to the body via the proximal lumen. In slow continuous ultrafiltration (SCU or SCUF), the process is performed so slowly that no fluid substitution is necessary. In addition to avoiding the expense and complexity of haemodialysis, this system enables continuous but gradual removal of fluid, thereby allowing very fine control of fluid balance in addition to electrolyte control and removal of metabolites. This control of fluid balance often facilitates the use of parenteral nutrition. Because of the advantages of haemofiltration over peritoneal dialysis and haemodialysis, continuous haemofiltration is currently the commonest type of renal replacement therapy used in patients in intensive care units.

Haemodiafiltration

Haemodiafiltration is a technique that combines the ability to clear small molecules, as in haemodialysis, with the large molecule clearance of haemofiltration. It is, however, more expensive than traditional haemodialysis, but does offer potential benefits. Whilst some studies suggest that haemodialfiltration may provide a clinical benefit compared to haemofiltration or haemodialysis, this is controversial (Rabindranath et al., 2006). However, enhanced combined control of fluid and solute removal provided by this technique is likely to be increasingly used over the next decade.

Acute peritoneal dialysis

Acute peritoneal dialysis is rarely used now for AKI except in circumstances where haemodialysis is unavailable. A semi-rigid catheter is inserted into the abdominal cavity. Warmed sterile peritoneal dialysis fluid (typically 1–2 L) is

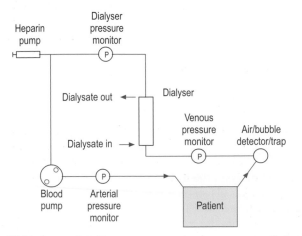

Fig. 17.5 A typical dialysis circuit representing emergency dialysis via a dialysis catheter.

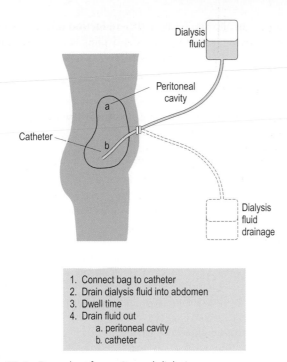

1. Connect bag to catheter
2. Drain dialysis fluid into abdomen
3. Dwell time
4. Drain fluid out
   a. peritoneal cavity
   b. catheter

Fig. 17.6 Procedure for peritoneal dialysis.

Table 17.5 Approximate clearances of common renal replacement therapies

Renal replacement therapy	Clearance rate (mL/min)
Intermittent haemodialysis	150–200
Intermittent haemofiltration	100–150
Acute intermittent peritoneal dialysis	10–20
Continuous haemofiltration	5–15

instilled into the abdomen, left for a period of about 30 min (dwell time) and then drained into a collecting bag (Fig. 17.6). This procedure may be performed manually or by semiautomatic equipment. The process may be repeated up to 20 times a day, depending on the condition of the patient.

Acute peritoneal dialysis is relatively cheap and simple, does not require specially trained staff or the facilities of a renal unit. It does, however, have the disadvantages of being uncomfortable and tiring for the patient. It is associated with a high incidence of peritonitis and permits protein loss, as albumin crosses the peritoneal membrane.

Drug dosage in renal replacement therapy

Whether a drug is significantly removed by dialysis or haemofiltration is an important clinical issue. Drugs that are not removed may well require dose reduction to avoid accumulation and minimise toxic effects. Alternatively, drug removal may be significant and require a dosage supplement to ensure an adequate therapeutic effect is maintained. In general, since haemodialysis, peritoneal dialysis and haemofiltration depend on filtration, the process of drug removal can be considered analoguous to glomerular filtration. Table 17.5 gives an indication of approximate clearances of common renal replacement therapies, which for continuous regimens provide an estimate for the creatinine clearance of the system.

Drug characteristics that favour clearance by the glomerulus are similar to those that favour clearance by dialysis or haemofiltration. These include:

- low molecular weight
- high water solubility
- low protein binding
- small volume of distribution
- low metabolic clearance

Unfortunately, a number of other factors inherent in the dialysis process affect clearance; they include:

- duration of dialysis procedure
- rate of blood flow to dialyser
- surface area and porosity of dialyser
- composition and flow rate of dialysate

For peritoneal dialysis other factors come into play and include:

- rate of peritoneal exchange
- concentration gradient between plasma and dialysate

In view of the above, it is usually possible to predict whether a drug will be removed by dialysis, but it is very difficult to quantify the process except by direct measurement, which is rarely practical. Consequently, a definitive, comprehensive guide to drug dosage in dialysis does not exist. However, limited data for specific drugs are available in the literature, while many drug manufacturers have information on the dialysability of their products and some include dosage recommendations in their summaries of product characteristics. The most practical method for treating patients undergoing dialysis is to assemble appropriate dosage guidelines for a range of drugs likely to be used in patients with renal impairment and attempt to restrict use to these.

As drug clearance by haemofiltration is more predictable than in dialysis, it is possible that standardised guidelines on drug elimination may become available. In the interim, a set of individual drug dosage guidelines similar to those described above would be useful in practice.

Factors affecting drug use

How the drug to be used is absorbed, distributed, metabolised and excreted, and whether it is intrinsically nephrotoxic are all factors that must be considered. The pharmacokinetic behaviour of many drugs may be altered in renal failure.

Absorption

Oral absorption in AKI may be reduced by vomiting or diarrhoea, although this is frequently of limited clinical significance.

Metabolism

The main hepatic pathways of drug metabolism appear unaffected in renal impairment. The kidney is also a site of metabolism in the body, but the effect of renal impairment is clinically important in only two situations. The first involves the conversion of 25-hydroxycholecalciferol to 1,25-dihydroxycholecalciferol (the active form of vitamin D) in the kidney, a process that is impaired in renal failure. Patients in AKI occasionally require vitamin D replacement therapy, and this should be in the form of 1α-hydroxycholecalciferol (alfacalcidol) or 1,25-dihydroxycholecalciferol (calcitriol). The latter is the drug of choice in the presence of concomitant hepatic impairment. The second situation involves the metabolism of insulin. The kidney is the major site of insulin metabolism, and the insulin requirements of diabetic patients in AKI are often reduced.

Distribution

Changes in drug distribution may be altered by fluctuations in the degree of hydration or by alterations in tissue or serum protein binding. The presence of oedema or ascites increases the volume of distribution while dehydration reduces it. In practice, these changes will only be significant if the volume of distribution of the drug is small, that is, less than 50 L. Serum protein binding may be reduced owing to either protein loss or alteration in binding caused by uraemia. For certain highly bound drugs the net result of reduced protein binding is an increase in free drug, and care is, therefore, required when interpreting serum concentrations. Most analyses measure the total serum concentration, that is, free plus bound drug. A drug level may, therefore, fall within the accepted concentration range but still result in toxicity because of the increased proportion of free drug. However, this is usually only a temporary effect. Since the unbound drug is now available for elimination, its concentration will eventually return to the original value, albeit with a lower total bound and unbound level. The total drug concentration may, therefore, fall below the therapeutic range while therapeutic effectiveness is maintained. It must be noted that the time required for the new equilibrium to be established is about four or five elimination half-lives of the drug, and this may be altered itself in renal failure. Some drugs that show reduced serum protein binding include diazepam, morphine, phenytoin, levothyroxine, theophylline and warfarin. Tissue binding may also be affected; for example, the displacement of digoxin from skeletal muscle binding sites by metabolic waste products that accumulate in renal failure result in a significant reduction in digoxin's volume of distribution.

Excretion

Alteration in renal clearance of drugs in renal impairment is the most important parameter to consider when considering dosage. Generally, a fall in renal drug clearance indicates a decline in the number of functioning nephrons. The glomerular filtration rate can be used as an estimate of the number of functioning nephrons. Thus, a 50% reduction in the glomerular filtration rate will suggest a 50% decline in renal clearance.

Renal impairment, therefore, often necessitates drug dosage adjustments. Loading doses of renally excreted drugs are often necessary in renal failure because of the prolonged elimination half-life which leads to an increased time to reach steady state. The equation for a loading dose is the same in renal disease as in normal patients, thus:

$$\text{loading dose (mg)} = \text{target concentration (mg/L)} \times \text{volume of distribution (L)}$$

The volume of distribution may be altered but generally remains unchanged.

It is possible to derive other formulae for dosage adjustment in renal impairment. One of the most useful is:

$$DR_{rf} = DR_n \times [(1 - F_{eu}) + (F_{eu} \times RF)]$$

where DR_{rf} is the dosing rate in renal failure, DR_n is the normal dosing rate, RF is the extent of renal impairment = patient's creatinine clearance (mL/min)/ideal creatinine clearance (120 mL/min) and F_{eu} is the fraction of drug normally excreted unchanged in the urine. For example, when RF = 0.2 and F_{eu} = 0.5, 60% of the normal dosing rate should be given.

An alteration in dosing rate can be achieved by either altering the dose itself or the dosage interval, or a combination of both as appropriate. Unfortunately, it is not always possible to obtain the fraction of drug excreted unchanged in the urine. In practice, it is simpler to use the guidelines for prescribing in renal impairment found in the British National Formulary. These are adequate for most cases, although the specialist may need to refer to other texts.

Nephrotoxicity

The list of potentially nephrotoxic drugs is long. Although the commonest serious forms of renal damage are interstitial nephritis and glomerulonephritis, the majority of drugs only cause damage by hypersensitivity reactions and are safe in many patients. Some drugs, however, are directly nephrotoxic, and their effects on the kidney are more predictable. Such drugs include aminoglycosides, amphotericin, colistin, the polymixins and ciclosporin. The use of any drug with recognised nephrotoxic potential should be avoided where possible. This is particularly true in patients with pre-existing renal impairment or renal failure. Figure 17.7 summarises the most important and common adverse effects of drugs on renal function, indicating the likely regions of the nephron in which damage occurs. Additional information on adverse effects can be found in Hems and Currie (2005).

Inevitably, occasions will arise when the use of potentially nephrotoxic drugs becomes necessary, and on these occasions constant monitoring of renal function is essential. In conclusion, when selecting a drug for a patient with renal failure, an agent should be chosen that approaches the ideal characteristics listed in Box 17.1.

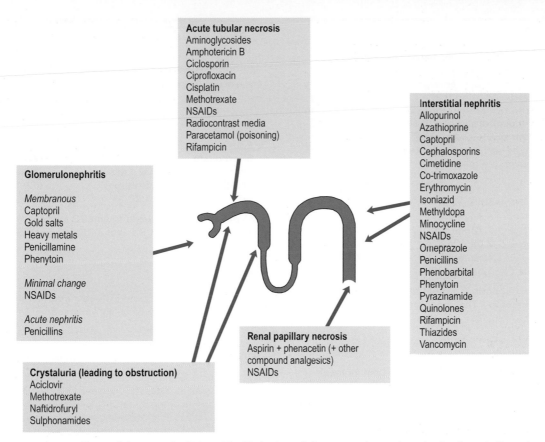

Acute tubular necrosis
Aminoglycosides
Amphotericin B
Ciclosporin
Ciprofloxacin
Cisplatin
Methotrexate
NSAIDs
Radiocontrast media
Paracetamol (poisoning)
Rifampicin

Interstitial nephritis
Allopurinol
Azathioprine
Captopril
Cephalosporins
Cimetidine
Co-trimoxazole
Erythromycin
Isoniazid
Methyldopa
Minocycline
NSAIDs
Omeprazole
Penicillins
Phenobarbital
Phenytoin
Pyrazinamide
Quinolones
Rifampicin
Thiazides
Vancomycin

Glomerulonephritis

Membranous
Captopril
Gold salts
Heavy metals
Penicillamine
Phenytoin

Minimal change
NSAIDs

Acute nephritis
Penicillins

Renal papillary necrosis
Aspirin + phenacetin (+ other
compound analgesics)
NSAIDs

Crystaluria (leading to obstruction)
Aciclovir
Methotrexate
Naftidrofuryl
Sulphonamides

Fig. 17.7 Common adverse effects of drugs on the kidney. The likely sites of damage to the nephron (stylised) are indicated.

Box 17.1 Characteristics of the ideal drug for use in a patient with renal failure

- No active metabolites
- Disposition unaffected by fluid balance changes
- Disposition unaffected by protein binding changes
- Response unaffected by altered tissue sensitivity
- Wide therapeutic margin
- Not nephrotoxic

Case studies

Case 17.1

Mrs J a 60-year-old widow, had long-standing hypertension that was unsatisfactorily controlled on a variety of agents. Her drug therapy included furosemide 40 mg once a day, amlodipine 10 mg daily and a salt restricted diet. Following a routine review of her therapy, ramipril 2.5 mg once daily was added to her treatment regimen in an attempt to improve blood pressure control.

Mrs J was recently diagnosed with gastroenteritis. A week after her diagnosis she presented to her local hospital accident and emergency unit, with ongoing diarrhoea. Her BP was found to be 100/60 mmHg and serum biochemistry revealed creatinine levels of 225 μmol/L (50–120 μmol/L, Na⁺ 125 mmol/L (135–145 mmol/l) and K⁺ 5.2 mmol/L (3.5–5.0 mmol/L).

Questions

1. What was the likely cause and underlying mechanism to this patients's problem?
2. What treatment should be given?

Answers

1. ACE inhibitors reduce angiotensin II production, thus, attenuate angiotensin II mediated vasoconstriction of the efferent arterioles that contributes to the high-pressure gradient across the glomerulus necessary for filtration. It is not usually a problem in the majority of individuals; however, in patients with pre-existing compromised renal blood flow, such as renal artery stenoses, the kidney relies more heavily on angiotensin-mediated vasoconstriction of the postglomerular arterioles to maintain renal function. Hypovolaemia caused, for example, by diuretic use and a diarrhoeal illness would tend to exacerbate this problem. Moreover, it is likely that sodium depletion would render the kidney even more dependent upon vasoconstriction of efferent arterioles through activation of the tubuloglomerular feedback system, further sensitising the kidney to the effects of ACE inhibitors.

   Mrs J might well have been suffering from incipient renal failure, but remained asymptomatic until her renal reserve diminished.
2. The inappropriate use of an ACE inhibitor should be stopped, as should the diuretic temporarily. Mrs J should be rehydrated using sodium chloride 0.9% and kidney function markers monitored in the hope that recovery will occur.
3. Investigations should be arranged to determine whether Mrs J has renal artery stenosis as a cause of her AKI after initiation of the ACE inhibitor (see Chapter 18).

Case 17.2

Mr B a known intermittent heroin and cocaine abuser, was discovered comatose in his room early in the morning. He was admitted to hospital as an emergency. An indirect history from an acquaintance indicated that Mr B had been drinking very heavily prior to the incident (probably more than a bottle of whisky in a 24-h period) and had smoked both heroin and cocaine of unknown source and purity.

On examination he was found to be dehydrated and serum biochemistry revealed the following:

		Reference range
Sodium	147 mmol/L	(135–145)
Potassium	6.1 mmol/L	(3.5–5.0)
Calcium	1.72 mmol/L	(2.20–2.55)
Phosphate	2.0 mmol/L	(0.9–1.5)
Creatinine	485 μmol/L	(50–120)
Creatinine kinase	120,000 IU/L	(<200)

Urine dipstick reacted positive for blood with no signs of red blood cells on microscopy. The urine was faintly reddish-brown in colour.

Question

What is likely to have occurred and how should it be treated?

Answer

Cocaine, heroin or alcohol abuse sometimes cause muscle damage resulting in rhabdomyolysis. The mechanism is unclear, but includes vasoconstriction, an increase in muscle activity, possibly because of seizures, self-injury, adulterants in the drug (e.g. arsenic, strychnine, amphetamine, phencyclidine, quinine) or compression (associated with long periods of inactivity). ATN may ensue from a direct nephrotoxic effect of the myoglobin released from damaged muscle cells, microprecipitation of myoglobin in renal tubules (as casts) or a reduction in medullary blood flow. The presence of myoglobin is suggested by the urine dipstick test, which reacts not only to red cells but also to free haemoglobin and myoglobin. Extremely high levels of myoglobinuria may result in urine the colour of Coca-Cola. High serum creatinine kinase levels are indicative of rhabdomyolysis together with the presence of free myoglobin in serum and urine. Serum levels of potassium and phosphate are elevated partly by the effects of incipient renal failure but also through tissue breakdown and intracellular release. Creatinine levels are often higher than expected because of muscle damage.

Treatment should involve fluid replacement with normal saline to reverse dehydration. Furosemide and other loop diuretics should be avoided as these decrease intra-tubular pH which may be a co-factor for cast precipitation. Indeed, in cases where urine pH is less than 6, administration of intravenous isotonic sodium bicarbonate may be of use. The patient's ECG should be monitored, because of the risks involved with rapid elevation in serum potassium. Timely, appropriate corrective therapy must be instigated where necessary. In 50–70% of cases with rhabdomyolysis, dialysis is required to support recovery.

Case 17.3

Mr D is a patient who has been admitted to an intensive care unit with AKI, which developed following a routine cholecystectomy. His electrolyte picture shows the following:

		Reference range
Sodium	138 mmol/L	(135–145)
Potassium	7.2 mmol/L	(3.5–5.0)
Bicarbonate	19 mmol/L	(22–31)
Urea	32.1 mmol/L	(3.0–6.5)
Creatinine	572 μmol/L	(50–120)
pH	7.28	(7.36–7.44)

The patient was connected to an ECG monitor and the resultant trace indicated absent P waves and a broad QRS complex.

Question

Explain the biochemistry and ECG abnormalities and indicate what therapeutic measures must be implemented.

Answer

Hyperkalaemia is one of the principal problems encountered in patients with renal failure. The increased levels of potassium arise from failure of the excretory pathway and also from intracellular release of potassium. Attention should also be paid to pharmacological or pharmaceutical processes that might lead to potassium elevation (e.g. inappropriate potassium supplements, ACE inhibitors, etc.). The acidosis noted in this patient, which is common in AKI, also aggravates hyperkalaemia by promoting leakage of potassium from cells. A serum potassium level greater than 7.0 mmol/L indicates that emergency treatment is required as the patient risks life-threatening ventricular arrhythmias and asystolic cardiac arrest. If ECG changes are present, as in this case, emergency treatment should be initiated when serum potassium rises above 6.5 mmol/L.

The emergency treatment should include:

1. Stabilisation of the myocardium by intravenous administration of 10–30 mL calcium gluconate 10% over 5–10 min. The effect is temporary but the dose can be repeated.
2. Intravenous administration of 10–20 units of soluble insulin with 50 mL of 50% glucose to stimulate cellular potassium uptake. The dose may be repeated. The blood glucose should be monitored for at least 6 h to avoid hypoglycaemia.
3. Acidosis may be corrected with an intravenous dose of sodium bicarbonate, preferably as an isotonic solution. Correction of acidosis stimulates cellular potassium re-uptake.
4. Intravenous salbutamol 0.5 mg in 100 mL 5% dextrose administered over 15 min has been used to stimulate the cellular Na-K ATPase pump and thus drive potassium into cells. This may cause disturbing muscle tremors at the doses required to reduce serum potassium levels.

References

Hems, S., Currie, A., 2005. Renal disorders. In: Lee, A. (Ed.), Adverse Drug Reactions, second ed. Pharmaceutical Press, London.

Kellum, J., Leblanc, M., Venkataraman, R., 2008. Acute Renal Failure Clinical Evidence 09 2001, BMJ Publishing Group, London. Available at http://clinicalevidence.bmj.com/ceweb/conditions/knd/2001/2001_contribdetails.jsp. Accessed Sep. 2010.

Rabindranath, K.S., Strippoli, G.F.M., Daly, C., et al., 2006. Haemodiafiltration, haemofiltration and haemodialysis for end-stage kidney disease. Cochrane Database of Systematic Reviews, Issue 4. Art No. CD006258. doi:10.1002/14651858. CD006258. Available at http://www2.cochrane.org/reviews/en/ab006258.html Accessed Sep. 2010.

Further reading

Dishart, M.K., Kellum, J.A., 2000. An evaluation of pharmacological strategies for the prevention and treatment of acute renal failure. Drugs 59, 79–91.

Short, A., Cumming, A., 1999. ABC of intensive care: renal support. Br. Med. J. 319, 41–44.

Steddon, S., Ashman, N., Chesser, A., Cunningham, J., 2007. Oxford Handbook of Nephrology and Hypertension. Oxford University Press, Oxford.

18 Chronic kidney disease and end-stage renal disease

J. Marriott, P. Cockwell and S. Stringer

Key points

- The prevalence of chronic kidney disease (CKD) increases with age and is greater in females and some ethnic populations.
- CKD is classified according to severity from 1 to 5, where 5 is the most advanced and 1 the least.
- CKD 1–3 is common and may not cause symptoms. It may progress to end-stage renal disease but frequently remains stable for many years.
- CKD is an important risk factor for cardiovascular disease.
- As CKD becomes more advanced (stages 4 and 5), virtually all body systems are adversely affected.
- Clinical signs and symptoms of severe CKD include oedema, anaemia, hypertension, bone pain, nocturia, neurological changes and disordered muscle function.
- The aims of treatment are to reverse or arrest the process responsible for CKD, relieve symptoms and reduce cardiovascular morbidity and mortality.
- To prevent further renal damage, adequate control of blood pressure and reduction of proteinuria are essential.
- Renal anaemia is common when the glomerular filtration rate (GFR) falls below 30 mL/min but can be corrected by erythropoietin in 90–95% of cases.
- End-stage renal disease is the point at which life can only be sustained by dialysis or transplantation. This may occur soon after presentation or after several years.
- The need for dialysis therapy is increasing at about 5% per annum with attendant resource implications.
- There are two principal types of dialysis: haemodialysis and peritoneal dialysis. In both, waste products and metabolites are transferred from the patient's blood across a semi-permeable membrane to a dialysis solution.
- Renal transplantation remains the treatment of choice for end-stage renal disease. However, up to 60% of patients on dialysis programmes are not fit enough to be put on the transplant list.

Chronic kidney disease (CKD) is defined by a reduction in the glomerular filtration rate (GFR) and/or urinary abnormalities or structural abnormalities of the renal tract. The severity of CKD is classified from 1 to 5 depending upon the level of GFR (Table 18.1). It is a common condition affecting up to 10% of the population in Western societies and is more common in some ethnic minority populations and in females. The incidence increases exponentially with age such that some degree of CKD is almost inevitable in persons over 80 years of age. Social deprivation is also associated with a higher prevalence of CKD. The scale of CKD and the consequences for the health service has been appreciated only in the last few years.

Estimates for the incidence of the various grades of CKD are shown in Table 18.1 and have been derived from large American studies, although data suggests the rates in the UK are similar (UK Renal Registry, 2008). In the past, patients with CKD were often unrecognised owing to difficulties in measuring or estimating the GFR and their health needs were largely unmet. The recent development of simple methods to estimate GFR has revealed a huge population of patients with significant kidney disease. This will pose a considerable challenge to health services in the future. National guidance on the management of CKD has been published (NICE, 2008) and includes management in primary and secondary care.

CKD differs from acute kidney injury (AKI) by virtue of chronicity and a different spectrum of causes. However, AKI and CKD are not mutually exclusive; patients with AKI may not recover renal function to their baseline and may be left with residual CKD. In addition, patients with CKD may experience episodes of AKI sometimes causing reversible step-wise declines in renal function.

Renin-angiotensin-aldosterone system

The renin-angiotensin-aldosterone system (RAAS) has a critical role in the progression of CKD and an awareness of this system is important for understanding the pathophysiology of CKD and the targets for therapeutic intervention. Most of the renal effects of this system are through regulating intraglomerular pressures and salt and water balance. Renin is an enzyme which is formed and stored in the juxtaglomerular apparatus and released in response to decreased afferent intra-arterial pressures, decreased glomerular ultrafiltrate sodium levels and sympathetic nervous system activation. In patients with CKD, intra-renal pressures are often low and sympathetic overactivity is common; these factors lead to increased renin secretion. This can occur with normal or elevated systemic blood pressure.

Table 18.1 Classification of chronic kidney disease

Stage of CKD	Glomerular filtration rate	Description	Prevalence in the UK (% of population)
1	≥90 mL/min + proteinuria/haematuria or structural damage	Kidney damage with normal or increased GFR but other evidence of kidney damage	3.3
2	60–89 mL/min + proteinuria/haematuria or structural damage	Slight decrease in GFR with other evidence of kidney disease	3.0
3a 3b	45–59 mL/min 30–44 mL/min	Moderate reduction in GFR With or without evidence of other kidney disease	4.3
4	13–29 mL/min	Severe reduction in GFR	0.2
5	<15 mL/min	Kidney failure, use suffix (D) if dialysis	0.1

GFR, glomerular filtration rate.
Use suffix (P) to denote proteinuria, suffix (D) to denote dialysis and suffix (T) to denote transplantation. For example, a patient with CKD 3a and proteinuria would be described as CKD 3A p. A patient with CKD 5 on dialysis would be CKD5 d

Renin promotes cleavage of the protein angiotensinogen, which is produced by the liver, to produce angiotensin I. Angiotensin I is converted to angiotensin II by angiotensin-converting enzyme (ACE). Angiotensin II has two major physiological effects. First, it acts on the zona glomerulosa of the adrenal cortex to promote production of the mineralocorticoid hormone aldosterone, with resultant increased distal tubular salt and water reabsorption. Furthermore, it promotes antidiuretic hormone (ADH) release, which increases proximal tubular sodium reabsorption and promotes thirst. In combination, these lead to salt and fluid retention, high intravascular volumes, hypertension and oedema. Second, it is a direct vasoconstrictor and promotes systemic and (preferential) renal hypertension. The renal effects are predominantly on the efferent glomerular arteriole. Vasoconstriction at this site is mediated by a high density of angiotensin II receptors. When these receptors are ligated by angiotensin II, there is increased intra-glomerular pressures. Whilst this leads to an overall increase in GFR in the short-term, over a longer period glomerular hypertension promotes accelerated glomerular scarring and worsening CKD. In addition to the vascular and endocrine effects of the RAAS, it is now recognised that there is a local immune modulatory role for this system. Both resident (e.g. tubular epithelial) cells and inflammatory (monocytes and macrophages) cells synthesise components of the RAAS and are themselves targeted by the system. For example, monocytes and macrophages express the angiotensin II receptor and activation through this receptor leads to an enhanced inflammatory and fibrotic phenotype of the cell. This raises the intriguing concept that some of the effects of blocking the RAAS are due to direct anti-inflammatory and anti-fibrotic effects. Figure 18.1 shows this pathway and identifies the points at which pharmacological interventions targeted for a biological effect translates into clinical outcomes.

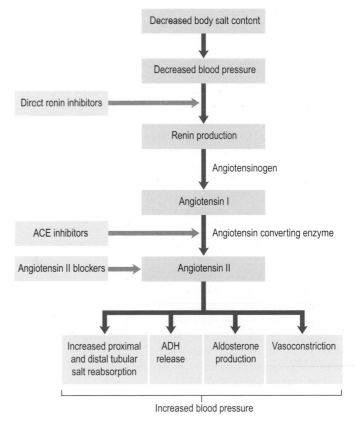

Fig. 18.1 The renin–angiotensin–aldosterone system and targets for pharmaceutical intervention.

Measurement of renal function

The scale of CKD has only been recognised in recent years because detection is dependent upon an accurate estimation of the GFR. The GFR is defined as the volume of filtrate produced by the glomeruli of both kidneys each minute and is a reliable indicator of renal function.

It is laborious and expensive to measure GFR by gold standard tests such as inulin or radiolabelled isotope clearance. These tests are only used when extremely accurate assessment of kidney function is required. An example of this is measurement of kidney function in a potential living kidney donor where an individual is proposing to donate a kidney to a family member or close friend.

As a consequence, a number of equations have been validated for use in the routine clinical setting. These equations provide an estimate of glomerular filtration rate (eGFR) based on the combination of serum or plasma creatinine and a number of variables which add precision to the estimation of kidney function. The commonest eGFR equation used in clinical practice is the four-variable MDRD (Modification of Diet in Renal Disease Study) equation. The biochemical variable that provides the basis of the MDRD and most other GFR equations is serum creatinine.

Serum creatinine

While serum creatinine concentration is related to renal function, it is also dependent upon the rate of production of creatinine by the patient. Creatinine is a by-product of normal muscle metabolism and is formed at a rate proportional to muscle mass (20 g muscle equates to approximately 1 mg creatinine production) and therefore is related to age, sex and ethnicity.

Creatinine is freely filtered by the glomerulus, so when muscle mass is stable any change in serum creatinine levels reflects a change in its renal clearance. Consequently, measurement of serum creatinine can be utilised to give an estimate of the kidney function. It is important to note, however, that creatinine also undergoes significant tubular secretion (~10–20%). This becomes important in advanced CKD (stages 4 and 5) and limits the value of measuring serum creatinine to determine renal function in advanced CKD.

MDRD glomerular filtration rate equation

Eight eGFR equations were validated for the MDRD study (Levey et al., 1999). These used demographic and serum variables (including serum creatinine level, age, gender, non-black ethnicity, higher serum urea levels, and lower serum albumin levels) in a series of equations. The four-variable equation (also known as the abbreviated (a)MDRD equation) has been adopted into clinical practice and incorporates age, creatinine, gender and ethnicity (Fig. 18.2).

The MDRD equation is more accurate than serum creatinine alone as an estimator of kidney function; however, it has not been validated in the elderly, those with creatinine levels within the normal range or transplant recipients. The CKD classification system is based on the aMDRD eGFR.

Other estimates of kidney function

Creatinine clearance

This is similar to the GFR as nearly all the filtered creatinine appears in the urine. It is a measurement of the volume of blood that is cleared of creatinine with time. Measurements of creatinine clearance (Cl_{Cr}) require accurate collection of 24 h urine samples with a serum creatinine sample midway through this period. This is time-consuming, inconvenient and prone to inaccuracy and as such is now rarely used in clinical practice. Figure 18.3 shows the equation for measuring creatinine clearance.

Cockroft–Gault equation

The Cockroft–Gault equation uses weight, sex and age to estimate creatinine clearance and was derived using average population data (Cockroft and Gault, 1976). The equation is shown in Fig. 18.4.

Estimates of glomerular filtration rate in paediatric patients

Estimates of GFRs in paediatric patients can be made using the Schwartz formula (Schwartz, 1985) or the Counahan–Barratt method (Counahan et al., 1976) which both rely upon inclusion of the height of the child in estimating creatinine clearance, since height correlates with muscle mass.

Urea

Urea is also used in the assessment of renal function despite a variable production rate and diurnal fluctuation in response to the protein content of the diet. Levels of urea

$$Cl_{Cr} = \frac{(U \times V)}{S}$$

where **U** is the urine creatinine concentration (µmol/L), **V** is the urine flow rate (mL/min) and **S** is the serum creatinine concentration (µmol/L)

Fig. 18.3   Creatinine clearance calculation.

$$Cl_{Cr} = \frac{F\,(140\,\text{age (years))} \times \text{weight (kg)}}{\text{Serum creatinine (µmol/L)}}$$

where **F** = 1.04 (females) or 1.23 (males)

Fig. 18.4   The Cockroft–Gault formula.

eGFR (mL/min/1.73m²) = 186 × [serum creatinine (µmol/L)/88.4]$^{-1.154}$ × [age]$^{-0.203}$ × [0.742 if **female**] × [1.212 if **African-American**]

Fig. 18.2   Four-variable MDRD equation used to calculate eGFR.

may also be elevated by dehydration or an increase in protein catabolism such as that accompanying gastro-intestinal haemorrhage, severe infection, trauma (including surgery) and high-dose steroid therapy. Serum urea levels are, therefore, an unreliable measure of renal function, but can be used as an indicator of the patient's general condition and state of hydration. A rapid elevation of serum urea, before any rise in corresponding creatinine levels, is often a sign of an impending deterioration in renal function or a marker for pre-renal failure associated with intravascular volume depletion.

Significance of CKD

CKD is significant as it indicates the possibility of progression to end-stage renal disease, and a strong association with accelerated cardiovascular disease, similar in magnitude to that observed in diabetics. The cardiovascular risk increases with the severity of CKD but is detectable at all levels. Thus, it is important to pay particular attention to traditional cardiovascular risk factors such as smoking, cholesterol and blood pressure in patients with CKD. However, it is known from previous studies that these risk factors only contribute around 50% of the total cardiovascular disease risk and recent interest has focused on the identification of novel risk factors to explain the remainder of the risk.

It is important to make a distinction between cardiovascular disease related to macrovascular atherosclerosis and that related to microvascular changes, often found in individuals with CKD. The cardiovascular disease found in CKD is more likely to be related to small vessel disease initiated by endothelial dysfunction rather than atherosclerotic disease. In addition, patients with CKD often have associated left ventricular hypertrophy which may be related to chronic volume overload and uraemia.

Progression to more advanced stages of CKD may occur, particularly if the blood pressure is inadequately controlled and there is significant proteinuria, but this is by no means the rule and many patients with CKD remain stable for years or even decades. These patients need to be followed up with regular blood and urine tests to detect progression, if it occurs. Low risk patients, that is, those with unchanging GFR over time, with controlled blood pressure and no proteinuria may not require long-term follow up by a kidney specialist and surveillance can be carried out satisfactorily in primary care.

Patients with CKD 1–3 (Table 18.1) are frequently asymptomatic. The reduction of GFR is insufficient to cause uraemic symptoms and any minor abnormalities in the urine such as proteinuria or haematuria are usually not noticed by patients. There is a frequent association with high blood pressure which may be the cause or a consequence of renal damage. Recognition of these patients is important as it allows early modification of traditional cardiovascular risk factors. These patients should be investigated to determine if there is a treatable cause for their CKD and followed up to identify those individuals with progressive disease.

Patients with CKD stages 4 and 5 (Table 18.1) should usually be followed up in a nephrology clinic because they will require specialist management of the complications of CKD such as anaemia and bone disease, whilst many will also be undergoing preparation for renal replacement therapy.

Causes of CKD

The reduction in renal function observed in CKD results from damage to the infrastructure of the kidney in discrete areas rather than throughout the kidney. The nephron is the functional unit of the kidney and while the mechanism of damage depends on the underlying cause of renal disease, as nephrons become damaged and fail, remaining nephrons compensate for loss of function by hyperfiltration secondary to raised intra-glomerular pressure. This causes 'bystander' damage with secondary nephron loss. This vicious cycle is illustrated in Fig. 18.5. The patient remains well until so many nephrons are lost that the GFR can no longer be maintained despite activation of compensatory mechanisms. As a consequence there is a progressive decline in kidney function.

CKD arises from a variety of causes (Table 18.2), although by the time a patient has established CKD it may not be possible to identify the exact cause. However, attempting to establish the cause is useful in the identification and elimination of reversible factors, to plan for likely outcomes and treatment needs, and for appropriate counselling when a genetic basis is established. The causes of CKD listed in Table 18.2 are ordered according to prevalence. It is important to note the prevalence of these factors is different in CKD and end stage renal disease. In end stage renal disease, diseases such as adult polycystic kidney disease (APKD) are overrepresented and ischaemic/hypertensive nephropathy underrepresented. The reasons for this are that individuals with APKD are likely to survive to reach end stage renal disease while those with diabetes or ischaemic renal damage may succumb to cardiovascular disease before end stage renal disease is reached.

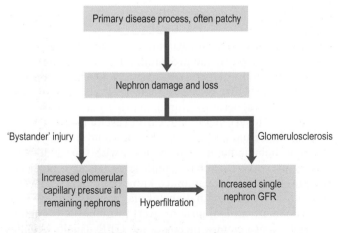

Fig. 18.5 Mechanism of progressive renal damage.

Table 18.2 Primary diagnosis in renal replacement therapy patients by age and gender (Renal Registry, 2008)

Primary diagnosis	% all patients	Inter-centre range (%)	% age <65	% age >65	% male:female ratio
Aetiology uncertain/ glomerulonephritis (not biopsy proven)	21.6	2.1–84.3	19.2	26.6	1.6
Glomerulonephritis (biopsy proven)	15.3	2.3–22.4	17.8	10.0	2.2
Pyelonephritis	11.9	3.2–19.4	13.6	8.3	1.1
Diabetes	13.2	2.8–26.0	12.3	15.1	1.6
Polycystic kidney	9.2	2.0–15.8	9.6	8.3	1.1
Hypertension	5.4	1.0–16.0	4.6	6.9	2.4
Renal vascular disease	3.5	0.3–16.1	1.1	8.2	2.0
Other	14.5	1.9–36.1	16.0	11.3	1.3
Not sent	5.5	0.1–46.2	5.7	5.2	1.5

Ischaemic/hypertensive renal disease

Ischaemic nephropathy has traditionally been referred to under perfusion of the kidneys caused by renal artery stenosis. This explanation has fallen from favour recently and this term is now taken to mean impairment of renal function beyond occlusion of the main renal arteries. Hypertension results in atherosclerosis which can cause occlusive renovascular disease and small vessel damage. In patients with significant large vessel occlusive disease arteriolar nephrosclerosis, interstial fibrosis and glomerular collapse may be present (Lerman and Textor, 2001). These diagnoses account for around 30% of CKD and a smaller proportion of end stage renal disease. The effective management of hypertension is crucial to reduce renal damage.

Metabolic diseases

Diabetes mellitus is the most common metabolic disease that leads to CKD, whilst the predominant lesion is glomerular and referred to as diabetic nephropathy. Diabetes accounts for around 13% of CKD (see Table 18.2) and is associated with faster renal deterioration than other pathologies: these patients are at very significant cardiovascular risk by virtue of both CKD and diabetes. Both type 1 and 2 diabetes can result in diabetic nephrophy, patients with type 1 diabetes usually present with renal complications at a younger age and may benefit from combined kidney and pancreas transplantation. Patients with diabetes may present with no proteinuria, micro albuminuria or overt proteinuria, though as the level of proteinuria increases the GFR usually declines and in many patients this represents an inexorable decline towards end stage renal disease.

Chronic glomerulonephritis

All types of chronic glomerulonephritis (GN) combined cause about 15% of cases of advanced CKD. The commonest cause of glomerulonephritis is IgA nephropathy which is characterised by deposition of polymeric IgA in the glomerulus with subsequent immune activation. Other patterns of glomerulonephritis include membranous nephropathy, where there is granular deposition of immunoglobulin on the glomerular capillary basement membrane. Systemic autoimmune diseases such as systemic lupus erythematosus can cause a variety of types of glomerulonephritis. Finally, some chronic forms of glomerulonephritis are pauci-immune, that is they have no immune deposition. This is seen in focal and segmental glomerulosclerosis.

Lower urinary tract disease

A variety of differing pathologies make up this group and together they represent 5–10% of all cases of CKD. The conditions include the following.

Reflux disease

This results from reflux of urine back up the renal tract towards the kidneys. This can result in recurrent infections and subsequent scarring.

Renal stone disease

Kidney stones are primarily formed of calcium oxalate and calcium phosphate. They can cause urinary tract obstruction and infection.

Chronic pyelonephritis

Recurrent urinary tract infection can result in renal scarring; this is often in the context of reflux disease but may occur without it.

Extrinsic renal tract obstruction

In males, the commonest cause of this is prostatic hypertrophy though there are many other causes.

Hereditary/congenital diseases

There are many inherited renal diseases and together they represent 5% of CKD cases. It is, however, important to remember that they make up a higher proportion of cases of end stage renal disease. The commoner inherited conditions are APKD and Alport's syndrome. Autosomal dominant polycystic kidney disease is an inherited condition which results in the formation of multiple cysts in both kidneys throughout life. The kidneys become enlarged and frequently fail in middle age. Alport's syndrome is a disorder of glomerular basement membranes caused by a mutation affecting type IV collagen; X-linked, autosomal dominant and autosomal recessive forms of inheritance are all seen. The clinical manifestations include progressive nephritis with haematuria, proteinuria and sensorineural deafness.

Unknown cause

It is not uncommon for the cause of CKD to be unknown and this is the case in around 30% of patients who typically present with small kidneys and unremarkable immunological investigations. When the kidneys are small it is often not possible to carry out a renal biopsy or if possible the histology often shows severe scarring with no indication of the underlying cause.

Clinical manifestations

While uraemic symptoms are rare in CKD stage 4, they become more apparent as the patient approaches end stage renal disease. The onset of symptoms is slow and insidious so that patients may not realise that they are unwell. It is not uncommon for patients to present in end stage renal disease and require immediate dialysis at their first contact with the medical profession.

End stage renal disease is characterised by the requirement of renal replacement therapy to sustain life and it is often accompanied by uraemia, anaemia, acidosis, osteodystrophy, neuropathy and is frequently accompanied by hypertension, fluid retention and susceptibility to infection (Fig. 18.6). It results from a significant reduction in the excretory, homeostatic, metabolic and endocrine functions of the kidney that occur over a period of months or years.

In the following section, the clinical features of CKD are described, along with the pathogenesis.

Urinary tract features

Both polyuria and nocturia are found in CKD though neither is universal and many patients with CKD have no urinary symptoms. Proteinuria is common in CKD and can be present

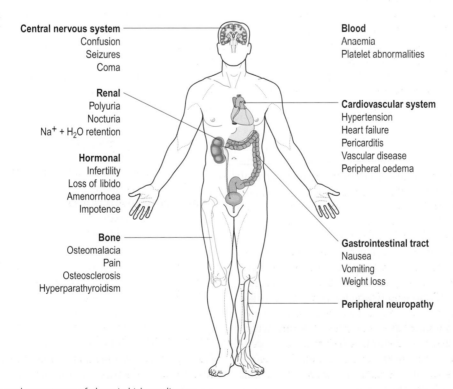

Fig. 18.6 Typical signs and symptoms of chronic kidney disease.

to varying degrees. Proteinuria is commonly measured using single urine samples to determine the albumin creatinine ratio (ACR). This method has almost entirely replaced the 24 h urine collection which was inconvenient and often unreliable. An ACR of 3-30 mg/mmol is described as microalbuminuria while in nephrotic-range proteinuria it is >250 mg/mmol. Haematuria may also be present and can reflect either glomerular or lower urinary tract pathology. The presence of blood and/or protein in the urine is described as an active urinary sediment. Whenever blood in the urine is detected an infection should be considered and excluded by urine microscopy for white cells and culture for organisms.

Polyuria and nocturia

Polyuria, where the patient frequently voids high volumes of urine, is often seen in CKD and results from medullary damage and the osmotic effect of a high serum urea level (>40 mmol/L). The ability to concentrate urine is also lost in CKD, which together with failure of physiological nocturnal antidiuresis, invariably results in nocturia, where the patient will be wakened two or three times a night with a full bladder.

Proteinuria

A degree of proteinuria is common in CKD and the prevalence of proteinuria increases with the severity of CKD. There are a number of precipitating factors including glomerular disease, failure of protein reabsorption in the tubules and rarely overflow of excess plasma proteins as seen in myeloma. Pronounced proteinuria (>1 g of protein in a 24-h collection, equivalent to an ACR >70 mg/mmol) usually indicates a glomerular aetiology. The presence and quantity of proteinuria are major determinants of progressive CKD.

Haematuria

Haematuria can be either macroscopic or microscopic; macroscopic haematuria is likely to result from lower urinary tract pathology (such as bladder lesions) and microscopic haematuria is most often of glomerular origin. Microscopy can identify the presence of casts which are also seen in glomerular diseases and allow the discrimination of the course of haematuria.

Hypertension and fluid overload

Most patients with CKD will have hypertension and this may be a cause or a consequence (or a combination of both) of their kidney disease. Furthermore, raised blood pressure may exacerbate renal damage and lead to accelerated deterioration of CKD.

Severe renal impairment leads to sodium retention, which in turn produces circulatory volume expansion with consequent hypertension. This form of hypertension is often termed 'salt-sensitive', as it may be exacerbated by salt intake. Lesser degrees of renal impairment reduce kidney perfusion,

which activates renin production, with subsequent angiotensin-mediated vasoconstriction. Treatment of blood pressure, irrespective of choice of therapy, generally improves the course of CKD. As the GFR falls to very low levels the kidneys are unable to excrete salt and water adequately, resulting in the retention of extravascular fluid. All patients with fluid overload will by definition also have salt retention, even if this is not manifest in the serum sodium concentration.

Clinical findings

Eye damage in the form of hypertensive retinopathy may be found in those patients whose blood pressure has not been adequately controlled. This can be prevented by appropriate and timely antihypertensive therapy. Fluid retention can manifest as peripheral and pulmonary oedema and ascites. Oedema may be seen around the eyes on waking, the sacral region in supine patients and from the feet upwards in ambulatory patients. Volume-dependent hypertension occurs in about 80% of patients with CKD and becomes more prevalent as the GFR falls.

Uraemia

Many substances including urea, creatinine and water are normally excreted by the kidney and accumulate as renal function decreases. Some of the substances responsible for the toxicity of uraemia are intermediate in size between small, readily dialysed molecules and large non-dialysable proteins. These are described as 'middle molecules' and include phosphate, guanidines, phenols and organic acids. Clearly, there are a wide range of uraemic toxins but it is the blood level of urea that is often used to estimate the degree of toxin accumulation in uraemia. True symptomatic uraemia only occurs in very advanced CKD.

Clinical findings

The symptoms of uraemia include anorexia, nausea, vomiting, constipation, foul taste and skin discolouration that is presumed to be due to pigment deposition compounded by the pallor of anaemia. The characteristic complexion is often described as 'muddy', and is frequently associated with severe pruritus without an underlying rash. In extremely severe cases, crystalline urea is deposited on the skin (uraemic frost).

In uraemia, there is also an increased tendency to bleed, which can exacerbate pre-existing anaemia because of impaired platelet adhesion and modified interaction between platelets and blood vessels resulting from altered blood rheology.

Anaemia

Anaemia is a common consequence of CKD and affects most people with CKD stages 4 and 5. The fall in haemoglobin level is a slow, insidious process accompanying the decline in renal function. A normochromic, normocytic pattern is usually seen with haemoglobin levels falling to around 8 g/dL by end stage renal disease.

Several factors contribute to the pathogenesis of anaemia in CKD, including shortened red cell survival, marrow suppression by uraemic toxins and iron or folate deficiency associated with poor dietary intake or increased loss, for example, from gastro-intestinal bleeding. However, the principal cause results from damage of peritubular cells leading to inadequate secretion of erythropoietin. This hormone, which is produced mainly, although not exclusively, in the kidney, is the main regulator of red cell proliferation and differentiation in bone marrow. Hyperparathyroidism also reduces erythropoiesis by damaging bone marrow and therefore exacerbates anaemia associated with CKD. The RAAS is also involved in erythropoiesis since renin increases erythropoietin production and this explains how ACE inhibitors can cause small reductions in haemoglobin.

Clinical findings

Anaemia in CKD is a major cause of fatigue, breathlessness at rest and on exertion, lethargy and angina. Patients may also complain of feeling cold, poor concentration and reduced appetite and libido. Compensatory haemodynamic changes occur with CKD, cardiac output is increased to improve oxygen delivery to tissues, although this may result in tachycardia and palpitations. The anaemia of CKD usually responds to treatment with erythropoietin-stimulating agents (ESAs).

Bone disease (renal osteodystrophy)

Renal osteodystrophy describes the four types of bone disease associated with CKD:

- secondary hyperparathyroidism
- osteomalacia (reduced mineralisation)
- mixed renal osteodystrophy (both hyperparathyroidism and osteomalacia)
- adynamic bone disease (reduced bone formation and resorption).

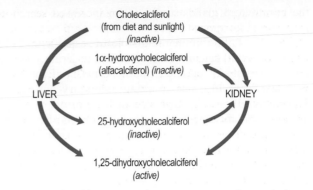

Fig. 18.7   Renal and hepatic involvement in vitamin D metabolism.

Cholecalciferol, the precursor of active vitamin D, is both absorbed from the gastro-intestinal tract and produced in the skin by the action of sunlight. Production of active vitamin D, 1,25-dihydroxycholecalciferol (calcitriol), requires the hydroxylation of the colecalciferol molecule at both the 1α and the 25 position (Fig. 18.7).

Hydroxylation at the 25 position occurs in the liver, while hydroxylation of the 1α position occurs in the kidney; this latter process is impaired in renal failure. The resulting deficiency in vitamin D leads to defective mineralisation of bone and subsequent osteomalacia which is almost inevitable in those with CKD stage 3 and beyond.

The deficiency in vitamin D with the consequent reduced calcium absorption from the gut in combination with the reduced renal tubular reabsorption results in hypocalcaemia (Fig. 18.8).

These disturbances are compounded by hyperphosphataemia caused by reduced phosphate excretion, which in turn reduces the concentration of ionised serum calcium by sequestering calcium phosphate in bone and in soft tissue. Hypocalcaemia, hyperphosphataemia and a reduction in the direct suppressive action of 1,25-dihydroxycholecalciferol on

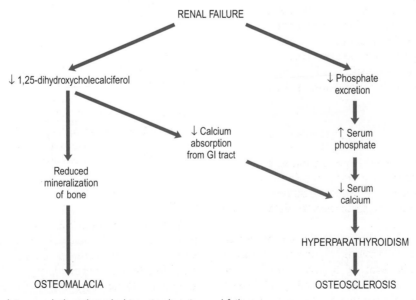

Fig. 18.8   Disturbance of calcium and phosphate balance in chronic renal failure.

the parathyroid glands results in an increased secretion of parathyroid hormone (PTH).

Since the failing kidney is unable to respond to PTH by increasing renal calcium reabsorption, the serum PTH levels remain persistently elevated, and hyperplasia of the parathyroid glands occurs. The resulting secondary hyperparathyroidism produces a disturbance in the normal architecture of bone and this is termed osteosclerosis (hardening of the bone). A further possible consequence of secondary hyperparathyroidism produced in response to hypocalcaemia is that sufficient bone reabsorption may be caused to maintain adequate calcium levels. This, in combination with hyperphosphataemia, may result in calcium phosphate deposition and soft tissue calcification.

Clinical findings

Bone pain is the main symptom, and distinctive appearances on radiography may be observed, such as 'rugger-jersey' spine, where there are alternate bands of excessive and defective mineralisation in the vertebrae (Fig. 18.9).

Neurological changes

The most common neurological changes are non-specific and include inability to concentrate, memory impairment, irritability and stupor probably caused by uraemic toxins.

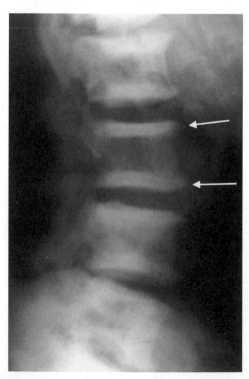

Fig. 18.9 Lateral radiograph of the spine in a patient with chronic renal failure. Characteristic endplate sclerosis (arrows) are referred to as 'rugger-jersey spine' (reproduced by kind permission of Dr M. J. Kline, Department of Diagnostic Radiology, Cleveland Clinic Foundation).

Clinical features

Fits owing to cerebral oedema or hypertension may occur. A 'glove and stocking' peripheral neuropathy can occur as can mono-neuritis multiplex.

Muscle function

Muscle symptoms are probably caused by general nutritional deficiencies and electrolyte disturbances, notably of divalent cations and especially by hypocalcaemia.

Clinical findings

Muscle cramps and restless legs are common and may be major symptoms causing distress to patients, particularly at night. Rarely a proximal myopathy of shoulder and pelvic girdle muscles may develop.

Electrolyte disturbances

Since the kidneys play such a crucial role in the maintenance of volume, extracellular fluid composition and acid–base balance, it is not surprising that disturbances of electrolyte levels are seen in CKD.

Sodium

Serum sodium levels can be relatively normal even when creatinine clearance is very low. However, patients may exhibit hypo- or hypernatraemia depending upon the condition and therapy employed (see Table 18.3).

Table 18.3 Causes and mechanism of serum sodium abnormalities in chronic kidney disease

	Mechanism	Cause/effect
Hypernatraemia	Sodium overload	Drugs, for example, antibiotic sodium salts
	Hypotonic fluid loss	Osmotic diuresis
	↓ Water intake	Sweating Unconsciousness
Hyponatraemia	Dilution by intracellular water movement	Mannitol
Hyperglycaemia	Water overload	Acute dilution by intravenous fluids, for example, 5% dextrose infusion Excessive intake Congestive cardiac failure Nephrotic syndrome

Potassium

Potassium levels can be elevated in CKD. Hyperkalaemia is a potentially dangerous condition as the first indication of elevated potassium levels may be life-threatening cardiac arrest. Potassium levels of over 7.0 mmol/L are life-threatening and should be treated as an emergency. Hyperkalaemia may be exacerbated in acidosis as potassium shifts from within cells.

ECG changes accompany any rise in serum potassium and become more pronounced as levels increase. T waves peak ('tenting'), there is a reduction in the size of P waves, an increase in the PR interval and a widening of the QRS complex. P waves eventually disappear and the QRS complex becomes even wider. Ultimately, the ECG assumes a sinusoidal appearance prior to cardiac arrest (see Fig. 18.10).

Hydrogen ions

Hydrogen ions (H^+) are a common end-product of many metabolic processes and about 40–80 mmol are normally excreted via the kidney each day. In renal failure, H^+ is retained, causing acidosis; the combination of H^+ with bicarbonate (HCO_3^-) results in the removal of some hydrogen as water, the elimination of carbon dioxide via the lungs, and a reduction in serum bicarbonate level.

A. Normal serum potassium (3.5–5.0) mmol/L

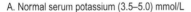
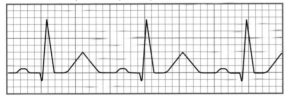

B. Serum potassium approximately 7.0 mmol/L

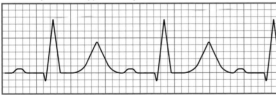

C. Serum potassium approximately 8.0–9.0 mmol/L

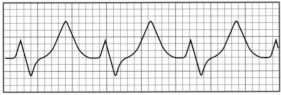

D. Serum potassium greater than 10.0 mmol/L

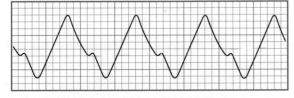

Fig. 18.10 Typical ECG changes in hyperkalaemia.

Diagnosis, investigations and monitoring

Although the diagnosis of CKD may be suspected because of signs and symptoms of renal disease, more often it is discovered incidentally. There are patients with CKD for whom no cause can be identified, often because they have two small kidneys which are not safe to biopsy. This appearance results from damage at some unspecified time in the past.

Family, drug and social histories are all important in elucidating the causes of renal failure, since genetics or exposure to toxins, including prescription, over-the-counter and herbal drugs, might be implicated.

Physical examination may be helpful. Signs of anaemia and skin pigmentation, excoriations owing to scratching and whitening of the skin with crystalline urea ('uraemic frost') may point to severe disease. Palpable or audible bruits over the femoral arteries are strongly associated with extensive arteriosclerosis and are commonly found in patients with renal vascular disease. Ankle oedema and a raised jugular venous pressure suggest fluid retention and in severe CKD a fishy smell on the breath known as 'uraemic foetor' is characteristic. In some patients, the kidneys may be palpable. Large irregular kidneys are indicative of polycystic disease, whereas smooth, tender enlarged kidneys are likely to be infected or obstructed. However, in the large majority of CKD the kidneys are small and are impalpable. A palpable bladder suggests outflow tract obstruction which is often due to prostatic hypertrophy in men.

Functional assessment of the kidney may be performed by testing serum and urine. The serum creatinine level is a more reliable indicator of renal function than the serum urea level though both are normally measured. Hyperkalaemia, acidosis with a correspondingly low serum bicarbonate level, hypocalcaemia and hyperphosphataemia are frequently present and can help to differentiate a new presentation of CKD from AKI.

Urine should be examined visually and microscopically and urinalysis performed for assessment of urinary sediment and a spot urine assessment of the ACR. The patient may report a change in urine colour, which might result from blood staining by whole cells or haemoglobin, drugs or metabolic breakdown products. Urine may also appear milky after connection with lymphatics, cloudy following infection, contain solid material such as stones, crystals, casts, or froth excessively in proteinuria.

Dipstick tests enable simple, rapid estimation of a wide range of urinary parameters including pH, specific gravity, leucocytes, nitrites, glucose, blood and protein. Positive results should, however, be quantified by more specific methods.

Structural assessments of the kidney may be performed using a number of imaging procedures, including:

- ultrasonography
- intravenous urography (IVU)
- plain abdominal radiography
- computed tomography (CT), magnetic resonance imaging (MRI) and magnetic resonance angiography (MRA).

Ultrasonography

This method produces two dimensional images using sound waves and is used as the first-line investigational tool in many hospitals. The technique is harmless, non-invasive, quick, inexpensive, enables measurements to be made and produces images in real time. The latter feature allows accurate and safe positioning of biopsy needles. Ultrasonography is particularly useful in the differentiation of renal tumours from cysts and in the assessment of renal tract obstruction. Doppler ultrasonography is a development that enables measurement of flow rate and direction of the intra- and extrarenal blood supply.

Intravenous urography

IVU is now used very infrequently because it uses high doses of radiation and contrast media, newer modalities such as CT scanning can provide more information. Timed serial radiographs are taken of the kidneys and the full length of the urinary tract following an intravenous injection of an iodine-based contrast medium that is filtered and excreted by the kidney. IVU will show the following:

- the presence, length and position of the kidneys; in CKD the kidneys generally shrink in proportion to nephron loss, the exception being the enlarged kidneys seen in polycystic disease
- the presence or absence of renal scarring and the shape of the calices and renal pelvis; renal cortical scarring and caliceal distortion indicate chronic pyelonephritis
- obstruction to the ureters, for example, by a stone, tumour or retroperitoneal fibrosis; these require surgical intervention
- the shape of the bladder and the presence of residual urine; enlargement and a post-micturition residue suggest urethral obstruction such as prostatic hypertrophy.

Nuclear medicine investigations

There are two commonly used nuclear medicine investigations, the first uses mercapto acetyl tri-glycerine (MAG3). This is used for assessment of renal perfusion and the identification of outflow obstruction. The other is a dimercapto succinic acid (DMSA) scan, the purpose of which is to ascertain the percentage that each kidney contributes to overall function.

The similar techniques of CT and MRI provide excellent structural information about the kidneys and urinary tract. They use less radiation (none in the case of MRI) and less contrast media than an IVU, although the machinery required is more expensive than that needed for traditional imaging methods. CT is particularly useful in the investigation of kidney stones, where it has superseded the IVU. MRA can also give information about renal blood supply; however, in recent years, concerns have arisen about the use of gadolinium as a contrast agent used in MRA. This has been associated with nephrogenic systemic fibrosis which results in death in a proportion of patients; those with CKD stages 4 and 5 are at highest risk

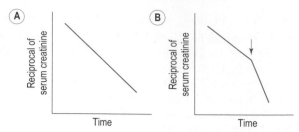

Fig. 18.11 Stylised reciprocal creatinine plots. (A) Linear, uniform progression in the decline in renal function. (B) Sudden decline in renal function (arrow).

of developing this condition. While the use of gadolinium is not contraindicated in this group, it must be used with great care and protocols will vary from unit to unit.

Renal biopsy

If imaging techniques fail to give a cause for the reduction in renal function, a renal biopsy may be performed, although in advanced disease extensive scarring of the renal tissue may obscure the original (primary) diagnosis. Also, the small shrunken kidneys often seen in CKD are difficult to biopsy and may subsequently bleed. Most clinicians do not biopsy in this setting. In patients whose GFR is below 30 mL/min, injection of vasopressin (ADH) might minimise bleeding following renal biopsy, although evidence for this is limited and use is not widespread.

Graphical plots of glomerular filtration rate

All patients with CKD should have their serum biochemistry and haematology monitored regularly to detect any of the sequelae of the disease. In some patients with CKD, the decline in renal function progresses at a constant rate and may be monitored by plotting the estimated GFR against time (Fig. 18.11). The intercept with the x-axis indicates the time at which renal function will fall to zero and can be used to predict when the GFR will reach approximately 10 mL/min, that is, the level at which renal replacement therapy should be initiated (Fig. 18.11A). If an abrupt decline in the slope of the reciprocal plot is noted (Fig. 18.11B), this indicates a worsening of the condition or the presence of an additional renal insult. The cause should be detected and remedied if possible. It is, however, increasingly recognised that most patients with CKD do not sustain a predictable decline. Many stabilise or follow a path of episodes of accelerated decline followed by months or years of stability. These observations are of great interest and are an increasing focus of clinical research.

Prognosis

When the GFR has declined to about 20 mL/min, a continuing deterioration in renal function to end stage renal disease is common even when the initial cause of the kidney damage has been removed and appropriate treatment instigated. The mechanisms for the decline in renal function include uncontrolled hypertension, proteinuria and damage resulting from hyperfiltration through the remaining intact nephrons. Serial GFR measurements should be monitored in conjunction with the patient's clinical condition to ensure the detection of the most appropriate point at which to commence renal replacement therapy. When a patient reaches an eGFR of 20 mL/min, plans should be in place for choice of renal replacement modality, transplantation or conservative management and where appropriate ongoing management of anaemia and bone disease.

Treatment

The aims of the treatment of CKD can be summarised as follows:

- Reverse or arrest the process causing the renal damage (this may not be possible)
- Avoid conditions that might worsen renal failure (Box 18.1)
- Treat the secondary complications of CKD (renal anaemia and bone disease)
- Relieve symptoms
- Implement regular dialysis treatment and/or transplantation at the most appropriate time.

Reversal or arrest of primary disease

By definition, CKD rarely has a readily reversible component, in contrast to acute renal failure. However, it is sometimes possible to identify a disease specific factor that is contributing to declining renal function and remove it. A postrenal lesion such as a ureter obstructed by a stone or a ureteric tumour may be successfully treated surgically. Glomerulonephritis may respond to immunosuppressants and/or steroids. Clearly, when drug-induced renal disease is suspected the offending agent should be stopped. These factors predominantly cause acute renal failure but they can cause acute on chronic failure and their reversal may prevent further deterioration.

Hypertension

Optimum control of blood pressure is one of the most important therapeutic measures since there is a vicious cycle of events whereby hypertension causes damage to the intrarenal vasculature resulting in thickening and hyalinisation of the

---

Box 18.1 Factors that might exacerbate established chronic renal failure

Reduced renal blood flow
Hypotension
Hypertension
Nephrotoxins including drugs
Renal artery disease
Obstruction, for example, prostatic hypertrophy

---

walls of arterioles and small vessels. This damage effectively reduces renal perfusion, contributing to stimulation of the RAAS. Arteriolar vasoconstriction, sodium and water retention result, which in turn exacerbates the hypertension.

Antihypertensive therapy with certain agents might produce a transient reduction in GFR over the first 3 months of treatment as the systemic and glomerular blood pressure drop; this is mainly seen with ACE inhibitors/angiotensin receptor blockers (ARBs). However, it is possible to ultimately halt or slow the decline in many cases.

The drugs used to treat hypertension in renal disease are generally the same as those used in other forms of hypertension, although allowance must be made for the effect of renal failure on drug disposition (NICE, 2008).

Calcium channel blockers

For patients without proteinuria, calcium channel blockers (CCBs) are the agents of choice. They produce vasodilatation principally by reducing Ca^{2+} influx into vascular muscle cells. CCBs also appear to promote sodium excretion in hypertension associated with fluid overload. The mechanism is unclear but may relate to the finding that high sodium levels can cause vasoconstriction by interfering with calcium transport.

Both verapamil and diltiazem (non-dihydropyridine CCBs) block conduction across the atrioventricular node and should not be used in conjunction with β-blockers. They are also negative cardiac inotropes. By contrast, dihydropyridines such as nifedipine and amlodipine produce less cardiac depression and differentially dilate afferent arterioles in the kidney. In theory, dihydropyridines can, therefore, cause intraglomerular hypertension and glomerular damage despite decreased systemic hypertension, the relevance of this to the history of CKD is uncertain.

CCBs can produce headache, facial flushing and oedema. The latter can be confused with the symptoms of volume overload but is resistant to diuretics. The mechanism via which these effects occur is related to a change in pre-capillary hydrostatic pressure, which forces fluid into the interstitial compartment. The oedema is not related to salt or water retention; hence, the lack of response to diuretic therapy.

Angiotensin-converting enzyme inhibitors and angiotensin receptor blockers

The role of ACE inhibitors in hypertensive patients with renal insufficiency is complicated, the current evidence base supports the principle that all diabetic patients with micro/macroalbuminuria and CKD should be treated with ACE inhibitors or ARBs regardless of blood pressure. There is also evidence that in non-diabetic patients with proteinuria, the use of these drugs can reduce proteinuria and thus reduce progression of CKD. ACE inhibitors reduce circulating angiotensin II and ARBs block binding to the angiotensin II receptor, which results in vasodilatation and reduced sodium retention.

These agents can produce a reduction in GFR by preventing the angiotensin II mediated vasoconstriction of the efferent glomerular arteriole. This contributes to the high-pressure gradient across the glomerulus, which is responsible for filtration and intra-glomerular hypertension. This problem may only be important in patients with renal vascular disease, particularly those with functionally significant renal artery stenoses where they should be avoided.

ACE inhibitors and ARBs preferentially protect the glomerulus over and above their effect as systemic hypertensive agents, through decreasing efferent glomerular arteriolar vasoconstriction and therefore intra-glomerular hypertension and hyperfiltration. Whilst the evidence for use of these drugs in patients with diabetic renal disease and proteinuric non-diabetic CKD is clear, care must be exercised in the following settings:

- Patients who sustain an early decline (in the first 7–10 days after ACE inhibitors/ARBs commencement) in kidney function. The drug should be stopped and potential renal artery stenosis investigated.
- Patients with non-proteinuric, non-diabetic CKD. These agents are overused in this setting. There is no evidence that they provide a real renal benefit over other anti-hypertensive drugs.
- Patients with an accelerated decline in kidney function in the months to years after commencement of ACE inhibitors/ARBs. This is increasingly described and may reflect a resetting of the intra-renal perfusion to a level that potentiates chronic renal ischaemia present in most cases of CKD irrespective of cause.
- Patients with an intercurrent acute illness, particularly those admitted to hospital. Hypotension or infection will put patients at an increased risk of AKI.

For long-term management, it is usually preferable to use an agent with a duration of action that permits once-daily dosing. There is little to choose clinically between the ACE inhibitors currently on the market; however, consideration should be given to the cost benefits of choosing an agent that does not require dose adjustment in renal failure.

It has been reported that ACE inhibitors may reduce thirst, which may be useful in those patients who have a tendency to fluid overload as a result of excessive drinking. ACE inhibitors are potassium sparing and therefore serum potassium should be monitored carefully. A low-potassium diet may be necessary.

ARBs have properties similar to ACE inhibitors with the advantage that, since they do not inhibit the breakdown of kinins such as bradykinin, they do not cause the dry cough associated with the ACE inhibitors. There is interest in the potential use of dual blockade of the RAAS using ACE inhibitors and ARBs to produce more complete blockade of angiotensin II. However, evidence to date has shown no added benefit and some evidence of adverse renal outcomes.

The observation that patients treated with ACE inhibitors initially have lower circulating angiotensin II but then experienced a rise in angiotensin II, known as the escape phenomenon, led to the expectation that dual blockade with ACE inhibitors and ARBs would resolve this. This has not been the case in practice and other solutions to this problem have been sought. Renin is the rate-limiting enzyme of the RAAS, and it has been suggested that interruption at this stage should provide complete RAAS blockade. The direct renin inhibitors (DRIs) are a new class of antihypertensive and the early evidence suggests a greater benefit when combined with an ARB than when used as monotherapy.

Diuretics

Diuretics are of use in patients with salt and volume overload, which is usually indicated by the presence of oedema. This type of hypertension may be particularly difficult to treat. The choice of agent is generally limited to a loop diuretic. Potassium sparing diuretics are usually contraindicated owing to the risks of developing hyperkalaemia, and thiazides become ineffective as renal failure progresses. In combination with ACE inhibitors, spironolactone can significantly reduce proteinuria; however, the combination of these agents clearly raises the risk of significant hyperkalaemia and care must be taken (Bianchi et al., 2005). The combination should be avoided when the eGFR falls to <30 mL/min.

As loop diuretics need to be filtered to exert an action, progressively higher doses are required as CKD worsens. Doses of more than 250 mg/day of furosemide may be required in advanced renal failure. Patients who do not respond to oral loop diuretic therapy alone may benefit from concomitant administration of metolazone, which acts synergistically to produce a profound diuresis. Alternatively, the loop diuretic may be given intravenously. Care must be taken to avoid hypovolaemia (by monitoring body weight) and electrolyte disturbances such as hypokalaemia and hyponatraemia.

Thiazide diuretics, with the notable exception of metolazone, are ineffective at a low GFR and may accumulate, causing an increased incidence of side effects.

β-Blockers

β-Blockers are commonly used in the treatment of hypertension in CKD. They exhibit a range of actions including a reduction of renin production. Consequently, β-blockers have a particular role in the rational therapy of hypertension without fluid overload. However, β-blockers can reduce cardiac output, cause peripheral vasoconstriction and exacerbate peripheral vascular disease.

It is advisable to use the more cardioselective β-blockers atenolol or metoprolol. Atenolol is excreted renally and consequently should require dosage adjustment in renal failure. In practice, however, atenolol is effective and tolerated well by renal patients at standard doses. However, metoprolol is theoretically a better choice since it is cleared by the liver and needs no dosage adjustment, although small initial doses are advised in renal failure since there may be increased sensitivity to its hypotensive effects.

Selective α1-blockers

These vasodilators produce a variety of actions that may be of benefit in hypertension associated with CKD. Sympathetic adrenergic activity can lead to sodium retention. Selective

α_1-blockers have also been shown to produce improvements in insulin sensitivity, adverse lipid profiles and obstruction caused by hypertrophy of the prostate, all of which might be associated with some forms of CKD. These agents are used less commonly since there is some evidence that, in comparison to other antihypertensives, use is associated with adverse cardiovascular outcomes, especially the development of heart failure.

Vasodilators

The vasodilators hydralazine and minoxidil have been used to treat hypertension in CKD with varying degrees of success but are usually only used when other measures inadequately control blood pressure. The sensitivity of patients to these drugs is often increased in renal failure, so, if used, therapy should be initiated with small doses. These agents cause direct peripheral vasodilation with resultant reflex tachycardia, which may require suppression by co-prescription of a β-blocker.

Centrally acting drugs

Methyldopa and clonidine are not commonly used as antihypertensives in CKD because of their adverse side effect profiles. If they are used in renal failure, initial doses should be small because of increased sensitivity to their effects.

Spironolactone

The potassium sparing diuretic spironolactone is an aldosterone receptor antagonist, and it is through this effect that it reduces proteinuria. Studies have suggested that it may be additionally effective in combination with either an ACE inhibitor or an ARB but not as triple therapy. Care needs to be taken to avoid hyperkalaemia in patients on these regimens.

Statins

Statins are known to have beneficial effects on endothelial function, improving renal perfusion while reducing abnormal permeability to plasma proteins. However, statins are not indicated for delaying the progression of CKD but are currently used for conventional indications only in such patients.

Management of symptoms associated with CKD

Gastro-intestinal symptoms

Nausea and vomiting may persist after starting a low-protein diet. Metoclopramide is useful to treat this, but sometimes accumulation of the drug and its metabolites may occur, leading to extrapyramidal side effects. Patients should be started on a low dose, which should then be increased slowly. Prochlorperazine or cyclizine may also be useful. The 5-HT$_3$ antagonists such as ondansetron have also been shown to be effective. The anaemic patient often becomes less nauseated when treated with an erythropoiesis stimulating agent.

Constipation is a common problem in patients with renal disease, partly as a result of fluid restriction and anorexia and partly as a consequence of drug therapy with agents such as phosphate binders. It is particularly important that patients managed with peritoneal dialysis do not become constipated, as this can reduce the efficacy of dialysis. Conventional laxative therapy may be used, such as bulk-forming laxatives or increased dietary fibre for less severe constipation. Alternatively, a stimulant such as senna with enemas or glycerine suppositories may be used for severe constipation. Higher doses of senna, typically 2–4 tablets at night, may be required. It should be noted that certain brands of laxatives that contain ispaghula husk may also contain significant quantities of potassium, and should be avoided in renal failure because of the risk of hyperkalaemia. Sterculia preparations are an effective alternative.

Pruritus

Itching associated with renal failure can be extremely severe, distressing and difficult to treat. It can also be disfiguring as a result of over-enthusiastic scratching. The exact mechanism responsible for the itching is not clear and several possibilities have been suggested including: xerosis (dry skin), skin micro-precipitation of divalent ions, elevated PTH levels and increased dermal mast cell activity. Generally, however, no underlying cause is found and it is likely that a multifactorial process is responsible.

Sometimes correction of serum phosphate or calcium levels improves the condition, as does parathyroidectomy. Conventionally, oral antihistamines are used to treat pruritus; however, topical versions should not be used owing to the risk of allergy. Non-sedating antihistamines such as loratidine are generally less effective than sedating antihistamines such as chlorphenamine or alimemazine which may be useful, particularly at night. Topical crotamiton lotion and creams may also be useful in some patients. Other non-drug therapies include either warming or cooling the skin using baths, three times weekly, UVB phototherapy and modified electrical acupuncture.

Dietary modifications for uraemic symptoms

Although urea is only one of the toxins encountered in uraemia, many patients experience a symptomatic improvement when dietary protein intake is reduced, presumably through a reduction in the output of nitrogenous waste. There is some evidence that, as well as reducing the symptoms of uraemia, protein restriction slows the progression of CKD, but this remains controversial. Protein-restricted diets have been used extensively in the past but they are unpalatable and the benefits marginal, so they are used infrequently in modern medical practice.

Dietary modifications in CKD

Low protein diets have already been discussed. Other dietary modifications include sodium and fluid restriction to reduce the risk of fluid overload, potassium restriction to reduce the risk of hyperkalaemia and vitamin supplementation. The dietary restrictions for patients with CKD can be arduous and difficult to follow.

Fluid retention

Oedema may occur as a result of sodium retention and the resultant associated water retention. Patients with CKD may also have hypoalbuminaemia following renal protein loss, and this can result in an osmotic extravasation of fluid and its retention in tissues. By end stage renal disease pulmonary and peripheral oedema is best controlled with dialysis but diuretics can be useful. The daily fluid intake should be restricted to between one and three litres, depending upon the volume of urine produced by the patient (if any). It is important to note that the fluid allowance must include fluids ingested in any form, including sauces, medicines and fruits, in addition to drinks. The fluid restriction is very difficult to maintain. Sucking ice cubes may relieve an unpleasantly dry mouth, but patients should be encouraged not to swallow the melted water.

Sodium restriction. Sodium intake can be reduced to a satisfactory level of 80 mmol/day by avoiding convenience foods and snacks or the addition of salt to food at the table. This is usually tolerable to patients. It is important to be aware of the contribution of sodium-containing medication, including some antibiotics, soluble or effervescent preparations, magnesium trisilicate mixture, Gaviscon, sodium bicarbonate and the plasma expanders hetastarch and gelatin.

Potassium restriction. Hyperkalaemia often occurs in CKD and may cause life-threatening cardiac arrhythmias. If untreated, asystolic cardiac arrest and death may result. Patients are often put on a potassium-restricted diet by avoiding potassium-rich foods such as fruit and fruit drinks, vegetables, chocolate, beer, instant coffee and ice cream. Many medicines have a high potassium content, for example, potassium citrate mixture, some antibiotics and ispaghula husk sachets. The use of these drugs is less of a problem in dialysed patients. Emergency treatment is necessary if the serum potassium level is above 7.0 mmol/L or if there are ECG changes. The most effective treatment is dialysis but if this is not available other measures may be tried (see Chapter 17).

The rationale and necessity for a renal diet and fluid restriction can be difficult for a patient to understand and adherence may be a problem. Consequently, the involvement of a specialist renal dietician can be valuable in optimising dietary therapies.

Anaemia

The normochromic, normocytic anaemia of CKD does not respond to iron or folic acid unless there is a coexisting deficiency. Traditionally, the only treatment available was to give red blood cell transfusions, but this is time-consuming, expensive, an infection risk, may lead to fluid and iron overload and promotes antibody formation, which may give problems if transplantation is subsequently attempted. The introduction of ESAs, initially as recombinant human erythropoietins (epoetin alfa and beta) have transformed the management of renal anaemia. Epoetin alfa and beta were thought to be indistinguishable in practical terms, as well as being immunologically and biologically indistinguishable from physiological erythropoietin. However, it has now been recognised that epoetins can be associated with the production of anti-erythropoietin antibodies leading to a severe anaemia which is unresponsive to exogenous epoetin. This is known as pure red cell aplasia (PRCA) and is more commonly associated with epoetin alfa when given by the subcutaneous route. The subcutaneous route is preferred as it provides equally effective clinical results while using similar or smaller doses (up to 30% less) when given three times a week. Most patients report a dramatically improved quality of life after starting epoetin therapy.

Darbepoetin alfa is a novel erythropoiesis-stimulating protein (NESP) that is a recombinant hyperglycosylated analogue of epoetin which stimulates red blood cell production by the same mechanism as the endogenous hormone. The terminal half-life in man is three times longer than that of epoetin and consequently requires a once weekly or alternate weekly dosing schedule. Recently, a longer acting ESA has been introduced (methoxy polyethylene glycol-epoetin beta, pegzerepoetin alfa). This is a continuous erythropoietin receptor activator (CERA), which can be used in a once monthly dosing schedule.

Iron and folate deficiencies must be corrected before therapy is initiated, while patients receiving epoetin generally require concurrent iron supplements because of increased marrow requirements. Supplemental iron is often given intravenously owing to bioavailability problems with oral forms. Maintaining iron stores ensures the effect of epoetin is optimised for minimum cost, as with insufficient iron stores a patient will not respond to treatment with epoetin.

Epoetin therapy should aim to achieve a slow rise in the haemoglobin concentration to avoid cardiovascular side effects associated with a rapidly increasing red cell mass, such as hypertension, increased blood viscosity/volume, seizures and clotting of vascular accesses. Blood pressure should be closely monitored.

An initial subcutaneous or intravenous epoetin dose of 50 units/kg body-weight three times weekly, increased as necessary in steps of 25 units/kg every 4 weeks, should be given to produce a haemoglobin increase of not more than 2 g/dL per month. The target haemoglobin concentration is commonly 10.5–12.5 g/dL with most aiming for a target around 11.5 g/dL. Once this has been reached, a maintenance dose of epoetin in the region of 33–100 units/kg three times a week or 50–150 units/kg twice weekly should maintain this level.

There have been several studies of ESAs which have shown an increased risk of cardiovascular morbidity and overall mortality in people treated to a target >12.5 g/dL (Phrommintikul et al., 2007). This has lead to more conservative dosing strategies and prompt discontinuation or reduction of dose in patients with Hb >12.5 g/dL.

Correcting anaemia usually helps control the symptoms of lethargy and myopathy, and often greatly reduces nausea. Improved appetite on epoetin therapy can, however, increase potassium intake, and may necessitate dietary control.

Acidosis

Since the kidney is the main route for excreting H^+ ions, CKD may result in a metabolic acidosis. This will cause a reduction in serum bicarbonate that may be treated readily with oral doses of sodium bicarbonate of 1–6 g/day. As the dose of bicarbonate is not critical, it is easy to experiment with different dosage forms and strengths to suit individual patients. If acidosis is severe and persistent then dialysis may be required. Correction of acidosis may slow the decline in renal function.

Neurological problems

Neurological changes are generally caused by uraemic toxins and improve on the treatment of uraemia by dialysis or diet. Muscle cramps are common and are often treated with quinine sulphate. Restless legs may respond to low doses of clonazepam or co-careldopa.

Osteodystrophy

The osteodystrophy of renal failure is due to three factors: hyperphosphataemia, vitamin D deficiency and hyperparathyroidism.

Hyperphosphataemia

The management of hyperphosphataemia depends initially upon restricting dietary phosphate. This can be difficult to achieve effectively, even with the aid of a specialist dietician, because phosphate is found in many palatable foods such as dairy products, eggs, chocolate and nuts. Phosphate-binding agents can be used to reduce the absorption of orally ingested phosphate in the gut, by forming insoluble, non-absorbable complexes when taken a few minutes before or with meals. Traditionally, phosphate-binders were usually salts of a di- or trivalent metallic ion, such as aluminium, calcium or occasionally magnesium. Whilst calcium containing phosphate binders remain in widespread use, sevelemar and lanthanum-based binders are increasingly used.

Calcium acetate is widely used as a phosphate binder. The capacity of calcium acetate and calcium carbonate to control serum phosphate appears similar. However, phosphate control is achieved using between half and a quarter of the dose of elemental calcium when calcium acetate is used. Whether this translates to a decreased likelihood of producing unwanted hypercalcaemia with calcium acetate therapy is as yet unclear.

Calcium carbonate has been used as a phosphate binder. Unfortunately, it is less effective as a phosphate binder than aluminium, and sometimes requires doses of up to 10 g daily. Calcium carbonate has advantages, however, in that correction of concurrent hypocalcaemia can be achieved.

Sevelamer, a hydrophilic but insoluble polymeric compound is used increasingly as a phosphate binder. Sevelamer binds phosphate with an efficacy similar to calcium acetate but with no risk of hypercalcaemia. Mean levels of total and low-density cholesterol are also reduced with sevelamer use. This compound does not appear to present any risk of toxicity but may cause bowel obstruction and is relatively expensive when compared to other phosphate binders.

Lanthanum, like sevelamer, is a non-calcium containing phosphate binder; there is therefore no resultant risk of hypercalcaemia but there are gastro-intestinal side effects and the drug is significantly more expensive than the alternatives. While both of the non-calcium containing phosphate binders available have been shown to reduce phosphate levels and keep calcium within acceptable levels, no improvements in cardiovascular endpoints have been demonstrated to date.

Historically, aluminium hydroxide was widely used as a phosphate binder owing to the avid binding capacity of aluminium ions. However, a small amount of aluminium may be absorbed by patients with CKD owing to poor clearance of this ion, which can produce toxic effects including encephalopathy, osteomalacia, proximal myopathy and anaemia. Dialysis dementia was a disease observed among haemodialysis patients associated with aluminium deposition in the brain and exacerbated by aluminium in the water supply and the use of aluminium cooking pans. Desferrioxamine (4–6 g in 500 mL of saline 0.9% per week) has been used to treat this condition by removing aluminium from tissues by chelation. The tendency of aluminium to cause constipation is an added disadvantage. Therefore, aluminium as a phosphate binder in CKD should be used with caution.

Vitamin D deficiency and hyperparathyroidism

Vitamin D deficiency may be treated with the synthetic vitamin D analogues 1α-hydroxycholecalciferol (alfacalcidol) at 0.25–1 μcg/day or 1,25-dihydroxycholecalciferol (calcitriol) at 1–2 μcg/day. The serum calcium level should be monitored, and the dose of alfacalcidol or calcitriol adjusted accordingly. Hyperphosphataemia should be controlled before starting vitamin D therapy since the resulting increase in the serum calcium concentration may result in soft tissue calcification.

A new agent, paricalcitol, has recently been suggested for use in patients who either do not respond to alfacalcidol or who need doses of alfacalcidol that are impractical because of hypercalcaemia. Paricalcitol is a synthetic, biologically active vitamin D analogue that selectively upregulates the vitamin D receptor in the parathyroid glands reducing PTH synthesis and secretion. It also upregulates the calcium sensing receptor in the parathyroids and reduces PTH by inhibiting parathyroid proliferation, PTH synthesis and secretion without affecting calcium or phosphorus levels.

The rise in 1,25-dihydroxycholecalciferol and calcium levels that result from starting vitamin D therapy usually suppresses the production of PTH by the parathyroids. If vitamin D therapy does not correct PTH levels then parathyroidectomy, to remove part or most of the parathyroid glands, may be needed. This surgical procedure was once commonly performed on CKD patients, but is now less frequent owing to effective vitamin D supplementation.

Cinacalcet is a calcimimetic which increases the sensitivity of calcium sensing receptors to extracellular calcium ion, this results in reduced PTH production. The benefit of this treatment is the suppression of PTH without resultant hypercalcaemia. It is recommended (NICE, 2007) for use as an alternative to parathyroidectomy for patients who are not fit enough to undergo this procedure. Common therapeutic problems in chronic renal failure are summarised in Table 18.4.

Renal transplantation

Renal transplantation has transformed the outlook for many patients with end stage renal disease. The clinical outcomes of renal transplantation are now excellent. One-year patient and graft survival is 98% and 90–95%, respectively, and most patients who receive a transplant will never need to return to dialysis treatment. A renal transplant performed today in the developed world will continue to function, on average, in excess of 15 years. However, an important consider-

ation is that renal transplantation is the treatment of choice for patients with end stage renal disease who are fit to receive a renal transplant; this recognises that many patients in end stage renal disease are frail and elderly and/or have a number of co-existing medical problems such that they are not fit to undergo a major operation (implantation of the kidney) or to tolerate the immunosuppressive drugs that are required to prevent the transplant rejecting. This means that at any given time the majority of patients are not actually on a national waiting list for a renal transplant.

For those patients who are fit enough to receive a renal transplant and are successfully transplanted, there is a profound survival benefit compared to remaining on dialysis treatment. The average transplant recipient lives two or three times as long as a matched dialysis patients who does not receive a renal transplant but remains on dialysis treatment. In addition, a transplant patient is less likely to be hospitalised and has a better quality of life than a dialysis patient. The secondary complications of CKD such as anaemia and bone disease resolve in many patients who are successfully transplanted. Furthermore, there are major health economic benefits to renal transplantation compared to dialysis. Transplantation is a far less expensive treatment than dialysis, particularly after the first year, when the large majority of the costs are limited to payment for the immunosuppressive drugs.

One of the major challenges for renal transplantation is the identification of a sufficient number of donor kidneys to fulfil demand. This is reflected in the increasing number

Table 18.4 Common therapeutic problems in chronic renal failure

Problem	Comment
Drug choice	Care with choice/dose of all drugs. Care to avoid renotoxic agents pre-dialysis to preserve function. Beware herbal therapies as some contain immune system boosters (reverse immunosuppressant effects) and some are nephrotoxic
Drug excretion	CKD will lead to accumulation of drugs and their active metabolites if they are normally excreted by the kidney
Dietary restrictions	Restrictions on patient often severe. Fluid allowance includes foods with high water content, for example, gravy, custard, and fruit
Hypertension	Frequently requires complex multiple drug regimens. CCBs can cause oedema that might be confused with fluid overload
Analgesia	Side-effects are increased. Initiate with low doses and gradually increase. Avoid pethidine as metabolites accumulate. Avoid NSAIDs unless specialist advice available
Anaemia	Epoetin requires sufficient iron stores to be effective. Absorption from oral iron supplements may be poor and i.v. iron supplementation might be required. Care required to make sure that epoetin use does not produce hypertension
Immunosuppression	Use of live vaccines should be avoided (BCG, MMR, mumps, oral polio, oral typhoid, smallpox, yellow fever)
Pruritis (itching)	Can be severe. Treat with chlorphenamine; less sedating antihistamines often less effective. Some relief with topical agents, for example, crotamiton
Restless legs	Involuntary jerks can prevent sleep. Clonazepam 0.5–1 mg at night may help

of people who are waiting for a kidney; in the UK the average time on the waiting list before transplantation is around 3 years. Kidneys donated for the national waiting list are harvested from deceased donors. At the time of donation, donors are classified as dead as a consequence of either brain stem or cardiac death; these are also called heart beating and non-heart beating donors, respectively.

The numbers of deceased donors as a proportion of those on the waiting list for a kidney transplant have fallen. Therefore, living donor transplantation has become increasingly common. In addition to part addressing the scarcity of donor organs, patients who receive kidney transplants from living donors have better outcomes than patients who receive deceased donor kidneys. This is due to a number of factors, including the quality of the organs, because living donors undergo a detailed health screening and if there is any indication that they have significant medical problems they are excluded from donation.

One of the major factors responsible for excellent outcomes for kidney transplant recipients is the use of immunosuppressive drugs to control the response the immune system of the recipient mounts against the donor kidney. This is called an alloresponse. Alloimmunity refers to an immune response against tissue derived from an individual of the same species as the recipient of the tissue.

The major disadvantage of all immunosuppressive agents is their relative non-specificity, in that they cause a general depression of the immune system. This exposes the patient to an increased risk of malignancy and infection, which is an important cause of morbidity and mortality.

Immunosuppressants

The major pharmacological groups of immunosuppressive agents are summarised in Table 18.5.

Transplant recipients receive a high load of immunosuppression at the time of transplantation; this is known as induction immunosuppression. Induction immunosuppression is to protect the transplant from the high immunological risk that is present in the first few weeks after surgery. In the months following the transplant, the immunosuppression load is then incrementally reduced. Most patients will reach long-term low dose maintenance immunosuppression sometime between 6 and 12 months after the transplant. However, whilst the transplant remains in the recipient it continues to represent an immunological risk; whilst overt,

Table 18.5 Mechanism of action of immunosuppressants commonly used following renal transplantation

Drug	Mechanism	Comment
Steroids	Bind to steroid receptors and inhibit gene transcription and function of T-cells, macrophages and neutrophils	Prophylaxis against and reversal of rejection
Ciclosporin	Forms complex with intracellular protein cyclophilin → inhibits calcineurin. Ultimately inhibits interleukin-2 synthesis and T-cell activation	Long-term maintenance therapy against rejection
Tacrolimus	Forms complex with an intracellular protein → inhibits calcineurin	Long-term maintenance therapy against rejection Rescue therapy in severe or refractory rejection
Sirolimus	Inhibits interleukin-2 cell signalling → blocks T-cell cycling and inhibits B-cells	Usually used in combination with ciclosporin ± steroids
Mycophenolate	Inhibits inosine monophosphate dehydrogenase → reduces nucleic acid synthesis → inhibits T- and B-cell function	Usually used in combination with ciclosporin/tacrolimus ± steroids
Azathioprine	Incorporated as a purine in DNA → inhibits lymphocyte and neutrophil proliferation	Usually used in combination with ciclosporin/tacrolimus ± steroids
Muromonab (OKT3, mouse monoclonal anti-CD3)	Binds to CD3 complex → blocks, inactivates or kills T-cell. Short $t_{1/2}$	Prophylaxis against rejection Reversal of severe rejection
Polyclonal horse/rabbit antithymocyte or antilymphocyte globulin (ATG, ALG)	Antibodies against lymphocyte proteins → alter T- and B-cell activity	Prophylaxis against rejection Reversal of severe rejection
Humanised or chimaeric anti-CD25 (basiliximab and daclizumab)	Monoclonal antibodies that bind CD25 in interleukin-2 complex → prevent T-cell proliferation	Prophylaxis against acute rejection in combination with ciclosporin and steroids

late rejection is uncommon, it can occur at any time if the patient stops taking their immunosuppressants. For a transplant to last many years, sustained day on day adherence with treatment is essential.

The commonest combination used at induction is the calcineurin inhibitor (CNI) tacrolimus, the anti-proliferative agent mycophenolate mofetil (MMF) and corticosteroids. Most patients also receive antibody induction. The antibody that is most commonly used is a monoclonal anti-CD25 antibody for people at low or medium immunological risk and anti-T-cell polyclonal antibodies (thymoglobulin or ATG) for people at high immunological risk. Patients at high immunological risk include: those who have lost a previous transplant because of rejection; the presence of preformed circulating anti-HLA antibodies at the time of transplantation (sensitisation); and major HLA mismatches (particularly at HLA-DR) between donor and recipient. Guidelines for the use of immunosuppressive therapy in kidney transplant patients have been issued (NICE, 2004). More recent international consensus guidelines recommend use of newer agents such as MMF and emphasise the use of tacrolimus (rather than ciclosporin) as the CNI of choice. Tacrolimus is associated with less acute rejection than ciclosporin and may be associated with better graft function at one year and less graft loss (Knoll and Bell, 1999). However, there is no overwhelming evidence as yet that patients who receive tacrolimus as a CNI from induction have a survival benefit compared to patients who receive ciclosporin. It should be noted that generic/proprietary formulations of some drugs (e.g. tacrolimus and ciclosporin) are not interchangeable.

Calcineurin inhibitors (ciclosporin and tacrolimus)

The discovery and development of ciclosporin and latterly tacrolimus has led to a step improvement in one-year renal transplant survival from 50–70% to 85–95%.

In T-cells that have been exposed to T-cell receptor (TCR) ligation (signal 1) and co-stimulation (signal 2), there is activation of intra-cytoplasmic signalling pathways that include mobilisation of a molecule called calcineurin. Calcineurin contributes to the activation of a molecule called nuclear factor of activated T-cells (NFAT). This factor then migrates to the nucleus and initiates transcription of IL-2 and other pro-inflammatory cytokines which are involved in driving an activated T-cell into a proliferative phase, so that it makes multiple copies of itself. Ciclosporin and tacrolimus affect calcineurin through blocking binding proteins (cyclophilin and tacrolimus-binding protein, respectively) that are important for calcineurin activity.

The action of CNIs is partially selective in that they predominantly target T-cells and have no direct effect on B cells; as a consequence, CNIs are associated with infections seen in people with deficiencies in the cellular limb of the immune response. These are predominantly intracellular infections such as viral, fungal, protozoal and mycobacterial infections.

Both ciclosporin and tacrolimus are critical dose drugs. That is, there is a narrow therapeutic window between underdosing and toxicity. Both drugs, therefore, require monitoring by serum levels. Trough levels are usually taken 12 h after the previous dose and immediately before the next dose.

Ciclosporin

Ciclosporin causes a wide range of side effects, including nephrotoxicity, hypertension, fine muscle tremor, gingival hyperplasia, nausea and hirsutism. Hyperkalaemia, hyperuricaemia, hypomagnesaemia and hypercholestraemia may also occur. Nephrotoxicity is a particularly serious side effect and occasionally necessitates the withdrawal of ciclosporin. There is tremendous inter- and intra-patient variation in absorption of ciclosporin. Blood level monitoring is required to achieve maximum protection against rejection and minimise the risk of side effects. The range regarded as acceptable varies between centres, but is commonly around 100–200 ng/mL in the first 6 months after transplantation and 80–150 ng/mL from 6 months onwards.

Ciclosporin interacts with a number of drugs that either lead to a reduction in ciclosporin levels, increase the risk of rejection or cause an elevation in ciclosporin levels leading to increased toxicity. Some drugs enhance the nephrotoxicity of ciclosporin (Box 18.2).

Ciclosporin should not be administered with grapefruit juice, which should also be avoided for at least an hour pre-dose, as this can result in marked increases in blood concentrations. This effect appears to be due to inhibition of enzyme systems in the gut wall resulting in transiently reduced ciclosporin metabolism.

Tacrolimus

Tacrolimus is not chemically related to ciclosporin, but acts by a similar mechanism. The side effect profile is similar to that of ciclosporin with some subtle differences. Disturbances of glucose metabolism leading to impaired glucose tolerance and new onset diabetes after transplantation (NODAT) occurs in around 10–15% of patients who receive tacrolimus, this is twice as common as the incidence seen in patients who receive ciclosporin. In contrast, hirsutism is less of a problem in patients who receive tacrolimus than those who receive ciclosporin. In patients who are commenced on ciclosporin and then develop an episode of acute rejection, conversion to tacrolimus lowers the risk of recurrent rejection. Tacrolimus is an easier drug to use than ciclosporin. Careful monitoring is required with a target level of 8–15 ng/mL in the first weeks following transplantation which is usually decreased in patients who follow an uncomplicated course to 5–8 ng/mL from 6 months.

Box 18.2 Examples of drug interactions involving ciclosporin

- Reduce ciclosporin serum levels (hepatic enzyme inducers): phenytoin, phenobarbital, rifampicin, isoniazid
- Increase ciclosporin serum levels (hepatic enzyme inhibitors): diltiazem, erythromycin, corticosteroids, ketoconazole
- Enhance ciclosporin nephrotoxicity: aminoglycosides, amphotericin, co-trimoxazole, melphalan

Steroids

Prednisolone is the oral agent commonly used for immunosuppression after renal transplantation, while high-dose intravenous methylprednisolone is given as a single dose at induction with further use limited for cases of acute rejection. The maintenance dose of prednisolone to minimise adrenal suppression is around 0.1 mg/kg/day given as a single dose in the morning. The use of steroid therapy often leads to complications, particularly if high doses are given for long periods. In addition to a cushingoid state, the use of steroids may cause gastro-intestinal bleeding, hypertension, dyslipidaemia, diabetes, osteoporosis and mental disturbances. Patients who are temporarily unable to take oral prednisolone should be given an equivalent dose of hydrocortisone intravenously.

In the past decade, there has been an increasing use of steroid avoidance regimens. This term is misleading as patients still receive steroids, but use is restricted to the first week of transplantation. Currently, there is no long-term evidence to show this approach provides equivalence to a continuous steroid dosing regimen, but one-year outcomes are comparable. If steroids are subsequently withdrawn months after the transplant, then outcomes with steroid avoidance regimens are worse.

Azathioprine

Azathioprine is derived from 6-mercaptopurine and is, therefore, an antimetabolite which reduces DNA and RNA synthesis-producing immunosuppression.

Azathioprine is given orally in a dose of up to 2 mg/kg/day. There is no advantage in giving it in divided doses. Since azathioprine interferes with nucleic acid synthesis, it may be mutagenic, and pharmacy and nursing staff should avoid handling the tablets. Azathioprine has a significant drug interaction with allopurinol, causing fatal marrow suppression and this combination should be avoided.

Mycophenolate mofetil (MMF)

MMF is a pro-drug of mycophenolic acid. It inhibits the enzyme inosine monophosphate dehydrogenase needed for guanosine synthesis which leads to reduced B-cell and T-cell proliferation. However, other rapidly dividing cells are less affected, as guanosine is produced in other cells. Consequently, mycophenolate has a more selective mode of action than azathioprine.

The drug is given in combination with tacrolimus at a dose of 1 g twice a day which can subsequently be reduced after 6 weeks to 750 mg twice a day. A dose of 1.5 g twice a day is prescribed when used in combination with ciclosporin because the ciclosporin interferes with enterohepatic recirculation of mycophenolate metabolites with consequent lower exposure at a similar dose.

Compared to azathioprine, MMF reduces the risk of acute rejection episodes and improves long-term graft survival. However, it is a more potent immunosuppressant than azathioprine and is associated with a significant increased risk of opportunistic infections.

Sirolimus (rapamycin)

Sirolimus is a macrolide antibiotic that binds to the FKBP-25 cellular receptor. This complex initiates a sequence that produces modulation of regulatory kinases that ultimately interfere with the proliferative effects of IL-2 on lymphocytes. The progression of T-cells from the G1 to S phase is blocked, so inhibiting cell division and therefore cell proliferation.

Adverse effects include hyperkalemia, hypomagnesemia, hyperlipidemia, hypertriglyceridemia, leukopenia, anemia, imp-aired wound healing, and joint pain. Currently, the role of sirolimus in renal transplantation has not been clearly defined. In combination with CNIs, it produces additive nephrotoxicity; when used with MMF it increases the risk of marrow suppression and mucosal side effects. Most experts currently limit the use of sirolimus to patients who have declining kidney function as a consequence of CNIs, but where graft function is still maintained to a GFR of >40 mL/min without significant proteinuria.

Monoclonal antibodies

The humanised or chimeric anti-CD25 monoclonal antibodies basiliximab and daclizumab are clinically similar and bind to CD25 in the IL-2 complex of activated T-lymphocytes. This renders all T-cells resistant to IL-2 and therefore prevents T-cell proliferation. They are used as prophylaxis against acute rejection in combination with CNIs and steroids (NICE, 2004). Daclizumab is currently not available in the UK.

Polyclonal antibodies

These were the first antibodies used as immunosuppressants and contain antibodies with a number of different antigen-combining sites. Polyclonal antibodies are used peri-operatively as prophylaxis against rejection and in some cases to reverse episodes of severe rejection. The main preparations are antithymocyte globulin (ATG) or antilymphocyte globulin (ALG).

ATG is produced from rabbit or equine serum immunised with human T-cells. It contains antibodies to human T-cells, which on injection will attach to, neutralise and eliminate most T-cells, thereby weakening the immune response. ALG is similar to ATG, is of equine origin, but is not specific to T-cells as it also acts on B-cells.

It is not certain how polyclonal antibodies act to inhibit T-cell mediated immune responses but depletion of circulating T-cells, modulation of cell surface receptor molecules, induction of energy and apoptosis of activated T-cells have all been proposed.

The main drawback to the use of anti-T-cell sera is the relatively high incidence of side effects, notably anaphylactic reactions including hypotension, fever and urticaria. These reactions are more frequently observed with the first dose and may require supportive therapy with steroids and antihistamines. Severe reactions may necessitate stopping treatment. Steroids and antihistamines may be given prophylactically to prevent or minimise allergic reactions. Pyrexia often occurs on the first day of treatment but usually subsides without requiring treatment. Tolerance testing by administration of a test dose is advisable, particularly in patients such as asthmatics who commonly experience allergic reactions. In the event of adverse reactions, ALG and ATG can be substituted for each other.

Other precautions

Transplant patients are given prophylactic antibiotic therapy for varying periods postoperatively owing to the risks of infection associated with immunosuppression. Treatment with co-trimoxazole to prevent *Pneumocystis carinii*, isoniazid and pyridoxine in high-risk patients to prevent tuberculosis, valganciclovir to prevent cytomegalovirus, and nystatin or amphotericin to prevent oral candidiasis are commonly used. Vaccination with live organisms (e.g. BCG, MMR, oral poliomyelitis, oral typhoid) must be avoided in the immunosuppressed patient.

Implementation of regular dialysis treatment

End stage renal failure is the point at which the patient will die without the institution of renal replacement by dialysis or transplantation.

The principle of dialysis is simple. The patient's blood and a dialysis solution are positioned on opposing sides of a semi-permeable membrane across which exchange of metabolites occurs. The two main types of dialysis used in CKD are haemodialysis and peritoneal dialysis. Neither has been shown to be superior to the other in any particular group of patients and so the personal preference of the patient is important when selecting dialysis modality. Haemodialysis and acute peritoneal dialysis are discussed in Chapter 17.

As patients with end stage renal failure may require dialysis treatment for many years, adaptations to the process of peritoneal dialysis have been made that enable the patient to follow a lifestyle as near normal as possible. Continuous ambulatory peritoneal dialysis (CAPD) involves a flexible non-irritant silicone rubber catheter (Tenckhoff catheter) that is surgically inserted into the abdominal cavity. Dacron cuffs on the body of the catheter become infiltrated with scar tissue during the healing process, causing the catheter to be firmly anchored in place. Such catheters may remain viable for many years. During the dialysis process thereafter, a bag typically containing 2.5 L of warmed dialysate and a drainage bag are connected to the catheter using aseptic techniques. Used dialysate is drained from the abdomen under gravity into the drainage bag, fresh dialysate is run into the peritoneal cavity and the giving set is disconnected. The patient continues his or her activities until the next exchange some hours later. The procedure is repeated regularly so that dialysate is kept in the abdomen 24 h a day. This is usually achieved by repeating the process four times a day with an average dwell time of 6–8 h. A number of different dialysis solutions are available of which the majority are glucose based.

Another form of peritoneal dialysis is known as automated peritoneal dialysis (APD) in which exchanges are carried out overnight while the patient sleeps. Dialysis fluid is exchanged – three to five times over a 10-h period with volumes of 1.5–3 L each time. During the day time the patient usually has a dwell of fluid within the abdominal cavity.

Since peritoneal dialysis is continuous and corrects fluid and electrolyte levels constantly, dietary and fluid restrictions are less stringent. Blood loss is also avoided, making the technique safer in anaemic patients. Unfortunately, peritoneal dialysis is not an efficient process; it only just manages to facilitate excretion of the substances required and, as albumin crosses the peritoneal membrane, up to 10 g of protein a day may be lost in the dialysate. It is also uncomfortable and tiring for the patient, and is contraindicated in patients who have recently undergone abdominal surgery.

Peritonitis is the most frequently encountered complication of peritoneal dialysis. Its diagnosis usually depends on a combination of abdominal pain, cloudy dialysate or positive microbiological culture. Empirical antibiotic therapy should, therefore, be commenced as soon as peritonitis is clinically diagnosed. Gram-positive cocci (particularly *Staphylococcus aureus*) and Enterobacteriaceae are the causative organisms in the majority of cases, while infection with Gram-negative species and *Pseudomonas* species are well recognised. Fungal infections are also seen, albeit less commonly.

Most centres have their own local protocol for antibiotic treatment of peritonitis. In one example, levofloxacin, a quinolone with good Gram-negative activity is given orally, in combination with vancomycin, which has excellent activity against Gram-positive bacteria, is administered via the intraperitoneal route. As in all situations, the antibiotic regimen should be adjusted appropriately after the results of microbiological culture and sensitivity have been obtained.

Haemodialysis is particularly suitable for patients producing large amounts of metabolites, such as those with high nutritional demands or a large muscle mass, where these substances are produced faster than peritoneal dialysis can remove them. It also provides a back-up for those patients in whom peritoneal dialysis has failed.

The various techniques of haemofiltration, a technique related to haemodialysis, are also discussed in detail in Chapter 17.

Case studies

Case 18.1

Mr D, a 19-year-old undergraduate student, visited his university health centre complaining of a 3-month history of fatigue, weakness, nausea and vomiting that he had attributed to 'examination stress'. His previous medical history indicated an ongoing history of bed wetting from an early age. Laboratory results from a routine blood screen showed the following:

		Reference range
Sodium	137 mmol/L	(135–145)
Potassium	4.8 mmol/L	(3.5–5.0)
Phosphate	2.5 mmol/L	(0.9–1.5)
Calcium	1.6 mmol/L	(2.20–2.55)
Urea	52 mmol/L	(3.0–6.5)
Creatinine	620 µmol/L	(50–120)
Haemoglobin	7.5 g/dL	(13.5–18.0)

Subsequent referral to a specialist hospital centre established a diagnosis of chronic renal failure secondary to reflux nephropathy.

Question

Explain the signs and symptoms experienced by Mr D and the likely course of his disease?

Answer

Mr D is suffering from the signs and symptoms of uraemia resulting from chronic renal failure. Mechanical reflux damage to his kidneys has compromised renal function and resulted in an accumulation of toxins, including urea and creatinine that, in turn, have contributed to his nausea, vomiting and general malaise. His biochemical results indicate other features typical of uraemic syndrome associated with chronic renal failure. The low haemoglobin is indicative of reduced erythropoetin production following progressive kidney damage. Renal osteodystrophy is also present, as inadequate vitamin D production and the raised serum phosphate have contributed to the hypocalaemia.

This patient is likely to have remained symptom free for a period of years despite progressively worsening renal function. The kidneys operate with a substantial functional reserve under normal conditions. Patients generally remain asymptomatic as their renal reserve diminishes. Eventually there is a failure in the ability of the damaged kidney to compensate and symptoms appear late in the condition.

Case 18.2

Mr K, a 43-year-old male with established CKD, had been maintained for 3 years on continuous ambulatory peritoneal dialysis. He was admitted to hospital for cadaveric renal transplantation. On examination he was found to have slight ankle oedema. He weighed 60 kg and his blood pressure was 135/90 mmHg and pulse rate 77 min^{-1}. He was administered the following immunosuppressants preoperatively: an anti-CD25 antibody, tacrolimus, mycophenolate and prednisolone.

Question

How should the immunosuppressants be administered to Mr K and how should immunosuppression be managed postoperatively?

Answer

Anti-CD25 antibodies and high-dose methylprednisolone are given intravenously at the time of the operation. Typically, tacrolimus at 200–300 μcg/kg/day as two split doses, it is important to note that there are two preparations of tacrolimus, a once daily dose and a divided dose preparation. The once daily preparation is called Advagraf® and the twice daily preparation is Prograf®, the preparations are not interchangeable and as a result they must be prescribed by brand name, changes between preparations must only be made by a transplant specialist. MMF at 1 g twice a day and prednisolone at 10 mg twice a day are given as oral doses to continue in the days and weeks following transplantation. These are commenced within 12 h of the operation. In living kidney donation where the transplant operation is planned, patients are preloaded for several days before the transplant. Intravenous tacrolimus is available, but should only be used in exceptional circumstances, usually when the gut is not working and all drugs and nutrition need to be given by the parenteral route.

Early dose adjustments in tacrolimus following transplantation are common and directed by drug levels. These are checked daily for the first week following transplantation; by 6 months they will be checked on alternate weeks. In the long-term, the median dose of tacrolimus is around 2 mg twice a day and the dose of MMF can be reduced to 500–750 mg twice a day in the large majority of patients. The dose of prednisolone is titrated down so that by 3 months it is 5–10 mg/day. Acute rejection episodes, diagnosed on a renal biopsy performed for a decline in graft function are treated with high-dose steroids. For antibody mediated (severe) rejection, plasma exchange and intravenous immunoglobulin are used.

Case 18.3

Mr A is a patient with CKD secondary to chronic interstitial nephritis. He complains of chronic fatigue, lethargy and breathlessness on exertion, palpitations and poor concentration. His recent haematological results were found to be:

		Reference range
Haemoglobin	5.6 g/dL	(13.5–17.5)
Red cell count	$2.92 \times 10^9 \ L^{-1}$	$(4.5–6.5 \times 10^9 \ L^{-1})$
Haematocrit	0.208	(0.40–0.54)
Serum ferritin	88.0 μcg/L	(15–300)

Question

Explain Mr A's symptoms and haematological results and outline the optimal treatment.

Answer

Mr A's symptoms are most likely to result from a normochromic, normocytic anaemia caused by renal failure. Levels of erythropoetin produced by the kidney are reduced in renal failure. Production of erythropoetin from extrarenal sites, for example, liver, are not sufficient to maintain erythropoesis, which is also inhibited by uraemic toxins and hyperparathyroidism. The anaemia associated with renal failure is further compounded by a reduction in red cell survival through low-grade haemolysis, bleeding from the gastro-intestinal tract and blood loss through dialysis, aluminum toxicity which interferes with haem synthesis, and iron deficiency, usually through poor dietary intake.

Therapy with epoetin is the treatment of choice. However, iron and folate deficiencies should be corrected if epoetin therapy is to be successful. Iron demands are generally raised during epoetin treatment and iron status should be regularly monitored. If serum ferritin falls below 100 μcg/L then iron supplementation should be started. Often intravenous iron is required to provide an adequate supply, despite the dangers associated with administration of iron by this route.

References

Bianchi, S., Bigazzi, R., Campese, V.M., 2005. Antagonists of aldosterone and proteinuria in patients with chronic kidney disease: a controlled pilot study. Am. J. Kidney Dis. 46, 45–51.

Cockroft, D., Gault, M., 1976. Predication of creatinine clearance from serum creatinine. Nephron 16, 31–34.

Counahan, R. Chantler, C., Ghazali, S., et al., 1976. Estimation of glomerular filtration from plasma creatinine concentration in children. Arch. Dis. Child 51, 875–878.

Knoll, G.A., Bell, R.C., 1999. Tacrolimus versus ciclosporin for immunosuppression in renal transplant: meta-analysis of randomized trials. Br. Med. J. 318, 1104–1107.

Lerman, L., Textor, S.C., 2001. Pathophysiology of ischaemic nephropathy. Urol. Clin. North Am. 28, 793–803.

Levey, A.S., Bosch, J.P., Lewis, J.B., et al., 1999. A more accurate method to estimate glomerular function rate from serum creatinine: a new prediction equation. Ann. Intern. Med. 130, 461–470.

National Institute for Health and Clinical Excellence, 2004. Immunosuppressive Therapy for Renal Transplantation in Adults. Technology Appraisal 85. NICE, London. Available at: http://guidance.nice.org.uk/TA85.

National Institute for Health and Clinical Excellence, 2007. Cinacalcet for the Treatment of Secondary Hyperparathyroidism in Patients with End Stage Renal Disease on Maintenance Dialysis Therapy. Technology Appraisal 117. NICE, London. Available at: http://guidance.nice.org.uk/TA117/Guidance/doc/English.

National Institute for Health and Clinical Excellence, 2008. Chronic Kidney Disease: Early Identification and Management of Chronic Kidney Disease in Adults in Primary and Secondary Care. Clinical Guideline 73. NICE, London. Available at: http://www.nice.org.uk/nicemedia/pdf/CG073NICEGuideline.pdf.

Phrommintikul A., Haas, S.J., Elsik, M., et al., 2007. Mortality and target haemoglobin concentrations in anaemic patients with chronic kidney disease treated with erythropoietin: a meta-analysis. Lancet 369, 381–388.

Schwartz, G.J., 1985. A simple estimate of glomerular filtration rate in adolescent boys. J. Pediatr. 106, 522–526.

UK Renal Registry, 2008. The 11th Annual Report. Renal Association, Bristol.

Further reading

Daugirdas, J.T., Blake, P.G., Ing, S.T., 2007. Handbook of Dialysis, fourth ed. Lippincott Williams & Wilkins, Philadelphia.

Feehally, J., Floege, J., Johnson, R.J., 2007. Comprehensive Clinical Nephrology, third ed. Mosby, London.

Go, A.S., Chertow, G.M., Fan, D., et al., 2004. Chronic kidney disease and the risks of death, cardiovascular events and hospitalisation. N. Engl. J. Med. 351, 1296–1305.

Steddon, S., Ashman, N., Chesser, A., et al., 2007. Oxford Handbook of Nephrology and Hypertension, Oxford University Press, Oxford.

The ONTARGET investigators, 2008. Telmisartan, ramipril, or both in patients at high risk of vascular events. N. Engl. J. Med. 358, 1547–1559.

Hypertension 19

A. G. Dyker

Key points

- Hypertension can be defined as a condition in which blood pressure is elevated to an extent where benefit is obtained from blood pressure lowering. There is no clear-cut blood pressure threshold separating normal from hypertensive individuals. The risk of complications is related to the levels that blood pressure is elevated.
- The World Health Organization has identified hypertension as one of the most important preventable causes of premature morbidity and mortality.
- Hypertension should not be seen as a risk factor in isolation and decisions on management should not focus on blood pressure alone but on total cardiovascular risk.
- The complications of hypertension include stroke, myocardial infarction, heart failure, renal failure and dissecting aortic aneurysm.
- Modest reductions in blood pressure result in substantial reductions in the relative risks of these complications.
- For correct diagnosis, careful measurement of blood pressure is necessary on several occasions using well-maintained and validated equipment.
- Non-pharmacological interventions are important and include weight reduction, avoidance of excessive salt and alcohol, increased intake of fruit and vegetables and regular aerobic exercise. Other cardiovascular risk factors such as smoking, dyslipidaemia and diabetes should be addressed.
- A large selection of antihypertensive drugs is available. It is important to use drugs that minimise patient side effects.
- The most appropriate choice of initial drug therapy depends on the age and racial origin of the patient, as well as the presence of other medical conditions. For younger white patients, an ACE inhibitor is recommended as first-line treatment. For older patients and black people, a calcium channel blocker or thiazide diuretic is an appropriate initial choice.
- Many people need combinations of drugs to achieve adequate blood pressure control. Medication should be convenient to take and adverse effects should be avoided.

Hypertension (high blood pressure) is an important risk factor for the future development of cardiovascular disease. It can be defined as a condition where blood pressure is elevated to an extent that clinical benefit is obtained from blood pressure lowering. Blood pressure measurement includes systolic and diastolic components, and both are important in determining an individual's cardiovascular risk.

Blood pressure is continuously distributed in the population and there is no clear cut-off point between hypertensive and normotensive subjects, although a figure of systolic/diastolic blood pressure of 140/90 mmHg is considered the upper limit of 'normal'. Such values that are used as treatment thresholds or targets are, however, largely arbitrary. Treatment decisions in milder hypertensive subjects should now be made on the basis of patients' overall future risk of vascular disease. There is, however, considerable evidence from clinical trials to demonstrate that treatment of subjects with blood pressures above the threshold currently used in clinical practice results in important clinical benefits. Hypertension is largely a condition of older individuals. While diastolic pressure peaks at age 50, systolic pressure continues to increase with advancing age, making isolated systolic hypertension a common feature of old age. Generally, the risk of cardiovascular disease doubles for every 20/10 mmHg rise in blood pressure.

The cardiovascular complications associated with hypertension are shown in Box 19.1. The most common and important of these are stroke and myocardial infarction. An increase of 5 mmHg in usual diastolic blood pressure is associated with a 35–40% increased risk of stroke. There is a similar but less steep association for coronary heart disease risk. The risk of heart failure is increased six-fold in hypertensive subjects. Meta-analysis of clinical trials has indicated that these risks are reversible with relatively modest reductions in blood pressure of 10/6 mmHg associated with a 38% reduction in stroke and 16% reduction in coronary events (Collins et al., 1990), while a 5 mmHg reduction in blood pressure is associated with a 25% reduction in risk of renal failure.

The absolute benefits of blood pressure lowering achieved as a result of these relative risk reductions depend on the underlying level of risk in an individual. High-risk subjects

---

Box 19.1 Complications of hypertension

- Myocardial infarction
- Stroke
  - Cerebral/brainstem infarction
  - Cerebral haemorrhage
  - Lacunar syndromes
  - Multi-infarct disease
- Hypertensive encephalopathy/malignant hypertension
- Dissecting aortic aneurysm
- Hypertensive nephrosclerosis
- Peripheral vascular disease

295

gain more benefit in terms of events saved per year of therapy. Absolute risk is highest in those who already have evidence of cardiovascular disease, such as previous myocardial infarction, transient ischaemic attack or stroke, or who have other evidence of cardiovascular dysfunction such as electrocardiogram (ECG) or echocardiograph abnormality. Risk is also increased in the elderly and in people with diabetes or renal failure and is further enhanced by other risk factors such as smoking, dyslipidaemia, obesity and sedentary lifestyle. In those under the age of 75, men are at greater risk than women. Cardiovascular risk in an individual who has no current cardiovascular disease can be estimated from coronary risk prediction charts (Joint British Societies, 2005; see Chapter 24).

Epidemiology

Between 10% and 25% of the population are expected to benefit from drug treatment of hypertension; the exact figure depending on the cut-off value for blood pressure and the age group considered for active treatment.

In 90–95% of cases of hypertension, there is no underlying medical illness to cause high blood pressure. This is termed 'essential' hypertension, so named because at one time it was erroneously believed to be an 'essential' compensation mechanism to maintain adequate circulation. The precise aetiology of essential hypertension is currently unknown. Genetic factors clearly play a part as the condition clusters in families, with hypertension being twice as common in subjects who have a hypertensive parent. Genetic factors account for about one-third of the blood pressure variation between individuals, although no single gene appears to be responsible except in some rare conditions such as polycystic kidney disease and other metabolic conditions such as Liddle's syndrome (Beevers et al., 2001). The remaining 5–10% of cases are secondary to some other disease process (Box 19.2).

Box 19.2 Causes of hypertension

Primary hypertension (90–95%)
- Essential hypertension

Secondary hypertension (5–10%)
- Renal diseases
- Endocrine diseases
  - *Steroid excess*: hyperaldosteronism (Conn's syndrome); hyperglucocorticoidism (Cushing's syndrome)
  - *Growth hormone excess*: acromegaly
  - *Catecholamine excess*: phaeochromocytoma
  - *Others*: pre-eclampsia
- Vascular causes
  - *Renal artery stenosis*: fibromuscular hyperplasia; renal artery atheroma; coarctation of the aorta
- Drugs
  - Sympathomimetic amines
  - Oestrogens (e.g. combined oral contraceptive pills)
  - Ciclosporin
  - Erythropoietin
  - NSAIDs
  - Steroids

Hypertension is more common in black people of African Caribbean origin, who are also at particular risk of stroke and renal failure. Hypertension is exacerbated by other factors, for example, high salt or alcohol intake or obesity.

Regulation of blood pressure

The mean blood pressure is the product of cardiac output and total peripheral resistance. In most hypertensive individuals, cardiac output is not increased and high blood pressure arises as a result of increased total peripheral resistance caused by constriction of small arterioles.

Control of blood pressure is important in evolutionary terms and a number of homeostatic reflexes have evolved to provide blood pressure homeostasis. Minute-to-minute changes in blood pressure are regulated by the baroreceptor reflex, while the renin–angiotensin–aldosterone system is important for longer term salt, water and blood pressure control. Long-term increases in shear stress can cause vascular remodelling of the endothelium which lead to the formation of a procoagulant rather than anticoagulant surface. At the same time, systems that lead to vascular relaxation, for example nitric oxide, are overcome by increased sensitivity to vasoconstricter substances such as endothelin which predispose to vascular disease and further increases in peripheral resistance which lead to a vicious cycle increasing blood pressure further due to the increase in vascular resistance. Other substances with a role in controlling blood pressure include atrial natriuretic peptide, bradykinin and antidiuretic hormone. Some new therapies seek to treat high blood pressure by modifying responses to these substances, for example, the endothelin antagonist darusentan.

Clinical presentation

Hypertension is often an incidental finding when subjects present for screening or with unrelated conditions. Severe cases may present with headache, visual disturbances or evidence of target organ damage (stroke, ischaemic heart disease or renal failure). In the UK, all patients under 80 years of age should have their blood pressure checked at least every 5 years, with an annual review for those with high normal values in the range 135–139 mmHg systolic or 85–89 mmHg diastolic.

Malignant (accelerated) hypertension

Malignant or accelerated hypertension is an uncommon condition characterised by greatly elevated blood pressure (usually >220/120 mmHg) associated with evidence of ongoing small vessel damage. Fundoscopy may reveal papilloedema, haemorrhages and/or exudates, while renal damage can manifest as haematuria, proteinuria and impaired renal function. The condition may be associated with hypertensive encephalopathy, which is caused by small vessel changes in the cerebral circulation associated with cerebral oedema. The clinical features are confusion, headache, visual loss, seizures and coma. Brain imaging (particularly MRI) usually demonstrates extensive white matter changes. Malignant hypertension is a medical emergency that requires hospital admission and rapid control of blood pressure over 12–24 h towards normal levels.

Management of hypertension

In the UK, the management of hypertension is guided by consensus guidelines produced by the British Hypertension Society (BHS) and the National Institute for Health and Clinical Excellence (NICE). In 2004, there were significant differences between NICE and BHS guidance but these were addressed in the form of modified joint guidance issued in 2006 which specifically addressed the areas of controversy (National Collaborating Centre for Chronic Conditions: Hypertension, 2006). The European Society of Hypertension also published a task force discussion document in January 2009 and formal guidance in 2007 (Mancia et al., 2009).

Diagnosis of hypertension

In the UK, it is recommended that all adults have their blood pressure measured every 5 years. Those with high normal (130–139 mmHg systolic or 85–89 mmHg diastolic) or previous high readings should have annual measurement.

Blood pressure should be measured using a well-maintained sphygmomanometer of validated accuracy. Blood pressure should initially be measured in both arms and the arm with the highest value used for subsequent readings. The subject should be relaxed and, at least at the first presentation, blood pressure should be measured in both the sitting and the standing positions. An appropriate sized cuff should be used since one that is too small will result in an overestimation of the patient's blood pressure. The arm should be supported level with the heart and it is important that the patient does not hold their arm out since isometric exercise increases blood pressure. Blood pressure is measured using the Korotkov sounds which appear (the first phase) and disappear (the fifth phase) over the brachial artery as pressure in the cuff is released. Cuff deflation should occur at approximately 2 mmHg/s to allow accurate measurement of the systolic and diastolic blood pressures. The fourth Korotkov phase (muffling of sound) has previously been used for diastolic blood pressure measurement but is not currently recommended unless Korotkov V cannot be defined. Having established that the blood pressure is increased, the measurement should be repeated several times over several weeks, unless the initial measurement is at dangerously high levels, in which case several measurements should be made during the same clinic attendance.

Home or ambulatory blood pressure measurements

Some people develop excessive and unrepresentative blood pressure rises when attending the doctor's surgery, so-called 'white coat' hypertension. These patients can be diagnosed if they use a blood pressure machine themselves at home or by 24-h ambulatory blood pressure monitoring. Home blood pressure measurement is inexpensive but it is important to have a machine of validated accuracy that the patient can use properly. Ambulatory blood pressure monitoring over 24 h is also useful for patients who have unusual variability in blood pressure, resistant hypertension or symptoms suggesting hypotension. Home or ambulatory blood pressure measurements are usually lower than clinic recordings, on average by 12/7 mmHg.

Assessment of the hypertensive patient

Secondary causes

It is important to take a careful history checking for features that might suggest a possible secondary cause of hypertension. Examples would be symptoms of renal disease, for example, haematuria, polyuria, etc., or the paroxysmal symptoms that suggest the rare diagnosis of phaeochromocytoma and include headache, postural dizziness, syncope. A careful physical examination should be performed for abdominal bruits, which suggest possible renal artery stenosis, radiofemoral delay which suggest coarctation of the aorta and palpable kidneys which suggest polycystic kidney disease. Laboratory analysis should include a full blood count, electrolytes, urea, creatinine and urinalysis. In some patients, further investigations may be appropriate, for example, ultrasound of the abdomen or isotope renogram where renal disease is suspected. A renin–angiotensin ratio is a useful screening test to investigate for possible hyperaldosteronism while serum metanephrine and urinary catecholamines may detect underlying phaeochromocytoma.

A low serum potassium may alert to the presence of hyperaldosteronism but it should be remembered that renin levels are suppressed by β-blockers and aldosterone by angiotensin converting enzyme inhibitors and receptor antagonists. A very high aldosterone/renin ratio may suggest Conn's syndrome or primary hyperaldosteronism. This is usually caused by a benign adenoma or simple hyperplasia within the zona glomerulosa of the adrenal gland, the presence of which may be demonstrated by CT or MRI scanning. The tumours may be surgically resected, but where there is a suggestion of hyperaldosteronism and no obvious tumour on imaging, patients may still respond to spironolactone, an aldosterone antagonist, while remaining relatively resistant to other antihypertensives.

Contributing factors

The patient should also be assessed for possible contributory factors to hypertension such as obesity, excess alcohol or salt intake and lack of exercise. Occasionally, hypertension may be provoked by the use of drugs (see Box 19.2), including over-the-counter medicines used as cold and flu remedies. Other risk factors should also be documented and addressed, for example, smoking, diabetes and hyperlipidaemia. It is important to establish whether there is a family history of cardiovascular disease.

Evidence of end-organ damage

The patient should also be examined carefully for evidence of end-organ damage from hypertension. This should include examination of the optic fundi to detect retinal changes.

An ECG should be performed to detect left ventricular hypertrophy or subclinical ischaemic heart disease. It is advisable to check the renal function and test the urine for signs of microalbuminutria which may be an indicator of a higher risk of future end-stage renal disease and overall vascular risk.

Determination of cardiovascular risk

An accurate assessment of cardiovascular disease risk is essential before recommending appropriate management in hypertension. Patients with documented atheromatous vascular disease, for example, previous myocardial infarction or stroke, angina or peripheral vascular disease are at high risk of recurrent events. Those with type 2 diabetes over 40 years of age are also at high risk and can be regarded as 'coronary equivalents', that is, with risks similar to non-diabetic patients with previous myocardial infarction. For non-diabetic patients without vascular disease it is necessary to estimate cardiovascular risk (see Chapter 24). A 10-year cardiovascular disease risk of 20% (equivalent to a 15% coronary heart disease risk) is regarded as an appropriate threshold for antihypertensive therapy in patients with moderate hypertension, as well as for lipid-lowering therapy. Treatment decisions based on these tables will favour treatment in elderly subjects. While a younger patient may be at lower absolute risk over 10 years and may not meet the criteria for blood pressure and lipid treatment, they may be at higher lifetime and longer term risk of premature death and vascular disease and, thus, still merit risk factor intervention.

Other factors to consider include microalbuminuria which increases cardiovascular risk by a factor of 2–3 and the combination of reduced GFR and microalbuminuria may increase risk by as much as six-fold (Cirillo et al 2008; Sehestedt et al., 2009).

Treatment

Non-pharmacological approaches

Non-pharmacological management of hypertension is important, although the effects are often disappointing. Patients with mild hypertension in the range 140–159/90–100 mmHg can be assessed for levels of risk while offered lifestyle advice. General health education is important to allow patients to make informed choices about management. In order to maximise potential benefit, patients should receive clear and unambiguous advice, including written information they can digest in their own time. Written advice for patients can be downloaded from the BHS website (http://www.bhsoc.org/).

In patients who are overweight, weight loss results in reduction in blood pressure of about 2.5/1.5 mmHg/kg. The DASH diet (Dietary Approaches to Stop Hypertension) was evaluated in a clinical trial and found to lower blood pressure significantly (4.5/2.7 mmHg) compared with a typical US diet. This diet emphasises fruit, vegetables, and low-fat dairy produce in addition to fish, low-fat poultry and whole grains while minimising red meat, confectionary and sweetened drinks (Appel et al., 1997). Subjects should reduce their salt intake, for example, by not adding salt to food on the plate. A daily sodium intake of <100 mmol (i.e. 6 g sodium chloride or 2.4 g elemental sodium) should be the aim. There is a significant amount of hidden salt in processed meat, ready meals, cheese and even bread. A dietary assessment may be required to accurately quantify a patient's salt intake and advise on how reductions might be made.

Most subjects will need to control their intake of calories and saturated fat. Regular aerobic exercise, at a level appropriate to the individual subject, at least 3 times a week for at least 30 min derives maximum benefit. This results in improved physical fitness as well as a reduction in blood pressure. Alcohol intake should be restricted to two (females) or three (males) units per day. Although smoking does not affect blood pressure, it increases cardiovascular risk and patients should quit or, if this is not possible, reduce their cigarette consumption.

Unless hypertension is severe, it is appropriate to observe the subject over several months while instituting non-pharmacological interventions. However, if there is a more urgent need for drug treatment, non-pharmacological interventions should occur in parallel.

Drug treatment

Treatment thresholds

Treatment thresholds are summarised in Table 19.1. Lifestyle advice should be provided to all patients with any degree of hypertension. Patients with severe hypertension (>220/120 mmHg confirmed on several readings on the same occasion) should be treated immediately and some guidance suggests that dual therapy should be commenced immediately in patients with blood pressure >20 mmHg above their target as monotherapy is unlikely to be fully effective (Mancia et al., 2007). Patients with blood pressures in the range 160–220/100–120 mmHg should be monitored over several weeks and treated if blood pressure remains in this range. The period of observation before starting treatment depends on the severity of the hypertension and the presence or absence of end-organ damage (see Table 19.1). Patients whose blood pressure is in the range 140–159/90–99 mmHg should be observed annually unless they have evidence of target organ damage, cardiovascular complications, diabetes or a calculated cardiovascular risk >20% over 10 years, in which case drug treatment should be offered. Patients with blood pressure in the range 135–139/85–89 mmHg should be reassessed annually, while those with blood pressure lower than this can be rechecked every 5 years.

Target blood pressures

Within the Hypertension Optimal Treatment (HOT) study (Hansson et al., 1998), patients were allocated diastolic target blood pressures of <90, 85, 80 mmHg. The study struggled to stratify patients effectively into these treatment groups but analysis suggested that the optimum target blood pressure was <140/85 mmHg with little benefit in lowering to lower levels of 120/70 mmHg but also little evidence of harm.

Table 19.1 Threshold blood pressures for intervention

Initial blood pressure		Management
Systolic (mmHg)	Diastolic (mmHg)	
Malignant hypertension		Admit and treat immediately
>220	>120	Repeat several times at the same attendance and treat immediately if blood pressure persists in this range
180–219	110–119	Confirm over 1–2 weeks and treat if blood pressure remains in this range
160–179	100–109	Repeat over 3–4 weeks (end-organ damage present) or 2–12 weeks (no end-organ damage), institute non-pharmacological measures and treat if blood pressure persists in this range
140–159	90–99	Repeat over several weeks. Institute non-pharmacological measures. Treat if remains in this range and patient has target organ damage, cardiovascular complications or an estimated 10-year cardiovascular risk >20%. Otherwise reassess annually
135–139	85–89	Reassess annually
<135	<85	Reassess in 5 years

The UK Prospective Diabetes Study Group (1998a,b) suggested 'tight' blood pressure control was better than less tight in patients with non-insulin-dependent diabetes. The targets in the UK Prospective Diabetes Study were 'tight' <150/85mmHg and 'less tight' <180/105mmHg but the actually achieved blood pressures were lower, for example, 154/87mmHg versus 144/82mmHg. Recommendations in diabetics have, therefore, suggested treating to a target of 140/80mmHg or less, although few studies have successfully lowered blood pressure to these levels.

A more recent study (Cardio-Sis) randomised non-diabetic subjects with systolic blood pressure >150mmHg to target systolic blood pressure of <140 or <130mmHg (Verdecchia et al., 2009). The primary end-point was left ventricular hypertrophy though the secondary end-point of a composite cardiovascular end-point was reduced (as well as the primary end-point) in the 130-mmHg group, with no increase in adverse events. This, however, is not robust enough evidence to recommend a reduction in blood pressure target levels and would require a larger study of hard clinical end-points to confirm these findings.

Achievement of target blood pressures is incorporated as a quality indicator for the General Medical Services Contract for primary care doctors in the UK. Diabetic patients are an exception and benefit from more aggressive blood pressure reduction. Target blood pressures for diabetic and non-diabetic subjects are summarised in Table 19.2. It should be emphasised that the audit standard will not be achieved in all patients.

Antihypertensive drug classes

β-Adrenoreceptor antagonists

The mode of action of β-adrenoreceptor antagonists in hypertension is uncertain. β-Adrenoreceptor blockade reduces cardiac output in the short term and during exercise. They also reduce renin secretion by antagonising β-receptors in the juxtaglomerular apparatus. Central actions may also be important for

Table 19.2 Target clinic blood pressures according to British Hypertension Society guidelines 2004 (Williams et al., 2004)

	Clinic blood pressure	
	No diabetes (mmHg)	Diabetes (mmHg)
Optimal treated blood pressure	<140/85	<130/80
Audit standard	<150/90	<140/80

some agents. Non-selective β-blockers may give rise to adverse effects as a result of antagonism of β_2-adrenoceptors, that is, asthma and worsened intermittent claudication. However, the so-called 'cardioselective' (β_1-selective) β-blockers are not entirely free of these adverse effects. Patients who develop very marked bradycardia and tiredness may tolerate a drug with partial agonist activity such as pindolol.

β-Adrenoreceptor antagonists also have substantial clinical trial evidence of benefit over placebo in hypertension, and are relatively inexpensive. However, their use is declining and they have been relegated to fourth-line therapy in the UK according to NICE guidance (Fig. 19.1). This recommendation largely stems from the evidence that they may be less effective at preventing stroke in conjunction with their diabetogenic effects. The Losartan For Endpoint reduction in hypertension (LIFE) study compared an atenolol/thiazide-based regime with a losartan-based regime and demonstrated equivalent levels of blood pressure reduction but with a small excess incidence of stroke in the atenolol arm (Dahlöf et al., 2002). In the Anglo Scandinavian Cardiac Outcomes Trial (ASCOT) study, the risk of diabetes was 2.5% higher in the atenolol arm compared with the amlodipine arm with similar increased risk of diabetes found within the atenolol arm of the LIFE study (Dahlöf et al., 2005). A Cochrane review

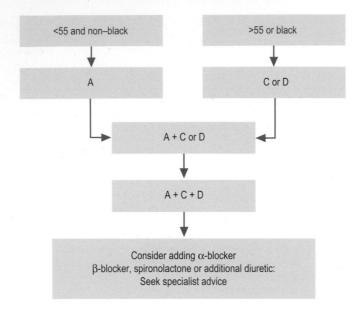

A = ACE inhibitor; C = calcium channel blocker; D = diuretic

Fig. 19.1 Algorithm for drug sequencing in hypertension.

warned of the excess risk in developing diabetes in patients prescribed combinations of thiazide diuretics and β-blockers. This would equate to one new case per 500 treated (Mason et al., 2004). The combination of thiazide and a β-blocker should, therefore, be avoided if possible, particularly in those who are at risk of developing diabetes (e.g. obese, strong family history of diabetes, South Asian origin).

To complicate matters, however, a long-term 20-year follow-up study of the UKPDS study found similar cardiovascular outcomes between patients on β-blockers and ACE inhibitors with a reduction in all causes of mortality which actually favoured β-blockers (Holman et al., 2008). β-Blockers do remain most suitable for younger hypertensives who have another indication for β-blockade, such as coronary heart disease. β-Blockers are also effective in suppressing atrial fibrillation and this may be one group of patients where first-line therapy with β-blockers is still merited.

It can be safely assumed that the place for β-blockers for patients with hypertension is likely to remain controversial.

Diuretics

There is substantial clinical trial evidence that benefit is obtained from the use of thiazide, for example, bendroflumethiazide, hydrochlorothiazide, or thiazide-like, for example, chlortalidone, indapamide, diuretics in hypertension; these drugs are both inexpensive and well tolerated by most patients. Their diuretic action is achieved by blockade of distal renal tubular sodium reabsorption. Initially, they reduce blood pressure by reducing circulating blood volume but in the longer term they reduce total peripheral resistance, suggesting a direct vasodilatory action.

Although generally well tolerated, thiazide and thiazide-like diuretics may cause hypokalaemia, small increases in LDL-cholesterol and triglyceride, and gout associated with impaired urate excretion. Erectile dysfunction is also common.

Most blood pressure lowering occurs with very low doses of thiazide diuretics. Increasing the dose substantially increases the risk of metabolic disturbance without causing further blood pressure reduction. For bendroflumethiazide it is rarely (if ever) appropriate to use doses greater than 2.5 mg/day and a dose of 1.25 mg daily is often effective. Most studies of diuretics have also incorporated β-blockers and this combination can have adverse metabolic consequences which may lead to new onset diabetes. Within the Anti-hypertensive and Lipid Lowering treatment to prevent Heart Attack Trial (ALLHAT), the absolute risk of developing diabetes was 3.5% higher in the chlortalidone group than the lisinopril group (ALLHAT Collaborative Research Group, 2002).

As with the β-blocker saga it remains an issue of contention as to whether this diabetic tendency is clinically significant. There was no reduction in efficacy associated with thiazide use in ALLHAT and indeed there were less heart failure outcomes in the diuretic-treated patients compared with those receiving calcium channel blockers or ACE inhibitors.

Loop diuretics are no more effective at lowering blood pressure than thiazides unless renal function is significantly impaired or the patient is receiving agents that inhibit the renin–angiotensin system. They are also a suitable choice if heart failure is present.

Spironolactone, an aldosterone antagonist, is not suitable for first-line therapy but is an increasingly important treatment option for patients with resistant hypertension. Where hyperaldosteronism is suspected, spironolactone may prove to be effective. Spironolactone is a potassium sparing diuretic and should be used with caution especially if used in combination with ACE inhibitors or angiotensin receptor blockers

(ARBs), and should almost always be avoided with other potassium sparing diuretics, for example, amiloride.

Renin-angiotensin-aldosterone antagonists

ACE inhibitors block the conversion of angiotensin I to angiotensin II, while ARBs block the action of angiotensin II at the angiotensin II type 2_1 receptor. Since angiotensin II is a vasoconstrictor and stimulates the release of aldosterone, antagonism results in vasodilation and potassium retention as well as inhibition of salt and water retention. ACE inhibitors also block kininase production and, thus, prevent the breakdown of bradykinin. This appears to be important in the aetiology of ACE inhibitor induced cough, which is a troublesome side effect in 10–20% of users. ARBs do not inhibit kininase and are an appropriate choice for patients who are intolerant of ACE inhibitors because of cough. ACE inhibitors are also associated with a significant incidence of angioedema, which can in severe cases cause dangerous swelling of the pharyngolargyngeal area leading to stridor, threatening the patient's airway. This adverse reaction is commoner in black subjects.

Calcium channel blockers

These agents block slow calcium channels in the peripheral blood vessels and/or the heart. The dihydropyridine group work almost exclusively on L-type calcium channels in the peripheral arterioles and reduce blood pressure by reducing total peripheral resistance. In contrast, the effect of verapamil and diltiazem are primarily on the heart, reducing heart rate and cardiac output. Long-acting dihydropyridines are preferred because they are more convenient for patients and avoid the large fluctuations in plasma drug concentrations that may be associated with adverse effects.

Although effective for lowering blood pressure and preventing cardiovascular events, adverse effects are common, for example, oedema and flushing. Gum hypertrophy may occur with dihydropyridines and constipation with verapamil. Concerns have previously been raised by observational studies (Psaty et al., 1995) and meta-analysis (Furberg et al., 1995) that there may be an increased risk of coronary heart disease in recipients of dihydropyridine calcium channel blockers. However, randomised clinical trials have not confirmed these observations (Gong et al., 1996, Staessen et al., 1997) and have indicated that dihydropyridines are of similar efficacy to thiazide diuretics in preventing cardiovascular events (Brown et al., 2000).

α-Adrenoreceptor blockers

Drugs of this class antagonise α-adrenoceptors in the blood vessel wall and, thus, prevent noradrenaline (norepinephrine)-induced vasoconstriction. As a result, they reduce total peripheral resistance and blood pressure. Prazosin was originally used but had the disadvantage of being short-acting and causing first-dose hypotension. Newer agents such as doxazosin and terazosin have a longer duration of action. There are concerns about the first-line use of β-blockers since the ALLHAT study has indicated that doxazosin is more often associated with heart failure and stroke than thiazide diuretics (ALLHAT Collaborative Research Group, 2000). However, they are an appropriate choice as add-in therapy for patients inadequately controlled using other agents. They can frequently cause postural hypotension but may alleviate symptoms in men with prostatic hyperterophy.

Centrally acting agents

Methyldopa and moxonidine inhibit sympathetic outflow from the brain, resulting in a reduction in total peripheral resistance. Methyldopa is not widely used because it has pronounced central adverse effects, including tiredness and depression. It continues to be used in pregnancy, since it does not cause fetal abnormalities. It is also occasionally used in patients with resistant hypertension. Moxonidine is a newer agent that blocks central imidazoline and α_2-adrenoceptors found within the medulla oblongata of the brain. It can cause side effects of dry mouth, headache, fatigue and dizziness, although it appears to have fewer central adverse effects than methyldopa. Other centrally acting agents such as clonidine and reserpine are almost never used in modern practice because of their pronounced adverse effects.

Other agents

Several other drugs are available for use for people with more resistant hypertension. Minoxidil is a powerful antihypertensive drug but its use is associated with severe peripheral oedema and reflex tachycardia. It should be restricted to patients with severe hypertension who are also taking β-blockers and diuretics. It causes pronounced hirsutism and is not a suitable treatment for women. Hydralazine can be used as add-on therapy for patients with resistant hypertension but is not well tolerated as it is a profound vasodilator and may occasionally be associated with drug-induced systemic lupus erythematosus. Sodium nitroprusside is a direct-acting arterial and venous dilator that is administered as an intravenous infusion for treating hypertensive emergencies and for the acute control of blood pressure during anaesthesia. Hypertension has previously been treated with ganglion blockers such as guanethidine but these drugs are now of historical interest only.

Recent additions to the licensed armory of antihypertensive agents include the renin antagonist aliskiren. There is evidence that this agent may have a similar blood pressure lowering effect to other agents and may be safely added to other inhibitors of the renin–angiotensin–aldosterone system to provide a greater level of inhibition (O'Brien et al., 2007). Due to its cost and a relative lack of experience in its use, it can only be suggested as an add-on therapy where other more established treatment options have failed to control blood pressure. It is generally well tolerated but may cause diarrhoea at higher doses.

The endothelin antagonist darusentan is undergoing clinical trials in resistant hypertension. Early studies show it may be effective in resistant cases but may be associated with a high incidence of fluid retention (Weber et al., 2009).

Drug selection

Drugs should be chosen on the basis of efficacy, safety, convenience to the patient and cost. For assessing efficacy, it is essential to use evidence from large-scale clinical trials that demonstrate measurable effects on hard end-points like incidence of stroke and other cardiovascular events or death. Smaller scale studies looking at the effects of drugs on blood pressure and surrogate markers such as left ventricular hypertrophy or carotid artery stenosis may generate a hypothesis of a future treatment strategy but should be used to change current strategies. When considering safety, it is important to recognise that these drugs will be taken in the long term and there are advantages to using drugs which have long-established safety records. It is also important to recognise the importance of symptomatic adverse effects since these may reduce adherence. Patients should feel as well during treatment of their blood pressure as they did before drug treatment was instituted. Patient convenience is another important factor and use of once-daily preparations will result in better adherence than more frequent regimens. Since the hypertensive population is very large it is necessary to be conscious of the cost of individual preparations. Combinations of low doses of antihypertensive drugs are often better tolerated than single drugs taken in high dose. The choice of drugs available for treating hypertension is shown in Table 19.3, and common therapeutic problems are noted.

Clinical trial evidence

Initial evidence of benefit in placebo-controlled clinical trials came from studies that primarily involved thiazide diuretics or β-blockers. However, there is increasing evidence of clinical benefit from newer drug classes including ACE inhibitors and calcium channel blockers.

The Blood Pressure Lowering Treatment Trialists Collaboration (2000) carried out a meta-analysis of old against new treatments. They concluded that newer treatments were no more effective than older therapies. Since this study was done several landmark comparative clinical trials have been published.

The Captopril Prevention Project (CAPPP) demonstrated that captopril was as effective as diuretics or β-blockers for preventing cardiovascular morbidity (Hansson et al., 1999a). However, captopril was associated with a 25% higher stroke risk, perhaps because it did not reduce blood pressure as effectively as conventional therapy in this particular study.

The LIFE study demonstrated that losartan was more effective at preventing vascular events, especially stroke, than atenolol in just over 9000 hypertensive patients with left ventricular hypertrophy, although reductions in blood pressure were similar. Losartan was also better tolerated (Dahlöf et al., 2002).

The ALLHAT study (ALLHAT Collaborative Research Group, 2002) involved over 40,000 older, high-risk hypertensive patients with the aim of determining whether the occurrence of fatal coronary heart disease or non-fatal myocardial infarction was lower in those treated with newer agents (amlodipine, lisinopril or doxazosin) compared with a thiazide-like diuretic (chlortalidone). The doxazosin arm was discontinued early because of a higher rate of events, especially heart failure, compared with the diuretic. For the remaining three drugs there was no difference in occurrence of the primary end-point. Chlortalidone was more effective than amlodipine and lisinopril in lowering blood pressure and preventing heart failure and was also marginally more effective than lisinopril in preventing stroke.

The second Australian National Blood Pressure Study Group (Wing et al., 2003) compared enalapril with hydrochlorthiazide in just over 6000 hypertensive subjects recruited in primary care. The primary end-point was any cardiovascular event or death from any cause. In this relatively small study, there was a trend in favour of the ACE inhibitor which was of borderline statistical significance.

The VALUE study (Julius et al., 2004) compared amlodipine and valsartan in high-risk hypertensive subjects. No differences in the primary composite cardiac end-point were observed, although non-fatal myocardial infarction was less common with amlodipine, which also lowered blood pressure to a greater extent. Conversely, onset of diabetes was less common with valsartan.

The ASCOT study (Dahlöf et al., 2005) compared a modern treatment regimen based on amlodipine and perindopril with a traditional regimen based on atenolol and bendroflumethiazide. The study involved over 20,000 high-risk hypertensives. The amlodipine-based therapy was associated with better blood pressure reduction and reductions in the occurrence of cardiovascular events, total mortality and diabetes, although the primary composite end-point was not significantly affected. It is uncertain how much of the benefit can be attributed to the better blood pressure control achieved in the amlodipine-based arm and how specific these findings are to the drug doses and sequencing specified in the trial protocol for each arm of the study.

These various trials have provided results that are conflicting, in part because of differences in trial design and quality. However, there is increasing evidence that β-blockers may be less effective at preventing cardiovascular end-points, as suggested by LIFE and ASCOT studies. In a meta-analysis (Lindholm et al., 2005), β-blockers were less effective than other antihypertensives at preventing stroke, although no significant differences were observed in effects on myocardial infarction or death. There is no consistent evidence that thiazides or thiazide-like drugs are less effective than newer agents in preventing cardiovascular events.

Recommendations for drug sequencing

In the UK, the BHS and NICE issued joint guidelines in 2006 on the order in which drugs should be used (National Collaborating Centre for Chronic Conditions, 2006). This replaced previous guidelines which differed between the two reflecting the ongoing controversy regarding the role of β-blockers. These recommend an initial choice of an

Table 19.3 Summary of antihypertensive drugs and common therapeutic problems

Class	Examples	Major adverse effects	Comment
Diuretics	Thiazides: bendroflumethiazide	Hypokalaemia Gout Glucose intolerance Hyperlipidaemia	Cheap, effective. Efficacy proven in clinical trials Concerns about long-term metabolic effects More appropriate in older patients
	Loops: furosemide K sparing: spironolactone	Impotence Uraemia Dehydration Hyperkalaemia Gynaecomastia	Especially for patients with cardiac failure Especially for resistant hypertension
β-Blockers	Atenolol Propranolol Metoprolol	Tiredness Reduced exercise tolerance Bradycardia	Cheap Adverse effects common Possibly less effective in preventing cardiovascular events
	Labetalol Celiprolol	Cold peripheries Claudication Wheezing Cardiac failure Impotence	Especially for patients with ischaemic heart disease
Calcium antagonists: dihydropyridine	Nifedipine	Flushing	Not well tolerated (especially early in treatment). Recent trials confirm reductions in stroke and myocardial infarction
	Amlodipine	Oedema Postural hypotension Headache	Similar efficacy to thiazides Especially for elderly patients and those with ischaemic heart disease or diabetes
Calcium antagonists: rate limiting	Verapamil	Bradycardia/heart block	Well tolerated. Suitable for patients with ischaemic heart disease who are unable to tolerate β-blockers
	Diltiazem	Constipation (verapamil only)	Caution needed when used in combination with β-blockers
ACE inhibitors	Captopril Enalapril Lisinopril Perindopril Ramipril	Cough Rash, taste disturbance Renal failure Angioedema	More expensive. Cough very common Appropriate for use in younger patients and those with cardiac failure or diabetes
α-Blockers	Prazosin Doxazosin	Oedema Postural hypotension	More expensive. Adverse effects common. No evidence to date of long-term efficacy. Less effective than thiazides at preventing heart failure and combined cardiovascular outcomes (ALLHAT study)
	Terazosin		Second line
Angiotensin receptor blockers	Losartan Valsartan	Renal failure Oedema	More expensive Especially for patients in whom ACE inhibitor indicated but not tolerated due to cough
	Irbesartan	Headache	More effective in preventing vascular events than atenolol in patients with LVH
Centrally acting vasodilators	Methyldopa	Tiredness	Poorly tolerated. Only used in severe hypertension or hypertension of pregnancy
	Moxonidine	Depression	Third line
Direct-acting vasodilators	Diazoxide Minoxidil Nitroprusside	Oedema Postural hypotension Headache	Poorly tolerated. Only used in severe hypertension

ACE inhibitor or ARB (A) as first-line therapy in younger (<55 years) non-black patients. The rationale for this is that these patients often have hypertension associated with high concentrations of renin. It is, therefore, logical to treat these patients with drugs that antagonise the renin–angiotensin system.

For patients >55 and black patients, who tend to have hypertension associated with low renin concentrations, calcium channel blockers (C) or thiazide diuretics (D) are advocated as first-line options. If initial drug therapy fails to control blood pressure, A and D or C is suggested. Subsequently, a combination of A plus C plus D may be used. After this, further therapies, for example, β-blocker, α-blocker, spironolactone, etc., could be added as necessary to achieve adequate control (Fig. 19.1). β-Blockers may be used in those patients with a high sympathetic drive, in pregnant women where labetolol has a good safety record or where other agents are not tolerated.

European guidance (Box 19.3) has eschewed a formal ranking of treatments and instead suggested a table of drugs and indications where they might be most appropriately indicated (Mancia et al., 2007).

Box 19.3 Conditions favouring use of particular antihypertensive agents (modified from Mancia et al., 2007)

Thiazide diuretics
  Systolic hypertension in the elderly
  Heart failure
  Black patients
ACE inhibitors
  Heart failure
  Left ventricular dysfynction
  Post-myocardial infarction
  Diabetic nephropathy
  Left ventricular hypertrophy
  Proteinuria
β-Blockers
  Angina
  Post-myocardial infarction
  Heart failure (stable)
  Atrial fibrillation
  Pregnancy
Calcium channel blockers (dihydropyridines)
  Systolic hypertension in the elderly
  Angina
  Pregnancy
  Black patients
Calcium channel blockers (verapamil/diltiazem)
  Angina
  Atrial fibrillation
Loop diuretics
  Renal impairment
  Heart failure
Aldosterone antagonists
  Heart failure
  Post-myocardial infarction
  Conn's syndrome

Special patient groups

Race

People of African Caribbean origin have an increased prevalence of hypertension and left ventricular hypertrophy and are at high risk of stroke and renal failure. They obtain particular benefit from reduced salt intake and are also sensitive to diuretic and calcium channel blockers, while β-blockers appear less effective, at least when used as monotherapy. African Caribbean people have reduced plasma renin activity and, as a result, ACE inhibitors and ARBs are also less effective. This was illustrated in the ALLHAT study where stroke and coronary events were more common in black patients randomised to lisinopril compared to those receiving chlortalidone.

British Asians also have an increased prevalence of hypertension, diabetes and insulin resistance and a particularly high risk of coronary heart disease and stroke. There is currently no evidence of a difference in drug response when compared with white Europeans. However, combinations of β-blockers and thiazides should be avoided when possible because of the higher risk of diabetes.

Elderly ✷

The elderly have a high prevalence of hypertension, with over 70% having blood pressures greater than 140/90 mmHg. They are also at high absolute risk of cardiovascular events. Therefore, the absolute benefits of blood pressure treatment are particularly large in this group. Antihypertensive therapy may also reduce the risk of heart failure and dementia. The Study of Cognition and Prognosis in the Elderly (SCOPE) study (Lithell et al., 2003) was designed to investigate the effects of candesartan on the occurrence of cognitive decline or dementia but revealed no benefit, probably because of the lack of difference in blood pressure between the two arms of the study

The elderly are at particular risk of certain adverse effects of treatment such as postural hypotension and it is important that both sitting and standing blood pressure are monitored. Nevertheless, the benefits of therapy are so great that treatment should be offered at any age unless the patient is very frail or their life expectancy is very short. Isolated systolic hypertension (systolic >160 mm Hg, diastolic <90 mmHg) is common in the elderly and there is irrefutable evidence that drug treatment is beneficial in this group (SHEP Co-operative Research Group, 1991, Staessen et al., 1997). The elderly have more variable blood pressure and larger numbers of measurements may be required to confirm hypertension.

Calcium channel blockers and low-dose thiazide diuretics are safe and effective treatments for elderly hypertensive people and their use is endorsed by large-scale clinical trials. β-Blockers are less effective at reducing blood pressure and preventing clinical end-points. The Swedish Trial in Old Patients with hypertension-2 (STOP-2) compared the effects of conventional (β-blocker or thiazide) and newer drugs (ACE inhibitors or calcium channel blockers) on cardiovascular morbidity in older subjects and did not detect significant differences (Hansson et al., 1999b).

In the Hypertension in the Very Elderly Trial (HYVET), 4000 patients with a mean age of 84, blood pressure 160–199 mmHg systolic at entry were treated to a target of systolic 150 mmHg for 1.8 years with indapamide (a thiazide-like diuretic) and if required the ACE inhibitor perindopril. There was a 30% reduction in fatal and non-fatal stroke, 21% reduction in death from all causes, and fewer adverse events in the actively treated group (Beckett, 2008).

The elderly certainly benefit from treatment of hypertension but the threshold and target for treatment has not been fully elucidated. Most studies in the elderly recruited patients with relatively high baseline targets (>160–190 mmHg systolic) achieving blood pressure on treatment of between 150 and 170 mmHg and only one achieved target blood pressure lower than 140 mmHg and in this study outcome was poorer in the treated group (JATOS Study Group, 2008). There may be little benefit in striving for strict systolic targets beyond 150 mmHg in these patients, particularly if control is being achieved to the detriment of overall patient well-being.

Diabetes

In type 1 diabetes, the presence of hypertension often indicates the presence of diabetic nephropathy. In this group, blood pressure reduction and ACE inhibition slow the rate of decline in renal function. To achieve adequate blood pressure control, combinations of drugs will be needed. Thiazides, β-blockers, calcium channel blockers and α-blockers are all suitable as add-on treatments to ACE inhibitors which should be first-line therapy. Target blood pressure should be <130/80 mmHg or <125/75 mmHg if there is diabetic nephropathy. The evidence supporting this recommendation is, however, limited and obtaining such levels of control in diabetics often impossible.

In type 2 (non-insulin dependent) diabetes, hypertension is particularly common, affecting 70% of people in this group. It is strongly associated with obesity and insulin resistance and control of blood pressure is more important for preventing complications than tight glycaemic control. There is no evidence that one group of drugs is more or less effective than any other. The ADVANCE trial treated diabetics with indapamide and perindopril in addition to prestudy antihypertensive agents. The active group was found to have a further reduction in blood pressure and a significant reduction in adverse renal outcomes (21%) (Patel et al., 2007). It remains a subject of debate whether ACE inhibitors and ARBs have specific renoprotective benefits over and above their effects on blood pressure.

Renal disease

In patients with chronic renal impairment, good blood pressure control slows the progression of renal dysfunction. ACE inhibition reduces the incidence of end-stage renal failure but it is not clear if this is a specific effect or non-specific action as a result of blood pressure lowering. ACE inhibitors also reduce 24-h protein loss and should be used in patients with 24-h protein excretion of >3 g or rapidly progressive renal dysfunction. ACE inhibitors may worsen renal impairment in patients with renal vascular disease and careful monitoring of electrolytes and creatinine is mandatory. Salt restriction is particularly important in managing hypertension in renal disease. Thiazide diuretics are ineffective in patients with significant renal dysfunction and loop diuretics should be used when a diuretic is needed.

A further note of caution regarding overtreatment of blood pressure to overaggressive targets comes from the ONTARGET study which randomised patients with vascular disease or high-risk diabetics to high-dose ramipril, telmisartan (ARB) or both. Many patients were already taking polypharmacy for hypertension and blood pressures at entry were approximately 142/82 mmHg in all groups. Treatment reduced blood pressure by 6.4/4.3 mmHg in the ramipril group, 7.4/5.0 mmHg in the telmisartan group and 9.8/6.3 mmHg in the combination group. This would give the combination group a post-treatment blood pressure of 132/76 mmHg. This combination group was associated with adverse renal outcomes, for example, renal failure and high potassium with no improvement in other cardiovascular outcomes (Yusuf et al., 2008a).

Stroke

Hypertension is the most important risk factor for stroke in patients with or without previous stroke. There is increasing evidence that in those with a previous stroke, blood pressure reduction reduces the risk of stroke recurrence as well as other cardiovascular events. The PROGRESS study, while clearly demonstrating a benefit of lowering blood pressure in patients with cerebrovascular disease, only demonstrated benefit in those whose blood pressure was >140 mmHg on entry or who were already on antihypertensives. The size of benefit was proportional to the size of the blood pressure reduction. The combination of perindopril and indapamide lowered systolic blood pressure by 12.3 mmHg and stroke incidence by an impressive 43%, while perindopril alone was associated with a small drop in systolic blood pressure and no reduction in stroke risk (PROGRESS Collaborative Group, 2001). On treatment, blood pressure in the actively treated group was 132 mmHg systolic which has led some to suggest a target of 130 mmHg for such patients but this is based on post hoc analysis and has not been recommended in formal guidance.

The PROFESS study randomised patients with cerebrovascular disease to telmistartan or placebo and obtained systolic blood pressure of 136 in the active group versus 140 mmHg in the placebo group with no difference in the vascular outcomes between the two groups. This may have been due to the relatively small difference in blood pressure between the two groups (Yusuf et al., 2008b).

The question 'what to do with blood pressure in the setting of acute stroke?' has remained an evidence-free zone until fairly recently. Blood pressure naturally rises then falls in the days and hours following acute stroke and some have argued that elevated levels are necessary to maintain brain circulation due to the failure of cerebral autoregulatory mechanisms around the time of stroke. The theory that lowering blood pressure could reduce cerebral perfusion due to a lack of the usual autoregulatory mechanisms is counterweighted by the potential for further damage due to cerebral oedema. The Control Hypertension and Hypotension Immediately Poststroke Study (CHHIPS) randomised acute stroke patients to placebo, lisinopril (sublingual) or intravenous bolus of labetolol and evaluated the incidence of neurological deterioration. There was no adverse outcome in any actively treated group despite reductions in blood pressure (21 vs. 11 mmHg for systolic blood pressure; Potter et al., 2009) This was a relatively small study and larger confirmatory studies are required before firm recommendations for patient management should be made.

In patients with intracerebral haemorrhage, acute reduction of blood pressure has also been demonstrated to be feasible and probably safe with reduced haematoma growth in the actively treated group (Anderson et al., 2008).

Pregnancy

An increased blood pressure before 20 weeks gestation usually indicates pre-existing chronic hypertension that may not have been previously diagnosed. As in all younger hypertensive patients, a careful assessment is needed to exclude possible secondary causes, although radiological and radionuclide investigations should usually be deferred until after pregnancy. Hypertension diagnosed after 20 weeks gestation may also indicate chronic hypertension, which may have been masked during early pregnancy by the fall in blood pressure that occurs at that time. Patients with elevated blood pressure in pregnancy are at increased risk of pre-eclampsia and intrauterine growth retardation. They need frequent checks of their blood pressure, urinalysis and fetal growth. Pre-eclampsia is diagnosed when the blood pressure increases by 30/15 mmHg from measurements obtained in early pregnancy or if the diastolic blood pressure exceeds 110 mmHg and proteinuria is present. There is consensus that blood pressure should be treated with drugs if it exceeds 150–160/100–110 mmHg, although some clinicians use a lower threshold, for example, 140/90 mmHg. Methyldopa is the most suitable drug choice for use in pregnancy because of its long-term safety record. Calcium channel blockers, hydralazine and labetalol are also used. β-Blockers, particularly atenolol, are used less often as they are associated with intrauterine growth retardation. Although diuretics reduce the incidence of pre-eclampsia they are little used in pregnancy because of concerns about decreasing maternal blood volume. ACE inhibitors and ARBs are contraindicated, as they are associated with oligohydramnios, renal failure and intrauterine death.

Meta-analysis of trials suggests that antihypertensive drugs reduce risk of progression to severe hypertension and reduce hospital admissions, although excessive blood pressure reduction may reduce fetal growth.

Oral contraceptives

Use of combined oral contraceptives results, on average, in an increase of 5/3 mmHg in blood pressure. However, severe hypertension can occur in a small proportion of recipients months or years into treatment. Progesterone-only preparations do not cause hypertension so often but are less effective for contraception, especially in younger women. Combined oral contraceptives are not absolutely contraindicated in hypertension unless other risk factors for cardiovascular disease, such as smoking, are present.

Hormone replacement therapy

There is little evidence that hormone replacement therapy is associated with an increase in blood pressure and women with hypertension should not be denied access to these agents if there is an appropriate indication. However, hormone replacement therapy itself does not reduce and may increase the risk of cardiovascular events. Large increases in blood pressure have occasionally been reported in individuals and it is important to monitor blood pressure during the first few weeks of therapy and 6-monthly thereafter. In women with resistant hypertension, during treatment with hormone replacement therapy, the effectiveness of discontinuing hormone replacement should be assessed.

A list of the indications and contraindications to the various antihypertensive agents can be found in Table 19.4.

Ancillary drug treatment

Aspirin

The use of aspirin reduces cardiovascular events at the expense of an increase in gastro-intestinal complications. Its use should be restricted to patients who have no contraindications and either:

- have evidence of established vascular disease or
- have no evident cardiovascular disease but who are over 50 years of age and have either evidence of target organ damage or a 10-year cardiovascular disease risk of >20%.

Blood pressure should be controlled (<150/90 mmHg) before aspirin is instituted.

Lipid-lowering therapy

There is increasing evidence from clinical trials of the benefit of lipid-lowering drug treatment in patients with hypertension. For example, in the ASCOT study lipid-lowering arm (ASCOT-LLA), treatment with atorvastatin 10 mg was associated with substantial reductions in coronary heart disease and stroke, in spite of the fact that those with total cholesterols initially higher than 6.5 mmol/L were excluded from the study (Sever et al., 2003). Lipid-lowering therapy, usually with a statin, should be prescribed to patients under 80 years of age with a total cholesterol >3.5 mmol/L who either have pre-existing vascular disease or a 10-year cardiovascular risk of >20%.

Table 19.4 Use of antihypertensive drugs adapted from British Hypertension Society guidelines

Class	Indications	Contraindications
Diuretics	Elderly ISH Heart failure Secondary stroke prevention	Gout
β-Blockers	Myocardial infarction Angina (Heart failure)	Asthma/chronic obstructive pulmonary disease Heart block (Heart failure) (Dyslipidaemia) (Peripheral vascular disease) (Diabetes, except with coronary heart disease)
Calcium antagonists: dihydropyridine	Elderly isolated systolic hypertension (Elderly) (Angina)	
Calcium antagonists (rate limiting)	Angina (Myocardial infarction)	Combination with β-blocker (Heart block) (Heart failure)
ACE inhibitors	Heart failure Left ventricular (LV) dysfunction Type 1 diabetic nephropathy Secondary stroke prevention (Chronic renal disease) (Type 2 diabetic nephropathy) (Proteinuric renal disease)	Pregnancy Renovascular disease (Renal impairment) (Peripheral vascular disease)
α-Blockers	Benign prostatic hypertrophy (Dyslipidaemia)	Urinary incontinence (Postural hypotension) (Heart failure)
Angiotensin receptor blockers	ACE inhibitor intolerance Type 2 diabetic nephropathy Hypertension with LVH Heart failure in ACE inhibitor-intolerant subjects Post-MI (LV dysfunction post-MI) (Intolerance of other antihypertensive drugs) (Proteinuric renal disease) (Chronic renal failure) (Heart failure)	As ACE inhibitors
Centrally acting vasodilators	Pregnancy (methyldopa only) Resistant hypertension unresponsive to first-line therapy	
Direct-acting vasodilators	Resistant hypertension, unresponsive to first-line therapy	

Note: Strong indications and contraindications are shown. Text in parentheses indicates weak/possible indications or contraindications.

Case studies

Case 19.1

A 55-year-old woman of African Caribbean origin is found to have consistently elevated blood pressure over several weeks, her lowest reading being 155/98 mmHg. She is overweight and has diabetes, and is being treated with metformin. Her renal function and urinalysis are both normal.

Questions

1. Should drug therapy be initiated for her hypertension?
2. If her hypertension was treated with drugs, which agents offer particular advantages, and which should be avoided?

Answers

1. Provided her blood pressure has been measured accurately over several weeks, it should be treated, since her diabetes is an important additional risk factor. It is important to ensure that an appropriately sized blood pressure cuff is being used, in view of her obesity. Non-pharmacological interventions should also take place in parallel. Restriction of salt intake may be particularly helpful in people of African Caribbean race and weight reduction would benefit her hypertension and diabetes.

2. ACE inhibitors are an attractive choice for diabetic patients who have nephropathy. However, there is no evidence of nephropathy in this patient and ACE inhibitors are less effective antihypertensives in people of African Caribbean origin. β-Blockers reduce hypoglycaemic awareness; this is not a contraindication in this case since metformin does not cause hypoglycaemia. However, β-blockers are also less effective in those of African Caribbean descent. Diuretics work well in African Caribbean patients with hypertension, but may worsen glucose tolerance and may not, therefore, be the most appropriate first choice. Calcium channel blockers do not have adverse metabolic effects and are effective in people of this origin and would, therefore, be an appropriate choice. Tight blood pressure control is important and several agents may be required, including diuretics, ACE inhibitors, β-blockers and α-blockers.

Case 19.2

Mr PT, a 35-year-old man, is overweight and has a blood pressure of 178/114 mmHg. He smokes 25 cigarettes daily and drinks 28 units of alcohol per week. He has a sedentary occupation. He eats excessive quantities of saturated fat and salt.

Questions

1. How should this patient be managed?
2. What pharmacological treatment for blood pressure would be appropriate if non-pharmacological treatment was unsuccessful?
   Mr PT subsequently stopped smoking and lost some weight but remained hypertensive. He was treated with atenolol 50 mg daily.
   His blood pressure fell to 136/84 mmHg but he developed tiredness and bradycardia and complained of erectile impotence.
3. What are the treatment options for Mr PT?

Answers

1. Since he is a young man, his absolute risk of cardiovascular events is low, at least for the time being. However, he has several additional risk factors that need to be addressed, including his sedentary lifestyle and his smoking. Non-pharmacological methods have the potential of reducing his blood pressure considerably, including reduction in weight and salt intake. Measurement of plasma cholesterol may help him modify his diet, although he is unlikely to qualify for lipid-lowering therapy in view of his young age.

2. If drug treatment was appropriate, initial treatment with an ACE inhibitor would be consistent with current guidance, in view of his age. This is likely to be more effective for blood pressure lowering than a calcium channel blocker or diuretic. β-Blockers have been recommended as an option in younger patients but are now considered less suitable as initial therapy. Other drugs could be added or substituted if he was intolerant to initial therapy or it did not reduce his blood pressure to target levels.

3. It is possible that he would feel less tired using a β-blocker with intrinsic sympathomimetic activity (e.g. pindolol) but this is by no means guaranteed. The effects on his sexual function are unpredictable. It would probably be better to change him to a drug of a different class such as an ACE inhibitor. A calcium channel blocker or thiazide diuretic (although these also commonly cause impotence) may be added if necessary.

Case 19.3

A 24-year-old woman with a family history of hypertension is prescribed an oral contraceptive. Six months after starting this, she is noted to have a blood pressure of 148/96 mmHg.

Question

How should this patient be managed?

Answer

If her blood pressure is consistently raised she may have either essential hypertension or hypertension induced by the oral contraceptive, or a combination. Her blood pressure may fall if her oral contraceptive is discontinued. She will, however, need advice on adequate contraceptive methods. A progesterone-only preparation would be one possibility. She would need careful counselling about the methods available and how successful they are. If her blood pressure remained elevated after discontinuing her oral contraception, she is likely to have underlying hypertension. This may be essential in nature, in view of the family history; however, because of her age she should undergo some investigations to exclude possible secondary causes of hypertension. She is at low risk of complications and there is no urgency to consider drug treatment. If there is a strong wish to use combined oral contraception, it would be important to control other risk factors as far as possible and to consider drug treatment for her hypertension.

Case 19.4

A 73-year-old lady has a long-standing history of hypertension and intolerance to antihypertensive drugs. Bendroflumethiazide was associated with acute attacks of gout, she developed breathlessness and wheezing while taking atenolol, nifedipine caused flushing and headache, and doxazosin was associated with intolerable postural hypotension. Four weeks earlier she had been started on enalapril but was now complaining of a dry persistent cough. Her blood chemistry has remained normal.

Questions

1. Is the patient's cough likely to be an adverse effect of enalapril?
2. What other options are available for controlling her blood pressure?

Answers

1. Yes it is. A dry cough is a common adverse effect of ACE inhibitors. It affects approximately 10–20% of recipients and is more common in women. Some patients are able to tolerate the symptom but in many the drug has to be discontinued.

2. Angiotensin receptor blockers can be used in patients intolerant of ACE inhibitors due to cough. They are unlikely to produce this symptom since they do not inhibit the metabolism of pulmonary bradykinin. Centrally acting agents such as methyldopa or moxonidine could also be considered. However, these are not well tolerated and side effects are quite likely in this patient. A non-dihydropyridine calcium channel blocker such as verapamil is another alternative. Measurement of plasma uric acid could also be considered followed by prophylactic treatment with allopurinol before introducing a diuretic. Alternatively, a trial of spironolactone or the renin antagonist aliskiren could be considered.

Case 19.5

A 23-year-old woman has a normal blood pressure (118/82 mmHg) when reviewed at 8 weeks of pregnancy. In the 24th week of pregnancy, she is reviewed by her midwife and found to have a blood pressure of 148/96 mmHg. Urinalysis is normal.

Questions

1. What is the likely diagnosis?
2. What complications does the patient's high blood pressure place her at increased risk of?
3. Should she receive drug treatment? If so, with which drug? If not, how should she be managed?

Answers

1. She may have gestation-induced hypertension or chronic hypertension that had previously been masked by the fall in blood pressure that happens in early pregnancy.
2. She is at increased risk of pre-eclampsia and intrauterine growth retardation.
3. There are differences of opinion between specialists as to whether blood pressure should be treated at this level during pregnancy. In favour of treatment is the substantial rise over the earlier blood pressure recording. Some specialists would not treat unless the blood pressure was >170/110 mmHg or other complications were present. If she were treated, methyldopa would be a suitable choice. In any event, she needs close monitoring of her blood pressure, urinalysis and fetal growth.

Case 19.6

An elderly patient comes to the pharmacy with a prescription for the following medications: salbutamol inhaler 200 μcg as required, beclometasone inhaler 200 μcg twice daily, bendroflumethiazide 2.5 mg daily, modified release diltiazem 180 mg once daily and atenolol 50 mg daily. The atenolol was being started by the patient's primary care doctor, apparently because of inadequate blood pressure control.

Question

What action should the pharmacist take?

Answer

There are two reasons to be concerned about the addition of atenolol to this patient's drug regimen. First, there is a potentially hazardous interaction with diltiazem which may result in severe bradycardia or heart block. Second, the patient is receiving treatment for obstructive airways disease and this may be worsened by the atenolol. Third, there is increasing evidence to demonstrate the combination of a thiazide and a β-blocker increases the risk of developing diabetes. The prescription should be discussed with the prescriber.

Case 19.7

A patient is admitted to hospital with a stroke. A CT scan of the brain shows a cerebral infarct. The patient's blood pressure is 178/102 mmHg and remains at this level over the first 6 h after admission to the ward.

Question

Should antihypertensive medication be prescribed?

Answer

There is no good evidence that antihypertensive drug treatment is beneficial in the early stages of acute stroke and there is a risk that lowering blood pressure may compromise cerebral perfusion further. However, in the longer term, blood pressure reduction is valuable for preventing further strokes and other cardiovascular events. It would be appropriate to monitor the blood pressure and start treatment after a few days if it remains persistently elevated. A thiazide diuretic and/or ACE inhibitor are commonly used under these circumstances, following the demonstration of benefit in the PROGRESS study (PROGRESS Collaborative Group, 2001).

Case 19.8

A 67-year-old man has been treated for hypertension with atenolol 50 mg daily for several years. He feels well and his blood pressure is controlled. He has read an article in the paper that suggests atenolol is not considered the most suitable drug for treating high blood pressure and enquires about changing his prescription.

Question

Should an alteration to his treatment be recommended?

Answer

There is increasing evidence that β-blockers, including atenolol, may be less effective at preventing cardiovascular events, especially stroke, than other drugs and are associated with a higher risk of development of diabetes, especially if used in combination with thiazide diuretics. They are also less effective at reducing blood pressure in older people. However, if his blood pressure is well controlled and the treatment suits him there is no strong reason to change his medication unless he is at particular risk of diabetes.

Case 19.9

A 58-year-old male patient is noted to have high blood pressure by his primary care doctor. There is no evidence of end-organ damage and he has no other cardiovascular risk factors. The blood pressure remains greater than 160/100 mmHg each time it is checked in the surgery over several weeks, in spite of salt and alcohol reduction. The patient buys a wrist blood pressure monitor in a pharmacy and takes several readings at home. These are all below 130/75 mmHg.

Question

What advice should he be given about the need for drug treatment?

Answer

He may have 'white coat' hypertension. Since this is associated with a lower risk than sustained hypertension he may not need drug treatment. However, before making this judgement it is important to check that his machine is accurate. This can be done by comparing readings with a validated machine, or by checking to see if the make of blood pressure monitor has been verified as accurate by the British Hypertension Study.

References

ALLHAT Collaborative Research Group, 2000. Major cardiovascular events in hypertensive patients randomised to doxazosin vs. chorthalidone. Antihypertensive and lipid lowering treatment to prevent heart attack trial (ALLHAT). J. Am. Med. Assoc. 283, 1967–1975.

ALLHAT Collaborative Research Group, 2002. Major outcomes in high-risk hypertensive patients randomized to angiotensin-converting enzyme inhibitor or calcium channel blocker vs. diuretic: the antihypertensive and lipid lowering treatment to prevent heart attack trial (ALLHAT). J. Am. Med. Assoc. 288, 2981–2997.

Anderson, C.S., Yining, H., Wang, J.G., et al., 2008. Intensive blood pressure reduction in acute cerebral haemorrhage trial (INTERACT): a randomised pilot trial. Lancet Neurol. 7, 391–399.

Appel, L.J., Moore, T.J., Obarzanek, E., et al., 1997. A clinical trial of the effects of dietary patterns on blood pressure. N. Engl. J. Med. 336, 1117–1124.

Beckett, N.S., Peters, R., Fletcher, A.E., et al., 2008. Treatment of hypertension in patients 80 years of age or older. N. Engl. J. Med. 358, 1887–1898.

Beevers, G., Lip, G.Y.H., O'Brien, E., 2001. The pathophysiology of hypertension. Br. Med. J. 322, 912–916.

Blood Pressure Lowering Treatment Trialists Collaboration, 2000. Effects of ACE inhibitors, calcium antagonists, and other blood pressure lowering drugs: results of prospectively designed overviews of randomized trials. Lancet 356, 1955–1964.

Brown, M.J., Palmer, C.R., Castaigne, A., et al., 2000. Morbidity and mortality in patients randomised to double blind treatment with a long acting calcium channel blocker or diuretic in the international nifedipine GITS study (INSIGHT). Lancet 356, 366–372.

Cirillo, M., Lanti, M.P., Menotti, A., et al., 2008. Definition of kidney dysfunction as a cardiovascular risk factor: use of urinary albumin excretion and estimated glomerular filtration rate. Arch. Int. Med. 168, 617–624.

Collins, R., Petro, R., MacMahon, S., et al., 1990. Blood pressure, stroke and coronary heart disease. Part 2. Short-term reductions in blood pressure: overview of randomised drugs trials in their epidemiological context. Lancet 335, 827–838.

Dahlöf, B., Devereux, R., Kjeldsen, S.E., et al., 2002. Cardiovascular morbidity and mortality in the Losartan For Endpoint reduction in hypertension study (LIFE): a randomised trial against atenolol. Lancet 359, 995–1003.

Dahlöf, B., Sever, P.S., Poulter, N.R., et al., ASCOT Investigators, 2005. Prevention of cardiovascular events with an antihypertensive regimen of amlodipine adding perindopril as required versus atenolol adding bendroflumethiazide as required, in the Anglo Scandinavian Cardiac Outcomes Trial – Blood Pressure Lowering Arm (ASCOT–BPLA). Lancet 366, 895–906.

Furberg, C.D., Psaty, B.M., Meyer, J.V., 1995. Nifedipine: dose-related increase in mortality in patients with coronary heart disease. Circulation 92, 1326–1331.

Gong, L., Zhang, W., Zhu, Y., et al., 1996. Shanghai Trial Of Nifedipine in the Elderly (STONE). J. Hypertens. 14, 1237–1245.

Hansson, L., Lindholm, L.H., Niskanen, L., et al., 1999a. Effect of angiotensin-converting-enzyme inhibition compared with conventional therapy on cardiovascular morbidity and mortality in hypertension. The Captopril Prevention Project (CAPPP). Lancet 353, 611–616.

Hansson, L., Lindholm, L.H., Ekbom, T., et al., 1999b. Randomised trial of old and new antihypertensive drugs in elderly patients: cardiovascular mortality and morbidity in the Swedish Trial in Old Patients with hypertension-2 study. Lancet 354, 1751–1756.

Hansson, L., Zanchetti, A., Carruthers, S.G., et al., for the HOT Study Group, 1998. Effects of intensive blood-pressure lowering and low-dose aspirin in patients with hypertension: principal results of the hypertension optimal treatment (HOT) randomised trial. Lancet 351, 1755–1762.

Holman, R.R., Paul, S.K., Bethel, M.A., et al., 2008. Long-term follow-up after tight control of blood pressure in type 2 diabetes. N. Engl. J. Med. 359, 1565–1576.

JATOS Study Group, 2008. Principal results of the Japanses trial to assess optimal systolic blood pressure in elderly hypertensive patients. Hypertens. Res. 31, 2115–2127.

Joint British Societies, 2005. JBS 2: Joint British Societies' guidelines on prevention of cardiovascular disease in clinical practice. Heart 91, v1–v52.

Julius, S., Kjeldsen, S.E., Weber, M., et al., 2004. Outcomes in hypertensive patients at high cardiovascular risk treated with regimens based on valsartan or amlodipine: the VALUE randomised trial. Lancet 363, 2022–2031.

Lindholm, L.H., Carlberg, B., Samuelsson, O., 2005. Should beta blockers remain first choice in the treatment of primary hypertension? A meta-analysis. Lancet 366, 1545–1553.

Lithell, H., Hansson, L., Skoog, I., et al., SCOPE Study Group, 2003. The Study of Cognition and Prognosis in the Elderly (SCOPE): principal results of a randomised double-blind intervention trial. J. Hypertens. 21, 875–1866.

Mancia, G., de Backer, G., Dominiczak, A., et al., 2007. Guidelines for the management of arterial hypertension. The Task Force for the Management of Arterial Hypertension of the European Society of hypertension (ESH) and of the European Society of Cardiology (ESC). J. Hypertens. 25, 1105–1187.

Mancia, G., Laurent, S., Agabiti-Rosei, E., et al., 2009. Reappraisal of European guidelines on hypertension management: a European Society of Hypertension Task Force document. J. Hypertens. 27, 2121–2158.

Mason, J., Dickinson, H., Nicolson, D., et al., 2004. The diabetogenic potential of thiazide diuretics and beta-blocker combinations in the management of hypertension. Available at: http://www2.cochrane.org/colloquia/abstracts/ottawa/P-097.htm.

National Collaborating Centre for Chronic Conditions, Hypertension. 2006, Management of hypertension in adults in primary care: partial update. Royal College of Physicians, London. Available at: http://www.nice.org.uk/page.aspx?o=CG034fullguideline.

O'Brien, E., Barton, J., Nussberger, J., et al., 2007. Aliskiren reduces blood pressure and suppresses plasma renin activity in combination with a thiazide diuretic, an angiotensin-converting enzyme inhibitor, or an angiotensin receptor blocker. Hypertension 49, 276–284.

Patel, A., MacMahon, S., Chalmers, J., et al., 2007. Effects of a fixed combination of perindopril and indapamide on macrovascular and microvascular outcomes in patients with type 2 diabetes mellitus (the ADVANCE trial): a randomised controlled trial. Lancet 370, 829–840.

Potter, J.F., Robinson, T.G., Ford, G.A., et al., 2009. Controlling hypertension and hypotension immediately post stroke (CHHIPS): a randomized, placebo-controlled, double-blind pilot trial. Lancet Neurol. 8, 48–56.

PROGRESS Collaborative Group, 2001. Randomised trial of a perindopril-based blood pressure lowering regimen among 6105 individuals with previous stroke or transient ischaemic attack. Lancet 358, 1033–1041.

Psaty, B.M., Heckbert, S.R., Kocpsell, T.D., et al., 1995. The risk of myocardial infarction associated with antihypertensive drug therapies. J. Am. Med. Assoc. 274, 620–625.

Sehestedt, T., Jeppesen, J., Hansen, T.W., et al., 2009. Which markers of subclinical organ damage to measure in individuals with high normal blood pressure? J. Hypertens. 27, 1165–1171.

Sever, P.S., Dahlof, B., Poulter, N.R., et al., 2003. Prevention of coronary and stroke events with atorvastatin in patients who have average or lower-than-average cholesterol concentrations in the Anglo Scandinavian Cardiac Outcomes Trial – Lipid Lowering Arm. Lancet 361, 1149–1158.

SHEP Co-operative Research Group, 1991. Prevention of stroke by antihypertensive drug treatment in older persons with isolated systolic hypertension: final results of the Systolic Hypertension in the Elderly Program (SHEP). J. Am. Med. Assoc. 265, 3255–3264.

Staessen, J.A., Fagard, R., Thijs, L., et al., for the Systolic Hypertension in Europe (Syst-Eur) Trial Investigators, 1997. Randomised double-blind comparison of placebo and active treatment for older patients with isolated systolic hypertension. Lancet 350, 757–764.

UK Prospective Diabetes Study Group, 1998a. Tight blood pressure control and risk of macrovascular and microvascular complications in type 2 diabetes: UKPDS 38. Br. Med. J. 317, 703–713.

UK Prospective Diabetes Study Group, 1998b. Efficacy of atenolol and captopril in reducing risk of macrovascular and microvascular complications in type 2 diabetes: UKPDS 39. Br. Med. J. 317, 713–726.

Verdecchia, P., Staessen J.A., Angeli, F., et al., on behalf of the Cardio-Sis investigators, 2009. Usual versus tight control of systolic blood pressure in non-diabetic patients with hypertension (Cardio-Sis): an open-label randomised trial. Lancet 374, 525–533.

Weber, M.A., Black, H., Bakris, G., et al., 2009. A selective endothelin-receptor antagonist to reduce blood pressure in patients with treatment-resistant hypertension: a randomised, double-blind, placebo-controlled trial. Lancet 374, 1423–1431.

Williams, B., Poulter, N.R., Brown, M.J., et al., 2004. Guidelines for the management of hypertension: report of the fourth working party of the British Hypertension Society, 2004 – BHS IV. J. Hum. Hypertens. 18, 139–185. Reprinted by permission from Macmillan Publishers Ltd.

Wing, L.M.H., Reid, C.M., Ryan, P., et al., 2003. A comparison of outcomes with angiotensin-converting-enzyme inhibitors and diuretics for hypertension in the elderly. N. Engl. J. Med. 348, 583–592.

Yusuf, S., Teo, K.K., Pogue, J., et al., 2008a. ONTARGET Investigators Telmisartan, ramipril, or both in patients at high risk for vascular events. N. Engl. J. Med. 358, 1547–1559.

Yusuf, S., Diener, H.C., Sacco, R.L., et al., PRoFESS Study Group, 2008b. Telmisartan to prevent recurrent stroke and cardiovascular events. N. Engl. J. Med. 359, 1225–1237.

Further reading

Brown, M.J., Cruickshank, J.K., Dominiczak, A.F., et al., 2003. Better blood pressure control: how to combine drugs. J. Hum. Hypertens. 17, 81–86.

Gradman, A.H., Basile, J.N., Carter, B.I., et al., 2010. Combination therapy in hypertension. J. Am. Soc. Hypertens. 4, 42–50.

Hollenberg, N.K., 2009. Atlas of Hypertension, sixth ed. Current Medicine, Philadelphia.

Ljungman, C., Mortensen, L., Kahan, T., et al., 2009. Treatment of mild to moderate hypertension by gender perspective: a systematic review. J. Womens Health 18, 1049–1062.

Mancia, G., Laurent, S., Agabiti-Rosei, E., et al., 2009. Reappraisal of European guidelines on hypertension management: a European Society of Hypertension Task Force document. J. Hypertens. 27, 2121–2158.

Messerli, F., Williams, B., Ritz, E., 2007. Essential hypertension. Lancet 370, 591–603.

Mohler, E.R., Townsend, R.R., 2005. Advanced Therapy in Hypertension and Vascular Disease. BC Decker Inc., Hamilton.

Safar, M., O'Rourke, M., 2006. Arterial Stiffness in Hypertension. Elsevier, Oxford.

20 Coronary heart disease

D. McRobbie

Key points

- Coronary heart disease (CHD) is common, often fatal and frequently preventable.
- High dietary fat, smoking and sedentary lifestyle are risk factors for CHD and require modification if present.
- Hypertension, hypercholesterolaemia and diabetes mellitus, obesity and personal stress are also risk factors and require optimal management.
- Stable angina should be managed with nitrates for pain relief and β-blockers, unless contraindicated, for long-term prophylaxis. Where β-blockers are inappropriate, the use of calcium channel blockers and/or nitrates may be considered.
- Acute coronary syndromes arise from unstable atheromatous plaques and may be classified as to whether there is ST elevation myocardial infarction (STEMI) or non-ST elevation myocardial infarction (NSTEMI).
- ST elevation on the ECG indicates an occluded coronary artery and is used to determine treatment with fibrinolysis or primary angioplasty.
- Patients with NSTEMI may have experienced myocardial damage, are at increased risk of death and may benefit from a glycoprotein IIb/IIIa inhibitor.

Coronary heart disease (CHD), sometimes described as coronary artery disease (CAD) or ischaemic heart disease (IHD), is a condition in which the vascular supply to the heart is impeded by atheroma, thrombosis or spasm of coronary arteries. This may impair the supply of oxygenated blood to cardiac tissue sufficiently to cause myocardial ischaemia which, if severe or prolonged, may cause the death of cardiac muscle cells. Similarities in the development of atheromatous plaques in other vasculature, in particular the carotid arteries, with the resultant cerebral ischaemia has resulted in the term cardiovascular disease (CVD) being adopted to incorporate CHD, cerebrovascular disease and peripheral vascular disease.

Myocardial ischaemia occurs when the oxygen demand exceeds myocardial oxygen supply. The resultant ischaemic myocardium releases adenosine, the main mediator of chest pain, by stimulating the A1 receptors located on the cardiac nerve endings. Myocardial ischaemia may be 'silent' if the duration is of insufficient length, the afferent cardiac nerves are damaged (as with diabetics) or there is inhibition of the pain at the spinal or supraspinal level.

Factors increasing myocardial oxygen demand often precipitate ischaemic episodes and are commonly associated with increased work rate (heart rate) and increased work load (force of contractility). Less commonly, myocardial ischaemia can also arise if oxygen demand is abnormally increased, as may occur in patients with thyrotoxicosis or severe ventricular hypertrophy due to hypertension. Myocardial oxygen supply is dependant on the luminal cross-sectional area of the coronary artery and coronary arteriolar tone. Atheromatous plaques decrease the lumen diameter and, when extensive, reduce the ability of the coronary artery to dilate in response to increased myocardial oxygen demand. Ischaemia may also occur when the oxygen-carrying capacity of blood is impaired, as in iron-deficiency anaemia, or when the circulatory volume is depleted.

CHD kills over 6.5 million people worldwide each year.

Epidemiology

Almost 200,000 people die from CVD in the UK each year with CHD accounting for almost a half of these. About 30% of premature deaths (below 75 years old) in men and 22% of premature deaths in women result from CVD.

The epidemiology of CHD has been studied extensively and risk factors for developing CHD are now well described. Absence of established risk factors does not guarantee freedom from CHD for any individual, and some individuals with several major risk factors seem perversely healthy. Nonetheless, there is evidence that in developed countries, education and publicity about the major risk factors have led to changes in social habits, particularly with respect to a reduction in smoking and fat consumption, and this has contributed to a decrease in the incidence of CHD.

The UK has seen a steady decline in deaths from CHD of about 4.5% per annum since the late 1970s. A recent study indicated that both reductions in major risk factors and improvements in treatment have contributed to this reduction (Unal et al., 2004). While impressive, this rate of decline has not been as great as in other countries like Australia and Finland. In Eastern European countries, the death rates from CHD have increased significantly during the same period.

The improvement in deaths from CHD has been chiefly among those with higher incomes; however, the less prosperous social classes continue to have almost unchanged levels of CHD. Better treatment has also contributed to a decrease

312

in cardiac mortality, although CHD still accounted for some 94,000 deaths in 2006 in the UK, including 70% of sudden natural deaths, 22% of male deaths and 16% of female deaths. In most developed countries, CHD is the leading cause of adult death but in the UK the poor outcome of lung cancer treatments makes cancer marginally the leading cause. In the UK, in comparison with Caucasians, people of South Asian descent have a 45–50% higher death rate from CHD, and Caribbeans and West Africans have a 35–50% lower rate.

Prevalence

About 3.5% of UK adults have symptomatic CHD. One-third of men aged 50–59 years of age have evidence of CHD, and this proportion increases with age. In the UK, there are about 1.3 million people who have survived a myocardial infarction and about 2 million who have, or have had, angina and this equates to about 5% of men and 3% of women. Approximately 260,000 people suffer a myocardial infarction in any year, of whom 40–50% die.

Mortality increases with age and is probably not due to a particular age-related factor but to the cumulative effect of risk factors that lead to atheroma and thrombosis and hence to CAD. In the USA, age-related death rates for CHD have fallen by 25% over a decade, but the total number of CHD deaths has fallen by only 10% because the population is ageing. Similarly, in the UK the death rates are falling but the numbers living with CHD are increasing.

Women appear less susceptible to CHD than men, although they seem to lose this protection after menopause, presumably because of hormonal changes. Race has not proved to be a clear risk factor since the prevalence of CHD seems to depend much more strongly on location and lifestyle than on ethnic origin or place of birth. It has been shown that lower social or economic class is associated with increased obesity, poor cholesterol indicators, higher blood pressure and higher C-reactive protein (CRP) measurements, an indicator of inflammatory activity.

Risk factors

Traditionally, the main potentially modifiable risk factors for CHD have been considered to be hypertension, cigarette smoking, raised serum cholesterol and diabetes. More recently psychological stress and abdominal obesity have gained increased prominence (Box 20.1). Patients with a combination of all these risk factors are at risk of suffering a myocardial infarction some 500 times greater than individuals without any of the risk factors. Stopping smoking, moderating alcohol intake, regular exercise and consumption of fresh fruit and vegetables were associated independently and additively with reduction in the risk of having a myocardial infarction.

Diabetes mellitus is a positive risk factor for CHD in developed countries with high levels of CHD, but it is not a risk factor in countries with little CHD. Insulin resistance, as defined by high fasting insulin concentrations, is an independent risk factor for CHD in men. In the UK, the mortality rates from CHD are up to five times higher for people with diabetes, while the risk of stroke is up to three times higher.

Box 20.1 Factors that increase or decrease the risk of developing CHD

Factors that increase the risk of CHD
Cigarette smoking
Raised serum cholesterol
Hypertension
Diabetes
Abdominal obesity
Increased personal stress

Factors that decrease the risk of CHD
Regular consumption of fresh fruit and vegetables
Regular exercise
Moderate alcohol consumption
Modification of factors that increase the risk of CHD

While unusual physical exertion is associated with an increased risk of infarction, an active lifestyle that includes regular, moderate exercise is beneficial, although the optimum level has not been determined and its beneficial effect appears to be readily overwhelmed by the presence of other risk factors. A family history of CHD is a positive risk factor, independent of diet and other risk factors. Hostility, anxiety or depression are associated with increased CHD and death, especially after myocardial infarction when mortality is doubled by anxiety and quadrupled by depression.

Epidemiological studies have shown associations between CHD and prior infections with several common microorganisms, including *Chlamydia pneumoniae* and *Helicobacter pylori*, but a causal connection has not been shown. The influence of fetal and infant growth conditions, and their interaction with social conditions in childhood and adult life, has been debated strongly for decades but it is clear that lower socio-economic status and thinness in very early life are linked to higher incidences of CHD.

Aetiology

The vast majority of CHD occurs in patients with atherosclerosis of the coronary arteries (see Fig. 20.1) that starts before adulthood. The cause of spontaneous artherosclerosis is unclear, although it is thought that in the presence of hypercholesterolaemia, a non-denuding form of injury occurs to the endothelial lining of coronary arteries and other vessels. This injury is followed by subendothelial migration of monocytes and the accumulation of fatty streaks containing lipid-rich macrophages and T-cells. Almost all adults, and 50% of children aged 11–14 years, have fatty streaks in their coronary arteries. Thereafter, there is migration and proliferation of smooth muscle cells into the intima with further lipid deposition. The smooth muscle cells, together with fibroblasts, synthesise and secrete collagen, proteoglycans, elastin and glycoproteins that make up a fibrous cap surrounding cells and necrotic tissue, together called a plaque. The presence of atherosclerotic plaques results in narrowing of vessels and a reduction in blood flow and a decrease in the ability of the

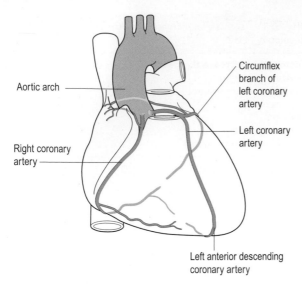

Fig. 20.1 Main coronary arteries.

coronary vasculature to dilate and this may become manifest as angina. Associated with the plaque rupture is a loss of endothelium. This can serve as a stimulus for the formation of a thrombus and result in more acute manifestations of CHD, including unstable angina (UA) and myocardial infarction. Plaque rupture caused by physical stresses or plaque erosion may precipitate an acute reaction. Other pathological processes are probably involved, including endothelial dysfunction which alters the fibrin–fibrinolysis balance and the vasoconstriction–vasodilation balance. There is interest in the role of statins and angiotensin-converting enzyme (ACE) inhibitors in modifying endothelial function.

There is also great interest in the role of inflammation, especially in acute episodes. At postmortem, many plaques are found to contain inflammatory cells and inflammatory damage is found at the sites of plaque rupture.

Measurement of acute phase inflammatory reactions, such as fibrinogen and CRP, has a predictive association with coronary events. High-sensitivity CRP assays have been used in populations without acute illness to stratify individuals into high-, medium- and low-risk groups. In patients with other risk factors, however, CRP adds little prognostic information. CRP is produced by atheroma, in addition to the major producer which is the liver, and is an inflammatory agent as well as a marker of inflammation. Evidence is emerging that drug therapy which reduces CRP in otherwise healthy individuals reduces the incidence of major cardiac events (Ridker, 2008).

Oxidative stress which involves the uncontrolled production of reactive oxygen species (ROS) or a reduction in antioxidant species has been linked in the laboratory to several aspects of cardiovascular pathogenesis including endothelial malfunction, lipid metabolism, atheroma formation and plaque rupture, but the clinical importance is unclear. The use of antioxidants has been disappointingly unsuccessful but there is interest in peroxisome proliferator-activated receptor (PPAR) agonists that modify ROS production; some of these are already in use for treating diabetes and are associated with favourable changes in many metabolic markers for CVD. Other agents that reduce ROS production include statins and drugs that reduce angiotensin production.

Modification of risk factors

Common to all stages of CHD treatment is the need to reduce risk factors (Table 20.1). The patient needs to appreciate the value of the proposed strategy and to be committed to a plan for changing their lifestyle and habits, which may not be easy to achieve after years of smoking or eating a particular diet. Preventing CHD is important but neither instant nor spectacular. It may require many sessions of counseling over several years to initiate and maintain healthy habits. It may also involve persuasion of patients to continue taking medication

Table 20.1 Effect of interventions on risk of myocardial infarction

Intervention	Control	Benefit of intervention
Stopping smoking for ≥5 years	Current smokers	50–70% lower risk
Reducing serum cholesterol		2% lower risk for each 1% reduction in cholesterol
Treatment of hypertension		2–3% lower risk for each 1 mmHg decrease in diastolic pressure
Active lifestyle	Sedentary lifestyle	45% lower risk
Mild to moderate alcohol consumption (approx. 1 unit/day)	Total abstainers	25–45% lower risk
Low-dose aspirin	Non-users	33% lower risk in men
Postmenopausal oestrogen replacement	Non-users	44% lower risk

The quality of data associated with these interventions varies greatly and figures may not apply to all patient groups.

for asymptomatic disorders such as hypertension or hyperlipidaemia. The general public, with government as its agent, need to agree that a reduction in the incidence of CHD is worth some general changes in lifestyle or liberty, for example, such as prohibiting the freedom to smoke in public. National campaigns to encourage healthy eating or exercise are expensive, as is the long-term medical treatment of hypertension or hyperlipidaemia, and such strategies must have the backing of governments to succeed. It has been argued that community-wide campaigns on cholesterol reduction have had measurable benefits in Finland, the USA and elsewhere, at least in high-risk, well-educated and affluent groups. It follows that the next challenge is to extend that success to poorer, ethnically diverse groups and to those portions of the population with mild-to-moderate risk.

For every individual there is a need to act against the causative factors of CHD. Thus, attempts should be made to control hypertension, heart failure, arrhythmias, dyslipidaemia, obesity, diabetes mellitus, thyroid disease, anaemia and cardiac valve disorders. Apart from medication, these will require careful attention to diet and exercise and will necessitate smoking cessation. Cardiac rehabilitation classes and exercise programmes improve many risk factors including obesity, lipid indices, insulin resistance, psychological state and lifestyle. They also impact on morbidity and mortality.

Epidemiological studies have suggested that antioxidants and hormone replacement therapy may be of benefit in preventing and treating coronary disease. Unfortunately, randomised clinical trials of vitamin E or hormone replacement therapy suggest that these agents are not of benefit and may indeed result in higher rates of cardiovascular events.

Clinical syndromes

The primary clinical manifestation of CHD is chest pain. Chest pain arising from stable coronary atheromatous disease leads to stable angina and normally arises when narrowing of the coronary artery lumen exceeds 50% of the original luminal diameter. Stable angina is characterised by chest pain and breathlessness on exertion; symptoms are relieved promptly by rest.

A stable coronary atheromatous plaque may become unstable as a result of either plaque erosion or rupture. Exposure of the subendothelial lipid and collagen stimulates the formation of thrombus which causes sudden narrowing of the vessel. The spectrum of clinical outcomes that result are grouped together under the term acute coronary syndrome (ACS) and characterised by chest pain of increasing severity either on minimal exertion or, more commonly, at rest. These patients are at high risk of myocardial infarction and death and require prompt hospitalisation. Many aspects of the treatment of stable angina and ACS are similar but there is a much greater urgency and intensity in the management of ACS.

Stable angina

Stable angina is a clinical syndrome characterised by discomfort in the chest, jaw, shoulder, back, or arms, typically elicited by exertion or emotional stress and relieved by rest or nitroglycerin. Characteristically, the discomfort (it is often not described by the patient as a pain) occurs after a predictable level of exertion, classically when climbing hills or stairs, and resolves within a few minutes on resting. Unfortunately, the clinical manifestations of angina are very variable. Many patients mistake the discomfort for indigestion. Some patients, particularly diabetics and the elderly, may not experience pain at all but present with breathlessness or fatigue; this is termed silent ischaemia.

Further investigations are needed to confirm the diagnosis and assess the need for intervention. The resting electrocardiogram (ECG) is normal in more than half of patients with angina. However, an abnormal ECG substantially increases the probability of coronary disease; in particular, it may show signs of previous myocardial infarction. Non-invasive testing is helpful. Exercise testing is useful both in confirming the diagnosis and in giving a guide to prognosis. Alternatives such as myocardial scintigraphy (isotope scanning) and stress echocardiography (ultrasound) provide similar information.

Coronary angiography is regarded as the gold standard for the assessment of CAD and involves the passage of a catheter through the arterial circulation and the injection of radio-opaque contrast media into the coronary arteries. The X-ray images obtained permit confirmation of the diagnosis, aid assessment of prognosis and guide therapy, particularly with regard to suitability for angioplasty and coronary artery bypass grafting.

Non-invasive techniques, including magnetic resonance imaging (MRI) and multi-slice CT scanning, are being developed and tested as alternatives to angiography.

Treatment of stable angina is based on two principles:

- Improve prognosis by preventing myocardial infarction and death.
- Relieve or prevent symptoms.

Pharmacological therapy can be considered a viable alternative to invasive strategies, providing similar results without the complications associated with percutaneous coronary intervention (PCI). An algorithm for addressing both these principles is outlined in Fig. 20.2. In addition, diabetes, hypertension and dyslipidaemia in patients with stable angina should be well controlled. Smoking cessation, without or with pharmacological support, and weight loss should be attempted.

Antithrombotic drugs

One of the major complications arising from atheromatous plaque is thrombus formation. This causes an increase in plaque size and may result in myocardial infarction. Antiplatelet agents, in particular aspirin, are effective in preventing platelet activation and thus thrombus formation. Aspirin is of proven benefit in all forms of established CHD, although the risk–benefit ratio in people at risk of CHD is less clear.

Aspirin. Aspirin acts via irreversible inhibition of platelet COX-1 and thus thromboxane production, which is normally complete with chronic dosing of 75 mg/day. This antiplatelet action is apparent within an hour of taking a dose of 300 mg. The effect on platelets lasts for the lifetime of the platelet.

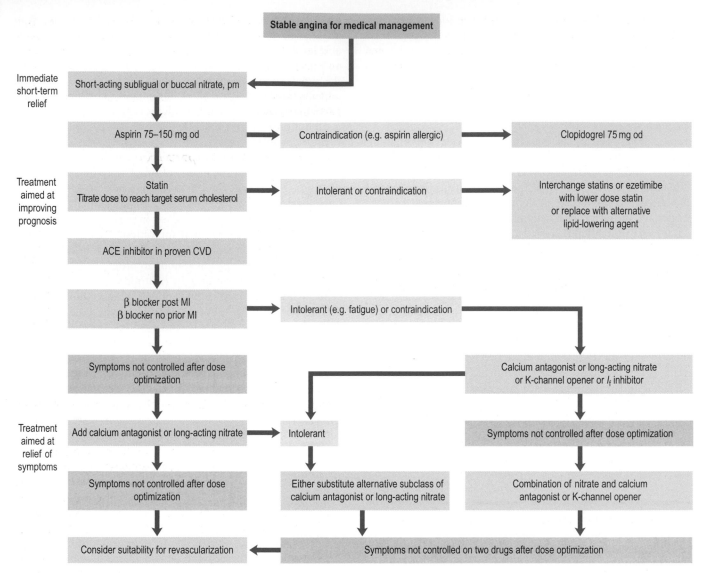

Fig. 20.2 Algorithm for the medical management of stable angina (Fox et al., 2006).

The optimal maintenance dose seems to be 75–150 mg day with lower doses having limited cardiac risk protection and higher doses increasing the risk of gastro-intestinal side effects. Dyspepsia is relatively common in patients taking aspirin and patients should be advised to take the medicine with or immediately after food. Enteric-coated preparations are no safer, and patients with ongoing symptoms of dyspepsia may require concomitant acid suppression with a proton pump inhibitor or switching to clopidogrel. Adverse reactions to aspirin include allergy, including bronchospasm. The benefits and risk of using aspirin in patients with asthma or a previous history of gastro-intestinal bleeding need to be carefully considered.

Clopidogrel. Clopidogrel inhibits ADP activation of platelets and is useful as an alternative to aspirin in patients who are allergic or cannot tolerate aspirin. Data from one major trial (CAPRIE Steering Committee, 1996) indicate that clopidogrel is at least as effective as aspirin in patients with stable

coronary disease. The usual dose is 300 mg once, then 75 mg daily. Although less likely to cause gastric erosion and ulceration, gastro-intestinal bleeding is still a major complication of clopidogrel therapy. There is evidence that the combination of a proton pump inhibitor and aspirin is as effective as using clopidogrel alone in patients with a history of upper gastro-intestinal bleeding.

COX-2 inhibitors. The analgesic and anti-inflammatory action of non-steroidal anti-inflammatory drugs (NSAIDs) is believed to depend mainly on their inhibition of COX-2, and the unwanted gastro-intestinal effects of NSAIDs on their inhibition of COX-1. COX-2 inhibition reduces the production of prostacyclin, which has vasodilatory and platelet-inhibiting effects. Studies have raised concern about the cardiovascular safety of NSAIDs. Initially, the concern was focussed on the selective cyclo-oxygenase-2 inhibitors and a link to an increased cardiovascular risk. Recently, evidence has shown the more traditional non-selective NSAIDs increase cardiovascular risk in both patients with established CVD and in the healthy population (Fosbol et al., 2010). NSAIDs with high COX-2 specificity increase the risk of myocardial infarction and should be avoided where possible in patients with stable angina.

ACE inhibitors

ACE inhibitors are established treatments for hypertension and heart failure, and have proven beneficial post myocardial infarction. In addition to the vasodilation caused by inhibiting the production of angiotensin II, ACE inhibitors have anti-inflammatory, antithrombotic and antiproliferative properties. Some of these effects are mediated by actions on vascular endothelium and might be expected to be of benefit in all patients with CAD. ACE inhibitors also reduce the production of ROS.

The use of ACE inhibitors in patients without myocardial infarction or left ventricular damage is based on two trials: the HOPE study (Yusuf et al., 2000) which studied ramipril and the EUROPA (2003) study which used perindopril. These trials also identified an incidental delay in the onset of diabetes mellitus in susceptible individuals which may be of long-term benefit to them. The HOPE study, a secondary prevention trial, investigated the effect of an ACE inhibitor on patients over 55 years old who had known atherosclerotic disease or diabetes plus one other cardiovascular risk factor. The use of ramipril decreased the combined endpoint of stroke, myocardial infarction or cardiovascular death by approximately 22%. The benefits were independent of blood pressure reduction. This has major implications for the management of CHD patients, both for the decision to treat all and the choice of treatment. At present the use of ACE inhibitors in patients with coronary disease, but without myocardial infarction, has general acceptance and is recommended in European guidelines.

Statins

Studies have repeatedly demonstrated the benefit of reducing cholesterol, especially low-density lipoprotein-cholesterol (LDL-C), in patients with CHD.

Earlier studies focused on patients with 'elevated' cholesterol, but all patients with coronary risk factors benefit from reduction of their serum cholesterol level. It is now clear that there is no 'safe' level of cholesterol for patients with CAD and that there is a continuum of risk down to very low cholesterol levels. Levels of LDL-C of <2mmol/L and total cholesterol <4mmol/L are recommended for patients with established CVD (NICE, 2008). Statins should be prescribed alongside lifestyle advice for both primary prevention of CVD and in those with established CVD (see Chapter 24 for more detail).

In addition to cholesterol-lowering properties, statins also have antithrombotic, anti-inflammatory and antiproliferative properties. They are also important in restoring normal endothelial function and inhibit the production of ROS in the vessel wall. There is some evidence that patients with elevated levels of CRP have better outcomes with statin therapy even if cholesterol levels are not raised. Most patients with stable angina will be on statins for their cholesterol-lowering effects. It is important, however, to recognise that these drugs may have beneficial effects independent of cholesterol lowering and this makes them valuable even in patients with 'normal' cholesterol levels.

Symptom relief and prevention

In stable angina, much of the drug treatment is directed towards decreasing the workload of the heart and, to a lesser extent, improving coronary blood supply; this provides symptomatic relief and improves prognosis. Therapy to decrease workload is targeted at both decreasing afterload and controlling heart rate. Recent evidence suggests a prognostic benefit when the resting heart rate is controlled below 70 beats/min. Drug treatment is initiated in a stepwise fashion according to symptom relief and side effects. A number of patients will require a number of anti-anginal medicine to control their angina symptoms.

β-Blockers

Various studies have demonstrated the beneficial effect of β-blockers in angina and they are now considered first-line agents. β-Blockers reduce mortality both in patients who have suffered a previous myocardial infarction and in those with heart failure. They reduce myocardial oxygen demand by blocking β-adrenergic receptors, thereby decreasing the heart rate and force of left ventricular contraction and lowering blood pressure. The decreased heart rate not only reduces the energy demand on the heart but also permits better perfusion of the subendocardium by the coronary circulation. β-Blockers may also reduce energy-demanding supraventricular or atrial arrhythmias and counteract the cardiac effects of hyperthyroidism or phaeochromocytoma.

β-Blockers are particularly useful in exertional angina. Patients treated optimally should have a resting heart rate of around 60 beats/min. Although many patients may dislike the side effects of β-blockers, they should be urged to continue wherever reasonable. β-Blockers should be used with caution in patients with diabetes as the production of insulin is under adrenergic system control and thus their concomitant use may worsen glucose control. β-Blockers can also mask the symptoms of hypoglycaemia and patients in whom the combination is considered of value should be warned of this; however, most clinicians now believe that the benefits of taking β-blockers, even in diabetics, outweigh the risks and they are frequently prescribed.

While β-blockers are widely used, their tendency to cause bronchospasm and peripheral vascular spasm means that they are contraindicated in patients with asthma, and used with caution in chronic obstructive airways diseases and peripheral vascular disease as well as in acute heart failure and bradycardia.

Cardioselective agents such as atenolol, bisoprolol and metoprolol are preferred because of their reduced tendency to cause bronchoconstriction, but no β-blocker is completely specific for the heart. Agents with low lipophilicity, for example, atenolol, penetrate the central nervous system (CNS) to a lesser extent than others, for example, propranolol, metoprolol, and do not so readily cause the nightmares, hallucinations and depression that are sometimes found with lipophilic agents, which should not be used in patients with psychiatric disorders. CNS-mediated fatigue or lethargy is found in some patients with all β-blockers, although it must be distinguished from that of myocardial suppression. β-Blockers should not be stopped abruptly for fear of precipitating angina through rebound receptor hypersensitivity. They are contraindicated in the rare Prinzmetal's angina where coronary spasm is a major factor.

All β-blockers tend to reduce renal blood flow, but this is only important in renal impairment. Drugs eliminated by the kidney (Table 20.2) may need to be given at lower doses in the renally impaired or in the elderly, who are particularly susceptible to the CNS-mediated lassitude. Drugs eliminated by the liver have a number of theoretical interactions with other agents that affect liver blood flow or metabolic rate, but these are rarely of clinical significance since the dose should be titrated to the effect. Likewise, although there is theoretical support for the use of agents with high intrinsic sympathomimetic activity (ISA) to reduce the incidence or severity of drug-induced heart failure, there is no β-blocker that is free from this problem, and clinical trials of drugs with ISA have generally failed to show any extra benefit.

Calcium channel blockers

Calcium channel blockers (CCBs) act on a variety of smooth muscle and cardiac tissues and there are a large number of agents which have differing specificities for different body tissues.

Table 20.2 Properties and pharmacokinetics of β-blockers

	Blockade	Lipophilicity	ISA	Oral absorption	Elimination
Acebutolol	β_1 (some β_2)	+	+	90%[a]	Active metabolite ($t_{1/2}$ 11–13 h, renal)
					Gut 50%, $t_{1/2}$ 3–4 h
Atenolol	β_1	–	–	50%	Renal $t_{1/2}$ 5–7 h
Betaxolol	β_1	+	–	100%	Hepatic + renal $t_{1/2}$ 15 h
Bisoprolol	β_1	+	–	90%	Hepatic + renal $t_{1/2}$ 10–12 h
Carteolol	$\beta_1\beta_2$	–	++	80%	Hepatic + renal $t_{1/2}$ 3–7 h
Carvedilol	$\beta_1\beta_2\alpha_1$	+	–	80%[a]	Hepatic + renal $t_{1/2}$ 4–8 h
Celiprolol	$\beta_1\alpha_2$	–	β_2+	30–70%	Renal + gut $t_{1/2}$ 5–6 h
Esmolol	β_1	–	–	i.v.	Blood enzymes $t_{1/2}$ 9 min
Labetalol	$\beta_1\beta_2\alpha_1$	–	–	100%[a]	Hepatic $t_{1/2}$ 6–8 h
Metoprolol	β_1	+	–	95%[a]	Hepatic $t_{1/2}$ 3–4 h
Nadolol	$\beta_1\beta_2$	–	–	30%	Renal $t_{1/2}$ 16–18 h
Nebivolol	β_1	+	–	12–96%[b]	Hepatic $t_{1/2}$ 8–27 h[b]
Oxprenolol	$\beta_1\beta_2$	+	++	90%[a]	Hepatic + $t_{1/2}$ 1–2 h
Pindolol	$\beta_1\beta_2$	+	+++	90%	Hepatic + renal $t_{1/2}$ 3–4 h
Propranolol	$\beta_1\beta_2$	+	–	90%[a]	Hepatic $t_{1/2}$ 3–6 h
Sotalol	$\beta_1\beta_2$	–	–	70%	Renal $t_{1/2}$ 15–17 h
Timolol	$\beta_1\beta_2$	+	–	90%[a]	Hepatic + renal $t_{1/2}$ 3–4 h

All figures are approximate and subject to interpatient variability. Therapeutic ranges are not well defined.
ISA, intrinsic sympathomimetic activity; $t_{1/2}$, elimination half-life.
[a]Extensive first-pass metabolism may result in a significant decrease in bioavailability.
[b]Genetically determined groups of slow and fast metabolisers have been identified.

While short-acting dihydropyridine CCBs have been implicated in the exacerbation of angina due to the phenomenon of 'coronary steal', longer acting dihydropyridines, for example, amlodipine and felodipine or longer acting formulations, for example, nifedipine LA, have demonstrated symptom-relieving potential similar to β-blockers. Dihydropyridines have no effect on the conducting tissues and are effective arterial dilators, decreasing afterload and improving coronary perfusion but also causing flushing, headaches and reflex tachycardia. This may be overcome by combination with a β-blocker. The use of dihydropyridines in angina is based on efficacy in trials that have used surrogate markers such as exercise tolerance rather than mortality as the endpoint.

CCBs with myocardial rate control as well as vasodilatory properties, for example, diltiazem, and those with predominantly rate-controlling effects, for example, verapamil, have also been shown to improve symptom control, reduce the frequency of anginal attacks and increase exercise tolerance. They should be avoided in patients with compromised left ventricular function and conduction abnormalities. Verapamil and diltiazem are suitable for rate control patients in whom β-blockers are contraindicated on grounds of respiratory or peripheral vascular disease. They should be used with caution in patients already receiving β-blockers, as bradycardia and heart block have been reported with this combination.

CCBs have a particular role in the management of Prinzmetal's (variant) angina which is thought to be due to coronary artery spasm.

Nitrates

Organic nitrates are valuable in angina because they dilate veins and thereby decrease preload, dilate arteries to a lesser extent thereby decreasing afterload, and promote flow in collateral coronary vessels, diverting blood from the epicardium to the endocardium. They are available in many forms but all relax vascular smooth muscle by releasing nitric oxide, which was formerly known as endothelium-derived relaxing factor, which acts via cyclic GMP. The production of nitric oxide from nitrates is probably mediated by intracellular thiols, and it has been observed that when tolerance to the action of nitrates occurs, a thiol donor (such as N-acetylcysteine) may partially restore the effectiveness of the nitrate. Antioxidants such as vitamin C have also been used. While clinical trials have not established any mortality gain from the use of oral nitrate preparations, their role in providing symptom relief is well established.

Tolerance is one of the main limitations to the use of nitrates. This develops rapidly, and a 'nitrate-free' period of a few hours in each 24-h period is beneficial in maintaining the effectiveness of treatment. The nitrate-free period should coincide with the period of lowest risk, and this is usually night time, but not early morning, which is a high-risk period for infarction. Many patients receiving short-acting nitrates two or three times a day would do well to have their doses between 7 a.m. and 6 p.m. (say, 8 a.m. and 2 p.m. for

isosorbide mononitrate), but this is generally not practised in UA where there is no low-risk period and where continuous dosing is used, with increasing doses if tolerance develops.

There are many nitrate preparations available, including intravenous infusions, conventional or slow-release tablets and capsules, transdermal patches, sublingual tablets and sprays and adhesive buccal tablets. Slow-release preparations and transdermal patches are expensive, do not generally offer such flexible dosing regimens as short-acting tablets. Sustained release tablets do not release the drug over the whole 24-h period producing a 'nitrate free period', whereas patches need to be removed for a few hours each day. Buccal tablets are expensive and offer no real therapeutic advantage in regular therapy. Like sublingual sprays and tablets, however, they have a rapid onset of action and the drug bypasses the liver, which has an extensive first-pass metabolic effect on oral nitrates. The sublingual preparations, whether sprays or suckable or chewable tablets, are used for the prevention or relief of acute attacks of pain but may elicit the two principal side effects of nitrates: hypotension with dizziness and fainting, and a throbbing headache. To minimise these effects, patients should be advised to sit down, rather than lie or stand, when taking short-acting nitrates, and to spit out or swallow the tablet once the angina is relieved. Sublingual glyceryl trinitrate (GTN) tablets have a very short shelf-life on exposure to air, need to be stored carefully and replaced frequently. As a consequence they are now little used. All nitrates may induce tachycardia.

Three main nitrates are used: GTN (mainly for sublingual, buccal, transdermal and intravenous routes), isosorbide dinitrate and isosorbide mononitrate. All are effective if given in appropriate doses at suitable dose intervals (Table 20.3). Since isosorbide dinitrate is metabolised to the mononitrate, there is a preference for using the more predictable mononitrate, but this is not a significant clinical factor. A more relevant feature may be that whereas the dinitrate is usually given three or four times a day, the mononitrate is given once or twice a day. Slow-release preparations exist for both drugs.

Nicorandil

Nicorandil is a compound that exhibits the properties of a nitrate but which also activates ATP-dependent potassium channels. The IONA Study Group (2002) compared nicorandil with placebo as 'add-on' treatment in 5126 high-risk patients with stable angina. The main benefit for patients in the nicorandil group was a reduction in unplanned admission to hospital with chest pain. The study did not tell us when to add nicorandil to combinations of antianginals such as β-blockers, CCBs and long-acting nitrates. There is a theoretical benefit from these agents in their action to promote ischaemic preconditioning. This phenomenon is seen when myocardial tissue is exposed to a period of ischaemia prior to sustained coronary artery occlusion. Prior exposure to ischaemia renders the myocardial tissue more resistant to permanent damage. This mechanism is mimicked by the action of nicorandil.

Table 20.3 Properties of commonly used nitrates

Drug	Speed of onset	Duration of action	Notes
Glyceryl trinitrate (GTN)			
Intravenous	Immediate	Duration of infusion	
Transdermal	30 min	Designed to release drug steadily for 24 h	Tolerance develops if applied continuously
SR tablets and capsules	Slow	8–12 h	
Sublingual tablets	Rapid (1–4 min)	<30 min	Inactivated if swallowed
			Less effective if dry mouth
Spray	Rapid (1–4 min)	<30 min	
Buccal tablets	Rapid (1–4 min)	4–8 h	Nearly as rapid in onset as sublingual tablets
Isosorbide dinitrate			
SR tablets	Similar to GTN		
Intravenous	Similar to GTN		
Sublingual	Slightly slower than GTN	As for GTN	
Chewable tablets	2–5 min	2–4 h	Less prone to cause headaches than sublingual tablets
Oral tablets	30–40 min	4–8 h	
Isosorbide mononitrate			
Oral tablets	30–40 min	6–12 h	
SR tablets or capsules	Slow	12–24 h	Some brands claim a nitrate-free period if given once daily

SR, sustained-release.

Ivabradine

Ivabridine represents a class of antianginal agents which block the I_f current. I_f is a mixed Na^+–K^+ inward current activated by hyperpolarisation and modulated by the autonomic nervous system. This regulates pacemaker activity in the sinoatrial node and controls heart rate. Inhibition, therefore, reduces heart rate without affecting the force of contraction. Ivabridine is similar in efficacy to atenolol and CCBs and may be of particular use in patients in whom β-blockers are contraindicated. The most frequent adverse drug reactions are dose-dependent transient visual symptoms that manifest as transient enhanced brightness commonly associated with abrupt changes in light intensity. They may be related to the action of ivabradine at hyperpolarisation-activated, cyclic nucleotide-gated cation current channels present in the retina. Visual symptoms may resolve spontaneously during therapy or after drug discontinuation.

Ranolazine

Ranolazine, a selective inhibitor of late sodium influx, attenuates the abnormalities of ventricular repolarisation and contractility associated with ischaemia. It has been shown to increase exercise tolerance, reduce anginal episodes and reduce the use of GTN. Side effects include dizziness, constipation, nausea, and the potential for prolongation of the QTc interval. Ranolazine seems to be a safe addition to current traditional drugs for chronic stable angina, especially in aggressive multidrug regimens.

Acute coronary syndrome

Definition and cause

The group of conditions referred to as ACS often present with similar symptoms of chest pain which is not, or only partially, relieved by GTN. These conditions include acute myocardial infarction (AMI), UA and non-ST-elevation myocardial infarction (NSTEMI). AMI with persistent ST segment elevation on the ECG usually develops Q waves, indicating transmural infarction. UA and NSTEMI present without persistent ST segment elevation and are managed differently, although a similar early diagnostic and therapeutic approach is employed. All patients with ACS should be admitted to hospital for evaluation, risk stratification and treatment. The spectrum of ACS is described in Fig. 20.3.

ACS arises from the rupture of an unstable atheromatous plaque. This exposes the cholesterol-rich plaque in the intima to the blood, initiating platelet activation and eventual thrombus formation. The volume of the eventual thrombus and the time the vessel is occluded determine the degree of myocardial necrosis that occurs. The major difference in approach to these patients arises from whether the coronary artery involved is felt to be occluded or open.

Patients with an occluded coronary artery suffer myocardial damage, the extent of which is determined by the duration and site of the occlusion. The primary strategy for these patients is the restoration of coronary flow with either a fibrinolystic agent or primary angioplasty. If the coronary artery is patent, however, then fibrinolysis is unnecessary and probably harmful, although

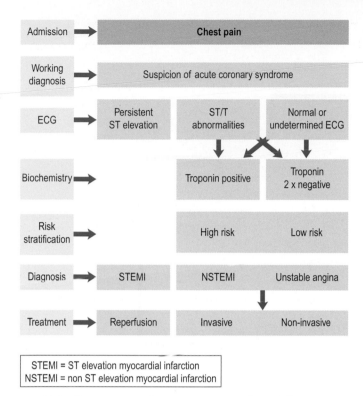

Admission	**Chest pain**		
Working diagnosis	Suspicion of acute coronary syndrome		
ECG	Persistent ST elevation	ST/T abnormalities	Normal or undetermined ECG
Biochemistry		Troponin positive	Troponin 2 x negative
Risk stratification		High risk	Low risk
Diagnosis	STEMI	NSTEMI	Unstable angina
Treatment	Reperfusion	Invasive	Non-invasive

STEMI = ST elevation myocardial infarction
NSTEMI = non ST elevation myocardial infarction

Fig. 20.3 The spectrum of acute coronary syndrome (Thygesen et al., 2007).

angioplasty may still be appropriate. When the vessel is open, for both groups, patient management focuses on the unstable coronary plaque and is, therefore, fundamentally similar.

Troponins (troponin I or troponin T) are cardiac muscle proteins which are released following myocardial cell damage and are highly sensitive and specific for myocardial infarction. They are useful in diagnosing patients with ACS and for predicting response to drug therapy; they are now key to the management of these patients and have replaced cardiac enzymes such as creatinine kinase (CK), aspartate transaminase (AST) and lactate dehydrogenase (LDH).

Diagnostic criteria for AMI have changed to incorporate the increasing availability of new diagnostic techniques with traditional symptoms and ECG changes. The following criteria for AMI, agreed by the European Society of Cardiology, rely on the rise of cardiac biomarkers (preferably troponin) with at least one value above the 99th percentile of the upper reference limit (URL) together with evidence of myocardial ischaemia with at least one of the following symptoms of ischaemia:

- ECG changes indicative of new ischaemia: new ST changes (STEMI or new left bundle branch block (LBBB))
- Development of pathological Q waves in the ECG
- Image evidence of new loss of viable myocardium or new regional wall motion abnormality.

Mortality rates of patients with presumed myocardial infarction or ACS in the first month is approximately 50% and of these deaths about half occur within the first 2 h. The

prognosis of an individual who has suffered a STEMI and receives hospital treatment has improved following the widespread use of thrombolytic therapy and primary percutaneous intervention

The most dangerous time after a myocardial infarction is the first few hours when ventricular fibrillation (VF) is most likely to occur.

Patients without persistent ST elevation on the ECG may still have experienced myocardial damage due to temporary occlusion of the vessel or emboli from the plaque-related thrombus blocking smaller distal vessels and will have raised levels of troponin. These patients have had a NSTEMI. Patients without ST elevation and without a rise in troponin or cardiac enzymes are defined as having UA. The long-term prognosis in NSTEMI is similar to that of STEMI. The early adverse event rate is lower but these patients are more likely to suffer death, recurrent myocardial infarction or recurrent ischaemia after hospital discharge than patients with STEMI. More emphasis is now placed on improving the treatment of patients with NSTEMI than was previously the case.

The Global Registry of Acute Coronary Events (GRACE; available at http://www.outcomes-umassmed.org/GRACE/) is an international registry which has enrolled patients with ACS (UA, NSTEMI and STEMI) since 1999. The registry indicates a similar incidence of UA, NSTEMI and STEMI.

The classification of ACS based on ECG findings and measurement of troponin is shown in Fig. 20.4.

Treatment of ST elevation myocardial infarction

Treatment of STEMI may be divided into three categories:

- provide immediate care to alleviate pain, prevent deterioration and improve cardiac function;
- manage complications, notably heart failure and arrhythmias;
- prevent further infarction or death (secondary prophylaxis).

The management of heart failure and arrhythmias are covered more extensively in Chapters 21 and 22, respectively, and will not be discussed here. The remaining therapeutic aims are to relieve pain, return patency to the coronary arteries, minimise infarct size, provide prophylaxis to arrhythmias and institute secondary prevention.

Immediate care to alleviate pain, prevent deterioration and improve cardiac function

Pain relief. Patients with suspected STEMI should receive sublingual GTN under the tongue, oxygen administered and intravenous access established immediately. If sublingual GTN fails to relieve the chest pain, intravenous morphine may be administered together with an antiemetic such as prochlorperazine or metoclopramide. There is no benefit in leaving a patient in pain while the diagnosis is considered. Pain is associated with sympathetic activation, which causes vasoconstriction, increases the workload of the heart and can exacerbate the underlying condition.

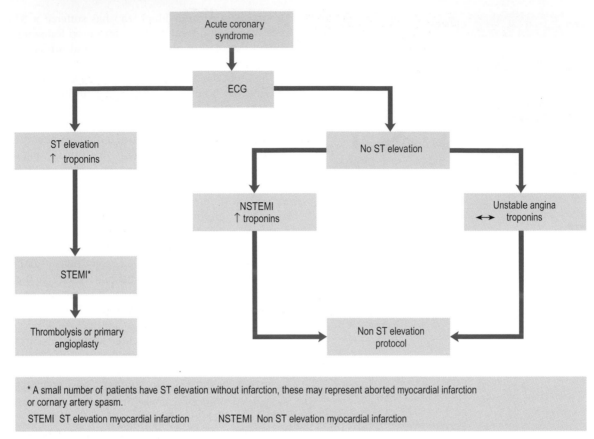

Fig. 20.4 Classification of ACS based on ECG and measurement of troponins.

Antiplatelet therapy. An aspirin tablet chewed as soon as possible after the infarct and followed by a daily dose for at least 1 month has been shown to reduce mortality and morbidity. Follow-up studies have demonstrated additional benefit in continuing to take daily aspirin, probably for life. The reduction in mortality is additional to that obtained from thrombolytic therapy (Table 20.4). Clopidogrel, given in addition to aspirin, can further improve coronary artery blood flow but the additional absolute reduction in mortality is small, at approximately 0.4% (Sabatine et al., 2005). In suspected heart attack patients in the UK, both aspirin and clopidogrel may be administered by the ambulance crew.

Restoring coronary flow and myocardial tissue perfusion

In patients with STEMI, early restoration of coronary artery patency results in an improved outcome; this may occur spontaneously in some patients but frequently only after substantial myocardial damage has occurred. Clinical trial data indicate that hospital mortality at 1 month has been reduced from 16% to 4–6% with the widespread use of coronary interventions, fibrinolytic agents and secondary prevention. In practice, available data suggest a higher mortality than that recorded in clinical trials.

The timing of treatment is vital, since myocardial damage after onset of an acute ischaemic episode is progressive and there are pathological data to suggest it is irreversible beyond 6 h. Clinical data from large studies of fibrinolysis have shown that the sooner treatment is started after the onset of pain, the better. All trials show that rapid treatment is important and this has a greater effect than the choice of drug; several studies indicate that giving fibrinolytics an average of 30–60 min earlier can save 15 lives per 1000 treated. Hospitals need to maintain fast-track systems to ensure maximum benefit, although there is still some worthwhile benefit up to 12 h after infarction.

Treatment within 1 h has been found to be particularly advantageous, although difficult to achieve, for logistical reasons, in anyone who has an infarct outside hospital. Prioritisation of ambulances to emergency calls for chest pain and appropriately equipped paramedics or primary care doctors administering fibrinolytics out of hospital have all helped reduce delay in fibrinolysis administration. Increased numbers of and direct access to hospitals offering primary angioplasty sites has further reduced the time to myocardial tissue reperfusion. Current reperfusion strategies are outlined in Fig. 20.5.

Table 20.4 Vascular deaths at 35 days in the ISIS-2 study (1990)	
Placebo	13.2%
Aspirin	10.7%
Streptokinase	10.4%
Aspirin + streptokinase	8.0%

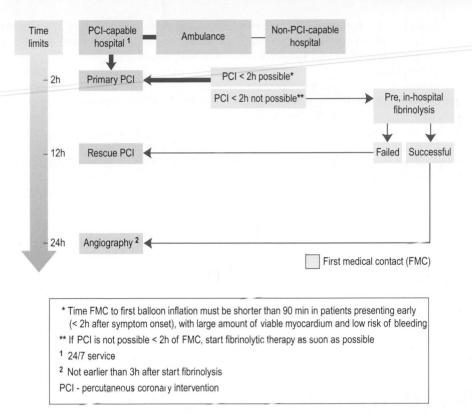

* Time FMC to first balloon inflation must be shorter than 90 min in patients presenting early
   (< 2h after symptom onset), with large amount of viable myocardium and low risk of bleeding

** If PCI is not possible < 2h of FMC, start fibrinolytic therapy as soon as possible

[1] 24/7 service

[2] Not earlier than 3h after start fibrinolysis

PCI - percutaneous coronary intervention

Fig. 20.5 Reperfusion strategies. The thick arrow (dark blue) indicate the preferred strategy (Van de Werf, 2008).

Fibrinolytics. Fibrinolytic agents (Table 20.5) have transformed the management of these patients by substantially improving coronary artery patency rates which has translated into a 25% relative reduction in mortality. The risk of haemorrhagic stroke (around 1%) and a failure to adequately reperfuse the affected myocardium in approximately 50% of cases have remained despite advances in fibrinolytics.

Percutaneous coronary intervention. The introduction of primary PCI (angioplasty and/or stent insertion without prior or concomitant fibrinolytic therapy) has demonstrated superiority to fibrinolysis when it can be performed expeditiously by an experienced team in a hospital with an established 24h a day interventional programme. In this context, primary angioplasty is better than fibrinolysis at reducing the overall short-term death, non-fatal reinfarction and stroke. The target for time from first medical contact to first balloon inflation should be less than 2h. If the delay to angioplasty is likely to be longer than 2h, facilitated PCI can be undertaken.

Facilitated PCI involves use of a fibrinolytic to achieve reperfusion prior to a planned PCI. This approach allows the clinical team to bridge an anticipated delay in undertaking a PCI.

Rescue PCI is performed on coronary arteries which remain occluded despite attempts at fibrinolysis. It has better outcomes than repeated fibrinolytic therapy or conservative management.

PCIs encompass various invasive procedures to improve myocardial blood delivery by opening up the blood vessels. PCIs open stenosed coronary vessels and are less invasive than coronary bypass surgery, where the coronary vessels are replaced.

A percutaneous (through the skin) transluminal (through the lumen of the blood vessels) coronary (into the heart) angioplasty (surgery or repair of the blood vessels) (PTCA) was first carried out on a conscious patient in 1977. Now over 2 million people a year undergo PCIs. The procedure is less invasive than coronary artery bypass graft (CABG) surgery.

PCI involves the passing of a catheter via the femoral or radial artery and aorta into the coronary vasculature under

Table 20.5 Fibrinolytic agents (thrombolytics)

	Fibrin specificity	Elimination	Half-life (min)	Dosing	Antigenic	Mode of action
Streptokinase		Hepatic	18–23	1h infusion	Yes	Activator complex
Alteplase	++	Hepatic	3–8	Bolus + 90 min infusion	No	Direct
Reteplase	+	Renal	15–18	Two boluses	No	Direct
Tenecteplase	+++	Hepatic	20–28	One bolus	No	Direct

radio-contrast guidance. Inflation of a balloon at the end of the catheter in the area of the atheromatous plaques opens the lumen of the artery. For patients undergoing PCI there is a small risk of death, myocardial infarction and long-term restenosis. This is reduced by insertion of a coronary artery stent and the use of pre- and peri-procedural antiplatelet therapy. Over the last 10 years the proportion of patients undergoing PCI and stent insertion has accounted for >95% of all PCI procedures.

Antiplatelet and anticoagulant therapy. After stent insertion there is a short-term risk of thrombus formation until the endothelial lining of the blood vessel has been re-established. The combination of clopidogrel (600 mg initiated pre-procedure and 75 mg daily thereafter) and aspirin has been shown to reduce the risk of myocardial infarction and need for reperfusion therapy and decrease the length of hospital stay.

Patients undergoing primary PCI should receive aspirin and clopidogrel as early as possible. Antiplatelet naïve patients should receive 300 mg of aspirin and 600 mg of clopidogrel. In the UK and elsewhere in Europe, these are administered by paramedics. Prasugrel has less metabolic activation steps and has a faster and more reliable onset of antiplatelet action. In combination with aspirin, it is recommended (NICE, 2009) for preventing atherothrombotic events in individuals undergoing PCI only when:

- immediate primary PCI for STEMI is necessary;
- stent thrombosis has occurred during clopidogrel treatment; and
- the individual has diabetes mellitus.

Heparin is routinely administered during the PCI procedure and is titrated to maintain an activated clotting time (ACT) of 250–350 s. Glycoprotein IIb/IIIa receptor antagonists, particularly abciximab, have been shown to reduce mortality if used during the procedure. These are used in combination with heparin, and a lower ACT (200–250 s) is targeted to reduce bleeding complications. Bivalirudin, a direct thrombin inhibitor, has demonstrated less bleeding compared to abciximab and may be useful in those at risk of increased bleeding.

Much of the evidence for the use of glycoprotein IIb/IIIa receptor antagonists was accumulated before high-dose clopidogrel or more potent antiplatelets were in routine practice. Current recommendations are that in the setting of dual-antiplatelet therapy with unfractionated heparin or bivalirudin as the anticoagulant, glycoprotein IIb/IIIa receptor antagonists can be useful at the time of primary PCI but cannot be recommended as routine therapy.

Intracoronary administration of vasodilators such as adenosine, verapamil, nicorandil, papaverine, and nitroprusside during and after primary PCI has been shown to improve flow in the infarct-related coronary artery and myocardial perfusion, and/or to reduce infarct size, but large prospective randomised trials with hard clinical outcomes are missing.

Fibrinolytics. Fibrinolytic agents fall into two categories: fibrin specific (alteplase, tenecteplase and reteplase) and fibrin non-specific (streptokinase). There are theoretical advantages for the fibrin-specific agents which are superior in terms of achieving coronary artery patency in angiographic studies. Angiographic patency has been shown to correlate well with outcome in thrombolytic trials but it has been difficult to prove that this benefit translates into an improvement in mortality. Studies have demonstrated considerable benefit from fibrinolytics given soon after the onset of pain but little difference between streptokinase and the more expensive tissue plasminogen activator (alteplase) in reducing mortality. Fast injection of fibrin-specific agents is better than slower infusion of streptokinase, especially in younger patients with anterior infarcts. Tenecteplase and reteplase have the advantage that they can be administered by bolus injection, which facilitates pre-hospital administration and reduces errors.

Patients receiving alteplase also receive a 5000 unit heparin bolus followed by a 48-h infusion adjusted to maintain the activated partial thromboplastin time (APTT) in the therapeutic range. Intravenous enoxaparin followed by subcutaneous injections may be an alternative. Heparin has not been compared to placebo in trials of tenecteplase or reteplase but it is standard practice to use heparin with these agents. Heparin has no advantage in addition to streptokinase, which has a longer lasting and less specific fibrinolytic action.

A low dose of fondaparinux, a synthetic, indirect anti-Xa agent, has been found to be superior to placebo or heparin in preventing death and reinfarction in patients who received fibrinolytic therapy (OASIS-6 Trial Group, 2006).

Bivalirudin, a direct thrombin inhibitor, reduces reinfarction rates compared to heparin when given with streptokinase but has not been studied with fibrin-specific agents. This combination resulted in a non-significant increase in non-cerebral bleeding complications (HERO-2 Trial Investigators, 2001).

Trials using various dosing combinations of glycoprotein IIb/IIIa inhibitors with newer fibrinolytic agents have not found a regimen that increases overall survival (Menon et al., 2004).

All fibrinolytics cause haemorrhage, which may present as a stroke or a gastro-intestinal bleed, and there is an increased risk with regimens that use intravenous heparin. Recent strokes, bleeds, pregnancy and surgery are contraindications to fibrinolysis. Streptokinase induces cross-reacting antibodies which reduce its potency and may cause an anaphylactoid response. Patients with exposure to streptokinase, or with a history of rheumatic fever or recent streptococcal infection, should not receive the drug. The use of hydrocortisone to reduce allergic responses has fallen out of favour, but patients should be carefully observed for hypotension during the administration of streptokinase.

Old age is no longer considered to be a contraindication to fibrinolysis. Although the risks are greater, the benefit is also greater, but the doses of alteplase and tenecteplase need to be adjusted for body weight.

All the major trials have used specific ECG criteria for entry, usually ST elevation in adjacent leads or LBBB, and eliminated patients with major contraindications to fibrinolysis (Box 20.2). Confusion often arises about the term 'relative contraindication'. For example, systolic hypertension is common in AMI, so most protocols recommend lowering the blood pressure with either a β-blocker or intravenous nitrates before commencing fibrinolysis. An increasing number of

> **Box 20.2** Contraindications to fibrinolysis (Van de Werf, 2008)
>
> **Absolute contraindications**
> - Haemorrhagic stroke of unknown origin at any time
> - Ischaemic stroke in preceding 6 months
> - CNS damage or neoplasms
> - Recent major trauma/surgery/head injury (within preceding 3 weeks)
> - Gastro-intestinal bleed within the last month
> - Known bleeding disorder
> - Non-compressible punctures
> - Aortic dissection
>
> **Relative contraindications**
> - Transient ischaemic attack in preceding 6 months
> - Oral anticoagulant therapy
> - Pregnancy or within 1 week postpartum
> - Advanced liver disease
> - Active peptic ulcer
> - Infective endocarditis
> - Traumatic resuscitation
> - Refractory hypertension (systolic blood pressure >180 mmHg)

patients are on warfarin and this again is regarded as a relative contraindication to fibrinolysis; thresholds for the use of fibrinolysis in patients on warfarin vary from an INR of 2–2.4. The use of fibrinolytic therapy in patients with relative contraindications should take into account the site of the myocardial infarction and the likely size of the infarction. For example, in patients with a large anterior myocardial infarction the benefits of fibrinolysis may outweigh risk. In patients where there is a serious concern regarding bleeding following fibrinolysis, primary angioplasty should be considered.

Management of complications

Heart failure. Heart failure during the acute phase of STEMI is associated with a poor short- and long-term prognosis. It should be managed with oxygen, intravenous furosemide and nitrates. More severe failure or cardiogenic shock (tissue hypoperfusion resulting from cardiac failure with symptoms of hypotension, peripheral vasoconstriction and diminished pulses, decreased urine output and decreased mental status) should be treated with inotropes and/or inter-aortic balloon pumps to maintain the systolic blood pressure above 90 mmHg. Invasive monitoring may be required.

Arrhythmias. Life-threatening arrhythmias such as ventricular tachycardia, sustained VF or atrio-ventricular block occur in about one fifth of patients presenting with a STEMI, although this is decreasing due to early reperfusion therapy. β-Blockers have been the subject of many studies because of their anti-arrhythmic potential and because they permit increased subendocardial perfusion. In studies undertaken prior to the widespread use of fibrinolytics, the early administration of an intravenous β-blocker was shown to limit infarct size and reduce mortality from early cardiac events. A post hoc analysis of the use of atenolol in the GUSTO-I trial and a systematic review (Freemantle et al., 1999) did not support the routine, early intravenous use of β-blockers and, therefore, oral β-blockers are started within 24 h of the event. If a β-blocker is contraindicated because of respiratory or vascular disorders, verapamil may be used, since it has been shown to reduce late mortality and reinfarction in patients without heart failure, although it shows no benefit when given immediately after an infarct. Diltiazem is less effective but may be used as an alternative. This is clearly not a class effect; other channel blockers have produced different results and nifedipine increases mortality in patients following a myocardial infarction.

Initially, magnesium infusions looked promising when given early after infarction. However, in large trials (ISIS-4), no reductions in mortality were found making the routine use of magnesium inappropriate. Magnesium infusions are used, however, to correct low serum magnesium levels if cardiac arrhythmias are present.

Sinus bradycardia and heart block may also occur after a myocardial infarction and patients may require temporary or permanent pacemaker insertion.

Blood glucose. Patients with a myocardial infarction are often found to have high serum and urinary glucose levels, usually described as a stress response. The CREATE-ECLA trial (Mehta et al., 2005) studied more than 20,000 patients and showed a neutral effect of insulin on mortality, cardiac arrest and cardiogenic shock. Current guidelines do not support the routine use of insulin in STEMI in patients not previously known to be diabetic.

Up to 20% of patients who have a myocardial infarction have diabetes. Moreover, diabetic patients are known to do poorly after infarction, with almost double the mortality rate of non-diabetics. In these patients, an intensive insulin regimen, both during admission and for 3 months after, was found to save lives (Malmberg, 1997). However, the follow-up study (Malmberg et al., 2005) did not show any mortality benefit from intensive insulin therapy compared to standard therapy. In patients with diabetes, it appears reasonable, however, to continue to control blood glucose levels within the normal range immediately post-infarct.

Prevention of further infarction or death (secondary prophylaxis)

Lipid-lowering agents. Reduction of cholesterol through diet and use of lipid-lowering agents are effective at reducing subsequent mortality and morbidity in patients with established CAD. Patients with established CHD should be treated to ensure LDL-C is less than 2 mmol/L and total cholesterol less than 4 mmol/L (see Chapter 24). In patients with AMI or high-risk NSTEMI, there was a reduction in the combination end point of death, myocardial infarction, or documented UA requiring hospitalisation, revascularisation or stroke when patients were treated with high intensity statin (atorvastatin 80 mg) compared to standard statin therapy (Cannon et al., 2004). A meta-analysis of studies (Josan et al., 2008) reaffirmed the benefit of high intensity statin therapy especially in those patients with ACSs. An additional finding of particular interest was that the results were significant for the high intensity treatment arms despite approximately half of patients not achieving LDL-C of less than 2 mmol/L.

β-Blockers. Long-term use of a β-blocker has been shown in several studies to decrease mortality in patients in whom there is no contraindication. β-Blockade should be avoided in individuals with heart block, bradycardia, asthma, obstructive airways disease or peripheral vascular disease. One large cohort study compared low and high doses of β-blockers with no therapy and found benefit in all treated patients with similar survival rates but a lower heart failure rate in the low-dose group (Rochon et al., 2000).

Angiotensin-converting enzyme inhibitors. ACE inhibitors have been tried in various doses and durations and have proved beneficial in reducing the incidence of heart failure and mortality. In all but the earliest trials, patients were given an ACE inhibitor for 4–6 weeks and treatment continued in patients with signs or symptoms of heart failure or left ventricular dysfunction. The HOPE study (Yusuf et al., 2000) found that ramipril improved survival in all groups of patients with CHD and this has led clinicians to continue ACE inhibitors in all patients with a myocardial infarction over the age of 55 and in younger patients with evidence of left ventricular dysfunction. Contraindications to their use include hypotension and intractable cough.

There is considerable interest in focusing on the possible benefits of combining ACE inhibition with angiotensin II receptor blockers. Angiotensin blockade alone does not cause the accumulation of bradykinins that may be part of the benefit of using ACE inhibitors. Clinical trials (OPTIMAAL Study Group, 2002; VALIANT Investigators, 2003) have failed to find a benefit over ACE inhibition. Nonetheless, angiotensin receptor blockers are probably suitable in patients who cannot tolerate an ACE inhibitor. The relative benefits of ACE inhibitors and other treatments are shown in Table 20.6.

Eplerenone. In patients with heart failure, post-AMI, an improvement in survival and decreased cardiovascular mortality and hospitalisation was seen in those taking the aldosterone antagonist eplerenone (EPHESUS Trial; Pitt et al., 2003). Serious hyperkalemia occurred more frequently in the eplerenone arm and monitoring of serum potassium is warranted when used in practice.

Antidepressants. Anxiety is almost inevitable and a quarter of patients who have suffered a myocardial infarction subsequently experience marked depression. Post-myocardial infarction depression is associated with poor medication compliance, a lower quality-of-life score and a four-fold increase in mortality (Januzzi et al., 2000). Antidepressant treatments have not been subjected to formal trials but it seems reasonable to try to reduce the depression. There is concern about the potential for older antidepressants, such as tricyclic antidepressants, to increase the QT interval and cause arrhythmias. Newer antidepressants are less prone to cause these arrhythmias and selective seretonin receptor inhibitors (SSRIs) are preferred.

Rehabilitation programmes, which include some measure of social interaction, physical activity and education, are also of proven benefit. Although psychological stress clearly worsens outcomes, stress reduction interventions have not been tested and proven to work independently of other measures.

Nitrates. Studies on nitrates in myocardial infarction were mostly completed before fibrinolysis was widely used.

Table 20.6 Relative benefits of treating 1000 patients for myocardial infarction (MI)

Intervention	Events prevented
Intravenous β-adrenoceptor blocker	6 deaths
ACE inhibitor	6 deaths
Aspirin	20–25 deaths
Streptokinase (in hospital)	20–25 deaths
Alteplase (in hospital)	35 deaths
Streptokinase (before hospital)	35–40 deaths
Fibrinolysis 4½–1 h earlier	15 deaths
Long-term aspirin	16 deaths/MI/strokes
Long-term β-blockade	18 deaths/MI
Long-term ACE inhibitor	21–45 deaths/MI
10% reduction in serum cholesterol	7 deaths/MI
Stopping smoking	27 deaths

Adapted from McMurray and Rankin (1994).

Nitrates improve collateral blood flow and aid reperfusion, thus limiting infarct size and preserving functional tissue. ISIS-4 (1993) and GISSI-3 (1994) demonstrated that nitrates did not confer a survival advantage in patients receiving fibrinolysis. Sublingual nitrates may be given for immediate pain relief, and the use of intravenous or buccal nitrates can be considered in patients whose infarction pain does not resolve rapidly or who develop ventricular failure.

Anticoagulants and antiplatelets. Anticoagulation with warfarin is not generally recommended following a myocardial infarction, despite promising results in trials that have practiced exceptionally good anticoagulant monitoring. This is partly because of the success of antiplatelet therapy with aspirin. Aspirin does not have the same need for expensive and time-consuming follow-up and monitoring as warfarin, and is associated with fewer drug interactions. Clopidogrel has been shown to be beneficial, in addition to aspirin, in patients who have had a myocardial infarction (COMMIT, 2005). As the number of patients who receive a stent increases, the combination of aspirin and clopidogrel for a year or longer is now more frequent. Routine use of dipyridamole and sulfinpyrazone is not recommended after a myocardial infarction.

Treatment of non-ST elevation acute coronary syndromes

ACS without ST elevation is classified as either UA or NSTEMI. UA is defined as angina that occurs at rest or with minimal exertion, or new (within 1 month) onset of severe angina or worsening of previously stable angina. NSTEMI (or non-Q wave MI) is the more severe manifestation of ACS.

There are about 115,000 new patients diagnosed each year with UA or NSTEMI in England and Wales. Despite the use of standard therapy the rate of adverse outcomes such as death, non-fatal MI or refractory angina requiring revascularisation, remains at 5–7% at 7 days and about 15–30% at 30 days; 5–14% of patient with UA or NSTEMI die within the first year of diagnosis.

There are extensive data for angioplasty following NSTEMI where patients frequently have significant residual coronary artery narrowing despite treatment with antiplatelet agents, heparin and glycoprotein IIb/IIIa antagonists.

Patients with NSTEMI may either be treated with an interventional strategy, where all patients undergo angiography and PCI following admission, or conservatively where they undergo angiography and intervention only if they remain unstable or have a positive exercise test. Initial trials of early intervention did not demonstrate any benefit but with the advent of advanced angioplasty techniques using stents and adjuvant drug therapies including clopidogrel and glycoprotein IIb/IIIa antagonists, there appears to be a clear advantage for an interventional strategy in high-risk patients (Fox et al., 2005).

Patients presenting with UA/NSTEMI can be classified into three categories depending on their risk of death or likelihood of developing an AMI. High-risk patients (those with ST segment changes during chest pain, chest pain within 48 h, troponin T-positive patients and those presenting already on intensive anti-anginal therapy) can be effectively managed with aggressive medical and interventional therapy. This results in fewer individuals progressing to AMI.

Various pharmacological agents such as antithrombin and antiplatelet drugs, and coronary revascularisation (particularly PCI) have been shown to improve the outcome of patients with UA or NSTEMI. These interventions are known to be associated with some treatment hazards, particularly bleeding complications. The risks must be balanced against potential treatment benefits for each individual patient. This balance is influenced by the patient's estimated risk of an adverse cardiovascular outcome as a consequence of the ACS. The absolute magnitude of benefit from an intervention is generally greatest in those at highest risk. A confounding issue is that treatment hazards, such as bleeding complications, are often also greatest in those at highest risk of an ischaemic event.

Measures of risk can be derived from the clinical assessment of a patient and the use of a formal risk scoring system, such as the GRACE, PURSUIT, PREDICT or TIMI scores. Scores based on clinical trial data generally exclude patients who are at high risk of an adverse cardiovascular outcome such as the elderly, or those with renal or heart failure, and as a consequence the evidence for clinical and cost-effectiveness of therapeutic interventions is confined to patients at lower to intermediate levels of risk. Risk score based on registry data, for example, GRACE, may provide a more realistic estimation of risk (Tables 20.7 and 20.8).

In patients with NSTEMI, the immediate administration of 300 mg aspirin can reduce mortality or subsequent myocardial infarction by 50%. Risk stratification according to a recognised tool should be used to guide the subsequent choice of pharmacological and/or surgical intervention. The exclusion of STEMI and confirmation of NSTEMI is important as the use of fibrinolysis in NSTEMI confers no benefit, and merely increases the risk of bleeding. In patients with NSTEMI, the preferred treatment normally involves a combination of antiplatelet agents to reduce the formation of a thrombus.

Antiplatelet and anticoagulant drugs

The current range of antiplatelet and anticoagulant drugs available for the reduction of thrombotic events in ACS leads to the potential for a large number of combinations. In all cases, the benefit of reducing thrombotic events must be balanced against the potential for an increased risk of bleeding.

In the early 1990s, unfractionated heparin, when combined with aspirin showed a reduction in death and subsequent myocardial infarction compared with aspirin alone. The use of the low molecular weight heparin (LMWH), enoxaparin, subsequently demonstrated superiority over unfractionated heparin, with both usually continued for 48 h, or until chest pain resolved or discharge. Both groups of drugs were tested in the era before PCI became part of routine practice.

The CURE study (2001) showed that clopidogrel, given as a loading dose of 300 mg followed by 75 mg daily in combination with aspirin and heparin, reduced the combined end point of death, myocardial infarction and revascularisation in all patients with NSTEMI. Clopidogrel needs to be continued for 12 months but should be stopped 5–7 days before any major surgery to reduce the risk of bleeding.

As PCI has become more routine as part of the management of high-risk NSTEMI patients, more aggressive antiplatelet treatment has been required to reduce both peri-procedural and post-procedural thromboembolic complications.

Expression of glycoprotein IIb/IIIa is one of the final steps in the platelet aggregation cascade. Inhibiting these receptors has been a strategy prior to, and during, PCI for some time. Glycoprotein IIb/IIIa inhibitors bind to the IIb/IIIa receptors on platelets (Fig. 20.6) and prevent cross-linking of platelets by fibrinogen. There are three classes of these agents: murine-human chimeric antibodies, for example, abciximab; synthetic peptides, for example, eptifibatide; and non-peptide synthetics, for example, tirofiban. Oral agents are ineffective and the murine-human chimeric antibodies appear to be effective only in the context of PCI.

In high-risk patients undergoing PCI and receiving background heparin, triple antiplatelet therapy (aspirin, clopidogrel and a glycoprotein IIb/IIIa inhibitors) has been shown to be superior to standard dose dual-antiplatelet therapy (aspirin and clopidogrel) particularly in troponin positive individuals (Kastrati et al., 2006). However, much of this evidence was generated before the introduction of higher doses of clopidogrel or more potent oral antiplatelet agents.

There is no clear benefit to giving glycoprotein IIb/IIIa inhibitors more than 4 h before PCI (upstream) compared to waiting until immediately before or during the procedure (deferred) (Stone et al., 2007).

Currently, all patients with a likely or definite diagnosis of NSTEMI should receive a loading dose of aspirin 300 mg (see Fig. 20.7). Patients undergoing PCI intervention should

Table 20.7 Classification of high-risk patients with NSTEMI as determined by the GRACE prediction score card and nomogram

GRACE Prediction Score Card

Risk calculator for in-hospital mortality for ACS with NSTEMI

Sum the points to calculate the total risk score. Correlate the score with the appropriate risk category (for all cause mortality during in-hospital stay as set out in Table 20.8).

Findings at initial hospital presentation					Findings during hospitalisation	
1		**3**			**6**	
Age (years)	Points	Resting heart rate (beats/min)	Points		Initial serum creatinine (µmol/L)	Points
<30	0	<50	0		0–34	1
30–39	8	50–69	3		35–70	4
40–49	25	70–89.9	9		71–105	7
50–59	41	90–109.9	15		106–140	10
60–69	58	110–149.9	24		141–176	13
70–79	75	150–199.9	38		177–353	21
80–89	91	>200	46		>354	28
>90	100					
2		**4**			**7**	
Killip class		Systolic blood pressure (mmHg)			Elevated cardiac enzymes	14
I. No clinical signs of HF	0	<80	58			
II. Rales and/or JVD	20	80–99.9	53			
III. Pulmonary oedema	39	100–119.9	43			
IV. Cardiogenic shock	59	120–139.9	34			
		140–159.9	24			
		160–199.9	10			
		>200	0			
		5			**8**	
		ST Segment deviation	28		Cardiac arrest on admission	39

(JVD, jugular venous distension)

have a higher loading dose of 600 mg of clopidogrel or 60 mg of prasugrel, unless contraindicated, to reduce events during and after PCI. Clopidogrel is often given as 300 mg on admission and a further 300 mg when the decision to intervene is made. Prasugrel, with its faster time to maximum effect, has demonstrated some benefit but routine use is not recommended (NICE, 2009). Patients who are not planned for intervention should receive a lower loading dose of clopidogrel 300 mg.

All patients should receive heparin, bivalirudin or fondaparinux. Unfractionated heparin is preferred for patients with compromised renal function. Fondaparinux, a synthetic pentasaccharide factor Xa inhibitor which has predictable and sustained anticoagulation with fixed dose, once-a-day subcutaneous administration, causes less bleeding than enoxaparin, an LMWH. Concerns over catheter related thrombus mean it should not be considered if patients are planned for PCI within 24 h of chest pain. Bivalirudin is a

Table 20.8 GRACE prediction nomogram for all cause mortality during in-hospital stay and up to 6 months post discharge

Risk category (tertiles)	GRACE risk score	In-hospital death (%)
Low	<109	<1
Intermediate	109–140	1–3
High	>140	>3

Risk category (tertiles)	GRACE risk score	Post-discharge to 6 months
Low	<89	<3
Intermediate	89–118	3–8
High	>118	>8

GRACE Registry. Available at www.outcomes-umassmed.org/GRACE/index.cfm.

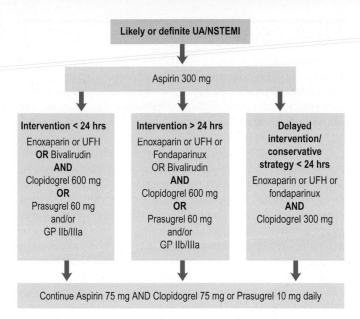

Fig. 20.7 Treatment options for patients with likely or definite unstable angina (UA) or NSTEMI in relation to time of PCI intervention.

synthetic analogue of hirudin that binds reversibly to thrombin and inhibits clot-bound thrombin and may be considered an alternative.

The decision to use glycoprotein IIb/IIIa inhibitors is dependant on the centre and operator and whether the planned intervention for the patient is to be surgical or pharmacological. The introduction of higher loading doses of clopidogrel and more potent oral agents, as well as an increased focus on the bleeding risks associated with combination therapy, has reduced the use of these agents in many centres.

Recommendation of an anticoagulant regimen has become more complicated by a number of new choices suggested by contemporary trials, some of which do not provide adequate comparative information for common practice settings.

Anti-ischaemic drugs

The use of both β-blockers and nitrates in the management of patients with NSTEMI is based on studies of their use in stable angina and AMI. Their use is, however, well established and based on a firm pathophysiological and pharmacological rationale.

Statins

High intensity statins have been shown to benefit patients when given early in ACS. They are usually started on admission if the diagnosis of CAD is definite, independent of the patient's cholesterol level. Treatment should aim to achieve total cholesterol of <4 mmol/L and an LDL-C of <2 mmol/L.

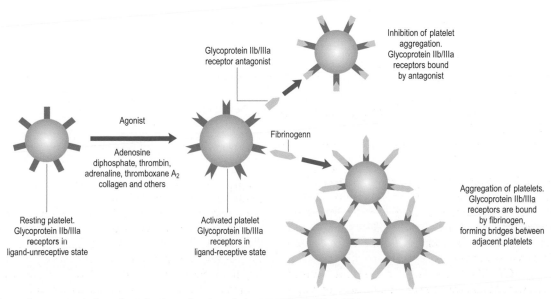

Fig. 20.6 Schematic representation of mechanism of action of glycoprotein IIb/IIIa inhibitors.

Patient care

Patients with CHD range from those who have investigational evidence of CHD but no symptoms to those who have major pain and exercise limitation. All need encouragement in adhering to preventive measures including diet, exercise and smoking cessation. Patients need to be able to discuss concerns about their health.

Exercise must be tailored according to the patient's threshold for angina. In general, although some patients are too cavalier, most are likely to err on the cautious side and may need to be encouraged to do more. Many centres now run cardiac rehabilitation classes to encourage patients to exercise and adopt a suitable lifestyle.

There are simple treatments and important lifestyle changes that can reduce cardiovascular risk and slow or even reverse progression of established coronary disease. The most important of these to address is smoking cessation. The risk of CHD is two to four times higher in heavy smokers (those who smoke at least 20 cigarettes/day) than in those who do not smoke. Other reports estimate the age-adjusted risk for smokers of more than 25 cigarettes/day is five to 21 times that of non-smokers. Smokers should be encouraged to quit. Within months of stopping smoking, CHD risk begins to decline. Within 5 years of smoking cessation the risk decreases to approximately the level found in people who have never smoked, regardless of the amount smoked, duration of the habit and the age at cessation. The use of nicotine replacement therapy almost doubles a smokers' chance of successfully stopping smoking (18% vs. 11%). All patients who smoke should be offered advice on cessation and encouraged to attend specialist smokers' clinics to further improve their chance of quitting.

Patient beliefs about medicines and medication-taking behaviour (and therefore adherence) are also important determinants of outcome and are influenced by many factors. These can largely be divided into beliefs about the importance of the medicine and concerns about the medicine's harmful effects. In order to assure the patient's concordance with medication regimens, it is necessary to address each individual patient's beliefs and concerns. One approach to counselling patients with CHD may be to divide the medication prescribed into those used to reduce risk of heart attacks and death, and those for symptom control. Key points to be discussed will relate to side effects and what to do if they occur, the need to continue medication until told otherwise and to ensure they do not run out of medication. Patients should be encouraged to identify their concerns and these should be addressed as openly and honestly as possible.

Patients also need up-to-date advice when faced with difficult choices regarding medical treatment, angiographic procedures or surgery. Patients have good reason to be anxious at times but some patients restrict their activities unnecessarily out of fear of angina and infarction.

Some of the common therapeutic problems encountered in the management of CHD are described in Table 20.9.

Table 20.9 Common therapeutic problems in coronary heart disease

Problem	Comment
Used incorrectly, nitrates may cause hypotensive episodes or collapse	Advise to sit down when using nitrate sprays or sublingual tablets
A daily nitrate-free period is required to maintain efficacy of nitrates	Avoid long-acting preparations and prescribe asymmetrically (e.g. 8 a.m. and 2 p.m.)
NSAIDs are associated with renal failure when given with ACE inhibitors	Warn patients to use paracetamol as their analgesic of choice
Speed is essential when patients need fibrinolytic drugs after infarction	Arrange emergency admission to hospital where fast-track systems should exist
Aspirin may cause gastro-intestinal bleeding	Advise on taking with food and water. Consider use of prophylactic agents in high-risk patients
β-Blockers are often considered unpleasant to take	Encourage patient to use regularly. Change the time of day. Consider a vasodilator if cold extremities are a problem. Consider verapamil or diltiazem
β-Blockers are contraindicated in respiratory and peripheral vascular disease	Consider verapamil or diltiazem. Pay strict attention to other treatments and removal of precipitating factors
Patients often receive multiple drugs for prophylaxis and for treatment of co-existing disorders	Use once-daily preparations, dosing aids and intensive social and educational support. Avoid all unnecessary drugs
ACE inhibitors are contraindicated in pregnancy, especially the first trimester	Advise women of child-bearing years to avoid conception or seek specialist advice first

Case studies

Case 20.1

A 55-year-old man presents to his primary care doctor complaining of tightness in his chest when he digs the garden. It eases when he has a rest. On investigation he has a raised serum glucose concentration and is considered to be a newly diagnosed non-insulin-dependent type II diabetic.

Question

What cardiovascular investigations and treatments should this patient receive?

Answer

The patient's blood pressure and ECG should be checked and he should be examined for signs of hypertensive or diabetic target organ damage, including albuminuria. His serum lipid profile should be measured.

He should receive GTN spray or sublingual tablets for the chest symptoms that are almost certainly angina. He should take aspirin daily and a statin if his lipid profile is abnormal. Some prescribers would give a statin in almost all diabetic, CHD patients and likewise an ACE inhibitor. Certainly, any hypertension should be treated aggressively so that the diastolic pressure is less than 80 mmHg. A β-blocker may also be useful to control blood pressure and prevent further episodes of angina, but many prescribers would wait until there was evidence of failure of the other therapies. In view of his relatively young age, a referral to a cardiologist for possible angiography would be considered. Dietary advice and help to stop smoking, if needed, would be given. Diabetic treatments should be given (see Chapter 44).

Case 20.2

The following patients are admitted for treatment of myocardial infarction:
1. an asthmatic
2. a man previously treated for infarction
3. a patient with rheumatoid arthritis.

Question

What contraindications, or possible contraindications, are there to standard treatments in the above patients?

Answers

1. An asthmatic should not receive a β-blocker without careful consideration and supervision because of the risk of bronchoconstriction; there is also a small risk of bronchoconstriction with aspirin.
2. A previous infarct may have been treated with streptokinase and a repeat dose should be avoided. Tissue plasminogen activator should be used instead.
3. Fibrinolytics are contraindicated if there is a serious risk of bleeding. A patient with rheumatoid arthritis may be receiving NSAIDs or steroids and enquiries must be made into any history of gastro-intestinal bleeding. NSAIDs would also not be prescribed with ACE inhibitors because of the risk of impaired renal function. Aspirin is not contraindicated with NSAIDs, and may be useful, but will increase the risk of gastro-intestinal bleeding.

Case 20.3

A patient with rheumatoid disease, treated with naproxen, has CHD.

Question

Is there any benefit or harm in adding aspirin to his treatment?

Answer

Aspirin is more beneficial than any other non-steroidal anti-inflammatory agent in modifying platelet activity and reducing mortality and morbidity in CHD. There is an increased risk of gastro-intestinal bleeding if two agents are given but at low doses of aspirin this should not be a major consideration. There is some evidence, however, that some NSAIDs interfere with the action of aspirin by blocking access to the active site on the COX-1 enzyme. Such agents should be avoided. Diclofenac does not block the receptor and ibuprofen has a short action and is acceptable if given 2 h after the daily dose of aspirin.

Acknowledgement

Permission to use material prepared for versions of this chapter which appeared in earlier editions of this textbook by D.K. Scott and J. Dwight is gratefully acknowledged.

References

Cannon, C.P., Braunwald, E., McCabe, C.H., et al., 2004. Intensive versus moderate lipid lowering with statins after acute coronary syndromes. N. Engl. J. Med. 350, 1495–1504.

CAPRIE Steering Committee, 1996. A randomised, blinded, trial of clopidogrel versus aspirin in patients at risk of ischaemic events (CAPRIE). Lancet 348, 1329–1339.

COMMIT (Clopidogrel and Metoprolol in Myocardial Infarction Trial) Collaborative Group, 2005. Addition of clopidogrel to aspirin in 45,852 patients with acute myocardial infarction: randomised placebo-controlled trial. Lancet 366, 1607–1621.

CURE (Clopidogrel in Unstable Angina to Prevent Recurrent Events) Trial Investigators, 2001. Effects of clopidogrel in addition to aspirin in patients with acute coronary syndromes without ST-segment elevation. N. Engl. J. Med. 345, 494–502.

EUROPA Study Investigators, 2003. The EURopean trial On reduction of cardiac events with perindopril in stable coronary artery disease investigators. Efficacy of perindopril in reduction of cardiovascular events among patients with stable coronary artery disease: randomised, double-blind, placebo-controlled, multicentre trial (the EUROPA study). Lancet 362, 782–788.

Fosbøl, E.L., Folke, F., Jacobsen, S., et al., 2010. Cause-specific cardiovascular risk associated with nonsteroidal anti-inflammatory drugs among healthy individuals. Circ. Cardiovasc. Qual. Outcomes. 3, 395–405. doi:10.1161/CIRCOUTCOMES.109.861104.

Fox, K.A.A., Poole-Wilson, P., Clayton, T., et al., 2005. Five-year outcome of an interventional strategy in non-ST-elevation acute coronary syndrome: the British Heart Foundation RITA 3 randomised trial. Lancet 366, 914–920.

Fox, K., Garcia, M.A.A., Ardissino, D., et al., 2006. The task force on the management of stable angina pectoris of the European Society of Cardiology. Guidelines on the management of stable angina pectoris. Eur. Heart J. 27, 1341–1381. doi:10.1093/eurheartj/ehl001.

Freemantle, N., Cleland, J., Young, P., et al., 1999. Beta blockade after myocardial infarction: systematic review and meta regression analysis. Br. Med. J. 318, 1730–1737.

GISSI-3 (Gruppo Italiano per lo Studio della Sopravvivenza nell'infarto Miocardico), 1994. Effects of lisinopril and transdermal glyceryl trinitrate singly and together on 6-week mortality and ventricular function after acute myocardial infarction. Lancet 343, 1115–1122.

HERO (Hirulog and Early Reperfusion or Occlusion)-2 Trial Investigators, 2001. Thrombin-specific anticoagulation with bivalirudin versus heparin in patients receiving fibrinolytic therapy for acute myocardial infarction: the HERO-2 randomised trial. Lancet 358, 1855–1863.

IONA Study Group, 2002. Effect of nicorandil on coronary events in patients with stable angina: the Impact of Nicorandil in Angina (IONA) randomised trial. Lancet 349, 1269–1275.

ISIS-2 (Second International Study of Infarct Survival) Collaborative Group, 1990. In-hospital mortality and clinical course of 20, 891 patients with suspected acute myocardial infarction randomised between tissue plasminogen activator or streptokinase with or without heparin. Lancet 336, 71–75.

ISIS-4 (Fourth International Study of Infarct Survival) Collaborative Group, 1995. A randomised factorial trial assessing early oral captopril, oral mononitrate, and intravenous magnesium sulphate in 58,050 patients with suspected acute myocardial infarction. Lancet 345, 669–685.

Januzzi, J.L., Stern, T.A., Pasternak, R.C., et al., 2000. The influence of anxiety and depression on outcomes of patients with coronary artery disease. Arch. Intern. Med. 160, 1913–1921.

Josan, K., Majumdar, S.R., McAlister, F.A., 2008. The efficacy and safety of intensive statin therapy: a meta-analysis of randomized trials. Can. Med. Assoc. J. 178, 576–584.

Kastrati, A., Mehilli, J., Neumann, F.J., et al., 2006. Abciximab in patients with acute coronary syndromes undergoing percutaneous coronary intervention after clopidogrel pretreatment: the ISAR-REACT 2 randomized trial. J. Am. Med. Assoc. 295, 1531–1538.

Malmberg, K., for the DIGAMI (Diabetes Mellitus Insulin Glucose Infusion in Acute Myocardial Infarction) Study Group, 1997. Prospective randomised study of intensive insulin treatment on long term survival after acute myocardial infarction in patients with diabetes mellitus. DIGAMI (Diabetes Mellitus, Insulin Glucose Infusion in Aacute Myocardial Infarction) Study Group. Br. Med. J. 314, 1512–1515.

Malmberg, K., Ryden, L., Wedel, H., et al., 2005. Intense metabolic control by means of insulin in patients with Diabetes Mellitus and Acute Myocardial Infarction (DIGAMI 2): effects on mortality and morbidity. Eur. Heart J. 26, 650–661.

McMurray, J.J.V., Rankin, A.C., 1994. Treatment of myocardial infarction, unstable angina and angina pectoris. Br. Med. J. 309, 1343–1350.

Mehta, S.R., Yusuf, S., Diaz, R., et al., 2005. Effect of glucose-insulin-potassium infusion on mortality in patients with acute ST-segment elevation myocardial infarction: the CREATE-ECLA randomized controlled trial. J. Am. Med. Assoc. 293, 437–446.

Menon, V., Harrington, R.A., Hochman, J.S., et al., 2004. Thrombolysis and adjunctive therapy in acute myocardial infarction. Chest 126, 549S–575S.

National Institute for Health and Clinical Excellence, 2008. Cardiovascular Risk Assessment and the Modification of Blood Lipids for the Primary and Secondary Prevention of Cardiovascular Disease. NICE, London. Available at: http://www.nice.org.uk/CG067.

National Institute for Health and Clinical Excellence, 2009. Prasugrel for the Treatment of Acute Coronary Syndromes with Percutaneous Coronary Intervention. NICE, London. Available at: http://guidance.nice.org.uk/TA182.

OASIS-6 Trial Group, 2006. Effects of fondaparinux on mortality and reinfarction in patients with acute ST-segment elevation myocardial infarction. J. Am. Med. Assoc. 295, 1519–1530.

OPTIMAAL Study Group, 2002. Effect of losartan and captopril on mortality and morbidity in high-risk patients after acute myocardial infarction: the OPTIMAAL randomized trial. Lancet 360, 752–780.

Pitt, B., Remme, W., Zannad, F., for the Eplerenone Post-Acute Myocardial Infarction Heart Failure Efficacy and Survival Study Investigators, et al., 2003. Eplerenone, a selective aldosterone blocker, in patients with left ventricular dysfunction after myocardial infarction. N. Engl. J. Med. 348, 1309–1321.

Ridker, P.M., Danielson, E., Fonseca, F.A.H., for the JUPITER Study Group et al., 2008. Rosuvastatin to prevent vascular events in men and women with elevated C-reactive protein. N. Engl. J. Med. 359, 2195–2207.

Rochon, P.A., Tu, J.V., Anderson, G.M., et al., 2000. Rate of heart failure and 1-year survival for older people receiving low-dose β-blocker therapy after myocardial infarction. Lancet 356, 639–644.

Sabatine, M.S., Cannon, C.P., Gibson, C.M., for the CLARITY-TIMI 28 Investigators et al., 2005. Addition of clopidogrel to aspirin and fibrinolytic therapy for myocardial infarction with ST-segment elevation. N. Engl. J. Med. 352, 1179–1189.

Stone, G.W., Bertrand, M.E., Moses, J.W., et al., 2007. Routine upstream initiation vs deferred selective use of glycoprotein IIb/IIIa inhibitors in acute coronary syndromes: the ACUITY Timing Trial. J. Am. Med. Assoc. 297, 591–602.

Thygesen, K., Alpert, J.S., White, H.D., et al., 2007. Joint ESC/ACCF/AHA/WHF Task Force for the redefinition of myocardial infarction. Universal definition of myocardial infarction. Eur. Heart J. 28, 2525–2538.

Unal, B., Critchley, J.A., Capewell, S., 2004. Explaining the decline in coronary heart disease mortality in England and Wales between 1981 and 2000. Circulation 109, 1101–1107.

VALIANT (VALsartan In Acute myocardial iNfarction Trial) Investigators, 2003. Valsartan, captopril, or both in myocardial infarction complicated by heart failure, left ventricular dysfunction, or both. N. Engl. J. Med. 349, 1893–1906.

Van de Werf, F., Bax, J., Betriu, A., et al., 2008. The task force on the management of ST-segment elevation acute myocardial infarction of the European Society of Cardiology. Management of acute myocardial infarction in patients presenting with persistent ST-segment elevation. Eur. Heart J. 29, 2909–2945.

Yusuf, S., Sleight, P., Pogue, J., et al., 2000. Effects of an angiotensin-converting-enzyme inhibitor, ramipril, on cardiovascular events in high-risk patients. The Heart Outcomes Prevention Evaluation (HOPE) Study Investigators. N. Engl. J. Med. 342, 145–153.

Further reading

Montalescot, G., Wiviott, S.D., Braunwald, E., et al., 2009. Prasugrel compared with clopidogrel in patients undergoing percutaneous coronary intervention for ST-elevation myocardial infarction (TRITON-TIMI 38): double-blind, randomised controlled trial. Lancet 373, 723–731.

National Institute for Health and Clinical Excellence, 2010. Unstable Angina and NSTEMI. The Early Management of Unstable Angina and Non-ST-Segment-Elevation Myocardial Infarction. NICE, London. Available at: http://www.nice.org.uk/guidance/CG94.

Chronic heart failure 21

S. A. Hudson, J. McAnaw and T. Dreischulte

Key points

- Heart failure is a common condition that affects the quality of life causing fatigue, breathlessness and oedema. It often has a poor prognosis.
- Heart failure is a maladaptive condition with haemodynamic and neurohormonal disturbances. Increased understanding of its pathophysiology and the strength of the evidence base allow a rational approach to therapeutic management.
- The aims of drug treatment are to control symptoms and to improve survival. By slowing disease progression the aim is to maintain quality of life.
- Diuretics are used for symptomatic management of heart failure, and are combined with other agents in the treatment of systolic dysfunction.
- Angiotensin converting enzyme (ACE) inhibitors and β-blockers are first-line agents in asymptomatic and symptomatic patients with systolic dysfunction.
- Angiotensin II receptor blockers (ARBs) are an alternative choice in patients intolerant of or resistant to ACE inhibitor therapy. Where use of an ARB is inappropriate, the combination of hydralazine and nitrate may still have a place.
- Aldosterone antagonists have been shown to improve morbidity and mortality when used as adjunctive therapy in patients with heart failure due to systolic dysfunction.
- Digoxin may still have a role in improving symptoms and reducing the rate of hospitalisation for patients with heart failure in sinus rhythm, but has not been demonstrated to affect mortality.
- Heart failure is a condition in which integration of pharmaceutical care within multidisciplinary models of patient care can improve clinical outcomes for patients and contribute to the continuity of care.

Chronic heart failure results from deficiency in the heart's function as a pump, where the delivery of blood, and therefore oxygen and nutrients, becomes inadequate for the needs of the tissues. Chronic heart failure is a complex condition associated with a number of symptoms arising from defects in left ventricular filling and/or emptying, of which shortness of breath (exertional dyspnoea, orthopnoea and paroxysmal nocturnal dyspnoea), fatigue and ankle swelling are the most common. The symptoms of heart failure are due to inadequate tissue perfusion, venous congestion and disturbed water and electrolyte balance. Impairment of renal function, and the associated water retention, adds to the burden placed on the heart. In chronic heart failure, the physiological mechanisms that aim to maintain adequate tissue perfusion become counterproductive and contribute to the progressive nature of the condition.

Treatment is aimed at improving left ventricular function, controlling the secondary effects that lead to the occurrence of symptoms, and delaying disease progression. Drug therapy is indicated in all patients with heart failure to control symptoms (where present), improve quality of life and prolong survival. Patients with heart failure usually have their functional status assessed and categorised using the New York Heart Association (NYHA) classification system shown in Table 21.1.

Epidemiology

Chronic heart failure is a common condition with a prevalence ranging from 0.3% to 2% in the population at large, 3–5% in the population over 65 years old, and between 8% and 16% of those aged over 75 years. Heart failure accounts for 5% of adult medical admissions to hospital. There is a loss of cardiac reserve with age, and heart failure may often complicate the presence of other conditions in the elderly. More than 10% of patients with heart failure also have atrial fibrillation as a contributory factor. This combination presents a risk of thrombo-embolic complications, notably stroke; the risk is 2% in patients in sinus rhythm, but may exceed 10% a year in patients with atrial fibrillation who are not anticoagulated and have attendant risk factors.

Table 21.1 New York Heart Association (NYHA) classification of functional status of the patient with heart failure

I	No symptoms with ordinary physical activity (such as walking or climbing stairs)
II	Slight limitation with dyspnoea on moderate to severe exertion (climbing stairs or walking uphill)
III	Marked limitation of activity, less than ordinary activity causes dyspnoea (restricting walking distance and limiting climbing to one flight of stairs)
IV	Severe disability, dyspnoea at rest (unable to carry on physical activity without discomfort)

333

Heart failure is a progressive condition with complex possible causes, and mortality varies according to aetiology and severity. The variable prognosis is represented by a median survival of about 5 years after diagnosis. The prognosis can be predicted according to the severity of the disease, with an overall annual mortality rate for patients with chronic heart failure estimated at 10%. Main causes of death are progressive pump failure, sudden cardiac death and recurrent myocardial infarction.

Aetiology

Heart failure may be a consequence of myocardial infarction, but as a chronic condition it is often gradual in onset with symptoms arising insidiously and without any specific cause over a number of years. The common underlying aetiologies in patients with heart failure are coronary artery disease and hypertension. The appropriate management of these predisposing conditions is also an important consideration in controlling heart failure in the community. Identifiable causes of heart failure include aortic stenosis, cardiomyopathy, mechanical defects such as cardiac valvular dysfunction, hyperthyroidism and severe anaemia. Conditions that place increased demands on the heart can create a shortfall in cardiac output and lead to intermittent exacerbation of symptoms. Symptoms of heart failure may occur as a consequence of hyperthyroidism, where the tissues place a greater metabolic demand, or severe anaemia, where there is an increased circulatory demand on the heart. Cardiac output may also be compromised by bradycardia or tachycardia, or by a sustained arrhythmia such as that experienced by patients in atrial fibrillation.

Atrial fibrillation often accompanies hyperthyroidism and mitral valve disease, where a rapid and irregular ventricular response can compromise cardiac efficiency. Improved management of the underlying causes, where appropriate, may alleviate the symptoms of heart failure, whereas the presence of mechanical defects may require the surgical insertion of prosthetic valve(s). While around 50% of patients with heart failure have significant left ventricular systolic dysfunction, the other half is comprised of patients who have either a normal or insignificantly reduced left ventricular ejection fraction (EF), although there is no consensus on the threshold for compromised EF and assessment of each patient relies mainly on clinical symptoms. These patients are referred to as having heart failure with preserved left ventricular ejection fraction (HFPEF). However, most of the available evidence from clinical trials regarding the pharmacological treatment of heart failure to date relates to those patients with heart failure due to left ventricular systolic dysfunction. Clinical symptomatic description of chronic heart failure is mild, moderate, or severe heart failure. 'Mild' is used for patients who are mobile with no important limitations of dyspnoea or fatigue, 'severe' for patients who are markedly symptomatic in terms of exercise intolerance and 'moderate' for those with restrictions in between. Trials tend to formalise these categories into NYHA Categories I–IV (Table 21.1).

Pathophysiology

In health, cardiac output at rest is approximately 5 L/min with a mean heart rate of 70 beats per minute and stroke volume of 70 mL. Since the filled ventricle has a normal volume of 130 mL, the fraction ejected is over 50% of the ventricular contents, with the remaining (residual) volume being approximately 60 mL. In left ventricular systolic dysfunction, the EF is reduced to below 45%, and symptoms are common when the fraction is below 35%, although some patients with a low EF can remain asymptomatic. When the EF falls below 10%, patients have the added risk of thrombus formation within the left ventricle and in most cases anticoagulation with warfarin is indicated.

Left ventricular systolic dysfunction can result from cardiac injury, such as myocardial infarction, or by exposure of the heart muscle to mechanical stress such as long-standing hypertension. This may result in defects in systolic contraction, diastolic relaxation, or both. Systolic dysfunction arises from impaired contractility, and is reflected in a low EF and cardiac dilation. Diastolic dysfunction arises from impairment of the filling process. Diastolic filling is affected by the rate of venous return, and normal filling requires active diastolic expansion of the ventricular volume. The tension on the ventricular wall at the end of diastole is called the preload, and is related to the volume of blood available to be pumped. That tension contributes to the degree of stretch on the myocardium. In diastolic dysfunction, there is impaired relaxation or reduced compliance of the left ventricle during diastole and, therefore, less additional blood is accommodated. In pure diastolic dysfunction, the EF can be normal but cardiac dilation is absent. Sustained diastolic dysfunction, which is a feature in a minority of patients with heart failure, may lead to systolic dysfunction associated with disease progression and left ventricular remodelling (structural changes and/or deterioration).

During systolic contraction, the tension on the ventricular wall is determined by the degree of resistance to outflow at the exit valve and that within the arterial tree, that is, the systemic vascular resistance. Arterial hypertension, aortic narrowing and disorders of the aortic valve increase the afterload on the heart by increasing the resistance against which the contraction of the ventricle must work. The result is an increased residual volume and consequently an increased preload as the ventricle overfills, and produces greater tension on the ventricular wall. In the normal heart, a compensatory increase in performance occurs as the stretched myocardium responds through an increased elastic recoil. In the failing heart, this property of cardiac muscle recoiling under stretch is diminished, with the consequence that the heart dilates abnormally to accommodate the increased ventricular load. With continued dilation of the heart the elastic recoil property can become much reduced. Failure of the heart to handle the increasing ventricular load leads to pulmonary and systemic venous congestion. At the same time, the increased tension on the ventricular wall in heart failure raises myocardial oxygen requirements, which increases the risk of an episode of myocardial ischaemia or arrhythmias.

The failing heart may show cardiac enlargement due to dilation, which is reversible with successful treatment. An irreversible increase in cardiac muscle mass, cardiac hypertrophy, occurs with progression of heart failure and is a consequence of long-standing hypertension. While hypertrophy may initially alleviate heart failure, the increased mass is pathologically significant because it ultimately increases the demands on the heart and oxygen consumption.

A reflex sympathetic discharge caused by the diminished tissue perfusion in heart failure exposes the heart to catecholamines where positive inotropic and chronotropic effects help to sustain cardiac output and produce a tachycardia. Arterial constriction diverts blood to the organs from the skin and gastro-intestinal tract but overall raises systemic vascular resistance and increases the afterload on the heart.

Reduced renal perfusion due to heart failure leads to increased renin release from the glomerulus in the kidney. Circulating renin raises blood pressure through the formation of angiotensin I and angiotensin II, a potent vasoconstrictor, and renin also prompts adrenal aldosterone release. Aldosterone retains salt and water at the distal renal tubule and so expands blood volume and increases preload. Arginine vasopressin released from the posterior pituitary in response to hypoperfusion adds to the systemic vasoconstriction and has an antidiuretic effect by retaining water at the renal collecting duct.

These secondary effects become increasingly detrimental to cardiac function as heart failure progresses, since the vasoconstriction adds to the afterload and the expanded blood volume adds to the preload. The expanded blood volume promotes the atrial myocytes to release a natural vasodilator, atrial natriuretic peptide (ANP), to attenuate the increased preload.

The compensatory mechanisms for the maintenance of the circulation eventually become overwhelmed and are ultimately highly counterproductive, leading to the emergence and progression of clinical signs and symptoms of heart failure. The long-term consequences are that the myocardium of the failing heart undergoes biochemical and histological changes that lead to remodelling of the left ventricle which further complicates disease progression. In those patients where the condition is severe and has progressed to an end stage, heart transplantation may be the only remaining treatment option.

Clinical manifestations

The reduced cardiac output, impaired oxygenation and diminished blood supply to muscles cause fatigue. Shortness of breath occurs on exertion (dyspnoea) or on lying (orthopnoea). When the patient lies down, the postural change causes abdominal pressure on the diaphragm which redistributes oedema to the lungs, leading to breathlessness. At night the pulmonary symptoms give rise to cough and an increase in urine production prompts micturition (nocturia), which adds to the sleep disturbance. The patient can be inclined to waken at night as gradual accumulation of fluid in the lungs may eventually provoke regular attacks of gasping (paroxysmal nocturnal dyspnoea). Characteristically the patient describes the need to sit or stand up to seek fresh air, and often describes a need to be propped up by three or more pillows to remedy the sleep disturbances that are due to fluid accumulation.

Table 21.2 Clinical manifestations of heart failure

Venous (congestion)	Cardiac (cardiomegaly)	Arterial (peripheral hypoperfusion)
Dyspnoea	Dilation	Fatigue
Oedema	Tachycardia	Pallor
Hypoxia	Regurgitation	Renal impairment
Hepatomegaly	Cardiomyopathy	Confusion
Raised venous pressure	Ischaemia, arrhythmia	Circulatory failure

Patients with heart failure may appear pale and their hands cold and sweaty. Reduced blood supply to the brain and kidney can cause confusion and contribute to renal failure, respectively. Hepatomegaly occurs from congestion of the gastro-intestinal tract, which is accompanied by abdominal distension, anorexia, nausea and abdominal pain. Oedema affects the lungs, ankles and abdomen. Signs of oedema in the lungs include crepitations heard at the lung bases. In acute heart failure, symptoms of pulmonary oedema are prominent and may be life-threatening. The sputum may be frothy and tinged red from the leakage of fluid and blood from the capillaries. Severe dyspnoea may be complicated by cyanosis and shock. Table 21.2 presents the clinical manifestations of heart failure.

Investigations

Patients with chronic heart failure are diagnosed and monitored on the basis of signs and symptoms from physical examination, history and an exercise tolerance test. On physical examination of the patient, a lateral and downward displacement of the apex beat can be identified as evidence of cardiac enlargement. Additional third and/or fourth heart sounds are typical of heart failure and arise from valvular dysfunction. Venous congestion can be demonstrated in the jugular vein of the upright reclining patient by an elevated jugular venous pressure (JVP), which reflects the central venous pressure. The JVP is measured by noting the visible distension above the sternum and may be accentuated in heart failure by the application of abdominal compression in the reclining patient. Confirmation of heart failure, however, should not be based on symptom assessment alone.

Echocardiography is important when investigating patients with a suspected diagnosis of heart failure. An echocardiogram allows visualisation of the heart in real time and will identify whether heart failure is due to systolic dysfunction, diastolic dysfunction or heart valve defects. With the provision of direct access echocardiography services to doctors in primary care, an increasing number of patients can now be quickly referred to confirm or exclude heart failure due to left ventricular systolic dysfunction or other structural abnormalities. Some reports suggest that between 50% and 75% of

Table 21.3 Investigations performed to confirm a diagnosis of heart failure

Investigation	Comment
Blood test	The following assessments are usually performed: • Blood gas analysis to assess respiratory gas exchange • Serum creatinine and urea to assess renal function • Serum alanine- and aspartate-aminotransferase plus other liver function tests • Full blood count to investigate possibility of anaemia • Thyroid function tests to investigate possibility of thyrotoxicosis • Serum BNP or NT pro-BNP to indicate likelihood of a diagnosis of heart failure (screening test) • Fasting blood glucose to investigate possibility of diabetes mellitus
12-lead electrocardiogram	A normal ECG usually excludes the presence of left ventricular systolic dysfunction. An abnormal ECG will require further investigation
Chest radiograph	A chest radiograph (X-ray) is performed to look for an enlarged cardiac shadow and consolidation in the lungs
Echocardiography	An echocardiogram is used to confirm the diagnosis of heart failure and any underlying causes, for example, valvular heart disease

patients referred to direct access clinics may have normal left ventricular function, which has important implications for the selection of appropriate drug treatment. Table 21.3 shows a number of investigations that are routinely performed in the assessment of heart failure symptoms. The use of serum natriuretic peptide measurement in the diagnosis of patients with heart failure is currently limited by the lack of defined cut-off values and, therefore, measurements are only considered in combination with ECG/chest X-ray data prior to echocardiography.

Treatment of heart failure

Until the 1980s, pharmacotherapy was driven by the aim to control symptoms, when diuretics and digoxin were the mainstay of treatment. While relieving the symptoms of heart failure remains decisive in improving a patient's quality of life, a better understanding of the underlying pathophysiology has led to major advances in the pharmacological treatment of heart failure. With the introduction of angiotensin converting enzyme (ACE) inhibitors, β-blockers, angiotensin II receptor blockers (ARBs) and aldosterone antagonists, delaying disease progression and ultimately improving survival have become realistic goals of therapy. An outline of the site of action of the various drugs is schematically presented in Fig. 21.1.

In heart failure patients with co-morbid conditions known to contribute to heart failure, such as hyperthyroidism, anaemia, atrial fibrillation and valvular heart disease, attention must be given to ensuring these underlying contributing factors are well controlled. Patients with atrial fibrillation may be candidates for electrocardioversion. Tachycardia from atrial fibrillation usually requires control of the ventricular rate through suppression of atrioventricular node conduction. In patients with heart failure, the use of digoxin and/or β-blockers is recommended in such circumstances. In these patients, the use

of either anticoagulant or antiplatelet agents is necessary and should be based on an assessment of stroke risk.

In patients with heart failure and preserved EF, diuretics are commonly used for symptom control and there is some limited evidence to suggest that ACE inhibitors can reduce hospitalisation. However, the use of all other agents of proven benefit in treating heart failure due to left ventricular systolic dysfunction are currently not supported by an evidence base.

There is consensus that all patients with left ventricular systolic dysfunction should be treated with both an ACE inhibitor and a β-blocker in the absence of intolerance or contraindications. The evidence base for treatment clearly shows that use of an ACE inhibitor (or angiotensin receptor blocker) and β-blocker therapy in patients with heart failure due to left ventricular systolic dysfunction leads to an improvement in symptoms and reduction in mortality. There is some evidence to suggest that either agent can be initiated first, as both appear to be just as effective and well tolerated (CARMEN 2004, CIBIS III, 2005). Beneficial effects on morbidity and mortality have also been shown for the use of ARBs, aldosterone antagonists and hydralazine/nitrate combinations when used in the treatment of chronic heart failure. Digoxin has been shown to improve morbidity and reduce the number of hospital admissions in patients with heart failure, although its effect on mortality has not been demonstrated. Table 21.4 describes the treatment of acute heart failure in the hospital setting, while Fig. 21.2 highlights the possible treatment options for patients with chronic heart failure due to left ventricular systolic dysfunction.

The selection of adjunctive therapy beyond the use of ACE inhibitor and β-blocker therapy is largely dependent on the nature of the patient and the preference of the heart failure specialist involved in the patient's care. It is accepted that there is a limit as to how many agents any one patient can tolerate; therefore, the selection of drug therapy will probably be tailored to each individual patient, meaning that treatment plans will vary.

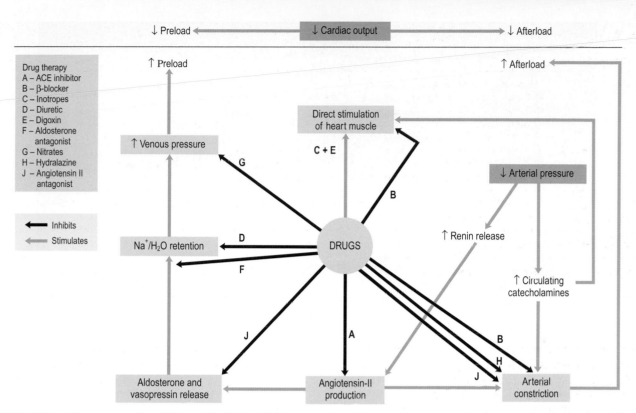

Fig. 21.1 Schematic representation of drug action in heart failure.

Table 21.4 Treatment of acute heart failure due to left ventricular systolic dysfunction in patients requiring hospitalisation

Problem	Drug therapy indicated
Anxiety	Use of intravenous opiates to reduce anxiety and reduce preload through venodilation
Breathlessness	High-flow oxygen (60–100%) may be required in conjunction with i.v. furosemide as either direct injection or 24-h infusion (5–10 mg/h). Venodilation with i.v. GTN is also effective at doses titrated every 10–20 min against systolic BP ≤ 110 mmHg
Arrhythmia	Digoxin useful in control of atrial fibrillation. Amiodarone is the drug of choice in ventricular arrhythmias
Expansion of blood volume following blood transfusion	An elevation in preload, such as can occur acutely by expansion of blood volume after a transfusion, can exacerbate the degree of systolic dysfunction. Therefore, it is necessary to continue or increase diuretic dosage during this time

Diuretics

In chronic heart failure, diuretics are used to relieve pulmonary and peripheral oedema by increasing sodium and chloride excretion through blockade of sodium re-absorption in the renal tubule. Normally, in the proximal tubule, about 70% of sodium is reabsorbed along with water. In mild heart failure, either a thiazide or more often a loop diuretic is chosen depending on the severity of the symptoms experienced by the patient and the degree of diuresis required. Thiazides are described as 'low-ceiling agents' because maximum diuresis occurs at low doses, and they act mainly on the cortical diluting segment (the point of merger of the ascending limb with the distal renal tubule) at which 5–10% of sodium is normally removed. Although thiazides have some action at this site, they fail to produce a marked diuresis since a compensatory increase in sodium re-absorption occurs in the loop of Henle, and consequently thiazides are ineffective in patients with moderate-to-severe renal impairment (eGFR <30 mL/min) or persisting symptoms. Additionally, doses above the equivalent of bendroflumethiazide 5 mg have an increased risk of adverse metabolic effects with no additional symptomatic benefit. Thiazides are, therefore, now rarely used as sole diuretic therapy and are reserved for cases where the degree of fluid retention is very mild, renal function is not compromised or as an adjunct to loop diuretics (see below).

Functional status of patient (NYHA)		Drug therapy indicated
Asymptomatic	I	In absence of contraindication or intolerance • ACE inhibitor (use Angiotensin II receptor blocker if not tolerated) • β-blocker In early post-MI patient with diabetes mellitus • Eplerenone*
Symptomatic	II–IV	As above, with addition of • Diuretic Where patient still symptomatic despite optimization of above therapy, consider addition of the following agents on specialist advice** • Candesartan • Digoxin (if patient in sinus rhythm) • Spironolactone (in moderate to severe heart failure) • Eplerenone* (if patient post-MI or spironolactone-intolerant) • Hydralazine/ISDN (beneficial in African-American patients)

* Therapy should be introduced within a month after acute MI
** Use of adjunctive therapy must be guided by a heart failure specialist/cardiologist, as there are certain combinations that require very close monitoring or complete avoidance according to current clinical evidence.

Fig. 21.2 Outline of treatment options for patients with chronic heart failure due to left ventricular systolic dysfunction.

Loop diuretics are indicated in the majority of symptomatic patients and most patients will be prescribed one of either furosemide, bumetanide or torasemide in preference to a thiazide. These agents are known as 'high-ceiling agents' because their blockade of sodium re-absorption in the loop of Henle continues with increased dose. They have a shorter duration of action (average 4–6 h) compared to thiazides (average 12–24 h), and produce less hypokalaemia. In high doses, however, their intensity of action may produce hypovolaemia with risk of postural hypotension, worsening of symptoms and renal failure. In practice, high doses of furosemide (up to 500 mg/day) may be required to control oedema in patients with poor renal function. In the acute situation, doses of loop diuretics are titrated to produce a weight loss of 0.5–1 kg per day.

In longer term use, patients with heart failure frequently develop some resistance to the effects of loop diuretic due to a compensatory rebound in sodium retention. In this situation, a combination of thiazide and loop diuretics has been shown to have a synergistic effect, even in patients with reduced renal function. In the UK, metolazone is also used as an adjunct to augment the effects of loop diuretics. The potentially profound diuresis produced by such a combination poses serious risks, such as dehydration and hypotension, and patients who are prescribed metolazone in addition to an existing loop diuretic must be carefully monitored. In practice, patients with oedema treated with loop diuretics may best be treated using a degree of self-management. Some patients are instructed to make upward adjustment of loop diuretic dose or to add metolazone therapy on particular days, for example, when they self-record a gain of 2 kg or more in their body weight over a short period of time.

Diuretics also have a mild vasodilator effect that helps improve cardiac function and the intravenous use of loop diuretics reduces preload acutely by locally relieving pulmonary congestion before the onset of the diuretic effect. Effective diuretic therapy is demonstrated by normalisation of filling pressure. Therefore, continued elevation of the JVP suggests a need for more diuretic unless otherwise contraindicated. Intravenous furosemide must be administered at a rate not exceeding 4 mg/min to patients with renal failure, since it can cause ototoxicity when administered more rapidly.

Details of diuretic therapy used in left ventricular systolic dysfunction are summarised in Table 21.5.

ACE inhibitors

ACE inhibitors are indicated as first-line treatment for all grades of heart failure due to left ventricular systolic dysfunction, including those patients who are asymptomatic. These agents exert their effects by reducing both the preload and afterload on the heart, thereby increasing cardiac output.

ACE inhibitors act upon the renin–angiotensin–aldosterone system, and they reduce afterload by reducing the formation of angiotensin II, a potent vasoconstrictor in the arterial system. These drugs also have an indirect effect on sodium and water retention by inhibiting the release of aldosterone and vasopressin, thereby reducing venous congestion and preload. The increase in cardiac output leads to an improvement in renal perfusion, which further helps to alleviate oedema. ACE

Table 21.5 Diuretics and aldosterone antagonists used in the treatment of heart failure

Class and agent	Onset and duration of effect		Comment
Thiazide and related	**Oral**		
Bendroflumethiazide	Onset 1–2 h		Thiazides are effective in the treatment of sodium and water retention, although there is generally a loss of action in renal failure (GFR <25 mL/min). Metolazone has an intense action when added to a loop diuretic and is effective at low GFR
	Duration 12–18 h		
Metolazone	Onset 1–2 h		
	Duration 12–24 h		
Loop	**Oral**	**Parenteral**	
Furosemide	Onset 0.5–1 h	Onset 5 min	Loop diuretics are preferred in the treatment of sodium and water retention where renal dysfunction is evident or more severe grades of heart failure present. Agents can be given orally or by infusion, and all are effective at low GFR
	Duration 4–6 h	Duration 2 h	
Bumetanide	As above	As above	
Torasemide	Onset <1 h	Onset 10 min	
	Duration <8 h	Duration <8 h	
Aldosterone antagonist	**Oral**		
Spironolactone	Onset 7 h		Can enhance diuretic effect of loop and/or thiazide. Due to slow onset of action needs 2–3 days before maximum diuretic effect reached. Spironolactone can improve survival when given as an adjunct to ACE inhibitor and diuretic therapy at a recommended dose of 25 mg daily (initial dose of 25 mg daily or on alternate days)
	Duration 24 h		
Aldosterone antagonist	**Oral**		
Eplerenone	Half-life 3–5 h		In early post-MI patients with symptomatic heart failure (or asymptomatic patients with diabetes mellitus), eplerenone 50 mg daily improved survival when added to optimal therapy (initial dose of 25 mg daily)

inhibitors also potentiate the vasodilator bradykinin and may intervene locally on ACE in cardiac and renal tissues.

ACE inhibitors are generally well tolerated by most patients and have been shown to improve the quality of life and survival in patients with mild-to-severe systolic dysfunction (CONSENSUS, 1987; CONSENSUS II, 1992; SOLVD-P, 1992; SOLVD-T, 1991; V-HeFT II, 1991), including those patients who have experienced a myocardial infarction (AIRE), 1993; SAVE, 1992; TRACE, 1995). When an ACE inhibitor is prescribed, it is important to ensure that the dose is started low and increased gradually, paying close attention to renal function and electrolyte balance. The dose should be titrated to achieve the target dose that has been associated with long-term benefits shown in clinical trials or (if not possible) the maximum tolerable dose. There is some evidence to suggest that high doses of ACE inhibitor are more effective than low doses in relation to reduction in mortality, although it is uncertain whether this is a general class effect (ATLAS, 1999). In clinical practice, it is possible that some patients may be treated with ACE inhibitors at doses below those used in clinical trials. As a consequence, actual outcomes in heart failure treatment may not be as good as expected from the trial findings.

The introduction of an ACE inhibitor may produce hypotension, which is most pronounced after the first dose and is sometimes severe. Patients at risk include those already on high doses of loop diuretics, where the diuretics cannot

be stopped or reduced beforehand, and patients who may have a low-circulating fluid volume (due to dehydration) and an activated renin–angiotensin system. Hypotension can also occur where the ACE inhibitor has been initiated at too high a dose or where the dose has been increased too quickly after initiation. In the primary care setting, treatment must be started with a low dose which is usually administered at bedtime. In patients at particular risk of hypotension, a test dose of the shorter-acting agent captopril can be given to assess suitability for treatment before commencing long-term treatment with a preferred ACE inhibitor. Once it has been established that the ACE inhibitor can be initiated safely, the preferred option would be to switch to a longer acting agent with once- or twice-daily dosing, starting with a low dose which would be gradually titrated upwards to the recommended target (Table 21.6). Monitoring of fluid balance, blood biochemistry and blood pressure are essential safety checks during initiation and titration of ACE inhibitor therapy.

One of the most common adverse effects seen with ACE inhibitors is a dry cough and this is reported in at least 10% of patients. However, since a cough can occur naturally in patients with heart failure it is sometimes difficult to determine the true cause. ACE inhibitor therapy can also compromise renal function, although in patients in whom there is a reduction in renal perfusion due to worsening heart failure or hypovolaemia,

Table 21.6 Vasodilators used in the treatment of heart failure

	Dose	Frequency	Half-life (h)	Comment
ACE inhibitor				
Captopril	Target: 50–100 mg Start: 6.25 mg	Three times daily	8	First-dose hypotension may occur. May worsen renal failure. Adjust dose in renal failure. Hyperkalaemia, cough, taste disturbance and hypersensitivity may occur particularly with captopril
Enalapril	Target: 10–20 mg Start: 2.5 mg	Twice daily	11	
Lisinopril	Target: 20–35 mg Start: 2.5–5 mg	Once daily	12	ACE inhibitors have been shown to improve survival, with starting and target dose for those agents used in clinical trials highlighted
Ramipril	Target: 10 mg Start: 2.5 mg	Once daily (or divided dose)	13–17	
Trandolapril	Target: 4 mg Start: 0.5 mg	Once daily	16–24	
Cilazapril		Once daily	9	
Fosinopril		Once daily	11–14	
Perindopril		Once daily	25	
Quinapril		Once daily	–	
β-Blocker				
Carvedilol	Target: 25–50 mg Start: 3.125 mg	Twice daily	6–10	May initially exacerbate symptoms but if initiated at low dose and slowly titrated can improve long-term survival, even in elderly patients with heart failure Metoprolol succinate is currently not licensed for use in the UK
Bisoprolol	Target: 10 mg Start: 1.25 mg	Once daily	10–12	
Metoprolol (succinate) CR/XL formulation	Target: 200 mg Start: 12.5–25 mg	Once daily	3–7	
Nebivolol	Target: 10 mg Start: 1.25 mg	Once daily	10	Half-life of nebivolol can be 3–5 times longer in slow metabolisers
Nitrates				
Glyceryl trinitrate			1–4 min	Isosorbide dinitrate metabolised to isosorbide mononitrate. High doses needed. Tolerance can be prevented by nitrate-free period of >8 h. Protective effect against cardiac ischaemia. GTN given intravenously for sustained effect in acute/severe heart failure but limited by tolerance
Isosorbide dinitrate			1	
Isosorbide mononitrate			5	
Nitroprusside			2 min	Light sensitive. Acts on veins and arteries. Cyanide accumulation and acidosis limit treatment duration
Angiotensin II receptor blocker				
Losartan			6–9	Comparable effectiveness to ACE inhibitor in patients with ACE inhibitor intolerance, although similar effect on renal function and blood pressure. Recent evidence suggests improved survival when ARB used as adjunctive therapy. However, increased potential for deterioration in renal function and/or hyperkalaemia
Candesartan	Target: 32 mg Start: 4–8 mg	Once daily	9	
Valsartan	Target: 160 mg Start: 40 mg	Twice daily	9	
Hydralazine			2–3	Hydralazine has a direct action on arteries. Tolerance occurs. May cause drug-induced lupus and sodium retention

renal dysfunction can also occur. Therefore, there are a number of instances where ACE inhibitor intolerance can be misdiagnosed in practice. Where ACE inhibitor intolerance is suspected, patients can usually be successfully rechallenged with an ACE inhibitor once their heart failure is more stable, although careful monitoring of the patient should be undertaken during initiation and subsequent dose titration. If the increase in the patient's serum creatinine is >100% from baseline, the ACE inhibitor should be stopped, intolerance confirmed and specialist advice sought. Where the increase from baseline is 50–100%, the ACE inhibitor dose should be halved and serum creatinine concentration rechecked after 1–2 weeks. If renal function is stable and no cough or other adverse effects are reported, therapy should be continued. Where the problem persists, an alternative treatment option might be required, for example, ARB (similar benefits on morbidity and mortality, but there is a possibility of similar adverse effects on blood pressure and renal function) or hydralazine–nitrate combination.

ACE inhibitors are potentially hazardous in patients with pre-existing renal disease, as blockade of the renin-angiotensin system may lead to reversible deterioration of renal function. In particular, ACE inhibitors are contraindicated in patients with bilateral renal artery stenosis, in whom the renin-angiotensin system is highly activated to maintain renal perfusion. Since most ACE inhibitors or their active metabolites rely on elimination via the kidney, the risk of other forms of dose-related toxicity is also increased in the presence of renal failure. Fosinopril, which is partially excreted by metabolism, may be the preferred agent in patients with renal failure. ACE inhibitors are also contraindicated in patients with severe aortic stenosis because their use can result in a markedly reduced cardiac output due to decreased filling pressure within the left ventricle. Table 21.6 summarises the activity and use of ACE inhibitors.

Angiotensin II receptor blockers

Although comparisons of ACE inhibitors and ARBs have shown similar benefits on morbidity and heart failure mortality, only ACE inhibitors have been shown to have positive effects on all cause mortality. ARBs should, therefore, not be used instead of ACE inhibitors, unless the patient experiences intolerable side effects.

The use of ARBs as an adjunct to ACE inhibitor and β-blocker therapy has been associated with significant reductions in cardiovascular events and hospitalisation rate (CHARM Added, 2003). Although this finding is encouraging, the impact on mortality alone remains inconsistent and there is no clear consensus on when to use an ARB as adjunctive therapy. In studies involving patients unable to tolerate an ACE inhibitor, ARBs have been shown to be comparable to ACE inhibitors in reducing the risk of cardiovascular death and rate of hospitalisation, and in the control of symptoms in heart failure patients (CHARM Alternative, 2003; Val-HeFT, 2002). Therefore, ARBs are recommended for use as an alternative to ACE inhibitor therapy where intolerance has been confirmed. It is important to note that in patients who have renal failure secondary to ACE inhibitors, switching to an ARB is of no theoretical or practical benefit, as similar adverse effects are likely.

A recent meta-analysis has raised concerns about a possible increase of cancer in people taking ARBs (Sipahi et al., 2010). Although the implications of this are unclear it adds weight to the recommendation that ACE inhibitors, not ARBs, should be the first-line agent when selecting a drug to act on the renin-angiotensin system.

β-Blockers

Formerly, β-blockers have been contraindicated in patients with heart failure. However, the sympathetic neurohormonal overactivity that occurs in response to the failing heart has been identified as a decisive factor in the progression of ventricular dysfunction. Consequently, β-blockers have been tested in a number of clinical trials. There is now substantial evidence that β-blockers reduce mortality among patients with mild-to-moderate symptomatic heart failure (ANZ Carvedilol, 1997; CAPRICORN, 2001; CIBIS II, 1999; MERIT-HF, 1999; US Carvedilol, 1996) and those with severe heart failure

(COPERNICUS, 2001). This beneficial effect also extends to the elderly heart failure population (SENIORS, 2005).

The use of β-blockers is, therefore, recommended for all patients with heart failure due to left ventricular systolic dysfunction, irrespective of age and the degree of dysfunction. However, due to their negative inotropic effects, β-blockers should only be initiated when the patient's condition is stable. There is insufficient evidence for a class effect to be assumed illustrated by the fact that in one trial, metoprolol tartrate was found to be inferior to carvedilol (COMET, 2003). Currently, nebivolol, bisoprolol and carvedilol are the only licensed β-blockers for the treatment of heart failure in the UK.

It is likely that patients will experience a worsening of symptoms during initiation of therapy and, therefore, patients are started on very low doses of β-blocker (e.g. carvedilol 3.125 mg daily) with careful titration occurring over a number of weeks or months with careful monitoring. The goal is to titrate the dose towards those used in clinical trials that have been associated with morbidity and mortality benefits (carvedilol 25–50 mg daily). Table 21.6 summarises the activity and use of β-blockers in heart failure.

Despite the demonstrated benefits, there is ongoing concern that certain subgroups of patients with heart failure continue to be undertreated with β-blockers. These groups include patients with chronic obstructive pulmonary disease (COPD), peripheral vascular disease, diabetes mellitus, erectile dysfunction and older adults. With the exception of patients with reversible pulmonary disease, who have typically been excluded from β-blocker trials (CIBIS II, 1999; MERIT-HF, 1999), there is now sufficient evidence to justify the use of β-blockers licensed for heart failure in these patients. In addition, a systematic review of trials on cardio-selective β-blockers found no clinically significant adverse respiratory effects in patients with reversible COPD, although it would be prudent to use these agents in such patients with caution and with appropriate monitoring in place (Salpeter S. et al., 2005).

Aldosterone antagonists

The use of aldosterone antagonists as an adjunct to standard treatment has been shown to have an effect on morbidity and mortality in patients with heart failure. Spironolactone has been shown to reduce mortality and hospitalisation rates in patients with moderate-to-severe heart failure (RALES, 1999). The use of eplerenone has also been shown to be associated with similar benefits in early post-MI patients with symptomatic heart failure or early post-MI diabetic patients with asymptomatic heart failure (EPHESUS, 2003, EMPHASIS-HF, 2010).

Aldosterone can cause sodium and water retention, sympathetic activation and parasympathetic inhibition, all of which are associated with harmful effects in the patient with heart failure. Aldosterone antagonists counteract these effects by directly antagonising the activity of aldosterone, providing a more complete blockade of the renin–angiotensin–aldosterone system when used in conjunction with an ACE inhibitor. Although the combination of spironolactone (at a dose of 50 mg daily or more) and an ACE inhibitor is associated with an increased risk of developing hyperkalaemia, the use of a 25-mg daily dose has been shown to have little effect on serum potassium and provides a significant reduction in mortality. The use of spironolactone is, however, contraindicated in those patients with a serum potassium >5.5 mmol/L or serum creatinine >200 µmol/L. With eplerenone, similar contraindications exist and, therefore, close monitoring of blood biochemistry and renal function must be undertaken for use of either agent. The activity and use of spironolactone and eplerenone are summarised in Table 21.5.

Currently, there is no evidence available regarding the effectiveness and safety of combining an ACE inhibitor, ARB and an aldosterone antagonist, and therefore it is recommended that this combination is avoided until more information about this particular combination becomes available.

Digoxin

Although digoxin has an established role in the control of atrial fibrillation, its place in the treatment of heart failure is still the subject of debate. There is evidence to show that when digoxin has been used to treat heart failure in patients in sinus rhythm, as an adjunct to ACE inhibitor and diuretic therapy, then worsening of symptoms occurs on withdrawal of digoxin (PROVED, 1993; RADIANCE, 1993). While the use of digoxin in heart failure in patients in sinus rhythm has no measurable impact on mortality, it reduces the number of hospital admissions (DIG, 1997). Consequently, digoxin is currently recommended for use as add-on therapy at low doses in patients with moderate-to-severe heart failure who remain symptomatic despite adequate doses of ACE inhibitor, β-blocker and diuretic treatment. Due to the lack of effect on mortality, it is unlikely that digoxin would be considered before the other adjunctive therapies available.

Digoxin is a positive inotropic agent and acts by increasing the availability of calcium within the myocardial cell through an inhibition of sodium extrusion, thereby increasing sodium–calcium exchange and leading to enhanced contractility of cardiac muscle. Digoxin increases cardiac output in patients with co-existing atrial fibrillation by suppressing atrioventricular conduction and controlling the ventricular rate. In patients with atrial fibrillation, the serum digoxin concentration usually needs to be at the higher end of the reference range (0.8–2 µcg/L) or beyond to control the arrhythmia. However, a high serum digoxin concentration is not necessarily required to achieve an inotropic effect in patients in sinus rhythm. Digoxin is also associated with both vagal stimulation and a reduction in sympathetic nerve activity, and these may play important roles in the symptomatic benefits experienced by those patients in sinus rhythm receiving lower doses. In practice, the dose prescribed will be judged appropriate by the clinical response expressed as relief of symptoms and control of ventricular rate. Routine monitoring of serum digoxin concentrations in the pharmaceutical care of the patient is not recommended, other than to confirm or exclude digoxin toxicity or investigate issues around patient compliance.

Digoxin treatment is potentially hazardous due to its low therapeutic index and so all patients receiving this drug should be regularly reviewed to exclude clinical signs or symptoms of adverse effects. Digoxin may cause bradycardia and lead to potentially fatal cardiac arrhythmias. Other symptoms associated with digoxin toxicity include nausea, vomiting, confusion and visual disturbances. Digoxin toxicity is more pronounced in the presence of metabolic or electrolyte disturbances and in patients with cardiac ischaemia. Those patients who develop hypokalaemia, hypomagnesaemia, hypercalcaemia, alkalosis, hypothyroidism or hypoxia are at particular risk of toxicity. Treatment may be required to restore serum potassium, and in emergency situations intravenous digoxin-specific antibody fragments can be used to treat life-threatening digoxin toxicity. Table 21.7 summarises the activity and use of digoxin.

Table 21.7 Inotropic agents used in the treatment of heart failure

Class and agent	Pharmacological half-life	Comment
Cardiac glycosides		
Digoxin	39 h	In renal failure, half-life of digoxin is prolonged. Dosage individualisation
Digitoxin	5–8 days	required. Serum drug concentration monitoring used to confirm or exclude toxicity or effectiveness. Dose of digitoxin unaffected by renal failure. CNS, visual and GI symptoms linked to digoxin toxicity. No benefit in terms of mortality, but use associated with improved symptoms and reduced hospitalisation for heart failure. Beneficial in AF, although risk of arrhythmias with high doses. If given i.v. must be administered slowly (20 min) to avoid cardiac ischaemia
Phosphodiesterase inhibitors		
Enoximone	4.2 h	Used only in severe heart failure as adjunctive therapy. Associated with
Milrinone	2.4 h	arrhythmias and increased mortality with chronic use
Sympathomimetics		
Dobutamine	2 min	Continuous intravenous use only. Require close monitoring in critical care setting
Dopamine	2 min	
Dopexamine	6–7 min	
Isoprenaline	>1 min	

Nitrates/hydralazine

Nitrates exert their effects in heart failure predominantly on the venous system where they cause venodilation, thereby reducing the symptoms of pulmonary congestion. The preferred use of nitrates is in combination with an arterial vasodilator such as hydralazine, which reduces the afterload, to achieve a balanced effect on the venous and arterial circulation. The combined effects of these two drugs lead to an increase in cardiac output, and there is evidence to show the combination is effective and associated with a reduction in mortality in patients with heart failure (V-HeFT I, 1986). Although the combination can improve survival, the reduction in mortality is much smaller than that seen with ACE inhibitors (V-HeFT II, 1991), especially in the white population. The combination has been shown to reduce mortality, heart failure hospitalisation rates and quality of life in patients of African descent, when added as an adjunct to optimum medical therapy (A-HeFT, 2004) and this benefit is sustained (A-HeFT, 2007).

The evidence supports the use of hydralazine 300 mg daily with isosorbide dinitrate (ISDN) 160 mg daily (although in practice an equivalent dose of isosorbide mononitrate, ISMN, is often used). Since the emergence of ACE inhibitors, with their superior effects on morbidity and mortality, the combination has mainly been reserved for patients unable to tolerate, or with a contraindication to, ACE inhibitor therapy.

Organic nitrate vasodilators work by interacting with sulphydryl groups found in the vascular tissue. Nitric oxide is released from the nitrate compound and this in turn activates soluble guanylate cyclase in vascular smooth muscle, leading to the vasodilatory effect. Plasma nitric oxide concentrations are not clearly related to pharmacological effects because of their indirect action on the vasculature. Depletion of tissue sulphydryl groupings can occur during continued treatment with nitrates, and is partly responsible for the development of tolerance in patients with sustained exposure to high nitrate doses. Restoration of sulphydryl groupings occurs within hours of treatment being interrupted; therefore, nitrate tolerance can be prevented by the use of an asymmetrical dosing regimen to ensure that the patient experiences a daily nitrate-free period of more than 8 h.

In the acute setting, glyceryl trinitrate (GTN) is frequently administered intravenously, along with a loop diuretic, to patients with heart failure to relieve pulmonary congestion. When using this route of administration, it is important that a Teflon-coated catheter is used to avoid adsorption of the GTN onto the intravenous line.

ISDN can be given orally and is completely absorbed; however, only 25% of a given dose appears as ISDN in serum with 60% of an oral dose being rapidly converted to ISMN. ISMN is longer acting and, therefore, most of the accumulated effects of a dose of ISDN are attributable to the 5-isosorbide mononitrate metabolite. Consequently, a 20-mg dose of ISDN is approximately equivalent to a 10-mg dose of ISMN. In practice, nitrate preparations are usually given orally in the form of ISMN, and intravenously in the form of GTN (see Table 21.6).

Hydralazine has a direct action on arteriolar smooth muscle to produce arterial vasodilation. Its use is associated with the risk of causing drug-induced systemic lupus erythematosus (SLE). SLE is an uncommon multisystem connective tissue disorder that is more likely to occur in patients classified as slow acetylators of hydralazine, which accounts for almost half the UK population.

Inotropic agents

The use of inotropic agents (except digoxin) is almost exclusively limited to hospital practice, where acute heart failure may require the use of one or more inotropic agents, particularly the sympathomimetic agents dobutamine and dopamine, in an intravenous continuous infusion. These agents have inotrope-vasodilator effects which differ according to their action on α, β_1, β_2 and dopamine receptors (β_1-agonists increase cardiac contractility, β_2-agonists produce arterial vasodilation, dopamine agonists enhance renal perfusion). With dopamine, low doses (0–2 µcg/kg/min) have a predominant effect on dopamine receptors within the kidneys to improve urine output, intermediate doses (2–5 µcg/kg/min) affect β_1-receptors, producing an inotropic effect, and high doses (10 µcg/kg/min) have a predominant action on α-adrenoreceptors. Dobutamine has a predominantly inotropic and vasodilator action due to the action of the (+) isomer selectively on β-adrenoreceptors (see Table 21.7). Tolerance to sympathomimetic inotropic agents may develop on prolonged administration, particularly in patients with underlying ischaemia, and is also associated with a risk of precipitating arrhythmias.

Noradrenaline (norepinephrine) is an α-adrenoreceptor agonist where its vasoconstrictor action limits its usefulness in severely hypotensive patients such as those in septic shock. Adrenaline (epinephrine) has β_1, β_2 and α-adrenoreceptor agonist effects and is used in patients with low vascular resistance. However, it is more arrhythmogenic than dobutamine and should be used with caution.

Phosphodiesterase inhibitors are rarely used in clinical practice as a consequence of trials showing an increased risk of mortality (PROMISE, 1991).

Other agents

Direct-acting vasodilators such as sodium nitroprusside are rarely used except in the acute setting when they are given by continuous infusion. Vasodilation occurs as a result of the catalysis of nitroprusside in vascular smooth muscle cells to produce nitric oxide. The fact that nitric oxide production in this instance is via a different route when compared to the catalysis of GTN (where there is a need for sulphydryl groups) may explain why there is little tolerance seen with nitroprusside. In patients with impaired renal function thiocyanate, a metabolic product of nitroprusside can accumulate over several days, causing nausea, anorexia, fatigue and psychosis.

Patients with coronary heart disease may be candidates for calcium-blocking antianginal vasodilators. However, some of these agents can exacerbate co-existing heart failure, since their negative inotropic effects offset the potentially beneficial arterial vasodilation. Amlodipine and felodipine have a more selective action on vascular tissue and, therefore, a less pronounced effect on cardiac contractility than other calcium antagonists and should be the agents of choice where appropriate.

In hospitalised patients in whom compromised respiratory function remains despite medical management of heart failure, the treatment options include mechanical ventilation, continuous positive airway pressure ventilation and the use of intra-aortic balloon pumping.

Guidelines

Several groups have produced evidence-based consensus clinical guidelines for the management of chronic heart failure. The focus of the various guidelines tends to be on chronic medication use (National Institute for Health and Clinical Excellence, 2010; American College of Cardiology/American Heart Association Task Force on Practice Guidelines, 2009; European Society of Cardiology, 2008; Scottish Intercollegiate Guidelines Network, 2007). All guidelines confirm that ACE inhibitors and β-blockers should be given to all patients with all grades of heart failure, whether symptomatic or asymptomatic, in the absence of contraindication or intolerance.

In ACE inhibitor-intolerant patients, the preferred alternative is an ARB. However, it should be remembered that where ACE inhibitor intolerance is due to renal dysfunction, hypotension or hyperkalaemia, similar effects could be expected with an ARB. If an ARB is an unsuitable alternative, the use of hydralazine/nitrate combination or digoxin could be considered, although the latter combination of agents has no effect on mortality. For patients with symptomatic heart failure, a loop diuretic is usually recommended to treat oedema and control symptoms. In heart failure patients who are still symptomatic despite being on optimum therapy (ACE inhibitor, β-blocker with/without a diuretic), the use of adjunctive therapies is recommended which can include ARB, aldosterone antagonists, hydralazine/nitrate combination and digoxin where the patient is still in sinus rhythm.

There is also debate as to whether diastolic dysfunction is a true diagnosis. The cause of 'apparent' heart failure symptoms can in many cases be attributed to another disease/condition such as respiratory disease, obesity or ischaemic heart disease. However, there may also be some patients in whom the cause of heart failure symptoms remains uncertain. Therefore, specific recommendations for the drug treatment of diastolic heart failure are still lacking.

Patient care

Heart failure remains poorly understood by the general public, amongst whom only 3% were able to identify the condition when presented with a list of typical symptoms. Patients with heart failure are often elderly and often include patients with co-morbidity such as coronary heart disease and hypertension. Other complications include renal impairment, polypharmacy and variable adherence to prescribed medication regimens. Where renal function is compromised, careful attention to dosage selection is required for drugs excreted largely unchanged in the urine. Patients with heart failure are at particular risk of fluid or electrolyte imbalance, adverse effects and drug interactions. Consequently, careful monitoring is indicated to help detect problems associated with suboptimal drug therapy, unwanted drug effects and poor patient adherence.

A number of therapeutic problems may be encountered by the patient with heart failure. Notably, heart failure often complicates other serious illness, and is a common cause of hospital admission. In addition to monitoring clinical signs and symptoms in the acute setting, there should be monitoring of fluid and electrolyte balance, assessment of renal and hepatic function, and performance of chest radiograph, electrocardiograph and haemodynamic measurements where appropriate.

Patient education and self-monitoring

The patient must be in a position to understand the need for treatment and the benefits and risks offered by prescribed medication before concordance with a treatment plan can be reached. Appropriate patient education is necessary to encourage an understanding of their condition, inform patients of the extent of their condition and how prescribed drug treatment will work and affect their daily lives. It is also important to encourage them to be an active participant in their care where appropriate. Specific advice should be given to reinforce the timing of doses and how each medication should be taken. Patients also need to be advised of potentially troublesome symptoms that may occur with the medication, and whether such effects are avoidable, self-limiting or a cause for concern.

Patients should be made aware that diuretics will increase urine production, and that doses are usually timed for the morning to avoid inconvenience during the rest of the day or overnight. However, there are cases where patients are advised that they can alter the timing of the dose(s) if required to suit their lifestyle or social commitments, with the agreement of their doctor. There are also some patients who use a flexible diuretic dosing regimen, where they can take an extra dose of diuretic in response to worsening signs or symptoms as part of an agreed self-management protocol. To use such a regimen, the patient has to monitor and record their weight on a daily basis, and have clear instructions to take an extra dose of diuretic when a notable increase in weight is detected as a result of fluid retention, and when to seek medical attention. It is also important for patients to be aware of signs and symptoms of drug toxicity with medicines such as digoxin, for example anorexia, diarrhoea, nausea and vomiting, and be aware of the action to be taken should these symptoms occur.

Timing of doses is also important. If a nitrate regimen is being used, then patients must be made aware that the last dose of the nitrate should be taken mid to late afternoon to ensure that a nitrate-free period occurs overnight, thus, reducing the risk of nitrate tolerance. However, patients with prominent nocturnal symptoms require separate consideration. Where β-blockers are introduced, it is important that the patient is aware of the need for gradual dose titration due to the risk of the medication aggravating heart failure symptoms. Certain medicines for the treatment of minor ailments that are available for purchase over the counter without a prescription can aggravate heart failure, such as ibuprofen, antihistamines and effervescent formulations. It is important that patients know what action to take if their symptoms become progressively worse, and whom to contact when necessary for advice. Table 21.8 provides a general patient education and self-monitoring checklist, highlighting the typical areas where advice should be given.

Monitoring effectiveness of drug treatment

Therapeutic effectiveness is confirmed by assessing the patient for improvements in reported symptoms such as shortness of breath and oedema, and for noticeable changes in exercise tolerance. Oedema is often visible and remarked upon by patients, especially in the feet (ankles) and hands (wrists and fingers). Increased oedema may be reflected by an increase in the patient's body weight, and can be more easily assessed if the patient routinely records their weight and reviews this on a daily basis. Questions about tolerance to exercise are also use-

ful in identifying patients who may be experiencing difficulties with their condition or where the treatment plan is suboptimal. Onset or deterioration of symptoms is often slow and patients are more inclined to adapt their lifestyle gradually by moderating daily activities to compensate. This should be borne in mind whenever a patient assessment is undertaken.

Identifying the symptoms of poor heart failure control can be complicated by many factors, such as the presence of conditions like arthritis and parkinsonism which can also affect a patient's mobility. Poor control of respiratory disease, presenting as an increased shortness of breath or exacerbation of other respiratory symptoms, can also be mistaken for loss of control of heart failure. Therefore, consideration of these and other factors is necessary in the interpretation of presenting symptoms, as a deterioration in symptoms may not be solely due to worsening heart failure or ineffective heart failure medication.

Dietary factors can lead to loss of symptom control, where failure to restrict sodium intake may contribute to an ongoing problem of fluid retention. Simple dietary advice to avoid processed foods and not to add salt to food should be reinforced.

Table 21.8 Patient education and self-monitoring in the treatment of heart failure

Topic	Advice	Comment
Diuretics	• Will cause diuresis • Timing of dose • Flexible dosing (where indicated)	Monitor for incontinence, muscle weakness, confusion, dizziness, gout, unusual gain in weight within very short time-period (few days). Use of diary to record and monitor daily weight can help identify when to take an agreed extra dose of diuretic. Patient also able to adjust time of dose to suit lifestyle where necessary
ACE inhibitors	• Improve symptoms • Avoid standing rapidly	Monitor for hypotension, dizziness, cough, taste disturbance, sore throat, rashes, tingling in hands, joint pain
β-Blockers	• Symptoms worsen initially • Gradual increase in dose	Monitor for hypotension, dizziness, headache, fatigue, gastro-intestinal disturbances, bradycardia
Cardiac glycosides	• Report toxic symptoms	Monitor for signs or symptoms of toxicity, such as anorexia, nausea, visual disturbances, diarrhoea, confusion, social withdrawal
Nitrates	• Timing of dose • Postural hypotension • Avoid standing rapidly	Monitor for headache, hypotension, dizziness, flushing (face or neck), gastro-intestinal upset. Ensure asymmetrical dosing pattern for nitrates to provide nitrate-free period and reduce risk of tolerance developing
Potassium salts	• Administration of dose (soluble + non-soluble)	Monitor for gastro-intestinal disturbances, swallowing difficulty, diarrhoea, tiredness, limb weakness. Ensure patient knows how to take their medication safely, for example, swallow whole immediately after food, or soluble forms to be taken with appropriate amount of water/fruit juice and allow fizzing to stop
Purchased medicines	• Choice of medicines	Ensure patient is aware of need to seek advice when purchasing medicines for minor ailments. Ask pharmacist to confirm suitability when selecting
Understanding the condition	• What heart failure is • Impact on lifestyle • Treatment goals	Ensure patient understands their condition, treatment goals and complications that may impact on their quality of life. Important to motivate the patient with respect to lifestyle modification and achievement of agreed treatment goals relative to the degree of heart failure present (asymptomatic, mild, moderate or severe symptoms)
Health issues	• Diet; sodium intake • Alcohol intake • Smoking • Exercise • Other risk factors	Issues related to diet, alcohol consumption, smoking habit, regular gentle exercise (walking). Other associated risk factors, for example, hypertension, ischaemic heart disease, need to be addressed where appropriate

According to some manufacturers, the absorption of ACE inhibitors, for example, captopril, perindopril, may be slowed by food or antacids and, therefore, patients should be advised to take the dose before food in the morning to ensure maximum effect.

Patients with heart failure may often receive suboptimal drug treatment, due to the fact that they are not prescribed first-line therapy, such as ACE inhibitors and β-blockers, and the dosage is below the recommended target dose. All patients at risk of suboptimal treatment need to be routinely identified, and this will require the involvement of health care professionals in the monitoring of symptoms and the individualisation of each patient's therapeutic plan.

In an effort to systematically identify whether a patient's therapeutic plan adheres to the current evidence base for treatment, and whether any changes might be required to optimise therapy, the audit tool shown in Box 21.1 could be used in routine practice. The tool has been derived from published consensus-based clinical guidelines, and could underpin a more comprehensive medication review.

Monitoring safety of drug treatment

A number of issues around the safe use of medication must be considered, especially in those patients with co-morbidity and/or a high number of prescribed medicines. In these patients there is an increased risk of drug–drug and drug–disease interactions (Tables 21.9-21.11). It is important to be aware of clinically important interactions and to investigate potentially problematic combinations, as well as to regularly assess the patient for any signs or symptoms of drug therapy problems. Monitoring for problems such as negative inotropic effects, excessive blood pressure reduction, and salt and fluid retention should be undertaken and, where appropriate, laboratory measurement of serum drug concentration (digoxin) or physiological markers (potassium, creatinine) should be performed to confirm or exclude adverse effects. Patients started on an ACE inhibitor should have renal function and serum electrolytes checked at 1 and 3 months after starting therapy, and 6 monthly once a maintenance dose is reached.

Potential problems with diuretic therapy

The use of diuretic therapy for sodium and water retention is common in the treatment of heart failure, although there can be a number of problems for the patient to contend with. Elderly patients in particular are at risk from the unwanted effects of diuretics. The increase in urine volume can worsen incontinence or precipitate urinary retention in the presence of an enlarged prostate, while overuse can lead to a loss of

Table 21.9 Monitoring the effectiveness of drug treatment in patients with heart failure

Consider	Monitor for	Comment
Clinical markers	• Poor symptom control • Achievement of agreed treatment goals	Signs or symptoms of undertreatment or advancing disease need to be addressed (dyspnoea, breathlessness and/or fatigue). The aim is for good symptom control and either maintenance or improvement in quality of life. Persisting symptoms or hospitalisation may indicate a revision of drug therapy or the addition of other agents where appropriate
Interactions	• Drug–drug interactions	Some interactions may result in reduced effectiveness and require dosage adjustment or change in choice of drug
Compliance	• Formulation acceptability • Dose timing and interval • Unusual time interval between requests for prescription medication	Poor adherence can result from drug being ineffective (over- or under-use), experience of side effects, a complicated drug regimen or patient behaviour (intentional non-adherence or forgetfulness). Reasons need to be identified and addressed where possible, for example, adjusting frequency and timing of doses, review choice of formulation, education. Initiation of devices to improve compliance should be considered where appropriate
Evidence-based prescribing	• Implementation of evidence-based guidelines • Audit of prescribed treatment for heart failure	The drug of choice for a particular patient may not reflect the evidence base for treatment for patients with heart failure. It is important to ensure evidence-based treatments are considered for every patient, and choices of medication confirmed or changed where appropriate. Audit of guideline recommendations to help confirm that treatment plans are optimal can be systematically applied to help assess appropriateness of treatment (see Box 21.1)
Multidisciplinary working	• Input from other health care professionals	It is important to be aware of what care has already been provided to minimise the risk of giving conflicting advice to the patient or duplicating work already done. It may also allow reinforcement of key information. There is an increasing evidence base for the benefits of multidisciplinary models of care for chronic heart failure patients

Box 21.1 Criteria for the assessment of drug treatment in a patient with chronic heart failure (Scottish Intercollegiate Guidelines Network, 2007)

Need for drug therapy (all patients)
1. Is an ACE inhibitor prescribed?
2. If intolerant to ACE inhibitor, is an ARB prescribed?
3. If intolerant to an ACE inhibitor and ARB, is H/ISDN prescribed?
4. Is a β-blocker prescribed?
5. Has patient received pneumococcal vaccination?
6. Has patient received influenza vaccination?

Need for drug therapy (as appropriate)
7. If symptomatic on optimised doses of ACE inhibitor and BB, is an aldosterone antagonist or candesartan prescribed?
8. If symptomatic on optimised therapy with ACE inhibitor I, BB and ARB/aldosterone antagonist, is digoxin prescribed?
9. If post-MI, is an antiplatelet and statin prescribed?
10. In AF, is thrombo-embolic prophylaxis prescribed?

Need for dose titration
11. If an ACE inhibitor I is prescribed, target dose achieved?
12. If an ARB is prescribed, target dose achieved?
13. If a BB is prescribed, target dose achieved?
14. If warfarin prescribed, is dose titrated to INR?

Medication safety
15. Aggravating drugs avoided (if possible):
    (a) NSAIDs
    (b) Tricyclic antidepressants
    (c) Some antihistamines (e.g. diphenhydramine)
    (d) Dihydropyridine calcium channel blockers (except amlodipine or felodipine)
    (e) Diltiazem, verapamil
    (f) Glitazone anti-diabetics
    (g) Minoxidil
    (h) Itraconazole and other azole antifungals
    (i) Macrolide antibiotics
    (j) Corticosteroids
    (k) Tadalafil
    (l) Lithium

ACE inhibitor, angiotensin converting enzyme inhibitor; AF, atrial fibrillation; ARB, angiotensin receptor blocker; BB, β-blocker; H, hydralazine; INR, international normalised ratio; MI, myocardial infarction.

control of heart failure and worsening of symptoms. Rapid diuresis with a loop diuretic leading to more than a 1-kg loss in body weight per day may exacerbate heart failure due to an acute reduction in blood volume, hypotension and diminished renal perfusion, with a consequent increase in renin release. Prolonged and excessive doses of diuretics can also contribute to symptoms of fatigue as a consequence of electrolyte disturbance and dehydration. The adverse biochemical effects of excessive diuresis include uraemia, hypokalaemia and alkalosis. Diuretic-induced glucose intolerance may affect diabetic control in type 2 diabetes, but more commonly diuretics reveal glucose intolerance in patients who are not diagnosed as being diabetic. Diuretics also increase serum urate leading to hyperuricaemia, although this may not require a change in drug therapy if symptoms of gout are absent (estimated incidence of 2%).

Hyponatraemia may occur with diuretics, and is usually due to water retention rather than sodium loss. Severe hyponatraemia (serum sodium concentration of less than 115 mmol/L) causes confusion and drowsiness. It commonly arises when potassium-sparing agents are used in diuretic combinations.

Diuretics may also lead to hypokalaemia as a result of urinary sodium increasing the rate of K^+/Na^+ exchange in the distal tubule. Serum potassium concentrations below 3.0 mmol/L occur in less than 5% of patients receiving diuretics. The occurrence of hypokalaemia is hazardous for patients receiving digoxin and also for those with ischaemic heart disease or conduction disorders. It is more commonly found with thiazide diuretics than loop agents, and is more likely to occur when diuretics are used for heart failure than for hypertension. This is probably due to the fact that higher doses are used and there is an associated activation of the renin angiotensin system. Patients with a serum potassium level of less than 3.5 mmol/L require treatment with potassium supplements or the addition of a potassium-sparing diuretic. The use of a potassium-sparing diuretic is considered to be more effective at preventing hypokalaemia than using potassium supplements. Prevention of hypokalaemia requires at least 25 mmol of potassium, while treatment requires 60–120 mmol of potassium daily. Since proprietary diuretic-potassium combination products usually contain less than 12 mmol in each dose, their use is often inappropriate.

Potassium supplements are poorly tolerated at the high doses often needed to treat hypokalaemia, and a liquid formulation is more preferable to a solid form. This is mainly due to the fact that solid forms can produce local high concentrations of potassium salts in the gastro-intestinal tract, with the risk of damage to the tract in patients with swallowing difficulties or delayed gastro-intestinal transit. In patients with deteriorating renal function or renal failure, the use of potassium supplements or potassium-sparing diuretics might cause hyperkalaemia, and therefore careful monitoring of these agents is essential.

Potential problems with ACE inhibitor and ARB therapy

ACE inhibitors are the cornerstone of the treatment of heart failure, but there are also risks associated with their use. ARBs, which also act on the renin–angiotensin–aldosterone system, pose similar risks to those recognised for ACE inhibitors. Both agents can predispose patients to hyperkalaemia through a reduction in circulating aldosterone; therefore, potassium supplements or potassium-retaining agents should be used with care when co-prescribed, and careful monitoring of serum potassium should be mandatory. Although potassium retention can be a problem with ACE inhibitors and ARBs, it can also be an advantage by helping to counteract the potassium loss that can result from the use of diuretic therapy. However, since this effect on potassium cannot be predicted, laboratory monitoring is still necessary to confirm that serum potassium concentration remains within safe limits.

The use of an aldosterone antagonist as adjunctive therapy with an ACE inhibitor (or ARB if the patient is ACE inhibitor intolerant) can be safely undertaken with minimal effects on the serum potassium concentration, provided that recommended target doses for the aldosterone antagonist are not

Table 21.10 Common drug–drug interactions with prescribed heart failure medication

Drug	Interacts with	Result of interaction
Diuretic	NSAIDs	Decreased effect of diuretic and increased risk of renal impairment
	Carbamazepine	Increased risk of hyponatraemia
	Lithium	Excretion of lithium impaired (thiazides worse than loop diuretics)
ACE inhibitor or ARB	NSAIDs	Antagonism of hypotensive effect. Increased risk of renal impairment
	Ciclosporin	Increased risk of hyperkalaemia
	Lithium	Excretion of lithium impaired
	Diuretics	Enhanced hypotensive effect. Increased risk of hyperkalaemia with potassium-sparing drugs
Digoxin	Amiodarone	Increased digoxin level (need to halve maintenance dose of digoxin)
	Propafenone	Increased digoxin level (need to halve maintenance dose of digoxin)
	Quinidine	Increased digoxin level (need to halve maintenance dose of digoxin)
	Verapamil	Increased risk of AV block
	Diuretics	Increased risk of hypokalaemia and therefore toxicity
	Amphotericin	Increased cardiac toxicity if hypokalaemia present
Nitrates	Sildenafil	Increased hypotensive effect
	Heparin	Increased excretion of heparin
Spironolactone	Digoxin	Spironolactone may interfere with measurement of digoxin serum levels, resulting in inaccurate interpretation
β-Blocker	Amiodarone	Increased risk of bradycardia
	Diltiazem	Increased risk of AV block and bradycardia
	Verapamil	Increased risk of hypotension, heart failure and asystole

Table 21.11 Common drug–disease interactions with prescribed heart failure medication

Drug	Concurrent disease	Potential outcome
Diuretic	Prostatism	Urinary retention/incontinence
	Hyperuricaemia	Exacerbation of gout
	Liver cirrhosis	Encephalopathy
ACE inhibitor	Renal artery stenosis	Renal failure
	Severe aortic stenosis	Exacerbation of heart failure
	Renal impairment	Renal failure
	Hypotension	Hypotension and cardiogenic shock
β-Blocker	Asthma	Bronchoconstriction/respiratory arrest
	Bradyarrhythmias	Exacerbation of heart failure
	Hypotension	Further hypotension and cardiogenic shock
Digoxin	Bradyarrhythmias	Exacerbation of heart failure
	Renal impairment	Exacerbation of heart failure and digoxin toxicity leading to cardiac arrhythmias

When initiating ACE inhibitor or ARB therapy, volume depletion due to prior use of a diuretic increases the risk of a large drop in blood pressure occurring following the first dose. As a consequence, diuretic treatment is usually withheld during the initiation phase of therapy in an effort to minimise this effect.

A dry cough, which may be accompanied by a voice change, occurs in about 10% of patients receiving an ACE inhibitor. It is more common in women and is associated with a raised level of kinins. Rashes, loss or disturbances of taste, mouth ulcers and proteinuria may also occur with ACE inhibitor therapy, particularly with captopril. These unwanted effects tend to be more common in patients with connective tissue disorders.

A number of ACE inhibitors are administered as pro-drugs, so close monitoring is advised in patients with liver dysfunction, as this could reduce the benefits associated with their use. Most ACE inhibitors are dependent on the kidney for excretion, and require careful dosage titration in patients with existing renal dysfunction. Differences in the pharmacokinetic characteristics do not fully explain the differences in duration of action seen with the ACE inhibitors, as this is also related to ACE binding affinity. Throughout treatment the dose must be individualised to obtain maximum benefit in relation to symptom relief and survival, with minimum side effects. When the experience of adverse effects requires a review of therapeutic alternatives, ARBs can be considered as an alternative treatment option. Although the side effect profile of ARB therapy is very similar to that of ACE inhibitors, it is not identical.

exceeded (see Table 21.5). Although this is usually the case, laboratory monitoring of potassium is mandatory to ensure patient safety. Heparin therapy has also been shown to increase the risk of hyperkalaemia when used alongside ACE inhibitor or ARB therapy, and therefore a similar approach to monitoring should be taken when co-prescribed.

Potential problems with β-blocker therapy

Until recently, the use of β-blockers was contraindicated in patients with heart failure due to negative inotropic and chronotropic effects. However, β-blockers have clearly been shown to be safe and effective in patients with heart failure and should be used in all patients in the absence of contraindications or intolerance. Initiation of treatment and titration of dose must be done under close supervision, with very small dose increments used to minimise transient worsening of heart failure symptoms. Titration of the dose to target is normally performed over a number of weeks or months, and close patient monitoring is required to ensure safety is not compromised. The maximum tolerable dose for a patient may be below the target dose and may limit further dose titration. Monitoring for excessive bradycardia or rapid deterioration of symptoms is necessary to ensure patient safety, while also monitoring the patient's prescribed dose to ensure that dosage increments are gradual and the patient is not subjected to an overall worsening of symptoms.

Potential problems with digoxin therapy

Although digoxin has been shown to reduce hospitalisation rates for patients with heart failure, its use is associated with a range of adverse effects including non-specific signs and symptoms of toxicity such as nausea, anorexia, tiredness, weakness, diarrhoea, confusion and visual disturbances. Digoxin also has the potential to cause fatal arrhythmias. It slows atrioventricular conduction and produces bradycardia, but it may also cause various ventricular and supraventricular arrhythmias. Digoxin toxicity typically causes conduction disturbances with enhanced automaticity leading to premature ventricular contractions. Patients at particular risk are those with myocardial ischaemia, hypoxia, acidosis or renal failure.

The appropriateness of digoxin dosage should be guided by assessment of the patient's renal function (from serum creatinine and creatinine clearance determinations) and from the patient's pulse rate. Renal function may also be affected by drug therapy or loss of control of heart failure; therefore, any medicine which affects in digoxin clearance will have an impact on the serum digoxin concentration. The possibility of a high serum digoxin concentration should also be considered in any patient whose health deteriorates or who shows signs and symptoms of potential digoxin toxicity.

Potential problems with other cardiovascular drugs

There are a number of other cardiovascular drugs that may be prescribed for patients with diseases or conditions other than heart failure, with some agents capable of worsening or aggravating symptoms. Patients with coronary artery disease may be candidates for calcium-blocking antianginal vasodilators. However, some of these agents, for example, diltiazem and verapamil, can exacerbate co-existing heart failure, since their negative inotropic effects offset the potentially beneficial arterial vasodilation. Second-generation dihydropyridines such as amlodipine and felodipine have a preferential action on the vasculature. They have less pronounced effects on cardiac contractility than other calcium antagonists, and this makes them the agents of choice where a limitation of the heart rate is not required.

Symptoms of fainting or dizziness on standing may indicate a need to review diuretic or vasodilator therapy. Patients should be reassured about mild postural effects and given advice to avoid standing from their chair too quickly. The patient and the health care team need to confirm the safety of the patient's treatment plan regularly, and be vigilant for any signs or symptoms suggesting otherwise.

A summary of monitoring activity required to ensure the safety of drug use is outlined in Table 21.12.

Table 21.12 Monitoring the safety of drug treatment in patients with heart failure

Consider	Monitor	Comment
Clinical markers	Side effects Toxicity Adverse drug reactions	There is a need to monitor for signs/symptoms of overtreatment with prescribed medication, such as diuretics (dehydration) and digoxin (nausea and vomiting). Look for signs of patient intolerance, allergy, serious adverse effects or troublesome side effects. Document unexpected adverse drug reactions if reported
Laboratory markers	Changes in organ function Biochemical changes Haematological changes Suspected digoxin toxicity	Renal function assessment and implications for drug choice and dosage individualisation required, especially in the elderly and for initiation or titration of ACE inhibitor therapy (creatinine, potassium, urea). Hypokalaemia can lead to digoxin toxicity, and serum drug concentration measurement may be performed to confirm or exclude toxicity. Haematological side effects with some drugs have been reported, for example, ACE inhibitors, therefore, laboratory checks may be required in response to clinical signs/symptoms presented
Interactions	Drug–drug interactions Drug–disease interactions	Some interactions may result in harm to the patient
Co-morbidity	Drug selection for concomitant conditions	The presence of heart failure may influence treatment choice for co-existing diseases or conditions, for example, coronary artery disease, thyroid disease, respiratory disease. Where possible, ensure drugs known to worsen heart failure are avoided or used with caution, for example, non-steroidal anti inflammatory agents or corticosteroids in rheumatoid arthritis

Potential problems with non-cardiovascular agents

A number of agents should be avoided or used with caution in patients with heart failure because of their known negative inotropic or pro-arrhythmic effects that may aggravate symptoms of heart failure (see Box 21.1). In particular, the use of non-steroidal anti-inflammatory drugs (NSAIDs) should be actively discouraged where possible. Not only do NSAIDs cause fluid retention and put patients at increased risk of bleeding, especially if they are already taking antiplatelets or anticoagulants, there is also an increased risk of acute renal failure, particularly in those on long-term use and in the elderly. Recent articles have described the synergistic/cumulative adverse renal effects of combinations of ACE inhibitors or ARBs with diuretics and NSAIDs, which are particularly common in patients with heart failure.

Case studies

Case 21.1

Mr GF, a 57-year-old, suffered a myocardial infarction 12 months ago and at the time was also found to have left ventricular systolic dysfunction on echocardiography. He is currently asymptomatic (NYHA I). At your request, he has agreed to see you for a medication review regarding his drug therapy. He has a history of type 2 diabetes mellitus (8 years) and his current prescription includes enalapril 10 mg twice daily, gliclazide 80 mg twice daily, bisoprolol 5 mg daily, aspirin 75 mg daily, and a glyceryl trinitrate spray to use when required.

Question

1. Is the current treatment plan for heart failure optimal?

Answer

1. Mr GF has echocardiographic evidence of left ventricular systolic dysfunction, but has no signs or symptoms of heart failure at present. Therefore, the absence of diuretic therapy is expected, although enquiry into the presence/absence of symptoms would form part of any review and would be included in the patient monitoring.

   He is prescribed an ACE inhibitor at the recommended target dose (enalapril 10–20 mg twice daily) and treatment with this agent is optimal at present. There is scope for a further increase in dose should the need arise. When we consider β-blocker therapy, the current dose of bisoprolol (5 mg daily) is below the recommended target and should, therefore, be titrated to a dose of 10 mg daily or maximum tolerable dose. This titration should be implemented gradually over a period of weeks or months with close monitoring of blood pressure and heart rate. Regular assessment of the patient for side effects or signs and symptoms of heart failure should also be undertaken, as each incremental rise in β-blocker dose may be accompanied by a worsening (or in this case, appearance) of heart failure symptoms. When considering other potential changes to the treatment plan for heart failure, there may have been an opportunity for the introduction of eplerenone at the time of his myocardial infarction provided this was done within 14 days of the event. However, given that the myocardial infarction was 12 months ago, the use of eplerenone would not be indicated based on the current evidence.

With Mr GF's history of myocardial infarction and type 2 diabetes mellitus, his cardiovascular risk is high and he should, therefore, also be prescribed lipid-lowering therapy (regardless of his serum cholesterol measurement), for example, a statin.

Case 21.2

Mrs JM, 66 years old, presents with a new prescription for candesartan 4 mg daily. On checking her medication record she has been prescribed lisinopril 20 mg daily, bisoprolol 10 mg daily and furosemide 40 mg daily for the last 6 months to treat her heart failure. Her blood pressure was measured 2 weeks ago and was 128/78 mmHg.

Question

1. How do you respond to the new prescription?

Answer

1. It is unclear from the information given whether candesartan is prescribed as an adjunct to ACE inhibitor therapy (provided the dose has been optimised) or as an alternative to ACE inhibitor due to intolerance. If being used as an adjunct, it is also unclear whether the patient also has an intolerance to aldosterone antagonists. Therefore, it is important to confirm the intended use of candesartan in this case through speaking to the patient and/or prescriber. If candesartan is being used as an alternative to either the ACE inhibitor or aldosterone antagonist, it is important to establish the reason for intolerance and ensure the therapeutic choice is appropriate for the patient. Patients are usually found to be intolerant of ACE inhibitors for three main reasons: dry cough, hypotension or compromised renal function. As heart failure can produce symptoms of a dry cough, it can sometimes be difficult to ascertain whether the ACE inhibitor or the heart failure is responsible. Dry cough occurs secondary to the inhibition of bradykinin metabolism and is generally identified shortly after initiation of an ACE inhibitor or after a dose increase; therefore, inquiry into the timing of symptoms attributed to ACE inhibitor intolerance is important. If the reason is due to persistent dry cough, an ARB would be a suitable alternative. However, if the ACE inhibitor intolerance is related to hypotension or renal dysfunction, it is likely an ARB would induce similar adverse effects and, therefore, other alternatives may need to be discussed with a heart failure specialist. In patient's intolerant of an aldosterone antagonist, the main reasons tend to be related to hyperkalaemia or unacceptable side effects such as gynaecomastia in men, gastro-intestinal intolerance and renal dysfunction.

   If candesartan is being used as adjunctive therapy, which is supported by the current evidence base for treatment, careful introduction and titration of dose must be undertaken due to the increased risk of hypotension, renal dysfunction and hyperkalaemia (ACE inhibitors and ARBs are both potassium conserving). The addition of candesartan would normally be under the guidance of a heart failure specialist, and should be initiated at a low dose and gradually titrated up to the target (32 mg daily) or maximum tolerable dose. It is important to note that dose increases during the titration period should be at least 2 weeks apart. Although Mrs JM has a normal blood pressure measurement at present, it is unclear whether renal function or blood biochemistry has previously been checked and it is important that this is confirmed prior to starting candesartan. The monitoring plan for Mrs JM should include regular checks of blood pressure, serum creatinine (and estimation of renal function), serum potassium and clinical assessment for any signs/symptoms of adverse effects/intolerance. This should be done

7–14 days after initiation and final dose titration. As the addition of candesartan should improve heart failure symptom control, regular patient monitoring will allow an assessment of the effectiveness of therapy.

Case 21.3

Mr HS, 72 years old, is admitted to hospital with increasing shortness of breath at rest. He has a previous medical history of severe left ventricular systolic dysfunction, confirmed by echocardiography, and angina. Before admission he had been taking the following medication: lisinopril 10 mg daily, furosemide 80 mg each morning and 40 mg at 2 pm, digoxin 62.5 μcg each morning, ISMN SR 60 mg daily, glyceryl trinitrate spray 1–2 doses as required, aspirin 75 mg dispersible each morning. His chest X-ray shows severe pulmonary oedema, his blood pressure is 110/70 mmHg and serum urea and electrolytes are within normal range. During the admission, carvedilol 3.125 mg twice daily is started.

Questions

1. What therapeutic options would you choose to treat the acute symptoms presented by Mr HS at the beginning of his admission?
2. Was the addition of bisoprolol appropriate for this patient?
3. What other drug treatment options might be considered for this patient in the longer term?

Answers

1. The administration of furosemide by the intravenous route is necessary as there is decreased absorption of oral furosemide secondary to gastro-intestinal oedema in acute heart failure. The administration of i.v. furosemide allows rapid serum levels to be achieved which has the benefit of producing venodilation (reducing the preload) which helps improve symptoms long before there is diuresis. Only after the oedema has resolved should the patient revert back to oral administration of diuretics. At this time, the dosage can be adjusted to maintain an appropriate fluid balance. Where diuresis is inadequate with an oral loop diuretic alone, the addition of a thiazide diuretic such as bendroflumethiazide or metolazone should be considered. Metolazone should be given initially at low dose of 2.5 mg daily, or less often if required, to avoid rapid diuresis leading to hypotension and/or renal failure.

2. Although there is good evidence to show that β-blocker therapy is safe and effective for patients with NYHA stage IV heart failure, it is not currently recommended that it should be initiated in patients with acute symptoms of heart failure. Where β-blocker therapy is indicated, initiation should occur when the patient's heart failure has been stable for at least 2 weeks and started at a very low dose on specialist advice (i.e. carvedilol 3.125 mg twice daily). The dose should be titrated gradually over a period of months towards the recommended target dose where appropriate, provided the patient tolerates each increment. In Mr HS's case, however, there is evidence to suggest that β-blocker use at discharge can be done safely in patients with heart failure, with positive effects on survival for both heart failure and coronary heart disease.

3. There is also scope to increase the dose of lisinopril to 20–35 mg daily provided the patient can tolerate the higher dose, as this is associated with greater benefits on morbidity and mortality. Based on his systolic blood pressure and assuming satisfactory renal function, there is no reason why this option cannot be explored and it would be reasonable to delay any titration of dosage until the symptoms become more stable. This is important since the use of large doses of loop diuretics in acutely ill patients

may predispose to ACE inhibitor-induced renal impairment. An aldosterone antagonist (or angiotensin receptor blocker if patient tolerance poor) could be added to Mr HS's existing drug therapy. If the patient is poorly controlled on optimised doses of ACE inhibitor and β-blocker. Either addition would show benefits on morbidity and mortality if added to the existing treatment plan. The decision to initiate the angiotensin receptor blocker would usually lie with a heart failure specialist based on the individual patient. As Mr HS approaches end-stage heart failure, there may be a need to focus solely on symptom relief.

Case 21.4

Mrs FM, a 70-year-old with chronic asthma and mild heart failure, has been prescribed naproxen 250 mg three times daily. On inspection of her medication record, it is discovered that she is also receiving:

Furosemide 40 mg each morning
Ramipril 5 mg in the morning
Prednisolone 5 mg daily
Salbutamol inhaler two puffs four times daily when required
Salmeterol 50 μcg inhaler one puff twice daily
Beclometasone 250 μcg inhaler two puffs twice daily
Omeprazole 10 mg daily

When asked her about symptom control she told that she is still breathless at night which, in addition to her painful knee, is keeping her awake.

Questions

1. Do you think Mrs FM should be taking naproxen?
2. What other aspects of this patient's medication regimen could be improved?
3. What is the likely effect of the prescribed therapy on serum potassium concentrations?

Answers

1. NSAIDs such as naproxen can exacerbate asthma and heart failure by inducing bronchospasm and by causing fluid retention, respectively. They can also lead to upper gastro-intestinal problems, particularly when co-prescribed with oral steroids. It would be worth checking what has been tried already. If the painful knee is responsive to a simple analgesic such as paracetamol, this would be the preferred option. Alternatively, if an NSAID is necessary and tolerated, the use of ibuprofen in low dosage would be slightly less likely to have an effect on respiratory and renal function, although it may still aggravate symptoms of heart failure. Further investigation into the persistence of respiratory symptoms is required as it is unclear whether the patient's breathlessness is due to an exacerbation of her asthma or a worsening of her heart failure, and therefore the interpretation of this symptom is difficult.

2. The clinical nature of the breathlessness is not easy to determine, and therefore makes the solution to this case uncertain at this stage. A number of issues, which also include confirming both diagnoses, should be considered. It is important to establish whether the patient is receiving maximum benefit from inhaled treatment. Inhaler technique must be checked and improved if necessary and the dose of beclometasone optimised. A regular regimen of salbutamol is not advisable since it may impair control of asthma by masking the onset of exacerbations. A review of the need for an oral steroid should be undertaken, and any reduction in the use of an oral steroid must be done gradually to avoid exacerbation of the asthma and ensure that the patient does not experience adrenal insufficiency.

Reduction of the oral steroid dose may benefit the heart failure. Although the prednisolone dose is low its impact on treated heart failure is probably low but nevertheless should be taken into account in the review of its use.

When considering the treatment of heart failure, application of the criteria set identified the following were not met in Mrs FMs treatment:

- **Not achieved target dose of ACE inhibitor**
- **Not prescribed any aldosterone antagonist**
- **Not prescribed candesartan**
- **Potentially aggravating drug prescribed (NSAID, naproxen)**

There is scope to increase the dose of ramipril to 5 mg twice daily if tolerated, which is the target dose in heart failure patients. However, as β-blocker is contraindicated in this patient, consideration may be given to an adjunctive therapy such as an aldosterone antagonist, for example spironolactone. If the patient was known to be intolerant of an aldosterone antagonist, an ARB, for example candesartan, could be added instead. The decision around which agent to select first may come down to personal choice if symptoms are moderate. An increase in the dose of furosemide could also be considered provided the breathlessness is due to heart failure.

3. Mrs FM is receiving a number of medications with the potential to affect serum potassium. Diuretics, oral and inhaled steroids (high dose) and β-agonists can reduce potassium, while ACE inhibitors can increase potassium. It is impossible to predict the extent to which each agent will affect potassium, especially with inhaled treatments as the dose normally needs to be high before there is any significant systemic absorption. Determination of serum potassium is necessary and if it remains low under the current treatment plan, or is at risk of being altered due to changes in drug dosage such as an increase in ramipril to 5 mg twice daily, then close observation will be required.

Case 21.5

Mr CH, a 78-year-old, regularly visits your pharmacy for his medication and has moderately symptomatic heart failure (NYHA III). During a recent review with his primary care doctor, Mr CH described worsening of his heart failure symptoms. His doctor has said he could take an extra dose of furosemide 40 mg if required, but Mr CH would need to be referred back to the hospital cardiology consultant before changing any other medication. He is currently prescribed ramipril 5 mg daily, nebivolol 2.5 mg daily and furosemide 40 mg daily. His blood pressure has been measured as 103/62 mmHg (heart rate 54 bpm) and he has an estimated creatinine clearance of 20 mL/min.

Questions

1. What is the rationale behind the decision to refer Mr CH to the cardiology consultant?
2. What other drug treatment options might be considered?

Answers

1. Mr CH is prescribed both ACE inhibitor and β-blocker therapy in accordance with the evidence base for treatment. As Mr CH has symptomatic heart failure (NYHA III), he is also prescribed furosemide in response to signs and symptoms of fluid retention. When Mr CH reports deterioration in the control of his heart failure symptoms, the prescriber must consider what treatment options are available for Mr CH and make any necessary changes.

   Neither the ACE inhibitor nor β-blocker is prescribed at the recommended target dose (see Table 21.6); therefore, there is scope to titrate the dose of either agent to the target dose which should result in improvement of symptoms and a reduced need for diuretic therapy. However, there may be reluctance to increase the dose of ACE inhibitor possibly due to the fact that Mr CH has a relatively low blood pressure and compromised renal function (estimated creatinine clearance 20 mL/min). However, it is unclear whether Mr CH is receiving maximally tolerated doses and whether his apparent hypotension is indeed symptomatic. Similarly, there may be reluctance to increase the dose of β-blocker due to a low blood pressure and heart rate (54 bpm). As both options may adversely affect the patient, the doctor has decided to treat the symptoms with additional diuretic when required as a short-term solution prior to Mr CH's appointment with the cardiology consultant. Advice should be sought from a heart failure specialist where a patient may be poorly tolerant of ACE inhibitor or β-blocker, or where there is a risk of hypotension or renal failure in susceptible individuals. In Mr CH's case, specialist supervision is required for optimisation of therapy.

2. It is unlikely that there will be much scope to add further medication, and optimising either ACE inhibitor or β-blocker therapy will be limited due to their effects on blood pressure and/or renal function. Mr CH may be a likely candidate for cardiac resynchronisation therapy (CRT) and should probably be assessed for this. An ECG would confirm his eligibility for therapy if his QRS duration was >120 ms, and would be likely to improve his symptoms and survival. It may also help increase his blood pressure and renal function to a point where further optimisation of ACE inhibitor and β-blocker dose might be possible.

Acknowledgements

The authors would like to thank Steve McGlynn and Carl Fenelon of NHS Greater Glasgow & Clyde (Pharmacy and Prescribing Support Unit) for helpful discussions of the case illustrations.

Special note: Sadly, Professor Steve Hudson passed away in November 2010. Steve was a pioneer in clinical pharmacy.

References

A-HeFT, Taylor, A.L., Ziesche, S., Yancy, C., et al., for the African-American Heart Failure Trial Investigators, 2004. Combination of isosorbide dinitrate and hydralazine in blacks with heart failure. N. Engl. J. Med. 351, 2049–2057.

A-HeFT, Taylor, A.L., Ziesche, S., Yancy, C., et al., for the African-American Heart Failure Trial Investigators, 2007. Early and sustained benefit on event-free survival and heart failure hospitalization from fixed-dose combination of isosorbide dinitrate/hydralazine: consistency across subgroups in the African-American Heart Failure Trial. Circulation 115, 1747–1753.

Acute Infarction Ramipril Efficacy (AIRE) Study Investigators, 1993. Effect of ramipril on mortality and morbidity of survivors of acute myocardial infarction with clinical evidence of heart failure. Lancet 342, 821–828.

American College of Cardiology/American Heart Association Task Force on Practice Guidelines, 2009. Guideline update for the diagnosis and management of chronic heart failure in the adult – summary article. Circulation 112, e154–235.

ANZ Carvedilol, 1997. Randomised, placebo-controlled trial of carvedilol in patients with congestive heart failure due to ischaemic heart disease. Australia/New Zealand Heart Failure Research Collaborative Group. Lancet 349, 375–380.

ATLAS, Packer, M., Poole-Wilson, P.A., Armstrong, P.W., et al., 1999. Comparative effects of low and high doses of the angiotensin-converting enzyme inhibitor, lisinopril, on morbidity and mortality in chronic heart failure. ATLAS Study Group Circ. 100, 2312–2318.

CAPRICORN Investigators, 2001. Effect of carvedilol on outcome after myocardial infarction in patients with left-ventricular dysfunction: the CAPRICORN randomised trial. Lancet 357, 1385–1390.

CARMEN, Komajda, M., Lutiger, B., Madeira, H., et al., 2004. Tolerability of carvedilol and ACE-inhibition in mild heart failure. Results of CARMEN (Carvedilol ACE-Inhibitor Remodelling Mild CHF Evaluation). Eur. J. Heart Fail. 6, 467–475.

CHARM Added, McMurray, J.J., Ostergren, J., Swedberg, K., et al., 2003. Effects of candesartan in patients with CHF and reduced left-ventricular systolic dysfunction taking angiotensin-converting-enzyme inhibitors: the CHARM Added trial. Lancet 362, 767–771.

CHARM Alternative, Granger, C.B., McMurray, J.J., Yusuf, S., et al., 2003. Effects of candesartan in patients with CHF and reduced left-ventricular systolic function intolerant to angiotensin-converting-enzyme inhibitors: the CHARM Alternative trial. Lancet 362, 772–776.

CIBIS II: Investigators Committees, 1999. The Cardiac Insufficiency Bisoprolol Study II (CIBIS II): a randomised trial. Lancet 353, 9–13.

CIBIS III, Willenheimer, R., van Veldhuisen, D.J., Silke, B., et al., 2005. Effect on survival and hospitalization of initiating treatment for chronic heart failure with bisoprolol followed by enalapril, as compared with the opposite sequence: results of the randomized Cardiac Insufficiency Bisoprolol Study (CIBIS) III. Circulation 112, 2426–2435.

COMET, Poole-Wilson, P.A., Swedberg, K., Cleland, J.G.F., et al., for the COMET Investigators, 2003. Comparison of carvedilol and metoprolol on clinical outcomes in patients with chronic heart failure in the Carvedilol Or Metoprolol European Trial (COMET): a randomised controlled trial. Lancet 362, 7–13.

CONSENSUS I: CONSENSUS Trial Study Group, 1987. Effects of enalapril on mortality in severe congestive heart failure. N. Engl. J. Med. 316, 1429–1435.

CONSENSUS II, Swedberg, K., Held, P., Kjekshus, J., et al., 1992. Effects of the early administration of enalapril on the mortality in patients with acute myocardial infarction. Results from the co-operative new Scandinavian enalapril survival study II. N. Engl. J. Med. 327, 678–684.

COPERNICUS, Packer, M., Coats, A.J., Fowler, M.B., et al., for the Carvedilol Prospective Randomized Cumulative Survival Study Group, 2001. Effect of carvedilol on survival in severe chronic heart failure. N. Engl. J. Med. 334, 1651–1658.

DIG: Digitalis Investigation Group, 1997. The effect of digoxin on mortality and morbidity in patients with heart failure. N. Engl. J. Med. 336, 525–533.

EPHESUS, Pitt, B., Remme, W., Zannad, F., et al., 2003. Eplerenone, a selective aldosterone blocker, in 38 patients with left ventricular dysfunction after myocardial infarction. N. Engl. J. Med. 348, 1309–1321.

European Society of Cardiology, 2008. Guidelines for the diagnosis and treatment of acute and chronic heart failure. The task force for the diagnosis and treatment of acute and chronic heart failure 2008 of the European Society of Cardiology. Developed in collaboration with the Heart Failure Association of the ESC (HFA) and endorsed by the European Society of Intensive Care Medicine (ESICM). Eur. J. Heart Fail. 10, 933–989.

MERIT-HF Study Group, 1999. Effect of metoprolol CR/XL in chronic heart failure: metoprolol CR/XL randomised intervention trial in congestive heart failure (MERIT-HF). Lancet 353, 2001–2007.

National Institute of Health and Clinical Excellence, 2010. Chronic heart failure CG108. NICE, London. Available at: http://www.nice.org.uk/nicemedia/live/13099/50514/50514.pdf.

PROMISE, Packer, M., Carver, J.R., Rodeheffer, R.J., et al., for the PROMISE Study Research Group, 1991. Effect of oral milrinone on mortality in severe chronic heart failure. N. Engl. J. Med. 325, 1468–1475.

PROVED, Uretsky, B.F., Young, J.B., Shahidi, F.E., et al., for the PROVED Investigative Group, 1993. Randomized study assessing the effect of digoxin withdrawal in patients with mild to moderate chronic congestive heart failure: results of the PROVED trial. J. Am. Coll. Cardiol. 22, 955–962.

RADIANCE, Packer, M., Gheorghiade, M., Young, J.B., et al., 1993. Withdrawal of digoxin from patients with chronic heart failure treated with angiotensin-converting-enzyme inhibitors. RADIANCE Study. N. Engl. J. Med. 329, 1–7.

RALES, Pitt, B., Zannad, F., Remme, W.J., et al., for the Randomized Aldactone Evaluation Study Investigators, 1999. The effect of spironolactone on morbidity and mortality in patients with severe heart failure. N. Engl. J. Med. 341, 709–717.

SAVE, Pfeffer, M.A., Braunwald, E., Moye, L.A., et al., 1992. Effect of captopril on mortality and morbidity in patients with left ventricular dysfunction after myocardial infarction. Results of the Survival and Ventricular Enlargement trial (SAVE). N. Engl. J. Med. 327, 669–677.

Scottish Intercollegiate Guidelines Network, 2007. Management of Chronic Heart Failure (Guidline 95). SIGN, Edinburgh. Available at www.sign.ac.uk.

SENIORS, Flather, M.D., Shibata, M.C., Coats, A.J., et al., 2005. Randomized trial to determine the effect of nebivolol on mortality and cardiovascular hospital admission in elderly patients with heart failure (SENIORS). Eur. Heart J. 26, 215–225.

Sipahi, I., Debanne, S.M., Rowland, D.Y., et al., 2010. Angiotensin-receptor blockade and risk of cancer: meta-analysis of randomised controlled trials. Lancet Oncol. 11, 627–636.

SOLVD-P: SOLVD Investigators, 1992. Effect of enalapril on mortality and the development of heart failure in asymptomatic patients with reduced left ventricular ejection fractions. N. Engl. J. Med. 327, 685–691.

SOLVD-T: SOLVD Investigators, 1991. Effect of enalapril on survival in patients with reduced left ventricular ejection fractions and congestive heart failure. N. Engl. J. Med. 325, 293–302.

TRACE: Trandolapril Cardiac Evaluation Study Group, 1995. A clinical trial of the angiotensin-enzyme inhibitor trandolapril in patients with left ventricular dysfunction after myocardial infarction. N. Engl. J. Med. 333, 1670–1676.

US Carvedilol, Packer, M., Bristow, M.R., Cohn, J.N., et al., 1996. The effect of carvedilol on morbidity and mortality in patients with chronic heart failure. US Carvedilol Heart Failure Study Group. N. Engl. J. Med. 334, 1349–1355.

V-HeFT I, Cohn, J.N., Archibald, D., Ziesche, S., et al., 1986. Effect of vasodilator therapy on mortality in chronic congestive heart failure. Results of a Veterans Administration Cooperative Study. N. Engl. J. Med. 314, 1547–1552.

V-HeFT II, Cohn, J.N., Johnson, G., Ziesche, S., et al., for the V-HeFT II Study, 1991. A comparison of enalapril with hydralazine-isosorbide dinitrate in the treatment of chronic congestive heart failure. N. Engl. J. Med. 325, 303–310.

Val-HeFT, Maggioni, A.P., Anand, I., Gottlieb, S.O., et al., 2002. Effects of valsartan on morbidity and mortality in patients with heart failure not receiving angiotensin-converting enzyme inhibitors. J. Am. Coll. Cardiol. 40, 1422–1424.

Zannad, F., McMurray, J.J.V., Krum, H., van Veldhuisen, D.J., et al., for the EMPHASIS-HF Study Group 2011. Eplerenone in patients with systolic heart failure and mild symptoms. N. Engl. J. Med. 364, 11–21.

Further reading

Koshman, S.L., Charrois, T.L., Simpson, S.H., et al., 2008. Pharmacist care of patients with heart failure. A systematic review of randomized trials. Arch. Intern. Med. 168, 687–694.

McMurray, J., Cohen-Solal, A., Dietz, R., et al., 2005. Practical recommendations for the use of ACE inhibitors, β-blockers, aldosterone antagonists and angiotensin receptor blockers in heart failure: putting guidelines into practice. Eur. J. Heart Fail. 7, 710–721.

22 Arrhythmias

S. Sporton and S. Antoniou

Normal cardiac electrophysiology

The normal cardiac rhythm, sinus rhythm, is characterised by contraction of first the atria and then the ventricles (systole) followed by relaxation (diastole) during which the heart refills with blood before the next cardiac cycle begins. This orderly sequence of contraction and relaxation is regulated by the heart's electrical activity. Heart muscle cells (myocytes) are electrically active and capable of generating action potentials, which initiate contraction of the myocyte through a process known as excitation–contraction coupling. Adjacent myocytes form electrical connections through protein channels called gap junctions. An action potential in one myocyte causes current flow between itself and adjacent myocytes which in turn generate their own action potentials and in this way an 'activation wavefront' spreads though the myocardium, resulting in a wave of contraction.

Cardiac action potential

An understanding of the ionic basis of the cardiac action potential is important because drugs used in the treatment of cardiac arrhythmias act by altering the function of trans-membrane ion channels. Inherited abnormalities of ion channel function ('channelopathies') are an important cause of sudden cardiac death due to arrhythmia and are increasingly implicated in the pathogenesis of other arrhythmias including atrial fibrillation (AF).

The phospholipid membrane of cardiac myocytes is spanned by numerous proteins known as ion channels, whose permeability to specific ions varies during the cardiac cycle resulting in a resting (diastolic) membrane potential, diastolic depolarisation in cells with pacemaker activity, and action potentials.

The resting membrane potential of −60 to −90 mV occurs because the intracellular potassium (K^+) concentration is much higher than the extracellular K^+ concentration as a result of a transmembrane pump known as Na^+–K^+–ATPase, which pumps K^+ ions into the cell in exchange for sodium (Na^+) ions. K^+ ions diffuse out of the cell through selective K^+ channels (the inward rectifier current or I_{K1}) unaccompanied by anions, resulting in a net loss of charge and thus a negative resting, diastolic or phase 4, transmembrane potential (Fig. 22.1A).

Certain specialised myocytes form the cardiac conduction system and these cells have pacemaker activity, that is, they are capable of generating their own action potentials due to gradual depolarisation of the transmembrane potential during diastole (phase 4), referred to as the pacemaker potential (Fig. 22.1B). The pacemaker potential occurs as a result of (i) a gradual reduction in an outward K^+ current called the delayed rectifier (I_K) current, (ii) increasing dominance of an inward current of Na^+ and some Ca^{2+} ions known as I_f (f stands for 'funny') and (iii) an inward calcium current I_{Ca} through voltage-gated calcium channels. As a result of the pacemaker potential, the transmembrane potential gradually becomes less negative until a threshold potential is reached at which an action potential is triggered. The rate of depolarisation of the pacemaker potential, and hence the heart rate, is influenced by the autonomic nervous system. Sympathetic nervous system activation and circulating catecholamines increase the heart rate by binding to ß₁-adrenoreceptors leading to an increase in intracellular cyclic AMP, which results in changes to the permeability of the various ion channels

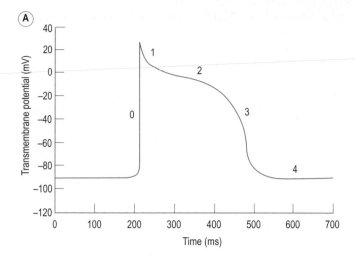

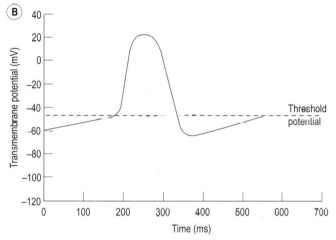

Fig. 22.1 The cardiac action potential. (A) An action potential from ventricular myocardium. During diastole (phase 4), the resting transmembrane potential is constant at −90 mV. The upstroke (phase 0) of the action potential is due to the rapid influx of Na⁺ ions. The early phase of repolarisation (phase 1) is due to efflux of K⁺ ions, followed by a plateau phase (phase 2) at about 0 mV during which influx of Ca^{2+} ions is balanced by efflux of K⁺ ions. Towards the end of diastole, influx of Ca^{2+} ions diminishes and efflux of K⁺ ions increases, resulting in repolarisation (phase 3) back to the negative resting membrane potential. (B) An action potential from the sinus node. During diastole (phase 4), there is progressive depolarisation towards a threshold potential at which an action potential is triggered. The upstroke (phase 0) of the action potential is less steep than in ventricular myocardial cells because the sinus node cells lack 'fast' Na⁺ channels and so depolarisation is dependent upon influx of Ca^{2+} ions.

responsible for the pacemaker current. Parasympathetic nervous system activation, mediated by muscarinic cholinergic receptors, has the opposite effect.

The rapid depolarisation of the cardiac action potential (Fig. 22.1A, phase 0) occurs because of a rapid increase in the permeability of the cell membrane to Na⁺ ions, which enter rapidly through 'fast' Na⁺ channels in a current known as I_{Na}. The I_{Na} current is brief as the 'fast' Na⁺ channels inactivate rapidly. The early phase of repolarisation (phase 1) is due to closure of the fast Na⁺ channels, an outward K⁺ current known as I_{to} (to – transient outward) and a further K⁺ current known as the ultra-rapid component of the delayed rectifier current or I_{Kur}. The plateau phase (phase 2) of the cardiac action potential occurs because the inward movement of Ca^{2+} ions (I_{Ca}) is balanced by the outward movement of K⁺ ions. Repolarisation (phase 3) occurs as I_{Ca} diminishes and two further components of the delayed rectifier (I_{K}) current known as the rapid (I_{Kr}) and slow (I_{Ks}) components predominate, with an important contribution from I_{K1}.

There is considerable variation in the expression of transmembrane ion channels in different parts of the heart, with corresponding variation in the morphology of the action potential. The most marked example is that myocytes in the sinus and AV nodes contain few Na⁺ channels. The upstroke of the action potential in these cells is due, predominantly, to the influx of Ca^{2+} ions and, therefore, is considerably slower than the upstroke in other myocytes (Fig. 22.1B). The variation in ion channel expression throughout the heart is essential for normal cardiac function, helps to explain the pathophysiology of many inherited and acquired diseases complicated by cardiac arrhythmia and accounts for the relative selectivity of antiarrhythmic and other drugs for certain parts of the heart.

Refractoriness

The action potential of cardiac myocytes differs from that seen in nerve cells by the presence of a plateau phase during which the myocyte is electrically inexcitable and refractory, that is, incapable of generating another action potential. It is only towards the end of repolarisation (phase 3) that the myocyte regains excitability. The time interval between the onset of the action potential and the regaining of electrical excitability is known as the refractory period. Under most circumstance the refractory period of a cardiac myocyte corresponds closely to the duration of the cardiac action potential and, therefore, drugs that prolong action potential duration (APD) prolong the refractory period.

Normal cardiac conduction

During normal sinus rhythm (Fig. 22.2), an activation wavefront begins in the sinus node, a group of cells with pacemaker activity on the upper free wall of the right atrium. The rate of diastolic depolarisation and hence the rate of discharge of the sinus node is increased by sympathetic nerve stimulation, circulating catecholamines or sympathomimetic drugs mediated by ß₁-adrenoreceptors on the cell membranes of the sinus node myocytes. Parasympathetic (vagus) nerve stimulation exerts the opposite effect, mediated by muscarinic cholinergic receptors.

An activation wavefront spreads across the atrial myocardium, leading to atrial contraction and generating the P wave on the surface electrocardiogram (ECG; Fig. 22.3). The last part of the atria to be activated is the atrioventricular (AV) node, the electrical and structural properties of which result in a slow conduction velocity, allowing atrial emptying to be completed before ventricular contraction begins

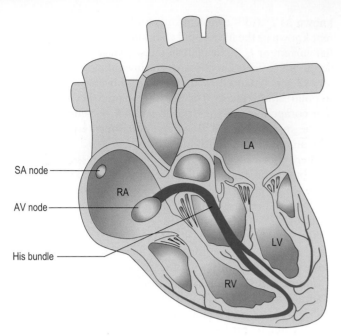

Fig. 22.2 The normal cardiac conduction system. During sinus rhythm, an activation wavefront spreads from the sinus (sinoatrial – SA) node across the atrial myocardium before entering the atrioventricular node. The activation wavefront then enters the bundle of His, which penetrates the annulus fibrosus and forms the only electrical connection between the atria and ventricles. The bundle of His divides into right and left bundle branches which ramify into a subendocardial network of Purkinje fibres that transmit the activation wavefront rapidly across the ventricles. Activation of the ventricles proceeds from endocardium to epicardium.

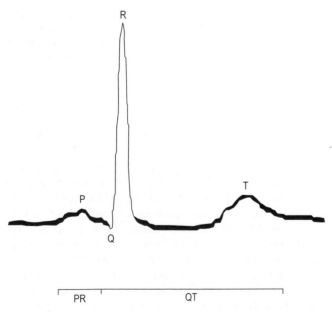

Fig. 22.3 The normal electrocardiogram (ECG). The P wave results from activation (depolarisation of the atria). The PR interval is isoelectric as the activation wavefront proceeds slowly through the atrioventricular node. The QRS complex reflects activation of the ventricles and is large compared to the P wave because of the much greater mass of the ventricular myocardium, and brief, reflecting extremely rapid conduction in the His–Purkinje system. The T wave represents ventricular repolarisation.

and represented by the PR interval on the ECG. Conduction velocity in the AV node is increased by sympathetic nerve stimulation, circulating catecholamines or sympathomimetic drugs, mediated by β_1-adrenoreceptors while parasympathetic (vagus) nerve stimulation exerts the opposite effect via muscarinic cholinergic receptors.

The atria and ventricles are electrically isolated from each other by the annulus fibrosus, the electrically non-conductive fibrous tissue forming the valve rings. In the normal heart, there is just one electrical connection between the atria and ventricles, the bundle of His, which conveys the activation wavefront from the AV node and penetrates the annulus fibrosus before dividing into the right and left bundle branches. The bundle branches ramify into a sub-endocardial network of Purkinje fibres, which convey the activation wavefront rapidly across the ventricles ensuring near-simultaneous contraction of the ventricular myocardium, and are represented by the narrow QRS complex of the ECG. Finally, the activation wavefront spreads from endocardium to epicardium. A wave of repolarisation then spreads across the ventricles resulting in the T wave. The QT interval on the ECG, therefore, represents the duration of ventricular depolarisation and repolarisation. There is an inverse relationship between the time to activation of different areas of the ventricular myocardium and APD such that the latest areas to be activated have the shortest APD. The purpose of this relationship is that repolarisation is rapid and uniform throughout the ventricular myocardium, which serves to maintain electrical stability.

Arrhythmia mechanisms

Cardiac arrhythmias occur because of abnormalities of impulse formation or propagation.

Abnormal impulse formation

Abnormal automaticity

Automaticity is another term for pacemaker activity, a characteristic possessed by all cells of the specialised cardiac conduction system during health and, potentially, by other cardiac myocytes during certain disease states. The rate of firing of a pacemaker cell is largely determined by the duration of the phase 4 diastolic interval (Fig. 22.4). This in turn is determined by (i) the maximum diastolic potential following repolarisation of the preceding action potential, (ii) the slope of diastolic depolarisation due to pacemaker currents and (iii) the threshold potential for generation of a new action potential. In the healthy state, there is a hierarchy of firing rates within the specialised conduction system with the highest rate in the sinus node followed by the AV node and then the His–Purkinje system. The sinus node is, therefore, the dominant pacemaker and determines the heart rate, while the pacemaker activity in the distal conduction system is 'overdriven' by the sinus node. Abnormal automaticity describes either accelerated pacemaker activity in cells of the distal cardiac conduction system such that they escape from overdrive

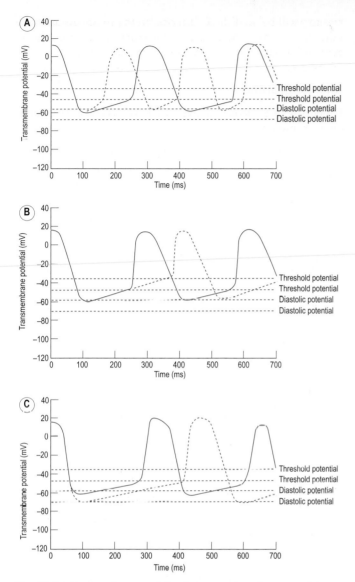

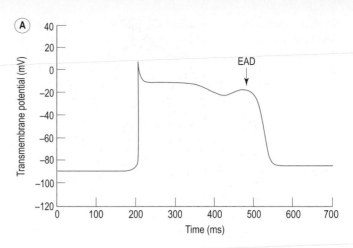

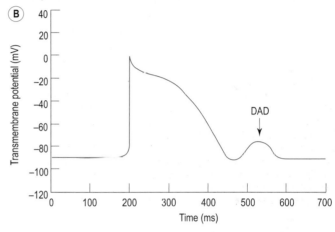

Fig. 22.5 Triggered activity. (A) An early afterdepolarisation (EAD) occurring at the start of phase 3 of the cardiac action potential. (B) A delayed afterdepolarisation (DAD) occurring after repolarisation, during phase 4. Either EADs or DADs may reach the threshold potential for generation of a further action potential.

Fig. 22.4 Abnormal automaticity. A sinus node action potential is shown (in bold) with a characteristic slow upstroke. Following repolarisation, gradual diastolic depolarisation occurs as a result of pacemaker currents. When the threshold potential is reached a further action potential is generated. The rate of firing of the pacemaker cell is governed largely by the duration of the diastolic interval which is in turn determined by (A) the slope of diastolic depolarisation, (B) the threshold potential and (C) the maximum diastolic potential. Each of these (shown by dotted lines) may be altered by disease states leading to abnormal automaticity.

suppression by the sinus node, or the development of pacemaker activity in cells that do not form part of the cardiac conduction system.

Triggered activity

Triggered activity describes impulse formation dependent upon afterdepolarisations. Early afterdepolarisations (EADs) occur during phase 2 or 3 of the cardiac action potential whereas delayed afterdepolarisations (DADs) occur during phase 4 (Fig. 22.5). In both cases, afterdepolarisation may reach the threshold potential required for generation of a new action potential.

EADs are characteristic of the congenital and acquired long QT syndromes. The prolonged APD promotes reactivation of the inward calcium current I_{Ca} which may directly cause EADs during phase 2. Furthermore, action potential prolongation and ß-adrenoreceptor stimulation promote calcium overload in the sarcoplasmic reticulum. This in turn leads to the spontaneous release of calcium in bursts by the sarcoplasmic reticulum. The resultant increase in intracellular calcium concentration activates the transmembrane Na^+/Ca^{2+} exchanger which moves one calcium ion out of the myocyte in exchange for three sodium ions and, therefore, results in an EAD during phase 3. In the long QT syndromes, an EAD may initiate a form of polymorphic ventricular tachycardia (VT) known as Torsade de Pointes. EADs are more prominent at slow heart rates.

DADs are seen during reperfusion following ischaemia, heart failure, digitalis toxicity and in catecholaminergic polymorphic VT. They occur because of spontaneous release of calcium in bursts by the sarcoplasmic reticulum, activating the

Na^+/Ca^{2+} exchanger as described for EADs and resulting in a DAD during phase 4. A DAD may result in a single extrastimulus ('ectopic beat') or in repetitive firing, that is, tachycardia. DADs are more prominent at rapid heart rates and during sympathetic nervous stimulation of ß-adrenoreceptors.

Abnormal impulse propagation

Re-entry

Many clinically important arrhythmias are due to re-entry, in which an activation wavefront rotates continuously around a circuit. Re-entry depends upon a trigger in the form of a premature beat, and a substrate, that is, the re-entry circuit itself. A precise set of electrophysiological conditions must be met in order for re-entry to occur (Fig. 22.6): (i) there must be a central non-conducting obstacle around which the re-entry circuit develops, (ii) a premature beat must encounter unidirectional conduction block in one limb (a) of the re-entry circuit, (iii) conduction must proceed slowly enough down the other limb (b) of the re-entry circuit that electrical excitability has returned in the original limb (a), allowing the activation wavefront to propagate in a retrograde direction along that limb, and (iv) the circulating activation wavefront must continue to encounter electrically excitable tissue. This is a function of the length of the re-entry circuit, the conduction velocity of the activation wavefront and the effective refractory period of the myocardium throughout the circuit. Class I antiarrhythmic drugs block sodium channels and, therefore, reduce the amplitude and rate of rise of the cardiac action potential and in so doing, reduce the conduction velocity of an activation wavefront. Class I antiarrhythmic drugs may exert their major antiarrhythmic effect by abolishing conduction altogether in areas of diseased myocardium forming part of a re-entry circuit in which conduction is already critically depressed. Class III antiarrhythmic drugs prolong cardiac APD and hence the refractory period. If previously activated cells in a re-entry circuit (the 'tail') remain refractory when the re-entrant wavefront (the 'head') returns to that area, conduction will fail and re-entry will be abolished. Drug-induced prolongation of the refractory period may, therefore, terminate and/or prevent re-entrant arrhythmias.

Clinical problems

Patients with a cardiac arrhythmia may present with a number of symptoms:

- The most common symptom is palpitation, an awareness of an abnormal heartbeat, although some patients with clearly documented arrhythmia have no palpitation. Arrhythmias start suddenly and, therefore, if the patient clearly describes palpitation of sudden onset ('like flicking a switch'), this is a useful pointer to an arrhythmia rather than heightened awareness of sinus tachycardia, which has a less sudden onset.
- The heart is designed to work most efficiently in sinus rhythm. Any arrhythmia compromises cardiac function. Classical symptoms that arise due to reduced cardiac output include reduced exercise capacity, breathlessness and fatigue.
- Angina may accompany tachycardia, even in the absence of coronary artery disease. Tachycardia increases the metabolic rate of cardiac muscle and hence its demand for blood flow. Myocardial perfusion occurs predominantly during diastole and during tachycardia proportionately less time is spent in diastole and so myocardial demand for blood can exceed supply, resulting in angina.
- A sudden drop in cardiac output may accompany either bradycardia or tachycardia, causing episodes of dizziness (presyncope), loss of consciousness (syncope) or, in extreme cases, sudden death from cardiac arrest.
- Atrial tachyarrhythmias such as atrial flutter and atrial fibrillation may be complicated by the development of intracardiac thrombus, usually within the left atrial appendage. This thrombus may embolise to any part of the body but the most common clinical presentation is with a transient ischaemic attack or stroke.

Arrhythmias may aggravate heart failure in two ways: (i) the haemodynamic effect of the arrhythmia may precipitate heart failure or aggravate existing heart failure and (ii) prolonged tachycardia of any type may lead to tachycardia-induced cardiomyopathy.

Diagnosis

A detailed history should be obtained, covering all of the symptoms listed above. A characteristic of cardiac arrhythmias is their random onset. Symptoms occurring under specific circumstances are less likely to be due to arrhythmia, but there are exceptions including certain uncommon types of VT, some cases of supraventricular tachycardia (SVT) due to an accessory pathway and vasovagal syncope (faints). Other key features of the history include:

- A history of cardiac disease
- Other diagnosed medical conditions

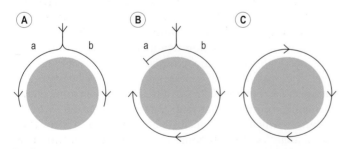

Fig. 22.6 Re-entry. During sinus rhythm, (A) an activation wavefront encounters a zone of fixed conduction block but can propagate anterogradely on either side of this zone, down limbs a and b of a potential re-entry circuit. A premature beat (B) encounters unidirectional conduction block in limb a but propagates anterogradely down limb b and re-enters limb a retrogradely. If limb a is now capable of retrograde conduction, the re-entry circuit is completed and re-entry continues (C) as long as the activation wavefront continually meets electrically excitable tissue.

- A full drug history, including over-the-counter medicines and recreational drugs including alcohol
- A family history of heart disease and of sudden unexpected death.

Physical examination is essential but often normal between episodes of arrhythmia. Mandatory investigation includes a 12-lead ECG and an echocardiogram to detect structural heart disease. Other investigations for structural and ischaemic heart disease may be indicated at this stage with the aim of detecting any underlying structural heart disease. If the history does not include sinister features such as syncope or a family history of sudden unexpected death at a young age, and the resting 12-lead ECG and echocardiogram are normal, then the patient can be reassured that they are extremely unlikely to have a serious heart rhythm disturbance. The extent of further investigation will be dictated by how troublesome the symptoms are.

The most certain way of reaching a firm diagnosis is a 12-lead ECG recorded during the patient's symptoms demonstrating arrhythmia. As many arrhythmias occur intermittently, some form of ECG monitoring is often necessary. This may include a continuous ambulatory ECG (Holter) recording for up to 7 days at a time if the symptoms occur frequently or, for less frequent symptoms an event recorder, which may store ECG strips automatically if it detects an arrhythmia or if activated by the patient during their symptoms. An insertable loop recorder may be implanted subcutaneously and is an ECG event recorder with a battery life of about 3 years, making it a useful tool for the diagnosis of infrequent arrhythmias.

Management

Pathological tachycardia is conventionally defined as a resting heart rate over 100 beats/min and can be classified according to whether it arises in or involves the atria (supraventricular tachycardias) or the ventricle (ventricular tachyarrhythmias).

Supraventricular tachycardias

These are tachycardias arising from or involving the atria.

Inappropriate sinus tachycardia

Although uncommon, inappropriate sinus tachycardia, that is, sinus tachycardia with no identifiable underlying cause, is one of the more difficult arrhythmias to treat. The presenting symptom is usually palpitation and the typical patient is a young, predominantly female, adult with no history of heart disease or other physical illness. The 12-lead ECG shows sinus tachycardia and ambulatory ECG monitoring demonstrates sinus tachycardia but with diurnal variation in heart rate. Echocardiography is required to exclude structural heart disease, and thyroid function and urinary catecholamine excretion should be measured to detect thyrotoxicosis and phaechromocytoma, respectively, as rare underlying causes

of sinus tachycardia. If treatment is required on symptomatic grounds, ß-blockers or verapamil are first line therapy. Ivabradine, a selective 'funny channel' blocker, has been used in resistant cases but is not currently licensed for this indication. Catheter ablation of the sinus node has been performed in highly symptomatic drug-resistant inappropriate sinus tachycardia but with limited success and risks including symptomatic sinus bradycardia and phrenic nerve palsy.

Atrial flutter

Atrial flutter is a right atrial tachycardia with a re-entry circuit around the tricuspid valve annulus. The atrial rate is typically 300 min^{-1}. The long refractory period of the AV node protects the ventricles from 1:1 conduction: In the presence of a healthy AV node and the absence of AV node-modifying drugs, there is usually 2:1 AV conduction resulting in a regular narrow-complex tachycardia with a ventricular rate of 150 min^{-1}.

Atrial flutter confers a risk of thromboembolism similar to that of AF and this risk should be managed in the same way. Emergency management of atrial flutter is dictated by the clinical presentation but may include d.c. cardioversion or ventricular rate control with drugs which increase the refractory period of the AV node such as ß-blockers, verapamil, diltiazem or digoxin. ß-Blockers, verapamil and digoxin may be given intravenously. As the re-entry circuit is confined to the right atrium and does not involve the AV node, adenosine will not terminate atrial flutter but will produce transient AV block, allowing the characteristic flutter waves to be seen on the ECG (Fig. 22.7).

There is a limited role for antiarrhythmic drugs, whether used acutely to achieve chemical cardioversion or in the longer term to maintain sinus rhythm. Class Ic antiarrhythmic drugs such as flecainide should be used only in conjunction with AV node-modifying drugs such as ß-blockers, verapamil, diltiazem or digoxin because they may otherwise cause slowing of the atrial flutter circuit and 1:1 conduction though the AV node which may be life-threatening. Sotalol and amiodarone have been used to restore and maintain sinus rhythm and have the advantage of controlling the ventricular rate where rhythm control is incomplete. Catheter ablation of atrial flutter is highly effective and safe and is increasingly used in preference to long-term drug treatment.

Focal atrial tachycardia

As its name implies, this relatively uncommon arrhythmia results from the repetitive discharge of a focal source within the atria or surrounding venous structures. The tachycardia mechanism may be caused by abnormal automaticity, triggered activity or microreentry. Management is as described for atrial flutter with three exceptions: (i) some focal atrial tachycardias terminate with adenosine, (ii) the potential for class Ic antiarrhythmic drugs to slow tachycardia and result in 1:1 AV conduction is lower than for atrial flutter, and (iii) catheter ablation of focal atrial tachycardia may be more challenging than that of atrial flutter, but is curative in a majority of cases.

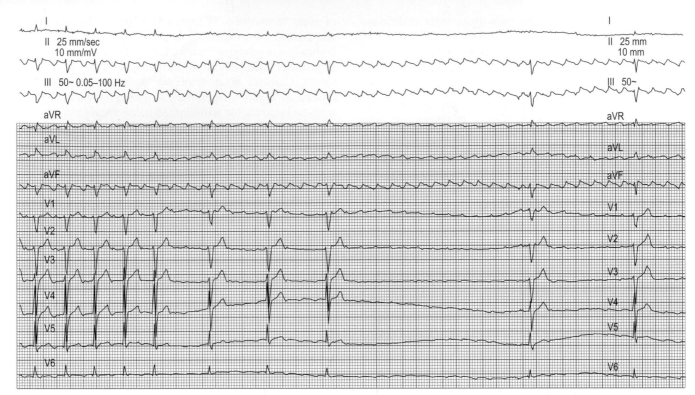

Fig. 22.7 A 12-lead electrocardiogram (ECG) recorded during the administration of intravenous adenosine. The initial rhythm is atrial flutter with 2:1 conduction from atria to ventricles. The QRS complexes obscure the atrial activity on the ECG. Adenosine does not terminate the atrial flutter but causes temporary atrioventricular block revealing the characteristic 'sawtooth' ECG morphology of typical atrial flutter.

Junctional re-entry tachycardia

The term 'supraventricular tachycardia' (SVT) is widely used to describe junctional re-entry tachycardias but is a misnomer because it implies any tachycardia arising from the atria. Junctional re-entry tachycardia is a more specific term and may be preferable.

Two mechanisms account for most junctional re-entry tachycardias: both involve a macroreentry circuit (Fig. 22.8). AV nodal re-entry tachycardia (AVNRT) rotates around a circuit including the AV node itself and the so-called AV nodal fast and slow pathways, which feed into the AV node. Atrioventricular re-entry tachycardia (AVRT) comprises a re-entry circuit involving the atrial myocardium, the AV node, the ventricular myocardium and an accessory pathway, a congenital abnormality providing a second electrical connection between the atria and ventricles in addition to the His bundle, thus forming a potential re-entry circuit.

Many accessory pathways conduct only retrogradely from the ventricles to the atrium. In these cases, the ECG during sinus rhythm appears normal and the accessory pathway is described as 'concealed'. Other accessory pathways conduct anterogradely and retrogradely. In these cases, the ECG during sinus rhythm is abnormal and is described as having a Wolff–Parkinson–White pattern (Fig. 22.9). This abnormality is characterised by a short PR interval as the conduction velocity of an accessory pathway is usually faster than that of the AV node, and a delta wave, a slurred onset to the QRS complex which occurs because an accessory pathway inserts into ventricular myocardium which conducts more slowly than the His–Purkinje system.

Junctional re-entry tachycardias are characterised by a history of discrete episodes of rapid regular palpitation that start and stop suddenly and occur without warning and apparently at random. The peak age range at which symptoms begin is from the mid-teens to the mid-thirties and the condition is more common in women. There are no symptoms between episodes, and cardiac examination and investigation at these times are usually normal. The diagnosis is usually made on the basis of the history, ideally confirmed by an ECG recorded during an episode showing a regular narrow-complex tachycardia with no discernible P waves or P waves occurring in a 1:1 relationship with the QRS complexes.

Acute treatment of junctional re-entry tachycardia aims to terminate the tachycardia by causing transient conduction block in the AV node, an obligatory part of the re-entry circuit. Vagotonic manoeuvres such as carotid sinus massage, a Valsalva manoeuvre or eliciting the diving reflex by immersion of the face in ice-cold water may all result in a brief vagal discharge sufficient to block conduction in the AV node, terminating tachycardia. The same effect may be achieved with intravenous adenosine given as a rapid bolus injection in doses up to 12 mg. Intravenous verapamil 5 mg also as a rapid bolus injection is a good alternative where adenosine is contraindicated.

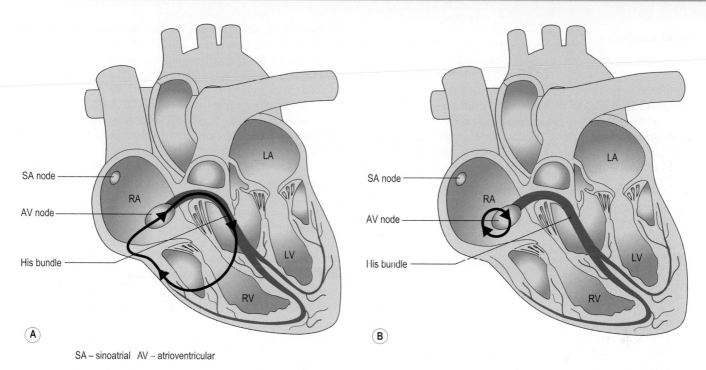

SA – sinoatrial   AV – atrioventricular

Fig. 22.8 The re-entry circuits of (A) AV nodal re-entry tachycardia (AVNRT) and (B) atrioventricular re-entry tachycardia (AVRT). (A) The AVNRT circuit comprises 'fast' and 'slow' pathways feeding into the AV node itself. The slow pathway is the target of catheter ablation. The AVRT circuit comprises atrial myocardium, the AV node and His bundle, ventricular myocardium and an accessory pathway, a small strand of muscle providing a second abnormal connection between atrium and ventricle, thus forming a potential re-entry circuit. The accessory pathway itself is the target of catheter ablation. SA, sinoatrial; AV, atrioventricular.

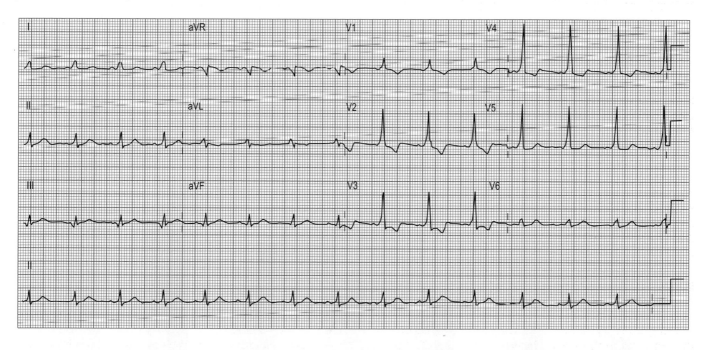

Fig. 22.9 An electrocardiogram showing a Wolff–Parkinson–White pattern. The PR interval is short and the QRS complex is abnormally broad, with a slurred upstroke or delta wave.

Junctional re-entry tachycardia is often recurrent. There is a limited role for prophylactic drug treatment as this is generally not a dangerous condition affecting young and otherwise healthy people. Among other factors, the efficacy, toxicity and acceptability of what may be long-term drug treatment require careful consideration. Options for prophylactic drug treatment include ß-blockers, verapamil, flecainide and sotalol. Particular importance should be given to discussion about the management of junctional re-entry tachycardia during pregnancy. Catheter ablation is curative in one sitting in a majority of cases.

Atrial fibrillation

AF is the most common sustained arrhythmia, affecting about 1% of the population. AF is rare before the age of 50 but its prevalence approximately doubles with each decade thereafter such that about 10% of those over 80 are affected. AF is characterised by extremely rapid and uncoordinated electrical activity in the atria and variable conduction through the AV node, resulting in irregular and usually rapid ventricular contraction.

The clinical importance of AF results from:

(i)   Symptoms including palpitation, reduced exercise capacity, breathlessness and fatigue
(ii) Increased risk of thomboembolic stroke
(iii) Exacerbation of heart failure through its direct haemodynamic effect and by causing tachycardia-induced cardiomyopathy
(iv) Increased all-cause mortality (odds ratio 1.5 for men and 1.9 for women)

AF may be classified as:

Paroxysmal: self-limiting episodes of AF lasting no more than 7 days

Persistent: AF lasting more than 7 days or requiring cardioversion

Longstanding persistent: continuous AF for more than 1 year

Permanent: where a decision has been made not to attempt cure of persistent AF.

Stroke risk. All patients presenting with AF (or atrial flutter) should undergo assessment of their risk of stroke. Although various risk stratification schemes exist, they are exemplified by the $CHADS_2$ score, which assigns one point each for Congestive cardiac failure, Hypertension, Age >75 years, and Diabetes mellitus and two points for if there is a history of previous Stroke. Surprisingly, the frequency of AF episodes does not seem to influence stroke risk. The risk of stroke is directly proportional to the $CHADS_2$ score. Meta-analysis of numerous trials of stroke prevention in AF has suggested a relative risk reduction for stroke of 64% with warfarin and 22% with aspirin (Fig. 22.10).

Warfarin is more difficult to take than aspirin because of the need for monitoring of the international normalised ratio (INR) and because of the potential for dietary and drug interactions with warfarin. Warfarin also increases the risk of serious bleeding. The absolute benefit of warfarin over aspirin for the prevention of stroke in AF is proportional to the $CHADS_2$ score and the point at which the benefit of warfarin is considered to outweigh the risk is an annual untreated stroke risk of 4%. For this reason, current guidelines recommend stroke prophylaxis with warfarin for those with a $CHADS_2$ score of ≥2, warfarin or aspirin for a $CHADS_2$ score of 1 and aspirin for those with a $CHADS_2$ score of 0.

While $CHADS_2$ is the most common guideline, in patients with AF and a $CHADS_2$ score of 1, a lower incidence of stroke and/or death from all causes has been found among patients treated with vitamin K antagonists (VKAs) when compared with no antithrombotic therapy. In contrast, prescription of an antiplatelet agent was not associated with a lower risk of events compared with no antithrombotic therapy.

Identification of the 'low risk' category clearly needed to be improved, so patients can be truly identified as low risk.

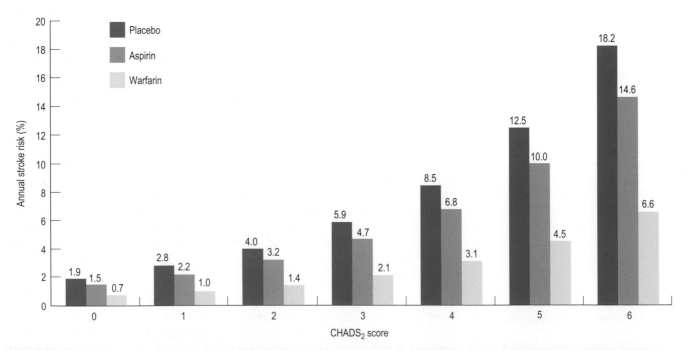

Fig. 22.10 Annual stroke risk is directly related to the $CHADS_2$ score (black bars). Aspirin reduces stroke risk by approximately 22% (dark blue bars) and warfarin by approximately 64% (light blue bars). This figure shows that, although the *relative* stroke risk reduction is higher with warfarin than with aspirin whatever the $CHADS_2$ score, the *absolute* difference is directly related to the $CHADS_2$ score. Warfarin is inconvenient to take and increases the risk of serious bleeding and, therefore, a clear benefit from taking warfarin rather than aspirin is apparent only for those with $CHADS_2$ scores of ≥2.

This can be achieved by using CHA2DS2–VASc [Cardiac failure, Hypertension, Age ≥75 (doubled), Diabetes, Stroke (doubled)–Vascular disease (prior myocardial infarction, peripheral artery disease, complex aortic plaque), Age 65–74 and Sex category (female =1, male = 0)]. This schema improves on $CHADS_2$ as it classifies a low proportion of subjects into the 'moderate risk' category, and helps better determine the truly 'low risk' patients who have very low event rates and no need for anticoagulation.

There is no evidence that any form of treatment for AF, other than warfarin or aspirin, reduces the risk of stroke regardless of how apparently successful it is in maintaining sinus rhythm. Current guidelines, therefore, recommend indefinite stroke prophylaxis with warfarin or aspirin on the basis of the risk stratification.

It is often difficult to maintain INR levels within the therapeutic range of 2.0 3.0. There is evidence that the INR may be outside of this range up to half of the time. A subtherapeutic INR substantially increases risk of stroke or arterial thromboembolism. Conversely, a high INR increases the risk of bleeding. The approximate annual frequency of major and minor bleeding with warfarin is 3% and 10%, respectively. Patients' and physicians' concern about the use of warfarin has resulted in its under-utilisation, particularly among elderly people, who are at the greatest risk of stroke. These difficulties have led to a search for alternative agents. The most advanced of these achieve their anticoagulant effect by inhibiting a single activated clotting factor, either thrombin (factor IIA) or factor XA. These drugs have a more predictable pharmacological profile that negates the need for frequent monitoring and may represent a step forward in the care of patients with AF. These agents are expected to offer advantages of enhanced or similar efficacy compared with warfarin without an increased risk of major bleeding.

Emergency management. AF associated with unstable angina, heart failure or hypotension requires emergency treatment. In most cases, the treatment of choice is d.c. cardioversion. Concerns about thromboembolism as the heart returns to sinus rhythm are valid but should not delay emergency treatment. Immediate d.c. cardioversion is appropriate when the onset of AF is clearly identified as within 48 h of presentation or when the patient is already taking warfarin and has had a therapeutic INR for at least 4 weeks. If facilities permit, a trans-oesophageal echocardiogram may be performed in patients not already on warfarin in order to exclude intracardiac thrombus. Heparin should then be given immediately and continued until the INR is within the therapeutic range. Anticoagulant therapy should be continued for at least 3 months following cardioversion. Long-term stroke prophylaxis is guided thereafter by the $CHADS_2$ score. If d.c. cardioversion is deemed inappropriate, rapid ventricular rate control may be achieved with intravenous ß-blockers, verapamil or digoxin.

Long-term management. There has been considerable debate about the pros and cons of a rate-control strategy, focusing on achieving adequate control of the ventricular rate with drugs modifying the AV node versus a rhythm-control strategy, in which an attempt is made to restore and maintain sinus rhythm with antiarrhythmic drugs ± d.c. cardioversion. These strategies have been compared in several large-scale prospective randomised trials, which have failed to demonstrate an advantage to a rhythm-control strategy. Sinus rhythm has been associated with a 47% reduction in all-cause mortality, although this benefit was offset by a 49% increase in mortality associated with antiarrhythmic drugs (AFFIRM investigators, 2004). In that study, a wide variety of antiarrhythmic drugs were used at the discretion of the investigator. These included several class I antiarrhythmic drugs, sotalol and amiodarone. A rhythm-control strategy may be more appropriate in (i) younger patients, (ii) those with paroxysmal AF, (iii) AF associated with heart failure and (iv) patients who remain symptomatic despite adequate ventricular rate control.

Ventricular rate control. The mainstay of a ventricular rate-control strategy is the use of drugs which prolong the AV nodal refractory period, thus reducing the ventricular rate. Digoxin may control the ventricular rate at rest but is less successful at controlling the rate during exertion. ß-Blockers or calcium channel blockers (verapamil or diltiazem) are generally effective both at rest and on exertion, although a combination of these drugs is occasionally necessary. Where ventricular rate control cannot be achieved with drugs, catheter ablation of the AV node in combination with permanent pacemaker implantation can provide excellent symptom relief. The adverse effects of right ventricular apical pacing may offset some of the benefit of a slower ventricular rate and regular rhythm and, therefore, biventricular pacing may be more appropriate in this situation.

Rhythm control. Rhythm control can be considered in terms of either restoration or maintenance of sinus rhythm. The most rapid and effective means of restoring sinus rhythm is d.c. cardioversion. Where AF is of short duration, well tolerated and not associated with structural heart disease, class IC antiarrhythmic drugs such as flecainide and class III drugs such as amiodarone may be used intravenously in order to achieve chemical cardioversion. Stroke risk should be managed in the same way as described for the emergency management of AF.

Although sinus rhythm can be restored in most patients through d.c. cardioversion or antiarrhythmic drugs, alone or in combination, most patients will revert to AF without further treatment. The SAFE-T trial examined 665 patients with AF of at least 72 h duration. Sinus rhythm was restored with antiarrhythmic drugs (sotalol or amiodarone) or placebo, supplemented where necessary by d.c. cardioversion (Singh et al., 2005). Patients were then maintained on placebo, sotalol or amiodarone. By 2 years, that probability of remaining in sinus rhythm was 10% (placebo), 30% (sotalol) and 50% (amiodarone). Another similar study (Roy et al., 2000) demonstrated equivalent efficacy of sotalol and the class Ic antiarrhythmic propafenone in the maintenance of sinus rhythm (40% at 2 years) and confirmed the superiority of amiodarone (60%). Most heart rhythm specialists consider that the toxicity of amiodarone precludes its long-term use for the management of AF. Dronedarone, it was hoped, would provide efficacy similar to amiodarone but it has been shown to be less effective, although it has far fewer side effects.

Modern strategies for curative catheter ablation of AF followed the discovery in 1998 that paroxysmal AF is due, in most cases, to rapid firing by the musculature surrounding the pulmonary veins close to their junctions with the left atrium. The cornerstone of most current ablation strategies for paroxysmal AF is complete electrical isolation of all four pulmonary veins from the left atrium, using either radiofrequency ablation (cautery) or cryoablation to ablate in rings around the pairs of ipsilateral veins. Catheter ablation can cure a majority of paroxysmal AF but needs to be repeated in 30–40% of patients and carries risk including stroke (3/1000) and pericardial effusion (1–2/100). Catheter ablation has been shown in small randomised studies to be superior to antiarrhythmic drug therapy in maintaining sinus rhythm and improving symptoms and quality of life. Catheter ablation has also been shown in non-randomised studies to improve left ventricular ejection fraction and heart failure symptoms. No benefit has been demonstrated in terms of reduced stroke risk or mortality. The natural history of AF is for episodes of AF to increase in frequency and duration until persistent AF supervenes. This progression appears to occur as a result of atrial remodelling, a complex and incompletely understood process involving electrical and structural changes in the whole atrial myocardium predisposing to the development of AF independent of the pulmonary veins. Catheter ablation strategies for persistent AF are more complex than those for paroxysmal AF with a correspondingly higher rate of repeat procedures and a lower overall success rate. For all of these reasons, drug therapy remains the first line treatment of AF with catheter ablation reserved for patients with symptomatic AF that cannot be managed satisfactorily with drugs and whose symptoms trouble them enough to wish to undergo ablation.

Ventricular tachyarrhythmias

Ventricular tachycardia

VT is a rapid heart rhythm originating in the ventricles. VT may present with palpitation, chest pain, breathlessness, presyncope, syncope or sudden cardiac death (death occurring suddenly and unexpectedly within 1 h of the onset of symptoms from a presumed cardiac cause). It is clinically useful to subdivide VT in the following ways:

VT complicating structural heart disease. Most VT occurs in patients with significant structural heart disease. Most of these are associated with a healed myocardial infarction but other important causes include hypertensive and valvular heart disease and a variety of cardiomyopathies including dilated, hypertrophic or arrhythmogenic right ventricular cardiomyopathy. VT of this type is usually due to re-entry. Scarring of ventricular myocardium creates the central obstacle around which potential re-entry circuits develop forming the VT 'substrate'. In this setting, a single ventricular premature beat, the VT 'trigger', may induce VT. The importance of VT complicating structural heart disease is that there is a high chance of the VT recurring and patients are at substantially increased risk of sudden cardiac death.

'Normal heart' VT. These uncommon VTs occur in the context of a structurally normal heart and a normal ECG in sinus rhythm and are exemplified by right ventricular outflow tract (RVOT) tachycardia and fascicular tachycardia. The importance of recognising these VTs is that unlike VT associated with structural heart disease, they are associated with a normal prognosis, may be managed successfully with drugs (ß-blockers, verapamil or flecainide for RVOT tachycardia, verapamil for fascicular tachycardia) and are curable by catheter ablation.

Ventricular fibrillation

Ventricular fibrillation (VF) comprises rapid and totally disorganised electrical activity in the ventricles such that effective contraction ceases and results in sudden death unless sinus rhythm is restored either spontaneously or by defibrillation. Acute myocardial ischaemia and infarction are probably responsible for most VF, although virtually any structural heart disease may also be complicated by VF. Other cases occur in the context of a group of conditions known as channelopathies:

Channelopathies. This is a group of inherited conditions characterised by abnormal function of the protein channels present in the cardiac myocyte cell membrane that regulate the flow of ions responsible for generating the resting transmembrane potential and the action potential. These include the long QT syndromes, short QT syndrome, early repolarisation syndrome, Brugada syndrome and catecholaminergic polymorphic VT. A detailed description of these conditions is beyond the scope of this chapter but there are certain key points:

- With the exception of catecholaminergic polymorphic VT, each is associated with characteristic abnormalities of the resting ECG in sinus rhythm.
- Each may be complicated by ventricular tachyarrhythmias and sudden cardiac death.
- ß-Blockers reduce the likelihood of arrhythmia in long QT syndromes and catecholaminergic polymorphic VT.
- Many drugs lengthen the QT interval (Box 22.1) and are contraindicated in patients with long QT syndromes.

Box 22.1 Drugs associated with prolonged QT intervals (adapted from Crouch et al., 2003)

Inhalational agents: halothane, isoflurane
Macrolide antibiotics: erythromycin, clarithromycin
Halofantrine
Lithium
Fosphenytoin
Mizolastine
Phenothiazines
Pentamidine
Sertindole
Antihistamines: terfenadine, astemizole, mizolastine
Antipsychotics: haloperidol, droperidol, pimozole
Tricyclic antidepressants: amitriptyline, imipramine
Class IA or III antiarrhythmics

A list of drugs known to prolong the QT interval can be found at http://www.azcert.org.

- Class I antiarrhythmic drugs and a variety of other drugs are contraindicated in Brugada syndrome. A list of drugs to avoid in the Brugada syndrome can be found at http://www.azcert.org.
- Most patients with these conditions who experience syncope, cardiac arrest or who develop spontaneous ventricular arrhythmias will be considered for an implantable cardioverter-defibrillator (ICD).

Emergency management of ventricular arrhythmias. VF and pulseless VT should be managed according to Resuscitation Council (UK) guidelines for advanced life support, which are updated periodically and can be found at http://www.resus.org.uk.

VT associated with a pulse is also the subject of guidelines by the Resuscitation Council (UK). If the patient is hypotensive in a low cardiac output state or has heart failure, the correct treatment is prompt d.c. cardioversion. If none of these features is present, chemical cardioversion may be attempted with intravenous amiodarone 300 mg over 20–60 min followed by 900 mg over the next 24 h. Amiodarone must be given via a central vein because it can cause thrombophlebitis when given peripherally and limb threatening soft tissue damage if extravasation occurs.

Ongoing management of ventricular arrhythmias. Once stabilised, patients presenting with VT or VF should remain in hospital and their management should be discussed at an early stage with a specialist cardiac electrophysiology service. Investigations should be performed to establish the nature and extent of underlying heart disease, with emphasis on detecting structural heart disease, coronary artery disease, inducible myocardial ischaemia and consideration of channelopathies in those with structurally normal hearts.

Most patients with ischaemic heart disease should be treated with aspirin, statins, angiotensin converting enzyme (ACE) inhibitors or angiotensin II receptor antagonists and ß-blockers. ß-Blockers and ACE inhibitors reduce somewhat the risk of sudden cardiac death. Although these patients remain at high risk of sudden cardiac death due to recurrent ventricular tachyarrhythmias, there is no role for the routine use of antiarrhythmic drugs. In patients with complex ventricular ectopy and impaired left ventricular systolic function following acute myocardial infarction, class IC antiarrhythmic drugs including flecainide were shown in the CAST study (Echt et al., 1991) to increase mortality while in other high-risk groups amiodarone has been shown to have no effect on all-cause mortality (Cairns et al., 1997; Julian et al., 1997). All patients should be considered for an ICD. These devices have been shown to improve prognosis following:

- Cardiac arrest due to VT or VF in the absence of a reversible underlying cause
- VT associated with syncope or significant haemodynamic compromise
- VT with a left ventricular ejection fraction of less than 35%.

Although ICDs treat further episodes of VT and VF, they do not prevent these arrhythmias from recurring and resulting in device therapies including shocks that are psychologically traumatic and lead to premature battery depletion. In the case of frequently recurring ventricular arrhythmias, patients should be on the maximum tolerated dose of a ß-blocker and there is a role for antiarrhythmic drugs including amiodarone and mexiletine. Catheter ablation of VT is an important adjunctive treatment in this situation.

Bradycardia

Bradycardia is conventionally defined as a resting heart rate below 60 min^{-1} when awake or 50 min^{-1} when asleep. Bradycardia can be classified as sinus bradycardia, where the sinus node discharges too slowly, or AV block ('heart block'), where conduction between the atria and ventricles is impaired. AV block may be subdivided into three classes:

First degree. Every P wave conducts to the ventricles but takes longer than normal to do so. The PR interval on the ECG is prolonged to greater than 200 ms (one large square on a standard ECG).

Second degree. Some but not all P waves conduct to the ventricles. Progressive PR interval prolongation followed by a non-conducted P wave is referred to as Mobitz type I or Wenckebach heart block and implies block occurring in the AV node. Mobitz type II heart block is the term used when a non-conducted P wave is not preceded by progressive PR interval prolongation and implies block occurring in the conducting system below the level of the AV node.

Third degree ('complete heart block'). No P waves conduct to the ventricles.

Bradycardia may be due to intrinsic cardiac disease or secondary to non-cardiac disease or drugs. In many cases, bradycardia due to intrinsic cardiac disease is idiopathic, that is, occurs without other identifiable heart disease. Bradycardia may also complicate acute myocardial infarction or virtually any form of structural heart disease and is also common following cardiac surgery. Non-cardiac causes of bradycardia include vasovagal syncope (faints), hypothyroidism, hyperkalaemia, hypothermia and raised intracranial pressure. Complete heart block may occur as a complication of Lyme disease (tick-borne borreliosis). Drugs commonly associated with bradycardia include ß-blockers, verapamil, diltiazem, digoxin and antiarrhythmic drugs of any class.

The management of bradycardia is as follows:

- Treat underlying medical conditions
- Consider stopping or reducing the dose of causative drugs
- Consider temporary or permanent pacemaker implantation. Permanent pacemaker implantation for sinus bradycardia is indicated for symptom relief whereas in the case of second and third degree AV block permanent pacemaker implantation is indicated on both symptomatic and prognostic grounds.

In an emergency situation, drugs may be used in an attempt to support the heart rate until trans-venous pacing can be established. The most useful drugs in this situation are atropine in 500 μcg boluses up to a total of 3 mg, adrenaline infused at a rate of 2–10 μcg/min or isoprenaline 1–10 μcg/min, titrated against heart rate. External pacing is another useful measure until transvenous pacing can be established. More detailed guidance on the emergency management of bradycardia may be viewed at http://www.resus.org.uk.

Drug therapy

Antiarrhythmic drug therapy is used to control the frequency and severity of arrythmias, with the aim of maintaining sinus rhythm where possible. Although antiarrhythmic drug treatment has been the mainstay of arrhythmia treatment, many of these drugs have limited efficacy and important toxicity. Many arrhythmias are now curable by catheter ablation. Implantable devices such as permanent pacemakers and ICDs have assumed an increasingly important role in the treatment of arrhythmias and, in many cases, antiarrhythmic drugs have an adjunctive role. Antiarrhythmic drugs can be grouped according to their electrophysiological effects at a cellular level, using the Vaughan–Williams classification. Alternatively, antiarrhythmic drugs may be classified according to their main sites of action within the heart.

Vaughan–Williams Classification

All antiarrhythmic drugs act by altering the movement of electrolytes across the myocardial cell membrane. The Vaughan–Williams classification groups drugs according to their ability to block the movement of one or more of these ions across the myocardial cell membrane. Most drugs have several modes of action, and their effectiveness as antiarrhythmic agents depends upon the summation of these effects. The effect of the different drug classes on the various phases of the action potential in His–Purkinje fibres are shown in Table 22.1. The choice of which drug to use is based upon the origin of the arrhythmia, regardless of its pattern. However, the preference of one class over another may vary, depending on a clinician's experience with particular drugs, on the presentation of the arrhythmia and on patient characteristics. Such factors also govern the choice of drug within a class. The drug chosen should have the dosing schedule and adverse effect

profile that best suit the patient or inconvenience them least (see Tables 22.2–22.4). Thus, for example, a patient with glaucoma or prostatism should not be given disopyramide which possesses marked anticholinergic properties, and a patient with obstructive airways disease should preferably not be prescribed a ß-blocker (class II), though if considered essential they could have a cardioselective agent.

The pharmacokinetic profiles of selected antiarrhythmics are presented in Table 22.5.

Class I

Class I drugs act by blocking the fast sodium channels that are responsible for the rapid depolarisation phase of the cardiac action potential, thus reducing the rate of depolarisation (the slope of phase 0) and the amplitude of the action potential. The conduction velocity of an activation wavefront is determined partly by the slope and amplitude of the cardiac action potential and partly by the resistance to current flow through the myocardium. The effect of sodium channel blockade is a decrease in conduction velocity. Certain re-entrant arrhythmias such as VT complicating previous myocardial infarction depend upon slow conduction in part of the re-entrant circuit. Class I antiarrhythmic drugs may critically slow or even abolish conduction in these areas, thus terminating and/or preventing re-entry.

The action potential in the sinoatrial and AV nodes does not depend on fast sodium channels for depolarisation; instead, phase 0 depolarisation is carried by calcium channels. Class I antiarrhythmic drugs, therefore, have no direct effect on nodal tissue.

In addition to their effect on depolarisation, class I antiarrhythmic drugs may also alter the APD and hence the

Table 22.1 Effect of different drug classes on phases of action potential in His–Purkinje fibres

Phase	Dominant ion movement	Drug class	Effect
0	Sodium inward	IA IB IC	Block ++ Block + Block +++
2	Calcium inward	IV	Block
3	Potassium outward	III	Marked slowing
4	Sodium inward, potassium outward	I, II, IV	Slows

Table 22.2 Electrophysiological effects of some antiarrhythmics

Class	Antiarrhythmic agents	Effects on duration of		Sinus rate
		QRS	QT	
IA	Quinidine, procainamide, disopyramide	+	+	+
IB	Lidocaine (lignocaine), mexiletine, phenytoin	0/−	−	0
IC	Flecainide, propafenone	++	0	−−
II	Atenolol, metoprolol, sotalol, esmolol	0	++	−−
III	Amiodarone, bretylium, sotalol	0	+++	−
IV	Verapamil, diltiazem, adenosine	0	0	−−

+, increased; −, decreased; 0, no change.

Table 22.3 Adverse effects of antiarrhythmic drugs (class I)

Drug	Cardiac	Non-cardiac	Caution or avoid in
Disopyramide	Torsade de Pointes Myodepressant	Anticholinergic (urinary retention, constipation, dry mouth, blurred vision)	Glaucoma, prostatism, hypotension
Procainamide		Lupus, nausea, diarrhoea	Myasthenia gravis, slow acetylators (increased risk of lupus)
Quinidine	Torsade de Pointes Vasodilation (i.v.)	Diarrhoea, nausea, tinnitus, headache, deafness, confusion, visual disturbances, blood dyscrasias	Myasthenia gravis
Lidocaine (lignocaine)		Convulsions in overdose, paraesthesiae	Liver failure (reduce dose)
Mexiletine		Nausea, paraesthesiae	Second or third degree heart block
Flecainide	Proarrhythmic Myodepressant	Paraesthesiae, tremor	Not recommended if any cardiac dysfunction
Propafenone	Proarrhythmic Myodepressant	Gastro-intestinal disturbances	Not recommended if any cardiac dysfunction

Table 22.4 Adverse effects of antiarrhythmic drugs (classes II–IV)

Drug	Cardiac	Non-cardiac	Caution or avoid in
ß-blockers (general)	Myodepressant Heart block	Bronchoconstriction (β_2) Vasoconstriction Hallucinations/vivid dreams (greater with more lipophilic agents) Decreased renal blood flow Changes in serum lipid profile Drowsiness, fatigue	Asthma, COPD, Raynaud's disease, diabetes mellitus, depression
Dofetilide	Torsade de Pointes		Combination with disopyramide or amiodarone or drugs in Table 22.1
Amiodarone	Torsade de Pointes	Hyper-/hypothyroidism, pneumonitis, myopathy, neuropathy, hepatitis, corneal deposits, photosensitivity	Thyroid disease, liver dysfunction, lung disease (e.g. pneumonectomy)
Bretylium	Hypotension	Initial sympathomimetic response, nausea	
Verapamil	Heart block	Constipation, headaches, flushing, ankle oedema, light-headedness	Myasthenia gravis
Adenosine	Heart block	Bronchoconstriction, flushing, chest pain	Asthma, COPD, combination with dipyridamole Decompensated heart failure, patients with a history of convulsions/seizures or recent heart transplant (<1 year)

effective refractory period (ERP) via an effect on potassium channels responsible for action potential repolarisation. Class I antiarrhymic drugs are subdivided into three groups according to their effect on APD: class IA drugs increase the APD, class IB drugs shorten the APD, and class IC drugs have no effect on APD. These effects may be assessed by measurement of the QT interval on the ECG, which reflects average ventricular APD.

The properties of class I antiarrhythmic drugs may be summarised as follows:

Table 22.5 Pharmacokinetics of selected antiarrhythmics

	Oral absorption	% protein binding	Elimination, metabolism, half-life (therapeutic range if recommended to be measured)
Amiodarone	Slow, variable	>95	Extensive metabolism, very variable rate, $t_{1/2}$ 2 days initially increasing to 40–60 days
Bretylium	Intravenous/intramuscular only	Unbound	Renal, $t_{1/2}$ 5–10 h
Digoxin	Variable, 70%	25	70% renal, variable, $t_{1/2}$ 36 h (0.8–2 ng/mL)
Diltiazem	40% absorbed	80	Hepatic, $t_{1/2}$ 3 h
Disopyramide	Rapid, >80%	30–90	50% renal, 15% bile, active metabolite, $t_{1/2}$ 4–10 h
Flecainide	Complete, slow	40	30% renal, $t_{1/2}$ 20 h
Lidocaine	Intravenous/intramuscular only	60–80	10% renal, rapid hepatic metabolism to CNS-toxic products, $t_{1/2}$ 8–100 min increases with duration of dosing
Mexiletine	>90%	60–70	10% renal, $t_{1/2}$ 10–12 h, hepatic metabolites mostly inactive
Procainamide	Rapid, >75%	15–20	50% renal, 25–40% converted to N-acetylprocainamide (active, $t_{1/2}$ 6 h), procainamide $t_{1/2}$ 2.5–4.5 h
Propafenone	Complete, rapid	>95	Extensive first-pass metabolism, capacity-limited, $t_{1/2}$ 2–12 h
Quinidine	Rapid, >80%	80–90	Mixed renal and hepatic, $t_{1/2}$ 6 h
Verapamil	Rapid, >90%	90	Hepatic, $t_{1/2}$ 4–12 h, marked first-pass effect

All values quoted are subject to marked interindividual variability. Most therapeutic ranges are poorly defined. Oral absorption does not account for drug lost by first-pass hepatic metabolism. Rapid absorption indicates a peak plasma concentration in less than 2 h.
$t_{1/2}$ elimination half-life at normal renal function.

Sodium channel blockade
IC > IA > IB
Effect on APD and ERP
IA prolong
IB shorten
IC no effect

Increasing the APD, and hence the effective refractory period, may terminate and prevent re-entry tachycardias by prolonging the duration that tissue is refractory and prevent re-entrant wavefronts from re-exciting the tissue. Although contributing to the antiarrhythmic effects of these drugs, APD prolongation is also responsible for one of their important adverse effects, Torsade de Pointes.

Class IA antiarrhythmic drugs have additional anticholinergic actions and oppose vagal activity. This can lead to both sinus tachycardia and a shortened refractory period of the AV node, as both the sinus and AV nodes are densely innervated and tonically inhibited by the vagus nerve. One consequence of this effect on the AV node is a more rapid ventricular rate during AF, necessitating co-treatment with drugs such as digoxin, ß-blockers or calcium channel blockers.

Class IA agents

Class IA antiarrhythmic drugs have been used for the treatment of a variety of atrial and ventricular arrhythmias but are now rarely used because of their proarrhythmic (Torsade de Pointes) and non-cardiac side effects and potential for drug interactions.

Quinidine was one of the earliest antiarrhythmic drugs developed. Quinidine, an alkaloid derived from the cinchona tree bark, had a significant role in the treatment of many arrhythmias. After concerns about increased risk of ventricular arrhythmia and death with quinidine emerged, the use of quinidine fell dramatically in favour of newer antiarrhythmic medications.

Disopyramide has been used to treat a wide variety of supraventricular and ventricular arrhythmias. The drug is given orally and excreted by the kidneys, with a half-life of 6–8 h, necessitating frequent dosing. Disopyramide has strong affinity for muscarinic cholinergic receptors (40 times that of quinidine) and commonly causes anticholinergic side effects such as blurred vision, dry mouth, constipation and urinary retention. Disopyramide may precipitate acute glaucoma in predisposed individuals. Disopyramide also causes sympathetic inhibition resulting in vasodilation. Other adverse effects occur less frequently than with quinidine (e.g. gastro-intestinal, QRS prolongation, Torsade de Pointes and hypotension) and there is no interaction with digoxin.

Procainamide has been used in an initial attempt at the pharmacologic cardioversion of AF of recent onset. Procainamide may be given orally or intravenously. Procainamide is metabolised to *n*-acetyl procainamide. Both have antiarrhythmic activity and are excreted mainly by the kidneys. The half-life of procainamide is short (3–4 h), necessitating frequent dosing. The half-life of *n*-acetyl procainamide is considerably longer than that of procainamide. The risk of a lupus-like syndrome comprising a rash, fever and arthralgia (likeliest in slow acetylators) is about one in three of those patients treated for longer than 6 months. Hypotension due to an inhibitory effect on sympathetic ganglia, QRS and QT interval prolongation are common adverse effects with intravenous administration.

Class IB agents

As a group, class IB agents inhibit the fast sodium current (typical class I effect) while shortening the APD in non-diseased tissue. The former has the more powerful effect, while the latter might actually predispose to re-entrant arrhythmias, but ensures that QT prolongation does not occur. Class IB agents act selectively on diseased or ischaemic tissue, where they are thought to promote conduction block in slowly conducting tissue critical to the maintenance of re-entry, thereby interrupting re-entry circuits.

Lidocaine was previously the standard intravenous agent for the suppression of serious ventricular arrhythmias associated with acute myocardial infarction and following cardiac surgery but has now been almost completely superseded by ß-blockers. Lidocaine acts preferentially on ischaemic myocardium and is more effective in the presence of a high external potassium concentration. Therefore, hypokalaemia must be corrected for maximum efficacy. The kinetics of lidocaine is such that it is rapidly de-ethylated by the liver precluding oral administration. The two critical factors governing lidocaine metabolism, and hence its efficacy, are liver blood flow (decreased in old age and by heart failure and ß-blockade) and drugs that induce or inhibit the enzyme of the cytochrome P450 system. Lidocaine is rapidly distributed within minutes after an initial intravenous loading dose, requiring the need for a continuous infusion or repetitive dosing to maintain therapeutic blood levels. Lidocaine has no value in treating supraventricular tachyarrhythmias.

Mexiletine may be administered intravenously or orally to control VT. Frequent gastro-intestinal and central nervous system (CNS) side effects (dizziness, light-headedness, tremor, nervousness, difficulty with coordination) limit the dose and possible therapeutic benefit.

Class IC agents

The major electrophysioloical effects of these agents are that they are powerful inhibitors of the fast sodium channel causing a marked depression of the upstroke of the cardiac action potential. In addition, they may variably prolong the APD by delaying inactivation of the slow sodium channel and inhibition of the rapid component of the repolarising delayed rectifier current (I_{kr}) which may explain the prolongation of the QRS complex and QT interval. Class IC agents are potent antiarrhythmics used largely in the control of paroxysmal supraventricular and ventricular tachyarrhythmias resistant to other drugs, although they have acquired a particularly bad reputation as a result of the proarrhythmic effects seen in CAST (Cardiac Arrhythmia Supression Trial) and the CASH (Cardiac Arrest Study Hamburg) studies. Faster heart rates, increased sympathetic activity, and diseased or ischaemic myocardium all contribute to the proarrhythmic effects of these drugs. This has led to these drugs being contraindicated in patients with structural heart disease as poor systolic function exaggerates the proarrhythmic effects. However, flecainide is effective for the treatment of both supraventricular and ventricular arrhythmias in patients without structural heart disease and is moderately successful for maintenance of sinus rhythm after cardioversion of AF. Propafenone has mild ß-blocking properties, especially in higher doses so should be avoided in patients with reversible obstructive airways disease.

Class II agents: ß-Adrenoreceptor antagonists (ß-blockers)

β_1- and β_2-adrenoreceptors are present in the cell membranes of myocytes throughout the heart. Activation of ß-adrenoreceptors by norepinephrine released from postganglionic sympathetic neurones and circulating norepinephrine and epinephrine increases the rate of discharge of the sinus node (positive chronotropy), increases the conduction velocity and shortens the refractory period of the AV node (positive dromotropy) and increases the force of contraction (contractility) of myocytes (positive inotropy).

ß-Adrenoreceptors are coupled to G proteins, which activate adenylyl cyclase to form cAMP from ATP. Increased cAMP directly activates the pacemaker current I_f to increase the rate of diastolic depolarisation and hence to increase the sinus rate. cAMP also activates a cAMP-dependent protein kinase (PK-A) that phosphorylates L-type calcium channels, which causes increased calcium entry into the cell. Increased calcium entry during the plateau phase of the action potential leads to enhanced release of calcium by the sarcoplasmic reticulum and hence an increase in contractility. Intracellular calcium overload predisposes to the development of early or late afterdepolarisations which may result in arrhythmias due to triggered activity.

ß-Blockers prevent the normal ligand (norepinephrine or epinephrine) from binding to the ß-adrenoreceptor by competing for the binding site. The antiarrhythmic properties of ß-blockers are probably the result of several mechanisms: (i) reducing the likelihood of arrhythmias due to triggered activity, (ii) opposing the increased sympathetic activity in patients with sustained VT and in patients with acute myocardial infarction and (iii) indirectly preventing arrhythmia via their antihypertensive and anti-ischaemic effect.

ß-Blockers licensed for the treatment of arrhythmias include propranolol, acebutol, atenolol, esmolol, metoprolol and sotalol. The antiarrhythmic activity of the various ß-blockers is reasonably uniform, the critical property being β_1-adrenoreceptor blockade. Atenolol, metoprolol propranolol and esmolol are available for intravenous use. Esmolol, a selective β_1-adrenoreceptor antagonist, has a half-life of 9 min with full recovery from its ß-blockade properties within 30 min. Esmolol is quickly metabolised in red blood cells, independent of renal and hepatic function, and due to its short half-life, can be useful in situations where there are relative contraindications or concerns about the use of a ß-blocker. Sotalol has some class III activity as well as class II effects and bretylium is considered to have class II activity in addition to class III.

The use of ß-blockers is somewhat constrained by their adverse effects. β_2-Adrenoreceptors on bronchial smooth muscle are tonically activated by circulating catecholamines to cause bronchodilation. ß-Blockers can, therefore, cause bronchoconstriction and are contraindicated in patients with asthma and should be used with caution in chronic obstructive pulmonary disease. β_2-Adrenoreceptors are also found on vascular smooth muscle and are tonically activated by circulating catecholamines to cause vasodilatation. ß-Blockers may, therefore, cause vasoconstriction and exacerbate the symptoms of peripheral vascular disease.

Cardiac adverse effects of ß-blockers include sinus bradycardia, exacerbation of AV conduction block, reduced exercise capacity and exacerbation of acute heart failure. In patients with chronic, stable heart failure, however, due to mild to moderate LV systolic dysfunction and already treated by ACE inhibitors and diuretics, ß-blockers improve both symptoms and prognosis. Other adverse effects of ß-blockers include nightmares and impotence.

ß-Blockers vary in their lipid solubility. Agents such as propranolol and carvedilol are highly lipid-soluble whilst others such as atenolol and nadolol are more hydrophilic. Lipid solubility determines the degree of drug penetration into the CNS and the utility of haemodialysis or haemofiltration. High lipid solubility is associated with a larger volume of distribution and better CNS penetration. Lipophilic ß-blockers are primarily metabolised by the liver. Conversely, hydrophilic ß-blockers have a small volume of distribution and are eliminated essentially unchanged by the kidneys; this property allows hydrophilic ß-blockers to be removed by haemodialysis.

Class III agents

Class III antiarrhythmic drugs prolong cardiac APD by inhibiting repolarising outward potassium currents I_{Kr} and/or I_{Ks}. This action prolongs the effective refractory period, reducing the likelihood of arrhythmias due to re-entry. Prolongation of cardiac APD is reflected by QT interval prolongation on the ECG. Primary indications for class III agents are AF, atrial flutter and ventricular tachyarrhythmias.

Class III drugs include amiodarone, sotalol and bretylium. Amiodarone has additional class I, II and IV activity while sotalol has marked class II activity. An important limitation of class III agents is that action potential prolongation may be complicated by Torsade de Pointes. The development of Torsade de Pointes is attributed to a combination of triggered activity as a result of EADs and increased transmural dispersion of repolarisation within the ventricles as action potential prolongation is not uniform across the ventricular wall. Hypokalaemia, hypomagnesaemia or bradycardia increase the likelihood of Torsade de Pointes and, therefore, sotalol, with marked class II activity, may be uniquely arrhythmogenic.

Amiodarone. Amiodarone is a potent antiarrhythmic drug that is effective in treating a wide variety of atrial and ventricular arrhythmias but its use is constrained by complex pharmacokinetics and concern about toxicity. Many heart rhythm specialists would consider that the side effect profile of amiodarone precludes its use for the long-term treatment of atrial arrhythmias. Amiodarone may be extremely effective in the emergency treatment of VT and ventricular fibrillation, especially where recurrent. Amiodarone may also reduce the likelihood of recurrent ventricular arrhythmias when taken on a long-term basis but confers no prognostic benefit and should be considered as an adjunct to treatment with an ICD.

When rapid control of an arrhythmia is needed, the intravenous route is preferred, with 300 mg given over 30 min to an hour followed by 900 mg over 23–24 h, administered through a central vein. Higher loading doses may cause hypotension. A concurrent oral loading regimen of up to 2400 mg daily in two to four divided doses is usually given for 7–14 days and then reduced to a maintenance dose of 200 mg daily or less.

During the early stages of therapy with amiodarone (whether intravenous or oral), the kinetics of the drug are different from those after chronic administration. Amiodarone is highly lipid soluble and so has a very large volume of distribution. As the slowly equilibrating tissue stores are penetrated to a minimal extent during the early days of therapy, the effective elimination half-life ($t_{1/2}$) is initially dependent upon a more rapidly exchanging compartment, with a $t_{1/2}$ of 10–17 h, substantially shorter than the $t_{1/2}$ seen during chronic administration. The short $t_{1/2}$ becomes important during the acute phase and any intravenous to oral changeover period because the absorption of oral amiodarone is very slow, taking up to 15 h. The combination of a relatively fast elimination and a poor rate of absorption could lead to a significant fall in serum amiodarone levels if intravenous therapy is stopped abruptly when oral therapy is initiated, with the period of maximum risk being the first 24 h of oral therapy. It is, therefore, advisable to phase out intravenous therapy gradually and allow an intravenous/oral overlap period of at least 24 h. Once amiodarone has reached saturation, amiodarone is eliminated very slowly, with a half-life of about 25–110 days. Due to amiodarone's long terminal half-life, there is a potential for drug interactions to occur several weeks (or even months) after treatment with it has been stopped. Common interactions include antibacterials, other antiarrhythmics, lipid-regulating drugs and digoxin.

Amiodarone has been associated with toxicity involving the lungs, thyroid gland, liver, eyes, skin, and peripheral nerves. The incidence of most adverse effects is related to total amiodarone exposure (i.e. dosage and duration of treatment). Therefore, practitioners must consider carefully the risk–benefit ratio of the use of amiodarone in each patient, use the lowest possible dose of amiodarone, monitor for adverse effects and, if possible, discontinue treatment if adverse effects occur.

Corneal microdeposits (reversible on withdrawal of treatment) develop in nearly all adult patients given prolonged amiodarone; these rarely interfere with vision, but drivers may be dazzled by headlights at night. However, if vision is impaired or if optic neuritis or optic neuropathy occur, amiodarone must be stopped to prevent blindness. Long-term administration of amiodarone is associated with a blue-grey discoloration of the skin. This is more commonly seen in individuals with lighter skin tones. The discoloration may revert upon cessation of the drug. However, the skin color may not return completely to normal.

Individuals taking amiodarone may become more sensitive to the harmful effects of UV-A light. Using sunblock that also blocks UV-A rays appears to prevent this side effect. Amiodarone contains iodine and can cause disorders of thyroid function. Both hypothyroidism and hyperthyroidism may occur. Clinical assessment alone is unreliable and laboratory tests should be performed before treatment and every 6 months including tri-iodothyronine (T3), T4 and thyroid stimulating hormone (TSH). A raised T3 and T4 with a very low or undetectable TSH concentration suggests the development of thyrotoxicosis. Amiodarone-associated thyrotoxicosis may be refractory to treatment and amiodarone should usually be withdrawn, at least temporarily, to help achieve control, although treatment with carbimazole is often required. Hypothyroidism can be treated safely with replacement therapy without the need to withdraw amiodarone if amiodarone is considered essential. Amiodarone is also associated with hepatotoxicity and treatment should be discontinued if severe liver function abnormalities or clinical signs of liver disease develop.

The most serious adverse effect of amiodarone therapy is pulmonary toxicity, typically acute pneumonitis or more insidious pulmonary fibrosis. In early studies, the frequency of pulmonary toxicity during amiodarone therapy was 2–17%. More recent studies have shown a lower incidence in patients receiving dosages of 300 mg/day or less. Although acute pneumonitis may respond to corticosteroids, pulmonary fibrosis is largely irreversible.

Class IV agents

The plateau phase of the cardiac action potential results from the inward movement of Ca^{2+} ions balanced by the outward movement of K^+ ions. Class IV agents (calcium channel blockers) block the inward movement of calcium ions during phase 2 by binding to L-type calcium channels on cardiac myocytes. The effect of class IV antiarrhythmic drugs is most marked in the sinoatrial and AV nodes, in which depolarisation is dependent upon calcium channels. Class IV antiarrhythmic drugs, therefore, cause sinus bradycardia (negative chronotropic effect), and, by reducing the conduction velocity and prolonging the AV nodal effective refractory period, reduce the ventricular rate during atrial tachyarrhythmias such as AF and flutter (negative dromotropic effect). By reducing intracellular calcium concentration class IV antiarrhythmic drugs also exert a negative inotropic effect. Only the non-dihydropyridine calcium channel blockers (verapamil and diltiazem) have direct cardiac effects.

Verapamil possesses a chiral carbon and is marketed as a racemic mixture of R- and S-stereoisomers. In humans, both isomers share qualitatively similar negative chronotropic and dromotropic effects on the sinoatrial and AV nodes, respectively, but the S-stereoisomer is 10–20 times more potent than the R with respect to these effects. Hence, the S-stereoisomer determines the negative chronotropic and dromotropic effects of verapamil, while the R-stereoisomer is of minor importance.

Verapamil also undergoes extensive stereoselective first-pass hepatic metabolism. S-verapamil is more rapidly metabolised than R-verapamil after oral administration, resulting in a lower bioavailability of the S-stereoisomer and a proportionally higher concentration of the R-stereoisomer in the systemic circulation (20% and 50%, respectively). However, because C_{max} is higher with the immediate-release formulation and S-verapamil is 10–20 times more potent than R-verapamil, it is unsurprising that this difference is also clinically significant. With the immediate-release formulation, a plot of PR-interval change versus time has the same shape as the concentration–time curve. The extended-release formulation does not have the same concentration–time effect relationship. This has been attributed to the difference in oral input rates, to the concentration-related saturable first-pass hepatic metabolism, or both.

Since the formulation of verapamil may play a role in the drug's complex pharmacokinetics and efficacy, one formulation of verapamil cannot be safely substituted for another. Immediate release preparations are preferred to maximise bioavailability of the S-stereoisomer.

Class IV antiarrhythmic drugs should be avoided in sick sinus syndrome or second- or third-degree heart block unless the patient has a permanent pacemaker. Combined therapy with a calcium channel blocker and ß-blocker should be instituted with caution because of the risk of excessive AV block, and should be used where only where monotherapy is insufficient to control ventricular rate during atrial flutter or fibrillation. Verapamil causes greater arterial vasoodilation than diltiazem and may be especially useful in patients with hypertension or angina. Both agents have a negative inotropic effect and are thus contraindicated in heart failure. Adverse effects are mostly predictable and include ankle oedema, flushing, dizziness, light-headedness and headache. Constipation is common in patients receiving verapamil whilst a rash is common with diltiazem.

Adenosine

The potassium channel opener adenosine and its pro-drug adenosine triphosphate (ATP) act as indirect calcium antagonists and resemble verapamil in their antiarrhythmic activity.

In cardiac tissue, adenosine binds to adenosine type 1 (A_1) receptors, which are coupled to Gi proteins. Activation of this pathway opens transmembrane potassium channels, which hyperpolarises the cell. Activation of the Gi protein also decreases cAMP, which inhibits L-type calcium channels and, therefore, calcium entry into the cell. In cardiac pacemaker cells located in the sinoatrial node, adenosine acting through A_1 receptors inhibits the pacemaker current (I_f), which decreases the slope of phase 4 of the pacemaker action potential thereby decreasing its spontaneous firing rate (negative chronotropy). Inhibition of L-type calcium channels also decreases conduction velocity of the AV node (negative dromotropy). Finally, adenosine, by acting on presynaptic purinergic receptors located on sympathetic nerve terminals, inhibits the release of norepinephrine.

The ultra-short duration of action (<10 s) of intravenous adenosine makes it very suitable as a diagnostic aid and for interrupting supraventricular arrhythmias in which the AV node is part of the re-entry pathway. Adenosine is, however, a bronchoconstrictor and causes dyspnoea, flushing, chest pain and further transient arrhythmias in a high proportion of patients, and its metabolism is inhibited by dipyridamole, a vasodilator drug that blocks adenosine uptake by cells, thereby reducing the metabolism of adenosine.

Digoxin

Digitalis compounds are potent inhibitors of transmembrane Na^+/K^+-ATPase. This ion transport system moves sodium ions out of the cell in exchange for potassium ions. The consequent rise in the intracellular sodium concentration increases the activity of a transmembrane Na^+/Ca^+ exchanger in cardiac myocytes as well as many other cells, which moves sodium out of the cell in exchange for calcium. The resulting increased intracellular calcium concentration stimulates calcium release from the sarcoplasmic reticulum which increases contractility (positive inotropic effect).

Digoxin also acts on the autonomic nervous system to increase vagal tone and reduce sympathetic nervous activity, reducing conduction velocity and increasing the effective refractory period of the AV node. Digoxin, therefore, reduces the ventricular rate during persistent atrial flutter and AF and may be particularly useful in patients with these arrhythmias in the context of congestive cardiac failure. Digoxin has limited efficacy in controlling the ventricular rate in situations where the sympathetic nervous system predominates such as during exercise. It is, therefore, only useful as monotherapy in sedentary patients. ß-Blockers and calcium channel blockers are more useful for controlling the ventricular rate on exertion as well as at rest.

Digoxin is no longer indicated for the treatment of paroxysmal AF as it has no direct antiarrhythmic effect and neither terminates an episode of AF nor reduces the likelihood of further episodes of AF occurring. Furthermore, digoxin has limited efficacy for ventricular rate control at the start of an episode of AF where sympathetic nervous system activity is often high.

The positive inotropic effect of digoxin has long been used in the treatment of patients with systolic heart failure and sinus rhythm. As evidence emerged that other positive inotropic agents such as milrinone increase mortality in heart failure the role of digoxin was reexamined. Perhaps the largest and best designed of these trials, the Digitalis Investigation Group (1997) trial, established that digoxin had no effect on all-cause mortality in patients with stable congestive cardiac failure, a left ventricular ejection fraction of under 45% and sinus rhythm but significantly reduced a combined endpoint of CHF mortality and hospitalisation due to heart failure. With a large body of evidence attesting to the morbidity and mortality benefits of ACE inhibitors, ß-blockers and spironolactone the role of digoxin has diminished. Digoxin may still be useful in patients who remain symptomatic despite comprehensive therapy with these drugs.

The long half-life of digoxin (about 36 h) warrants special consideration when treating arrhythmias as several days of constant dosing would be required to reach steady-state. Therefore, loading doses of up to 1.5 mg may be used rapidly to increase digoxin serum levels. Digoxin is given once daily thereafter, usually in 125 or 250 μcg doses and has a narrow therapeutic window with the ideal blood concentration regarded as 1–2 μcg/L. Since digoxin is excreted predominantly by the kidney (70% renal elimination in normal renal function), renal function is the most important determinant of the daily digoxin dosage. Importantly, in severe renal insufficiency, there is also a decrease in the volume of distribution of digoxin and, therefore, lower loading doses should be used.

Both the therapeutic and toxic effects of digoxin are potentiated by hypokalaemia and hypercalcaemia. There are also numerous drug interactions (Table 22.6), some of which are pharmacokinetic and some of which are pharmacological.

The occurrence of adverse drug reactions is common, owing to the narrow therapeutic index of digoxin. Adverse effects are concentration-dependent, and are rare when serum digoxin concentration is less than 0.8 μcg/L. Common adverse effects

Table 22.6 Interactions involving digoxin

Effect	Offending agent or condition
Serum level increased by	Amiodarone, verapamil, diltiazem, quinidine, propafenone, clarithromycin, broad-spectrum antibiotics (erythromycin, tetracyclines), decreased renal blood flow (ß-blockers, NSAIDs), renal failure, heart failure
Serum level decreased by	Colestyramine, sulfasalazine, neomycin, rifampicin, antacids, improved renal blood flow (vasodilators), levothyroxine (thyroxine)
Therapeutic effect increased by	Hypokalaemia, hypercalcaemia, hypomagnesaemia, antiarrhythmic classes IA, II, IV, diuretics that cause hypokalaemia, corticosteroids, myxoedema, hypoxia (acute or chronic), acute myocardial ischaemia or myocarditis
Therapeutic effect decreased by	Hyperkalaemia, hypocalcaemia, thyrotoxicosis

include loss of appetite, nausea, vomiting and diarrhoea as gastro-intestinal motility increases. Other common effects are blurred vision, visual disturbances (yellow-green halos and problems with colour perception), confusion and drowsiness. The often described adverse effect of digoxin, xanthopsia, the disturbance of colour vision (mostly yellow and green colour) is rarely seen.

Patient care

Patients with arrhythmias may experience considerable anxiety about the possibility that they will have a serious arrhythmia at any moment and may, therefore, require considerable reassurance with regular follow-up. The patient's family and friends may need to be advised on what to do in the event of an acute arrhythmia. An individual's anxiety may not be helped by the fact that most antiarrhythmic drugs work in only a proportion of patients and several treatment options may be tried before the most appropriate one is identified.

Patients should give informed consent for all interventions, and prescribers must be prepared for a patient to have a different view on the use of a medicine compared to their own. This was illustrated in a study of patients' and prescribers' attitudes to the use of aspirin and warfarin for stroke prevention in AF. Not only did prescribers differ markedly on the balance of risks between stroke prevention and bleeding caused by treatment but patients feared a stroke more than doctors. Prescribers should seek and respect patients' views on such treatment choices, rather than assume all patients are the same or that they will always agree with their own views.

Examples of some common therapeutic problems that may occur during the management of arrhythmias are set out in Table 22.7.

Table 22.7 Common therapeutic problems in the management of arrhythmias

Problem	Comment
All antiarrhythmics are proarrhythmic	Prevention is better than cure. Minimise the requirement for drugs by careful attention to precipitating factors. Consider use of pacemakers or non-pharmacological therapies if appropriate
Nausea and vomiting with blurred vision and visual discolouration on digoxin	Symptoms and signs of digoxin toxicity noting digoxin has a narrow therapeutic range. Poor renal function may have also contributed
ß-Blockers are generally contraindicated in bronchial and peripheral vascular disease	Consider verapamil or diltiazem
Calcium channel blockers-induced constipation	If it occurs, give regular osmotic laxatives
Torsade de Pointes may be precipitated by taking other medication with amiodarone or disopyramide	Patients should remind members of health care team that they are taking antiarrhythmic drugs, as well as consider electrolyte disturbance such as hypokalaemia
Patients experiencing myopathy	Healthcare professionals involved in screening prescriptions for antiarrhythmics should be aware of the clinically relevant interactions and how to manage these. Patients who are taking statins will need regular monitoring for signs of myopathy, particularly those on high-intensity statin therapy
Severe asthmatic patient admitted with SVT	Adenosine is contraindicated due to the risk of bronchospasm. Verapamil is a suitable alternative
Amiodarone is commonly associated with an increased tendency to sunburn	Warn all patients to stay covered up when outdoors, use sun block or stay indoors
Acutely treated patient with AF cardioverted initially with i.v. amiodarone, but on converting to oral therapy, converted back to AF	While amiodarone has a long terminal half-life once saturated, amiodarone has a very large volume of distribution and since tissue stores are penetrated to a minimal extent during the early days of therapy, the effective elimination half-life ($t_{1/2}$) is initially dependent upon a more rapidly exchanging compartment, with a $t_{1/2}$ of 10–17 h, substantially shorter than the $t_{1/2}$ seen during chronic administration. The shorter $t_{1/2}$ becomes important during the acute phase and any intravenous to oral changeover period because the absorption of oral amiodarone is very slow, taking up to 15 h. The combination of a relatively fast elimination and a poor rate of absorption could lead to a significant fall in serum amiodarone levels if intravenous therapy is stopped abruptly when oral therapy is initiated, with the period of maximum risk being the first 24 h of oral therapy. It is, therefore, advisable to phase out intravenous therapy gradually and allow an intravenous/oral overlap period of at least 24 h

SVT, supraventricular tachycardia; AF, atrial fibrillation.

Case studies

Case 22.1

A 25-year-old female presents to the hospital emergency department with a 2-h history of palpitation and chest tightness. She has experienced several similar episodes in the past, all of which have started abruptly at rest, and consisted of rapid, regular palpitations. Previous episodes have all stopped after a few minutes and between events she has been entirely well. She has no history of heart disease or other ongoing medical problems and is on no regular drug treatment. She drinks alcohol within recommended weekly limits and takes no other recreational drugs. On examination she is anxious, has a slightly cool periphery, her pulse is 190 bpm and regular and blood pressure is 130/90 mmHg. The remainder of the examination is unremarkable. A 12-lead ECG demonstrates a regular narrow-complex tachycardia with no discernible P waves.

Question

What is the most likely diagnosis and how should she be managed?

Answer

The patient has the signs and symptoms of SVT. Non-pharmacological means of restoring sinus rhythm include carotid sinus massage, subjecting the patient to the Valsalva manoeuvre or eliciting the diving reflex by immersion of the face in ice-cold water. Either approach should result in a brief vagal discharge sufficient to block conduction in the AV node and terminate the tachycardia. If these manoeuvres are unsuccessful, intravenous adenosine can be given in doses of up to 12 mg as a rapid bolus injection followed quickly by a saline flush. Intravenous verapamil 5 mg may also be administered as a rapid bolus injection and is a good alternative where adenosine is contraindicated.

Case 22.2

Mr DS was admitted to hospital for an emergency laparotomy for a perforated gut. He has a history of paroxysmal atrial fibrillation (AF) for which he is on long-term amiodarone 200 mg once daily.

Following the laparotomy he has new onset AF which the medical team would like to treat pharmacologically. His only other current medication is thromboprophylaxis with enoxaparin 20 mg once daily.

Questions

1. What treatment plan would you initially suggest?
2. What long-term monitoring would be appropriate for Mr DS?

Answers

1. If Mr DS has any electrolyte abnormalities these should be corrected. If he remains in AF he should be prescribed amiodarone by IV infusion, as the long-term maintenance dose is clearly no longer adequate following the laparotomy.

   The reduced dose of enoxaparin should be noted. This is because Mr DS is a post surgical patient and at high risk of bleeding.
   Mr DS cardioverts back to sinus rhythm following a bolus dose of 300 mg amiodarone. The plan is to maintain him on amiodarone long term.

2. Given that Mr DS is to continue amiodarone long term the following monitoring would be appropriate:

Chest X-ray: pulmonary	Baseline and if symptoms present
Thyroid panel	Baseline and every 3–6 months
Liver panel	Baseline and every 3–6 months
Eye examination	Baseline and every 12 months
ECG	Baseline and as required
Clinical evaluation	Baseline and every 3 months

Case 22.3

Mr SB is 77 years of age who attends the hospital emergency department with worsening shortness of breath. His previous medical history includes a myocardial infarction 10 years ago which left him with left ventricular dysfunction (ejection fraction < 40%). He also has hypertension. His current medication includes:

   Bisoprolol 5 mg daily
   Ramipril 5 mg daily
   Aspirin 75 mg daily
   Furosemide 80 mg each morning.

   His heart rate is 65 bpm and irregular, and he has a blood pressure of 160/85 mmHg. Mr SB's ECG shows atrial fibrillation (AF). It was decided to control his AF with bisoprolol with no alteration of dose.

Questions

1. What drug is most appropriate for stroke prevention in Mr SB?
2. The junior doctor asks you whether warfarin should be initiated along with aspirin or in place of it.

Answers

1. All patients presenting with AF (or atrial flutter) should undergo assessment of their risk of stroke. Although various risk stratification schemes exist, the $CHADS_2$ score is widely used. For Mr SB the following is determined:

   Congestive cardiac failure 1
   Hypertension 1
   Age >75 years 1
   Diabetes mellitus 0
   Stroke 0
   Given Mr SB has a $CHADS_2$ score of 3 this suggests an annual stroke risk of 5.9% if no therapy is prescribed. This risk will reduce to 4.7% if he is prescribed aspirin, or 2.1% if he is prescribed warfarin. Assuming no contraindications or concerns, warfarin should be prescribed.

2. In patients with stable vascular disease, such as those with no acute ischaemic events or PCI/stent procedure in the preceding year, warfarin monotherapy should be used. Concomitant antiplatelet therapy should not be prescribed. Published data support the use of warfarin for secondary prevention in patients with coronary artery disease. Warfarin is at least as effective as aspirin. It should be noted that any combination of an antiplatelet agent with a vitamin K antagonist such as warfarin will significantly increase the risk of a major bleed.

References

AFFIRM investigators, 2004. Relationship between sinus rhythm, treatment, and survival in the atrial fibrillation follow-up investigation of rhythm management (AFFIRM) study. Circulation 109, 1509–1513.

Cairns, J.A., Connolly, S.J., Roberts, R., et al., 1997. Randomised trial of outcome after myocardial infarction in patients with frequent or repetitive ventricular premature depolarisations: CAMIAT Canadian Amiodarone Myocardial Infarction Arrhythmia Trial Investigators. Lancet 349, 675–682.

Crouch, M.A., Limon, L., Cassano, A.T., 2003. Drug-related QT interval prolongation: drugs associated with QT prolongation. Pharmacotherapy 23, 802–805.

Digitalis Investigation Group, 1997. The effect of digoxin on mortality and morbidity in patients with heart failure. N. Engl. J. Med. 336, 5325–5333.

Echt, D.S., Liebson, P.R., Mitchell, L.B., et al., 1991. Mortality and morbidity in patients receiving encainide, flecainide, or placebo: the Cardiac Arrhythmia Suppression Trial. N. Engl. J. Med. 324, 781–788.

Julian, D.G., Camm, A.J., Frangin, G., et al., 1997. Randomised trial of effect of amiodarone on mortality in patient with left ventricular dysfunction after recent myocardial infarction: EMIAT. European Myocardial Infarct Amiodarone Trial Investigators. Lancet 349, 667–674.

Roy, D., Talajic, M., Doran, P., 2000. Amiodarone to prevent recurrence of atrial fibrillation. N. Engl. J. Med. 342, 913–920.

Singh, B.N., Singh, S.N., Reda, D.J., 2005. Amiodarone versus sotalol for atrial fibrillation. N. Engl. J. Med. 352, 1861–1872.

Further reading

Billman, G.E. (Ed.), 2010. Novel Therapeutic Targets for Antiarrhythmic Drugs. Wiley, Hoboken.

Fogoros, R.N., 2007. Antiarryhthmic Drugs: A Practical Guide, second ed. Wiley-Blackwell, Oxford.

Lip, G., Nieuwlaat, R., Pisters, R., et al., 2010. Refining clinical risk stratification for predicting stroke and thromboembolism in atrial fibrillation using a novel risk factor based approach: the Euro Heart Survey on Atrial Fibrillation. Chest 137, 263–272.

23 Thrombosis

P. A. Routledge and H. G. M. Shetty

Key points

Venous thromboembolism (VTE)

- VTE has an incidence of 2–5%.
- Combinations of sluggish blood flow and hypercoagulability are the commonest causes of VTE. Vascular injury is also a recognised causative factor.
- Treatment of VTE involves the use of anticoagulants and, in severe cases, thrombolytic drugs.
- Anticoagulant therapy usually involves an immediate-acting agent such as heparin followed by maintenance treatment with warfarin.
- Unfractionated heparins increase the rate of interaction of thrombin with antithrombin III 1000-fold and prevent the production of fibrin from fibrinogen.
- Low molecular weight heparins inactivate factor Xa, have a longer half-life and produce a more predictable response than unfractionated heparins.
- Warfarin is the most widely used coumarin because of potency, reliable bioavailability and an intermediate half-life of elimination (36 h).
- Warfarin consists of an equal mixture of two enantiomers, (*R*)- and (*S*)-warfarins, that have different anticoagulant potencies and routes of metabolism.

Arterial thromboembolism

- Arterial thromboembolism is normally associated with vascular injury and hypercoagulability.
- Acute myocardial infarction is the commonest form of arterial thrombosis.
- Arterial thromboembolism affecting the cerebral circulation results in either transient ischaemic attacks (TIAs) or, in severe cases, cerebral infarction (stroke).

Thrombosis is the development of a 'thrombus' consisting of platelets, fibrin, red cells and white cells in the arterial or venous circulation. If part of this thrombus in the venous circulation breaks off and enters the right heart, it may be lodged in the pulmonary arterial circulation, causing pulmonary embolism (PE). In the left-sided circulation, an embolus may result in peripheral arterial occlusion, either in the lower limbs or in the cerebral circulation (where it may cause thromboembolic stroke). Since the pathophysiology of each of these conditions differs, they will be discussed separately under the headings 'Venous thromboembolism' (VTE) and 'Arterial thromboembolism'.

Venous thromboembolism

Epidemiology

VTE is common, with an incidence of 2–5%. PE is now the commonest cause of maternal death, and deep vein thrombosis may result in not only PE but also subsequent morbidity as a result of the post-phlebitic limb. Thromboembolism appears to increase in prevalence over the age of 50 years, and the diagnosis is more often missed in this age group.

Aetiology

VTE occurs primarily due to a combination of stagnation of blood flow and hypercoagulability. Vascular injury is also a recognised causative factor but is not necessary for the development of venous thrombosis. In VTE, the structure of the thrombus is different from that in arterial thromboembolism. In the former, platelets seem to be uniformly distributed through a mesh of fibrin and other blood cell components, whereas in arterial thromboembolism the white platelet 'head' is more prominent and it appears to play a much more important initiatory role in thrombus.

Sluggishness of blood flow may be related to bed rest, surgery or reduced cardiac output, for example in heart failure. Factors increasing the risk of hypercoagulability include surgery, pregnancy, oestrogen administration, malignancy, myocardial infarction and several acquired or inherited disorders of coagulation (for further detail of genetic factors, see Rosendaal and Reitsma, 2009).

Protein C deficiency

Protein C deficiency is inherited by an autosomal dominant transmission. Such patients are at increased risk not only of VTE but also of warfarin skin necrosis. This occurs because protein C (and its closely related co-factor, protein S) is a vitamin K-dependent antithrombotic factor that can be further suppressed by the administration of warfarin. Thrombosis in the small vessels of the skin may occur if large loading (induction) doses of warfarin are given to such patients when the suppression of the antithrombotic effects of these factors occurs before the antithrombotic effects of blockade of vitamin K-dependent clotting factor (II, VII, IX and X) production has occurred. Although the prevalence of protein C deficiency is 0.2%, only one subject in 70 (i.e. 0.0003%) will be symptomatic, and the condition accounts for around 4% of patients presenting with thromboembolic disease before the age of 45 years.

Protein S deficiency

Protein S deficiency is probably even rarer than protein C deficiency, but the familial form, inherited in an autosomal dominant fashion, is a high-risk state, accounting for possibly 5–8% of cases of thromboembolism in patients less than 45 years old.

Factor V Leiden

The presence of factor V Leiden, a point mutation in the factor V gene, causes the activated factor V molecule to be resistant to deactivation by activated protein C (APC). This defect may have a prevalence of 5% in Caucasian populations, and higher in patients with thromboembolic disease, and may in itself be of little consequence until there is another risk factor, such as immobility and use of the contraceptive pill. In these circumstances, the combination of risks may be responsible for the increased predisposition to thromboembolism in a high proportion of affected individuals.

Antithrombin III deficiency

Antithrombin III deficiency is a rare autosomal dominantly inherited abnormality associated with a reduced plasma concentration of this protein. The defect may not result in clinical problems until pregnancy or until patients enter their fourth decade, when venous and (to a lesser extent) arterial thrombosis becomes more common. Nevertheless, it has been estimated to be responsible for between 2% and 5% of thromboembolism occurring before age 45.

Lupus anticoagulant

Lupus anticoagulant, an antibody against phospholipid, is so named because it increases the clotting time in blood when measured by some standard coagulation tests. Patients affected are more prone to thromboembolism. This factor is found in 10% of patients with systemic lupus erythematosus (SLE) where it is associated with a threefold increase in thromboembolic risk; it is also found in the primary antiphospholipid syndrome (PAPS), where it may signify an increased risk of venous and arterial thrombosis and of recurrent miscarriage.

Prothrombin 20210 mutation

A mutation in part of the prothrombin gene (prothrombin 20210A) results in increased prothrombin concentrations and an increased risk of venous thrombosis. Carriers have a two- to threefold increased risk of venous thrombosis, and the variant is found with similar frequency as factor V Leiden in Caucasian populations.

Fibrinogen gamma 10034T

Approximately 6% of individuals carry this variant gene, which increases thrombotic risk approximately twofold.

Oestrogens

Oestrogens increase the circulating concentrations of clotting factors I, II, VII, VIII, IX and X and reduce fibrinolytic activity. They also depress the concentrations of antithrombin III, which is protective against thrombosis. This effect is dose-related, and venous thrombosis was more often seen with the high (50 μcg) oestrogen-containing contraceptive pill than with the present lower dose preparations. Hormonal replacement therapy, pregnancy and the puerperium (up to 6 weeks after delivery) are also recognised risk factors for VTE.

Malignancy

VTE is also commoner in malignancy (the risk may be up to fivefold greater). Although first described in association with carcinoma of the pancreas, all solid tumours seem to be associated with this problem. This may be related to the expression of tissue factor or factor X activators, but several other mechanisms may also be responsible. Cancer treatment also appears to be a risk factor.

Surgery

The increased risk of VTE in surgery is related in part to stagnation of venous blood in the calves during the operation and also to tissue trauma, since it appears to be more common in operations that involve marked tissue damage, such as orthopaedic surgery. This may in turn be related to release of tissue thromboplastin and to reduced fibrinolytic activity. The most important risk factors associated with clinical thromboembolism after surgery are age, varicose veins with associated phlebitis and obesity (body mass index > 30 kg/m²), prolonged immobility or continuous travel of greater than 3 h approximately 4 weeks before or after surgery.

Other risk factors

There are several other patient-related risk factors for VTE. Age over 60 years is an important factor. Critical care admission, dehydration, and one or more significant medical comorbidities such as heart disease, metabolic, endocrine or respiratory pathologies, acute infectious diseases and inflammatory conditions are all important risk factors for VTE. A full list can be found in the relevant National Institute for Health and Clinical Excellence (2010) guideline.

Clinical manifestations

In 90% of patients, deep vein thrombosis occurs in the veins of the lower limbs and pelvis. In up to half of cases, this may not result in local symptoms or signs, and the onset of PE may be the first evidence of the presence of VTE. In other cases, patients classically present with pain involving the calf or thigh associated with swelling, redness of the overlying skin and increased warmth. In a large deep venous thrombosis that prevents venous return, the leg may become discolored and oedematous. Massive venous thrombus can occasionally result in gangrene, although this occurs very rarely now that effective drug therapies are available.

PE may occur in the absence of clinical signs of venous thrombosis. It may be very difficult to diagnose because of the non-specificity of symptoms and signs. Clinical diagnosis is often made because of the presence of associated risk factors. Obstruction with a large embolus of a major pulmonary artery may result in acute massive PE, presenting with sudden shortness of breath and dull central chest pain, together with marked haemodynamic disturbance, for example severe hypotension and right ventricular failure, sometimes resulting in death due to acute circulatory failure unless rapidly treated.

Acute submassive pulmonary embolus occurs when less than 50% of the pulmonary circulation is occluded by embolus, and the embolus normally lodges in a more distal branch of the pulmonary artery. It may result in some shortness of breath but if the lung normally supplied by that branch of the pulmonary artery becomes necrotic, pulmonary infarction results with pleuritic pain and haemoptysis (coughing up blood), and there may be a pleural 'rub' (a sound like Velcro® being torn apart when the patient breathes in) as a result of inflammation of the lung. Patients may, rarely, develop recurrent thromboembolism. This may not result in immediate symptoms or signs but the patient may present with increasing breathlessness and signs of pulmonary hypertension (right ventricular hypertrophy) and, if untreated, progressive respiratory failure.

Investigations

Deep vein thrombosis

Although several conditions may mimic deep vein thrombus, such as a Baker's cyst, which involves rupture of the posterior aspect of the synovial capsule of the knee, deep vein thrombosis is the commonest cause of pain, swelling and tenderness of the leg. The clinical diagnosis of venous thrombosis is relatively unreliable, and venography is the most specific diagnostic test.

Venography. Venography involves injection of radio-opaque contrast medium, normally into a vein on the top of the foot, and subsequent radiography of the venous system.

Ultrasound. Ultrasound is a non-invasive alternative to venography that does not involve exposure to ionizing radiation or potentially allergenic contrast media. It is now the initial investigation of choice in clinically suspected deep vein thrombosis, although it is less sensitive for below-knee and isolated pelvic deep vein thrombosis.

Magnetic resonance imaging (MRI). MRI is also non-invasive and avoids radiation exposure. When used with direct thrombus imaging (DTI), which detects methaemoglobin in the clot, MRI DTI is sensitive and specific, even with below-knee and isolated pelvic deep vein thrombosis. However, it is not widely clinically available and ultrasound remains the primary initial investigation.

Pulmonary embolism

Pulmonary arteriography. The diagnosis of PE is most often made using one of two techniques: pulmonary arteriography or ventilation–perfusion scanning. Pulmonary arteriography is the most specific test. This requires catheterisation of the right side of the heart and an injection of contrast medium into the pulmonary artery. Adequate facilities and experienced personnel are, therefore, required and it is now generally reserved for those situations where massive or submassive PE is suspected but non-invasive tests have given indeterminate results.

Ventilation–perfusion scanning. Ventilation–perfusion scanning involves the injection of a radiolabelled substance into the vein and measurement of perfusion via the pulmonary circulation, using a scintillation counter. This is often combined with a ventilation scan in which radiolabelled gas, normally xenon, is inhaled by the patient. PE classically results in an area of under- or non-perfusion of a part of the lung that, nevertheless, because the airways are patent, ventilates normally. This pattern is called ventilation–perfusion mismatch and is a specific sign of PE.

Spiral computed tomography. Computed tomography angiography (CT angiography) using helical or spiral CT (sCT) is now being increasingly used in some centres and has a high accuracy rate. Although subsegmental emboli can be missed, visualisation of smaller arterial branches, and therefore detection of small emboli, may improve with the availability of multidetector scanners. Not only does sCT enable direct visualisation of emboli, but also visualisation of the lung parenchyma and mediastinum may help in the differential diagnosis in non-embolic cases. MRI is also being developed for the diagnosis of PE and early results are promising.

Other findings. Other findings occur in PE, such as changes in the chest radiograph, for example a raised right hemidiaphragm as a result of loss of lung volume (PE more commonly affects the right than the left lung). Hypoxia is also seen, and the larger the pulmonary embolus the worse this is. The electrocardiogram may show signs of right ventricular strain. The echocardiogram may show right ventricular overload and dysfunction in massive PE. However, all these changes are relatively non-specific and do not obviate the need for the specific tests mentioned above.

Treatment

The aim of treatment of venous thrombosis is to allow normal circulation in the limbs and, wherever possible, to prevent damage to the valves of the veins, thus reducing the risk of the swollen post-phlebitic limb. Second, it is important to try to prevent associated PE and also recurrence of either venous thrombosis or PE in the risk period after the initial episode.

In acute massive PE, the initial priority is to correct the circulatory defect that has caused the haemodynamic upset, and in these circumstances, rapid removal of the obstruction using thrombolytic drugs or surgical removal of the embolus may be necessary. In acute submassive PE, the goal of treatment is to prevent further episodes, particularly of the more serious acute massive PE. In both deep vein thrombosis and PE, a search must be made for underlying risk factors, such as carcinoma, which may occur in up to 10% of patients, and particularly in those with repeated episodes of VTE.

The treatment of VTE consists of the use of anticoagulants and, in severe cases, thrombolytic drugs. Anticoagulant therapy involves the use of immediate-acting agents (particularly heparin) and oral anticoagulants, the commonest of which is warfarin. Not only do these treat the acute event, but they also prevent recurrence and may be necessary for some time after the initial event, depending on the persistence of risk factors for recurrent thromboembolism.

Prophylaxis

Prevention of initial episodes of VTE in those at risk is clearly of great importance. It was estimated that around 25,000 people in the UK die from preventable hospital-acquired VTE annually, including patients admitted to hospital for medical care as well as surgery. There is also widespread evidence of inconsistent use of prophylactic measures for VTE in hospital patients, including mechanical as well as pharmacological means of VTE prophylaxis. Some of the medicines described below contribute to those pharmacological measures. Guidelines on this are available (National Institute for Health and Clinical Excellence, 2010).

Heparins

Conventional or unfractionated heparin (UFH) is a heterogeneous mixture of large mucopolysaccharide molecules ranging widely in molecular weight between 3000 and 30,000, with immediate anticoagulant properties. It acts by increasing the rate of the interaction of thrombin with antithrombin III by a factor of 1000. It, thus, prevents the production of fibrin (factor I) from fibrinogen. Heparin also has effects on the inhibition of production of activated clotting factors IX, X, XI and XII, and these effects occur at concentrations lower than its effects on thrombin.

Unlike UFH, low molecular weight heparins (LMWHs) contain polysaccharide chains ranging in molecular weight between 4000 and 6000. Whereas UFH produces its anticoagulant effect by inhibiting both thrombin and factor Xa, LMWHs predominantly inactivate only factor Xa. In addition, unlike UFH, they inactivate platelet-bound factor Xa and resist inhibition by platelet factor 4 (PF4), which is released during coagulation. Bemiparin, dalteparin, enoxaparin, reviparin and tinzaparin are LMWHs with similar efficacy and adverse effects.

Because UFH and LMWHs all consist of high molecular weight molecules that are highly ionised (heparin is the strongest organic acid found naturally in the body), they are not absorbed via the gastro-intestinal tract and must be given by intravenous infusion or deep subcutaneous (never intramuscular) injection. UFH is highly protein-bound and it appears to be restricted to the intravascular space, with a consequently low volume of distribution. It does not cross the placenta and does not appear in breast milk. Its pharmacokinetics are complex, but it appears to have a dose-dependent increase in

half-life. The half-life is normally about 60 min, but is shorter in patients with PE. It is removed from the body by metabolism, possibly in the reticuloendothelial cells of the liver, and by renal excretion. The latter seems to be more important after high doses of the compound.

LMWHs have a number of potentially desirable pharmacokinetic features compared with UFH. They are predominantly excreted renally and have longer and more predictable half-lives than UFH and so have a more predictable dose response than UFH. They can, therefore, be given once or, at the most, twice daily in a fixed dose, sometimes based on the patient's body weight, without the need for laboratory monitoring, except for patients given treatment doses and at high risk of bleeding.

The major adverse effect of all heparins is haemorrhage, which is commoner in patients with severe heart or liver disease, renal disease, general debility and in women aged over 60 years. The risk of haemorrhage is increased in those with prolonged clotting times and in those given heparin by intermittent intravenous bolus rather than by continuous intravenous administration. UFH is monitored by derivatives of the activated partial thromboplastin time (APTT), for example the kaolin–cephalin clotting time (KCCT); in those patients with a KCCT three times greater than control, there is an eightfold increase in the risk of haemorrhage. The therapeutic range for the KCCT during UFH therapy, therefore, appears to be between 1.5 and 2.5 times the control values. Rapid reversal of the effect of heparin can be achieved using protamine sulphate, but this is rarely necessary because of the short duration of action of heparin. LMWHs may produce fewer haemorrhagic complications, and monitoring of effect is not routinely required. At doses normally used for treatment, they do not significantly affect coagulation tests and routine monitoring is not necessary (British Committee for Standards in Haematology, 2006a).

Heparins, particularly UFH, may also cause thrombocytopenia (low platelet count). This may occur in two forms. The first occurs 3–5 days after treatment and does not normally result in complications. The second type of thrombocytopenia occurs after about 6 days of treatment and often results in much more profound decreases in platelet count and an increased risk of thromboembolism. LMWHs are thought to be less likely to cause thrombocytopenia but this complication has been reported, including in individuals who had previously developed thrombocytopenia after UFH. For these reasons, patients should have a platelet count on the day of starting UFH and the alternate-day platelet counts should be performed from days 4 to 14 thereafter. For patients on LMWH, the platelet counts should be performed at 2–4 day intervals from day 4 to 14 (British Committee for Standards in Haematology, 2006b). If the platelet count falls by 50% and/or the patient develops new thrombosis or skin allergy during this period, heparin-induced thrombocytopenia (HIT) should be considered, and if strongly suspected or confirmed, heparin should be stopped and an alternative agent such as a heparinoid or hirudin commenced.

Heparin-induced osteoporosis is rare but may occur when the drug is used during pregnancy, and may be dose-related.

The exact mechanism is unknown. Other adverse effects of heparin are alopecia, urticaria and anaphylaxis, but these are also rare.

It has been shown that there is a non-linear relationship between the dose of UFH infused and the KCCT. This means that disproportionate adjustments in dose are required depending on the KCCT if under- or over-dosing is to be avoided (Box 23.1). Since the half-life of UFH is 1 h, it would take 5 h (five half-lives of the drug) to reach a steady state. A loading dose is, therefore, administered to reduce the time to achieve adequate anticoagulation. UFH in full dose can also be given by repeated subcutaneous injection, and in these circumstances the calcium salt appears to be less painful than the sodium salt. Opinions differ as to whether the subcutaneous or intravenous route is preferable. The subcutaneous route may take longer to reach effective plasma heparin concentrations but avoids the need for infusion devices.

Heparin is normally used in the immediate stages of venous thrombosis and PE until the effects of warfarin become apparent. In the past, it has been continued for 7–10 days, but recent evidence indicates that around 5 days of therapy may be sufficient in many instances. This shorter treatment may also reduce the risk of the rare but potentially very serious complications of severe HIT, which normally occurs after the sixth day. LMWH should be administered for at least 5 days or until the INR has been in the therapeutic range for two successive days, whichever is the longer. They have largely replaced UFH, since they can be given subcutaneously (without a loading dose), and without routine monitoring. A full blood count should be ordered after 5 days on LMWH and throughout the duration of LMWH treatment to monitor for heparin-related thrombocytopenia. Patients with previous exposure to heparin within the past 100 days should also have a platelet count performed before the second dose of heparin is administered (Winter et al., 2005).

Heparinoids

Danaparoid is a heparinoid that is licensed for prophylaxis of deep vein thrombosis in patients undergoing general or orthopaedic surgery. It is a mixture of the low molecular weight sulphated glycosaminoglycuronans: heparin sulphate, dermatan sulphate and a small amount of chondroitin sulphate. It acts by inhibiting factor Xa and, like LMWHs, is given by subcutaneous injection. It normally has a low cross-reactivity rate with heparin-associated antiplatelet antibodies and if this is not present can be used in the treatment of individuals who develop HIT but still need ongoing anticoagulation. It is administered intravenously, with monitoring of anti-Xa activity only required in those at high risk of bleeding, for example renal insufficiency. It should be avoided in severe renal insufficiency and severe hepatic insufficiency.

Hirudins

Lepirudin, a recombinant hirudin, is licensed for anticoagulation in patients with type II (immune) HIT who require parenteral antithrombotic treatment. The dose of lepirudin is adjusted according to the APTT, and it is given intravenously by infusion. Haemorrhage is greater in those with poor renal function. Severe anaphylaxis occurs rarely in association with lepirudin treatment and is more common in previously exposed patients (British Committee for Standards in Haematology, 2006b). Bivaluridin is an analogue of hirudin, but acts as a direct thrombin inhibitor. It is licensed for anticoagulation in patients undergoing percutaneous coronary intervention (PCI). It has to be administered parenterally and the activated clotting time (ACT) is used to assess its activity. Haemorrhage is also an important adverse effect of this agent.

Fondaparinux

Fondiparinux sodium is a synthetic pentasaccharide that binds to antithrombin III, thus inhibiting factor Xa but without effect on factor IIa. Therefore, at doses normally used for treatment, it does not significantly affect coagulation tests and routine monitoring of these is not necessary. It has to be given parenterally. It is used for prophylaxis of VTE in high-risk situations and for treatment of acute deep vein thrombosis and treatment of acute PE, except in haemodynamically unstable patients or patients who require thrombolysis or pulmonary embolectomy. It also has an indication for the treatment of unstable angina or non-ST-segment elevation myocardial infarction (NSTEMI) and for treatment of ST-segment elevation myocardial infarction (STEMI). Haemorrhage is the most important adverse effect.

Box 23.1 Guidelines to control unfractionated heparin (UFH) treatment

Loading dose
5000 iu over 5 min

Infusion
Start at 1400 iu/h (e.g. 8400 iu in 100 mL of normal saline over 6 h). Check after 6 h. Adjust dose according to ratio of the KCCT to the control value using the values below

KCCT ratio	Infusion rate change
>7.0	Discontinue for 30 min to 1 h and reduce by >500 iu/h
>5.0	Reduce by 500 iu/h
4.1–5.0	Reduce by 300 iu/h
3.1–4.0	Reduce by 100 iu/h
2.6–3.0	Reduce by 50 iu/h
1.5–2.5	No change
1.2–1.4	Increase by 200 iu/h
<1.2	Increase by 400 iu/h

After each dose change, wait 10 h before next KCCT estimation unless KCCT >5, when more frequent (e.g. 4-hourly) estimation is advisable. Developed using Diogen (Bell and Alton); local validation may be necessary.

Source: Modified from Fennerty et al. (1986) and reproduced in British Committee for Standards in Haematology (1998).

KCCT, Kaolin–cephalin clotting time.

Oral anticoagulants

Warfarin. Although not the only coumarin anticoagulant available, warfarin is by far the most widely used drug in this group because of its potency, duration of action and more reliable bioavailability. Acenocoumarol (nicoumalone) has a much shorter duration of action and phenindione may be associated with a higher incidence of non-haemorrhagic adverse effects. When given by mouth, warfarin is completely and rapidly absorbed, although food decreases the rate (but not the extent) of absorption. It is extremely highly plasma protein-bound (99%) and, therefore, has a small volume of distribution (7–14 L). It consists of an equal mixture of two enantiomers, (*R*)- and (*S*)-warfarins. They have different anticoagulant potencies and routes of metabolism.

Both enantiomers of warfarin act by inducing a functional deficiency of vitamin K and thereby prevent the normal carboxylation of the glutamic acid residues of the amino-terminal ends of clotting factors II, VII, IX and X. This renders the clotting factors unable to cross-link with calcium and thereby bind to phospholipid-containing membranes. Warfarin prevents the reduction of vitamin K epoxide to vitamin K by epoxide reductase. (*S*)-warfarin appears to be at least five times more potent in this regard than (*R*)-warfarin. Since warfarin does not have any effect on already carboxylated clotting factors, the delay in onset of the anticoagulant effect of warfarin is dependent on the rate of clearance of the fully carboxylated factors already synthesised. In this regard, the half-life of removal of factor VII is approximately 6 h, that of factor IX 24 h, factor X 36 h and factor II 50 h. Some of the variability in response to warfarin may be related to genetic variations in the gene encoding the vitamin K epoxide reductase multiprotein complex (*VKORC1* gene).

The effect of warfarin is monitored using the one-stage prothrombin time, for example the international normalised ratio (INR). This test is sensitive chiefly to factors VII, II and X (and to a lesser extent factor V, which is not a vitamin K-dependent clotting factor). However, factor VII, to which the INR is sensitive, is the most important factor in the extrinsic pathway of clotting. The optimum therapeutic range for the INR differs for different clinical indications since the lowest INR consistent with therapeutic efficacy is the best in reducing the risk of haemorrhage. Examples of therapeutic ranges recommended for certain indications are given in Table 23.1 (British Committee for Standards in Haematology, 1998, 2006c).

Warfarin is metabolised by the liver via the cytochrome P450 system. Only very small amounts of the drug appear unchanged in the urine. The average clearance is 4.5 L/day and the half-life ranges from 20 to 60 h (mean 40 h). It, thus, takes approximately 1 week (around five half-lives) for the steady state to be reached after warfarin has been administered. The enantiomers of warfarin are metabolised stereo-specifically, (*R*)-warfarin being mainly reduced at the acetyl side chain into secondary warfarin alcohols while (*S*)-warfarin is predominantly metabolised at the coumarin ring to hydroxywarfarin. The clearance of warfarin may be reduced in liver disease as well as during the administration of a variety of drugs known to inhibit either the (*S*) or (*R*), or both, enantiomers. These are shown in Table 23.2 which is not exhaustive. The number of possible interactions and the potential severity of their outcome mean that it is essential not to prescribe any medicine concomitantly with warfarin until a thorough check on all possible interactions has been undertaken. The British National Formulary contains comprehensive tables listing possible interactions between warfarin and other medicines.

Renal function is thought to have little effect on the pharmacokinetics of, or anticoagulant response to, warfarin. Some of the variability in warfarin dose requirement is related to genetic polymorphisms of the cytochrome (CYP2C9) mediating the rate of hepatic metabolism of (*S*)-warfarin. Individuals with the variant isoform (either heterozygotes or in particular homozygotes) metabolise this more active enantiomer more slowly and so require lower doses.

The major adverse effect of warfarin is haemorrhage, which often occurs at a predisposing abnormality such as an ulcer and a tumour. The risk of bleeding is increased by excessive anticoagulation, although this may not need to be present for severe haemorrhage to occur. Close monitoring of the degree of anticoagulation of warfarin is, therefore, important, and guidelines for reversal of excessive anticoagulation are shown in Table 23.3.

It is also important to reduce the duration of therapy of the drug to the minimum effective period to reduce the period of risk.

Skin reactions to warfarin may also occur but are rare. The most serious skin reaction is warfarin-induced skin necrosis, which may occur over areas of adipose tissue such as the breasts, buttocks or thighs, especially in women, and which is related to relative deficiency of protein C or S. This is important because these deficiencies result in an increased risk of thrombosis, and therefore warfarin may more often be used in such subjects. Preventing excessive anticoagulation in the initial stages of induction of therapy may reduce the severity of the reaction. A dosing schedule which helps to achieve this is shown in Table 23.4.

Warfarin may also be teratogenic, producing in some instances a condition called chondrodysplasia punctata. This is associated with 'punched-out' lesions at sites of ossification, particularly of the long bones but also of the facial bones, and may be associated with absence of the spleen. Although it has been associated predominantly with warfarin anticoagulation during the first trimester of pregnancy, other abnormalities, including cranial nerve palsies, hydrocephalus and microcephaly, have been reported at later stages of pregnancy if the child is exposed.

Although other coumarin anticoagulants are available, in the vast majority of cases these have not been shown to have any clear benefits over warfarin. They may be used occasionally where a patient does not tolerate warfarin. The necessary duration of anticoagulation in venous thrombosis and pulmonary embolus is still uncertain. On the basis of the available evidence, therapy may be required for approximately 6 months after the first deep vein thrombosis or pulmonary embolus. It may be possible to reduce the duration of therapy in patients who have

Table 23.1 Recommended target INRs for different conditions and grade of recommendation

Indication	Target INR	Grade of recommendation
Pulmonary embolus	2.5	A
Proximal deep vein thrombosis	2.5	A
Calf vein thrombus	2.5	A
Recurrence of venous thromboembolism when no longer on warfarin therapy	2.5	A
Recurrence of venous thromboembolism while on warfarin therapy	3.5	C
Symptomatic inherited thrombophilia	2.5	A
Antiphospholipid syndrome	3.5	A
Non-rheumatic atrial fibrillation	2.5	A
Atrial fibrillation due to rheumatic heart disease, congenital heart disease, thyrotoxicosis	2.5	C
Cardioversion	2.5	B
Mural thrombus	2.5	B
Cardiomyopathy	2.5	C
Mechanical prosthetic heart valve (caged ball or caged disk), aortic or mitral[a]	3.5	B
Mechanical prosthetic heart valve (tilting disc or bileaflet), mitral[a]	3.0	B
Mechanical prosthetic heart valve (tilting disc), aortic[a]	3.0	B
Mechanical prosthetic heart valve (bileaflet), aortic[a]	2.0	B
Bioprosthetic valve	2.0 (if anticoagulated)	A
Ischaemic stroke without atrial fibrillation	Not indicated	C
Retinal vessel occlusion	Not indicated	C
Peripheral arterial thrombosis and grafts	Not indicated	A
Arterial grafts	2.5 (if anticoagulated)	
Coronary artery thrombosis	2.5 (if anticoagulated)	
Coronary artery graft	Not indicated	A
Coronary angioplasty and stents	Not indicated	A

Source: British Committee for Standards in Haematology (1998, 2006c).
INR, international normalised ratio; A, at least one randomised controlled trial (RCT); B, well-conducted clinical trials but no RCT; C, expert opinion but no studies.
[a]If the valve type is not known, a target INR of 3.0 is recommended for valves in the aortic position and 3.5 in the mitral position.

had a postoperative episode since it is likely that the risk factor has been reversed (unless immobility continues). In patients with a second episode, therapy may be required for even longer and in patients with more than two episodes, life-long treatment may be necessary to reduce the risk of recurrence (British Committee for Standards in Haematology, 1998).

Dabigatran. Dabigatran is an orally active inhibitor of both free and clot-bound thrombin (Wittkowsky, 2010). It has a rapid onset of action and does not require laboratory monitoring. Dabigatran etexilate is a pro-drug which is hydrolysed to active dabigatran in the liver. Since 80% of activated dabigatran is excreted unchanged through the kidneys, it

Table 23.2 Some clinically important drug interactions with warfarin

Interacting drug	Effect of interaction on anticoagulant effect	Probable mechanism(s)
Colestyramine Colestipol	Reduced anticoagulant effect	Impaired absorption and increased elimination of warfarin. N.B. Long-term treatment may cause impaired vitamin K absorption and enhance anticoagulant effect
Barbiturates Carbamazepine Griseofulvin Phenytoin (see also below) Primidone Rifampicin Rifabutin St John's wort	Reduced anticoagulant effect	Induction of warfarin metabolism
Amiodarone Azapropazone Chloramphenicol Cimetidine Ciprofloxacin Clarithromycin Dextropopoxyphene Erythromycin Fluconazole Fluvastatin Itraconazole Ketoconazole Mefenamic acid Metronidazole Miconazole Nalidixic acid Norfloxacin Ofloxacin Phenylbutazone Sulfinpyrazone Sulphonamides (e.g. in co-trimoxazole) Voriconazole Zafirlukast	Increased anticoagulant effect	Inhibition of warfarin metabolism
Anabolic steroids Bezafibrate Danazol Gemfibrozil Levothyroxine Phenytoin (see also above) Salicylates/aspirin (high dose) Stanozolol Tamoxifen Testosterone	Increased anticoagulant effect	Pharmacodynamic potentiation of anticoagulant effect
Cranberry juice	Increased anticoagulant effect	Mechanism unknown
NSAIDs (including aspirin at all doses) Clopidogrel	Increased risk of bleeding	Additive effects on coagulation and haemostasis
Oral contraceptives, oestrogens and progestogens	Reduced anticoagulant effect	Pharmacodynamic antagonism of anticoagulant effect
Vitamin K (e.g. in some enteral feeds)		

Table 23.3 Recommendations for management of bleeding and excessive anticoagulation in patients receiving warfarin

Cause	Recommendation
3.0<INR<6.0 (target INR 2.5) 4.0<INR<6.0 (target INR 3.5)	1. Reduce warfarin dose or stop 2. Restart warfarin when INR <5.0
6.0<INR<8.0, no bleeding or minor bleeding	1. Stop warfarin 2. Restart when INR <5.0
INR>8.0, no bleeding or minor bleeding	1. Stop warfarin 2. Restart warfarin when INR <5.0 3. If other risk factors for bleeding give 0.5–2.5 mg of vitamin K (oral)
Major bleeding	1. Stop warfarin 2. Give prothrombin complex concentrate 50 units/kg or FFP 15 mL/kg 3. Give 5 mg of vitamin (oral or i.v.)

Source: British Committee for Standards in Haematology (1998).
INR, international normalised ratio; FFP, fresh frozen plasma.

Table 23.4 Suggested warfarin induction schedule

Day	INR	Warfarin dose (mg)
First	<1.4	10
Second	<1.8	10
	1.8	1
	>1.8	0.5
Third	<2.0	10
	2.0–2.1	5
	2.2–2.3	4.5
	2.4–2.5	4
	2.6–2.7	3.5
	2.8–2.9	3
	3.0–3.1	2.5
	3.2–3.3	2
	3.4	1.5
	3.5	1
	3.6–4.0	0.5
	>4.0	0 (predicted maintenance dose)
Fourth	<1.4	>8
	1.4	8
	1.5	7.5
	1.6–1.7	7
	1.8	6.5
	1.9	6
	2.0–2.1	5.5
	2.2–2.3	5
	2.4–2.6	4.5
	2.7–3.0	4
	3.1–3.5	3.5
	3.6–4.0	3
	4.1–4.5	Miss out next day's dose then give 2 mg
	>4.5	Miss out 2 days' doses then give 1 mg

Source: Modified from Fennerty et al. (1984).
INR, international normalised ratio.

should be avoided in patients with severe renal impairment (creatinine clearance < 30 mL/min) and the dose should be reduced in moderate renal impairment (creatinine clearance 30–50 mL/min). Dabigatran is a substrate for the transport protein p-glycoprotein (p-GP), which facilitates renal elimination of certain drugs. Amiodarone, an inhibitor of p-GP, reduces the clearance of dabigatran and so doses should be reduced in patients who are on concurrent treatment with amiodarone. In patients who are on strong p-GP inhibitors such as verapamil and clarithomycin, dabigatran should be used with caution and it should not be used together with quinidine. Drugs such as rifampicin and St John's Wort, which are potent p-GP inducers, may potentially reduce its efficacy. Dabigatran can be used for prophylaxis of VTE in adults after total hip replacement or total knee replacement surgery (National Institute for Health and Clinical Excellence, 2008). Haemorrhage is the major adverse effect.

Rivaroxaban. Rivaroxaban is an orally active inhibitor of both the 'free' and prothombinase complex-bound forms of activated factor X (Xa) (Wittkowsky, 2010). Two thirds of the dose is metabolised, principally by CYP450 enzymes and the remaining third is excreted unchanged in the urine. Like dabigatran, rivaroxaban also appears to be a p-GP substrate and it should be used with caution when prescribed concomitantly with p-GP inhibitors and potent p-GP inducers. It should also be used with caution in patients with creatinine clearance less than 30 mL/min (severe renal impairment) and is contraindicated in those with creatinine clearance less than 15 mL/min. Several CYP3A4 inhibitors and inducers have been shown to affect its metabolism. Some CYP3A4 inhibitors significantly increase the AUC of rivaroxaban, particularly ketoconazole and other azole-antimycotics such as itraconazole, voriconazole and posaconazole and also HIV protease inhibitors such as ritonavir. Therefore, the use of rivaroxaban is not recommended in patients receiving concomitant systemic treatment with these agents. The CYP3A4 inducer rifampicin (and possibly other inducers of this cytochrome) reduces the AUC for rivaroxaban. It is recommended as an option for prophylaxis of VTE in adults after hip or knee replacement surgery (National Institute for Health and Clinical Excellence, 2009). It also does not require laboratory monitoring. Haemorrhage is the major adverse effect.

Fibrinolytic drugs

Thrombolytic therapy is used in life-threatening acute massive pulmonary embolus. It has been used in deep vein thrombosis, particularly in those patients where a large amount of clot exists and venous valvular damage is likely. However, fibrinolytic drugs are potentially more dangerous than anticoagulant drugs, and evidence is not available in situations other than acute massive embolism to show a sustained benefit from their use.

Streptokinase. Streptokinase was the first agent available in this class. It was produced from streptococci and is a large protein that binds to and activates plasminogen, thus encouraging the breakdown of formed fibrin to fibrinogen degradation products. It also acts on the circulating fibrinogen to produce a degree of systemic anticoagulation. Since it is a large protein molecule, it cannot be administered orally and has to be given by intravenous infusion. The half-life of removal from the body is 30 min. It is cleared chiefly by the reticuloendothelial system in the liver.

Its major adverse effect is to increase the risk of haemorrhage but it may also be antigenic and produce an anaphylactic reaction. It may also cause hypotension during infusion and in some patients, particularly those who have been administered the drug within the previous 12 months, a relative resistance to the drug may occur. Thrombolytic therapy is contraindicated in patients who have had major surgery or with active bleeding sites in the gastro-intestinal or genitourinary tract, those who have a history of stroke, renal or liver disease, and those with hypertension. It should also be avoided during pregnancy and the postpartum period.

Alteplase. Tissue plasminogen activator (rt-PA) or alteplase was developed using recombinant DNA technology. Although this agent is much more expensive than streptokinase, it can be used in those situations where streptokinase may be less effective because of development of antibodies, for example within 1 year of previous streptokinase use or where allergy to streptokinase has previously occurred. Because it produces a lesser degree of systemic anticoagulation (it is more active against plasminogen associated with the clot), immediate use of heparin subsequently is necessary to prevent recurrence of thrombosis. Alteplase is also used for acute ischaemic stroke, where its prompt use may improve outcome in carefully selected individuals (National Institute for Health and Clinical Excellence, 2007). At the time of writing, it is the only thrombolytic licensed for this indication (see arterial thromboembolism).

Reteplase and tenecteplase. Reteplase, and more recently tenecteplase, are also fibrin-specific agents and so heparin is required to prevent rebound thrombosis. They are indicated for the treatment of acute myocardial infarction. In this clinical situation, reteplase is administered as an intravenous bolus, followed by a second bolus 30 min later (double bolus), and tenecteplase is given as a single intravenous bolus. They, therefore, have the advantage of convenience of administration compared with alteplase, and are the preferred option in pre-hospital settings, particularly when administered by paramedics (National Institute for Health and Clinical Excellence, 2002a).

Urokinase. Urokinase, like alteplase and streptokinase, can be used for the treatment of deep vein thrombosis and PE. It is also licensed to restore patency in intravenous catheters and cannulas blocked by fibrin thrombi.

Patient care

The patient on oral anticoagulants should be given full information on what to do in case of problems and what circumstances and drugs to avoid. An anticoagulant card with previous INR values and doses should also be provided. The patient should be told of the colour code for the different strengths of warfarin tablet and advised to carry their treatment card at all times. The likely duration of anticoagulant therapy should be made clear to the patient to avoid unnecessary and potentially dangerous prolongations of treatment. Patients who have received a fibrinolytic agent should also carry a card identifying the drug given and the date of administration.

Arterial thromboembolism

Acute myocardial infarction is the commonest clinical presentation of acute arterial thrombosis. Stroke is commonly caused by atherothromboembolism from the great vessels or embolism arising from the heart (approximately 80% of strokes). These two conditions are discussed elsewhere. Peripheral arterial thrombosis or thromboembolism may also occur, most often in the lower limb. Antiplatelet drugs are often used for prophylaxis, but surgical embolectomy and/or fibrinolytic therapy may be needed for treatment of acute thrombotic or thromboembolic events to avoid consequent ischaemic damage.

Aetiology

Arterial thromboembolism is normally associated with vascular injury and hypercoagulability. Vascular injury is most often due to atheroma, itself aggravated by smoking, hypertension, hyperlipidaemia or diabetes mellitus. Although the exact mechanism is not clear, it is thought that platelet aggregation may be induced by the sheer stresses caused by stenosis of an atherosclerotic vessel. This thrombotic material may embolise to cause occlusion further downstream. Hypercoagulability is also a risk factor. It may be associated with increased plasma fibrinogen levels and an increase in circulating cellular components, for example polycythaemia or thrombocythaemia. As mentioned earlier, the thrombus formed in the artery contains a much larger proportion of platelets, possibly reflecting the fact that other blood components that are not as readily adherent may be dissipated by the higher flow rates in the arterial circulation. Oestrogens, by the mechanisms described earlier, are likely to increase the risk of arterial as well as venous thrombosis. Hyperlipidaemia may also increase the risk of hypercoagulability as well as enhancing thrombotic risk through its role in the progression of atheroma and vascular injury.

Treatment and prevention

Aspirin

Aspirin (acetylsalicylic acid) is a potent inhibitor of the enzyme cyclo-oxygenase, which catalyses the production of prostaglandins. It reduces the production of pro-aggregatory prostaglandin, thromboxane A_2 in the platelet, an effect that lasts for the life of the platelet.

Aspirin is well absorbed after oral administration. It is rapidly metabolised by esterases in the blood and liver (so that its half-life is only 15–20 min) to salicylic acid and other metabolites that are excreted in the urine. In the doses used in prophylaxis against thromboembolism, aspirin is largely metabolised by the liver but in overdose, urinary excretion of salicylate becomes a limiting factor in drug elimination.

The major adverse effect of aspirin is gastro-intestinal irritation and bleeding. This problem is much more common with higher doses of aspirin (300 mg or more) that were once used in the prevention of arterial thromboembolism but are less common with the doses (e.g. 75 mg) now recommended. There is evidence that concomitant use of ulcer-healing drugs, particularly proton pump inhibitors, can reduce the risk of non-steroidal anti-inflammatory drug (NSAID)-induced peptic ulceration in patients susceptible to the problem, but haemorrhagic risk may not be significantly reduced. There is also little evidence that buffered or enteric-coated preparations of aspirin are safer in this respect. However, the vast majority of patients tolerate low-dose aspirin well, and it is normally given as a single oral dose of soluble aspirin. Aspirin may also, rarely, induce asthma, particularly in patients with co-existing reversible airway obstruction. Other patients have a form of aspirin hypersensitivity that may result in urticaria and/or angioedema. In this situation, there may be cross-reactivity with other NSAIDs.

Haemorrhagic stroke is a rare but a very serious complication of therapy with aspirin (and with other antiplatelet agents). Recent evidence examining risks and benefits of aspirin has resulted in the recommendation that while long-term use of aspirin, in a dose of 75 mg daily, is of benefit for all patients with established cardiovascular disease, use of aspirin in primary prevention, in those with or without diabetes, is of unproven overall benefit. It must not be given to children or young people under 16 years of age because of the risk of the rare but life-threatening possibility of Reye's Syndrome (which may cause liver and renal failure).

Clopidogrel

Clopidogrel is a pro-drug that is metabolised in part to an active thiol derivative. The latter inhibits platelet aggregation by rapidly and irreversibly inhibiting the binding of adenosine diphosphate (ADP) to its platelet receptor, thus preventing the ADP-mediated activation of the glycoprotein IIb/IIIa receptor for the life of the platelet. It is an orally active pro-drug and is given once daily for the reduction of atherosclerotic events in those with pre-existing atherosclerotic disease. In this respect, it may be a useful alternative to aspirin in aspirin-allergic subjects but haemorrhage occurs with the same frequency as aspirin, and thrombocytopenia (sometimes severe) may be commoner than with aspirin therapy. Activation to its active metabolite may be subject to a genetic polymorphism of CYP450 2C19 and may also be reduced by the proton pump inhibitor, omeprazole or esomeprazole; so use of alternative gastroprotective agents may need to be considered if required.

Clopidogrel is also licensed for combination use with low-dose aspirin in the management of acute coronary syndrome without ST-segment elevation, when it is given for up to 12 months after the initial event (National Institute for Health and Clinical Excellence, 2004, 2005). Most benefit is obtained in the first 3 months and there is no evidence of benefit of clopidogrel after 12 months in this indication. In combination with low-dose aspirin, clopidogrel is also licensed for acute myocardial infarction with ST-segment elevation. It is recommended for at least 4 weeks in this indication, but the optimum treatment duration has not been established. Finally clopdogrel is sometimes used (with aspirin) in stenting procedures and this sometimes results in long-term use.

Prasugrel

Prasugrel inhibits platelet activation and aggregation. Its active metabolite binds to the $P2Y_{12}$ class of ADP receptors on platelets. It is recommended for use in combination with aspirin as an option for the prevention of atherothrombotic events in patients with acute coronary syndromes undergoing PCI, only when immediate primary PCI is necessary for STEMI, *or* stent thrombosis occurred during treatment with clopidogrel, or the patient has diabetes mellitus (National Institute for Health and Clinical Excellence, 2009).

Dipyridamole

Dipyridamole is used by mouth as an adjunct to oral anticoagulation for prophylaxis of thromboembolism associated with prosthetic heart valves. Modified-release preparations are licensed (alone or preferably in combination with low-dose aspirin) for secondary prevention of ischaemic stroke and TIAs (see treatment of stroke). There is evidence that the combination of modified-release dipyridamole and low-dose aspirin may reduce the risk of recurrent stroke and other cardiovascular events compared to aspirin alone. It is a phosphodiesterase inhibitor and, thus, elevates concentrations of cyclic AMP. It may also block the uptake of adenosine by erythrocytes and other cells. Adverse effects include headache (to which tolerance may gradually develop) gastro-intestinal problems, flushing and hypotension.

Glycoprotein IIb/IIIa inhibitors

Glycoprotein IIb/IIIa inhibitors prevent platelet aggregation by blocking the binding of fibrinogen to receptors on platelets.

Abciximab. Abciximab is a monoclonal antibody which binds to coronary glycoprotein IIb/IIIa receptors and to other related sites. It is licensed as an adjunct to heparin and aspirin for the prevention of ischaemic complications in high-risk patients undergoing percutaneous transluminal coronary intervention. Abciximab should be used once only to avoid further risk of thrombocytopenia.

Eptifibatide and tirofiban. Eptifibatide and tirofiban also inhibit glycoprotein IIb/IIIa receptors; they are licensed for use with heparin and aspirin to prevent early myocardial infarction in patients with unstable angina or non-ST-segment elevation myocardial infarction (NSTEMI).

Abciximab, eptifibatide and tirofiban all have to be administered parenterally and should be used by specialist clinicians only (National Institute for Health and Clinical Excellence, 2002b).

Patient care

Aspirin is normally well tolerated at the doses used for stroke prevention. However, it should not be given to patients with a history of gastro-intestinal ulceration. Since it may induce bronchospasm in susceptible individuals, it should be used cautiously in such circumstances. It is best tolerated if taken once daily as soluble aspirin after food.

Case studies

Case 23.1

A 75-year-old patient receiving warfarin to prevent deep vein thrombosis and previously well controlled comes to the clinic with an INR of 12, despite taking the same dose of drug. There is no evidence of bleeding.

Question

What should be done?

Answer

Since the patient's INR is >8 (even if there is no bleeding), the national guidelines recommend that warfarin be stopped. The patient should then be given phytomenadione (vitamin K₁) 2.5–5 mg by mouth using the intravenous preparation orally [unlicensed use], or 0.5–1 mg by slow intravenous injection (if complete reversal required 5–10 mg by slow intravenous injection). The dose of phytomenadione should be repeated if the INR is still too high after 24 h. The warfarin can be restarted when the INR is <5.0. However, a single dose often helps the INR to return to close to the target level at 24 h without causing warfarin resistance subsequently. A search for clinical conditions or drugs which might cause warfarin sensitivity should also be made. Measurement of plasma warfarin concentration may help in difficult cases.

Case 23.2

A patient receiving heparin for 7 days for extensive VTE develops arterial thrombosis.

Question

What would you suspect in this situation and what should be done?

Answer

The rare but serious HIT may be responsible. The platelet count should be measured immediately and if HIT is strongly suspected or confirmed, the heparin should be discontinued immediately. An alternative anticoagulant should be started in full dosage whilst specific confirmatory tests are being performed unless there are significant contraindications. Danaparoid and lepirudin may be considered as alternative anticoagulants in these circumstances.

Case 23.3

A patient admitted to an acute hospital with suspected myocardial infarction says that he had a myocardial infarction 4 years ago and was treated with a drug to 'dissolve the clot in the coronary artery'. The chest pain started 4 h earlier and his electrocardiogram shows ST-segment elevation in the anterior leads.

Question

What relevance may his previous treatment and present history and findings have to his management on this occasion?

Answer

Thrombolytic drugs are indicated for any patient with acute myocardial infarction, provided the likely benefits outweigh the possible risks. Trials have shown that the benefit is greatest in those with ECG changes that include ST-segment elevation, especially in those with anterior infarction, and in patients with bundle branch block. The patient has received a thrombolytic, possibly streptokinase, in the past. He should be asked if he was given a card with the identity of the therapy to carry with him. If the prior treatment was with streptokinase or anistreplase (no longer available), prolonged persistence of antibodies to streptokinase may reduce the effectiveness of subsequent treatment. Therefore, streptokinase should not be used again beyond 4 days of first administration of streptokinase (or anistreplase) and urgent consideration should be given to the use of an alternative thrombolytic agent such as alteplase, reteplase and tenecteplase.

Case 23.4

A 64-year-old male patient is to be prescribed aspirin therapy following an acute myocardial infarction.

Question

What questions should you ask the patient before starting treatment with aspirin?

Answer

The patient should be asked if he has had aspirin before and, if so, whether he tolerated it. Caution is necessary in patients with a previous history of gastro-intestinal ulceration, with uncontrolled hypertension; active peptic ulceration is also a contraindication. Other contraindications include severe hepatic impairment and severe renal failure. It may induce bronchospasm or angioedema in susceptible individuals, for example in asthmatics, and caution should be exercised in these circumstances.

Case 23.5

A 56-year-old woman on warfarin therapy for atrial fibrillation with mitral stenosis appears to become resistant to warfarin after previously good control on 5 mg daily. Her INR does not rise above 1.4 even when her warfarin dose is increased to 20 mg daily.

Question

What can be done to find the cause of the resistance?

Answer

The patient should be asked about any new medications which might have been introduced recently, including over-the-counter and herbal preparations. Some proprietary medicines may contain vitamin K which could cause resistance by pharmacodynamic mechanisms. Other medicines, including the herbal medicine St John's wort, might induce warfarin metabolism and result in resistance as a result of a pharmacokinetic interaction (see Table 23.2). One other cause of apparent resistance to warfarin is poor adherence and this should, therefore, be considered. Supervised administration of the dose and/or measurement of plasma warfarin concentrations may be of value if the latter is suspected.

References

British Committee for Standards in Haematology, 1998. Guidelines on oral anticoagulation (warfarin): third edition. Br. J. Haematol. 132, 277–285.

British Committee for Standards in Haematology, 2006a. Guidelines on the use and monitoring of heparin. Br. J. Haematol. 133, 19–34.

British Committee for Standards in Haematology, 2006b. The management of heparin induced thrombocytopenia. Br. J. Haematol. 133, 259–269.

British Committee for Standards in Haematology, 2006c. Guidelines on oral anticoagulation (warfarin): third edition, 2005 update. Br. J. Haematol. 132, 277–285.

Fennerty, A., Dolben, J., Thomas, P., et al., 1984. Flexible induction dose regimen for warfarin and prediction of maintenance dose. Br. Med. J. 288, 1268–1270. Available at: http://www.ncbi.nlm.nih.gov/pmc/articles/PMC1441080/?tool=pubmed.

Fennerty, A.G., Renowden, S., Scolding, N., et al., 1986. Guidelines for the control of heparin treatment. Br. Med. J. 292, 579–580. Available at: http://www.ncbi.nlm.nih.gov/pmc/articles/PMC1339561/?tool=pubmed.

National Institute for Health and Clinical Excellence, 2002a. The Clinical Effectiveness and Cost Effectiveness of Early Thrombolysis for Treatment of Myocardial Infarction. Technology appraisal 52. NICE, London. Available at: http://www.nice.org.uk/guidance/index.jsp?action=byID&r=true&o=11480.

National Institute for Health and Clinical Excellence, 2002b. Acute Coronary Syndromes – Glycoprotein IIb/IIIa Inhibitors (Review). Technology appraisal 47. NICE, London. Available at: http://www.nice.org.uk/guidance/index.jsp?action=byID&r=true&o=11470.

National Institute for Health and Clinical Excellence, 2004. Clopidogrel in the Treatment of Non-ST-Segment-Elevation Acute Coronary Syndrome. Technology appraisal 80. NICE, London. Available at: http://www.nice.org.uk/guidance/index.jsp?action=byID&r=true&o=11536.

National Institute for Health and Clinical Excellence, 2005. Clopidogrel and Dipyridamole for the Prevention of Atherosclerotic Events. Technology appraisal 90. NICE, London. Available at: http://www.nice.org.uk/guidance/index.jsp?action=byID&r=true&o=11558.

National Institute for Health and Clinical Excellence, 2007. Alteplase for the Treatment of Acute Ischaemic Stroke. Technology Appraisal TA122. NICE, London. Available at: http://guidance.nice.org.uk/TA122.

National Institute for Health and Clinical Excellence, 2008. Dabigatran Etexilate for the Prevention of Venous Thromboembolism After Hip or Knee Replacement Surgery in Adults. Technology Appraisal TA157. NICE, London. Available at: http://guidance.nice.org.uk/TA157.

National Institute for Health and Clinical Excellence, 2009. Prasugrel for the Treatment of Acute Coronary Syndromes with Percutaneous Coronary Intervention. Technology Appraisal TA182. NICE, London. Available at: http://guidance.nice.org.uk/TA182.

National Institute for Health and Clinical Excellence, 2010. Reducing the Risk of Venous Thromboembolism (Deep Vein Thrombosis and Pulmonary Embolism) in Patients Admitted to Hospital. Clinical guideline 92. NICE, London. Available at: http://guidance.nice.org.uk/CG92.

Rosendaal, F.R., Reitsma, P.H., 2009. Genetics of venous thrombosis. J. Thromb. Haemostasis 7 (Suppl. 1), 301–304.

Winter, M., Keeling, D., Sharpen, F., et al., 2005. Procedures for the outpatient management of patients with deep vein thrombosis. Clin. Lab. Haematol. 27, 61–66.

Wittkowsky, A.K., 2010. New oral anticoagulants: a practical guide for clinicians. J. Thromb. Thrombolysis 29, 182–191.

Dyslipidaemia 24

R. Walker and H. Williams

Key points

- Elevated concentrations of total cholesterol (TC) and low-density lipoprotein cholesterol (LDL-C) increase the risk of cardiovascular disease (CVD), while high-density lipoprotein cholesterol (HDL-C) confers protection.
- Two-thirds of the UK adult population have a serum TC above 5 mmol/L. The average TC concentration is 5.6 mmol/L.
- Dyslipidaemia may develop secondary to disorders such as diabetes mellitus, hypothyroidism, chronic renal failure, nephrotic syndrome, obesity, high alcohol intake and some drugs.
- Androgens, β-blockers, ciclosporin, oral contraceptives, diuretics, glucocorticoids and vitamin A derivatives are examples of drugs that can have an adverse effect on the lipid profile.
- There are five main classes of lipid-lowering agents: statins, fibrates, resins, nicotinic acid derivatives and absorption blockers.
- Statins are generally the drugs of choice in the treatment of primary prevention and secondary prevention of CVD.
- The aim of treatment in primary prevention (>20% risk of cardiovascular disease over 10 years) is to reduce overall cardiovascular risk by treatment with simvastatin 40 mg/day or a suitable alternate generic agent. No target treatment levels for TC or LDL cholesterol are recommended in primary prevention.
- In secondary prevention, treatment should be started with simvastatin 40 mg/day or a suitable alternate generic agent. If serum TC remains above 4 mmol/L or LDL-C remains above 2 mmol/L, the dose of statin can be increased, but this may increase the likelihood of side effects.

Disorders of lipoprotein metabolism together with high fat diets, obesity and physical inactivity have all contributed to the current epidemic of atherosclerotic disease seen in developed countries. Disorders of lipoprotein metabolism that result in elevated serum concentrations of total cholesterol (TC) and low-density lipoprotein cholesterol (LDL-C) increase the risk of an individual developing cardiovascular disease (CVD). In contrast, high-density lipoprotein cholesterol (HDL-C) confers protection against CVD, with the risk reducing as HDL-C increases. It is, therefore, clear that the term hyperlipidaemia, which was formerly used to describe disorders of lipoprotein metabolism, is inappropriate. It is more appropriate to use the term dyslipidaemia, which encompasses both abnormally high levels of specific lipoproteins, for example,

LDL-C, and abnormally low levels of other lipoproteins, for example, HDL-C, as well as disorders in the composition of the various lipoprotein particles. It is particularly appropriate when considering the individual at risk of CVD with a normal or high TC and low HDL-C (total cholesterol:HDL-C ratio).

Epidemiology

Lipid and lipoprotein concentrations vary among different populations, with countries consuming a Western type of diet generally having higher TC and LDL-C levels than those where regular consumption of saturated fat is low.

The ideal serum lipid profile is unknown and varies between different populations, even across Europe, and also within a given population. For practical purposes the values presented in Table 24.1 represent the target levels for TC and LDL-C in the UK for adults receiving treatment for secondary prevention of CVD. For completeness, the values for triglycerides and HDL-C are also presented, although the benefit of achieving the stated targets is less clear.

Despite a 50% reduction in the death rate from CVD over the past 25 years, it remains the leading cause of premature

Table 24.1 Optimal serum lipid profile

Total cholesterol (TC)[a]	<4.0 mmol/L
LDL cholesterol (LDL-C)[a]	<2.0 mmol/L
Triglycerides[b]	<1.7 mmol/L
HDL cholesterol (HDL-C)	>1.0 mmol/L in men
	>1.2 mmol/L in women

[a]Target levels in individuals with established atherosclerotic disease, coronary heart disease, stroke, peripheral arterial disease, diabetes mellitus or where there is a cardiovascular disease risk >20% over 10 years. In these identified individuals, the aim is to achieve the value stated in the table or a 25% reduction in total cholesterol and a 30% reduction in LDL-C from their baseline levels should these set target levels lower than those stated in the table.
[b]Fasting levels.

389

death and morbidity in the UK (British Heart Foundation, 2008), and the higher the levels of TC in an individual the greater the chance of developing CVD. At the individual level there appears no level below which a further reduction of TC or LDL-C is not associated with a lower risk of CVD. The death rate from CVD is threefold higher in males than females, but because women live longer and are at increased risk of stroke after the age of 75 years their lifetime risk of disease is greater (National Institute of Health and Clinical Excellence, 2008a).

TC levels tend to increase with age such that 80% of British men aged 45–64 years have a level that exceeds 5 mmol/L and the population average is 5.6 mmol/L. In contrast, in rural China and Japan, the average is 4 mmol/L.

Population-based approaches to vascular screening have the potential to provide significant health gain for society as most deaths from CVD occur in individuals who are not yet identified as at increased risk. Moreover, a small reduction in average population levels of TC and LDL-C can potentially prevent many deaths. In England, a scheme was introduced in 2009 for everyone between 40 and 74 years of age to receive a free health check to include measurement of TC and the TC:HDL-C ratio. The intention was that individuals would be given the necessary information about their health to make changes to lifestyle and avoid preventable disease.

Lipid transport and lipoprotein metabolism

The clinically important lipids in the blood (unesterified and esterified cholesterol and triglycerides) are not readily soluble in serum and are rendered miscible by incorporation into lipoproteins. There are six main classes of lipoproteins: chylomicrons, chylomicron remnants, very low-density lipoproteins (VLDL-C), intermediate-density lipoproteins (IDL-C), low-density lipoproteins (LDL-C) and high-density lipoproteins (HDL-C).

The protein components of lipoproteins are known as apoproteins (apo), of which apoproteins A-I, E, C and B are perhaps the most important. Apoprotein B exists in two forms: B-48, which is present in chylomicrons and associated with the transport of ingested lipids, and B-100, which is found in endogenously secreted VLDL-C and associated with the transport of lipids from the liver (Fig. 24.1).

When dietary cholesterol and triglycerides are absorbed from the intestine they are transported in the intestinal lymphatics as chylomicrons. These are the largest of the lipoprotein particles of which triglycerides normally constitute approximately 80% of the lipid core. The chylomicrons pass through blood capillaries in adipose tissue and skeletal muscle where the enzyme lipoprotein lipase is located, bound to the endothelium. Lipoprotein lipase is activated by apoprotein C-II on the surface of the chylomicron. The lipase catalyses the breakdown of the triglyceride in the chylomicron to free fatty acid and glycerol, which then enter adipose tissue and muscle. The cholesterol-rich chylomicron remnant is taken up by receptors on hepatocyte membranes, and in this way dietary cholesterol is delivered to the liver and cleared from the circulation.

VLDL-C is formed in the liver and transports triglycerides, which again make up approximately 80% of its lipid core, to the periphery. The triglyceride content of VLDL-C is removed by lipoprotein lipase in a similar manner to that described for chylomicrons above, and forms IDL-C particles. The core of IDL-C particles is roughly 50% triglyceride and 50% cholesterol esters, acquired from HDL-C under the influence of the enzyme lecithin-cholesterol acyltransferase (LCAT). Approximately 50% of the body's IDL particles are cleared from serum by the liver. The other 50% of IDL-C are further hydrolysed and modified to lose triglyceride and apoprotein E1 and become LDL-C particles. LDL-C is the major cholesterol-carrying particle in serum.

LDL-C provides cholesterol, an essential component of cell membranes, bile acid and a precursor of steroid hormones to those cells that require it. LDL-C is also the main lipoprotein involved in atherogenesis, although it only appears to take on this role after it has been modified by oxidation. For reasons that are not totally clear, the arterial endothelium becomes permeable to the lipoprotein. Monocytes migrate through the permeable endothelium and engulf the lipoprotein, resulting in the formation of lipid-laden macrophages that have a key role in the subsequent development of atherosclerosis. The aim of treatment in dyslipidaemia is normally to reduce concentrations of LDL-C (and consequently atherogenesis) and thus reduce TC at the same time.

While VLDL-C and LDL-C are considered the 'bad' lipoproteins, HDL-C is often considered to be the 'good' anti-atherogenic lipoprotein. In general, about 65% of TC is carried in LDL-C and about 25% in HDL.

High-density lipoprotein

HDL-C is formed from the unesterified cholesterol and phospholipid removed from peripheral tissues and the surface of triglyceride-rich proteins. The major structural protein is apoA-I. HDL-C mediates the return of lipoprotein and cholesterol from peripheral tissues to the liver for excretion in a process known as reverse cholesterol transport.

Reverse cholesterol transport pathway

The reverse cholesterol transport pathway (Fig. 24.2) controls the formation, conversion, transformation and degradation of HDL-C and is the target site for a number of new, novel drugs and has recently been described (Chapman et al., 2010).

The reverse cholesterol transport system involves lipoprotein-mediated transport of cholesterol from peripheral, extra-hepatic tissues and arterial tissue (potentially including cholesterol-loaded foam cell macrophages of the atherosclerotic plaque) to the liver for excretion, either in the form of biliary cholesterol or bile acids. The ATP-binding cassette transporters, ABCA1 and ABCG1, and the scavenger receptor B1, are all implicated in cellular cholesterol efflux mechanisms to specific apoA-1/HDL acceptors. The progressive action of lecithin:cholesterol

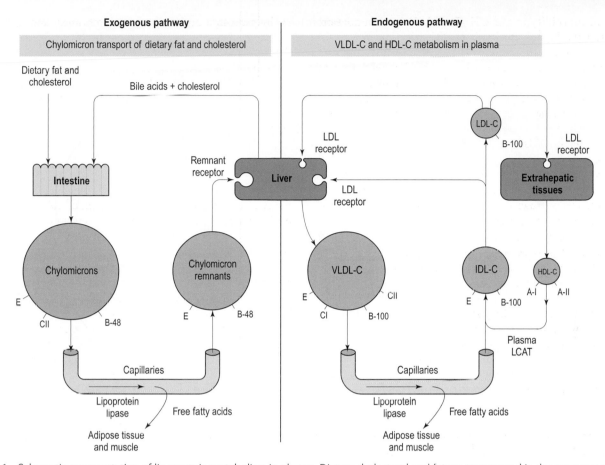

Fig. 24.1 Schematic representation of lipoprotein metabolism in plasma. Dietary cholesterol and fat are transported in the exogenous pathway. Cholesterol produced in the liver is transported in the endogenous pathway.

acyl transferase on free cholesterol in lipid-poor, apolipoprotein A-I-containing nascent high-density lipoproteins, including pre-β-HDL, gives rise to the formation of a spectrum of mature, spherical high-density lipoproteins with a neutral lipid core of cholesteryl ester and triglyceride. Mature high-density lipoproteins consist of two major subclasses, large cholesteryl ester-rich HDL_2 and small cholesteryl ester-poor, protein-rich HDL_3 particles; the latter represent the intravascular precursors of HDL_2. The reverse cholesterol transport system involves two key pathways: (a) the direct pathway (blue lines), in which the cholesteryl ester content (and potentially some free cholesterol) of mature high-density lipoprotein particles is taken up primarily by a selective uptake process involving the hepatic scavenger receptor B1 and (b) an indirect pathway (dotted blue lines) in which cholesteryl ester originating in HDL is deviated to potentially atherogenic VLDL, IDL and LDL particles by cholesteryl ester transfer protein. Both the cholesteryl ester and free cholesterol content of these particles are taken up by the liver, predominantly via the LDL receptor which binds their apoB100 component. This latter pathway may represent up to 70% of cholesteryl ester delivered to the liver per day. The hepatic LDL receptor is also responsible for the direct uptake of high-density lipoprotein particles containing apoE; apoE may be present as a component of both HDL_2 and HDL_3 particles, and may be derived either by transfer from triglyceride-rich lipoproteins, or from tissue sources (principally liver and monocyte-macrophages). Whereas HDL uptake by the LDL receptor results primarily in lysosomal-mediated degradation of both lipids and apolipoproteins, interaction of HDL with scavenger receptor B1 regenerates lipid-poor apoA-I and cholesterol-depleted HDL, both of which may re-enter the HDL/apoA-I cycle.

From the above it is evident that HDL-C plays a major role in maintaining cholesterol homeostasis in the body. As a consequence it is considered desirable to maintain both levels of the protective HDL-C and the integrity of the reverse cholesterol transport pathway. Low levels of HDL-C are found in 17% of men and 5% of women and may be a risk factor for atherogenesis that is comparable in importance to elevated levels of LDL-C. Drugs that reduce HDL-C levels are considered to have an undesirable effect on lipid metabolism and increase the risk of developing CVD.

Triglycerides

The role of hypertriglyceridaemia as an independent risk factor for coronary heart disease (CHD) is unclear because triglyceride levels are confounded by an association with low HDL-C, hypertension, diabetes and obesity, and a synergistic effect with LDL-C and/or low HDL-C. An isolated elevation of triglyceride may be the consequence of a primary disorder of lipid metabolism, it may be secondary to the use of medicines or it may be a component of the metabolic syndrome or type 2

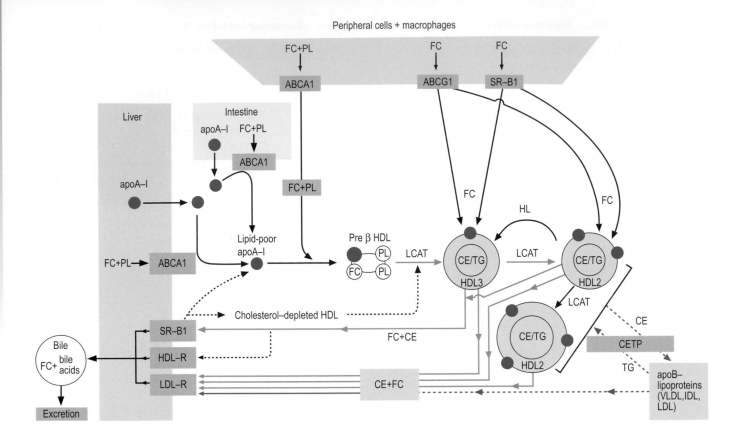

Peripheral cells + macrophages

ABC A1 = ATP binding cassette transporter A1; ABC G1 = ATP binding casssette transporter G1; CE = cholesterol ester; CETP = cholesteryl ester transfer protein; FC = free cholesterol; HDL–R = holo HDL receptor; HL = hepatic lipase; LCAT = lecithin cholesterol acyltransferase; LPL = lipoprotein lipase; PL = phospholipids; SR–B1 = hepatic scavenger receptor B1; TG = triglycerides

Fig. 24.2 Pathways of reverse cholesterol transport in man (Chapman et al., 2010 with kind permission from Oxford University Press, Oxford).

diabetes mellitus. Many individuals have a mixed dyslipidaemia that includes elevated levels of triglycerides and LDL-C, but reduction of LDL-C normally remains the primary focus of treatment. A recent analysis, in over 73,000 individuals, of a genetic variant which regulates triglyceride concentrations has demonstrated a causal association between triglycerides and CHD (Triglyceride Coronary Disease Genetics Consortium and Emerging Risk Factors Collaboration, 2010).

Aetiology

Primary dyslipidaemia

Up to 60% of the variability in cholesterol fasting lipids may be genetically determined, although expression is often influenced by interaction with environmental factors. The common familial (genetic) disorders can be classified as:

- the primary hypercholesterolaemias such as familial hypercholesterolaemias in which LDL-C is raised
- the primary mixed (combined) hyperlipidaemias in which both LDL-C and triglycerides are raised

- the primary hypertriglyceridaemias such as type III hyperlipoproteinaemia, familial lipoprotein lipase deficiency and familial apoC-II deficiency.

Familial hypercholesterolaemia

Heterozygous familial hypercholesterolaemia (often referred to as FH) is an inherited metabolic disease that affects approximately 1 in 500 of the population. In the UK, this represents about 110,000 individuals. Familial hypercholesterolaemia is caused by a range of mutations, which vary from family to family, in genes for the pathway that clear LDL-C from the blood. The most common mutation affects the LDL receptor gene. Given the key role of LDL receptors in the catabolism of LDL-C, patients with FH may have serum levels of LDL-C two to three times higher than the general population. It is important to identify and treat these individuals from birth, otherwise they will be exposed to high concentrations of LDL-C and will suffer the consequences. Familial hypercholesterolaemia is transmitted as a dominant gene, with siblings and children of a parent with FH having a 50% risk of inheriting it. It is important to suspect FH in people that present with TC >7.5 mmol/L, particularly where there is evidence of premature CV disease within the family. Guidance on diagnosis, identifying affected relatives and management are available but it is important to seek specialist advice for this group of high-risk patients (National Institute of Health and Clinical Excellence, 2008b).

In patients with heterozygous FH, CVD presents about 20 years earlier than in the general population, with some individuals, particularly men, dying from atherosclerotic heart disease often before the age of 40 years. The adult heterozygote typically exhibits the signs of cholesterol deposition such as corneal arcus (crescentic deposition of lipids in the cornea), tendon xanthoma (yellow papules or nodules of lipids deposited in tendons) and xanthelasma (yellow plaques or nodules of lipids deposited on eyelids) in their third decade.

In contrast to the heterozygous form, homozygous FH is extremely rare (1 per million) and associated with an absence of LDL receptors and almost absolute inability to clear LDL-C. In these individuals, involvement of the aorta is evident by puberty and usually accompanied by cutaneous and tendon xanthomas. Myocardial infarction has been reported in homozygous children as early as 1.5–3 years of age. Up to the 1980s, sudden death from acute coronary insufficiency before the age of 20 years was normal.

Familial combined hyperlipidaemia

Familial combined hyperlipidaemia has an incidence of 1 in 200 and is associated with excessive synthesis of VLDL-C. In addition to increases in triglyceride and LDL-C levels, patients also typically have raised levels of apoB and elevated levels of small, dense LDL particles. It is associated with an increased risk of atherosclerosis and occurs in approximately 15% of patients who present with CHD before the age of 60 years.

Familial type III hyperlipoproteinaemia

Familial type III hyperlipoproteinaemia has an incidence of 1 in 5000. It is characterised by the accumulation of chylomicron and VLDL remnants that fail to get cleared at a normal rate by hepatic receptors due to the presence of less active polymorphic forms of apoE. Triglycerides and TC are both elevated and accompanied by corneal arcus, xanthelasma, tuberoeruptive xanthomas (groups of flat or yellowish raised nodules on the skin over joints, especially the elbows and knees) and palmar striae (yellow raised streaks across the palms of the hand). The disorder predisposes to premature atherosclerosis.

Familial lipoprotein lipase deficiency

Familial lipoprotein lipase deficiency is characterised by marked hypertriglyceridaemia and chylomicronaemia, and usually presents in childhood. It has an incidence of 1 per million and is due to a deficiency of the extrahepatic enzyme lipoprotein lipase, which results in a failure of lipolysis and the accumulation of chylomicrons in plasma. The affected patient presents with recurrent episodes of abdominal pain, eruptive xanthomas, lipaemia retinalis (retinal deposition of

lipid) and enlarged spleen. This disorder is not associated with an increased susceptibility to atherosclerosis; the major complication is acute pancreatitis.

Familial apolipoprotein C-II deficiency

In the heterozygous state, familial apoC-II deficiency is associated with reduced levels of apoC-II, the activator of lipoprotein lipase. Typically, levels of apoC-II are 50–80% of normal. This level of activity can maintain normal lipid levels. In the rare homozygous state, there is an absence of apolipoprotein C-II and despite normal levels of lipoprotein lipase, it cannot be activated. Consequently, homozygotes have triglyceride levels from 15 to above 100 mmol/L (normal range <1.7 mmol/L) and may develop acute pancreatitis. Premature atherosclerosis is unusual but has been described.

Lipoprotein(a)

There are many other familial disorders of lipid metabolism in addition to those mentioned above but most are very rare. However, a raised level of lipoprotein(a), otherwise known as Lp(a), appears to be a genetically inherited determinant of CVD. Lp(a) is a low-density lipoprotein-like particle synthesised by the liver and first described more than 40 years ago. It is found in the serum of virtually everyone in a wide concentration range (0.01–2 g/L) with up to 70% of the variation in concentration being genetically determined. The concentration of Lp(a) is not normally distributed and the contribution of inheritance to circulating Lp(a) levels is more pronounced than for any other lipoprotein or apoprotein. A parental history of early-onset CVD is associated with raised concentrations of Lp(a), and these appear to play a role in both atherogenesis and thrombosis. An important component of Lp(a) is apo(a), which is structurally and functionally similar to plasminogen and may competitively bind to fibrin and impair fibrinolysis.

Concentrations of Lp(a) above 0.3 g/L occur in about 20% of caucasians and increase the risk of coronary atherosclerosis and stroke. Under a wide range of circumstances, there are continuous, independent, and modest associations of Lp(a) concentration with the risk of CHD and stroke (Emerging Risk Factors Collaboration, 2009).

Secondary dyslipidaemia

Dyslipidaemias that occur secondary to a number of disorders (Box 24.1), dietary indiscretion or as a side effect of drug therapy (Table 24.2) account for up to 40% of all dyslipidaemias. Fortunately, the lipid abnormalities in secondary dyslipidaemia can often be corrected if the underlying disorder is treated, effective dietary advice implemented or the offending drug withdrawn.

On occasion, a disorder may be associated with dyslipidaemia but not the cause of it. For example, hyperuricaemia (gout) and hypertriglyceridaemia co-exist in approximately 50% of men. In this particular example, neither is the cause

Box 24.1 Examples of disorders known to adversely affect the lipid profile

Anorexia nervosa
Bulimia
Type 1 diabetes
Type 2 diabetes
Hypothyroidism
Pregnancy
Inappropriate diet
Alcohol abuse
Chronic renal failure
Nephrotic syndrome
Renal transplantation
Cardiac transplantation
Hepatocellular disease
Cholestasis
Myeloma

Table 24.2 Typical effects of selected drugs on lipoprotein levels

Drug	VLDL-C	LDL-C	HDL-C
Alcohol	↑	0	↑
Androgens, testosterone	↑	↑	↓
ACE-inhibitors	0	0	0
β-Blockers	↑	0	↓
Calcium channel blockers	0	0	0
Ciclosporin	↑	↑	↑
Oestrogens, oestradiol	↑	↓	↓
Glucocorticoids	↑	0	↑
Isotretinoin	↑	0	↓
Progestins	↓	↑	↓
Protease inhibitors	↑	0	0
Sertraline	↑	↑	0
Tacrolimus	↑	↑	↑
Thiazide diuretics	↑	↑	↓
Valproate	↑	0	↓

Effect seen may vary depending on dose, duration of exposure and drugs within same class.
↓, reduction; ↑, increase; 0, no change.

of the other and treatment of one does not resolve the other. There are, however, two notable exceptions to the rule with this example: nicotinic acid and fenofibrate. Both drugs reduce triglyceride levels but nicotinic acid increases urate levels while fenofibrate reduces them by an independent uricosuric effect.

Some of the more common disorders that cause secondary dyslipidaemias include the following.

Diabetes mellitus

Premature atherosclerotic disease is the main cause of reduced life expectancy in patients with diabetes. The atherosclerotic disease is often widespread and complications such as plaque rupture and thrombotic occlusion occur more often and at a younger age. The prevalence of CHD is up to four times higher among diabetic patients with more than 80% likely to die from a cardiovascular event. LDL levels are a stronger predictor of CV risk in diabetic patients than blood glucose control or blood pressure.

Type 1 diabetes. In patients with type 1 diabetes, HDL-C may appear high but for reasons which are unclear, it does not impart the same degree of protection against CVD as in those without diabetes. It is, therefore, not appropriate to use cardiovascular risk prediction charts that utilise the TC:HDL-C ratio in patients with type 1 diabetes. Patients with type 1 diabetes have a two- to three-fold increased risk of developing CVD.

Type 2 diabetes. Patients with type 2 diabetes typically have increased triglycerides and decreased HDL-C. Levels of TC may be similar to those found in non-diabetic individuals but the patient with type 2 diabetes often has increased levels of highly atherogenic small dense LDL particles.

Individuals with type 2 diabetes and aged over 40 years, but without CVD, are often considered to have the same cardiovascular risk as patients without diabetes who have survived a myocardial infarction. This assumption is generally appropriate but influenced by patient age, duration of diabetes and gender and holds better for women than men. This probably occurs because the impact of type 2 diabetes is more marked in women than men. In some guidelines, the criteria for at risk is age above 40 years but with one other risk factor present, for example, hypertension, obesity, smoker, etc.

National Institute of Health and Clinical Excellence (2008a) consider an individual with type 2 diabetes to be at high premature cardiovascular risk for their age unless he or she:

- is not overweight
- is normotensive (<140/80 mmHg in the absence of antihypertensive therapy)
- does not have microalbuminuria
- does not smoke
- does not have a high-risk lipid profile
- has no history of CVD and
- has no family history of CVD.

Where the individual is found to be at risk the patient is typically started on 40 mg simvastatin (or equivalent generic statin). Current guidance indicates the dose can be titrated up to simvastatin 80 mg a day if lipid levels are not reduced to less than 4 mmol/L for TC and less than 2 mmol/L for LDL-C on 40 mg simvastatin. In those who do not reach target with 80 mg simvastatin, 80 mg atorvastatin may be tried. However, with both drugs at the higher dose there is increasing concern about their side effect profile and consequently use is limited at these doses.

Individuals aged 18–39 with type 2 diabetes may also be at high risk and in need of treatment with a statin. Again at-risk individuals typically receive 40 mg simvastatin, or equivalent alternate statin, a day titrated up to 80 mg a day if levels for TC of less than 4 mmol/L and less than 2 mmol/L for LDL-C are not achieved. Again there are emerging concerns about use of these higher doses.

Hypothyroidism

Abnormalities of serum lipid and lipoprotein levels are common in patients with untreated hypothyroidism. Hypothyroidism may elevate LDL-C because of reduced LDL receptor activity and it frequently causes hypertriglyceridaemia and an associated reduction in HDL-C as a result of reduced lipoprotein lipase activity. Remnants of chylomicrons and VLDL-C may also accumulate. However, once adequate thyroid replacement has been instituted the dyslipidaemia should resolve.

Chronic renal failure

Dyslipidaemia is frequently seen in patients with renal failure in the predialysis phase, during haemodialysis or when undergoing chronic ambulatory peritoneal dialysis. The hypertriglyceridaemia that most commonly occurs is associated with reduced lipoprotein lipase activity and often persists despite starting chronic maintenance renal dialysis.

Nephrotic syndrome

In patients with the nephrotic syndrome, dyslipidaemia appears to be caused by an increased production of apoB-100 and associated VLDL-C along with increased hepatic synthesis of LDL-C and a reduction in HDL-C. The necessary use of glucocorticoids in patients with the nephrotic syndrome may exacerbate underlying lipoprotein abnormality.

Obesity

Chronic, excessive intake of calories leads to increased concentrations of triglycerides and reduced HDL-C. Obesity *per se* can exacerbate any underlying primary dyslipidaemia. Individuals with central obesity appear to be at particular risk of what has become known as the metabolic or DROP (*d*yslipidaemia, insulin *r*esistance, *o*besity and high blood *p*ressure) syndrome which represents a cluster of risk factors. Obesity and sedentary lifestyle coupled with inappropriate diet and genetic factors interact to produce the syndrome (Kolovou et al., 2005).

Alcohol

In the heavy drinker, the high calorie content of beer and wine may be a cause of obesity with its associated adverse effect on the lipid profile. In addition, alcohol increases hepatic triglyceride synthesis, which in turn produces hypertriglyceridaemia.

Light to moderate drinkers (1–3 units/day) have a lower incidence of CVD and associated mortality than those who do not drink. This protective effect is probably due to an increase in HDL-C, and appears independent of the type of alcohol. Men should be advised to limit their alcohol intake to 3–4 units a day, and not exceed 21 units a week. For women, the equivalent recommendation is 2–3 units a day with a maximum intake of 14 units a week. Everyone should be advised not to binge drink and have one or two alcohol free days a week.

Drugs

A number of drugs can adversely affect serum lipid and lipoprotein concentrations (see Table 24.2).

Antihypertensive agents. Hypertension is a major risk factor for atherosclerosis, and the beneficial effects of lowering blood pressure are well recognised. It is, however, a concern that, although treatment of patients with some antihypertensives has reduced the incidence of cerebrovascular accidents and renal failure, there has been no major impact in reducing the incidence of CHD. It has been suggested that some of these antihypertensive agents have an adverse effect on lipids and lipoproteins that override any beneficial reduction of blood pressure.

Diuretics. Thiazide and loop diuretics increase VLDL-C and LDL-C by mechanisms that are not completely understood. Whether these adverse effects are dose dependent is also unclear. Use of a thiazide for less than 1 year has been reported to increase TC by up to 7% with no change in HDL-C. However, there is evidence that the short-term changes in lipids do not occur with the low doses in current use. Studies of 3–5 years' duration have found no effect on TC.

β-Blockers. The effects of β-blockers on lipoprotein metabolism are reflected in an increase in serum triglyceride concentrations, a decrease in HDL-C, but with no discernible effect on LDL-C. β-Blockers with intrinsic sympathomimetic activity appear to have little or no effect on VLDL-C or HDL-C. Pindolol has intrinsic sympathomimetic activity but is rarely used as an antihypertensive agent since it may exacerbate angina. Alternatively, the combined α- and β-blocking effect of labetalol may be of use since it would appear to have a negligible effect on the lipid profile.

Overall, the need to use a diuretic or a β-blocker must be balanced against patient considerations. A patient in heart failure should receive a diuretic if indicated regardless of the lipid profile. Likewise, the patient with heart failure may also benefit from a β-blocker such as bisoprolol or carvedilol. Patients who have had a myocardial infarction should be considered for the protective effect of a β-blocker and again the benefits of use will normally override any adverse effects on the lipid profile.

If an antihypertensive agent is required, that is, without adverse effects on lipoproteins, many studies would suggest that angiotensin converting enzyme (ACE) inhibitors, angiotensin II receptor antagonists, calcium channel blockers or α-adrenoceptor blockers could be used.

Oral contraceptives. Oral contraceptives containing an oestrogen and a progestogen provide the most effective contraceptive preparations for general use and have been well studied with respect to their harmful effects.

Oestrogens and progestogens both possess mineralocorticoid and glucocorticoid properties that predispose to hypertension and diabetes mellitus, respectively. However, the effects of the two hormones on lipoproteins are different. Oestrogens cause a slight increase in hepatic production of VLDL-C and HDL-C, and reduce serum LDL-C levels. In contrast, progestogens increase LDL-C and reduce serum HDL-C and VLDL-C.

The specific effect of the oestrogen or progestogen varies with the actual dose and chemical entity used. Ethinyloestradiol at a dose of 30–35 μcg or less would appear to create few problems with lipid metabolism, while norethisterone is one of the more favourable progestogens even though it may cause a pronounced decrease in HDL-C.

Corticosteroids. The effect of glucocorticoid administration on lipid levels has been studied in patients treated with steroids for asthma, rheumatoid arthritis and connective tissue disorders. Administration of a glucocorticoid such as prednisolone has been shown to increase TC and triglycerides by elevating LDL-C and, less consistently, VLDL-C. The changes are generally more pronounced in women. Alternate-day therapy with glucocorticoids has been suggested to reduce the adverse effect on lipoprotein levels in some patients.

Ciclosporin. Ciclosporin is primarily used to prevent tissue rejection in recipients of renal, hepatic and cardiac transplants. Its use has been associated with increased LDL-C levels, hypertension and glucose intolerance. These adverse effects are often exacerbated by the concurrent administration of glucocorticoids. The combined use of ciclosporin and glucocorticoid contributes to the adverse lipid profile seen in transplant patients. Unfortunately, the administration of a statin to patients treated with ciclosporin increases the incidence of myositis, rhabdomyolysis (dissolution of muscle associated with excretion of myoglobin in the urine) and renal failure. Use of a statin is, therefore, contraindicated in patients receiving ciclosporin.

Case reports of similar interactions between statins and other drugs used to prevent tissue rejection, including tacrolimus and sirolimus, have also been reported.

Hepatic microsomal enzyme inducers. Drugs such as carbamazepine, phenytoin, phenobarbital, rifampicin and griseofulvin increase hepatic microsomal enzyme activity and can also increase serum HDL-C. The administration of these drugs may also give rise to a slight increase in LDL-C and VLDL-C. The overall effect is one of a favourable increase in the TC:HDL-C ratio. It is interesting to note that patients treated for epilepsy have been reported to have a decreased incidence of CVD.

Risk Assessment

Primary prevention

In patients with no evidence of CHD or other major atherosclerotic disease, there are a number of CVD risk prediction charts, including those produced by the Joint British Societies

(JBS2) (British Hypertension Society, 2009) for males (Fig. 24.3) and females (Fig. 24.4). JBS2 recommends that all adults from the age of 40 years, with no history of CVD or diabetes, and not receiving treatment for raised blood pressure or dyslipidaemia, should receive opportunistic screening every 5 years in primary care. The cardiovascular risk calculated using the JBS2 charts is based on the number of cardiovascular events expected over the next 10 years in 100 women or men with the same risk factors as the individual being assessed. Those with a cardiovascular risk >20% over 10 years are deemed to require treatment according to current national and international guidelines, although individuals with a risk as low as 8% over 10 years will gain some benefit, this will be small.

Risk assessment is not required when the individual is 75 years of age or older, or they have pre-existing CVD. These individuals are already assumed to have a 10-year risk of at least 20%.

When using the JBS2 risk prediction charts a number of factors need to be taken into account at screening and include:

- *Age:* in individuals under 40 years of age the charts overestimate risk; over the age of 70 years risk is underestimated by the charts and most have a 10-year risk >20%.
- *Gender:* there are separate charts for men and women.
- *Ethnicity:* the risk prediction charts have only been validated in white caucasians and underestimate risk in individuals from the Indian subcontinent (India, Pakistan, Bangladesh and Sri Lanka) by a factor of 1.5.
- *Smoking history:* individuals who have stopped smoking within 5 years of assessment should be considered as current smokers.
- *Family history:* risk increases by a factor of 1.5 when CHD has occurred in a first-degree relative (parent, offspring, sibling) male <55 years or female <65 years, when a number of family members have developed CHD risk increases by a factor of 2 (Box 24.2).
- *Body mass index (BMI) and waist circumference:* the charts do not adjust for either BMI or waist circumference; these factors need to be taken into account in the clinical decision-making process.
- *Non-fasting blood glucose:* if non-fasting glucose >6.1 mmol/L, the individual should be assessed for impaired glucose regulation or diabetes.

Individuals with type 2 diabetes aged over 40 years and with an additional cardiovascular risk factor are considered to be at greater than 20% risk over 10 years and eligible for treatment. In those who are 40 years of age or older but without any additional risk factor, a specific risk engine is available (http://www.dtu.ox.ac.uk/riskengine/) based on data from the United Kingdom Prospective Diabetes Study.

Framingham

Up to 2008, risk charts and calculators based on Framingham data were the most widely used and researched approach for calculating cardiovascular risk, and are the data on which the risk

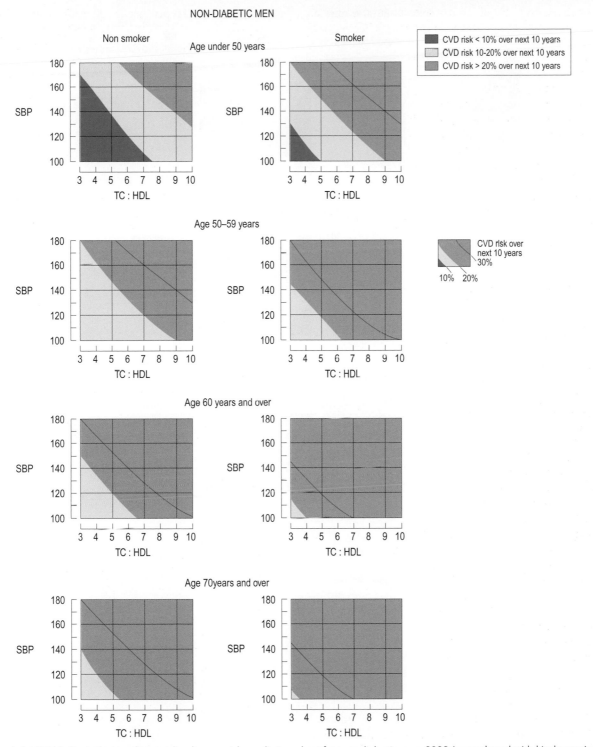

Fig. 24.3 Joint British Societies' cardiovascular disease risk prediction chart for non-diabetic men 2009 (reproduced with kind permission of University of Manchester). SBP, systolic blood pressure mmHg; TC:HDL, serum total cholesterol to HDL cholesterol ratio.

charts discussed above are based. The Framingham data derive from a North American population studied in the 1960s to 1980s. The data generally overestimate risk in the UK population but underestimate risk, as discussed, in those with a family history of premature CVD, South Asian men, people with diabetes and those from a deprived socioeconomic background.

Assign

This is a risk calculator based on data from a Scottish population and includes many of the variables utilised in the Framingham-based model. It also takes into account social status, determined by postcode of residence in Scotland, and

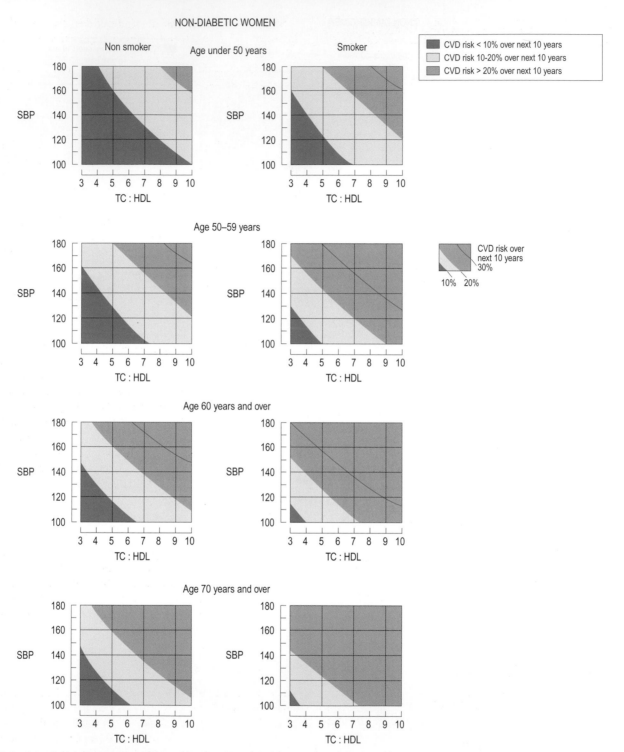

Fig. 24.4 Joint British Societies' cardiovascular disease risk prediction chart for non-diabetic women 2009 (reproduced with kind permission of University of Manchester). SBP, systolic blood pressure mmHg; TC:HDL, serum total cholesterol to HDL cholesterol ratio.

family history of CVD (Woodward et al., 2007). The calculator can be found at: http://www.assign-score.com.

QRISK2

This is a relatively new CVD risk calculator, based on a database of anonymised UK primary care patients established in 2003. It contains over 10 million sets of encrypted patient records. A cohort of 1.28 million patients without evidence of diabetes mellitus or CVD was identified, and followed up for more than 5 years looking for the first development of CVD as an endpoint.

The current version of the calculator (QRISK2) uses the following parameters with any missing values calculated by a complex averaging procedure:

Box 24.2 Criteria that indicate familial hypercholesterolaemia

Family history of dyslipidaemia or cardiovascular disease:
- in first-degree female relative less than 65 years old
- in first-degree male relative less than 55 years old

Xanthelasma or corneal arcus under the age of 45

[a]Tendon xanthomata + TC >7.5 mmol/L at any age
[a]Tendon xanthomata + LDL-C >4.9 mmol/L

[a]Tendon xanthomata may not be readily apparent in younger people

- Patient age (35–74)
- Patient gender
- Current smoker (yes/no)
- Family history of heart disease aged <60 (yes/no)
- Existing treatment with blood pressure agent (yes/no)
- Postcode (postcode is linked to Townsend score measure of deprivation)
- BMI (height and weight)
- Systolic blood pressure (use current not pre-treatment value)
- Total and HDL cholesterol
- Self-assigned ethnicity (not nationality)
- Rheumatoid arthritis
- Chronic kidney disease
- Atrial fibrillation.

The QRISK2 calculator is available at http://www.qrisk.org/

The Department of Health and NICE endorse the use of either Framingham-based risk prediction tools or QRISK2.

Secondary prevention

Patients with CVD and levels of TC >4 mmol/L and LDL-C >2 mmol/L are the ones most likely to benefit from treatment with lipid-lowering agents. Typical of individuals who fall into this category are patients with a history of angina, myocardial infarction, acute coronary syndrome, coronary artery bypass grafting, coronary angioplasty or cardiac transplantation as well as patients with evidence of atherosclerotic disease in other vascular beds such as patients post-stroke or TIA, and those with peripheral arterial disease.

As in the situation with primary prevention outlined above, if an individual is to receive a lipid-lowering agent as part of a secondary prevention strategy, the possibility of a familial dyslipidaemia and the need to assess other family members must not be overlooked (National Institute of Health and Clinical Excellence, 2008b).

Treatment

Lipid profile

When a decision has been made to determine an individual's lipid profile, a random serum TC and HDL-C will often suffice. If a subsequent decision is made to commence treatment and monitor outcome, a more detailed profile that includes triglycerides is required. Treatment should not be initiated on the basis of a single random sample.

Serum concentrations of triglycerides increase after the ingestion of a meal and, therefore, patients must fast for 12–15 h before they can be measured. Patients must also be seated for at least 5 min prior to drawing a blood sample. TC level and HDL are little affected by food intake, and this is, therefore, not a consideration if only these are to be measured. However, it is important that whatever is being measured reflects a steady-state value. For example, during periods of weight loss, lipid concentrations decline as they do following a myocardial infarction. In the case of the latter, samples drawn within 24 h of infarct onset will reflect the preinfarction state. In general, measurement should be deferred for 2 weeks after a minor illness and for 3 months after a myocardial infarction, serious illness or pregnancy.

Once the TC, HDL-C and triglyceride values are known it is usual to calculate the value for LDL-C using the Friedewald equation:

$$LDL\text{-}C = (Total\ cholesterol - HDL\text{-}C) - (0.45 \times triglyceride)\ mmol/L.$$

The Friedewald equation should not be used in non-fasting individuals, it is less reliable in individuals with diabetes and is not valid if the serum triglyceride concentration >4 mmol/L.

Although lipid target levels are normally only defined for TC and LDL-C, increasingly non-HDL-C is measured. The value for non-HDL-C is obtained by subtracting the value for HDL-C from TC. Non-HDL-C consequently represents the total of cholesterol circulating on apoprotein B particles, that is, both LDL and triglyceride-rich lipoproteins, and represents the main atherogenic particles. A desirable value is <3 mmol/L.

Lifestyle

When a decision is made to start treatment with a lipid-lowering agent, other risk factors must also be tackled as appropriate, such as smoking, obesity, high alcohol intake and lack of exercise (Box 24.3). Underlying disorders such as diabetes mellitus and hypertension should be treated as appropriate. Issues around body weight, diet and exercise will be briefly covered in the following sections.

Body weight and waist measurement

The overweight patient is at increased risk of atherosclerotic disease and typically has elevated levels of serum triglycerides, raised LDL-C and a low HDL-C. This adverse lipid profile is often compounded by the presence of hypertension and raised blood glucose, that is, the metabolic syndrome. A reduction in body weight will generally improve the lipid profile and reduce overall cardiovascular risk.

It is useful to classify the extent to which an individual is overweight by calculating their BMI. The BMI (kg/m^2) in all but the most muscular individual gives a clinical measure of adiposity.

- BMI 18.5: underweight
- BMI 18.6 to 24.9: ideal
- BMI 25 to 29.9: overweight (low health risk)

- BMI 30 to 40: obese (moderate health risk)
- BMI >40: morbidly obese (high health risk)

The distribution of body fat is also recognised as a factor that influences CVD risk. Measurement of waist circumference is perhaps the easiest and most practical indicator of central obesity and correlates well with CVD risk. Target waist circumference should be <102 cm in white caucasian men, <88 cm in white caucasian females and in Asians <90 cm in men and <80 cm in females.

Diet

Diet modification should always be encouraged in a patient with dyslipidaemia but is rarely successful alone in bringing about a significant improvement in the lipid profile. Randomised controlled trials of dietary fat reduction or modification have shown variable results on cardiovascular morbidity and mortality. In pragmatic, community-based studies, reductions in TC of only 3–6% have been achieved. The overall picture is that patients with dyslipidaemia should receive dietary advice and a small number of those who adhere to the advice will experience a fall in TC.

There is a common misconception that a healthy diet is one that is low in cholesterol. However, generally it is the saturated fat content that is important, although many components of a healthy diet are not related to fat content. For example, the low incidence of cardiovascular disease in those who consume a Mediterranean-type diet suggests an increased intake of fruit and vegetables is also important. The typical Mediterranean diet has an abundance of plant food (fruit, vegetables, breads, cereals, potatoes, beans, nuts and seeds) minimally processed, seasonally fresh, and locally grown; fresh fruit as the typical daily dessert, with sweets containing concentrated sugars or honey consumed a few times per week; olive oil as the principal source of fat; dairy products (principally cheese and yoghurt) consumed daily in low to moderate amounts; 0–4 eggs consumed weekly; and red meat consumed in low to moderate amounts. This diet is low in saturated fat (<8% of energy) and varies in total fat content from <25% to >35% of energy.

Fish. Regular consumption of the long chain omega-3 fatty acids, principally ecosapentaenoic acid and docosahexaenoic acid, typically found in fatty fish and fish oils, has been linked to the low levels of CHD seen in Inuits (Eskimos). The risk of fatal myocardial infarction in those with CVD has been shown to be reduced by consuming omega-3 fatty acids. Consumption of omega-3 fatty acids decrease triglyceride levels but have little effect on LDL-C or HDL-C. The proposed mechanisms is thought to involve the omega-3 fatty acids and their antiarrhythmic properties, ability to reduce blood pressure and heart rate, lower triglyceride levels, stimulate endothelial-derived nitric oxide, increase insulin sensitivity, decrease platelet aggregation and decrease proinflammatory eicosanoids. There would appear to be benefits in consuming at least two portions (portion = 140 g) of fish per week, including a portion of oily fish, particularly in those who have had a myocardial infarction. Pregnant women are advised to limit their intake of oily fish to two portions per week because of the potential accumulation of low level pollutants in the fish.

Trans fats. Trans fats are unsaturated fatty acids with at least one double bond in the trans configuration. They are formed when vegetable oils are hydrogenated to convert them into semisolid fats that can be incorporated into margarines or used in commercial manufacturing processes. Trans fats are typically found in deep fried fast foods, bakery products, packaged snack foods, margarines and crackers. When the calorific equivalent of saturated fats, cis unsaturated fats and trans fats are consumed, trans fats raise LDL-C, reduce HDL-C and increase the ratio of TC:HDL-C. In addition to these harmful effects, trans fats also increase the blood levels of triglycerides, increase levels of Lp(a) and reduce the particle size of LDL-C, all of which further increase the risk of CHD. It is, therefore, necessary to reduce the dietary intake of trans fatty acids to less than 0.5% of total energy intake and this has led to calls for a complete ban on trans fats in foods.

Stanol esters and plant sterols. The availability of margarines and other foods enriched with plant sterols or stanol esters appears to increase the likelihood that LDL-C can be reduced by dietary change. Both stanol esters and plant sterols at a maximum effective dose of 2 g/day inhibit cholesterol absorption from the gastro-intestinal tract and reduce LDL-C by an average of 10%. They compete with cholesterol for incorporation into mixed micelles, thereby impairing its absorption from the intestine. However, as with other dietary changes, the reduction seen varies between individuals and is probably dependent on the initial cholesterol level. There is currently no evidence that ingestion lowers the risk of cardiovascular events.

Antioxidants. Antioxidants occur naturally in fruit and vegetables and are important components of a healthy diet. Their consumption is thought to be beneficial in reducing the formation of atherogenic, oxidised LDL-C. Primary and secondary prevention trials with antioxidant vitamin supplements, however, have not been encouraging. Neither vitamin E nor beta-carotene supplements would appear to reduce the risk of CHD but likewise have not been shown to be harmful.

Salt. Dietary salt (sodium) has an adverse effect on blood pressure and, therefore, a potential impact on CHD and stroke. As part of dietary advice the average adult intake of sodium should be reduced from approximately 150 mmol (9 g)–100 mmol (6 g) of salt or even lower. This intake can be reduced by consuming fewer processed foods, avoiding many ready meals and not adding salt to food at the table.

Exercise

Moderate amounts of aerobic exercise (brisk walking, jogging, swimming, cycling) on a regular basis have a desirable effect on the lipid profile of an individual. These beneficial effects have been demonstrated within 2 months in middle-aged men exercising for 30 min, three times a week. Current advice for adults who are not routinely active is to undertake 30 min of moderate-intensity activity on at least 5 days of the week. This can be undertaken in bouts of 10 min. For active individuals, additional aerobic exercise of vigorous intensity is recommended for 20–30 min three times a week. Exercise *per se* probably has little effect on TC levels in the absence of a reduction in body weight, body fat or dietary fat. Perhaps the most important effect of regular exercise is to raise levels of HDL-C in a dose-dependent manner according to energy expenditure.

Overall, comprehensive dietary and lifestyle changes (stopping smoking, stress management training and moderate exercise) can bring about regression of coronary atherosclerosis. Unfortunately, many find it difficult to attain or sustain the necessary changes. In others, dietary and lifestyle changes alone will never be adequate or will not bring about the necessary improvement in lipid profile quickly enough. As a consequence, the use of lipid-lowering drugs is widespread.

Drugs

If an individual is found to be at risk of CVD (primary prevention) it may be appropriate to give a trial of dietary and lifestyle changes for 3–6 months. This rarely achieves the required effect on the lipid profile and drug therapy is required. This must not, however, negate a sustained effort by the individual to make appropriate dietary and lifestyle adjustments. In an individual requiring treatment for secondary prevention, a delay of several months in starting treatment is not appropriate and treatment will normally be commenced immediately with a lipid-lowering agent.

Primary prevention

In primary prevention, dyslipidaemia should not be treated in isolation and management must be embarked upon with clear goals. In addition to lifestyle advice, this will not only address management of dyslipidaemia but will also seek to optimise use of antihypertensive agents, other cardiovascular protective therapies and achieve tight blood glucose control as appropriate. In patients without evidence of arterial disease, treatment must be considered if the risk of CVD is >20% or more over 10 years. Although some dispute the benefit of statins in primary prevention (Kausik et al., 2010), treatment will normally include:

- a lipid-lowering agent such as simvastatin 40 mg/day (or alternative) but no treatment targets are set
- personalised information on modifiable risk factors including physical activity, diet, alcohol intake, weight and tight control of diabetes
- advice to stop smoking
- advice and treatment to achieve blood pressure below 140 mmHg systolic and 90 mmHg diastolic.

Some also consider an isolated raised TC:HDL ratio >6.5 warrants treatment regardless of the risk assessment outcome, but this approach has received little support in national treatment guidelines.

Secondary prevention

In individuals diagnosed with CVD or other occlusive arterial disease, treatment should include:

- a lipid-lowering agent to lower TC aiming towards a TC <4 mmol/L and LDL-C <2 mmol/L
- advice to stop smoking
- personalised information on modifiable risk factors including physical activity, diet, alcohol intake, weight and diabetes
- advice and treatment to achieve blood pressure at least below 140 mmHg systolic and 90 mmHg diastolic
- tight control of blood pressure and glucose in those with diabetes
- low-dose aspirin (75 mg daily)
- ACE inhibitors especially for those with left ventricular dysfunction, heart failure, diabetes, hypertension or nephropathy
- β-blocker for those who have had a myocardial infarction and in those with heart failure
- warfarin (or aspirin) for those with atrial fibrillation and additional stroke risk factors.

Lipid-lowering therapy

There are five main classes of lipid-lowering agents available:

- Statins
- Fibrates
- Bile acid binding agents
- Cholesterol absorption inhibitors
- Nicotinic acid and derivatives.

Agents such as soluble fibre and fish oils have also been used to reduce lipid levels. A number of new agents are also under investigation for their novel effect on different parts of the cholesterol biosynthesis pathway (Table 24.3).

Table 24.3 Mechanism of lipid-lowering agents under investigation

Drug group	Mechanism
Acyl-coenzyme A: cholesterol acyltransferase (ACAT) inhibitors	ACAT esterifies excess intracellular cholesterol. Inhibition of ACAT prevents transport of cholesterol into the arterial wall and thereby prevents atheroma developing. Lowers VLDL-C and triglycerides
Bile acid sequestrants	Related to first-generation resins but improved patient tolerance. Sequester bile acids and prevent re-absorption. Reduce LDL-C while HDL-C and triglycerides increase or remain unchanged
Cholesteryl ester transfer protein (CETP) inhibitors	CETP is responsible for the transfer of cholesteryl ester from HDL-C to the atherogenic LDL-C and VLDL-C
Lipoprotein lipase (LPL) activity enhancers	LPL is responsible for VLDL-C catabolism with subsequent loss of triglycerides and increase in HDL-C. Protects against atherosclerosis
Microsomal triglyceride transfer protein (MTP) inhibitors	Inhibit absorption of lipid and reduce hepatic secretion of lipoproteins, thereby reducing atherosclerotic plaque formation
Peroxisome proliferator-activated receptor (PPAR) activators	PPAR-α and -γ regulate the expression of genes involved in lipid metabolism and inhibit atherosclerotic plaque rupture. They reduce entry of cholesterol into cells, lower LDL-C and triglycerides, and increase HDL-C
Squalene synthase inhibitors	Inhibit squalene synthase, upregulate LDL receptor activity and enhance removal of LDL-C

The choice of lipid-lowering agent depends on the underlying dyslipidaemia, the response required and patient acceptability. The various groups of drugs available have different mechanisms of action and variable efficacy depending on the lipid profile of an individual. Statins are currently the drugs of choice in the majority of patients with dyslipidaemia due to the overwhelming evidence that treatment with these agents reduces cardiovascular events.

Statins

The discovery of a class of drugs, the statins, which selectively inhibit 3-hydroxy-3-methylglutaryl-CoA reductase (HMG-CoA reductase) was a significant advance in the treatment of dyslipidaemia. Their primary site of action is the inhibition of HMG-CoA reductase in the liver and the subsequent inhibition of the formation of mevalonic acid, the rate-limiting step in the biosynthesis of cholesterol. This results in a reduction in intracellular levels of cholesterol, an increase in expression of hepatic LDL receptor, and enhanced receptor-mediated catabolism and clearance of LDL-C from serum. Production of VLDL-C, the precursor of LDL-C, is also reduced. The overall effect is a reduction in TC, LDL-C, VLDL-C and triglycerides with an increase in HDL-C. The reduction in LDL-C occurs in a dose-dependent manner, with a lesser and dose-independent effect on VLDL-C and triglycerides.

Simvastatin was the first member of the group to be marketed in the UK and it was followed by pravastatin, fluvastatin, atorvastatin, cerivastatin and rosuvastatin. Cerivastatin was withdrawn from the market in 2001 due to an observed increased risk of fatal rhabdomyolysis whilst rosuvastatin, the newest member of the group, was launched in March 2003. Lovastatin has been available in the USA for many years

whilst pitavastatin, likewise, has been available in Japan since 2003 with little attempt, until recently, to market in the UK.

The efficacy of statins has been demonstrated in a number of landmark, randomised placebo-controlled trials. A greater absolute benefit was seen in those trials that involved established CVD, that is, secondary prevention studies, compared to those that involved individuals without established CVD, that is, primary prevention studies. Statins are currently the lipid-lowering agents of choice in both primary and secondary prevention of CVD.

There is much debate around the statin of choice. Simvastatin is currently the preferred agent because of its relatively low cost, safety profile and evidence of efficacy (see Table 24.4). Perhaps more important is the need to identify patients who need treatment, ensure they receive an appropriate, effective dose of a statin and adhere to treatment. Despite overwhelming evidence of benefit, effectiveness is frequently compromised by poor adherence with up to 50% of patients discontinuing treatment within 12 months and 75% within 3 years. Patient factors that influence this include perception of risk, side effects of medication, expected treatment duration and socio-demographic factors.

Rosuvastatin is the most potent of the statins with evidence of impact on morbidity and mortality. It is normally reserved for those individuals that have had an inadequate response to their first-line statin. There remain concerns about its safety profile, and rhabdomyolysis in particular, when used at the higher dose of 40 mg/day. It is recommended that this dose should only be used in individuals with severe FH and at high cardiovascular risk under specialist supervision. In patients of Asian origin (Japanese, Chinese, Filipino, Vietnamese, Korean and Indian), the maximum dose should not exceed 20 mg/day because of their increased predisposition to myopathy and rhabdomyolysis.

Table 24.4 Typical recommendations for use of lipid-lowering agents (UKMI, 2009) (LDL-C, low-density lipoprotein cholesterol; TG, triglycerides; TC, total cholesterol)

Drug therapy	Primary prevention (If >40 years and 10-year risk ≥ 20%)		Secondary prevention (All adults with CVD)		Acute coronary syndrome	Familial hypercholesterolaemia (adults)
	WITHOUT diabetes	WITH diabetes (any age)	WITHOUT diabetes	WITH diabetes		
FIRST LINE						
Simvastatin dose	40mg	40mg	40mg	40mg	High intensity statin*	40mg
SECOND-LINE AFTER INITIAL TREATMENT WITH SIMVASTATIN 40MG (OR EQUIVALENT)						
High-intensity statin (simvastatin 80mg or equivalent alternative)	No recommendations	Consider if TC >4.0mmol/L AND LDL-C >2mmol/L	Consider if TC >4.0mmol/L AND LDL-C >2mmol/L	Corsider if TC >4.0mmol/L AND LDL-C >2mmol/L	*Simvastatin 80mg or atorvastatin 80mg	Give if needed to achieve a reduction in LDL-C of >50% from baseline
OTHER TREATMENT OPTIONS						
Ezetimibe	Only if statin not tolerated	No recommendations	Only if statin not tolerated	Add to statin if there is ex sting or newly diagnosed CVD or increased albumin excretion rate	Only if statin not tolerated	Use as monotherapy if: statins contraindicated or not tolerated, OR combined with a statin if: TC or LDL-C not controlled
Fibrates	Only if statin not tolerated	Add to statin if: TG > 4.5mmol/L despite optimised glycaemic control TG 2.3 – 4.5mmol/L and high CVD risk	Only if statin not tolerated	Add to statin if TG remains >4.5mmol/L despite optimised glycaemic control	Only if statin not tolerated	Use only on the acvice of a specialist: if statins or ezetimibe are contraindicated or not tolerated, in combination with a statin on specialist advice
Bile acid sequestrants	Only if statin not tolerated	No recommendations	Only if statin not tolerated	No recommendations	Only if statin not tolerated	
Nicotinic acid	No recommendations	Do not use routinely	Only if statin not tolerated	Do not use routinely	Only if statin not tolerated	

All the statins require the presence of LDL receptors for their optimum clinical effect, and consequently they are less effective in patients with heterozygous FH because of the reduced number of LDL receptors. However, even in the homozygous patient where there are no LDL receptors they can bring about some reduction of serum cholesterol, although the mechanism is unclear.

Adverse effects

Many side effects appear mild and transient. The commonest include gastro-intestinal symptoms, altered liver function tests and muscle aches. Less common are elevation of liver transaminase levels in excess of three times the upper limit of normal, hepatitis, rash, headache, insomnia, nightmares, vivid dreams and difficulty concentrating.

Myopathy (unexplained muscle soreness or weakness) leading to myoglobulinuria secondary to rhabdomyolysis is also a rare but serious potential adverse effect of all the statins that can occur at any dose. The risk of myopathy is increased:

- when there are underlying muscle disorders, a family history of muscle disorders, renal impairment, untreated hypothyroidism, alcohol abuse, or the recipient is aged over 65 years or female
- where statins are co-prescribed with other lipid-lowering drugs, for example, fibrates, nicotinic acid
- when there is a past history of myopathy with another lipid-lowering drug or statin
- where there is co-prescription of simvastatin or atorvastatin with drugs that inhibit CYP3A4.

The statins are a heterogeneous group metabolised by different CYP450 isoenzymes. Simvastatin, atorvastatin and lovastatin are metabolised by CYP3A4, fluvastatin is metabolised by CYP 2C9, and pravastatin and rosuvastatin are eliminated by other metabolic routes and less subject to interactions with CYP450 isoenzymes than other members of the family. Nevertheless, caution is still required as a 5- to 23-fold increase in pravastatin bioavailability has been reported with ciclosporin. Simvastatin and atorvastatin do not alter the activity of CYP3A4 themselves, but their serum levels are increased by known inhibitors of CYP3A4 (Table 24.5). Advice has been published for the prescribing of simvastatin and atorvastatin with inhibitors of CYP3A4 (Table 24.6).

Pleiotropic properties

While the effect of statins on the lipid profile contributes to their beneficial outcome in reducing morbidity and mortality from CVD, other mechanisms, known as pleiotropic effects, may also play a part. These effects include plaque stabilisation, inhibition of thrombus formation, reduced serum viscosity and anti-inflammatory and antioxidant activity. These pleiotropic properties, that is, cholesterol-independent effects, are far reaching and reveal a clinical impact beyond a process of reducing TC. For example, lowering TC produces only modest reductions of a fixed, atherosclerotic, luminal stenosis but results in a qualitative change of the plaque and helps stabilise it. This protects the plaque from rupturing and triggering further coronary events.

Table 24.5 Examples of drug interactions involving statins and the cytochrome P450 enzyme pathway

CYP 450 isoenzyme	Inducers	Inhibitors
CYP3A4		
Atorvastin	Phenytoin	Ketoconazole
Lovastatin	Barbiturate	Itraconazole
Simvastatin	Rifampicin	Fluconazole
	Dexamethasone	Erythromycin
	Cyclophosphamide	Clarithromycin
	Carbamazepine	Tricyclic
	Omeprazole	antidepressants
		Nefazodone
		Venlafaxine
		Fluoxetine
		Sertraline
		Ciclosporin
		Tacrolimus
		Diltiazem
		Verapamil
		Protease inhibitors
		Midazolam
		Corticosteroids
		Grapefruit juice
		Tamoxifen
		Amiodarone
CYP2C9		
Fluvastatin	Rifampicin	Ketoconazole
	Phenobarbitone	Fluconazole
	Phenytoin	Sulfaphenazole

Table 24.6 Advice for prescribing simvastatin or atorvastatin with inhibitors of CYP3A4

Avoid simvastatin with potent inhibitors of CYP3A4:	HIV protease inhibitors, azole, antifungals, erythromycin, clarithromycin, telithromycin
Do not exceed the following doses:	Simvastatin 10 mg daily with ciclosporin, gemfibrozil or niacin (>1 g/day) Simvastatin 20 mg daily with verapamil or amiodarone Simvastatin 40 mg daily with diltiazem
Avoid grapefruit juice when taking simvastatin	
Atorvastatin to be used cautiously with CYP3A4 inhibitors:	Additional care required at high doses of atorvastatin; avoid drinking large quantities of grapefruit juice

Inflammation is thought to play a prominent part in the development of atherosclerosis and increased levels of C-reactive protein have been used to identify individuals at risk of plaque rupture and consequent myocardial infarction and stroke. Statins have been shown to reduce the levels of C-reactive protein in several trials.

An important aspect of vascular endothelium dysfunction is the impaired synthesis, release and activity of endothelial-derived nitric oxide, an important and early marker of atherosclerosis. After the administration of a statin, one of the earliest effects observed (within 3 days) is an increased endothelial nitric oxide release, thereby mediating an improvement in vasodilation of the endothelium.

For some while it has been thought that part of the beneficial effect of statins on CVD could be attributed to an effect on blood coagulation. It is now evident that statins, amongst their many actions, decrease platelet activation and activity, reduce prothrombin activation, factor Va generation, fibrinogen cleavage and factor XIII activation, and increase factor Va inactivation.

Over-the-counter sale

Low-dose (10 mg) simvastatin can be purchased from community pharmacies in the UK to treat individuals at moderate cardiovascular risk. Men aged 55–70 years with or without risk factors and men aged 45–54 years or women aged 55–70 years with at least one risk factor (smoker, obese, family history of premature CHD or of South Asian origin) are eligible for treatment. Simvastatin cannot be sold to individuals who have CVD, diabetes or familial dyslipidaemia or are taking lipid-lowering agents or medication that may interact with simvastatin. The rationale for over-the-counter sale is to reduce the risk of a first major coronary event in adults at moderate risk but sales have been low. Moreover, the evidence base to support the use of 10 mg simvastatin and achieve long-term cardiovascular benefit is limited.

Patient counselling

In patients receiving a statin, a once-daily regimen involving an evening dose is often preferred. Several of the statins (fluvastatin, pravastatin, simvastatin) are claimed to be more effective when given as a single dose in the evening compared to a similar dose administered in the morning. This has been attributed to the fact that cholesterol biosynthesis reaches peak activity at night. However, atorvastatin and rosuvastatin may be taken in the morning or evening with similar efficacy. A reduction in TC and LDL-C is usually seen with all statins within 2 weeks, with a maximum response occurring by week 4 and maintained thereafter during continued therapy.

Fibrates

Members of this group include bezafibrate, ciprofibrate, fenofibrate and gemfibrozil. They are thought to act by binding to peroxisome proliferator-activated receptor α (PPAR-α) on hepatocytes. This then leads to changes in the expression of genes involved in lipoprotein metabolism. Consequently, fibrates reduce triglyceride and, to a lesser extent, LDL-C levels while increasing HDL-C. Fibrates take 2–5 days to have a measurable effect on VLDL-C, with their optimum effect present after 4 weeks. In addition to their effects on serum lipids and lipoproteins, the fibrates may also have a beneficial effect on the fibrinolytic and clotting mechanisms. The fibrates also produce an improvement in glucose tolerance, although bezafibrate probably has the most marked effect.

In the patient with elevated triglycerides and gout, only fenofibrate has been reported to have a sustained uricosuric effect on chronic administration. Overall, there appears little to differentiate members of the group with regard to their effect on the lipid profile, with fenofibrate and ciprofibrate being the most potent members of the group.

In patients with diabetes, the typical picture of dyslipidaemia is one of raised triglycerides, reduced HDL-C and near normal LDL-C. Despite the effect of fibrates to reduce triglycerides and increase HDL-C, statins are first-line lipid-lowering agent in most guidelines because of a lack of clear evidence that fibrates prevent CVD in diabetes. It was hoped that a 5-year study of fenofibrate in individuals with type 2 diabetes (FIELD Investigators, 2005) would clarify the issue. However, in the final analysis the results provided little convincing evidence to change from recommending a statin, although they did confirm the safety of using a combination of a statin and fenofibrate. In contrast, gemfibrozil should not be used with a statin.

Overall, fibrates should not be used first line to reduce lipid levels in either primary or secondary prevention. Fibrates can be used first line in patients with isolated severe hypertriglyceridaemia. In individuals with mixed hyperlipidaemia, fibrates may be considered when a statin or other agent is contraindicated or not tolerated.

Adverse effects

Overall, the side effects of fibrates are mild and vary between members of the group. Their apparent propensity to increase the cholesterol saturation index of bile renders them unsuitable for patients with gallbladder disease. Gastro-intestinal symptoms such as nausea, diarrhoea and abdominal pain are common but transient, and often resolve after a few days of treatment. Myositis has been described, and is associated with muscle pain, unusual tiredness or weakness. The mechanism is unclear but it is thought fibrates may have a direct toxic action on muscle cells in susceptible individuals.

Fibrates have been implicated in a number of drug interactions (Table 24.7), of which two in particular are potentially serious. Fibrates are known to significantly increase the effect of anticoagulants, while concurrent use with a statin is associated with an increased risk of myositis and, rarely, rhabdomyolysis. Concurrent use of cerivastatin and gemfibrozil was noted to cause rhabdomyolysis and this contributed to the withdrawal of cerivastatin from clinical use in 2001.

Bile acid binding agents

The three members of this group in current use are colestyramine, colestipol and colesevelam. Both colestyramine and colestipol were formerly considered first-line agents in the management of patients with FH but now have limited use. Colesevelam is the most recent of the bile acid binding agents to receive marketing authorisation (in 2004) and consequently has never had a first-line indication. Each of the bile acid binding agents reduce TC and increase triglyceride levels.

Table 24.7 Typical drug interactions involving bile acid binding agents and fibrates[a]

Drug group	Interacting drug	Comment
Bile acid binding agents Colestyramine/colestipol		All medication should be taken 1 h before or at least 4 h after colestyramine/colestipol to reduce absorption caused by binding in the gut
	Acarbose	Hypoglycaemia enhanced by colestyramine
	Digoxin	Absorption reduced
	Diuretics	Absorption reduced
	Levothyroxine	Absorption reduced
	Mycophenolate mofetil	Absorption reduced
	Paracetamol	Absorption reduced
	Raloxifene	Absorption reduced
	Valproate	Absorption reduced
	Statins	Absorption reduced
	Vancomycin	Effect of oral vancomycin antagonised by colestyramine
	Warfarin	Increased anticoagulant effect due to depletion of vitamin K or reduced anticoagulant effect due to binding or warfarin in gut
Colesevelam		All medication should be taken at least 4 h before or 4 h after colesevelam to reduce absorption caused by binding in the gut
	Ciclosporin	Absorption reduced
	Digoxin	Absorption unchanged
	Glyburide	Absorption reduced
	Levothyroxine	Absorption reduced
	Oral contraceptive	Absorption reduced
	Statins	Absorption unchanged
	Valproate	Absorption unchanged
	Warfarin	Absorption unchanged. Increased anticoagulant possible due to depletion of vitamin K
Fibrates	Antidiabetic agents	Improvement in glucose tolerance
	Ciclosporin	Increased risk of renal impairment
	Colestyramine/colestipol	Reduced bioavailability of fibrate if taken concomitantly
	Statin	Increased risk of myopathy
	Warfarin	Increased anticoagulant effect

[a]Absorption studies involve concomitant administration.

Following oral administration, neither colestyramine, colestipol nor colesevelam are absorbed from the gut. They bind bile acids in the intestine, prevent re-absorption and produce an insoluble complex that is excreted in the faeces. The depletion of bile acids results in an increase in hepatic synthesis of bile acids from cholesterol. The depletion of hepatic cholesterol upregulates the hepatic enzyme 7-α-hydoxylase which increases the conversion of cholesterol to bile acids. This increases LDL receptor activity in the liver and removes LDL-C from the blood. Hepatic VLDL-C synthesis also increases and it is this which accounts for the raised serum triglycerides.

Colestyramine has a starting dose of one 4 g sachet twice a day. Over a 3- to 4-week period the dose should normally be built up to 12–24 g daily taken in water or a suitable liquid as a single dose, or up to four divided doses each day. Occasionally, 36 g a day may be required, although the benefits of increasing the dose above 16 g a day are offset by gastro-intestinal disturbances and poor patient adherence.

Colestipol is also available in a granular formulation and can be mixed with an appropriate liquid at a dose of 5 g once or twice daily. This dose can be increased every 1–2 months to a maximum of 30 g in a single- or twice-daily regimen.

Colesevalam is up to six times as potent as the other bile acid binding agents, probably because of a greater binding to glycocholic acid. Whether this translates into better clinical outcomes or more, or less, problems with drugs administered concurrently is unclear. Colesevalam is administered as a 625-mg tablet to a maximum dose of 4.375 g/day (7 tablets). There is limited evidence to suggest it may achieve a higher adherence than colestyramine or colestipol. It can be taken as a single- or twice-daily regimen.

Adverse effects

With all three agents, side effects are more likely to occur with high doses and in patients aged over 60 years. Bloating, flatulence, heartburn and constipation are common complaints. Constipation is the major subjective side effect, and although usually mild and transient, it may be severe.

Colestyramine, colestipol and colesevelam are known to interact with many drugs primarily by interfering with absorption (Table 24.7). Whether these absorption-type interactions are qualitatively and quantitatively similar between the different agents is unclear and the picture is confused when the absorption of a given drug is known to interact with one bile acid binding agent but has not been tested with other members of the group.

Long-term use of bile acid binding agents may also interfere with the absorption of fat soluble vitamins and supplementation with vitamins A, D and K is recommended.

Patient counselling

Palatability is often a major problem with the bile acid binding agents and patients need to be well motivated and prepared for the problems they may encounter.

Both colestyramine and colestipol are available in an orange flavour and/or as a low sugar (aspartame-containing) powder. Colestipol is without taste and is odourless. Each sachet of colestyramine or colestipol should be added to at least 150 or 100 mL of liquid, respectively, and stirred vigorously to avoid the powder clumping. The powder does not dissolve but disperses in the chosen liquid, which may be water, fruit juice, skimmed milk or non-carbonated beverage. Both may also be taken in soups, with cereals, and with pulpy fruits with high moisture content, such as apple sauce.

All patients receiving a bile acid binding agent should be advised that reduced absorption with co-administered drugs should be anticipated. Medication that has to be taken should be administered 1 h before (at least 4 h for colesevelam) or at least 4 h after the bile acid binding agent. As a consequence, for individuals on multiple drug therapy, bile acid binding agents may not be appropriate for this reason alone.

Cholesterol absorption inhibitors

Ezetimibe is a 2-azetidinone derivative that interacts with a putative cholesterol transporter in the intestinal brush border membrane and thereby blocks cholesterol re-absorption from the gastro-intestinal tract. It can reduce LDL-C by 15–20% when added to diet. Ezetimibe also brings about a small increase in HDL-C and a reduction in triglycerides. When added to a statin, ezetimibe lowers LDL-C more than with a statin alone.

Ezetimibe should be prescribed either with a statin, a fibrate or a nicotinic acid derivative and rarely by itself, and then only in statin intolerant individuals. Although apparently well tolerated, no long-term trials (Kastelein et al., 2008; Rossebø et al., 2008) have demonstrated an additional reduction in cardiovascular morbidity or mortality that could be attributed to ezetimibe.

Nicotinic acid and derivatives

Nicotinic acid in pharmacological doses (1.5–6 g) lowers serum LDL-C, TC, VLDL-C, apolipoprotein B, triglycerides and Lp(a) and increases levels of HDL-C (particularly the beneficial HDL$_3$ subfraction). It clearly has a range of beneficial effects on the lipid profile and is licensed for use in combination with a statin, or by itself if the patient is statin-intolerant or a statin is inappropriate.

The commonest side effect of nicotinic acid is flushing which is most prominent in the head, neck and upper torso and occurs in over 90% of patients. It is cited as the major reason for discontinuation of treatment in 25–40% of patients. A number of strategies have been devised to overcome this, including co-administration of a cyclo-oxygenase inhibitor such as aspirin. Other strategies include regular consistent dosing, the use of extended-release formulations, patient education, dosing with meals or at bedtime, and the avoidance of alcohol, hot beverages, spicy foods, and hot baths or showers close to or after dosing. Less common side effects of nicotinic acid include postural hypotension, diarrhoea, exacerbation of peptic ulcers, hepatic dysfunction, gout and increased blood glucose levels.

Acipimox is structurally related to nicotinic acid, has similar beneficial effects on the lipid profile and a better side effect profile but appears to be less potent. An extended-release preparation of nicotinic acid has also been marketed to reduce the incidence of side effects, but up to 30% of users still report problems.

The most recent nicotinic acid-based product to be marketed is a fixed dose combination of nicotinic acid with laropriprant marketed as Tredaptive® in 2008. It is licensed for use in combination with a statin or as monotherapy when a statin is inappropriate or not tolerated. Tredaptive® possesses the general benefit of nicotinic acid whilst the laropriprant is a potent, selective antagonist of the prostaglandin D$_2$ receptor subtype 1 (DP$_1$). Given that prostaglandin D$_2$ mediates the flushing associated with nicotinic acid the rationale for the combination is sound, but there are currently no long-term trials of efficacy and tolerability.

Fish oils

Fish oil preparations rich in omega-3 fatty acids have been shown to markedly reduce serum triglyceride levels by decreasing VLDL-C synthesis, although little change has been observed in LDL-C or HDL-C levels. The effect is, however, inconsistent and significant increases in LDL-C have also been reported to accompany the use of fish oils. Data from several studies suggest that omega-3 fatty acids protect against CHD mortality, particularly sudden death, rather than non-fatal events, but this may not be due to the lipid-lowering efficacy. Commercial products available contain omega-3-acid ethyl esters (Omacor®) and omega-3-marine triglycerides (Maxepa®). Either can be used as an alternative to a fibrate or in combination with a statin.

Soluble fibre

Preparations containing soluble fibre, such as ispaghula husk, have been shown to reduce lipid levels. The fibre is thought to bind bile acids in the gut and increase the conversion of cholesterol to bile acids in the liver. However, their role in the management of dyslipidaemia is unclear and they are much less effective than statins in reducing TC and LDL-C.

Cholesterol ester transfer protein (CETP) inhibitors

Low levels of CETP are associated with increased levels of HDL-C and reduced cardiovascular risk. CETP transfers cholesterol from HDL-C to LDL-C and VLDL-C, thereby altering the HDL-C:LDL-C ratio in a potentially unfavourable manner. As a consequence, inhibitors of CETP are expected to have a beneficial cardiovascular effect. Torcetrapib was a potent inhibitor of CETP and in trials demonstrated a dose-dependent ability to increase HDL-C, with little effect on LDL-C or triglycerides. Increases in serum HDL-C of more than 100% were reported. Unfortunately, the side effect profile of torcetrapib included an increase in cardiovascular events and all cause mortality thereby preventing it reaching the market. Newer inhibitors of CETP include dalcetrapib and anacetrapib and these look more promising.

Case studies

Case 24.1

Mr DF is a 43-year-old man who has been relatively fit and well for the past 20 years during which he has rarely visited his primary care doctor. Two weeks ago he was admitted to hospital having suffered a myocardial infarction. On questioning it was revealed that his brother had died in a road traffic accident at the age of 19 and his father had died from CHD aged 54 years.

Examination of Mr DF revealed a corneal arcus and tendon xanthomas. Blood drawn within 2h of the onset of his myocardial infarction revealed TC 7.8 mmol/L, HDL-C 0.9 mmol/L and triglycerides 2.3 mmol/L.

Questions

1. What is the likely diagnosis of Mr DF?
2. What are the treatment options?
3. Mr DF wants to know why he was not identified as being at high risk of CHD before he suffered his myocardial infarction.

Answers

1. Mr DF has the signs and family history of classic heterozygous FH, most likely due to a genetic defect in the LDL receptor on hepatocytes. His presentation with an acute cardiac event at such an early age is indicative of the raised cardiovascular risk present for individuals with FH.
2. Mr DF has a high level of LDL-C and action is required to reduce it. Appropriate lifestyle advice is necessary but a statin will be required to achieve the desired outcome of at least a 50% reduction in LDL-C. In addition, this patient has recently suffered a myocardial infarction, which in itself is an indication for a high intensity statin first line, such as atorvastatin 80 mg daily. This patient should be managed by a specialist in the first instance and relatives, including any children, should be screened for the presence of FH to allow initiation of early lipid-lowering therapy.
3. Unfortunately, Mr DF's father probably died of heart disease at a time when the practice of detecting affected families and screening first-degree relatives was not widespread. The early, unrelated death of his brother and Mr DF's previous good health would not have given an opportunity to identify any underlying familial disorder.

   From population data it is known that the prevalence of heterozygous FH is about 1 in 500. Consequently, 120,000 cases would be expected in the UK. However, far fewer cases are known and screening programmes to track cases in affected families are now in place. A family history of elevated TC or death

from CHD before the age of 55 in a first-degree male relative, as in the case of Mr DF, is an important sign that should highlight the potential risk to other family members.

Case 24.2

Mr PT is a 52-year-old active school teacher. Four years ago he was found to have a raised TC and elevated blood pressure for which he was started on 10 mg simvastatin and 2.5 mg bendroflumethiazide. Over the years his dose of simvastatin has been gradually increased to 40 mg a day, but apart from this his medication has remained unchanged. He presents at the clinic complaining of aches and pains in his legs over the past 10 days. On questioning he reveals that over recent months he has been eating fresh grapefruit and consuming the occasional glass of grapefruit juice. A tentative diagnosis of myopathy is initially made.

Questions

1. What is the likelihood that grapefruit juice has contributed to Mr PT's problem?
2. Are any additional biochemical tests warranted?
3. Would atorvastatin, rosuvastatin or pravastatin be a more appropriate statin to prescribe if Mr PT wanted to continue with the occasional glass of grapefruit juice?

Answers

1. Grapefruit juice is known to interact with statins through its inhibition of the cytochrome P450 CYP3A4 enzyme. It has been suggested that it is the furanocoumarin in the grapefruit juice which binds to CYP3A4 and inactivates it in both the liver and the gastro-intestinal tract. As little as 200 mL of grapefruit juice may inhibit CYP3A4, thereby prolonging the half-life of the statin and increasing serum levels. When taken on a regular basis this can increase the risk of dose-related side effects such as rhabdomyolysis and increase the risk of myopathy. Current advice is that grapefruit juice should be avoided altogether when taking simvastatin, regardless of whether it is fresh grapefruit or grapefruit juice, grapefruit juice diluted from concentrate or frozen grapefruit juice.
2. A creatine kinase (CK) level should be checked in patients complaining of significant muscle pain to exclude overt myopathy.
   - If CK is raised significantly (>5 times upper normal level), temporary withdrawal of the statin is warranted. Once the CK falls to normal levels, and in view of the suspicion that grapefruit intake was a precipitating factor, the statin could be reinitiated and the patient warned to avoid grapefruit and seek advice promptly should the muscle aches recur.
   - If the CK is normal, then this is a simple myalgia. Grapefruit should be avoided and hopefully the symptoms resolve. If the pain does not resolve this may have an impact on adherence and an alternate statin should be considered. Of all the agents currently on the UK market, simvastatin is more likely to cause myalgia and myopathy.
3. Atorvastatin is also metabolised by CYP3A4. Although the effect is less dramatic than with simvastatin, the concurrent intake of large quantities of grapefruit juice with atorvastatin is not recommended. Neither pravastatin nor rosuvastatin is substantially metabolised by P450 and may be better alternatives. However, when there is a past history of myopathy the need for caution remains as the risk of recurrence is enhanced whatever lipid-lowering agent is prescribed. It should also be noted that rosuvastatin, unlike pravastatin, has no clinical outcome data and would not be appropriate for use in this

patient. There are also separate concerns regarding the muscle toxicity of rosuvastatin, especially when used at the higher dose of 40 mg. This again would indicate that rosuvastatin is not the best option for Mr PT.

As this patient is being treated with a statin for primary prevention, National Institute of Health and Clinical Excellence (2008a) guidelines suggest that only generic statin agents are cost-effective and, therefore, pravastatin should be considered as a first-line alternative for this patient.

Case 24.3

Mrs MC is a very active, 51-year-old caucasian lady who for the past 6 months has been suffering from the classic symptoms of the menopause. Six months ago on a routine visit to her doctor she had her lipid profile measured and this revealed an HDL-C of 0.8 mmol/L and TC of 5 mmol/L. Her blood pressure was 140/80 mmHg. She is currently prescribed no medication but is receiving intensive lifestyle support to lower her cholesterol. She has no other medical history of note other than a record that her mother died at the age of 66 years from a heart attack.

Mrs MC would like to be prescribed hormone replacement therapy to control her menopausal symptoms and reduce her risk of CVD.

Questions

1. Is it appropriate to prescribe hormone replacement therapy to reduce Mrs MC's cardiovascular risk?
2. What is the value of measuring HDL-C?
3. Does Mrs MC have a risk of CVD that requires treatment with a lipid-lowering agent?

Answers

1. Most epidemiological studies have demonstrated a beneficial effect of hormone replacement therapy on the development of CHD in postmenopausal women. However, randomised controlled trials with defined clinical endpoints have failed to support a reduction in cardiovascular events. Whether this has arisen because of how the body responds to hormone replacement therapy, the age of the women studied or the influence of the type of hormone replacement therapy, the dose, route of administration and duration of treatment is unclear. At present there are no compelling data to justify the use of hormone replacement therapy for the prevention or treatment of CVD in postmenopausal women. In fact, current evidence indicates that HRT may increase the risk of breast cancer, ovarian cancer, CVD and thromboembolic disease. If Mrs MC is to be prescribed HRT, then this should be based on the need to control her menopausal symptoms and improve her quality of life.
2. HDL-C is a major fraction of cholesterol in serum and an important determinant of cardiovascular risk in men and women, even when the level of TC appears to be within the normal range. The incidence of myocardial infarction is positively correlated with the cholesterol concentration and inversely related to the concentration of HDL-C. The TC:HDL-C ratio is another way to represent this risk and has been shown to have good predictive capabilities in women. Until the menopause, women generally have high levels of HDL-C as a result of the circulating oestrogen. However, following the menopause, HDL-C levels fall rapidly. Lifestyle advice may improve the TC/HDL ratio, especially via increased physical activity.

3. With reference to the Joint British Societies risk prediction charts, it can be determined that with a TC:HDL-C ratio of 6.25 (5/0.8) and a systolic blood pressure of 140 mmHg, Mrs MC has a 10–20% risk of developing CVD over the next 10 years. This would not automatically make her a candidate for treatment with a lipid-lowering agent as her 10-year cardiovascular risk is not >20%. Knowledge of Mrs MC's BMI and blood glucose level would be useful additional information, as would a more detailed insight into her family history of CVD. It is only when all the relevant information has been gathered that a final decision on the use of a lipid-lowering agent can be made. It would also be of interest to determine whether the lifestyle support has brought about any improvement in Mrs MC's lipid profile or blood pressure.

Case 24.4

Mr EC is a 48-year-old executive for a large multinational company who works long hours and frequently has to travel abroad. He has a family history of CHD and 9 months ago he attended a coronary screening clinic for a health check. At the clinic he was found to have a normal blood pressure but a blood screen revealed a TC of 5.7 mmol/L and triglycerides of 11.8 mmol/L. When he revisited the clinic 4 weeks later after trying to follow dietary advice, a fasting blood sample revealed a TC of 5 mmol/L and triglycerides of 2.7 mmol/L. Liver function tests were normal. He is a non-smoker and claims never to drink more than 10 units of alcohol per week.

After repeated requests to revisit the clinic he eventually turned up stating he had been away from home for 6 months on a series of business trips. He was trying to keep to a low-fat diet and his blood profile revealed TC 5.7 mmol/L, triglycerides 4.3 mmol/L, HDL-C 0.8 mmol/L and LDL-C 3 mmol/L.

Questions

1. Is Mr EC at high risk of CHD?
2. Is Mr EC a candidate for lipid-lowering therapy?
3. Should Mr EC's children be screened for dyslipidaemia?

Answers

1. Mr EC has a TC:HDL-C ratio of 7.1 (5.7/0.8). If the Joint British Societies risk charts were used they would indicate he has a 10-year risk of CHD of 10–20% and does not require lipid-lowering treatment. However, the tables underestimate the risk of CHD in those with familial hyperlipidaemia or a history of premature CHD.

   Mr EC would appear to have a mixed lipaemia, although it is difficult to interpret non-fasting triglycerides because of the influence of food intake. The low HDL-C suggests he is overweight and/or has a non-ideal lifestyle. Exclusion of diabetes, high alcohol intake, liver and renal impairment is necessary. The possibility of impaired glucose tolerance should not be overlooked and a glucose tolerance test should be performed.
2. Given the elevated triglycerides and TC, Mr EC is certainly a candidate for lifestyle advice. The use of a statin may be considered if the lifestyle changes do not bring about the necessary improvements in the lipid profile. However, the dyslipidaemia may be secondary to obesity, alcoholism, diabetes or hypothyroidism. If any of these disorders are present the appropriate treatment may correct the underlying dyslipidaemia.

3. The family history of CHD is important but is only significant if the age of onset in a parent or sibling was under 55 years of age for an affected male or under 65 years for an affected female. A rare familial disorder, for example, familial dysbetalipoproteinaemia, may be the causative factor. If this was confirmed his children should be screened after puberty as the offending gene may not express itself in the younger child.

Mr EC was subsequently found to have diabetes for which he initially received metformin together with a statin. In this scenario where a patient is diagnosed with type 2 diabetes, it is also important to consider advising children about lifestyle issues and the need to control weight throughout life.

Case 24.5

Mr JT is a 68-year-old man with stable angina. He is currently receiving simvastatin 40 mg daily with well controlled lipid levels (TC 3.8 mmol/L; LDL-C 1.8 mmol/L; HDL-C 0.9 mmol/L, triglycerides 1.3 mmol/L). He has been on simvastatin for the past 7 years, and has complained previously about muscle aches, but on this visit he states that his muscle pain has become more troublesome, to the extent that he wishes to come off the statin. He asks if there is nothing else he can take to control his cholesterol.

Questions

1. What action would you take immediately?
2. What options are available for Mr JT?
3. What would you recommend to Mr JT?

Answers

1. A CK level should be checked to exclude myopathy in this patient, as this can occur at any time during statin treatment. Assuming the CK is normal and this is myalgia, then it is still essential to address this patient's concerns, as this muscle pain is likely to impact on patient adherence over time.

An important issue is to ensure that the patient understands why they are taking a statin. The emphasis should be on the expected reduction in the risk of death, heart attack or stroke; rather than on simply achieving cholesterol treatment targets.

It may be worth temporarily stopping the statin to demonstrate the causal relationship. If the aches and pains remain despite cessation of simvastatin, then this is unlikely to be a statin-related issue. Many people complain of aches and pains, particularly as they get older and it is easy to blame the statin for all these complaints.

2. Options for Mr JT include:
   a. Reducing the dose of simvastatin

   Mr JT has been on simvastatin for many years and a simple reduction in dose to 20 mg may improve tolerability without compromising the lipid control substantially. While an increase in TC and LDL-C is expected with dose reduction, this is usually small (in the order of 6%) and should have little overall impact on risk.
   b. Substituting an alternative statin

   Simvastatin causes more myalgia and myopathy than other statins; therefore, an alternative agent may be better-tolerated. Pravastatin is particularly well tolerated and may be a suitable alternative in this patient where potency is less of an issue. Where greater potency is required, atorvastatin (starting at a dose of 10–20 mg daily and increasing as required to control lipids) or rosuvastatin are a possibility.
   c. Switching to an alternative agent, such as ezetimibe

   Non-statin agents could be used to lower cholesterol but should be reserved for patients unable to tolerate statins. Ezetimibe monotherapy may be a suitable alternative, although use is not supported by cardiovascular outcome data.
   d. Using a low dose of statin plus an alternative agent, such as ezetimibe

   This may be a suitable option if this patient can only tolerate small doses of statins, and the ezetimibe is introduced to increase the degree of cholesterol lowering achieved. This is a useful combination in some patients, but every effort should be made to maximise the statin dose prior to adding ezetimibe to ensure maximal outcome benefits.

3. In this patient, a good starting point would be a reduction in the dose of simvastatin to 20 mg daily, providing the patient is willing to continue to take this drug. Myalgia appears to be dose related and the symptoms may resolve with the lower dose. An alternative is to try pravastatin, perhaps at a starting dose of 20 mg to see if this is better tolerated. The dose will probably need increasing to give adequate control of lipid levels. The use of ezetimibe should be reserved as an add-in if only low doses of statins can be tolerated or for monotherapy if that patient cannot be persuaded to take any statin at all. This patient should be reviewed regularly over the next few months until his concerns regarding his lipid-lowering therapy have been addressed, to encourage on-going adherence.

References

British Heart Foundation, 2008. Coronary Heart Disease Statistics Book. BHF, London.

British Hypertension Society, 2009. Proposed Joint British Societies Cardiovascular Disease Risk Assessment Charts. Available at: http://www.bhsoc.org/Cardiovascular_Risk_Prediction_Chart.stm.

Chapman, M.J., Le Goff, W., Guerin, M., et al., 2010. Cholestery ester transfer protein: at the heart of the action of lipid modulating therapy with statins, fibrates, niacin, and cholesteryl ester transfer protein inhibitors. Eur. Heart J. 31, 149–164.

Emerging Risk Factors Collaboration, 2009. Lipoprotein(a) concentration and the risk of coronary heart disease, stroke, and nonvascular mortality. J. Am. Med. Assoc. 302, 412–423.

FIELD Investigators, 2005. Effects of long-term fenofibrate therapy on cardiovascular events in 9795 people with type 2 diabetes mellitus (the FIELD study): randomised controlled trial. Lancet 366, 1849–1861.

Kastelein, J.J., Akdim, F., Stroes, E.S., et al., 2008. Simvastatin with or without ezetimibe in familial hypercholesterolemia. The ENHANCE study. N. Engl. J. Med. 358, 1431–1443.

Kausik, R.K., Sreenivasa, R.K.S., Erqou, S., et al., 2010. Statins and all-cause-mortality in high-risk primary prevention: a meta-analysis of 11 randomized controlled trials involving 65,229 participants. Arch. Intern. Med. 170, 1024–1031.

Kolovou, G.D., Anagnostopoulou, K.K., Cokkinos, D.V., 2005. Pathophysiology of dyslipidaemia in the metabolic syndrome. Postgrad. Med. J. 81, 358–366.

National Institute of Health and Clinical Excellence, 2008a. Cardiovascular Risk Assessment and the Modification of Blood Lipids for the Primary and Secondary Prevention of Cardiovascular Disease. NICE, London. Available at: http://www.nice.org.uk/CG067.

National Institute of Health and Clinical Excellence, 2008b. Identification and Management of Familial Hypercholesterolaemia. NICE, London. Available at: http://guidance.nice.org.uk/CG71/Guidance/pdf/English.

Rossebø, A.B., Pedersen, T.R., Boman, K., et al., for the SEAS Investigators, 2008. Intensive lipid lowering with simvastatin and ezetimibe in aortic stenosis. N. Engl. J. Med. 359, 1343–1356.

Triglyceride Coronary Disease Genetics Consortium and Emerging Risk Factors Collaboration, 2010. Triglyceride-mediated pathways and coronary disease: collaborative analysis of 101 studies. Lancet 375, 1634–1639.

UKMI, 2009. Lipid Modification. North West Medicines Information Service, Liverpool. Available at: http://www.nelm.nhs.uk/en/ NeLM-Area/Health-In-Focus/NICE-Bites--August-0908/.

Woodward, M., Brindle, P., Tunstall-Pedoe, H., 2007. Adding social deprivation and family history to cardiovascular risk assessment: the ASSIGN score from the Scottish Heart Health Extended Cohort (SHHEC). Heart 93, 172–176.

Further reading

Brinton, E.A., 2008. Does the addition of fibrates to statin therapy have a favourable risk to benefit ratio. Curr. Atherosclerosis Rep. 10, 25–32.

Cannon, C.P., Steinberg, B.A., Murphy, S.A., et al., 2006. Meta-analysis of cardiovascular outcomes trials comparing intensive versus moderate statin therapy. J. Am. Coll. Cardiol. 48, 438–445.

Genest, J., McPherson, R., Frohlich, J., et al., 2009. Canadian Cardiovascular Society/Canadian guidelines for the diagnosis and treatment of dyslipidaemia and prevention of cardiovascular disease in the adult – 2009 recommendations. Can. J. Cardiol. 25, 567–579.

Kearney, P.M., Blackwell, L., Collins, R., et al., 2008. Cholesterol Treatment Trialists' (CTT) collaborators: efficacy of cholesterol-lowering therapy in 18,686 people with diabetes in 14 randomised trials of statins: a meta-analysis. Lancet 371, 117–125.

Mills, E.J., Rachlis, B., Wu, P., et al., 2008. Primary prevention of cardiovascular mortality and events with statin treatment. J. Am. Coll. Cardiol. 52, 1769–1781.

Ray, K.K., Seshasai, S.R., Erqou, S., et al., 2010. Statins and all-cause mortality in high-risk primary prevention: a meta-analysis of 11 randomized controlled trials involving 65,229 participants. Arch. Intern. Med. 170, 1024–1031.

25 Asthma

K. P. Gibbs and D. Cripps

Key points

- Asthma is a common and chronic inflammatory condition of the airways whose cause is not completely understood.
- Common symptoms are caused by hyperresponsive airways and include coughing, wheezing, chest tightness and shortness of breath.
- The only reliable, simple and objective way to diagnose asthma is to demonstrate reversible airflow limitation.
- In the UK, there are approximately 1400 deaths from asthma each year.
- Asthma is still a poorly controlled disease despite effective treatments.
- Asthma triggers should be avoided or controlled.
- Pharmacological therapy should involve early anti-inflammatory treatment in all but the mildest asthmatics and follow national, evidence-based guidance.
- Optimum treatment involves the lowest doses of therapy that provide good symptom control with minimal or no side effects, and the best drug delivery device is one that the patient can use correctly.
- Patients should be encouraged and educated to take an active role in their disease management, be given individualised self-management plans and be regularly supervised by the health care team.

Asthma means 'laboured breathing' in Greek and was first described 3000 years ago. It is a broad term used to refer to a disorder of the respiratory system that leads to episodic difficulty in breathing. The national UK guidelines (BTS/SIGN, 2009) define asthma as 'a chronic inflammatory disorder of the airways which occurs in susceptible individuals; inflammatory symptoms are usually associated with widespread but variable airflow obstruction and an increase in airway response to a variety of stimuli. Obstruction is often reversible either spontaneously or with treatment'.

Epidemiology

The exact prevalence of asthma remains uncertain because of the differing ways in which airway restriction is reported, diagnostic uncertainty (especially for children under 2 years) and the overlap with other conditions such as chronic obstructive pulmonary disease (COPD). Over 5 million people in the UK have asthma (Asthma UK, 2001) and around 300 million worldwide. Mortality from asthma is estimated at approximately 0.4 per 100,000 with around 1400 deaths per annum in the UK. Most deaths occur outside hospital; the most common reasons for death are thought to be inadequate assessment of the severity of airway obstruction by the patient and/or clinician and inadequate therapy with inhaled or oral steroids.

The probability of children having asthma-like symptoms is estimated to be between 5% and 12%, with a higher occurrence in boys than girls and in children whose parents have an allergic disorder. Between 30% and 70% of children will become symptom free by adulthood. Individuals who develop asthma at an early age, however, do have a poorer prognosis.

The prevalence of asthma actually appears to be rising despite advances in therapy. There is some doubt about this, however, due to the differing criteria for the diagnosis of asthma used in different studies. Asthma is considered to be one of the consequences of Western civilisation and appears to be related to a number of environmental factors. Air pollution resulting from industrial sources and transport may be interacting with smoking, dietary and other factors to increase the incidence of this debilitating problem.

Aetiology

The two main causes of asthma symptoms are airway hyperresponsiveness and bronchoconstriction. Hyperresponsiveness is an increased tendency of the airway to react to stimuli or triggers to cause an asthma attack. Bronchoconstriction is a narrowing of the airways that causes airflow obstruction. Possible triggers are listed in Table 25.1. One of the most common trigger factors is the allergen found in the faeces of the house dust mite, which is almost universally present in bedding, carpets and soft furnishing. Pollen from grass (prevalent in June and July) can lead to seasonal asthma. The role of occupation in the development of asthma has become apparent with increased industrialisation. There are many causes of occupational asthma, and bronchial reactivity may persist for years after exposure to the trigger factor. Drug-induced asthma can be severe and the most common causes are β-blocker drugs and prostaglandin synthetase inhibitors. The administration of β-adrenoceptor blockers to a patient, even in the form of eye drops, can cause β_2-receptor

Table 25.1 Examples of asthma triggers

Trigger	Examples
Allergens	Pollens, moulds, house dust mite, animals (dander, saliva and urine)
Industrial chemicals	Manufacture of, for example, isocyanate-containing paints, epoxy resins, aluminium, hair sprays, penicillins and cimetidine
Drugs	Aspirin, ibuprofen and other prostaglandin synthetase inhibitors, β-adrenoceptor blockers
Foods	A rare cause but examples include nuts, fish, seafood, dairy products, food colouring, especially tartrazine, benzoic acid and sodium metabisulfite
Environmental pollutants	Traffic fumes. cigarette smoke, sulphur dioxide
Other industrial triggers	Wood or grain dust, colophony in solder, cotton, dust, grain weevils and mites
Miscellaneous	Cold air, exercise, hyperventilation, viral respiratory tract infections, emotion or stress, swimming pool chlorine

blockade and consequent bronchoconstriction. Selective β-adrenoceptor blockers are thought to pose slightly less risk, but as these lose their selectivity at higher doses, it is generally recommended that this group of drugs is avoided altogether in asthma patients. Aspirin and related non-steroidal anti-inflammatory drugs can cause severe bronchoconstriction in susceptible individuals. Aspirin inhibits the enzyme cyclo-oxygenase, which normally converts arachidonic acid to (bronchodilatory) prostaglandins. When this pathway is blocked, an alternative reaction predominates, leading to an increase in production of bronchoconstrictor (cys-) leukotrienes. Figures from differing studies vary, but between 2% and 20% of the adult asthma population are thought to be sensitive to aspirin.

Pathophysiology

Asthma can be classified according to the underlying pattern of airway inflammation with the presence or absence of eosinophils in the airways (eosinophilic vs. non-eosinophilic). Traditionally patients are described as having 'extrinsic asthma' when an allergen is thought to be the cause of their asthma. This is more common in children with a history of atopy, where triggers, such as dust mite, cause IgE production. Other environmental factors are also important, such as exposure to rhinovirus during the first 3 years of life (Holgate et al., 2010). 'Intrinsic asthma' develops in adulthood, with symptoms triggered by non-allergenic factors such as a viral

infection, irritants which cause epithelial damage and mucosal inflammation, emotional upset which mediates excess parasympathetic input or exercise which causes water and heat loss from the airways, triggering mediator release from mast cells. In practice, patients often have features of both types of asthma and the classification is unhelpful and oversimplifies the pathogenesis of asthma.

Mast cell components are released as a result of an IgE antibody-mediated reaction on the surface of the cell. Histamine and other mediators of inflammation are released from mast cells, for example, leukotrienes, prostaglandins, bradykinin, adenosine and prostaglandin-generating factor of anaphylaxis, as well as various chemotactic agents that attract eosinophils and neutrophils. Macrophages release prostaglandins, thromboxane and platelet-activating factor (PAF). PAF appears to sustain bronchial hyperreactivity and cause respiratory capillaries to leak plasma, which increases mucosal oedema. PAF also facilitates the accumulation of eosinophils within the airways, a characteristic pathological feature of asthma. Eosinophils release various inflammatory mediators such as leukotriene C_4 (LTC_4) and PAF. Epithelial damage results and thick viscous mucus is produced that causes further deterioration in lung function. These cell-derived mediators also play a role in causing marked hypertrophy and hyperplasia of bronchial smooth muscle (these structural changes are described as 'airway remodelling'), mucus gland hypertrophy leading to excessive mucus production and airway plugging, airway oedema, acute bronchoconstriction and impaired mucociliary clearance.

Mucus production is normally a defence mechanism, but in asthma patients, there is an increase in the size of bronchial glands and goblet cells that produce mucus. Mucus transport is dependent on its viscosity. If it is very thick, it plugs the airways, which also become blocked with epithelial and inflammatory cell debris. Mucociliary clearance is also decreased due to inflammation of epithelial cells. The environmental insults causing asthma are also thought to affect the structure and function of the airway epithelium. The exact role of these cytokines, cellular mediators and the interrelationships with each other and with the causative allergenic or non-allergenic mechanisms has, however, yet to be fully determined and may vary over time (Douwes et al., 2002; Holgate et al., 2010). Fig. 25.1 outlines the main cellular mechanisms involved.

Clinical manifestations

Asthma can present in a number of ways. It may manifest as a persistent cough, but most commonly, it is described as recurrent episodes of difficulty in breathing (dyspnoea) associated with wheezing (a high-pitched noise due to turbulent airflow through a narrowed airway). Diagnosis is usually made from the clinical history confirmed by demonstration of reversible airflow obstruction and measures of lung function. The history of an asthma patient often includes the presence of atopy and allergic rhinitis in the close family. Symptoms of asthma are often intermittent, and the frequency and severity of an episode can vary from individual to individual. Between periods

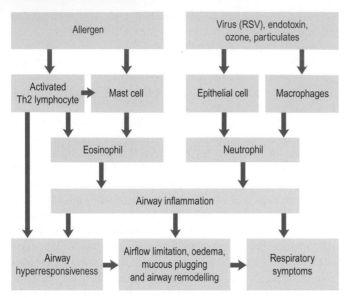

Fig. 25.1 Postulated cellular mechanisms involved in airway inflammation (adapted from Douwes et al., 2002).

of wheezing and breathlessness, patients may feel quite well. The absence of an improvement in ventilation, however, cannot rule out asthma, and in younger children, it is sometimes very difficult to perform lung function tests; in this case, diagnosis relies on subjective symptomatic improvement in response to bronchodilator therapy.

Acute severe asthma is a dangerous condition that requires hospitalisation and immediate emergency treatment. It occurs when bronchospasm has progressed to a state where the patient is breathless at rest and has a degree of cardiac stress. This is usually progressive and can build up over a number of hours or even days. The breathlessness, with a peak flow rate <100 L/min, is so severe that the patient often cannot talk or lie down. Expiration is particularly difficult and prolonged as air is trapped beneath mucosal inflammation. The pulse rate can give an indication of severity; severe acute asthma can increase the pulse rate to more than 110 beats/min in adults. It is common to see hyperexpansion of the thoracic cavity and lowering of the diaphragm, which means that accessory respiratory muscles are required to try to inflate the chest. Breathing can become rapid (>30 breaths/min) and shallow, leading to low oxygen saturation ($SpO_2 < 92\%$) with the patient becoming fatigued, cyanosed, confused and lethargic. The arterial carbon dioxide tension ($PaCO_2$) is usually low in acute asthma. If it is high, it should respond quickly to emergency therapy. Hypercapnia (high $PaCO_2$ level) that does not diminish is a more severe problem and indicates progression towards respiratory failure.

Some patients remain difficult to control with persistent symptoms and/or despite treatment at BTS/SIGN step 4 or 5. This is known as 'refractory' or 'difficult to treat' asthma. These patients must be carefully evaluated by a respiratory specialist; this will include confirming an accurate diagnosis of asthma, adherence to therapy and individual psychological factors.

Investigations

The function of the lungs can be measured to help diagnose and monitor various respiratory diseases. A series of routine tests has been developed to assess asthma as well as other respiratory diseases such as COPD.

The most useful test for abnormalities in airway function is the forced expiratory volume (FEV). This is measured by means of lung function assessment apparatus such as a spirometer. The patient inhales as deeply as possible and then exhales forcefully and completely into a mouthpiece connected to a spirometer. The FEV_1 is a measure of the FEV in the first second of exhalation. The forced vital capacity (FVC) can also be measured, which is an assessment of the maximum volume of air exhaled with maximum effort after maximum inspiration. The FEV_1 is usually expressed as a percentage of the total volume of air exhaled, reported as the FEV_1/FVC ratio. This ratio is a useful and highly reproducible measure of the capabilities of the lungs. Normal individuals can exhale at least 70% of their total capacity in 1 s. In obstructive lung disorders, such as asthma, the FEV_1 is usually decreased, the FVC normal or slightly reduced and the FEV_1/FVC ratio decreased, usually <0.7 (Fig. 25.2).

A peak flow meter is a useful means of self-assessment for the patient. It gives slightly less reproducible results than the spirometer but has the advantage that the patient can do regular tests at home with a hand-held meter. The peak flow meter measures peak expiratory flow (PEF) rate, the maximum flow rate that can be forced during expiration. The PEF can be used to assess the improvement or deterioration in the disease as well as the effectiveness of treatment. For all three measurements (FEV_1, FVC and PEF), there are normal values with which the patient's results can be compared. However, these normal values vary with age, race, gender, height and weight. The measurement of FEV_1, FVC or PEF does not detect early deterioration of lung function such as bronchospasm and mucus plugging in the smaller airways.

The diagnosis of asthma can be confirmed by measuring the response to a bronchodilator or by examining a patient's day-to-day variation in PEF readings. A diurnal variability of 60 L/min (or more than 20%) is highly suggestive of asthma

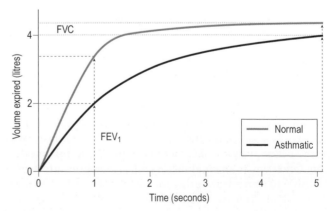

Fig. 25.2 Typical lung spirometry in normal subjects and asthma patients.

(GINA, 2009). However, individuals may not have airflow obstruction at the time of the test, so the absence of an improvement does not rule out asthma. In this situation, peak flow readings can be done at home with repeated pre- and post-bronchodilator readings taken at various times of the day.

Treatment

As asthma involves inflammation and bronchoconstriction, treatment should be directed towards reducing inflammation and increasing bronchodilation. Treatment aims should include a lack of day and nighttime symptoms, no asthma exacerbations, no need for rescue medication, normal PEFs and no unwanted side effects from medication (BTS/SIGN, 2009; GINA, 2009). Anti-inflammatory drugs should be given to all but those with the mildest of symptoms. Other measures, such as avoidance of recognised trigger factors, may also contribute to the control of this disease. The lowest effective dose of drugs should be given to minimise short-term and long-term side effects. It should, however, always be remembered that asthma is a potentially life-threatening illness, is often undertreated and not all patients will achieve optimal control. Common therapeutic and practice problems encountered in the management of asthma are outlined in Box 25.1.

Chronic asthma

The pharmacological management of asthma depends upon the frequency and severity of a patient's symptoms. Infrequent attacks can be managed by treating each attack when it occurs, but with more frequent attacks, preventive therapy needs to be used.

Box 25.1   Management of common practice problems

- Reducing exposure to trigger risk factors may help to improve asthma control.
- Successful management of asthma requires a partnership between the patient and the health care provider.
- Aim to give patients the ability to control their asthma by supporting guided self-management.
- Individualised action plans improve health outcomes, particularly in moderate to severe disease.
- Increased use of reliever medication is a warning of deterioration of asthma control.
- Assessment of asthma control is essential when deciding to step up or step down treatment.
- At each treatment review, inhaler technique and adherence to treatment should be checked.
- The main treatments for exacerbations of asthma include repeated β_2-agonists, early use of corticosteroids and oxygen to raise S_aO_2 above 92%.
- Mild exacerbations (PEF reduction of <20%) can often be managed in community settings.
- After exacerbations, patients should be reviewed early to identify possible triggers and review the action plan.

S_aO_2, arterial oxygen concentration.

The preferred route of administration of the agents used in the management of asthma is by inhalation. This allows the drugs to be delivered directly to the airways in smaller doses and with fewer side effects than if systemic routes were used. Inhaled bronchodilators also have a faster onset of action than when administered systemically and give better protection from bronchoconstriction.

Treatment of chronic asthma should be managed in a stepwise progression. This section concentrates on management in adults, as outlined in Fig. 25.3, but corresponding management steps for children are available (BTS/SIGN, 2009). Therapy is moved up the steps according to the severity of the patient's asthma symptoms and response to current treatment. When a patient has been stable for at least 3 months (GINA, 2009), therapy should be stepped back down; for example, by halving the inhaled corticosteroid (ICS) dose. International guidelines aim for management to achieve and maintain clinical control, which is defined in Table 25.2. A model for patient review and adjustment of therapy, based on assessment of asthma control, has been suggested (Crompton et al., 2006) and is shown in Fig. 25.4. To help in patient education, the terms used to describe the effects of asthma medication are similar across all manufacturers and sources of education. 'Reliever' is used for agents that give immediate relief of symptoms. Agents that act to reduce inflammation or give long-term bronchodilation are referred to as 'controllers' or 'preventers'.

Reliever medication

Short-acting β-adrenoceptor agonist bronchodilators. β-Adrenoceptor agonists are the mainstay of asthma management. Salbutamol and terbutaline are selective β_2-agonists and have few β_1-mediated side effects such as cardiotoxicity. β_2-Receptors are, however, also present in myocardial tissue; cardiovascular stimulation resulting in tachycardia and palpitations is still the main dose-limiting toxicity with these agents when used in high dosage.

An inhaled β_2-agonist is the first-line agent in the management of asthma. This is used as required by the patient for the symptomatic relief of breathlessness and wheezing, for example, salbutamol 200 μcg when required. This may be the only treatment necessary for those with infrequent symptoms. There is no advantage to regular administration.

Additional bronchodilators. Additional bronchodilators may be required if the above therapy does not adequately control symptoms (Tables 25.3 and 25.4).

Inhaled anticholinergic agents. These block muscarinic (M1, M2, M3) receptors in bronchial smooth muscle but are generally of little additional value in asthma management. Ipratropium has a slower onset of action than β_2-agonists but a longer duration of action. Anticholinergics may be helpful in patients who also have a degree of obstructive airways disease.

Long acting β-adrenoreceptor agonist bronchodilators. When low-dose inhaled steroids fail to control asthma symptoms adequately at step 3, long-acting β_2-agonists should be added instead of increasing the steroid dose. Symptom relief after a trial period, for example, 4–6 weeks, must then be assessed to

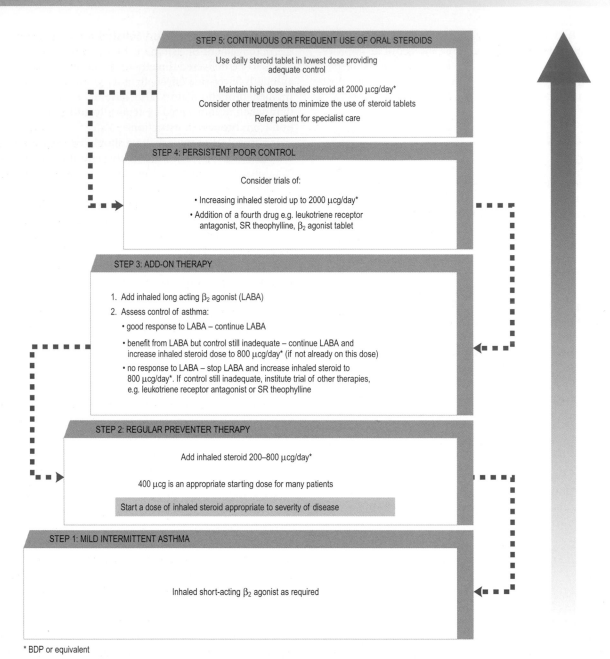

STEP 5: CONTINUOUS OR FREQUENT USE OF ORAL STEROIDS

Use daily steroid tablet in lowest dose providing adequate control

Maintain high dose inhaled steroid at 2000 μcg/day*

Consider other treatments to minimize the use of steroid tablets

Refer patient for specialist care

STEP 4: PERSISTENT POOR CONTROL

Consider trials of:

• Increasing inhaled steroid up to 2000 μcg/day*

• Addition of a fourth drug e.g. leukotriene receptor antagonist, SR theophylline, β₂ agonist tablet

STEP 3: ADD-ON THERAPY

1. Add inhaled long acting β₂ agonist (LABA)
2. Assess control of asthma:
   • good response to LABA – continue LABA
   • benefit from LABA but control still inadequate – continue LABA and increase inhaled steroid dose to 800 μcg/day* (if not already on this dose)
   • no response to LABA – stop LABA and increase inhaled steroid to 800 μcg/day*. If control still inadequate, institute trial of other therapies, e.g. leukotriene receptor antagonist or SR theophylline

STEP 2: REGULAR PREVENTER THERAPY

Add inhaled steroid 200–800 μcg/day*

400 μcg is an appropriate starting dose for many patients

Start a dose of inhaled steroid appropriate to severity of disease

STEP 1: MILD INTERMITTENT ASTHMA

Inhaled short-acting β₂ agonist as required

* BDP or equivalent

Fig. 25.3 Summary of stepwise management in adults (reproduced by permission of the BMJ Publishing Group, from BTS/SIGN, 2009).

Table 25.2 Levels of asthma control (GINA, 2009)

Characteristic	Controlled all of the following	Partly controlled any measure present in any week	Uncontrolled
Daytime symptoms	Twice or less/week	More than twice/week	
Limitation of activities	None	Any	Three or more features of partly controlled asthma present in any week
Nocturnal symptoms/awakening	None	Any	
Need for reliever/rescue treatment	Twice or less/week	More than twice/week	
Lung function (PEF or FEV₁)	Normal	<80% predicted or personal best (if known)	
Any exacerbation should prompt a review of maintenance treatment to ensure that it is adequate.			

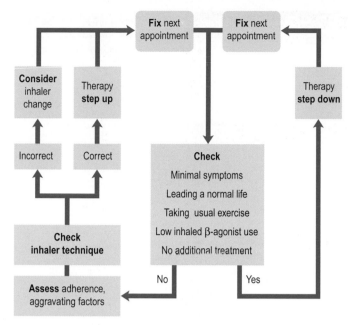

Fig. 25.4 Adjusting therapy to achieve asthma control (from Crompton et al., 2006 reproduced by permission. Copyright Elsevier publishing).

see if the LABA has been effective and whether further treatment needs to be added to or existing treatment changed.

Meta-analysis of LABA trials has shown a potential increase in asthma deaths of 1 death in 1000 patient-years of use, but this increased risk is lessened when used alongside ICSs (Saltpeter et al., 2006). Taking this evidence into account, it is advised that LABAs should

- only be added if regular use of standard-dose ICS has failed to control asthma adequately
- not be initiated in patients with rapidly deteriorating asthma
- be introduced at a low dose and the effect properly monitored before considering dose increase
- be discontinued in the absence of benefit
- be reviewed as appropriate; stepping down therapy should be considered when good long-term asthma control has been achieved (MHRA, 2008).

Combination ICS/LABA inhalers are available which may improve adherence compared to separate inhalers; as adherence to ICS is generally poor, using combination inhalers may ensure that the LABA is not used alone for variable periods of time.

A formoterol and budesonide combination inhaler can be given both as maintenance therapy and for symptomatic relief. Current trial evidence shows that this dosing method is an alternative at step 3 for adults who are poorly controlled on SABA and ICS, have experienced one or more severe exacerbations in the previous 12 months, or as an alternative to increasing the ICS dose to above 2 mg/day at step 4 (NPC, 2008).

Oral bronchodilators. Oral bronchodilators can also be added, for example, theophylline at steps 3–4 or β_2-agonists at step 4 for additional symptom control. Slow-release forms should be used, usually twice daily, although these can be used in a single night-time dose if nocturnal symptoms are troublesome.

Theophylline should be started at a dose of 400–500 mg/day in adults and, if required, increased after 7 days to 800–1000 mg/day. In children, higher doses may be required but this will be determined by the age of the child (see Chapter 10).

Theophylline has a narrow therapeutic index and its hepatic metabolism varies greatly between individuals. Theophylline clearance is affected by a variety of factors, including disease states and concurrent drug therapy. The dose used should, therefore, take into account these factors, which are listed in Table 25.5. Plasma levels may be taken after 3–4 days at the higher dose, and it has been normal practice to adjust the dose to keep the plasma level within a therapeutic window of 10–20 mg/L, although improvements in respiratory function are seen at levels as low as 5 mg/L in some patients. As the bronchodilating effects of theophylline are proportional to the log of the plasma concentrations, there is proportionally less bronchodilation as the plasma level increases. The mild side effects such as nausea and vomiting are seen at concentrations as low as 13 mg/L but are more common over 20 mg/L. Significant cardiac symptoms, tachycardia and persistent vomiting are usually seen at concentrations of 40 mg/L while severe CNS effects, such as seizures, have been seen at 30 mg/L but are more common above 50 mg/L.

Table 25.3 Comparison of inhaled bronchodilators

Drug	Onset of action (min)	Peak action (min)	Duration of action (h)
Ipratropium	3–10	60–120	4–6
Formoterol	2–3		12
Salbutamol	5–15	60[a]	4–6
Salmeterol	10-14	150[a]	12[a]
Terbutaline	5–30	60–120	3–6

[a]Approximate or median value.

Table 25.4 Daily dose range for selected bronchodilators

Drug and route	Age and total daily dosage range		
Aminophylline			
Intravenous injection	Adult; 5 mg/kg (single dose)	1 month–18 years; 5 mg/kg (single dose) up to 500 mg maximum	
Intravenous infusion	16 years–adult; 500 mg/kg/h	9–16 years; 800 mg/kg/h	1 month–9 years; 1 mg/kg/h
Oral	Child over 40 kg–adult; 225–450 mg m/r twice a day		
Formoterol			
Inhaled	6 years–adult; 12–24 μcg twice a day		
Ipratropium bromide			
Inhaled	12 years–adult; 20–40 μcg 3–4 times daily	6–12 years; 20–40 μcg 3 times daily	1 month–6 years; 20 μcg 3 times daily
Nebulised for acute bronchospasm	Adult; 500 μcg repeated as necessary	6–12 years; 250–500 μcg repeated as necessary (max. 1 mg daily)	Under 5 years; 125–250 μcg repeated as necessary (max. 1 mg daily)
Salbutamol			
Inhaled	5 years–adult; 200 μcg when required, up to 4 times a day	Child, 100 μcg when required, up to 4 times a day	
Nebulised for acute bronchospasm	Adult; 2.5–5 mg repeated as necessary	6–18 years; 2.5–5 mg repeated every 20–30 min if necessary	2–5 years; 2.5 mg repeated every 20–30 min if necessary
Salmeterol			
Inhaled	12 years–adult; 50–100 μcg twice a day	4–12 years; 50 μcg twice a day	2–4 years; 25 μcg twice a day
Terbutaline			
Inhaled	5 years–adult; 500 μcg when required, up to four times a day		
Nebulised for acute bronchospasm	Adult; 5–10 mg repeated as necessary	6–18 years; 5–10 mg repeated every 20–30 min if necessary	2–5 years; 5 mg repeated every 20–30 min if necessary
Theophylline			
Oral	12 years–adult; 175–500 mg (m/r) twice a day	6–12 years; 175–250 mg (m/r) twice a day	

Note: The Salbutamol and Terbutaline nebulised rows also list an "Under 2 years" column: Salbutamol — Under 2 years; 2.5 mg repeated every 20–30 min if necessary; Terbutaline — Under 2 years; 5 mg repeated every 20–30 min if necessary.

Differing brands of theophylline have differing bioavailabilities, so brands should not be interchanged.

High-dose β_2-*agonists.* High-dose β_2-agonists are only considered if conventional doses do not achieve adequate symptom control. Nebulised drugs such as salbutamol 2.5–5 mg per dose are given.

Terbutaline has been given by continuous subcutaneous infusion in the maintenance treatment of difficult to treat asthma.

Preventer medication

Anti-inflammatory agents. Regular anti-inflammatory treatment should be used for patients who are not controlled on a SABA alone (BTS/SIGN, 2009). Corticosteroids are the most commonly used anti-inflammatory agents (Table 25.6), but others such as the cromones are available.

Inhaled corticosteroids. Corticosteroids suppress the chronic airway inflammation associated with asthma. At present, ICSs are the initial drugs of choice, with a starting dose for an adult of beclometasone or budesonide 400 μcg/day (or an equivalent) given in divided doses.

The threshold frequency of β_2-agonist use which prompts the start of ICSs has not been fully established but national guidance (BTS/SIGN, 2009) recommends considering ICS for patients with any of the following:

- Exacerbations of asthma in the past 2 years
- Using inhaled β_2-agonists three times a week or more
- Symptoms three times a week or more
- Waking one night a week with symptoms

Table 25.5 Factors affecting theophylline clearance

Decreased clearance	Increased clearance
Congestive cardiac failure	Cigarette smoking
Cor pulmonale	Children 1–12 years
Chronic obstructive pulmonary disease	High-protein, low-carbohydrate diet
Viral pneumonia	Barbecued meat
Acute pulmonary oedema	Carbamazepine
Cirrhosis	Phenobarbital
Premature and term babies	Phenytoin
Elderly	Sulfinpyrazone
Obesity	
High-carbohydrate, low-protein diet	
Cimetidine	
Erythromycin	
Oral contraceptives	
Ciprofloxacin	
Propranolol	

If symptoms persist, the ICS dose is increased stepwise accordingly. The ICS dose should be reduced, if possible, once symptoms and PEF rates have improved and stabilised. If a patient's asthma cannot be controlled by the above ICS dose and the inhaler technique and adherence are adequate, the dose can be increased to a maximum of 1.5–2 mg a day.

All ICSs have dose-related side effects. Adrenal suppression occurs at around doses of >1500 μcg/day of beclometasone in adults. In children, doses of 400 μcg/day of beclometasone or more are associated with growth failure and adrenal suppression; children treated at these doses should be under the care of a specialist paediatrician. Oropharyngeal side effects such as candidiasis are also more common at higher doses (Box 25.2). Measures to minimise this can be tried, such as using a large-volume spacer device and rinsing the mouth with water or brushing teeth after inhalation, but there is little evidence to confirm how effective these are.

Cromones. Inhaled sodium cromoglicate and nedocromil sodium are less effective than corticosteroids in asthma. Although rarely used, they may be possible alternatives if corticosteroids cannot be tolerated.

Leukotriene receptor antagonists. Two leukotriene receptor antagonists, montelukast and zafirlukast, are currently licensed in the UK. Leukotriene receptor antagonists are included in step 4 as add-on therapy for adult patients but are less effective than LABAs in controlling asthma when added to ICSs. If these agents are initiated, then a 4–6 week trial should be undertaken; if there is no improvement in control, the drug should be stopped. They seem to be of particular value in aspirin-induced asthma, possibly due to the role of leukotrienes in this form of asthma.

Anti-IgE monoclonal antibodies. The first of these, omalizumab, is used for the treatment of severe persistent IgE (30–1500 iu/mL)-mediated asthma as add-on therapy to existing optimised therapy in adults and individuals over 12 years of age who have severe unstable disease (NICE, 2007). Patient response should be measured and omalizumab discontinued after 16 weeks if no adequate response is seen.

Oral corticosteroids. Oral corticosteroids should only be used, at step 5, if symptom control cannot be achieved with maximum doses of inhaled bronchodilators and steroids. They should be given as a single morning dose to minimise adrenal suppression. Alternate-day dosing produces fewer side effects but is less effective in controlling asthma.

Short courses (of up to 3 weeks) of high-dose oral steroids, 40–50 mg daily, can be safely used during exacerbations of asthma.

Steroid-sparing agents. Immunosuppressive agents can be tried in an attempt to reduce a regular steroid dose. Methotrexate, ciclosporin and gold have been tried with varying

Table 25.6 Inhaled corticosteroids used for the prophylaxis of asthma

Drug and age range	Total daily dosage range (MDI)	
	Standard dose	High dose
Beclometasone diproprionate or budesonide[a]		
Adult	100–400 μcg twice a day	400–1000 μcg twice a day
12–18 years	100–400 μcg twice a day	400–1000 μcg twice a day
Under 12 years	100–200 μcg twice a day	200–400 μcg twice a day
Ciclesonide		
Adult	80 μcg once daily	160 μcg once daily
Fluticasone		
Adult	50–200 μcg twice a day	400–1000 μcg twice a day
12–18 years	50–200 μcg twice a day	200–500 μcg twice a day
4–12 years	50–100 μcg twice a day	100–200 μcg twice a day
Mometasone		
Adult	200–400 μcg once daily	400 μcg twice a day
12-18 years	200 μcg twice a day	Up to 400 μcg twice a day

[a]There are bioavailability differences between CFC-free steroid inhalers. Always check dosing for specific brands.

Box 25.2 Adverse reactions associated with drugs used in the management of asthma

β₂-Agonists
- *By inhalation*: adverse drug reactions are uncommon
- *Nebulisation, orally or parenterally*: fine tremor (usually the hands), nervous tension, headache, peripheral vasodilation, tachycardia. The adverse reactions often diminish as tolerance develops with continued administration
- *High doses*: hypokalaemia, aggravation of angina

Inhaled corticosteroids
- Hoarseness, oral or pharyngeal candidiasis
- Adrenal suppression may occur with high doses, for example, beclometasone diproprionate above 1500 μcg daily

Oral corticosteroids
- Prolonged use of these results in exaggeration of some of the normal physiological effects of steroids
- Mineralocorticoid effects include: hypertension, potassium loss, muscle weakness, and sodium and water retention. These effects are most notable with fludrocortisone, are significant with hydrocortisone, occur only slightly with prednisolone and methylprednisolone and are negligible with dexametasone and betametasone
- Glucocorticoid effects include: precipitation of diabetes, osteoporosis, development of a paranoic state, depression, euphoria, peptic ulceration, immunosuppression, Cushing's syndrome (moon face, striae and acne), growth suppression in children, worsening of infection, skin thinning, striae atrophicae, increased hair growth, perioral dermatitis and acne
- Adrenal suppression occurs with high doses and/or prolonged treatment. Steroid therapy must be gradually withdrawn in these patients to avoid precipitating an adrenal crisis of hypotension, weight loss, arthralgia and, sometimes, death

Ipratropium bromide
- Occasionally: dry mouth
- Precipitation of acute glaucoma with nebulised therapy, possibly worsened by co-administration of salbutamol. A mouthpiece should be used to minimise the exposure of the eyes to the nebulised drug
- Rarely: systemic anticholinergic effects such as urinary retention and constipation

Methotrexate
- Myelosuppression, mucositis and, rarely, pneumonitis

Nedocromil sodium
- Mild and transient nausea, coughing, transient bronchospasm, throat irritation, headache and a bitter taste

Sodium cromoglicate
- Coughing, transient bronchospasm and throat irritation due to inhalation of the powder

Theophylline
- Although about 5% of the population experience minor adverse effects (nausea, diarrhoea, nervousness and headache), increasing the plasma concentration results in more serious effects. The following is a guide to the plasma levels at which the adverse reactions usually occur:
  - Above 20 mg/L: persistent vomiting, insomnia, gastro-intestinal bleeding, cardiac arrhythmias
  - Above 35 mg/L: hyperglycaemia, hypotension, more serious cardiac arrhythmias, convulsions, permanent brain damage and death
- Individual patients may suffer these effects at plasma levels other than those quoted, for example, convulsions have occurred in patients at 25 mg/L

Leukotriene receptor antagonists
- Abdominal pain, headache, diarrhoea, dizziness, upper respiratory tract infections. Rarely: acute hepatitis (associated with zafirlukast), Churg–Strauss syndrome

---

success. All have potentially toxic side effects and need to be closely monitored.

Acute severe asthma

The management of acute asthma depends on the severity of the attack and its response to treatment, as well as an appreciation of the patient's past history and present treatment. If an acute attack becomes persistent and difficult to treat, it is known as acute severe asthma. The aims of treatment are to prevent any deterioration in the patient's condition and hasten recovery.

Prevention. The ideal way of treating an acute attack is to empower patients to recognise when their condition is deteriorating so they can initiate treatment to prevent the attack becoming severe. This can be achieved with an individualised self-management plan.

The dose of inhaled β₂-agonist should be increased, and a short course of oral steroids commenced, for example, prednisolone at a dose of 40–50 mg every morning for 1 week. The dose of ICS is often also increased, but there is limited evidence to support this.

If the condition deteriorates further, hospital admission may become necessary. This could be a self-referral from the patient, responding to criteria drawn up by the doctor, such as their PEF falling below 50% of their usual best. The education of patients and their relatives in the management of acute attacks should always stress the prompt initiation of further treatment and early referral.

Immediate management. The immediate treatment of acute severe asthma should take place in the patient's home if a moderate attack. Admission to hospital is considered if PEF drops below 50% predicted or normal, or the patient cannot complete sentences in one breath or is too breathless to talk, or if life-threatening features are present. A suggested treatment protocol for management in hospital is outlined in Fig. 25.5.

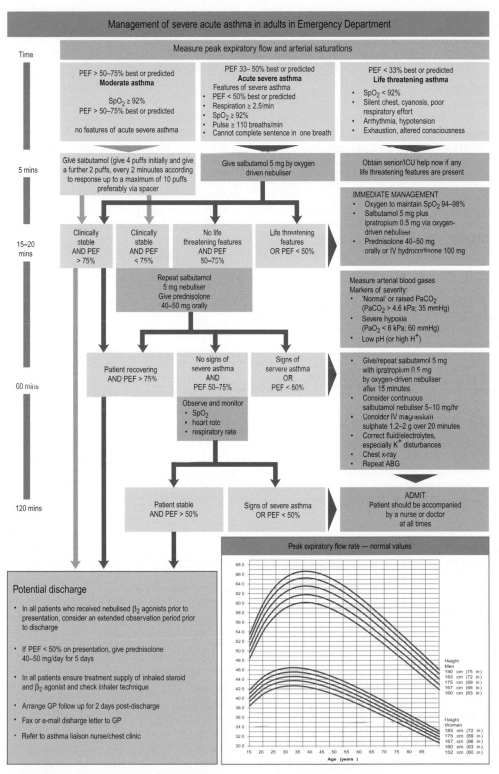

Fig. 25.5 Management of acute severe asthma in adults in hospital reproduced by permission of the Scottish Intercollegiate Guidelines Network from BTS/SIGN, 2009.

Oxygen is administered to achieve an oxygen saturation of 92% or more. A β_2-agonist is administered by metered dose inhaler (MDI) with a spacer attachment (4 puffs, then 2 puffs every 2 min until 10 mg or symptom relief) as there is no demonstrable difference between this and using a nebuliser. With more severe symptoms, or during an admission to hospital, nebulisers are used because they permit a high dose (10–20 times the dose of a MDI) and they require no co-ordination on the part of the patient between inspiration and actuation, which is helpful in those distressed. Patients undergoing an acute attack often have an inspiratory rate that is too low to use an MDI effectively.

Corticosteroids are also given in the acute attack; oral prednisolone (40–50 mg daily, for 5 days). Intravenous hydrocortisone (100 mg) should only be required if the patient cannot take oral medication. This reduces and prevents the inflammation that causes oedema and hypersecretion of mucus and hence helps to relieve the resultant smooth muscle spasm. The clinical response to both oral and parenteral steroids has an onset at 1–2 h with a peak effect at 6–8 h. If life-threatening features are present, such as cyanosis, bradycardia, confusion, exhaustion or unconsciousness, higher dose bronchodilators are used: nebulised salbutamol 5 mg with ipratropium bromide 500 μcg, repeated after 15 min; with subsequent consideration to continuous nebulisation of salbutamol at 5–10 mg/h. The addition of an anticholinergic such as ipratropium often gives a response that is greater than that of the two agents used alone.

Intravenous aminophylline can be given with a bolus dose of 250 mg over 30 min, followed by a continuous infusion of 500 μcg/kg/h. The bolus should be omitted if the patient is known to take oral theophylline or aminophylline. The choice between intravenous aminophylline and β_2-agonist depends on concurrent therapy and side effect profiles. The dose of intravenous aminophylline used must also take into account recent theophylline therapy in addition to other factors (Table 25.7). Serious toxicity can occur with parenteral aminophylline and patients must be carefully monitored for nausea and vomiting, the most common early signs of toxicity.

If the aminophylline infusion is continued for more than 24 h, the plasma theophylline concentration may be measured to guide any necessary alteration in infusion rate in order to maintain the level in the optimum range of 10–20 mg/L.

Intravenous magnesium sulphate, 1.2–2 g as a 20-min infusion, has been shown to help in some patients who have not had a good response to initial treatment. There is, however, no evidence to support repeated dosing regardless of therapeutic outcome.

Further deterioration in condition may require assisted mechanical ventilation on an intensive care unit. Regular monitoring of arterial blood gases and oxygen saturation is performed to help detect any deterioration in condition.

Antibiotics are only indicated where there is evidence of a bacterial infection.

Ongoing management. The subsequent management of acute severe asthma depends on the patient's clinical response. All patients should be monitored throughout their treatment with objective measures of their PEFs before and after bronchodilator treatment and with continual monitoring of their arterial blood gas concentrations to ensure adequate oxygen is being given.

As the patient responds to treatment, infusions can be stopped and other treatment changed or tailed off as described above. As improvement continues, an inhaled β_2-agonist is substituted for the nebulised form and the oral corticosteroids stopped or reduced to a maintenance dose if clinically necessary. Throughout the treatment programme, potential drug interactions should be anticipated and managed appropriately (Table 25.8).

All patients should have a follow-up after an acute attack with symptoms monitored, reasons for admission addressed and inhaler technique checked. A self-management plan should be drawn up and discussed with each patient.

Patient care

The correct use of drugs and the education of patients are the cornerstones of asthma management. There are three main steps in the education of the asthmatic patient.

1. The patient should have an understanding of the action of each of the medicines they use.
2. The appropriate choice of inhalation device(s) should be made and the patient educated to use them correctly.
3. An individualised action (self-management) plan should be developed for each patient.

All members of the health care team should provide education and support for the asthmatic patient at regular intervals. The need for each patient to understand their asthma and its management must be balanced against the dangers of overwhelming the patient with information, particularly when the asthma has been newly diagnosed. To try to overcome this, a 'ladder of asthma knowledge' has been proposed. Patients are counseled in a gradual manner, each session adding to the previous one in content and reinforcing existing knowledge (Box 25.3).

Table 25.7 Intravenous aminophylline dosing in acute severe asthma

	Aminophylline dose	Patient characteristics
Loading dose	5 mg/kg over 20–30 min	Adults and children
	3 mg/kg over 10–15 min	Previous theophylline therapy (although some authorities do not use a loading dose in these patients)
Maintenance dose	500 μcg/kg/h	Non-smoking adults
	700 μcg/kg/h	Children under 12 or smokers
	200 μcg/kg/h	Cardiac failure, liver impairment, pneumonia

Table 25.8 Common clinically significant interactions with drugs used in the management of asthma

Drug	Interacting drug	Probable mechanism and clinical result
β_2-Agonists	Methyldopa	Acute hypotension possible with β_2-agonist infusions
Corticosteroids	Anticoagulants	High-dose steroids enhance anticoagulant effect of coumarins
	Antifungals	Metabolism of steroids possibly affected by antifungal agents
	Barbiturates	Accelerates steroid metabolism
	β_2-Agonists	Increased risk of hypokalaemia with high doses
	Carbamazepine	Reduced steroid effect due to increased metabolism
	Ciclosporin	Increases plasma concentration of prednisolone
	Methotrexate	Increased risk of haematological toxicity
	Phenytoin	Reduced steroid effect due to increased metabolism
	Rifampicin	Reduced steroid effect due to increased metabolism
Theophylline	Azithromycin	May increase theophylline plasma levels
	β_2-Agonists (high dose)	Increased risk of hypokalaemia
	Carbamazepine	Induction of theophylline metabolism resulting in decreased plasma levels
	Clarithromycin	Inhibition of theophylline metabolism resulting in increased plasma levels
	Cimetidine	Inhibition of theophylline metabolism resulting in increased plasma levels
	Ciprofloxacin	Increased plasma concentration. Possible risk of convulsions
	Diltiazem	Increased theophylline plasma levels
	Erythromycin (oral)	Inhibition of theophylline metabolism resulting in increased plasma levels
	Fluconazole	Possible increase in theophylline plasma level
	Dihydropyridine calcium antagonists	May increase theophylline plasma levels
	Fluvoxamine	Increased theophylline plasma levels, halve theophylline dose
	Isoniazid	May increase theophylline plasma levels
	Ketoconazole	Possible increase in theophylline plasma level
	Lithium carbonate	Reducing plasma lithium concentrations as theophylline enhances lithium renal clearance
	Norfloxacin	Increased plasma concentration. Possible risk of convulsions
	Phenytoin	Plasma concentrations of theophylline and phenytoin both reduced
	Primidone	Induction of theophylline metabolism resulting in decreased plasma levels
	Rifampicin	Induction of theophylline metabolism resulting in decreased plasma levels
	Ritonavir	Metabolism of theophylline increased
	Smoking (tobacco)	Induction of theophylline metabolism resulting in decreased plasma levels
	St John's wort	Reduced theophylline plasma levels
	Verapamil	Increased theophylline plasma levels

Box 25.3 Ladder of asthma knowledge for patients

Step 1: Patient/carer understands what relief medication does, side effects which may occur, aims of treatment, what is happening to them and their chest. Education material is made available
Step 2: Patient/carer accepts and agrees about use of medication, importance of preventers and recognition of symptoms
Step 3: Patient/carer knows how to monitor PEF and symptoms, when to increase dose of inhaled steroids and contact their medical practice
Step 4: Patient/carer confident to manage own medication, increasing and decreasing dose using PEF or symptom monitoring, start oral steroids and attend their medical practice

Knowledge

Increasing the patients' knowledge about their asthma therapy is a necessary component of asthma management. However, education alone has not been shown to have a beneficial effect on morbidity. Education programmes must, therefore, also look at modifying their behaviour and attitude to asthma. Counselling should lead to increased patient confidence in the ability to self-manage asthma, thereby decrease hospital admission rates and emergency visits by primary care doctors, increase adherence and improve quality of life.

Specific counselling on drug therapy should concentrate on three areas: drugs used to relieve symptoms, drugs used to prevent asthma attacks, and drugs which are given only as reserve treatment for severe attacks.

Inhalation device

The choice of a suitable inhalation device is vital in asthma management. The incorrect use of inhalers will lead to suboptimal treatment. A review of inhaler technique studies has concluded that up to 50% of patients in Europe are unable to use their inhaler correctly (Crompton et al., 2006). There is no demonstrable difference in efficacy between the various devices available. Other factors, therefore, need to be considered when choosing the appropriate device, including the patient's age, severity of disease, manual dexterity, co-ordination and personal preference. The range of different devices available for the drugs commonly used in asthma is shown in Table 25.9.

Table 25.9 Inhalation devices and spacer devices available

Drug	Type of inhaler device						
	Metered dose	Breath-actuated spacer for MDI	Single-dose spacer for MDI	Multiple-dose dry powder inhaler	Nebuliser dry powder inhaler	Large-volume	Small-volume
Salbutamol	✓	✓	✓	✓	✓	✓	✓
Ipratropium	✓		✓		✓		✓
Terbutaline				✓	✓		
Salmeterol	✓			✓			✓
Formoterol			✓				
Tiotropium[a]	✓[b]		✓				
Beclometasone	✓	✓	✓	✓			✓
Budesonide	✓			✓	✓	✓	✓
Ciclesonide	✓						✓
Fluticasone	✓			✓	✓	✓	✓
Mometasone				✓			
Cromoglicate	✓	✓	✓		✓		✓
Nedocromil	✓						✓

[a]Only licensed for use in COPD.
[b]Delivers a soft aerosol 'mist'.

Metered dose aerosol inhalers

The pressurised MDI is the most widely prescribed inhalation device in the UK (Fig. 25.6). It usually contains a solution or suspension of active drug, with a typical particle size of 2–5 μm, in a liquefied propellant. Operation of the device releases a metered dose of the drug with a droplet size of 35–45 μm. The increased droplet size is due to the propellant, which evaporates when expelled from the inhaler. Inhalers have now been switched from chlorofluorocarbon (CFC) propellants to newer, non-CFC, hydrofluoroalkanes.

MDIs have the advantage of being multidose, small and widely available for most drugs used in asthma management. Their main disadvantage is that correct use requires a good technique. A particular problem for many patients is co-ordinating the beginning of inspiration with the actuation of the inhaler. Even when this is done correctly, MDIs only deliver about 10% of drug to the airways, with 80% deposited in the oropharynx. Corticosteroids administered by MDIs can cause dysphonia and oral candidiasis. The candidiasis can be minimised either by advising patients to gargle with water after using the inhaler and to expel the water from the mouth afterwards, or by using a spacer device. Newer devices are utilising other mechanisms to produce an aerosol such as a soft mist inhaler (SMI) which may give benefits in lung deposition and ease of use.

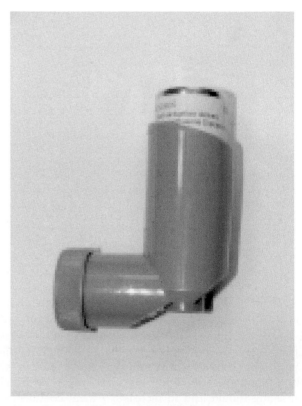

Fig. 25.6 Pressurised metered dose inhaler.

Table 25.10 Inhaler device choice for children

Age group	Drug group	First choice device	Second choice device
0–2 years	All	MDI + spacer + facemask	Nebuliser
3–4 years	All	MDI + spacer	Nebuliser or dry powder
5–15 years	Bronchodilators	MDI or dry	Powder or breath-actuated MDI
5–15 years	Corticosteroids	MDI + spacer	Dry powder or breath-actuated MDI

Younger children, in particular, find MDIs difficult to use and the addition of a spacer device can make this easier, allowing inhalation over several ambient breaths.

The correct technique for using MDIs is as follows:

1. MDIs have a mouthpiece dust cap which has to be removed before use (patients may fail to remove this). The cap must be replaced after use to prevent subsequent inhalation of foreign bodies.
2. The MDI must be vigorously shaken. This distributes the drug particles uniformly throughout the propellant (newer CFC-free inhalers may be solutions and not require shaking – see manufacturer's literature). The MDI must be held upright.
3. The patient should breathe out gently, but not fully.
4. The tongue should be placed on the floor of the mouth and the inhaler placed between the lips, which are then closed round the mouthpiece.
5. The patient should now start to breathe in slowly and deeply through the mouth.
6. The canister is pressed to release the dose while the patient continues to breathe in. This synchronisation of inspiration and actuation, so that there is a supporting stream of air to carry the drug to the lungs, is probably the most common point of failure in those with bad inhalation technique. Patients who are very short of breath, for example, during a severe asthma attack, find this particularly difficult.
7. The breath is held for at least 10 s. This allows the drug particles reaching the periphery of the lung to settle under gravity. Using this technique, about 15% of a dose may reach the lungs. Exhalation should be through the nose.
8. If a second dose is required, 30–60 s should elapse before repeating the inhalation procedure to allow the dosing chamber to re-fill.

Studies indicate that personal tuition improves inhaler technique, particularly if regularly repeated. Other methods of instruction include videos (see http://medguides.medicines. org.uk/demonstrations.aspx), package inserts and information leaflets or booklets provided by organisations such as Asthma UK and the pharmaceutical industry. Regular patient review, at least annually, is recommended. This can be used as an opportunity to check technique, along with assessment of the ability to generate the appropriate inspiratory flow for the device (Broeders et al., 2009).

Metered dose inhaler with a spacer extension

Extension devices allow greater evaporation of the propellant, so reducing particle size and velocity. This also reduces oropharyngeal deposition and potentially increases lung deposition. Oral candidiasis and dysphonia (impaired voice) from ICSs may also be reduced by using these devices. Spacers are useful for people who have poor co-ordination between inspiration and actuation and several types of spacer are available. In younger children, these offer advantages over MDIs alone with respect to adherence. Recommendations (see Table 25.10) have been published regarding device choice (NICE, 2000, 2002).

Large-volume (750 mL) spacers are available such as the Volumatic® (Fig. 25.7); these are manufacturer specific and have not been assessed or licensed for use with devices of other companies. These spacers have one-way valves that allow several inhalations of one dose from the spacer's chamber. No co-ordination is required between actuation of the MDI and inhalation. A large-volume spacer can be used instead of a nebuliser to deliver high doses of a β_2-agonist in acute severe asthma attacks. Disadvantages of these spacers include their large size, which renders them less portable, and their proven efficacy only with inhalers from the same manufacturer. Spacers should be washed regularly in warm, soapy water and left to drip dry without rinsing. Cloths should not be used for drying a spacer as this affects the antistatic coating of plastic spacers. All spacers should be replaced every 6–12 months. Facemasks are available for young children.

Small- and medium-volume spacer devices are available, either as an integral part of the design of some MDIs or as

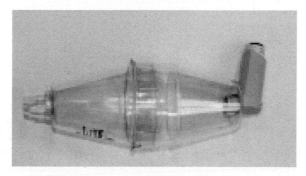

Fig. 25.7 Large-volume spacer (Volumatic®).

a separate device (Fig. 25.8). These spacers have also been used to compensate for poor inhaler technique in adults and reduce the oropharyngeal deposition of steroids. These are more convenient to carry around than the larger spacers. The published evidence of additional benefit from these devices in either increasing efficacy or decreasing adverse effects is more limited than with large volume spacers.

Breath-actuated metered dose inhalers

These MDIs are actuated automatically by inspiratory flow rates of about 22–36 L/min. A breath-actuated MDI is illustrated in Fig. 25.9. These eliminate the need for the correct co-ordination of inspiration and actuation but require priming before each actuation.

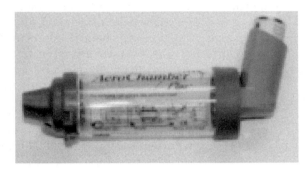

Fig. 25.8 Medium-volume spacer (Aerochamber Plus®).

Dry powder inhalers

Several types of dry powder inhalers (DPIs) are available. These are propellant free and are designed to be easier to use than conventional MDIs. They are useful for those who have difficulty co-ordinating an MDI and can be used by children as young as 4 years old. Table 25.10 sets out the recommendations for device choice in children.

DPIs are available as either single-dose or multiple-dose devices (Fig. 25.10). Single-dose devices pierce or break a gelatin capsule to release the contents and must be regularly cleaned to avoid powder clogging the device. Multiple-dose devices are preferred by many patients since they avoid having to reload for each dose. Care must be taken to hold these devices in the correct orientation to avoid the powder falling out of the device before inhalation. Patients commenced on DPIs are sometimes concerned at the absence of any taste or spray plume which they have become accustomed to when using an MDI; reassurance that this is perfectly normal and that correct use of the DPI (including a check that the device is not empty) will ensure that the required dose is delivered should overcome this problem.

Nebulisers

A nebuliser produces an aerosol by blowing air or oxygen through a solution to produce droplets of 5 μm or less in size. Nebulisers require little co-ordination from the patient as any drug is inhaled through a facemask or mouthpiece using normal tidal breathing. Only about 13%

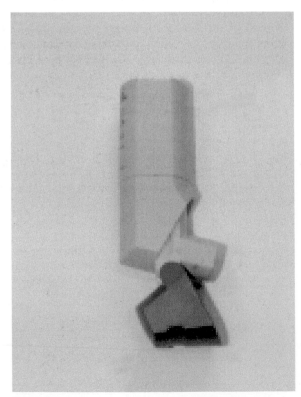

Fig. 25.9 Breath-actuated metered dose inhaler (Easi-breathe®).

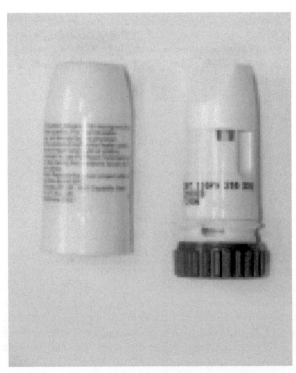

Fig. 25.10 Multiple-dose dry powder inhaler (Turbohaler®).

of the dose used is deposited in the lungs, but because the doses used are higher than those used in other aerosol devices, patients will generally receive a higher dose than from an MDI. However, in mild and moderate exacerbations of asthma, no benefit has been shown over using 4–6 puffs of a MDI.

Nebulisers are useful in patients who are unable to use conventional inhalers, for example, children under 2 years old, patients with severe attacks of asthma unable to produce sufficient inspiratory effort and those lacking the co-ordination to use other inhalers. Nebulised bronchodilators can be used in acute severe asthma attacks, often avoiding the need for intravenous drugs.

Most of the short-acting β_2-agonists, as well as ipratropium bromide, fluticasone, budesonide and sodium cromoglicate, are available for nebulisation.

The safe and correct use of nebulisers requires careful counselling, especially if they are to be used in the home. The following points are critical for the correct use of a nebuliser.

1. Nebulisers should only be driven by compressed air or by oxygen at flow rates of at least 5–6 L/min to ensure that droplets of the correct size are produced.
2. To maximise nebulised drug, a minimum volume of 3–4 mL should be nebulised. This volume is required to reduce the amount of drug that is unavoidably left in the 'dead-space' (typically about 1 mL) at the end of nebulisation. This 'dead space' is less with newer nebulisers and no further dilution of commercial nebuliser solutions is used. Sodium chloride 0.9% must be used if solutions are diluted.
3. Most nebuliser chambers are disposable but will last 3–4 months when used by a patient at home. The chamber must be emptied after use, and each day, the chamber should be rinsed in hot water and dried by blowing air through the device. Several centres advocate that once a week the chamber

should be sterilised using 0.02% hypochlorite to prevent bacterial contamination; the chamber is then thoroughly rinsed to remove all traces of hypochlorite and then dried.
4. The nebuliser should be serviced at least once a year.

There are disadvantages with the use of nebulisers. Of particular concern is the overreliance on the nebuliser by some patients which results in a delay in seeking medical advice. The high doses of bronchodilators used can also increase the incidence of side effects, and these vary depending on the drug nebulised.

Self-management programmes

Every individual with asthma should be considered for a self-management education programme. These programmes will contain structured education along with an individualised action plan. They aim to give the individual more confidence by involving them in the management of their own asthma. The individual should then be able to deal with any fluctuation in their condition and know when to seek medical advice. Personalised action plans have been shown to improve health outcomes in individuals with asthma (Gibson et al., 2002).

Key elements of an action plan include being able to monitor symptoms, measure peak flow, understand their medicine and how it should be used, and knowing how to deal with fluctuations in severity of asthma according to written guidance. Symptom diaries, management guidance cards and peak flow reading diary cards are available from organisations such as Asthma UK and pharmaceutical companies who manufacture asthma products.

An action plan can also include details of when to increase the dose of an inhaled steroid, when to take a short course of oral corticosteroids and when to self-refer to a general medical practitioner or local hospital (Table 25.11).

Table 25.11 Example of a personalised action plan setting out the action required in response to a given peak flow reading and/or symptoms

Peak flow	Example of symptoms	Action
>80% of personal best value	Intermittent or few symptoms	When required, β_2-agonist for symptom relief, continue regular inhaler corticosteroid, consider reducing the dosage every 3 months if stable
61–80% of best	Waking at night Symptoms of a cold	Double dose of inhaled corticosteroid if taking <400 μcg day BDP Start oral corticosteroid if taking >400 μcg/day BDP
40–60% of best	Increasing breathlessness or using a β_2-agonist every 2–3 h	Start oral corticosteroid course. Contact a doctor
<40% of best	Severe attack Poor response to β_2-agonist	Call emergency doctor or ambulance urgently

BDP, equivalent dose of beclometasone dipropionate.

Case studies

Case 25.1

Mr GT is 54 years old and has been diagnosed with asthma for 4 years. He is 180 cm tall and weighs 95 kg. He has recently been admitted to hospital with an acute exacerbation of his asthma, precipitated by a lower respiratory tract infection. During his admission, his steroid medication was altered from Qvar Easi-breathe® 100 μcg twice daily to Symbicort 400/12 Turbohaler® 1 puff twice daily. He also takes Salbutamol Easi-breathe® inhaler 200 μcg when required.

Questions

1. By how much has his ICSs dose been increased?
2. Should Mr GT be reviewed after discharge?
3. Would Mr GT benefit from self-management information and a personalised action plan?
4. Four months after his discharge, Mr GT has had no further exacerbations and his daily best PEF reading is around 520 L/min; he has no limitations of activity because of his asthma and uses his salbutamol inhaler between two and three times a week. How can Mr GT's level of asthma control be determined?
5. You determine that Mr GT's asthma is now controlled. Could his therapy now be stepped down? If so, how should this be done?

Answers

1. Qvar® is a hydrofluoroalkane CFC-free inhaler with microfine particles of a mass median diameter of 1.1 μm. Clinical studies show that adult patients require approximately half the dose of Qvar® to achieve the same degree of asthma control as with CFC-containing beclometasone inhalers. Care must always be taken when switching between ICS brands (see http://www.mhra.gov.uk/). Tables exist to help with determining equivalent doses (BTS/SIGN, 2009). Qvar® 200 μcg daily is equivalent to 400 μcg of other beclometasone/budesonide preparations, so Mr GT's ICS dose has been doubled.
2. He should be reviewed within 1 month of hospital discharge. This has been associated with a reduced risk of further acute episodes.
3. He would benefit from self-management information and a personalised action plan. The evidence of improved health outcomes for asthmatic patients is particularly good for those with moderate to severe disease and those who have had recent exacerbations.

   A personalised action plan should contain:

   - Advice about recognising loss of asthma control, as assessed by symptoms and PEF readings
   - The action to take if asthma deteriorates, including when and how to seek emergency help and when to commence a course of emergency oral steroids, which should be prescribed in advance.

4. Asthma control is usually assessed on the basis of clinical history, symptoms, inhaler usage and technique. An acute exacerbation is often indicative of poor control over a period of time.

   The level of asthma control for Mr GT can be determined by utilising tools such as the levels of asthma control in the GINA guidelines (GINA, 2009; Table 25.2) and the commonly used Royal College of Physicians, '3 questions':

- Have you had difficulty sleeping because of your asthma symptoms (including cough)?
- Have you had your usual asthma symptoms during the day (cough, wheeze, chest tightness or breathlessness)?
- Has your asthma interfered with your usual activities (e.g. housework, work/school, etc.)?

Management issues should also be discussed:

- Any issues of importance to the patient
- Inhaler technique must be checked, any deficiencies corrected, and if necessary a different device tried
- Adherence to prescribed medication should be assessed
- Mr GT has to be willing to try a step-down in his therapy. His ICS dose can be reduced slowly; a reduction of between 25% and 50% is usually tried every 3 months. A reduction to Symbicort® 200/6 1 puff twice daily could be attempted at this stage. The potential for worsening symptoms and the increased risk of exacerbation should be explained when step-down is attempted, particularly as the LABA dose is also being reduced. Opportunity should be taken to also promote general lifestyle advice:

  – Mr GT's body mass index is 29.3 and he is classed as overweight. He should be advised that a healthy diet and regular exercise will help with weight reduction and improve asthma control
  – Offer stop smoking advice if relevant
  – Advise him to avoid exposure to tobacco smoke
  – Provide allergen avoidance advice

Mr GT should be asked to keep twice daily PEF readings and a symptom diary. He will need to be reviewed again in 3 months unless symptoms deteriorate before then. Mr GT should be advised to consider increasing his medication again if his asthma deteriorates; his action plan can be adjusted accordingly.

Case 25.2

Mrs LJ is 32 years old and was recently diagnosed on hospital admission with breathlessness following exposure to cold air. You are conducting a follow-up review after her hospital admission.

Questions

1. What advice should you cover in your consultation with Mrs LJ? Mrs LJ tells you that she has a cat and wonders if this could be affecting her asthma.
2. What information can you give Mrs LJ on allergen avoidance?

Answers

1. Effective management of asthma requires a partnership between the patient and the health care professionals involved in providing the care. The aim is to enable and empower the patient to gain the confidence, skills and knowledge to take a major role in the management of their asthma (GINA, 2009). Open-ended questions such as 'If we could make one thing better about your asthma what would it be?' may help to elicit a patient-centred agenda (BTS/SIGN, 2009). Topics that should be covered in this and subsequent consultations include:

   - Nature of the disease
   - Nature of the treatment
   - Identification of areas where the patient most wants treatment to have effect
   - How to use the treatment, particularly inhaler technique. Websites with video instruction, such as http://www.medicines.org.uk/Guides/Pages/how-to-use-your-inhaler-videos can be used to reinforce verbal instruction and demonstration.

- Develop self-monitoring/self-assessment skills
- Negotiate a personalised action plan in light of identified patient goals
- Recognise and manage acute exacerbations
- Appropriate allergen or trigger avoidance, for example, smoking, pollen, exercise, air pollution and stress
- Ensure Mrs LJ has received a current influenza vaccination

Practical information and treatment plans should be reinforced with written instruction; this can also be from patient support groups such as Asthma UK http://www.asthma.org.uk/. Every subsequent consultation with any health care professional should be an opportunity to review reinforce and extend both knowledge and skills.

2. There is no doubt that increased allergen exposure in sensitised individuals is associated with an increase in asthma symptoms, bronchial hyperresponsiveness and deterioration in lung function (BTS/SIGN, 2009); this includes animal allergens. However, the removal of cats from the home has not been shown to always benefit individuals with asthma. The reduction of exposure to other allergens, such as house dust mite, may also be considered for their potential effect on asthma symptoms. There is no evidence for the effectiveness of dust mite reduction strategies (Getzsche and Johansen, 2008).

If Mrs LJ wishes to try and reduce the burden of allergens in her home, then the following can be considered:

- Complete barrier bed-covering systems
- Remove carpets
- Remove soft toys from beds for children
- High temperature washing of bed linen
- Use acaricides on soft furnishings
- Ensure good ventilation with or without dehumidification
- Use a high-efficiency vacuum cleaner with an inbuilt air filter to reduce cat allergens.

If these measures provide no benefit to asthma symptoms or quality of life after a trial of a few months, they should be stopped.

Case 25.3

Mr KM is a 49-year-old man who has been diagnosed with asthma since childhood. He also suffers from allergic rhinitis with symptoms following exposure to grass pollen in the early summer. He is also allergic to cats. Over the past 2 years his asthma has been steadily deteriorating with a marked reduction in his ability to walk without becoming breathless. He now experiences daily symptoms and is woken up at night several times a week with shortness of breath which is temporarily relieved using a salbutamol inhaler. His current medication is:

Salbutamol DPI 200 μcg when required (currently using three or four times every day)

Seretide-250® evohaler® 2 puffs twice daily
Montelukast 10 mg at night
Aminophylline m/r (Phyllocontin®) 450 mg twice daily

He has had five exacerbations in the past 18 months, requiring hospitalisation. His last admission was 1 month ago with a severe exacerbation requiring a short period of ventilation support. He was discharged with a course of prednisolone 40 mg daily for 14 days but has had to continue taking prednisolone and currently takes 10 mg daily.

Questions

1. At which step of the BTS/SIGN guidelines is Mr KM, and what is his likely diagnosis?
2. What should be the next step in his management?
3. Is there a link between asthma and allergic rhinitis?
4. Mr KM has a positive skin prick test for animal dander and his IgE titre measures 425 IU/L. Is Mr KM suitable for treatment for omalizumab and, if so, for how long should this be given?

Answers

1. He is at step 5, with uncontrolled asthma despite taking 1000 μcg of inhaled fluticasone daily (equivalent to 2000 μcg of beclometasone), a LABA, and three other medications, including oral steroids. It is likely that Mr KM has 'difficult to treat' asthma.
2. Mr KM should be referred to a respiratory specialist. He requires careful assessment which will include:

   - Confirmation or verification of the diagnosis of asthma, including asthma subsets such as steroid-resistant asthma (PEF increase less than 15% after 2 weeks of steroids), psychosocial asthma, premenstrual asthma, aspirin-induced asthma, rhinitis, occupational asthma, allergic bronchopulmonary aspergillosis
   - Identification of preventable causes of persistent symptoms
   - A review of inhaler technique
   - An assessment of adherence to treatment. A significant proportion of patients who may be considered difficult to treat are non-adherent with their corticosteroid therapy. The number of ICS and SABA inhalers dispensed per year can be an indicative measure of non-adherence
   - IgE titre.

3. Allergic rhinitis co-exists with asthma in the majority of patients. The rhinitis should be treated with intranasal steroids as this has been demonstrated to improve asthma morbidity.
4. Mr KM meets the criteria for omalizumab to be given. Omalizumab takes between 12 and 16 weeks to demonstrate effectiveness. Mr KM should be reviewed at 16 weeks and omalizumab only continued if there is a marked improvement in symptoms.

References

Asthma UK, 2001. Out in the open. A true picture of asthma in the United Kingdom today. National Asthma Campaign asthma audit 2001. Asthma J. 6, 1–14.

British Thoracic Society/Scottish Intercollegiate Guidelines Network (BTS/SIGN), 2009. Update: British guideline on the management of asthma. Available at http://www.sign.ac.uk/guidelines/fulltext/101/index.html.

Broeders, M., Sanchis, J., Levy, M., et al., 2009. The ADMIT series – Issues in inhalation therapy. 2. Improving technique and clinical effectiveness. Primary Care Respir. J. 18, 76–82 Available at http://www.thepcrj.org/journ/view_article.php?article_id=627.

Crompton, G.K., Barnes, P.J., Broeders, M., et al., 2006. The need to improve inhalation technique in Europe: a report from the Aerosol Drug Management Improvement Team. Respir. Med 100, 1479–1494.

Douwes, J., Gibson, P., Pekkanen, J., et al., 2002. Non-eosiniphilic asthma: importance and possible mechanisms. Thorax 57, 643–648.

Getzsche, P.C., Johansen, H.K., 2008. House dust mite control measures from asthma. Cochrane Database of Systematic Reviews. Issue 2 Art No. CD001187. doi:10.1002/14651858. CD001187.

Gibson, P.G., Powell, H., Wilson, A., et al., 2002. Self-management education and regular practitioner review for adults with asthma.

Cochrane Database of Systematic Reviews. Issue 3. Art. No. CD001117. doi:10.1002/14651858. CD001117.

GINA Global Initiative for Asthma, 2009. Global strategy for asthma management and prevention. GINA. Available at http://www. ginasthma.com/GuidelinesResources.asp?l1=2&l2=0.

Holgate, S., Arshad, H.S., Roberts, G.C., et al., 2010. A new look at the pathogenesis of asthma. Clin. Sci. 118, 439–450.

Medicines and Healthcare products Regulatory Agency, 2008. Asthma: Long-Acting β_2-Agonists. MHRA, London. Available at http://www. mhra.gov.uk/Safetyinformation/Generalsafetyinformationandadvice/ Product-specificinformationandadvice/Asthma/index.htm.

National Institute for Health and Clinical Excellence, 2000. Guidance on the Use of Inhaler Systems (Devices) in Children Under 5 Years with Chronic Asthma. Technology Appraisal 10. NICE, London. Available at http://guidance.nice.org.uk/TA10.

National Institute for Health and Clinical Excellence, 2002. Inhaler Devices for Routine Treatment of Chronic Asthma in Older Children (Aged 5–15 Years). Technology Appraisal 38. NICE, London. Available at http://guidance.nice.org.uk/TA38.

National Institute for Health and Clinical Excellence, 2007. Omalizumab for Severe Persistent Allergic Asthma. Technology Appraisal 133. NICE, London. Available at http://guidance.nice.org.uk/TA133.

National Prescribing Centre (NPC), 2008. Current issues in the Drug Treatment of Asthma. MeReC Bull. 19, 1–6. Available at http://www.npc.co.uk/ebt/merec/resp/asthma/merec_bulletin_ vol19_no2.html.

Saltpeter, S.R., Buckley, N.S., Ormiston, T.M., et al., 2006. Meta-analysis: effect of long-acting β-agonists on severe asthma exacerbations and asthma-related deaths. Ann. Intern. Med. 144, 904–912.

Further reading

Asthma UK. Available at http://www.asthma.org.uk/index.html.

Chanez, P., Wenzel, S.E., Anderson, G.P., et al., 2007. Severe asthma in adults: what are the important questions? J. Allergy Clin. Immunol. 119, 1337–1348.

Dolovici, M.B., Ahrens, R.C., Hess, D.R., et al., 2005. Device selection and outcomes of aerosol therapy: evidence-based guidelines. Chest 127, 335–371. Available at http://chestjournal.chestpubs.org/ content/127/1/335.long.

Fitzgerald, J.M., Gibson, P.G., 2006. Asthma exacerbations – 4: prevention. Thorax 61, 992–999.

Murphy, A., 2007. Asthma in Focus. Pharmaceutical Press, London.

National Institute for Health and Clinical Excellence, 2002. Corticosteroids for the Treatment of Chronic Asthma in Adults and Children Aged 12 Years and Over. Technology Appraisal 138. NICE, London. Available at http://guidance.nice.org.uk/TA138.

Pedersen, S., 2010. From asthma severity to control: a shift in clinical practice. Primary Care Respir. J. 19, 3–9. Available at http://www. thepcrj.org/journ/view_article.php?article_id=666.

Pinnock, H., Fletcher, M., Holmes, S., et al., 2010. Setting the standard for routine asthma consultations: a discussion of the aims, process and outcomes of reviewing people with asthma in primary care. Primary Care Respir. J. 19, 75–83. Available at http://www.thepcrj. org/journ/view_article.php?article_id=684.

Chronic obstructive pulmonary disease 26

D. Cripps and K. P. Gibbs

Key points

- Chronic obstructive pulmonary disease (COPD) is a leading cause of morbidity and mortality worldwide.
- COPD is the most prevalent manifestation of obstructive lung disease and mainly comprises chronic bronchitis and emphysema.
- The reduction of exposure to tobacco smoke, occupational dusts, chemicals and pollutants is an important goal to prevent the onset and progression of COPD.
- Risk factors for COPD include host factors (α_1-antitrypsin deficiency and airway hyper-responsiveness) and exposures (tobacco smoke, occupational dusts and chemicals, indoor and outdoor pollutants, infections) and socio-economic status.
- Smoking cessation is the single most effective intervention to reduce the risk of developing COPD and slow disease progression. This should be the primary focus of management.
- The management of COPD should follow both national and international guidance.
- COPD care should be delivered by a multidisciplinary team; assessing and managing patients, advising patients on self-management strategies and exercise, identifying and monitoring patients at high risk of exacerbations and educating patients and other health professionals.
- Patients should undergo non-pharmacological pulmonary rehabilitation, such as breathing exercises.

Chronic obstructive pulmonary disease (COPD) is a disease state characterised by airflow limitation that is not fully reversible. The airflow limitation is usually both progressive and associated with an abnormal inflammatory response of the lungs to noxious particles or gases (GOLD, 2009).

COPD is a general term that covers a variety of other disease labels including chronic obstructive airways disease (COAD), chronic obstructive lung disease (COLD), chronic bronchitis and emphysema.

COPD has been defined (National Institute for Health and Clinical Excellence, 2010) as:

- Airflow obstruction with a reduced FEV_1/FVC ratio of less than 0.7.
- If FEV_1 is $\geq$80% of predicted normal, a diagnosis of COPD should only be made in the presence of respiratory symptoms, for example breathlessness or cough.

Epidemiology

COPD is the fifth leading cause of death in the UK and the fourth in the world. It is expected to rise to third position by 2020. It is estimated that over 3 million people have the disease in the UK, with 2 million having undiagnosed COPD (National Clinical Guideline Centre, 2010). COPD is the largest single cause of lost working days in the UK. It is accountable for more than 10% of all hospital admissions and directly costs the NHS around £491 m/year. The burden of COPD on the UK healthcare system exceeds that of asthma and is outlined in Table 26.1.

Respiratory diseases including chronic bronchitis are more common in areas of high atmospheric pollution and in people with dusty occupations such as foundry workers and coal miners. Areas that are highly industrialised generally have the highest incidence of COPD. The UK has around twice the rate of mortality from respiratory disease compared to the European average.

Pathology

The major pathological changes in COPD affect four different compartments of the lung and all are affected in most individuals to varying degrees (American Thoracic Society/European Respiratory Society Task Force, 2004).

Central airways (<2 mm diameter, cartilaginous)

The bronchial glands hypertrophy and goblet cell proliferation occurs. This results in excessive mucus production (chronic bronchitis). Epidemiologically chronic bronchitis is defined as a chronic or recurrent cough with sputum production on most days for at least 3 months of the year during at least 2 consecutive years, in the absence of other diseases recognised to cause sputum production. There is a loss of ciliary function with increase in inflammatory cells, notably lymphocytes, macrophages and, later in the disease, neutrophils.

Table 26.1 Annual morbidity and mortality from COPD (National Clinical Guideline Centre, 2010)

	Hospital admissions	GP consultations	Deaths
England and Wales	130,000	1.4 million	30,000

431

Peripheral airways (<2 mm diameter, non-cartilaginous)

Bronchiolitis is present from early disease with a pathological increase in goblet cells and in inflammatory cells in the airway walls. With disease progression, fibrosis develops along with increased deposition of collagen in the airway walls.

Lung parenchyma (respiratory bronchioles, alveoli and capillaries)

In emphysema, elastases destroy elastin, thus resulting in dilation and destruction of the respiratory bronchioles and alveolar sacs and ducts. Because of this there is a loss of the alveolar wall attachments and peripheral airway collapse.

Emphysema is defined as an abnormal enlargement of the air spaces distal to the terminal bronchioles. There are two main forms: (1) centrilobular emphysema which involves dilation and destruction of respiratory bronchioles, alveolar ducts and alveoli and (2) panacinar emphysema which involves destruction of the whole acinus. The former predominates in COPD, the latter in patients with α_1-antitrypsin deficiency.

Pulmonary vasculature

Vessel walls thicken early in the course of the disease along with endothelial dysfunction. The vessel walls become infiltrated by inflammatory cells, including macrophages and lymphocytes, and there is increased vascular smooth muscle which can lead to pulmonary hypertension. In advanced disease, there is emphysematous destruction of the vascular bed and collagen deposition.

Aetiology

Tobacco smoking is the most important and dominant risk factor in the development of COPD but other noxious particles also contribute, such as occupational exposure to chemical fumes, irritants, dust and gases. A person's exposure can be thought of in terms of the total burden of inhaled particles. These cause a (normal) inflammatory response in the lungs. Smokers, however, seem to have an exaggerated response which eventually causes tissue destruction and impaired repair mechanisms. In addition to inflammation, the other main processes involved in the pathogenesis of COPD are an imbalance of proteinases and antiproteinases in the lungs, and oxidative stress.

Not all smokers go on to develop clinically significant COPD; genetic factors seem to modify each individual's risk. The age at which an individual begins smoking, total pack-years smoked and current smoking status are predictive of COPD mortality. Passive exposure to cigarette smoke may also contribute to respiratory symptoms and COPD by increasing the lungs' total burden of inhaled particles and gases (GOLD, 2009). Tobacco exposure is quantified in 'pack-years':

$$\text{Total pack years} = \frac{\text{Number of cigarettes smoked per day}}{20} \times \text{number of years of smoking}$$

Additional risk factors include the natural ageing process of the lungs. Males are currently more at risk of developing chronic bronchitis, but as the number of women who smoke increases, the incidence of chronic bronchitis in females will also rise. The major risk factors are summarised in Table 26.2.

Table 26.2 Risk factors for the development of COPD

Risk factor	Comment
Smoking	Risk increases with increasing consumption but there is also large interindividual variation in susceptibility
Age	Increasing age results in ventilatory impairment; most frequently related to cumulative smoking
Gender	Male gender was previously thought to be a risk factor but this may be due to a higher incidence of tobacco smoking in men. Women have greater airway reactivity and experience faster declines in FEV_1, so may be at more risk than men
Occupation	The development of COPD has been implicated with occupations such as coal and gold mining, farming, grain handling and the cement and cotton industries
Genetic factors	α_1-Antitrypsin deficiency is the strongest single genetic risk factor, accounting for 1–2% of COPD. Other genetic disorders involving tissue necrosis factor and epoxide hydrolase may also be risk factors
Air pollution	Death rates are higher in urban areas than in rural areas. Indoor air pollution from burning biomass fuel is also implicated as a risk factor, particularly in underdeveloped areas of the world
Socio-economic status	More common in individuals of low socio-economic status
Airway hyper-responsiveness and allergy	Smokers show increased levels of IgE, eosinophils and airway hyper-responsiveness but how these influence the development of COPD is unknown

Inflammation

COPD is characterised by chronic inflammation throughout the airways, parenchyma and pulmonary vasculature. This is a different pattern of inflammation from that of asthma, with an increase in neutrophils, macrophages and T-lymphocytes (particularly CD8[+]); increased eosinophils occur in some patients during exacerbations. These inflammatory cells cause the release of inflammatory mediators and cytokines such as leukotriene B4, interleukin-8 and tumour necrosis factor-α (TNF-α). Over time the actions of these mediators damages the lungs and leads to the characteristic pathological changes observed.

Proteinase and antiproteinase imbalance

The observation that α_1-antitrypsin-deficient individuals are at increased risk of developing emphysema has led to the theory that an imbalance between proteinases and antiproteinases leads to lung destruction. In COPD, there is either an increased production/activity of proteinases or a decreased production/activity of antiproteinases. The main proteinases, proteolytic enzymes such as neutrophil elastin are released by macrophages or neutrophils. The antiproteinases inhibit the damage caused by the proteolytic enzymes. The main antiproteinase is α_1-antitrypsin, also known as α_1-proteinase inhibitor. Cigarette smoke has been shown to inactivate this protein. Oxidative stress also decreases the activity of antiproteinases.

Oxidative stress

An imbalance of oxidants and antioxidants exists in COPD with the balance in favour of the oxidants. This state of oxidative stress contributes to the development of the disease by damaging the intracellular matrix, oxidising biological molecules which cause cell destruction and promoting histone acetylation. There also seems to be a link between oxidative stress and the poor response to corticosteroids seen in COPD. To work, corticosteroids must recruit histone deacetylase to switch off the transcription of inflammatory genes. In COPD, the activity of histone deacetylase is impaired by the oxidative stress, thereby reducing the responsiveness to corticosteroids. Cigarette smoke also impairs the function of histone deacetylase.

Pathophysiology

The pathogenic mechanisms and pathological changes described above lead to the physiological abnormalities of COPD: mucus hypersecretion, ciliary dysfunction, airflow limitation and hyperinflation, gas exchange abnormalities, pulmonary hypertension and systemic effects (American Thoracic Society/European Respiratory Society Task Force, 2004).

Mucus hypersecretion, ciliary dysfunction and complications

Enlarged mucus glands cause hypersecretion of mucus and the squamous metaplasia of epithelial cells results in ciliary dysfunction. These are typically the first physiological abnormalities in COPD.

Normally, cilia and mucus in the bronchi protect against inhaled irritants, which are trapped and expectorated. The persistent irritation caused by cigarette and other smoke causes an exaggeration in the response of these protective mechanisms and leads to inflammation of the small bronchioles (bronchiolitis) and alveoli (alveolitis). Cigarette smoke also inhibits mucociliary clearance, which causes a further build-up of mucus in the lungs. As a result, macrophages and neutrophils infiltrate the epithelium and trigger a degree of epithelial destruction. This, together with a proliferation of mucus-producing cells, leads to plugging of smaller bronchioles and alveoli with mucus and particulate matter.

This excessive mucus production causes distension of the alveoli and loss of their gas exchange function. Pus and infected mucus accumulate, leading to recurrent or chronic viral and bacterial infections. The primary pathogen is usually viral but bacterial infection often follows. Common bacterial pathogens include *Streptococcus pneumoniae*, *Moraxella catarrhalis* and *Haemophilus influenzae*.

Bronchiectasis is a pathological change in the lungs where the bronchi become permanently dilated. It is common after early attacks of acute bronchitis during which mucus both plugs and stretches the bronchial walls. In severe infections, the bronchioles and alveoli can become permanently damaged and do not return to their normal size and shape. The loss of muscle tone and loss of cilia can contribute to COPD because mucus has a tendency to accumulate in the dilated bronchi.

Airflow limitation and hyperinflation

Fibrosis and narrowing (airway remodelling) of the smaller conducting airways (<2 mm diameter) is the main site of expiratory airflow limitation in COPD. This is compounded by the loss of elastic recoil (destruction of alveolar walls), destruction of alveolar support/attachments and the accumulation of inflammatory cells mucus and plasma exudates during exercise. The degree of airflow limitation is measured by spirometry.

This progressive destructive enlargement of the respiratory bronchioles, alveolar ducts and alveolar sacs is referred to as emphysema. Adjacent alveoli can become indistinguishable from each other, with two main consequences. The first is loss of available gas exchange surfaces, which leads to an increase in dead space and impaired gas exchange. The second consequence is the loss of elastic recoil in the small airways, vital for maintaining the force of expiration, which leads to a tendency for them to collapse, particularly during expiration. Increased thoracic gas volume and hyperinflation of the lungs result. The causes of airflow limitation in COPD are summarised in Box 26.1.

Box 26.1	Causes of airflow limitation in COPD (GOLD, 2009)
Irreversible	• Fibrosis and narrowing of the airways • Loss of elastic recoil due to alveolar destruction • Destruction of alveolar support that maintains patency of small airways
Reversible	• Accumulation of inflammatory cells, mucus and plasma exudates in the bronchi • Smooth muscle contraction in peripheral and central airways • Dynamic hyperinflation during exercise

Gas exchange abnormalities

This occurs in advanced disease and is characterised by arterial hypoxaemia with or without hypercarbia. The anatomical changes during COPD result in an abnormal distribution of ventilation and perfusion within the lungs and create the abnormal gaseous exchange.

Pulmonary hypertension and cor pulmonale

Pulmonary hypertension develops late in COPD after gas exchange abnormalities have developed. The thickening of the bronchiole and alveolar walls resulting from chronic inflammation and oedema leads to blockage and obstruction of the airways. Alveolar distension and destruction result in distortion of the blood vessels that are closely associated with the alveoli. This causes a rise in the blood pressure in the pulmonary circulation. Reduction in gas diffusion across the alveolar epithelium leads to a low partial pressure of oxygen in the blood vessels (hypoxaemia) due to an imbalance between ventilation and perfusion. By a mechanism that is not clearly established, chronic vasoconstriction results and causes a further increase in blood pressure and further compromises gas diffusion from air spaces into the bloodstream. The chronic low oxygen levels lead to polycythaemia, thereby increasing blood viscosity. In advanced disease, persistent hypoxaemia develops along with pathological changes in the pulmonary circulation. Sustained pulmonary hypertension results in a thickening of the walls of the pulmonary arterioles, with associated pulmonary remodelling and an increase in right ventricular pressure within the heart.

The consequence of continued high right ventricular pressure is eventual right ventricular hypertrophy, dilation and progressive right ventricular failure (cor pulmonale). Pulmonary oedema develops as a result of physiological changes subsequent to the hypoxaemia and hypercapnia, such as activation of the renin–angiotensin system, salt and water retention and a reduction in renal blood flow.

Systemic effects

Systemic inflammation and skeletal muscle wasting can occur in COPD which limit exercise capacity and worsen prognosis. Osteoporosis, depression, normocytic normochromic anaemia are potential sequelae, as well as increased risk of cardiovascular disease associated with elevated levels of C-reactive protein.

Clinical manifestations

Diagnosis

A diagnosis of COPD should be considered in any patient who has symptoms of cough, wheeze, regular sputum production or exertional dyspnoea and/or a history of exposure to COPD risk factors (see Table 26.2). Spirometry is then used to confirm the diagnosis. There is no single diagnostic test for COPD.

Clinical features

COPD is a progressive disorder, which passes through a potentially asymptomatic mild phase, before the moderate phase and then severe disease. The traditional description of COPD symptoms, particularly in severe disease, depends on whether bronchitis or emphysema predominate. Chronic bronchitic patients exhibit excess mucus production and a degree of bronchospasm, resulting in wheeze and dyspnoea. Hypoxia and hypercapnia (high levels of carbon dioxide in the tissues) are common. This type of patient has a productive cough, is often overweight and finds physical exertion difficult due to dyspnoea. The bronchitic patient is sometimes referred to as a 'blue bloater'. This term is used because of the tendency of the patient to retain carbon dioxide caused by a decreased responsiveness of the respiratory centre to prolonged hypoxaemia that leads to cyanosis, and also the tendency for peripheral oedema to occur. Bronchitic patients lose the ability to increase the rate and depth of ventilation in response to persistent hypoxaemia. The reason for this is not clear, but decreased ventilatory drive may result from abnormal peripheral or central respiratory receptors. As the disease progresses, patients will experience an increasing frequency of exacerbations of acute dyspnoea triggered by excess mucus production and obstruction. In severe disease, the chest diameter is often increased, giving the classic barrel chest. As obstruction worsens, hypoxaemia increases, leading to pulmonary hypertension. Right ventricular strain leads to right ventricular failure, which is characterised by jugular venous distension, hepatomegaly and peripheral oedema, all of which are consequences of an increase in systemic venous blood pressure. Recurrent lower respiratory tract infections can be severe and debilitating. Signs of infection include an increase in the volume of thick and viscous sputum, which is yellow or green in colour and may contain bacterial pathogens, squamous epithelial cells, alveolar macrophages and saliva, but pyrexia may not be present. Eventually, cardiorespiratory failure with hypercapnia will occur, which may be severe, unresponsive to treatment and result in death.

The clinical features of emphysema are different from those of bronchitis. A patient with emphysema will experience increasing dyspnoea even at rest, but often there is minimal cough and the sputum produced is scanty and mucoid. Generally, bronchial infections tend to be less common in emphysema. The patient with emphysema is sometimes referred to as a 'pink puffer' because he or she hyperventilates to compensate for hypoxia by breathing in short puffs. As a result, the patient appears pink with little carbon dioxide retention and little evidence of oedema. The patient will breathe rapidly (tachypnoea), because the respiratory centres are responsive to mild hypoxaemia, and will have a flushed appearance. Typically, a patient with emphysema will be thin and have pursed lips in an effort to compensate for a lack of elastic recoil and exhale a larger volume of air. Such a patient will tend to use the accessory muscles of the chest and neck to assist in the work of breathing. Hypoxaemia is not a problem until the disease has progressed. Emphysema patients will become progressively dyspnoeic, without exacerbations triggered by increased sputum production. Eventually, cor pulmonale will develop very rapidly, usually in the late stages of the disease, leading to intractable hypercapnia and respiratory arrest. The bronchitic 'blue bloater' and emphysemic 'pink puffer' represent two ends of the COPD spectrum. In reality, the underlying pathophysiology may well be a mixture, and the resulting signs and symptoms somewhere between the two extremes described.

The clinical progress of COPD depends on whether bronchitis or emphysema predominates.

Additional specific problems are also common in patients with COPD:

- Obstructive sleep apnoea hypopnoea syndrome (OSAHS)
- Acute respiratory failure

The sleep apnoea syndrome is a respiratory disorder characterised by frequent or prolonged pauses in breathing during sleep. It leads to a deterioration in arterial blood gases and a decrease in the saturation of haemoglobin with oxygen. Hypoxaemia is often accompanied by pulmonary hypertension and cardiac arrhythmias, which may lead to premature cardiac failure.

Acute respiratory failure is said to have occurred if the PaO_2 suddenly drops and there is an increase in $PaCO_2$ that decreases the pH to 7.3 or less. The most common cause is an acute exacerbation of chronic bronchitis with an increase in volume and viscosity of sputum. This further impairs ventilation and causes more severe hypoxaemia and hypercapnia. The clinical signs and symptoms of acute respiratory failure include restlessness, confusion, tachycardia, cyanosis, sweating, hypotension and eventual unconsciousness.

Investigations

Lung function tests are used to assist in diagnosis. A spirometer is used to measure lung volumes and flow rates. The main measurement made is the forced expiratory volume in the first second of exhalation (FEV_1). Other tests can be performed, such as:

- *Vital capacity (VC)*: the volume of air inhaled and exhaled during maximal ventilation;

- *Forced vital capacity (FVC)*: the volume of air inhaled and exhaled during a forced maximal expiration after full inspiration;
- *Residual volume (RV)*: the volume of air left in the lungs after maximal exhalation.

Airflow obstruction is defined as:

- FEV_1 less than 80% of that predicted for the patient and
- FEV_1/FVC less than 0.7.

VC decreases in bronchitis and emphysema. RV increases in both cases but tends to be higher in patients with emphysema due to air being trapped distal to the terminal bronchioles. Total lung capacity is often normal in patients with bronchitis but is usually increased in emphysema, again due to air being trapped. Smoking increases the normal deterioration in FEV_1 over time, from about 30 mL/year to about 45 mL/year. The major criticism of measuring FEV_1 and FVC is that they detect changes only in airways greater than 2 mm in diameter. As airways less than 2 mm in diameter contribute only 10–20% of normal resistance to airflow, there is usually severe obstruction and extensive damage to the lungs by the time the lung function tests (FEV_1 and FVC) detect abnormalities. Additionally, lung function tends to deteriorate with age even in the absence of COPD, and so use of FEV_1/FVC can lead to overdiagnosis in the elderly. Underdiagnosis may also be a problem in patients under 45 years of age.

Both UK and international COPD guidelines use spirometry to categorise the severity of COPD. These are summarised in Table 26.3. Testing should be carried out after a dose of inhaled bronchodilator to prevent overdiagnosis or overestimation of severity.

At diagnosis and evaluation, patients may receive other investigations as outlined in Table 26.4.

Chest radiographs reveal differences between the two disease states. A patient with emphysema will have a flattened diaphragm with loss of peripheral vascular markings and the appearance of bullae. These are indicative of extensive trapping of air. A patient with bronchitis will have increased bronchovascular markings and may also have cardiomegaly (increased cardiac size due to right ventricular failure) with prominent pulmonary arteries.

Table 26.3 Assessment of severity of airflow obstruction (adapted from National Institute for Health and Clinical Excellence, 2010; GOLD, 2009)

FEV_1	Severity (NICE)	Severity (GOLD)
Greater than 80% predicted		Stage I: Mild
50–80% predicted	Mild	Stage II: Moderate
30–49% predicted	Moderate	Stage III: Severe
Less than 30% predicted	Severe	Stage IV: Very severe

Table 26.4 Additional investigations at the diagnosis of COPD

Investigation	Note
Chest X-ray	To exclude other pathologies
Full blood count	To identify anaemia or polycythaemia
Serial domiciliary peak flow measurements	To exclude asthma if there is a doubt about diagnosis
α_1-Antitrypsin	Particularly with early-onset disease or a minimal smoking/family history
Transfer factor for carbon monoxide	To investigate symptoms that seem disproportionate to the spirometric impairment
CT scan of the thorax	To investigate symptoms that seem disproportionate to the spirometric impairment To investigate abnormalities seen on the chest X-ray To assess suitability for surgery
ECG	To assess cardiac status if features of cor pulmonale
Echocardiogram	To assess cardiac status if features of cor pulmonale
Pulse oximetry	To assess need for oxygen therapy If cyanosis or cor pulmonale is present or if FEV_1 <50% of predicted value
Sputum culture	To identify organisms if sputum is persistently present and purulent

Treatment

Stable COPD

Drug treatments, together with other measures such as physiotherapy and artificial ventilation, have not been shown to improve the natural progression of COPD. Quality of life and symptoms will, however, improve with suitable treatment and it is likely that the correct management of the patient will lead to a reduction in hospital admissions and prevent premature death. In patients with severe COPD and hypoxaemia, long-term oxygen therapy (LTOT) is the only treatment known to improve the prognosis.

The aims of treatment for patients with COPD are shown in Box 26.2 and the common therapeutic problems associated with COPD in Box 26.3. Drug treatment itself can only relieve symptoms; it does not modify the underlying pathology. Most patients with COPD are considered to have irreversible obstruction, in contrast to patients with asthma, but a significant number do seem to respond to bronchodilators.

Smoking cessation

Smoking is the most important factor in the development of obstructive airways disease. All COPD patients who are still smoking, regardless of age, should be encouraged to stop and be offered help to do so, at every opportunity. Unless contraindicated, all patients who are planning to stop smoking should be offered nicotine replacement therapy (NRT), varenicline or bupropion, as appropriate along with a support programme (NRT) (National Institute for Health and Clinical Excellence, 2010). Individually targeted advice may prove to be more successful in persuading individuals to give up, especially in those who are well.

Bronchodilators

Bronchodilators in COPD are used to reverse airflow limitation. As the degree of limitation varies widely, their effectiveness should be assessed in each patient using respiratory function tests and by assessing any subjective improvement reported by the patient. Patients may experience

---

Box 26.2 Treatment aims for patients with COPD

- Prevent disease progression
- Relieve symptoms
- Improve exercise tolerance
- Improve health status
- Prevent and treat complications such as hypoxaemia and infections
- Prevent and treat exacerbations
- Reduce mortality

Box 26.3 Common therapeutic problems associated with COPD

- Failure of patient to stop smoking
- Inadequate inhaler technique leading to subtherapeutic dosing
- Poor adherence with treatment regimen
- Inappropriate prescribing of antibiotics in an acute exacerbation of COPD
- Failure to properly assess a patient for home nebuliser therapy
- Failure to ensure adherence to 15 h a day of home oxygen therapy

improvements in exercise tolerance or relief of symptoms such as wheeze and cough. Treatment options for the use of bronchodilators and inhaled corticosteroids (ICSs) are outlined in Fig. 26.1.

Initial empiric therapy with short-acting bronchodilators, prescribed 'when required', for the relief of breathlessness and exercise limitation are recommended for initial use (National Institute for Health and Clinical Excellence, 2010). If patients remain breathless or have exacerbations despite short-acting bronchodilators then maintenance therapy is recommended, with:

- FEV_1 ≥50% predicted: long-acting β_2-adrenoceptor agonist (LABA) or long-acting antimuscarinic (LAMA)
- FEV_1 <50% predicted: a combination of either LABA and ICSs or LABA and LAMA

If the patient remains breathless, or has exacerbations, then triple therapy should be considered (i.e. ICS and LABA in a combination inhaler together with a LAMA).

Short-acting bronchodilators (short-acting β_2-adrenoceptor agonist or short-acting antimuscarinic). Selective β_2-agonists provide rapid relief and have a low incidence of side effects. Inhaled treatment is as efficacious as oral agents and is, therefore, preferred because of fewer side effects. The dose response curve for β_2-agonists in COPD is almost flat and there is little

benefit in giving more than 1 mg. The effects of short-acting β_2-agonists last for 4 h and they should be used 'as required' for symptom relief. Used before exercise, they can improve exercise tolerance. Poor patient response to bronchodilators may be due to poor inhalation technique, so this should be checked as often as possible and the inhaler device changed if necessary.

In patients with COPD, parasympathetic (vagal) airway muscle tone is the major reversible component. Inhaled anticholinergic drugs reverse this vagal tone and have a significant bronchodilator effect, especially in the elderly.

Long-acting bronchodilators. Long-acting bronchodilators include LAMAs and LABAs. The only LAMA in the UK, tiotropium, has a 24-h duration of action and can reduce exacerbation rates, increase exercise tolerance and reduce rates of hospital admissions, though not the rate of decline in lung function. There is no strong evidence to favour either a LABA or LAMA for monotherapy (National Clinical Guideline Centre, 2010).

High-dose bronchodilators. Some patients with distressing or debilitating breathlessness despite maximal inhaled therapy may benefit from higher doses, either by inhaler or via a nebuliser. These patients should have their inhaled therapy optimised, possibly using a protocol as outlined in Box 26.4.

Theophylline. Theophylline is a weak bronchodilator but seems to have useful additional physiological effects in COPD

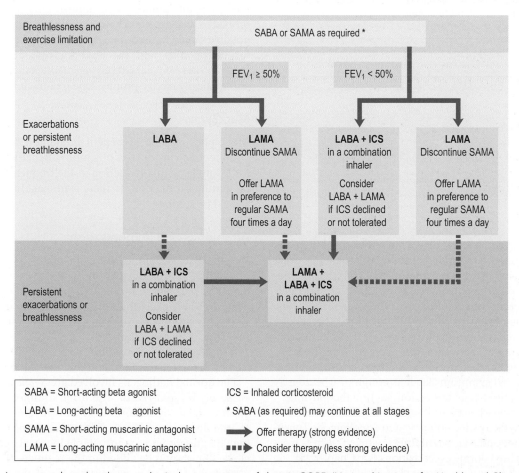

Fig. 26.1 Stepwise approach to the pharmacological management of chronic COPD (National Institute for Health and Clinical Excellence, 2010; with kind permission from National Institute for Health and Clinical Excellence).

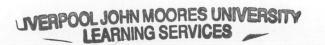

Box 26.4 Optimisation of high dose inhaled and nebulised therapy for patients with severe COPD (adapted from Boe et al., 2001; National Institute for Health and Clinical Excellence, 2010; O'Driscoll, 1997)

1. Assessment by a respiratory specialist. Check diagnosis and confirm severity. Ensure optimal inhaler technique

2. Ensure all other therapies have been tried

3. Optimise hand-held inhaler dosing, for example:
   - Salbutamol 200–400 μcg four times a day
   - Ipratropium bromide 40 μcg four times a day or tiotropium 18 μcg once daily

   or a combination of these agents

4. Try further increasing the dose of the hand-held inhaler to:
   - Salbutamol up to 1 mg four times a day, and/or
   - Ipratropium bromide up to 160 μcg four times a day (although the effect of alternative use of tiotropium at this stage is unknown)

   These doses are unlicensed in the UK

5. If a poor response at step 4, consider a period of home nebulizer therapy with careful examination of patient response, over at least 2 weeks
   - Reduction in symptoms
   - An increase in the patient's ability to undertake activities of daily living
   - An increase in exercise capacity
   - An improvement in lung function
   - The occurrence of side effects such as tachycardia and tremor

6. Initial therapy: try nebulised salbutamol 2.5 mg or terbutaline 5 mg four times a day and assess response at 2 weeks

7. If the response to monotherapy is poor, consider one or more of the following:
   - Salbutamol 5 mg or terbutaline 10 mg four times a day, or
   - Ipratropium bromide 250–500 μcg four times a day, or the combination
   - Salbutamol 2.5–5 mg and ipratropium 500 μcg four times a day

8. Decide which treatment in step 7 was the most beneficial

---

such as increased respiratory drive, improved diaphragmatic function and improved cardiac output, although the exact clinical benefits have not been quantified. The use of theophylline should only be considered after a trial of short acting with long-acting bronchodilators. Whenever theophylline is tried in the management of COPD, an initial therapeutic trial of several weeks should be carried out. If subjective and objective measures of lung function show an improvement, then theophylline can be continued as maintenance therapy. Persistent nocturnal symptoms such as cough or wheeze may be helped by the night-time use of long-acting theophylline.

Care must be taken when prescribing theophylline. Its clearance is affected by many factors, including cigarette smoking, viral pneumonia, heart failure and concurrent drug treatment, such as macrolide antibiotics used during exacerbations (see Chapter 25).

Theophylline is being investigated in low concentrations for its ability to reverse the decrease in histone deacetylase activity associated with oxidative stress. This may prove to be of benefit in reversing corticosteroid resistance.

Corticosteroids

Patients with COPD show a poor response to corticosteroids and have a largely steroid-resistant pattern of inflammation (Barnes, 2004). It is postulated that the oxidative stress of COPD inhibits the mechanism by which corticosteroids, acting through histone deacetylase, switch off activated inflammatory genes.

The long-term benefits of ICSs in COPD have only been shown in patients with moderate-to-severe disease, with an FEV_1 less than 50% of predicted value and who are having exacerbations requiring treatment with antibiotics and oral corticosteroids (National Institute for Health and Clinical Excellence, 2010). A reduction in the number of exacerbations and a slowing of the decline in health status have been shown, but these have no effect on improving lung function and result in an increased risk of pneumonia.

ICSs should be used, although there is no consensus over the minimum effective dose. In the UK, no inhaled steroid is licensed for use in COPD except when used with LABA in combination devices.

There is little place for oral steroids in stable COPD. Some patients with advanced disease may require maintenance oral therapy if this cannot be withdrawn after a short course prescribed to treat an exacerbation. In this instance, the lowest dose possible should be used. The patient should be regularly assessed for osteoporosis and the need for osteoporosis prevention. Patients over 65 years receiving maintenance therapy should automatically receive prophylactic treatment for osteoporosis.

Mucolytics

Mucolytics may be of benefit in stable COPD if there is a chronic cough productive of sputum. Benefit must be assessed, for example, with a reduction in the frequency of cough and/or sputum production. If there is no benefit, then mucolytics should be stopped.

Antibiotics and immunisation

Prophylactic antibiotics have no place in the management of COPD. Antibiotic therapy is, however, vital if a patient develops purulent sputum. If a patient frequently develops acute infective exacerbations of bronchitis then they should be given a supply of antibiotics to keep at home to start at the first sign of an exacerbation.

Initial routine sputum cultures are unhelpful in these patients as they are unreliable in identifying the pathogenic organisms.

The normal pathogens involved are *S. pneumoniae*, *H. influenzae* or *M. catarrhalis*. The usual antibiotics of choice are co-amoxiclav, amoxicillin, erythromycin or doxycycline. If the infection follows influenza, *Staphylococcus aureus* may be present and an anti-staphylococcal agent such as flucloxacillin should be added to the regimen. If the infection is considered atypical in presentation or if the purulent sputum is still present after 1 week of treatment, then sputum cultures should be taken to try to identify the pathogenic organisms. A single dose of pneumococcal vaccine and annual influenza vaccinations have been shown to reduce hospitalisations and the risk of death in the elderly with chronic lung disease, and should be offered to those with chronic airflow obstruction. The prevalent strains of influenza change, so the vaccine composition is, correspondingly, altered annually.

Acute exacerbations of COPD

Patients with COPD suffer acute worsenings of the disease, referred to as acute exacerbations. These exacerbations can be spontaneous but are often precipitated by infection and lead to respiratory failure with hypoxaemia and retention of carbon dioxide. Many patients can be managed at home (see National Institute for Health and Clinical Excellence, 2010) but some will require admission to hospital.

Bronchodilators

Bronchodilators are used to treat the increased breathlessness that is associated with exacerbations. These can be given by metered-dose inhaler (MDI) or nebuliser, although practically breathless patients are often unable to use MDIs effectively. A β_2-agonist can be given with or without an anticholinergic agent, depending on the benefits obtained.

Antibiotics

Bacteria can be isolated from the sputum of patients with stable COPD but antibiotics can be used to treat exacerbations of COPD associated with a history of more purulent sputum. The choice of antibiotic should be dependent on local policy, sensitivity patterns and any previous treatments. An amino-penicillin or a macrolide with increased activity against *H. influenzae* or oxytetracycline is generally suitable as a first-line agent. Sputum should be sent for culture in order to check the appropriateness of initial therapy, and the antibiotic changed if necessary.

Corticosteroids

A short course of oral steroids has been shown to benefit FEV_1 and reduce the duration of hospitalisation. Patients managed at home who have increased breathlessness which interferes with daily activities and all those admitted to hospital should be treated. A suitable course is prednisolone 30 mg every morning, given for 7–14 days.

Other treatment

Intravenous aminophylline can be considered, if there is an inadequate response to bronchodilators. The loading dose and maintenance dose required should be carefully chosen as these depend on various factors (see Chapter 25).

Oxygen therapy is necessary to improve hypoxia. In about a quarter of patients with COPD, a predisposition to carbon dioxide retention will be present. Administration of high concentrations of oxygen to these individuals can lead to an increase in retention of carbon dioxide and, thus, to respiratory acidosis. The widely held view that this effect is due to loss of hypoxic ventilatory drive has been questioned; a more complex process involving a mismatch between ventilation and perfusion is now thought to play a significant role. The goal is an initial oxygen saturation of between 88% and 92% to avoid respiratory acidosis but to allow enough oxygen to be administered to overcome potentially life-threatening hypoxia (O'Driscoll et al., 2008). The initial concentration used should be 24–28% and then titrated to oxygen saturation. Arterial blood gases should be monitored regularly.

During an acute attack, pyrexia, hyperventilation and the excessive work of breathing can result in an inability to eat or drink. This can lead to dehydration which requires treatment with intravenous hydration.

Chest physiotherapy is employed to mobilise secretions, promote expectoration and expand collapsed lung segments. Nebulised 0.9% sodium chloride has also been used to help.

Although largely superseded by non-invasive ventilatory support, doxapram (as a continuous infusion at a rate of 1–4 mg/min) can be tried in patients with acute respiratory failure, carbon dioxide retention and depressed ventilation. Doxapram stimulates the respiratory and vasomotor centres in the medulla, increases the depth of breathing and may slightly increase the rate of breathing. Arterial oxygenation is usually not improved because of the increased work of breathing induced by doxapram. This agent has a narrow therapeutic index with side effects such as arrhythmias, vasoconstriction, dizziness and convulsions and may be harmful if used when the $PaCO_2$ is normal or low.

Treatment of hypoxaemia and cor pulmonale

COPD is responsible for over 90% of cases of cor pulmonale. Although patients often tolerate mild hypoxaemia, once the resting PaO_2 drops below 8 kPa signs of cor pulmonale develop. Treatment is symptomatic and involves managing the underlying airways obstruction, hypoxaemia and any pulmonary oedema that develops. Peripheral oedema is managed using thiazide or loop diuretics, although there are concerns over their metabolic effects reducing respiratory drive. Oxygen is used to treat hypoxaemia, and this should also promote a diuresis. All patients should be assessed for the need for LTOT.

Domiciliary oxygen therapy

The aim of therapy is to improve oxygen delivery to the cells, increase alveolar oxygen tension and decrease the work of breathing to maintain a given PaO_2. Domiciliary oxygen therapy can be given in two ways.

Intermittent (short burst) administration. Intermittent administration is used to increase mobility and capacity for exercise and to ease discomfort. Intermittent administration is of most benefit in patients with emphysema.

Continuous LTOT. LTOT for at least 15 h/day has been shown to improve survival in patients with severe, irreversible airflow obstruction, hypoxaemia and peripheral oedema (MRC Working Party, 1981). LTOT can only be prescribed if specific conditions are met, as described in Box 26.5. The main aim of treatment is to achieve a PaO_2 of at least 8 kPa without causing a rise in $PaCO_2$ of more than 1 kPa, achieved by adjusting the oxygen flow rate. Before LTOT can be prescribed each individual must be assessed accordingly (see Box 26.5).

Oxygen can be prescribed as oxygen cylinders but 15 h/day at 2 L/min requires ten 1340-L cylinders a week. A more convenient system is to use a concentrator, which converts ambient air to 90% oxygen using a molecular sieve. The concentrator is sited in a well-ventilated area in the home with plastic tubing to terminals in rooms such as the living room and bedroom. Tubing from the terminals delivers oxygen to the patient, who wears a mask or uses the more convenient nasal prongs. This tubing should be long enough to allow some mobility.

Patient care

Pulmonary rehabilitation

Early pulmonary rehabilitation should be considered for patients at all stages of disease progression when symptoms and disability are present. Patients should participate in a co-coordinated programme of non-pharmacological treatment including:

- advice and support to stop smoking
- nutritional assessment
- aerobic exercise training to increase capacity and endurance for exercise
- strength training for upper and lower limbs
- relaxation techniques
- breathing retraining, for example, diaphragmatic and pursed lips breathing to improve the ventilatory pattern and improve gas exchange
- education about their medicines, nutrition, self-management of their disease and lifestyle issues
- psychological support because COPD patients often have decreased capacity to participate in social and recreational activities and can become anxious, depressed or fatigued.

A multidisciplinary team should deliver these programmes and should include a minimum of 6 and a maximum of 12 weeks of physical exercise, disease education, psychological and social interventions (National Institute for Health and Clinical Excellence, 2010).

Pulmonary rehabilitation programmes that include at least 4 weeks exercise training have been shown to improve dyspnoea and exercise capacity. The long-term effects, however, of these programmes has yet to be established, although personalised education to COPD patients about their condition has been shown to reduce their need for health services.

Stopping smoking

The health hazards associated with smoking are well known and publicised. To give up smoking, which has been described as a form of drug addiction, requires self-motivation. Stopping smoking does not, however, have an immediate effect. A reduction in COPD mortality is not seen until about 10 years or more after cessation of smoking.

Members of the healthcare team can educate smokers about the dangers and actively encourage and motivate those who want to give up. Brief conversations between individuals and health professionals about stopping smoking are both effective and cost-effective in encouraging individuals to quit (National Institute for Health and Clinical Excellence, 2006).

Once a decision to quit has been made, it is the degree of dependence rather than the level of motivation that will influence the success rate. Smokers need both initial advice from all healthcare professionals and follow-up support. For example, especially in the early stages, symptoms such as coughing increase after the cigarettes are stopped. The patient must be closely supported to avoid a return to the habit. Strategies such as individual behavioural counselling, group behaviour therapy and use of self-help materials and telephone counselling and 'quit lines' have been advocated as effective interventions.

There are a number of therapeutic options to help an individual to stop smoking and these include NRT, bupropion and varenicline.

Nicotine replacement

The major mode of action of NRT is thought to involve stimulation of nicotine receptors in the brain and the subsequent release of dopamine. This, together with the peripheral effects of nicotine, leads to a reduction in nicotine withdrawal symptoms. NRT may also act as a coping mechanism, making cigarette smoking less rewarding. NRT does not, however, completely eliminate the effects of withdrawal as none of the available products reproduces the rapid and high levels of nicotine obtained from cigarettes.

There is little research comparing the relative effectiveness of NRT products, but all seem to have similar success rates. Choice of product should be made on the number of cigarettes smoked (irrespective of the nicotine content), the smoker's personal preference and tolerance to side effects. An individual is more likely to adhere to the cessation programme if using a product which suits him or her. The types of NRT available are summarised in Table 26.5.

NRT approximately doubles smoking cessation rates compared with controls (either placebo or no NRT), irrespective of the intensity of adjunctive therapy. The strongest evidence is

Table 26.5 Comparison of selected nicotine replacement products

Formulation	Use and comments	Specific side effects
Patch: 24 h: 7, 14 and 21 mg; 16 h: 5, 10, 15 and 25 mg	One daily on clean, non-hairy, unbroken skin. Remove before morning (16 h) or next morning (24 h). Apply to fresh site or non-hairy skin, usually at the hip, trunk or upper arm. Should not be applied to broken skin	Local skin irritation and rashes, insomnia. Do not use with generalised skin disease
Gum: 2 and 4 mg	Chew until taste is strong then rest gum between gum and cheek; chew again when taste has faded. Repeat this for 30 min or until taste dissipates. Avoid acidic drinks for 15 min before and during chewing the gum	Jaw ache, headache and dyspnoea. Mild burning sensation in the mouth and throat
Sublingual tablet: 2 or 4 mg each	Rest under tongue until dissolved	
Lozenge: 1, 2 or 4 mg each	Place between gum and cheek and allow to dissolve. Delivers slightly more nicotine than the equivalent gum	Nasal irritation, rhinorrhoea, sneezing, throat irritation and cough. This usually dissipates with continued use
Inhalator: 10 mg per cartridge	Inhale as required. Helps to satisfy the hand-to-mouth ritual of using a cigarette which may help some people. The nicotine is absorbed through the mouth rather than the lungs. Use with caution in people with asthma	Nasal irritation, rhinorrhoea, sneezing, throat irritation and cough. This usually dissipates with continued use
Nasal spray: 500 μcg per spray	One spray into each nostril as needed. More rapidly absorbed than other forms of NRT so often used for acute relief of cravings. Not recommended for people with nasal or sinus conditions, allergies or asthma	

for use of patches and gum. The choice of product and initial dose is also influenced by the degree of tobacco dependence; heavy smokers (15 to 20+ cigarettes a day and/or smoking within 30 min of waking) will require higher NRT doses. The available types of NRT product are set out below:

Long acting. Long-acting transdermal patches are considered to be most suitable for people who smoke regularly through the day. The 24-h patch, worn overnight, is better for people who crave nicotine first thing in the morning. Use of the patch can cause insomnia or vivid dreams and so can either be removed before bedtime or a 16-h patch used instead. Heavy smokers should be started on the high-dose patches.

Short acting. There are several short-acting products available:

Gum. It is important to chew nicotine gum correctly. The gum should be chewed slowly until the taste becomes strong and then allowed to rest between the cheek and teeth to allow absorption. When the taste has faded the gum should be chewed again. Nicotine gum is not a good choice for people with dentures or other vulnerable dental work. Most gum users do not consume enough in a day to match the nicotine levels from smoking. Patients should be encouraged to use 10–15 pieces of gum a day, for example, as one piece an hour.

Lozenge. These are allowed to dissolve in the mouth and periodically moved around, until completely gone. One lozenge per hour is recommended during the initial period of use to provide adequate nicotine absorption.

Inhalator. Inhalators may be particularly useful for people who miss the physical act of smoking. Nicotine is absorbed via the buccal mucosa, peaking in 20–30 min. To achieve sufficient blood levels, the user should puff on the inhalator for 2 min each hour, changing the cartridge after three 20-min sessions.

Nasal spray. A nasal spray is most useful for people who smoke 20 or more cigarettes per day. The side effects of sneezing and a burning sensation in the nose usually wear off after a day or two, so patients should be encouraged to persevere.

Sublingual tablets. These tablets dissolve under the tongue and may be useful for people with dentures who have difficulty using nicotine gum. Hourly use should be recommended.

Bupropion (amfebutamone)

Originally used as an antidepressant, bupropion has been licensed for use in smoking cessation. It inhibits neuronal noradrenaline and dopamine uptake, reducing tobacco withdrawal symptoms by increasing CNS dopamine levels. Treatment should be started while the patient is still smoking with a target date to stop smoking set during the second week of use. The total treatment period should be for 7–9 weeks. The initial dose should be 150 mg daily for 6 days, increasing to 150 mg twice a day thereafter (with at least 8 h between doses). Bupropion is as effective as NRT and intensive behavioural support. There is no clear evidence of benefit over NRT but there is some evidence of better results if used in combination with NRT.

Bupropion should not be used in patients with a current or previous seizure disorder or in patients with bulimia, anorexia nervosa, bipolar disorder, severe hepatic cirrhosis or those taking monoamine oxidase inhibitors; nor is it appropriate for use in smokers under the age of 18. Bupropion inhibits cytochrome P450 enzymes and so may inhibit the metabolism of other drugs. The main side effects experienced include dry mouth, insomnia (avoid bedtime dosing), headache, dizziness, allergic reactions, taste disorder and seizures.

Varenicline

Varenicline is an oral selective partial $\alpha_4\beta_2$ agonist at the neuronal nicotinic acetylcholine receptor. Varenicline alleviates the symptoms of craving and withdrawal, whilst reducing the rewarding and reinforcing effects of smoking by preventing nicotine binding to $\alpha_4\beta_2$ receptors. Trial evidence suggests use may result in a higher abstinence rate than either bupropion or NRT, although this may not be sustained after 12 months. Use is recommended as an option for smokers aged 18 or over wishing to quit, ideally in the context of a behavioural support programme (National Institute for Health and Clinical Excellence, 2007). Varenicline should be started 1–2 weeks before stopping smoking. The main side effects are nausea, vomiting, abnormal dreams and insomnia. Fears over a possible increased risk of depression and suicide have been allayed (Gunnell et al., 2009), although individuals who develop agitation, depressed mood or suicidal thoughts are required to seek prompt medical advice.

Combination therapy involving varenicline and bupropion (either with each other or in conjunction with NRT) is not recommended.

Use of inhaled therapy

For individuals suffering from obstructive airways disease with a degree of reversibility, the correct use of inhaled therapy is a vital part of overall management.

Medication counselling needs to highlight the modes of action of the bronchodilators, particularly the more rapid onset of the β_2-agonists to relieve breathlessness rather than the slower-acting anticholinergics. If inhaled steroids are prescribed, the importance of regular administration must be stressed. The incorrect use of any inhaler will lead to subtherapeutic dosing. The correct use of inhalers is, therefore, as vital in the management of COPD patients as it is for patients with asthma (see Chapter 25). The advantages and disadvantages of each type of inhaler device are summarised in Table 26.6.

Domiciliary oxygen therapy

Studies have shown that only about 50% of patients on LTOT comply with the requirement for 15 h of treatment a day. Counselling will be required to persuade the patient to comply with this minimum figure. Emphasis must be given to the improvement in quality of life gained from treatment rather than the idea of being continually 'tied' to the oxygen supply. If an oxygen concentrator is used, limited mobility can be gained by installing at least two terminals for the unit (usually in the living room and bedroom) with long tubing between the terminal and nasal prongs.

Patients should be actively encouraged to stop smoking if they still do; because of the fire risk if they use LTOT. Moreover, the carbon monoxide present in tobacco smoke binds to haemoglobin and forms carboxy-haemoglobin, which decreases the amount of oxygen that can be transported by the blood and will partially or completely negate the beneficial effects of LTOT.

The long-term, chronic nature of COPD may leave a patient with a fear of exercise as this will cause dyspnoea (breathlessness). Thus, the patient with COPD may decide not to undertake any exercise. Ambulatory oxygen cylinders can be used to encourage mobility and increase exercise tolerance during travel outside the home.

Patients using domiciliary oxygen are followed up to provide education and support, to assess the oxygen saturation of the patient and to assess the suitability of the delivery device for ambulatory oxygen if provided. Suitable devices have been suggested (National Institute for Health and Clinical Excellence, 2010) depending on the amount of time required for use (Table 26.7).

Table 26.6 Comparison of inhaler devices

Inhaler type	Compact	Hand–lung co-ordination required	Easy to use	Reduces oropharynx deposition
MDI	+	+	−	−
MDI + small spacer	+	±	±	+
MDI + large spacer	−	−	±	+
Breath-actuated MDI	+	−	+	−
Dry powder	+	−	±	−
Breath-actuated dry powder	+	−	+	−
Nebuliser	−	−	±	−

MDI, metered-dose inhaler; +, feature present; ±, feature present for some patients; −, feature absent.

Table 26.7 Oxygen delivery for ambulatory oxygen therapy (National Institute for Health and Clinical Excellence, 2010)

How long is the oxygen used by the patient?	Best type of delivery device
Less than 90 min	Small cylinder
90 min to 4 h	Small cylinder with oxygen-conserving device
More than 4 h	Liquid oxygen
More than 30 min, with flow rates greater than 2 L/min	Liquid oxygen

Case studies

Case 26.1

Mr JF, a 74-year-old man, has a long-standing history of COPD. He has a 70-pack-year history of smoking, but finally managed to give up 4 years ago, after numerous admissions to hospital for infective exacerbations. He is recovering on the respiratory ward from his first admission for 6 months. His consultant believes he may be a candidate for long-term oxygen therapy.

Questions

1. What criteria should Mr JF fill in order to be eligible for long-term oxygen therapy?
2. How is long-term oxygen therapy delivered?
3. Why might Mr JF be anxious about starting long-term oxygen therapy?
4. How would you allay these concerns?
5. What is the intended outcome of using long-term oxygen therapy?

Answers

1. In order to be eligible for long-term oxygen therapy, patients should have, when stable and on two separate occasions at least 3 weeks apart:

   pO_2 <7.3 kPa
   or
   pO_2 >7.3 kPa and <8.0 kPa as well as at least one of the following:

   - secondary polycythaemia
   - nocturnal hypoxaemia (O_2 saturations <90% for >30% of the time)
   - peripheral oedema
   - pulmonary hypertension

2. It is impractical to deliver long-term oxygen therapy using cylinders. Instead, an oxygen concentrator, a device which increases the relative concentration of oxygen in environmental air via a molecular 'sieving' process, is used. In most cases, a flow rate of 2 L/min is delivered via nasal cannulae. Patients must use the concentrator for at least 15 h, and preferably over 20 h a day to achieve intended therapeutic outcomes (see below).

3. Mr JF may be concerned for several reasons listed:

   - the length of time he will be tied to the machine each day
   - restrictions on leaving the house once he starts his 15 h a day
   - the cost of the electricity required to drive the concentrator
   - loss of supply if there is a power cut

4. Mr JF's concerns are logical but he can be reassured. The concentrator can be used while he is asleep (generally two outlets are installed, one in the living room and the other in the bedroom) and so this leaves him up to 9 h a day where he does not need to be using oxygen. The 15-h minimum does not have to be continuous, and so he can leave the house or interrupt the oxygen delivery as necessary to carry out activities of daily living. The cost of the electricity is covered by the oxygen contractor, who will monitor usage using a meter. Contractors are required to install a backup power supply which will continue to drive the concentrator for a minimum of 8 h should the mains supply fail.

5. Provided patients receive the required duration of therapy each day, beneficial effects on life expectancy, exercise tolerance and mental capacity can be anticipated.

Case 26.2

Mrs VL, a 58-year-old lady, has been brought into hospital by ambulance having been struggling with dyspnoea and significantly reduced exercise tolerance for several days. You review her chart and medical notes on the hospital admissions ward. The working diagnosis is an infective exacerbation of COPD. The patient presents with:

Thick green sputum which the patient reports is usually clear/white.

O_2 saturation of 82% on 28% oxygen delivered via a Venturi mask

Arterial blood gases (ABG):

    pH 7.33 (7.35–7.45)
    pO_2 7.24 kPa (10.7 kPa)
    pCO_2 7.1 kPa (4.7–6.0 kPa)
    Bicarbonate 46 mmol/L (22–26 mmol/L)
    D-dimer negative

Drug history:

    Salbutamol 2.5 mg via a nebuliser four times a day
    Symbicort® 200/6 2 puffs twice a day
    Tiotropium 18 μcg daily
    Furosemide 40 mg twice a day
    Ramipril 5 mg daily
    Alendronate 70 mg weekly on Saturdays
    Adcal D3 2 tablets daily

Mrs VL is commenced on:

    Salbutamol 5 mg via a nebuliser 4 hourly
    Ipratropium bromide 500 μcg via a nebuliser 6 hourly
    Prednisolone 30 mg daily
    Co-amoxiclav 1.2 g i.v. three times a day
    Doxycycline 200 mg stat then 100 mg od thereafter.

Questions

1. Explain the arterial blood gas profile.
2. What is the significance of the negative D-dimer result?

3. If she does not respond to initial therapy, what might it be appropriate to change or introduce?

Answers

1. The low pO_2 indicates significant hypoxia. A slightly low pH and slightly elevated pCO_2 suggest a respiratory acidosis. The high bicarbonate level indicates that this acid/base disturbance is compensated at this level. The bicarbonate is likely to have accumulated over a relatively prolonged period.

2. A negative D-dimer is a strong indicator that Mrs VL's dyspnoea is not as a result of a pulmonary embolism. Although a raised D-dimer is not a reliable means of confirming thromboembolic disease (low specificity – frequent false positives), it is far more reliable in excluding such conditions where the result falls within the normal range (high sensitivity – rare false negatives). It is important to exclude conditions such as pulmonary embolism or acute left ventricular failure when patients with COPD present with increased shortness of breath to avoid missed diagnoses.

3. The concentration of oxygen could be increased to 35%. Mrs VL may be at risk of developing hypercapnia as a result of her COPD, and so her arterial blood gases should be rechecked 30–60 min after the change in her oxygen therapy. Particular attention should be made to any increase in the carbon dioxide concentration. If Mrs VL's respiratory rate exceeds 30 breaths/min while using a Venturi mask, the oxygen flow rate should be increased by 50%. The target for oxygen therapy is to achieve a saturation of 88–92%.

   Inadequate response to nebulised bronchodilators is an indication where intravenous aminophylline should be considered. A loading dose of 5 mg/kg over at least 20 min followed by a continuous infusion of 500 μcg/kg/h can be administered. Levels should be checked within the first 24 h of therapy.

   There is no evidence that use of mucolytics at this acute stage will be of benefit.

Case 26.3

Mrs SS is a 61-year-old retired factory worker who has been recently diagnosed with COPD after admission to hospital. She was discharged a few days ago having been started on a nicotine patch, 14 mg every 24 h. She asks you for advice on the best way to give up smoking as she has tried several times in the past and failed to quit. She smokes around 25 cigarettes a day and has been smoking since she was 17. She has a history of oesophageal reflux and also has epilepsy.

Questions

1. Why is it important for Mrs SS to give up smoking?
2. How many pack-years has she smoked?
3. What aspects should be discussed when helping someone to stop smoking?
   When you question Mrs SS about her previous attempts to stop smoking, she confides that her husband smokes in the house and she finds it difficult not to smoke when he does. She has tried nicotine gum but finds it difficult to use with her dentures. Her current patch does not seem to be helping, it has reduced her craving but not eliminated it, especially when she wakes up in the morning.
4. Is the current management of Mrs SS appropriate?
5. What non-pharmacological support should be offered to Mrs SS?

Answers

1. Stopping smoking is the single most important way of affecting a patient's outcome at all stages of COPD. Giving up smoking will slow down the gradual decline in FEV_1 that is seen in smokers.

2.
$$\text{Total pack years} = \frac{\text{Number of cigarettes smoked per day}}{20} \times \text{number of years of smoking}$$

   Mrs SS has smoked approximately 55 pack-years.

3. There are five key steps in helping a smoker to stop smoking, the 'five As':

   - Ask about tobacco use. This should include an assessment of the degree of addiction
   - Advise to quit
   - Assess willingness to make an attempt
   - Assist in quit attempt
   - Arrange follow-up.

   Motivation from the patient is the key to giving up smoking but is related to the degree of dependence on tobacco. Heavy smokers may exhibit low motivation to quit as they lack confidence in their ability to do so.

4. Nicotine replacement patches are considered to be most suitable for people who smoke regularly through the day but a 21- to 25-mg patch would have been a more appropriate starting dose for someone smoking 20 or more cigarettes a day. Two of the most common side effects are insomnia or vivid dreams, if these occur the patch can either be removed before bedtime or a 16-h patch used. A suitable alternative would be the short-acting gum, lozenge or nasal spray. Mrs SS would require the 4-mg gum and should be encouraged to use the 8- to 12-pieces of gum a day to provide approximately 20 mg of absorbed nicotine per day. As the nasal spray is most useful for people who smoke 20 or more cigarettes per day, this may be the preferred formulation.
   Mrs SS may benefit from a combination of products. Although this practice is not specifically recommended by product manufacturers, it is considered suitable in highly dependent patients, or in those who have had unsuccessful quit attempts using a single nicotine replacement therapy preparation. If breakthrough cravings are felt despite a background patch then the addition of short-acting dosage forms may be used as 'rescue' medication.
   A date on which to quit smoking should be set. Nicotine replacement therapy should be prescribed in blocks of 2 weeks. Mrs SS should be seen and helped regularly throughout this process, before and after her quit date. The duration of nicotine replacement therapy in people who maintain an abstinence is usually 8–12 weeks, depending on the product, followed by a dose reduction.
   Another option would be to try varenicline. This may be more effective in achieving continuous abstinence (National Institute for Health and Clinical Excellence, 2007) than either nicotine replacement therapy or bupropion. Varenicline should be started 1–2 weeks before Mrs SS's quit date and is continued for a total of 12 weeks, although an additional 12 weeks' therapy may be required. Bupropion is contraindicated as this may increase Mrs SS's risk of seizures.

5. It is thought that around 3% of smokers quit every year on their own but that percentage increases when they are given simple advice whilst encouraging the quit attempt. Several non-pharmacological strategies exist to help:

   - Written self-help material.
   - Counselling and behavioural therapy. These aim to motivate the smoker and help with the skills and strategies required to cope with nicotine withdrawal, psychological pressures to smoke and situations of temptation to smoke.

In all cases, pharmacological therapy should also be offered as appropriate.

Several NHS, patient and charitable organisations can provide help and support to people wishing to stop smoking. Information can be obtained from the followed web sites:

http://smokefree.nhs.uk/
http://www.quit.org.uk/
http://www.patient.co.uk/health/Smoking-Tips-to-Help-you-Stop.htm

References

American Thoracic Society/European Respiratory Society Task Force, 2004. Standards for the Diagnosis and Management of Patients with COPD Version 1.2. American Thoracic Society, New York [updated 8 September 2005]. Available at: http://www.thoracic.org/go/copd.

Barnes, P.J., 2004. Corticosteroid resistance in airway disease. Proc. Am. Thorac. Soc. 1, 264–268.

Boe, J., Dennis, J.H., O'Driscoll, B.R., for the European Respiratory Society Task Force, 2001. European Respiratory Society guidelines on the use of nebulizers. Eur. Respir. J. 18, 228–242. Available at: http://erj.ersjournals.com/cgi/content/full/18/1/228.

GOLD, 2009. Global Strategy for the Diagnosis, Management, and Prevention of Chronic Obstructive Pulmonary Disease. Medical Communication Resources Inc. Available at: http://www.goldcopd.org/Guidelineitem.asp?l1=2&l2=1&intId=2003.

Gunnell, D., Irvine, D., Wise, L., et al., 2009. Varenicline and suicidal behaviour: a cohort study based on data from the general practice research database. Br. Med. J. b3805, 339.

MRC Working Party, 1981. Long-term domiciliary oxygen therapy in chronic hypoxic cor pulmonale complicating chronic bronchitis and emphysema. Lancet 1, 681–686.

National Clinical Guideline Centre, 2010. Chronic Obstructive Pulmonary Disease: Management of Chronic Obstructive Pulmonary Disease in Adults in Primary and Secondary Care. National Clinical Guideline Centre, London. Available at: http://guidance.nice.org.uk/CG101/Guidance/pdf/English.

National Institute for Health and Clinical Excellence, 2006. Brief Interventions and Referral for Smoking Cessation in Primary Care and Other Settings. Public Health Intervention Guidance 1. NICE, London. Available at: http://www.nice.org.uk/nicemedia/pdf/SMOKING-ALS2_FINAL.pdf.

National Institute for Health and Clinical Excellence, 2007. Varenicline for Smoking Cessation. Technology Appraisal 123. NICE, London. Available at: http://www.nice.org.uk/TA123.

National Institute for Health and Clinical Excellence, 2010. Chronic Obstructive Pulmonary Disease. Clinical Guideline 101. NICE, London. Available at: http://www.nice.org.uk/guidance/index.jsp?action=byID&o=13029.

O'Driscoll, B.R., 1997. Nebulisers for chronic obstructive pulmonary disease. Thorax 52 (Suppl. 2), S49–S52.

O'Driscoll, B.R., Howard, L.S., Davison, A.G., on behalf of the British Thoracic Society Emergency Oxygen Guideline Development Group, 2008. Guideline for emergency oxygen use in adult patients. Thorax 63(Suppl. VI), vi69–vi73. doi:10.1136/thx.2008.102947.

Further reading

Barnes, P., Shapiro, S.D., Pauwels, R.A., 2003. Chronic obstructive pulmonary disease: molecular and cellular mechanisms. Eur. Respir. J. 22, 672–688.

Braman, S., 2006. Chronic cough due to acute bronchitis: ACCP evidence-based clinical practice guidelines. Chest 129(Suppl. 1), 95S–103S.

Henningfield, J.E., Fant, R.V., Buchalter, A.R., et al., 2005. Pharmacotherapy for nicotine dependence. CA Cancer J. Clin. 55, 281–299.

Molyneux, M., 2004. ABC of smoking cessation: nicotine replacement therapy. Br. Med. J. 328, 454–456.

Morgan, M.D., Britton, J.R., 2003. Chronic obstructive pulmonary disease 8: non-pharmacological management of COPD. Thorax 58, 453–457.

Srivastava, P., Currie, G.P., Britton, J., 2006. ABC of chronic obstructive pulmonary disease: smoking cessation. Br. Med. J. 332, 1324–1326.

27 Insomnia

S. Bleakley and M. Sie

Key points

- Hypnotic drugs do not cure insomnia but can provide useful short-term symptomatic treatment.
- Before starting medication, the primary cause of insomnia should be investigated and treated appropriately where possible.
- Hypnotic drugs should only be used short-term (2–4 weeks); long-term regular use leads to tolerance, dependence and other adverse effects.
- Sleep hygiene, relaxation techniques and psychological methods are more appropriate than hypnotics as long-term treatment for patients with insomnia.
- Non-benzodiazepine hypnotics such as zopiclone, zolpidem and zaleplon have similar pharmacological and adverse effects to benzodiazepines, offer few advantages and are more expensive.
- A melatonin preparation is available for primary insomnia. Its place in therapy is yet to be determined but it does not cause tolerance or dependence.

Definitions and epidemiology

Insomnia refers to difficulty in either falling asleep, remaining asleep or feeling refreshed from sleep. Complaints of poor sleep increase with increasing age and are twice as common in women as in men (Sateia and Nowell, 2004). Thus, by the age of 50, a quarter of the population are dissatisfied with their sleep, the proportion rising to 30–40% (two-thirds of them women) among individuals over 65 years.

Pathophysiology

Insomnia reflects a disturbance of arousal and/or sleep systems in the brain. These systems are functionally interrelated and their activity determines the degree and type of alertness during wakefulness and the depth and quality of sleep.

Sleep systems

The phenomenon of sleep is actively induced and maintained by neural mechanisms in several brain areas, including the lower brainstem, pons and parts of the limbic system. These mechanisms have reciprocal inhibitory connections with arousal systems, so that the activation of sleep systems inhibits waking and vice versa. Normal sleep includes two distinct levels of consciousness, orthodox sleep and paradoxical sleep, which are promoted from separate neural centres.

Orthodox sleep normally takes up about 75% of sleeping time. It is somewhat arbitrarily divided into four stages (1–4) which merge into each other, forming a continuum of decreasing cortical and behavioural arousal (see Fig. 27.1). Stages 3 and 4 represent the deepest phase of sleep and are also termed slow-wave sleep (SWS).

Paradoxical sleep, rapid eye movement (REM) sleep, normally takes up about 25% of sleeping time and has quite different characteristics to non-rapid eye movement (NREM) sleep. The EEG shows unsynchronised fast activity similar to that found in the alert conscious state and the eyes show rapid jerky movements. Peripheral autonomic activity is increased during REM sleep and there is an increased output of catecholamines and free fatty acids. Vivid dreams and nightmares most often occur during REM sleep, although brief frightening dreams (hypnagogic hallucinations) can occur in orthodox sleep, especially at the transition between sleeping and waking. Normally, stage 4 sleep occurs primarily in the first few hours of the night, while REM sleep is most prominent towards the morning. Brief awakenings during the night are normal. Both SWS and REM sleep are thought to be essential for brain function and both show a rebound after a period of deprivation, usually at the expense of lighter (stage 1 and 2) sleep which appears to be expendable. Many drugs can affect the different stages of sleep.

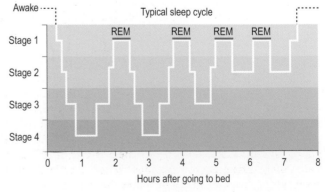

Fig. 27.1 The five stages of sleep. REM, rapid eye movement.

Benzodiazepines suppress stages 3 and 4 of sleep, but only cause a slight decrease in REM sleep. Z-hypnotics shorten stage 1 of sleep and prolong stage 2 of sleep but have little effect on stages 3, 4 and REM sleep. Chloral derivatives do not affect sleep architecture.

Aetiology and clinical manifestations

Insomnia may be caused by any factor which increases activity in arousal systems or decreases activity in sleep systems. Many causes act on both systems (Morin, 2003). Increased sensory stimulation activates arousal systems, resulting in difficulty in falling asleep. Common causes include chronic pain, gastric reflux, uncontrolled asthma and external stimuli such as noise, bright lights and extremes of temperature. Anxiety may also delay sleep onset as a result of increased emotional arousal.

Drugs are an important cause of insomnia. Difficulty in falling asleep may result directly from the action of stimulants, including caffeine, nicotine, theophylline, sympathomimetic amines, some antidepressants, levothyroxine and antimuscarinics. Some illicit substances, cocaine, amphetamines and anabolic steroids can also cause insomnia. Drug withdrawal after chronic use of central nervous system depressants, including hypnotics, anxiolytics and alcohol, commonly causes rebound insomnia with delayed or interrupted sleep, increased REM sleep and nightmares. With rapidly metabolised drugs, such as alcohol or short acting benzodiazepines, this rebound may occur in the latter part of the night, resulting in early waking. Certain drugs, including antipsychotics, tricyclic antidepressants and propranolol, may occasionally cause nightmares.

Difficulty in staying asleep is characteristic of depression. Patients typically complain of early waking but sleep records show frequent awakenings, early onset of REM sleep and reduced NREM sleep. Alteration of sleep stages, increased dreaming and nightmares may also occur in schizophrenia, while recurring nightmares are a feature of post-traumatic stress disorder (PTSD). Interference with circadian rhythms, as in shift work or rapid travel across time zones, can cause difficulty in falling asleep or early waking.

Frequent arousals from sleep are associated with myoclonus, 'restless legs syndrome', muscle cramps, bruxism (tooth grinding), head banging and sleep apnoea syndromes. Reversal of the sleep pattern, with a tendency for poor nocturnal sleep but a need for daytime naps, is common in the elderly, in whom it may be associated with cerebrovascular disease or dementia. In general, decreased duration of sleep has been shown to increase the risk of obesity (Kripke et al., 2002) and hypertension (Gangwisch et al., 2006). Sleep disturbances in the elderly are also associated with increased falls, cognitive decline and a higher rate of mortality (Cochen et al., 2009). There is growing concern that daytime sleepiness resulting from insomnia increases the risk of industrial, traffic and other accidents

Investigations and differential diagnosis

Many patients complaining of insomnia overestimate their sleep requirements. Although most people sleep for 7–8 h daily, some healthy subjects require as little as 3 h of sleep and sleep requirements decline with age. Such 'physiological insomnia' does not usually cause daytime fatigue, although the elderly may take daytime naps. If insomnia is causing distress, primary causes such as pain, drugs which disturb sleep, psychiatric disturbance including anxiety and depression and organic causes such as sleep apnoea should be identified and treated before hypnotic therapy is prescribed.

Treatment

Non-drug therapies

Explanation of sleep requirements, attention to sleep hygiene (see Box 27.1), reduction in caffeine or alcohol intake and the use of analgesics where indicated may obviate the need for hypnotics (Anon, 2004). Medications that cause insomnia should also be avoided if possible. Psychological techniques such as relaxation therapy and cognitive behavioural therapy (CBT) are also helpful (Kierlin, 2008). However, studies comparing psychological approaches to hypnotics are scarce (Riemann and Perlis, 2009).

Hypnotic drugs

Hypnotic drugs provide only symptomatic treatment for insomnia. Although often efficacious in the short-term, they do little to alter the underlying cause which should be sought and treated where possible. About 20 million prescriptions for hypnotics are issued each year in the UK and these drugs can improve the quality of life if used rationally.

Box 27.1 Principles of typical advice for good sleep hygiene (Anon, 2004)

- Have a good bed time routine, go to bed and get up at the same time every day and avoid daytime naps.
- Avoid stimulants such as caffeine, nicotine, chocolate and alcohol 6 h before bedtime.
- Take regular exercise during the day, but avoid strenuous exercise within 4 h of bedtime.
- Avoid large meals close to bedtime.
- Associate bed with sleep. Do not watch TV or listen to music when retiring to bed.
- The bedroom should be a quiet, relaxing place to sleep; make sure the room is not too hot or too cold.
- If after 30 min you cannot get off to sleep, then get up. Leave the bedroom and try to do something else, return to bed when sleepy. This can be repeated as often as necessary until you are asleep.

The ideal hypnotic would

- gently suppress brain arousal systems while activating systems that promote deep and satisfying sleep,
- have a rapid onset of action with a duration of less than 8 h,
- have no hangover effect the next day,
- not induce tolerance or dependence if used long-term,
- not cause withdrawal effects when stopped,
- not depress respiration,
- be safe for use in the elderly patient.

Unfortunately, no such hypnotic exists; most available hypnotics are general central nervous system depressants which inhibit both arousal and sleep mechanisms. Thus, they do not induce normal sleep and often have adverse effects, including daytime sedation ('hangover') and rebound insomnia on withdrawal. They are unsuitable for long-term use because of the development of tolerance and dependence.

Benzodiazepines

By far the most commonly prescribed hypnotics are the benzodiazepines. A number of different benzodiazepines are available (see Table 27.1). These drugs differ considerably in potency (equivalent dosage) and in rate of elimination but only slightly in clinical effects. All benzodiazepines have sedative/hypnotic, anxiolytic, amnesic, muscular relaxant and anticonvulsant actions with minor differences in the relative potency of these effects.

Pharmacokinetics

Most benzodiazepines marketed as hypnotics are well absorbed and rapidly penetrate the brain, producing hypnotic effects within half an hour after oral administration. Rates of elimination vary, however, with elimination half-lives from 6 to 100 h (see Table 27.1). These drugs undergo hepatic metabolism via oxidation or conjugation and some form pharmacologically active metabolites with even longer elimination half-lives. Oxidation of benzodiazepines is decreased in the elderly, in patients with hepatic impairment and in the presence of some drugs, including alcohol.

Pharmacokinetic characteristics are important in selecting a hypnotic drug. A rapid onset of action combined with a medium duration of action (elimination half-life about 6–8 h) is usually desirable. Too short a duration of action may lead to, or fail to control, early morning waking, while a long duration of action (e.g. nitrazepam) may produce residual effects

Table 27.1 Overview of the medication used for insomnia

Drug	Usual dose at night (adult) (mg)	Half life in adults (h)	Licensed indication	Tolerance	Dependence
Benzodiazepines					
Diazepam	2–5	24–36	Insomnia (short-term use)	Yes	Yes
Loprazolam	1	11	Insomnia (short-term use)	Yes	Yes
Lorazepam	1	12–16	Insomnia (short-term use)	Yes	Yes
Lormetazepam	0.5–1.5	10	Insomnia (short-term use)	Yes	Yes
Nitrazepam	5–10	18–36	Insomnia (short-term use)	Yes	Yes
Temazepam	10–20	5–11	Insomnia (short-term use)	Yes	Yes
Z-Hypnotics					
Zaleplon	10	2	Insomnia (short-term use up to 2 weeks)	Yes	Yes
Zolpidem	5–10	2–3	Insomnia (short-term use up to 4 weeks)	Yes	Yes
Zopiclone	3.75–7.5	3.5–6	Insomnia (short-term use up to 4 weeks)	Yes	Yes
Chloral and Derivatives (rarely used)					
Cloral Betaine	707	Unclear	Insomnia (short-term use)	Yes	Yes
Clomethiazole					
Clomethiazole	192–384	4–5	Severe insomnia in elderly (short-term use)	Yes	Yes
Antihistamines					
Promethazine	25–50	10–19	Night sedation and insomnia (short-term use)	Yes	No
Melatonin					
Melatonin Circadin® Unlicensed products also available	2	3.5–4	Insomnia in adults over 55 years (short-term use)	No	No

the next day and may lead to accumulation if the drug is used regularly. However, frequency of use and dosage are also important. For example, diazepam (5–10 mg) produces few residual effects when used occasionally, despite its slow elimination, although chronic use impairs daytime performance. Large doses of short acting drugs may produce hangover effects, while small doses of longer acting drugs may cause little or no hangover.

Mechanism of action

Most of the effects of benzodiazepines result from their interaction with specific binding sites associated with postsynaptic $GABA_A$ receptors in the brain. All benzodiazepines bind to these sites, although with varying degrees of affinity, and potentiate the inhibitory actions of GABA at these sites.

$GABA_A$ receptors are multi-molecular complexes (see Figs. 27.2 and 27.3) that control a chloride ion channel and contain specific binding sites for GABA, benzodiazepines and several other drugs, including many non-benzodiazepine hypnotics and some anticonvulsant drugs (Haefely, 1990). The various effects of benzodiazepines (hypnotic, anxiolytic, anticonvulsant, amnesic, muscle relaxant) result from GABA potentiation in specific brain sites and at different types of $GABA_A$ receptor. There are multiple subtypes of $GABA_A$ receptor which may contain different combinations of at least 18 sub-units (including α_{1-6}, β_{1-3}, γ_{1-3} and others) and the subtypes are differentially distributed in the brain.

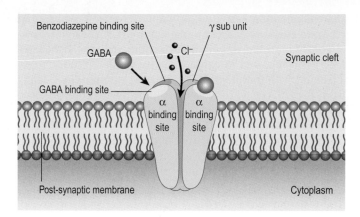

Fig. 27.3 *Schematic representation of the $GABA_A$ receptor.* GABA is the major inhibitory neurotransmitter in the central nervous system. The $GABA_A$ receptor is composed of five sub-units – two α, two β and one γ sub-unit. Two molecules of GABA activate the receptor by binding to the α sub-units. Once activated the receptor allows the passage of negatively charged ions (Cl–) into the cytoplasm, which results in hyper-polarisation and the inhibition of neurotransmission. Source: www.CNSforum.com.

Benzodiazepines bind to three or more subtypes and it appears that their combination with α_2-containing subtypes mediates their anxiolytic effects, α_1-containing subtypes their sedative and amnesic effects, and α_1 as well as α_2 and α_5 their anticonvulsant effects (Rudolph et al., 2001).

Zopiclone

In 1988, zopiclone, a cyclopyrrolone, was the first non-benzodiazepine to be approved for the treatment of insomnia in the European market. Although classed as a non-benzodiazepine, it still binds to benzodiazepine receptors but is said to be more selective for the α_1 subtype. It has hypnotic effects similar to benzodiazepines and carries a similar potential for adverse effects including tolerance, dependence and abstinence effects on withdrawal. Psychiatric reactions, including hallucinations, behavioural disturbances and nightmares, have been reported to occur shortly after the first dose. Other common adverse reactions include a bitter taste, a dry mouth and difficulty arising in the morning (Zammit, 2009). This drug appears to have no particular advantages over benzodiazepines, although it may cause less alteration of sleep stages and does not have the controlled drug requirements of the benzodiazepines. Eszopiclone the S- (+) isomer of zopiclone is available in the USA but there are no current plans to launch in the UK. What advantage, if any, the isomer incurs over zopiclone is unclear.

Zolpidem

Zolpidem is an imidazopyridine that binds preferentially to the α_1 benzodiazepine receptor sub-unit thought to mediate hypnotic effects. It is an effective hypnotic with only weak anticonvulsant and muscle relaxant properties. As it has a

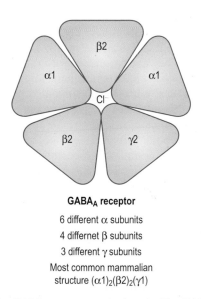

GABA$_A$ receptor

6 different α subunits

4 differnet β subunits

3 different γ subunits

Most common mammalian structure $(\alpha1)_2(\beta2)_2(\gamma1)$

Fig. 27.2 *The $GABA_A$ receptor and sub-units.* The $GABA_A$ receptor is a heteropentameric glycoprotein. A total of five distinct polypeptide sub-units have been cloned to date; α, β, γ, d and r, and multiple isoforms of these sub-units are reported in the literature. Different confirmations of the $GABA_A$ receptor are found throughout the brain, and the most common mammalian arrangements of sub-units is $(\alpha1)_2(\beta2)_2(\gamma1)$. The specific sub-units in the $GABA_A$ receptor confer functional diversity on the receptor. For example, the γ sub-unit needs to be co-expressed with the α and β sub-units to observe the potentiation of the $GABA_A$ receptor by benzodiazepines.

short elimination half-life (2 h) hangover effects are rare but rebound effects may occur in the later part of the night, causing early morning waking and daytime anxiety. High doses have been reported to cause brief psychotic episodes, tolerance and withdrawal effects. Anecdotal case reports (mainly from the USA) have associated zolpidem with complex sleep related behaviours. These have included 'sleep-driving', making phone calls, preparing food and eating while asleep. The majority of these cases also involved ingestion of alcohol and should be interpreted with caution because they are not replicated in the wider medical literature (Zammit, 2009). A controlled release version of zolpidem (zolpidem-CR) is available in some countries.

Zaleplon

Zaleplon is a pyrazolopyrimidine which, like zolpidem, binds selectively to the α_1 benzodiazepine receptor. It is an effective hypnotic, has a very short elimination half-life (1 h) and appears to cause minimal residual effects on psychomotor or cognitive function after 5 h. There is little evidence of tolerance or withdrawal effects in short-term use and the drug appears suitable for use in the elderly (Doble et al., 2004).

All the 'Z-hypnotics' are recommended for short-term use only (2–4 weeks) and are more expensive than benzodiazepines. There is no compelling evidence to distinguish them from the shorter acting benzodiazepine hypnotics (National Institute of Health and Clinical Excellence, 2004). Patients who do not respond to either a benzodiazepine or z-hypnotic should not be prescribed the other.

Melatonin

Melatonin is a naturally occurring hormone, produced by the pineal gland, which regulates the circadian rhythm of sleep. It begins to be released once it becomes dark, and continues to be released until the first light of day. Melatonin release decreases with age which may in-part explain why older adults require less sleep. Melatonin supplementation promotes sleep initiation and helps to reset the circadian clock allowing uninterrupted sleep. It has also been shown to improve next day functioning. Contrary to most other hypnotics melatonin shows no abuse or tolerance potential and appears to have no next day sedation problems. Prolonged release melatonin (Circadin®) was launched in June 2008 and is available at a dose of 2 mg at night for up to 3 weeks. It is licensed as monotherapy in primary insomnia for adults over 55 years old. Whilst the adverse effect profile looks advantageous there are currently no trials comparing melatonin against psychological or other hypnotic treatments. Circadin® is also much more expensive than other currently prescribed hypnotics (Anon, 2009).

Other hypnotic drugs

The risk of adverse effects, including dependence and dangerous respiratory depression in overdose, generally outweighs the potential benefits of the older hypnotics, chloral derivatives, clomethiazole and barbiturate. Therefore, these drugs are best avoided. Antidepressants with sedative properties, such as amitriptyline, mirtazapine, trazodone and agomelatine may be helpful if sleep disturbance is secondary to depression. Sedative antihistamines, such as promethazine, diphenhydramine and chlorphenamine, which can be purchased over-the-counter, have mild-to-moderate hypnotic efficacy but commonly produce hangover effects and rebound insomnia can occur after prolonged use (Anon, 2004).

Potential adverse effects of hypnotic use

Tolerance and dependence

Tolerance to the hypnotic effects of benzodiazepines and probably z-hypnotics develops rapidly and may lead to dosage escalation. Nevertheless, poor sleepers may report continued efficacy and the drugs are often used long-term because of difficulties on withdrawal.

Rebound insomnia

Rebound insomnia, in which sleep is poorer than before drug treatment, is common on withdrawal of benzodiazepines. Sleep latency (time to onset of sleep) is prolonged, intra-sleep wakenings become more frequent and REM sleep duration and intensity are increased, with vivid dreams or nightmares which may add to frequent awakenings. These symptoms are most marked when the drugs have been taken in high doses or for long periods, but can occur after only a week of low dose administration. They are prominent with moderately, rapidly eliminated benzodiazepines (temazepam, lorazepam) and may last for many weeks. With slowly eliminated benzodiazepines (diazepam), SWS and REM sleep may remain depressed for some weeks and then slowly return to the baseline, sometimes without a rebound effect. Tolerance and rebound effects are reflections of a complex homeostatic response to regular drug use, involving desensitisation, uncoupling and internalisation of certain GABA/benzodiazepine receptors and sensitisation of receptors for excitatory neurotransmitters (Allison and Pratt, 2003). These changes encourage continued hypnotic usage and contribute to the development of drug dependence.

Oversedation and hangover effects

Many benzodiazepines used as hypnotics can give rise to a subjective 'hangover' effect and after most of them, even those with short elimination half-lives, psychomotor performance, including driving ability and memory, may be impaired on the following day. Over sedation is most likely with slowly eliminated benzodiazepines, especially if used chronically, and is most marked in the elderly in whom drowsiness, incoordination and ataxia, leading to falls and fractures, and acute confusional states may result even from small doses. Chronic use can cause considerable cognitive impairment, sometimes suggesting dementia. Paradoxical excitement may occasionally occur.

Some benzodiazepines in hypnotic doses may decrease alveolar ventilation and depress the respiratory response to hypercapnia, increasing the risk of cerebral hypoxia, especially in the elderly and in patients with chronic respiratory disease.

Drug interactions

Benzodiazepines have additive effects with other central nervous system depressants. Combinations of benzodiazepines with alcohol, other hypnotics, sedative tricyclic antidepressants, antihistamines or opioids can cause marked sedation and may lead to accidents or severe respiratory depression.

Rational drug treatment of insomnia

A hypnotic drug may be indicated for insomnia when it is severe, disabling, unresponsive to other measures or likely to be temporary. In choosing an appropriate agent, individual variables relating to the patient and to the drug need to be considered (see Table 27.1).

Patient care

Type of insomnia

The duration of insomnia is important in deciding on a hypnotic regimen. Transient insomnia may be caused by changes of routine such as overnight travel, change in time zone, alteration of shift work or temporary admission to hospital. In these circumstances, a hypnotic with a rapid onset, medium duration of action and few residual effects could be used on one or two occasions.

Short-term insomnia may result from temporary environmental stress. In this case, a hypnotic may occasionally be indicated but should be prescribed in low dosage for 1 or 2 weeks only, preferably intermittently, on alternate nights or one night in three.

Chronic insomnia presents a much greater therapeutic problem. It is usually secondary to other conditions (organic or psychiatric) at which treatment should initially be aimed. In selected cases, a hypnotic may be helpful but it is recommended that such drugs should be prescribed at the minimal effective dosage and administered intermittently (one night in three) or temporarily (not more than 2 or 3 weeks). Occasionally it is necessary to repeat short, intermittent courses at intervals of a few months.

The elderly

The elderly are especially vulnerable both to insomnia and to adverse effects from hypnotic drugs. They may have reduced metabolism of some drugs and may be at risk of cumulative effects. They are also more susceptible than younger people to central nervous system depression, including cognitive impairment and ataxia (which may lead to falls and fractures). They are sensitive to respiratory depression, prone to sleep apnoea and other sleep disorders and are more likely to have 'sociological', psychiatric and somatic illnesses which both disturb sleep and may be aggravated by hypnotics. For some of these elderly patients, hypnotics can improve the quality of life but the dosage should be adjusted (usually half the recommended adult dose) and hypnotics with long elimination half-lives or active metabolites should be avoided.

A considerable number of elderly patients give a history of regular hypnotic use going back for 20 or 30 years. In many of these patients, gradual reduction of hypnotic dosage or even withdrawal may be indicated and can be carried out successfully, resulting in improved cognition and general health with no impairment of sleep or escalation of other symptoms (Curran et al., 2003).

The young

Traditional benzodiazepine-like are generally contraindicated for children. Where sedation is required, sedative antihistamines or melatonin are usually recommended.

Disease states

Hypnotics are contraindicated in patients with acute pulmonary insufficiency, significant respiratory depression, obstructive sleep apnoea or severe hepatic impairment. In patients with chronic pain or terminal conditions, suitable analgesics including non-steroidal anti-inflammatory agents or opiates, sometimes combined with neuroleptics, usually provide satisfactory sedation. In such patients, the possibility of drug dependence becomes a less important issue and regular use of hypnotics with a medium duration of action should not be denied if they provide symptomatic relief of insomnia.

Choice of drug

There is little difference in hypnotic efficacy between most of the available agents. The main factors to consider in the rational choice of a hypnotic regimen are duration of action and the risk of adverse effects, especially over sedation and the development of tolerance and dependence. Cost may also be a factor when prescribing melatonin.

Rate of elimination

Slowly eliminated drugs should be avoided because of the risk of over sedation and hangover effects. Very short acting drugs such as zaleplon carry the risk of late night rebound insomnia and daytime anxiety. Drugs with a medium elimination half-life (6–8 h) appear to have the most suitable profile for hypnotic use. These may include temazepam and loprazolam, as these are the drugs of first choice in most situations where hypnotics are indicated. Zopiclone is a reasonable second choice and sedative antihistamine such as promethazine is a safe third choice. These are useful in children, although sedative antihistamine may produce daytime drowsiness.

Duration and timing of administration

To prevent the development of tolerance and dependence, the maximum duration of treatment should be limited to 2 or 3 weeks and treatment should, where possible, be intermittent (one night in two or three). Dosage should be tapered slowly if hypnotics have been taken regularly for more than a few weeks. Doses should be taken 20 min before retiring in order to allow dissolution in the stomach and absorption to commence before the patient lies down in bed.

Case studies

Case 27.1

Mr PH, aged 24, was hospitalised for 3 months after a serious motorcycle injury followed by painful complications. While in hospital he developed panic attacks and insomnia. He received no psychological support but was prescribed temazepam, initially in 20 mg doses but later increased to 60 mg because of continued insomnia. After discharge from hospital Mr PH continued to receive temazepam from his primary care doctor and the dosage was increased over a period of years until he was taking 80 mg temazepam each night and 40–80 mg during the day. At the age of 30, Mr PH was removed from the practice list of his doctor after he altered a prescription. He later attended several different primary care doctors, obtaining multiple temazepam prescriptions. When he could no longer satisfy his need from prescriptions he took to obtaining temazepam on the street, taking large and irregular doses by mouth. All this time, his anxiety levels increased. His behaviour became chaotic and he was twice imprisoned for credit card fraud but he was able to obtain temazepam and other drugs from his co-prisoners. When last heard of, Mr PH, aged 35, was again buying temazepam illicitly, as well as other addictive drugs, had started injecting intravenously and was involved in a court case for obtaining money under false pretences.

Question

How could this tragedy have been prevented?

Answer

Mr PH's downfall could have been averted at several stages.

- The hospital staff should not have allowed the temazepam dosage to escalate and should have provided psychological/psychiatric help for what was probably PTSD or panic disorder.
- An antidepressant drug could have been prescribed, along with psychological measures, instead of prolonged treatment with excessive doses of temazepam.
- On discharge from hospital, Mr PH's doctor should have been warned of his temazepam intake and a slow withdrawal schedule suggested.
- The series of primary care doctors who gave Mr PH prescriptions should have been aware that he was likely to obtain illicit supplies and should have referred him to a withdrawal clinic or drugs unit.

Case 27.2

Mrs AK, a recently widowed lady aged 65, had difficulty sleeping after her bereavement. She was prescribed nitrazepam in a bedtime dose of 5 mg, which was very effective and was continued for over 4 weeks. Mrs AK lived alone but was visited occasionally by her daughter. On a visit 2 weeks after the nitrazepam was started, Mrs AK seemed calm and said that she was sleeping well but the daughter noticed her mother was unsteady on her feet. A week later the daughter visited again and found her mother lying on the bedroom floor, in pain and unable to move. She said that she had lost her balance on getting out of bed. An ambulance was called and it was found in hospital that Mrs AK had broken her hip.

Question

Should the doctor have prescribed nitrazepam for this lady?

Answers

- Long acting benzodiazepines should be avoided in the elderly. The elimination half-life of nitrazepam is 15–38 h and the recommended dose for the elderly is 2.5–5 mg. Temazepam, loprazolam or lormetazepam would have been a better choice but for short-term use only (preferably only 2 weeks).
- The elderly are particularly prone to ataxia and light-headedness with benzodiazepines and this can lead to falls and fractures.
- Benzodiazepines are not recommended, except acutely, for bereavement. Their amnesic effects may interfere with subsequent psychological adjustment.

References

Allison, C., Pratt, J.A., 2003. Neuroadaptive processes in GABAergic and glutamatergic systems in benzodiazepine dependence. Pharmacol. Ther. 98, 171–195.

Anon, 2004. What's wrong with prescribing hypnotics? Drug Ther. Bull. 42, 89–93, Available at: http://dtb.bmj.com/content/42/12/89.full.pdf. Accessed March 2010.

Anon, 2009. Melatonin for primary insomnia. Drug Ther. Bull. 47, 74–77. Available at: http://dtb.bmj.com/content/47/7/74.full.pdf. Accessed March 2010.

Cochen, V., Arbus, C., Soto, M.E., et al., 2009. Sleep disorders and their impact on healthy, dependent and frail older adults. J. Nutr. Health. Aging 13, 322–330.

Curran, H.V., Collins, R., Fletcher, S., 2003. Older adults and withdrawal from benzodiazepine hypnotics in general practice: effects on cognitive function, sleep, mood and quality of life. Psychosom. Med. 33, 1223–1237.

Doble,, A., Martin,, I.L., Nutt,, D., 2004. Calming the brain: benzodiazepines and related drugs from laboratory to clinic. Martin Dunitz, London.

Gangwisch, J., Heymsfield, S., Boden-Albala, B., et al., 2006. Short sleep duration as a risk factor for hypertension. Hypertension 47, 833–839.

Haefely, W., 1990. Benzodiazepine receptor and ligands: structural and functional differences. In: Hindmarch, I., Beaumont, G., Brandon,

S. et al. (Eds.), Benzodiazepines: Current Concepts. John Wiley, Chichester, pp. 1–18.

Kierlin, L., 2008. Sleeping without a pill: non-pharmacologic treatments for insomnia. J. Psychiatr. Pract. 14, 403–407.

Kripke, D., Garfinkel, L., Wingard, D., et al., 2002. Mortality associated with sleep duration and insomnia. Arch. Gen. Psychiatry 59, 131–136.

Morin, C.M., 2003. Treating insomnia with behavioural approaches: evidence for efficacy, effectiveness and practicality. In: Szuba, M.P., Kloss, J.D., Dinges, D.F. (Eds.), Insomnia: Principles and Management. Cambridge University Press, Cambridge, pp. 83–95.

National Institute of Health and Clinical Excellence, 2004. Guidance on the use of Zaleplon, Zolpidem and Zopiclone for the short-term management of insomnia. Technology Appraisal 77. NICE, London, Available at: http://guidance.nice.org.uk/TA77/Guidance/pdf/English. Accessed March 2010.

Riemann, D., Perlis, M.L., 2009. The treatments of chronic insomnia: a review of benzodiazepine receptor agonists and psychological and behavioral therapies. Sleep Med. Rev. 13, 205–214.

Rudolph, U., Crestani, F., Mohler, H., 2001. $GABA_A$ receptor subtypes: dissecting their pharmacological functions. Trends Pharmacol. Sci. 22, 188–194.

Sateia, M.J., Nowell, P.D., 2004. Insomnia. Lancet 364, 1959–1973.

Zammit, G., 2009. Comparative tolerability of newer agents for insomnia. Drug Saf. 32, 735–738.

Further reading

Bloom, H.G., Ahmed, I., Alessi, C.A., et al., 2009. Evidence-based recommendations for the assessment and management of sleep disorders in older persons: supplement. J. Am. Geriatr. Soc. 57, 761–789.

Parish, J., 2009. Sleep-related problems in common medical conditions. Chest 135, 563–572.

Sullivan, S.S., Guilleminault, C., 2009. Emerging drugs for insomnia: new frontiers for old and novel targets. Expert Opin. Emerg. Drugs 14, 411–422.

28 Anxiety disorders

S. Bleakley and D. Baldwin

Key points

- Benzodiazepines should only be used short-term (2–4 weeks) as long-term regular use can lead to tolerance, dependence and other adverse effects.
- If benzodiazepines are indicated, the smallest effective dose should be used along with intermittent dosing where possible. Start with small doses, increase if necessary. Use half the adult dose in elderly patients.
- Psychological therapies (talking therapies) are generally considered first-line treatments in all anxiety disorders because they may provide a longer lasting response and lower relapse rates than pharmacotherapy.
- Some antidepressants are appropriate long-term treatment for anxiety disorders.
- Selective serotonin reuptake inhibitors (SSRIs) are the recommended antidepressants in anxiety disorders but can worsen symptoms at the beginning of treatment and, therefore, should be initiated at half the usual dose used.

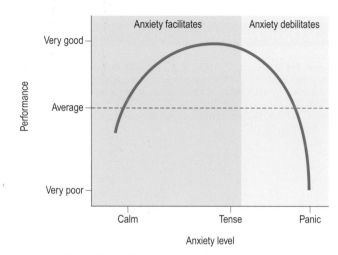

Fig. 28.1 The Yerks Dodson curve.

Definitions and epidemiology

Anxiety is a normal, protective, psychological response to an unpleasant or threatening situation. Mild to moderate anxiety can improve performance and ensure appropriate action is taken. However, excessive or prolonged symptoms can be disabling, lead to severe distress and cause much impairment to social functioning. Figure 28.1 shows that as anxiety levels increase performance/actions increase. However, as the anxiety level increases beyond acceptable or tolerated levels, the performance declines.

The term 'anxiety disorder' encompasses a variety of complaints which can either exist on their own or in conjunction with another psychiatric or physical illness. Symptoms of anxiety vary but generally present with a combination of psychological, physical and behavioural symptoms (Fig. 28.2). Some of these symptoms are common to many anxiety disorders while others are distinctive to a particular disorder. Anxiety disorders are broadly divided into generalised anxiety disorder (GAD), panic disorder, social phobia, specific phobias, post-traumatic stress disorder (PTSD) and obsessive-compulsive disorder (OCD), see Table 28.1. Patient testimonials are presented in Box 28.1. Approximately two-thirds of sufferers of an anxiety disorder will have another psychiatric illness. This is most commonly depression and often successful treatment of

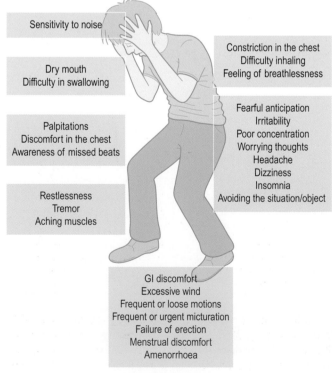

Fig. 28.2 The symptoms of anxiety.

Table 28.1 A brief description of the common anxiety disorders

Symptoms common to all anxiety disorders	Fear or worry, sleep disturbances, concentration problems, dry mouth, sweating, palpitations, GI discomfort, restlessness, shortness of breath, avoidance behaviour
Generalised anxiety disorder (GAD)	Persistent (free floating), excessive and inappropriate anxiety on most days for at least 6 months. The anxiety is not restricted to a specific situation
Panic disorder (with or without agoraphobia)	Recurrent, unexplained surges of severe anxiety (panic attack). Most patients develop a fear of repeat attacks or the implications of an attack. Often seen in agoraphobia (fear in places or situations from which escape might be difficult)
Social phobia (or social anxiety disorder)	A marked, persistent and unreasonable fear of being observed, embarrassed or humiliated in a social or performance situation (e.g. public speaking or eating in front of others)
Specific phobia	Marked and persistent fear that is excessive or unrealistic, precipitated by the presence (or anticipation) of a specific object or situation (e.g. flying, spiders). Sufferers avoid the feared object/subject or endure it with intense anxiety
Post-traumatic stress disorder (PTSD)	Can occur after an exposure to a traumatic event which involved actual or threatened death, or serious injury or threats to the physical integrity of self or others. The person responds with intense fear, helplessness or horror. Sufferers can re-experience symptoms (flashbacks) and avoid situations associated with the trauma. Usually occurs within 6 months of the traumatic event
Obsessive-compulsive disorder (OCD)	Persistent thoughts, impulses or images (obsessions) that are intrusive and cause distress. The person attempts to get rid of these obsessions by completing repetitive time-consuming purposeful behaviours or actions (compulsions). Common obsessions include contamination while the compulsion may be repetitive washing or cleaning

Box 28.1 Patient testimonies (NICE, 2005a,b)

Symptoms described by a sufferer of post-traumatic stress disorder:

> I would feel angry at the way the crash happened and that there was nothing I could do to stop it or help. I was physically exhausted, but was finding it hard to sleep. As soon as the bedroom light went out at night a light would come on in my head and all I could do was lie there and think. When I would eventually fall asleep, I would wake up with nightmares of the crash. I could not get away from it. It was all I could think about in the day and all I would dream about at night.

Thoughts from a sufferer of obsessive-compulsive disorder:

> I've just arrived home from work. Tired and tense, I'm convinced my hands are contaminated with some hazardous substance and my primary concern now is to ensure that I don't spread that contamination to anything that I, or others, may subsequently touch. I will wash my hands, but first I will need to put a hand in my pocket to get my door keys, contaminating these, the pocket's other contents, and everything else I touch on my way to the sink. It will be late evening before I will have completed the whole decontamination ritual.

A slow recovery described by a post-traumatic stress disorder and panic attack sufferer:

> Slowly I gained ground and as each new insight came I was able to see my symptoms diminish. The panic attacks tapered off, the intensity of the flashbacks dwindled, and my irritable bowel began to loosen some of its hold on me. I was able to breathe again.

an underlying depression will significantly improve the symptoms of anxiety. Many patients will also present with more than one anxiety disorder at the same time which can further complicate treatment. Anxiety disorders are the most commonly reported mental illness and as a whole have a lifetime prevalence of 21% (Baldwin et al., 2005) with specific phobias the most commonly reported.

For all anxiety disorders together the overall female to male ratio is 2:1. The age of onset of most anxiety disorders is in young adulthood (20s and 30s), although the maximum prevalence of generalised anxiety and agoraphobia in the general population is in the 50–64 year age group.

Pathophysiology

Anxiety occurs when there is a disturbance of the arousal systems in the brain. Arousal is maintained by at least three interconnected systems: a general arousal system, an 'emotional' arousal system and an endocrine/autonomic arousal system (Fig. 28.3). The general arousal system, mediated by the brainstem reticular formation, thalamic nuclei and basal forebrain bundle, serves to link the cerebral cortex with incoming sensory stimuli and provides a tonic influence on cortical reactivity or alertness. Excessive activity in this system, due to internal or external stresses, can lead to a state of hyperarousal as seen in anxiety. Emotional aspects of arousal, such as fear and anxiety, are contributed by the limbic system which also serves to focus attention on selected aspects of the environment. There is evidence that increased activity in certain limbic pathways is associated with anxiety and panic attacks.

These arousal systems activate somatic responses to arousal, such as increased muscle tone, increased sympathetic activity and increased output of anterior and posterior pituitary hormones. Inappropriate increases in autonomic activity are

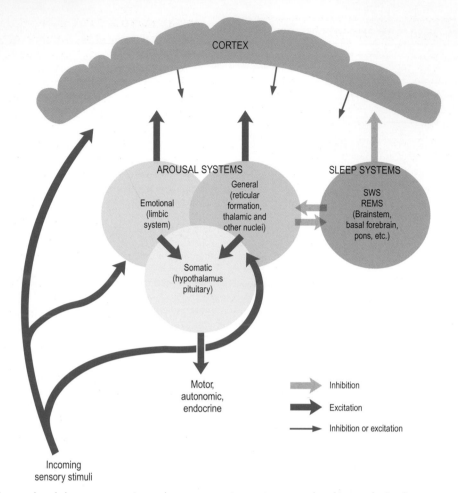

Fig. 28.3 Diagram of arousal and sleep systems. Arousal systems receive environmental and internal stimuli, cause cortical activation and mediate motor, autonomic and endocrine responses to arousal. Reciprocally connected sleep systems generate slow-wave sleep (SWS) and rapid eye movement sleep (REMS). Either system can be excited or inhibited by cognitive activity generated in the cortex.

often associated with anxiety states; the resulting symptoms (palpitations, sweating, tremor, etc.) may initiate a vicious circle that increases the anxiety.

Several neurotransmitters have been implicated in the arousal systems. Acetylcholine is the main transmitter maintaining general arousal but there is evidence that heightened emotional arousal is particularly associated with noradrenergic and serotonergic activity. Drugs which antagonise such activity have anxiolytic effects. In addition, the inhibitory neurotransmitter γ-aminobutyric acid (GABA) exerts an inhibitory control on other transmitter pathways and increased GABA activity may have a protective effect against excessive stress reactions. Many drugs which increase GABA activity, such as the benzodiazepines, are potent anxiolytics.

Aetiology and clinical manifestations

Anxiety is commonly precipitated by stress but vulnerability to stress appears to be linked to genetic factors such as trait anxiety. Many patients presenting for the first time with anxiety symptoms have a long history of high anxiety levels going back to childhood. Anxiety may also be induced by central stimulant drugs (caffeine, amphetamines), withdrawal from chronic use of central nervous system depressant drugs (alcohol, hypnotics, anxiolytics) and metabolic disturbances (hyperventilation, hypoglycaemia, thyrotoxicosis). It may form part of a depressive disorder and may occur in temporal lobe lesions and in rare hormone-secreting tumours such as phaeochromocytoma or carcinoid syndrome.

Apart from the psychological symptoms of apprehension and fear, somatic symptoms may be prominent in anxiety and include palpitations, chest pain, shortness of breath, dizziness, dysphagia, gastro-intestinal disturbances, loss of libido, headaches and tremor. Panic attacks are experienced as storms of increased autonomic activity combined with a fear of imminent death or loss of control. If panic becomes associated with a particular environment, commonly a crowded place with no easy escape route, the patient may actively avoid similar situations and eventually become agoraphobic. When anxiety is precipitated by a specific cause then behaviour can become altered to ensure the sufferer avoids the cause. This avoidance behaviour can maintain the often irrational fear and strengthen the desire to avoid the threat.

Investigations and differential diagnosis

In patients presenting with symptoms and clinical signs of anxiety, it is important to exclude organic causes such as thyrotoxicosis, excessive use of stimulant drugs such as caffeine and the possibility of alcoholism or withdrawal effects from benzodiazepines. However, unnecessary investigations should generally be avoided if possible. Extensive gastroenterological, cardiological and neurological tests may increase anxiety by reinforcing the patient's fear of a serious underlying physical disease.

Treatment

Treatment for anxiety disorders often requires multiple approaches. The patient may need short-term treatment with an anxiolytic, such as a benzodiazepine, to help reduce the immediate symptoms combined with psychological therapies and an antidepressant for longer term treatment and prevention of symptoms returning.

Psychotherapy

Psychological therapies (talking therapies) are generally considered first-line treatments in all anxiety disorders because they may provide a longer lasting response and lower relapse rates than pharmacotherapy. Psychotherapy, however, is less available, more demanding and takes longer time to work than pharmacotherapy. If the patient is unable to tolerate the anxiety or associated distress, then medicines are often used before psychotherapy or while awaiting psychotherapy. The ideal treatment should be tailored to the individual and may involve a combination of both psychotherapy and pharmacotherapy. The type of treatment should depend on symptoms, type of anxiety disorder, speed of response required, long-term goals and patient preference.

The specific psychotherapy with the most supporting evidence in anxiety disorders is cognitive behavioural therapy (CBT). Cognitive behaviour therapy focuses on the 'here and now' and explores how the individual feels about themselves and others and how behaviour is related to these thoughts. Through individual therapy or group work the patient and therapist identify and question maladaptive thoughts and help develop an alternative perspective. Individual goals and strategies are developed and evaluated with patients encouraged to practise what they have learned between sessions. Therapy usually lasts for around 60–90 minutes every week for 8–16 weeks, or longer in more resistant cases. Cognitive behavioural therapists are usually health professionals such as mental health nurses, psychologists, general practitioners, social workers, counsellors or occupational therapists who have undertaken specific training and supervision.

In PTSD, CBT is trauma focused, with the therapist helping the patient confront their traumatic memory and people or objects associated with this trauma. At the same time, patients are taught skills to help them cope with the emotional or physical response of this trauma. One such skill includes relaxation training which may involve systematically relaxing major muscle groups in a way that decreases anxiety. Another psychotherapy sometimes recommended in PTSD is eye movement desensitisation and reprocessing (EMDR). This involves briefly recounting the trauma or objects associated with the trauma to the therapist who will then simultaneously initiate another stimulus, for example, moving a finger continuously in front of the patient's eyes or hand tapping. Over time it enables the patient to focus on alternative thoughts when associations with the trauma occur. A single session of debriefing following a traumatic event is not thought effective to prevent PTSD and, therefore, not recommended.

In OCD, CBT includes exposure and response prevention (ERP). This involves the therapist and the patient repeatedly facing the fears, beginning with the easiest situations and progressing until all the fears have been faced. At the same time the person must not perform any rituals or checks.

Specific phobias are also almost exclusively treated using exposure techniques and most patients will respond to this treatment. Only a very few will require additional drug therapy.

Other psychotherapies, although occasionally tried, have a poorer evidence base than CBT and are, therefore, not usually recommended. Self-help is one alternative technique which is recommended (NICE, 2007) for GAD and panic disorder. It involves using materials either alone or in part under professional guidance to learn skills to help cope with the anxiety. The materials such as books, tapes or computer packages can be accessed at home and in the patients' own time. Some self-help material, however, is of poor quality, so it is probably best used in those who have mild symptoms and who do not need more intensive treatments.

Pharmacotherapy

Benzodiazepines

Benzodiazepines are commonly prescribed to provide immediate relief of the symptoms of severe anxiety. A number of different benzodiazepines are available (Table 28.2). These drugs differ considerably in potency (equivalent dosage) and in rate of elimination but only slightly in clinical effects. All benzodiazepines have sedative/hypnotic, anxiolytic, amnesic, muscular relaxant and anticonvulsant actions with minor differences in the relative potency of these effects.

Pharmacokinetics. Most benzodiazepines are well absorbed and rapidly penetrate the brain, producing an effect within half an hour after oral administration. Rates of elimination vary; however, with elimination half-lives from 8 to 35 h (see Table 28.2). The drugs undergo hepatic metabolism via oxidation or conjugation and some form pharmacologically active metabolites with even longer elimination half-lives. Oxidation of benzodiazepines is decreased in the elderly, in patients with hepatic impairment and in the presence of some drugs, including alcohol. Benzodiazepines are metabolised through the cytochrome P450 3A4/3 enzyme system in the liver, so

Table 28.2 Profile of selected benzodiazepines (Bazire, 2009; Taylor et al., 2009)

Drug	Usual daily dose (mg)	Half-life hours (range)	Equivalent dose to diazepam 10 mg
Alprazolam	0.5–1.5	13 (12–15)	Unknown
Chlordiazepoxide	30	12 (6–30)	30 mg
Clonazepam	2–4	35 (20–60)	1–2 mg
Diazepam	5–30	32 (21–50)	–
Lorazepam	1–4	12 (8–25)	1 mg
Oxazepam	30	8 (5–15)	30 mg
Temazepam	10–20	8 (5–11)	20 mg

significant enzyme inducers (such as carbamazepine) may reduce levels while enzyme inhibitors (e.g. erythromycin) may increase levels (Bazire, 2009).

Mechanism of action. Most of the effects of benzodiazepines result from their interaction with specific binding sites associated with postsynaptic $GABA_A$ receptors in the brain. All benzodiazepines bind to these sites, although with varying degrees of affinity, and potentiate the inhibitory actions of GABA at these sites. GABA is the most important inhibitory neurotransmitter in the central nervous system (CNS). Neuronal activity in the CNS is regulated by the balance between GABA inhibitory activity and excitatory neurotransmitters such as glutamate. If the balance swings towards more GABA activity, sedation, ataxia and amnesia occur. Conversely, when GABA is reduced arousal, anxiety and restlessness occur. $GABA_A$ receptors are multimolecular complexes that control a chloride ion channel and contain specific binding sites for GABA, benzodiazepines and several other drugs, including many non-benzodiazepine hypnotics and some anticonvulsant drugs (Haefely, 1990) (Fig. 28.4). The various effects of benzodiazepines (hypnotic, anxiolytic, anticonvulsant, amnesic, myo-relaxant) result from GABA potentiation in specific brain sites and at different $GABA_A$ receptor types There are multiple subtypes of $GABA_A$ receptor which may contain different combinations of at least 17 subunits (including α_{1-6}, β_{1-3}, γ_{1-3} and others) and the subtypes are differentially distributed in the brain (Christmas et al., 2008). Benzodiazepines bind to two or more subtypes and it appears that combination with α_2-containing subtypes mediates their anxiolytic effects and α_1-containing subtypes their sedative and amnesic effects. There is some evidence that patients with anxiety disorders

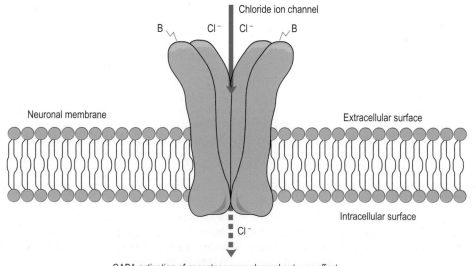

GABA activation of receptor opens channel gate, an effect enhanced by benzodiazepine binding to receptor subunits

Fig. 28.4 Schematic diagram of the $GABA_A$ receptor. This consists of five subunits arranged around a central chloride ion channel (one subunit has been removed in the diagram to reveal the ion channel, shown in the closed position). Some of the subunits have binding sites for benzodiazepines (B) and other hypnotics and anticonvulsants. Activation of the receptor by GABA opens the chloride channel, allowing chloride ions (Cl^-) to enter the cell, resulting in hyperpolarisation (inhibition) of the neurone. Occupation of the benzodiazepine site, along with GABA, potentiates the inhibitory actions of GABA.

have reduced numbers of benzodiazepine receptors in key brain areas that regulate anxiety responses (Roy-Byrne, 2005). Secondary suppression of noradrenergic and/or serotonergic and other excitatory systems may also be of importance in relation to the anxiolytic effects of benzodiazepines.

Role in treating anxiety. The benzodiazepines have been used for over 40 years in the treatment of anxiety and can provide rapid symptomatic relief from acute anxiety states. Concerns over dependence and tolerance restrict use to short-term use only. Many clinical trials have shown short-term efficacy in patients with anxiety disorders, although the efficacy shown is in part dependent on the year of publication of the study. Older randomised controlled trials appear to show a larger effect than more recent ones (Martin et al., 2007). Anxiolytic effects have also been reported in normal volunteers with high trait anxiety and in patients with anticipatory anxiety before surgery. However, in subjects with low trait anxiety and in non-stressful conditions, benzodiazepines may paradoxically increase anxiety and impair psychomotor performance.

Although useful for many anxiety disorders, benzodiazepines are not generally recommended for those with panic disorder as the long-term outcome is poor (NICE, 2007). Some patients report worse panic attacks after the benzodiazepines are stopped. Benzodiazepines are also useful at the start of SSRI treatment in OCD and as hypnotics in PTSD (NICE, 2005a,b). They should, however, be used at the lowest effective dose prescribed intermittently where possible and used for no longer than 2–4 weeks.

Choice of benzodiazepine in anxiety. The choice of benzodiazepine depends largely on pharmacokinetic characteristics. Potent benzodiazepines such as lorazepam and alprazolam (Table 28.2) have been widely used for anxiety disorders but are probably inappropriate. Both are rapidly eliminated and need to be taken several times a day. Declining blood concentrations may lead to interdose anxiety as the anxiolytic effect of each tablet wears off. The high potency of lorazepam (~10 times that of diazepam), and the fact that it is available only in 1 and 2.5 mg tablet strengths, has often led to excessive dosage. Similarly, alprazolam (~20 times more potent than diazepam) has often been used in excessive dosage, particularly in the USA. Such doses lead to adverse effects, a high probability of dependence and difficulties in withdrawal.

A slowly eliminated benzodiazepine such as diazepam is more appropriate in most cases. Diazepam has a rapid onset of action and its slow elimination ensures a steady blood concentration. Clonazepam, although long acting, is more potent than diazepam and in practice is often difficult to withdraw from. It is only indicated for epilepsy in the UK, but is commonly used as an anxiolytic.

Parenteral administration of lorazepam or diazepam may occasionally be indicated for severely agitated psychiatric patients.

Adverse effects. Adverse effects include drowsiness, lightheadedness, confusion, ataxia, amnesia, a paradoxical increase in aggression, an increased risk of falls and fractures in the elderly and an increased risk of road traffic accidents. They are also widely acknowledged as addictive and cause tolerance after more than 2–4 weeks of continuous use (Taylor et al.,

2009). Respiratory depression is rare, but possible following high oral doses or parenteral use. Flumazenil, a benzodiazepine receptor antagonist, can reverse the effects of severe reactions but requires repeated dosing and close monitoring because of its short half-life.

Psychomotor and cognitive impairment. Although oversedation is not usually a problem in anxious patients, there is evidence that long-term use of benzodiazepines results in psychomotor impairment and has adverse effects on memory. Many patients on long-term benzodiazepines complain of poor memory and incidents of shoplifting have been attributed to memory lapses caused by benzodiazepine use. In elderly patients, the amnesic effects may falsely suggest the development of dementia. There is some evidence that benzodiazepines also inhibit the learning of alternative stress-coping strategies, such as behavioural treatments for agoraphobia. Additive effects with other CNS depressants including alcohol occur and may contribute to road traffic and other accidents.

Disinhibition, paradoxical effects. Occasionally, benzodiazepines produce paradoxical stimulant effects. These effects are most marked in anxious subjects and include excitement, increased anxiety, irritability and outbursts of rage. Violent behaviour has sometimes been attributed to disinhibition by benzodiazepines. This behaviour is normally suppressed by social restraints, fear or anxiety. Increased day-time anxiety can also occur with rapidly eliminated benzodiazepines and may be a withdrawal effect.

Affective reactions. Chronic use of benzodiazepines can aggravate depression, may sometimes provoke suicide attempts in impulsive patients, and can cause depression in patients with no previous history of depressive disorder. Aggravation of depression is a particular risk in anxious patients who often have mixed anxiety/depression. Benzodiazepines are taken alone or in combination with other drugs in 40% of self-poisoning incidents. Although relatively non-toxic in overdose, they can cause fatalities as a result of drug interactions and in those with respiratory disease.

Some patients on long-term benzodiazepines complain of 'emotional anaesthesia' with inability to experience either pleasure or distress. However, in some patients, benzodiazepines induce euphoria and they are occasionally used as drugs of abuse.

Dependence. The greatest drawback of chronic benzodiazepine use is the development of drug dependence. It is generally agreed that the regular use of therapeutic doses of benzodiazepines as hypnotics or anxiolytics for more than a few weeks (2–4 weeks) can give rise to dependence, with withdrawal symptoms on cessation of drug use in over 40% of patients. It is estimated that there are about 1 million long-term benzodiazepine users in the UK and many of these are likely to be dependent. People with substance misuse histories, anxious or 'passive-dependent' personalities seem to be most vulnerable to dependence and withdrawal symptoms. Such individuals make up a large proportion of anxious patients in psychiatric practice, are often described as suffering from 'chronic anxiety' and are the type of patient for whom benzodiazepines are most likely to be prescribed.

Such patients often continue to take benzodiazepines for many years because attempts at dosage reduction or drug withdrawal result in abstinence symptoms, which they are unable to tolerate. Nevertheless, these patients continue to suffer from anxiety symptoms despite continued benzodiazepine use, possibly because they have become tolerant to the anxiolytic effects and may also suffer from other adverse effects of long-term benzodiazepine use such as depression or psychomotor impairment.

Abuse. In the last 15 years, there has been much concern about benzodiazepine abuse. Some patients escalate their prescribed dosage and may obtain prescriptions from several doctors. These tend to be anxious patients with 'passive-dependent' personalities who may have a history of alcohol misuse; they often combine large doses of benzodiazepines with excessive alcohol consumption. In addition, a high proportion (30–90%) of illicit recreational drug abusers also use benzodiazepines and some take them as euphoriants in their own right. Recreational use of most benzodiazepines has been reported in various countries; in the UK, temazepam is most commonly abused. Exceedingly large doses (over 1 g) may be taken and sometimes injected intravenously. Benzodiazepines became easily available due to widespread prescribing which favoured their entrance into the illicit drug scene. Abusers become dependent and suffer the same adverse effects and withdrawal symptoms as prescribed dose users.

Benzodiazepine withdrawal. Many patients on long-term benzodiazepines seek help with drug withdrawal. Clinical experience shows that withdrawal is feasible in most patients if carried out with care. Abrupt withdrawal in dependent subjects is dangerous and can induce acute anxiety, psychosis or convulsions. However, gradual withdrawal, coupled where necessary with psychological treatments, can be successful in the majority of patients. The duration of withdrawal should be tailored to individual needs and may last many months. Dosage reductions may be of the order of 1–2 mg of diazepam per month. Even with slow dosage reduction, a variety of withdrawal symptoms may be experienced, including increased anxiety, insomnia, hypersensitivity to sensory stimuli, perceptual distortions, paraesthesia, muscle twitching, depression and many others (Box 28.2). These may last for many weeks, though diminishing in intensity, but occasionally the withdrawal syndrome is protracted for a year or more. Transfer to diazepam, because of its slow elimination and availability as a liquid and in low dosage forms, may be indicated for patients taking other benzodiazepines. Useful guidelines for benzodiazepine withdrawal are given in the British National Formulary and detailed withdrawal schedules are also available (Lader et al., 2009).

The eventual outcome does not appear to be influenced by dosage, type of benzodiazepine, duration of use, personality disorder, psychiatric history, age, severity of withdrawal symptoms or rate of withdrawal. Hence, benzodiazepine withdrawal is worth attempting in patients who are motivated to stop and most patients report that they feel better after withdrawal than when they were taking the benzodiazepine. Community pharmacists may be ideally suited to advise doc-

---

Box 28.2 Some common benzodiazepine withdrawal symptoms

Symptoms common to anxiety states	Symptoms relatively specific to benzodiazepine withdrawal
Anxiety, panic	Perceptual distortions, sense of movement
Agoraphobia	
Insomnia, nightmares	Depersonalisation, derealisation
Depression, dysphoria	Hallucinations
Excitability, restlessness	Distortion of body image
Poor memory and concentration	Tingling, numbness, altered sensation
Dizziness, light-headedness	Skin prickling (formication)
Weakness, 'jelly legs'	Sensory hypersensitivity
Tremor	Muscle twitches, jerks
Muscle pain, stiffness	Tinnitus
Sweating, night sweats	Psychosis[a]
Palpitations	Confusion, delirium[a]
Blurred or double vision	Convulsions[a]
Gastro-intestinal and urinary symptoms	

[a]Usually only on rapid or abrupt withdrawal from high doses.

---

tors and patients on the management of benzodiazepine withdrawal. Leading a benzodiazepine withdrawal clinic may also be a useful role for pharmacist or nurse prescribers.

Drug interactions. In addition to the pharmacokinetic interactions listed earlier, benzodiazepines have additive effects with other CNS depressants. Combinations of benzodiazepines with alcohol, other hypnotics, sedative tricyclic antidepressants (TCAs), antihistamines or opioids can cause marked sedation and may lead to accidents, collapse or severe respiratory depression.

Pregnancy and lactation. The regular use of benzodiazepines is not recommended in pregnancy since the drugs are concentrated in fetal tissue where hepatic metabolism is minimal. They have been associated with an increased risk of oral clefts following first trimester exposure, a low birth weight, neonatal depression, feeding difficulties and withdrawal symptoms if given in late pregnancy. They also enter breast milk and may cause sedation, lethargy and weight loss in the infant. Long-acting benzodiazepines should particularly be avoided during lactation because of the potential for the infant to accumulate the drug. Short- to medium-acting benzodiazepines are occasionally used with enhanced monitoring of the infant.

Antidepressant drugs

Antidepressants can provide a long-term treatment option for those with an anxiety disorder. They are generally recommended for those who are unable to commit to or have not responded to psychological therapies. In addition, antidepressants are considered first-line treatment option either alone or in combination with CBT in patients suffering from OCD with moderate or severe impairment (NICE, 2005a). The number needed to treat (NNT) to see one benefit with antidepressants is around five in PTSD and GAD (NICE, 2005b, 2007).

The response rate to antidepressants in anxiety is often lower and takes longer than that seen in depression. Initial worsening of symptoms can occur and high therapeutic doses are often required to improve response (Baldwin et al., 2005).

Selective serotonin reuptake inhibitors. The selective serotonin reuptake inhibitors (SSRIs) have a broad anxiolytic effect and are considered the first drug options in GAD, panic disorder, social phobia, PTSD and OCD (NICE, 2005a,b, 2007; Baldwin et al., 2005). Individual SSRIs have varying licensed indications across the anxiety disorders but this does not necessarily mean others have no supporting evidence. Where more than one SSRI is licensed in a particular disorder it is not possible to conclude which SSRI would be more effective because of the lack of direct head to head trials. The SSRIs do differ in their interaction potential, side effect profile and ease of discontinuation. Initial worsening of symptoms is common when starting an SSRI in anxiety, so beginning with half the dose than that used in depression is recommended as is reassuring the patient that this is usually only experienced for the first few weeks of treatment. In view of these concerns, the NICE (2007) guidelines for GAD and panic disorder recommend that patients are reviewed every 2 weeks for the first 6 weeks of treatment to monitor for efficacy and tolerability.

Tricyclic antidepressants. Certain TCAs such as clomipramine, imipramine and amitriptyline are efficacious in some anxiety disorders. They are, however, associated with a greater burden of adverse reactions such as anticholinergic effects, hypotension and weight gain. Of particular concern is the TCAs' cardiac toxicity in overdose which relegates their use to second line following the failure of an SSRI. They should be avoided in any patient at risk of suicide or those with an underlying cardiac disease. TCAs commonly cause sedation which occasionally can prove useful in anxiety disorders. Clomipramine may also be slightly more effective in OCD compared with SSRIs.

Monoamine-oxidase inhibitors. The monoamine-oxidase inhibitors (MAOIs) are rarely used in practice because of their potential interactions with other medicines and tyramine in the diet. Moclobemide is a reversible MAOI, so causes fewer problematic interactions. Phenelzine and moclobemide are occasionally used by specialists in social phobia following the failure of an SSRI. Phenelzine is also recommended as a third-line treatment option in PTSD (NICE, 2005b).

Other antidepressants. The selective and noradrenaline reuptake inhibitor (SNRI) venlafaxine has some evidence to support its use in almost all the anxiety disorders, but it is only licensed for use in GAD and social phobia at a dose of 75 mg/day in the extended release form. Discontinuation symptoms are common following venlafaxine withdrawal and can be experienced after missing a single dose. Patients prescribed venlafaxine should be reminded of the importance of a slow withdrawal (over at least 4 weeks) when discontinuation is necessary. Venlafaxine can increase blood pressure at higher doses and so is contraindicated in patients with a very high risk of cardiac ventricular arrhythmia or uncontrolled hypertension. Duloxetine, another SNRI, is also licensed in GAD and can similarly increase blood pressure.

Mirtazapine, an α_2-adrenoreceptor antagonist, is recommended as an option for PTSD if patients do not wish to participate in trauma focused CBT (NICE, 2005b). Mirtazapine has a lower incidence of nausea, vomiting and sexual dysfunction than the SSRIs but can commonly cause weight gain and sedation.

No other antidepressants are routinely recommended for anxiety disorders, although some such as agomelatine are under clinical trials in anxiety to investigate potential future uses. To reduce the risk of symptoms returning patients should be advised to continue the antidepressant for at least 6 months following improvement of symptoms in GAD and panic disorder and for 12 months in PTSD, OCD and social phobia (NICE, 2005a, 2007; Baldwin et al., 2005). Those with an enduring and recurrent illness, however, may continue for many years, depending on the risk of relapse and severity of symptoms.

For a complete review of the antidepressants, including adverse effects and interactions, see Chapter 29.

Other medications occasionally used in anxiety

Hydroxyzine, a sedating antihistamine, is licensed for the short-term treatment of anxiety in adults at a dose of 50–100 mg four times a day. The clinical evidence only supports its use in GAD (for up to 4 weeks) if sedation is required. NICE supports the use of a sedating antihistamine in the immediate management of GAD but state they should not be used in panic disorders (NICE, 2007).

Antipsychotics have limited evidence and a high side effect burden when used in anxiety disorders. The first-generation (typical) antipsychotics are associated with movement disorders such as akathisia and tardive dyskinesia and so are rarely used in anxiety. The second-generation (atypical) antipsychotics are less likely to cause movement disorders but can have other physical health concerns. The majority of the evidence only supports antipsychotics (specifically risperidone and quetiapine) in combination with an SSRI in OCD in those who have failed to respond to the SSRI alone. Olanzapine augmentation has also been used in PTSD and social phobia.

Pregabalin is licensed for GAD and has shown an anxiolytic effect over placebo after 1 week in adults or 2 weeks in the elderly (Montgomery et al., 2008). Two short-term studies (4 and 6 weeks) suggest that pregabalin 400–600 mg/day is as effective but better tolerated than venlafaxine 75 mg/day XL or lorazepam 6 mg/day. Pregabalin, however, commonly causes dizziness, somnolence and nausea and is more expensive than other medication options in GAD and should be limited to specialist use only after other treatments have failed.

Buspirone, a $5HT_{1A}$ partial agonist, is licensed for short-term use in anxiety. It is not a benzodiazepine and so does not treat or prevent benzodiazepine withdrawal problems. In GAD, buspirone and other azapirones are superior to placebo in short-term studies (4–9 weeks) but less effective or acceptable than benzodiazepines (Chessick et al., 2006). NICE have said the evidence for buspirone in GAD is equivocal and, therefore, presumably not recommended (NICE, 2007). There is no evidence supporting buspirone in other anxiety disorders.

Table 28.3 Overview of the recommended drug treatments in anxiety

	Generalised anxiety disorder (GAD)	Panic disorder	Social phobia (social anxiety disorder)	Obsessive-compulsive disorder (OCD)	Post-traumatic stress disorder (PTSD)
Immediate management/ short-term treatment	Benzodiazepines (2–4 weeks only) Hydroxyzine	Benzodiazepines not recommended by NICE	Benzodiazepines (2–4 weeks only)	Benzodiazepines (only to counter initial worsening of symptoms with SSRIs)	Hypnotics may be considered for short-term use for insomnia
First-line pharmacotherapy[a]	SSRI Escitalopram Paroxetine Sertraline	SSRI Citalopram Escitalopram Paroxetine	SSRI Escitalopram Paroxetine	SSRI Escitalopram Fluoxetine Fluvoxamine Paroxetine Sertraline	SSRI Paroxetine Sertraline
Other drug treatments with some supporting evidence	Buspirone Duloxetine Imipramine Pregabalin[c] Venlafaxine	Clomipramine[b] Imipramine[b] Mirtazapine Moclobemide Venlafaxine	Moclobemide[c] Phenelzine[c] Venlafaxine	Clomipramine Augmentation with quetiapine or risperidone[c]	Amitriptyline[c] Augmentation with olanzapine or risperidone[c] Imipramine Mirtazapine[b] Phenelzine[c] Venlafaxine

[a]The licensed SSRI is indicated but other SSRIs may also be beneficial.
[b]Unlicensed but recommended by NICE (2005a,b, 2007).
[c]Usually prescribed by mental health specialists only.

Propranolol and oxprenolol are both licensed for anxiety symptoms but are probably only useful for physical symptoms such as palpitations, tremor, sweating and shortness of breath. β-Blockers do not have sufficient evidence to support their inclusion in NICE guidelines but intriguingly small pilot studies indicate that giving an immediate course of propranolol following a traumatic event may prevent emerging PTSD (Pitman et al., 2002; Vaiva et al., 2003).

An overview of the recommended drug treatments in anxiety is provided in Table 28.3.

Case studies

Case 28.1

Mrs DW is a 32-year-old with a 10-year history of 'emotional problems'. These have largely been dealt with by her primary care doctor who has prescribed low dose TCAs for the last 3 years. Mrs DW's life is severely restricted by a number of rituals which she obsessively carries out. They include washing of sinks, baths and toilets, disinfection of kitchen surfaces, and vacuuming. These activities occupy up to 8 hours a day.

Current prescribed medication:
Diazepam 10 mg three times a day
Amitriptyline 25 mg twice a day
Both have been prescribed for 3 years

Mrs DW is concerned about possible addiction to her medication, as previous attempts to stop it have been unsuccessful. In addition, both she and her family feel that more can be achieved and are willing to work at solving the problems faced by Mrs DW.

Questions

1. Is this appropriate therapy for OCD and if not what would be a better first choice?
2. Suggest possible drug therapies for Mrs DW and indicate for how long they should be continued?
3. Providing an alternative therapy is commenced, recommend an appropriate scheme for withdrawal of the diazepam.

Answers

1. Benzodiazepines are not recommended in OCD. First choice is cognitive behaviour therapy or an SSRI.
2. Potential drug treatments include high dose SSRIs or clomipramine. Augmentation strategies (e.g. antipsychotics) would also be a possibility. Treatment may need to be continued for a year before a dose reduction is tried.
3. As Mrs DW is on a dose of 30 mg diazepam daily, it would be appropriate to consider reducing the diazepam by 2 mg/day every 1–2 weeks until 20 mg/day dose is reached. Further reductions may need to be 1 mg every 1–2 weeks until stopped. Longer intervals between dose reduction may be necessary as the dose reduces towards zero. Patient may wish to adopt faster withdrawal and accept the consequences. All patients should be monitored for increased anxiety, restlessness, agitation, etc., and may need slow withdrawal.

Case 28.2

Mrs AB, a previously well 30-year-old woman, had been treated with paroxetine 40 mg daily for anxiety/depression which had been precipitated by a traumatic marriage break-up. After taking paroxetine for 18 months, Mrs AB's problems had mainly resolved and she was feeling well. She decided that she no longer needed the drug and stopped taking it. Within 3 days her anxiety/depression returned with insomnia and nightmares. Her mood lowered and she became irritable and found herself weeping for no reason. A week later she returned to her doctor complaining of these symptoms as well as depersonalisation and strange electric shock sensations. The doctor thought the original depression had returned and reinstated paroxetine which cleared up her symptoms within a few days.

Questions

1. What alternative explanation could there be for Mrs AB's symptoms and what other decision could the doctor have made?
2. What would be a suitable withdrawal schedule for her paroxetine?

Answers

1. All antidepressants can cause a discontinuation reaction. Mrs AB's symptoms were typical of SSRI withdrawal. This occurs most commonly with paroxetine, perhaps partly due to its rapid rate of elimination (half-life 21 h in chronic users).
2. In this previously well lady no longer under marital stress, the doctor, after reinstating paroxetine, could have supplied a gradual tapering schedule of drug withdrawal, that is, reducing the dose by 10 mg/week, aiming to withdrawal in 4 weeks.

Case 28.3

Mr SB is a 22-year-old soldier. He has recently returned from his second active tour where he was injured by a roadside bomb. Two of his squad were killed in the same blast and, although his physical injuries healed quickly, he has persistent and intense episodes of panic and flashbacks. He is especially aroused at night and has great difficulty getting to sleep. An initial prescription of an SSRI has proved ineffective and he is currently on the waiting list for psychological therapies.

Question

1. What alternative drug treatment may be appropriate?

Answer

1. A sedating antidepressant such as mirtazapine or amitriptyline may be appropriate, ensuring adequate duration of therapy and effective dose. A short cause of a benzodiazepine may prove useful but for no longer than 2–4 weeks. Alternatively, augmenting the antidepressant with a sedating antipsychotic such as olanzapine may be useful. For prolonged symptom treatment and relapse prevention it is likely that the patient will need to fully engage with psychological therapies.

Case 28.4

Ms AC is a 32-year-old personal assistant to a director of a leading investment company. She has recently been promoted to this role and is now expected to entertain potential clients by dining out with the director at local restaurants. She has always preferred eating alone in the comfort of her own home and the thought of eating in public while promoting the business fills her with dread, which brings on palpitations and shortness of breath.

Questions

1. What drug therapy is available which may provide some immediate relief of her anxiety symptoms?
2. What would be an appropriate choice of treatment for long-term control and prevention of symptoms?

Answers

1. β-Blockers such as propranolol may help with the shortness of breath and palpitations but will not treat the fear and dread. Benzodiazepines may be appropriate but may affect her performance and cause other adverse reactions.
2. For long-term control, a course of cognitive behavioural therapy including exposure techniques is appropriate or treatment with an SSRI such as escitalopram.

References

Baldwin, D., Anderson, I., Nutt, D., et al., 2005. Evidence-based guidelines for the pharmacological treatment of anxiety disorders: recommendations from the British Association for Psychopharmacology. J. Psychopharmacol. 19, 567–596.

Bazire, S., 2009. Psychotropic Drug Directory. HealthComm UK, Aberdeen.

Chessick, C.A., Allen, M.H., Thase, M.E., et al., 2006. Azapirones for generalized anxiety disorder. Cochrane Database of Systematic Reviews Issue 3, Art No. CD006115. doi:10.1002/14651858.CD006115.

Christmas, D., Hood, S., Nutt, D., 2008. Potential novel anxiolytic drugs. Curr. Pharm. Des. 14, 3534–3546.

Haefely, W., 1990. Benzodiazepine receptor and ligands: structural and functional differences. In: Hindmarch, I., Beaumont, G., Brandon, S., et al. (Eds.), Benzodiazepines: Current Concepts. John Wiley, Chichester, pp. 1–18.

Lader, M., Tylee, A., Donoghue, J., 2009. Withdrawing benzodiazepines in primary care. CNS Drugs 23, 19–34.

Martin, J., Sainz-Pardo, M., Furukawa, T., et al., 2007. Review: benzodiazepines in generalized anxiety disorder: heterogeneity based on systematic review and meta-analysis of clinical trials. J. Psychopharmacol. 21, 774–782.

Montgomery, S.A., Chatamra, K., Pauer, L., et al., 2008. Efficacy and safety of pregabalin in elderly people with generalised anxiety disorder. Br. J. Psychiatry 193, 389–394.

National Institute for Health and Clinical Excellence, 2005a. Obsessive compulsive disorder. Clinical Guideline 31. Available at: http://www.nice.org.uk/Guidance/CG31. Accessed March 2010.

National Institute for Health and Clinical Excellence, 2005b. Post traumatic stress disorder (PTSD). Clinical Guideline 26. Available at: http://www.nice.org.uk/CG26. Accessed March 2010.

National Institute for Health and Clinical Excellence, 2007. Anxiety: management of anxiety (panic disorder, with or without agoraphobia, and generalised anxiety disorder) in adults in primary, secondary and community care. Clinical Guideline 22 (amended). Available at: http://www.nice.org.uk/nicemedia/pdf/CG022NICEguidelineamended.pdf. Accessed March 2010.

Pitman, R., Sanders, K., Zusman, R., et al., 2002. Pilot study of secondary prevention of posttraumatic stress disorder with propranolol. Biol. Psychiatry 51, 189–192.

Roy-Byrne, P.P., 2005. The GABA-benzodiazepine receptor complex: structure, function and role in anxiety. J. Clin. Psychiatry 66 (Suppl. 2), 14–20.

Taylor, D., Paton, C., Kapur, S., 2009. The Maudsley Prescribing Guidelines, 10th ed. Informa Healthcare, London.

Vaiva, G., Ducrocq, F., Jezequel, K., et al., 2003. Immediate treatment with propranolol decreases posttraumatic stress disorder two months after trauma. Biol. Psychiatry 54, 947–949.

Further reading

Baldwin, D., 2008. Room for improvement in the pharmacological treatment of anxiety disorders. Curr. Pharm. Des. 14, 3482–3491.

Garner, M., Mohler, H., Stein, D., et al., 2009. Research in anxiety disorders: from the bench to the bedside. Eur. Neuropsychopharmacol. 19, 381–390.

Katzman, M., 2009. Current considerations in the treatment of generalized anxiety disorder. CNS Drugs 23, 103–120.

Useful resources

The British Association for Behavioural and Cognitive Psychotherapies has a list of therapists, training resources and general information for the public.
www.babcp.com

Anxiety UK: a national charity for anyone affected by an anxiety disorder.
www.anxietyuk.org.uk

No Panic: a national charity offering support for suffers of panic attacks, phobias, Obsessive Compulsive Disorder and Generalised Anxiety Disorder.
www.nopanic.org.uk

Affective disorders 29

J. P. Pratt

Key points

- Diagnosis should be made using standardised criteria, for example, DSM IV, ICD 10.
- Target symptoms should be recorded and response to treatment monitored against these symptoms.
- In patients with depression of mild severity, non-pharmacological strategies should be considered as first-line intervention.
- The evidence base for determining the use of a particular antidepressant in an individual patient does not exist. For most patients, when an antidepressant is indicated, a generic SSRI should be considered as a first-line treatment option.
- Currently, all antidepressants are considered equally effective but differ in their side effect profile, toxicity in overdose, need for dose titration and monitoring.
- In the absence of a previous response or contraindication, antidepressant choice should be guided by evidence-based clinical guidelines and the clinician and the patient's perception of the risks and benefits of available options. Resource implications should not be ignored.
- Emerging evidence and a greater understanding of the clinical application of pharmacogenomics may increase the ability to individualise treatments in the future.
- Comprehensive assessment, accurate diagnosis, adequate duration of pharmacotherapy and involvement of the patient in the treatment regimen are the cornerstones of effective management of affective disorders.
- Valproate, antipsychotics and benzodiazepines, sometimes in combination, are the treatments of choice in acute mania.
- Either lithium, valproate or specific antipsychotics may be considered to be the first-line prophylactic agent of choice in bipolar I disorder.

This chapter focuses on affective disorders in adults. The issues of affective disorders in children and adolescents are more complex and beyond the scope of this section.

The central feature of an affective disorder is an alteration in mood. The most common presentation is that of a low mood or depression. Less commonly, the mood may become high or elated, as in mania.

Classification

Depression

The term 'depression' can in itself be misleading. Everyone in the normal course of daily life will experience alterations in mood. Depressed mood in this context does not represent a disorder or illness; in fact, lowered mood as a response to the ups and downs of living is considered normal and termed sadness or unhappiness. Sometimes clinical depression may present in a mild form, so it is important to differentiate this from normal unhappiness.

Mania

If the mood becomes elated or irritable this may be a symptom of mania. The term 'mania' is used to describe severe cases, frequently associated with psychotic symptoms. Hypomania describes a less severe form of the disorder. In clinical practice, this distinction often becomes blurred, with hypomania being seen as patients develop, or recover from, mania.

Bipolar and unipolar disorders

If a patient develops one or more severe episodes of a mood disorder which includes a manic episode, the condition may be termed a bipolar disorder. The existence of repeated manic episodes alone is sufficient to be termed a bipolar disorder. The disorder can be further categorised as bipolar I, where full-blown episodes of mania occur, and bipolar II, where depressive episodes are interspersed with less severe hypomanic episodes. The term 'manic-depressive' is now outdated. Rapid cycling describes the existence of four or more episodes within a year. Unipolar mood disorder is used to describe single episodes of depression.

Epidemiology

Differences in diagnosis, particularly of depression, make it difficult to estimate the true incidence of affective disorders. The lifetime risk of developing a bipolar I disorder is said to be about 1% (0.3–1.5%). An accurate estimate for the more broadly defined bipolar II disorder is more difficult and it may be much more common, with studies suggesting a lifetime prevalence of between 0.2% and 10.9%. The incidence of bipolar I is generally reported to be the same for both men and women, whereas some studies suggest that bipolar II may be slightly more common in women. By comparison, the overall incidence of depression is much higher and there does appear to be a significant difference between the sexes. Studies from America and Europe, using standard assessment tools, found a lifetime prevalence of between 16% and 17%,

465

with a 6-month prevalence of about 6%. Higher rates are consistently found in women but social, economic and ethnic factors are also likely to be influential. Although depression may occur at any age, including early childhood, it is estimated that the average age of onset of depression is in the mid-20s. Some earlier studies found the incidence and prevalence of depression in women peaking at the age of 35–45 years. In bipolar disorder, an earlier age of onset is suggested, perhaps in late adolescence, with most people experiencing their first episodes before 30 years of age.

Aetiology

Like most psychiatric disorders, the causes of affective disorders remain unknown. In depression, it is likely that genetic, hormonal, biochemical, environmental and social factors all have some role in determining an individual's susceptibility to developing the disorder, with major life events sometimes, but not always, acting as a precipitant for a particular episode. Although pharmacological treatments are clearly effective, there is no simple relationship between biochemical abnormalities and affective disorders.

Genetic causes

In depression, one theory suggests that a variant of the gene responsible for encoding the serotonin transporter protein could account for early childhood experiences being translated into an increased risk of depression through stress sensitivity in adulthood. In bipolar disorder, some genetic linkage has been proposed, but a precise marker remains elusive.

The incidence of affective disorder in first-degree relatives of someone with severe depression may be about 20%, which is almost three times the risk for relatives in control groups. Comparisons of the risk of affective disorder in the children of both parents with an affective disorder show a four times greater risk, and the risk is doubled in children with one parent with an affective disorder. Studies looking at twins have found fairly strong evidence for a genetic factor. Evidence of a genetic link has also been found in studies of children from parents with affective disorder who were adopted by healthy parents. A higher incidence of affective disorder was found in the biological parents of adopted children with affective disorder than in the adoptive parents.

Environmental factors

Although environmental stresses can often be identified prior to an episode of mania or depression, a causal relationship between a major event in someone's life and the development of an affective disorder has not been firmly established. It may be that life events described as 'threatening' are more likely to be associated with depression. The lack of prospective studies makes it difficult to interpret data linking early life events, such as loss of a parent, to the development of an affective disorder. The fact that specific environmental stresses have not been identified should not lead to the conclusion that the environment or lifestyle is irrelevant to the course or development of affective disorders. Employment, higher socio-economic status and the existence of a close and confiding relationship have been consistently noted to offer some protection against the development of an episode.

Biochemical factors

In its simplistic form, the biochemical theory of depression postulates a deficiency of neurotransmitter amines in certain areas of the brain. This theory has been developed to suggest that receptor sensitivity changes may be important. Alternative propositions suggest a central role of acetylcholine arising from dysregulation of the cholinergic and noradrenergic neurotransmitter systems. Although many neurotransmitters may be implicated, the theory focuses on an involvement of the neurotransmitters noradrenaline (norepinephrine), serotonin (5-hydroxytryptamine) and dopamine. This theory emerged from the findings that both monoamine oxidase inhibitors (MAOIs) and tricyclic antidepressants appeared to increase neurotransmitter amines, particularly noradrenaline (norepinephrine), at important sites in the brain. When it was found that reserpine, previously used as an antihypertensive, caused both a depletion of neurotransmitter and also induced depression, this was taken as an apparent confirmation of the theory.

Although less attention has been paid to dopaminergic activity, some studies have found reduced activity in depressed patients, and an overactivity has been postulated in mania.

The concept of noradrenergic (norepinephrinergic) and serotonergic forms of depression has not gained widespread support, and there is no justification in measuring the activity of neurotransmitters such as noradrenaline (norepinephrine) or serotonin metabolites in routine clinical practice.

Endocrine factors

The endocrine system, particularly the hypothalamic-pituitary-adrenal (HPA) axis and the hypothalamic-pituitary-thyroid (HPT) axis, is felt to be implicated in the development of affective disorders. Some endocrine disorders such as hypothyroidism and Cushing's syndrome have also been associated with changes in mood. People with depression have been found to have increased cortisol levels, which also supported the proposition that mood disorders may be linked to dysfunction within the HPA axis. This led to the development of a dexamethasone suppression test for depression in the 1970s. The relationship between cortisol and symptoms of depression is complex which severely limits the clinical utility of such a test.

Physical illness and side effects of medication

Disorders of mood, particularly depression, have been associated with several types of medication and a number of physical illnesses (Box 29.1). Depression can affect the outcome in people with a range of physical problems. An increase in death rates has been found in those patients with co-morbid depression.

Box 29.1 Drugs and physical illnesses implicated in disorders of mood

Drugs
Analgesics
Antidepressants
Antihypertensives
Anticonvulsants
Opiate withdrawal
Amfetamine withdrawal
Benzodiazepine withdrawal
Antipsychotics
Benzodiazepines
Antiparkinsonism agents
Steroids
Oral contraceptives

Physical illness
Viral illness
Carcinoma
Neurological disorders
Diabetes
Multiple sclerosis
Thyroid disease
Addison's disease
Systemic lupus erythematosus
Pernicious anaemia

Box 29.2 ICD 10 diagnostic criteria for bipolar affective disorder (WHO, 1992)

Characterised by repeated (at least two) episodes in which the patient's mood and activity levels are significantly disturbed. This disturbance consisting on some occasions of an elevation in mood and increased energy and activity (mania or hypomania), and on others of a lowering of mood and decreased energy and activity (depression).

Manic episodes usually begin abruptly and last for between 2 weeks and 4–6 months (median 4 months). Depression tends to last longer (median about 6 months). Episodes of both kinds often follow stressful life events or other mental trauma, but the presence of such stress is not essential for the diagnosis.

Clinical manifestations

Depression

A low mood is the central feature of depression. This is often accompanied by a loss of interest or pleasure in normally enjoyable activities. Thinking is pessimistic and in some cases suicidal. A depressed person may complain they have little or no energy. In severe cases, psychotic symptoms such as mood congruent hallucination or delusion may be present. Anxiety or agitation frequently accompany the disorder, and the so-called biological features of sleep disturbances, weight loss and loss of appetite are often present. Depressed people typically complain of somatic symptoms, particularly gastric problems, and non-specific aches are common. Sexual drive is often reduced, and some people may lose interest in sex altogether. In some cases, the biological symptoms are reversed and excessive eating and sleeping may occur. In contrast to agitation, psychomotor retardation may be a presenting feature.

Bipolar disorder

Standardised diagnostic criteria vary. For an ICD 10 diagnosis of bipolar disorder, at least two mood episodes must occur, one of which must be manic or hypomanic (Box 29.2). According to DSM IV, at least one episode of mania must have occurred for a diagnosis of bipolar I disorder to be made; depression may also occur, but it is not essential.

Mania

In mania, the mood is described as elated or irritable and the accompanying overactivity is usually unproductive. Disinhibition may result in excessive spending sprees, inappropriate sexual activity and other high-risk behaviours. Driving may be particularly dangerous. Manic people may describe their thoughts as racing, with ideas rapidly changing from one topic to another. Speech may be very rapid with frequent punning and rhyming. Ideas may become grandiose with patients embarking on fantastic projects which lead nowhere and inevitably are left incomplete and disjointed. Clothing is usually flamboyant, and if make-up is worn it is usually excessive and involves bright colours.

Severity

The severity of the disorder may vary from mild through moderate to severe. In most circumstances, it would be inappropriate for people with mild forms of the disorders to be seen by specialist services and treated with pharmacotherapy. In the absence of a risk of serious self-harm, people with less severe forms of the disorder should be treated by the primary health care team. Guidelines advise that a stepwise approach is taken on the management of depression, with increasing evidence supporting the fact that antidepressant therapy is more likely to be effective in the more severe episodes (NICE, 2009).

If left untreated, it is important to remember that affective disorders carry a risk of mortality. In addition to suicidal attempts by someone who is depressed, the lack of self-care and physical exhaustion resulting from mania may be life-threatening. The social and financial consequences can have a devastating effect on both the patient with mania or hypomania and their family. Depression may also contribute to exacerbation of physical problems such as increased pain and worsening outcomes from cardiac disease (Nicholson et al., 2006).

Investigations

There are no universally accepted biochemical or genetic tests which will confirm the presence of an affective disorder. Various rating scales have been developed that may help to demonstrate the severity of depressive disorder or distinguish a predominantly anxious patient from a depressed patient. Within the limits of our current understanding of the technology, biochemical or genetic tests are unlikely to be helpful in determining the treatment plan or management of affective disorders.

In the UK, mental and behavioural disorders are commonly classified using the *International Classification of Diseases*, ICD 10 (WHO, 1992). The American Psychiatric Association has developed a precise system of diagnosis, based on the description of symptoms in the *Diagnostic and Statistical Manual of Mental Disorders* (DSM IV TR), now in its revised, fourth edition (American Psychiatric Association, 2000).

A systematic approach to the diagnosis of affective disorders is important when considering the effectiveness of medication. Most new clinical trials for antidepressants or antipsychotics require a DSM diagnosis as an entry criterion. In the UK, the ICD 10 classification is commonly used, with the severity of depression determined by the presence of the number of symptoms (see Boxes 29.2 and 29.3). More recently, use of the symptom count as a single factor upon which to base treatment decisions has been cautioned against (NICE, 2009). Account should also be taken of the extent of impairment and disability associated with depression.

National guidelines provide a sound framework for the management of depression (NICE, 2009) and bipolar disorder (NICE, 2006). It is important that people with depression are identified. A simple screening process for the presence of depression could involve asking the patient two questions about their mood and interest. For example, the patient could be asked 'During the last month, have you often been bothered by feeling down, depressed or hopeless?' and 'During the last month, have you often been bothered by having little interest or pleasure in doing things?'. If the answer to either question is 'no', it is unlikely the patient will be considered to have a depressive disorder. Patients who answer 'yes' warrant further investigation.

Identification of target symptoms may be useful in evaluating the response to treatment. In routine clinical practice, antidepressant medication should not generally be used to treat patients with mild depression. Non-pharmacological strategies are preferable in this group.

Rating scales

Various rating scales can be used to assist with the assessment of the severity of the disorder. Two of the more commonly used rating scales are the Beck Depression Inventory and the Hamilton Depression Rating Scale.

Beck Depression Inventory

This is a self-reporting scale looking at 21 depressive symptoms. The subject is asked to read a series of statements and mark on a scale of 1–4 how severe their symptoms are.

Box 29.3 ICD 10 diagnostic criteria for a depressive episode (WHO, 1992)

Usual symptoms
Depressed mood, loss of interest and enjoyment, and reduced energy leading to increased fatiguability and diminished activity

Common symptoms
Reduced concentration and attention
Reduced self-esteem and self-confidence
Ideas of guilt and unworthiness (even in a mild type of episode)
Bleak and pessimistic views of the future
Ideas or acts of self-harm or suicide
Disturbed sleep
Diminished appetite

In a depressive episode, the mood varies little from day to day and is often unresponsive to circumstances, yet may show characteristic diurnal variation as the day goes on. The clinical picture shows marked individual variations, and atypical presentations are particularly common in adolescence. In some cases, anxiety, distress and motor agitation may be more prominent at times than the depression.

For depressive episodes of all grades of severity, a duration of 2 weeks is usually required for diagnosis, but shorter periods may be reasonable if symptoms are unusually severe and of rapid onset.

Mild depressive episode: For at least 2 weeks, at least two of the usual symptoms of a depressive episode plus at least two of the common symptoms listed above.

An individual with a mild depressive episode is usually distressed by the symptoms and has some difficulty in continuing with ordinary work and social activities, but will probably not cease to function completely.

Moderate depressive episode: For at least 2 weeks, at least two or three of the usual symptoms of a depressive episode plus at least three (preferably four) of the common symptoms listed above.

An individual with moderately severe depressive episode will have these symptoms to a marked degree, but this is not essential if a particularly wide variety of symptoms is present overall. They will usually have considerable difficulties in continuing with social, work or domestic activities.

Severe depressive episode: For at least 2 weeks, all three of the usual symptoms of a depressive episode plus at least four of the common symptoms listed above, some of which should be of severe intensity.

An individual with severe depressive episode may be unable or unwilling to describe many symptoms in detail, but an overall grading of severe may still be justified. They will usually show considerable distress or agitation, unless retardation is a marked feature. Loss of self-esteem or feelings of uselessness or guilt are likely to be prominent. Suicide is a distinct danger, particularly in severe cases.

The higher the score, the more severely depressed a person may be.

Hamilton Depression Rating Scale

This rating scale is used by a health care professional at the end of an interview to rate the severity of depression.

Treatment

The aim of treatment is to prevent harm and to relieve distress or to be prophylactic. It is important to differentiate symptoms of the disorder from the premorbid personality. In general, the drugs which are used to control the symptoms of mania are not specifically antimanic. These agents are also used to treat other disorders. This means the diagnosis will primarily influence the way in which these drugs are used rather than the choice of drug per se. Clinicians should be aware of the licensed indication of treatments, so that any 'off label' use is done knowingly and in line with current best practice.

In the treatment of depression, all the antidepressants currently available in the UK may be considered to be equally effective. There is increasing evidence that patients with more severe episodes of depression are more likely to respond to antidepressant drugs, as opposed to placebo, than those with less severe forms of the disorder (Fournier et al., 2010). There is also some evidence to suggest that sertraline and escitalopram may have a more favourably risk/benefit profile than some other antidepressants (Cipriani et al., 2009). However, it is unclear if the magnitude of the difference between these drugs is sufficient to direct treatment choice for most depressed patients.

There are some generalisations which may help individualise the choice of antidepressant. Females may have a poorer tolerance of migraine than males and tricyclic antidepressants are less well tolerated and more likely to be toxic in overdose than the selective serotonin reuptake inhibitors (SSRIs). Patients may prefer one drug over another based on their past experience of benefit or side effects. Overall, the major difference between antidepressant agents is in their side effect profile and toxicity in overdose. There can also be significant variations in the costs of different agents.

Treatment of depression

In moderate and severe depression, pharmacological intervention is important, but this should never be considered in isolation from the social, cultural and environmental influences on the patient. Non-pharmacological therapies are effective and in mild depression they are considered preferable to drug treatment. Non-drug treatments and antidepressant medication are not mutually exclusive and in some cases it is preferable to use both in combination.

Drug treatment

Despite the availability of many new antidepressants, the therapeutic effectiveness of these agents has changed little since the discovery of the antidepressant properties of drugs used to prevent migraine in the late 1950s. Further research may reveal differences between antidepressants. Advances in the clinical utility of pharmacogenomics may, in time, provide clinicians with a tool to individualise pharmacotherapy. Overall, the SSRI antidepressants appear to be better tolerated than tricyclics and their safety profile in overdose should be an important consideration for use.

A strong response to placebo is found in most of the studies of antidepressants. Tolerability is, therefore, an important factor in the choice of drug; patients who are unable to tolerate the side effects of antidepressants are likely to discontinue these drugs. Antidepressants should be taken in adequate doses for some 4–6 weeks, and up to 12 weeks in older people, to achieve a full response. Following a single episode of depression, treatment should be continued for 6 months, at the same dose at which the patient achieved remission, before attempting withdrawal. In patients experiencing multiple episodes of depression, treatment should be continued for longer periods (2 years).

Withdrawal of antidepressants should normally be undertaken gradually. Following abrupt discontinuation, patients may experience symptoms of withdrawal that include gastro-intestinal symptoms, together with headache, giddiness, sweating, shaking and insomnia. In addition, extrapyramidal reactions may be associated with abrupt withdrawal from some of the SSRI antidepressants. Following successful treatment, antidepressants should be gradually reduced over a period of 4 weeks. This period should be increased if patients experience problems, or where medication has been given for extended periods.

Generally, the long half-life of fluoxetine enables the drug to be stopped without the need for tapering from the standard antidepressant dose of 20 mg. Patients taking MAOIs may experience psychomotor agitation following discontinuation.

As patients do not experience the craving typically associated with drugs of addiction, most health care professionals do not class antidepressants as addictive. Patients should be warned that there is a risk of problems with abrupt discontinuation, but use of emotive words like addiction or dependence is best avoided. In moderate or severe depression, the balance of risks and benefits is usually in favour of using antidepressants. Occasionally, some patients report that they have become dependent on their antidepressants and feel unable to stop taking them. These concerns should not be dismissed lightly, but the focus of discussion with the patient should be on the overall risks and benefits of the treatment in the context of their individual circumstances.

As discussed earlier, there is no strong evidence for the existence of a particular biochemical subtype of depression. However, some patients do respond better to particular antidepressants. This has led to the widely held view that previous response to treatment is a strong indication to use that particular drug in the treatment of a future episode.

In addition to previous response, the other important considerations to take into account when selecting an antidepressant are side effects, contraindications, toxicity in overdose, patient preference and clinician familiarity.

Generally speaking, the older drugs have a poorer side effect (Barbui et al., 2001; Geddes et al., 2002) and toxicity profile than the more recently introduced agents. Traditionally, the antidepressant drugs are categorised by their chemical structure, for example, tricyclic, or their predominant pharmacological action, for example, MAOI, SSRI.

Tricyclic antidepressants. A greater understanding of the pharmacology of antidepressants has given much support to the so-called biochemical theory of depression. Although substantial data on the pharmacological effects of the tricyclic antidepressants exist, it is still not clear how the drugs relieve the symptoms of depression. This is an important point often overlooked when discussing the issue with patients. The notion that depression is a simple lack of, or imbalance of, chemicals has little basis in fact. It merely provides a useful framework from which to discuss the benefits and harms of antidepressants.

It was thought originally that the primary effect of these drugs was related to their ability to block the reuptake of noradrenaline (norepinephrine) and/or 5HT following their release and action as neurotransmitters. As this effect occurs some weeks before the antidepressant response, clearly this is not the whole story. Following chronic administration, further biochemical changes take place, particularly with pre- and postsynaptic receptor sensitivity. Reduction of presynaptic α_2-inhibitory receptor sensitivity occurs, and this increases the production of noradrenaline (norepinephrine). Other effects which may be relevant include an increase in α_1 and β_1 receptor sensitivity. It is now felt that these receptor changes in the cerebral cortex and hippocampus may be more relevant to the antidepressant response than simple reuptake inhibition.

There are a number of tricyclic antidepressants in current clinical use. The basic chemical structures of these compounds are similar but there are differences between them. All the tricyclic antidepressants block the reuptake of noradrenaline (norepinephrine) and 5HT to a greater or lesser degree. In view of the risks associated with cardiac abnormalities, an ECG is advised prior to initiating treatment with this group of drugs.

Imipramine. The antidepressant effect of imipramine was demonstrated around 50 years ago and it has been widely prescribed in subsequent years. Although imipramine is less sedating than other tricyclic drugs, some patients may still experience problems. As well as cardiovascular problems, significant antimuscarinic effects such as dry mouth, blurred vision and constipation occur. Females tend to tolerate imipramine less well than males. At one time it was felt to be important that the drug should be prescribed at the full therapeutic dose. Recent analysis of clinical trials suggests this is not the case. If patients respond to lower doses, there is no rationale for increasing the dose further. Tolerance may develop to some of the unpleasant side effects, and this may be facilitated by starting with a lower dose of the drug and gradually increasing the dose over a week.

In addition to the unpleasant side effect profile, imipramine is toxic following overdose. Considering that the drug is used to treat a disorder which involves suicide, this relative lack of safety is an important disadvantage. As with all tricyclics, imipramine should only be used in circumstances where cardiac tolerability can be assured and intentional overdose can be prevented. Imipramine is metabolised by demethylation to an active metabolite, desipramine. Both the parent drug and its metabolite have long half-lives, of 9–20 and 10–35h, respectively, that permit single daily dosing.

Amitriptyline. Also developed in the late 1950s, amitriptyline has a similar poor side effect and toxicity profile to imipramine but is more sedative. Additional sedative properties are sometimes considered an advantage in selected patients. The widespread use of low doses of amitriptyline commonly relate to its use in the management of pain, rather than depressive disorders. Like imipramine, the drug and its active metabolite (nortriptyline) have long half-lives, of 9–46 and 18–56h, respectively. The dose range is similar to imipramine.

Clomipramine. This was one of the first antidepressants found to be a potent 5HT reuptake inhibitor. Some clinicians believed that the drug was more effective than other antidepressants, but little evidence exists to support this anecdotal view. However, the effects on 5HT may explain the benefit of this drug in the management of obsessive-compulsive disorder.

Data from a fatal toxicity index (Buckley and McManus, 2002) show clomipramine to have a lower than expected toxicity index. It is unlikely that clomipramine is inherently less toxic than other antidepressants, so this finding could be accounted for by other factors, such as the relatively high rate of prescribing in non-depressive states.

Dosulepin. Guidelines for the management of depression (NICE, 2009) advise that dosulepin should not be prescribed because of the risks associated with cardiac problems and toxicity in overdose compared to other available treatments.

Doxepin. Doxepin has similar effects and side effects to the traditional tricyclics. Limited evidence suggests that it may have fewer cardiac effects in patients with pre-existing cardiac disease than other traditional tricyclics. However, direct comparisons do not exist and a newer, alternative agent should be considered in preference to doxepin in patients with cardiac disease.

Lofepramine. Although desipramine is a metabolite of lofepramine, the latter should not be considered purely as a pro-drug. Important differences exist between lofepramine and the other traditional tricyclics. Antimuscarinic effects do occur with lofepramine, but these are less severe than with other tricyclics. In addition, despite being metabolised to desipramine, lofepramine is significantly safer in overdose than the traditional agents. This may be due to lofepramine antagonising the cardiac effects of desipramine. Lofepramine does not have a significant sedative effect, which may be an advantage in some patients, but in others the lack of sedation may be seen as a disadvantage. Some patients may complain of an alerting effect from lofepramine, particularly if the majority of the dose is given at bedtime. Despite a few reports of hepatic problems, given the favourable side effect profile and low toxicity in overdose, lofepramine may be considered as a reasonable option if an SSRI is ineffective or not tolerated.

Nortriptyline. Nortriptyline is the major metabolite of amitriptyline, but appears to have little effect on blood pressure. Nortriptyline shares many of the properties of the traditional tricyclic antidepressants.

Trimipramine. This is a particularly sedative tricyclic antidepressant with few differences from the rest of the traditional tricyclics.

Monoamine oxidase inhibitors. Two types of MAOI are available: the traditional MAOIs, which are both non-selective and irreversible, and moclobemide, which is a selective reversible inhibitor of monoamine oxidase type A (RIMA). In clinical practice, the traditional MAOIs are not widely prescribed. If patients are able to tolerate adequate doses, they are effective antidepressants, particularly in patients with atypical symptoms of depression. Due to the potential for drug and food interactions, MAOIs should be reserved for use in situations where a first-line SSRI antidepressant has failed. The potential for MAOIs to interact with other drugs and tyramine-containing foods has been well known since the 1960s. It is important that patients are made aware of the dietary restrictions and potential for serious drug interactions. These can be found in standard texts such as the British National Formulary.

Although the inhibitory effect of these drugs on monoamine oxidase is well understood, as with other antidepressants it is still not clear exactly how the MAOIs exert their antidepressant effect. MAOIs inhibit the enzymes responsible for the oxidation of noradrenaline (norepinephrine), 5HT and other biogenic amines. Two forms of monoamine oxidase have been found to exist, MAO-A and MAO-B. The traditional MAOIs are all non-selective and inhibit both forms of the enzyme.

Inhibition of MAO-A is thought to be responsible for the antidepressant effects. It is also responsible for metabolising tyramine and producing the cheese interaction. Moclobemide is an antidepressant that acts as a reversible inhibitor of MAO-A. As tyramine is metabolised by both forms of the enzyme, if tyramine-containing foods are consumed, tyramine is metabolised by MAO-B enzymes as well as being able to reverse the inhibition of MAO-A. Unless very large quantities of tyramine are ingested, this appears to prevent the typical hypertensive reaction seen with conventional MAOIs and tyramine-containing foods.

Traditional MAOIs. The traditional MAOIs and moclobemide have little anticholinergic effect. Nevertheless, some patients do experience dry mouth, constipation and urinary retention. In contrast to the hypertension which follows the interaction of tyramine-rich foods with the traditional MAOIs, these drugs are liable to cause postural hypotension as a side effect. This side effect may be particularly problematic with phenelzine and may prevent adequate dosages being achieved.

Tranylcypromine. Tranylcypromine has a structure that closely resembles amfetamine. It has a significant stimulant effect, and because of this could be more likely to give rise to problems around dependence. Unlike the other MAOIs, it does not irreversibly inhibit monoamine oxidase, which is said to recover some 5 days after withdrawal of the drug. Even so, the precautions associated with the MAOIs must still be continued for 2 weeks after discontinuing the drug. Due to the amfetamine-like alerting effect of tranylcypromine, the last dose should not be given after about 3 p.m. The risk of severe interaction is also said to be greater with tranylcypromine than with other MAOIs.

Phenelzine. Phenelzine has a hydrazine structure and because hydrazines have been associated with hepatocellular jaundice, it is recommended that phenelzine should be avoided in patients with hepatic impairment or abnormal liver function tests.

Reversible inhibitors of monoamine oxidase. Although moclobemide is an effective antidepressant, with less propensity for interactions with tyramine-rich foods, caution should

still be exercised as other drug interactions do occur. It could be considered, after a suitable wash-out period, as an option if a first- or second-line SSRI is ineffective.

Selective serotonin reuptake inhibitors. These agents were developed in an attempt to reduce some of the problems associated with the tricyclic antidepressants. Overall, the SSRIs are better tolerated by most patients and coupled with the fact that they are considerably less toxic in overdose; this means that they should be the first-line choice for the pharmacological management of moderate or severe depression (NICE, 2009). As generic versions of the drugs are available, the financial impact of using SSRIs first line has reduced in recent years. The SSRIs have a broadly similar range of side effects, but there are variations in the intensity or duration. The degree of specificity for serotonin reuptake differs between the SSRIs, but this does not correlate with clinical efficacy. If given in adequate doses for an adequate period of time, all the drugs in this class appear to be equally effective.

They do not appear to be significantly more or less effective than traditional tricyclics. They are, however, better tolerated than tricyclics and importantly much less toxic if taken in overdose. There are differences between SSRI's effect on the cytochrome P450 isoenzyme system. This may also be an important factor to consider when individualising treatment.

Fluvoxamine. Although patients experience few antimuscarinic side effects, other problems related to serotonergic enhancement such as nausea, headache and nervousness have been reported.

Fluoxetine. The main difference between fluoxetine and the other SSRIs is the long half-lives of both the parent drug and its primary active metabolite, desmethylfluoxetine. In the initial stages of treatment, some patients may experience a greater feeling of nervousness with fluoxetine than with the other SSRIs, but in most cases tolerance to this develops. The long half-life of fluoxetine and its major metabolite is a problem if severe side effects develop. In other situations, the long half-life means that the risks of discontinuation syndrome is reduced. Formulations of fluoxetine that can be taken on a weekly basis are available in some parts of the world.

Paroxetine. Although all the SSRIs have been reported to cause extrapyramidal-type movements, paroxetine appears to be more commonly implicated. The problem may be particularly severe following abrupt discontinuation of high doses.

Sertraline. Like the other SSRIs, sertraline is an effective antidepressant. Although doses of up to 200 mg have been used, doses of 150 mg and above should not be given for longer than 8 weeks.

Citalopram. The efficacy and side effect profile of citalopram appear similar to the other agents but, like sertraline, the reduced propensity for interactions with drugs metabolised by the cytochrome P450 2D6 isoenzyme may be an advantage in some cases.

Escitalopram. Escitalopram is thought to be the active *S* enantiomer of citalopram, which is a racemic mixture of *R*- and *S*-citalopram. The use of escitalopram has been advocated on the basis that the *R* enantiomer has no antidepressant effect, and may even counteract some of the antidepressant effects of the *S* enantiomer of escitalopram.

Lithium. Lithium does have antidepressant properties but will be discussed in more detail in the antimanic section.

Other drugs

Trazodone. *In vitro*, trazodone appears to operate as a mixed serotonin agonist/antagonist, but clinically it is thought to operate as a serotonin agonist. Trazodone is much safer than the tricyclics following overdose but causes pronounced sedative and hypotensive effects in some patients. Priapism has also been noted as a rare but distressing side effect. This is probably due to its potent α-receptor blocking properties.

Mianserin. Mianserin was one of the first antidepressants to demonstrate an improved toxicity profile following overdose. Like many of the newer drugs, it has fewer antimuscarinic side effects than the traditional tricyclics. One drawback in using mianserin is the need for monthly blood counts during the first 3 months of treatment, due to a high reported incidence of blood dyscrasias, particularly in the elderly. Mianserin is no longer widely prescribed in the UK.

Venlafaxine. Venlafaxine was reported to be the first in a new class of antidepressants, the serotonin-noradrenaline reuptake inhibitors (SNRIs). These antidepressants were developed in an attempt to improve efficacy over the standard agents. As the name suggests, they prevent the reuptake of both serotonin and noradrenaline (norepinephrine), a mechanism they have in common with the tricyclic antidepressants. It was hoped this would result in a drug with similar efficacy to the tricyclics in more severe cases but without the antimuscarinic, cardiac or toxic effects of the older drugs. Guidelines for depression (NICE, 2009) highlight the relative poor tolerability and increased risks of toxicity compared to the SSRIs. In view of this, venlafaxine is not recommended as a first-line treatment for patients with moderate or severe depression.

Duloxetine. Like venlafaxine, duloxetine is an SNRI. It weakly inhibits dopamine reuptake and may be less well tolerated than SSRIs. Given the relative benefit/tolerability profile, the drug is considered to be a second-line treatment option.

Reboxetine. Reboxetine is a specific noradrenergic (norepinephrinergic) reuptake inhibitor (NARI). Response rates appear similar to other antidepressants. This casts further doubt on the existence of particular subtypes of depression likely to respond to particular antidepressants. Patients experiencing problems with serotonergic-related side effects may benefit from a switch to reboxetine.

Mirtazapine. Mirtazapine is a noradrenergic and specific serotonergic antidepressant (NaSSA). It enhances both noradrenergic (norepinephrinergic) and $5HT_1$ serotonergic transmission. Specific $5HT_1$ neurotransmission is achieved as the drug also acts as a $5HT_2$ and $5HT_3$ antagonist. The receptor-specific effects of mirtazapine may explain some reduction in sexual dysfunction and nausea compared to other SSRIs. Despite this novel pharmacology, mirtazapine appears little different from other antidepressants in terms of efficacy.

Agomelatine. Agomelatine is structurally related to melatonin, it gained regulatory approval for use as an antidepressant in Europe in 2009. It is thought to act as an agonist at melatonin MT_1 and MT_2 and antagonist at $5HT_{2c}$ (Kasper and Hamon, 2009). In contrast to other antidepressants, it has no effect on monoamine uptake systems. Liver function tests are required prior to commencement and at intervals during treatment as rare cases of hepatic dysfunction have been reported. As yet there is insufficient evidence to comment on the place of this drug in the management of depression, but its relatively high cost may limit its use within the UK.

Choice of antidepressant. Whilst it has been suggested (Cipriani et al., 2009) that sertraline and escitalopram should be considered first-choice antidepressants for the majority of patients, it is unclear whether this will be translated into routine practice. The severity of the disorder, patient preference and previous experience should also play a part as they are also likely to affect outcome. In some areas, cost has become a critical factor in choice. For most people with moderate-to-severe depression, unless otherwise contraindicated, the use of a generic SSRI as the first-line choice is appropriate. Previous response, tolerance and the likelihood of drug interactions should also be considered.

In clinical practice, the identification of patients at high risk of suicide is difficult, and all patients with severe depression should be considered at risk of self-harm. The quantities of medication supplied to these patients should be carefully monitored.

Other treatments

Non-drug treatments. In addition to drug treatment, it is important to consider the patient's wider social, cultural and environmental circumstances. Although most patients with moderate to severe symptoms of depression will be offered pharmacological treatment, all patients and their close family should be offered help and support to cope with depression. Specific non-pharmacological interventions such as cognitive behaviour therapy (CBT) can be as effective as drug treatments. For people with more severe symptoms of depression, a combination of antidepressants and CBT is recommended. For mild-to-moderate forms of depression or persistent subthreshold symptoms, then non-drug strategies based on the principals of CBT should be considered as the first-line treatment (NICE, 2009).

The basis of CBT was developed over 50 years ago and subsequently refined into a specific therapy in the 1970s. This type of treatment helps patients to address their unhelpful thoughts and actions associated with depression. Over a series of up to 20 sessions the CBT therapist works with the patient either alone or in groups, to replace negative or self-critical thoughts and actions with more positive and helpful ones. CBT is not a 'quick fix' solution to depression, patients are often given 'homework' between sessions to try and put their positive actions into place. Interpersonal psychotherapy (IPT) is another form of psychotherapy which may help patients overcome symptoms of depression. This type of therapy aims to improve the patient's social functioning by linking their mood with interpersonal contacts so that their depressive mood and relationships can simultaneously improve.

Electroconvulsive therapy. Electroconvulsive therapy (ECT) would only be considered after referral to a psychiatrist. Although it is said to have a faster onset of action, its effects are fairly short-lived and antidepressants are normally required to prevent relapse. Although the treatment itself is considered safe, there are risks from the anaesthetic agent, and some patients suffer short-term memory loss following treatment.

St John's wort (*Hypericum perforatum*). Extracts of hypericum have been shown to be as effective as standard antidepressants in the management of major depression (Linde et al., 2008). In England and Wales, prescribers are advised against prescribing hypericum because of uncertainty about appropriate doses and persistence of effect. Problems can also be caused due to the variation in the nature of preparations available and the potential for serious interactions with other drugs.

Treatment of mania

Valproate semisodium (divalproate) is licensed in the UK as a specific treatment for mania associated with bipolar disorder. Other antipsychotics, including lithium and benzodiazepines, may also have a role in the management of mania. There appears to be insufficient evidence to differentiate between the various antipsychotics licensed for use in the acute management of mania and as a consequence the side effect profile, tolerability, previous experience and patient preference should all be considered when selecting the agent to use. Short-term adjunctive treatment with a benzodiazepine may be also be required.

Lithium may be used as an antimanic agent but it takes longer than other agents to produce its full effect and few would consider lithium as their agent of choice for acute antimanic treatment. However, it remains a drug of choice for long-term use to prevent recurrence or relapse. Valproate, certain antipsychotics, carbamazepine and lamotrigine (off-label use) may also be considered for this indication. In the future, further evidence or new technologies may emerge that permit better individualisation of treatment.

When used prophylactically the antimanic agents are commonly referred to as mood stabilisers.

If an episode of mania occurs in patients taking antidepressants, the antidepressant should be withdrawn. If mania occurs in patients already taking an antimanic agent for prophylaxis, attention should be given to maximising the dose and, if necessary, adding a second agent.

Valproate semisodium

This is a 1:1 molar combination of sodium valproate and valproic acid. Following administration, valproate ion is released and subsequently absorbed. The therapeutic differences between sodium valproate and valproate semisodium have not been established. However, the latter is the only form of valproate licensed for the acute treatment of mania. The mechanism of action in mania is unclear but may be related to increased levels of GABA. The antimanic effects of valproate are seen within 3 days, but the full benefit of treatment may not be apparent for up to 3 weeks. Dose should be rapidly titrated to between 1000 and 2000 mg per day. Routine valproate serum levels are not necessary, but levels between 50 and 100 mg/L have been reported to be associated

with optimal response in some patients. Although the risks of liver damage are greater in young children, liver function tests should be performed prior to initiation of therapy and periodically thereafter in all patients. In addition, the patient must be instructed to report any problems, such as unexplained bruising, that may indicate abnormalities in coagulation. Although valproate is well established as a prophylactic treatment to prevent relapse, this is an off-label use and should not be used in patients likely to become pregnant because of its teratogenic potential.

Antipsychotics

All the antipsychotics share a common effect of blocking dopamine D_2 postsynaptic receptors to some degree. Most of the newer antipsychotics, for example olanzapine, risperidone, quetiapine and aripiprazole, are licensed for use in the management of acute mania and prevention of new manic episodes.

Concerns about the side effect profiles of antipsychotic drugs often limit use, but in reality individual patients vary in their concern for and susceptibility to different side effects. Therefore, it is important that treatment choices are individualised and patients monitored regularly for side effects. Haloperidol, in an appropriate dose, is still commonly prescribed as part of the acute management of mania. It is less sedating than other antipsychotics which means it may occasionally be necessary to control severe behaviour disturbances with additional sedatives such as lorazepam, either orally or by injection. When a single agent is not considered to be effective, consideration should be given to augmenting the antipsychotic with valproate. Dose and duration of treatment are important considerations when treating acute mania. The dose of antipsychotic should be reviewed as the patient improves and where necessary consideration given to switching to an alternative prophylactic agent or continuing treatment to prevent relapse.

Lithium

Although lithium is effective in the acute management of mania, other treatments are generally preferred. This is due to the delay in response and variability of physical exertion and fluid intake which may compromise the safe use of lithium. In the acute situation, lithium may take up to 10–14 days to exert an effect. Dose is adjusted to achieve a target serum lithium concentration of 0.8–1 mmol/L for the management of acute episodes of mania, and for patients who have previously or have subsyndromal symptoms.

Antipsychotics or valproate semisodium, either alone or in combination, along with benzodiazepines should be considered the first-line treatment in the acute phase of mania.

Following an acute episode, lithium is a well-established treatment that may be considered as a first-line option for prophylaxis (Baldessarini and Tondo, 2000). Continuation therapy with a prophylactic mood stabiliser should be considered in all bipolar patients who have had two or more acute episodes within 2–4 years. It may also be reasonable to consider prophylaxis in any patient following a severe manic episode. As treatment is long term, the cooperation of the patient is essential and so a thorough explanation of the risks and benefits of the treatment is vital.

Before lithium treatment is initiated, an assessment of the patient's physical state is essential. Thyroid, renal and cardiac function should all be within normal limits. It is, however, still possible to use lithium, with caution, in patients with mild-to-moderate renal failure or cardiovascular impairment. Any thyroid deficiency should be corrected before lithium treatment is commenced. Patients should be informed of the need for monitoring and cautioned about the consequences of dehydration and risks of drug interactions.

Serum levels. There is a narrow therapeutic window for lithium serum levels and variation in the reference ranges reported. Some of this variation can be accounted for by variation in dose schedules. In the main, 12-h (post-dose) levels above 1.2 mmol/L are considered to be toxic and levels below 0.4 mmol/L are not considered to be effective. In adults, if lithium serum levels are kept in the range 0.4–0.8 mmol/L, then lithium is usually well tolerated with minimal side effects. Levels at or above 0.7 mmol/L are reported as being more effective than lower doses.

For most patients the range of 0.4–0.8 mmol/L is appropriate for prophylaxis, but if lithium is used to control the acute phase, levels may need to be around 1.0 mmol/L. To accurately interpret lithium levels, it is important that the correct schedule is followed and to establish consistent results, the 12-h standard serum lithium protocol has been devised. This means that lithium levels should be taken in the morning as near as possible to 12 h after the last dose of lithium.

As the absorption and bioavailability of lithium may vary from brand to brand, it is important that patients do not inadvertently change brands or dosage forms without levels being checked. Lithium not only has a narrow therapeutic range but is particularly toxic in overdose. Common side effects reported by patients are gastro-intestinal disturbances, tremor, thirst, polyuria, weight gain and lethargy. In addition to complaints of side effects, some patients prefer to remain untreated as they feel lithium 'damps down' their creativity and they miss the slight 'highs' that occur as part of their illness.

Patients taking a prophylactic mood stabiliser may occasionally stop taking their medication when they feel they no longer need it, or want to see if they can overcome the disorder without the need for drugs. Patients commonly have several trials on a mood stabiliser before they accept that the balance of risks and benefits is usually in favour of longer term treatment. There is a significant risk of relapse if lithium is discontinued abruptly.

Other anticonvulsants

Carbamazepine is generally considered as a second-line prophylactic treatment, when first-line therapy is either not tolerated or is ineffective. Emerging evidence continues to support the use of lamotrigine as an alternative in patients with bipolar depression (Geddes et al., 2009).

Treatment combinations

In patients who cannot be controlled on a single mood stabiliser, consideration should be given to combining treatments. Although not entirely without risks, all the above drugs have been used in various combinations in resistant cases.

Patient care

In the acute phase of an affective disorder, a patient will have little or no insight into his or her condition. This often makes it difficult to prescribe medication following an informed discussion on the risks and benefits of treatment. Depressed patients may say they are not worth treating; most manic patients will find it impossible to engage in meaningful dialogue, or they may insist they do not need medication and consistently refuse treatment. Thus, in the initial stages of treatment, some patients are treated against their will. As patients respond to treatment, it is crucial that the benefits and risks of treatment are explained. This may need to be repeated and backed up by written information. Engaging the patient and including them in the choice of treatment not only supports their basic human rights but is also likely to lead to a better therapeutic outcome. The discussion should also allow the patient to record their preference for future treatment. This may include drug regimens they would prefer to receive should they relapse as well as medication they would find objectionable.

During the acute phase of their illness, patients may often forget what they have been told about their medication. It is, therefore, important to regularly offer information or reassurance about medication, even if the patient is reported to have fully discussed the actions and effects with a health care professional.

Many patients are frightened by the notion of taking medication that will affect their mind. Taking an antidepressant is often felt to be a sign of failure or weakness by the patient as well as their family and friends. This often leads people to try and deal with their depression without medication. This is fine for the milder forms of the disorder and is sometimes referred to as 'watchful waiting'. In more severe cases, such an approach could have life-threatening consequences for the patient.

Patients should always be offered the opportunity of discussing their medication. The use of patient information leaflets and the involvement of the family or close friends may help patients understand the risks and benefits of their treatment. Many of the drugs used in the treatment of affective disorders have the potential to interact with other drugs that have been prescribed or purchased. Some of these are summarised in Table 29.1.

Common therapeutic problems in the management of affective disorder are outlined in Table 29.2.

Table 29.1 Examples of important drug interactions with drugs used in the management of affective disorders

Antidepressant	Interacting drug	Effect
Tricyclics	Adrenaline (epinephrine) and other directly acting sympathomimetics	Greatly enhances effect. Dangerous acting sympathomimetics
	Alcohol	Enhanced sedation
	Antiarrhythmics	Risk of ventricular arrhythmias
	Anticonvulsants	Lowered seizure threshold and possible lowered tricyclic levels
	MAOIs	Severe hypertension
	Fluoxetine	Increased tricyclic serum levels
SSRIs	Anticoagulants	Enhanced effects
	MAOIs	Dangerous
	Lithium	Possible serotonin syndrome
MAOIs	Alcohol, fermented beverages, tyramine-rich foods	Hypertensive crisis
	Antihypertensives	Increased effect
	Anticonvulsants	Lowered seizure threshold
	Levodopa	Hypertensive crisis
	Sympathomimetics	Hypertensive crisis
Antipsychotics	Anaesthetic agents	Hypotension
	Anticonvulsants	Lowered seizure threshold
	Antiarrhythmics	Risk of ventricular arrhythmias
	Astemizole and terfenadine	Risk of ventricular arrhythmias
Lithium	Non-steroidal anti-inflammatory drugs (NSAIDs)	Enhanced lithium serum levels
	SSRIs	Possible serotonin syndrome
	Diuretics	Enhanced lithium serum levels particularly with thiazides
	Angiotensin-converting enzyme (ACE) inhibitors	Enhanced lithium serum levels
	Sumatriptan	Possible central nervous system toxicity
St John's wort	Induces cytochrome P450 enzymes, particularly 1A2, 2C9 and 3A4	
	Indinavir	Reduced serum concentration (avoid)
	Warfarin	Reduced anticoagulant effect (avoid)
	SSRIs	Increased serotonergic effect (avoid)
	Carbamazepine (and other anticonvulsants)	Reduced serum concentrations (avoid)
	Digoxin	Reduced serum concentration (avoid)
	Oestrogens and progestogens	Reduced contraceptive effect (avoid)
	Theophylline	Reduced serum concentration (avoid)
	Ciclosporin	Reduced serum concentration (avoid)

Table 29.2 Common therapeutic problems in the management of affective disorder

Problem	Possible solution
Antidepressants	
Treatment failure (30–40% of patients will not respond to first antidepressant)	Ensure adequate dose and duration of treatment
	Check adherence, engage the patient, develop therapeutic alliance
	Reassess response against target symptoms
Risk of self-harm	Reconfirm diagnosis and identify compounding factors, for example, high levels of alcohol consumption in unsupervised situations
Withdrawal reactions	Ensure gradual withdrawal
Relapse on discontinuation	Consider long-term treatment
Intolerance	Consider changing to a different class
Antimanic agents	
Treatment failure	Ensure adequate dose, check serum levels and adherence; consider drug combinations
Toxicity adverse effects	Determine dose by clinical response, guided by serum levels
	Ensure patient is well informed and able to recognise impending toxicity and adverse effects of treatment
Weight gain	Dietary advice; consider alternative pharmacotherapy
Lithium levels	Ensure serum levels are 12 h post-dose, taken in the morning. Regular monitoring is important

Case studies

Case 29.1

Ms PS is a 17-year-old woman who presented to her primary care doctor with a 2-month history of difficulty in getting to sleep. She described herself as feeling generally unhappy. She had lost interest in socialising but was able to perform most of her usual daily routines. She sometimes felt as though she had little energy and was spending more time just watching the television.

Question

What diagnosis is likely to be given to Ms PS and what are the important factors to take into account when advising on treatment?

Answer

On further questioning by her primary care doctor, Ms PS does not reveal any ideas of self-harm. She is in a supportive relationship and, although she has some financial concerns, these are not excessive. It is likely that her depression is sub-threshold or of mild severity. Referral to specialist services is not appropriate. The patient should be given advice on sleep hygiene, including the removal of the television from her bedroom. A watching brief should be maintained and the patient asked to attend for a follow-up appointment within 2 weeks.

Antidepressants should not be prescribed. The risk/benefit balance is generally against prescribing antidepressants in people under 18 years of age. There is also little evidence to support the use of antidepressants in this case. More appropriate treatment options to consider would be a structured group exercise programme, guided self-help based on the principles of cognitive behavioural therapy or computerised cognitive behavioural therapy. The specific intervention should be guided by Ms PS's preferences.

Case 29.2

Mr DD is a 50-year-old unemployed man with a long-standing history of bipolar I disorder. He was admitted, as a voluntary patient, to an acute psychiatric ward by his community psychiatric nurse (CPN). The admission followed a short period of increasingly disturbed behaviour. Mr DD's daughter had contacted the CPN when she discovered that her father had just spent over £5000 on scientific instruments from an Internet auction site. Over the same period she had noticed that her father had lost interest in his self-care and become elated at the prospect of being on the verge of developing a special formula to solve the fuel crisis. On the ward Mr DD said he felt 'fine, fine all the time'. He told staff on the ward that he didn't need to be in hospital and it was keeping him away from his top secret mission. He also told ward staff that they could not keep him on the ward and insisted he was within his rights to go home. Mr DD's speech was sometimes very rapid, and it was sometimes difficult to understand what he was saying. His records showed that on his last admission he had been treated with haloperidol.

Question

What treatment is appropriate for Mr DD?

Answer

Before initiating treatment it is important to rule out any organic or physical causes for Mr DD's presentation. Following a thorough physical and psychiatric examination, it was established that Mr DD had been relatively well since commencing treatment with lithium almost 4 years previously.

It is important that symptoms of mania are brought under control. Haloperidol would be a suitable choice, in view of his previous response. However, a review of Mr DD's medication history revealed that he had experienced several acute dystonic reactions to haloperidol during previous admissions. His daughter also reported that her father had commented on how awful it felt being given haloperidol during his last admission. Mr DD was, therefore, given the option to discuss alternative antipsychotic treatment. He agreed to take olanzapine which was prescribed at a dose of 15 mg daily.

When Mr DD's manic symptoms are controlled, prophylactic treatment should be discussed with him. This should include a discussion about why he had discontinued lithium several months earlier. The opportunity should be taken to provide written information with the offer of a further discussion that should include his daughter.

Mr DD had stopped lithium as he felt he no longer needed it but after discussion was prepared to restart treatment. Renal, thyroid and cardiac function should be assessed, and if within normal limits, lithium carbonate 400 mg at night may be prescribed.

One week later a 12-h standard serum lithium level should be performed and the dose of lithium adjusted to achieve the same lithium levels as before (0.6 mmol/L).

The side effects and signs of impending toxicity from lithium should be explained to Mr DD and if possible his daughter. They should be given written information about the side effects, potential interactions, signs of toxicity and provided with a booklet to enable them to record the results of regular investigation. The arrangements for future prescribing and monitoring of lithium should be clarified so that Mr DD's care is not compromised by moving across organisational boundaries.

Case 29.3

Mrs FA is a 40-year-old designer. She was admitted to an acute psychiatric unit from the emergency department of the local hospital. She had taken an overdose of 32 co-codamol tablets when her husband told her he was going to leave her. On the ward she told staff she hated her life, and that everything was going wrong. She was angry that she had not been successful in killing herself as there was no point in living. She could see no hope for the future and had no interest in anything, not even eating.

Question

What course of action would you advise?

Answer

Mrs FA has a severe episode of depression. Antidepressant drug treatment should be initiated immediately. In line with guidelines for the management of depression, one of the SSRIs, for example, citalopram, should be considered as a suitable choice. Although Mrs FA may be reluctant to take medication, it should be explained that the drug does relieve the symptoms of depression. As soon as practical, the explanation should be followed up by discussing the importance of taking treatment for 4–6 weeks before the full benefit is realised and the likely time course of antidepressant treatment being in the region of 6 months. Mrs FA should also be given the opportunity to discuss any concerns she may have about becoming dependent on the antidepressant as well as a general explanation about possible side effects.

Case 29.4

Mr MA is a 49-year-old unemployed man. He was admitted to a psychiatric unit at the request of the crisis intervention team. Mr MA had been prescribed fluoxetine 20 mg 2 months ago, and after no apparent response the prescriber in the crisis team had changed this to citalopram 4 weeks earlier. On admission he was noted to be withdrawn, lacking motivation and just gave 'yes' or 'no' in response to questioning. He reported no interests in his life, and it was noted that he had attempted to harm himself in the past. Two weeks after admission there was no significant improvement in his symptoms.

Question

What treatment options are appropriate for Mr MA?

Answer

Before considering a change in treatment, it should be confirmed that Mr MA has regularly taken his antidepressant medication. Serum levels are not generally available, or particularly helpful. Scrutiny of the medicine charts, discussion with nursing staff, relatives, key workers and the patient will enable a reasonable judgement to be reached. A dose increase could be considered if the patient had shown a limited response. In this case, the patient had received no apparent benefit and a change in treatment was warranted.

An in-depth review of his physical condition and previous medication should be undertaken. This should include discussion with the patient about any previous antidepressant treatment he had found to be particularly effective, or troublesome.

This review revealed that Mr MA had received several different antidepressants over the past 20 years. Three years ago he was treated with venlafaxine S/R 75 mg twice daily. The medical records confirmed Mr MA's view that this medication had helped him in the past, but on further questioning he stated that he had not taken medication for long after discharge from hospital as he did not want to get 'hooked' on it.

The importance of long-term treatment and the proposed treatment plan should be discussed with Mr MA. Particular issues to be addressed include an assessment of physical functioning including base line blood pressure and the need for ongoing periodic monitoring. In view of Mr MA's concerns about dependence, particular attention should be given to discussion around this issue. Based on Mr MA's agreement to the treatment plan, his previous response, the lack of any physical contraindication and the ability to organise ongoing, periodic blood pressure monitoring would be a reasonable treatment option.

Case 29.5

Ms YS is a 28-year-old student with a history of bipolar I disorder. She had recently moved to the area in the hope of continuing her studies. She was admitted to an acute psychiatric unit at the request of her key worker who reported that Ms YS had recently become increasingly elated and her partner was very concerned about the increased credit card bills she was incurring.

Whilst on the ward she attempted to develop sexual relationships with several young male patients.

Question

Describe the treatment options available for Ms YS.

Answer

There is insufficient information to determine whether or not Ms YS was being treated adequately with a prophylactic mood stabiliser. It is important to determine if the current episode was related to inadequate prophylactic treatment.

The current episode of hypomania must be treated. She is currently at risk through her promiscuity and the excessive use of her credit card. Both behaviours are likely to affect her ability to maintain a relationship with her partner.

As Ms YS was taking adequate contraceptive precautions and was adamant that she had no intention or desire to become pregnant, initially treatment with valproate semisodium should be considered. Olanzapine or another antipsychotic could also be considered, but Ms YS did not want to be treated with an antipsychotic. An assessment of liver function, prothrombin rate and full blood count should be performed prior to initiating therapy.

The patient should be informed of the important adverse effects of therapy. In particular, she should be advised to report any unexplained bruising and to avoid the use of salicylates. Treatment should be commenced at 250 mg three times daily and increased in accordance with response and tolerability. Benzodiazepines may also be considered as a short-term adjunct if additional sedation is required.

Following resolution of the acute episode, long-term prophylaxis must be considered. In this case, Ms YS had previously been treated with lithium, but had refused to continue as this had caused significant weight gain.

In view of the patient's refusal to consider lithium, prophylactic options include carbamazepine or valproate semisodium (valproate semisodium is not licensed for prophylactic use in the UK). Little hard evidence currently exists to guide the choice. It is important to take the patient's view into account. Even though valproate does not have a UK marketing authorisation for prophylaxis in bipolar disorder, on the basis of informed choice, prophylactic treatment with valproate was agreed with Ms YS.

Case 29.6

Ms AB is a 55-year-old unemployed lady with a long-standing history of depression. She has been treated with several antidepressants over the years and is currently under the care of the community mental health team.

The only treatment that appears to have had any effect on her depressive episodes has been dosulepin. She has taken several overdoses in the past and her psychiatrist is reluctant to prescribe this drug.

Question

What measures could be taken to enable Ms AB to be treated effectively?

Answer

Ms AB does not have treatment-resistant depression. She has been successfully treated with dosulepin in the past, but impulsively takes an overdose as a way of dealing with difficult circumstances even when she is not depressed.

Non-drug strategies by the mental health team should be directed at enabling Ms AB to find alternative ways of dealing with these difficulties.

In view of the obvious risk of fatality, alternative antidepressant treatment should be considered. Dosulepin could remain as an option for Ms AB due to her previous response to this drug and the lack of response to other antidepressants, but this would fall outside current guidance for the management of depression (NICE, 2009). Practical measures of controlling the quantities of medication should be introduced such as ensuring she only receives sufficient medication for 2 or 3 days treatment.

Communication between all those involved in the care of Ms AB is crucial. When individualizing the supply of medication in this way, all those involved must be alert to the possibility that the system of supply may break down. In this case, an apparently routine prescription for 1 month's supply of medication may have fatal consequences.

References

American Psychiatric Association, 2000. Diagnostic and Statistical Manual of Mental Disorders, fourth ed. Text Revision (DSM-IV-TR) American Psychiatric Publishing Inc., Washington, DC.

Baldessarini, R.J., Tondo, L., 2000. Does lithium treatment still work? Evidence of stable responses over three decades. Arch. Gen. Psychiatry 57, 187–908.

Barbui, C., Hotopf, M., Freemantle, N., et al., 2001. Selective serotonin re-uptake inhibitors versus tricyclic and heterocyclic antidepressants: comparison of drug adherence. Cochrane Review Cochrane Library, Issue 2. Update Software, Oxford.

Buckley, N.A., McManus, P.R., 2002. Fatal toxicity of serotoninergic and other antidepressant drugs: analysis of United Kingdom mortality data. Br. Med. J. 325, 1332–1333.

Cipriani, A., Furukawa, T.A., Salanti, G., et al., 2009. Comparative efficacy and acceptability of 12 new-generation antidepressants: a multiple-treatments meta-analysis. Lancet 373, 746–758.

Fournier, J., DeRubeis, R.J., Hollon, S., et al., 2010. Antidepressant drug effects and depression severity A patient-level meta-analysis. J. Am. Med. Assoc. 303, 47–53.

Geddes, J.R., Freemantle, N., Mason, J., et al., 2002. Selective serotonin reuptake inhibitors (SSRIs) for depression. Cochrane Review. Cochrane Library, Issue 1. Update Software, Oxford.

Geddes, J.R., Calabrese, J.R., Goodwin, G.M., 2009. Lamotrigine for treatment of bipolar depression: independent meta-analysis and meta-regression of individual patient data from five randomised trials. Br. J. Psychiatry 194, 4–9.

Kasper, S., Hamon, M., 2009. Beyond the monoaminergic hypothesis: agomelatine, a new antidepressant with an innovative mechanism of action. World J. Biol. Psychiatry 10, 117–126.

Linde, K., Berner, M.M., Kriston, L., 2008. St John's wort for major depression. Cochrane Database of Systematic Reviews. Issue 4, Art No. CD000448. doi:10.1002/14651858.CD000448.pub3.

National Institute for Clinical Excellence, 2006. Bipolar Disorder. The Management of Bipolar Disorder in Adults, Children and Adolescents in Primary and Secondary Care. Clinical Guideline 38. NICE, London. Available at: http://www.nice.org.uk/nicemedia/live/10990/30193/30193.pdf Accessed 13 April. 2011.

National Institute for Clinical Excellence, 2009. Depression. The Treatment and Management of Depression in Adults (Partial Update of NICE Clinical Guideline 23 on in Primary and secondary Care). Clinical Guideline 90. NICE, London. Available at: http://www.nice.org.uk/nicemedia/live/12329/45888/45888.pdf. Accessed 13 April 2011.

Nicholson, A., Kuper, H., Hemingway, H., 2006. Depression as an aetiologic and prognostic factor in coronary heart disease: a meta-analysis of 6362 events among 146 538 participants in 54 observational studies. Eur. Heart J. 27, 2763–2774.

World Health Organization, 1992. International Classification of Diseases and Related Health Problems, 10th Revision (ICD 10). World Health Organisation, Geneva.

Further reading

Cipriani, A., Santilli, C., Furukawa, T.A., et al., 2009. Escitalopram versus other antidepressive agents for depression. Cochrane Database of Systematic Reviews. Issue 2. Art. No.: CD006532. doi:10.1002/14651858.CD006532.pub2.

Geddes, J.R., Burgess, S., Hawton, K., et al., 2004. Long term lithium therapy for bipolar disorder: systematic review and meta-analysis of randomized controlled trials. Am. J. Psychiatry 161, 217–222.

Gelder, M., Andreasen, N., Lopez-Ibor, J., et al., 2009. Oxford Textbook of Psychiatry, second ed. Oxford University Press, Oxford.

Goodwin, G., 2009. Evidence-based guidelines for treating bipolar disorder: revised second edition–recommendations from the British Association for Psychopharmacology. J. Psychopharmacol. 23, 346–388.

Mann, J.J., 2005. The medical management of depression. N. Engl. J. Med. 353, 1819–1834.

Scottish Intercollegiate Guidelines Network, 2005. Bipolar Affective Disorder. SIGN, Edinburgh. Available at www.sign.ac.uk/pdf/sign82.pdf. Accessed 13 April 2011.

Shiloh, R., Stryjer, R., Weizman, A., et al., 2006. Atlas of Psychiatric Pharmacotherapy, second ed. Informa Healthcare, Abingdon.

Walden, J., Heinz, G. (Eds.), 2004. Bipolar Affective Disorders: Etiology and Treatment. Thieme Publishing Group, Stuttgart.

Schizophrenia 30

D. Branford

Key points

- Schizophrenia is a complex illness which varies greatly in presentation.
- Positive symptoms such as hallucinations, delusions and thought disorder, which commonly occur in the acute phase of the illness, usually respond to treatment with antipsychotic drugs.
- Negative symptoms such as apathy, social withdrawal and lack of drive, which occur commonly in the chronic phase of the illness, are more resistant to drug treatment.
- The term 'atypical' is used to describe the newer antipsychotic drugs that do not cause extrapyramidal side effects.
- The atypical antipsychotics are associated with a range of metabolic side effects including weight gain and diabetes.
- Typical antipsychotic drugs are often associated with anticholinergic, sedative and cardiovascular side effects in addition to extrapyramidal side effects.
- Long-term treatment with typical antipsychotic drugs is associated with the development of tardive dyskinesia.
- Most typical and atypical antipsychotic drugs have similar efficacy in the treatment of schizophrenia.
- Decisions about which antipsychotic drug to use should be a mutual decision based on an informed discussion involving individual preference, previous efficacy and side effects.
- Clozapine has a broader spectrum of activity than traditional antipsychotic drugs with some efficacy for treatment-resistant schizophrenia and negative symptoms.

The concept of schizophrenia can be difficult to understand. People who do not suffer from schizophrenia can have little idea of what the experience of hallucinations and delusions is like. The presentation of schizophrenia can be extremely varied, with a great range of possible symptoms. There are also many misconceptions about the condition of schizophrenia that have led to prejudice against sufferers of the illness. People with schizophrenia are commonly thought to have low intelligence and to be dangerous. In fact, only a minority shows violent behaviour, with social withdrawal being a more common picture. Up to 10% of people with schizophrenia commit suicide.

Classification

Since the late nineteenth century there have been frequent attempts to define the illness we now call schizophrenia. Kraepelin, in the late 1890s, coined the term 'dementia praecox' (early madness) to describe an illness where there was a deterioration of the personality at a young age. Kraepelin also coined the terms 'catatonic' (where motor symptoms are prevalent and changes in activity vary), 'hebephrenic' (silly, childish behaviour, affective symptoms and thought disorder prominence) and 'paranoid' (clinical picture dominated by paranoid delusions). A few years later Bleuler, a Swiss psychiatrist introduced the term 'schizophrenia', derived from the Greek words *skhizo* (to split) and *phren* (mind), meaning the split between the emotions and the intellect.

Two systems for the classification of schizophrenia are widely used: the *Diagnostic and Statistical Manual of Mental Disorders*, 4th edition (DSM IV; American Psychiatric Association, 1994) and the *International Classification of Diseases*, 10th edition (ICD 10; World Health Organization, 1992).

Symptoms and diagnosis

Acute psychotic illness

To establish a definite diagnosis of schizophrenia it is important to follow the diagnostic criteria in either DSM IV or ICD 10, but symptoms which commonly occur in the acute phase of a psychotic illness include the following:

- awkward social behaviour, appearing preoccupied, perplexed and withdrawn, or showing unexpected changes in behaviour
- initial vagueness in speech which can progress to disorders of the stream of thought or poverty of thought
- abnormality of mood such as anxiety, depression, irritability or euphoria
- auditory hallucinations, the most common of which are referred to as 'voices'; such voices can give commands to patients or may discuss the person in the third person, or comment on their actions
- delusions, of which those relating to control of thoughts are the most diagnostic; for example, patients feel that thoughts are being inserted into or withdrawn from their mind
- lack of insight into the illness.

These symptoms are commonly called positive symptoms.

Factors affecting diagnosis and prognosis

There is a reluctance to classify people as suffering schizophrenia on the basis of one acute psychotic illness, but there are a number of features which aid prediction of whether an acute illness will become chronic. These features include:

- age of onset, which, typically for schizophrenia, is late teenage to 30 years
- reports of a childhood which indicate the individual did not mix or was a rather shy and withdrawn personality
- a poor work record
- a desire for social isolation
- being single and not seeming to have sexual relationships
- a gradual onset of the illness and deterioration from the previous level of functioning
- grossly disorganised behaviour

Treatment

There is a wide range of antipsychotic drugs available for the treatment of a psychotic illness. Although most antipsychotic drugs are equally effective in the treatment of psychotic symptoms, some individuals respond better to one drug than another.

There is controversy over how long people should remain on an antipsychotic drug following their first acute illness. Some would argue that, if the prognosis is poor, long-term therapy should be advocated. Others would want to see a second illness before advocating long-term therapy.

Chronic schizophrenia

Between 60% and 80% of patients who suffer from an acute psychotic illness will suffer further illness and become chronically affected. For these patients the diagnosis of schizophrenia can be applied.

As schizophrenia progresses, there may be periods of relapse with acute symptoms but the underlying trend is towards symptoms of lack of drive, social withdrawal and emotional apathy. Such symptoms are sometimes called negative symptoms and respond poorly to most antipsychotic drugs.

Causes of schizophrenia

Although the cause of schizophrenia remains unknown, there are many theories and models.

Vulnerability model

The vulnerability model postulates that the persistent characteristic of schizophrenia is not the schizophrenic episode itself but the vulnerability to the development of such episodes of the disorder. The episodes of the illness are time limited but the vulnerability remains, awaiting the trigger of some stress. Such vulnerability can depend on premorbid personality, the individual's social network or the environment. Manipulation and avoidance of stress can abort a potential schizophrenic episode.

Developmental model

The developmental model postulates that there are critical periods in the development of neuronal cells which, if adversely affected, may result in schizophrenia. Two such critical periods are postulated to occur when migrant neural cells do not reach their goal in fetal development and when supernumerary neural cells slough off at adolescence. This model is supported by neuroimaging studies which show structural brain abnormalities in patients with schizophrenia.

Ecological model

The ecological model postulates that external factors involving social, cultural and physical forces in the environment, such as population density, individual space, socio-economic status and racial status, influence the development of the disorder. The evidence in support of such a model remains weak.

Genetic model

There is undoubtably a genetic component to schizophrenia, with a higher incidence in the siblings of schizophrenics. However, even in monozygotic twins there are many cases where only one sibling has developed schizophrenia.

Transmitter abnormality model

The suggestion that schizophrenia is caused primarily by an abnormality of dopamine receptors and, in particular, D_2 receptors, has largely emerged from research into the effect of antipsychotic drugs. Such a theory is increasingly being questioned.

Other factors

Numerous other factors have been implicated in the development and cause of schizophrenia. These include migration, socio-economic factors, perinatal insult, infections, season of birth, viruses, toxins and family environment.

In reality, all of these factors may influence both the development and progression of schizophrenia. Social, familial and biological factors may lead to premorbid vulnerability and subsequently influence both the acute psychosis and the progression to chronic states. What is then likely is that the illness will feed back to influence social, familial and biological factors, thus leading to future vulnerability.

Drug treatment

Mode of action of antipsychotic drugs

Although the cause of schizophrenia is the subject of controversy, an understanding of the mode of action of antipsychotic drugs has led to the dopamine theory of schizophrenia. This theory postulates that the symptoms experienced in schizophrenia are caused by an alteration to the level of dopamine activity in the brain. It is based on knowledge that dopamine receptor antagonists are often effective antipsychotics while drugs which increase dopamine activity, such as amfetamine, can either induce psychosis or exacerbate a schizophrenic illness.

At least six dopamine receptors exist in the brain, with much activity being focused on the D_2 receptor as being responsible for antipsychotic drug action. However, drugs such as pimozide, that claim to have a more specific effect on D_2 receptors, do not appear superior in antipsychotic effect when compared to other agents.

Research into the mode of action of clozapine has caused a change of attention to the mesolimbic system in the brain and to different receptors. Clozapine does not chronically alter striatal D_2 receptors but does appear to affect striatal D_1 receptors. It also appears to have more effect on the limbic system and on serotonin ($5HT_2$) receptors, which may explain its reduced risk of extrapyramidal symptoms. The term 'atypical' is used to categorise those antipsychotic drugs that, like clozapine, rarely produce extrapyramidal side effects (EPSEs).

Although the reason for the superiority of clozapine in schizophrenia treatment remains an enigma, a variety of theories have led to the development of a new family of antipsychotic drugs. Some mimic the impact of clozapine on a wide range of dopamine and serotonin receptors, for example, olanzapine, others mimic the impact on particular receptors, for example, $5HT_2/D_2$ receptor antagonists such as risperidone, others focus on limited occupancy of D_2 receptors, for example, quetiapine, while others focus on alternative theories such as partial agonism (aripiprazole).

Rationale for use of drugs

Although a variety of social and psychological therapies are helpful in the treatment of schizophrenia, drugs form the essential cornerstone. The aim of all therapies is to minimise the level of handicap and achieve the best level of mental functioning. Drugs do not cure schizophrenia and are only partially effective at eradicating some symptoms such as delusions and negative symptoms. At the same time, benefits have to be balanced against side effects and whether the need to suppress particular symptoms is important. For example, if the person has a delusion that he or she is responsible for famine in Africa, but this does not in any way influence that person's behaviour or mood, a common view would be that there would be little point in increasing antipsychotic drug therapy. However, others would argue that this 'untreated' delusion would make the person stand out or be subject to social stigma and the delusion should be more aggressively treated. If, on the other hand, this delusion led to great distress, or violent or dangerous behaviour, then an increase in antipsychotic drugs would usually be indicated.

It is now accepted that antipsychotic drugs can control or modify symptoms such as hallucinations and delusions that are evident in the acute episode of illness. Except for clozapine and the other atypicals, there is little evidence for antipsychotic drugs being of value in the treatment of the negative symptoms, although the matter remains controversial (Chakos et al., 2001). Antipsychotic drugs increase the length of time between breakdowns and shorten the length of the acute episode in most patients.

Drug selection and dose

Over the years there have been many changes to the range of antipsychotic drugs available. Despite the availability of newer agents many of the issues relevant to drug selection and dose have remained similar for the last 50 years and include:

Individual response

Drug selection should not be based on chemical group alone, since individual response to a particular drug or dose may be more important.

Side effects

For older, typical antipsychotic drugs, side effects such as hypotension, extrapyramidal symptoms and anticholinergic effects are key factors in the choice of drug. In contrast, with the newer atypical drugs, side effects such as diabetes, sexual dysfunction and weight gain affect adherence in many patients. Sedation remains a factor for all antipsychotic drugs.

The key side effects of concern are those categorised as EPSEs. Those that caused these side effects were called typical antipsychotic drugs and those that did not were called atypical. This classification system, however, has always remained subject to criticism as some atypicals will cause EPSEs when used at higher doses and the side effects of the different atypicals can vary considerably. EPSEs include:

Akathisia or motor restlessness. This causes patients to pace up and down, constantly shift their leg position or tap their feet.

Dystonia is the result of sustained muscle contraction. It can present as grimacing and facial distortion, neck twisting and laboured breathing. Occasionally the patient may have an oculogyric crisis in which, after a few moments of fixed staring, the eyeballs move upwards and then sideways, remaining in that position. In addition to these eye movements, the mouth is usually wide open, the tongue protruding and the head tilting backwards.

Parkinson-like side effects usually present as tremor, rigidity and poverty of facial expression. Drooling and excessive salivation are also common. A shuffling gait may be seen and the patient may show signs of fatigue when performing repetitive motor activities.

Another movement disorder more commonly associated with typical antipsychotics is tardive dyskinesia. Tardive dyskinesia normally affects the tongue, facial and neck muscles but can also affect the extremities. Individuals with tardive dyskinesia often have abnormalities of posture and movement of the fingers in addition to the oral-lingual-masticatory movements.

Epidemiological studies support the association between the prescribing of typical antipsychotic drugs and the development of tardive dyskinesia. Other factors which also appear to be associated include the duration of exposure to antipsychotic drugs, the co-prescribing of anticholinergic drugs, the co-prescribing of lithium, advanced age, prior experience of acute extrapyramidal symptoms and brain damage. Many other factors have been postulated to be associated with tardive dyskinesia such as depot formulations of antipsychotic drugs, dosage of antipsychotic drug and antipsychotic drugs with high anticholinergic activity, but such associations remain unproven.

Although the mechanism by which tardive dyskinesia arises is unclear, the leading hypothesis is that after prolonged blockade of dopamine receptors, there is a paradoxical increase in the functional activity of dopamine in the basal ganglia occurs. This increased functional state is thought to come about through a phenomenon_of disuse supersensitivity of dopamine receptors. The primary clinical evidence to support this theory arises because tardive dyskinesia is late in onset following prolonged exposure to antipsychotic drugs and has a tendency to worsen upon abrupt discontinuation of the antipsychotic drug.

Attempts to treat tardive dyskinesia have been many and varied. Treatments include use of dopamine-depleting agents such as reserpine and tetrabenazine, dopamine-blocking agents such as antipsychotic drugs, interference with catecholamine synthesis by drugs such as methyldopa, cholinergic agents such as choline and lecithin, use of GABA mimetic agents such as sodium valproate and baclofen, and the provision of drug holidays. Rarely are these strategies successful. Most successful strategies currently involve a gradual withdrawal of the typical antipsychotic drug and replacement with an atypical antipsychotic drug.

Concerns about the EPSEs and toxicity of typical antipsychotic drugs led to calls over the past 10 years for the 'atypicals' to be prescribed more widely. This approach was supported in national guidance which advocated that atypical antipsychotic drugs should be used for the treatment of a first illness. However, increasing concern about the side effects of the atypical antipsychotic drugs, which includes weight gain, diabetes and sexual dysfunction, has led many clinicians to question the benefits of the newer and more expensive atypical antipsychotics. In more recent guidance (National Institute for Health and Clinical Excellence, 2009), it has been advocated that:

- Oral antipsychotic medication should be offered to people with newly diagnosed schizophrenia.
- Information on the benefits and side effects of each antipsychotic agent should be provided and discussed with the patient.
- The decision as to which antipsychotic to use should be made in partnership with the patient and carer as appropriate.
- When deciding on the most suitable medication, the relative potential of the individual antipsychotics to cause EPSEs such as akathisia, metabolic side effects such as weight gain and other side effects including unpleasant subjective experiences should be considered.
- Combined antipsychotic medication should not be started, except for short periods (e.g. when changing medication).

Information on the advantages and disadvantages of the various antipsychotic drugs can be found in Table 30.1.

A significant factor that has influenced prescribing practice in schizophrenia in recent years has been an improved understanding of the role of clozapine in treatment-resistant schizophrenia.

Clozapine and refractory illness

Clozapine was developed as an antipsychotic drug during the 1960s. Unfortunately, use is associated with a 1–2% incidence of neutropenia and this initially resulted in the withdrawal of the drug from clinical practice. However, it was noted even at an early stage in the drug's history that it was free of the extrapyramidal side frequently seen with the other antipsychotic drugs. In the 1980s, clozapine was demonstrated to have a greater efficacy than other antipsychotics (Kane et al., 1988; Lieberman et al., 1994) and was subsequently reintroduced into clinical practice but with routine monitoring of blood mandatory.

Clozapine is now established as the drug of choice in treatment-resistant schizophrenia but it is not without problems (Tuunainen et al., 2000). In addition to neutropenia, it is associated with a greater risk of seizures, particularly if doses are above 600 mg daily. Some guidelines recommend the co-prescribing of sodium valproate to reduce this risk. In addition, use is associated with excessive drooling, hypotension and sedation during the early stages of treatment, requiring slow dose increases initially.

A regimen of gradual dose increases starting at 12.5 mg twice daily aiming to reach 300 mg in 2–3 weeks is normally recommended. However, this rate of dose increase is frequently too rapid, with tachycardia being a particular problem. In such cases, it is usual to slow down the rate of dose increase to a half or a quarter of that recommended. Although tachycardia is a common problem with clozapine initiation, if use is associated with fever, chest pain or hypotension this may indicate a high risk of myocarditis and the drug should be stopped (Committee on Safety of Medicines, 2002).

Polypharmacy

Polypharmacy remains a matter of concern in the management of individuals with schizophrenia. It usually arises because:

- There is a poor response to standard drug treatment.
- There are unrealistic expectations about the onset of action and the extent of treatment control.
- Prescribers feel inhibited about using high doses and resort to prescribing two or more antipsychotic drugs to achieve control, particularly in the acute situation. The consensus is that very high doses of antipsychotics do not improve the overall level of response (Royal College of Psychiatrists, 2006). Increasingly, though, prescribers are being encouraged to use clozapine at an earlier stage for patients who do not fully respond to treatment.

Table 30.1 Neuroleptics/antipsychotics and their commonly associated attributes and problems

Drug group	Drug	Comment
Butyrophenones	Haloperidol	Regarded as the gold standard reference antipsychotic Extrapyramidal side effects of parkinsonian rigidity, dystonia, akathisia Tardive dyskinesia with long-term use Drug most associated with neuroleptic malignant syndrome Sedation common Hormonal effects common Wide range of formulations including long-acting injection
	Benperidol	As haloperidol Claimed to reduce sexual drive, although little evidence to support the claim
Phenothiazines Piperidine	Pericyazine	Marked anticholinergic side effects of dry mouth, blurred vision and constipation Postural hypotension and falls in the elderly Lower incidence of extrapyramidal side effects
	Pipotiazine	As pericyazine but only available as depot formulation
Aliphatic	Chlorpromazine	As haloperidol but in addition postural hypotension, low body temperature, rashes and photosensitivity Increased sedative effects
	Promazine	As chlorpromazine but low potency Considered by some to have weak antipsychotic effect
	Levomepromazine (methotrimeprazine)	Very sedative and postural hypotension common Mostly used in terminal illness
Piperazine	Trifluoperazine	As chlorpromazine but greater incidence of extrapyramidal side effects and lower incidence of anticholinergic effects Tardive dyskinesia with long-term use Some antiemetic properties
	Fluphenazine	As trifluoperazine but also available as depot formulation
	Perphenazine	As trifluoperazine
Thioxanthines	Flupentixol	Similar to fluphenazine but also available as depot formulation
	Zuclopenthixol	Similar to chlorpromazine but also available as depot formulation
Diphenylbutylpiperidines	Pimozide	As haloperidol but concerns about cardiac effects at high dose limits use
Benzamides	Sulpiride	Lower incidence of extrapyramidal effects Few anticholinergic effects Useful adjunct to clozapine in refractory illness
	Amisulpride	As sulpiride
Dibenoxazepine tricyclics	Clozapine	Drug of choice for treatment-resistant schizophrenia Low incidence of extrapyramidal side effects or tardive dyskinesia Neutropenia in 1–2% of cases Enhanced efficacy against both positive and negative symptoms Sedation, dribbling, drooling, weight gain and diabetes
Thienobenzodiazepines	Olanzapine	Sedation, weight gain and diabetes Low incidence of extrapyramidal side effects and low impact on prolactin
	Quetiapine	Low incidence of extrapyramidal side effects and low impact on prolactin
	Zotepine	Similar to olanzapine but higher rate of prolactin elevation and higher rate of drug-induced seizures
Serotonin–dopamine antagonists	Risperidone	Extrapyramidal side effects at higher doses. High rate of prolactin elevation
	Paliperidone	As risperidone
	Ziprasidone	As risperidone
	Sertindole	Available on named patient basis only due to risk of sudden cardiac events
Partial dopamine agonist	Aripiprazole	Low level of side effects but light-headedness and blurred vision common

- Once control has been achieved there may be reluctance to reduce either dose or the number of drugs an individual is receiving for fear of re-emergence of symptoms.
- There is an imbalance between the perceived need in the hospital ward setting for sedation rather than an antipsychotic effect. The sedating side effects of antipsychotic drugs may be evident within hours; they are rapid in onset but may begin to wear off after 2–3 weeks. The antipsychotic effects on thought disorder, hallucinations and delusions may take some weeks to appear, although if there has been no response within 2–3 weeks a change of antipsychotic or change of dose may be indicated.

Neuroleptic equivalence

Although antipsychotic drugs vary in potency, studies on relative dopamine receptor binding have led to the concept of chlorpromazine equivalents as a useful method of transferring dosage from one product to another. Concern has been expressed about the variation between sources for such values, in particular about the quoted chlorpromazine equivalents of the butyrophenones and the conversion of depot doses to oral doses (Table 30.2). Likewise, there is no agreement on the equivalent doses of the atypicals.

For research purposes the concept of proportion of the maximum dose stated in the British National Formulary (BNF) has been developed as a standardised method for calculating average doses used in practice. However, this may not be a useful way of determining a dose when transferring a patient from one antipsychotic to another.

Table 30.2 Equivalence of typical antipsychotic drugs to 100 mg chlorpromazine (from Foster, 1989)

Drug	Usual dose (mg) equivalent of to 100 mg chlorpromazine	Variations in quoted dosage (mg) equivalent to 100 mg of chlorpromazine
Oral antipsychotics		
Promazine	200	100–250
Thioridazine	100	50–120
Trifluoperazine	5	3.5–7.5
Haloperidol	2	1.5–5
Sulpiride	200	–
Depot antipsychotics administered every 2 weeks (all administered as the decanoate)		
Zuclopenthixol	200	80–200
Flupentixol	40	16–40
Fluphenazine	25	10–25
Haloperidol	20	–

Augmentation strategies and polytherapy

Schizophrenia is a complex illness with a very varied presentation. In addition to the core symptoms, elements of other mental illnesses such as mania, depression and anxiety may predominate. Controversy remains about whether these associated symptoms should be treated separately or as a part of schizophrenia. In addition, there is debate about whether these presentations represent an alternative diagnosis, for example, schizoaffective disorder when the mood disorder is a primary component of the presentation. The current fashion is for these components of the illness to be treated separately, with much resulting polytherapy with SSRI antidepressants and antiepileptic drugs for mood control.

In addition to the above, complex prescriptions can arise when treatment with clozapine is perceived to be inadequate or doses are limited due to side effects. The theory behind the addition of a further drug can be either that the plasma concentration of the clozapine will be enhanced by the addition of another drug, or the second drug will enhance a particular receptor blockade which may be considered necessary in a specific patient (Cipriani et al., 2009; Paton et al., 2007). The augmentation strategy with the best evidence to support its use is the addition of sulpiride or amisulpride to clozapine. Other strategies include the addition of risperidone, lamotrigine or Ω3 fatty acids. However, many of the trials that support these augmentation strategies are small scale and a meta-analysis concluded that no single strategy was superior to another (Paton et al., 2007).

Long-acting formulations of antipsychotic drugs

Most long-acting (depot) formulations, including the long-acting olanzapine formulation, are synthesised by esterification of the hydroxyl group of the antipsychotic drug to a long chain fatty acid such as decanoic acid. The esters which are more lipophilic and soluble are dissolved in an oily vehicle such as sesame oil or a vegetable oil (viscoleo). Once the drug is injected into muscle it is slowly released from the oil vehicle. Active drug becomes available following hydrolysis for distribution to the site of the action. A long-acting injection of olanzapine has been marketed which contains a salt of olanzapine and pamoic acid suspended in an aqueous vehicle. This also is designed for intramuscular injection every 2–4 weeks.

Although the ideal long-acting antipsychotic formulation should release the drug at a constant rate so that plasma level fluctuations are kept to a minimum, all the available products produce significant variations (Table 30.3). This can result in increased side effects at the time of peak plasma concentrations, usually after 5–7 days, for oil-based depots and increased patient irritability towards the end of the period, as plasma concentrations decline. For many patients though, oil-based long-acting formulations result in a very slow decline in drug availability after a period of chronic administration (Altamura et al., 2003). When transferring a patient from depot formulations to oral administration, it may be many months before the effect of the depot finally wears off.

Table 30.3 Comparison of depot antipsychotics

Drug	Ester	Vehicle	Time to peak (days) from single dose	Half-life (days)
Haloperidol	Decanoate	Sesame oil	3–9	21
Flupentixol	Decanoate	Viscoleo oil	7	17
Zuclopenthixol	Decanoate	Viscoleo oil	4–7	19
Fluphenazine	Decanoate	Sesame oil	0.3–1.5	6–9
Pipotiazine	Palmitate	Sesame oil	10–15	15
Risperidone		Microspheres	32	8–9
Olanzapine	Pamoate	Aqueous	3	10
Paliperidone	Palmitate	Microspheres	13	25–49

Long-acting risperidone injection involves a microsphere formulation. The microspheres delay the release of risperidone for 3–4 weeks. Once release has commenced, the risperidone reaches a maximum concentration 4–5 weeks after the injection with a decline over the subsequent 2–3 weeks. This more rapid decline has an advantage that by 2 months after the last injection, little of the risperidone will remain. The delay in onset is often a reason for relapse as it is necessary to maintain oral supplementation for at least 6 weeks and this may be overlooked.

In addition to the principles of drug choice and dosage selection that apply to oral drugs, with depot therapy there is also a need to consider the future habitation of the patient. If the patient is to live an independent lifestyle, depot formulations are indicated, but if the person is to remain in staffed accommodation and receive other medicines routinely administered by a nurse, the use of depot formulations may not be logical.

Advantages and disadvantages of long-acting formulations

Non-adherence with oral medicines is a major problem in patients with any long-term illness and the administration of depot formulations guarantees drug delivery. It has been argued that, although depot injections are expensive, they have economic advantages because they reduce hospital admissions, improve drug bioavailability by avoiding the deactivating processes which occur in the gut and liver, and result in more consistent plasma levels of drug.

Depot formulations have the disadvantage of reduced flexibility of dosage, the painful nature of administration and, for the older depots, a high incidence of EPSEs. In addition, risperidone long-acting injection has the disadvantage of considerable delay in onset, whilst the olanzapine depot is associated with a post-injection syndrome consistent with olanzapine overdose. Although this side effect is relatively rare there is a requirement for patients to be observed for 3 hours following injection thereby limiting its acceptability.

Anticholinergic drugs

Anticholinergic drugs are prescribed to counter the EPSEs of typical antipsychotics, and at one time were routinely prescribed. It is generally accepted that, with the possible exception of the first few weeks of treatment with antipsychotic drugs known to have a high incidence of EPSEs, anticholinergic drugs should only be prescribed when a need has been shown. A number of studies have looked at the discontinuation of anticholinergic agents and reported re-emergence of the symptoms. Up to 60% of patients may be affected by re-emergence of symptoms and between 25% and 30% of patients will have a continuing need for anticholinergic drugs. The anticholinergic drugs are not without problems, having their own range of side effects that include dry mouth, constipation and blurred vision. Trihexyphenidyl in particular, is renowned for its euphoric effects and withdrawal problems can include cholinergic rebound. One of the benefits of the atypical antipsychotic drugs is the reduced need for co-prescription of anticholinergic drugs. However, EPSEs can still occur with atypical antipsychotic drugs, particularly at high dose.

Interactions and antipsychotic drugs

There are claimed to be many interactions involving antipsychotic drugs but few appear to be clinically significant. Propranolol increases the plasma concentration of chlorpromazine, and carbamazepine accelerates the metabolism of haloperidol, risperidone and olanzapine. When tricyclic antidepressants are administered with phenothiazines, increased antimuscarinic effects such as dry mouth and blurred vision can occur and most antipsychotic drugs increase the sedative effect of alcohol. The SSRI antidepressants fluvoxamine, fluoxetine and paroxetine interact with clozapine, resulting in increases in clozapine plasma concentration.

Therapeutic drug monitoring

Therapeutic drug monitoring is only of value if there is a reliable laboratory assay and a correlation exists between the concentration of the drug in any particular body compartment, usually blood/plasma, and its clinical effectiveness. Unfortunately, this is not the case for most antipsychotic drugs and the measurement of drug concentrations is not a part of routine clinical practice. In recent years, however, it has become common to measure clozapine levels although even with this drug there is only a weak correlation between plasma levels and clinical effect. The general guidance is that individuals who have not adequately responded to clozapine and have a plasma level below 350–500 µcg/L may benefit from a dose increase and those who suffer side effects and have a plasma level above this range may benefit from a dose reduction. Those with a plasma level above 1000 µcg/L are more likely to suffer seizures and cover using sodium valproate should be considered.

Adverse effects and antipsychotic medicines

There are a large number of adverse effects associated with antipsychotic medicines. Some of these effects, such as sedation, antilibido effects and weight gain may be considered to be of value with particular patients, but the susceptibility to such adverse effects is often a major factor in determining drug choice. Prescribing guidelines are available (Bazire, 2009; Taylor et al., 2009) which provide details of the relative likelihood of side effects with the various antipsychotic drugs. The major side effects are set out below.

Sedation

Although sedation is most commonly associated with chlorpromazine and clozapine, it is primarily related to dosage with other antipsychotics. Products claiming to be less sedating can often only substantiate this when used at low doses.

Weight gain and diabetes

Weight gain was a common feature of the first phenothiazine antipsychotics. It was originally thought this side effect was caused by a direct effect on metabolism. This side effect has also become a feature of some of the newer atypical antipsychotic medicines, particularly olanzapine and clozapine. This re-emergence of an old side effect with the new drugs has rekindled interest in the cause, which is now thought to be more associated with loss of control of food intake, rather than a direct effect on food metabolism. In addition to weight gain, these two atypical antipsychotic drugs have also been associated with increased incidence of diabetes. Controversy remains about whether there is a link between the weight gain and onset of diabetes, and whether the development of diabetes is more associated with the illness of schizophrenia than the drugs. Whatever the link, the controversy has led to the acceptance that people with schizophrenia often suffer poor physical health in addition to poor mental health and require regular monitoring of physical health risk factors. Increased concern about the physical and metabolic side effects of the antipsychotic medicines has led to increased requirements to monitor urea and electrolytes, blood lipids, full blood count, plasma glucose and blood pressure.

QT prolongation and cardiac risk

Some antipsychotic drugs are associated with changes to the QT interval measured on the elecrocardiogram (ECG) and, if given in high doses, may increase the risk of sudden cardiac death. Although, overall, the risk is low, monitoring the ECG has become part of normal practice, especially if high doses are used.

Anticholinergic side effects

Side effects such as dry mouth, constipation and blurred vision are particularly associated with piperidine phenothiazines.

Extrapyramidal side effects

Side effects such as akathisia, dystonia and parkinsonian effects are associated with typical antipsychotic drugs and occur frequently, particularly with depot antipsychotics, piperazine phenothiazines such as trifluoperazine and fluphenazine, and butyrophenones such as haloperidol. These side effects are reversible by using anticholinergic drugs or by dosage reduction. The common extrapyramidal effects include akathisia, dystonia and parkinson-like side effects (see the previous section)

Hormonal effects and sexual dysfunction

These side effects are primarily influenced by the effect on prolactin. This may result in galactorrhoea, missed menstrual periods and loss of libido. Some studies have suggested very high levels of sexual dysfunction with some antipsychotic drugs such as typical antipsychotic drugs and the atypical antipsychotics risperidone and amisulpride. However, in many of these studies the background level of such dysfunction is unclear. In addition, there has been a debate about the extent to which the long-term elevation of prolactin, particularly in the young, may be a cause of osteoporosis. What remains controversial though is at what point an elevated prolactin level should result in a discussion about choosing an alternative antipsychotic.

Postural hypotension and photosensitivity

Postural hypotension and photosensitivity are particularly associated with the aliphatic phenothiazines such as chlorpromazine.

Neuroleptic malignant syndrome (NMS)

The NMS is a rare but serious complication of antipsychotic drug treatment. The primary symptoms are rigidity, fever, diaphoresis, confusion and fluctuating consciousness. Confirmation can be sought through detection of elevated levels of creatinine kinase. The onset is particularly associated with high-potency typical drugs such as haloperidol, recent and rapid changes to dose and abrupt withdrawal of anticholinergic drugs. Treatment usually requires admission to a medical ward and withdrawal of all antipsychotic drugs.

Case studies

Case 30.1

Lee is a 20-year-old man. His childhood was disrupted by constant changes to family membership. From an early age his behaviour was difficult but despite such changes by the age of 16 he was achieving well at school. Aged 17, he became involved with the illicit drug culture and increasingly lost interest in his studies. His parents became concerned as he appeared to undergo a change of personality, communicating with them very little. He eventually dropped out of school and took various short-term jobs. He was unable to sustain any long-term employment. He moved into a flat and seemed to live a twilight existence involving illicit drugs and all-night raves. Police were called to his flat following a violent disturbance. They found Lee living in squalor. He was surrounded by pieces of paper containing incomprehensible messages and was incoherent. He sat with a fixed stare, appearing quite inaccessible. He kept laughing and responding to imaginary people. He was very resistant to hospital admission, and had to be admitted under a section of the Mental Health Act 2007. On the ward he has remained quiet but appears to be in conversation with people who are not there.

Questions

1. Outline the drug(s) of choice for Lee and the rationale for selection.
2. What factors would influence the likely prognosis?
3. Outline the drug(s) of choice if there is the need to control aggressive behaviour.

Answers

1. The first need is to ascertain whether the patient's behaviour results from abuse of illicit substances or the onset of a schizophrenic illness. If the former, he would be expected to recover within a few days with little or no drug treatment. If, however, this is the first presentation of a schizophrenic illness, the symptoms are likely to persist and it would be appropriate to prescribe an antipsychotic drug. The choice of antipsychotic drug for first-illness psychosis may partly depend on the formulation acceptable to the situation but would usually be an atypical antipsychotic drug. If oral medicines were refused the intramuscular formulation of olanzapine may be the drug of choice. If there were concerns that he may not swallow the drug, aripiprazole, olanzapine and risperidone are formulated as orodispersible formulations.
2. A number of factors in Lee's history indicate a poor prognosis:
   - there has been a deterioration in function
   - his age, which is typical for a first breakdown
   - his poor work record
   - grossly disorganised behaviour
   - a number of positive symptoms such as hallucinations
3. If Lee becomes aggressive and there was a need to use medicines to control the aggression a decision would have to be made about whether to use antipsychotic drugs or benzodiazepines. In the past, sedative antipsychotic drugs such as chlorpromazine, haloperidol or zuclopenthixol were favoured, but increasing concern about sudden death has led to a move to use benzodiazepines such as lorazepam or diazepam. However, the introduction of intramuscular olanzapine has resulted in some swing back to using antipsychotic drugs for the control of violent and aggressive behaviour.

Case 30.2

Gordon has relapsed for the third time this year, the pattern for the last two relapses being the same. His positive symptoms responded rapidly on both previous occasions. On the first he suffered severe extrapyramidal side effects with 30 mg daily of haloperidol and was subsequently stabilised and discharged on sulpiride 400 mg twice daily and procyclidine 5 mg twice daily. He almost immediately stopped taking the sulpiride, claiming not to be ill. During his second relapse he was successfully treated with risperidone 4 mg daily but again stopped the medicine.

Questions

1. Was Gordon's drug treatment appropriate?
2. What strategies could be adopted to maintain Gordon in treatment?

Answers

1. Gordon's initial treatment was not according to current guidelines. The initial treatment with a large dose of haloperidol in a drug-naive patient would now be regarded as excessive. The initial choice of a low-dose typical antipsychotic followed by a second choice of an atypical after the patient suffered extrapyramidal side effects was common practice prior to the publication of national guidance (National Institute for Health and Clinical Excellence, 2009). An atypical antipsychotic would be regarded as the drug of choice for first illness.
2. Gordon has no insight into his illness or the need for continuing treatment. This could be for a number of reasons:
   - It is part of the illness, and his failure to gain insight is symptomatic of incomplete recovery.
   - He lacks a supportive environment to ensure that he takes medicines.
   - He is suffering from side effects that deter him from taking the medicines.

   In most cases, the use of a depot antipsychotic injection would be the easiest way to ensure adherence, although if Gordon is determined to avoid drug treatment this strategy is unlikely to be successful. In his case, the history of good response to oral risperidone and severe extrapyramidal side effects with a typical antipsychotic drug would indicate that the long-acting intramuscular formulation of risperidone may be a good choice.

Case 30.3

Sharon, aged 25, has a 3-year history of schizophrenia with many admissions to hospital. Throughout the period of her illness she has received a range of different oral antipsychotic drugs including chlorpromazine, haloperidol, sulpiride, risperidone and olanzapine, as well as the depot formulations of haloperidol and zuclopenthixol. For most of this time she has had a fixed belief that she is involved with a range of mythical beasts that sexually assault her. When she is ill these beings torment her. She currently receives zuclopenthixol decanoate 500 mg by intramuscular injection every week, olanzapine 10 mg at night, carbamazepine 200 mg three times daily, haloperidol 10 mg four times daily, and procyclidine 10 mg three times daily. She has remained on the ward for the last 4 months with no sign of improvement. She has greatly increased in weight, now approaching 20 stone. The team wishes to consider clozapine for Sharon.

Questions

1. Comment on the current drug therapy Sharon is receiving.
2. What action is required before Sharon can receive clozapine?

Answers

1. Although it is not uncommon for polypharmacy to occur when there has been poor response, the practice is frowned upon. Additional medicines are often added in a crisis or in the hope of achieving a greater degree of response. As in this case, the strategy is often unsuccessful. The particular issues of note with this patient's drug regimen are

   - The combination of a typical and an atypical antipsychotic drug reduces the potential benefit of using a drug with a low incidence of extrapyramidal side effects because the patient still suffers extrapyramidal side effects, requires procyclidine, and is at risk of developing tardive dyskinesia.
   - The very large total dose she is receiving from the combination of antipsychotic drugs.
   - The dose of anticholinergic drug (procyclidine) is high and likely to result in its own side effects.

   - The need for such frequent dosing of the intramuscular depot might not be necessary; administration at 2-week intervals would normally be appropriate.
   - There is little evidence to support the value of carbamazepine, either for schizophrenia or as an adjunctive treatment.
   - She is suffering severe weight gain.
   - The interaction between carbamazepine and the antipsychotic drugs may be reducing their potential efficacy.

2. The preparation for treatment with clozapine involves a number of steps. These include

   - registration with the clozapine monitoring scheme
   - background blood tests to ensure that the patient is not already suffering from neutropenia or another blood disorder
   - stopping the depot antipsychotic drug; this would usually occur some weeks before starting clozapine
   - stopping carbamazepine as this interacts with clozapine
   - slowly reducing haloperidol
   - gradually stopping procyclidine

   Ideally all other treatments would be stopped and clozapine prescribed alone. Sometimes the final step of withdrawing other medicines may occur during the initiation phase with clozapine.

References

Altamura, A., Sassella, F., Santini, A., et al., 2003. Intramuscular preparations of antipsychotics uses and relevance in clinical practice. Drugs 63, 493–512.

American Psychiatric Association, 1994. Diagnostic and Statistical Manual of Mental Disorders, fourth ed. American Psychiatric Association, Washington.

Bazire, S., 2009. Psychotropic Drug Directory: The Professionals' Pocket Handbook and Aide Memoire. Fivepin Ltd, Salisbury.

Chakos, M., Lieberman, J.A., Hoffman, E., et al., 2001. Effectiveness of second-generation antipsychotics in patients with treatment-resistant schizophrenia: a review and meta-analysis of randomized trials. Am. J. Psychiatry 158, 518–526.

Cipriani, A., Boso, M., Barbui, C., 2009. Clozapine combined with different antipsychotic drugs for treatment resistant schizophrenia. Cochrane Database Syst. Rev. 3. Art. No. CD006324 doi: 10.1002/14651858.CD006324.pub2. Available at: http://www2.cochrane.org/reviews/en/ab006324.html.

Committee on Safety of Medicines, 2002. Clozapine and cardiac safety: updated advice for prescribers. Curr. Probl. Pharmacovigil. 28, 8.

Kane, J., Honigfield, G., Singer, J., et al., 1988. Clozapine for the treatment-resistant schizophrenic; a double blind comparison with chlorpromazine (clozaril collaborative study). Arch. Gen. Psychiatry 45, 789–796.

Lieberman, J.A., Safferman, A.Z., Pollack, S., et al., 1994. Clinical effects of clozapine in chronic schizophrenia: response to treatment and predictors of outcome. Am. J. Psychiatry 15, 1744–1752.

National Institute for Health and Clinical Excellence, 2009. Schizophrenia: Core Interventions in the Treatment and Management of Schizophrenia in Adults in Primary and Secondary Care. Clinical guideline 82 update http://www.nice.org.uk/nicemedia/live/11786/43608/43608.pdf.

Paton, C., Whittington, C., Barnes, T., 2007. Augmentation with a second antipsychotic in patients with schizophrenia who partially respond to clozapine: a meta-analysis. J. Clin. Psychopharmacol. 27, 198–204.

Royal College of Psychiatrists, 2006. Consensus Statement on High-Dose Antipsychotic Medication. CR138, RCP, London.

Taylor, D., Paton, C., Kapur, S., 2009. The Maudsley Prescribing Guidelines, 10th ed. Informa Healthcare, London.

Tuunainen, A., Wahlbeck, K., Gilbody, S., 2000. Newer atypical antipsychotic medication versus clozapine for schizophrenia. Cochrane Database Syst. Rev. 1 Art No. CD000966. doi: 10.1002/14651858.CD000966.

World Health Organization, 1992. International Classification of Diseases and Related Health Problems, 10th ed (ICD 10), World Health Organization, Geneva.

Further reading

Barbui, C., Signoretti, A., Mule, S., et al., 2009. Does the addition of a second antipsychotic drug improve clozapine treatment? Schizophr. Bull. 35, 458–468.

Bobo, W.V., Stovall, J.A., Knostman, M., et al., 2010. Converting from brand-name to generic clozapine: a review of effectiveness and tolerability data. Am. J. Health Syst. Pharm. 67, 27–37.

Gao, K., Gajwani, P., Elhaj, O., Calabrese, J.R., 2005. Typical and atypical antipsychotics in bipolar depression. J. Clin. Psychiatry 66, 1376–1385.

Lang, U., Willbring, M., von Golitschek, R., et al., 2008. Clozapine-induced myocarditis after long-term treatment: case presentation and clinical perspectives. J. Psychopharmacol. 22, 576–580.

Leucht, S., Komossa, K., Rummel-Kluge, C., et al., 2009. A meta-analysis of head-to-head comparisons of second-generation antipsychotics in the treatment of schizophrenia. Am. J. Psychiatry 166, 152–163.

Lieberman, J.A., Stroup, T.S., McEvoy, J.P., et al., for the Clinical Antipsychotic Trials of Intervention Effectiveness (CATIE) Investigators, 2005. Effectiveness of antipsychotic drugs in patients with chronic schizophrenia. N. Engl. J. Med. 353, 1209–1223.

National Collaborating Centre for Mental Health, 2010. Schizophrenia: The NICE Guideline on Core Interventions in the Treatment and Management of Schizophrenia in Adults in Primary and Secondary Care. British Psychological Society, London.

Epilepsy **31**

J. W. Sander and S. Dhillon

Key points

- An epileptic seizure is a transient paroxysm of uncontrolled discharges of neurones causing an event which is discernible by the person experiencing the seizure and/or an observer.
- The incidence of epileptic seizures is around 50 cases per 100,000 of the population.
- About 70–80% of all those who develop epilepsy will become seizure free on treatment and about 50% will eventually withdraw their medication successfully.
- Generalised seizures result in impairment of consciousness from the onset; they include tonic clonic convulsions, absence attacks and myoclonic seizures.
- Focal seizures include simple partial seizures, complex partial seizures and secondarily generalised seizures.
- Treatment of epilepsy is usually for at least 3 years and, depending on circumstances, sometimes for life.
- Treatment aims to control seizures using one drug without causing side effects and minimising the use of polypharmacy.
- Management of epilepsy requires empowering patients to understand their condition and medication and helping them develop effective partnerships with health professionals.

An epileptic seizure is a transient paroxysm of uncontrolled discharges of neurones causing an event that is discernible by the person experiencing the seizure and/or by an observer. The tendency to have recurrent attacks is known as epilepsy; by definition, a single attack does not usually constitute epilepsy. Epileptic seizures or attacks are a symptom of many different diseases, and the term epilepsy is loosely applied to a number of conditions that have in common a tendency to have recurrent epileptic attacks. A patient with epilepsy will show recurrent epileptic seizures that occur unexpectedly and stop spontaneously.

Epidemiology

There are problems in establishing precise epidemiological information for a heterogeneous condition such as epilepsy. Unlike most ailments, epilepsy is episodic; between seizures, patients may be perfectly normal and have normal investigations. Thus, the diagnosis is essentially clinical, relying heavily on eyewitness descriptions of the attacks. In addition, there

are a number of other conditions in which consciousness may be transiently impaired and which may be confused with epilepsy. Another problem area is that of case identification. Sometimes the person may be unaware of the nature of the attacks and so may not seek medical help. People with milder epilepsy may also not be receiving ongoing medical care and so may be missed in epidemiological surveys. Furthermore, since there is some degree of stigma attached to epilepsy, people may sometimes be reluctant to admit their condition. Indeed, epilepsy is still one of the world's most stigmatised conditions. In today's society, in both developed and developing countries, fear, misunderstanding, discrimination and social stigma still exist and these affect the quality of life for people with the disorder and their families.

Epilepsy does impact on an individual's human rights, for example, access to health and life insurance is affected. A person who suffers from epilepsy may not be able to obtain a driving licence and it has an impact on the choice of career. In addition, legislation can impact on the life of individuals with epilepsy, for example, in some countries epilepsy may deter marriages. Legislation based on internationally accepted human rights standards can prevent discrimination and rights violations, improve access to health care services and raise quality of life (WHO, 2009). A global campaign has been established to raise awareness about epilepsy, provide information and highlight the need to improve care and reduce the disorder's impact through public and private collaboration. This is supported through a partnership established between WHO, the International League Against Epilepsy (ILAE) and the International Bureau for Epilepsy (IBE).

Epilepsy is recognised as a priority in effective health care delivery and there are still a number of issues that health professionals should consider:

- Epilepsy is a chronic neurological disorder that affects people of all ages.
- Around 50 million people worldwide have epilepsy.
- Nearly 90% of the people with epilepsy are found in developing regions.
- Epilepsy responds to treatment 70% of the time. Despite this, approximately 75% of affected people in developing countries do not get the treatment they need.
- People with epilepsy and their families suffer from stigma and discrimination in many parts of the world.

Incidence and prevalence

Epileptic seizures are common. The incidence (number of new cases per given population per year) has been estimated at between 20 and 70 cases per 100,000 persons, and the cumulative incidence (the risk of having the condition at some point in life) at 2–5%. The incidence is higher in the first two decades of life but falls over the next few decades, only to increase again in late life, due mainly to cerebrovascular diseases. Currently, the elderly are the group in the populations with the highest incidence of epilepsy. Most studies of the prevalence of active epilepsy (the number of cases in the population at any given time) in developed countries cite figures of 4–10 per 1000 with a rate of 5 per 1000 population most commonly quoted. In developed countries, annual new cases are between 0.4 and 0.7 per 1000 general population.

In developing countries, the prevalence of epilepsy is higher with rates of 6–10 per 1000 population cited and reported annual new cases twice those seen in developed countries, presumably due to the higher risk of experiencing conditions that can lead to permanent brain damage. Overall, nearly 90% of epilepsy cases worldwide are found in developing regions.

Prognosis

Up to 5% of people will suffer at least one seizure in their lifetime. The prevalence of active epilepsy is, however, much lower and most patients who develop seizures have a very good prognosis. About 70–80% of all people developing epilepsy will eventually become seizure free, and about half will successfully withdraw their medication. Once a substantial period of remission has been achieved, the risk of further seizures is greatly reduced. A minority of people (20–30%) will develop chronic epilepsy and in such cases, treatment is more difficult. People with symptomatic epilepsy, more than one seizure type, associated learning disabilities or neurological or psychiatric disorders are more likely to have a poor outcome. Of people with chronic epilepsy, fewer than 5% will be unable to live in the community or will depend on others for their day-to-day needs. Most people with epilepsy are entirely normal between seizures but a small minority of patients with severe epilepsy may suffer physical and intellectual deterioration.

Mortality

People with epilepsy, especially younger patients and those with severe epilepsy are at an increased risk of premature death. Most studies have given overall standardised mortality ratios between two and three times that of the general population. Common causes of death in people with epilepsy include accidents such as drowning, head injury, road traffic accidents, status epilepticus, tumours, cerebrovascular disease, pneumonia and suicide. Sudden unexpected death, an entity which remains unexplained, is common in chronic epilepsy, particularly among the young who have convulsive forms of epilepsy.

Aetiology

Epileptic seizures are produced by abnormal discharges of neurones that may be caused by any pathological process which affects the cortical layer of the brain. The idiopathic epilepsies are those in which there is a clear genetic component, and they probably account for a third of all new cases of epilepsy. In a significant proportion of cases, however, no cause can be determined and these are known as the cryptogenic epilepsies. Possible explanations for cryptogenic epilepsy include as yet unexplained metabolic or biochemical abnormalities and microscopic lesions in the brain resulting from brain malformation or trauma during birth or other injury. The term 'symptomatic epilepsy' indicates that a probable cause has been identified.

The likely aetiology of epilepsy depends upon the age of the patient and the type of seizure. The commonest causes in young infants are hypoxia or birth asphyxia, intracranial trauma during birth, metabolic disturbances and congenital malformations of the brain or infection. In young children and adolescents, idiopathic seizures account for the majority of the epilepsies, although trauma and infection also play a role. In this age group, particularly in children aged between 6 months and 5 years, seizures may occur in association with febrile illness. These are usually short, generalised tonic clonic convulsions that occur during the early phase of a febrile disease. They must be distinguished from seizures that are triggered by central nervous system infections which produce fever, for example, meningitis or encephalitis. Unless febrile seizures are prolonged, focal, recurrent or there is a background of neurological handicap, the prognosis is excellent and it is unlikely that the child will develop epilepsy.

The range of causes of adult-onset epilepsy is very wide. Both idiopathic epilepsy and epilepsy due to birth trauma may also begin in early adulthood. Other important causes are head injury, alcohol abuse, cortical dysplasias, brain tumours and cerebrovascular diseases. Brain tumours are responsible for the development of epilepsy in up to a third of patients between the ages of 30 and 50 years. Over the age of 50 years, cerebrovascular disease is the commonest cause of epilepsy, and may be present in up to half of patients.

Pathophysiology

Epilepsy differs from most neurological conditions as it has no pathognomonic lesion. A variety of different electrical or chemical stimuli can easily give rise to a seizure in any normal brain. The hallmark of epilepsy is a rather rhythmic and repetitive hyper-synchronous discharge of neurones, either localised in an area of the cerebral cortex or generalised throughout the cortex, which can be observed on an electroencephalogram (EEG).

Neurones are interconnected in a complex network in which each individual neurone is linked through synapses with hundreds of others. A small electrical current is discharged by neurones to release neurotransmitters at synaptic levels to permit communication with each other. Neurotransmitters fall into two basic categories: inhibitory or excitatory. Therefore, a neurone discharging can either excite or inhibit neurones connected to it. An excited neurone will activate the next neurone whereas an inhibited neurone will not. In this manner, information is conveyed, transmitted and processed throughout the central nervous system.

A normal neurone discharges repetitively at a low baseline frequency, and it is the integrated electrical activity generated by the neurones of the superficial layers of the cortex that is recorded in a normal EEG. If neurones are damaged, injured or suffer a chemical or metabolic insult, a change in the discharge pattern may develop. In the case of epilepsy, regular low-frequency discharges are replaced by bursts of high-frequency discharges usually followed by periods of inactivity. A single neurone discharging in an abnormal manner usually has no clinical significance. It is only when a whole population of neurones discharge synchronously in an abnormal way that an epileptic seizure may be triggered. This abnormal discharge may remain localised or it may spread to adjacent areas, recruiting more neurones as it expands. It may also generalise throughout the brain via cortical and subcortical routes, including collosal and thalamocortical pathways. The area from which the abnormal discharge originates is known as the epileptic focus. An EEG recording carried out during one of these abnormal discharges may show a variety of atypical signs, depending on which area of the brain is involved, its progression and how the discharging areas project to the superficial cortex.

Clinical manifestations

The clinical manifestation of a seizure will depend on the location of the focus and the pathways involved in its spread. An international seizure classification scheme based on the clinical features of seizures combined with EEG data is widely used to describe seizures. It divides seizures into two main groups according to the area of the brain in which the abnormal discharge originates. If it involves initial activation of both hemispheres of the brain simultaneously, the seizures are termed 'generalised'. If a discharge starts in a localised area of the brain, the seizure is termed 'partial' or 'focal'.

Generalised seizures

Generalised seizures result in impairment of consciousness from the onset. There are various types of generalised seizures.

Tonic clonic convulsions

Often called 'grand mal' attacks, these are the commonest of all epileptic seizures. Without warning, the patient suddenly goes stiff, falls and convulses, with laboured breathing and salivation. Cyanosis, incontinence and tongue biting may occur. The convulsion ceases after a few minutes and may often be followed by a period of drowsiness, confusion, headache and sleep.

Absence attacks

Often called 'petit mal', these are a much rarer form of generalised seizure. They happen almost exclusively in childhood and early adolescence. The child goes blank and stares; fluttering of the eyelids and flopping of the head may occur. The attacks last only a few seconds and often go unrecognised even by the child experiencing them.

Myoclonic seizures

These are abrupt, very brief involuntary shock-like jerks, which may involve the whole body, or the arms or the head. They usually happen in the morning, shortly after waking. They may sometimes cause the person to fall, but recovery is immediate. It should be noted that there are forms of non-epileptic myoclonic jerks that occur in a variety of other neurological diseases and may also occur in healthy people, particularly when they are just going off to sleep.

Atonic seizures

These comprise a sudden loss of muscle tone, causing the person to collapse to the ground. Recovery afterwards is quick. They are rare, accounting for less than 1% of the epileptic seizures seen in the general population, but much commoner in patients with severe epilepsy starting in infancy.

Partial or focal seizures

Simple partial seizures

In these seizures, the discharge remains localised and consciousness is fully preserved. Simple partial attacks on their own are rare and they usually progress to the other forms of partial seizure. What actually happens during a simple partial seizure depends on the area of the discharge and may vary widely from person to person but will always be stereotyped in one person. Localised jerking of a limb or the face, stiffness or twitching of one part of the body, numbness or abnormal sensations are examples of what may occur during a simple partial seizure. If the seizure progresses with impairment of consciousness, it is termed a complex partial seizure. If it develops further and a convulsive seizure occurs, it is then called a partial seizure with secondary generalisation. In attacks which progress, the early part of the seizure, in which consciousness is preserved, may manifest as a sensation or abnormal feeling and is called the aura or warning.

Complex partial seizures

The person may present with altered or 'automatic' behaviour: plucking his or her clothes, fiddling with various objects and acting in a confused manner. Lip smacking or chewing movements, grimacing, undressing, performing aimless activities, and wandering around in a drunken fashion may occur on their own or in different combinations during complex partial seizures. Most of these seizures originate in the frontal or temporal lobes of the brain and can sometimes progress to secondarily generalised seizures.

Secondarily generalised seizures

These are partial seizures, either simple or complex, in which the discharge spreads to the entire brain. The person may have a warning, but this is not always the case. The spread of the discharge can occur so quickly that no feature of the localised onset is apparent to the person or an observer, and only an EEG can demonstrate the partial nature of the seizure. The involvement of the entire brain leads to a convulsive attack with the same characteristics as a generalised tonic clonic convulsion.

There have been recent proposals to revise the concepts, terminology and approaches for classifying seizures and forms of epilepsy (Berg et al., 2010). In this proposal, the so-called natural classes, for example, specific underlying cause, age at onset, associated seizure type; or pragmatic groupings, for example, epileptic encephalopathies, self-limited electroclinical syndromes, serve as the basis for classification.

Diagnosis

Diagnosing epilepsy can be difficult as it is first necessary to demonstrate a tendency to recurrent epileptic seizures. The one feature that distinguishes epilepsy from all other conditions is its unpredictability and transient nature. The diagnosis of epilepsy is clinical and depends on a reliable account of what happened during the attacks, if possible both from the patient and from an eyewitness. Investigations may help and the EEG is usually one of them. These investigations, however, cannot conclusively confirm or refute the diagnosis of epilepsy.

There are other conditions that may cause impairment or loss of consciousness and which can be misdiagnosed as epilepsy; these include syncope, breath-holding attacks, transient ischaemic attacks, psychogenic attacks, etc. In addition, people may present with acute symptomatic seizures or provoked seizures as a result of other problems such as drug intake, metabolic dysfunction, infection, head trauma or flashing lights (photosensitive seizures). These conditions have to be clearly ruled out before a diagnosis of epilepsy is made. Epilepsy must only be diagnosed when seizures occur spontaneously and are recurrent. The diagnosis must be accurate since the label 'suffering with epilepsy' carries a social stigma that has tremendous implications for the person.

The EEG is often the only examination required, particularly in generalised epilepsies, and it aims to record abnormal neuronal discharges. EEGs have, however, limitations that should be clearly understood. Up to 5% of people without epilepsy may have non-specific abnormalities in their EEG recording, while up to 40% of people with epilepsy may have a normal EEG recording between seizures. Therefore,

the diagnosis of epilepsy should be strongly supported by a bona fide history of epileptic attacks. Nevertheless, the EEG is invaluable in classifying seizures.

The chance of recording the discharges of an actual seizure during a routine EEG, which usually takes 20–30 min, is slight and because of this, ambulatory EEG monitoring and EEG video-telemetry are sometimes required. Ambulatory EEG allows recording in day-to-day circumstances using a small cassette recorder. EEG video-telemetry is useful in the assessment of difficult cases, particularly if surgery is considered. The person is usually admitted to hospital and remains under continuous monitoring. This is only helpful in a very few cases, and it is best suited for people who have frequent seizures.

Neuroimaging with magnetic resonance imaging (MRI) is the most valuable investigation when structural abnormalities such as stroke, tumour, congenital abnormalities or hydrochephalus are suspected. MRI should be carried out in anyone presenting with partial seizures or where a structural lesion on the brain may be responsible for seizures.

Treatment

National Institute for Health and Clinical Excellence (2004a) issued guidance on the diagnosis and treatment of the epilepsies in adults and children in primary and secondary care. The guidance covered issues such as when a person with epilepsy should be referred to a specialist centre, the special considerations concerning the care and treatment of women with epilepsy and the management of people with learning disabilities. The key points of the guidance are summarised in Box 31.1.

Box 31.1 Key points on the diagnosis and management of epilepsy (National Institute for Health and Clinical Excellence, 2004a)

- Diagnosis to be made urgently by a specialist with an interest in epilepsy
- EEG to be used to support diagnosis
- MRI to be used in people who develop epilepsy as adults, in whom focal onset is suspected, or in whom seizures persist
- Seizure type(s) and epilepsy syndrome, aetiology and co-morbidity to be determined
- Initiation of appropriate treatment to be recommended by a specialist
- Treatment individualised according to seizure type, epilepsy syndrome, co-medication and co-morbidity, the individual's lifestyle and personal preferences
- The individual with epilepsy, and their family and/or carers, to participate in all decisions about care, taking into account any specific need
- Comprehensive care plans to be agreed
- Comprehensive provision of information about all aspects of condition
- Regular structured review at least once a year
- Patient to be referred back to secondary or tertiary care if:
  - Epilepsy inadequately controlled
  - Pregnancy considered or pregnant
  - Antiepileptic drug withdrawal considered
- MRI, magnetic resonance imaging; EEG, electroencephalogram.

Treatment during seizures

Convulsive seizures may look frightening but the person is not in pain, will usually have no recollection of the event afterwards and is usually not seriously injured. Emergency treatment is seldom necessary. People should, however, be made as comfortable as possible, preferably lying down (ease to the floor if sitting), cushioning the head and loosening any tight clothing or neckwear. During seizures, people should not be moved unless they are in a dangerous place, for example, in a road, by a fire or hot radiator, at the top of stairs or by the edge of water. No attempt should be made to open the person's mouth or force anything between the teeth. This usually results in damage, and broken teeth may be inhaled, causing secondary lung damage. When the seizure stops, people should be turned over into the recovery position and the airway checked for any blockage.

Partial attacks are usually less dramatic. During automatisms, people may behave in a confused fashion and should generally be left undisturbed. Gentle restraint may be necessary if the automatism leads to dangerous wandering. Attempts at firm restraint, however, may increase agitation and confusion. No drinks should be given after an attack, nor should extra antiepileptic drugs (AEDs) be administered. It is commonly felt that seizures may be life-threatening, but this is seldom the case. After a seizure, it is important to stay with the person and offer reassurance until the confused period has completely subsided and the person has recovered fully.

If a seizure persists for more than 10 min, if a series of seizures occur or if the seizure is particularly severe, then intravenous or rectal administration of 10–20 mg diazepam for adults, with lower doses being used in children, is advisable.

Status epilepticus

Initial management of status epilepticus is supportive and may include:

- positioning the person to avoid injury
- supporting respiration
- maintaining blood pressure
- correcting hypoglycaemia

Drugs used include intravenous lorazepam or diazepam. Alternative medicines include midazolam in cases where the person has not responded to first-line drugs. Alternatively, buccal midazolam has been advocated and is increasingly being used, although it is not licensed in the UK. In severe cases, phenytoin, clonazepam or phenobarbital sodium may be required.

Febrile convulsions

Convulsions associated with fever are termed febrile convulsions and may occur in the young. Brief febrile convulsions are managed conservatively with the primary aim of reducing the temperature of the child. Tepid sponging and use of paracetamol is usual. Prolonged febrile convulsions lasting 10–15 min or longer or in a child with risk factors require active management to avoid brain damage. The drug of choice is diazepam by intravenous or rectal (rectal solution) administration. Prophylactic management of febrile convulsions may be required in some children, such as those with pre-existing risk factors or a history of previous prolonged seizures.

Long-term treatment

In most cases, epilepsy can only be treated by long-term, regular drug therapy. The objective of therapy is to suppress epileptic discharges and prevent the development of epileptic seizures. In the majority of cases, full seizure control can be obtained, and in other patients drugs may reduce the frequency or severity of seizures.

Initiating treatment with an AED is a major event in the life of a person, and the diagnosis should be unequivocal. Treatment options must be considered with careful evaluation of all relevant factors, including the number and frequency of attacks, the presence of precipitating factors such as alcohol, drugs or flashing lights, and the presence of other medical conditions (Feely, 1999). Single seizures do not require treatment unless they are associated with a structural abnormality in the brain, a progressive brain disorder or there is a clearly abnormal EEG recording. If there are long intervals between seizures (over 2 years), there is a case for not starting treatment. If there are more than two attacks that are clearly associated with a precipitating factor, fever or alcohol for instance, then treatment may not be necessary.

Therapy is long-term, usually for at least 3 years and, depending on circumstances, sometimes for life. A full explanation of all the implications must be given to the person and they must be involved in all stages of the treatment plan. It is vital that the person understands the implications of treatment and agrees with the treatment goals. Empowerment of the person with epilepsy to be actively involved in the decision-making process will encourage adherence and is essential for effective clinical management. Support for people so that they understand the implications of the condition and why drug therapy is so important is crucial to ensure effective clinical management.

Health professionals have a key role in supporting people with epilepsy to ensure they are able to manage their medicines appropriately. AED treatment will fail unless the patient fully understands the importance of regular therapy and the objectives of treatment. Poor adherence is still a major factor which results in hospital admissions and poor seizure control and leads to the clinical use of multiple AEDs.

General principles of treatment

Therapy aims to control seizures using one drug, with the lowest possible dose that causes the fewest side effects possible. The established AEDs, carbamazepine, ethosuximide and sodium valproate, are still important parts of the antiepileptic armamentarium. Acetazolamide, clobazam, clonazepam, phenobarbital phenytoin and primidone are also still used. In the last two decades, new AEDs such as vigabatrin, lamotrigine, gabapentin, topiramate, tiagabine, oxcarbazepine, levetiracetam, pregabalin, zonisamide, lacosamide and eslicarbazepine acetate have been introduced. The choice of drugs depends largely on the seizure type, and so correct diagnosis and classification are essential. Table 31.1 lists the main indications for the more commonly used AEDs, and Table 31.2 summarises the clinical use of the newer AEDs.

Initiation of therapy in newly diagnosed patients

The first-line AED most suitable for the person's seizure type should be introduced slowly, starting with a small dose. This is because too rapid an introduction may induce side effects that will lose the person's confidence. For most drugs, this gradual introduction will produce a therapeutic effect just as fast as a rapid introduction, and the person should be reassured about this.

Maintenance dosage

There is no single optimum dose of any AED that suits all patients. The required dose varies from person to person, and from drug to drug. Drugs should be introduced slowly and then increased incrementally to an initial maintenance dosage. Seizure control should then be assessed, and the dose of drug changed if necessary. For most AEDs, dosage increments are constant over a wide range. More care is, however, needed with phenytoin as the serum level–dose relationship is not linear, and small dose changes may result in considerable serum level changes. Generic prescribing for epilepsy remains controversial. Most specialists would prefer people to remain on the same brand of medication, and this is also preferred by the majority of people with epilepsy. This is obviously important in those people in whom the dosage has been carefully titrated to achieve optimal control.

Altering drug regimens

If the maximal tolerated dose of a drug does not control seizures, or if side effects develop, the first drug can be replaced with another first-line AED. To do this, the second drug should be added gradually to the first. Once a good dose of the new drug is established, the first drug should then slowly be withdrawn.

Withdrawal of drugs

AEDs should not be withdrawn abruptly. With barbiturates and benzodiazepines, in particular, rebound seizures may occur. Withdrawal of individual AEDs should be carried out in a slow stepwise fashion to avoid the precipitation of withdrawal seizures (e.g. over 2–3 months). This risk is particularly great with barbiturates, for example, phenobarbital and primidone, and benzodiazepines, for example, clobazam and clonazepam. If a drug needs to be withdrawn rapidly, for example, if there are life-threatening side effects, then diazepam or another benzodiazepine can be used to cover the withdrawal phase.

Examples of withdrawal regimens are given below.

- Carbamazepine
  100–200 mg every 2 weeks (as part of a drug change)
  100–200 mg every 4 weeks (total withdrawal)

- Phenobarbital
  15–30 mg every 2 weeks (as part of a drug change)
  15–30 mg every 4 weeks (total withdrawal)

- Phenytoin
  50 mg every 2 weeks (as part of a drug change)
  50 mg every 4 weeks (total withdrawal)

- Sodium valproate
  200–400 mg every 2 weeks (as part of a drug change)
  200–400 mg every 4 weeks (total withdrawal)

- Ethosuximide
  125–250 mg every 2 weeks (as part of a drug change)
  125–250 mg every 4 weeks (total withdrawal)

Variations in the above regimens may be used in different settings. People must be monitored closely for any change in seizure frequency. The pace of withdrawal may be slower if the person is within the higher end of the quoted dose range. The pace of withdrawal may be faster if the person is an inpatient.

When to make dose changes

Some AEDs have long half-lives and it may, therefore, take some time, normally five half-lives, before a change in dose results in a stable blood level. For example, phenobarbital has a half-life of up to 6 days and will take more than 4 weeks to

Table 31.1 Antiepileptic drugs for different seizure types

Seizure type	First-line treatment	Second-line treatment
Partial seizures		
	Carbamazepine	Topiramate
	Lamotrigine	Valproate
	Oxcarbazepine	Clobazam
	Levetiracetam	Zonisamide
		Pregabalin
		Phenytoin
		Gabapentin
		Lacosamide
		Eslicarbazepine
Generalised seizures		
Tonic clonic	Valproate sodium	Lamotrigine
Tonic	Carbamazepine	Clobazam
Clonic	Lamotrigine	Phenobarbital
Absence	Ethosuximide	Clonazepam
	Sodium valproate	Lamotrigine
Atypical absences	Sodium valproate	
Atonic	Clonazepam	Lamotrigine
	Clobazam	Carbamazepine
		Phenytoin
		Acetazolamide
		Topiramate
Myoclonic	Sodium valproate	Levetiracetam
	Clonazepam	Acetazolamide
		Topiramate

Table 31.2 Summary of newer antiepileptic agents

Antiepileptic drugs	Clinical use	Available formulation	Side effect profile
Lamotrigine	Monotherapy and adjunctive treatment of partial seizures, primary and secondary generalised tonic clonic seizure, Lennox–Gastaut syndrome	Tablets: 25, 50, 100, 200 mg Dispersible tablets: 5, 25, 100 mg	Dizziness, headache, diplopia, ataxia, nausea, somnolence, vomiting, rash. Rare: Stevens–Johnson syndrome, hematological
Vigabatrin	Adjunctive treatment of partial seizures with or without secondary generalisation, monotherapy for West's syndrome	Tablets: 500 mg Powder: 500 mg/sachet	Drowsiness, fatigue, dizziness, visual field defects nystagmus, abnormal vision, agitation, amnesia, depression, psychosis, increased weight, withdrawal seizures
Gabapentin	Adjunctive treatment of partial seizures with or without secondary generalisation, neuropathic pain	Capsules: 100, 300, 400 mg Tablets: 600, 800 mg	Somnolence, dizziness, ataxia, headache, fatigue, nystagmus, tremor, nausea, vomiting, increased weight
Tiagabine	Adjunctive treatment of partial seizures with or without secondary generalisation	Tablets: 5, 10, 15 mg	Dizziness, asthenia, nervousness, tremor, diarrhoea, depression, emotional liability, confusion, abnormal thinking, decreased weight
Topiramate	Adjunctive treatment of partial seizures with or without secondary generalisation, Lennox–Gastaut syndrome, primary generalised tonic clonic seizures	Tablets: 25, 50, 100, 200 mg Sprinkle capsules: 15, 25 mg	Dizziness, abnormal thinking, somnolence, ataxia, fatigue, confusion, impaired concentration, paresthesia, decreased weight, nephrolithiasis (1.5%)
Zonisamide	Adjunctive therapy in treatment of partial seizures with or without secondary generalisation	Capsule: 25, 50, 100 mg	Somnolence, anorexia, dizziness, headache, nausea, agitation/irritability, confusional state, depression
Lacosamide	Adjunctive for partial epilepsy with or without secondary generalisation	Tablets: 50, 100, 150, 200 mg Syrup: 15 mg/mL	Dizziness, headache, depression, diplopia nystagmus, impaired co-ordination, impaired memory, drowsiness, tremor, fatigue, pruritus

produce a stable blood level. For this reason an assessment of the effectiveness of any dose change should be undertaken several weeks after the dose change has been made and be informed by knowledge of the half-life of the drug.

Newer AEDs

The newer AEDs are generally used as second-line drugs when treatment with established first-line drugs has failed. Exceptions to this are lamotrigine, levetiracetam, topiramate and oxcarbazepine, which have indications for first-line use in the UK. Lamotrigine is considered the first-line option in women of child-bearing potential who have idiopathic generalised epilepsy because of the teratogenic profile of sodium valproate, otherwise the first-line drug for this indication. Oxcarbazepine has the same indications as carbamazepine, although the latter is probably more cost-effective.

There is no evidence that the newer AEDs are more effective than the established drugs, although it could be argued that they might be better tolerated. The chronic side effect profile of the new AEDs has not yet been fully established and this is the main reason why use should be reserved for those cases where benefit outweighs risk. Guidance has been issued that covers the use of the newer AEDs in adults (National Institute for Health and Clinical Excellence, 2004b):

- Newer drugs, for example, lamotrigine, oxcarbazepine and topiramate, suitable for the type of epilepsy to be treated can be used in patients where older drugs, for example, sodium valproate or carbamazepine, do not provide effective clinical control or cause untolerable side effects.
- Gabapentin, levetiracetam, tiagabine and vigabatrin are generally used in combination with another drug.
- Newer drugs can be used where older drugs are unsuitable for the person, for example, liver disease, or where unwanted effects cannot be tolerated.
- The aim should be to treat people with just one AED where possible.

The guidance for adults was followed up by advice for use of the newer AEDs in children (National Institute for Health and Clinical Excellence, 2004c). This advice reflected that issued for adults and included:

- Lamotrigine, oxcarbazepine or topiramate can be given to children as sole treatment for epilepsy.
- Gabapentin, tiagabine and vigabatrin are generally used as combination therapy with another drug.
- Vigabatrin is suitable for first-line treatment of young children with a rare type of infantile spasm called West's syndrome.
- Newer drugs are indicated if older drugs are unsuitable, for example, in liver disease, or if patients cannot tolerate unwanted effects.
- Children should be treated with just one AED where possible.

A third set of national guidance was issued on the diagnoses and management of the epilepsies in adults and children in primary and secondary care (National Institute for Health and Clinical Excellence, 2004a). A recent report on the implementation of this guidance (National Institute for Health and Clinical Excellence, 2009) revealed:

- No major change was noticed in the rate of increase for prescriptions for newer AEDs.
- Use of the newer AEDs had increased at a faster rate than the older drugs.
- Over 70% of patients received mono-therapy for their epilepsy during the period monitored. Of these patients, 60% received an 'old' epilepsy drug. Of newly diagnosed patients, 80% received mono-therapy as their treatment.
- 68% of adults received a medication review within 12 months of being prescribed a drug for their epilepsy.

Follow-up and monitoring of treatment

It is essential to follow up patients in whom AED treatment has been started. The reason for this is essentially to monitor the efficacy and side effects of treatment, upon which drug dosage will depend, but also to encourage good adherence to the treatment. This follow-up is particularly important in the early stages of treatment, when an effective maintenance dose may not have been fully established, when the importance of regular adherence may not have been recognised by the person, and when the psychological adjustment to regular treatment may not be resolved.

Chronic epilepsy

The drug treatment of people with established epilepsy that is uncontrolled despite initial attempts is much more difficult than that of newly diagnosed patients. Prognosis is worse, drug resistance may have developed, and there may be additional neurological, psychological or social problems.

Assessment. The diagnosis of epilepsy should be reassessed before assuming seizures are intractable. A significant proportion of patients may have been incorrectly diagnosed. The aetiology of the epilepsy should also be considered, and the question of a progressive neurological condition addressed. A treatment history should be obtained and note made of

previous drugs used which were helpful, unhelpful or of uncertain benefit. Serum level measurements should be obtained where appropriate and drugs not previously tried should be identified.

Choice of drug and dosage. Treatment should always be started with one AED appropriate for seizure type and suitable for the individual. Only when attempts at monotherapy fail should a combination of two AEDs be tried. In the majority of patients, there is no place for therapy with more than two drugs. The choice of drugs should be made according to seizure type and previous treatment history. Drugs that were helpful in the past or found to be of uncertain benefit, or which have not been used before, should be tried if appropriate to seizure type. The use of sedative AEDs should be minimised where possible.

Intractable epilepsy. It is important to realise that there are limits to AED treatment and that in some people, albeit a small group, seizure control is not possible with the drugs currently available. In such cases, the goal of drug treatment changes, and the objectives are to reduce medication to minimise toxicity while providing partial control. The sedative drugs, for example, barbiturates or benzodiazepines, should be used only where absolutely necessary. In these persons, surgical treatment or the use of experimental antiepileptic agents may be considered. However, only a relatively small number of people with partial epilepsy are suitable for curative surgical treatment.

Stopping treatment

Withdrawing therapy should be considered in people who have been seizure free for a considerable period of time. In no individual case, however, can the safety of drug withdrawal be guaranteed, and the risk of relapse on withdrawal of medication in a person who has been seizure free for more than 2 years is about 40%. The longer the person has been free of seizures, the lower the risk of seizure recurrence when drugs are withdrawn. If a person has a learning disability, partial seizures or symptomatic epilepsy, neurological signs or other evidence of cerebral damage, this risk is much higher and in such cases it may be best to continue drug treatment indefinitely. Drug withdrawal should be carried out only very slowly in staged decrements, and only one drug at a time should be withdrawn.

The risks of drug withdrawal should be clearly explained to the person, and the possible medical and social implications taken into account. There may be serious social or domestic consequences should seizures recur, and the attacks may be subsequently difficult to control, even if the original AED regimen is re-established. In the final analysis, the decision to withdraw therapy is an individual one, and the person should be made aware of the risks and benefits of withdrawal.

Monitoring antiepileptic therapy

Therapeutic drug monitoring (TDM) involves the measurement of serum drug levels and their pharmacokinetic interpretation. It is an integral component in the management of people taking phenytoin and carbamazepine but is less useful in people receiving other AEDs. Indeed, TDM has a very limited use for new AEDs except in people who are acutely unwell, pregnant or elderly. It is also very useful to document AED side effects and in managing drug interactions. Adherence may also be a problem in these patients and hence TDM may be useful to establish adherence with the treatment.

TDM is indicated:

- at the onset of therapy
- if seizure control is poor or sudden changes in seizure control occur
- if toxicity is suspected
- if poor or non-adherence is suspected
- to monitor the time-scale of drug interactions
- when changing AED therapy or making changes to other aspects of a person's drug regimen that may interact with the AED.

The frequency of undertaking TDM varies. Stabilised patients may require their serum levels to be checked only once or twice a year. TDM may be used more often in some people, for one or more of the above indications. A number of the newer AEDs do not require routine TDM. However, since most are used as adjuvant therapy, it is useful to establish baseline levels of existing drugs before the new agent is introduced. Clinical effects should be monitored and TDM, where appropriate, carried out at 6–12 month intervals.

Drug development and action

The older, more established AEDs were developed in animal models in which the potential drugs were assessed in terms of their ability to raise seizure threshold or prevent spread of seizure discharge. The animals involved in these tests would not have epilepsy but would have seizures induced by, for instance, maximal electroshock or subcutaneous pentylenetetrazole. As a consequence the relevance of these models to epilepsy can be questioned.

Established AEDs such as phenytoin, phenobarbital, sodium valproate, carbamazepine, ethosuximide, clonazepam and diazepam are effective but have poor side effect profiles, are involved in many interactions and have complex pharmacokinetics. Over the past 10–15 years, there has been renewed interest in the development of new AEDs, based on a better understanding of excitatory and inhibitory pathways in the brain. The main mechanisms of current drugs are thought to involve enhancement of the inhibitory GABA-ergic system, for example, benzodiazepines, barbiturates, tiagabine, vigabatrin or use-dependent blockers of sodium channels, for example, carbamazepine, oxcarbazepine, lamotrigine and phenytoin (Fig. 31.1).

New drugs include lamotrigine, pregabalin, levetiracetam, topiramate, felbamate, lacosamide, oxcarbazepine, eslicarbazepine and zonisamide. Unlike most of the older agents, vigabatrin, lamotrigine, levetiracetam, lacosamide, gabapentin, pregabalin and zonisamide are devoid of clinically significant enzyme-inhibiting or enzyme-inducing properties. Oral contraceptives may increase the metabolism of lamotrigine and topiramate, and oxcarbazepine may induce cytochrome P450 CYP3A4 which is responsible for the metabolism of oral contraceptives (Sabers and Gram, 2000).

AED profiles

The maintenance doses for the more widely used AEDs are given in Table 31.3, while their pharmacokinetic profile is presented in Table 31.4. Drug interactions are summarised in Table 31.5, and common side effects in Table 31.6.

Acetazolamide

Acetazolamide is occasionally used as an AED. It can be prescribed as a second-line drug for most types of seizures, but particularly for partial seizures, absence seizures and myoclonic seizures. Its intermittent use in catamenial seizures has also been suggested. Acetazolamide has only limited use as long-term therapy because of the development of tolerance in the majority of patients. Side effects include skin rashes, weight loss, paraesthesia, drowsiness and depression. Routine TDM is not available for this drug.

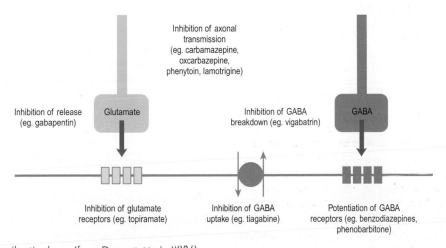

Fig. 31.1 Action of antiepileptic drugs (from Duncan et al., 2006).

Table 31.3 Commonly used starting and maintenance doses of antiepileptic drugs for adults

Antiepileptic drug	Starting dose (mg)	Average maintenance	Doses/day (total mg/day)
Acetazolamide	250	500–1500	2
Carbamazepine	100	600–2400	2–4 (retard 2)
Clobazam	10	10–30	1–2
Clonazepam	0.5	0.5–3	1–2
Ethosuximide	250	500–1500	1–2
Gabapentin	300	900–1200	3
Lacosamide	50	200–400	2
Lamotrigine	50[a]	100–500[a]	2
Levetiracetam	1000	2000–3000	2
Oxcarbazepine	300	900–1800	2–3
Phenobarbital	60	60–180	1
Phenytoin	200–300	200–400	1–2
Sodium valproate	500	2000–2500	1–2
Tiagabine	5[b]	30–45	3
Vigabatrin	500	2000–4000	1–2
Zonisamide	50	300–500 or 200–300[c]	2

[a]Reduce by 50% if on sodium valproate.
[b]If taking enzyme inducer.
[c]If taking enzyme inducer or have impaired renal or liver function.

Carbamazepine

Carbamazepine is a drug of first choice in tonic clonic and partial seizures, and may be of benefit in all other seizure types except generalised absence seizures and myoclonic seizures. Tolerance to its beneficial effect does not usually develop. Adverse events may occur in up to a third of patients treated with carbamazepine but only about 5% of these events will require drug withdrawal, usually due to skin rash, gastro-intestinal disturbances or hyponatraemia. Dose-related adverse reactions including ataxia, dizziness, blurred vision and diplopia are common. Serious adverse events including hepatic failure and bone marrow depression are extremely uncommon.

Carbamazepine exhibits autoinduction, that is, induces its own metabolism as well as inducing the metabolism of other drugs. It should, therefore, be introduced at low dosage and this should be steadily increased over a period of a month. The target serum concentration therapeutic range is 4–12 μcg/mL. In addition, a number of clinically important pharmacokinetic interactions may occur, and caution should be exercised when co-medication is instituted (see Table 31.5). For patients requiring higher doses, the slow-release preparation of carbamazepine has distinct advantages, allowing twice-daily ingestion and avoiding high peak serum concentrations. A 'chewtab' formulation is also available and pharmacokinetic studies have shown that it performs well even if inadvertently swallowed whole. Carbamazepine retard offers paediatric patients in particular a dosage form that reduces fluctuations in the peak to trough serum levels and hence allows a twice-daily regimen, which can assist compliance.

Clobazam

Clobazam is a 1,5-benzodiazepine that is said to be less sedative than 1,4-benzodiazepine drugs such as clonazepam and diazepam. Although the development of tolerance is common, clobazam is used as an adjunctive therapy for patients

Table 31.4 Pharmacokinetic data of antiepileptic drugs

Drug	Absorption			Protein binding (% bound)	Elimination		
	F (%)	T_{peak} (h)	V_d (L/kg)		$T_{1/2}$ (h)	Renal excretion (%)	Active metabolite
Carbamazepine	75–85	1–5 (chronic dose)	0.8–1.6	70–78	24–45 (single), 8–24 (chronic)	<1	Yes
Diazepam	90	1–2	1–2	96	20–95	2	Yes
Clonazepam	80–90	1–2	2.1–4.3	80–90	19–40	2	–
Gabapentin	51–59	2–3	57.7	0	5–7	100	No
Lamotrigine	100	2–3	0.92–1.22	55	24–35 (induces its own metabolism)	<10	No
Ethosuximide	90–95	3–7	0.6–0.9	0	20–60	10–20	No
Phenobarbital	95–100	1–3	0.6	40–50	50–144	20–40	No

Table 31.4 Pharmacokinetic data of antiepileptic drugs—cont'd

Drug	Absorption			Protein binding (% bound)	Elimination		
	F (%)	T_{peak} (h)	V_d (L/kg)		$T_{1/2}$ (h)	Renal excretion (%)	Active metabolite
Phenytoin	85–95	4–7	0.5–0.7	90–95	9–40 (non-linear kinetics)	<5	No
Primidone	90–100	1–3	0.4–1.1	20–30	3–19	40	Yes
Sodium valproate	100	0.5–1.0	0.1–0.5	88–92	7–17	<5	No
Vigabatrin	60–80	2	0.6–1.0	0	5–7	100	No
Zonisamide	100	2–4	1.1–1.7	40	52–69	30	Yes

F, bioavailability; T_{peak}, time to peak; V_d, volume of distribution.

Table 31.5 Examples of drug interactions involving antiepileptic drugs

Drug affected	Effect on serum level	Drug implicated	Possible mechanism
Carbamazepine	Increase	Valproate sodium Cimetidine Dextropropoxyphene Erythromycin Isoniazid Troleandomycin Danazol	Enzyme inhibition
	Decrease	Phenytoin, phenobarbital	Enzyme induction
Ethosuximide	Increase	Valproate sodium	Enzyme inhibition
	Decrease	Carbamazepine	Enzyme induction
Lamotrigine	Increase	Valproate sodium	Enzyme inhibition
	Decrease	Phenytoin, carbamazepine	Enzyme induction
Phenobarbital	Increase	Valproate sodium	Enzyme inhibition
	Decrease	Rifampicin	Enzyme induction
Phenytoin	Increase	Valproate sodium Chloramphenicol Isoniazid Disulfiram Fluconazole Flu vaccine Amiodarone Fluoxetine	Enzyme inhibition Mechanism unclear
	Decrease	Phenobarbital Rifampicin Carbamazepine Furosemide Acetazolamide	Enzyme induction Decreased responsiveness of renal tubules. Increased osteomalacia
Sodium valproate	Increase	Salicylates	Displacement from protein binding sites and possible enzyme inhibition
Topiramate	Decrease	Phenytoin, carbamazepine	Enzyme induction
	Decrease	Potential enzyme inducers	Enzyme induction
Zonisamide	Decrease	Carbamazepine, phenytoin, phenobarbital and primidone	Enzyme induction

Table 31.6 Side effect profile of antiepileptic drugs

Drug	Dose related (predictable)	Non-dose related (idiosyncratic)
Carbamazepine	Diplopia, drowsiness, headache, nausea, orofacial dyskinesia, arrhythmias	Photosensitivity, Stevens–Johnson syndrome, agranulocytosis, aplastic anaemia, hepatotoxicity
Clonazepam	Fatigue, drowsiness, ataxia	Rash, thrombocytopenia
Ethosuximide	Nausea, vomiting, drowsiness, headache, lethargy	Rash, erythema multiforme, Stevens–Johnson syndrome
Gabapentin	Drowsiness, diplopia, ataxia, headache	Not reported
Lacosamide	Nausea, vomiting, dizziness, headache, drowsiness, depression, diplopia (double vision), impaired memory, impaired coordination, tremor, fatigue (tiredness), asthenia (muscle weakness), pruritus (itching).	Not reported
Lamotrigine	Headaches, drowsiness, diplopia, ataxia	Liver failure, disseminated intravascular coagulation
Levetiracetam	Dizziness, drowsiness, irritability, behavioural problems, insomnia, ataxia (unsteadiness), tremor, headache, nausea	Not reported
Oxcarbazepine	Diplopia (double vision), ataxia (unsteadiness), headache, nausea, confusion and vomiting	Skin rash
Phenobarbital	Fatigue, listlessness, depression, poor memory, impotence	Maculopapular rash, exfoliation, hepatotoxicity hypocalcaemia, osteomalacia, folate deficiency
Phenytoin	Ataxia, nystagmus, drowsiness, gingival hyperplasia, hirsutism, diplopia, asterixis, orofacial dyskinesia, folate deficiency	Blood dyscrasias, rash, Dupuytren's contracture, hepatotoxicity
Sodium valproate	Dyspepsia, nausea, vomiting, hair loss, anorexia, drowsiness	Acute pancreatitis, aplastic anaemia, thrombocytopenia, hepatotoxicity
Tigabine		Dizziness, fatigue (tiredness), nervousness, tremor, concentration difficulties, depression of mood, agitation
Topiramate	Dizziness, drowsiness, nervousness, fatigue, weight loss	Not reported
Vigabatrin	Drowsiness, dizziness, weight gain	Behavioural disturbances, severe psychosis
Zonisamide	Ataxia, dizziness, somnolence, anorexia	Hypersensitivity, weight decrease, rash, gastro-intestinal problems

with partial or generalised seizures who have proved unresponsive to other antiepileptic medication. Its intermittent use in catamenial epilepsy has also been suggested. Clobazam may produce less sedation than other benzodiazepines, but otherwise its adverse effects are similar, including dizziness, behavioural disturbances and dry mouth. Withdrawal may be difficult.

Clonazepam

Clonazepam, a 1,4-benzodiazepine, is a second-line drug for generalised tonic clonic seizures, absences, myoclonic seizures and as adjunctive therapy for partial seizures but, as with clobazam, effectiveness often wears off with time as tolerance develops. Parenteral clonazepam is useful in status epilepticus. It has an adverse effect profile similar to that of clobazam, but may be more sedating.

Diazepam

Diazepam is used mainly in the treatment of status epilepticus, intravenously or in the acute management of febrile convulsions as a rectal solution. Absorption from suppositories or following intramuscular injection is slow and erratic. The rectal solution may also be useful in status epilepticus if it is not possible to give the drug intravenously.

Eslicarbazepine acetate

Eslicarbazepine acetate is a drug which is similar to oxcarbazepine and which is licensed as a second-line treatment for partial seizures. As with oxcarbazepine, its mode of action is thought to be by interacting with voltage-gated sodium channels. Currently it is only available in a 800-mg tablet. It has a long half-life and can be used once per day. Its pharmacokinetics profile and side effects are also similar to those of oxcarbazepine.

Ethosuximide

Ethosuximide is a drug of first choice for generalised absence seizures, and has no useful effect against any other seizure type. Tolerance does not seem to be a problem. The most commonly encountered adverse effects are gastro-intestinal symptoms, which occur frequently at the beginning of therapy. Behaviour disorders, anorexia, fatigue, sleep disturbances and headaches may also occur. The therapeutic range commonly quoted is 40–100 μcg/mL, but some patients may require higher concentrations, sometimes as high as 150 μcg/mL. The absorption of ethosuximide is complete, the bioavailability of the syrup and capsule formulations being equivalent. An increase in daily dose may lead to disproportionately higher increases in average serum concentrations; therefore, careful monitoring is indicated at high doses.

Felbamate

Felbamate may be used as a drug of last resort in people with intractable epilepsy. It is licensed in the USA and most countries of the European Union but not in the UK. Its mechanism of action is unknown. The usual dose is between 1200 and 3600 mg/day. Felbamate exhibits significant pharmacokinetic interactions with phenytoin, carbamazepine and valproic acid. Side effects of felbamate include diplopia, insomnia, dizziness, headache, ataxia, anorexia, nausea and vomiting. A major limiting problem is its potential to cause aplastic anaemia and liver failure, affecting up to 1 in 4000 patients exposed to the drug. It, therefore, seems prudent to limit use to specialist centres and severe intractable cases.

Gabapentin

Gabapentin is occasionally used as a second-line treatment of partial seizures. Although initially developed as an AED, its main use currently is for the treatment of neuropathic pain. In view of its pharmacokinetic profile, a three times daily dosage must be used. To date, no clinically significant interactions with other AEDs, or other drugs, have been reported. The most frequently reported side effects are drowsiness, dizziness, diplopia, ataxia and headache.

Lacosamide

Lacosamide, a functionalised amino acid, is a second-line drug for partial epilepsy in patients over the age of 16 years. Its putative mode of action is not shared with any other currently available AEDs. It is said to enhance the slow inactivation of sodium channels and to modulate collapsing response mediator protein-2 (CRMP-2), although it is not known how this contributes to its antiepileptic action. The recommended doses are between 200 and 400 mg/day divided in two doses. It should be started at 50–100 mg/day and increased by 50 mg/day every 1 or 2 weeks. No drug–drug interactions are known. Its commonest side effects are dizziness, headaches, nausea and diplopia. No idiosyncratic side effects have yet been associated with this drug. The drug should be used with caution in patients with a history of cardiac conduction problems as it is know to increase the PR interval in some patients.

Lamotrigine

Lamotrigine may be used as a first-line drug in patients with partial seizures, with or without secondary generalisation, and in tonic clonic convulsions. The recommended starting dose is 50 mg when used as monotherapy, and 25 mg when used as an add-on therapy; the latter dose is given on alternate days in patients receiving concomitant sodium valproate and daily in patients receiving other AEDs, with a maximum recommended dose of 400 mg/day in two divided doses. It should be slowly titrated as too rapid a titration may be associated with an increased incidence of skin rash. Lamotrigine does not seem to interact with other concomitantly administered AEDs. However, hepatic enzyme inducers increase the metabolism of lamotrigine, reducing its half-life. Therefore, higher doses of lamotrigine need to be administered if it is used in conjunction with enzyme inducers such as phenytoin and carbamazepine. Inhibitors of hepatic enzymes such as sodium valproate block the metabolism of lamotrigine and reduced doses of lamotrigine need to be used if both drugs are given in combination.

Headaches, drowsiness, ataxia and diplopia, usually transient, are the most commonly reported acute adverse effects, particularly during dose escalation. A skin rash is the commonest idiosyncratic side effect of lamotrigine and affects up to 3% of patients.

Levetiracetam

Levetiracetam is indicated for the treatment of refractory partial epilepsy. Placebo-controlled trials in refractory partial epilepsy have shown a 50% seizure reduction in up to 40% of patients. In these trials, 8% of participants became seizure free compared to none on placebo. The usual dose is between 1500 and 3000 mg a day. It is usually started at 500 mg a day and the dose titrated upwards in incremental steps of 500 mg every 1 or 2 weeks. It is well tolerated and the most frequent central nervous system adverse events are dizziness, irritability, asthenia and somnolence. No idiosyncratic adverse events have yet been reported.

Oxcarbazepine

Oxcarbazepine is an analogue of carbamazepine. It is an inactive pro-drug that is converted in the liver to the active 10-hydroxy metabolite and bypasses the 10,11-epoxide, the primary metabolite of carbamazepine. The usual dose is between 900 and 2400 mg/day. The spectrum of efficacy and side effects is broadly comparable to carbamazepine. The principal advantage of oxcarbazepine over carbamazepine is the lack of induction of hepatic enzymes, with the consequence that there is no auto-induction of the metabolism of the drug and fewer pharmacokinetic interactions. In addition, two-thirds of patients who are allergic to carbamazepine can tolerate oxcarbazepine.

Phenobarbital

Phenobarbital, a barbiturate, may be used for the treatment of tonic clonic, tonic and partial seizures. It may also be used in other seizure types. Its antiepileptic efficacy is similar to that of phenytoin or carbamazepine. Adverse effects on cognitive function, the propensity to produce tolerance and the risk of serious seizure exacerbation on withdrawal make it an unattractive option, and it should be used only as a last resort. In addition to cognitive effects, barbiturates may cause skin rashes, ataxia, folate deficiency, osteomalacia, behavioural disturbances (particularly in children) and an increased risk of connective tissue disorders such as Dupuytren's contracture and frozen shoulder. Phenobarbital is a potent enzyme inducer and is implicated in several clinically important drug interactions (see Table 31.5).

Phenytoin

In current practice, phenytoin is now a second-line drug for partial seizures, tonic clonic seizures as well atonic seizures and atypical absences. It is not effective in typical generalised absences and myoclonic seizures. Tolerance to its antiepileptic action does not usually occur. Phenytoin has non-linear kinetics and a low therapeutic index, and in some patients frequent drug serum level measurements may be necessary. Drug interactions (see Table 31.5) are common as phenytoin metabolism is very susceptible to inhibition by some drugs, while it may enhance the metabolism of others. Caution should be exercised when other medication is introduced or withdrawn.

Adverse events may occur in up to a half of patients treated with phenytoin, but only about 10% will necessitate drug withdrawal, most commonly due to skin rash. Dose-related adverse reactions including nystagmus, ataxia and lethargy are common. Cosmetic effects such as gum hypertrophy, hirsutism and acne are well-recognised adverse effects, and should be taken into account when prescribing for children and young women. Chronic adverse effects include folate deficiency, osteomalacia, Dupuytren's contractures and cerebellar atrophy. Serious idiosyncratic adverse events, including hepatic failure and bone marrow depression, are extremely uncommon.

Pregabalin

This drug has been licensed for the adjunctive treatment of refractory partial epilepsy. It is closely related to gabapentin and a structural analogue of the neurotransmitter GABA but does not seem to affect transmitter response. It modulates calcium channels by binding to a subunit of Ca^{2+} and this action is thought to be the basis of its antiepileptic mechanism. The recommended doses for pregabalin are between 150 and 600 mg divided into two doses, although some people may respond to doses outside this range. Pregabalin would normally be started at 50 or 75 mg twice daily and increased in incremental steps of 50 mg every 2 weeks up to 600 mg according to clinical need. Pregabalin is available in 25, 50, 75, 100, 150, 200 and 300 mg tablets.

Overall, pregabalin is well tolerated and so far no idiosyncratic side effects have been described. Dizziness, drowsiness, ataxia, tremor and diplopia are the most common side effects. Weight gain, particularly with higher doses, seems to be a chronic side effect of this medication. No pharmacokinetic interactions have yet been identified. In addition to its use in epilepsy, pregabalin has also been indicated for neuropathic pain and there are studies to suggest that it might be useful in generalised anxiety disorders.

Primidone

Primidone is principally metabolised to phenobarbital *in vivo* and has similar effects but a more severe side effect profile than phenobarbital. There is nothing to recommend primidone as an AED over phenobarbital.

Rufinamide

Rufinamide is licensed as an orphan drug for the adjunctive treatment of seizures in Lennox-Gastaut syndrome. It is a triazole derivative and is structurally unrelated to any other AED. Its mode of action is unknown. A serious hypersensitivity syndrome that may include rash, fever, lymphadenopathy, hepatic dysfunction, haematuria and multi-organ dysfunction has been reported upon initiation of therapy. Individuals should be warned to seek immediate medical assistance if signs or symptoms of hypersensitivity develop.

Sodium valproate

Sodium valproate is a drug of first choice for the treatment of generalised absence seizures, myoclonic seizures and generalised tonic clonic seizures, especially if these occur as part of the syndrome of primary generalised epilepsy. Tolerance to its anti-epileptic action does not usually occur. Drug interactions with other AEDs may be problematic. Phenobarbital levels increase following co-medication with valproate, and a combination of these two drugs may result in severe sedation. Sodium valproate may also inhibit the metabolism of lamotrigine, phenytoin and carbamazepine. Enzyme-inducing drugs enhance the metabolism of sodium valproate, so caution should be exercised when other AEDs are introduced or withdrawn.

Up to a third of patients may experience adverse effects, but fewer than 5% will require the drug to be stopped. Adverse effects include anorexia, nausea, diarrhoea, weight gain, alopecia, skin rash and thrombocytopenia. Confusion, stupor, tremor and hyper-ammonaemia are usually dose related. Serious adverse events, including fatal pancreatic and hepatic failure, are extremely uncommon. In children under 2 years, on other AEDs and with pre-existing neurological deficit, the risk of this is 1/500. In adults on valproate monotherapy, the risk is 1/37,000.

The usual therapeutic range quoted is 50–100 μcg/mL, although because of the lack of a good correlation between total valproate concentrations and effect, serum level monitoring of the drug has limited use. TDM should only be performed in cases of suspected toxicity, deterioration in seizure control, to check adherence or to monitor drug interactions. Routine monitoring of this drug is not necessary. Sodium valproate is more teratogenic than other commonly used AEDs and should be used cautiously in women of child-bearing age.

Stiripentol

Stiripentol is licensed as an orphan drug for severe myoclonic epilepsy of infancy (SMEI) when used in conjunction with sodium valproate and clobazam. It is an aromatic alcohol and is unrelated to any other AED. Its mode of action is unknown.

Tiagabine

Tiagabine is a drug with mild efficacy in seizure control. It is used as a second-line drug in partial seizures with or without secondary generalisation. The usual dose is between 30 and 45 mg a day, and it is normally started at 10 mg/day in two divided doses, with incremental steps of 5 mg every 2 weeks. The most common adverse events are on the central nervous system and consist of sedation, tremor, headache, mental slowing, tiredness and dizziness. Confusion, irritability and depression may occur. Increases in seizure frequency and episodes of non-convulsive status have also been reported.

So far, no life-threatening idiosyncratic reactions have been reported. Use in pregnancy is not recommended, although no teratogenicity has been reported in humans.

Topiramate

Topiramate is chemically unrelated to other AEDs and is used as a second-line drug for patients with partial seizures. Usual doses are between 200 and 600 mg/day. It has to be titrated slowly, and the recommended starting dose is 25 mg once daily, titrating upwards in 25 mg/day increments every 2 weeks up to 200 mg/day in two divided doses. After that the dose should be increased by 50 mg every 2 weeks until seizure control is achieved or side effects develop. It has no clinically significant interactions with other AEDs, although hepatic enzyme inducers accelerate its metabolism and topiramate doses need to be adjusted downwards if patients are coming off carbamazepine or phenytoin.

Side effects of topiramate include dizziness, drowsiness, nervousness, impaired concentration, paraesthesias, nephrolithiasis and fatigue. Patients starting topiramate should increase their fluid intake to reduce the risk of kidney stones. Weight loss is seen in up to 30% of patients receiving topiramate.

Vigabatrin

Vigabatrin is an inhibitor of GABA transaminase but because of a poor safety profile, it is a last resort drug for partial seizures. Vigabatrin may also be useful in West's syndrome, particularly if associated with tuberous sclerosis. Vigabatrin does not interact with other drugs apart from decreasing phenytoin levels, probably by blocking its absorption. The most common adverse events associated with vigabatrin are behavioural disturbances, ranging from agitation and confusion to frank psychosis and visual field defects. Other known adverse effects include drowsiness, headaches, ataxia, weight gain, depression and tremor. Careful monitoring for side effects, particularly ophthalmological, on initiation of therapy is essential. Routine TDM is not available for this drug.

Zonisamide

Zonisamide, a sulphonamide analogue which inhibits carbonic anhydrase, is a potent blocker of the spread of epileptic discharges. This effect is believed to be mediated through action at voltage-sensitive sodium channels.

It is used as a second-line drug for patients with partial seizures with or without secondary generalisation. Anecdotal reports of its efficacy in other seizure types, particularly myoclonic seizures, need to be formally tested. Recommended doses are between 200 and 500 mg/day, although some patients may derive benefit from doses outside this range. The recommended starting dose for most patients is 100 mg once daily, titrating upwards every 2 weeks in 100 mg/day increments until seizure control is achieved or side effects develop. Its long elimination half-life allows once-daily dosing.

Zonisamide does not affect levels of carbamazepine, barbiturates or valproate, but may increase the serum concentration of phenytoin by about 10–15%. Zonisamide metabolism is, however, induced by carbamazepine, barbiturates and phenytoin and higher zonisamide doses may be necessary during co-administration with these AEDs.

Side effects of zonisamide include dizziness, drowsiness, headaches, hyporexia, nausea and vomiting, weight loss, skin rashes, irritability, impaired concentration and fatigue. These are mostly transient and seem to be related to the dose and rate of titration. Nephrolithiasis has also been reported, particularly in caucasians. It is not recommended for women of child-bearing age as there are issues about its teratogenic potential (Table 31.7).

Evidence for clinical use of newer drugs

The evidence for the efficacy, tolerability, and safety of seven new AEDs (gabapentin, lamotrigine, topiramate, tiagabine, oxcarbazepine, levetiracetam and zonisamide) in the treatment

Table 31.7 Common therapeutic problems in epilepsy

Problem	Comment
Hepatic enzyme induction	Enzyme induction occurs with carbamazepine, phenytoin, phenobarbital, primidone and topiramate Interactions occur with a large number of drugs including oral contraceptives
Use of progesterone-only contraceptives with enzyme-inducing antiepileptic drug	Best avoided. If no acceptable alternative, patient should take at least double usual dose of progesterone-only pill
Use of combined oral contraceptive with enzyme-inducing antiepileptic drug	Preparations containing 50 µcg of oestrogen should be used
Continuation of antiepileptic drug during pregnancy	Ideally review before attempting pregnancy to determine if reducing or discontinuing treatment is possible
Use of phenytoin as monotherapy	Less frequently considered first-line monotherapy due to poor side effect profile, narrow therapeutic index and saturation pharmacokinetics
Prescribing of branded antiepileptic drugs	Debate continues about whether significant differences exist between generic and branded antiepileptic drugs

of children and adults with refractory partial and generalised epilepsies was assessed by French et al. (2004). All drugs demonstrated efficacy as add-on therapy in patients with refractory partial epilepsy. The relative efficacy of the various agents could not, however, be determined due to the differing populations and dose ranges employed in the various studies. The analysis did, however, show that for all drugs, efficacy and side effects increased with increasing dose. A slower titration of dosage improved tolerability and hence the guidance remains to start with a low dose and increase slowly until side effects occur. For efficacy it appears useful to push to maximal tolerated dose.

Wilby et al. (2005) evaluated the clinical effectiveness, tolerability and cost-effectiveness of gabapentin, lamotrigine, levetiracetam, oxcarbazepine, tiagabine, topiramate and vigabatrin for epilepsy in adults. They included randomised controlled trials (RCTs) and systematic reviews for the newer AEDs when used in the treatment of adults with newly diagnosed or refractory epilepsy and relevant comparator studies which employed older AEDs, other newer AEDs and placebo. The overall findings revealed the following:

- Minimal good-quality evidence exists to support the use of newer AEDs as part of monotherapy or adjunctive therapy over older AEDs, or to support the use of one new AED in preference to another.
- Data relating to clinical effectiveness, safety and tolerability failed to demonstrate consistent and statistically significant differences between the newer and older drugs. The exception being comparisons between newer adjunctive AEDs and placebo, where a significant difference favoured use of the newer AEDs.
- Newer AEDs used as monotherapy may be cost-effective for the treatment of patients who have experienced adverse events with older AEDs, who have failed to respond to the older drugs, or where such drugs are contraindicated.

- An integrated economic analysis suggested that newer AEDs used as adjunctive therapy were cost-effective when compared with continuing current treatment alone.

Case studies

Case 31.1

JB is a 31-year-old woman with a history of early morning myoclonic jerks starting at the age of 16. When she was 18 years old she had her first generalised tonic clonic convulsive seizure. A diagnosis of juvenile myoclonic epilepsy was made and she was started on sodium valproate 1200 mg a day which controlled her seizures.

At the age of 21 the patient had a healthy baby and experienced no problems with epilepsy control. Aged 22, she had her second pregnancy and delivered a healthy baby girl. Three weeks after delivery early morning myoclonic seizures returned. The dose of sodium valproate was increased to 1500 mg to control jerks. However, 6 months later she experienced a recurrence of her convulsive attacks with no clear precipitating factor. Sodium valproate was increased to 2000 mg a day. Early morning myoclonic seizures crept back and she had further convulsive seizures. Lamotrigine was started at 200 mg daily. She has been completely seizure-free for the last 2 years and is now driving again.

JB wants to discuss her medication with you and would like to stop treatment. She has no plans to increase her family.

Question

What advice would you give JB?

Answers

JB should be advised to continue on medication. She has juvenile myoclonic epilepsy, which tends to recur when medication is withdrawn. The patient has no intention of having further children and, therefore, pregnancy need not be a consideration in the choice of her continued drug therapy. She is generally well and hence it would be sensible to advise her to continue with the present regimen, as sodium valproate and lamotrigine have a synergistic effect in juvenile myoclonic epilepsy. If, however, she wants to reduce medication, then a slow decrease of valproate with optimisation of treatment with lamotrigine should be considered.

Case 31.2

Mr OB is a 44-year-old man who suffers from partial epilepsy. An MRI scan shows a choroid cyst on the right temporal lobe, bilateral hippocampal sclerosis and cerebral atrophy. Seizures take the form of complex partial attacks and at night secondary generalisations occur. He has had trials of treatment with every single drug in the book and almost every combination.

Six months ago, he was taking 225 mg of topiramate (could not tolerate more), 400 mg of phenytoin and 10 mg of clobazam each day. At this point levetiracetam was added and titrated up to 2000 mg a day. This led to a significant improvement in seizure control. Indeed, seizures have almost completely been abolished and he is only having occasional nocturnal events. He is, however, complaining of drowsiness and periods of unsteadiness.

Question

What treatment is appropriate for this patient?

Answer

Mr OB needs his drug regimen optimising. The decision should be made to reduce either the dose of topiramate or that of phenytoin. The consensus view is that phenytoin should probably be reduced first. However, this patient had a bad experience in the past when an attempt was made to discontinue phenytoin, at which time he had a significant increase in seizure frequency. It would, therefore, be more appropriate to discontinue topiramate in Mr OB. This was done and his improvement has been maintained.

Case 31.3

Ms GD is a 28-year-old woman with a history of early morning myoclonic jerks since age 14 years. At 16 years of age she presented with her first generalised tonic clonic convulsive seizure and was referred to a hospital specialist who diagnosed juvenile myoclonic epilepsy. At that time Ms GD was started on sodium valproate 1200 mg a day and within a few weeks her seizures were totally controlled. Ms GD has since remained on the same medication and has been well controlled. However, she now wishes to start a family and is concerned about the effects of the valproate on her baby.

Question

What advice would you give Ms GD?

Answer

The available evidence indicates sodium valproate is teratogenic, with the most common malformation reported being neural tube defects. Ms GD has had no seizures for over 5 years and it must, therefore, be determined whether she still needs medication. The risk of recurrence is low since she has been fit free for well over 5 years. An important consideration is whether or not she is a driver since if she is taken off medication and has a seizure, she will be unable to hold a licence. The other issue is the effect of pregnancy on her seizure threshold as there is some evidence that up to 20% of women may experience an increase in fits during pregnancy. The

options that need to be considered include change of medication. The following medicines need to be reviewed: lamotrigine, topiramate and levetiracetam.

Case 31.4

TD is a 41-year-old patient who has cryptogenic partial epilepsy. He experienced his first seizure at age 14 and this was diagnosed as a secondary generalised attack, although discussing his history revealed he might have had complex partial seizures. Two years ago TD was referred for assessment but it was felt that he was not a candidate for surgery. TD was taking carbamazepine 1200 mg a day and could not tolerate higher doses. Previous trials of valproate, phenytoin, phenobarbital, vigabatrin, lamotrigine, oxcarbazepine and topiramate had demonstrated little benefit. Levetiracetam was started and increased to 2500 mg. Improvement in seizure control has been noted over the past 2 years with only two nocturnal complex partial seizures recorded. His current medication is levetiracetam 2500 mg/day and carbamazepine 1200 mg/day.

Question

What should be done next? Should TD's therapy be reduced to levetiracetam monotherapy?

Answer

There is a need to discuss with TD whether he wishes to continue with his medication. Issues of relevance include a long history of epilepsy, the diagnosis and the range of drugs previously tried. It also needs to be clear whether he wishes to drive or not. If patients have been seizure free for 2 years, it is usual to review therapy.

Case 31.5

Mr FD is a 23-year-old student who was involved in a road traffic accident and admitted to hospital with a head trauma. He was stabilised but during his admission had a seizure and was then discharged on no medication. At 3 months he attends an out-patient hospital follow-up appointment and has had no further seizures.

Question

With regard to his clinical management was this appropriate; is there a role for prophylactic anticonvulsant medication?

Answer

Mr FD requires a full neurological review. The long-term use of antiepileptics following head injury is not indicated unless the patient has a history of seizures and Mr FD has had no seizures post-discharge.

Case 31.6

RA is a 75-year-old retired teacher who lives alone. He has long-standing epilepsy and his current medication includes phenytoin 300 mg daily. RA is in general good health but suffered a recent fall and was rushed to hospital with a suspected fractured neck of femur. On admission he was stabilised and found not to have sustained a fracture. His other medication included furosemide 40 mg mane and enalapril 5 mg twice daily. Routine blood levels of the anticonvulsants revealed a toxic level of phenytoin of 40 mg/L (normal therapeutic range 10–20 mg/L).

Question

How long will it take for the toxic levels of phenytoin to fall within the therapeutic range?

Answer

Phenytoin exhibits non-linear pharmacokinetics. Usual management will involve withholding phenytoin and monitoring serum levels each day. One assumption that can be made is that if the hepatic enzymes are fully saturated with phenytoin then at maximum metabolic capacity, approximately 10 mg/L of the drug will be eliminated each day. Initially, however, the drug will redistribute into serum so for the first few days phenytoin levels will fall slowly. It is usual for the levels to take 6–7 days to fall within the therapeutic range. Therapy will then need to be reviewed. On further investigation it was revealed the patient had a severe chest infection and was prescribed ciprofloxacin. His antibiotic regimen was completed 5 days ago. He was suffering from phenytoin toxicity which may have resulted in ataxia and contributed to his fall.

References

Berg, A.T., Berkovic, S.F., Brodie, M.J., et al., 2010. Revised terminology and concepts for organization of seizures and epilepsies: report of the ILAE commission on classification and terminology, 2005–2009. Epilepsia 51, 676–685.

Duncan, J.S., Sander, J.W., Sisodiya, S.M., et al., 2006. Adult epilepsy. Lancet 367, 1087–1100.

Feely, M., 1999. Drug treatment of epilepsy. Br. Med. J. 318, 106–109.

French, J.A., Kanner, A.M., Bautista, J., et al., 2004. Efficacy and tolerability of the new antiepileptic drugs, II: treatment of refractory epilepsy. Epilepsia 45, 410–423.

National Institute for Health and Clinical Excellence, 2004a. The epilepsies: the diagnosis and management of the epilepsies in adults and children in primary and secondary care. Clinical Guideline 20. NICE, London. Available at: http://www.nice.org.uk/page. aspx?o=CG020&c=cns.

National Institute for Health and Clinical Excellence, 2004b. New drugs for epilepsy in adults. Technology Appraisal 76. NICE, London. Available at: http://www.nice.org.uk/download. aspx?o=ta076guidance.

National Institute for Health and Clinical Excellence, 2004c. Newer drugs for epilepsy in children. Technology Appraisal 76. NICE, London. Available at: http://www.nice.org.uk/page. aspx?o=ta079guidance.

National Institute for Health and Clinical Excellence, 2009. Implementation uptake report: the epilepsies, the diagnosis and management of the epilepsies in adults and children in primary and secondary care. NICE, London. Available at: http://www.nice.org.uk/media/250/28/ImpUptakeReportCG20.pdf.

Sabers, A., Gram, L., 2000. Newer anticonvulsants: comparative review of drug interactions and adverse effects. Drugs 60, 23–33.

WHO, 2009. Epilepsy, Key Facts. Fact Sheet Number 999. Available at: http://www.who.int/mediacentre/factsheets/fs999/en/.

Wilby, J., Kainth, A., Hawkins, N., et al., 2005. Clinical effectiveness, tolerability and cost-effectiveness of newer drugs for epilepsy in adults: a systematic review and economic evaluation. Health Technology Assessment 9 (15). Available at: http://www.hta.ac.uk/1304.

Further reading

Brodie, M.J., Kwan, P., 2005. Epilepsy in elderly people. Br. Med. J. 331, 1317–1322.

Nair, D.R., Nair, R., O'Dyer, R. (Eds.), 2010. Epilepsy. Clinical Publishing, Oxford.

Shorvon, S.D. (Ed.), 2009. Epilepsy. Oxford University Press, Oxford.

Takahashi, K. (Ed.), 2008. Epilepsy Research Progress. Nova Science Publishers Inc. New York.

Tebb, Z., Tobias, J.D., 2006. New anticonvulsants – new adverse effects. South Med. J. 99, 375–379.

Parkinson's disease 32

D. J. Burn

Key points

- Parkinson's disease is the second most common neurodegenerative disease, affecting 1% of the population over the age of 65.
- Parkinson's disease is characterised by bradykinesia, rest tremor, rigidity and, later in the disease course, postural instability.
- Neuronal loss in the brainstem (substantia nigra) leads to a profound dopamine deficiency in the striatum. This provides the rationale for dopaminergic replacement therapies.
- Depression is common in Parkinson's disease. It is the major determinant of quality of life and is often missed. The depression of Parkinson's disease can be readily treated.
- Levodopa, coupled with a dopa-decarboxylase inhibitor, remains the most potent oral treatment for Parkinson's disease. There is debate as to whether levodopa should be deferred in biologically young patients, in an attempt to delay the onset of motor complications.
- Several other drug treatments are available for the management of Parkinson's disease. When given as adjunctive therapy to levodopa, the primary aim of these agents is to smooth out motor fluctuations.
- End-of-dose deterioration and the on–off phenomenon are motor complications synonymous with the use of levodopa, usually after a number of years. Despite advances in oral pharmacotherapy, the on–off phenomenon remains difficult to treat effectively.
- Surgical treatments of Parkinson's disease, using deep brain stimulation, are effective in highly selected cases.
- Advanced Parkinson's disease is difficult to manage, particularly dementia and neuropsychiatric problems. Reduction of dopaminergic therapy may be the best compromise. Rivastigmine may be useful for dementia associated with Parkinson's disease.

Parkinson's disease is the most common cause of Parkinsonism and is the second most common neurodegenerative disease, after Alzheimer's disease. Although descriptions of the condition appeared before the nineteenth century, it was James Parkinson's eloquent account in 1817 that fully documented the clinical features of the illness now bearing his name. The identification of dopamine deficiency in the brains of people with Parkinson's disease and the subsequent introduction of replacement therapy with levodopa represent a considerable success story in the treatment of neurodegenerative illness in general. There remain, however, a number of significant management problems in Parkinson's disease, particularly in the advanced stages of the condition.

Epidemiology

Parkinson's disease affects 1% of the population over 65 years of age, rising to 2% over the age of 80. One in 20 patients is, however, diagnosed before their 40th year. It is estimated that 110,000 people have Parkinson's disease in the UK. The condition is found worldwide, with variability in prevalence estimates most likely reflecting study methodology, rather than real differences. Most epidemiological studies have indicated a small male-to-female predominance.

Other causes of Parkinsonism include neurodegenerative conditions, multiple system atrophy and progressive supranuclear palsy. The prevalence for these conditions is approximately 5.0 per 100,000. Drug-induced Parkinsonism is a common form of so-called symptomatic Parkinsonism. It affects 10–15% of individuals exposed to dopamine receptor-blocking agents including neuroleptics and some labyrinthine sedatives.

Aetiology

Both genetic and environmental factors have been implicated as a cause of Parkinson's disease. While opinions were initially polarised, it now seems probable that in the majority of cases there is an admixture of influences, with environmental factors precipitating the onset of Parkinson's disease in a genetically susceptible individual.

Environmental factors became pre-eminent in the 1980s, when drug addicts attempting to manufacture pethidine accidently produced a toxin called MPTP (1-methyl-4-phenyl-1,2,3,6-tetrahydropyridine). Ingestion or inhalation of MPTP rapidly produced a severe Parkinsonian state, indistinguishable from advanced Parkinson's disease. Notably, not all individuals exposed to MPTP developed Parkinsonism, either acutely or on subsequent follow-up, suggesting inter-individual susceptibility to the toxic effects. MPTP is a relatively simple compound and is quite similar to paraquat. The more recent demonstration that chronic systemic exposure to the pesticide rotenone can reproduce the clinical and pathological features of Parkinson's disease in rats has generated considerable interest.

In a small number of patients, genetic factors are dominant. The discovery of a mutation in the gene coding for a synaptic protein called α-synuclein has provided tremendous impetus for further research. Such mutations have been described in fewer than 10 families worldwide. Nevertheless, because α-synuclein is a major component of the pathological hallmark of Parkinson's disease, the Lewy body (see below), the challenge is to discover how a mutation in this protein in a tiny minority can relate to the formation of Lewy bodies in the vast majority. In recent years, eight genetic loci and a further four genes (*parkin*, *DJ-1*, *PINK1* and *LRRK-2*) have been identified (Healy et al., 2004). The intriguing thing is that the protein products of these genes are involved in a cellular system called the ubiquitin-proteasome system, which plays a crucial role in removing and recycling abnormal or damaged proteins. Current thinking is that abnormalities in the way in which the cell handles mutated or abnormal proteins may ultimately lead to its death, through increased oxidative stress and/or reduced mitochondrial energy production. The Lewy body may actually represent a defence mechanism by the cell to 'parcel up' potentially damaging proteinaceous material (Olanow et al., 2004).

More recently, cell-to-cell transfer of α-synuclein has been demonstrated *in vitro* and also in engrafted stem cell tissue. This suggests that the pathology of Parkinson's disease may be propagated between neurones and could have major implications for the spread of Lewy body pathology within the brain, as well as its treatment (Olanow and Prusiner, 2009) (Fig. 32.1).

Pathophysiology

The characteristic pathological features of Parkinson's disease are neuronal loss in pigmented brainstem nuclei, together with the presence of eosinophilic inclusion bodies, called Lewy bodies, in surviving cells. The pars compacta of the substantia nigra in the midbrain is particularly affected. Dopaminergic neurones within this nucleus project to the striatum, which is, therefore, deprived of the neurotransmitter dopamine. In Parkinson's disease, there is a loss of

over 80% of nigral neurones before symptoms appear. The 'Braak hypothesis' has been proposed to account for spread of pathology within the Parkinsonian brain and suggests that α-synuclein may first accumulate in the lower brainstem and then gradually ascend rostrally to affect critical brain regions including the substantia nigra and ultimately the cerebral cortex (Braak et al., 2003).

Dopaminergic neurones are not the only cells to die within the brainstem, and a plethora of other nuclei and neurotransmitter systems are also involved. For example, cholinergic neurones within the pedunculopontine nucleus degenerate, providing potential clinicopathological correlates with postural instability, swallowing difficulty (dysphagia) and sleep disturbance (REM sleep behavioural disturbance). The involvement of this nucleus in Parkinson's disease may explain why dopaminergic therapy is relatively ineffective in treating these particular clinical problems. Within the striatum, changes occur within γ-aminobutyric acid-containing neurones, as a consequence of nigrostriatal dopaminergic deficiency and also non-physiological dopaminergic replacement. These changes are thought to play a key role in mediating the development of involuntary movements (dyskinesias) which develop after a number of years of levodopa treatment. The loss of noradrenergic and serotonergic neurones within the locus coeruleus and the raphé nucleus, respectively, may provide a pathophysiological basis for depression, which is common in Parkinson's disease.

Clinical features

Motor features

Bradykinesia is a sine qua non for Parkinsonism in general. If a person does not have slowness of movement, they cannot have either Parkinsonism or Parkinson's disease. Rest tremor, extrapyramidal rigidity (so-called lead pipe and/or cog-wheel) and postural instability comprise the remaining classic tetrad of clinical features for Parkinson's disease. Asymmetry of signs at disease onset is very common. The rest tremor is a rhythmic movement with a frequency of 4–6 Hz (cycles/s), typically noticed with the patient at rest. It is sometimes described as 'pill-rolling' in nature, from the movement of the thumb across the fingers. However, 15–20% of patients do not develop a tremor. Further, up to 60% of people with Parkinson's disease may have a dominant postural tremor, worse with the arms held outstretched, which can cause diagnostic confusion with essential tremor (see below). Postural instability is a late feature of Parkinson's disease and comprises an impairment of righting reflexes with a tendency to fall. There may be a flexed truncal posture and loss of arm swing when walking. There is reduced blink frequency and facial expression, which, together with rather reduced volume (hypophonic) and monotonous speech, may lead to significant difficulties in communication. Writing becomes small (micrographia) and barely legible.

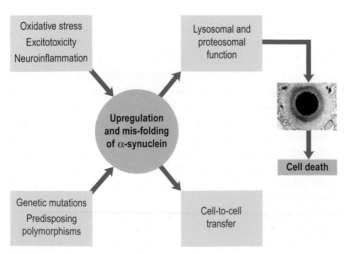

Fig. 32.1 Summary of pathophysiological processes believed to be central to Parkinson's disease.

Non-motor features

Autonomic dysfunction may occur in Parkinson's disease. The patient may drool and have greasy skin (seborrhoea). Urogenital difficulties, with erectile dysfunction in males and urinary urgency in both sexes, are commonly encountered. Frank incontinence is, however, rare. Constipation is invariable and is multifactorial in origin. Falling blood pressure on standing (postural hypotension) may contribute to falls later in the disease course. Depression affects approximately 40% of people with Parkinson's disease and is a major determinant of both carer stress and nursing home placement. It can be a very early feature, and may precede the onset, of Parkinson's disease. Recent studies have demonstrated that depression, above any other factor, is the most significant determinant of quality of life in the person with Parkinson's disease, yet it is generally underdiagnosed. The occurrence of dementia in Parkinson's disease is related predominantly to the age of the patient. Longitudinal community-based studies indicate that dementia may ultimately develop in 80% of people with Parkinson's disease. The cognitive impairment may be accompanied by hallucinations that are often visual, delusional misinterpretation, including paranoid ideation, and rapid fluctuations in attention.

Differential diagnosis

It is important to remember that, while Parkinson's disease is a common form of Parkinsonism, there are numerous other degenerative and symptomatic causes. Further, 'all that shakes is not Parkinson's disease'. Table 32.1 gives a differential diagnosis for causes of Parkinsonism. These are separated into degenerative and symptomatic categories. The list is not exhaustive and excludes, for instance, rare Parkinsonian manifestations in uncommon diseases. A detailed description of these different causes of Parkinsonism is beyond the scope of this chapter, but a few points should be highlighted. Essential tremor is not included in Table 32.1, as this common condition does not cause bradykinesia. Nevertheless, it may be very difficult to differentiate from tremor-dominant Parkinson's disease. A positive family history and good response to alcohol may provide vital clues towards the diagnosis of essential tremor, although in practice these are not always reliable.

Several clinical and clinicopathological series have confirmed our fallibility in not making a correct diagnosis of Parkinson's disease. If clinical criteria, such as those produced by the UK Parkinson's Disease Brain Bank, are not applied, then the error rate (false-negative diagnosis) may be as high

as 25–30%. These criteria are listed in Box 32.1. Degenerative conditions commonly masquerading as Parkinson's disease include progressive supranuclear palsy, multiple system atrophy and Alzheimer's disease.

Drug-Induced Parkinsonism

Perhaps the most important differential diagnosis to consider when a patient presents with Parkinsonism is whether their symptoms and signs may be drug induced. This is because drug-induced Parkinsonism is potentially reversible upon cessation of the offending agent. Reports linking drug-induced Parkinsonism with the neuroleptic chlorpromazine were first published in the 1950s. Since then, numerous other agents have been associated with drug-induced Parkinsonism. Many of these are widely recognised, although others are not (Box 32.2). Compound antidepressants were a problem in the past because they contained neuroleptic drugs. For example, fluphenazine was found with nortriptyline in Motival® (discontinued in the UK in 2006) and often overlooked as a potential culprit. Repeat prescription of vestibular sedatives and anti-emetics

---

Box 32.1 Clinical criteria for diagnosis of Parkinson's disease

Step 1 Diagnosis of Parkinsonian syndrome
The patient has bradykinesia, plus one or more of the following:
(a) classic rest tremor
(b) muscular rigidity
(c) postural instability, without other explanation

Step 2 Exclusion criteria for Parkinson's disease
(a) history of repeated strokes
(b) history of repeated head injury
(c) history of definite encephalitis
(d) oculogyric crises
(e) dopamine receptor blocking agent exposure at onset of symptoms
(f) more than one affected relative
(g) sustained remission
(h) strictly unilateral features after 3 years
(i) supranuclear gaze palsy
(j) cerebellar signs
(k) early severe autonomic involvement
(l) early severe dementia
(m) extensor plantar
(n) cerebral tumour or hydrocephalus on CT
(o) negative response to large doses of levodopa
(p) MPTP exposure

Step 3 Supportive prospective positive criteria for Parkinson's disease (three or more required for diagnosis of definite Parkinson's disease)
(a) unilateral onset
(b) rest tremor present
(c) progressive disorder
(d) progressive persistent asymmetry
(e) an excellent (>70%) response to levodopa
(f) a sustained (>5 years) response to levodopa
(g) severe levodopa-induced dyskinesias
(h) clinical course >10 years

CT, computed tomography.

Table 32.1 Differential diagnosis of Parkinsonism

Degenerative causes	Symptomatic causes
Parkinson's disease	Dopamine receptor blocking agents

Box 32.2 Examples of non-neuroleptic drugs associated with drug-induced Parkinsonism

Sodium valproate
Tetrabenazine
Calcium channel blockers (e.g. cinnarizine)
Amiodarone
Lithium[a]
Phenelzine[b]
Amphotericin B[c]
5-Fluorouracil[b]
Vincristine–adriamycin[b]
Pethidine[b]

[a]Lithium causes postural tremor. Reports of Parkinsonism occurring with lithium have usually been in the context of prior exposure to neuroleptics.

[b]Only single case reports of drug-induced Parkinsonism with these drugs.

[c]One case report of drug-induced Parkinsonism in a child after bone marrow transplantation and a second in association with cytosine arabinoside therapy.

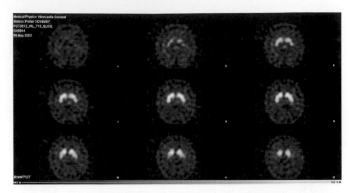

Fig. 32.2 A normal FP-CIT SPECT scan image, showing symmetric tracer uptake in both striata (mirror image commas). In Parkinson's disease, the tail of the comma is lost at an early stage, with the most severe loss being contralateral to the side most affected clinically.

such as prochlorperazine and cinnarizine are other commonly encountered causes of drug-induced Parkinsonism. The pathogenesis of drug-induced Parkinsonism is unlikely to be only due to dopamine receptor blockade. If this were the case, the incidence and severity should correlate with the drug dosage and length of exposure, and this is not clearly observed. Sodium valproate is also now recognised to cause an encephalopathy dominated by Parkinsonism and cognitive impairment which is reversible upon drug cessation. Again, there is considerable idiosyncrasy in who develops this encephalopathy when exposed to valproate.

Drug-induced Parkinsonism is more common in the elderly and in women. The clinical features can be indistinguishable from Parkinson's disease, although the signs in drug-induced Parkinsonism are more likely to be bilateral at the onset. Withdrawal of the offending agent will lead to improvement and resolution of symptoms and signs in approximately 80% of patients within 8 weeks of discontinuation. Drug-induced Parkinsonism may, however, take up to 18 months to fully resolve in some cases. Further, in other patients, the Parkinsonism may improve after stopping the drug, only to then deteriorate. In this situation, the drug may have unmasked previously latent Parkinson's disease. This contention is supported by a study which noted an increased risk of Parkinson's disease in subjects who had experienced a previous reversible episode of drug-induced Parkinsonism.

Investigations

The diagnosis of Parkinson's disease is a clinical one and should be based, preferably, upon validated criteria. In young-onset or clinically atypical Parkinson's disease, a number of investigations may be appropriate. These include copper studies and DNA testing to exclude Wilson's disease and Huntington's

disease, respectively. Brain imaging by computed tomography (CT) or magnetic resonance imaging (MRI) may be necessary to exclude hydrocephalus, cerebrovascular disease or basal ganglia abnormalities suggestive of an underlying metabolic cause. When there is difficulty in distinguishing Parkinson's disease from essential tremor, a form of functional imaging called FP-CIT SPECT (also known as *DaTSCAN*) may be useful, as this technique can sensitively identify loss of nigrostriatal dopaminergic terminals in the striatum (Fig. 32.2). Thus, in essential tremor, the SPECT scan is normal, whereas in Parkinson's disease, reduced tracer uptake is seen (Jennings et al., 2004).

Differentiating Parkinson's disease from multiple system atrophy and progressive supranuclear palsy is a not uncommon clinical problem and may be very difficult, particularly in the early disease stages. FP-CIT SPECT cannot differentiate Parkinson's disease from these other forms of degenerative Parkinsonism. MRI brain scanning, anal sphincter electromyography, tilt table testing for orthostatic hypotension and eye movement recordings may all be of some help, although they are rarely diagnostic in their own right.

Treatment

General approach

When treatment becomes necessary, it is impossible to generalise about which drug should be commenced. All currently available drugs for Parkinson's disease are symptomatic, as no agent has yet been shown, beyond reasonable doubt, to have disease-modifying or neuroprotective properties. There is no accepted algorithm for the treatment of Parkinson's disease, although a clinical management guideline has been produced (NICE, 2006).

A number of factors, including patient preference, age, severity and type of disease (tremor-dominant versus bradykinesia-dominant) and co-morbidity, need to be taken into account. The efficacy and tolerability of levodopa in Parkinson's disease was first described 1967, when the drug was started in low doses and gradually increased thereafter (Cotzias et al., 1967).

Unfortunately, despite dramatic initial benefits, the limitations of levodopa treatment were quickly realised and a phenomenon termed the 'long-term levodopa syndrome' was recognised. This syndrome comprises premature wearing off of the anti-Parkinsonian effects of levodopa, and response fluctuations. The wearing-off effect is the time before a patient is due their next dose of medication, during which they become increasingly bradykinetic. Response fluctuations can include dramatic swings between gross involuntary movements (dyskinesias) and a frozen, immobile state. The rapid and sudden switching between the dyskinetic state and profound akinesia is also termed the 'on–off' phenomenon. If this occurs rapidly and repeatedly, the term 'yo-yo-ing' is sometimes used. These problems emerge at a rate of approximately 10% per year, so that by 10 years into their illness all Parkinson's disease patients can expect to experience such unpredictable responses. Notably, however, levodopa-induced dyskinesias and fluctuations develop earlier in younger Parkinson's disease patients than in older patients. On–off episodes may be extremely disabling and remain a major therapeutic challenge in the management of Parkinson's disease.

Current management trends have, therefore, shifted towards either later administration of levodopa, provided alternative treatments can give adequate symptomatic control, or the use of combination therapies, in an effort to reduce the cumulative dose of levodopa given. The benefit for such 'levodopa-sparing' strategies beyond 5 years into the illness remains a matter of debate.

Drug treatment

Levodopa preparations

Immediate-release levodopa. Irrespective of the debate regarding early or late levodopa therapy, there is no doubt that levodopa remains the most effective oral symptomatic treatment for Parkinson's disease. It is administered with the peripheral dopa-decarboxylase inhibitors carbidopa or benserazide, where carbidopa plus levodopa is known as co-careldopa (Sinemet®) and benserazide plus levodopa is co-beneldopa (Madopar®). The decarboxylase inhibitor blocks the peripheral conversion of levodopa to dopamine and thereby allows a lower dose of levodopa to be administered. Levodopa readily crosses the blood–brain barrier and is converted by endogenous aromatic amino acid decarboxylase to dopamine and then stored in surviving nigrostriatal nerve terminals.

Immediate-release levodopa is usually commenced in a dose of 50 mg/day, increasing every 3–4 days until a dose of 50 mg three times daily is reached. The patient should be instructed in the early stage of the illness to take the drug with food to minimise nausea. Paradoxically, in more advanced Parkinson's disease, it may be beneficial to take levodopa 30 min or so before food, as dietary protein can critically interfere with the absorption of the drug. If there is little or no response to 50 mg three times daily, the unit dose may be doubled to 100 mg. Should the patient's levodopa dose escalate to 600 mg/day with no significant response, the diagnosis of Parkinson's disease should be reviewed. Levodopa, commenced in the above way, is usually well tolerated. Nausea, vomiting and orthostatic hypotension are the most commonly encountered side effects. These adverse events may be circumvented by increasing the levodopa dose even more slowly, or co-prescribing domperidone 10 or 20 mg three times daily. Later in the illness, and in common with all anti-Parkinsonian drugs, levodopa may cause vivid dreams, nightmares or even a toxic confusional state.

Clinically relevant drug interactions with levodopa include hypertensive crises with monoamine oxidase type A inhibitors. Levodopa should, therefore, be avoided for at least 2 weeks after stopping the inhibitor. Levodopa can also enhance the hypotensive effects of antihypertensive agents and may antagonise the action of antipsychotics. The absorption of levodopa may be reduced by concomitant administration of oral iron preparations.

Controlled-release levodopa. Both Sinemet® and Madopar® are available as controlled-release (CR) preparations. The nomenclature for Sinemet CR® is confusing, as the drug is marketed as Sinemet CR® (carbidopa/levodopa 50/200) and also as Half Sinemet CR® (carbidopa/levodopa 25/100). Trying to prescribe Half Sinemet CR® unambiguously can be difficult. If the instruction is misinterpreted and a tablet of Sinemet CR® is halved, the slow-release mechanism is actually disrupted.

Levodopa in controlled release preparations has a bioavailability of 60–70%, which is less than the 90–100% obtained from immediate-release formulations. Controlled release preparations have a response duration of 2–4 h, compared with 1–3 h for immediate release.

Two large studies in early Parkinson's disease over 5 years have not shown any benefit for controlled release use over immediate-release levodopa in terms of dyskinesias and response fluctuation frequency. However, controlled release preparations may be of help in simplifying drug regimens, in relieving nocturnal akinesia, and in co-prescribing with immediate-release levodopa during the day to relieve end-of-dose deterioration.

Two commonly encountered problems with controlled release preparations are, first, changing the patient from all immediate release to all controlled release levodopa. This is poorly tolerated, as controlled release levodopa has a longer latency than immediate-release levodopa to turn the patient 'on' (typically 60–90 vs. 30–50 min), and the patient's perception is that the quality of their 'on' period is poorer. Second, controlled release preparations should not be prescribed more than four times a day, as the levodopa may accumulate, causing unpredictable motor fluctuations.

Co-careldopa intestinal gel. An intestinal gel preparation of levodopa and carbidopa (Duodopa®) is available that is administered directly into the small bowel (specifically, the jejunum) via a percutaneous route, using a portable electronic pump. Through continuous delivery in this way, motor fluctuations may be significantly reduced. Although effective, this treatment modality requires careful patient selection. The endoscopic insertion of a percutaneous jejunostomy carries a definite morbidity and mortality. The treatment is also very expensive while mechanical problems with tube detachment and blockage have been reported.

Dopamine agonists

In theory, dopamine agonists, which stimulate dopamine receptors both post- and presynaptically, would seem to be a very attractive therapeutic option in Parkinson's disease, as they may bypass the degenerating nigrostriatal dopaminergic neurones. Unfortunately, experience to date with the oral agents available has usually shown them to be less potent than levodopa and less well tolerated. One drug in this class, apomorphine, is used in a parenteral form. It is particularly potent and is described in detail below.

Dopamine agonists differ in their affinity for a number of receptors, including the dopamine receptor family. It is not known whether these differences are clinically significant, but experience to date would suggest not. Cabergoline is an ergot dopamine agonist with a much longer plasma half-life of 63–68 h than other agents in this class. This means that once-daily dosing is possible. Ropinirole and pramipexole are non-ergot derivatives that originally had to be administered three times daily. Slow release preparations of ropinirole (XL) and pramipexole (PR) are now available for once-daily dosing. A transdermally administered non-ergot dopamine agonist, rotigotine, is also available as a 24-h adhesive patch.

Four double-blind, randomised and controlled studies of up to 5 years duration have compared the use of a dopamine agonist (cabergoline, ropinirole, pramipexole and pergolide) with levodopa in the treatment of early Parkinson's disease. Although the studies differed in a number of ways, such as levodopa supplementation not being permitted in the pergolide study, the results produced a consistent message that use of dopamine agonists in early Parkinson's disease is associated with a lower incidence of dyskinesias when compared with levodopa. Supplementary levodopa was, however, required in a significant number of patients in the cabergoline (65% of patients initially randomised to cabergoline), ropinirole (66% of patients initially randomised to ropinirole) and pramipexole (53% of patients initially randomised to pramipexole) studies, suggesting that only a subgroup of patients derive adequate benefit from agonist monotherapy alone. Follow-up studies suggest that the addition of levodopa is required in the vast majority of patients and that any initial benefits in terms of lower dyskinesia incidence on agonist alone may be lost when levodopa is then introduced.

There have been very few comparative studies performed between the dopamine agonists, so it is not possible to be definitive as to which drug should be recommended. In practice, it is often worth changing from one agonist to another if side effects are a problem, since there is variability in a given patient's tolerance to the different drugs.

Dopamine agonist side effects. The principal side effect of the dopamine agonists are nausea and vomiting, postural hypotension, hallucinations and confusion, and exacerbation of dyskinesias. Ergot derivatives run the risk of causing pleuropulmonary fibrosis, which occurs in 2–6% of patients on long-term bromocriptine treatment. Annual monitoring with chest X-ray and erythrocyte sedimentation rate (ESR) has been suggested for patients taking ergot derivative agonists, although the utility and cost-effectiveness of this recommendation have not been established. More recently, concern has been expressed over the high frequency of cardiac valvulopathy, notably of the tricuspid valve, found in patients exposed to the ergot derivatives pergolide and cabergoline. Neither drug should be used as first-line agonists in Parkinson's disease. If prescribed, regular echocardiographic monitoring should be undertaken. There is also an increased risk of toxicity when erythromycin is co-prescribed with a dopamine agonist.

Ropinirole and pramipexole were previously implicated in causing 'sleep attacks', with sudden onset of drowsiness, leading to driving accidents in some cases. The term 'sleep attack' is almost certainly a misnomer, however, as patients do have warning of impending sleepiness, although they may subsequently be amnesic for up to several minutes while in this state. Excessive sleepiness attributable to anti-Parkinsonian drugs is actually not a new phenomenon and is almost certainly a 'class effect' of all dopaminergic therapies. It is essential to advise patients taking all anti-Parkinsonian agents that they may be prone to excessive drowsiness. This may be compounded by the use of other sedative drugs and alcohol.

Dopamine agonists have also been associated with impulse control disorders (ICDs). These disorders include pathological gambling, hypersexuality and excessive shopping. The onset may relate to dopamine D2/3 receptor stimulation in predisposed individuals. The patient and their carer should be warned about these potential problems before the drug is prescribed and regularly screened for abnormal behaviours while taking the agonist.

Catechol-O-methyl transferase inhibitors

Inhibitors of the enzyme catechol-O-methyl transferase (COMT) represent a novel addition to the range of therapies available for Parkinson's disease (Schrag, 2005). Use of the first agent in this class, tolcapone, was originally suspended in Europe because of fears over hepatotoxicity, although the drug became available again in 2005, accompanied by strict prescribing and monitoring guidelines. Entacapone is also available and studies have not shown derangement of liver function with this drug.

COMT itself is a ubiquitous enzyme, found in gut, liver, kidney and brain among other sites. In theory, COMT inhibition may occur both centrally, where the degradation of dopamine to homovanillic acid is inhibited, and peripherally, where conversion of levodopa to the inert 3-O-methyldopa is inhibited, to benefit the patient with Parkinson's disease. In practice, both tolcapone and entacapone act primarily as peripheral COMT inhibitors.

Placebo-controlled studies in patients with fluctuating Parkinson's disease have confirmed the efficacy of entacapone in decreasing 'off' time and permitting a concomitant reduction in levodopa dose. A 20% reduction in 'off' time is reported, translating into nearly 1.5 h less immobility per day. This reduction tends to occur towards the end of the day, a time when many Parkinson's disease patients are at their worst in terms of motor function. A comparison of entacapone and tolcapone suggested that tolcapone may be the more potent COMT inhibitor, achieving up to an extra 1.5 h of 'on' time per day.

When entacapone is prescribed, a 200 mg dose is used with each dose of levodopa administered, up to a frequency of 10 doses/day. Because of increased dyskinesias, an overall reduction of 10–30% in the daily dose of levodopa may be anticipated. Entacapone can be employed with any other anti-Parkinsonian drug, although caution may be needed with apomorphine. More recently, entacapone has been marketed as a compound tablet with levodopa and carbidopa (Stalevo®). Although each tablet contains 200 mg of the COMT inhibitor, there are six different doses of levodopa available (50, 75, 100, 125, 150 and 200 mg), to provide flexibility. The compound tablet may help adherence by significantly reducing the total daily number of tablets a patient needs to take.

Tolcapone is prescribed as a fixed 100 mg three times a day regimen, increasing if necessary to 200 mg three times a day. It may only be used after the patient has tried and failed entacapone and where provision for 2-weekly monitoring of liver function tests for the first 12 months, reducing in frequency thereafter, is available. Again, a concomitant reduction in levodopa may be necessary to offset an increase in dyskinesias.

The optimal way to use COMT inhibition is unknown. A patient experiencing end-of-dose deterioration, or generally underdosed, would seem to be the ideal candidate. However, there are few comparative studies of COMT inhibitors versus dopamine agonists available to provide guidance as to which class of drug is best to use, and when. The STRIDE-PD study (Stocchi et al., 2010) assessed the potential benefit of combined treatment with levodopa and entacapone in *de novo* Parkinson's disease patients to address whether this combined treatment was associated with a lower incidence of dyskinesias. Unfortunately, the opposite was actually found, with a higher incidence of dyskinesias in patients randomised to levodopa and entacapone compared with levodopa alone.

Other than exacerbation of dyskinesias, COMT inhibitors may also cause diarrhoea, abdominal pain and dryness of the mouth. Urine discolouration is reported in approximately 8% of patients taking entacapone.

It is best to avoid non-selective monoamine oxidase inhibitors or a daily dose of selegiline in excess of 10 mg when using entacapone. In addition, the co-prescribing of venlafaxine and other noradrenaline (norepinephrine) reuptake inhibitors is best avoided. Entacapone may potentiate the action of apomorphine. Patients taking iron preparations should be advised to separate this medication and entacapone by at least 2 h.

Monoamine oxidase type B inhibitors

The propargylamines selegiline and rasagiline are inhibitors of monoamine oxidase type B. Inhibition of this enzyme slows the breakdown of dopamine in the striatum. These agents effectively have a 'levodopa-sparing' effect and may delay the onset of, or reduce existing, motor complications. Both drugs may also have an antiapoptotic effect (apoptosis is a form of programmed cell death thought to be important in several neurodegenerative conditions, including Parkinson's disease). Whether or not the drugs have a neuroprotective effect by this or some other means remains controversial. A recent study suggested that 1 mg of rasagiline may have a disease-modifying benefit in early Parkinson's disease, although this study was difficult to interpret since the same effect was not seen with the 2 mg dose (Olanow et al., 2009). Further, the magnitude of effect was very modest and of uncertain clinical relevance. The findings, therefore, need to be interpreted with caution but do offer some cause for optimism.

A single daily dose of 5 or 10 mg of selegiline is prescribed. Higher doses are associated with only minimal additional inhibition of monoamine oxidase. Selegiline may also be administered as a lyophilised freeze-dried buccal preparation. The dose of rasagiline is 1 mg daily.

Both selegiline and rasagiline may be used as *de novo* or adjunctive treatments in Parkinson's disease, although trial data for the latter indication are strongest for rasagiline and buccal selegiline.

Following publication of a study (Lees, 1995) which showed excess mortality in a group of patients taking selegiline, it was suggested that the drug was best avoided in patients with falls, confusion and postural hypotension. A subsequent meta-analysis, including nine trials of selegiline, did not, however, identify any excess mortality in patients taking selegiline (Ives et al., 2004). Selegiline can cause hallucinations and confusion, particularly in moderate-to-advanced disease. The withdrawal of selegiline may then be associated with significant deterioration in motor function. Unlike selegiline, rasagiline is not metabolised to amfetamine-like products, so neuropsychiatric side effects are less frequent. Selegiline should not be co-prescribed with selective serotonin reuptake inhibitors, as a serotonin syndrome, including hypertension and neuropsychiatric features, has been reported in a small minority of cases. Caution is also required for rasagiline when co-prescribing with a selective serotonin reuptake inhibitor.

Amantadine

Amantadine was introduced as an anti-Parkinsonian treatment in the late 1960s. It has a number of possible modes of action, including facilitation of presynaptic dopamine release, blocking dopamine reuptake, an anticholinergic effect, and also as a *N*-methyl-D-aspartate (NMDA) receptor antagonist. Initially employed in the early stages of treatment, where its effects are mild and relatively short-lived, interest has focused more recently upon the use of amantadine as an antidyskinetic agent in advanced disease (Blanchet et al., 2003).

Daily doses of 100–300 mg amantadine may be used. Some recommend even higher doses for improved antidyskinetic effect, although side effects become much more frequent at higher doses. These side effects include a toxic confusional state, peripheral oedema and livedo reticularis (a persistent patchy reddish-blue mottling of the legs, and occasionally the arms). There may be significant rebound worsening of Parkinsonism when amantadine is withdrawn. The mechanism for this is unknown.

Anticholinergic drugs

The availability of anticholinergic drugs such as trihexyphenidyl and orphenadrine predated the introduction of levodopa by nearly 90 years. Anticholinergic drugs have a moderate effect in reducing tremor but do not have any significant benefit upon bradykinesia.

The use of anticholinergic agents has declined because of troublesome side effects, including constipation, urinary retention, cognitive impairment and toxic confusional states. In selected younger patients, an anticholinergic drug may still be helpful but close monitoring is advised. Postmortem studies have suggested that long-term anticholinergic use may have adverse disease-modifying effects in Parkinson's disease, by increasing cortical levels of Alzheimer-type pathology (Perry et al., 2003).

Tricyclic antidepressants have anticholinergic properties, normally regarded as a disadvantage in the treatment of depression. These drugs are generally longer acting than other anticholinergic agents and may have a potential benefit in Parkinson's disease, both for their anticholinergic effects and also their effect in inhibiting monoamine reuptake at adrenergic nerve endings. A low dose of a tricyclic antidepressant, for example, amitriptyline 10–25 mg, at night is sometimes useful in alleviating nocturnal akinesia, improving sleep and improving performance early in the morning.

Apomorphine

Apomorphine is a specialised, but almost certainly underused, drug in the treatment of Parkinson's disease. It is the most potent dopamine agonist available and is administered either by bolus subcutaneous injection or by continuous subcutaneous infusion. The drug is acidic and is generally difficult to administer in a stable form which does not lead to irritation of skin or mucosal surfaces. Alternative methods of administration, including transdermal and intranasal routes and the use of an implantable copolymer-based apomorphine matrix, are being evaluated.

The drug produces a reliable 'on' effect with short latency of action. A single bolus lasts for up to 60 min, depending upon the dose given. Continuous subcutaneous apomorphine may significantly improve dyskinesias in advanced Parkinson's disease, as well as lessening akinesia and rigidity. This may allow oral anti-Parkinsonian medications to be reduced.

Apomorphine causes profound nausea, vomiting and orthostatic hypotension. These problems are counteracted by pre-dosing for 2–3 days with domperidone 20 mg three times daily. Neuropsychiatric disturbance, probably at a lower frequency than with oral agonists, and skin reactions, including nodule formation, are other potential side effects. Apomorphine, in conjunction with levodopa, may cause a Coomb's positive haemolytic anaemia, which is reversible. It is recommended that patients be screened before beginning treatment and at 6-monthly intervals thereafter.

Surgical treatment

There has been renewed interest in the use of neurosurgical techniques for the treatment of Parkinson's disease (Walter and Vitek, 2004). This has resulted not only from recognition of the shortcomings of medical treatment currently available but also from an improved understanding of basal ganglia circuitry and better neuroimaging methods. Table 32.2. summarises techniques currently being employed and evaluated. The functional effects of lesioning (-otomy) and the use of deep brain stimulation are similar, in that the high frequency used in stimulation is believed to act by blocking, or 'jamming' neurones. Deep brain stimulation has the advantage of being reversible but is costly, and programming the stimulator may be very time consuming.

The subthalamic nucleus target is the current target of choice in most centres and the number of published patient-years experience with this surgical approach has increased rapidly over the past decade. Several randomised controlled studies have confirmed the benefits that may be gained from deep brain stimulation of the subthalamic nucleus, in terms of impairment, activities of daily living, and quality of life. Careful case selection is essential for all forms of surgical intervention for Parkinson's disease: older and less biologically fit patients, those with active cognitive and/or neuropsychiatric problems, and patients with a suboptimal levodopa response are generally regarded as poor surgical candidates.

Surgery may also play a role in neurorestorative treatments. Such approaches include stem cell and fetal cell transplantation, and also gene transfer using viral vectors. To date, there have been conflicting results regarding the efficacy of fetal cell

Table 32.2 Summary of anatomical targets for surgical treatment of Parkinson's disease

Target	Bradykinesia	Tremor	Dyskinesia	Comments
Thalamus	–	+++	–	Bilateral thalamotomy is not recommended because of a high incidence of bulbar dysfunction
Globus pallidus	++	++	+++	10–15% incidence of persistent adverse events with unilateral pallidotomy; no reliable data for bilateral procedures
Subthalamic nucleus	+++	+++	++	Weight gain, contralateral dyskinesia, involuntary eyelid closure and speech disturbance reported

+ to +++ refers to the relative efficacy of the procedure for the clinical feature; – refers no benefit for the procedure for the clinical feature.
For each of the three targets listed, both ablation and stimulation procedures have been evaluated.

transplants. These differences may well reflect transplantation technique, the nature of the tissue being implanted, whether immunosuppression is prescribed, and how patients are selected and assessed. Despite the negative results from two double-blind studies of embryonic cell implantation, researchers continue to explore the potential benefits from this approach.

Patient care

Common therapeutic solutions to problems encountered in the management of people with Parkinson's disease are presented in Table 32.3. After diagnosis, the provision of an explanation of the condition, education and support are essential. The Parkinson's Disease Society (www.parkinsons. org.uk) produces an excellent range of literature to help the newly diagnosed patient come to terms with the condition. In accordance with advice given by the Society itself, patients who drive are advised to inform their insurance company and also the Driver and Vehicle Licensing Agency.

A doctor will record impairments in the clinic, while the patient is more concerned with their disability and handicap. Thus, a patient can be noted to have seemingly marked impairment and yet may not complain about significant disability. The converse may also be true. Not all patients, therefore, require immediate treatment. Further, concomitant depression may distort the patient's perception of their disability, leading to inappropriate prescribing of anti-Parkinsonian therapy. In this situation, the use of an antidepressant may be more helpful. There is no good evidence base for which antidepressant should be used, and both the tricyclic agents and selective serotonin reuptake inhibitors have their advocates.

Accurate adherence with the timing of therapy may be particularly important in patients who are beginning to develop long-term treatment complications. It can be helpful for patients to keep diary cards when they begin to experience problems with either bradykinesia or dyskinesia, so that these symptoms can be related to drug and food intake. Careful changes in timing of drug therapy or meals may initially be sufficient to reduce variation in performance. Some patients experience troublesome early morning bradykinesia. It may then be beneficial to prescribe an initial dose of a rapidly acting agent, such as dispersible oral co-beneldopa, to take on first wakening so that the patient can then get up and dress. A combination of levodopa with dopamine agonists, which are more slow acting, may be useful in the patient with motor fluctuations. A combination of levodopa and a COMT inhibitor may be more appropriate in a patient with end-of-dose deterioration.

Other factors that need to be considered in patients with Parkinson's disease are the benefits of adequate sleep and rest at night, which may be made more difficult if they have urinary frequency or problems with nocturnal bradykinesia. Judicious use of hypnotic therapy may be appropriate, while a tricyclic antidepressant may offer the dual benefit of sedation with anti-cholinergic effect. Low friction sheets to assist turning in bed and encouragement of mobility through physiotherapy may also be helpful. The treatment of the patient with severe disease remains one of the greatest challenges in the management of Parkinson's disease. On–off fluctuations may be refractory to oral dopaminergic therapies. Sudden freezing episodes compound failing postural stability, leading

Table 32.3 Common therapeutic solutions in the management of Parkinson's disease

Problem	Cause	Possible Solution
Early-onset dyskinesias in young Parkinson's disease patient	Exposure to levodopa? Biological factors?	Delay introduction of levodopa, or use lowest possible dose, or use alternative agent (e.g. agonist, MAOB inhibitor)
One dose of levodopa does not last until the next (wearing off)	Advanced disease (pre- and post-synaptic changes)	More frequent, smaller doses of levodopa, COMT inhibitor, dopamine agonist or MAOB-inhibitor
Pain and immobility during the night	Evening dose of levodopa not lasting long enough	Use slow release levodopa preparation or dopamine agonist
Freezing episodes and/or unpredictable motor fluctuations	Advanced disease (pre- and post-synaptic changes)	Apomorphine, duodopa or surgery Physiotherapy helpful for freezing
Mismatch between patient's symptoms and signs	Underlying depression?	Consider antidepressant
Confusion and hallucinations with preserved cognition	Toxic (drug-related) psychosis	Exclude intercurrent infection or other medical problem Review and reduce anti-Parkinsonian therapy Consider atypical anti-psychotic agent
Confusion and hallucinations with impaired cognition	Underlying brain pathology, and cholinergic deficit	Reduce anti-Parkinsonian therapy Cholinesterase inhibitor

to increasing falls and injuries. In select patients, the use of apomorphine, either as bolus injection (via a 'Penject' device) or as a continuous subcutaneous infusion, may be helpful.

The presence of reduced dexterity in virtually all people with Parkinson's disease means that thought needs to be given to the way in which medication is dispensed and stored. If the patient is taking a complex regimen of drugs or has early cognitive problems, the use of pre-packaged therapies may improve adherence.

Patients' relatives also need emotional and social support through what can be a very demanding period. The loss of physical mobility, together with a personality change, can be very difficult for relatives to cope with. The involvement of occupational therapists, social workers and specialists in palliative care in this situation is important.

Psychosis and dementia

When cognitive impairment is problematic, the use of conventional antipsychotic medication is inappropriate because such drugs can precipitate a catastrophic worsening of Parkinsonism. Behavioural disturbances require discussion with carers and, if possible, with the patient him- or herself. A graded withdrawal of anti-Parkinsonian drugs is often indicated, aiming to simplify the regimen to levodopa monotherapy. In rare cases, it may be necessary to reduce the dose or even completely withdraw levodopa therapy in order to control aggressive, sexually demanding or psychotic features. When reduction in dopaminergic therapy is ineffective or not tolerated because of unacceptable immobility, an atypical antipsychotic drug may be considered. In practice, the choice narrows down to quetiapine or clozapine, since risperidone and olanzepine are associated with worsening Parkinsonism, even in low doses. Further, both risperidone and olanzepine should not be used in cognitively impaired elderly people because of an increased risk of stroke. Clozapine is difficult to use for Parkinson's disease-associated psychosis because of the need to register the patient with a blood-monitoring programme. When quetiapine is used, it should be commenced in a low dose of 25 or 50 mg at night and increased slowly. The sedative effects may be helpful in promoting sleep.

Cholinesterase inhibitors have shown promise in treating the neuropsychiatric features of Parkinson's disease and may also have modest cognitive-enhancing benefits. Visual hallucinations, delusions, apathy and depression seem to be particularly responsive to these agents. These effects have been demonstrated for rivastigmine in dementia associated with Parkinson's disease in a large, multicentre, double-blind, placebo-controlled study (Emre et al., 2004). A randomised controlled trial of memantine in dementia associated with Parkinson's disease (and also patients with the closely related dementia with Lewy bodies) showed a modest benefit for memantine in the primary end-point, the Clinician's Global Impression of Change (Aarsland et al., 2009).

Autonomic problems

Other complications that may need attention include disorders of gut motility, which present as constipation or difficulty with swallowing, disturbances of micturition, sometimes presenting as nocturia, and postural hypotension. Constipation can be managed in the usual way with bulking agents and, if necessary, stimulant laxatives and stool-softening agents. The management of postural hypotension includes assessment of the patient's autonomic function in order to establish whether this is primarily drug related or associated with autonomic neuropathy. If the patient is dizzy on standing, simple measures such as advice on rising slowly may be adequate. The use of elastic stockings, to reduce pooling of the blood in the lower limbs, is sometimes helpful. Pharmacological approaches include the use of fludrocortisone or occasionally midodrine (a selective α_1-adrenergic agonist). It is also important to consider other therapies the patient is receiving that might contribute to such symptoms, for example, diuretics, and to stop these if possible.

Case studies

Case 32.1

A 48-year-old man, Mr V, has a 2-year history of Parkinson's disease. He is still working in an office. His wife confides in the Parkinson's Disease Nurse Specialist that she is concerned about his gambling. Whilst never a problem before his diagnosis, he is now spending huge sums of money on on-line casinos. They are getting into financial difficulties on account of this habit. She is upset and desperate for help.

Questions

1. What might be responsible for this gentleman's behaviour?
2. What would be the most appropriate management?

Answers

1. The most likely cause of Mr V's pathological gambling (so-called because of the adverse effect this is having on his family and life in general) relates to his medication. He was, in fact, taking the dopamine agonist pramipexole, as well as rasagiline to control his Parkinsonian symptoms. Dopamine agonists have been associated with impulse control disorders.
2. Mr V's dopamine agonist should be withdrawn as quickly as possible, via down-titration of the dose over a few weeks. This will, of course, worsen his motor symptoms. In Mr V's case, he required the use of co-careldopa to regain adequate control of his Parkinsonism, but off the agonist his gambling habit ceased completely. His wife was delighted. Had the patient and his wife been warned of this possible problem prior to starting the agonist the situation may not have got to such a near-disastrous social level. It is, therefore, essential to warn all patients starting dopamine agonists about the risk of impulse control disorders and to document this in writing in the medical records.

Case 32.2

A 70-year-old man, Mr W, was diagnosed as having mild Parkinson's disease 6 months ago. This did not require any treatment. He has no past medical history of note. He returns to clinic and it is clear that both his impairment and disability have worsened.

Questions

1. What initial treatment options should be considered for Mr W?
2. What considerations should be given to the initial drug choice?

Answers

1. There is no evidence to suggest that Mr W is depressed; a masked depression should always be considered when there is a 'mismatch' between impairment and reported disability. This was not the case here. A number of first-line anti-Parkinsonian drugs might, therefore, be considered, including immediate-release levodopa preparations, dopamine agonists and monoamine oxidase type B inhibitors.
2. Co-morbid illness or a life-shortening problem, such as cancer, usually mean that levodopa would be first choice, simply because it is most potent, with a good risk:benefit ratio. If the patient is biologically fit, then either a dopamine agonist or a monoamine oxidase type B inhibitor might be appropriate, so long as the disability is not too severe and there are no other contraindications. Dopamine agonists and selegiline, in particular, have the potential to cause or exacerbate neuropsychiatric problems and the patient and their family should be warned of such side effects. In particular, the patient and their family should be informed of the risk of impulse control disorders, generally associated with dopamine agonists, and this warning recorded in the medical records. By using these 'levodopa-sparing' agents, the onset of dyskinesias may be delayed by several years.

Case 32.3

A 59-year-old gentleman, Mr X, has had Parkinson's disease for 8 years. This was initially treated with selegiline and ropinirole. Due to progressive functional disability and his wish to keep working, levodopa was introduced 5 years previously. He is now experiencing severe motor fluctuations during the day, with periods of marked dyskinesia and also increasingly unpredictable 'off' periods, during which he is stiff, immobile and anxious. Unsuccessful attempts to smooth out these fluctuations have been made by manipulating his levodopa unit dose and frequency, the use of entacapone, and changing his dopamine agonist.

Questions

1. What therapeutic options could be considered in Mr X's case?
2. What factors would influence the choice of treatment?

Answers

1. A relatively simple option that has not yet been considered is amantadine. This agent may have useful antidyskinetic effects in advanced Parkinson's disease. It is usually administered as 100 mg daily initially, increasing gradually to two or three times daily. The dose of levodopa therapy is left unchanged, to avoid worsening 'off' periods. Neuropsychiatric problems and/or a livedinous rash may complicate the use of amantadine, although younger patients are often able to tolerate the drug better. An alternative approach which may well be required is the use of continuous subcutaneous apomorphine with or without amantadine, as this may have a significant antidyskinetic effect and also effectively manage freezing episodes. Duodopa® therapy, administered via a percutaneous jejunostomy, may also be a consideration. Finally, deep brain stimulation of the subthalamic nucleus may be appropriate for Mr X.

2. Patient choice, after being given the relevant options, is clearly important, as the treatments involved are potentially invasive and associated with morbidity. A previous history of neuropsychiatric problems, active psychosis or severe depression, or cognitive impairment would be relative contraindications to surgery. Severe needle phobia or the lack of an appropriately experienced and committed local nurse specialist would compromise the effective administration of apomorphine.

Case 32.4

A 63-year-old lady, Mrs Y, is referred by a colleague because of suspected Parkinson's disease. There is also evidence of some cognitive decline in the past 12 months. She has a background history of epilepsy which was quiescent until three years ago. At that stage, she presented to the neurology department, and her anticonvulsant regimen adjusted to good effect. Examination confirms a mini-mental state examination (MMSE) score of 22/30, symmetric bradykinesia and some rigidity.

Questions

1. Which question might give additional diagnostic help in this lady's history?
2. What would be the best management?

Answers

1. Given this lady's history of epilepsy, and the subsequent evolution of Parkinsonism and cognitive decline, one would be suspicious of the change in her anticonvulsant medication. A drug history confirmed that she had been switched from phenytoin to sodium valproate, raising the possibility of a 'valproate encephalopathy'.
2. Discontinuation of the valproate is definitely worth attempting and converting to an alternative anticonvulsant. If there is doubt over the diagnosis, an FP-CIT SPECT scan can be helpful; in Parkinson's disease, the scan is abnormal, whereas in drug-induced Parkinsonism, because the problem is caused by postsynaptic blockade of dopamine receptors, tracer uptake will be normal. In this case, Mrs Y's Parkinsonism resolved completely and on repeat testing 6 months later her MMSE had risen to 29/30. She was taking lamotrigine to control her seizures at review.

Case 32.5

Mr Z has an 8-year history of Parkinson's disease. He is 77 years old. His motor symptoms are well controlled on a combination of one tablet of co-careldopa (25/100), three times a day and selegiline 10 mg daily. His wife comes to clinic with him and reports that he has recently been confused at night. Further, he has been hallucinating, seeing his long-dead mother at the bottom of the bed.

Question

What should be done?

Answer

The problem here is to what extent the features of Mr Z's psychosis relates to his drugs or to the underlying disease process. Dementia associated with Parkinson's disease is more common in the older patient with long-standing disease.

An MMSE to assess cognitive function in more detail would be appropriate (although note that this scale is relatively insensitive in detecting dementia associated with Parkinson's disease). Intercurrent infection and metabolic derangements, for example, hypothyroidism, should also be excluded.

Selegiline is best avoided in cases like this and should be discontinued. This may lead to an improvement in Mr Z's psychotic features, without any other action being necessary. The use of a typical antipsychotic agent for Mr Z is absolutely contraindicated, as it will only serve to worsen his Parkinson's disease. If cognitive function is well preserved and discontinuing selegiline fails to improve the situation, then a low dose of the atypical antipsychotic quetiapine could be considered. If there is evidence of dementia, a cholinesterase inhibitor would be a better therapeutic choice.

References

Aarsland, D., Ballard, C., Walker, Z., et al., 2009. Memantine in patients with Parkinson's disease dementia or dementia with Lewy bodies: a double-blind, placebo-controlled, multicentre trial. Lancet Neurol. 8, 613–618.

Blanchet, P.J., Verhagen-Metman, L., Chase, T.N., 2003. Renaissance of amantadine in the treatment of Parkinson's disease. Adv. Neurol. 91, 251–257.

Braak, H., Del Tredici, K., Rüb, U., et al., 2003. Staging of brain pathology related to sporadic Parkinson's disease. Neurobiol. Aging 24, 197–211.

Cotzias, G.C., Van Woert, M.H., Schiffer, L.M., 1967. Aromatic amino acids and modification of parkinsonism. N. Engl. J. Med. 276, 374–379.

Emre, M., Aarsland, D., Albanese, A., et al., 2004. Rivastigmine for dementia associated with Parkinson's disease. N. Engl. J. Med. 351, 2509–2518.

Healy, D.G., Abou-Sleiman, P.M., Wood, N.W., 2004. PINK, PANK or PARK. A clinician's guide to familial parkinsonism. Lancet Neurology 3, 652–662.

Ives, N., Stowe, R.L., Marro, J., et al., 2004. Monoamine oxidase type B inhibitors in early Parkinson's disease: meta-analysis of 17 randomised trials involving 3525 patients. Br. Med. J. 329, 593–596.

Jennings, D.L., Seibyl, J.P., Oakes, D., et al., 2004. (123I)beta-CIT and single-photon emission computed tomographic imaging vs. clinical evaluation in Parkinsonian syndrome: unmasking an early diagnosis. Arch. Neurol. 61, 1224–1229.

Lees, A.J., on behalf of the Parkinson's Disease Research Group of the United Kingdom 1995. Comparison of therapeutic effects and mortality data of levodopa and levodopa combined with selegiline in patients with early, mild Parkinson's disease. Br. Med. J. 311, 1602–1607.

National Institute for Health and Clinical Excellence, 2006. Parkinson's disease: diagnosis and management in primary and secondary care. Clinical Guideline 35. NICE, London. Available at: http://www.nice.org.uk/page.aspx?o=CG035.

Olanow, C.W., Perl, D.P., DeMartino, G.N., et al., 2004. Lewy-body formation is an aggresome-related disorder: a hypothesis. Lancet Neurol. 3, 496–503.

Olanow, C., Rascol, O., Hauser, R., et al., the ADAGIO Study Investigators 2009. A double-blind, delayed-start trial of rasagiline in Parkinson's disease. N. Engl. J. Med. 361, 1268–1278.

Olanow, C.W., Prusiner, S.B., 2009. Is Parkinson's disease a prion disorder? Proc. Natl. Acad. Sci. 106, 12571–12572.

Perry, E.K., Kilford, L., Lees, A.J., et al., 2003. Increased Alzheimer pathology in Parkinson's disease related to antimuscarinic drugs. Ann. Neurol. 54, 235–238.

Schrag, A., 2005. Entacapone in the treatment of Parkinson's disease. Lancet Neurol. 4, 366–370.

Stocchi, F., Rascol, O., Kieburtz, K., et al., 2010. Initiating levodopa/carbidopa therapy with and without entacapone in early Parkinson disease: the STRIDE-PD study. Ann. Neurol. 68, 18–27.

Walter, B.L., Vitek, J.L., 2004. Surgical treatment for Parkinson's disease. Lancet Neurol. 3, 719–728.

Further reading

Chaudhuri, K.R., Healy, D.G., Schapira, A.V.H., 2006. Non-motor symptoms of Parkinson's disease: diagnosis and management. Lancet Neurol. 5, 235–245.

Clarke, C.E., 2007. Parkinson's disease. Br. Med. J. 335, 441–445.

Hauser, R.A., 2009. Levodopa: past, present and future. Eur. J. Neurol. 62, 1–8.

Lees, A.J., Hardy, J., Revesz, T., 2009. Parkinson's disease. Lancet 373, 2055–2066.

Olanow, C.W., Stern, M.B., Sethi, K., 2009. The scientific and clinical basis for the treatment of Parkinson's disease. Neurology 72, (21 Suppl 4): S1–136.

Pain 33

R. D. Knaggs and G. J. Hobbs

Key points

- Pain is multifactorial in its aetiology.
- Treatment often requires use of a combination of drugs with different mechanisms of action.
- For cancer pain, the World Health Organization (WHO) analgesic ladder forms the basis for the use of analgesic drugs. Some clinicians prefer to omit weak opioids and start strong opioid therapy earlier.
- Opioids are not effective for all types of pain. Adjuvant drugs, such as tricyclic antidepressants or anti-epileptic drugs, should be considered.
- Breakthrough pain is treated with doses of immediate-release opioids, usually prescribed in addition to modified release opioids.
- Antiemetics and laxatives may need to be prescribed for patients taking opioids.
- Cancer pain may vary as the disease progresses. Drug therapy should be reviewed regularly to ensure that the most appropriate agent is being used for the type, site and intensity of pain.
- Most drugs exist in a range of different formulations but, whenever possible, the oral route should be used.

Pain can be defined as:

'An unpleasant sensory and emotional experience associated with actual or potential tissue damage, or described in terms of such damage'.

Acute pain may be thought of as a physiological process having a biological function, allowing the patient to avoid or minimise injury. Persistent pain, on the other hand, may be described more as a disease than a symptom (Woolf, 2004).

Aetiology and neurophysiology

Neuroanatomy of pain transmission

The majority of tissues and organs are innervated by special sensory receptors (nociceptors) connected to primary afferent nerve fibres of differing diameters. Small myelinated Aδ fibres and unmyelinated C fibres are responsible for the transmission of painful stimuli to the spinal cord where these afferent primary fibres terminate in the dorsal horn.

Pain transmission further within the Central Nervous System (CNS) is far more complex and understood less well.

The most important parts of this process are the wide dynamic range cells in the spinothalamic tract that project to the thalamus and to the somatosensory cortex beyond. Modulation or inhibition of these neurones within the spinal cord result in less activity in the pain pathway. This modulatory action can be activated by stress or certain analgesic drugs such as morphine and is an important component of the gate theory of pain (Fig. 33.1). The gate control theory recognises the pivotal role the spinal cord plays in the continual modulation of neuronal activity by the relative activity of large (Aβ) and small (Aδ and C) fibres and by descending messages from the brain. Conversely, other influences can lead to an increased sensitivity to noxious stimuli. The most important of these is pain itself and further painful stimuli can lead to increased pain from relatively trivial insults. This occurs through neurochemical and anatomical changes within the CNS that have been termed central sensitisation.

Neurotransmitters and pain

Various neurotransmitters in the dorsal horn of the spinal cord are involved in pain modulation. These include amino acids such as glutamate and γ-aminobutyric acid (GABA), monoamines such as noradrenaline and 5-hydroxytryptamine (5-HT, serotonin) and peptide molecules, of which the opioid peptides are the most important. Opioid receptors are found in both the CNS and the periphery; in the CNS they are found in high concentrations in the limbic system, the brainstem and the spinal cord. The natural ligands (molecules that bind to

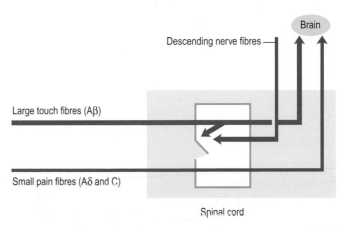

Fig. 33.1 Gate control theory of pain.

the receptor) at opioid receptors are a group of neuropeptides including the endorphins. Opioid analgesics mimic the actions of these natural ligands and exert their effect through the μ, δ and, to a lesser extent, the κ receptors. These receptors mediate the analgesic effect of morphine-like drugs.

Assessment of pain

Evaluation of pain should include a detailed description of the pain and an assessment of its consequences. There should be a full history, psychosocial assessment, medication history and assessment of previous pain problems, paying attention to factors that influence the pain. Diagnostic laboratory tests, imaging, including plain radiography, computer tomography (CT) and magnetic resonance imaging (MRI), and diagnostic nerve blocks may aid confirmation of the diagnosis.

Pain is a subjective phenomenon and quantitative assessment is difficult (Breivik et al., 2008). The most commonly used instruments are visual analogue and verbal rating scales. Visual analogue scales are 10 cm long lines labelled with an extreme at each end; usually 'no pain at all' and 'worst pain imaginable'. The patient is required to mark the severity of the pain between the two extremes of the scale. Verbal rating scales use descriptors such as 'none', 'mild', 'moderate' and 'excruciating'. More elaborate questionnaires such as the Brief Pain Inventory and the McGill Pain Questionnaire help to describe other aspects of the pain, and pain diaries record the influence of activity and medication on pain.

Management

Acute pain usually results from noxious stimulation as a result of tissue damage or injury. It can be managed effectively using analgesic drugs and is often self-limiting.

Persistent pain may be considered as pain which continues beyond the usual time required for tissue healing. Treatment may involve specialist pain management services, hospices and a multidisciplinary approach that assesses and manages patients using a biopsychosocial approach. Initial treatment is usually directed at the underlying disease process where possible, for example, medication, surgery or anti-tumour therapy. However, non-medical treatments such as physical therapy and various psychological techniques including cognitive behavioural therapy may also form part of a multimodal treatment programme. Pain can be modulated using non-pharmacological techniques: for example, stimulation-produced analgesia such as transcutaneous electrical nerve stimulation (TENS), acupuncture and massage, or invasive procedures such as neurosurgery or neurolytic nerve blocks.

Analgesic ladder

The World Health Organization (WHO) analgesic ladder (Fig. 33.2) forms the basis of many approaches to the use of analgesic drugs. There are essentially three steps: non-opioid

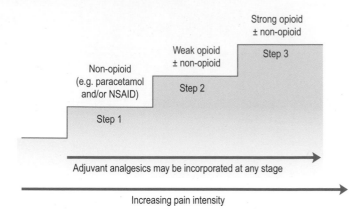

Fig. 33.2 WHO three-step analgesic ladder.

analgesics, weak opioids and strong opioids. The analgesic efficacy of non-opioids, such as paracetamol and non-steroidal anti-inflammatory drugs (NSAIDs) (e.g. aspirin, ibuprofen and diclofenac), is limited by side effects and ceiling effects, that is, beyond a certain dose, no further pharmacological effect is seen. If pain remains uncontrolled, then a weak opioid, such as codeine or dihydrocodeine, may be helpful. There may be additional benefit in combining a weak opioid with a non-opioid drug, although many commercial preparations contain inadequate quantities of both components and are no more effective than a non-opioid alone. Strong opioids, of which morphine is considered the gold standard, have no ceiling effect and therefore increased dosage continues to give increased analgesia but side effects often limit effectiveness. Adjuvant drugs, such as corticosteroids, antidepressants or anti-epileptics, may be considered at any step of the ladder.

Analgesic drugs

Paracetamol

Despite being used in clinical practice for over 50 years and much investigation, the mechanism by which paracetamol exerts its analgesic effect remains uncertain. Inhibition of prostaglandin synthesis within the CNS has been proposed, although this is probably not the only mechanism. Interaction with the serotonin (Tjolsen et al., 1991) and endocannabinoid (Högestätt et al., 2005) neurotransmitter systems have been demonstrated in animal models.

Following oral administration the bioavailability of paracetamol is around 60%, but if given by the rectal route it is much lower and much more variable. A formulation for intravenous infusion has been promoted over the last few years and this has largely replaced the rectal route of administration. Therapeutic plasma levels are reached within 30 min of oral administration. The elimination half-life of paracetamol is relatively short ($t_{1/2} = 2$–4 h); hence, frequent dosing is required to maintain its analgesic effect.

With normal doses, the majority of paracetamols are metabolised and inactivated in the liver, undergoing a phase II conjugation reaction with glucuronic acid (Fig. 33.3). A small

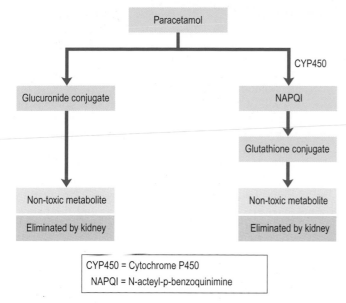

CYP450 = Cytochrome P450
NAPQI = N-acteyl-p-benzoquinimine

Fig. 33.3 Paracetamol metabolism in humans.

proportion of a dose is metabolised using a cytochrome P450 mediated reaction that forms a reactive intermediate, *N*-acteyl-*p*-benzoquinimine (NAPQI). Usually, NAPQI can be deactivated by conjugation with glutathione in the liver. However, following ingestion of a large amount of paracetamol the hepatic stores of both glucuronic acid and glutathione become depleted leaving free NAPQI, which causes liver damage.

The usual therapeutic dose for adults is paracetamol 1 g taken four times daily. It is very important that this dose is not exceeded, otherwise hepatotoxicity is more common. This may be particularly problematic for malnourished adults with low body weight (Claridge et al., 2010). A reduced maximum daily infusion dose (3 g/24 hours) is recommended for patients with hepatocellular insufficiency, chronic alcoholism or dehydration. Paracetamol is also available as an over-the-counter (OTC) medicine and is a component of many cold and influenza remedies. Compared with other analgesics, paracetamol is not as potent; however, when taken in combination with a NSAID or opioid, there is an additive analgesic effect.

Non-steroidal anti-inflammatory drugs

Mode of action

NSAIDs exert their analgesic and anti-inflammatory effects through inhibition of the enzyme cyclo-oxygenase. NSAIDs are used widely to relieve pain, with or without inflammation, in people with acute and persistent musculoskeletal disorders. In single doses, NSAIDs have superior analgesic activity compared to paracetamol (Hyllested et al., 2002). In regular higher dosages, they have both analgesic and anti-inflammatory effects, which makes them particularly useful for the treatment of continuous or regular pain associated with inflammation. NSAIDs have been shown to be suitable for the relief of pain in dysmenorrhoea, toothache and some headaches and to treat pain caused by secondary bone tumours, which result from lysis of bone and release of prostaglandins.

Clinical considerations

Differences in anti-inflammatory activity between NSAIDs are small, but there is considerable variation in individual patient response as well as the incidence and type of side effects. About 60% of patients will respond to any NSAID. Of the remaining patients, those who do not respond to one NSAID may well respond to another. An analgesic effect should normally be seen within a week, whereas an anti-inflammatory effect may not be achieved or assessable clinically for up to 3 weeks.

The potential treatment benefits of an NSAID must be weighed against the risks. NSAIDs are contraindicated in patients with known active peptic ulceration and should be used with caution in the elderly and in those with renal impairment or asthma.

COX-2 selective drugs

Cyclo-oxygenase exists in two forms: cyclo-oxygenase-1 (COX-1) and cyclo-oxygenase-2 (COX-2). COX-1 is a constitutive enzyme that is expressed under normal conditions in a variety of tissues, including the gastro-intestinal tract and kidney, where it catalyses the formation of prostaglandins required for homeostatic functions. It does not have a role in nociception or inflammation. COX-2 is an inducible enzyme that appears in damaged tissues shortly after injury and leads to the formation of inflammatory prostaglandins within these tissues. COX-2 selective NSAIDs should, theoretically, inhibit the formation of inflammatory prostaglandins without affecting the activity of COX-1 in areas such as the gut. In practice, use of COX-2 specific drugs is associated with reduced risks of gastro-intestinal side effects when compared with non-selective drugs. However, their use has also been linked with adverse effects including ischaemic cardiac events and this now limits their use.

Guidance on NSAID use

The lowest effective dose of NSAID or COX-2 selective inhibitor should be prescribed for the shortest time necessary. The need for long-term treatment should be reviewed periodically. Prescribing should be based on the safety profiles of individual NSAIDs or COX-2 selective inhibitors, on individual patient risk profiles, for example, gastro-intestinal and cardiovascular. Prescribers should not switch between NSAIDs without careful consideration of the overall safety profile of the products and the patient's individual risk factors, as well as the patient's preference (Medicines and Healthcare Regulatory Agency, 2006).

Concomitant aspirin, and possibly other antiplatelet drugs, greatly increases the gastro-intestinal risks of NSAIDs and severely reduces any gastro-intestinal safety advantages of COX-2 selective inhibitors. Aspirin should only be co-prescribed if absolutely necessary.

Weak opioids

Weak opioids are prescribed frequently, either alone or in combination with other analgesics, for a wide variety of painful disorders. There are three major drugs in this group, codeine, dihydrocodeine and dextropropoxyphene, which are recommended as step 2 of the WHO analgesic ladder for pain that has not responded to non-opioid analgesics. Despite this recommendation, there is little data which demonstrates that weak opioids are of any benefit in the relief of persistent pain, and it may be more beneficial to use a smaller dose of a strong opioid.

Co-proxamol, a combination of dextropropoxyphene and paracetamol, was withdrawn in the UK in 2007 following safety concerns, particularly toxicity in overdose. An unlicensed product remains available for patients who find it difficult to change to alternative treatment.

Codeine

Codeine is the prototypical drug in this group. It is structurally similar to morphine and about 10% of the codeine is demethylated to form morphine, and the analgesic effect may be due to this, at least in part. It is a powerful cough suppressant as well as being very constipating. In combination with NSAIDs, the analgesic effects are usually additive but the variability in response is considerable. A degree of genetic polymorphism occurs within the population such that the hepatic microsomal enzyme CYP2D6 that is responsible for the conversion of codeine to morphine does not catalyse this conversion in approximately 8% of the Caucasian population. The duration of analgesic action is about 3 h.

Dihydrocodeine

Dihydrocodeine is only available in a few countries and is chemically similar to codeine. It has similar properties to codeine when used at the same dosage and may be slightly more potent.

Dextropropoxyphene

Historically, dextropropoxyphene was prescribed in combination with other analgesics such as paracetamol (co-proxamol). There are few data on its therapeutic value, and at least one review concluded that analgesic efficacy is less than aspirin and barely more than placebo. At best, dextropropoxyphene failed to show any superiority over paracetamol (Li Wan Po and Zhang, 1997). At worst, it is a dangerous drug which has the potential for steadily developing toxicity. Patients with hepatic dysfunction and poor renal function are particularly at risk. It is associated with problems in overdose, notably a non-naloxone reversible depression of the cardiac conducting system. Dextropropoxyphene interacts unpredictably with a number of drugs, including carbamazepine and warfarin. In 2005, the Medicines and Healthcare products Regulatory Agency (MHRA) announced concerns about the safety and effectiveness of co-proxamol and directed that it should be withdrawn from clinical use in the UK; however, it still remains available as an unlicensed medicine for the small number of patients who do not obtain analgesia with other analgesic medicines.

Strong opioids

Morphine

Morphine is the 'gold standard' strong opioid analgesic. It is available for administration by a range of administration routes, including oral, rectal and injectable formulations and has a duration of action of about 4 h after oral administration. There is no ceiling effect when the dose is increased. A general protocol for morphine use to obtain rapid relief from acute pain is to use intravenous bolus doses of 2–5 mg titrated until pain relief is achieved. In the initial management of persistent non-cancer pain or cancer pain, an oral regimen is more appropriate using an immediate-release formulation. A usual starting dose is 5–10 mg every 4 h, and the patient should be advised to take the same dose as often as is necessary for breakthrough pain. It may be necessary to double the dose every 24 h until pain relief is achieved, although a slower dose escalation will often suffice. After control is achieved, it is usual to change to an oral modified release formulation, which allows less frequent dosing, either daily or twice-daily. There is no ceiling dose for the analgesic effect of morphine; daily doses of up to 1 or 2 g of morphine may be required for some cancer patients, but relatively few require more than about 200 mg daily. Morphine is metabolised in the liver and one metabolite, morphine 6-glucuronide, is pharmacologically active and this should be taken into consideration in patients who have renal failure.

Other strong opioids

Opioids such as pethidine and dextromoramide offer little advantage over morphine in that they are generally weaker in action with a relatively short duration of action (2 h). Dipipanone is only available in a preparation which contains an antiemetic (cyclizine), and increasing doses lead to sedation and the risk of developing a tardive dyskinesia with long-term use. Methadone has a long elimination half-life of 15–25 h, and accumulation occurs in the early stages of use. It has minimal side effects with long-term use and some patients who experience serious adverse effects with morphine may tolerate methadone.

Hydromorphone and oxycodone are synthetic opioids that have been used for many years in North America and more recently in Europe. They are available in both immediate and modified release preparations. Some patients appear to tolerate hydromorphone or oxycodone better than morphine but there is no evidence to suggest which patients achieve the best effect with either of these drugs.

Fentanyl is available as a transdermal formulation for long-term use. The patch is designed to release the drug continuously over 3 days. When starting the drug, alternative analgesic therapy should be continued for at least the first 12 h until therapeutic levels are achieved, and an immediate acting opioid should be available for breakthrough pain. Patches are replaced every 72 h.

The relative potencies of the commonly used opioids are summarised in Table 33.1.

Table 33.1 Relative potencies of opioid drugs

Drug	Potency (morphine = 1)
Codeine	0.1
Dihydrocodeine	0.1
Tramadol	0.2
Pethidine	0.1
Morphine	1
Diamorphine	2.5
Hydromorphone	7
Methadone	2–10 (with repeat dosing)
Fentanyl (transdermal)	150

Clinical considerations

Use of opioids is almost universally accepted in cancer pain but many patients with persistent non-cancer pain can find considerable relief with strong opioids; however, barriers to their use in this context appear to be based more on ignorance and political fashions than clinical evidence (Ballantyne and Mao, 2003). As a general rule, strong opioids effective in the management of neuropathic and musculoskeletal pain, including osteoarthritis, are less effective for sympathetically maintained pain.

Agonist-antagonist and partial agonists

Most of the drugs in this category are either competitive antagonists at the μ opioid receptor, where they can bind to the site but exert no action, or they exert only limited actions; that is, they are partial agonists. Those that are antagonists at the μ opioid receptor can provoke a withdrawal syndrome in patients receiving concomitant opioid agonists such as morphine. These properties make it difficult to use these agents in the control of persistent pain, and the process of conversion from one group of drugs to another can be complex.

Buprenorphine

Buprenorphine is a semi-synthetic, highly lipophilic opioid that is a partial agonist at the μ opioid receptor and an antagonist at both the δ and κ receptors. It undergoes extensive metabolism when administered orally and to avoid this effect, it is given sublingually. It has high receptor affinity and, through this property, a duration of action of 6 h.

A long duration of action and high bioavailability would suggest a role for buprenorphine in the management of persistent pain. Relatively recently, buprenorphine has been marketed as a transdermal formulation and may be an effective alternative to other strong opioids for persistent non-cancer pain. There is limited evidence of efficacy in osteoarthritis and low back pain. Following sublingual or intravenous administration the incidence of nausea and vomiting appears to be substantially higher than with morphine; however, respiratory depression and constipation are less frequent.

Pentazocine

Pentazocine, a benzomorphan derivative, is an agonist and at the same time a very weak antagonist at the μ opioid receptor. This drug became popular in the 1960s, when it was thought it would have little or no abuse potential. This is now known to be untrue, although its abuse potential is less than that of the conventional agonists such as morphine. It produces analgesia that is clearly different from morphine and is probably due to agonist actions at the κ-receptor. There are no detailed studies of its use in persistent pain, but its short duration of action (about 3 h) and the high incidence of psychomimetic side effects make it a totally unsuitable drug for such use.

Tramadol

Tramadol is a centrally acting analgesic that has opioid agonist activity and also has potent monoamine reuptake properties similar to many antidepressants. Indeed, tramadol appears to have intrinsic antidepressant activity. It is not as potent as morphine and efficacy is limited by side effects, including an unfavourably high risk of drowsiness and nausea and vomiting. Its monoaminergic activity appears to be valuable in the management of neuropathic pain and hence may be an acceptable alternative to a weak opioid.

Adverse effects of opioids

The adverse effects of opioids are nearly all dose related, and tolerance develops to the majority with long-term use.

Respiratory depression

Respiratory depression is potentially dangerous in patients with impaired respiratory function, but tolerance develops rapidly with regular dosing. It can be reversed by naloxone.

Sedation

Sedation is usually mild and self-limiting. Smaller doses, given more frequently, may counteract the problem. Rarely, dexamfetamine or methylphenidate has been used to counteract this effect.

Nausea and vomiting

Antiemetics should be co-prescribed routinely with opioids for the first 10 days. Choice of antiemetic will depend upon the cause, and a single drug will be sufficient in two-thirds of patients. Where nausea is persistent, additional causes should be sought and prescribing reviewed. If another antiemetic is used, it should have a different mode of action.

Constipation

Opioids reduce intestinal secretions and peristalsis, causing a dry stool and constipation. Unlike other adverse effects constipation tends not to improve with long-term use, and when opioids are used on a long-term basis most patients need a stool softener (e.g. docusate sodium) and a stimulant laxative (e.g. senna) regularly. Dosage should be titrated to give a comfortable stool. High-fibre diets and bulking agents do not work very well in preventing constipation in patients on opioids. Co-danthrusate (dantron + docusate sodium) and co-danthramer (dantron + poloxamer 188) are alternatives; however, because of the potential carcinogenicity and genotoxicity of dantron, they are only indicated for use in terminal care.

Tolerance, dependence and addition

Persistent treatment with opioids often causes tolerance to the analgesic effect, although the mechanism remains unclear (Holden et al., 2005). When this occurs the dosage should be increased or, alternatively, another opioid can be substituted, since cross-tolerance is not usually complete. Addiction is very rare when opioids are prescribed for pain relief.

Smooth muscle spasm

Opioids cause spasm of the sphincter of Oddi in the biliary tract and may cause biliary colic, as well as urinary sphincter spasm and urinary retention. Thus, in biliary or renal colic, it may be preferable to use another drug without these effects. Pethidine was believed to be the most effective in these circumstances but the evidence for this has been questioned (Thompson, 2001).

There is increasing evidence that long-term use of potent opioids may cause clinically significant adverse effects on the endocrine system, namely testosterone deficiency. Effects on the immune system are also under scrutiny.

Special techniques of opioid drug delivery

Patient-controlled analgesia (PCA)

PCA is a system which allows the patient to titrate the dose of opioid to suit their individual analgesic requirements. The drug is delivered using a syringe attached to an electronic or elastomeric pump, which delivers a preset dose when activated by the patient depressing a button. A lock-out period, during which the machine is programmed not to respond, ensures that a second dose is not delivered before the previous one has had an effect. Some devices allow an additional background infusion of drug to be delivered continuously. A maximum dose facility ensures that the machine does not deliver more than a preset dose over a given time. PCA is a useful technique for the management of pain after surgery. The system is convenient and enjoys a high degree of patient acceptability.

The traditional intermittent intramuscular injection of opioids can be effective but is less versatile than titrated intravenous administration. The subcutaneous route is subject to most of the problems associated with intramuscular administration but tends to be less painful.

Opioid use via any route is associated with nausea, and antiemetics should be prescribed routinely. Administration of compound preparations containing both opioids and antiemetics is not recommended as few preparations contain drugs with similar pharmacokinetic profiles and accumulation, usually of the antiemetic, may occur.

Epidural analgesia

Epidural injections and infusions may be effective in relieving pain arising from both malignant causes and non-cancer diseases and are very effective in postoperative and labour pain. Various combinations of local anaesthetics, opioids or steroids can be administered into the epidural space near to the spinal level of the pain.

Epidural opioids

Effective analgesia can be obtained by administering small doses of opioids to the epidural space. As there are opioid receptors in the spinal cord, smaller doses than administered by other parenteral routes are required and may be given with and without long acting local anaesthetic drugs. However, severe respiratory depression, nausea and vomiting, urinary retention and pruritus can occur after their use. Life threatening respiratory depression can occur when additional opioids are given by other routes to patients already receiving epidural opioids, and this practice should be actively discouraged. Respiratory depression which occurs soon after administration, due to intravascular absorption, is relatively common and simple to detect and treat. However, respiratory depression can also occur many hours after opioid administration. This is most common with morphine, probably because of its lower lipophilicity compared with fentanyl and diamorphine. Fentanyl has much greater stability than diamorphine and it can be prepared with bupivacaine in a terminally sterilised formulation which minimises the risk of adding the incorrect dose to an infusion fluid in a clinical environment and maintains sterility.

Local anaesthetics

Local anaesthetic drugs, such as lidocaine and bupivacaine, produce reversible blockade of neural transmission in automonic, sensory and motor nerve fibres by binding to sodium channels in the axon membrane from within, preventing sodium ion entry during depolarisation. The threshold potential is not reached, and consequently the action potential is not propagated. The concentration of local anaesthetic and dose used determine the onset, density and duration of the block. There are marked differences in the recommended maximum safe doses of different local anaesthetic agents. If the maximum dose is exceeded, serious cardiovascular (arrhythmias) and CNS effects (convulsions) may be observed.

Local anaesthetic drugs injected close to a sensory nerve or plexus will block the conduction of nerve impulses, including pain from sensory fibres and provide excellent analgesia. Some local anaesthetics are given with adrenaline (epinephrine) to reduce systemic toxicity and increase the duration of action.

Local anaesthetics can be applied directly to wounds or by local infiltration to produce postoperative analgesia; however, these approaches will not normally block pain arising from deep internal organs. Local anaesthetic techniques are particularly useful in day-stay surgery and children. Continuous infusions via a catheter will allow prolonged analgesia. More permanent neural blockade for the control of cancer pain may be achieved by using a neurolytic agent such as absolute alcohol or phenol.

A topical formulation of lidocaine has been marketed for the management of neuropathic pain caused by post-herpetic neuralgia. Up to three plasters may be worn for a 12-h period each day.

Epidural local anaesthetics

Long acting local anaesthetic drugs such as bupivacaine are most effective in relieving pain after major surgery. They work by blocking nerves in the spinal canal serving both superficial and deep tissues, and thus analgesia can be obtained in deep internal organs. Sensory and sympathetic nerves that maintain smooth muscle tone in blood vessels are blocked. As a result, vasodilation can occur, which may result in significant hypotension. Epidural catheters allow continuous infusions and long-term therapy by this route. Adverse effects may include muscle weakness in the area supplied by the nerve and, rarely, infection and haematomas.

Non-opioid analgesics

The pharmacological actions and use of the conventional non-opioids such as paracetamol, aspirin and NSAIDs are well known and will not be discussed further here.

Nefopam is a drug which is chemically related to orphenadrine and diphenhydramine, however, it is neither an opioid, anti-inflammatory drug nor an antihistamine. The mechanism of analgesic action remains unclear. As a non-opioid, it is not associated with the problems of dependence and respiratory depression. The drug has a very high number of dose-related side effects in clinical use that may be linked to its anti-cholinergic actions. Nefopam may be useful in asthmatic patients and in those who are intolerant of NSAIDs.

Adjuvant medication

To be an analgesic, a drug must relieve pain in animal models and give demonstrable and reliable pain relief in patients. Drugs such as the opioids and the NSAIDs clearly are analgesics. In some types of pain, such as cancer pain or neuropathic pain, the addition of non-analgesic drugs to analgesic therapy can enhance pain relief. A list of some adjuvant drugs is given in Table 33.2. It should be remembered that some drugs such as tricyclic antidepressants (TCAs) have intrinsic analgesic

Table 33.2 Adjuvant drugs used in the treatment of pain

Drug class	Type of pain	Example
Anti-epileptics	Neuropathic pain Migraine Cluster headache	Carbamazepine Sodium valproate Gabapentin Pregabalin Lamotrigine
Antidepressants	Neuropathic pain Musculoskeletal pain	Amitriptyline Imipramine Venlafaxine Duloxetine
Intravenous anaesthetic agents	Neuropathic pain Burn pain Cancer pain	Ketamine
Skeletal muscle relaxants	Muscle spasm Spasticity	Baclofen Dantrolene Botulinum toxin (type A)
Steroids	Raised intracranial pressure Nerve compression	Dexamethasone Prednisolone
Antibiotics	Infection	As indicated by culture and sensitivity
Antispasmodics	Colic Smooth muscle spasm	Hyoscine butylbromide Loperamide
Hormones/ hormonal analogues	Malignant bone pain Spinal stenosis Intestinal obstruction	Calcitonin Octreotide
Bisphosphonates	Bone pain (caused by cancer or osteoporosis)	Pamidronate (for cancer pain) Alendronate

activity, perhaps related to their ability to affect 5-HT and noradrenergic neurotransmission.

Antidepressants

Persistent pain is accompanied frequently by anxiety and depression. Thus, it is not surprising that the use of antidepressants and other psychoactive drugs is a routine component of pain management. There is evidence that some of these drugs have analgesic properties independent of their psychotropic effects.

The TCAs are frequently used for the treatment of persistent pain conditions with and without the anti-epileptics, and there is a substantial body of literature about their analgesic action (McQuay et al., 1996).

The biochemical activity of the TCAs suggests that their main effect is on serotonergic and noradrenergic neurones. The TCAs inhibit the reuptake of the monoamines, 5-HT and/or noradrenaline in neurones found within in the brain and spinal cord. Through a rather complex mechanism, this causes an initial fall in the release of these transmitters followed by a sustained rise in the concentration of neurotransmitter at synapses in the pain neural pathways. This rise usually takes 2–3 weeks to develop. Tricyclic antidepressants are effective analgesics in headache, facial pain, low back pain, arthritis, and, to a lesser degree, cancer pain.

Clinical use of antidepressants in persistent pain

When used in pain management, it is usual to start with a very low TCA dose, for example, amitriptyline 10–25 mg at night and to titrate upwards according to response and adverse effects. Within clinical trials TCA doses have varied considerably but most are lower than used in psychiatry, in the order of amitriptyline 50–75 mg/day. Under specialist supervision higher doses, for example, amitriptyline 150–200 mg/day may be appropriate.

Tricyclic antidepressants have a wide range of adverse effects due to interaction with histamine and muscarinic acetylcholine receptors and these may cause a marked reduction in patient adherence. Newer antidepressant drugs have generally been disappointing from the analgesic perspective. However, much of the research has looked at the selective serotonin reuptake inhibitors (SSRIs). Scientific (Sindrup and Jensen, 1999) and clinical evidence (Sindrup et al., 2005) suggest that a combination of noradrenergic and serotonergic transmission both need to be enhanced for an analgesic effect to be seen. The serotonin/noradrenaline reuptake inhibitors (SNRIs) venlafaxine and duloxetine have effects on both monoamines and appear to possess analgesic activity in neuropathic pain models. A number of antidepressant compounds, including trazodone and mirtazepine, do not act via monoamine reuptake inhibition and do not appear to possess intrinsic analgesic activity. They are effective antidepressants and may have a place in the treatment of co-existing depression but analgesia should be treated separately.

Anti-epileptics

The usefulness of this group of drugs is well established for the treatment of neuropathic pain (McQuay et al., 1995). Conditions which may respond to anti-epileptics include trigeminal neuralgia, glossopharyngeal neuralgia, various neuropathies, lancinating pain arising from conditions such as postherpetic neuralgia and multiple sclerosis and similar pains that may follow amputation or surgery. Several classes of drugs show anti-epileptic activity and these can be broadly classed as sodium channel blockers (carbamazepine, phenytoin), glutamate inhibitors (lamotrigine), voltage gated calcium channel ligands (gabapentin, pregabalin), GABA potentiators (sodium valproate, tiagabine) or drugs showing a mixture of these effects (topiramate). Failure to respond to one particular drug does not indicate that anti-epileptics as a broad class will be ineffective. A drug with a different mechanism of action or combination therapy could be considered.

Anti-epileptics are surprisingly effective in the prophylaxis of migraine and cluster headache. Their mode of action is unclear but both of these conditions are associated with abnormal excitability of certain groups of neurones and the neuronal depression caused by anti-epileptics is probably important.

Ketamine

Ketamine is an intravenous anaesthetic agent with a variety of actions within the CNS. Many of its effects are related to its activity at central glutamate receptors, although it also has actions at certain voltage-gated ion channels and opioid receptors. Low doses of ketamine (0.1–0.3 mg/kg/h via the intravenous route) can produce profound analgesia, even in situations where opioids have been ineffective, such as neuropathic pain. Despite its variable oral availability, oral administration of ketamine can be surprisingly effective (Annetta et al., 2005; Mercadante, 1996). Its usefulness is limited by troublesome psychotropic side effects, although the simultaneous administration of benzodiazepines or antipsychotics can reduce these problems.

Anxiolytics

Benzodiazepines may be used for short-term pain relief in conditions associated with acute muscle spasm and are sometimes prescribed to reduce the anxiety and muscle tension associated with persistent pain conditions. Many authorities believe that they reduce pain tolerance and there is good evidence that they can reduce the effectiveness of opioid analgesics, although the mechanism by which this occurs is unclear. Clonazepam has been used in the management of neuropathic pain. Diazepam can be used to control painful spasticity, due to acute or spinal cord injury, but sedation may be troublesome and baclofen (see below) is probably a more suitable choice.

Antihistamines

These agents were introduced into the management of persistent pain because of their sedative muscle relaxant properties. These actions are non-specific and it is not clear whether the clinical effect is mediated centrally or peripherally. Most clinical studies have been carried out with hydroxyzine, which has shown benefit in acute pain, tension headache and cancer pain, but is not commonly used in current clinical practice.

Skeletal muscle relaxants

Drugs described in this section are used for the relief of muscle spasm or spasticity. It is essential that the underlying cause of the spasticity and any aggravating factors such as pressure sores or infections are treated. Skeletal muscle relaxants usually help spasticity but this may be at the cost of decreased muscle tone elsewhere, which may lead to a decrease in patient mobility, which may make matters worse.

The drug of first choice is probably baclofen, which has a peripheral site of action, working directly on skeletal muscle. Baclofen is a derivative of the inhibitory neurotransmitter GABA and appears to be an agonist at the $GABA_B$ receptor. It is used commonly in the treatment of spasticity caused by multiple sclerosis or other diseases of the spinal cord, especially traumatic lesions.

Dantrolene is an alternative that is effective orally and which may have fewer, but potentially more serious, adverse effects. Its effect is due to a direct action on skeletal muscle and takes several weeks to develop.

The α_2-adrenergic agonist tizanidine has potent muscle relaxant activity and is an alternative to baclofen. It may also have some direct analgesic effects.

Botulinum toxin

The bacterium *Clostridium botulinum* produces a potent toxin that interferes directly with neuromuscular transmission. Purified preparations of the type A toxin produce long-lasting relaxation of skeletal muscle. The effect often lasts in excess of 3 months and avoids the systemic side effects of agents such as baclofen. Great care must be taken in administering this drug as spread may occur to adjacent muscle groups, producing excessive weakness. Overdosage, with systemic absorption, may lead to generalised muscle weakness and even respiratory failure.

Clonidine

The α-adrenergic agonist clonidine has been shown to produce analgesia, and there is evidence that both morphine and clonidine produce a dose-dependent inhibition of spinal nociceptive transmission that is mediated through different receptors for each drug. This may explain why clonidine has been shown to work synergistically with morphine when given by the intrathecal or epidural routes. Clonidine also appears to be effective when given by other routes or even topically, but may cause severe hypotension by any route.

Cannabinoids

Cannabis has been used as an analgesic for hundreds of years. Problems concerning the legal status of cannabis in most countries have hindered scientific investigation of its analgesic properties. The active ingredient in preparations made from the hemp plant, *Cannabis sativa,* is δ-9 tetrahydrocannabinol. This compound has analgesic activity in animal models of experimental pain as well as in the clinical situation (Burns and Ineck, 2006). Overall, analgesic activity appears relatively weak and it has not been possible to separate the analgesic activity from the potent psychotropic effects characteristic of these drugs but a commercial preparation is now licensed for the management of spasticity in multiple sclerosis. There may be a clearer analgesic effect in neuropathic pain but the evidence for this remains anecdotal.

Stimulation-produced analgesia

Stimulation-produced analgesia can be used for trauma, postoperative pain, labour pain and various persistent pains.

TENS and acupuncture

TENS machines are portable battery-powered devices that generate a small current to electrodes applied to the skin. The electrodes are placed at the painful site or close to the course of the peripheral nerve innervating the painful area, and the current is increased until paraesthesia is felt at the site of the pain. The current stimulates the large, rapidly conducting (Aβ) fibres which close the gating mechanism in the dorsal horn cells, and this inhibits the small, slowly conducting (Aδ and C) fibres. TENS, in particular, offers the patient a simple, non-invasive, self-controlled method of pain relief with relatively few adverse effects.

Acupuncture also works using a similar manner, although additional mechanisms, including stimulation of endogenous opioid release, may be involved. Acupuncture has been recommended for the treatment of low back pain (National Institute for Health and Clinical Excellence, 2009).

Treatment of selected pain syndromes

Postoperative pain

The majority of patients experience pain following surgery. The site and nature of surgery influences the severity of pain, although individual variation between patients does not allow prediction of the severity of pain by the type of operation.

Apart from the obvious humanitarian benefit of relieving suffering, pain relief is desirable for a number of physiological reasons after surgery or any form of major tissue injury. For example, poor-quality analgesia reduces respiratory function, increases heart rate and blood pressure, and amplifies the stress response to surgery. The use of intermittent and patient-controlled intermittent intravenous opioids injections has been described earlier in this chapter. However, opioids themselves may delay recovery and are associated with adverse events in the postoperative period (Kehlet et al., 1996). It is now common to treat postoperative pain using a 'multimodal approach', consisting of paracetamol, NSAIDs, opioids and local anaesthetic blocks or wound infiltration. NSAIDs such as diclofenac and ketorolac are used frequently, but must be used with caution in the postoperative period where there is a possibility of renal stress, such as blood loss, and the normal protective effect of prostaglandins on the kidney will be lost, culminating in acute renal failure. There is no evidence to support the pre-emptive use of either NSAIDs or local anaesthetic techniques, although there is some theoretical and clinical evidence suggesting that opioids given prior to surgery may be more effective than when given postoperatively.

Cancer pain

Cancer and pain are not synonymous. One-third of patients with cancer do not experience severe pain. Of the remaining two-thirds that do, about 88% can be controlled using basic principles of pain management (Scottish Intercollegiate Guidelines Network, 2008). Pain associated with cancer may arise from many different sources, and may exhibit the characteristics of both acute and persistent pain. The mechanisms and sources of cancer pain may change with time and regular assessment is required. Cancer occurs more frequently in the elderly, who may have a larger proportion of painful conditions than the general population. Pain may be arising from these sources too, and these require treatment at the same time.

Cancer pain can be treated both with drugs and other interventional techniques, such as radiotherapy and nerve blocks. Usually, drug treatment is based on the WHO analgesic ladder together with the use of adjuvant analgesics. Opioids are the mainstay for the treatment of cancer pain, although increasingly some clinicians progress from non-opioid drugs to a strong opioid such as morphine, omitting the middle step of the analgesic ladder.

Although this chapter is concerned only with the management of pain, care of the patient with a terminal illness requires management of all aspects of the patient. The Liverpool Care Pathway (LCP) is a resource recommended to promote high-quality care in the last days of life (Ellershaw and Wilkinson, 2003). At a basic level, the LCP is a way of acknowledging that death is imminent and ensuring the patient's comfort by omitting long-term non-essential medication and anticipatory prescribing in case the patient experiences pain, delirium, vomiting or breathlessness.

Opioid use in cancer pain

Morphine is the first-line opioid used for the management of cancer pain and may be given in immediate or modified release oral formulations. If not tolerated, alternatives such as oxycodone or hydromorphone, both having relatively long half-lives, may be considered. Optimal dosage is determined on an individual basis for each patient by titration against the pain. Patients requiring long-term modified release opioids should have additional oral doses of rapidly acting opioid to act as an 'escape' medicine for incident or breakthrough pain. The British National Formulary recommends that the standard dose of a strong opioid for breakthrough pain is one-tenth to one-sixth of the regular 24 hour total daily dose. Methadone should not be used as first-line treatment of cancer pain, but may be useful when alternatives have failed or the patient has experienced intolerable adverse effects.

When the oral route is unavailable, other routes of administration such as the buccal, rectal, transdermal or parenteral (subcutaneous, intravenous) or spinal (epidural or intrathecal) routes may be considered. Syringe drivers or implanted pumps may be used to provide analgesia in cases where conventional opioid delivery is ineffective. Morphine and oxycodone are available for parenteral administration and in the UK, diamorphine is also suitable and readily available. Diamorphine hydrochloride has the advantage of being very water soluble, so a high dose may be given in a small volume, which reduces the frequency of changes of syringes and refills necessary to provide adequate pain relief. The proportion of patients who need an implanted pump for intrathecal drug delivery is extremely small and is confined largely to those who are persistently troubled with unacceptable adverse effects. Such patients may achieve pain relief with lower equivalent opioid doses and have few problems with side effects. Long-term maintenance of indwelling lines and catheters requires training for the patient and specialist expertise from physicians and nursing teams, but excellent long-term results are possible.

Use of adjuvant drugs and treatments for cancer pain

Neuropathic pain is common in cancer. As many as 40% of cancer patients may have a neuropathic component to their pain. Tricyclic antidepressants and anti-epileptic drugs should be introduced early but where these are ineffective, ketamine may have an important role.

Levomepromazine, a phenothiazine with analgesic activity, is a useful alternative when opioids cannot be tolerated. It causes neither constipation nor respiratory depression and has antiemetic and anxiolytic activity. It is sedative, which may be either a virtue or a problem in palliative care.

Corticosteroids are useful in managing certain aspects of acute and persistent cancer pain. They are particularly useful for raised intracranial pressure and for relieving pressure caused by tumours on the spinal cord or peripheral nerves. Dexamethasone is the most commonly used steroid to ameliorate raised intracranial pressure in patients with brain tumours. High steroid doses given for 1 or 2 weeks do not require a reducing-dosage regimen. Also, they may produce a feeling of well-being, increased appetite and weight gain, all beneficial for cancer patients, although these effects are usually transient.

It is essential that underlying causes of pain be treated; therefore, it is appropriate to use antibiotics to treat infections, radiotherapy to reduce tumour bulk or control bone pain, or surgery to achieve fracture fixation or to relieve bowel obstruction in conjunction with antispasmodics such as hyoscine butylbromide.

Specific cancer pain syndromes

Three types of malignant pain are briefly outlined below to indicate various therapeutic approaches.

Cancer of the pancreas. Pain is caused by infiltration of the tumour into the pancreas as well as by obstruction of the bowel and biliary tracts and metastases in the liver. Patients may experience anorexia, nausea, vomiting and diarrhoea, and also are often depressed. Surgery, radiotherapy and chemotherapy may relieve pain for long periods, as does neurolytic blockade of the coeliac plexus. Opioid analgesics are useful and may be administered intravenously or epidurally by either bolus injection or continuous infusion.

Mesothelioma of the lung. Mesothelioma causes pain when the tumour penetrates surrounding tissues such as the pleura, chest wall and nerve plexuses. The WHO analgesic ladder should be used first, but it should be remembered that a NSAID may be beneficial as inflammation is often a component of the chest wall involvement. Adjuvants such as TCAs or steroids may be helpful. As the tumour progresses, nerve blocks or neurosurgery may be necessary, and invasion of the vertebrae can lead to nerve root or spinal cord compression. In the latter case, high dose steroids such as dexamethasone may be given intravenously, but radiotherapy is also useful in reducing the size of the tumour.

Metastatic bone pain. Metastatic bone pain is usually treated with courses of chemotherapy and radiotherapy, but analgesics may also be beneficial. A prostaglandin-like substance has been isolated from bone metastases and therefore NSAIDs and, more recently, bisphosphonates are often used in bone pain. Steroids also interfere with prostaglandin formation and dexamethasone, therefore, has a role, especially where there is nerve root or spinal cord compression.

Neuropathic pain

Neuropathic pain may be defined as 'pain arising as a direct consequence of a disease or lesion affecting the somatosensory system' and may occur as a result of pathological damage to nerve fibres in a peripheral nerve or in the CNS (see Table 33.3). Neuropathic pain may be spontaneous in nature

Table 33.3 Examples of causes of neuropathic pain

Cause of neuropathy	Examples
Trauma	Phantom limb Peripheral nerve injury Spinal cord injury Surgical
Infection/inflammation	Post-herpetic neuralgia HIV
Compression	Trigeminal neuralgia Sciatica
Cancer	Invasion/compression of nerve tissue by tumour
Ischaemia	Post-stroke pain Metabolic neuropathies (e.g. diabetic peripheral neuropathy)
Demyelination	Multiple sclerosis
Drugs	Vinca alkaloids Ethanol Taxols Anti-bacterials for TB and HIV

(continuous or paroxysmal) or evoked by sensory stimuli. As the underlying aetiology is different to inflammatory types of pain, patients typically present with disturbances in sensory function often describing their pain as tingling, shooting or electric shocks. It is possible for patients to present with pain in the context of sensory loss. Unlike inflammatory pain, neuropathic pain serves no biological advantage and can be described as an illness in its own right.

Typically, neuropathic pain does not respond as well to conventional analgesics, such as paracetamol and NSAIDs. Guidelines for the pharmacological management of neuropathic pain in the non-specialist setting have been published (National Institute for Health and Clinical Excellence, 2010).

Specific neuropathic pain syndromes

Postherpetic neuralgia. The pain associated with herpes zoster infection is severe, continuous and often described as burning and lancinating. Antiviral therapy, such as aciclovir, initiated at the first sign of the rash can reduce the duration of the pain, particularly postherpetic pain, which follows the disappearance of the rash. Tricyclic antidepressants such as amitriptyline are the mainstay of treatment, commencing with low doses (e.g. amitriptyline 10–25 mg at night) and gradually increased according to pain relief (usual dose amitriptyline 50–75 mg at night). This may be combined with anti-epileptic drugs if the response is poor or incomplete. Carbamazepine is historically important but newer anti-epileptic drugs, such as gabapentin and pregabalin, are considered first-line therapy and may be better tolerated. One study has demonstrated a significant difference in the incidence, and to a lesser extent the intensity, of pain in patients who received a single epidural methylprednisolone and bupivacaine injection, compared with those who received antiviral therapy and analgesia as 'standard care' (van Wijck et al., 2006). However, given the modest clinical effects on acute pain and no effect on the incidence of postherpetic neuralgia, the routine use of epidural local anaesthetic and steroid injection is not widely supported.

Diabetic peripheral polyneuropathy. Nerve damage and neuropathy is one of the long-term complications of diabetes mellitus (see Chapter 44) and is most prevalent in elderly patients with type II diabetes. Often patients describe numbness but also experience a burning sensation on their feet. The sensory loss can result in painless foot ulcers. Tricyclic antidepressants or serotonin noradrenaline reuptake inhibitors (duloxetine or venlafaxine), and anti-epileptics, such as gabapentin and pregabalin, have been demonstrated to be beneficial.

Trigeminal neuralgia. Trigeminal neuralgia presents as abrupt, intense bursts of severe, lancinating pain, provoked by touching sensitive trigger areas on one side of the face. The disorder may spontaneously remit for periods of several weeks or months. Anti-epileptic drugs, particularly carbamazepine, have been used successfully. If drug therapy is ineffective, neurosurgical techniques such as decompression of the fifth cranial nerve may be considered. If surgery is successful, anti-epileptics should be withdrawn gradually afterwards.

Peripheral nerve injury and neuropathy. Damage to, or entrapment of, nerves can cause pain, unpleasant sensations and paraesthesiae. Tricyclic antidepressants and anti-epileptic drugs, such as gabapentin, have been used with some success to treat neuropathic pain (Moore et al., 2011). A neuroma occurs when damaged or severed nerve fibres sprout new small fibres in an attempt to regenerate. Pain develops several weeks after the nerve injury, and is often due to the neuroma growing into scar tissue, causing pain as it is stretched or mobilised. Treatment of neuroma is very difficult and few treatments are successful. Options include surgery and injections of steroid and local anaesthetic agents.

Complex regional pain syndromes

These are an important group of painful conditions that may follow trauma or damage to nerves and are characterised by neuropathic pain, trophic changes and motor dysfunction. The key elements of successful treatment are effective multi-modal analgesia, including drugs with efficacy for neuropathic pain, and aggressive physiotherapy to facilitate a return to normal function. Sympathetic blockade using local anaesthetics may have a therapeutic role.

Back and neck pain

Back pain is one of the commonest reasons for presentation to a medical practitioner. Despite this, the problem is poorly understood. The most practical classification is based on the duration of symptoms (BenDebba et al., 1997). Acute low pain is generally defined as pain that lasts for a few days or weeks. The majority of these problems tend to be self-limiting and resolve spontaneously. Typical treatments include rest, adequate analgesia with paracetamol, combined with a NSAID and/or a weak opioid, and physiotherapy.

Persistent back pain lasts for much longer and progressively leads to a chronic state associated with pain, depression, anxiety and disability. Early intervention is necessary to ensure good functional and vocational outcomes. If a patient is off work for as much as 6 months, then there is a less than 50% chance of them ever returning to work. The likelihood of returning to work falls to less than 25% after 1 year and is almost zero after 2 years. Although pharmacological therapies may aid rehabilitation, other treatment strategies have a greater role to play in the management of persistent back pain. Guidelines for the management of non-specific persistent low back pain have been developed (National Institute for Health and Clinical Excellence, 2009). It is essential for the patient to develop self-management skills, and current recommendations emphasise the importance of using a biopsychosocial approach to manage this problem. Other treatment options include exercise programmes, manual therapy and acupuncture.

Osteoarthritis and rheumatoid arthritis

Pain often is a presenting symptom in osteoarthritis or the inflammatory arthritidies, which include rheumatoid arthritis. The pathophysiology and management of osteoarthritis and rheumatoid arthritis is covered in Chapter 53.

Myofascial pain

Myofascial pain is pain arising from muscles and is associated with stiffness and neuropathic symptoms such as tingling and paraesthesiae. It may occur spontaneously or following trauma, such as whiplash injury. Myofascial pain syndrome is sometimes also termed myositis, fibrositis, myalgia and myofasciitis. Acute muscle injury can be treated using first aid techniques with the application of a cooling spray or ice to reduce inflammation and spasm, followed by passive stretching of the muscle to restore its full range of motion. Injection therapy with local anaesthetic or saline may be used to disrupt sensitive muscle trigger points. Local injections of botulinum toxin have also been shown to be effective where muscle spasm is prolonged and severe. TENS and acupuncture have an important role to play in reducing pain and muscle spasm. Treatment of persistent myofascial syndromes should always include a programme of physical therapy.

Postamputation and phantom limb pain

The majority of amputees suffer significant stump or phantom limb pain for at least a few weeks each year. Pain will be present in the immediate postoperative period in the stump, and this may be caused by muscle spasm, nerve injury and sensitivity of the wound and surrounding skin. As the wound heals, the pain generally subsides. If it does not, the reason may be vascular insufficiency or infection. Pain occurring some number of years after amputation may be caused by changes in the structure of the bones or skin in the stump. Reduction in the thickness of overlying tissue with age may expose nerve endings to increased stimuli or ischaemia. Usually, conventional analgesics are beneficial for stump pain, although sometimes relatively high doses may be required. Tricyclic antidepressants may also be helpful for stump pain, and surgery may be necessary to restore the vascular supply or reduce trauma to nerve endings.

Phantom pain is a referred pain which produces a burning or throbbing sensation, felt in the absent limb. Cramping sensations are caused by muscular spasm in the stump. The patient with phantom limb pain is often anxious, depressed and frightened, all of which exacerbate the pain. Conventional analgesic drugs alone are generally not adequate for phantom pain, but TCAs and anti-epileptic drugs are useful adjuvants. Other therapy which can be effective includes TENS and sympathetic blockade. These patients frequently require management at specialist pain centres.

Headache

Everybody experiences the occasional tension headaches. They are caused by muscle contraction over the neck and scalp. Often they respond to simple analgesics available over-the-counter, such as paracetamol and NSAIDs. They may also respond to TCA drugs given as a single dose at night as well as non-pharmacological treatments, such as TENS. NSAIDs may be indicated if the headache is associated with cervical spondylosis or neck injury.

Migraine

Most migraine attacks respond to simple analgesics such as aspirin or paracetamol. Soluble preparations are best, as gut motility is reduced during a migraine attack and absorption of oral medication may be delayed. Migraine treatment has improved markedly with the development of the triptan drugs such as almotriptan, eletriptan, rizatriptan, sumatriptan, naratriptan and zolmitriptan (Goadsby, 2005). These are $5HT_{1B/1D}$-agonists that will often abort an attack, especially when given by the subcutaneous route. Their vaso-constrictor activity precludes their use in patients with angina or cerebrovascular disease but side effects are less serious than with the ergot derivatives they have replaced.

Prophylactic drug treatment of migraine includes α-adrenergic blockers, anti-epileptics and TCAs. Persistent treatment is undesirable.

Cluster headache

Cluster headache is a disabling condition characterised by severe unilateral head pain occurring in clusters of attacks varying from minutes to hours. It shares some pathological features with migraine and treatment is similar, although high-resolution MRI studies have shown specific anatomical differences in the brains of people with cluster headache. Triptans are effective in acute attacks, as is inhalation of 100% oxygen. Prophylaxis is similar to that of migraine.

Dysmenorrhoea

Dysmenorrhoea is a common cause of pelvic pain in women. NSAIDs are effective as first-line therapy due to their effect on cyclo-oxygenase inhibition but it can be helped also by the prescription of oral contraceptives, since pain is absent in anovulatory cycles. Dysmenorrhoea due to endometriosis may require therapy with androgenic drugs such as danazol or regulators of the gonadotrophins such as norethisterone.

Burn pain

Patients with burns may require a series of painful procedures such as physiotherapy, debridement or skin grafting. Premedication with a strong opioid before the procedure and the use of Entonox® (premixed 50% nitrous oxide and 50% oxygen) may be necessary to control the pain. Regular opioid administration may be useful to prevent the pain induced by movement or touch in the affected area. The anaesthetic drug ketamine (see above) has potent analgesic activity when used in subhypnotic doses. Its short duration of action may be beneficial to reduce the pain of dressing changes or other forms of incident pain. Even with low doses, a significant proportion of patients will experience side effects of dysphoria or hallucinations. These can be treated with benzodiazepines or antipsychotic compounds, such as haloperidol.

A summary of medicine indications and common therapeutic problems associated with analgesic use are presented in Table 33.4.

Table 33.4 Common therapeutic problems

Problem	Solution	Example
Neuropathic pain	Anti-epileptics	Carbamazepine Sodium valproate Gabapentin Lamotrigine
	Antidepressants	Amitriptyline Imipramine
	Intravenous anaesthetic agents	Ketamine
Malignant bone pain	Bisphosphonates	Pamidronate Calcitonin
Muscle spasm/ spasticity	Skeletal muscle relaxants	Baclofen Dantrolene Botulinum toxin (type A)
Raised intracranial pressure	Corticosteroids	Dexamethasone Prednisolone
Nausea with morphine	Antiemetic	Cyclizne Droperidol Ondansetron
	Use an alternative route of administration	Topical or subcutaneous
Constipation	Determine if drug induced, for example, opioids or tricyclic antidepressant	Co-prescribe laxatives (e.g. docusate sodium and senna)
Antidepressants in patients with ischaemic heart disease	Use a less cardiotoxic antidepressant	Duloxetine, venlafaxine
Drug interactions with carbamazepine	Use an anti-epileptic which does not affect hepatic enzymes	Gabapentin
Renal failure	Morphine accumulates; use lower dose Use a drug which is not eliminated by kidney	Fentanyl Buprenorphine
Sedation/ impaired cognition	Identify any drug-related causes and adjust dose or stop drug	

Case studies

Case 33.1

Mrs NP is a 55-year-old care home assistant who has type 2 diabetes. Her current prescription is for metformin 500 mg three times a day and amitriptyline 50 mg. When collecting her repeat prescription she mentions that she 'Can't get on with the new tablets' because they make her very drowsy in the mornings. You invite Mrs NP to attend to review her medication. During the consultation Mrs NP explains that for some time she has suffered from constant tingling and occasional shooting pain in her legs and feet and 3 months ago amitriptyline 10 mg daily was prescribed. About 1 month ago the dose of amitriptyline was increased to 50 mg daily. She takes the dose at night, as advised by her primary care doctor. When she works an early shift (about three times a week) she usually omits the dose of amitriptyline to be sure that she wakes up in time to get to work. Mrs NP says that she takes the metformin regularly and has no associated problems. She is keen to be fit enough to work because she is supporting her youngest son who is studying to be a doctor.

Question

What advice should you give to this patient?

Answer

Mrs NP has developed diabetic peripheral neuropathy, a type of neuropathic pain. She is experiencing intolerable side effects from the increased dose of amitriptyline and therefore does not take it regularly. There are several options to improve tolerability. Firstly, Mrs NP should consider increasing the dose of amitriptyline more slowly. She may also benefit from taking her amitriptyline dose earlier in the evening, approximately 60–90 min before retiring to bed, so that it results in less hangover effect the following day. If neither of these strategies is beneficial, she should consult her primary care doctor about switching to an alternative drug to manage her neuropathic symptoms. Recent guidance (National Institute for Health and Clinical Excellence, 2010) recommends either pregabalin or duloxetine as alternatives to a tricyclic anti-depressant as first-line therapy for neuropathic pain in the non-specialist setting.

Case 33.2

A 55-year-old lady with metastatic abdominal cancer from a probable primary in the pelvis presents with an abdominal mass. Her pain is uncontrolled despite regular prescription of oral opioids, and she has been sick for a week. Subacute bowel obstruction is present.

Question

How should this lady be managed?

Answer

Management should begin with admission and rehydration. She may be dehydrated and have marked electrolyte abnormalities which would need to be corrected. The oral route is unavailable for the delivery of adequate analgesia, and thus consideration should be given to the use of parenteral administration, either by the subcutaneous route or using patient-controlled analgesia. The sickness should be treated, and an underlying cause sought. This may be subacute obstruction which, in turn, may be due to constipation caused by the opioids or by the disease process. Abdominal masses that indent on palpation are faeces (not tumour). Abdominal radiographs would show fluid levels if there was obstruction rather than constipation. Other possible causes of vomiting are recent anticancer therapy, anxiety, dyspepsia from NSAIDs, raised intracranial pressure and vertigo.

Surgery may be needed to relieve the obstruction, but the need may be avoided by use of hyoscine butylbromide, which may control colic with little additional sedation. If the problem is one of constipation, rectal measures may be necessary to re-establish function. These may include suppositories, enemas or digital disimpaction. Once control of pain has been achieved and bowel function has returned to normal, she must receive regular combination laxative therapy, ideally a stimulant laxative such as senna, and a faecal softener, such as docusate sodium. A high fluid intake and increased dietary fibre should be encouraged, as this will help prevent stool from becoming hard.

There has been interest in the use of peripheral opioid receptor antagonists to reduce opioid-induced constipation. As they have higher affinity for the opioid receptor than the agonist, they bind preferentially to opioid receptors in the gastro-intestinal tract, allowing the agonist to continue to have its desired effect in the CNS. A combination of prolonged-release oxycodone and prolonged release naloxone (Targinact®) may be an alternative if maximal laxative therapy does not help this patient.

Attention should be paid to Mrs NP's emotional and spiritual needs at all times.

Case 33.3

A 28-year-old man had a crush fracture of his ankle after falling from a roof. Fixation 9 months ago was described as satisfactory, but his leg is now very painful to even small stimuli and he cannot use it or bear weight. The lower leg has muscle wasting and is much colder than the opposite limb. The skin is very sensitive to touch, shiny and has a poor circulation.

Question

What is this condition and how should this pain be treated?

Answer

The patient presents with a complex regional pain syndrome. Management should be aggressive and directed towards functional restoration. Use of effective multi-modal analgesia using pharmacological and non-pharmacological treatments is required. The aim is to facilitate aggressive physiotherapy and occupational therapy. There may be a burning component to the pain, which may respond to low doses of TCAs such as amitriptyline (10–25 mg at night initially, increased in small increments to 50–75 mg at night).

Aggressive treatment early in the course of the disease can reduce the length of time that patients have this problem, and early referral to seek specialised help is recommended. A small percentage of patients continue to have problems whatever treatment is given.

Case 33.4

An 85-year-old man is admitted to hospital after falling down a flight of stairs and landing heavily on his right side. On admission, he is in severe pain and finds breathing, and especially coughing, unbearably painful. A chest X-ray reveals that he has fractures of the 5th to 8th ribs on the right side.

Question

How should his pain be managed and what are the risks of under treatment?

Answer

Multiple rib fractures are potentially very serious and good analgesia can prevent potentially dangerous complications. Initial analgesia should include both potent opioids and NSAIDs (unless contraindicated). Opioids should be administered parenterally in the first instance and subsequent use of patient-controlled analgesia would allow the patient to titrate their own analgesic requirements. The chest injury may well result in damage to the underlying lung and it is essential to administer unrestricted high-flow oxygen to the patient as the combination of lung injury and ventilatory suppression secondary to either pain or the effects of opioids could lead to dangerous hypoxia. TENS may also prove helpful.

Arterial oxygen saturation (and preferably arterial blood gases) should be monitored. If pain remains poorly controlled or the patient's oxygenation deteriorates, thoracic epidural analgesia using a mixture of local anaesthetic and opioid may be considered.

Failure to treat pain adequately in this situation may lead to a reduction in the patient's ability to cough and clear secretions from the chest. This can lead to respiratory failure and even death. Analgesia should be sufficient to allow regular physiotherapy in order to minimise the risk of such complications.

Case 33.5

A 45-year-old woman presents to her primary care doctor with a 2-day history of back pain following a lifting injury at work. The pain is constant and aching in character with radiation into the posterior aspect of both thighs as far as the knee. Physical examination shows her to be maintaining a very rigid posture with some spasm of the large muscles of the back. Her range of movement is very poor but there are no neurological signs in the legs.

Question

Which drugs may help this lady's pain? What other advice should be given?

Answer

Acute back pain is very common and is rarely associated with serious spinal pathology. The absence of neurological signs is reassuring and indicates that early activity, possibly aided by a short course of analgesics, is the best way forward. Regular paracetamol every 6 h should be first-line treatment. This may be combined with NSAIDs, if tolerated. A muscle relaxant such as baclofen 20–40 mg/day in divided doses may be beneficial for short-term use only. The role of opioids is less clear. Short-term (7–14 days) use of a weak opioid such as codeine or tramadol is probably safe. Longer term use is less satisfactory as

there is no clear evidence of their efficacy and sedative side effects may reduce the patient's capacity and motivation to remain active.

The patient should be advised to remain active and accept that some pain is likely during the recovery phase. Failure to remain active and, in particular, excessive bed rest are both associated with worse outcomes.

Case 33.6

A 50-year-old man is admitted to hospital with an acute onset of severe mid-thoracic spinal pain. He is found to be anaemic and investigations show that he has multiple myeloma with widespread bony lesions, including fresh spinal fractures.

Question

Which drugs may help this man's pain? What particular hazards may occur in this condition?

Answer

This patient is extremely ill and even with aggressive chemotherapy, he is unlikely to survive more than a few months. Most of his pain will be related to the destruction of bone and the aim should be to provide pain relief via a 'central' mechanism through the use of opioids as well as reducing the rate of bone destruction and associated inflammatory responses. A potent opioid will be required and oral morphine would usually be the drug of first choice. In this situation, a combination of a modified release preparation together with liberal 'as required' dosing would be appropriate. The correct dose is the dose required to produce adequate pain relief without producing excessive sedation. Inflammatory pain may be improved by the use of NSAIDs and these should be given regularly, although they may be contraindicated in this condition (see below). High dose corticosteroids may achieve a similar effect and may also reduce the hypercalcaemia that is often seen in myeloma. Bone destruction and its associated pain may be reduced by the use of bisphosphonate compounds. In this case, intravenous pamidronate should be given.

Renal failure is common in myeloma. This may be due to obstruction of renal tubules by myeloma proteins or the effects of some chemotherapeutic agents. If renal impairment occurs, opioids should be used with caution so as to avoid problems with accumulation. Transdermal fentanyl may be a more appropriate drug. NSAIDs can precipitate acute renal failure in the presence of reduced renal blood flow. Finally, platelet function is often poor in patients with myeloma. This can be due to direct effects of myeloma proteins on platelets, bone marrow replacement by myeloma or the effects of chemotherapy. Use of NSAIDs may be associated with increased risk of gastro-intestinal haemorrhage.

Acknowledgement

The authors would like to acknowledge the contribution of S. Woolfrey and D. Kapur to previous versions of this chapter which appeared in earlier editions of this book.

References

Annetta, M.G., Iemma, D., Garisto, C., et al., 2005. Ketamine: new indications for an old drug. Curr. Drug Targets 6, 789–794.

Ballantyne, J.C., Mao, J., 2003. Opioid therapy for chronic pain. N. Engl. J. Med. 349, 1943–1953.

BenDebba, M., Torgerson, W.S., Long, D.M., 1997. Personality traits, pain duration, and severity, functional impairment, and psychological distress in patients with persistent low back pain. Pain 72, 115–125.

Breivik, H., Borchgrevink, P.C., et al. 2008. Assessment of pain. British Journal of Anaesthesia 101, 17–24.

Burns, T.L., Ineck, J.R., 2006. Cannabinoid analgesia as a potential new therapeutic option in the treatment of persistent pain. Ann. Pharmacother. 40, 251–260.

Claridge, L.C., Eksteen, B., Smith, A., et al., 2010. Acute liver failure after administration of paracetamol at the maximum recommended daily dose in adults. Br. Med. J. 341, c6764, doi: 10.1136/bmj.c6764.

Ellershaw, J., Wilkinson, S., 2003. Care of the Dying: A Pathway to Excellence. Oxford University Press, Oxford.

Goadsby, P.J., 2005. Advances in the understanding of headache. Br. Med. Bull. 73, 83–92.

Högestätt, E.D., Jonsson, B.A., Ermund, A., et al., 2005. Conversion on acetaminophen to the bioactive N-acylphenolamine AM404 via fatty acid hydrolase-dependent arachadonic acid conjugation in the nervous system. J. Biol. Chem. 280, 405–412.

Holden, J.E., Jeong, Y., Forrest, J.M., 2005. The endogenous opioid system and clinical pain management. AACN Clin. Issues 16, 291–301.

Hyllested, M., Jones, S., Pedersen, J.L., et al., 2002. Comparative effect of paracetamol, NSAIDs or their combination in postoperative pain management: a qualitative review. Br. J. Anaesth. 88, 199–214.

Kehlet, H., Rung, G.W., Callesen, T., 1996. Postoperative opioid analgesia: time for a reconsideration? J. Clin. Anesth. 8, 441–445.

Li Wan Po, A., Zhang, W.Y., 1997. Systematic overview of co-proxamol to assess analgesic effects of addition of dextropropoxyphene to paracetamol. Br. Med. J. 315, 1565–1571.

McQuay, H., Carroll, D., Jadad, A.R., et al., 1995. Anticonvulsant drugs for management of pain: a systematic review. Br. Med. J. 311, 1047–1052.

McQuay, H.J., Tramer, M., Nye, B., et al. 1996. A systematic review of antidepressants in neuropathic pain. Pain 68, 217–227.

Medicines and Healthcare Regulatory Agency, 2006. Updated safety information for non-steroidal anti-inflammatory drugs (NSAIDs). Available at http://www.mhra.gov.uk/NewsCentre/Pressreleases/CON2025039

Mercadante, S., 1996. Ketamine in cancer pain: an update. Palliat. Med. 10, 225–230.

Moore, R.A., Wiffen, P.J., Derry, S., McQuay, H.J. Gabapentin for chronic neuropathic pain and fibromyalgia in adults. Cochrane Database of Systematic Reviews 2011, Issue 3. Art. No.: CD007938. DOI: 10.1002/14651858.CD007938.pub2.

National Institute for Health and Clinical Excellence, 2009. Low back pain. Early management of persistent non-specific low back pain. Clinical Guideline 88. NICE, London. Available at http://www.nice.org.uk/nicemedia/pdf/CG88NICEGuideline.pdf.

National Institute for Health and Clinical Excellence, 2010. Neuropathic pain: the pharmacological management of neuropathic pain in adults in non-specialist setting. Clinical Guideline 96. NICE, London. Available at http://www.nice.org.uk/nicemedia/live/12948/47949/47949.pdf.

Scottish Intercollegiate Guidelines Network, 2008. Control of pain in adults with cancer. SIGN, Edinburgh. Available at http://www.sign.ac.uk/pdf/SIGN106.pdf.

Sindrup, S.H., Jensen, T.S., 1999. Efficacy of pharmacological treatments of neuropathic pain: an update and effect related to mechanism of drug action. Pain 83, 389–400.

Sindrup, S.H., Otto, M., Finnerup, N.B., et al., 2005. Antidepressants in the treatment of neuropathic pain. Basic Clin. Pharmacol. Toxicol. 96, 399–409.

Tjolsen, A., Lund, A., Hole, K., 1991. Antinociceptive effect of paracetamol in rats is partly dependent on spinal serotonergic systems. Eur. J. Pharmacol. 193, 193–201.

Thompson, D.R., 2001. Narcotic analgesic effects on the sphincter of Oddi: a review of the data and therapeutic implications in treating pancreatitis. Am. J. Gastroenterol. 96, 1266–1272.

van Wijck, A.J., Opstelten, W., Moons, K.G., et al., 2006. The PINE study of epidural steroids and local anaesthetics to prevent postherpetic neuralgia: a randomised controlled trial. Lancet 367, 219–224.

Woolf, C.J., 2004. Pain: moving from symptom control toward mechanism-specific pharmacologic management. Ann. Intern. Med. 140, 441–451.

Further reading

British Association for the Study of Headache, 2007. Guidelines for all healthcare professionals in the diagnosis and management of migraine, tension-type, cluster and medication-overuse headache. Available at http://216.25.88.43/upload/NS_BASH/BASH_guidelines_2007.pdf.

MacIntyre, P., Schug, S.A., 2007. Acute Pain Management: A Practical Guide, third ed. Elsevier, Philadelphia.

Macintyre, P.E., Scott, D.A., Schug, S.A., et al. (Eds.), 2010. Acute Pain Management: Scientific Evidence, third ed. Australia and New Zealand College of Anaesthetists and Faculty of Pain Medicine, Melbourne. Available at http://www.nhmrc.gov.au/_files_nhmrc/file/publications/synopses/cp104_3.pdf.

Marcus, D.A. (Ed.), 2005. Chronic Pain: A Primary Care Guide to Practical Management. Humana Press, Totowa.

McMahon, S., Koltzenburg, M. (Eds.), 2005. Melzack and Wall's Textbook of Pain, fifth ed. Churchill Livingstone, Edinburgh.

Melzack, R., Wall, P.D., 2003. Handbook of Pain Management: A Clinical Companion to Melzack and Wall's Textbook of Pain. Churchill Livingstone, Edinburgh.

Moore, R.A., McQuay, H.J., 2005. Prevalence of opioid adverse events in persistent non-malignant pain: systematic review of randomized trials of oral opioids. Arthritis Res. Therapy 7, R1046–R1051.

National Institute for Health and Clinical Excellence, 2004. Improving supportive and palliative care for adults with cancer. NICE, London. Available at http://www.nice.org.uk/nicemedia/live/10893/28816/28816.pdf.

Useful websites

The Radar Approach to Pain, http://www.painradar.co.uk/acute-pain-management-consensus.aspx.

Oxford Pain Internet site, http://www.medicine.ox.ac.uk/bandolier/booth/painpag/index.html.

Change Pain, http://www.change-pain.co.uk/

PalliativeDrugs.com, http://www.palliativedrugs.com/

The British Pain Society, http://www.britishpainsociety.org.

Nausea and vomiting 34

E. Mason and P. A. Routledge

Key points

- Patients must be assessed carefully, and often reassessed frequently, to identify the primary underlying cause of their nausea and/or vomiting.
- Antiemetics are symptomatic treatments only and do not treat the underlying cause.
- Drug choice is based on an understanding of the likely pathophysiology, the receptors involved, the available route of administration and drug side effects.
- In certain situations, prophylactic regimens are beneficial, for example, motion sickness, post-operative nausea and vomiting, chemotherapy-induced nausea and vomiting.
- Simple regimens are used where possible to prevent postoperative nausea and vomiting, such as parenteral cyclizine or prochlorperazine administered at induction. These and other antiemetics can be used for rescue therapy if vomiting occurs post-operatively.
- The choice of antiemetic to use in conjunction with cytotoxic chemotherapy depends on the emetogenicity of the cytotoxic drugs used. The $5HT_3$ antagonists such as ondansetron are very effective antiemetic drugs when highly emetogenic chemotherapy is used. The addition of dexametasone may provide further benefit.
- Anticipatory emesis associated with chemotherapy can be treated with benzodiazepine and dexametasone is useful in alleviating delayed emesis.

Nausea and vomiting are commonly (but not universally) associated symptoms. The word nausea is derived from the Greek *nautia*, meaning sea-sickness, while vomiting is derived from the Latin *vomere*, meaning to discharge. Nausea is a subjective sensation whereas vomiting is the reflex physical act of expulsion of gastric contents. Retching is defined as 'spasmodic respiratory movements' against a closed glottis with contractions of the abdominal musculature without expulsion of any gastric contents, that is, 'dry heaves' (American Gastroenterological Association, 2001). It is important to differentiate vomiting from regurgitation, rumination and bulimia. Regurgitation is the return of oesophageal or gastric contents into the hypopharynx with little effort. Rumination is the passive regurgitation of recently ingested food into the mouth followed by re-chewing, re-swallowing or spitting out. It is not preceded by nausea and does not include the various physical phenomena associated with vomiting. Bulimia involves overeating followed by self induced vomiting.

Epidemiology

Nausea and vomiting from all causes have significant associated social and economic costs in terms of loss of productivity and extra medical care. In the community, nausea (with or without vomiting) is most likely to be associated with infection, particularly gastro-intestinal infection. Vestibular disorders may cause vomiting as can motion sickness. Nausea and vomiting may be associated with pain, for example, migraine and severe cardiac pain. Many medicines also cause nausea and occasionally vomiting as a common dose-related (Type A) adverse effect. This is particularly common with opioid use in palliative care. Nausea and vomiting also occur post-operatively or in association with cytotoxic chemotherapy, or radiotherapy. These and other causes of nausea and vomiting are listed in Table 34.1.

Pathophysiology

Complex interactions between central and peripheral pathways occur in the production of the clinical features of nausea and vomiting. The most important areas involved peripherally are the gastric mucosa and smooth muscle (the enteric brain) and the afferent pathways of the vagus and sympathetic nerves. Centrally the significant areas involved are the area postrema, the chemoreceptor trigger zone (CTZ), the nucleus tractus solitarus (NTS) and the vomiting centre.

From a pharmacotherapeutic point of view, the most important aspect of this complex pathophysiology is the variety of receptors involved, including histaminergic (H_1), cholinergic (muscarinic M_1), dopaminergic (D2), serotonergic ($5HT_3$) and neurokinin-1 (NK_1) receptors. In the clinical situation, these become targets for various drugs directed at controlling the symptoms.

There are 10^8 neurons in the intestine and a complex interaction occurs between these, the mucosa, the smooth muscle in the intestine, the parasympathetic (vagus nerve) and sympathetic nerves and the higher centres in the spinal cord and brain to result in normal gastro-intestinal peristaltic activity. The enteric brain and the vagus nerve monitor stimuli from mucosal irritation and smooth muscle stretch which may result in nausea and/or vomiting.

The area postrema in the floor of the fourth ventricle contains the CTZ and is a special sensory organ rich in

Table 34.1 Selected causes of nausea and vomiting (adapted from Quigley et al., 2001)

Central	
i. Intracranial	Migraine
	Raised intracranial pressure (tumour, infection, haemorrhage, hydocephalus, etc.)
ii. Labyrinthine Iatrogenic	Labyrinthitis, motion sickness, Ménière's disease, otitis media
	Cancer chemotherapy
	Many other medicines (e.g. opioids)
	Radiotherapy
	Post-operative
Endocrine/ metabolic	Pregnancy, uraemia, diabetic ketoacidosis, hyperthyroidism, hyperparathyroidism, hypoparathyroidism, Addison's disease, acute intermittent porpyhria
Infectious	Gastroenteritis (viral or bacterial)
	Other infections elsewhere
Gastro-intestinal disorders	Mechanical obstruction (gastric outlet or small bowel)
	Organic gastro-intestinal disorders (e.g. cholecystitis, pancreatitis, hepatitis, etc.)
	Functional gastro-intestinal disorders (e.g. non-ulcer dyspepsia, irritable bowel syndrome, etc.)
Psychogenic disorders	Psychogenic vomiting, anxiety, depression
Pain related	Myocardial infarction

dopaminergic, serotonergic, histaminergic and muscarinic receptors. It is located outside the blood–brain barrier (BBB) and it is likely that chemicals, toxins, peptides, drugs and neurotransmitters in the cerebrospinal fluid (CSF) and bloodstream interact with this area to cause nausea and vomiting. However, the precise mechanism is not known.

The vomiting centre is situated in the dorsolateral reticular formation close to the respiratory centre and receives impulses from higher centres, visceral efferents, the eighth (auditory) nerve (the latter two through the nucleus tractus solitarius) and from the CTZ (Fig. 34.1). It includes a number of brainstem nuclei required to integrate the responses of the gastrointestinal tract, pharyngeal muscles, respiratory muscles and somatic muscles to result in a vomiting episode. The vomiting centre may be stimulated in association with, or in isolation from, the nausea process.

The vomiting reflex can be elicited either directly via afferent neuronal connections, especially from the gastro-intestinal tract and is probably dependent on the integrity of the nucleus tractus solitarius, or from humoral factors dependent on the integrity of the area postrema. The sequence of muscle excitation and inhibition necessary for the act of vomiting is probably controlled by a central pattern generator located in the nucleus tractus solitarius, and information from the CTZ and vagus nerve converges at this point.

The central causes of nausea and vomiting include increased intracranial pressure, dilation of cerebral arteries during migraine and stimulation of the labyrinthine mechanism or of the senses of sight, smell and taste.

The peripheral causes of nausea and vomiting include motion sickness, delayed gastric emptying and gastric mucosal irritation (ulceration, NSAIDs). These mechanisms are all mediated through the vagal afferent neurons. The vomiting associated with distension or obstruction of the gastro-intestinal tract is mediated through both the sympathetic and vagal afferent neurons.

Patient management

Management of the patient with nausea and vomiting is approached in three steps.

1. Recognise and correct any complications. This includes correction of dehydration, hypokalaemia and metabolic alkalosis in the acute situation with symptoms of less than 4 weeks duration. Weight loss and malnutrition are features of chronic nausea/vomiting, that is, when symptoms have been present for 4 weeks or longer.
2. Where possible, identify the underlying cause (see Table 34.1) and institute appropriate treatment. Here it is important to be aware that metabolic or endocrine conditions such as hypercalcaemia, hyponatraemia and hyperthyroidism can result in vomiting.
3. Implement therapeutic strategies to suppress or eliminate symptoms (these depend on the severity and clinical context). Ideally, antiemetic drugs are prescribed only when the cause of the nausea and/or vomiting is known, since by suppressing symptoms, they may otherwise delay diagnosis. This is especially true in children. However, they may sometimes be necessary temporarily in situations when directly addressing the underlying cause will not bring symptom relief sufficiently rapidly.

Some scenarios illustrating common therapeutic problems in the management of nausea and vomiting are outlined in Table 34.2.

Antiemetic drugs

Several classes of antiemetic drugs are available that antagonise the neurotransmitter receptors involved in the pathophysiology of nausea and vomiting. These classes of drugs are generally distinguished from each other by the identity of their main target receptor, although some act at more than one receptor.

Antihistamines

This group of medicines includes cinnarizine, cyclizine, diphenhydramine, diphenhydrinate and promethazine. They have some efficacy in nausea and vomiting caused by a wide

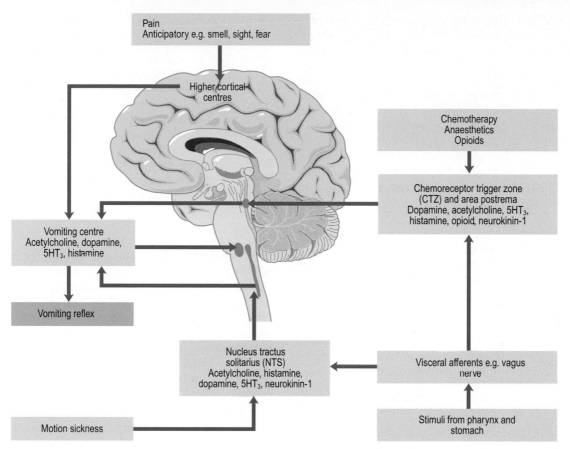

Fig. 34.1 Schematic representation of pathways involved in nausea and vomiting.

Table 34.2 Common therapeutic problems in managing patients with nausea and vomiting

Problem	Possible cause/solution
Persistent nausea and vomiting despite treatment	Is the cause correctly diagnosed? Review the antiemetic agent and the dose: if both correct, change to or add a second agent
Patient with PONV is vomiting despite suitable antiemetic regimen	Check analgesia: pain may be causing nausea and vomiting, or patient-controlled analgesia may require adjustment downwards to reduce analgesic dose
Patient with bowel obstruction is passing flatus	Prokinetic drug is first-choice antiemetic. $5HT_3$ antagonists may also be effective
Patient with bowel obstruction is not passing flatus	Spasmolytic drug is first choice. Prokinetic drugs are contraindicated. Similarly, bulk-forming, osmotic and stimulant laxatives are inappropriate; phosphate enemas and faecal softeners are better
A terminally ill patient receiving diamorphine is vomiting, despite use of haloperidol	Levomepromazine given as a 24-h subcutaneous infusion can be very effective
A patient with renal failure (uraemia) is vomiting	Consider a $5HT_3$ antagonist
A patient develops an acute dystonic reaction to metoclopramide	Give an intramuscular injection of an antihistamine. Such extrapyramidal reactions to metoclopramide are more common in young adults (especially females) and this agent is best avoided in this group

PONV, post-operative nausea and vomiting.

range of conditions, including motion sickness and postoperative nausea and vomiting (PONV). They are thought to block H_1 receptors in the CTZ and possibly elsewhere. However, several of these agents also have potent anticholinergic (M_1) receptor antagonist activity, which may contribute significantly to their efficacy as well as their adverse effect profile (see Section 'Anticholinergics'). The sedative effects of some antihistamines may also contribute to antiemetic activity, although this property appears not to be essential and it can be a particular problem when skilled tasks, such as driving, need to be performed. Nevertheless, the newer non-sedating antihistamines, for example, fexofenadine, are of limited value in nausea and vomiting.

Anticholinergics

This is one of the oldest classes of antiemetics, of which many members are potent inhibitors of muscarinic receptor (M_1) activity both peripherally and centrally. Anticholinergic drugs such as atropine, hyoscine and glycopyrronium have been used preoperatively to inhibit salivation and excessive respiratory secretions during anaesthesia. Anticholinergics act by inhibiting cholinergic transmission from the vestibular nuclei to higher centres within the cerebral cortex, thereby explaining their predominant use in the treatment of motion sickness. Hyoscine hydrobromide (scopolamine hydrobromide) is the most widely used agent and it can be given orally, by subcutaneous or intramuscular injection, or transdermally for motion sickness. Inhibition of peripheral muscarinic receptors can cause drowsiness, dry mouth, dilated pupils and blurred vision, decreased sweating, gastro-intestinal motility and gastro-intestinal secretions and difficulty with micturition. Anticholinergic agents may also precipitate closed-angle glaucoma in susceptible individuals.

Antidopaminergics

Phenothiazines and butyrophenones

Phenothiazines (e.g. prochlorperazine, perphenazine, and trifluoperazine) and butyrophenones (e.g. haloperidol and droperidol) act as antagonists at dopamine (D2) receptors in the CTZ, but may also have cholinergic (M_1) and histaminergic (H_1) receptor antagonist activity. As a consequence they share several adverse effects with antihistamines and anticholinergics, including drowsiness. In addition, the dopamine-blocking effects may be associated with acute dystonia (especially in children), and tardive dyskinesias or parkinsonism when used for prolonged periods. Prochlorperazine is less sedating and available as a buccal tablet and suppository for use when vomiting precludes oral administration. Phenothiazines are sometimes used for drug-associated emesis, including chemotherapy-induced nausea and vomiting (CINV), but like the butyrophenones, have in many situations been superseded by more specific agents such as metoclopramide and the selective $5HT_3$ antagonists. Levomepromazine is sometimes used to relieve nausea and vomiting in terminal care.

Metoclopramide

At lower doses, metoclopramide acts as a selective D2 antagonist at the CTZ and its effects mirror those of the phenothiazines and butyrophenones. However, it also exerts peripheral D2 antagonism at these doses, and stimulates cholinergic receptors in gastric smooth muscle, thus stimulating gastric emptying. It may, therefore, be more effective than phenothiazines and butyrophenones when nausea is related to gastro-intestinal or biliary disease. At higher doses, it may exert some $5HT_3$-receptor antagonism but at these doses, the incidence of acute dystonic reactions, particularly in young women and the elderly, may limit its usefulness in CINV.

Domperidone

Although domperidone does not readily cross the BBB, it is a selective antagonist of D2 receptors at the CTZ, which lies outside the BBB in the area postrema. It may also have peripheral effects that result in increased gastro-intestinal motility and faster gastric emptying. It is used in drug-associated vomiting, including CINV, and is relatively non-sedating. It can be given orally or by suppository. Acute dystonic reactions occur less frequently than with metoclopramide. It prevents nausea and vomiting during treatment with apomorphine and other dopamine agonists in Parkinson's disease and is also used to treat vomiting associated with emergency hormonal contraception.

Selective $5HT_3$-receptor antagonists

Serotonin or 5-hydroxytryptamine (5HT) plays an important role in nausea and vomiting. The subtype $5HT_3$-receptors, which mediate the vomiting pathway, are located peripherally on vagal nerve endings in the gastro-intestinal tract and centrally in the brain, with high concentrations found in the area postrema and nucleus tractus solitarius. Highly emetogenic agents such as cisplastin are thought to disrupt gastric mucosa and initiate the release of 5HT from enterochromaffin cells, which stimulate the $5HT_3$-receptors on afferent vagal nerve endings and thus trigger the emetic reflex. Selective $5HT_3$-receptor antagonists that act centrally and peripherally are now commonly used to treat or prevent CINV (with drugs of moderate to high emetogenic potential) and PONV. They are also effective in radiotherapy-induced nausea and vomiting. Selective $5HT_3$ antagonists are generally well tolerated, with the most common adverse effects being constipation, headache, dizziness and sensation of warmth or flushing. Some available agents include granisetron, ondansetron and palonosetron. They are all more expensive than antihistamines, phenothiazines, anticholinergics or dopamine antagonists.

Neurokinin-1 (NK_1) receptor antagonists

Substance P is a bioactive peptide that shares a common amino acid sequence with other bioactive peptides known as tachykinins. It appears to play an important role as a neurotransmitter in emesis as well as in pain and a number of other inflammatory processes. Substance P binds to the subtype neurokinin-1, or NK_1 receptors, which are found in the area postrema and nucleus tractus solitarius. Selective NK_1 receptor antagonists, aprepitant and fosaprepitant (a prodrug of aprepitant), are now available for use as an adjunct to dexametasone and a $5HT_3$ antagonist in preventing, but not treating, nausea and vomiting associated with moderately and highly emetogenic chemotherapy. They appear to be well tolerated but it is an inhibitor (and sometimes inducer) of cytochrome P450 (CYP3A4) and inducer of CYP2C9 and glucuronidation, so potential drug interactions with chemotherapeutic agents as well as other concomitantly administered agents, for example, possibly warfarin, may occur.

Cannabinoids

It is likely that the antiemetic activity of cannabinoids is related to stimulation of central and peripheral cannabinoid (CB1) receptors. Cannabinoids have modest antiemetic activity that is of similar magnitude to prochlorperazine in CINV, but they can cause a range of central nervous adverse effects, including drowsiness and sometimes behavioural disturbances, which may at times be severe. Thus, while the synthetic cannabinoid nabilone is indicated for nausea and vomiting caused by cytotoxic chemotherapy unresponsive to conventional antiemetics, it is recommended that patients are made aware of possible changes in their mood and other unwanted effects on their behaviour. In addition, nabilone should be used under close supervision, preferably in a hospital setting.

Corticosteroids

Corticosteroids are known to have antiemetic effects. Their mechanism of action is unclear but steroid receptors are thought to exist in the area postrema. As single agents, they appear to be at least as effective as prochlorperazine in preventing nausea and vomiting associated with mild to moderately emetogenic cytotoxic chemotherapy. Dexametasone, the most widely used corticosteroid in this context, improves the antiemetic activity of prochlorperazine and metoclopramide and may reduce some of the side effects associated with the latter. When combined with $5HT_3$ antagonists, corticosteroids are particularly effective in CINV associated with moderately emetogenic chemotherapy, or when used in delayed emesis. The same combination of dexametasone and a $5HT_3$ antagonist, and sometimes with aprepitant, may also be effective in CINV associated with highly emetogenic chemotherapy regimens.

Complementary and alternative medicines

Systematic reviews support the use of stimulating wrist acupuncture point P6 for preventing PONV in combination with, or as an alternative to, conventional antiemetics (Lee and Done, 2004). A systematic review of randomised trials has also demonstrated the efficacy of ginger (at least 1 g preoperatively) in PONV. Ginger has also been claimed to be beneficial in motion sickness and pregnancy-associated nausea, but the evidence for each is limited to single randomised trials (Ernst and Pittler, 2000).

Drug treatment in selected circumstances

Post-operative nausea and vomiting

Around 25% of patients experience PONV within 24 h of surgery (Gan et al., 2003). The aetiology is complex and multifactorial and includes patient-, medical-, surgical- and anaesthetic-related factors. Management is multimodal and involves strategies to reduce baseline risk such as using less emetogenic induction agents, anaesthetic agents and analgesics, consideration of the use of regional rather than general anaesthesia, adequate hydration and intraoperative supplemental oxygen use and avoidance of high-dose neostigmine.

Many antiemetic agents have some efficacy in post-operative nausea and vomiting but combination therapy with drugs from different classes may be needed in patients at high risk, such as those with a previous history of post-operative nausea and vomiting or motion sickness, or after high-risk procedures, for example, prolonged operations. Prophylactic treatments include dexametasone before induction or $5HT_3$ antagonists, antihistamines or phenothiazines at the end of surgery. Metoclopramide and cannabinoids appear to be of limited value in the management of post-operative nausea and vomiting.

Premedication with opioids increases the incidence of post-operative nausea and vomiting and this may be reduced by concurrent administration of either atropine or hyoscine, which are primarily used as anti-secretory drugs at premedication.

Risk scores

Prophylaxis is preferable to treatment and this can often be achieved not only by use of antiemetic drugs but also by suitable planning. For example, not all patients undergoing surgery will experience post-operative nausea and vomiting and universal prophylaxis is not cost-effective (Habib and Gan, 2004). A simple risk scoring system has been devised in which the score increases relative to the presence or absence of four factors:

- female gender
- history of motion sickness or PONV
- non-smoker
- opioid use during operation.

The incidence of post-operative nausea and vomiting with the presence of none, one, two, three or all four of these risk factors has been shown to be 10%, 20%, 40%, 60% and 80%, respectively (Apfel et al., 1999). Use of risk scores based on these criteria helps to appropriately tailor antiemetic use and can significantly reduce the incidence of nausea and vomiting in clinical practice (Apfel et al., 2002; Pierre et al., 2004).

Chemotherapy-induced nausea and vomiting

Three different types of CINV have been identified: acute, delayed and anticipatory. Acute emesis begins within 1 or 2 h of treatment and peaks in the first 4–6 h. Delayed emesis occurs more than 24 h after treatment, peaks at 48–72 h and then subsides over 2–3 days. It occurs characteristically after high-dose cisplatin but may also occur after the related agent carboplatin, as well as cyclophosphamide or an anthracycline. Anticipatory emesis occurs in patients who have developed significant CINV during previous cycles of therapy. Acute CINV is often associated with an increase in plasma serotonin concentrations for the most emetogenic agents, while delayed and anticipatory vomiting seem to be mediated by serotonin-independent pathways.

Management of CINV depends on the emetogenicity of the chemotherapy regimen and the use of combinations of antiemetic drugs based on their varying target receptors. Chemotherapy agents are divided into four emetogenic levels (Table 34.3) defined by expected frequency of emesis (Kris et al., 2006).

In high-level acute emesis, a single dose of a $5HT_3$ antagonist given before chemotherapy is therapeutically equivalent to a multidose regimen with these agents. Odansetron and granisetron appear to be equally effective in CINV and only one study suggests palonosetron is superior to granisetron when given in combination with dexametasone (Billio et al., 2010). Oral formulations of antiemetics are often as effective as intravenous ones. In lower level acute emesis, the cost of the $5HT_3$ antagonists is prohibitive and metoclopramide or prochlorperazine are commonly used and are sufficiently effective.

Dexametasone is the most extensively evaluated steroid in the management of CINV. Used alone, it is not sufficiently potent in CINV. However, it enhances the effect of other agents such as $5HT_3$ antagonists in high-risk situations and, together with metoclopramide, it also appears to be useful in treating delayed emesis.

The best management for anticipatory emesis is the avoidance of acute and delayed emesis during previous cycles. However, when anticipatory nausea and vomiting are a problem, a low dose of a benzodiazepine such as lorazepam is often effective.

When apparently appropriate antiemesis regimens fail, consideration should be given to the possibility of other underlying disease- and medication-related issues (Box 34.1).

Pregnancy-associated nausea and vomiting

Pregnancy-associated nausea and/or vomiting occurs in about 70% of women during the first trimester. Risk factors for vomiting include a personal history of previous pregnancy-associated nausea/vomiting or motion sickness or migraine-associated nausea/vomiting, a family history of hyperemesis gravidarum or a large placental mass, for example, due to multiple pregnancy. Symptoms usually begin 4 weeks after the last menses and in 80% of cases end at 12 weeks, having peaked at 9 weeks. In some women, the problem may persist

Table 34.3 Relative emetogenicity of chemotherapy drugs (from Kris et al., 2006)

Emetic risk (incidence of emesis without antiemetics)	Agent
High (>90%)	Cisplatin Mechlorethamine Streptozotocin Cyclophosphamide ≥1500 mg/m² Carmustine Dacarbazine Dactinomycin
Moderate (30–90%)	Oxaliplatin Cytarabine >1000 mg/m² Carboplatin Ifosfamide Cyclophosphamide <1500 mg/m² Doxorubicin Daunorubicin Epirubicin Idarubicin Irinotecan
Low (10–30%)	Paclitaxel Docetaxel Mitoxantrone Topotecan Etoposide Pemetrexed Methotrexate Mitomycin Gemcitabine Cytarabine ≤1000 mg/m² Flurouracil Bortezomib Cetuximab Trastuzumab
Minimal (<10%)	Bevacizumab Bleomycin Busulfan 2-Chlorodeoxyadenosine Fludarabine Rituximab Vinblastine Vincristine Vinrelbine

Box 34.1 Factors that cause nausea and vomiting in their own right and may contribute to the failure of apparently appropriate prophylactic regimens for chemotherapy-induced nausea and vomiting (CINV)

Hypercalcaemia or other metabolic or endocrine disturbance
CNS metastases
Antibiotics such as erythromycin/clarithromycin
Gastro-intestinal obstruction
Radiotherapy enteropathy

until 16–20 weeks. First-trimester nausea and vomiting are not usually harmful to either the fetus or the mother and is not generally associated with a poor pregnancy outcome.

In contrast, hyperemesis gravidarum is a condition of intractable vomiting complicating between 1% and 5% of pregnancies and sometimes resulting in serious fluid and electrolyte disturbance and nutritional deficits.

In first-trimester nausea and vomiting, simple measures such as small frequent carbohydrate-rich meals and reassurance are sufficient to control symptoms. Ginger and P6 acupressure have also been advocated, although the evidence base is equivocal in early pregnancy (Jewell and Young, 2003). More recent studies on the use of acupuncture in pregnancy-associated nausea and vomiting remain unclear (King and Murphy, 2009). It is important to avoid antiemetic drugs when possible, but promethazine has been recommended in severe vomiting, with prochorperazine or metoclopramide as second line agents. In Canada and the USA, a combination of pyridoxine (vitamin B_6) and an antihistamine (doxylamine) is approved for the treatment of nausea in pregnancy but this combination treatment appears to be less effective for controlling vomiting.

In the serious condition of hyperemesis gravidarum, drug therapy may be used, although no trials have shown clear benefit (Jewell and Young, 2003). Fluid and electrolyte replacement, rest and if necessary postpyloric or parenteral feeding to provide nutritional support and vitamins (e.g. thiamine to reduce the risk of Wernicke's encephalopathy) supplementation should be considered. There are few safety or efficacy data on which to select the most appropriate treatments so the agents recommended for vomiting of pregnancy mentioned above are generally used in the first instance in the UK.

Migraine

Migraine is a paroxysmal disorder with attacks of headaches, nausea, vomiting, photophobia and malaise. Treatment is directed at:

- prophylaxis: avoid triggers, try β-blockers, pizotifen and in severe cases a $5HT_{1B/D}$-receptor agonist such as sumatriptan
- analgesia, including aspirin, paracetamol, opioids, NSAIDs
- antiemetics.

Nausea and vomiting in migraine are associated with headache intensity, and the concomitant gastric stasis aggravates the nausea and vomiting and may also delay absorption of oral analgesics. Metoclopramide and domperidone attenuate the autonomic dysfunction and promote gastric emptying but the risk of acute dystonic crisis, especially with metoclopramide therapy should be borne in mind, especially in young women and children, but also in the elderly.

Labyrinthitis

Labyrinthine dysfunction results in vertigo, nausea and vomiting. Episodes may last a few hours or days. Causes include labyrinth viral infections, tumours and Ménière's disease. The onset of episodes is often unpredictable and disabling.

Betahistine sometimes has some benefit. The anticholinergics, antihistamines, phenothiazines or benzodiazepines can be used to suppress the vestibular system. Usually hyoscine is sufficient but if there is severe vomiting, prochlorperazine or metoclopramide may be of value.

Motion sickness

Motion sickness is a syndrome, a collection of symptoms without an identifiable cause. It is brought on by chronic repetitive movements which stimulate afferent pathways to the vestibular nuclei and lead to activation of the brainstem nuclei. Histaminergic and muscarinic pathways are involved. The symptoms include vague epigastric discomfort, headache, cold sweating and nausea which may culminate in vomiting. This is often followed by marked fatigue which can last hours or days. Onset of symptoms may be abrupt or gradual.

The anticholinergic agent hyoscine is the prophylactic drug of choice, although there is no evidence of its benefit once motion sickness is established (Spinks et al., 2004). Antihistamine drugs may also be effective. The less sedating antihistamines cinnarizine or cyclizine are used. Promethazine, an antihistamine with sedative effects, is also effective but phenothiazines, domperidone, metoclopramide and $5HT_3$-receptor antagonists appear to be ineffective in this situation. Treatment should be started before travel; for long journeys, promethazine or transdermal hyoscine may be preferred for their longer duration (24h and 3 days, respectively). Otherwise, repeated doses will be needed.

The most important adverse effect of many drugs used is sedation, whilst for anticholinergic drugs it is blurred vision, urinary retention and constipation. In laboratory studies, the degree to which these effects impair performance, for example, driving a car, is highly variable but subjects who take antimotion sickness drugs should normally be deemed unfit for such tasks. These drugs also potentiate the effects of alcohol.

Many non-drug treatments have been advocated for alleviation of motion sickness, including wristbands, which act on acupuncture points, variously positioned pieces of coloured paper or card, as well as plant extracts such as ginger. The evidence base for these interventions remains very limited.

Drug-associated nausea and vomiting

As well as chemotherapeutic agents, many commonly used medications for other disorders can cause nausea and vomiting (Quigley et al., 2001). Opioids are perhaps the most important group clinically, but dopamine agonists (used in Parkinson's disease), theophylline, digoxin and macrolide antibiotics such as erythromycin can all cause nausea and/or vomiting, often in a dose-related manner (Type A toxicity). High-dose oestrogen, used in postcoital contraception, can produce these symptoms. Consideration should be given to altering the dose of the offending agent when possible, and administering the medication with food. With some agents, tolerance may develop. Thus, tolerance to the emetic effects of opioids often develops within 5–10 days and, therefore, antiemetic therapy is not generally needed for long-term opioid use.

Palliative care-associated nausea and vomiting

Nausea and vomiting are common and distressing symptoms in cancer patients. In most cases, the causes of nausea and vomiting are due to multiple factors such as the tumour itself, concurrent infection, drugs and metabolic disturbances such as renal failure.

It is important to determine the predominant underlying cause for patients' symptoms by taking a careful history, examination and appropriate investigations so that potentially reversible causes of nausea and vomiting can be treated (Box 34.2) and the most suitable antiemetic prescribed.

Oral antiemetic therapy is effective for treatment of nausea in patients with advanced cancer but the subcutaneous route is preferred for those with severe persistent vomiting, either as a single dose injection or a continuous infusion via a syringe driver. When patients' symptoms improve, switching from subcutaneous injection to oral route might be preferable. Non-pharmacological interventions such as avoidance of certain food smells or unpleasant odours, relaxation techniques and use of acupuncture should be considered.

CINV is described in detail elsewhere in the chapter. Strong opioids such as morphine, diamorphine, oxycodone and fentanyl cause nausea and/or vomiting in up to one-third of patients following initiation of treatment but the incidence is lower for weaker opioids such as codeine. Metoclopramide, cyclizine or haloperidol are often given for the relief of the nausea and vomiting induced by opioids.

Gastroduodenal or intestinal obstructions in advanced malignancy are usually caused by occlusion to the lumen (intrinsically and/or extrinsically) or by absence of normal peristaltic propulsion. Surgery remains the definitive treatment for luminal occlusion due to cancer but this is often inappropriate for patients who are frail or with advanced malignancy. The main aim of pharmacological interventions is symptom control. A prokinetic dopamine (D2) antagonist such as metoclopramide or domperidone should be used for patients with nausea and vomiting associated with functional gastric or intestinal stasis. Prokinetics are also used in patients with partial gastric outlet obstruction but can worsen patients' symptoms of abdominal pain in complete gastric outlet obstruction. As prokinetics can exacerbate abdominal colicky pain associated with intestinal obstruction, their use should be avoided in that situation and antiemetics such as cyclizine or haloperidol should be used for symptom control.

Box 34.2 Potentially treatable causes of nausea and vomiting in palliative care

---

Hypercalcaemia
Constipation
Renal failure
Raised intracranial pressure
Infection
Bowel obstruction
Peptic ulcer disease
Drugs
Anxiety

Dexametasone has also been used for control of symptoms in malignant intestinal obstruction, not only for any antiemetic effect but also to reduce inflammatory tumour oedema around the obstructive lesion. Anticholinergics such as hyoscine butylbromide and somatostatin analogues such as octreotide have been used for symptom relief in intestinal obstruction by reducing gastro-intestinal secretion and motility and thus reducing the frequency and volume of vomitus.

Biochemical disturbances such as hypercalcaemia and renal failure can be a cause of nausea and vomiting in patients with advanced malignancy. However, aggressive treatment with bisphosphonates or insertion of nephrostomy tubes, respectively, would not be appropriate for those who are in the terminal stages of their disease. Haloperidol and cyclizine appear to be effective for biochemical causes of nausea and vomiting. Levomepromazine has antidopaminergic, antihistaminergic, antimuscarinic and antiserotonergic activity. It is effective for most causes of nausea and vomiting and may help alleviate restlessness. It can also be given intramuscularly, intravenously or subcutaneously, including by continuous subcutaneous infusion. It may be considered if first line antiemetics are insufficiently effective. Unfortunately, sedation and postural hypotension can be a problem in association with this agent.

Conclusion

Nausea and vomiting are symptoms caused by a variety of underlying causes. Thorough clinical assessment and appropriate investigations should be undertaken when prescribing a therapeutic trial of an antiemetic. The choice of agent(s) should be based upon the likely cause and severity of the symptoms, the possible underlying pathophysiology, and the recommendations of evidence-based guidelines which take into account clinical effectiveness and cost-effectiveness.

Case studies

Case 34.1

A 30-year-old man presents seeking a remedy for vomiting which had an acute onset, 12 h previously.

. . . .

Question

What questions should be asked to determine the nature, cause and seriousness of these symptoms?

. . . .

Answer

The cause of vomiting needs to be determined where possible to allow appropriate treatment to be initiated. The following questions should be asked.

- Are there symptoms or signs of infection, such as diarrhoea, sore throat, dysuria, photophobia, fever? (Infection, often of the gastro-intestinal tract, is one of the commonest causes of vomiting.)

- Is there headache? (Raised intracranial pressure and meningitis can present with vomiting as an early symptom, usually without any nausea.)
- Is there abdominal pain? (Abdominal pain before vomiting usually means an organic gastro-intestinal cause. Pain after vomiting may be due to muscle tenderness.)
- Has the patient started any new drugs (opioids, chemotherapeutic agents, digoxin, nicotine, NSAIDs, oral hypoglycaemics and some antibiotics are common causes) or drunk excess alcohol?
- Is there vertigo? (If present, this is suggestive of a labyrinthine cause.)

Case 34.2

A 19-year-old girl who is 12 weeks pregnant presents to hospital with intractable nausea and vomiting which has not responded to home therapy and which has resulted in hypotension and dehydration.

Question

List, in order of importance, the therapeutic strategies for this problem.

Answer

Treatment would normally involve:

- intravenous rehydration and electrolyte replacement
- bed rest
- antiemetics, such as promethazine; these are likely to be effective and there is little evidence to suggest that they have teratogenic effects
- postpyloric feeding
- steroids
- parenteral nutrition.

Case 34.3

A 45-year-old woman presents with ovarian carcinoma for which she is due to receive a course of cancer chemotherapy.

Question

What drugs might be appropriate, when should they be given, and what advice should be given to the patient regarding monitoring of symptoms after treatment with the chemotherapy?

Answer

This woman is likely to receive repeated cycles of emetic chemotherapy with carboplatin (moderate emetic risk) or cisplatin (high emetic risk) and, therefore, should be given prophylactic antiemetics before the start of chemotherapy. The choice of drug lies between metoclopramide combined with dexametasone for some moderate emetic risk situations, and one of the $5HT_3$-receptor antagonists (granisetron, ondansetron, or palonosetron) for high-risk situations, with dexametasone to provide additional benefit. The monitoring of emesis and nausea both within and outside hospital for up to 5 days after treatment is a useful exercise in deciding which patients may need other therapies. It is also important to remember that patients should be given appropriate doses of antiemetics as rescue therapy to cover delayed-onset nausea.

Case 34.4

A hospital with a large number of surgical specialties, including major inpatient thoraco-abdominal and day care procedures, wishes to update its PONV programme.

Question

What principles for a PONV programme should be taken into account?

Answer

The programme should contain a PONV risk score which can be used in preoperation assessment. A simplified score has been devised, adding one point for each of the following: female gender, non-smoking status, history of PONV, and opioid use. In low-risk individuals scoring 0 or 1 (<10% risk), prophylactic antiemetic therapy is unnecessary. Moderate-risk subjects (score 1, risk 10–30%) may require single-agent antiemetic prophylaxis, while in high-risk subjects (score 3, risk 30–60%) two agents (one of them often dexamethasone) may be needed if intravenous anaesthesia is not possible. In very high-risk subjects (score 4, risk > 60%), intravenous anaesthesia should be considered when possible and dexametasone and another antiemetic agent administered. PONV rescue therapy should be chosen depending on the post-operative clinical situation.

References

American Gastroenterological Association, 2001. AGA medical position statement: nausea and vomiting. Gastroenterology 120, 261–262.

Apfel, C.C., Laara, E., Koivuranta, M., et al., 1999. A simplified risk score for predicting postoperative nausea and vomiting. Anesthesiology 91, 693–700.

Apfel, C.C., Kranke, P., Eberhart, L.H., et al., 2002. Comparison of predictive models for postoperative nausea and vomiting. Br. J. Anaesth. 88, 234–240.

Billio, A., Morello, E., Clarke, M.J., 2010. Serotonin receptor antagonists for highly emetogenic chemotherapy in adults. Cochrane Database Syst. Rev. 1. Art. No.: CD006272.pub2. doi: 10.1002/14651858. Available at: http://www2.cochrane.org/reviews/en/ab006272.html.

Ernst, E., Pittler, M.H., 2000. Efficacy of ginger for nausea and vomiting: a systematic review of randomized clinical trials. Br. J. Anaesth. 84, 367–371.

Gan, T.J., Meyer, T., Apfell, C.C., et al., 2003. Consensus guidelines for managing postoperative nausea and vomiting. Anesth. Analg. 97, 62–71.

Habib, A., Gan, T.J., 2004. Evidence-based management of postoperative nausea and vomiting: a review. Can. J. Anaesth. 51, 326–341.

Jewell, D., Young, G., 2003. Interventions for nausea and vomiting in early pregnancy. Cochrane Database Syst. Rev. 4. Art. No.: CD000145. doi: 10.1002/14651858.

King, T.L., Murphy, P.A., 2009. Evidence-based approaches to managing nausea and vomiting in early pregnancy. J. Midwifery Womens Health 54, 430–444.

Kris, M.G., Hesketh, P.J., Somerfield, M.R., et al., 2006. American Society of Clinical Oncology guideline for antiemetics in oncology: update. J. Clin. Oncol. 24, 2932–2947.

Lee, A., Done, M.L., 2004. Stimulation of the wrist acupuncture point P6 for preventing postoperative nausea and vomiting. Cochrane Database Syst. Rev. 3 Art. No.: CD003281. doi: 10.1002/14651858.

Pierre, S., Corno, G., Benais, H., et al., 2004. A risk score-dependent antiemetic approach effectively reduces postoperative nausea and vomiting – a continuous quality improvement initiative. Can. J. Anaesth. 51, 320–325.

Quigley, E.M., Hasler, W.L., Parkman, H.P., 2001. A technical review on nausea and vomiting. Gastroenterology 120, 263–268.

Spinks, A.B., Wasiak, J., Villanueva, E.V., et al., 2004. Scopolamine for preventing and treating motion sickness. Cochrane Database Syst. Rev. 3 Art No CD002851.

Further reading

Berger, A., 2004. Prevention of Chemotherapy-Induced Nausea and vomiting. PRRR Inc, New York.

Gan, T.J., 2006. Risk factors for postoperative nausea and vomiting. Anesth. Analg. 102, 1884–1898.

Hatfield, A., Tronson, M. (Eds.), 2008. The Complete Recovery Room. fourth ed. Oxford University Press, Oxford.

Mannix, K., 2006. Palliation of nausea and vomiting in malignancy. Clin. Med. 6, 144–147.

Spinks, A., Wasiak, J., Bernath, V., Villanueva, E., 2007. Scopolamine (hyoscine) for preventing and treating motion sickness. Cochrane Database Syst. Rev. 3. Art. No.: CD002851. doi: 10.1002/14651858.CD002851.pub3 Available at: http://www2.cochrane.org/reviews/en/ab002851.html.

Respiratory infections 35

A. Robb and A. W. Berrington

Key points

- Oral cephalosporins have better clinical efficacy than penicillins in the treatment of streptococcal pharyngitis.
- There is controversy about whether otitis media should be treated with antibiotics or allowed to run its course.
- Viral respiratory tract infections are usually mild and self-limiting, but influenza and severe acute respiratory syndrome (SARS) can have severe consequences for individuals, for public health and for economic activity.
- Exacerbations of chronic bronchitis are not always infective in origin; antibiotics are used where appropriate but other therapeutic modalities are also valuable.
- *Streptococcus pneumoniae* remains the single most common cause of community-acquired pneumonia (CAP). Reduced susceptibility to penicillin can complicate the management of serious pneumococcal infections, but more significant degrees of resistance are currently not widespread among UK strains.
- CAP can be caused by a variety of pathogens, and this is reflected in the antimicrobial regimens recommended for initial treatment.
- There are many potential causes of hospital-acquired (nosocomial) pneumonia and each unit with patients at risk will have its own resident bacterial flora. This will strongly influence the choice of antibiotics for empiric therapy.
- *Pseudomonas aeruginosa* remains the most important respiratory pathogen in infections complicating cystic fibrosis; antibiotic treatment is targeted at this organism.
- Immunocompromised patients are at risk from a variety of opportunistic respiratory infections, for example, pneumocystis pneumonia in AIDS and invasive aspergillosis in neutropenic states.
- Health care-associated infections such as meticillin-resistant *Staphylococcus aureus* (MRSA) infection and *Clostridium difficile* infection (CDI) remain prevalent and should always be considered when choosing antibiotics.

Respiratory tract infections are the most common group of infections seen in the UK. Most are viral, for which (with some exceptions) only symptomatic therapy is available. In contrast, bacterial infections are a major cause of treatable respiratory illness.

The respiratory tract is divided into upper and lower parts: the upper respiratory tract consists of the sinuses, middle ear, pharynx, epiglottis and larynx, while the lower respiratory tract consists of the structures below the larynx, the bronchi, bronchioles and alveoli. Although there are anatomical and functional divisions both within and between these regions, infections do not always respect such boundaries. Nevertheless, it is clinically and bacteriologically convenient to retain a distinction between upper respiratory tract infections (URTIs) and lower respiratory tract infections (LRTIs).

Upper respiratory tract infections

Colds and flu

Viral URTIs causing coryzal symptoms, rhinitis, pharyngitis and laryngitis, and associated with varying degrees of systemic symptoms, are extremely common. These infections are usually caused by viruses from the rhinovirus, coronavirus, parainfluenza virus, respiratory syncytial virus, influenza virus and adenovirus families, although new viruses continue to be identified. For instance, in 2001, a novel respiratory pathogen was described that has become known as human *metapneumovirus* (hMPV). This causes a spectrum of respiratory illnesses particularly in young children, the elderly and the immunocompromised (Van Den Hoogen et al., 2001).

Colloquially, milder infections are called 'colds', while more severe infections may be known as 'flu'. This term should be distinguished from true influenza, reserved for infection caused by the influenza virus. In general, the management of these infections is symptomatic and consists of rest, adequate hydration, simple analgesics and antipyretics. Apart from one or two exceptional situations, antiviral drugs are not indicated and in most cases are not active. Antibacterial drugs have no activity against viral infections, although in the past they were widely prescribed, sometimes with spurious rationale such as prophylaxis against bacterial superinfection, sometimes simply because patients demanded them. In recent years, heightened awareness of the adverse consequences of antibiotic overuse has led to national campaigns aimed at discouraging the public from seeking antibiotic treatment for viral infections.

Influenza

True influenza is caused by one of the influenza viruses (influenza A, B or rarely C). It can be a serious condition characterised by severe malaise and myalgia and potentially complicated by life-threatening secondary bacterial infections such as staphylococcal pneumonia. Coryzal symptoms are not usually a feature of influenza, but the patient may have a cough. Influenza tends to occur during the winter months, providing an opportunity to offer preventive vaccination in the autumn. In the UK, influenza vaccine is normally targeted at three groups:

- those at risk of severe infection, for example, people aged 65 years and over, and younger patients in special disease risk groups
- those living in long-stay care facilities in which the infection might spread particularly rapidly, and
- those in whom infection would be problematic for other reasons, such as carers and health care workers.

Unfortunately, the virus mutates so rapidly that the circulating strains tend to change from season to season, necessitating annual revaccination against the prevailing virus.

Influenza A and B infections are amenable to both prevention and treatment with neuraminidase inhibitors (NAIs) and include agents such as zanamivir and oseltamivir, although there is controversy about whether the benefits justify the costs involved. Zanamivir is administered by dry powder inhalation, whereas oseltamivir is given orally. Clinical trials on parenteral administration for use in individuals with life-threatening infections are underway.

National guidelines for the UK recommend NAIs should only be used when influenza is circulating in the community (which is carefully defined), and in patients who are both at risk of developing complications and can commence treatment within a defined time window of onset or exposure (NICE, 2008, 2009). Individuals at risk and eligible for treatment include those:

- with chronic lung disease including asthma and chronic obstructive pulmonary disease (COPD)
- with heart disease (excluding uncomplicated hypertension)
- with chronic kidney disease
- with diabetes mellitus
- with chronic liver disease
- with chronic neurological disease
- who might be immunosuppressed
- aged 65 years or older
- in long-term residential or nursing homes during local outbreaks.

The anti-Parkinsonian drug amantadine, which has activity against influenza A virus, is not recommended for the treatment or prophylaxis of influenza due to emergence of resistance and the high incidence of adverse effects.

Pandemics (or global epidemics) of influenza A occur around every 25 years and affect huge numbers of people. The 1918 'Spanish flu' pandemic is estimated to have killed 20 million people. Further pandemics have taken place in 1957–1958 (Asian flu), 1968–1969 (Hong Kong flu) and 1977 (Russian flu). An avian strain, H5N1, emerged in South East Asia in 2003 and is now considered endemic in many parts of South East Asia and remains a concern for public health (WHO, 2010).

The World Health Organisation declared a worldwide influenza pandemic in June 2009 following the emergence of a novel H1N1 strain of swine lineage. In the UK, NICE guidance was superseded during the pandemic and NAIs were given to all individuals with flu-like illness. A vaccine was also developed. Pandemic planning had been in operation for many years with plans for rapid vaccine development and stockpiling of antivirals. However, in retrospect, infections caused by the pandemic strain were generally associated with much milder disease than seen in previous pandemics, and some authorities have been accused of over-reaction.

The widespread use of NAIs during the 2009 pandemic brought its own problems. Resistance to oseltamivir emerged (Gulland, 2009), and some argued that the cure was worse than the disease (Strong et al., 2009). Further, a Cochrane review (Jefferson et al., 2009) found no good evidence that oseltamivir prevents secondary complications such as pneumonia, one of the main justifications for its widespread use in pandemic influenza. However, the relatively benign course of the 2009 pandemic should not provide false reassurance as to the risks associated with future pandemics.

Sore throat (pharyngitis)

Causative organisms

Pharyngitis is a common condition. In most cases, it never comes to medical attention and is treated with simple therapy directed at symptom relief. Many cases are not due to infection at all but are caused by other factors such as smoking. Where infection is the cause, most cases are viral and form part of the cold-and-flu spectrum. Epstein–Barr virus (EBV), which causes glandular fever (infectious mononucleosis), is a less common but important cause of sore throat since it may be confused with streptococcal infection.

The only common bacterial cause of sore throat is *Streptococcus pyogenes*, the Lancefield group A β-haemolytic streptococcus. Infrequent causes include β-haemolytic streptococci of groups C and G, *Arcanobacterium haemolyticum*, *Neisseria gonorrhoeae* and mycoplasmas. *Corynebacterium diphtheriae*, the cause of diphtheria, is rare in the UK but should be borne in mind when investigating travellers returning from parts of the world where diphtheria is common. *C. ulcerans* is as common a cause of clinical diphtheria in the UK as *C. diphtheriae* but usually runs a more benign course.

Clinical features

The presenting complaint is sore throat, often associated with fever and the usual symptoms of the common cold. It is standard teaching that sore throats of different aetiology cannot be distinguished clinically. Nevertheless, more severe cases are more likely to be caused by EBV or *S. pyogenes*, and in these patients, there may be marked inflammation of the pharynx with a whitish exudate on the tonsils, plus enlarged and tender cervical lymph nodes.

Group A streptococcal infection has a number of potential complications. Pharyngeal infection may occasionally give rise to disseminated infection elsewhere, but this is rare. More frequent accompaniments are otitis media, peritonsillar abscess and sinusitis. These should be distinguished from the non-suppurative complications of streptococcal infection, rheumatic fever and glomerulonephritis, which are mediated immunologically. Occasional cases are still seen in the UK and remain important causes of renal and cardiac disease in developing countries. Scarlet fever, a toxin-mediated manifestation of streptococcal infection, is associated with a macular rash and sometimes considerable systemic illness.

In the UK, there has been a recent increase in rates of group A streptococcal infection. This includes invasive group A streptococcal infection (iGAS), associated with infection in normally sterile sites such as blood or tissue. The most common serotypes seen in England and Wales are *emm* 1, 3, and 89; *emm* 3 infections are associated with higher case fatality rates. The cause of the upsurge is unknown but may represent a natural periodic increase or alternatively excess transmission associated with high rates of influenza in 2008 (Lamagni et al., 2009).

Diagnosis

In most cases of pharyngitis, a bacteriological diagnosis cannot be made and thereby these are presumed to be viral in origin. The aim of any diagnostic procedure is to distinguish the streptococcal sore throat, which is amenable to antibiotic treatment, from viral infections, which are not. If a definite bacterial diagnosis is required, a throat swab should be taken for culture and, unless the details of a particular case prompt a search for more unusual organisms, culture techniques are directed towards detecting β-haemolytic streptococci. If bacterial culture is negative and glandular fever is suspected, blood should be taken for serological confirmation using either the non-specific 'monospot test' for atypical lymphocytes or specific tests for antibodies to EBV. Other viruses may be diagnosed by viral culture or serology, but this does not usually contribute to management. Rapid bedside tests are available that detect group A streptococcal antigens in the throat, but there are concerns about their sensitivity and specificity and they have not been widely introduced in the UK.

Treatment

Treatment of viral sore throat is directed at symptomatic relief, for example with rest, antipyretics and aspirin gargles. Streptococcal sore throat is usually treated with antibiotics although the extent to which they shorten the duration of symptoms and reduce the incidence of suppurative complications is modest (Del Mar et al., 2004). Antibiotic treatment also reduces the incidence of non-suppurative complications so is likely to be of greater benefit where these are common. There is also an argument that treating to eradicate streptococcal carriage might reduce the risk of relapse or later streptococcal infection at other sites.

Broadly, there are three treatment strategies:

1. give antibiotics to all patients with suspected streptococcal infection and do not investigate unless symptoms persist
2. give antibiotics to all patients with suspected streptococcal infection but stop them if a throat swab is negative, or
3. wait for throat swab culture results before starting antibiotics.

There is no correct approach and each has its advocates, although the problem of resistance has led to increasing pressure on prescribers to restrict empirical antibiotic use particularly for conditions such as pharyngitis that are frequently viral. The prevailing view is that antibiotics should not be routinely prescribed except where there is a high risk of severe infection, for instance, in immunocompromised patients (NICE, 2010).

Antibiotics effective against *S. pyogenes* include penicillins, cephalosporins and macrolides. Resistance to penicillins and cephalosporins has not (yet) been described in group A streptococci, although about 4% of isolates are resistant to erythromycin. Even against sensitive strains, macrolides such as erythromycin are demonstrably less effective than β-lactams.

Penicillins such as benzylpenicillin (penicillin G) or phenoxymethylpenicillin (penicillin V) have traditionally been regarded as the treatment of choice for streptococcal sore throat, but there is now convincing evidence that cephalosporins are more effective in terms of both clinical response and eradication of the organism from the oropharynx. This was summarised in a large meta-analysis of 40 studies in which 10-day courses of oral cephalosporins and penicillins were compared in the management of children with streptococcal pharyngitis (Casey and Pichichero, 2004). Bacteriological and clinical cure significantly favoured cephalosporins over penicillins, perhaps because penicillins are hydrolysed by β-lactamases produced by organisms such as anaerobes naturally resident in the oropharynx, whereas cephalosporins are not. The 10-day course length became accepted following earlier studies that compared the effect of different durations of penicillin treatment on bacteriological colonisation, but a recent systematic review (Atamimi et al., 2009) found comparable efficacy with shorter courses of newer antibiotics such as azithromycin.

However, despite the therapeutic superiority, it remains debatable whether the extra expense of cephalosporins is justified. Cefalexin is the preferred cephalosporin. Penicillin or amoxicillin is the preferred penicillin, with the proviso that amoxicillin and other aminopenicillins should not be used unless EBV infection is unlikely, since for reasons that are not understood, these drugs often cause skin rashes if used in this condition.

Acute epiglottitis

Acute epiglottitis is a rapidly progressive cellulitis of the epiglottis and adjacent structures. Local swelling has the potential to cause rapid-onset airway obstruction, so the condition is a medical emergency. Previously, almost all childhood cases and a high proportion of adult cases were caused by *Haemophilus influenzae* type b (Hib), with the rest being caused by other organisms such as pneumococci, streptococci and staphylococci. With the advent of routine vaccination against *H. influenzae* type b in October 1992, this disease has become uncommon.

The typical patient is a child between 2 and 4 years old with fever and difficulty speaking and breathing. The patient may drool because of impaired swallowing. The diagnosis is made clinically and the initial management is concentrated upon establishing or maintaining an airway. This takes priority over all other diagnostic and therapeutic manoeuvres. Thereafter, the diagnosis may be confirmed by visualisation of the epiglottis, typically described as 'cherry-red'. Microbiological confirmation may be obtained by culturing the epiglottis and the blood, but not until the airway is secure.

In view of the high prevalence of amoxicillin resistance among encapsulated *H. influenzae*, the treatment of choice is a cephalosporin. It is customary to use a third-generation cephalosporin such as cefotaxime or ceftriaxone, but there is no reason why the infection should not respond to a second-generation agent such as cefuroxime. If a sensitive organism is recovered, high-dose parenteral amoxicillin may be substituted.

Otitis media

Causative organisms

Inflammation of the middle ear (otitis media) is a common condition seen most frequently in children under 3 years of age. Most cases are due to bacteria, although viruses such as influenza virus and rhinoviruses have been implicated in a sizeable minority. *S. pneumoniae* and *H. influenzae* are the two most commonly encountered bacterial pathogens. *Moraxella catarrhalis* and *S. pyogenes* account for a smaller proportion of cases, perhaps 10%, and other bacteria are seen only rarely.

Clinical features

Classically, otitis media presents with ear pain, which may be severe. If the drum perforates, the pain is relieved and a purulent discharge may follow. There may be a degree of hearing impairment plus non-specific symptoms such as fever or vomiting. Complications include mastoiditis (which is now rare), meningitis and, particularly in the case of *H. influenzae* infection, septicaemia and disseminated infection. With the advent of routine vaccination against *H. influenzae* type b, these complications have become uncommon.

Diagnosis

The diagnosis of otitis media is essentially made clinically and laboratory investigations have little role to play. Unless the drum is perforated, there is little sense in sending a swab of the external auditory canal, the results of which are likely to be unhelpful or misleading. For this reason, a causative organism is rarely isolated and treatment has to be given empirically.

Treatment

There has been much debate about whether or not antibiotics should be used for the initial treatment of acute otitis media. A meta-analysis combined seven clinical trials involving 2202 children and concluded that, although antibiotics confer a modest reduction in pain at 2–7 days, they do not reduce the incidence of short-term complications such as hearing problems and they do cause side effects (Glasziou et al., 2004). The benefit of antibiotic treatment may be greater in children under two than in older children (Damoiseaux et al., 2000), but in any case about 80% of cases treated without antibiotics will resolve spontaneously within 3 days. If antibiotic treatment is to be given, it should be effective against the three main bacterial pathogens: *S. pneumoniae*, *H. influenzae* and *S. pyogenes*. The streptococci are usually sensitive to penicillins, but these are much less active against *H. influenzae*, so the broader spectrum agents amoxicillin or ampicillin are preferred. These drugs have identical antibacterial activity, but amoxicillin is recommended for oral treatment since it is better absorbed from the gastro-intestinal tract. Patients with penicillin allergy may be treated with a later-generation cephalosporin (see later).

About 20% of *H. influenzae* strains are resistant to amoxicillin due to production of β-lactamase, so if there is no response to amoxicillin, an alternative agent should be chosen. Both erythromycin and the earlier oral cephalosporins such as cefalexin are insufficiently active against *H. influenzae* and should not be used. Alternatives include co-amoxiclav (a combination of amoxicillin and the β-lactamase inhibitor clavulanic acid) or an orally active later-generation cephalosporin such as cefixime. Cefuroxime axetil, while active *in vitro*, is poorly absorbed and often causes diarrhoea.

Pneumococcal conjugate vaccines, which are currently given routinely in the childhood vaccination schedule, may reduce the incidence of acute otitis media, although a recent review (Jansen et al., 2009) found only modest benefit. No benefit was found for influenza vaccination (Hoberman et al., 2003). Long-term antibiotic prophylaxis might have a role in some children (Leach and Morris, 2006), but any benefit has to be balanced against the risks.

Acute sinusitis

Causative organisms

Normally, the paranasal sinuses are sterile but they can become infected following damage to the mucous membrane which lines them. This usually occurs following a viral URTI but is sometimes associated with the presence of dental disease. Acute sinusitis is usually caused by the same organisms which cause otitis media, but occasionally other organisms such as *S. aureus*, viridans streptococci (a term used to describe α-haemolytic streptococci other than *S. pneumoniae*) and anaerobes may be found. Viruses are occasionally found in conjunction with the bacteria.

Clinical features

The main feature of acute sinusitis is facial pain and tenderness, often accompanied by headache and a purulent nasal discharge. Complications include frontal bone osteomyelitis, meningitis and brain abscess. The condition may become chronic with persistent low-grade pain and nasal discharge, sometimes with acute exacerbations.

Diagnosis

As with otitis media, this is a clinical diagnosis and obtaining specimens for bacteriological examination is not usually practicable. In patients with chronic sinusitis, therapeutic sinus washouts may yield specimens for microbiological culture.

Treatment

Since the causative organisms are the same as those found in otitis media, the same recommendations for treatment apply. Proximity to the mouth means that anaerobes are implicated quite frequently in acute sinusitis, particularly if associated with dental disease, and in such cases, the addition of metronidazole may be worthwhile. Amoxicillin/clavulanate (co-amoxiclav) has also demonstrated effectiveness. Doxycycline has proved popular due to its broad spectrum of activity and once-daily dosage.

Lower respiratory infections

Acute bronchitis and acute exacerbations of COPD

Bronchitis means inflammation of the bronchi. It is important to distinguish between acute bronchitis, which is usually, if not always, infective, and chronic bronchitis, which is a chronic inflammatory condition characterised by thickened, oedematous bronchial mucosa with mucus gland hypertrophy and usually caused by smoking. Chronic bronchitis often co-exists with emphysema, both of which lead to airflow limitation and the clinical syndrome of COPD.

The importance of chronic bronchitis is that it renders the patient more susceptible to acute infections and more likely to suffer respiratory compromise as a result. These acute exacerbations of COPD are a frequent cause of morbidity and admission to hospital. An exacerbation is defined as 'a sustained worsening of the patient's symptoms from his or her usual stable state that is beyond normal day-to-day variations, and is acute in onset' (NICE, 2004). Common symptoms include worsening breathlessness, cough, increased sputum production and change in sputum colour. It is important to remember that not all acute exacerbations of COPD have an infective aetiology since atmospheric pollutants are sometimes implicated.

Causative organisms

In otherwise healthy patients, the causes of acute bronchitis include viruses such as rhinovirus, coronavirus, adenovirus and influenza virus, and bacteria such as *Bordetella pertussis*, *Mycoplasma pneumoniae* and *Chlamydophila pneumoniae* (formerly *Chlamydia pneumoniae*). The role of bacteria such as *S. pneumoniae* and *H. influenzae* is uncertain because these organisms are nasopharyngeal commensals and their isolation can be misleading, but there is a presumption that they account for at least a proportion of infections.

In patients with acute exacerbations of chronic bronchitis, sputum culture frequently yields potential pathogens such as *S. pneumoniae*, *H. influenzae* and *M. catarrhalis*. However, these organisms are also found in the sputum at much the same frequencies between exacerbations, so it is unclear to what extent (if at all) they play a pathogenic role. A considerable proportion of acute exacerbations is associated with viral infections such as colds or influenza, or might even be non-infective.

Clinical features

The characteristic feature of acute bronchitis is a cough productive of purulent sputum, that is, phlegm that is yellow or green, the colour reflecting the presence of pus cells, sometimes with wheezing and breathlessness. In patients with pre-existing lung disease, the lack of reserve may lead to respiratory compromise, which in turn may exacerbate, or be exacerbated by, cardiac failure. Sometimes, the condition progresses to frank bronchopneumonia (see later), although the dividing line between a severe exacerbation of COPD and bronchopneumonia is often unclear.

Diagnosis

The diagnosis of acute bronchitis or acute exacerbation of COPD is made clinically and does not depend on the results of investigations. If antibiotics are to be given, a sputum sample should be sent for bacteriology, as this will allow antibiotic sensitivity tests to be performed on potential pathogens. However, the decision to treat should not be based on the results of sputum culture alone.

Treatment

Younger patients without pre-existing respiratory disease are likely to recover rapidly and might not require specific treatment. For more severe cases, including exacerbations of COPD, the two main arms of treatment are airflow optimisation and antibiotic therapy. Airflow optimisation consists of physiotherapy to aid expectoration of secretions, adjunctive oxygen if appropriate, bronchodilators and sometimes short-course corticosteroids. In severe cases, a period of artificial ventilation may be required, an intervention which has become more common with the advent of non-invasive ventilation techniques.

Despite the reservation that many cases are non-infective, current guidelines recommend that antibiotics are prescribed when an exacerbation is associated with more purulent sputum (NICE, 2004). There is no unequivocal evidence that one antibiotic is better than another, so recommendations for empiric treatment are based generally upon spectrum, side effects and cost. Most authorities favour either a tetracycline such as doxycycline or an aminopenicillin such as amoxicillin, since these agents cover most strains of *S. pneumoniae* and *H. influenzae*. Some people argue in favour of co-amoxiclav, which covers β-lactamase producing strains of *H. influenzae* and *M. catarrhalis* that are therefore resistant to amoxicillin, but this agent is more expensive and has a greater incidence of side effects. For penicillin-allergic patients for whom tetracyclines are contraindicated, neither the macrolide erythromycin nor the earlier oral cephalosporins such as cefalexin or cefradine are sufficiently active against *H. influenzae* for empiric use. However, both clarithromycin and newer oral cephalosporins such as cefixime are active against haemophili while retaining activity against pneumococci.

The following recommendations can be made for the empiric antibiotic treatment of acute bronchitis and exacerbations of COPD. If a plausible pathogen is isolated, treatment can be modified accordingly.

First-line agents

- Doxycycline
- Amoxicillin

Second-line agents

- Co-amoxiclav
- Clarithromycin
- Cefixime

A number of other drugs are promoted for the treatment of COPD exacerbations. Of these, azithromycin is not recommended, as it is less active than clarithromycin against *S. pneumoniae*. The activity of ciprofloxacin against *S. pneumoniae* is insufficient to justify its use as monotherapy against pneumococcal infections (although it has useful activity against *H. influenzae* and *M. catarrhalis*), and levofloxacin (which is the active isomer of ofloxacin) does not seem to offer any great microbiological advantage. Moxifloxacin is a quinolone that retains activity against Gram-negative organisms such as *Haemophilus* and *Moraxella* but has greater activity against Gram-positives such as *S. pneumoniae*. It has been favourably compared to standard treatment in exacerbations of COPD (Wilson et al., 2004). However, its use has been limited by the high incidence of *Clostridium difficile* infection (CDI) associated with quinolone use, and rarely the development of life-threatening hepatic toxicity.

Bronchiolitis

Bronchiolitis is characterised by inflammatory changes in the small bronchi and bronchioles, but not by consolidation. It is particularly recognised as a disease of infants in the first year of life, in whom a small degree of airway narrowing can have a dramatic effect on airflow, but the causal organisms are equally capable of infecting adults, who may then act as reservoirs of infection. Most cases are caused by respiratory syncytial virus (RSV), which occurs in annual winter epidemics, but hMPV, parainfluenzaviruses, rhinoviruses, adenoviruses and occasionally *M. pneumoniae* have also been implicated.

Bronchiolitis is characterised by a prodrome of fever and coryzal symptoms which progresses to wheezing, respiratory distress and hypoxia of varying degrees. Aetiological confirmation may be made by immunofluorescence and/or viral culture of respiratory secretions, although increasingly the diagnosis of respiratory syncytial virus is made using rapid antigen detection tests.

The treatment of bronchiolitis is mainly supportive and consists of oxygen, adequate hydration and ventilatory assistance if required. Severe cases of respiratory syncytial virus disease may be treated with ribavirin, a synthetic nucleoside administered by nebuliser. There is limited evidence for its efficacy and it is currently only recommended for use in immunocompromised patients to reduce the duration of viral shedding (Yanney and Vyas, 2008).

Babies born earlier than 35 weeks of gestation or those less than 6 months of age at the onset of the respiratory syncytial virus season are at high risk of the disease. Likewise, infants under two years of age with chronic lung disease or severe immunodeficiency, or under 6 months of age with congenital heart disease are similarly at high risk, and all are candidates for prophylactic treatment with palivizumab. This is a humanised monoclonal antibody used for passive immunisation against respiratory syncytial virus (JCVI, 2005). There is currently no vaccine against RSV.

Pneumonia

Pneumonia is defined as inflammation of the lung parenchyma, that is, of the alveoli rather than the bronchi or bronchioles, of infective origin and characterised by consolidation. Consolidation is a pathological process in which the alveoli are filled with a mixture of inflammatory exudate, bacteria and white blood cells that on chest X-ray appear as an opaque shadow in the normally clear lungs.

A wide range of organisms can cause pneumonia, so it is useful to apply some kind of classification system, at least until the aetiology of a particular case has been determined. Pneumonia is often classified clinically into lobar pneumonia, bronchopneumonia or atypical pneumonia, but this does not correlate entirely with the bacteriological cause and in any case the distinctions are often blurred. It is more practical to classify pneumonia according to the nature of its acquisition, the usual terms being community-acquired pneumonia (CAP) and hospital-acquired pneumonia (HAP).

Community-acquired pneumonia

Causative organisms. The causes of CAP are summarised in Table 35.1. The most common vegetative bacterial causes are *S. pneumoniae*, the pneumococcus, which can cause both lobar and bronchopneumonia, and non-capsulate strains of *H. influenzae* which usually give rise to bronchopneumonia.

The so-called atypical pneumonias are a heterogeneous group of diseases which nevertheless have several clinical features in common and which are clinically distinct from the classic picture of pneumococcal pneumonia. Aetiological agents include *Legionella pneumophila*, *M. pneumoniae*, *C. pneumoniae*, *Chlamydophila psittaci*, *Coxiella burnetii* and viruses. *L. pneumophila* is the cause of Legionnaire's disease which occurs sporadically and in outbreaks often associated with contaminated air-conditioning or water systems. From 2002 to 2008, there were 300–600 new cases a year reported in England and Wales.

Table 35.1 Causes of community-acquired pneumonia

Organism	Comments
Streptococcus pneumoniae	Classically causes lobar pneumonia, bronchopneumonia now common
Haemophilus influenzae	Cause of bronchopneumonia, usually non-capsulate strains
Staphylococcus aureus	Severe pneumonia with abscess formation, typically following influenza
Klebsiella pneumoniae	Friedlander's bacillus, causing an uncommon but severe necrotising pneumonia
Legionella pneumophila	Particularly serogroup 1; causes Legionnaire's disease, usually acquired from aquatic environmental sources
Mycoplasma pneumoniae	Cause of acute pneumonia in young people, respiratory symptoms often overshadowed by systemic upset
Chlamydophila pneumoniae	Mild but prolonged illness usually seen in older people, respiratory symptoms often overshadowed by systemic upset
Chlamydophila psittaci	Causes psittacosis, a respiratory and multisystem disease acquired from infected birds
Coxiella burnetii	Causes Q fever, a respiratory and multisystem disease acquired from animals such as sheep
Viruses	Several viruses can cause pneumonia in adults, including influenza, parainfluenza and varicella zoster viruses

Legionnaire's disease may be rapidly progressive with very extensive consolidation and consequent respiratory failure.

Viral infections should not be forgotten as causes of pneumonia, although in practice it is unusual to make a definitive early diagnosis, so most cases are treated with antibacterials. Influenza can cause a primary viral pneumonia as well as be complicated by secondary bacterial (particularly staphylococcal) pneumonia, chickenpox can be complicated by primary varicella pneumonia particularly in adults, and cytomegalovirus is capable of causing a variety of infections, including pneumonia, in patients with compromised cell-mediated immunity.

Clinical features. Pneumococcal lobar pneumonia presents with a cough, initially dry but later producing purulent or blood-stained, rust-coloured sputum, together with dyspnoea, fever and pleuritic chest pain. The peripheral white blood cell count is usually raised and the patient may be bacteraemic. The chest X-ray shows consolidation confined to one or more lobes (or segments of lobes) of the lungs. This classic picture is now quite rare perhaps because the early use of antibiotics modifies the natural history of the disease.

Bronchopneumonia presents more non-specifically with productive cough and breathlessness, and patchy consolidation on the chest X-ray usually in the bases of both lungs. This disease is very common and is typically seen in patients with severe COPD or in those who are frail and terminally ill. In fact, pneumonia has been described as the old man's friend because it is a relatively painless cause of death.

The atypical pneumonias are characterised clinically by fever, systemic symptoms and a dry cough, radiologically by widespread patchy consolidation in both lungs and biochemically by abnormalities in liver enzymes and perhaps evidence of inappropriate antidiuretic hormone secretion, evident as a low plasma sodium.

Despite the differences described, clinical features alone are not usually sufficient to make a confident bacteriological diagnosis, a fact that has major implications for the empirical treatment of pneumonia.

Diagnosis. Sputum culture is the mainstay of diagnosis for pneumonia caused by pneumococci and *H. influenzae*. Sputum microscopy is unreliable because oropharyngeal contaminants are often indistinguishable from pathogens. The success of sputum culture is very dependent upon the quality of the specimen, which may be inadequate either because the patient is unable to expectorate or because the nature of the disease is such that sputum production is not a major feature. A more sensitive (although more invasive) technique is to perform bronchoscopy and bronchoalveolar lavage. Lavage fluid, being uncontaminated by mouth flora, is suitable for microscopy as well as culture.

In pneumococcal disease, blood cultures are frequently positive and national guidance (Lim et al., 2009) suggests that laboratories should also offer plasma and urine testing for pneumococcal antigen. *Legionella* infection may be diagnosed by culture (if appropriate media are used) or by urinary antigen testing, but culture of *Mycoplasma* and *Chlamydophila* species is beyond the scope of most routine diagnostic laboratories. Viruses may be detected by immunofluorescence, by viral culture or by polymerase chain reaction (PCR), but timely diagnosis requires a good specimen such as bronchoalveolar lavage fluid. In practice, the aetiology of atypical pneumonia is usually determined serologically (for instance, by acute and convalescent antibody testing), if at all.

Targeted treatment. The treatment of choice for pneumococcal pneumonia is benzylpenicillin or amoxicillin. Erythromycin monotherapy may be used in penicillin-allergic patients, but resistance rates are rising, macrolides are bacteriostatic rather than bactericidal and the comparative efficacy of this approach is not known. There is retrospective evidence that combination therapy using both a β-lactam and a macrolide can reduce mortality in patients whose pneumonia is complicated by pneumococcal bacteraemia (Martinez et al., 2003).

Pneumococci with reduced susceptibility to penicillin are becoming increasingly common, particularly in continental Europe and the USA. In the UK, about 5–10% of strains express 'intermediate susceptibility' (minimum inhibitory concentration; MIC 0.1–1 mg/L), but high-level resistance (MIC >1 mg/L) remains uncommon. Intermediate susceptibility may result in treatment failure in conditions such as otitis media or meningitis, infections at sites where antibiotic penetration is reduced, but antibiotic penetration into the lungs is sufficiently good that penicillin and amoxicillin remain effective for pneumonia. Strains expressing high-level resistance are unlikely to respond to penicillins, however. Such strains are often co-resistant to macrolides and other first-line agents, and may require treatment with a later-generation cephalosporin or a glycopeptide.

The sensitivity of *H. influenzae* to antibiotics has been discussed above. Amoxicillin is the agent of choice, with co-amoxiclav, parenteral cefuroxime, cefixime or ciprofloxacin as alternatives. Erythromycin is poorly active, but the newer macrolide clarithromycin and the azalide azithromycin possess more activity.

M. pneumoniae does not possess a cell wall and is therefore not susceptible to β-lactam agents. A tetracycline or a macrolide are suitable alternatives. Tetracyclines are also effective against *C. pneumoniae, C. psittaci* and *C. burnetii*, but erythromycin is probably less effective. Quinolones are also highly active against these organisms.

Staphylococcal pneumonia is usually treated with flucloxacillin plus a second agent such as rifampicin or fusidic acid, although there is no good clinical evidence that combination treatment is better than a single agent. MRSA (meticillin-resistant *S. aureus*) pneumonia is being seen more commonly in the community as well as in hospital. Strains of *S. aureus* expressing Panton-Valentine Leukocidin, an exotoxin, are capable of causing a severe necrotising pneumonia and if clinically suspected should warrant urgent critical care and specialist microbiological input.

Treatment recommendations for Legionnaire's disease are based on a retrospective review of the famous Philadelphia outbreak of 1976 (Fraser et al., 1977), in which two deaths occurred among the 18 patients who were given erythromycin, compared to 16 deaths in 71 patients treated with penicillin or amoxicillin. This observation accords with the facts that *Legionella* is an intracellular pathogen and that macrolides penetrate more efficiently than β-lactams into cells. Azithromycin is probably the most effective of the macrolide/azalide derivatives, but clinical evidence to confirm this is lacking. Other agents with proven clinical efficacy and good intracellular activity against *Legionella* include rifampicin and quinolones. There have been no randomised controlled clinical trials, nor are there likely to be. Guidance, based on observation studies, suggests non-severe cases should be treated with an oral fluoroquinolone (with a macrolide as an alternative), and severe cases treated with a combination of a fluoroquinolone plus either a macrolide or rifampicin, de-escalating to a fluoroquinolone as the sole agent after the first few days (Lim et al., 2009). Treatment is not recommended for the non-pneumonic form of legionellosis (Pontiac fever) which presents as a self-limiting flu-like illness.

Empiric treatment. All of the foregoing recommendations presuppose that the infecting organism is known before treatment is commenced. In practice, this is rarely the case and therapy will initially be empirical or best-guess in nature (Table 35.2). The most authoritative recommendations for the initial treatment of CAP are those produced by the British Thoracic Society (Lim et al., 2009). For mild disease, these recommend treatment with amoxicillin, providing activity against pneumococci and most strains of *H. influenzae*, with doxycycline or clarithromycin being the preferred alternatives in penicillin-allergic patients. However, for moderate or severe disease requiring admission to hospital, they take the view that, until the aetiology is known, treatment should cover both 'typical' causes (such as *S. pneumoniae* and *H. influenza*) and atypical causes (such as *M. pneumoniae, Chlamydophila* species and *Legionella*). For patients with moderate or severe CAP, the guidelines therefore recommend a combination of a β-lactam drug plus a macrolide, the exact choice of agent and route being decided according to the clinical severity of the infection. In practice, this is usually interpreted as amoxicillin plus a macrolide for less severe disease, and co-amoxiclav plus a macrolide (or cefuroxime plus a macrolide) for more severe disease. Severity is assessed according to clinical parameters and outcome predicted by use of one of a number of assessment tools such as CURB-65, based on the onset of *C*onfusion, the serum *U*rea, the *R*espiratory rate, the *B*lood pressure and age >65 years.

Moxifloxacin, a newer fluoroquinolone, is licensed in the UK for treatment of non-severe pneumonia where other antibiotics cannot be used. Currently, it is licensed only in oral form.

Pressure to treat pneumonia (much of which is pneumococcal and would respond to penicillin) with broad-spectrum empiric regimens, in particular, with cephalosporins and fluoroquinolones, has been cited as a factor in the rising incidence of *Clostridium difficile* and MRSA infections. The treatment of pneumonia illustrates many of the dilemmas and conflicting priorities of modern antimicrobial prescribing.

Prevention. Pneumococcal 23-valent polysaccharide vaccine and influenza vaccine should be offered to all those at risk of infection. For pneumococcal infection, this includes patients who fulfil the following criteria:

- asplenia or dysfunction of the spleen
- chronic respiratory disease
- chronic heart disease
- chronic renal disease
- chronic liver disease
- diabetes
- immunosuppressed
- aged 65 years or older
- cochlear implants
- cerebrospinal fluid leaks.

Hospital-acquired (nosocomial) pneumonia

Causative organisms. The most frequent causes of HAP are Gram-negative bacilli (Enterobacteriaceae, *Pseudomonas* spp. and *Acinetobacter* spp.) and *S. aureus*, including MRSA (Box 35.1). However, it is important to remember that pneumococcal pneumonia may develop in hospitalised patients and also that hospital water supplies have been implicated in outbreaks and sporadic cases of *Legionella* infection. Further, it must be recognised that the common Gram-negative causes of nosocomial pneumonia will vary between

Table 35.2 Treatment of community-acquired pneumonia

Scenario	Typical regimen	Comments
Mild to moderate pneumonia, organism unknown	Amoxicillin plus a macrolide	Amoxicillin covers *S. pneumoniae* and most *H. influenzae* while macrolide provides cover against atypical pathogens. It is debatable whether clinical outcomes are improved by using antibiotics active against atypical pathogens in all-cause non-severe community-acquired pneumonia
Severe pneumonia, organism unknown	Co-amoxiclav plus a macrolide Cefuroxime plus a macrolide in penicillin allergy	Co-amoxiclav and cefuroxime provide cover against *S. aureus*, coliforms and β-lactamase producing haemophili while retaining the pneumococcal cover of amoxicillin
Pneumococcal pneumonia	Penicillin or amoxicillin or a macrolide	High-level penicillin resistance remains uncommon in the UK.
H. influenzae	Non-β-lactamase producing: amoxicillin β-lactamase producing: cefuroxime or co-amoxiclav	Also sensitive to quinolones
Staphylococcal pneumonia	Non-MRSA: flucloxacillin +/– a second agent such as rifampicin or fusidic acid MRSA: requires microbiology input, options include linezolid or glycopeptides	Isolation of *S. aureus* from sputum may reflect contamination with oropharyngeal commensals and should be interpreted cautiously. MRSA pneumonia may also be treated with linezolid
Mycoplasma pneumoniae	Macrolide or tetracycline	Treat for 14 days
Chlamydophila spp.	Tetracycline preferred	Treat for 14 days
Legionella spp.	A fluoroquinolone such as ciprofloxacin. A macrolide such as clarithromycin is an alternative if intolerant.	Addition of a macrolide or rifampicin in severe cases

Box 35.1 Causes of hospital-acquired pneumonia

Common organisms
1. Gram-negative bacteria:
   Pseudomonas aeruginosa
   E. coli
   Klebsiella spp.
2. Gram-positive bacteria:
   S. pneumoniae
   S. aureus including MRSA

Less common organisms
1. Other 'coliforms' such as *Enterobacter* spp., *Serratia marcescens*, *Citrobacter* spp., etc.
   Acinetobacter spp.
   Other *Pseudomonas* and related species, such as
   S. maltophilia
   L. pneumophila (and other species)
2. Anaerobic bacteria
3. Fungi:
   Candida albicans (and other species)
   Aspergillus fumigatus (particularly following prolonged episodes of neutropenia)
4. Viruses:
   Cytomegalovirus
   Herpes simplex virus

hospitals and even between different units within the same hospital. This is especially true of ventilator-associated pneumonia, which for obvious reasons is usually acquired on intensive care units where broad-spectrum antibiotics are frequently used, and where there may be a particular 'resident flora' with an established antibiotic resistance pattern.

Clinical features. Nosocomial pneumonia accounts for 10–15% of all hospital-acquired infections, usually presenting with sepsis and/or respiratory failure. Up to 50% of cases are acquired on intensive care units. Predisposing features include stroke, mechanical ventilation, chronic lung disease, recent surgery and previous antibiotic exposure.

Diagnosis. Sputum is commonly sent for culture but is sometimes unhelpful as it may be contaminated by mouth flora. If the patient has received antibiotics, the normal mouth flora is often replaced by resistant organisms such as staphylococci or Gram-negative bacilli, making the interpretation of culture results difficult. Bronchoalveolar lavage is often more helpful. Blood cultures may be positive.

Treatment. The range of organisms causing nosocomial pneumonia is very large, so broad-spectrum empiric therapy is indicated. The choice of antibiotics will be influenced by preceding antibiotic therapy, the duration of hospital admission and above all by the individual unit's

Table 35.3 Treatment regimens for hospital-acquired pneumonia (HAP)

Regimen	Comments
Co-amoxiclav	Good activity against community-associated pathogens, many Enterobacteriaceae and *S. aureus*. Recommended for early-onset HAP (within 5 days of admission) in antibiotic naïve patients without other risk factors
Ureidopenicillin plus aminoglycoside (e.g. piperacillin plus gentamicin)	Good activity against Gram-negative bacilli such as *P. aeruginosa* and also against pneumococci. Combination of piperacillin with the β-lactamase inhibitor tazobactam, currently the only ureidopenicillin product marketed in the UK, extends the spectrum to include *S. aureus* (not MRSA), anaerobes and some strains of *E. coli*, *Klebsiella*, etc. that are resistant to piperacillin alone. Piperacillin-tazobactam can also be used reliably as monotherapy
Cephalosporin plus an aminoglycoside (e.g. cefuroxime plus gentamicin)	Good activity against Gram-negative bacilli such as *E. coli*, *Klebsiella*, and Gram-positive organisms, but poor against *P. aeruginosa* and anaerobes
Clindamycin plus aminoglycoside	Good activity against Gram-positive organisms and anaerobes but much less so against Gram-negatives. Favoured in the USA where metronidazole is unpopular for the treatment of anaerobic infections
Ciprofloxacin plus glycopeptide (vancomycin or teicoplanin)	Ciprofloxacin provides good activity against most Gram-negative bacilli including *P. aeruginosa*. Glycopeptide provides activity against *S. aureus* (including MRSA) and pneumococci, although its penetration into the respiratory tract is relatively poor
Meropenem (monotherapy)	Broad-spectrum agent including activity against Extended Spectrum Beta Lactamase (ESBL) producing Enterobacteriaceae. Not active against MRSA. Ertapenem does not cover *Pseudomonas* spp. or *Acinetobacter* spp. so is unsuitable
Linezolid combinations	It is increasingly necessary to cover MRSA in empiric or targeted treatment of hospital-acquired pneumonia. Traditional options include glycopeptides and, where the prevailing strains are sensitive, aminoglycosides, but there are concerns about penetration into the lung. Linezolid, an oxazolidinone, provides reliable activity
Aztreonam combinations	Good activity against gram-negative bacilli Including *Pseudomonas* but offers no activity against anaerobic or Gram-positive organisms. Expensive. A β-lactam agent that can be used safely in patients with history of severe penicillin allergy
Temocillin	Excellent activity against Gram-negative organisms including ESBL-producing Enterobacteriaceae. No activity against Gram-positive organisms and *Pseudomonas*
Ceftazidime (monotherapy)	Very active against Gram-negative bacilli including *Pseudomonas* but less so against Gram-positive organisms and anaerobes. Due to the high incidence of *Clostridium difficile* infection and selection of multi-resistant organisms associated with its use, this agent has largely been superseded by other newer agents

experience with hospital bacteria. The combinations shown in Table 35.3 have all been used at some time and all have advantages and disadvantages. Several of the combinations include an aminoglycoside, and this may not be desirable in all patients. Single-agent therapy is attractive for ease of administration, and agents such as piperacillin-tazobactam and meropenem have suitably broad spectra that include activity against *P. aeruginosa*. Currently licensed β-lactam agents are inactive against MRSA infections; in such cases specialist management advice is required.

In all cases, a macrolide would be added if Legionnaire's disease was suspected and, if not already covered by the regimen, metronidazole would be required for suspected anaerobic infection.

Prevention. General strategies for minimising the incidence of HAP include early postoperative mobilisation, analgesia, physiotherapy and promotion of rational antibiotic prescribing. The Department of Health's Saving Lives programme makes specific recommendations for the prevention of ventilator-associated pneumonia (DoH, 2007), including head of bed elevation, sedation holding to reduce the duration of mechanical ventilation and good general hygiene of tubing management and suction.

Another strategy proposed for the prevention of ventilator-associated pneumonia is selective decontamination of the digestive tract (SDD), based on the premise that the infecting organisms initially colonise the patient's oropharynx or intestinal tract (Kallett and Quinn, 2005). By administering non-absorbable antibiotics such as an aminoglycoside or colistin to the gut, and applying a paste containing these agents to the oropharynx, it is proposed that the potential causative organisms will be eradicated and the incidence of pneumonia thereby reduced. In some centres, an antifungal agent such as amphotericin B is added; others also advocate addition of a systemic broad-spectrum agent such as cefotaxime.

The role of selective decontamination of the digestive tract remains controversial. Recent guidelines (Masterton et al., 2008) recommend its consideration in patients in whom mechanical ventilation is anticipated for more than 48 h. Whether any benefits really outweigh the risks is unclear.

Another suggestion is prophylactic administration of aerosolised antibiotics to ventilated patients (and perhaps other patients at risk). Agents suitable for aerosolised delivery and with the appropriate antimicrobial spectrum include aminoglycosides (particularly tobramycin) and the polymyxin drug colistin. There are no published data available at present and therefore this approach cannot be universally recommended.

Aspiration pneumonia

One further condition which may be seen either in hospital or in the community is aspiration pneumonia, initiated by inhalation of stomach contents contaminated by bacteria from the mouth. Risk factors include alcohol, hypnotic drugs and general anaesthesia, all of these being factors that may make a patient vomit while unconscious. Gastric acid is very destructive to lung tissue and leads to severe tissue necrosis. Damaged tissue is then prone to secondary infection often with abscess formation. Anaerobic bacteria are particularly implicated, but these are often accompanied by aerobic organisms such as viridans streptococci. Treatment with metronidazole plus amoxicillin is usually adequate, but broader spectrum drugs may be used if there are reasons to suspect Gram-negative involvement, for instance, if the patient has been in hospital or previously exposed to antibiotics.

Severe acute respiratory syndrome

Severe acute respiratory syndrome (SARS) is caused by a coronavirus (SARS-associated coronavirus or SARS CoV). Clinically it causes pneumonitis, presenting with a flu-like prodrome and progressing to dyspnoea, dry cough and often adult respiratory distress syndrome, requiring ventilatory support. Treatment is largely supportive. It was first described in 2003 (Drosten et al., 2003) after a large outbreak originating in China spread throughout the Americas, Europe and Asia. The outbreak terminated in that year, with only small numbers of cases occurring since. Many experts predict that SARS will re-emerge.

Cystic fibrosis

Cystic fibrosis (CF) is an inherited, autosomal recessive disease which at the cellular level is due to a defect in the transport of ions in and out of cells. This leads to changes in the consistency and chemical composition of exocrine secretions, which in the lungs is manifest by the production of very sticky, tenacious mucus which is difficult to clear by mucociliary action. The production of such mucus leads to airway obstruction with resulting infection. Repeated episodes of infection lead eventually to bronchiectasis and permanent lung damage, which in turn predisposes the patient to further infection.

Infecting organisms

In infants and young children, *S. aureus* is the most common pathogen. *H. influenzae* is sometimes encountered, but from the age of about 5 years onwards *P. aeruginosa* is seen with increasing frequency until, by the age of 18, most patients are chronically infected with this organism, which once present is never completely eradicated. An important feature of those *P. aeruginosa* strains which infect patients with cystic fibrosis is their production of large amounts of alginate, a polymer of mannuronic and glucuronic acid. This seems to be a virulence factor for the organism in that it inhibits opsonisation and phagocytosis and enables the bacteria to adhere to the bronchial epithelium, thus inhibiting clearance. It does not confer additional antibiotic resistance. Strains which produce large amounts of alginate have a wet, slimy appearance on laboratory culture media and are termed 'mucoid' strains.

Occasionally, other Gram-negative bacteria are seen, such as *Escherichia coli*, which interestingly may also produce alginate in these patients, a characteristic which is otherwise very rare, or *Stenotrophomonas maltophilia*. Many centres worldwide have also experienced problems with members of the *Burkholderia cepacia* complex, which previously were known as plant pathogens. The most frequent culprits are *B. cenocepacia* (formerly *B. cepacia* genomovar III) and *B. multivorans* (formerly *B. cepacia* genomovar II). These organisms are often exceptionally resistant to antibiotics, and their acquisition may be associated with rapidly progressive respiratory failure. Patients colonised with *P. aeruginosa* and *B. cepacia* complex should be isolated to prevent transmission to other CF patients.

Clinical features

CF is characterised by persistent cough and copious sputum production. Many patients are chronically breathless. At times, acute exacerbations occur in which there is fever, increased cough with purulent sputum and increased dyspnoea. Systemic sepsis, however, is very rare. Eventually, chronic pulmonary infection leads to respiratory insufficiency, cardiac failure and death.

Treatment

Although this section will concentrate on antibiotic therapy, it should not be forgotten that other means of treatment such as physiotherapy play a vital part, while lung transplantation can be life saving. Even regarding antibiotics, there are fundamental questions that remain to be addressed; for instance, it is not known whether it is best to give antibiotics according to a planned, regular schedule or in response to exacerbations, and practice varies.

The treatment of infection in a child with cystic fibrosis will probably be directed against staphylococci, for which the usual anti-staphylococcal antibiotics such as flucloxacillin or erythromycin can be used. Once the patient is colonised by *P. aeruginosa*, treatment depends on early and vigorous therapy with antipseudomonal antibiotics (see Table 35.4). At first isolation of *P. aeruginosa*, eradication is attempted with oral ciprofloxacin and a nebulised antibiotic such as colistin.

Table 35.4 Antipseudomonal antibiotics

Antibiotic	Comment
Ticarcillin	One of the first β-lactam agents effective against *Pseudomonas* but now considered insufficiently active. In combination with the β-lactamase inhibitor clavulanic acid, it may be active against some otherwise resistant strains
Ureidopenicillins	Piperacillin, formulated in combination with the β-lactamase inhibitor tazobactam, is the only one of these agents now available in the UK
Monobactams	Aztreonam offers good activity against Gram-negative organisms but no activity against Gram-positive organisms
Cephalosporins	Ceftazidime is the most active antipseudomonal cephalosporin and is very active against other Gram-negative bacilli. It has rather lower activity against Gram-positive bacteria. *Pseudomonas* may develop resistance during treatment
Aminoglycosides	Gentamicin and tobramycin have very similar activity against *Pseudomonas*; tobramycin is perhaps slightly more active. Netilmicin is less active, while amikacin may be active against some gentamicin-resistant strains
Quinolones	Ciprofloxacin can be given orally and parenterally but as with ceftazidime, resistance can develop while the patient is on treatment. Other quinolones such as ofloxacin, its L-isomer levofloxacin, and moxifloxacin have better Gram-positive spectrum but concomitantly less activity against *Pseudomonas*
Polymyxins	These peptide antibiotics are considered too toxic for systemic use in all but the most desperate cases, but colistin (polymyxin E) can be given by inhalation
Carbapenems	Broad-spectrum agents with good Gram-negative activity. Imipenem was the first of these drugs, but CNS toxicity and its requirement for combination with the renal dipeptidase inhibitor cilastatin have largely led to its replacement by meropenem. Doripenem is a newer carbapenem with similar activity to meropenem. Ertapenem has poor activity against *P. aeruginosa*

For chronically colonised patients, regular prophylactic intravenous treatment is given with a β-lactam/aminoglycoside combination such as ceftazidime plus tobramycin. Agents such as meropenem or a quinolone are usually reserved for treatment failures or when resistant organisms are encountered. The prolonged use of ceftazidime or ciprofloxacin alone should be avoided if possible since strains of *P. aeruginosa* and some other Gram-negative bacilli may become resistant to these agents while the patient is receiving treatment. Other treatment modalities are emerging: in a multi-centre, randomised controlled trial, long-term low-dose azithromycin was associated with improvements in lung function in patients chronically infected with *P. aeruginosa* (Saiman et al., 2003).

Interestingly, patients with cystic fibrosis have a more rapid clearance of some antibiotics than other patients. This is particularly noticeable with the aminoglycosides and larger doses are often required to achieve satisfactory plasma levels.

Children with cystic fibrosis are admitted to hospital very frequently, sometimes for long periods of time, and it is not surprising that some of these children develop an intense dislike of hospitals. This has encouraged the use of long-term indwelling central venous cannulae to allow administration of intravenous antibiotics at home by the parents. Ciprofloxacin can be given orally and offers the possibility of treatment for less severe exacerbations at home, perhaps after a brief time in hospital for parenteral therapy.

B. cepacia is often very difficult to treat and strains may be resistant to all available antibiotics. Under these circumstances, combination therapy is often used.

There is some evidence that *in vitro* resistance in some Gram-negative organisms such as *P. aeruginosa* and *B. cepacia* complex does not correlate with treatment failure in the patient.

The use of inhaled (usually nebulised) antibiotics as an adjunct to parenteral therapy has attracted attention, both for treatment of acute exacerbations and for longer-term use in an attempt to reduce the *Pseudomonas* load. Agents which have been administered in this way include colistin, tobramycin and other aminoglycosides, carbenicillin and ceftazidime. The best evidence that long-term administration can be beneficial comes from a large multi-centre trial of nebulised tobramycin (Moss, 2001) in which 520 patients were randomised to receive once-daily nebulised tobramycin or placebo in on–off cycles for 24 weeks, followed by open-label tobramycin to complete 2 years of study. Nebulised tobramycin was safe and well tolerated and was associated with a reduction in hospitalisation and improvements in lung function. This was at the expense of a degree of tobramycin resistance, although this did not seem to be clinically significant.

Respiratory infection in the immunocompromised

The increased use of immunosuppressive agents, and to a lesser extent, the spread of HIV infection, has led to increasing numbers of immunocompromised individuals. Respiratory tract infections, in general, and pneumonia, in particular, are

Table 35.5 Basic causes, defects and infections in immunocompromised individuals

Principal defect	Causative illnesses, diseases or agents	Pathogens causing chest problem (defect related)			
		Bacteria	Viruses	Fungi	Others
Phagocytes	Acute leukaemia, bone marrow failure and chronic granulomatous disease	Staphylococci, aerobic Gram-negative bacilli, *Nocardia asteroides*		*Candida* and *Aspergillus* species	
Antibody (B-cell) immunity	X-linked agammaglobulinaemia, multiple myeloma, Waldenstrom's macroglobulinaemia and chronic lymphocytic leukaemia	Encapsulated bacteria such as *S. pneumoniae, H. influenzae, S. aureus*		*Pneumocystis jiroveci*	
Complement system		Encapsulated bacteria, and *N. meningitidis*			
Cell-mediated (T-cell) immunity	Di George syndrome, lymphoma, hairy cell leukaemia, medications (ciclosporin, steroids), AIDS, CMV and EBV infection	Intracellular micro-organisms, for example, mycobacteria, *Nocardia asteroides*	Varicella zoster virus, herpes simplex virus, cytomegalovirus, EBV	*Cryptococcus neoformans, Histoplasma capsulatum, Pneumocystis jiroveci*	*Toxoplasma gondii*
Defects caused by splenectomy or hyposplenism		Encapsulated bacteria such as *S. pneumoniae, H. influenzae, N. meningitidis* and *Capnocytophaga canimorsus*			

Most agents currently used in mainstay immunosuppression regimens to prevent graft rejection, in organ transplantation, interfere with discrete sites in the T- and B-cell activation cascades.

frequent complications. Morbidity and mortality are high; so rapid recognition, accurate diagnosis and correct treatment are of prime importance. Diagnosis may be complicated by the sheer number of potential pathogens, the problem of distinguishing infection from non-infective conditions such as malignant infiltration or radiation pneumonitis, and non-specific or delayed presentation. The nature, duration and severity of the underlying immune defect, together with specific epidemiologic or environmental factors, influence the risk of infection by different organisms. These are summarised briefly in Table 35.5. Common therapeutic problems are summarised in Table 35.6.

Table 35.6 Common therapeutic problems

Problem	Comments
No pathogens isolated on sputum culture	Possibilities include an inadequate specimen such as saliva, non-infected or sterilised sputum, or a pathogen that cannot be cultured on routine media such as *Chlamydophila pneumoniae* or *Mycobacterium tuberculosis*. Pneumococci are susceptible to autolysis and may fail to grow even from a well-taken specimen, particularly if transport to the laboratory is delayed
Staphylococcus aureus isolated (including MRSA)	*S. aureus* pneumonia is a severe disease with characteristic clinical features, often associated with bacteraemia. However, the organism is frequently isolated from the sputum of patients with bronchitis or bronchopneumonia. In these instances, it usually reflects contamination of the specimen with oropharyngeal commensals although some patients undoubtedly have a clinical infection requiring anti-staphylococcal antibiotics
Candida spp. isolated	Unless there are reasons to suspect *Candida* pneumonia (as a consequence of neutropenia, for example), the isolation of yeasts is likely to reflect oropharyngeal contamination of the specimen. Yeasts can be carried commensally in the mouth, particularly in the presence of dentures, but a search for clinically apparent mucocutaneous candidiasis should be made
Aspergillus spp. isolated	Invasive aspergillosis, allergic bronchopulmonary aspergillosis and aspergilloma should be considered. Alternatively, the finding might reflect inconsequential oropharyngeal carriage

Continued

Table 35.6 Common therapeutic problems—cont'd

Problem	Comments
Penicillin-resistant pneumococci isolated	Respiratory infections caused by strains with low-level resistance (MIC 0.1–1 mg/L) may be treated with penicillins. Strains with high-level resistance should be treated according to their sensitivity profile, for example, using a later-generation cephalosporin or a macrolide
Coliforms isolated	Significance depends on the clinical context: unlikely to be responsible for community-acquired infection unless there is bronchiectasis, but may be relevant to hospital-acquired infections particularly if present in pure culture
Failure of a chest infection to respond to antibiotics	Consider poor compliance, inadequate dosage, viral or otherwise insensitive aetiology. Remember that β-lactam drugs are ineffective against *Chlamydophila*, *Mycoplasma* and *Legionella* infections
Sore throat, no pathogens isolated	Consider viral aetiology, particularly glandular fever in teenagers and young adults
Persistent illness following treatment for pneumococcal pneumonia	Consider the possibility of an empyema (pus in the pleural space), a condition which usually requires surgical drainage

Case studies

Case 35.1

A 40-year-old woman presents to her GP with a 1-week history of sore throat. She is normally fit and well and has had no other symptoms other than some lethargy.

Questions

1. What are the likely causes of the sore throat?
2. Should antibiotics be prescribed?

   The GP decides to prescribe a 10-day course of penicillin V to cover possible streptococcal infection. Two weeks later the patient returns. She is feeling worse and now experiencing difficulty in swallowing. Examination of the throat reveals widespread white plaques.
3. What is the likely diagnosis?
4. What other investigations might be indicated?

Answers

1. A viral aetiology is the most likely cause. These are usually the same viruses that cause colds. Bacterial infection with group A streptococci usually presents with a more severe infection, but where there is doubt a throat swab can establish if bacteria are responsible.
2. Antibiotics are not recommended for routine use. Treatment is directed at symptomatic relief.
3. The likely cause is oral candidiasis. The presence of dysphagia raises the question of oesophageal involvement and hospital admission may be indicated.
4. Underlying immunocompromise must be considered. All patients with oral candidiasis should be offered HIV testing.

Case 35.2

A 61-year-old man is found collapsed at home and taken to hospital. His family report him complaining of a sore throat a few days before admission. On examination, he is pyrexial, hypoxic and tachycardic with reduced air entry to auscultation at the right base. Chest X-ray reveals a right basal pneumonia.

Questions

1. What is the likely diagnosis?
2. What are the possible infecting organisms?
3. What empirical antibiotics would you choose?

   The next day, his sputum yields a growth of beta haemolytic streptococci group A.
4. How should the patient be treated now?

Answers

1. Community-acquired pneumonia.
2. *S. pneumoniae*, *H. influenzae*; sore throat should alert to the possibility of iGAS.
3. Treatment should be guided by the CURB65 score, which assesses severity. Generally, a beta lactam antibiotic and a macrolide are used in combination.
4. There has been no reported resistance of group A streptococci to penicillins, so beta lactam agents should be appropriate. Patients should be isolated until they have received 24 h of treatment. However, this period has often elapsed by the time the diagnosis is made. Blood culture samples should also have been received as invasive infection may often cause an associated bacteraemia.

Case 35.3

A 72-year-old man with a known history of COPD presents to the hospital accident and emergency department with increasing breathlessness. He has a cough productive of cream coloured sputum which is normal for him. He has not noticed an increase in purulence or volume. Chest X-ray showed hyperinflated lungs but no focal consolidation, and a diagnosis of acute exacerbation of COPD was made.

Questions

1. How should this patient be managed?
2. What investigations would inform the diagnosis?

Answers

1. Many exacerbations of COPD are non-infective. Antibiotics should be reserved for where sputum has become more purulent.
2. The diagnosis of exacerbation of COPD is clinical. Sputum cultures should only be performed where antibiotics are being prescribed.

Case 35.4

A 7-year-old girl is seen in the hospital paediatric outpatient clinic. She is known to have cystic fibrosis and has had several exacerbations in the past which have been treated with flucloxacillin. On this visit she is stable, but a report of sputum culture received two days after the clinic shows a growth of *P. aeruginosa*.

Questions

1. What treatment should be started?
2. What other options are available?

    One week later, you receive a telephone call from the parents that she has become unwell and they suspect she has another chest infection.
3. What agents might be appropriate in treating the infection?

Answers

1. Eradication treatment should be commenced, with oral ciprofloxacin plus a nebulised antibiotic such as colistin.
2. In patients with chronic *Pseudomonas* carriage, there are other options to help reduce the frequency of infections. These include regular low-dose azithromycin and nebulised antibiotics such as tobramycin. Non-pharmacological measures such as physiotherapy should also be included.

3. Combination treatment is usually favoured, depending on individual susceptibility results, but might include a beta lactam antibiotic such as ceftazidime or piperacillin-tazobactam in combination with an aminoglycoside such as tobramycin.

Case 35.5

A 70-year-old man who is a lifelong non-smoker presents to his GP with recurrent chest infections. He has been experiencing a cough productive of sputum which is occasionally blood-stained for several months. He also complains of increasing breathlessness. He has had no relief from several courses of antibiotics. Chest examination is unremarkable. The following day the local microbiology laboratory reports the presence of acid-fast bacilli in the sputum.

Questions

1. What is the likely diagnosis?
2. What are the next steps in the management of this patient?

Answers

1. Acid-fast bacilli are consistent with the presence of *Mycobacterium* species in the sputum. This may indicate TB but does not confirm this, as other non-tuberculous mycobacteria may be present. The culture result will confirm the identity.
2. TB is best managed by a specialist in respiratory medicine and this patient should be referred for further investigation. Community infection control teams should be made aware of this result as this patient might have infective TB and may have come into contact with at risk individuals.

References

Atamimi, S., Khalil, A., Khalaiwi, ct al., 2009. Short versus standard duration antibiotic therapy for acute streptococcal pharyngitis in children. Cochrane Database of Systematic Reviews Issue 1, CD004872 Available at http://www.cochrane.org/reviews/en/ab004872.html.

Casey, J.R., Pichichero, M.E., 2004. Meta-analysis of cephalosporin versus penicillin treatment of Group A streptococcal tonsillopharyngitis in children. Pediatrics 113, 866–882.

Damoiseaux, R.A.M., Van Balen, F.A.M., Hoes, A.W., et al., 2000. Primary care based randomised, double blind trial of amoxicillin versus placebo for acute otitis media in children aged under 2 years. Br. Med. J. 320, 350–354.

Del Mar, C.B., Glasziou, P.P., Spinks, A.B., 2004. Antibiotics for sore throat. Cochrane Database of Systematic Reviews Issue 2, CD000023.

Department of Health, 2007. Saving Lives: Reducing Infection, Delivering Clean and Safe Care. High Impact Intervention No 5: Care Bundle for Ventilated Patients (or Tracheostomy Where Appropriate). Available at http://www.dh.gov.uk/prod_consum_dh/groups/dh_digitalassets/@dh/@en/documents/digitalasset/dh_078124.pdf.

Drosten, C., Gunther, S., Preiser, W., et al., 2003. Identification of a novel coronavirus in patients with severe acute respiratory syndrome. N. Engl. J. Med. 348, 1967–1976.

Fraser, D.W., Tsai, T.R., Orenstein, W., et al., 1977. Legionnaire's disease: description of an epidemic of pneumonia. N. Engl. J. Med. 297, 1189–1197.

Glasziou, P.P., Del Mar, C.B., Sanders, S.L., et al., 2004. Antibiotics for acute otitis media in children. Cochrane Library Issue 1, CD000219.

Gulland, A., 2009. Oseltamivir resistant swine flu spreads in Welsh hospital. Br. Med. J. 339, b4975.

Health Protection Agency, Legionnaires' disease in Residents of England and Wales – Nosocomial, Travel or Community Acquired Cases, 1980–2008. Available at http://www.hpa.org.uk/web/HPAweb&HPAwebStandard/HPAweb_C/1195733748327.

Hoberman, A., Greenberg, D.P., Paradise, et al., 2003. Effectiveness of inactivated influenza vaccine in preventing acute otitis media in young children. J. Am. Med. Assoc. 290 (12), 1608–1616.

Joint Committee on Vaccination and Immunisation, 2004. Minutes of the JCVI RSV sub-group on Thursday 11, November 2004. Available at http://www.advisorybodies.doh.gov.uk/jcvi/mins111104rvi.htm.

Kallet, R.H., Quinn, T.E., 2005. The gastro-intestinal tract and ventilator-associated pneumonia. Respir. Care 50, 910–923.

Jansen, A.G., Hak, E., Veenhoven, R.H., et al., 2009. Pneumococcal conjugate vaccines for preventing otitis media. Cochrane Database Systematic Reviews Issue 2, CD001480.

Jefferson, T., Jones, M., Doshi, P., et al., 2009. Neuraminidase inhibitors for preventing and treating influenza in healthy adults: systematic review and meta-analysis. Br. Med. J. 339, b5106.

Lamagni, T.L., Efstratiou, A., Dennis, J., et al., 2009. Increase in invasive group A streptococcal infections in England, Wales and Northern Ireland, 2008–2009. Eurosurveillance 14, 1–2.

Leach, A.J., Morris, P.S., 2006. Antibiotics for the prevention of acute and chronic suppurative otitis media in children. Cochrane Database Systematic Reviews Issue 4, CD004401.

Lim, W.S., Baudouin, S.V., George, R.C., et al., 2009. British Thoracic Society guidelines for the management of community acquired pneumonia in adults: update 2009. Thorax 64, (Suppl. III), iii1–iii55.

Martinez, J.A., Horcajada, J.P., Almeda, M., et al., 2003. Addition of a macrolide to a beta-lactam based empirical antibiotic regimen is associated with lower in-hospital mortality for patients with bacteraemic pneumococcal pneumonia. Clin. Infect. Dis. 36, 389–395.

Masterton, R.G., Galloway, A., French, G., et al., 2008. Guidelines for the management of hospital-acquired pneumonia in the UK: report of the Working Party on Hospital-Acquired Pneumonia of the British Society for Antimicrobial Chemotherapy. J. Antimicrob. Chemother. 62, 5–34.

Moss, R.B., 2001. Administration of aerosolized antibiotics in cystic fibrosis patients. Chest 120, 107–113.

National Institute for Health and Clinical Excellence, 2008. Oseltamivir, Amantadine and Zanamavir for the Prophylaxis of Influenza. TA 158, NICE, London. Available at http://guidance.nice.org.uk/TA158.

National Institute for Health and Clinical Excellence, 2009. Amantadine, Oseltamavir and Zanamavir for the Treatment of Influenza. TA 168, NICE, London. Available at http://guidance.nice.org.uk/TA168.

National Institute for Health and Clinical Excellence, 2004. Management of chronic obstructive pulmonary disease in adults in primary and secondary care. Clinical Guidance 12. NICE, London. Available at http://guidance.nice.org.uk/CG12.

NICE Clinical Knowledge Summaries 2010. Sore throat. Available at http://www.cks.nhs.uk/sore_throat_acute/management/detailed_answers/when_to_admit#-329330

Saiman, L., Marshall, B.C., Mayer-Hamblett, N., et al., 2003. Azithromycin in patients with cystic fibrosis chronically infected with *Pseudomonas aeruginosa*. J. Am. Med. Assoc. 290, 1749–1756.

Strong, M., Burrows, J., Redgrave, P., 2009. A/H1N1 pandemic: Oseltamivir's adverse events. Br. Med. J. 449, b3172.

Van Den Hoogen, B.G., De Jong, J.C., et al., 2001. A newly discovered human pneumovirus isolated from young children with respiratory tract disease. Nat. Med. 7, 719–724.

Wilson, R., Allegra, L., Huchon, G., et al., 2004. Short-term and long-term outcomes of moxifloxacin compared to standard antibiotic treatment in acute exacerbations of chronic bronchitis. Chest 125, 953–964.

World Health Organisation, 2010. Update on human cases of highly pathogenic avian influenza A (H5N1) infection: 2009. Wkly Epidemiol. Rec. 85, 49–51.

Yanney, M., Vyas, H., 2008. The treatment of bronchiolitis. Arch. Dis. Child 93, 793–798.

Further reading

Durrington, H.J., Summers, C., 2008. Recent changes in the management of community acquired pneumonia in adults. Br. Med. J. 336, 1429–1433.

Falk, G., Fahey, T., 2009. C-reactive protein and community-acquired pneumonia in ambulatory care: systematic review of diagnostic accuracy studies. Fam. Pract. 26, 10–21.

Moberley, S., Holden, J., Tatham, D., et al., 2008. Vaccines for preventing pneumococcal infection in adults. Cochrane Database Systematic Reviews Issue 1, CD000422.

Nightingale, C.H., Ambrose, P.G., File, T.M. (Eds.), 2003. Community-Acquired Respiratory Tract Infections: Antimicrobial Management. Taylor and Francis, Abingdon.

Santiago, E., Mandell, L., Woodhead, M., et al., 2006. Respiratory Infections. Holder Education, London.

Useful website

Health Protection Agency, http://www.hpa.org.uk/.

Urinary tract infections 36

N. J. B. Carbarns

Key points

- Urinary tract infection (UTI) is one of the most common complaints seen in general practice and accounts for about one-third of hospital-acquired infections.
- UTI is one of the commonest reasons for prescribing antibiotics.
- *Escherichia coli* is the most frequent pathogen, accounting for more than three-quarters of community-acquired urinary tract infections.
- Symptoms are variable; many UTIs are asymptomatic and some present atypically, particularly in children and the elderly.
- The concept of significant bacteriuria (at least 100,000 organisms/mL of urine) is generally used to distinguish between contamination and infection, but lower counts than this can cause symptoms and disease.
- Asymptomatic UTI should be treated in children and pregnant women.
- Catheter-related UTI should be treated only when the patient has systemic evidence of infection.
- Antimicrobial sensitivity patterns are changing. *E. coli* is becoming increasingly resistant to amoxicillin, cephalosporins, trimethoprim and the quinolones.
- A 3-day treatment course is usually sufficient in uncomplicated lower UTI in women. Longer, 7–14-day courses are recommended for men, children and pregnant women.
- While it is not always necessary to send urine samples for laboratory analysis unless empirical treatment fails, they provide local epidemiology and antibiotic resistance data.
- Antibiotic prophylaxis may be beneficial in women with recurrent UTIs and in children with structural or functional abnormalities.

The term urinary tract infection (UTI) usually refers to the presence of organisms in the urinary tract together with symptoms, and sometimes signs, of inflammation. However, it is more precise to use one of the following terms.

- *Significant bacteriuria:* defined as the presence of at least 100,000 bacteria/mL of urine. A quantitative definition such as this is needed because small numbers of bacteria are normally found in the anterior urethra and may be washed out into urine samples. Counts of fewer than 1000 bacteria/mL are normally considered to be urethral contaminants unless there are exceptional clinical circumstances, such as a sick immunosuppressed patient.

- *Asymptomatic bacteriuria:* significant bacteriuria in the absence of symptoms in the patient.
- *Cystitis:* a syndrome of frequency, dysuria and urgency, which usually suggests infection restricted to the lower urinary tract, that is, the bladder and urethra.
- *Urethral syndrome:* a syndrome of frequency and dysuria in the absence of significant bacteriuria with a conventional pathogen.
- *Acute pyelonephritis:* an acute infection of one or both kidneys. Usually, the lower urinary tract is also involved.
- *Chronic pyelonephritis:* a potentially confusing term used in different ways. It can refer to continuous excretion of bacteria from the kidney, to frequent recurring infection of the renal tissue or to a particular type of pathology of the kidney seen microscopically or by radiographic imaging, which may or may not be due to infection. Although chronic infections of renal tissue are relatively rare, they do occur in the presence of kidney stones and in tuberculosis.
- *Relapse and reinfection:* recurrence of urinary infection may be due to either relapse or reinfection. Relapse is recurrence caused by the same organism that caused the original infection. Reinfection is recurrence caused by a different organism, and is therefore a new infection.

Epidemiology

UTIs are among the most common infectious diseases occurring in either the community or health care setting. Uncomplicated UTIs typically occur in healthy adult non-pregnant women, whereas complicated UTIs are found in either sex and at any age, frequently associated with structural or functional urinary tract abnormalities.

Babies and infants

UTI is a problem in all age groups, although its prevalence varies markedly. In infants up to the age of 6 months, symptomatic UTI has a prevalence of about two cases per 1000 and is much more common in boys than in girls. In addition to these cases, asymptomatic UTI is much more common than this, occurring in around 2% of boys in their first few months of life.

Children

In preschool children, UTIs become more common and the sex ratio reverses, such that the prevalence of bacteriuria is 4.5% in girls and 0.5% in boys. In older children, the prevalence of bacteriuria falls to 1.2% among girls and 0.03% among boys. Overall, about 3–5% of girls and 1–2% of boys will experience a symptomatic UTI during childhood. However, in girls, about two-thirds of UTIs are asymptomatic. The occurrence of bacteriuria during childhood appears to correlate with a higher incidence of bacteriuria in adulthood.

Adults

When women reach adulthood, the prevalence of bacteriuria rises to between 3% and 5%. Each year, about a quarter of these bacteriuric women clear their infections spontaneously and are replaced by an equal number of newly infected women, who are often those with a history of previous infections. On average, about one in eight adult women has a symptomatic UTI each year and over half of adult women report that they have had a symptomatic UTI at some time, 20% recurrently, with the peak age incidence in their early 20s. UTI is uncommon in young healthy men, with 0.5% of adult men having bacteriuria. The rate of symptomatic UTI in men rises progressively with age, from 1% annually at age 18 to 4% at age 60.

Elderly

In the elderly of both sexes, the prevalence of bacteriuria rises dramatically, reaching 20% among women and 10% among men. In hospitals, a major predisposing cause of UTI is urinary catheterisation. With time, even with closed drainage systems and scrupulous hygiene, bacteria can be found in almost all catheters and this is a risk for the development of symptomatic infection.

Aetiology and risk factors

In acute uncomplicated UTI acquired in the community, *Escherichia coli* is by far the most common causative bacterium, being responsible for about 80% of infections. The remaining 20% are caused by other Gram-negative enteric bacteria such as *Klebsiella* and *Proteus* species, and by Gram-positive cocci, particularly enterococci and *Staphylococcus saprophyticus*. The latter organism is almost entirely restricted to infections in young, sexually active women.

UTI associated with underlying structural abnormalities, such as congenital anomalies, neurogenic bladder and obstructive uropathy, is often caused by more resistant organisms such as *Pseudomonas aeruginosa*, *Enterobacter* and *Serratia* species. Organisms such as these are also more commonly implicated in hospital-acquired urinary infections, including those in patients with urinary catheters.

Rare causes of urinary infection, nearly always in association with structural abnormalities or catheterisation, include anaerobic bacteria and fungi. Urinary tract tuberculosis is an infrequent but important diagnosis that may be missed through lack of clinical suspicion. A number of viruses are excreted in urine and may be detected by culture or nucleic acid amplification methods, but symptomatic infection is confined to immunocompromised patients, particularly children following bone marrow transplantation, in whom adenoviruses and polyomaviruses such as BK virus are associated with haemorrhagic cystitis.

Pathogenesis

There are three possible routes by which organisms might reach the urinary tract: the ascending, blood-borne and lymphatic routes. There is little evidence for the last route in humans. Blood-borne spread to the kidney can occur in bacteraemic illnesses, most notably *Staphylococcus aureus* septicaemia, but by far the most frequent route is the ascending route.

In women, UTI is preceded by colonisation of the vagina, perineum and periurethral area by the pathogen, which then ascends into the bladder via the urethra. Uropathogens colonise the urethral opening of men and women. That the urethra in women is shorter than in men and the urethral meatus is closer to the anus are probably important factors in explaining the preponderance of UTI in females. Further, sexual intercourse appears to be important in forcing bacteria into the female bladder, and this risk is increased by the use of diaphragms and spermicides, which have both been shown to increase *E. coli* growth in the vagina. Whether circumcision reduces the risk of infection in adult men is not known, but it markedly reduces the risk of UTI in male infants.

Organism

E. coli causes most UTIs and although there are many serotypes of this organism, only a few of these are responsible for a disproportionate number of infections. While there are as yet no molecular markers that uniquely identify uropathogenic *E. coli*, some strains possess certain virulence factors that enhance their ability to cause infection, particularly infections of the upper urinary tract. Recognised factors include bacterial surface structures called P-fimbriae, which mediate adherence to glycolipid receptors on renal epithelial cells, possession of the iron-scavenging aerobactin system, and increased amounts of capsular K antigen, which mediates resistance to phagocytosis.

Host

Although many bacteria can readily grow in urine, and Louis Pasteur used urine as a bacterial culture medium in his early experiments, the high urea concentration and extremes of osmolality and pH inhibit growth. Other defence mechanisms include the flushing mechanism of bladder emptying, since small numbers of bacteria finding their way into the bladder are likely to be eliminated when the bladder is emptied. Moreover, the bladder mucosa, by virtue of a surface glycosaminoglycan, is intrinsically resistant to bacterial adherence. Presumably, in sufficient numbers, bacteria with strong adhesive properties can overcome this defence. Finally, when the bladder is infected, white blood cells are mobilised to the bladder surface to ingest and destroy invading bacteria. The role of humoral antibody-mediated immunity in defence against infection of the urinary tract remains unclear. Genetic susceptibility of individual patients to UTI has been reviewed (Lichtenberger and Hooton, 2008).

Abnormalities of the urinary tract

Any structural abnormality leading to the obstruction of urinary flow increases the likelihood of infection. Such abnormalities include congenital anomalies of the ureter or urethra, renal stones and, in men, enlargement of the prostate. Renal stones can become infected with bacteria, particularly *Proteus* and *Klebsiella* species, and thereby become a source of 'relapsing' infection. Vesicoureteric reflux (VUR) is a condition caused by failure of physiological valves at the junction of the ureters and the bladder which allows urine to reflux towards the kidneys when the bladder contracts. It is probable that VUR plays an important role in childhood UTIs that lead to chronic renal damage (scarring) and persistence of infection. If there is a diminished ability to empty the bladder such as that due to spinal cord injury, there is an increased risk of bacteriuria.

Clinical manifestations

Most UTIs are asymptomatic. Symptoms, when they do occur, are principally the result of irritation of the bladder and urethral mucosa. However, the clinical features of UTI are extremely variable and to some extent depend on the age of the patient.

Babies and infants

Infections in newborn babies and infants are often overlooked or misdiagnosed because the signs may not be referable to the urinary tract. Common but non-specific presenting symptoms include failure to thrive, vomiting, fever, diarrhoea and apathy. Further, confirmation may be difficult because of problems in obtaining adequate specimens. UTI in infancy and childhood is a major risk factor for the development of renal scarring, which in turn is associated with future complications such as chronic pyelonephritis in adulthood, hypertension and renal failure. It is therefore vital to make the diagnosis early, and any child with a suspected UTI should receive urgent expert assessment.

Children

Above the age of 2, children with UTI are more likely to present with some of the classic symptoms such as frequency, dysuria and haematuria. However, some children present with acute abdominal pain and vomiting, and this may be so marked as to raise suspicions of appendicitis or other intra-abdominal

pathology. Again, however, it is extremely important that the diagnosis of UTI is made promptly to pre-empt the potential long-term consequences. National guidance has been published in the UK on paediatric UTIs to promote a more consistent clinical practice by ensuring prompt, accurate diagnosis and appropriate management (NICE, 2007). A key feature of the guidance is that children with unexplained fever should have their urine tested within 24 h and attention is given to avoiding over- or underdiagnosis, appropriate investigation and the prompt start of antibiotic treatment.

Adults

In adults, the typical symptoms of lower UTI include frequency, dysuria, urgency and haematuria. Acute pyelonephritis (upper UTI) usually causes fever, rigors and loin pain in addition to lower tract symptoms. Systemic symptoms may vary from insignificant to extreme malaise. Importantly, untreated cystitis in adults rarely progresses to pyelonephritis, and bacteriuria does not seem to carry the adverse long-term consequences that it does in children.

In about 40% of women with dysuria, urgency and frequency, the urine sample contains fewer than 100,000 bacteria/mL. These patients are said to have the urethral syndrome. Some have a true bacterial infection but with relatively low counts (100–1000 bacteria/mL). Some have urethral infection with *Chlamydia trachomatis*, *Neisseria gonorrhoeae*, mycoplasmas or other 'fastidious' organisms, any of which might give rise to symptoms indistinguishable from those of cystitis. In others, no known cause can be found by conventional laboratory techniques. It is important to consider the possibility of urinary tract tuberculosis, as special methods are necessary for its detection. Sometimes, the symptoms are of non-infectious origin, such as menopausal oestrogen deficiency or allergy. However, most cases of urethral syndrome will respond to standard antibiotic regimens as used for treating confirmed UTI.

Elderly

Although UTI is frequent in the elderly, the great majority of cases are asymptomatic, and even when present, symptoms are not diagnostic because frequency, dysuria, hesitancy and incontinence are fairly common in elderly people without infection. Further, there may be non-specific systemic manifestations such as confusion and falls, or alternatively the infection may be the cause of deterioration in pre-existing conditions such as diabetes mellitus or congestive cardiac failure, whose clinical features might predominate. UTI is one of the most frequent causes of admission to hospital among the elderly.

Investigations

The key to successful laboratory diagnosis of UTI lies in obtaining an uncontaminated urine sample for microscopy and culture. Contaminating bacteria can arise from skin, vaginal flora in women and penile flora in men. Patients therefore need to be instructed in how to produce a midstream urine sample (MSU). For women, this requires careful cleansing of the perineum and external genitalia with soap and water. Uncircumcised men should retract the foreskin. This is followed by a controlled micturition in which about 20 mL of urine from only the middle portion of the stream is collected, the initial and final components being voided into the toilet or bedpan. Understandably, this is not always possible and many so-called MSUs are in fact clean-catch specimens in which the whole urine volume is collected into a sterile receptacle and an aliquot transferred into a specimen pot for submission to the laboratory. These are more likely to contain urethral contaminants. In very young children, special collection pads for use inside nappies or stick-on bags are useful ways of obtaining a urine sample. Occasionally, in-and-out diagnostic catheterisation or even suprapubic aspiration directly from the bladder is necessary.

For primary care doctors located some distance from a laboratory, transport of specimens is a problem. Specimens must reach the laboratory within 1–2 h or should be refrigerated; otherwise, any bacteria in the specimen will multiply and might give rise to a false-positive result. Methods of overcoming bacterial multiplication in urine include the addition of boric acid to the container and the use of dipslides, in which an agar-coated paddle is dipped into the urine and submitted directly to the laboratory for incubation. Both of these alternatives have difficulties. For the boric acid technique, it is important that the correct amount of urine is added to the container to achieve the appropriate concentration of boric acid (1.8%, w/v), as the chemical has significant antibacterial activity when more concentrated. When the dip-slide is used, no specimen is available on which to do cell counts.

Concerns about the relative expense and slow turn-around time of urine microscopy and culture have stimulated interest in alternative diagnostic strategies. Some advocate a policy of empirical antimicrobial treatment in the first instance, and reserve investigation only for those cases that do not respond. Others are in favour of using cheaper, more convenient screening tests, for example, urine dipsticks. It is important to be aware that there is no rapid screening test that will reliably detect all UTIs. Urine microscopy and culture remain the standard by which other investigations are measured.

Dipsticks

Dipsticks for rapid near-patient testing for urinary blood, protein, nitrites and leucocyte esterase are usually used, although there are concerns that these are reliable only when applied to fresh urine samples tested at the point of care. Assessment of colour changes on dipsticks can be subjective and automated reading systems have been developed to assist interpretation. Generally, the negative predictive value is better than the positive predictive value, so their preferred use is as screening tests to identify those specimens which are least likely to be infected and which therefore do not require culture. A perfectly valid alternative is just to hold the specimen up to the light: specimens that are visibly clear are very likely to be sterile.

The leucocyte esterase test detects enzyme released from leucocytes in urine and is ~90% sensitive at detecting white blood cell counts of >10 mm^{-3}. It will be positive even if the cells have been destroyed due to delays in transport to a laboratory. However, vitamin C and antibiotics in the urine such as cephalosporins, gentamicin and nitrofurantoin may interfere with the reaction. Although the presence of leucocytes is common in UTIs, it may also occur in other conditions. Particularly in children, white blood cells can be present for many reasons, including fever alone.

The nitrite test (also called the Griess test) detects urinary nitrite made by bacteria that can convert excreted dietary nitrate used as a food preservative to nitrite. Although the coliform bacteria that commonly cause UTI can be detected in this way, some organisms cannot, for example, enterococci, group B streptococci, *Pseudomonas*, because they do not contain the converting enzyme. In addition, the test depends on sufficient nitrate in the diet and on allowing enough time, at least 4 h, for the chemical conversion to occur in the urine. Performance of the dipstick test is generally less diagnostic in infants and younger children than in the older age groups, and this may relate in part to the small capacity and frequent emptying of the infant bladder, resulting in lower numbers of organisms and less pyuria. The use of dipsticks alone for the diagnosis of UTI is not recommended for children under 3 years of age (NICE, 2007). The inability of the test to detect group B streptococci also makes it a relatively inappropriate test for screening for asymptomatic bacteriuria in pregnancy, in which this organism assumes particular importance as a cause of neonatal sepsis.

Although a negative dipstick test for leucocytes and nitrites can quite accurately predict absence of infection, their absence does not necessarily predict non-response to antibiotic treatment and further research is needed on this (Richards et al., 2005). Some experts consider that detection of nitrites in a symptomatic patient should prompt initiation of treatment (Gopal Rao and Patel, 2009). An algorithm for the use of dipstick testing in uncomplicated UTI in adult women is set out in Fig. 36.1.

There are other rapid methods for detecting bacteriuria, such as tests for interleukin-8, and no shortage of data concerning their sensitivity and specificity, but the optimal strategy will always be a compromise between accuracy, speed, convenience and cost, and is likely to be very different for different settings and populations.

Microscopy

Microscopy is the first step in the laboratory diagnosis of UTI and can be readily performed in practice. A drop of uncentrifuged urine is placed on a slide, covered with a coverslip and examined under a 40× objective. Excess white cells are usually seen in the urine of patients with symptomatic UTI, and more than 10 per high-power field is abnormal. It should be noted that there are other methods in common use, and laboratories may report white cell counts per microlitre (cubic millimetre) of urine or per millilitre. Automated machinery for microscopy of urine is increasingly used and

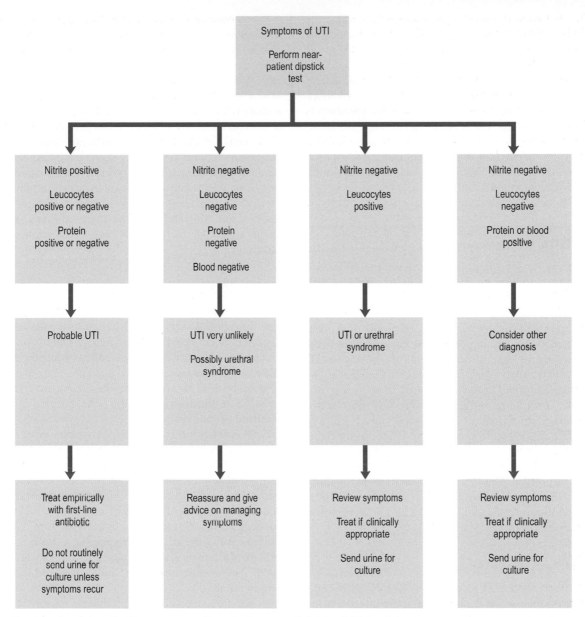

Fig. 36.1 Algorithm for diagnosis of acute uncomplicated urinary tract infection (UTI) in adult women.

offers increased precision and handling capacities of over 100 specimens/h. Although there is a substantial capital cost to such equipment, it is offset by savings in labour and bacterial culture materials. One feature of this equipment is that it is generally much more sensitive in detecting cells, so much so that laboratories using such systems will have a much higher number for significant results (e.g. >50 rather than >10 white cells/mm^3).

It is important not to be too rigid in the interpretation of the white cell count. UTI may occur in the absence of pyuria, particularly at the extremes of age, in pregnancy and in pyelonephritis. Red blood cells may be seen, as may white cell casts, which are suggestive of pyelonephritis. As a rule of thumb, the presence of at least one bacterium per field correlates with 100,000 bacteria/mL.

Culture

Bladder urine is normally sterile, but when passed via the urethra, it is inevitable that some contamination with the urethral bacterial flora will occur. This is why it is important that laboratories quantify the number of bacteria in urine specimens. In work carried out over 40 years ago, it was demonstrated that patients with UTI usually have at least 100,000 bacteria/mL, while in patients without infection, the count is usually below 1000 bacteria/mL. Between these figures lies a grey area, and it should be appreciated that the MSU is not an infallible guide to the presence or absence of urinary infection. True infections may be associated with low counts, particularly when the urine is very dilute because of excessive fluid intake or where the pathogen is slow growing. While the quantitative criterion for 'significant' bacteriuria is generally taken as >100,000/mL, in some specific groups, it is less: for men, >1000/mL and for women with symptoms of UTI, it is >100/mL (SIGN, 2006).

Most genuine infections are caused by one single bacterial species; mixed cultures usually suggest contamination. If a patient is taking an antibiotic when a urine specimen is obtained for culture, growth of bacteria may be inhibited. The laboratory may perform a test to detect antimicrobial substances in the urine, and this may be useful information to clarify circumstances in which the culture is negative but a significant pyuria is present.

Treatment

Although many, and perhaps most, cases clear spontaneously given time, symptomatic UTI usually merits antibiotic treatment to eradicate both symptoms and pathogen. Asymptomatic bacteriuria may or may not need treatment depending upon the circumstances of the individual case. Bacteriuria in children and in pregnant women requires treatment, as does bacteriuria present when surgical manipulation of the urinary tract is to be undertaken, because of the potential complications. On the other hand, in non-pregnant, asymptomatic bacteriuric adults without any obstructive lesion, screening and treatment are probably unwarranted in most circumstances (Nicolle et al., 2005). Unnecessary treatment will lead to selection of resistant organisms and puts patients at risk of adverse drug effects including bowel infection with *Clostridium difficile*, which has been particularly associated with the use of cephalosporins and quinolones. A number of common management problems are summarised in Table 36.1.

Non-specific treatments

Advising patients with UTI to drink a lot of fluids is common practice on the theoretical basis that more infected urine is removed by frequent bladder emptying. This is plausible, although not evidence based. Some clinicians recommend urinary analgesics such as potassium or sodium citrate, which alkalinise the urine, but these should be used as an adjunct to antibiotics. They should not be used in conjunction with nitrofurantoin, which is active only at acidic pH.

Antimicrobial chemotherapy

The principles of antimicrobial treatment of UTI are the same as those of the treatment of any other infection: from a group of suitable drugs chosen on the basis of efficacy, safety and cost, select the agent with the narrowest possible spectrum and administer it for the shortest possible time. In general, there is no evidence that bactericidal antibiotics are superior to bacteriostatic agents in treating UTI, except perhaps in relapsing infections. Blood levels of antibiotics appear to be unimportant in the treatment of lower UTI; what matters is the concentration in the urine. However, blood levels probably

are important in treating pyelonephritis, which may progress to bacteraemia. Drugs suitable for the oral treatment of cystitis include trimethoprim, the β-lactams, particularly amoxicillin, co-amoxiclav and cefalexin, fluoroquinolones such as ciprofloxacin, norfloxacin and ofloxacin, and nitrofurantoin. Where intravenous administration is required, suitable agents include β-lactams such as amoxicillin and cefuroxime, quinolones, and aminoglycosides such as gentamicin.

In renal failure, it may be difficult to achieve adequate therapeutic concentrations of some drugs in the urine, particularly nitrofurantoin and quinolones. Further, accumulation and toxicity may complicate the use of aminoglycosides. Penicillins and cephalosporins attain satisfactory concentrations and are relatively non-toxic, and are therefore the agents of choice for treating UTI in the presence of renal failure.

Antibiotic resistance

Antimicrobial resistance is a major concern worldwide. The susceptibility profile of commonly isolated uropathogens has been constantly changing. Coliform bacteria of many species that produce extended-spectrum β-lactamase (ESBL) enzymes have emerged in recent years, particularly as a cause of UTI in community-based patients. Before 2003, most ESBL-producing bacteria were hospital acquired and occurred in specialist units.

ESBL-producing bacteria are clinically important as they produce enzymes that destroy almost all commonly used β-lactams except the carbapenem class, rendering most penicillins and cephalosporins largely useless in clinical practice. Some ESBL enzymes can be inhibited by clavulanic acid, and combinations of an agent containing it, for example, co-amoxiclav, with other oral broad-spectrum β-lactams, for example, cefixime or cefpodoxime, have been used to treat UTIs caused by ESBL-producing *E. coli* (Livermore et al., 2008). These combinations are unlicensed and their effectiveness is variable.

In addition, many ESBL-producing bacteria are multiresistant to non-β-lactam antibiotics too, such as quinolones, aminoglycosides and trimethoprim, narrowing treatment options. ESBL-*E. coli* is often pathogenic and a high proportion of infections result in bacteraemia with resultant mortality (Tumbarello et al., 2007). Some strains cause outbreaks both in hospitals and in the community. Empirical treatment strategies may need to be reviewed in settings where ESBL-producing strains are prevalent, and it may be considered appropriate to use a carbapenem in seriously ill patients until an infection has been proved not to involve an ESBL producer.

Recently, even more resistant strains have emerged in India and Pakistan, with subsequent transfer to the UK, that carry a gene for a novel New Delhi metallo-β-lactamase-1 that also confers resistance to carbapenems. This bla_{NDM-1} gene was mostly found among *E. coli* and *Klebsiella*, which were highly resistant to all antibiotics except to colistin and tigecycline, which is not effective for UTI as it is chemically unstable in the urinary tract (Kumarasamy et al., 2010).

Table 36.1 Common management problems with urinary tract infections (UTI)

Problem	Comments
Asymptomatic infection	Asymptomatic bacteriuria should be treated where there is a risk of serious consequences (e.g. in childhood), where there is renal scarring, and in pregnancy. Otherwise, treatment is not usually required
Catheter *in situ*, patient unwell	Systemic symptoms may result from catheter-associated UTI, and should respond to antibiotics although the catheter is likely to remain colonised. Local symptoms such as urgency are more likely to reflect urethral irritation than infection
Catheter *in situ*, urine cloudy or smelly	Unless the patient is systemically unwell, antibiotics are unlikely to achieve much and may give rise to resistance. Interventions of uncertain benefit include bladder wash-outs or a change of catheter
Penicillin allergy	Clarify 'allergy': vomiting or diarrhoea are not allergic phenomena and do not contraindicate penicillins. Penicillin-induced rash is a contraindication to amoxicillin, but cephalosporins are likely to be tolerated. Penicillin-induced anaphylaxis suggests that all β-lactams should be avoided
Symptoms of UTI but no bacteriuria	Exclude urethritis, candidosis, etc. Otherwise likely to be urethral syndrome, which usually responds to conventional antibiotics
Bacteriuria but no pyuria	May suggest contamination. However, pyuria is not invariable in UTI and may be absent particularly in pyelonephritis, pregnancy, neonates, the elderly, and *Proteus* infections
Pyuria but no bacteriuria	Usually, the patient has started antibiotics before taking the specimen. Rarely, a feature of unusual infections (e.g. anaerobes, tuberculosis, etc.)
Urine grows *Candida*	Usually reflects perineal candidosis and contamination. True candiduria is rare, and may reflect renal candidosis or systemic infection with candidaemia
Urine grows two or more organisms	Mixed UTI is unusual – mixed cultures are likely to reflect perineal contamination. A repeat should be sent unless this is impractical (e.g. frail elderly patients), in which case best-guess treatment should be instituted if clinically indicated
Symptoms recur	May represent relapse or reinfection. A repeat urine culture should be performed shortly after treatment

Uncomplicated lower UTI

The problem with empirical treatment is that over 10% of the healthy adult female population would receive an antibiotic each year. The use of antibiotics to this extent in the population has implications for antibiotic resistance, a major focus of public health policy worldwide. This highlights the tension between maximising the benefit for individuals and minimising antibiotic resistance at a population level. Strategies have included diagnostic algorithms to predict more precisely who has a UTI, as well as issuing delayed prescriptions (Mangin, 2010).

Therapeutic decisions should be based on accurate, up-to-date antimicrobial susceptibility patterns. Data have been published from a European multicentre survey that examined the prevalence and antimicrobial susceptibility of community-acquired pathogens causing uncomplicated UTI in women (Kahlmeter, 2003). Among almost 2500 *E. coli* isolates, the resistance rates were 30% for amoxicillin, 15% for trimethoprim, 3.4% for co-amoxiclav, 2.3% for ciprofloxacin, 2.1% for cefadroxil and 1.2% for nitrofurantoin. These figures are lower than most routine laboratory data would suggest, but it should be remembered that the experience of diagnostic laboratories is likely to be biased by the overrepresentation of specimens from patients in whom empirical treatment has

already failed. It is important to be aware of local variations in sensitivity pattern and to balance the risk of therapeutic failure against the cost of therapy.

Adults

The preference for best-guess therapy would seem to be a choice between trimethoprim, an oral cephalosporin such as cefalexin, co-amoxiclav or nitrofurantoin, with the proviso that therapy can be refined once sensitivities are available. The quinolones are best reserved for treatment failures and more difficult infections, since overuse of these important agents is likely to lead to an increase in resistance, as has been seen in countries such as Spain and Portugal. These recommendations are summarised in Table 36.2.

Other drugs that have been used for the treatment of UTI include co-trimoxazole, pivmecillinam, fosfomycin and earlier quinolones such as nalidixic acid. Co-trimoxazole is now recognised as a cause of bone marrow suppression and other haematological side effects, and in the UK, its use is greatly restricted. Further, despite superior activity *in vitro*, there is no convincing evidence that it is clinically superior to trimethoprim alone in the treatment of UTI caused by strains susceptible to both. Pivmecillinam is an oral pro-drug that is metabolised

Table 36.2 Oral antibiotics used for lower urinary tract infections

Antibiotic	Dose (adult)	Side effects	Contraindications	Comments
Amoxicillin	250–500 mg three times a day	Nausea, diarrhoea, allergy	Penicillin hypersensitivity	High levels of resistance (>50%) in *E. coli*. Not used empirically
Co-amoxiclav	375–625 mg three times a day	See amoxicillin	See amoxicillin	Amoxicillin and clavulanic acid
Cefalexin	250–500 mg four times a day	Nausea, diarrhoea, allergy	Cephalosporin hypersensitivity, porphyria	
Trimethoprim	200 mg twice a day	Nausea, pruritus, allergy	Pregnancy, neonates, folate deficiency, porphyria	
Nitrofurantoin	50 mg four times a day	Nausea, allergy, rarely pneumonitis, pulmonary fibrosis, neuropathy	Renal failure, neonates, porphyria, G6PD deficiency	Modified-release form may be given twice daily. Inactive against *Proteus*
Ciprofloxacin	100–500 mg twice a day	Rash, pruritus, tendinitis	Pregnancy, children	Reserve for difficult cases

G6PD, glucose-6-phosphate dehydrogenase.

to mecillinam, a β-lactam agent with a particularly high affinity for Gram-negative penicillin-binding protein 2 and a low affinity for commonly encountered β-lactamases, and which therefore has theoretical advantages in the treatment of UTI. Pivmecillinam has been extensively used for cystitis in Scandinavian countries, where it does not seem to have led to the development of resistance, and for this reason, there have been calls for wider recognition of its usefulness, particularly for UTI caused by ESBL-producing strains. Fosfomycin is a broad-spectrum antibiotic with pharmacokinetic and pharmacodynamic properties that favour its use for treatment of cystitis with a single oral dose (Falagas et al., 2010). Finally, older quinolones such as nalidixic acid and cinoxacin were once widely used, but generally these agents have given ground to the more active fluorinated quinolones.

Duration of treatment

The question of duration of treatment has received much attention. Traditionally, a course of 7–10 days has been advocated, and this is still the recommendation for treating men, in whom the possibility of occult prostatitis should be borne in mind. For women, though, there has been particular emphasis on the suitability of short-course regimens such as 3-day or even single-dose therapy. The consensus of an international expert working group was that 3-day regimens are as effective as longer regimens in the cases of trimethoprim and quinolones. β-Lactams have been inadequately investigated on this point but short courses are generally less effective than trimethoprim and quinolones, and nitrofurantoin requires further study before definite conclusions can be drawn. Single-dose therapy, with its advantages of cost, adherence and the minimisation of side effects, has been used successfully in many studies but in general is less effective than when the same agent is used for longer.

In the urethral syndrome, it is worth trying a 3-day course of one of the agents mentioned earlier. If this fails, a 7-day course of tetracycline could be tried to deal with possible chlamydia or mycoplasma infection.

Children

In children, the risk of renal scarring is such that UTI should be diagnosed and treated promptly, even if asymptomatic. The drugs of choice include β-lactams, trimethoprim and nitrofurantoin. Quinolones are relatively contraindicated in children because of the theoretical risk of causing cartilage and joint problems. Children should be treated for 7–10 days.

Renal scarring occurs in 5–15% of children with UTI, who should be identified so that appropriate treatment can be instituted. Unfortunately, the subgroup at high risk cannot be predicted, and for this reason, many clinicians choose to investigate all children with UTI, for example, using ultrasound and radioisotope scanning.

Acute pyelonephritis

Patients with pyelonephritis may be severely ill and, if so, will require admission to hospital and initial treatment with a parenteral antibiotic. Suitable agents with good activity against *E. coli* and other Gram-negative bacilli include cephalosporins such as cefuroxime and ceftazidime, some penicillins such as co-amoxiclav, quinolones, and aminoglycosides such as gentamicin (Table 36.3). A first-choice agent would be parenteral cefuroxime, gentamicin or ciprofloxacin. When the patient is improving, the route of administration may be switched to oral therapy, typically using a quinolone. Conventionally, treatment is continued for 10–14 days.

Patients who are less severely ill at the outset may be treated with an oral antibiotic, and possibly with a shorter course of

Table 36.3 Parenteral antibiotics used for pyelonephritis

Antibiotic	Dose (adult)	Side effects	Contraindications	Comments
Cefuroxime	750 mg three times a day	Nausea, diarrhoea, allergy	Cephalosporin hypersensitivity, porphyria	Implicated in *Clostridium difficile*
Ceftazidime	1 g three times a day	See cefuroxime	See cefuroxime	See cefuroxime
Co-amoxiclav	1.2 g three times a day	Nausea, diarrhoea, allergy	Penicillin hypersensitivity	
Gentamicin	80–120 mg three times a day or 5 mg/kg once daily	Nephrotoxicity, ototoxicity	Pregnancy, myasthenia gravis	Monitor levels
Ciprofloxacin	200–400 mg twice a day	Rash, pruritus, tendinitis	Pregnancy, children	Implicated in *Clostridium difficile*
Piperacillin with tazobactam	4.5 g three times a day	Nausea, allergy	Penicillin hypersensitivity	
Meropenem	500 mg three times a day	Nausea, rash, convulsions		Reserve for multiresistant cases

treatment. The safety of this approach has been demonstrated in a study of adult women with acute uncomplicated pyelonephritis (Talan et al., 2000). Among 113 patients treated with oral ciprofloxacin 500 mg twice daily for 7 days (± an initial intravenous dose), the cure rate was 96%.

In hospital-acquired pyelonephritis, there is a risk that the infecting organism may be resistant to the usual first-line drugs. In such cases, it may be advisable to start a broad-spectrum agent such as ceftazidime, ciprofloxacin or meropenem.

Relapsing UTI

The main causes of persistent relapsing UTI are renal infection, structural abnormalities of the urinary tract and, in men, chronic prostatitis. Patients who fail on a 7–10-day course should be given a 2-week course, and if that fails, a 6-week course can be considered. Structural abnormalities may need surgical correction before cure can be maintained. It is essential that prolonged courses (i.e. more than 4 weeks) are managed under bacteriological control, for example, with monthly cultures. In men with prostate gland infection, it is appropriate to select antibiotics with good tissue penetration such as trimethoprim and the fluoroquinolones.

Catheter-associated infections

In most large hospitals, 10–15% of patients have an indwelling urinary catheter. Even with the very best catheter care, most will have infected urine after 10–14 days of catheterisation, although most of these infections will be asymptomatic. Antibiotic treatment will often appear to eradicate the infecting organism, but as long as the catheter remains in place, the organism, or another more resistant one, will quickly return. The principles of antibiotic therapy for catheter-associated UTI are therefore as follows:

- Do not treat asymptomatic infection.
- If possible, remove the catheter before treating symptomatic infection.

Although it often prompts investigation, cloudy or strong-smelling urine is not *per se* an indication for antimicrobial therapy. In these situations, saline or antiseptic bladder washouts are often performed, but there is little evidence that they make a difference. Similarly, encrusted catheters are often changed on aesthetic grounds, but it is not known whether this reduces the likelihood of future symptoms.

Following catheter removal, bacteriuria may resolve spontaneously but more often it persists (typically for over 2 weeks in over half of patients) and may become symptomatic, though usually it will respond well to short-course treatment.

Antimicrobial catheters

Several different types of novel catheters with anti-infective properties have been developed with the aim of reducing the ability of bacteria to adhere to the material, which should lead to a decreased incidence of bacteriuria and symptomatic infection. Several studies of the effect of incorporating antibiotics such as rifampicin and minocycline or silver-based alloys into the catheter have shown benefit. Although clearly more costly than standard catheters, economic evaluation shows silver alloy catheters to be cost efficient when used in patients needing catheterisation for several days. The effect of these catheters on clinical outcomes such as bacteraemia remains to be determined.

Bacteriuria of pregnancy

The prevalence of asymptomatic bacteriuria of pregnancy is about 5%, and about a third of these women proceed to develop acute pyelonephritis, with its attendant consequences for the health of both mother and pregnancy. Further, there is evidence that asymptomatic bacteriuria is associated with low birth weight, prematurity, hypertension and pre-eclampsia. For these reasons, it is recommended that screening be carried out, preferably by culture of a properly taken MSU, which should be repeated if positive for confirmation (National Collaborating Centre for Women's and Children's Health, 2003).

Rigorous meta-analysis of published trials has shown that antibiotic treatment of bacteriuria in pregnancy is effective at clearing bacteriuria, reducing the incidence of pyelonephritis and reducing the risk of preterm delivery. The drugs of choice are amoxicillin or cefalexin or nitrofurantoin, depending on the sensitivity profile of the infecting organism. Co-amoxiclav is cautioned in pregnancy because of lack of clinical experience in pregnant women. Trimethoprim is contraindicated (particularly in the first trimester) because of its theoretical risk of causing neural tube defects through folate antagonism. Nitrofurantoin should be avoided close to the time of expected delivery because of a risk of haemolysis in the baby. Ciprofloxacin is contraindicated because it may affect the growing joints. There are insufficient data concerning short-course therapy in pregnancy, and 7 days of treatment remains the standard. Patients should be followed up for the duration of the pregnancy to confirm cure and to ensure that any reinfection is promptly addressed.

Prevention and prophylaxis

There are a number of folklore and naturopathic recommendations for the prevention of UTI. Most of these have not been put to statistical study, but at least are unlikely to cause harm.

Cranberry juice

Cranberry juice (*Vaccinium macrocarpon*) has long been thought to be beneficial in preventing UTI, and this has been studied in a number of clinical trials. Cranberry is thought to inhibit adhesion of bacteria to urinary tract cells on the surface of the bladder. In sexually active women, a daily intake of 750 mL cranberry juice was associated with a 40% reduction in the risk of symptomatic UTI in a double-blinded 12-month trial. Many studies have been criticised for methodological flaws, and currently there is only limited evidence that cranberry juice is effective at preventing recurrent UTI (McMurdo et al., 2009). There have been no randomised controlled trials of the use of cranberry products (juice, tablets or capsules) in the treatment of established infection, or comparing it with established therapies such as antibiotics for preventing infection.

A hypothetical benefit in using cranberry instead of antibiotics for this purpose is a reduced risk of the development of antibiotic-resistant bacteria. A significant hazard is an interaction of cranberry with warfarin, with a risk of bleeding episodes, and available products are not available in standardised formulations. Further, cranberry juice is unpalatable unless sweetened with sugar and therefore carries a risk of tooth decay, although ironically it is reported to prevent dental caries by blocking adherence of plaque bacteria to teeth.

Antibiotic prophylaxis

In some patients, mainly women, reinfections are so frequent that long-term antimicrobial prophylaxis with specific antibiotics is indicated. If the reinfections are clearly related to sexual intercourse, then a single dose of an antibiotic after intercourse is appropriate. In other cases, long-term, low-dose prophylaxis may be beneficial. One dose of trimethoprim (100 mg) or nitrofurantoin (50 mg) at night will suffice. These drugs are unlikely to lead to the emergence of resistant bacteria, although breakthrough infection with strains intrinsically resistant to the chosen prophylactic antibiotic is possible.

Children

In children, recurrence of UTI is common and the complications potentially hazardous, so many clinicians recommend antimicrobial prophylaxis following documented infection. The evidence in favour of this practice is not strong (Le Saux et al., 2000), and although it has been shown to reduce the incidence of bacteriuria, there is no good-quality evidence that prophylactic antibiotics are effective in preventing further symptomatic UTIs and they have not been shown to reduce the incidence of renal scarring complications, which are the most important outcomes for the patient (Mori et al., 2009). Further, important variables remain to be clarified, such as when to begin prophylaxis, which agent to use and when to stop. Recent guidelines have abandoned the time-honoured recommendation for routine antibiotic prophylaxis following a first infection, although it may be considered when there is recurrent UTI (NICE, 2007).

Although evidence is limited for some recommendations, there are many common-sense general measures aimed at reducing the risk of recurrence of infection, particularly in girls. They include advice on regular bladder emptying, cleaning the perineal/anal area from front to back after toilet, treating constipation adequately and avoiding both bubble baths and washing the hair in the bath.

Case studies

Case 36.1

A 70-year-old man has consulted his primary care doctor three times in the past 3 months and seems to have the same *E. coli* infection on each occasion. A short course of antibiotics clears up the symptoms, but a clinical relapse is soon apparent. He is admitted to hospital for transurethral resection of the prostate and 2 days after the operation he becomes unwell with rigors, fever and loin pain. Microscopy of his urine shows over 200 white cells/mm³. Blood cultures are taken and rapidly become positive, with Gram-negative bacilli seen on microscopy.

Question

Is there any way of predicting which UTIs are likely to go on to cause further problems such as pyelonephritis or prostatitis? What antibiotic therapy is indicated now?

Answer

Progression of a simple UTI is much more common in patients other than young women. Foreign bodies such as catheters and stents, or physiological problems such as neurogenic bladder, increase the risk of a complicated UTI. In men, persistent or recurrent infection with the same organism is highly suggestive of prostatitis and should prompt an extended course of treatment. Pyelonephritis is more difficult to predict. Frequency, dysuria and haematuria indicate lower tract infection. Fever, vomiting, rigors and flank pain are more suggestive of upper renal tract involvement.

The patient should be started on intravenous antibiotic therapy for presumed prostatitis or pyelonephritis and consequent bacteraemia. The antibiotic should cover Gram-negative organisms found in the hospital environment such as *Klebsiella*, *Enterobacter* and *Pseudomonas*. Appropriate agents would be piperacillin-tazobactam, ceftazidime, ciprofloxacin or meropenem. An alternative would be an aminoglycoside such as gentamicin, provided the patient has satisfactory renal function.

Case 36.2

A pregnant woman aged 26 years is found to have bacteriuria at her first antenatal visit. There are no white or red cells seen in her urine. Urine culture demonstrates *E. coli* at a count of more than 100,000 bacteria/mL, sensitive to trimethoprim, nitrofurantoin and cefalexin but resistant to amoxicillin. Other than a degree of urinary frequency, which she ascribes to the pregnancy itself, the patient does not complain of any urinary symptoms.

Question

Does this patient need antibiotic treatment, and if so, which drugs could be safely used?

Answer

The patient may be correct that her urinary frequency is a consequence of pregnancy. However, because of the consequences of untreated infection during pregnancy, even asymptomatic bacteriuria should be treated. A repeat urine specimen should be obtained to confirm the finding, and treatment started with either cefalexin or co-amoxiclav for 7 days. Trimethoprim should be avoided during early pregnancy because of its theoretical risk of teratogenicity, and nitrofurantoin should be avoided in late pregnancy as it may cause neonatal haemolysis. Following treatment, she should be reviewed throughout the pregnancy to ensure eradication of the bacteriuria, and to permit early treatment of any relapse or reinfection.

Case 36.3

A 2-year-old boy is admitted to hospital with vomiting and abdominal pain. His mother reports that he was treated for UTI 6 months previously, but was not investigated further at the time. A clean catch urine sample shows over 50 white cells/mm³ and bacteria are seen on microscopy.

Question

What action should be taken?

Answer

It seems that this child is suffering from a recurrent UTI. An intravenous antibiotic such as cefuroxime should be started, since the child will not tolerate oral antibiotics at present. If the organism proves to be sensitive to amoxicillin, the treatment could be changed accordingly. Further investigations, for example, ultrasonography and radioisotope scan, may be carried out to determine any underlying cause of the infection and to look for already established renal scarring. The child may require long-term prophylaxis to prevent a further recurrence.

Case 36.4

A 62-year-old lady has been troubled by recurrent symptoms of UTI. She has been taking an oral oestrogen preparation for menopausal symptoms for some years. She is currently on an orthopaedic ward and catheterised because of incontinence. She is afebrile but has been confused since her hip replacement 5 days earlier, and remains on cefuroxime, which was started as prophylaxis at the time of the operation. The urine in her catheter bag is cloudy, has a high white cell count, and grows *Enterococcus faecalis* sensitive to amoxicillin but resistant to cephalosporins.

Question

How should this patient be managed? In older women, is there any association with the use of different types of oestrogen delivery systems and UTIs?

Answer

The patient's confusion may have a number of causes, including her recent surgery, sleep disturbance, drug toxicity, deep venous thrombosis or infection. If, following clinical examination and investigation, which should include blood cultures, her catheter-associated infection is thought to be contributing to her systemic problems, it should be treated with amoxicillin. If possible, the catheter should be removed, even if this is inconvenient for the nursing staff. Unless it has been prescribed for another indication, the cefuroxime is achieving nothing and may be stopped.

In post-menopausal women, there have been trials assessing the merits of topical oestrogen creams. Topical intravaginal oestriol cream has significant benefits in reducing the number of UTIs in those suffering recurrent infections. In a placebo-controlled trial, the rate of UTI was 12-fold less in the group receiving active oestrogen cream. This effect is not seen with oral oestrogens (Perrotta et al., 2008).

Case 36.5

A 45-year-old woman suffers from recurrent episodes of cystitis. Examination is unremarkable. On the occasions when a specimen has been sent, the urine has contained few white cells and no significant growth of organisms.

Question

How should the patient be managed?

Answer

This patient is suffering from the urethral syndrome, in which symptoms of infection are not associated with objective evidence of UTI. It may be felt necessary to investigate her to exclude less common causes of UTI such as herpes simplex virus, *Chlamydia trachomatis*, *Neisseria gonorrhoeae*, *Gardnerella vaginalis*, *Mycoplasma hominis* and *Lactobacilli*. Otherwise, her symptoms are likely to respond to conventional courses of antibiotics. Consider non-infective causes, for example, psychological factors, trauma from intercourse.

Case 36.6

A 23-year-old woman has recurrent symptoms of UTI temporally related to sexual intercourse, despite following advice to empty her bladder as soon as possible after sex.

Question

What do you think of the use of antibiotics such as trimethoprim for women who get recurrent problems after sexual intercourse?

Answer

Post-coital voiding does not have any prospective data to support it, but it is a simple, harmless intervention. Long-term continuous antimicrobial prophylaxis is unquestionably an effective treatment but may be overtreating those in whom UTIs follow intercourse. Post-coital prophylaxis, a single dose within 2 h of intercourse, has the advantage of using less antibiotic overall. One small placebo-controlled double-blind trial assessed the efficacy of post-coital co-trimoxazole in preventing recurrent UTI and found that 12% of the active-treatment patients developed a UTI in 6 months, compared to 82% of the control group. Other studies have shown nitrofurantoin, cefalexin and ciprofloxacin also to be effective.

References

Falagas, M.E., Vouloumanou, E.K., Togias, A.G., et al., 2010. Fosfomycin versus other antibiotics for the treatment of cystitis: a meta-analysis of randomized controlled trials. J. Antimicrob. Chemother. 65, 1862–1877.

Gopal Rao, G., Patel, M., 2009. Urinary tract infection in hospitalized elderly patients in the United Kingdom: the importance of making an accurate diagnosis in the post broad-spectrum antibiotic era. J. Antimicrob. Chemother. 63, 5–6.

Kahlmeter, G., 2003. An international survey of the antimicrobial susceptibility of pathogens from uncomplicated urinary tract infections: the ECO•SENS Project. J. Antimicrob. Chemother. 51, 59–76.

Kumarasamy, K.K., Toleman, M.A., Walsh, T.R., et al., 2010. Emergence of a new antibiotic resistance mechanism in India, Pakistan, and the UK: a molecular, biological, and epidemiological study. Lancet Infect. Dis. 10, 597–602.

Le Saux, N., Pham, B., Moher, D., 2000. Evaluating the benefits of antimicrobial prophylaxis to prevent urinary tract infections in children: a systematic review. Can. Med. Assoc. J. 163, 523–529.

Lichtenberger, P., Hooton, T.M., 2008. Complicated urinary tract infections. Curr. Infect. Dis. Rep. 10, 499–504.

Livermore, D.M., Hope, R., Mushtaq, S., et al., 2008. Orthodox and unorthodox clavulanate combinations against extended-spectrum β-lactamase-producers. Clin. Microbiol. Infect. 14 (Suppl. 1), 198–202.

Mangin, D., 2010. Urinary tract infection in primary care. Br. Med. J. 340, 373–374.

McMurdo, M.E.T., Argo, I., Phillips, G., et al., 2009. Cranberry or trimethoprim for the prevention of recurrent urinary tract infections? A randomized controlled trial in older women. J. Antimicrob. Chemother. 63, 389–395.

Mori, R., Fitzgerald, A., Williams, C., et al., 2009. Antibiotic prophylaxis for children at risk of developing a urinary tract infection: a systematic review. Acta Paediatr. 98, 1781–1786.

National Collaborating Centre for Women's and Children's Health, 2003. Antenatal Care: Routine Care for the Healthy Pregnant Woman. Royal College of Obstetricians and Gynaecologists Press, London, pp. 79–81.

National Institute for Health and Clinical Excellence, 2007. Urinary Tract Infection in Children: Diagnosis, Treatment and Long-Term Management. NICE, London. Available at http://www.nice.org.uk/nicemedia/pdf/CG54fullguideline.pdf. (1 October 2010, date last accessed).

Nicolle, L.E., Bradley, S., Colgan, R., et al., 2005. Infectious Diseases Society of America guidelines for the diagnosis and treatment of asymptomatic bacteriuria in adults. Clin. Infect. Dis. 40, 643–654.

Perrotta, C., Aznar, M., Mejia, R., et al., 2008. Oestrogens for preventing recurrent urinary tract infection in postmenopausal women. Cochrane Database of Systematic Reviews Issue 2 Art No. CD 005131 doi:10.1002/14651858.CD005131.pub2.

Richards, D., Toop, L., Chambers, S., et al., 2005. Response to antibiotics of women with symptoms of urinary tract infection but negative dipstick urine test results: double blind randomised controlled trial. Br. Med. J. 331, 143–146.

Scottish Intercollegiate Guidelines Network, 2006. Management of Suspected Bacterial Urinary Tract Infection in Adults. SIGN, Edinburgh. Available at http://www.sign.ac.uk/guidelines/fulltext/88/index.html. (1 October 2010, date last accessed).

Talan, D.A., Stamm, W.E., Hooton, T.M., 2000. Comparison of ciprofloxacin (7 days) and trimethoprim-sulfamethoxazole (14 days) for acute uncomplicated pyelonephritis in women: a randomized trial. J. Am. Med. Assoc. 283, 1583–1590.

Tumbarello, M., Sanguinetti, M., Montuori, E., et al., 2007. Predictors of mortality in patients with bloodstream infections caused by extended-spectrum β-lactamase-producing Enterobacteriaceae: importance of inadequate initial antimicrobial treatment. J. Antimicrob. Chemother. 51, 1987–1994.

Further reading

Anonymous, 2005. Cranberry and urinary tract infection. Drug Ther. Bull. 43, 17–19.

Hooton, T.M., 2010. Nosocomial urinary tract infections. In: Mandell, G.L., Bennett, J.E., Dolin, R. (Eds.), Principles and Practice of Infectious Diseases. Elsevier, London, pp. 3725–3737.

Pallett, A., Hand, K., 2010. Complicated urinary tract infections: practical solutions for the treatment of multiresistant Gram-negative bacteria. J. Antimicrob. Chemother. 65 (Suppl. 3), iii25–iii33.

Sobel, J.D., Kaye, D., 2010. Urinary tract infections. In: Mandell, G.L., Bennett, J.E., Dolin, R. (Eds.), Principles and Practice of Infectious Diseases. Elsevier, London, pp. 957–985.

Stamm, W.E., 2005. Urinary tract infections and pyelonephritis. In: Kasper,, D.L., Braunwald, E., Fauci, A.S., et al. (Eds.), Harrison's Principles of Internal Medicine. McGraw-Hill, New York, pp. 1715–1721.

Gastro-intestinal infections 37

J.W. Gray

Key points

- There are many different microbial causes of gastro-intestinal infections.
- Gastroenteritis is the most common syndrome of gastro-intestinal infection, but some gastro-intestinal pathogens can cause systemic infections.
- Fluid and electrolyte replacement is the mainstay of management of gastroenteritis.
- Most cases of gastroenteritis that occur in developed countries are mild and self-limiting, and do not require antibiotic therapy.
- Antibiotic therapy should be considered for patients with underlying conditions that predispose to serious or complicated gastroenteritis, or where termination of faecal excretion of pathogens is desirable to prevent further spread of the infection.
- *Clostridium difficile* is a very important cause of diarrhoea in hospitals. Strict control measures are required, and cases should be treated with oral metronidazole or vancomycin.
- Antibiotic therapy is also essential for life-threatening systemic infections, such as enteric fever.
- Where possible, antibiotic therapy should be delayed until a microbiological diagnosis has been established.
- The fluoroquinolones, for example, ciprofloxacin, are currently the most useful antibiotics for treating most bacterial gastro-intestinal infections, but resistance rates are increasing in many pathogens.
- Antibiotic resistance in gastro-intestinal pathogens is an escalating problem.

Gastro-intestinal infections represent a major public health and clinical problem worldwide. Many species of bacteria, viruses and protozoa cause gastro-intestinal infection, resulting in two main clinical syndromes. Gastroenteritis is a non-invasive infection of the small or large bowel that manifests clinically as diarrhoea and vomiting. Other infections are invasive, causing systemic illness, often with few gastro-intestinal symptoms. *Helicobacter pylori*, and its association with gastritis, peptic ulceration and gastric carcinoma, is discussed in Chapter 12.

Epidemiology and aetiology

In Western countries, the average person probably experiences one or two episodes of gastro-intestinal infection each year. Infections are rarely severe and the vast majority of cases never reach medical attention. Nevertheless, they are of considerable economic importance. In the UK, viruses such as rotaviruses, adenoviruses and noroviruses are probably the most common causes of gastroenteritis. *Campylobacter*, followed by non-typhoidal serovars of *Salmonella enterica*, are the most common reported causes of bacterial gastroenteritis. Cryptosporidiosis is the most commonly reported parasitic infection. In developing countries, the incidence of gastro-intestinal infection is at least twice as high and the range of common pathogens is much wider. Infections are more often severe and represent a major cause of mortality, especially in children.

Gastro-intestinal infections can be transmitted by consumption of contaminated food or water or by direct faecal–oral spread. Air-borne spread of viruses that cause gastroenteritis also occurs. The most important causes of gastro-intestinal infection, and their usual modes of spread, are shown in Table 37.1. In developed countries, the majority of gastro-intestinal infections are food borne. Farm animals are often colonised by gastro-intestinal pathogens, especially *Salmonella* and *Campylobacter*. Therefore, raw foods such as poultry, meat, eggs and unpasteurised dairy products are commonly contaminated and must be thoroughly cooked to kill such organisms. Raw foods also represent a potential source of cross-contamination of other foods, through hands, surfaces or utensils that have been inadequately cleaned. Food handlers who are excreting pathogens in their faeces can also contaminate food. This is most likely when diarrhoea is present, but continued excretion of pathogens during convalescence also represents a risk. Food handlers are the usual source of *Staphylococcus aureus* food poisoning, where toxin-producing strains of *S. aureus* carried in the nose or on skin are transferred to foods. Bacterial food poisoning is often associated with inadequate cooking and/or prolonged storage of food at ambient temperature before consumption. Water-borne gastro-intestinal infection is primarily a problem in countries without a sanitary water supply or sewerage system, although outbreaks of water-borne cryptosporidiosis occur from time to time in the UK. Spread of pathogens such as *Shigella* or enteropathogenic *Escherichia coli* by the faecal–oral route is favoured by overcrowding and poor standards of personal hygiene. Such infections in developed countries are most common in children and can cause troublesome outbreaks in paediatric wards, nurseries and residential children's homes.

Treatment with broad-spectrum antibiotics alters the bowel flora, creating conditions that favour superinfection with micro-organisms (principally *Clostridium difficile*) that can cause diarrhoea. *C. difficile* infection (CDI) may be associated

Table 37.1 Important causes of gastro-intestinal infection, their modes of spread and pathogenic mechanisms

Causative agent	Chief mode(s) of spread	Pathogenic mechanisms
Bacteria		
Campylobacter	Food, especially poultry, milk	Mucosal invasion Enterotoxin
Salmonella enterica, non-typhoidal serovars	Food, especially poultry, eggs, meat	Mucosal invasion Enterotoxin
Salmonella enterica serovars Typhi and Paratyphi	Food, water	Systemic invasion
Shigella	Faecal–oral	Mucosal invasion Enterotoxin
Escherichia coli		
Enteropathogenic	Faecal–oral	Mucosal adhesion
Enterotoxigenic	Faecal–oral, water	Enterotoxin
Enteroinvasive	Faecal–oral, food	Mucosal invasion
Verotoxin-producing	Food, especially beef	Verotoxin
Staphylococcus aureus	Food, especially meat, dairy produce	Emetic toxin
Clostridium perfringens	Food, especially meat	Enterotoxin
Bacillus cereus		
Short incubation period	Food, especially rice	Emetic toxin
Long incubation period	Food, especially meat and vegetable dishes	Enterotoxin
Vibrio cholerae O1, O139	Water	Enterotoxin
Vibrio parahaemolyticus	Seafoods	Mucosal invasion Enterotoxin
Clostridium difficile	Faecal–oral (nosocomial)	Cytotoxin Enterotoxin
Clostridium botulinum	Inadequately heat-treated canned/preserved foods	Neurotoxin
Protozoa		
Giardia lamblia	Water	Mucosal invasion
Cryptosporidium	Water, animal contact	Mucosal invasion
Entamoeba histolytica	Food, water	Mucosal invasion
Viruses	Food, faecal–oral, respiratory secretions	Small intestinal mucosal damage

with any antibiotic but clindamycin, the cephalosporins and the fluoroquinolones are most commonly implicated. CDI is most common in patients with serious underlying disease and in the elderly. Although some sporadic cases are probably due to overgrowth of endogenous organisms, person-to-person transmission also occurs in hospitals and care homes, sometimes resulting in large outbreaks.

Pathophysiology

Development of symptoms after ingestion of gastro-intestinal pathogens depends on two factors. First, sufficient organisms must be ingested and then survive host defence mechanisms,

and second, the pathogens must possess one or more virulence mechanisms to cause disease.

Host factors

Healthy individuals possess a number of defence mechanisms that protect against infection by enteropathogens. Therefore, large numbers of many pathogens must be ingested for infection to ensue; for example, the infective dose for *Salmonella* is typically around 10^5 organisms. Other species, however, are better able to survive host defence mechanisms; for example, infection with *Shigella* or verotoxin-producing *E. coli* (VTEC) can result from ingestion of fewer than 100 organisms. VTEC (principally *E. coli* O157) are especially important because of the risk of a life-threatening complication, haemolytic uraemic syndrome (HUS).

Gastric acidity

Most micro-organisms are rapidly killed at normal gastric pH. Patients whose gastric pH is less acidic, as for example, following treatment with antacids or ulcer-healing drugs, are more susceptible to gastro-intestinal infections. There is a particularly strong association between proton pump inhibitor use and CDI.

Intestinal motility

It is widely held that intestinal motility helps to rid the host of enteric pathogens, and that anti-motility agents are therefore potentially hazardous in patients with infective gastroenteritis. Despite this, self-medication with antidiarrhoeals is commonly practised, and in otherwise healthy individuals is probably safe.

Resident microflora

The resident microflora of the lower gastro-intestinal tract, largely composed of anaerobic bacteria, help to resist colonisation by enteropathogens.

Immune system

Phagocytic, humoral and cell-mediated elements are important in resistance to different pathogens. Individuals with inherited or acquired immunodeficiencies are therefore susceptible to specific gastro-intestinal infections, depending on which components of their immune system are affected.

Organism factors

The first requirement of gastro-intestinal pathogens is that they are able to adhere to the gut wall and colonise the intestine. The symptoms of gastro-intestinal infection can then be mediated by various mechanisms (see Table 37.1).

Toxins

Toxins produced by gastro-intestinal pathogens can be classified as enterotoxins, neurotoxins and cytotoxins. Enterotoxins act on intestinal mucosal cells to cause net loss of fluid and electrolytes. The classic enterotoxin-mediated disease is cholera, the result of infection with toxigenic serotypes of *Vibrio cholerae*. Many other bacteria produce enterotoxins, including enterotoxigenic *E. coli* and *Clostridium perfringens*. The emetic toxins of *S. aureus* and *Bacillus cereus* are neurotoxins that induce vomiting by an action on the central nervous system. The symptoms of botulism are mediated by a neurotoxin that blocks release of acetylcholine at nerve endings. Cytotoxins cause mucosal destruction and inflammation (see later). The pathogenicity of *C. difficile* is mediated by two exotoxins, TcdA and TcdB, both of which are potent cytotoxic

enzymes that damage the human colonic mucosa. Verotoxins are potent cytotoxins that cause direct damage to small-vessel endothelial cells, which is exacerbated by stimulation of production of inflammatory mediators by non-endothelial cells. This causes multiorgan microvascular injury, expressed most commonly as haemorrhagic colitis and HUS.

Mucosal damage

Cytotoxins are important in mediating mucosal invasion, but other mechanisms are also involved. Enteropathogenic *E. coli* causes diarrhoea by damaging microvilli when it adheres to the intestinal mucosa. Organisms such as *Shigella* and enteroinvasive *E. coli* express surface proteins that facilitate mucosal invasion. Diarrhoea due to mucosal damage may be due to reduction in the absorptive surface area or the presence of increased numbers of immature enterocytes which are secretory rather than absorptive.

Systemic invasion

The lipopolysaccharide outer membrane and possession of an antiphagocytic outer capsule are important virulence factors in invasive *Salmonella* infections.

Clinical manifestations

Many cases of gastro-intestinal infection are asymptomatic or cause subclinical illness. Gastroenteritis is the most common syndrome of gastro-intestinal infection, presenting with symptoms such as vomiting, diarrhoea and abdominal pain. The term 'dysentery' is sometimes applied to infections with *Shigella* (bacillary dysentery) and *Entamoeba histolytica* (amoebic dysentery), where severe colonic mucosal inflammation causes frequent diarrhoea with blood and pus. Table 37.2 shows the most important causative agents of gastroenteritis together with a brief description of the typical illness that each causes. However, the symptoms experienced by individuals infected with the same organism can differ considerably. This is important because it means that it is rarely possible to diagnose the cause of gastroenteritis on clinical grounds alone.

Gastro-intestinal manifestations of infection with VTEC range from non-bloody diarrhoea to haemorrhagic colitis. In addition, VTEC are the most important cause of HUS, a serious complication which is most common in young children and the elderly. HUS is defined by the triad of microangiopathic haemolytic anaemia, thrombocytopenia and acute renal dysfunction. The mortality is about 5% and up to half the survivors suffer long-term renal damage.

The clinical spectrum of CDI ranges from asymptomatic carriage to life-threatening pseudomembranous colitis (so-called because yellow-white plaques or membranes consisting of fibrin, mucus, leucocytes and necrotic epithelial cells are found adherent to the inflamed colonic mucosa).

Enteric fever, resulting from infection with *S. enterica* serovars Typhi and Paratyphi, presents with symptoms such as headache, malaise and abdominal distension after an incubation

Table 37.2 Characteristic clinical features of various causes of gastroenteritis

Causative agent	Incubation period	Symptoms (syndrome)
Campylobacter	2–5 days	Bloody diarrhoea Abdominal pain Systemic upset
Salmonella	6–72 h	Diarrhoea and vomiting Fever; may be associated bacteraemia
Shigella	1–4 days	Diarrhoea, fever (bacillary dysentery)
Escherichia coli Enteropathogenic Enterotoxigenic Enteroinvasive	 12–72 h 1–3 days 1–3 days	 Infantile diarrhoea Traveller's diarrhoea Similar to Shigella
Verotoxin-producing	1–3 days	Bloody diarrhoea (haemorrhagic colitis) Haemolytic uraemic syndrome
Staphylococcus aureus	4–8 h	Severe nausea and vomiting
Clostridium perfringens	6–24 h	Diarrhoea
Bacillus cereus Short incubation period Long incubation period	 1–6 h 6–18 h	 Vomiting Diarrhoea
Vibrio cholerae O1, O139	1–5 days	Profuse diarrhoea (cholera)
Vibrio parahaemolyticus	12–48 h	Diarrhoea, abdominal pain
Clostridium difficile	Usually occurs during/just after antibiotic therapy	Diarrhoea, abdominal pain, pseudomembranous enterocolitis
Giardia lamblia	1–2 weeks	Watery diarrhoea
Cryptosporidium	2 days–2 weeks	Watery diarrhoea
Entamoeba histolytica	2–4 weeks	Diarrhoea with blood and mucus (amoebic dysentery), liver abscess
Viruses	1–2 days	Vomiting, diarrhoea Systemic upset

period of 3–21 days. During the first week of the illness, the temperature gradually increases, but the pulse characteristically remains slow. Without treatment, during the second and third weeks, the symptoms become more pronounced. Diarrhoea develops in about half of cases. Examination usually reveals splenomegaly, and a few erythematous macules (rose spots) may be found, usually on the trunk. Serious gastro-intestinal complications such as haemorrhage and perforation are most common during the third week. Symptoms begin to subside slowly during the fourth week. In general, paratyphoid fever is less severe than typhoid fever.

Botulism typically presents with autonomic nervous system effects, including diplopia and dysphagia, followed by symmetrical descending motor paralysis. There is no sensory involvement.

Gastro-intestinal infections are often followed by a period of convalescent carriage of the pathogen. This usually lasts for no more than 4–6 weeks but can be for considerably longer, especially for *Salmonella*.

Investigations

Many cases of gastroenteritis outside hospital are mild and short lived, and microbiological investigation may not be necessary. However, investigations are always recommended where antibiotic therapy is being considered (Fig. 37.1), where there are public health concerns (e.g., if the sufferer works in the food industry) and for gastro-intestinal infections in hospitalised patients.

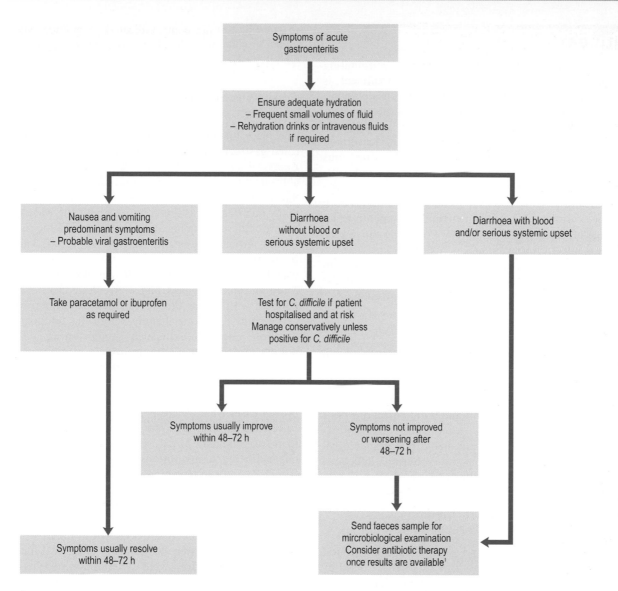

¹ Antibiotic therapy may have to be commenced empirically if patient has serious systemic upset

Fig. 37.1 Pathway for the investigation and management of patients with symptoms of acute gastroenteritis.

The mainstay of investigation of diarrhoeal illness is examination of faeces. Bacterial infections are usually diagnosed by stool culture. Various selective culture media designed to suppress growth of normal faecal organisms and/or enhance the growth of a particular pathogen are used. When sending specimens to the laboratory, it is important that details of the age of the patient, the clinical presentation and recent foreign travel are provided so that appropriate media for the likely pathogens can be selected. Several tests are available for rapid detection of *C. difficile* toxin, or of toxigenic *C. difficile*, in faeces: early and accurate diagnosis is crucial for the control of *C. difficile* in hospitals. Sigmoidoscopy is used to diagnose pseudomembranous colitis.

Various other procedures are sometimes useful in investigating patients with suspected bacterial gastroenteritis. Blood cultures should be taken from patients with severe systemic upset and are especially important when enteric fever is suspected. In enteric fever, the causative organism may also be cultured from urine or bone marrow. In *S. aureus* and *B. cereus* food poisoning, the pathogen can sometimes be isolated from vomitus. In cases of food poisoning, suspect foods may also be cultured. In general, serological investigations are of little value in the diagnosis of bacterial gastroenteritis. However, demonstration of serum antibodies to *E. coli* O157 can be helpful in confirming the cause of the HUS. Serological tests for typhoid and paratyphoid fever are available, but the results must be interpreted with caution. Botulism is diagnosed by demonstration of toxin in serum.

Parasitic infestations are usually detected by microscopic examination of faeces. Electron microscopy has been largely superseded by immunological and molecular-based detection techniques for detection of enteric viruses.

Treatment

Many gastro-intestinal infections are mild and self-limiting and never reach medical attention. Where treatment is required, there are three main therapeutic considerations. Fluid and electrolyte replacement is the cornerstone of treatment of diarrhoeal disease. Most patients can be managed with oral rehydration regimens, but severely dehydrated patients require rapid volume expansion with intravenous fluids. Symptomatic treatment with antiemetics and anti-motility (antidiarrhoeal) agents is sometimes used, especially as self-medication. Antimicrobial agents may be useful both in effecting symptomatic improvement and in eliminating faecal carriage of pathogens and therefore reducing the risk of transmitting infection to others.

Antiemetics and antidiarrhoeal drugs are discussed in Chapters 34 and 14, respectively. This chapter focuses on the place of antibiotic therapy in gastro-intestinal infections.

Antibiotic therapy

The requirement for antibiotic treatment in gastro-intestinal infection depends on the causative agent, the type and severity of symptoms and the presence of underlying disease. Antibiotics are ineffective in some forms of gastroenteritis, including bacterial intoxications and viral infections. For many other infections, such as salmonellosis and campylobacteriosis, effective agents are available, but antimicrobial therapy is often not clinically necessary. Serious infections such as enteric fever always require antibiotic therapy.

Conditions for which antibiotic therapy is not available or not usually required

The symptoms of *S. aureus* and short incubation period *B. cereus* food poisoning and botulism are usually caused by ingestion of preformed toxin, and therefore antibiotic therapy would not influence the illness. Pathogens such as *C. perfringens*, *Vibrio parahaemolyticus* and enteropathogenic *E. coli* usually cause a brief self-limiting illness that does not require specific treatment.

None of the presently available antiviral agents are useful in viral gastroenteritis. While most viral infections are self-limiting, chronic viral gastroenteritis can occur in immuno-compromised patients. Where possible, immunosuppression should be reduced. Immunoglobulin-containing preparations, administered orally or directly into the duodenum via a naso-gastric tube, have also been reported to be effective in managing chronic viral gastroenteritis in immunocompromised patients. As well as human serum immunoglobulin, antibodies from other species (e.g. immunised bovine colostrum) have been used. Immunotherapy of viral gastroenteritis remains experimental, and dosages and frequency of administration of immunoglobulin preparations cannot be recommended (Mohan and Haque, 2002).

At least one study has found that the risk of HUS in children with diarrhoea due to VTEC was much higher in those who received antibiotics. On that basis, it is advised in the UK that antibiotics are contraindicated in children with VTEC infection (National Collaborating Centre for Women's and Children's Health, 2009).

Conditions for which antimicrobial therapy may be considered

The place for antibiotics in the management of uncomplicated gastroenteritis due to bacteria such as *Salmonella* and *Campylobacter* is not clear cut. Certain antibiotics are reasonably effective in reducing the duration and severity of clinical illness and in eradicating the organisms from faeces. However, many microbiologists are cautious about the widespread use of antibiotics in diarrhoeal illness because of the risk of promoting antibiotic resistance (Sack et al., 1997). Another difficulty with respect to antibiotic prescribing is that it is not usually possible to determine the aetiological agent of diarrhoea on clinical grounds, and stool culture takes at least 48 h. Patients with severe illness, especially systemic symptoms, may require antibiotic therapy before the aetiological agent has been established. In such circumstances, a fluoroquinolone antibiotic such as ciprofloxacin would usually be the most appropriate empiric agent, at least in patients in whom CDI is considered unlikely or has been excluded. Otherwise, it is reasonable to limit antibiotic use to microbiologically proven cases where there is serious underlying disease and/or continuing severe symptoms. Antibiotics may also be used to try to eliminate faecal carriage, for example, in controlling outbreaks in institutions, or in food handlers who may be prevented from returning to work until they are no longer excreting gastro-intestinal pathogens.

Campylobacteriosis. Erythromycin is effective in terminating faecal excretion of *Campylobacter*. Some studies have shown that treatment commenced within the first 72–96 h of illness can also shorten the duration of clinical illness, especially in patients with severe dysenteric symptoms. The recommended dosage for adults is 250–500 mg four times a day orally for 5–7 days, and for children 30–50 mg/kg/day in four divided doses. Clarithromycin 250–500 mg (children under 1 year, 7.5 mg/kg; 1–2 years, twice a day; 3–6 years, 125 mg; 7–9 years, 5–7 days) or azithromycin 500 mg (children 10 mg/kg) once daily for 3 days are also effective. Ciprofloxacin, at a dose of 500 mg twice daily orally for adults, may also be effective in *Campylobacter* enteritis. However, whereas resistance rates to erythromycin have generally remained below 5%, resistance to ciprofloxacin has emerged, exceeding 10% in the UK and 50% in some countries (Dingle et al., 2005).

Salmonellosis. Most cases of *Salmonella* gastroenteritis are self-limiting and antibiotic therapy is unnecessary. However, antimicrobial therapy of salmonellosis is routinely recommended for infants aged under 6 months and immunocompromised patients, who are susceptible to complicated infections. Most antibiotics, even those with good *in vitro* activity, do not alter the course of uncomplicated *Salmonella* gastroenteritis. However, the fluoroquinolones, such as ciprofloxacin, can often shorten both the symptomatic period and the duration of faecal carriage. Ciprofloxacin resistance is now seen in up to 10% of non-typhoidal serovars of *S. enterica* in some countries but is still uncommon in the UK (Murray et al., 2005). The recommended dose of ciprofloxacin for adults is 500 mg twice daily orally for 1 week. Fluoroquinolones are not licensed for this indication in children, although there is increasing evidence that they can safely be given to children. The recommended dose of ciprofloxacin in childhood is 7.5 mg/kg twice daily orally. Trimethoprim at a dose of 25–100 mg twice daily orally may be used in children if it is preferred not to use a fluoroquinolone.

Ciprofloxacin given orally at a dose of 500–750 mg twice daily in adults (7.5–12.5 mg/kg twice daily in children) or 200 mg intravenously twice daily in adults (5–7.5 mg/kg twice daily in children) is recommended for invasive salmonellosis. Alternative agents include ampicillin or amoxicillin, trimethoprim or chloramphenicol (see under enteric fever). However, resistance to these agents is more common than resistance to ciprofloxacin, and they are not recommended as empiric therapy.

***E. coli* infections.** While most infections with enteropathogenic *E. coli* can be managed conservatively, small trials suggest that trimethoprim may be effective, especially in controlling nursery or hospital outbreaks. On the basis that enteroinvasive *E. coli* are closely related to *Shigella* and cause a similar clinical syndrome, similar therapy may be appropriate. Antibiotic therapy for traveller's diarrhoea caused by enterotoxigenic *E. coli* infection is often unnecessary, but troublesome symptoms will often respond to a single dose of ciprofloxacin or azithromycin, the need for further doses depending on clinical response. Alternatively, a 3–5 day course of trimethoprim may be given, although resistance is becoming increasingly common in some areas. Rifaximin is a new non-absorbable antibiotic that is available in a number of countries. It appears to be as effective as ciprofloxacin in treating *E. coli*-predominant traveller's diarrhoea but is ineffective in patients with inflammatory or invasive enteropathogens (Robins and Wellington, 2005). The dose for adults is 200 mg three times per day for 3 days.

Conditions for which antimicrobial therapy is usually indicated

Shigellosis. *Shigella sonnei*, which accounts for most cases of shigellosis in the UK and most other industrialised countries, usually causes a mild self-limiting illness. Even if not required on clinical grounds, antibiotic therapy for shigellosis is usually recommended in order to eliminate faecal carriage, and therefore prevent person-to-person transmission. In contrast to salmonellosis, a number of antibiotics may be effective in shortening the duration of illness and terminating faecal carriage. This is especially true of strains of *S. sonnei* that are endemic in industrialised countries, whereas in developing countries, *Shigella* species that are multiple antibiotic resistant are an increasing problem. The fluoroquinolones are highly effective in shigellosis and resistance is rare; therefore, they are often considered to be the treatment of choice, especially in adults and/or for treating imported infections. The dose of ciprofloxacin is 500 mg twice daily orally in adults (7.5 mg/kg twice daily in children). Amoxicillin is an alternative first-line

drug for *S. sonnei* infections acquired in the UK, where around 90% of isolates are susceptible. The dose of amoxicillin is 250 500 mg three times daily in adults, and 62.5–125 mg three times daily in children. Azithromycin (doses as for campylobacteriosis) is increasingly recommended as an alternative agent for shigellosis, especially in children (Jain et al., 2005). Third-generation cephalosporins such as ceftriaxone are another option for severe shigellosis. Trimethoprim resistance is now common, so this agent can no longer be recommended as empiric therapy. Antibiotic therapy is usually given for a maximum of 5 days.

Enteric fever. Treatment should be commenced as soon as a clinical diagnosis of enteric fever is made. Fluoroquinolones remain widely used as the first-choice treatment for typhoid and paratyphoid fevers. When treating isolates that are fully sensitive, the clinical response is at least as rapid as with the older treatments, there is a lower relapse rate, and convalescent faecal carriage is shortened. However, the proportion of isolates with reduced susceptibility to fluoroquinolones has increased to around 75%. Although most of these isolates have minimum inhibitory concentration (MIC) values below those regarded as fully resistant, treatment failures have been reported. Resistance to other antibiotics that have been commonly used to treat enteric fever, such as co-trimoxazole, chloramphenicol and ampicillin, is now frequent. These agents therefore cannot be recommended as alternatives to fluoroquinolones for empiric treatment of enteric fever, but may be useful in patients with bacterial isolates that are confirmed as sensitive. Doses of ciprofloxacin are as outlined for non-typhoidal salmonellosis. The usual dose of chloramphenicol is 50 mg/kg/day in four divided doses, and for ampicillin 100 mg/kg/day in four divided doses. Two weeks of antibiotic therapy is usually recommended, although shorter courses of ciprofloxacin (7–10 days) may be as effective.

Alternative agents that have been reported to be successful where treatment failure with fluoroquinolones has occurred include intravenous carbapenems or third-generation cephalosporins (e.g. ceftriaxone 75 mg/day; maximum dose 2.5 g/day) or oral azithromycin at a dose of 20 mg/kg/day (maximum 1000 mg) for at least 5 days. Time taken for clearance of bacteraemia may be longer with azithromycin, but the relapse rate appears to be lower than with β-lactam antibiotics such as ceftriaxone. There is some evidence that gatifloxacin, a new-generation fluoroquinolone, may be more effective than ciprofloxacin or ofloxacin in the treatment of infections where isolates have decreased fluoroquinolone susceptibility.

Chronic carriers of Salmonella. Patients may become chronic carriers after *Salmonella* infection, especially in the presence of underlying biliary tract disease. Oral ciprofloxacin 500–750 mg twice daily continued for 2–6 weeks is usually effective in eradicating carriage and has largely superseded the use of oral amoxicillin at a dose of 3 g twice daily.

Cholera. Fluid and electrolyte replacement is the key aspect of the management of cholera. However, antibiotics do shorten the duration of diarrhoea and therefore reduce the overall fluid loss, and also rapidly terminate faecal excretion of the organism. Effective agents include tetracyclines, erythromycin, trimethoprim, ampicillin or amoxicillin, chloramphenicol, ciprofloxacin and furazolidine. However, antibiotic resistance is being increasingly seen, and in particular, *V. cholerae* O139 is intrinsically resistant to furazolidine and trimethoprim. Choice of antibiotics is therefore governed by knowledge of local resistance patterns, which may vary between outbreaks. Tetracycline 250 mg four times daily, or doxycycline 100 mg once daily by mouth, is probably the most widely used therapy in adults. Ampicillin, amoxicillin or erythromycin are generally the preferred agents for children. Although clinical cure can be achieved after a single dose of antibiotics, treatment is usually given for 3–5 days to ensure eradication of *V. cholerae* from faeces.

C. difficile **infection.** The first objective is to diagnose CDI as soon as possible so that appropriate treatment and infection control measures can be put in place. Clinicians must consider the diagnosis in any patient where there is no clear alternative diagnosis for their diarrhoea. Stool samples must be sent to the laboratory immediately, and the laboratory must make testing available 7 days per week. Once the diagnosis is confirmed, attention must be paid to the patient's hydration and nutrition, non-essential antibiotic therapy or gastro-intestinal active drugs must be stopped and the patient's condition closely monitored. Although mild cases may resolve without specific therapy, treatment of all hospitalised patients with diarrhoea due to *C. difficile* is recommended, to shorten the duration of illness and to reduce environmental contamination and therefore the risk of nosocomial transmission.

Oral metronidazole 400 mg three times daily for 10 days is the treatment of choice for mild to moderate CDI. For severe CDI, oral vancomycin is recommended at a dose of 125 mg four times daily for 10 days. In patients unable to take oral medication, either drug can be administered via a nasogastric tube. Where there is no response to initial treatment, the dose of vancomycin can be increased to up to 500 mg four times daily, together with intravenous metronidazole 500 mg three times daily. Addition of oral rifampicin (300 mg twice daily) or administration of intravenous immunoglobulin (400 mg/kg) can also be considered.

Recurrence of symptoms occurs in about 20% of patients treated for CDI. Although some recurrences are due to germination of spores that have persisted in the colon since the original infection, it is recognised that some of these cases are due to reinfection, rather than relapse caused by the original strain (Loo et al., 2004). Most recurrences respond to a further 10–14 day course of metronidazole or vancomycin, but a few patients experience repeated recurrences. There is no reliable means of managing these patients. Options include:

- a supervised trial of anti-motility agents alone (if there are no abdominal symptoms or signs of severe CDI)
- tapering or pulse therapy with oral vancomycin given for 4–6 weeks
- a 2-week course of oral vancomycin 125 mg four times daily and oral rifampicin 300 mg twice daily
- intravenous immunoglobulin, especially if the patient's albumin status worsens
- donor stool transplant.

Trial data do not currently support the use of probiotics for the treatment or prevention of CDI (Department of Health and Health Protection Agency, 2009).

Cryptosporidiosis. Cryptosporidiosis in immunocompetent individuals is generally self-limiting. However, in immunosuppressed patients, severe diarrhoea can persist indefinitely and can even contribute to death. HIV-infected patients on highly active antiretroviral therapy (HAART) now have a much lower incidence of cryptosporidiosis due to immune reconstitution, and possibly a direct anti-cryptosporidium effect of protease inhibitors. There is no reliable antimicrobial therapy. Azithromycin, which is readily prescribable, is partially effective at a dose of 500 mg once daily (10 mg/kg once daily in children). Treatment should be continued until *Cryptosporidium* oocysts are no longer detectable in faeces (typically 2 weeks), to minimise the risk of relapse post-treatment. Occasionally, therapy has to be continued indefinitely to prevent relapse. Most other agents that have been recommended for treatment of cryptosporidiosis, for example, nitazoxanide, spiramycin, paromomycin and letrazuril, are not licensed in the UK. These can usually be sourced from special order manufacturing or importing companies (Smith and Corcoran, 2004). Of these agents, nitazoxanide has FDA approval in the USA, and has been shown to be effective in clinical trials at a dose of 500 mg twice daily (adults and children aged 12 years and over) for 3 days (children 1–3 years 100 mg bd; 4–11 years 200 mg bd). However, it is not effective unless the patient is able to mount an appropriate immune response.

Giardiasis. Metronidazole is the treatment of choice for giardiasis. Various oral regimens are effective, for example, 400 mg three times daily (7.5 mg/kg in children) for 5 days, or 2 g/day (children 500 mg to 1 g) for 3 days. Alternative treatments are tinidazole 2 g as a single dose, or mepacrine hydrochloride 100 mg (2 mg/kg in children) three times daily for 5–7 days. Nitazoxanide is a new thiazolide antiparasitic drug (discussed under cryptosporidiosis) that has also been licensed for treatment of giardiasis in some countries, but is not currently available in the UK. A single course of treatment for giardiasis has a failure rate of up to 10%. A further course of the same or another agent is often successful. Sometimes, repeated relapses are due to reinfection from an asymptomatic family member. In such cases, all affected family members should be treated simultaneously.

Amoebiasis. The aim of treatment in amoebiasis is to kill all vegetative amoebae and also to eradicate cysts from the bowel lumen. Metronidazole is highly active against vegetative amoebae and is commonly the treatment of choice for acute amoebic dysentery and amoebic liver abscess. The dose for adults is 800 mg (children 100–400 mg) three times daily for 5–10 days. To eradicate cysts, metronidazole therapy is followed by a 5-day course of diloxanide furoate 500 mg three times daily (20 mg/kg daily in three divided doses for children). Tinidazole has recently been shown to reduce clinical failure and be better tolerated than metronidazole (Gonzales et al., 2009). The dose of tinidazole for adults is 2 g daily for 2–3 days, and for children, 50–60 mg/kg daily for 3 days.

Asymptomatic excretors of cysts living in areas with a high prevalence of *E. histolytica* infection do not merit treatment because most individuals quickly become reinfected. However, asymptomatic excretors of cysts in Europe or North America are usually treated with diloxanide furoate for 5–10 days: metronidazole and tinidazole are relatively ineffective in this situation.

Patient care

People excreting gastro-intestinal pathogens are potentially infectious to others. Liquid stools are particularly likely to contaminate the hands and the environment. All cases of gastro-intestinal infection should be excluded from work or school at least until the patients are symptom free; hospitalised patients should be isolated in a single room. Patients should be advised on general hygiene, and in particular, on thorough handwashing and drying after visiting the toilet and before handling food.

In most countries, many gastro-intestinal infections are statutorily notifiable. Following notification, the authorities will judge whether the implications for public health merit investigation of the source of infection, contact screening or follow-up clearance stool samples from the original case.

Common therapeutic problems in the management of gastro-intestinal infection are summarised in Table 37.3. Problems associated with specific gastro-intestinal infections are summarised in Table 37.4.

Table 37.3 Practice points: general problems with treatment of gastro-intestinal infections

Problems	Resolution
Difficult or impossible to make a rapid aetiological diagnosis	Hospital laboratories are expected to offer rapid testing for *C. difficile* 7 days per week
New, more accurate, diagnostic tests for viral gastroenteritis are becoming more widely available	Few other recent improvements in the diagnosis of bacterial or parasitic infections
Clinical effectiveness and cost-effectiveness of antibiotic therapy for many bacterial gastro-intestinal infections are not clearly established	Without reliable data showing benefit, antimicrobial therapy is not used in the majority of infections
No specific therapies for viral gastroenteritis	Infections in otherwise healthy individuals are generally self-limiting Various non-evidence-based experimental treatments have been used to manage immunocompromised patients with protracted diarrhoea
Acute illness may be followed by a period of non-infective diarrhoea	Cautious use of antidiarrhoeal medication may be indicated at this stage

Table 37.4 Practice points: problems with treatment of specific gastro-intestinal infections

Infection	Antibiotic	Problems	Resolution
Campylobacteriosis	Erythromycin	Not always effective, especially if commenced >72 h after onset of symptoms	Reserve therapy for cases where symptoms are severe or worsening at time of diagnosis
	Ciprofloxacin[a]	Up to 50% of strains are resistant	Use only as a second-line agent for isolates that have been shown to be sensitive
Salmonellosis	Ciprofloxacin[a]	Not always effective Resistance is increasing	Reserve therapy for cases where symptoms are severe or worsening at time of diagnosis
Enteric fever	Ciprofloxacin[a]	Resistance is increasing	Alternative therapies must be guided by antibiotic sensitivities of the isolate
	Ampicillin or amoxicillin	Resistance to these agents now common	Ciprofloxacin[a] now generally regarded as treatment of choice
	Chloramphenicol	Higher incidence of chronic carriage and relapse than with ciprofloxacin	
Shigellosis	Trimethoprim	Resistance is increasing	Therapy should be guided by antibiotic sensitivities of the isolate. Most trimethoprim-resistant strains are ciprofloxacin sensitive

Continued

Table 37.4 Practice points: problems with treatment of specific gastro-intestinal infections—cont'd

Infection	Antibiotic	Problems	Resolution
Clostridium difficile	Metronidazole	Relapse rate up to 20%	Repeat course of treatment, or treatment with vancomycin
	Vancomycin	May be more effective, but much more expensive, than metronidazole Risk of promoting emergence and spread of vancomycin-resistant enterococci Relapse may occur	Generally reserved as a second-line agent, for example, where no response to metronidazole, or for patients with severe infection Repeat course of treatment; various treatment options for patients with repeated relapse
Cryptosporidiosis	Azithromycin	Not always effective Recommended only for patients who are immunocompromised or have unusually severe or protracted symptoms	Long-term therapy may be required to control symptoms Possible alternative agents are not licensed in UK

aCiprofloxacin is not licensed for general paediatric use; it is widely used to treat gastro-intestinal infections in children.

Case studies

Case 37.1

A 12-year-old boy is admitted to hospital with a history of fever, weight loss and malaise 1 week after returning from visiting relatives in Pakistan. Whilst there he was diagnosed as having typhoid fever, and although details are sketchy, it seems that he received treatment with ciprofloxacin. The only other medical history of note is that he experienced an anaphylactic reaction after taking penicillin 4 years ago. Twenty-four hours after admission, *S. enterica* serovar Typhi is isolated from a blood culture.

Questions

1. Why might the patient not have responded fully to the treatment given in Pakistan?
2. Which antibiotic would now be most appropriate as empiric therapy?

Answers

1. Strains of *S. enterica* serovar Typhi that have reduced susceptibility to fluoroquinolones are common in the Indian subcontinent. Although these strains are not usually fully fluoroquinolone resistant, treatment failures have been reported, even when an appropriate dose regimen has been used: in this case, there is not even any assurance that the treatment regimen in Pakistan was adequate.
2. Given the lack of assurance of the adequacy of the ciprofloxacin treatment in Pakistan, one option would be to re-treat with ciprofloxacin. However, given the high likelihood that the strain will have reduced susceptibility to ciprofloxacin, it would be more logical to use an alternative agent. Of those, carbapenems and cephalosporins are beta-lactam antibiotics that would be best avoided, given

the history of anaphylaxis following penicillin exposure. Azithromycin would appear, therefore, to be the empiric treatment of choice in this case.

Case 37.2

A mother brings her 6-year-old daughter to her primary care doctor because she has a 2-day history of bloody diarrhoea and abdominal pain. The family had been on a farm visit the previous weekend and had eaten food when there. The mother is anxious for her child to be treated with antibiotics because they will be going on their summer holiday in one week.

Questions

1. Give three possible infective causes of the girl's symptoms.
2. How should the clinician respond to the mother's request for antibiotics?

Answers

1. The two commonest bacterial gastro-intestinal infections, campylobacteriosis and salmonellosis, can both present in this way. Many other bacterial and protozoan causes of gastroenteritis can also cause similar symptoms. One bacterium that is especially important to consider in this case, where there is a history of a farm visit, is *E. coli* O157. Every effort should be made to obtain a stool sample from the patient for microbiological examination.
2. It would not be appropriate to treat this girl's symptoms empirically with antibiotics for a number of reasons. First, antibiotic therapy may make no difference to the speed of clinical resolution; second, where antibiotics are justified, the choice of drug will depend on the aetiological agent; and third, antibiotics are contraindicated in infection with *E. coli* O157, which must feature in the differential diagnosis in this case.

Case 37.3

A businessman is planning a short trip to Egypt. During previous visits to the area, he has experienced troublesome diarrhoea despite being careful about hygiene. Although the diarrhoea has not made him seriously unwell, it has caused him considerable inconvenience during business discussions.

Question

Are there any antimicrobials that he could take to prevent this problem?

Answer

Although traveller's diarrhoea is not usually serious, it can cause considerable inconvenience whether the sufferer is travelling for leisure or business reasons. Simple measures that can help prevent traveller's diarrhoea include taking care with food and drinks (only bottled water from reputable sources should be used). There are two approaches to antibiotic use in traveller's diarrhoea. Either the drug can be taken prophylactically to try to prevent diarrhoea developing, or treatment can be commenced with the onset of diarrhoea. The latter approach is generally preferred because it limits unnecessary exposure to antibiotics and the response to treatment is usually rapid. However, there are instances such as in this case where the inconvenience of even short-lived diarrhoea may be great enough to justify use of prophylaxis.

The choice of antibiotics for traveller's diarrhoea has been made more complicated by the increasing prevalence of antibiotic resistance in many developing countries. Drugs such as amoxicillin or trimethoprim no longer have a role. A fluoroquinolone, such as ciprofloxacin, still represents a reasonable first choice, with azithromycin as a possible alternative in areas where fluoroquinolone resistance is known to be common. For travellers from countries where it can be prescribed, rifaximin may be the agent of choice. For travellers to areas where infections such as amoebic dysentery or giardiasis are common, it may be appropriate to take a supply of metronidazole that can be started if there is no response to the first-line antibacterial prophylaxis.

Case 37.4

An 80-year-old woman on an elderly care ward develops watery diarrhoea and abdominal pain 4 days after commencing therapy with ciprofloxacin for a urinary tract infection. *C. difficile* toxin is detected in a stool sample. Five patients on that ward have also had *C. difficile*-associated diarrhoea during the past 2 months.

Questions

1. How should this patient be managed?
2. What measures might be taken to try to reduce the number of cases of *C. difficile*-associated diarrhoea on the ward?

Answers

1. Treatment with ciprofloxacin should be discontinued. Four-day antibiotic therapy for a urinary tract infection will often suffice, but if further treatment is required, an antibiotic that is less likely to disturb the bowel flora should be prescribed. Metronidazole is the preferred first-line treatment for mild to moderate CDI. The patient should be closely monitored for the frequency and severity of the diarrhoea. Oral vancomycin might be indicated later if her illness became more severe. The patient should be isolated to reduce the risk of spread of the infection.
2. There are two elements to control of *C. difficile* in hospitals. First, it is necessary to ensure that antibiotic prescribing is rational. There should be an antibiotic-prescribing policy that minimises use of antibiotics in general, and in particular, restricts use of antibiotics that are associated with a high risk of *C. difficile* (2nd- and 3rd-generation cephalosporins, clindamycin and fluoroquinolones). Compliance with the policy must be assured through measures such as checking of prescriptions, multidisciplinary antibiotic ward rounds, education of prescribers, and audits of antibiotic prescribing. Second, strict infection control precautions must be enforced, along with improved standards of environmental cleanliness, to reduce the risk of patients being exposed to the bacterium.

References

Dingle, K.E., Clarke, L., Bowler, I.C., 2005. Ciprofloxacin resistance among human *Campylobacter* isolates 1991–2004: an update. J. Antimicrob. Chemother. 55, 395–396.

Department of Health and Health Protection Agency, 2009. Clostridium Difficile Infection: How to Deal with the Problem. Department of Health, London.

Gonzales, M.L.M., Dans, L.F., Martinez, E.G., 2009. Antiamoebic drugs for treating amoebic colitis. Cochrane Database of Systematic Reviews. Issue 2 Art No. CD006085. doi:10.1002/14651858.CD006085.

Jain, S.K., Gupta, A., Glanz, B., et al., 2005. Antimicrobial-resistant *Shigella sonnei*: limited antimicrobial treatment options for children and challenges of interpreting in vitro azithromycin susceptibility. Pediatr. Infect. Dis. J. 24, 494–497.

Loo, V.G., Libman, M.D., Miller, M.A., et al., 2004. *Clostridium difficile*: a formidable foe. Can. Med. Assoc. J. 171, 47–48.

Mohan, P., Haque, K., 2002. Oral immunoglobulin for the prevention of rotavirus infection in low birth weight infants. Cochrane

Database of Systematic Reviews. Issue 3. Art. No.: CD003740. doi:10.1002/14651858.CD003740.

Murray, A., Coia, J.E., Mather, H., et al., 2005. Ciprofloxacin resistance in non-typhoidal *Salmonella* serotypes in Scotland, 1993–2003. J. Antimicrob. Chemother. 56, 110–1104.

National Collaborating Centre for Women's and Children's Health, 2009. Diarrhoea and Vomiting Caused by Gastroenteritis: Diagnosis, Assessment and Management in Children Younger Than 5 Years. RCOG Press, London.

Robins, G.W., Wellington, K., 2005. Rifaximin: a review of its use in the management of traveller's diarrhea. Drugs 65, 1697–1713.

Sack, R.B., Rahman, M., Yunus, M., et al., 1997. Antimicrobial resistance in organisms causing diarrheal disease. Clin. Infect. Dis. 24 (Suppl. 1), S102–S105.

Smith, H.V., Corcoran, G.D., 2004. New drugs and treatment for cryptosporidiosis. Curr. Opin. Infect. Dis. 17, 557–564.

Further reading

Bhan, M.K., Bahl, R., Bhatnagar, S., 2005. Typhoid and paratyphoid fever. Lancet 366, 749–762.

DuPont, H.L., 2005. What's new in enteric infectious diseases at home and abroad. Curr. Opin. Infect. Dis. 18, 407–412.

Loeb, M., Smaill, F., Smieja, M. (Eds.), 2009. Evidence-Based Infectious Diseases. Wiley-Blackwell, Oxford.

Starr, J., 2005. *Clostridium difficile* associated diarrhoea: diagnosis and treatment. Br. Med. J. 331, 498–501.

Townes, J.M., 2004. Acute infectious gastroenteritis in adults. Seven steps to management and prevention. Postgrad. Med. 115, 11–19.

Yoshikawa, T.T., Norman, D.C. (Eds.), 2009. Diseases in the Ageing. A Clinical Handbook. Springer, New York.

38 Infective meningitis

J. W. Gray

The brain and spinal cord are surrounded by three membranes, which from the outside inwards are the dura mater, the arachnoid mater and the pia mater. Between the arachnoid mater and the pia mater, in the subarachnoid space, is found the cerebrospinal fluid (CSF) (Fig. 38.1). This fluid, of which there is ~150 mL^{-1} in a normal individual, is secreted by the choroid plexuses and vascular structures which are in the third, fourth and lateral ventricles. CSF passes from the ventricles via communicating apertures to the subarachnoid space, after which it flows over the surface of the brain and the spinal cord (see Fig. 38.1). The amount of CSF is controlled by resorption into the bloodstream by vascular structures in the subarachnoid space, called the arachnoid villi. Infective meningitis is an inflammation of the arachnoid and pia mater

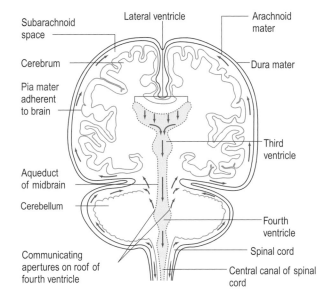

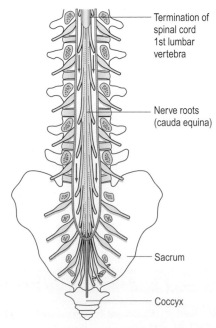

Fig. 38.1 The meninges covering the brain and spinal cord and the flow of cerebrospinal fluid (arrowed) (modified from Ross and Wilson (1981), by permission of Churchill Livingstone).

associated with the presence of bacteria, viruses, fungi or protozoa in the CSF. Meningitis is one of the most emotive of infectious diseases, and for good reason: even today, infective meningitis is associated with significant mortality and risk of serious sequelae in survivors.

Aetiology and epidemiology

In the UK, around 1500 cases of meningitis are notified annually. However, this almost certainly under represents the true incidence of meningitis. Viruses are the most common cause of meningitis, and are often less serious than bacterial or fungal forms of the disease.

Bacterial meningitis

Although bacterial meningitis occurs in all age groups, it is predominantly a disease of young children, with 40–50% of all cases occurring in the first 4 years of life. Two bacteria, *N. meningitidis* and *S. pneumoniae*, account for about 75% of cases. However, the pattern of micro-organisms causing meningitis is related to the age of the patient and the presence of underlying disease.

N. meningitidis is the most common cause of bacterial meningitis from infancy through to middle age, with peaks of incidence in the under-5-year age group and in adolescents. There are several serogroups of *N. meningitidis*, including A, B, C, W135 and Y. In the late twentieth century, serogroups B and C accounted for 60–65% and 35–40% of infections in the UK, respectively. However, with the introduction of vaccination against *N. meningitidis* serogroup C (MenC) into the routine immunisation programme in 1999, serogroup B now accounts for well over 80% of all meningococcal disease. There is currently no vaccine available for *N. meningitidis* serogroup B. Serogroups A and W135 predominate in Africa and the Middle East. A quadrivalent vaccine against serogroups A, C, W135 and Y is available to protect travellers to countries of risk. *S. pneumoniae* is the most common cause of meningitis in adults aged over 45 years, but almost half of all cases of pneumococcal meningitis occur in children aged under 5 years. It has a poorer outcome than meningococcal meningitis. Vaccination against the most common serotypes of *S. pneumoniae* using a conjugate vaccine was added to the routine childhood immunisation programme in the UK in 2006: the original 7-valent vaccine was then replaced by a 13-valent vaccine in Spring 2010. A different 23-valent polysaccharide vaccine is available for certain patient groups at risk of pneumococcal infection.

Haemophilus influenzae type b (Hib) was once the major cause of bacterial meningitis in children aged 3 months to 5 years, but introduction of routine immunisation in 1992 has almost eliminated Hib disease in the UK and other developed countries.

Although patients with meningococcal or Hib meningitis are potentially infectious, most cases of meningitis due to these bacteria are acquired from individuals who are asymptomatic nasopharyngeal carriers. People living in the same household

as a patient with meningococcal disease have a 500–1200-fold increased risk of developing infection if they do not receive chemoprophylaxis (see later). Susceptible young children who are household contacts of a case of Hib disease have a similarly increased risk of becoming infected. Epidemics of meningococcal disease sometimes occur. In developed countries, these take the form of clusters of cases among people living in close proximity (e.g. in schools or army camps) or in a particular geographical area. In Africa, large epidemics with many thousands of cases occur, usually during the dry season.

In the neonatal period, group B streptococci are the most common cause of bacterial meningitis. Other causes of neonatal meningitis include *Escherichia coli* and other *Enterobacteriaceae, Listeria monocytogenes, Staphylococcus aureus* and enterococci. In most cases, infection is acquired from the maternal genital tract around the time of delivery, but transmission between patients can also occur in hospitals.

L. monocytogenes is also an occasional cause of meningitis in immunocompromised patients. Meningitis can also occur as a complication of neurosurgery, especially in patients who have ventriculoatrial or ventriculoperitoneal shunts. Coagulase-negative staphylococci are the major causes of shunt-associated meningitis, but other bacteria are important, including *Enterobacteriaceae* and *S. aureus*. Meningitis due to *S. aureus* may also be secondary to trauma, or local or haematogenous spread from another infective focus. Meningitis may also be a feature of multisystem bacterial diseases such as syphilis, leptospirosis and Lyme disease.

The decline in the incidence of tuberculous meningitis in developed countries has mirrored the fall in the incidence of tuberculosis in these countries. Tuberculous meningitis may occur as part of the primary infection or as a result of recrudescence of a previous infection.

Viral meningitis

Human enteroviruses such as echoviruses and Coxsackie viruses account for about 70% of cases of viral meningitis in the UK. Herpes simplex and varicella zoster viruses account for most other cases. Occasional causes of viral meningitis include mumps virus and human immunodeficiency viruses.

Fungal meningitis

In Europe, fungal meningitis is rare in individuals without underlying disease. *Candida* species are an occasional cause of shunt-associated meningitis. *Cryptococcus neoformans* has emerged as an important cause of meningitis in patients with late-stage HIV infection and other severe defects of T-cell function. With greater use of fluconazole for oral candidiasis, and especially the advent of highly active antiretroviral therapy, cryptococcosis has become much less common in developed countries. However, in sub-Saharan African countries with the highest HIV prevalence, cryptococcus is the leading cause of infective meningitis. In certain other areas of the world, infections with fungi such as *Coccidioides immitis* and *Histoplasma capsulatum* are endemic.

Pathophysiology

Most cases of bacterial meningitis are preceded by nasopharyngeal colonisation by the causative organism. In most colonised individuals, infection will progress no further, but in susceptible individuals the organism invades the submucosa by circumventing host defences (e.g. physical barriers, local immunity, phagocytes) and gains access to the CNS by invasion of the bloodstream and subsequent haematogenous seeding of the CNS. Other less common routes by which micro-organisms can reach the meninges include:

- direct spread from the nasopharynx
- blood-borne spread from other foci of colonisation or infection
- abnormal communications with the skin or mucous membranes, for example skull fractures, anatomical defects or a meningocoele
- spread from an infected adjacent focus, for example brain abscess, tuberculoma, infected paranasal air sinus or infection of the middle ear.

Once in the subarachnoid space, the infection spreads widely and incites a cascade of meningeal inflammation. The cerebral tissue is not usually directly involved although cerebral abscess may complicate some types of meningitis.

The micro-organisms that most frequently cause meningitis are capable of doing so because they have a variety of virulence factors, including mechanisms for:

- attachment to host mucosal surfaces
- evasion of phagocytosis and other host defences
- meningeal invasion
- disruption of the blood–brain barrier
- induction of pathophysiological changes in the CSF space
- secondary brain damage.

Overall, the net result of infection is vascular endothelial injury and increased blood–brain barrier permeability leading to the entry of many blood components into the subarachnoid space. This contributes to cerebral oedema and elevated CSF protein levels. In response to the cytokine response, neutrophils migrate from the bloodstream into the CSF. Cerebral oedema contributes to intracranial hypertension and a consequent decrease in cerebral blood flow. Anaerobic metabolism ensues, which contributes to increased lactate and decreases glucose concentrations. If this uncontrolled process is not modulated by effective treatment, transient neuronal dysfunction or permanent neuronal injury results.

Clinical manifestations

Acute bacterial meningitis usually presents with sudden-onset headache, neck stiffness, photophobia, fever and vomiting. On examination, Kernig's sign may be positive. This is resistance to extension of the leg when the hip is flexed, due to meningeal irritation in the lumbar area. Where meningitis is complicated by septicaemia, there may be septic shock. The presence of a haemorrhagic skin rash is highly suggestive, but not pathognomic, of meningococcal infection. Untreated patients with bacterial meningitis deteriorate rapidly, with development of seizures, focal cerebral signs and cranial nerve palsies. Finally, obtundation and loss of consciousness herald death.

In infants with meningitis, the early physical signs are usually non-specific and include fever, diarrhoea, lethargy, feeding difficulties and respiratory distress. Focal signs such as seizures or a bulging fontanelle usually only occur at a late stage.

Viral meningitis usually presents with acute onset of low-grade fever, headache, photophobia and neck stiffness. Unless they develop encephalitis, patients usually remain alert and oriented.

Although tuberculous and fungal meningitis sometimes present acutely, these infections typically have a more indolent course. The early stages of the diseases are dominated by general symptoms such as malaise, apathy and anorexia. As they progress, symptoms and signs more typical of meningitis usually appear.

Diagnosis

The definitive diagnosis of meningitis is established by detection of the causative organism and/or demonstration of biochemical changes and a cellular response in CSF. CSF is obtained by lumbar puncture, where a needle is inserted between the posterior space of the third and fourth lumbar vertebrae into the subarachnoid space. Before performing lumbar puncture, the possibility of precipitating or aggravating existing brain herniation in patients with intracranial hypertension must be considered. A CT scan should be performed before undertaking lumbar puncture if any neurological abnormalities are present.

In health, the CSF is a clear colourless fluid which, in the lumbar region of the spinal cord, is at a pressure of $50–150\,mmH_2O$. There may be up to 5 cells/μL, the protein concentration is up to 0.4 g/L and the glucose concentration is at least 60% of the blood glucose (usually 2.2–4.4 mmol/L). Table 38.1 shows how the cell count and biochemical measurements can be helpful in determining the type of organism causing meningitis.

In bacterial and fungal meningitis, organisms may be visible in Gram-stained smears of the CSF. The common causes of bacterial meningitis are easily distinguished from each other by their Gram stain appearance. Special stains, such as the Ziehl–Neelsen method, are necessary to visualise mycobacteria. However, only small numbers of mycobacteria are present in the CSF in tuberculous meningitis and direct microscopy is often unrevealing. Although cryptococci can be visualised by Gram staining, they are often more easily seen with India ink staining, which highlights their prominent capsules.

Regardless of the microscopic findings, CSF should be cultured to try to confirm the identity of the causative organism and to facilitate further investigations such as antibiotic sensitivity testing and typing. Special cultural techniques are required for mycobacteria, fungi and viruses. Cultures of other

Table 38.1 Cellular and biochemical responses in different forms of infective meningitis

Type of meningitis	Cell count	Protein (g/L)	Glucose
Bacterial	Predominantly polymorphs, 500–2000 µL^{-1} (lymphocytes may predominate in early or partially treated cases)	1–3	<50% blood glucose
Tuberculous	Predominantly lymphocytes, 100–600 µL^{-1}	1–6	<50% blood glucose
Viral	Predominantly lymphocytes, 50–500 µL^{-1}	0.5–1	Usually normal
Cryptococcal	Predominantly lymphocytes, 50–1000 µL^{-1}	1–3	<50% blood glucose

sites are sometimes helpful. In suspected bacterial meningitis, blood for culture should always be obtained. Bacteraemia occurs in only 10% of patients with meningococcal meningitis but is more common in most other forms of meningitis. In suspected meningococcal disease, culture of a nasopharyngeal swab may be helpful because antibiotic penetration at this site is less. It increases the chances of isolating meningococci when antibiotics were administered to the patient before presentation to hospital.

Non-culture-based methods are increasingly used to investigate the aetiology of meningitis. In particular, molecular amplification techniques such as polymerase chain reaction (PCR) are now widely used to detect meningococci, pneumococci, *Mycobacterium tuberculosis* and various viruses, including herpes simplex viruses and enteroviruses.

Serum antibodies to *N. meningitidis* and various viruses may be detected, but these investigations usually depend on demonstration of seroconversion between two samples collected a week or more apart, and are therefore undertaken more for public health than clinical reasons. Patients with tuberculous meningitis may have a positive Mantoux test or an interferon-gamma release assay.

Drug treatment

Acute bacterial meningitis is a medical emergency that requires urgent administration of antibiotics. Other considerations in some forms of meningitis include the use of adjunctive therapy such as steroids, and the administration of antibiotics to prevent secondary cases.

Antimicrobial therapy

Pharmacokinetic considerations

The antimicrobial therapy of meningitis requires attainment of adequate levels of bactericidal agents within the CSF. The principal route of entry of antibiotics into CSF is by the choroid plexus; an alternative route is via the capillaries of the central nervous system into the extracellular fluid and hence into the ventricles and subarachnoid space (see Fig. 38.1). The passage of antibiotics into CSF is dependent on the degree of meningeal inflammation and integrity of the blood–brain barrier created by capillary endothelial cells, as well as the following properties of the antibiotic:

- lipid solubility (the choroidal epithelium is highly impermeable to lipid-insoluble molecules)
- ionic dissociation at blood pH
- protein binding
- molecular size
- concentration of the drug in the serum.

Antimicrobials fall into three categories according to their ability to penetrate the CSF:

- those that penetrate even when the meninges are not inflamed, for example chloramphenicol, metronidazole, isoniazid and pyrazinamide
- those that generally penetrate only when the meninges are inflamed, and used in high doses, for example most β-lactam antibiotics, the quinolones and rifampicin
- those that penetrate poorly under all circumstances, including the aminoglycosides, vancomycin and erythromycin.

Recommended regimens

Clinical urgency determines that empirical antimicrobial therapy will usually have to be prescribed before the identity of the causative organism or its antibiotic sensitivities are known. Consideration of the epidemiological features of the case, together with microscopic examination of the CSF, is often helpful in identifying the likely pathogen. However, empiric therapy is usually with broad-spectrum antimicrobial therapy to cover all likely pathogens, at least until definitive microbiological information is available. For the purpose of selecting empiric antimicrobial therapy, patients with acute bacterial meningitis can be categorised into four broad groups: neonates and infants aged below 3 months; immunocompetent older infants, children and adults; immunocompromised patients; and those with ventricular shunts.

Antibiotics for meningitis in neonates and infants aged below 3 months. The most important pathogens in neonates include group B streptococci, *E. coli* and other *Enterobacteriaceae*, *L. monocytogenes*. In many centres, a third-generation cephalosporin such as cefotaxime or ceftazidime, along with amoxicillin or ampicillin, is the empiric therapy of choice for neonatal meningitis (Galiza and Heath, 2009). Cephalosporins penetrate into CSF better than aminoglycosides, and their use in Gram-negative bacillary meningitis has contributed to a reduction in mortality to less than 10%. Other centres continue to use an aminoglycoside, such as gentamicin, together with benzylpenicillin, ampicillin or amoxicillin as empiric therapy. This approach remains appropriate, especially in countries such as the UK where group B streptococci are by far the predominant cause of early-onset neonatal meningitis. Whichever empiric regimen is used, therapy can be altered as appropriate once the pathogen has been identified. Suitable dosages are shown in Table 38.2.

In infants outside the immediate neonatal period, the classic neonatal pathogens account for a decreasing number of cases of meningitis and the common bacteria of meningitis in childhood (see later) become increasingly important. Amoxicillin or ampicillin plus cefotaxime or ceftriaxone is the recommended treatment. Therapy with amoxicillin or ampicillin and gentamicin is unsuitable for this age group because it provides inadequate cover against *H. influenzae*.

Antibiotics for meningitis in older infants, children and adults. Antimicrobial therapy has to cover *S. pneumoniae*, *N. meningitidis* and, in children aged below 5 years, *H. influenzae* (Yogev and Guzman-Cottrill, 2005). Achievable antibiotic CSF concentrations are compared with the susceptibilities of the common agents of meningitis in Table 38.3.

Third-generation cephalosporins, such as cefotaxime, are now widely used in place of the traditional agents of choice, chloramphenicol, ampicillin, amoxicillin and penicillin (see Table 38.2). This change has stemmed from concern over the rare but potentially serious adverse effects of chloramphenicol and the emergence of resistance to penicillin, ampicillin and chloramphenicol among *S. pneumoniae* and *H. influenzae* in particular. Chloramphenicol resistance and reduced susceptibility to penicillin have also been reported in *N. meningitidis*. The third-generation cephalosporins have a broad spectrum of activity that encompasses not only the three classic causes of bacterial meningitis but also many other bacteria that are infrequent causes of meningitis. However, cephalosporins are inactive against *L. monocytogenes*, and amoxicillin or ampicillin should be added where it is possible that the patient may have listeriosis, for example in elderly patients, or where Gram-positive bacilli are seen on Gram stain. Although earlier-generation cephalosporins such as cefuroxime achieve reasonable CSF penetration and are active against the agents of meningitis *in vitro*, they do not effectively sterilise the CSF and should not be used to treat meningitis.

Ceftriaxone is a third-generation cephalosporin with a spectrum of activity comparable to that of cefotaxime. However, because of the potential for calcium chelation *in vivo*, ceftriaxone must not be administered within 48 h of the completion

Table 38.2 Suitable antibiotic regimens for treatment of acute bacterial meningitis in different age groups

Age group	First-choice antibiotic therapy	Alternative therapies
Neonates, aged <8 days	Ampicillin, 50 mg/kg twice daily or amoxicillin 25 mg/kg twice daily and cefotaxime 50 mg/kg twice daily or ceftazidime 50 mg/kg twice daily	Benzylpenicillin 50 mg twice daily and ampicillin 50 mg/kg twice daily or amoxicillin 25 mg/kg twice daily and gentamicin 2.5 mg/kg twice daily
Neonates, aged 8–28 days	Ampicillin 50 mg/kg four times daily or amoxicillin 25 mg/kg three times daily and cefotaxime 50 mg/kg three times daily or ceftazidime 50 mg/kg three times daily	Benzylpencillin 50 mg three or four times daily or ampicillin 50 mg/kg three or four times daily or amoxicillin 25 mg/kg three times daily and gentamicin 2.5 mg/kg three times daily
Infants, aged 1–3 months	Ampicillin 50 mg/kg four times daily or amoxicillin 25 mg/kg three times daily and cefotaxime 50 mg/kg three times daily or ceftriaxone 75–100 mg/kg once daily	
Infants and children aged >3 months[a]	Cefotaxime 50 mg/kg three times daily or ceftriaxone[b] 75–100 mg/kg once daily	Ampicillin 50 mg/kg four times daily or amoxicillin 25 mg/kg three times daily or benzylpenicillin[c] 30 mg/kg 4-hourly and chloramphenicol[d] 12.5–25 mg/kg four times daily
Adults	Cefotaxime[e] 2 g three times daily or ceftriaxone[b,e] 2–4 g once daily	Benzylpenicillin 2.4 g 4-hourly or ampicillin 2–3 g four times daily or amoxicillin 2 g three or four times daily and chloramphenicol[d] 12.5–25 mg/kg four times daily

[a]Calculated doses for children should not exceed maximum recommended doses for adults.
[b]Ceftriaxone should not be administered to neonates within 48 h of completion of infusions of calcium-containing solutions; caution should be exercised in older age groups.
[c]Benzylpenicillin is inactive against *H. influenzae* and should therefore not be used in children aged <5 years.
[d]Monitoring of serum chloramphenicol levels is recommended, especially in children aged ≤4 years.
[e]Add ampicillin or amoxicillin to cover *L. monocytogenes* in elderly patients or where Gram-positive bacilli seen in CSF.

Table 38.3 Achievable CSF concentrations of antibiotics in meningitis and MIC values for common central nervous system pathogens

Antibiotic	CSF:serum ratio	Peak CSF level (mg/L)	MIC$_{90}$ (mg/L) values for		
			N. meningitidis	*H. influenzae*	*S. pneumoniae*
Ampicillin	1:10	10	0.02	0.25	0.05
Benzylpenicillin	1:20	1.5	0.02	1.0	0.02
Cefotaxime	1:20	10	0.01	0.06	0.25
Ceftriaxone	1:15	15	0.01	0.06	0.12
Chloramphenicol	1:2	15	1.0	1.0	2.5
Ciprofloxacin	1:5	0.6	0.004	0.015	1.0
Daptomycin	1:20	3.0	>4.0	>4.0	0.25
Gentamicin	1:40	<0.5	2.0	0.5	16
Imipenem	1:15	2.0	0.1	1.0	0.05
Linezolid	1:1.25	5.0	>8.0	>8.0	2.0
Meropenem	1:15	4.0	0.03	0.1	0.1
Rifampicin	1:20	1.0	0.5	1.0	2.0
Vancomycin	1:40	1.0	>4.0	>4.0	0.2

MIC$_{90}$, minimum concentration of antibiotic that is inhibitory for 90% of isolates; CSF, cerebrospinal fluid.

of infusions of calcium-containing solutions in neonates. The risk of precipitation is much lower in patients >28 days of age. Nevertheless, caution should still be exercised when treating older age groups, especially in the early treatment of meningococcal infections (where calcium-containing products are commonly used for resuscitation).

In meningitis due to *N. meningitidis* and *H. influenzae*, prompt administration of chemoprophylaxis to eliminate nasopharyngeal carriage can reduce the risk of secondary cases in close contacts of the case.

N. meningitidis. In view of the potentially rapid clinical progression of meningococcal disease, it is recommended that treatment should begin with the emergency administration of benzylpenicillin. Primary care clinicians should give penicillin while arranging transfer of the patient to hospital. The dose is 1200 mg for adults and children aged 10 years and above, 600 mg for children aged 1–9 years and 300 mg for children aged below 1 year. Ideally, this should be given intravenously. The intramuscular route is less likely to be effective in shocked patients but can be used if venous access cannot be obtained. The only contraindication is allergy to penicillin, where cefotaxime (1 g for adults, 50 mg/kg for children aged <12 years) or chloramphenicol (1.2 g for adults, 25 mg/kg for children aged <12 years) may be given, if available. However, it is not recommended that primary care clinicians routinely carry these alternative antibiotics.

Strains of *N. meningitidis* with reduced sensitivity to penicillin are well known and presently account for 5–10% of isolates in Europe and the USA. In general, these cases respond to treatment with adequate doses of benzylpenicillin, and failure of penicillin treatment has rarely been reported. Nevertheless, cefotaxime and ceftriaxone are now widely used in preference to benzylpenicillin or chloramphenicol.

S. pneumoniae. Benzylpenicillin was once widely regarded as the treatment of choice for pneumococcal meningitis. However, pneumococci resistant to penicillin have emerged across the world, presenting a major therapeutic challenge in view of the severity of pneumococcal meningitis.

Although currently only about 5% of pneumococci in the UK are penicillin resistant, the frequency of resistance is increasing, and resistance rates of more than 50% have been reported in other countries, including Spain, Hungary and South Africa. Penicillin resistance in pneumococci is defined in terms of the minimum inhibitory concentration (MIC) of penicillin. Most strains have a MIC value of 0.1–2.0 mg/L and are defined as having moderate resistance; strains with an MIC value of more than 2 mg/L are considered highly resistant. This distinction is relevant for less serious infections with moderately resistant strains, which may still respond to adequate doses of some β-lactam antibiotics, such as cefotaxime, ceftriaxone or a carbapenem. However, the clinical outcome of meningitis with penicillin-resistant pneumococci treated with a β-lactam antibiotic as monotherapy is less good. For this reason, many guidelines, including those produced by the Infectious Diseases Society of America, now recommend therapy with a combination of a third-generation cephalosporin and vancomycin (McIntosh, 2005). This approach has not been adopted universally in the UK but should certainly be considered for patients who might have acquired their infection in a location where the incidence of penicillin resistance is high. Where vancomycin is given intravenously to treat meningitis, it is important to aim for trough serum levels of 15–20 mg/L because of the limited CSF penetration of vancomycin. Another problem is the emergence of pneumococci that are tolerant to vancomycin, that is, they are able to survive, but not proliferate, in the presence of vancomycin. Although such strains are uncommon, the outcome of meningitis treated with vancomycin is poor (Cottagnoud and Tauber, 2004).

Other antibiotics may be useful in treating pneumococcal meningitis. Use of rifampicin in combination with a cephalosporin and/or vancomycin is sometimes recommended, but there are few data confirming this can improve the response rate in either penicillin-sensitive or -resistant pneumococcal meningitis. The dose of rifampicin is 600 mg twice daily in adults or 10 mg/kg (maximum 600 mg) twice daily in children. Chloramphenicol is a suitable alternative to penicillin for treatment of meningitis due to penicillin-sensitive strains, for example in patients who are penicillin allergic. However, chloramphenicol is not recommended for treating penicillin-resistant pneumococcal meningitis: although isolates may appear sensitive to chloramphenicol on routine laboratory testing, bactericidal activity is often absent and the clinical response is usually poor.

Consideration of alternative antibiotics for treatment of penicillin-resistant pneumococcal meningitis is largely based on case reports rather than clinical trials. Success has been reported with meropenem as monotherapy, and in conjunction with rifampicin. Moxifloxacin is a new-generation quinolone antibiotic with enhanced activity against Gram-positive bacteria, including *S. pneumoniae*, which has shown promise in experimental pneumococcal meningitis. Linezolid has excellent CSF penetration but does not have bactericidal activity, and clinical experience in treating meningitis has been variable (Rupprecht and Pfister, 2005).

Daptomycin is an interesting option that has potent bactericidal activity against penicillin-sensitive and -resistant pneumococci, but without being bacteriolytic. This may be an advantage in that bacterial intracellular components that contribute to the inflammatory response are not liberated by bacterial killing. Indeed, in treating experimental pneumococcal meningitis, daptomycin gives a better clinical outcome than conventional treatment.

The unpredictable nature of the response to therapy of penicillin-resistant pneumococcal meningitis means that patients require close observation during treatment, for example monitoring of C-reactive protein (CRP). Repeat examination of CSF during therapy should also be considered.

H. influenzae. A third-generation cephalosporin such as cefotaxime or ceftriaxone is generally the treatment of choice for *H. influenzae* meningitis. These agents have superseded the traditional therapies of chloramphenicol and/or ampicillin or amoxicillin.

Other bacteria. Meningitis in immunocompetent individuals is rarely due to other bacteria. The definitive treatment for these individuals should be determined on an individual basis in the light of careful clinical and microbiological assessment.

Chemoprophylaxis against meningocococcal and Hib infection. In meningococcal meningitis, spread between family members and other close contacts is well recognised; these individuals should receive chemoprophylaxis as soon as possible, preferably within 24 h. Sometimes, chemoprophylaxis may be indicated for other contacts, but the decision to offer prophylaxis beyond household contacts should only be made after obtaining expert advice (Box 38.1). Of the antibiotics conventionally used to treat meningococcal infections, only ceftriaxone reliably eliminates nasopharyngeal carriage; where another antibiotic has been used for treatment, the index case also requires chemoprophylaxis. A number of antibiotics are suitable as prophylaxis (Box 38.2).

Box 38.1 Indications for chemoprophylaxis in contacts of cases of infection with *N. meningitidis* or *H. influenzae* type b

---

Neisseria meningitidis
Household and other close contacts: prophylaxis usually initiated as soon as possible by clinicians caring for the patient

- Persons who have slept in the same house as the patient at any time during the 7 days before the onset of symptoms
- Boy/girl friends of the patient
- Unless treated with ceftriaxone (which reliably eliminates nasopharyngeal carriage), the index patient should also receive antibiotic prophylaxis as soon as he or she is able to take oral medication

Healthcare workers: prophylaxis should only be initiated after consultation with hospital infection control team or public health doctor

- Individuals who have administered mouth-to-mouth resuscitation or had some other form of prolonged close face-to-face contact with the patient
- Other contacts: prophylaxis should be initiated by a public health doctor
- Schools, nurseries, universities and other closed communities where two or more linked cases have occurred

---

Invasive *Haemophilus influenzae* type b infection
Household and other close contacts: prophylaxis usually initiated as soon as possible by clinicians caring for the patient

- Indicated only where there is another child aged less than 4 years who has not been immunised in the same household as the index patient. In such circumstances, prophylaxis should be given to all household contacts aged 1 month or older, unless there are contraindications. The index patient should also receive antibiotic prophylaxis as soon as he or she is able to take oral medication

Other contacts: prophylaxis very rarely necessary and should only be initiated by a public health physician

Box 38.2 Recommended prophylactic regimens for contacts of cases of infection with *N. meningitidis* or *H. influenzae* type b

Meningococcal infection

Ciprofloxacin[a] (oral)

Children aged 1 month – 4 years	125 mg as a single dose
Children aged 5–12 years	250 mg as a single dose
Adults	500 mg as a single dose

Rifampicin (oral)

Children aged <1 year	5 mg/kg twice daily on 2 consecutive days
Children aged 1–12 years	10 mg/kg (max 600 mg) twice daily on 2 consecutive days
Adults	600 mg twice daily on 2 consecutive days

Azithromycin[a] (oral)

Pregnant women	500 mg as a single dose

Ceftriaxone[a] (intramuscular)

Children aged <12 years	125 mg as a single dose
Adults	250 mg as a single dose

Invasive *Haemophilus influenzae* type b infection

Rifampicin (oral)

Children aged 1–3 months	10 mg/kg once daily for 4 days
Children aged >3 months	20 mg/kg once daily (max 600 mg) for 4 days
Adults[b]	600 mg once daily for 4 days

[a]Not licensed for this indication.
[b]For pregnant women, obtain expert advice.

Ciprofloxacin is now widely recommended for contacts of all ages (including pregnant and breast-feeding women) because of the convenience of single-dose administration and, unlike rifampicin, it does not interact with oral contraceptives and is readily available in community pharmacies. Although anaphylactoid reactions have been reported to occur in individuals receiving ciprofloxacin as chemoprophylaxis, none of these reactions has been fatal. If the strain is confirmed as group C (or A, W135 or Y), vaccination is normally offered to contacts who were given prophylaxis. There is no need to vaccinate the patient. There is currently no vaccine that protects against group B disease, which accounts for about 70% of cases of meningococcal disease in Europe.

Chemoprophylaxis against Hib infection is usually only indicated where there is an unimmunised child in the vulnerable age group in the household (see Box 38.1). Only rifampicin has been proved to be effective in eliminating nasopharyngeal carriage (see Box 38.2). Unimmunised household contacts aged below 4 years should also receive Hib vaccine. The index case should also receive rifampicin in order to eliminate nasopharyngeal carriage, and should be immunised, irrespective of age.

Antibiotics for meningitis in special groups

Immunocompromised host. In the immunocompromised neutropenic patient, the meninges can become infected. Possible causes of meningitis include *Enterobacteriaceae* and *Pseudomonas aeruginosa*, as well as the classic bacterial causes of meningitis. The choice of therapy is governed by the need to attain broad-spectrum coverage, using agents with good CSF penetration. Meropenem may now be the drug of choice for meningitis in this setting, although many other regimens are also appropriate.

Patients with cellular immune dysfunction are vulnerable to meningitis due to *L. monocytogenes* and *C. neoformans*. Ampicillin or amoxicillin, along with cefotaxime or ceftriaxone, is recommended as empirical antibacterial therapy for meningitis in these patients. Definitive treatment of listeria meningitis is normally with high-dose ampicillin (3 g four times daily) or amoxicillin (2 g four times daily), with the addition of gentamicin in order to obtain a synergistic effect. The most appropriate treatment for patients who are penicillin allergic, or in the rare circumstance of infection with a strain that is ampicillin resistant, is uncertain and specialist microbiological advice should be sought. Specific therapies for cryptococcal meningitis are described in detail as follows.

Splenectomised patients are susceptible to invasive infections with encapsulated bacteria, including *S. pneumoniae* and Hib. Standard therapy with either cefotaxime or ceftriaxone is appropriate.

Shunt-associated meningitis. Patients who have a ventricular shunt are at increased risk of meningitis. Shunt-associated infections are classified according to the site of initial infection. Internal infections, where the lumen of the shunt is colonised, constitute the majority of cases. External shunt infections involve the tissues surrounding the shunt. Most internal shunt infections are caused by coagulase-negative staphylococci. *S. aureus* and *Enterobacteriaceae* account for most external infections. It is generally held that management of shunt infections should include shunt removal, as well as antibiotic therapy (Infection in Neurosurgery Working Party, 2000), although the need for this has been questioned (Arnell et al., 2007). Appropriate antimicrobial regimens are shown in Table 38.4.

Tuberculous meningitis. The outcome in tuberculous meningitis relates directly to the severity of the patient's clinical condition on commencement of therapy. A satisfactory response demands a high degree of clinical suspicion such that appropriate chemotherapy is initiated early, even if tubercle bacilli are not demonstrated on initial microscopy. Most currently used antituberculous agents achieve effective concentrations in the CSF in tuberculous meningitis. Detailed discussion of antituberculous therapy is given in Chapter 40. Adjunctive steroid therapy is of value in patients with more severe disease, particularly those who suddenly develop cerebral oedema soon after starting treatment or who appear to be developing a spinal block. However, routine use of steroids is not recommended. They may suppress informative changes in the CSF and interfere with antibiotic penetration by restoring the blood–brain barrier. Early neurosurgical management of hydrocephalus by means of a ventriculoperitoneal or ventriculoatrial shunt is also important in improving the prospects for neurological recovery.

Cryptococcal meningitis. The standard treatment of cryptococcal meningitis is amphotericin B, given intravenously at a dose of 0.7–1.0 mg/kg/day, with or without flucytosine 100 mg/kg/day, for 6–10 weeks. Addition of flucytosine results in quicker clearance of yeasts from the CSF, although it is debatable whether this results in improved clinical outcome. Lipid formulations of amphotericin B, such as liposomal

Table 38.4 Antimicrobial regimens for treatment of shunt meningitis

Type of infection	First-choice antibiotic regimen	Other antibiotic regimens	Duration of therapy before reshunting
Internal shunt infection caused by Gram-positive bacteria	Intraventricular vancomycin + intravenous or oral rifampicin	Substitute flucloxacillin or intravenous vancomycin for rifampicin in cases of rifampicin resistance, except in the case of enterococci, where an aminoglycoside (e.g. gentamicin) should be used	7–10 days intravenous
External shunt infection caused by S. Aureus	As earlier, with the addition of intravenous flucloxacillin	Substitute intravenous vancomycin for flucloxacillin in the case of methicillin resistance (MRSA)	12–14 days
Enterobacteriaceae	Intravenous cefotaxime ± an aminoglycoside + intraventricular aminoglycoside	Substitute ceftazidime or meropenem for cefotaxime in the case of cefotaxime resistance	14 days
Polymicrobial ventriculoperitoneal shunt infections	Intravenous amoxicillin, metronidazole, cefotaxime ± an aminoglycoside + intraventricular aminoglycoside	Seek specialist advice	14 days
Candida	Intravenous amphotericin B + flucytosine	Intravenous fluconazole	10–14 days (antifungal fungal therapy should continue for 1 week after reshunting)

amphotericin B, at doses of 4–6 mg/kg/day have comparable efficacy to, and fewer side effects than, conventional amphotericin B at a dose of 0.7 mg/kg. As an alternative to prolonged therapy with two potentially toxic drugs, 2 weeks therapy with amphotericin B and flucytosine may be given, followed by consolidation therapy with fluconazole 400 mg/day for at least 10 weeks. Initial treatment with fluconazole 400–800 mg/day plus flucytosine is clinically inferior to amphotericin B-based regimens, and in any case is no better tolerated than amphotericin B-based regimens. Regular haematological and biochemical monitoring is recommended during treatment, along with measurement of serum concentrations of flucytosine (which should not exceed 80 mg/L).

The clinical response to treatment of cryptococcal meningitis is slow, and it often takes 2 or 3 weeks to sterilise the CSF. Monitoring of intracranial pressure is essential, with large-volume CSF drainage indicated if the opening pressure reaches 250 mmHg. Serial CSF cultures are occasionally helpful in following the response to treatment, but monitoring of cryptococcal antigen titres in serum or CSF is of little value.

Patients with HIV infection treated for cryptococcal meningitis should then receive fluconazole indefinitely, or at least until immune reconstitution occurs. The dose of fluconazole may be reduced to 200 mg/day, depending on the patient's clinical condition (Bicanic and Harrison, 2004). Itraconazole offers less good CSF penetration than fluconazole, but is a suitable alternative as maintenance therapy at a dose of 200–400 mg/day for patients unable to tolerate fluconazole. Clinical data with newer triazoles such as voriconazole and posaconazole remain limited, but these agents may be useful, especially in the rare situation of fluconazole-resistant cryptococcal meningitis. The echinocandin class of antifungals does not possess useful activity against Cryptococcus.

Viral meningitis. None of the currently available antiviral agents has useful activity against human enteroviruses, the commonest causes of viral meningitis (Big et al., 2009). Fortunately, however, the condition is usually self-limiting. The viruses that commonly cause this condition, herpes simplex and varicella zoster meningoencephalitis, are treated with high-dose aciclovir, 10 mg/kg three times daily for at least 10 days (adults and children aged 12 years and over). For younger children, the recommended doses are 20 mg/kg three times daily for infants up to age 3 months, and 500 mg/m² three times daily for those aged 3 months to 12 years.

Steroids as adjunctive therapy in bacterial meningitis. In pharmacological doses, corticosteroids, and in particular dexamethasone, regulate many components of the inflammatory response and also lower CSF hydrostatic pressure. However, by reducing inflammation and restoring the blood–brain barrier, they may reduce CSF penetration of antibiotics. The benefits of steroids in the initial management of meningitis due to M. tuberculosis and Hib are well established, although in other forms of bacterial meningitis the evidence has been less compelling. Methodological flaws have been identified in older studies where no benefit was seen from use of adjunctive steroid therapy. Recent work has found that adjunctive dexamethasone therapy reduces the rate of unfavourable outcomes from 25% to 15% in adults with bacterial meningitis. In this series, adjunctive treatment with dexamethasone was given before or with the first dose of antibiotics, without serious adverse effects. Overall, corticosteroids significantly reduce rates of mortality, severe hearing loss and neurological sequelae. The use of adjunctive dexamethasone is now recommended for children and adults with community-acquired bacterial meningitis, regardless of bacterial aetiology (Brouwer et al., 2010). Adjunctive therapy should be initiated before or with the first dose of antibiotics and continued for 4 days. The recommended dose for adults is 10 mg four times daily for 4 days (children 0.15 mg/kg four times daily for 4 days).

Intrathecal and intraventricular administration of antibiotics. Intrathecal administration, that is, administration into the lumbar subarachnoid space, of antibiotics was once widely used to supplement levels attained by concomitant systemic therapy. However, there is little evidence for the efficacy of this route of delivery, and it is now rarely used. In particular, it produces only low concentrations of antibiotic in the ventricles and therefore does little to prevent ventriculitis, one of the most serious complications of meningitis. Direct intraventricular administration of antibiotics in meningitis is important in certain types of meningitis, especially where it is necessary to use an agent, for example vancomycin or an aminoglycoside, that penetrates CSF poorly (Shah et al., 2004). The most common situation is in shunt-associated meningitis, where multiple antibiotic-resistant coagulase-negative staphylococci are the major pathogens, and where conveniently the patient will often have an external ventricular drain through which antibiotics can be administered.

There are considerable differences in recommended doses of antibiotics for intrathecal or intraventricular administration. A dose of 15–20 mg vancomycin per day is recommended for treatment of shunt-associated meningitis in adults with an extraventricular drain, and 10 mg/day for neonates and children. The paediatric dose may need to be reduced to 5 mg/day if ventricular size is reduced, or increased to 15–20 mg/day if the ventricular size is increased. In all patients, the dose frequency should be decreased to once every 2–3 days if CSF is not draining freely. The CSF vancomycin concentration should be measured after 3–4 days, aiming for a trough concentration of <10 mg/L. Recommended doses of antibiotics are otherwise largely based on anecdotal experience (Table 38.5).

Patient care

Common problems in the treatment of meningitis are set out in Table 38.6.

Table 38.5 Daily[a] doses (mg) of gentamicin and vancomycin for intraventricular administration

Antibiotic	Adult	Child ≥2 years	Child <2 years
Gentamicin	1.0[b]	1.0	1.0
Vancomycin	15–20	10[c]	10[c]

[a]If CSF is not draining freely, reduce dose frequency to once every 2–3 days.
[b]Dose can be increased to up to 5 mg in the most severe cases.
[c]Reduce dose to 5 mg if ventricular size is reduced, or increase to 15–20 mg/day if ventricular size is increased.

Table 38.6 Practice points in infective meningitis

Infection	Antibiotic	Common problems	Resolution
Bacterial meningitis	Chloramphenicol	Risk of serious toxicity, especially in neonates	Avoid use if possible Close monitoring of serum levels where use essential
Neonatal meningitis	Aminoglycosides (e.g. gentamicin)	Poor CSF penetration provides unreliable activity against Gram-negative bacteria Unpredictable neonatal pharmacokinetics (especially preterm neonates)	Substitute with, or add, an antibiotic with better CSF penetration (e.g. a cephalosporin) Close monitoring of serum levels
S. pneumoniae meningitis	Penicillin Cefotaxime or ceftriaxone Vancomycin (intravenous)	Resistance is increasing Treatment failure in meningitis due to penicillin Resistant strains Unreliable CSF penetration	Use cefotaxime or ceftriaxone ± vancomycin as empiric therapy Add rifampicin or vancomycin Consider one of the newer antibiotics with good activity against multiresistant Gram-positive bacteria
L. monocytogenes meningitis	Any	Relapse rate up to 10% after short courses of therapy	Give prolonged therapy (usually 3–4 weeks)
Cryptococcal meningitis	Amphotericin B Flucytosine Fluconazole	High incidence of side effects, for example fever, nausea, vomiting, anaemia, hypokalaemia, impaired renal function Risk of side effects, for example deranged liver function, bone marrow depression Low cure rate when used as monotherapy (except as consolidation therapy)	Change to lipid-based preparation of amphotericin B, or replace with fluconazole Close monitoring of serum levels Combine with flucytosine

Prevention of person-to-person transmission

Patients with meningitis may be infectious to others. Neonates with meningitis usually have generalised infections, and the causative organisms can often be isolated from body fluids and faeces. Babies with meningitis should therefore be isolated to prevent infection spreading to other patients. Patients with meningococcal or Hib meningitis should be isolated until after at least 48 h of antibiotic therapy. Contacts of these patients may be asymptomatic carriers and potentially infectious to others and/or at risk of developing invasive infection themselves. Chemoprophylaxis and vaccination can reduce these risks (see earlier). Patients with most other types of meningitis do not represent a significant infectious hazard, and enhanced infection control precautions are not usually necessary.

Case studies

Case 38.1

A 4-week-old premature infant presents on the hospital neonatal unit with poor feeding, fever and increasing drowsiness. Lumbar puncture reveals 1200 WBC/μL (80% of which are polymorphs), and low glucose and elevated protein levels. No organisms are seen on a Gram-stained smear of the CSF. The diagnosis is acute purulent meningitis.

Questions

1. What are the likely aetiological agents?
2. Which other investigations other than CSF culture might help in establishing the aetiological diagnosis?
3. What empiric antibiotic therapy should be commenced?

Answers

1. At 4 weeks of age, the possible causes include neonatal pathogens (group B streptococci, *Escherichia coli* and *Listeria monocytogenes*), nosocomial pathogens such as *Staphylococcus aureus* and Gram-negative bacilli and the usual causes of meningitis in older infants (especially *Neisseria meningitidis* and *Streptococcus pneumoniae*). Most group B streptococcal disease presents in the first few days of life, whilst listeria meningitis is very uncommon, meaning that of the neonatal pathogens there is a greater likelihood of Gram-negative bacillary meningitis.
2. It is important to collect blood cultures because neonatal meningitis is not uncommonly accompanied by bacteraemia. Molecular tests on CSF may be undertaken, but the commonly used tests are not directed against the most likely pathogens in this case. The results of any recent cultures from other anatomic sites may also be useful, especially in ensuring that empiric antibiotic therapy is active against potential pathogens the baby is known to harbour.
3. Given the range of potential pathogens, a combination of ampicillin or amoxicillin plus cefotaxime or ceftazidime would be the treatment of choice, unless the patient is known to be colonised with antibiotic-resistant bacteria such as MRSA or Gram-negative bacteria.

Case 38.2

A 70-year-old man is being treated for meningitis due to *Streptococcus pneumoniae* that is moderately resistant to penicillin (MIC value 0.75 mg/L). Despite 7 days' treatment with intravenous vancomycin and cefotaxime, there has been little improvement in his clinical condition. A CT scan has shown meningeal inflammation consistent with meningitis, but no evidence of intracranial complications that might explain his poor clinical response. The most recent trough (predose) serum vancomycin concentration was 5.3 mg/L.

Questions

1. Why might there have been an inadequate response to treatment with cefotaxime and vancomycin?
2. What options are there to modify his antimicrobial therapy?

Answers

1. CSF penetration of vancomycin is poor and the serum vancomycin concentration in any case low. It is therefore doubtful that the vancomcyin concentration in the CSF would be bactericidal. Even if the vancomycin concentration in CSF were adequate, the infection may be due to a vancomycin-tolerant strain of *S. pneumoniae*. Tolerant strains appear fully sensitive to vancomycin by routine laboratory antimicrobial susceptibility sensitivity testing. Cefotaxime alone may not adequately treat infections with penicillin-resistant pneumococci.
2. It is important to optimise the patient's treatment as quickly as possible. He might respond to increasing the dose of vancomycin with or without addition of rifampicin. However, these strategies give little assurance of success. It would probably be preferable to switch to an alternative agent. Meropenem is probably the agent with which there is most experience, which could continue to be combined with an increased dose vancomycin for extra assurance. Linezolid or daptomycin would be alternative options.

Case 38.3

An 18-year-old man is referred as an emergency with suspected meningitis. He was given intravenous penicillin by the primary care doctor before admission to hospital. On examination he is fully conscious, and neck stiffness is elicited. He is haemodynamically stable and no rash is present.

Questions

1. What investigations would you undertake to establish the diagnosis?
2. What treatment would you give?
3. What further action will be required if a diagnosis of meningococcal meningitis is likely?

Answers

1. Blood cultures and a nasopharyngeal swab for culture should be collected. There are no clinical contraindications to lumbar puncture, and in most centres this would be undertaken without a prior CT scan. The white cell count and glucose and protein concentrations in the CSF should be measured. A Gram stain should be undertaken, which may give immediate information on the likely identity of the pathogen, as well as culture and PCR. Some laboratories might also undertake antigen testing to try to establish an early aetiological diagnosis.

2. Antibiotic treatment should be with a third-generation cephalosporin (cefotaxime or ceftriaxone). The latter should be entirely safe to use in this situation given that it sounds unlikely that the patient will have required resuscitation with calcium-containing fluids. In addition, adjunctive therapy with dexamethasone, for which there appear to be no contraindications, should be considered.

3. Meningitis is a notifiable disease. If a diagnosis of meningococcal meningitis is considered likely, then prophylaxis should be offered to the patient and to close contacts as soon as possible to eliminate nasopharyngeal carriage and prevent secondary cases.

Case 38.4

A 46-year-old renal transplant recipient received 2 weeks treatment with amphotericin and flucytosine, and was then switched to fluconazole which he has received for a further 6 weeks (latterly as a hospital out-patient). However, after complaining of headaches, a repeat lumbar puncture has been undertaken and has shown that cryptococci are still present in the CSF.

Questions

1. Give three reasons why his treatment to date might have failed.
2. How would you now manage the situation?

Answers

1. It may be that the patient has not been adherent with his medication; the initial 2-week course of treatment with amphotericin may have been too short; or the infecting strain of *Cryptococcus* may be fluconazole resistant.
2. The first step should be to readmit the patient and recommence treatment with amphotericin and flucytosine. The microbiology laboratory should be asked to determine the sensitivity of the patient's isolate to fluconazole. Once that result has been ascertained, it will be possible to plan the patient's longer term management. Options would include completing a full course of amphotericin and flucytosine, or switching to one of the new triazoles such as posaconazole at some point. Close monitoring of the patient's response will be required.

References

Arnell, K., Enblad, P., Wester, T., et al., 2007. Treatment of cerebrospinal fluid shunt infections in children using systemic and intraventricular antibiotic therapy in combination with externalization of the ventricular catheter: efficacy in 34 consecutively treated infections. J. Neurosurg. 107, 213–219.

Bicanic, T., Harrison, T.S., 2004. Cryptococcal meningitis. Br. Med. Bull. 72, 99–118.

Big, C., Reineck, L.A., Aronoff, D.M., 2009. Viral infections of the central nervous system: a case-based review. Clin. Med. Res. 7, 142–146.

Brouwer, M.C., McIntyre, P., de Gans, J., et al., 2010. Corticosteroids for acute bacterial meningitis. Cochrane Database of Systematic Reviews. Issue 9. Art No. CD004405.

Cottagnoud, P.H., Tauber, M.G., 2004. New therapies for pneumococcal meningitis. Expert Opin. Investig. Drugs 13, 393–401.

Galiza, E.P., Heath, P.T., 2009. Improving the outcome of neonatal meningitis. Curr. Opin. Infect. Dis. 22, 229–234.

Health Protection Agency Meningococcus and Haemophilus Forum. Guidance for Public Health Management of Meningococcal Disease in the UK, updated January 2011. Health Protection Agency, London.

Infection in Neurosurgery Working Party of the British Society for Antimicrobial Chemotherapy, 2000. The management of neurosurgical patients with postoperative bacterial or aseptic meningitis or external ventricular drain-associated ventriculitis. Br. J. Neurosurg. 14, 7–12.

McIntosh, E.D., 2005. Treatment and prevention strategies to combat pediatric pneumococcal meningitis. Expert Rev. Anti-Infect. Ther. 3, 739–750.

Ross, J.S., Wilson, K.J.W., 1981. Foundations of Anatomy and Physiology, fifth ed. Churchill Livingstone, Edinburgh, pp. 172–173.

Rupprecht, T.A., Pfister, H.W., 2005. Clinical experience with linezolid for the treatment of central nervous system infections. Eur. J. Neurol. 12, 536–542.

Shah, S.S., Ohlsson, A., Shah, V.S., 2004. Intraventricular antibiotics for bacterial meningitis in neonates. Cochrane Database of Systematic Reviews . Issue 4. Art. No. CD004496. doi:10.1002/14651858. CD004496.pub2. Available at http://www2.cochrane.org/reviews/en/ab004496.html. Accessed 20 April 2011.

Yogev, R., Guzman-Cottrill, J., 2005. Bacterial meningitis in children: critical review of current concepts. Drugs 65, 1097–1112.

Further reading

Chang, L., Phipps, W., Kennedy, G., et al., 2005. Antifungal interventions for the primary prevention of cryptococcal disease in adults with HIV. Cochrane Database of Systematic Reviews. Issue 3. Art. No. CD004773.pub2. doi:10.1002/14651858. CD004773.pub2.

Chaudhuri A., Martinez-Martin P., Kennedy P.G., et al., 2008. EFNS guideline on the management of community-acquired bacterial meningitis: report of an EFNS Task Force on acute bacterial meningitis in older children and adults. Eur. J. Neurol. 15, 649–659

Chavez-Bueno, S., McCracken, G.H., 2005. Bacterial meningitis in children. Pediatr. Clin. North Am. 52, 795–810.

Correia, J.B., Hart, C.A., 2004. Meningococcal disease. Clin. Evid. 12, 1164–1181.

Riordan, A., 2010. The implications of vaccines for prevention of bacterial meningitis. Curr. Opin. Neurol. 23, 319–324.

Tunkel, A.R., Hartman, B.J., Kaplan, S.L., et al., 2004. Practice guidelines for the management of bacterial meningitis. Clin. Infect. Dis. 39, 1267–1284.

Zunt, J.R., 2010. Infections of the central nervous system in the neurosurgical patient. Handb. Clin. Neurol. 96, 125–141.

39 Surgical site infection and antimicrobial prophylaxis

P. Howard and J. A. T. Sandoe

Key points

- Surgical site infection is a major cause of mortality and morbidity.
- Development of surgical site infection is a complex process influenced by host, operative and microbial factors.
- The microbial cause of surgical site infection varies with type of procedure but *Staphylococcus aureus* remains the most commonly implicated pathogen.
- Surveillance of surgical site infection is necessary to benchmark and improve prevention strategies.
- Antimicrobial prophylaxis is just one of many approaches to reduce surgical site infection.
- Not all operations require antimicrobial prophylaxis.
- Antimicrobial prophylaxis should be used only where there is evidence of efficacy or expert consensus that benefits outweigh risks.
- The choice of antimicrobial prophylaxis depends on the operation, pharmacokinetics, pharmacodynamics and patient factors.
- The timing of antimicrobial administration is key to reducing surgical site infection.
- Pharmacists are unlikely to see many patients before surgery; they must therefore develop systems to ensure that appropriate antimicrobial prophylaxis is given at the right time.

Epidemiology

In England, there are over nine million operations and interventions undertaken each year. Over 50% of these are performed as day cases and many patients are admitted on the day of surgery (Health and Social Care Information Centre, 2009). Healthcare-associated infections (HCAIs), including surgical site infections, complicate around 7% of all hospital admissions (HIS/ICNA, 2007). Surgical site infections are of major clinical importance because they account for 14–16% of all healthcare-associated infections (HPS, 2009; Public Accounts Committee, 2009) and are associated with considerable morbidity and mortality. One-third of peri-operative deaths are related to surgical site infections (Astagneau et al., 2001). It has been estimated that surgical site infections double the length of hospital stay (Coello et al., 2005). While surgical site infections can be common in some procedures, the incidence can be minimised by the care provided before and after the operation, together with the skill of the surgeon (HPS, 2009).

Surveillance

Monitoring the incidence of surgical site infections is hampered by the lack of agreed measuring systems. In particular, to monitor the rates of surgical site infection within an organisation, or to benchmark between organisations, there needs to be a standard approach to diagnosis. Criteria for such a definition have been developed by the Centres for Disease Control and Prevention (CDC) (Mangram et al., 1999) and these are presented in Table 39.1. More detailed surgical site infection scoring systems have been developed but these are time consuming to use.

Mandatory surveillance for surgical site infections in orthopaedic surgery in the UK was introduced in 2003. In addition, Scotland monitors most other common procedures (http://www.hps.scot.nhs.uk) while in Wales caesarian section is also monitored (http://www.wales.nhs.uk). England has a voluntary reporting system for a broader range of operations (http://www.hpa.org.uk). All report their findings annually. Many surgical site infections, for example, those involving

Surgery is the branch of medical science that treats injury or disease or improves bodily function through operative procedures. Surgery has been used for thousands of years but has always been complicated to some extent by infection. Currently, surgery is an integral part of the management of many medical conditions and remains the definitive treatment for many cancers. Infections developing at the site of invasive surgical procedures are frequently referred to as surgical site infections. Surgical site infections occur when pathogenic micro-organisms contaminate a surgical wound, multiply and cause tissue damage. The term 'surgical site infection' encompasses not only infection at the site of incision but also infections of implants, prosthetic devices and adjacent tissues involved in the operation.

Table 39.1 Criteria for defining surgical site infection (Mangram et al., 1999)

Type	Level	Signs and symptoms
Superficial incisional	Skin and subcutaneous tissue	Localised (Celsian) signs such as redness, pain, heat or swelling at the site of the incision or by the presence of pus within 30 days
Deep incisional	Fascial and muscle layers	Presence of pus or an abscess, fever with tenderness of the wound, or a separation of the edges of the incision exposing the deeper tissues within 30 days (or 1 year if an implant used)
Organ or space infection	Any part of the anatomy other than the incision that is opened or manipulated during the surgical procedure, for example, joint or peritoneum	Loss of function of a joint, abscess in an organ, localised peritonitis or collection. Ultrasound or CT scans confirm infection. Within 30 days (or 1 year if implant is used)

prosthetic joints, often develop late (>28 days post-operation), so post-discharge surveillance schemes are essential. Patients need to be aware how a surgical site infection may present after discharge from hospital. Surveillance of surgical site infections and feedback to the surgical team has been shown to reduce rates of infection (Gastmeier et al., 2005).

Risk factors

Surgical site infections can be categorised into three groups: superficial incisional, deep incisional and organ or space (Fig. 39.1) Whether a wound infection occurs after surgery depends on a complex interaction between the following:

- Procedure-related factors, for example, implantation of foreign bodies, degree of trauma to host tissues and experience of surgeon

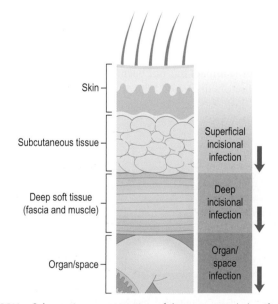

Fig. 39.1 Schematic representation of the anatomical classification of surgical site infection (Horan et al., 1992). Reproduced with permission from the University of Chicago Press.

- Patient related factors, for example, host immunity, nutritional status and the presence or absence of diabetes
- Microbial factors (tissue adherence and invasion)
- Peri-operative antimicrobial prophylaxis.

A system to stratify operative wounds by the expected level of bacterial contamination (Table 39.2) was developed to help predict likely infection rates (Mangram et al., 1999). A number of other factors have also been found to affect the incidence of surgical site infection and are discussed below.

Prosthetic implants

Medical implants have a detrimental effect on host defences such that a lower bacterial count is needed to initiate infection. Hence, there is a greater risk of infection during implant surgery. Bacteria growing on an abiotic surface, such as a prosthetic hip implant or heart valve, together with a protective layer of microbial polymers are known as a biofilm (Donlan and Costerton, 2002). Antimicrobials are frequently ineffective against micro-organisms growing in biofilms, making treatment of implant infections problematic and their prevention even more important.

Duration of surgery

The longer the operation, the greater is the risk of wound infection. This, in turn, may be influenced by the experience (Fig. 39.2) speed and skill of the surgeon and is additional to the classification of the operation by risk of infection, for example, clean, contaminated, dirty or infected.

Patient related factors

A number of patient related factors are known to influence the likelihood of developing a surgical site infection and include the following:

- Wound potential for infection, for example, clean, contaminated, dirty or infected site
- Physical status of patient (Table 39.3)
- Duration of procedure.

Table 39.2 Classification of surgical procedures by risk of infection (Mangram et al., 1999)

Type of procedure	Definition	Wound infection rate (%)	Example	Need for prophylaxis
Clean	Atraumatic; no inflammation encountered, no break in technique; gastro-intestinal, genitourinary and respiratory tracts not entered	1.5–4.2	Inguinal hernia repair	Not usually required
Contaminated	Gastro-intestinal or respiratory tract entered but without spillage; oropharynx, appendectomy, sterile genitourinary or biliary tract entered; minor break in technique	<10	Cholecystectomy (no spillage)	Usually required
Clean-contaminated	Acute inflammation; infected bile or urine; gross spillage from gastro-intestinal tract; major lapse in technique; fresh traumatic wound (12–24 h)	10–20	Appendicectomy	Required
Dirty and infected	Established infection; transection of clean tissues to enable collection of pus; traumatic wound with retained devitalised tissue; faecal contamination; delayed treatment	20–40	Sigmoid colectomy (Hartmann's procedure) for faecal peritonitis	Treatment required (not prophylaxis)

For each surgical procedure, a score of 0–3 is allocated to represent the number of risk factors present. Patients with a score of 0 are at the lowest risk of developing a surgical site infection, while those with a score of 3 have the greatest risk (Table 39.4). Use of this risk index allows comparison of similar patient groups in terms of surgical site infection risk over time. The risk index is a significantly better predictor of surgical-wound risk than the traditional wound classification system and performs well across a broad range of operative procedures.

Other factors

There are a number of other risk factors that may increase the risk of a surgical site infection (Table 39.5) for an individual patient but the impact has not been quantified to the extent of those risk factors discussed above.

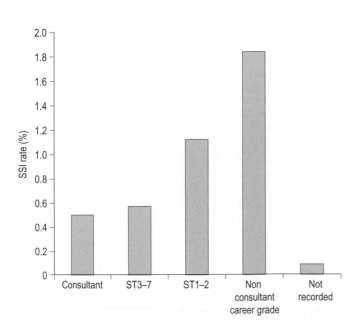

Fig. 39.2 Surgical site infection rate by grade of operator for orthopaedic surgery 2008 (Health Protection Scotland, 2009). Reproduced with kind permission from Health Protection Scotland.

Table 39.3 American Society of Anesthesiology (ASA) classification of physical status (Mangram et al., 1999)

ASA score	Physical status
1	A normal healthy patient
2	A patient with mild systemic disease
3	A patient with a severe systemic disease that limits activity but is not incapacitating
4	A patient with an incapacitating systemic disease that is a constant threat to life
5	A moribund patient that is not expected to survive 24 h with or without operation

Table 39.4 Risk index based on presence of co-morbidity and duration of operation (Culver et al., 1991)

Risk index	Infection rate (%)
0	1.5
1	2.9
2	6.8
3	13.0

Table 39.5 Patient and operative risk factors for surgical site infection

Patient risk factors	Operative risk factors
Advanced age	Tissue ischaemia
Malnutrition	Lack of haemostasis
Obesity	Tissue damage, for example, crushing by surgical instruments
Concurrent infection	Presence of necrotic tissue
Diabetes mellitus	Presence of foreign bodies including surgical materials
Liver impairment	
Renal impairment	
Immune deficiency states	
Prolonged preoperative stay	
Blood transfusion	
Smoking	

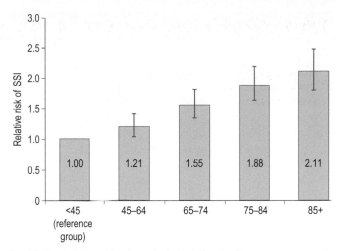

Fig. 39.3 Relative risk of surgical site infection by age group, 2003–2007, adjusted for surgical category (reference age group <45 years) (HPA, 2008). Reproduced with kind permission from Health Protection Agency.

Smoking

Smoking increases the risk of developing a wound infection (Myles et al., 2002). The mechanism is not known but tobacco use may delay wound healing via the vasoconstricting effects of nicotine and thus increase the risk of infection (Myles et al., 2002).

Diabetes mellitus

Long-term diabetes does not appear to have any impact on the risk of developing a surgical site infection. However, perioperative fluctuations in blood glucose for up to 48 h have been shown to double the infection risk in cardiac patients (Latham et al., 2001).

Age

Increasing age is associated with an increased risk of surgical site infection. However, there is debate whether age serves simply as a marker for underlying disease or whether the decline in immune function with age is the significant factor. A study of 72,000 patients in the USA, which adjusted for hospital type, procedure, duration, wound class and physical status of the patient, showed a 1.1% increase in surgical site infection per year of age from the age of 18 to 65 years, but a 1.2% decrease in individuals over 65 years (Kaye et al., 2005). In contrast, the findings of the English surgical site infection surveillance scheme (Fig. 39.3) indicated that the chance of getting a surgical site infection were 37% higher for a 65-year-old person compared to a 45-year-old person (HPA, 2008).

Pathogenesis

Most surgery involves an incision through one of the body's protective barriers, typically the skin or other epithelial surface such as the conjunctiva or tympanic membrane. When intact, these provide an excellent barrier to entry of both exogenous and endogenous bacteria into other epithelial surfaces including the mucosal surfaces of the gastro-intestinal and genitourinary tracts, which, when intact, prevent entry of the luminal contents into the surrounding tissues and organs.

Any surgical operation will breach at least one of the surfaces mentioned and allow entry of bacteria. Whether an infection follows depends on the ability of other defences to kill the invading bacteria. Important host mechanisms include antibodies, complement and phagocytes.

Development of a surgical site infection depends on survival of the contaminating micro-organism in a wound site at the end of a surgical procedure; the pathogenicity and number of these micro-organisms; and the host's immune response. Most micro-organisms are from the host (endogenous), but are occasionally introduced via surgical instruments, the environment or contaminated implants (exogenous). The likely invading micro-organism varies according to the type of surgery (Table 39.6). Data for

Table 39.6 Likely pathogens in post-operative wound infections

Category of surgery	Most likely pathogen(s)
Clean	
Cardiac/vascular/orthopaedic	Coagulase-negative staphylococci, *S. aureus*, Gram-negative bacilli
Breast	*S. aureus*
Clean-contaminated	
Burns	*S. aureus, Pseudomonas aeruginosa*
Head and neck	*S. aureus, Streptococcus* spp., anaerobes (from oral cavity)
Gastro-intestinal tract	Coliforms, anaerobes (*Bacteroides fragilis*)
Urogenital tract	Coliforms, *Enterococcus* spp.
Dirty	
Ruptured viscera	Coliforms, anaerobes (*B. fragilis*) *S. aureus*
Traumatic wound	*Streptococcus pyogenes, Clostridium* spp.

England from 2003 to 2007 has shown that the predominant organism was *Staphylococcus aureus*, which accounted for 38% of all surgical site infections (Fig. 39.4); 64% of these were caused by a meticillin-resistant strain (MRSA). The proportion of surgical site infections caused by *S. aureus*

was highest in hip hemiarthroplasty (57%), followed by limb amputation (54%) and open reduction of long bone fracture (52%). *Enterobacteriaceae* (coliforms) caused the second largest group of infections, accounting for 21% of all surgical site infections. These were the prominent causes of surgical site infections in three categories: large bowel surgery (33%), coronary artery bypass graft (32%) and small bowel surgery (30%).

Although there was a significant reduction in the risk of a surgical site infection for all categories over the 5 year period monitored, there was no change in the proportion of *S. aureus*, infections that were due to MRSA. Infection control measures including the introduction of mandatory MRSA screening for elective patients in 2009 should improve this. Known or previous MRSA carriers can be 'decolonised' and appropriate prophylactic antimicrobials administered that cover MRSA (e.g. teicoplanin).

Prevention of surgical site infection

The evidence that supports interventions to minimise surgical site infection has been highlighted in national guidelines (NICE, 2008a) and categorised into four areas: information to patients, preoperative phase, peri-operative phase and post-operative phase (Table 39.7). When selecting antimicrobial prophylaxis regimens or evaluating potential prophylaxis failures, it is important to ensure that all four aspects of prevention have been addressed.

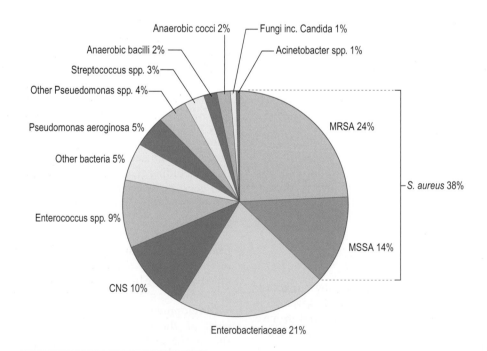

Anaerobic cocci 2% — Fungi inc. Candida 1%
Anaerobic bacilli 2% — Acinetobacter spp. 1%
Streptococcus spp. 3%
Other Pseuedomonas spp. 4%
Pseudomonas aeroginosa 5%
Other bacteria 5%
Enterococcus spp. 9%
CNS 10%
Enterobacteriaceae 21%
MRSA 24%
S. aureus 38%
MSSA 14%

CNS = coagulase negative staphylococci
MSSA = meticillin-sensitive *S. aureus*
MRSA = meticillin-resistant *S. aureus*
Total number of organisms reported = 5178

Fig. 39.4 Surgical site infection isolated organisms 2003–2007 (HPA, 2008).

Table 39.7 Recommendations for the prevention and treatment of surgical site infections (NICE, 2008a)

Category	Recommendation
Information for patients and carers	How to recognise a surgical site infection and what to do
Preoperative phase	Patient preparation: pre-op washing, hair removal, nasal MRSA decontamination and bowel preparation Antimicrobial prophylaxis guidance Staff preparation and theatre movement
Intra-operative phase	Operating team preparation Patient skin preparation Maintaining patient homeostasis Wound dressings
Post-operative phase	Dressing and cleansing the wound Antimicrobial treatment for surgical site infection Debridement of surgical site infections

Antimicrobial prophylaxis

In the early 1960s, it was demonstrated, using a guinea-pig model, that surgical-wound infection could be reduced by administration of an antimicrobial just before an incision was made, but the beneficial effect disappeared if antimicrobial administration was delayed by 3–4 h after the incision (Burke, 1961). Since then, many clinical trials have indicated the benefit of maintaining adequate antimicrobial tissue levels from the time of initial surgical incision until closure.

There are potential adverse consequences to the administration of antimicrobials for both the individual and the population. For the individual, side effects, ranging from antimicrobial associated diarrhoea or thrush to life-threatening allergic reactions, may arise. From the population perspective, the development of antimicrobial resistant bacteria is a concern. Antimicrobial prophylaxis should, therefore, only be offered to patients where there is evidence or, in the absence of evidence, expert consensus that the potential benefits of prophylaxis outweigh the risks.

The number of patients that need to be treated with antimicrobial agents to prevent one infection in the different types of surgery are presented in Table 39.8.

The infection risk associated with a particular surgical procedure and evidence of efficacy should be used to determine whether antimicrobial prophylaxis is to be administered. Not all surgical procedures warrant antimicrobial prophylaxis.

Choice of antimicrobial

Once it has been determined that antimicrobial prophylaxis is required, the next step is to select an appropriate agent(s). The choice of antimicrobial should take into account the following:

- Likely infecting organisms (procedure specific)
- Local susceptibility of potential pathogens to antimicrobials
- Pharmacokinetics, for example, penetration of antimicrobial to the site(s) in question
- Patient allergy to penicillins or other antimicrobials
- Administration time (bolus better than infusion)
- Drug cost
- Carriage of resistant organisms, for example, methicillin-resistant *S. aureus* (MRSA)
- Prevalence of *Clostridium difficile* infection in the hospital.

The majority of clinical trials that have demonstrated the benefit of antimicrobial prophylaxis are outdated, and probably do not reflect current surgical practice. First and second generation cephalosporins (cefazolin and cefuroxime) have been the mainstay of agents studied (Bratzler and Houck, 2004). There are advantages and disadvantages with using cephalosporins. The advantages include a low anaphylaxis risk, but they have the disadvantage of excessive or inadequate spectrum of cover depending on the operation (Morgan, 2006) and a strong association with *Clostridium difficile* infection. Many antimicrobials used in prophylaxis have not been extensively studied in clinical trials, but are selected on a theoretical basis of their antimicrobial spectrum (see Tables 39.9–39.11).

Table 39.8 Example of number needed to treat (NNT) for antimicrobial prophylaxis (SIGN, 2008)

Type of surgery	Operation	NNT	Outcome
Upper GI surgery	Stomach and duodenal surgery	5	Wound infection
Lower GI surgery	Colorectal surgery	4	Wound infection and intra-abdominal abscesses
Gynaecological	Caesarian section	19	Wound infection
Orthopaedic	Arthroplasty (hip replacement)	42	Hip infection

NNT is the number of patients that need to be treated to prevent one infection compared to receiving no antimicrobials.

Table 39.9 Antimicrobial susceptibility of common pathogens (adapted from SIGN, 2008)

Surgical site infection for a skin wound at any site

S. aureus	Highly variable (30–60% susceptible) to flucloxacillin therefore MRSA screening essential
Beta haemolytic Streptococci (BHS)	90% susceptible to penicillins, macrolides or clindamycin

Additional pathogens by site of infection
Head and neck surgery

Oral anaerobes	95% susceptible to metronidazole or co-amoxiclav

Operations below the diaphragm

Anaerobes	95% susceptible to metronidazole or co-amoxiclav
E. coli and other Enterobacteriaceae	80–90% of E. coli sensitive to cefuroxime, co-amoxiclav (or other β-lactam with inhibitor combination) or gentamicin

Insertion of a prosthesis, graft or shunt

Coagulase-negative Staph (CNS) S. aureus, diphtheroids	Two-thirds of CNS are methicillin-resistant, but β-lactams may still be used but preferably with a second agent with staphylococcal cover, for example, gentamicin, or a glycopeptide used instead. See above for S. aureus.

Timing and duration

Timing of antimicrobial administration is one of the most important aspects of prophylaxis regimens. Animal studies and latterly clinical observational studies have shown that prophylaxis is most effective when given immediately before an operation (within 30 min of induction of anaesthesia), so that antimicrobial activity is present for the duration of the operation and for about 4 h afterwards. Antimicrobials given too early prior to surgery are associated with prophylaxis failure, presumably because serum and tissue levels are not sustained during the surgical procedure. Similarly, for each hour antimicrobial administration was delayed after the start of the operation there was an increased rate of wound infection. This suggests bacterial replication, once commenced, cannot be eliminated by antimicrobial regimens designed for prophylaxis. The microbiological basis for these observations is likely to be that bacterial reproduction at a logarithmic rate follows a lag phase of relatively little increase in bacterial population. The lag phase for wound infection bacteria lasts typically 3–4 h. If bacteria inoculated into a wound can be killed or inhibited by antimicrobials given early, the immune system can kill the remaining organisms. However, if antimicrobials are given only when the growth curve has entered the logarithmic phase, the chances of successful prophylaxis are reduced.

Formerly, protocols for prophylaxis extended for several post-operative days. Now, single dose schedules are increasingly common with greater emphasis on ensuring immediate preoperative administration. As surgery may

Table 39.10 Micro-organisms commonly isolated from surgical site infections and prophylactic antimicrobials used in common surgical procedures (Prtak and Ridgway, 2009)

Surgical procedure	Most common micro-organisms	Examples of prophylactic IV antimicrobials
Gastro-intestinal	Bowel flora	
• Upper gastro-intestinal tract	S. aureus, Gram-negative bacilli	Co-amoxiclav or cefuroxime or gentamicin
• Biliary	S. aureus, Gram-negative bacilli (enterococci, anaerobes)	Co-amoxiclav or cefuroxime and metronidazole or gentamicin and metronidazole
• Colorectal/appendicectomy	S. aureus, Gram-negative bacilli, anaerobes	Co-amoxiclav or cefuroxime and metronidazole or gentamicin and metronidazole
Urogenital		
• Transrectal biopsy	S. aureus, Gram-negative bacilli, anaerobes	Co-amoxiclav or cefuroxime and metronidazole or gentamicin and metronidazole
• Transurethral resection of prostate	S. aureus, Gram-negative bacilli, enterococci	Co-amoxiclav or cefuroxime or gentamicin
Obstetric/gynaecological		
• Caesarean section	S. aureus, Gram-negative bacilli, streptococci (anaerobes)	Co-amoxiclav or cefuroxime and metronidazole
• Hysterectomy	S. aureus, Gram-negative bacilli, anaerobes	Co-amoxiclav or cefuroxime and metronidazole
Vascular		
• Reconstructive arterial surgery	Skin flora: primarily staphylococci	Co-amoxiclav or cefuroxime
• Amputation	S. aureus, anaerobes if gangrenous	Co-amoxiclav or cefuroxime and metronidazole or vancomycin and metronidazole
Orthopaedic		
• Joint replacement surgery	Skin flora: primarily staphylococci	Co-amoxiclav or cefuroxime or flucloxacillin and gentamicin

If patient has previously had MRSA or is at high risk (e.g. nursing home resident), use teicoplanin or other gylcopeptide.
For β-lactam allergy, replace co-amoxiclav or cefuroxime with teicoplanin +/− ciprofloxacin.

Table 39.11 Suggested cephalosporin-free antimicrobial prophylaxis for surgical site infection (adapted from SIGN, 2008)

Type of surgery	Suggested antimicrobials	Alternatives for penicillin allergy
Cardiothoracic	Flucloxacillin +/− gentamicin	Teicoplanin or Co-trimoxazole
ENT, maxillofacial and oral	Amoxicillin + metronidazole or Co-amoxiclav	Clarithromycin +/− metronidazole or Clindamycin
Gynaecology	Gentamicin + metronidazole	
Lower GI	Gentamicin + metronidazole	
Obstetrics	Co-amoxiclav	Clarithromycin +/− metronidazole or Clindamycin
Orthopaedic	Flucloxacillin +/− gentamicin	Teicoplanin or Co-trimoxazole
Thoracic	Flucloxacillin or Co-amoxiclav	
Upper GI	Gentamicin	
Urology	Gentamicin	
Vascular	Flucloxacillin +/− gentamicin (+metronidazole for amputations)	Co-trimoxazole or Teicoplanin

GI = gastro-intestial

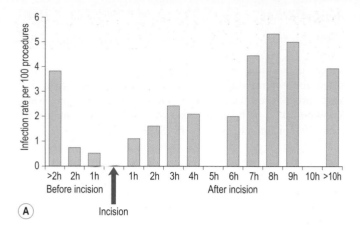

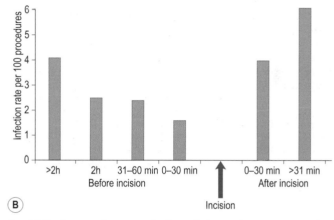

Fig. 39.5 Timing of antimicrobial prophylaxis administration and infection rate. Study A: The timing of prophylactic administration of antibiotics and the risk of surgical-wound infection (Classen et al., 1992). Study B: Trial to reduce antimicrobial prophylaxis errors (Steinberg et al., 2009). Taken from Mandell et al. (2010). Reproduced with kind permission from Elsevier.

be delayed at short notice, sometimes between the time the patient leaves the ward and arrives at the theatre, it is sensible for the administration of antimicrobials to be transferred from ward staff to the operating team when prophylaxis can be given around the time of induction of anaesthesia.

The optimum time to administer prophylactic antimicrobials before incision is probably 30 min, but national recommendations vary from less than 30 min (SIGN, 2008) to 60 min (NICE, 2008a) prior to incision. Figure 39.5 represents the two major studies undertaken to identify the optimum time for administration of prophylaxis. Both studies determined that post-incision administration of antimicrobials significantly increased the risk of surgical site infection.

Historically, the only occasion where antimicrobial administration has been delayed to after the incision is Caesarian section, where antimicrobials are given after cross clamping the umbilical cord to prevent drug delivery to the neonate. However, it is recognised that this does not provide the mother with adequate tissue levels at the time of incision and two studies have shown that antimicrobials can be given

safely before incision without adversely affecting the neonate (Sullivan et al., 2007; Thigpen et al., 2005).

When a tourniquet is used during orthopaedic procedures to minimise bleeding, the antimicrobial should be infused before inflating the tourniquet. This ensures adequate tissue levels are achieved at the site of surgery (Bratzler and Houck, 2004).

Certain practical issues should be considered when selecting an antimicrobial, for example, the requirement for intravenous infusion or safe intravenous bolus administration. An antimicrobial, which requires to be administered over a long period, for example, vancomycin 1 g over nearly 2 h, is much less likely to be given completely compared to teicoplanin, which is administered as a bolus.

To improve the timing of antimicrobial prophylaxis administration, the World Health Organisation (WHO) have introduced a question in their surgical safety checklist. The question *'Has antimicrobial prophylaxis been given within the last 60 minutes?'* is to be asked aloud before incision.

Repeat doses

Although single dose prophylaxis regimens are widely advocated (DH/HPA, 2008; NICE, 2008a; SIGN, 2008), many surgeons continue to use prolonged courses of 'prophylaxis' often for several days, without a clear evidence base. For some procedures, the optimum duration of prophylaxis is not known and 24–48 h prophylaxis is considered acceptable, for example, for open heart surgery (SIGN, 2008).

Where single dose prophylactic regimens have been adopted, the need for dosage adjustment in patients with reduced ability to excrete the drug (usually due to renal impairment) becomes unnecessary. This is because it is unlikely that single doses will have significant dose related adverse effects and idiosyncratic reactions are dose independent. Although the half-life of many drugs used is relatively short (1–2 h in normal volunteers), surgical patients often have slower clearance of antimicrobials from the blood. This concept will probably also hold true for prophylactic regimens lasting up to 48 h.

There are some situations in which it is necessary to prescribe additional doses of antibiotics to achieve the aim of adequate tissue levels at the time of wound closure. The additional doses may be needed when there is significant blood loss (>1500 mL) as plasma is effectively diluted by intra-operative transfusions and fluid replacement. Long operations may also need extra antimicrobial doses during the operation, but additional doses post-operatively do not provide an additional prophylactic benefit.

Antimicrobial administration by hospital theatre staff has practical implications for the route of administration. Ward-based administration of prophylaxis can be given orally if appropriate preparations exist, but this is impractical in sedated or unconscious patients. The oral route tends to suffer from variable absorption, especially in the presence of anaesthetic premedication, and this also makes it unsatisfactory. The intravenous route is the most reliable way of ensuring effective serum levels and is the only route supported by a substantial body of evidence.

A schematic model for the tissue concentration time profile of an antimicrobial agent used to prevent surgical site infection is presented in Fig. 39.6. After an initial dose of the antimicrobial agent, tissue concentrations reach their peak rapidly, with a subsequent decline over time. The goal of prophylaxis is for the antimicrobial tissue concentration to remain above the minimum inhibitory concentration (MIC) for the specific pathogens at the time of incision and throughout the procedure. The antimicrobial should be readministered during prolonged procedures to prevent a period where tissue concentrations are below the MIC (grey area). Failure to readminister antimicrobials appropriately may result in a period during which the wound is vulnerable. Recommendations for peri-operative re-dosing schedules are presented in Table 39.12. General guidance is to repeat doses of antimicrobials at intervals of 1–2 half-lives.

β-Lactam allergy

Penicillin and cephalosporin antibiotics have been the cornerstone of antimicrobial prophylaxis to prevent surgical site infections. Patients reported to be allergic to β-lactam

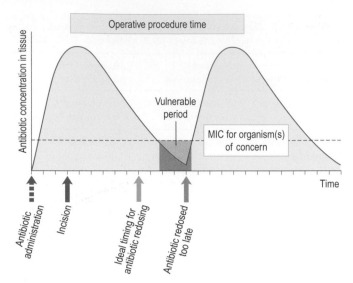

Fig. 39.6 Schematic presentation of tissue antibiotic concentration over time (Mandell et al., 2010). Reproduced with kind permission from Elsevier.

antibiotics or other antimicrobials need to be carefully assessed, as alternatives may not be optimal. Alternatives are often glycopeptides, for example, teicoplanin or vancomycin, which are more expensive, often need to be given by infusion (vancomycin) and can increase selection for resistant bacteria. The prevalence of penicillin allergy in the general population is unknown. The incidence of self reported penicillin allergy ranges from 1% to 10%, with the frequency of life-threatening anaphylaxis estimated at 0.01–0.05% (or 1–5 in 10,000). More than 80% of patients with a self reported allergy to penicillin have no evidence of IgE antibodies on skin testing. Important details of an allergic reaction include signs, symptoms, severity, history of prior reaction, time course of allergic event, temporal proximity to administered drug, route of administration, other medication being taken and adverse events to other medication (Park and Li, 2005). Reactions to penicillins and other β-lactams occur because of allergy to the parent compound or the metabolites. The cross sensitivity between penicillins and cephalosporins is unknown, but has been variably reported to be up to 10%. Early cephalosporin preparations were contaminated with penicillins probably leading to an over estimate of cross sensitivity (Saxon et al., 1987). As the generation of the cephalosporin increases, the likelihood of cross sensitivity decreases (Pichichero and Casey, 2007). Those with a penicillin allergy showed an increased risk of allergic reaction to a first generation cephalosporin. First generation cephalosporins share a similar side chain to penicillin and amoxicillin. However, cross sensitivity to second and third generation cephalosporins was lower. The different side chains appear to play a more dominant role than the β-lactam ring in allergy.

Recent prospective studies have shown that the cross-reactivity to carbapenems and monobactams is very small. It is around 1% for imipenem and meropenem, and no cross-reaction has been reported for aztreonam (Frumin and Gallagher, 2009).

Table 39.12 Time for peri-operative re-dosing of antimicrobials (adapted from Bratzler and Houck, 2004; Gilbert et al., 2009)

Antimicrobials	Peak serum level (mg/L)	Half-life (h)	Time to redose
Cefuroxime 1.5 g IV	100	1.5	3 to 4 h
Ciprofloxacin 400 mg IV	4.6	4	4 to 8 h
Co-amoxiclav 1.2 g	Unknown	1.4 AM/1.1 CL	3 to 4 h
Co-trimoxazole 960 mg IV	9 TMP/105 SMX	7–12 TMP/8–15 SMX	8 to 12 h
Flucloxacillin 1 g IV	120–350	0.5	3 h
Gentamicin	N/A as many doses used	2.5	3 to 6 h unless >2 mg/kg; then do not redose
Metronidazole 500 mg IV	20–25	6–14	6 to 8 h
Vancomycin 1 g IV	20–50	4–6	6 to 12 h
Teicoplanin 200 mg IV	20	90–157	12 h

AM, amoxicillin; CL, clavulanic acid; TMP, trimethoprim; SMX, sulphamethoxazole.

The increased use of penicillins rather than first or second generation cephalosporins for surgical site infection prophylaxis is increasing the potential for adverse reactions. In addition, the current nomenclature for penicillin combinations, for example, co-amoxiclav, can often make it more difficult for staff to recognise penicillin containing antimicrobials. Current guidance on the use of β-lactams in patients with penicillin allergy is detailed in Table 39.13.

Topical or local antimicrobial prophylaxis

Many surgical procedures involving the use of implants or prostheses now use topical antimicrobials to prevent late surgical site infection. Examples include antimicrobial loaded cement for fixing hip and knee joint replacements into bone. Gentamicin is the only antimicrobial in commercially available products in the UK. Surgeons do add other antimicrobial agents, especially if replacing an infected prosthesis with choice based on culture and sensitivities.

In vascular surgery, synthetic grafts bonded with or soaked in rifampicin are frequently used, despite evidence showing that there was no decrease in infection rates at 1 month and

2 years (Stewart et al., 2006). There is some evidence to support the local delivery of gentamicin into wounds via collagen fleece impregnated with gentamicin and further research into this was recommended (NICE, 2008a); however, two recent randomised controlled trials have shown it not to be efficacious (Bennett-Guerrero et al., 2010a,b) The use of topical cefotaxime in contaminated surgery has been shown not to decrease peritonitis, and should not be used.

Case Studies

Case 39.1

A patient is due to have an elective total hip replacement. As part of the routine, pre-admission screening is done, during which swab samples are taken. The patient is identified as being MRSA positive. The patient receives a five-day course of nasal mupirocin and topical chlorhexidine washes as 'decolonisation therapy' prior to the admission. The unit normally uses single dose co-amoxiclav as prophylaxis.

Question

Should there be a change to the routine antimicrobial prophylaxis for this patient?

Answer

A change to the routine antimicrobial prophylaxis should be recommended because co-amoxiclav is not active against MRSA. The commonly used terms 'decolonisation therapy' and 'MRSA eradication' falsely give the impression that this regimen eradicates MRSA carriage. In reality, it should be called 'suppression therapy' because these agents reduce the numbers of bacteria present

Table 39.13 Guidance on the use of β-lactam antibiotics in patients with penicillin allergy recommended by BNF (Joint Formulary Committee, 2010)

Allergic reaction	Action
Immediate hypersensitivity reaction to a penicillin	Avoid penicillins and cephalosporins
Minor rash – localised or widespread but delayed (>72 h)	Avoid penicillins, but cephalosporins are safe to use

but often fail to eradicate MRSA carriage. *S. aureus* is still the predominant cause of surgical site infection and this patient remains at risk of an MRSA surgical site infection. As a consequence an agent that is active against MRSA should be used. Glycopeptides are the recommended antimicrobial class in this situation and there are two options: teicoplanin and vancomycin. Vancomycin needs to be given as an infusion at a maximum rate of 10 mg/min, which means that administering a 1-g dose will take nearly 2 h and may be impractical before skin incision. Teicoplanin can be given as a bolus, so is the best choice. Teicoplanin 400 mg intravenously can therefore be used instead of vancomycin 1 g intravenous. Where bone cement is required to secure the prosthesis, a commercially prepared bone cement containing gentamicin should also be used. Ideally, all antimicrobial prophylaxis guidelines or protocols should contain an option for MRSA positive patients. Administration of appropriate regimens is facilitated by MRSA screening of all elective patients.

Case 39.2

A patient with a severe allergy to penicillin is admitted for a hemicolectomy for cancer of the colon. The unit uses a single dose co-amoxiclav regime as antimicrobial prophylaxis for large bowel surgery.

Question

The junior hospital doctor asks your advice as to the antimicrobials to use instead of co-amoxiclav? What advice would you give?

Answer

Colorectal surgery still carries one of the highest surgical site infection rates of up to 10% for elective procedures. The usual bacteria found in these surgical site infections are *S. aureus*, gram-negative bacilli (e.g. *E. coli*) and anaerobes. Options for treatment include gentamicin and metronidazole, or ciprofloxacin and metronidazole. Centres that have a problem with *Clostridium difficile* infection may prefer to use gentamicin and metronidazole. There is evidence for the use of single dose regimes.

Case 39.3

A 73-year-old lady is seen in pre-admission clinic for assessment prior to a knee replacement. She has recently had *Clostridium difficile* infection in the community after being treated with

a 1-week course of co-amoxiclav. She is asymptomatic now. The surgical team is reluctant to use its usual antimicrobial prophylaxis regime of co-amoxiclav, or cefuroxime or ciprofloxacin.

Question

The anaesthetist assessing the patient in pre-assessment clinic asks your advice on what to prescribe. The lady is currently being screened for MRSA. What advice would you give?

Answer

The most common pathogens in knee replacement surgical site infections are *S. aureus* and coagulase-negative staphylococci, although infection rates are low (0.2%, e.g. in Scotland). Depending on the result of the MRSA screening test, there will be different answers. If the lady is colonised with MRSA, she could receive a single dose of teicoplanin. Options for prophylaxis include flucloxacillin with gentamicin or teicoplanin, although the latter does not cover gram-negative bacteria. The use of gentamicin-containing cement would be recommended.

Case 39.4

A 72-year-old man is due for elective transurethral resection of the prostate (TURP) and is currently well with no signs of a urinary tract infection. Routine prophylaxis for surgical site infections on the unit is co-amoxiclav. The patient is known to have had a mitral valve replacement 2 years ago.

Question

You are asked whether the antimicrobial prophylaxis should be amended to cover this? What advice would you give?

Answer

NICE guidelines no longer recommend prophylaxis for patients at risk of endocarditis undergoing investigations involving the oral, gastro-intestinal or urogenital tract, in the absence of local infection (NICE, 2008b). The usual prophylaxis for this regimen should be recommended. If the patient had a urinary tract infection, this should ideally be treated before surgery.

References

Astagneau, P., Rioux, C., Golliot, F., et al., 2001. Morbidity and mortality associated with surgical site infections: results from the 1997–1999 INCISO surveillance. J. Hosp. Infect. 48, 267–274.

Bennett-Guerrero, E., Pappas, T.N., Koltun, W.A., et al., 2010a. Gentamicin-collagen sponge for infection prophylaxis in colorectal surgery. N. Engl. J. Med. 363, 1038–1049.

Bennett-Guerrero, E., Ferguson, T.B., Lin, M., et al., 2010b. Effect of an implantable gentamicin-collagen sponge on sternal wound infections following cardiac surgery: a randomized trial. J. Am. Med. Assoc. 304, 755–762.

Bratzler, D.W., Houck, P.M., 2004. Antimicrobial prophylaxis for surgery: an advisory statement from the National Surgical Infection Prevention Project. Clin. Infect. Dis. 38, 1706–1715.

Burke, J., 1961. The effective period of preventative antibiotic action in experimental incisions and dermal lesions. Surgery 50, 161–168.

Classen, D., Evans, R.S., Pestotnik, S.L., et al., 1992. The timing of prophylactic administration of antibiotics and the risk of surgical-wound infection. N. Engl. J. Med. 326 (5) 281–286.

Coello, R.C.A., Wilson, J., Ward, V., et al., 2005. Adverse impact of surgical site infections in English hospitals. J. Hosp. Infect. 60, 93–103.

Culver, D.H., Horan, T.C., Gaynes, R.P., et al., 1991. Surgical wound infection rates by wound class, operative procedure, and patient risk index. Am. J. Med. 91, S152–S157.

Department of Health and Health Protection Agency, 2008. *Clostridium difficile* infection: how to deal with the problem. DH/HPA, London. Available at http://www.hpa.nhs.uk/web/HPAwebFile/HPAweb_C/1232006607827.

Donlan, R.M., Costerton, J.W., 2002. Biofilms: survival mechanisms of clinically relevant microorganisms. Clin. Microbiol. Rev. 15, 167–193.

Frumin, J., Gallagher, J.C., 2009. Allergic cross-sensitivity between penicillin, carbapenem, and monobactam antibiotics: what are the chances? Ann. Pharmacother. 43, 304–315.

Gastmeier, P.S.D., Brandt, C., et al., 2005. Reduction of orthopaedic wound infections in 21 hospitals. Arch. Orthop. Trauma Surg. 125, 526–530.

Gilbert, D.N., Moellering, R.C., Eliopoulos, G.M., et al., 2009. Sanford Guide to Antimicrobial Therapy, 39th ed. Sperryville, Virginia.

Health and Social Care Information Centre, 2009. Hospital episodes statistics (England): main procedures and interventions: Summary, 2008–09. Department of Health, London. Available at http://www.hesonline.nhs.uk.

Health Protection Scotland, 2009. Surveillance of surgical site infection. 2009 Annual report. Health Protection Scotland, Glasgow. Available at http://www.documents.hps.scot.nhs.uk/hai/sshaip/publications/ssi/ssi-2008.pdf.

HIS/ICNA, 2007. The third prevalence survey of healthcare associated infections in acute hospitals 2006. Hospital Infection Society and Infection Control Nurses Association. Available at http://www.dh.gov.uk/prod_consum_dh/groups/dh_digitalassets/documents/digitalasset/dh_078389.pdf.

Health Protection Agency, 2008. Surveillance of healthcare associated infections report 2008. HPA, London. Available at http://www.hpa.nhs.uk/web/HPAwebFile/HPAweb_C/1216193833496.

Horan, T.C., Culver, D.H., Gaynes, R.P., 1993. Surgical Site Infection (ssi) risk stratum rates: What they are and how to compare them using aggregated data from the National Nosocomial Infections Surveillance (NNIS) System. Am. J. Infect. Control 21(2), 99.

Joint Formulary Committee, 2010. British National Formulary, 60th ed. British Medical Association and Royal Pharmaceutical Society, London.

Kaye, K.S., Schmit, K., Pieper, C., et al., 2005. The effect of increasing age on the risk of surgical site infection. J. Infect. Dis. 191, 1056–1062.

Latham, R., Lancaster, A.D., Covington, J.F., et al., 2001. The association of diabetes and glucose control with surgical site infections among cardiothoracic surgery patients. Infect. Control Hosp. Epidemiol. 22, 607–612.

Mandell, G.L., Bennett, J.E., Dolin, R., 2010. Principles and Practice of Infectious Diseases, seventh ed. Elsevier, Philadelphia.

Mangram, A.J.H.T., Pearson, M.L., et al., 1999. Guideline for prevention of surgical site prevention, 1999. Hospital Infection Control Practices Advisory Committee. Infect. Control Hosp. Epidemiol. 20, 250–255.

Morgan, M., 2006. Surgery and cephalosporins: a marriage made in heaven or time for divorce? Intern. J. Surg. 8. Available at http://www.ispub.com/journal/the_internet_journal_of_surgery/volume_8_number_1/article/surgery_and_cephalosporins_a_marriage_made_in_heaven_or_time_for_divorce.html.

Myles, P.S., Iacono, G.A., Hunt, J.O., et al., 2002. Risk of respiratory complications and wound infection in patients undergoing ambulatory surgery: smokers versus nonsmokers. Anesthesiology 97, 842–847.

National Institute for Health and Clinical Excellence, 2008a. Surgical site infection: prevention and treatment of surgical site infection. Clinical Guideline 74, NICE, London. Available at http://www.nice.org.uk/nicemedia/pdf/CG74NICEGuideline.pdf.

National Institute for Health and Clinical Excellence, 2008b. Prophylaxis against infective endocarditis: antimicrobial prophylaxis against infective endocarditis in adults and children undergoing interventional procedures. NICE, London. Available at http://www.nice.org.uk/nicemedia/pdf/CG64NICEguidance.pdf.

Park, M.A., Li, J.T., 2005. Diagnosis and management of penicillin allergy. Mayo Clin. Proc. 80, 405–410.

Pichichero, M.E., Casey, J.R., 2007. Safe use of selected cephalosporins in penicillin-allergic patients: a meta-analysis. Otolaryngol. Head Neck Surg. 136, 340–347.

Prtak, L.E., Ridgway, E.J., 2009. Prophylactic antibiotics in surgery. Surgery (Oxford) 27, 431–434.

Publics Account Committee, 2009. Reducing healthcare associated infections in hospitals in England. House of Commons, Hansard, London.

Saxon, A., Beall, G.N., Rohr, A.S., et al., 1987. Immediate hypersensitivity reactions to beta-lactam antibiotics. Ann. Intern. Med. 107, 204–215.

Scottish Intercollegiate Guideline Network, 2008. Antibiotic prophylaxis in surgery. SIGN, Edinburgh. Available at http://www.sign.ac.uk/pdf/sign104.pdf.

Steinberg, J.P., Braun, B.I., Hellinger, W.W., et al., 2009. Timing of antimicrobial prophylaxis and the risk of surgical site infections: results from the trial to reduce antimicrobial prophylaxis errors. Annals of Surgery 250 (1), 10–16.

Stewart, A., Eyers, P.S., Earnshaw, J.J., 2006. Prevention of infection in arterial reconstruction. Cochrane Database of Systematic Reviews, Issue 3, Art No. CD003073. DOI: 10.1002/14651858.CD003073.pub2. Available at http://onlinelibrary.wiley.com/o/cochrane/clsysrev/articles/CD003073/frame.html.

Sullivan, S.A., Smith, T., Chang, E., et al., 2007. Administration of cefazolin prior to skin incision is superior to cefazolin at cord clamping in preventing postcesarean infectious morbidity: a randomized, controlled trial. Am. J. Obstet. Gynecol. 196, 455e1–455e5.

Thigpen, B.D., Hood, W.A., Chauhan, S., et al., 2005. Timing of prophylactic antibiotic administration in the uninfected laboring gravida: a randomized clinical trial. Am. J. Obstet. Gynecol. 192, 1864–1868. Discussion pp. 1868–1871.

Further references

Anderson, D.J., Kaye, K.S., Classen, D., et al., 2008. Strategies to prevent surgical site infections in acute care hospitals. Infect. Control Hosp. Epidemiol. 29 (s1), S51–S56.

Nelson, R.L., Glenny, A.M., Song, F., 2009. Antimicrobial prophylaxis for colorectal surgery. Cochrane Database of Systematic Reviews, Issue 1, Art No. CD001181. DOI: 10.1002/14651858.CD001181.pub3. Available at http://onlinelibrary.wiley.com/o/cochrane/clsysrev/articles/CD001181/frame.html.

40 Tuberculosis

L. K. Nehaul

Key points

- In 2008, there were an estimated 9 million cases of tuberculosis (TB) and 2 million deaths from the disease worldwide.
- One-third of the world's population is infected with the tubercle bacillus.
- Adequate and effective treatment is essential to treat the individual, control the spread of TB and minimise the occurrence of drug-resistant disease.
- TB is caused by infection with *Mycobacterium tuberculosis*, *M. bovis* and *M. africanum*. *M. tuberculosis* accounts for around 99% of isolates in the UK.
- TB infection usually occurs by the respiratory route.
- People with HIV infection have an increased risk of developing active TB disease if co-infected with tubercle bacilli.
- Certain medical risk factors increase the risk of TB.
- Most treatment regimens in the developed world are of 6 months' duration and contain isoniazid, rifampicin and pyrazinamide, with ethambutol or streptomycin.
- Rifampicin, isoniazid and pyrazinamide are all potentially hepatotoxic. Isoniazid may cause a dose-dependent peripheral neuropathy, while ocular toxicity is the most important side effect of ethambutol.
- Multidrug-resistant TB is a problem in many parts of the world; extensively-drug-resistant TB was first reported in 2006.

Introduction

Tuberculosis (TB) is a bacterial infection, treatable by anti-TB drugs. It is a global problem, with the incidence varying across the world. In 1993, an increase in reported cases of TB in countries across all continents led the World Health Organization (WHO) to declare TB a global emergency. The burden of TB in many countries is compounded in those who have co-infection with the human immunodeficiency virus (HIV). Of additional concern has been the increase in multidrug-resistant tuberculosis (MDR-TB), with outbreaks in different parts of the world. In 2006, the emergence of extensively drug-resistant tuberculosis (XDR-TB) was first reported. The treatment of drug-resistant TB is complex, costlier and of a longer duration than drug-susceptible cases.

Adequate and effective treatment is essential, both clinically for patients and also to control TB, as the BCG vaccine does not prevent infection. Successful control depends on a close working collaboration between clinical, microbiological, pharmacy, infection control and public health teams in managing patients and their contacts, and a shared understanding with primary care teams as to the role of all health professionals involved in TB.

Clinical and public health practice for bringing TB under control in the UK is underpinned by guidance from National Institute for Health and Clinical Excellence (2006) and the Joint Committee on Vaccination and Immunisation (Department of Health, 2006).

Aetiology

TB is caused by tubercle bacilli, which belong to the genus *Mycobacterium*. These form a large group but only three relatives are obligate parasites that can cause TB disease. They are part of the *Mycobacterium tuberculosis* complex. The UK data for 2008 show that *M. tuberculosis* was isolated in 99% of confirmed cases, *M. bovis* in 0.4% and *M. africanum* in 0.5% that year (Health Protection Agency, 2009).

Mycobacterium species include:

- *M. tuberculosis* complex*: M. tuberculosis, M. bovis, M. africanum*
- *Mycobacteria other than tuberculosis:* Around 15 are recognised *as pathogenic to humans and some cause* pulmonary disease resembling TB. They have been found in soil, milk and water. They are also referred to as atypical mycobacteria.
- *Mycobacterium leprae:* The cause of leprosy.

Clinical aspects

Infection with tubercle bacilli occurs in the vast majority of cases by the respiratory route. The lung lesions caused by infection commonly heal, leaving no residual changes except occasional pulmonary or tracheobronchial lymph node calcification (Heymann, 2004). About 5% of those initially infected will develop active primary disease (Hawker et al., 2005). This can include pulmonary disease, through local progression in the lungs, or by lymphatic or haematogenous spread of bacilli, to pulmonary, meningeal or other extrapulmonary involvement, or lead to disseminated disease (miliary TB). In the other 95%, the primary lesion heals without intervention but in at least one-half of patients, the bacilli survive in a latent form, which may then reactivate later in life. Infants, adolescents and immunosuppressed people are more susceptible to the more serious forms of TB such as miliary or meningeal TB.

Pulmonary (respiratory) TB is more common in the UK than extrapulmonary (non-respiratory) TB. Sites of extrapulmonary disease include the pleura, lymph nodes, pericardium, kidneys, meninges, bones and joints, larynx, skin, intestines, peritoneum and eyes. In the UK, the lymph nodes are the most common site for extrapulmonary disease. In 2008, 55% of cases were pulmonary and 21% involved the extrathoracic lymph nodes.

Pulmonary TB may arise from exogenous reinfection or endogenous reactivation of a latent focus remaining from the initial infection. If untreated, about 65% of patients will die within 5 years, the majority of these within 2 years. Completion of chemotherapy using drugs to which the tubercle bacilli are sensitive almost always results in a cure, even with HIV infection.

Incubation period

The incubation period from infection to demonstrable primary lesion or significant tuberculin reaction ranges from 2 to 10 weeks. Latent infection may persist for a lifetime. HIV infection appears to shorten the interval for the development of clinically apparent TB.

Transmission

Transmission occurs through exposure to tubercle bacilli in air-borne droplet nuclei produced by people with pulmonary or respiratory tract TB during expiratory efforts such as coughing or sneezing. In general, only the respiratory forms of TB (tuberculosis of the larynx is highly contagious but rarely seen in the UK) are infectious. Most infections are acquired from adults with post-primary pulmonary TB. The greatest risk of infection is to close, prolonged contacts, mainly household contacts. Between 90% and 95% of cases of TB in children are non-infectious (Davies, 2003). TB cannot be acquired from individuals with latent TB infection (LTBI).

Patients should be considered infectious if they have sputum smear-positive pulmonary disease (i.e. they produce sputum containing sufficient tubercle bacilli to be seen on microscopic examination of a sputum smear) or laryngeal TB. Patients with smear-negative pulmonary disease (three sputum samples) are less infectious than those who are smear positive. The relative transmission rate from smear-negative compared with smear-positive patients has been estimated to be 0.22 (British Thoracic Society, 2000).

Risk groups

Certain groups are at increased risk of LTBI and possibly TB disease if exposed. These include:

- close contacts of patients with TB, especially those with sputum smear-positive pulmonary disease

> **Box 40.1** Examples of factors that increase risk of developing active tuberculosis if infected
>
> - HIV positive
> - Injecting drug users
> - Solid organ transplantation, jejunoileal bypass or gastrectomy
> - Haematological malignancy, for example leukaemia and lymphomas
> - Chronic renal failure or receiving haemodialysis
> - Receiving anti-TNFα treatment
> - Silicosis

- casual contacts (e.g. work colleagues) if they are immunosuppressed
- people from countries with a high incidence of TB (40/100,000 population or greater).

People with certain medical conditions are at increased risk of developing active TB if they have LTBI. These medical risk factors are set out in Box 40.1.

Impact of HIV infection

People with HIV infection have an increased risk of developing TB if exposed to infection. The estimated annual risk of TB in those with HIV infection and TB co-infection is around 10% as opposed to a 10% lifetime chance in someone infected with TB, but not HIV.

Drug-resistant TB

MDR-TB is caused by bacteria that are resistant to at least isoniazid and rifampicin, the most effective anti-TB drugs. MDR-TB results from either primary infection with resistant bacteria or may develop in the course of a patient's treatment.

XDR-TB is a form of TB caused by bacteria that are resistant to isoniazid and rifampicin, that is, MDR-TB, as well as any fluoroquinolone and any of the second-line anti-TB injectable drugs including amikacin, kanamycin or capreomycin (WHO, 2010).

Epidemiology

Epidemiology is a measure of the occurrence of a disease in different populations. It helps to identify population groups at increased risk of TB. The key measures for TB are the number of new cases in a specified period of time, usually 1 year, and the incidence rates, that is, new cases per 100,000 of the population. Incidence rates are a good comparative measure of differences in the occurrence of TB between countries or different sub-groups in the population, as they take into account the size of those groups. TB surveillance, which involves monitoring its occurrence and epidemiology, is an essential component of TB control programmes, because it helps to evaluate their effectiveness in reducing disease rates.

Global

Globally, it is estimated that TB causes about 2 million deaths worldwide each year. One-third of the world's population is infected with the tubercle bacillus. It is becoming the leading cause of death among HIV-positive people. Over 4 million cases of TB disease are notified annually although the estimated number of new cases is put at 9 million. The majority of cases occur in poor countries in the southern hemisphere (WHO, 2009).

The numbers of cases estimated to have occurred in 2008, globally and by WHO region, is presented in Table 40.1. Most cases of TB are in South East Asia, although the highest rates are in Africa.

In 2008, it was estimated that 440,000 people had MDR-TB worldwide, and one-third of these died. The brunt of the MDR-TB epidemic is borne by Asia, with almost 50% of cases worldwide estimated to occur in China and India. However, in some areas of the world, up to one in four people have drug-resistant TB. For example, 28% of all people newly diagnosed with TB in one region of North-Western Russia had the multidrug-resistant form of the disease (WHO, 2010).

UK

In the UK, since the late 1980s, there have been changes in the epidemiology of TB. Following a decrease in notifications over several decades, from the late 1980s cases of TB started to increase again.

A total of 8655 cases were reported in 2008 (Health Protection Agency, 2009). The overall rate across all population groups was 14.1 per 100,000 population. Of all cases, 39% occurred in the London region, where the rate was 44.3 per 100,000 population. Nineteen primary care organisations in England had a rate of 40 per 100,000 or over, all of which were in major urban areas. Rates of TB in England outside London varied from 5.7 per 100,000 in South-West England to 18.7 per 100,000 in the West Midlands. Incidence rates per 100,000 population were 8.7 in Scotland, 5.8 in Wales and 3.3 in Northern Ireland. The majority of cases (72%) were in the population born outside the UK and in those aged 16–44 years (61%). The TB rate was higher in those born abroad than among those born in the UK (86 compared with 4.4 per 100,000). This reflected higher rates of TB in people from high-incidence countries, mainly South Asia. The risk of TB is highest in the 5 years after arrival in the UK. TB can also occur as a travel-related disease in UK residents from high-incidence countries, who return to visit their country of birth and are exposed to TB. The numbers of cases by region in England, Wales and Northern Ireland, in 2008, is shown in Table 40.2.

Diagnosis

Symptoms

The symptoms and signs of TB include:

- Cough for 3 weeks or more/productive cough
- Sputum usually mucopurulent or purulent
- Haemoptysis not always a feature
- Fever may be associated with night sweats
- Tiredness
- Weight loss variable
- Anorexia variable
- Malaise.

Awareness of the disease

Awareness of TB on the part of health care professionals and of people in high-risk communities is essential to its control. Early diagnosis, especially of pulmonary TB, followed by prompt commencement of treatment can reduce the period of infectivity to other people, especially susceptible contacts, who might be at risk of the more serious forms of TB disease. Such contacts can include children in nurseries or schools or immunosuppressed patients in a hospital setting. Health care

Table 40.1 Estimated epidemiological burden of tuberculosis incidence globally and by WHO region (*Source*: WHO, 2010)

WHO region	Numbers (000s), 2008 (lower and upper bounds)	Rates per 100,000 population, 2008 (lower and upper bounds)
Africa	2800 (2700–3000)	350 (330–370)
Americas	280 (260–300)	31 (29–33)
Eastern Mediterranean	650 (580–740)	110 (99–130)
Europe	430 (400–460)	48 (45–51)
South-East Asia	3200 (2800–3700)	180 (160–210)
Western Pacific	1900 (1700–2200)	110 (95–130)
Global	9400 (8900–9900)	140 (130–150)

Table 40.2 Tuberculosis case reports and rates by UK region/country 2008 (adapted from Health Protection Agency, 2009)

UK region/country	Number of cases	Rate per 100,000 population
London	3376	44.3
West Midlands	1012	18.7
North West	745	10.8
Yorkshire and the Humber	647	12.4
East Midlands	517	11.7
South East	719	8.6
East of England	478	8.3
South West	297	5.7
North East	179	7.0
England	7970	15.5
Scotland	452	8.7
Wales	174	5.8
Northern Ireland	59	3.3

professionals should be particularly alert to symptoms suggestive of TB in health care workers or people working in childcare or institutional settings, and initiate investigations at the earliest possible opportunity. Such action can lead to the diagnosis of TB before it becomes infectious, thereby protecting vulnerable contacts.

TB should be considered in the differential diagnoses of patients with a chronic cough for which there is no other likely cause, or in individuals with chest infections not responding to treatment.

Clinical diagnosis

The clinical diagnosis of TB disease is based on the symptoms and signs in the patient together with chest radiography, microscopy of sputum (for acid-fast bacilli) followed by culture and tuberculin skin testing. Blood-based immunological tests, introduced in the last few years, will play an increasingly important role in TB diagnosis. These tests can distinguish between TB infection and previous BCG vaccination.

Investigations

Investigations are essential to confirm clinically suspected TB and should be arranged even if the diagnosis is strongly suspected on clinical grounds. Microbiological tests are crucial, especially for pulmonary disease, as they facilitate both the clinical and public health management of TB and ensure the appropriate implementation of infection control procedures for cases managed in healthcare settings.

Microbiological

Microbiological investigations are undertaken to assess the infectious state of the patient, and distinguish between infection with mycobacteria causing TB and other mycobacteria. They also determine the drug-susceptibility patterns of the infecting organisms, to ensure that the drugs prescribed will be effective in treating the individual patient. Investigations comprise microscopy, culture, drug-susceptibility testing and strain typing.

Direct microscopy of sputum is the simplest and quickest method of detecting the infectious patient, by looking for acid-fast bacilli. A minimum of three sputum samples, one of which should be early morning, should be collected from patients with suspected respiratory TB.

Direct microscopy is not as useful in non-pulmonary disease, any specimens taken should be sent for culture.

If conventional culture methods are used, such as the Lowenstein–Jensen medium, growth may take up to 6 weeks. Modern liquid cultures can produce results more quickly. Polymerase chain reaction (PCR)-based tests can also detect *M. tuberculosis* complex in clinical specimens.

A rapid test is available for assessing rifampicin resistance in individuals thought to have drug-resistant TB. A positive result indicates the need to assess susceptibility to other first-line anti-TB drugs. Drug-susceptibility testing still needs to be done on isolates grown on culture media.

DNA fingerprinting, or strain typing, is useful in the public health management of TB. In 2010, a new method, mycobacterial interspersed repetitive unit/variable number of tandem repeats (MIRU/VNTR) 24-loci strain typing, became available in the UK. Strain typing will help in establishing links between cases not previously identified, disproving links between apparent clusters of cases, and also in detecting cross-contamination in laboratories.

Tuberculin testing

Tuberculin testing is used to detect LTBI. Only the Mantoux test is now used but it should be carried out by health care professionals trained and experienced in its use. The standard Mantoux test consists of an intradermal injection of 2 TU of Statens Serum Institute (SSI) tuberculin RT23 in 0.1 mL solution for injection. In this test, 0.1 mL of the appropriate solution is injected intradermally, usually on the forearm, so that a bleb of around 7 mm is produced. The results are read 48–72 h later, although a valid reading can be obtained up to 96 h later. The transverse diameter of the area of induration is measured with a ruler and the result recorded in millimetres.

The interpretation of the test will depend on the clinical circumstances, including a past history of TB or exposure to TB. A diameter of induration of less than 6 mm is negative, that is, there is no significant hypersensitivity to tuberculin protein.

In the absence of specific risk factors for TB, induration of between 6 and 15 mm diameter may be due to previous TB infection, or BCG vaccination or exposure to non-tuberculous mycobacteria. An induration of more than 15 mm is strongly suggestive of TB infection or disease.

Chest radiography

The chest radiograph is a non-specific diagnostic tool, as TB may present as virtually any abnormality on chest radiography. This is why microbiological evidence of confirmation should be sought. Pulmonary TB may appear as broncho-pneumonia with confluent shadowing, without cavitation. Cavitation may be seen, the incidence can vary between 10% and 30%. Uncharacteristic radiological patterns may occur in the presence of HIV infection (Davies, 2003).

Diagnosis in people with HIV

TB can occur early in the course of HIV infection and may therefore be diagnosed before the patient is known to be HIV positive. The possibility of HIV infection in people with TB should therefore be considered, and testing for the virus is appropriate in those with risk factors for HIV.

Early in the course of HIV infection, before serious immunodeficiency occurs, TB is more likely to present with typical clinical features, and a positive tuberculin skin test, with cavitation and/or pleural disease on chest radiography. In the late stages of HIV infection, atypical presentations are more likely with unusual chest findings and extrapulmonary disease. The chest radiograph may be normal in up to 40% of cases.

Public health action

TB is a statutorily notifiable communicable disease in the UK. Cases should be notified on clinical suspicion by the attending doctor to the 'Proper Officer' for communicable disease control of the local authority where the patient resides. This is usually the local Consultant in Communicable Disease Control. In Scotland, notifications are made to the Health Board. Notification enables public health action to be initiated and involves investigation of prolonged, close contacts who might be at risk of infection, mainly those living in the same household as the patient, to assess them for LTBI or active TB disease. It may also enable the source of the infection to be found and treated.

Latent TB infection (LTBI) is not notifiable. Public health action is not taken for infections caused by 'mycobacteria other than TB'.

Treatment

In treating TB, a number of factors are important:

- Choice of drugs
- Length of treatment

- Co-morbidity especially HIV infection, liver and renal diseases
- Adherence to treatment by the patient.

It is important to tailor the management of the patient according to his or her situation, rather than just focus on the drug treatment of TB, as other factors in the patient's life may affect adherence.

Drug treatment

Treatment with anti-TB drugs has two main purposes:

- to cure people with TB, provided the bacilli are drug sensitive;
- to control TB, by either preventing the development of infectious forms or reducing the period of infectivity of people with infectious disease.

TB had started to decline in the UK before the advent of chemotherapy, probably due to improved nutrition and social conditions. With the advent of effective anti-TB chemotherapy, patients no longer needed treatment in a sanatorium. Results with regimens containing isoniazid together with *p*-aminosalicylate (PAS) or ethambutol, and sometimes streptomycin, gave excellent results. Treatment was required for 18–24 months if relapse was to be prevented. The availability of pyrazinamide and, more importantly, rifampicin made shorter courses of treatment a possibility. Most regimens in the developed world now contain isoniazid and rifampicin, which are the two most important drugs. These are prescribed together with pyrazinamide and possibly with another agent, such as ethambutol.

Bacterial characteristics

There are three populations of the *M. tuberculosis* (MTB) organism. The first population is that of the actively growing extracellular bacilli. Large numbers of bacilli can grow extracellularly in pulmonary cavities within liquefied caseous debris. This is the population in which drug resistance develops most rapidly. The second population consists of slow-growing or intermittently growing bacilli, which are inside macrophages. These are fewer in number, but the intracellular environment is acidic and many drugs are not active in these conditions. The third population is made up of slower-growing bacilli, which grow in solid caseous material. This environment is neutral in pH, but the penetration of drugs into this area can be compromised by a poor blood supply.

Rifampicin is the only drug that is bactericidal against all three populations. Isoniazid, streptomycin and the other aminoglycosides are bactericidal against extracellular bacilli. Isoniazid is also bactericidal against intracellular organisms. Pyrazinamide is bactericidal only against intracellular organisms and works well in an acidic pH. All other first-line TB drugs are bacteriostatic. Of the alternative drugs, which can be used in the treatment of drug-resistant TB, the quinolones have the highest bactericidal activity against *M. tuberculosis*.

When considering a treatment regimen for TB, it must be remembered that viable bacilli for slow-growing or intermittently growing populations may persist if drugs are not continued for an adequate period of time. The patient's condition can then relapse after chemotherapy is completed.

Treatment

The recommended standard treatment regimen for respiratory and most other forms of TB in the UK is:

- rifampicin, isoniazid, pyrazinamide and ethambutol for the initial 2 months (initial phase)
- a further 4 months of rifampicin and isoniazid (continuation phase).

A longer period of treatment than the standard 6 months is needed for meningeal TB and where there is direct spinal cord involvement.

Patients should be started on the standard treatment regimen on clinical diagnosis and the doses of the first-line anti-tuberculous agents are shown in Table 40.3. The drugs used can be changed if drug-susceptibility testing shows evidence of resistance.

The purpose of the concurrent use of four drugs in the initial phase is to reduce the bacterial population as rapidly as possible and prevent the emergence of drug-resistant bacteria. In general, daily dosing schedules are recommended. Combination tablets can be used and have the advantage of preventing accidental or inadvertent single drug therapy, which can lead to acquired drug resistance within weeks in active TB. It is important, however, to ensure the combination product contains the required dose of the constituent drugs.

Patients with suspected drug reactions or drug-resistant TB should always be referred back to the specialist physician and the healthcare team supervising their treatment.

Respiratory TB

Respiratory TB is defined as active TB affecting any of the following:

- lungs
- pleural cavity
- mediastinal lymph nodes
- larynx.

The standard 6-month regimen, as set out earlier, is recommended for the treatment of active respiratory TB in:

- adults not known to be HIV positive
- adults who are HIV positive
- children.

Table 40.3 Dosages of first-line anti-tuberculous agents[a]

Drug	Forms available	Adults daily	Adults intermittent (doses per week)	Children daily	Children intermittent (doses per week)	Renal failure	Liver failure
Rifampicin	Capsules 150 mg, 300 mg[b] Liquid 100 mg in 5 mL Injection for infusion 300 mg	450 mg/kg (<50 kg) 600 mg (>50 kg)	15 mg/kg (3)	10 mg/kg	15 mg/kg (3)	No	Only in severe liver failure
Isoniazid	Tablets 50 mg[b] Injection 25 mg/mL Elixir (special order)[c]	300 mg	15 mg/kg (3)	5–10 mg/kg	15 mg/kg (3)	Only in severe liver failure	In patients with acute or chronic liver disease
Ethambutol[f]	Tablets 100 mg, 400 mg[b] Mixture[c]	15 mg/kg[d]		As adult dose	30 mg/kg (3)	Yes	No
Pyrazinamide	Tablets 500 mg	1.5 g (<50 kg) 2.0 g (≥50 kg)	2.0 g[d] (<50 kg) (3) 2.5 g[a] (≥50 kg)	35 mg/kg		Yes	No
Streptomycin	Injection 1 g	750 mg (<50 kg) 1 g (<50 kg)	750 mg–1 g[e]	15 mg/kg		Yes	No

[a]Some of the doses quoted are not licensed but have been recommended by the British Thoracic Society.
[b]Also available as combined oral preparations.
[c]Mixture may be prepared extemporaneously.
[d]Doses refer to patients under 50 kg. Reduce by 500 mg for patients weighing less than 50 kg.
[e]Drug levels should be monitored to prevent toxicity.
[f]Acute calculation is required to reduce the risk of toxicity.

TB of peripheral lymph nodes

Trials have shown that 6 months of treatment are just as effective as 9 months for fully susceptible bacilli. The standard 6-month treatment regimen is recommended.

Meningeal TB

Patients with active meningeal TB (tuberculous meningitis) should be treated with rifampicin and isoniazid for 12 months together with pyrazinamide, and normally ethambutol, for the first 2 months. Ethambutol (and streptomycin if used in preference) only reach cerebrospinal fluid through inflamed meninges.

Care must be exercised when ethambutol is used in unconscious patients as a decline in visual acuity, a known side effect of ethambutol, cannot be assessed.

Meningeal TB is a serious disease and treatment must be started promptly. The stage at which the disease is diagnosed, and treatment started, most affects prognosis. Therefore, it is often justified to start a therapeutic trial of anti-TB drugs in the absence of a definite diagnosis.

The use of glucocorticoids is also recommended in the management of meningeal TB and is commenced at the same time as anti-tuberculous drugs. Consideration should be given to their gradual withdrawal within 2–3 weeks of initiation. The recommended doses (National Institute for Health and Clinical Excellence, 2006) are:

- Adults: equivalent to prednisolone 20–40 mg if on rifampicin, otherwise 10–20 mg
- Children: equivalent to prednisolone 1–2 mg/kg, maximum 40 mg.

The more recent British Infection Society (BIS) guidelines for the diagnosis and treatment of TB of the central nervous system (CNS) in adults and children (Thwaites et al., 2009) recommend all patients with meningeal TB should receive adjunctive corticosteroids (dexamethasone) regardless of disease severity at presentation.

Bone and joint TB

The spine is the most common site for bone TB. Bone and joint TB are treated effectively with standard agents such as isoniazid and rifampicin for 6 months, together with pyrazinamide and a fourth drug, usually ethambutol in the initial phase (for 2 months). This recommendation covers active spinal TB and active TB at other bone and joint sites. Occasionally, surgery may be needed to either relieve spinal cord compression or correct spinal deformities.

Disseminated TB

Generalised (disseminated or miliary) TB must be treated promptly as there is appreciable mortality from delayed diagnosis and treatment. The standard 6-month regimen containing both isoniazid and rifampicin, with pyrazinamide and ethambutol in the first 2 months, is used. If there is evidence of CNS involvement, treatment should be the same as for meningeal TB.

Pericardial TB

Although TB of the pericardium is rare in the UK, it is potentially important because of the possibility of cardiac tamponade and constrictive pericarditis, which are associated with a significant morbidity and mortality. The standard 6-month treatment regimen is recommended for patients with active pericardial disease. Glucocorticoids should also be prescribed at the following doses (National Institute for Health and Clinical Excellence, 2006):

- Adults: a glucocorticoid equivalent to prednisolone at 60 mg/day
- Children: a glucocorticoid equivalent to prednisolone 1 mg/kg/day (maximum 40 mg/day), with gradual withdrawal of the glucocorticoid, starting within 2–3 weeks of initiation.

Treatment of TB in special circumstances

TB in children

The doses of drugs used in children are shown in Table 40.3. Doses are generally estimated to facilitate prescription of easily administered volumes of liquid or tablets of appropriate strength. Ethambutol should not routinely be used in young children, who would be unable to report visual disturbances should they occur. However, it may be used if there is toxicity or resistance to other agents.

Pregnancy

As there is a risk of TB to the fetus, treatment should be commenced whenever it is moderately or highly probable that a pregnant woman has TB. Standard therapy should be given, although streptomycin should not be used as it may be ototoxic to the fetus. It is considered safe for mothers to breast feed while taking anti-tuberculous treatment. Pyridoxine (vitamin B_6) supplementation (10–25 mg/day) is recommended for breastfeeding women taking isoniazid. Patients should be warned of the reduced effectiveness of oral contraceptives in regimens containing rifampicin, and advised to use other, non-hormonal contraceptives.

Renal disease

Patients with renal disease may be given isoniazid, rifampicin and pyrazinamide in standard doses as these drugs are predominantly eliminated by non-renal routes. Ethambutol undergoes extensive renal elimination and therefore dose reduction is needed. Monitoring serum concentrations has been suggested, but this might not be readily available in many centres. Streptomycin must be used with considerable caution to prevent toxicity and is best avoided in renal failure. Rifampicin may be given in standard doses to patients on dialysis. However, doses of the other agents need to be modified, and a number of different regimens have been suggested.

Liver disease

Monitoring of liver enzymes is recommended in patients with liver failure or in alcoholics because rifampicin, isoniazid and pyrazinamide are all potentially hepatotoxic. However, increases in transaminases at the start of anti-tuberculous treatment occur frequently. These are usually transient and not a reason for stopping treatment unless frank jaundice or hepatitis develops, in which case all drugs should be stopped. It is usually possible to restart treatment when transaminases have returned to pre-treatment levels.

Immunocompromised patients

Patients who are immunocompromised, including those with HIV infection, should be treated with normal first-line agents unless multidrug-resistant TB is suspected. Theoretically, these patients have a greater risk of relapse and may need to be treated for longer than the normal 6 months.

TB and HIV co-infection

Guidelines for the treatment of TB/HIV co-infection (Pozniak et al., 2009) recommend that co-infected patients are managed by a multidisciplinary team which includes physicians with expertise in the treatment of both TB and HIV.

If patients on anti-tuberculous therapy are started on highly active antiretroviral therapy (HAART), then antiretrovirals should be chosen to avoid interactions with TB therapy. The treatment for TB should only be modified when drug interactions with antivirals do not allow the optimal TB treatment regimen. In some cases, a longer duration of treatment for the TB may be needed.

Chemo-preventive therapy for TB is not recommended in HIV-infected patients. However, as HIV-infected people with LTBI are more likely to progress to active TB disease than people without HIV, the detection and treatment of a latent infection is important.

HAART is effective at reducing the incidence of new TB in HIV-infected people. HIV-positive patients should therefore be offered HAART.

Drug-resistant TB

Drug-resistant TB is a considerable problem worldwide. In the UK, however, the proportion of TB isolates showing resistance is low (in 2008, 6% were resistant to isoniazid, 1.5% resistant to rifampicin, and 6.8% resistant to any first-line drug). Drug resistance is an important issue in the management of TB as it may compromise the effectiveness of treatment and prolong the period during which patients are infectious to others. Isoniazid is the most usual agent to which resistance is seen. Multi-drug resistance is important because the main bactericidal drugs, isoniazid and rifampicin, are ineffective. Treatment has to be individualised, requires a complex regimen involving the use of multiple reserve drugs and can cost at least £50,000 to £70,000 each to treat (Table 40.4). It is recommended that treatment of these individuals is only carried out by physicians with experience in drug-resistant TB; in hospitals, when inpatient treatment is necessary, with appropriate isolation facilities (negative pressure rooms); and in close conjunction with specialist centres.

Monitoring treatment

In pulmonary TB, sputum examination and culture are the most sensitive markers of treatment success. Patients taking regimens containing rifampicin and isoniazid should be non-infectious within 2 weeks. If a patient does not become culture negative, it may be due to either drug resistance or non-adherence, the latter being more likely. Good adherence is essential if treatment is to be successful and checking this can be difficult, especially when a patient is unwilling to cooperate.

Adverse reactions

The major adverse reactions of the first-line drugs are shown in Table 40.5. Rifampicin, isoniazid and pyrazinamide are all potentially hepatotoxic, and liver function should be checked before treatment commences with these drugs. Transient increases in transaminases and bilirubin commonly occur at the start of treatment although there is no need to continue to monitor liver function in patients where pre-treatment liver function was normal. However, liver function tests must be measured if fever, malaise, vomiting or jaundice develop and all drugs should be stopped. Liver function should be allowed to return to normal, at which time treatment can be recommenced one drug at a time. Clinical hepatitis is rare although patients may complain of vague symptoms such as abdominal pain and malaise which may indicate impending hepatitis.

Rifampicin is usually well tolerated, but gastro-intestinal upsets, fever and rash can occur. It interacts with many medications, including methadone, protease inhibitors and non-nucleoside reverse transcriptase inhibitors used to treat HIV infection, macrolide antibiotics, warfarin and hormonal contraceptives. It will colour the urine orange-red within approximately 4 h of a dose.

Hypersensitivity reactions or rashes may occur with any of the drugs. However, the most important, although rare, is caused by rifampicin and can be quite severe. It is more prevalent during intermittent treatment and presents as a flu-like syndrome, sometimes with abdominal pain and respiratory symptoms. This usually resolves on reverting to a daily dosage. However, if more serious effects occur, such as renal impairment or haematological abnormalities, the drug should be stopped and never restarted.

Isoniazid can cause fever, skin rashes and a dose-dependent peripheral neuropathy, probably due to depletion of vitamin B_6. This reaction is rare at recommended doses, but certain patient groups which include problem drinkers ('alcoholics') and pregnant women are at greater risk and should receive pyridoxine supplementation at a dose of 10–25 mg/day.

Pyrazinamide can cause hepatitis. This is not increased when the drug is given with isoniazid and rifampicin in the standard 6-month treatment regimen. However, when hepatic

Table 40.4 Reserve drugs: dosages and side effects (British Thoracic Society Joint Tuberculosis Committee, 1998)

Drug (once daily)	Children	Adults	Main side effects
Streptomycin	15 mg/kg	15 mg/kg (max dose 1 g daily)	Tinnitus, ataxia, vertigo, renal impairment
Amikacin	15 mg/kg	15 mg/kg	As for streptomycin
Capreomycin		15 mg/kg	As for streptomycin
Kanamycin		15 mg/kg	As for streptomycin
Ethionamide or prothianamide	15–20 mg/kg	<50 kg, 375 mg twice a day ≥50 kg, 500 mg twice a day	Gastro-intestinal, hepatitis; avoid in pregnancy
Cycloserine		250–500 mg twice a day	Depression, fits
Ofloxacin		400 mg twice a day	Abdominal distress, headache, tremulousness
Ciprofloxacin		750 mg twice a day	As ofloxacin plus drug interactions
Azithromycin		500 mg	Gastro-intestinal upset
Clarithromycin		500 mg twice a day	As for azithromycin
Rifabutin		300–450 mg	As for rifampicin; uveitis can occur with drug interactions, for example macrolides. Often cross-resistance with rifampicin
Thiacetazone	4 mg/kg	150 mg	Gastro-intestinal, vertigo, conjunctivitis, rash. Avoid if HIV positive (Stevens–Johnson syndrome)
Clofazimine		300 mg	Headache, diarrhoea, red skin discolouration
PAS sodium	300 mg/kg	10 g every morning or 5 g twice a day	Gastro-intestinal, hepatitis, rash, fever

PAS, *p*-aminosalicylate.

Table 40.5 Major adverse reactions of first-line anti-tuberculous drugs

Drug	Common reaction	Uncommon reaction
Isoniazid		Hepatitis, cutaneous hypersensitivity, peripheral neuropathy
Rifampicin		Hepatitis, cutaneous reactions, gastro-intestinal reactions, thrombocytopaenic purpura, febrile reactions, 'flu syndrome'
Pyrazinamide	Anorexia, nausea, flushing	Hepatitis, vomiting, arthralgia, hyperuricaemia, cutaneous hypersensitivity
Ethambutol		Retrobulbar neuritis, arthralgia

toxicity occurs, liver enzymes are elevated for a longer time than with rifampicin or isoniazid. If patients have known pre-existing hepatic dysfunction, the use of pyrazinamide should be carefully considered.

Ethambutol ocular toxicity (optic neuritis) is by far the most important side effect of ethambutol. Some patients with pre-existing ocular problems, for example those with diabetes, may be at greater risk of toxicity. Daily doses of 30 mg/kg or more increase the likelihood of toxicity, as does the administration of standard daily doses (15–25 mg) to patients with impaired renal function.

Patients should be tested for both visual acuity and red-green colour discrimination before treatment. If toxicity develops, the drug must be stopped promptly. This should lead to a gradual improvement in vision. Permanent damage may occur if the drug is continued.

In children older than 5 years of age, a dose of ethambutol of 15 mg/kg has been shown to be safe (Trebucq, 1997). A baseline ophthalmological assessment is important in children as in adults and should be repeated after 1–2 months.

Chemoprophylaxis

The use of chemoprophylaxis is important in preventing vulnerable individuals with LTBI from developing active TB disease. Without chemoprophylaxis, 40–50% of infants and 15% of older children with LTBI will develop active TB disease in 1–2 years. Prophylaxis is usually with isoniazid alone for 6 months or rifampicin and isoniazid for 3 months. Detailed guidance as to when isoniazid or rifampicin and isoniazid should be used has been produced by National Institute for Health and Clinical Excellence (2006).

BCG vaccine

BCG vaccine contains a live, attenuated strain derived from *M. bovis*. It does not protect against infection, but it prevents the more serious forms of disease such as miliary TB and meningeal TB. The BCG immunisation programme in the UK is now a risk-based programme, the key part being a neonatal programme targeted at protecting those children most at risk of exposure to TB, particularly from the more serious forms of the disease (Department of Health, 2006). Most age groups require a Mantoux test prior to being offered BCG vaccine.

Patient care

It is possible to cure virtually all patients with TB infection or disease provided that an adequate regimen, to which the bacilli are susceptible, is prescribed and the patient complies with treatment. By far the largest cause of treatment failure is non-adherence by the patient. This has serious consequences: treatment may fail and disease may relapse, in some cases with resistant organisms. A patient with infectious TB who does not adhere to treatment is a public health hazard.

Factors affecting adherence

A number of studies have shown that adherence falls as the number of tablets to be taken per day increases, and falls still further if doses have to be taken frequently through the day. Ideally, the least number of tablets should be given. Patients may fail to adhere because they feel better and do not appreciate the need to continue with their medication. Lack of clarity of instructions, written, verbal or other, may compromise adherence, particularly if the patient is confused by conflicting advice from different health care professionals. Finally, adverse effects, or symptoms perceived to be adverse effects, may reduce adherence.

Improving patient adherence

Anti-TB therapy should be prescribed once a day using as few tablets as possible. Single daily dosing enables patients to fit their medication into their daily routine. Rifampicin and isoniazid are both well absorbed when taken on an empty stomach. However, absorption is reduced and delayed when taken with or after food. It is therefore recommended that both should be taken 1 h before food to rapidly achieve peak blood levels. It is usually recommended that patients take their medication before breakfast. Cueing tablet taking to a regular activity may improve adherence in some patients.

The number of tablets to be taken each day may be reduced by using combination preparations of which several are available. Some, for example Rifater®, contain ratios of rifampicin, isoniazid and pyrazinamide that differ slightly from the dosages recommended by the British Thoracic Society. Combination preparations may not be suitable for use in children as the required dose regimens differ from those of adults.

Formulation

With the exception of streptomycin, first-line agents are usually administered orally. There is a liquid preparation of rifampicin available for patients who cannot take tablets or capsules. In patients who are severely ill, and cannot take oral medication, rifampicin may be given intravenously, and isoniazid can be administered by both the intravenous and intramuscular routes.

Information for patients

Written instructions and/or patient information leaflets (PILs) may be offered to support verbal counselling if there is any doubt as to the patient's understanding. It should be emphasised that the disease will be cured, but this will take some months and the tablets will need to be taken as prescribed even if the patient feels better. Some patients will adhere initially while they are unwell but will fail to adhere later as they begin to feel better.

The occurrence of some adverse effects may require discontinuation of a drug, but others are harmless. The patient should be told which side effects to expect and which require referral to a member of the healthcare team. Again, written instructions may be helpful.

A number of patients from abroad have a poor command of English. TB Alert has produced leaflets on the treatment of TB for patients. These can be found at the TB Alert website (http://www.tbalert.org/), and are available in languages other than English.

On occasion, drugs which are not licensed for use in the UK although licensed abroad are prescribed for TB. These may be obtained on a named-patient basis through recognised specialist wholesalers. Patients who receive these medicines require specific counselling to help them understand the special circumstances surrounding their use and receive appropriate patient information.

Directly observed therapy (DOT)

DOT, where the patient is observed taking their anti-tuberculous medication by a health care professional, is not needed for most cases of active TB. A risk assessment for treatment adherence should be undertaken in all patients, and

DOT regimens considered where non-adherence to treatment might be a problem, for example in street- or shelter-dwelling homeless people with active TB and patients with a history of non-adherence. This latter group includes individuals with chronic alcohol or other social problems.

DOT regimens may be fully or partially intermittent. In the latter, four drugs (isoniazid, rifampicin, pyrazinamide and either ethambutol or streptomycin) are given daily for 2 months followed by rifampicin and isoniazid two or three times weekly for the subsequent 4 months. For most drugs, the doses are increased when given intermittently and these are shown in Table 40.3. Trials of intermittent regimens have shown treatment is as effective when given intermittently as when given daily.

Counselling points

It is now a requirement for patients to be provided with a PIL for medication they are taking. Patients should be advised to read the PIL. The TB doctor, nurse and pharmacist should provide them with other relevant information orally. Patients taking rifampicin should be told that the drug will cause a harmless discolouration of their urine and other body fluids, for example sweat and tears. The staining of tears is important if the patient uses soft contact lenses as these may be permanently stained. Gas-permeable and hard lenses are unaffected. Women using the oral contraceptive pill should be advised to use other non-hormonal methods of contraception for the duration of rifampicin treatment and for 8 weeks afterwards as the effectiveness of hormonal contraceptives is reduced by rifampicin.

Although ocular side effects are rare when ethambutol is taken in normal dosages, patients should be warned of this potentially serious side effect. They should be advised to stop the drug and report to their doctor if they notice any changes in vision, such as a reduction in visual acuity or changes in colour vision. This is especially important because visual changes are usually reversible on discontinuation of the drug but may be permanent if the drug is not stopped.

Case studies

Case 40.1

A man in his 40s is referred to a chest physician with a cough productive of sputum and a fever. A chest x-ray indicates bilateral pneumonia with apical involvement. A sputum smear reveals the presence of acid, alcohol-fast bacilli. His physician considers that TB is the most likely clinical diagnosis. This is subsequently confirmed microbiologically. The patient does not comply with treatment and needs to be admitted to hospital, but refuses. There are indications he might be disruptive if admitted into hospital.

Questions

1. What form of TB does this patient have?
2. What can be done to compel his admission to hospital?
3. Which groups of healthcare staff should be involved in arrangements for his admission to hospital?

Answers

1. This man has sputum smear-positive pulmonary TB, the infectious form of the disease, and poses a risk of infection to others.
2. Legal measures should be considered to have the patient compulsorily admitted to hospital. These are set out in the Public Health (Control of Diseases) Act 1984 for England and Wales, and the Health Protection Regulations 2010. This will involve an application to the magistrates court for compulsory admission to hospital under a legally binding order, to be signed by the magistrates. The hospital will need to have agreed to his admission.
3. He will need to be admitted to a side room. Given that he may be disruptive, a multidisciplinary team meeting should be held to agree a care plan in preparation for his admission. This should be discussed with the patient, including the reasons why he will need to be kept in isolation. This should take place prior to an application for a court order if the patient refuses admission to hospital.

Case 40.2

A woman in her 40s is admitted to hospital with shortness of breath. She has lived in sub-Saharan Africa. She subsequently develops a non-productive cough. Bronchial washings are smear negative for acid-fast bacilli, but *M. tuberculosis* is isolated from the sample. Early sputum samples are smear negative, but later samples are smear positive.

Questions

1. What form of TB does this patient have?
2. Should she be in isolation?
3. What treatment should she receive for her TB?
4. Is she at low or high risk for drug-resistant TB?
5. What further microbiological investigations would be essential?

Answers

1. She has pulmonary TB, indicated by her symptoms and chest x-ray.
2. She should be in isolation in a single room. If a risk assessment suggests she may have MDR-TB, advice should be sought from the Infection Prevention and Control Team as to whether she should be transferred to a negative pressure room.
3. She should be commenced on standard quadruple therapy, comprising rifampicin and isoniazid, supplemented with pyrazinamide and ethambutol for the first 2 months.
4. A history of residence in sub-Saharan Africa suggests she could be at risk of drug-resistant TB, in particular multiple drug-resistant TB. The change in sputum smear status, despite being on standard quadruple therapy, would certainly suggest drug resistance.
5. A PCR test should be done on the isolate to determine whether her infecting strains of tubercle bacilli are resistant to rifampicin. Tests should also be done to assess susceptibility to other drugs.

Case 40.3

A woman in her mid-20s is diagnosed as having sputum smear-negative pulmonary TB. Although she initially takes her anti-TB drugs, she does not attend follow-up clinics and her condition deteriorates. Her primary care doctor collects a sputum sample from her and persuades her to attend the chest clinic. The sputum smear is now positive and it is found she has continued to work, despite being advised not to do so.

Questions

1. What type of treatment regimen should be offered to this patient?
2. Who should be involved in planning this treatment regimen, and what arrangements should be put in place to ensure this works?
3. Should the patient's work contacts be screened?

Answers

1. Patients like this should receive supervised treatment (DOTS) three times a week in a convenient setting, such as at home.
2. There needs to be close collaboration between the physician responsible for treatment, the patient's primary care physician, TB nurse, pharmacist, the public health team and the health care professionals (often district nurses or health visitors in the UK) who will supervise treatment. The patient needs to be involved in discussions about these arrangements, as treatment will not be successful without her cooperation.

   The physician will need to adjust the treatment dosage in line with the thrice-weekly regimen, inform the general practitioner and ensure the correct prescriptions are issued. Those supervising treatment need a clear explanation of what is expected of them, including details of the drugs and dose, and duration of treatment. They also need to know what to do if the patient does not adhere.
3. The question of whether work contacts should be screened must be dealt with on an individual case basis. This usually involves the health protection (public health) team informing the patient of the need to inquire into work contacts, and getting the patient's agreement to approach a supervisor or manager in the workplace. A telephone conversation will provide initial information on the working environment and should be followed up by a visit if initial inquiries indicate a possible need to screen workplace contacts.

Case 40.4

A 40-year-old man with young children aged under 5 is diagnosed with infectious pulmonary TB, but is not taking his anti-tuberculous drugs. He has mental health problems for which he is on treatment and is a drug misuser. Arrangements are made for him to have home-based directly observed treatment (DOT) for TB, but these break down.

Questions

1. What other arrangements should be considered for his treatment?
2. What other options could be pursued if alternative arrangements cannot be put in place?
3. Might a community pharmacist have a role in assisting with the treatment of such a patient?

Answers

1. The mental health team responsible for his care could be asked if they would observe him taking treatment. However, they may be concerned about the possible risk to themselves from exposure to someone with infectious TB. The same difficulties could arise if admission to a secure mental health facility is considered. If the patient is not in contact with the drug service, their involvement is only possible if the patient agrees to engage with them.
2. If none of the options in (1) are possible in practice, the patient remains an infectious risk, especially to his children. The advice of child protection professionals should therefore be sought, and if necessary a referral made to social services. The children will not necessarily be taken into care, alternative ways of supporting child care will be sought but their safety is paramount.
3. Community pharmacists could have a role to play in supervising treatment and this should be discussed with them where appropriate. If they agree, arrangements can be put in place, including a discussion between the pharmacist and the patient as to the 'rules of engagement', that is what the patient can expect from the pharmacist and what the pharmacist expects from the patient.

Acknowledgement

The help from TB physicians, specialist TB nurse and pharmacy colleagues in Gwent for advice on the practical and clinical aspects of treatment and assistance with the case studies is gratefully acknowledged.

References

British Thoracic Society, 2000. Control and prevention of tuberculosis in the United Kingdom. Thorax 55, 887–901.

British Thoracic Society Joint Tuberculosis Committee, 1998. Chemotherapy and management of tuberculosis in the United Kingdom: recommendations. Thorax 53, 536–548. With permission from BMJ Publishing Group Ltd.

Davies, P.D.O. (Ed.), 2003. Clinical Tuberculosis. Arnold, London.

Department of Health, 2006. Immunisation Against Infectious Disease. Chapter 32, Tuberculosis: BCG Immunisation DH, London. Available at: http://www.dh.gov.uk/en/Publicationsandstatistics/Publications/PublicationsPolicyAndGuidance/DH_113027.

Hawker, J., Begg, N., Blair, I., et al. (Eds.), 2005. Communicable Disease Control Handbook. Blackwell, Oxford.

Health Protection Agency, 2009. Tuberculosis in the UK: Annual Report on Tuberculosis Surveillance in the UK 2009. Health Protection Agency Centre for Infections, London.

Heymann, D.L. (Ed.), 2004. Control of Communicable Diseases Manual. American Public Health Association, Washington, DC.

National Institute for Health and Clinical Excellence, 2006. Tuberculosis – Clinical Diagnosis and Management of Tuberculosis and Measures for Its Prevention and Control. CG 33. NICE, London. Available at: http://guidance.nice.org.uk/CG33.

Pozniak, A.L., Collins, S., Coyne, K.M., et al., on behalf of the BHIVA Guidelines Writing Committee, 2009. Guidelines for the Treatment of TB/HIV Co-infection. British HIV Association, London. Available at:

http://bhiva.org/documents/Guidelines/Treatment%20Guidelines/
Current/TreatmentGuidelines2009.pdf.

Thwaites, G., Fisher, M., Hemingway, C., et al., 2009. The British Infection Society guidelines for the diagnosis and treatment of tuberculosis of the central nervous system in adults and children. J. Infect. 59, 167–187.

Trebucq, A., 1997. Should ethambutol be recommended for routine treatment of tuberculosis in children? A review of the literature. Int. J. Tuberc. Lung Dis. 1, 12–15.

WHO, 2009. Multidrug and Extensively Drug-Resistant TB (M/XDR-TB): 2010 Global Report on Surveillance and Response. WHO, Geneva. Available at: http://whqlibdoc.who.int/publications/2010/9789241599191_eng.pdf.

World Health Organization, 2009. Global Tuberculosis Control. A Short Update to the 2009 Report. WHO, Geneva. Available at: http://whqlibdoc.who.int/publications/2009/9789241598866_eng.pdf.

Further reading

American Thoracic Society, CDC, and Infectious Diseases Society of America, 2003. Treatment of Tuberculosis. MMWR 152: RR-11.

Campbell, I.A., Bah-Sow, O., 2006. Pulmonary tuberculosis: diagnosis and treatment. Br. Med. J. 332, 1194–1197.

Health Protection Scotland, 2009. Tuberculosis: Clinical Diagnosis and Management of Tuberculosis and Measures for Its Prevention and Control in Scotland. Health Protection Scotland, Glasgow.

Schlossberg, D. (Ed.), 2006. Tuberculosis and Nontuberculous Mycobacterial Infections. McGraw-Hill, New York.

World Health Organization, 2010. Treatment of Tuberculosis Guidelines. WHO, Geneva. Available at: http://whqlibdoc.who.int/publications/2010/9789241547833_eng.pdf.

Useful websites

Immunisation against infectious disease 'The Green Book' http://www.dh.gov.uk/en/Publicationsandstatistics/Publications/PublicationsPolicyAndGuidance/DH_079917.

The truth about TB http://www.thetruthabouttb.org/.

HIV infection 41

H. Leake Date and M. Fisher

Key points

- Untreated infection with the human immunodeficiency virus (HIV) leads to a progressive deterioration in the cellular immune response. After initial seroconversion, the infected individual may appear asymptomatic for a number of years, before developing symptomatic disease and/or acquired immune deficiency syndrome (AIDS).

- Complications arising from HIV infection can manifest in a variety of ways, usually as opportunistic infections or malignancies that are uncommon in the immunocompetent population.

- The aim of the treatment of HIV infection is to reconstitute, or prevent further deterioration of the immune system, with the intention of improving the quality and quantity of life. Management of HIV-related complications primarily involves the treatment and prophylaxis of opportunistic diseases.

- Currently available antiretroviral (ARV) agents are classified by their mechanism of actions as nucleoside or nucleotide analogue reverse transcriptase inhibitors (NRTIs), non-nucleoside reverse transcriptase inhibitors (NNRTIs), protease inhibitors (PIs), integrase inhibitors and entry inhibitors.

- Antiretroviral agents are given in combination, usually of at least three agents, to improve efficacy and reduce the development of viral resistance.

- Treatment regimens are frequently complex and many of the drugs have significant toxicities and interactions with other drugs and with food. A high level of adherence to therapy is vital to ensure efficacy and prevent the emergence of resistant virus.

Epidemiology

In June 1981, five cases of *Pneumocystis jiroveci* (formerly known as *carinii*) pneumonia (PCP) were described in homosexual men in the USA. Reports of other unusual conditions, such as Kaposi's sarcoma (KS), followed shortly. In each of these patients, there was found to be a marked impairment of cellular immune response, and so the term acquired immune deficiency syndrome, or AIDS, was coined. In 1984, a new human retrovirus, subsequently named human immunodeficiency virus (HIV), was isolated and identified as the cause of AIDS.

Although initially described in homosexual men, it soon became apparent that other population groups were affected, including intravenous drug users and haemophiliacs. During the first decade, the epidemic grew and the importance of transmission via heterosexual intercourse and from mother to child (vertical transmission) was increasingly recognised.

In the UK, since 1999 the number of new HIV diagnoses has been higher in heterosexuals than in men who have sex with men (MSM), although more recently this trend has been reversing, due to a decline in diagnoses among people infected heterosexually abroad (particularly from Sub-Saharan Africa). The majority of heterosexuals with HIV have acquired their infection in countries of high prevalence, whilst the majority of ongoing transmission within the UK is still amongst men who have sex with men. Additionally, there is an increasing proportion of individuals with HIV who are living into older age. It is postulated that the ageing process is accelerated in the context of HIV infection, with a resultant increase in co-morbidities, such as cardiovascular disease, osteoporosis and osteopaenia, cancer, cognitive impairment, and hepatic and renal dysfunction.

The impact of treatment advances on the incidence of AIDS-related illnesses and mortality has been dramatic. However, the absolute number of new AIDS diagnoses and HIV-related deaths in the UK has plateaued, largely due to late presentation and the failure to diagnose HIV infection amongst the asymptomatic population.

Although the number living with HIV globally continues to rise, there are encouraging trends (including in many low- and middle-income countries) of declining prevalence and a slower rate of increase in new infections. Significant progress has been made since 2000 in increasing access to antiretroviral therapies in resource-poor settings. Although choice of agents and facilities for monitoring may be limited, and locally produced generic formulations are often used, the resultant impact on mortality has been as dramatic as that seen previously in resource-rich countries.

The virus has been isolated from a number of body fluids, including blood, semen, vaginal secretions, saliva, breast milk, tears, urine, peritoneal fluid and cerebrospinal fluid (CSF). However, not all of these are important in the spread of infection and the predominant routes of transmission remain: sexual intercourse (anal or vaginal); sharing of unsterilised needles or syringes; blood or blood products in areas where supplies are not screened or treated; and vertical transmission *in utero*, during labour or through breast feeding.

Pathogenesis

HIV, in common with other retroviruses, possesses the enzyme reverse transcriptase and consists of a lipid bilayer membrane surrounding the capsid (Fig. 41.1). Its surface glycoprotein molecule

621

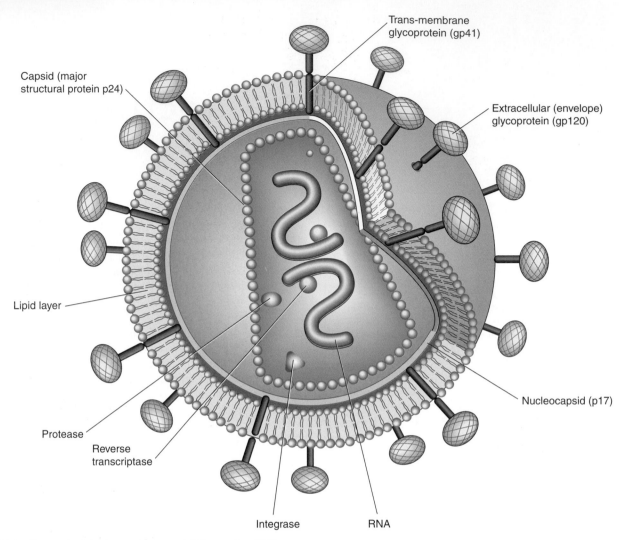

Fig. 41.1 Structure of the human immunodeficiency virus (HIV).

(gp120) has a strong affinity for the CD4 receptor protein found predominantly on the T-helper/inducer lymphocytes. Monocytes and macrophages may also possess CD4 receptors in low densities and can therefore also be infected. The process of HIV entry is more complex than originally thought, and in addition to CD4 attachment, subsequent binding to co-receptors such as CCR-5 or CXCR-4 and membrane fusion also occur (Fig. 41.2).

After penetrating the host cell, the virus sheds its outer coat and releases its genetic material. Using the reverse transcriptase enzyme, the viral RNA is converted to DNA using nucleosides. The viral DNA is then integrated into the host genome in the cell nucleus, where it undergoes transcription and translation, enabling the production of new viral proteins. New virus particles are then assembled and bud out of the host cell, finally maturing into infectious virions under the influence of the protease enzyme.

Immediately after primary HIV Infection (PHI, also known as 'seroconversion'), there is a very high rate of viral turnover. Equilibrium is then reached, at which stage the infection may appear to be clinically latent, but in fact, as many as 10,000 million new virions are produced each day.

Over time, as chronic infection ensues, cells possessing CD4 receptors, particularly the T-helper lymphocytes, are depleted

from the body. The T-helper cell is often considered to be the conductor of the 'immune orchestra' and thus, as this cell is depleted, the individual becomes susceptible to a myriad of infections and tumours. The rate at which this immunosuppression progresses is variable and the precise interaction of factors affecting it is still not fully understood. It is well recognised that some individuals rapidly develop severe immunosuppression, whilst others may have been infected with HIV for many years whilst maintaining a relatively intact immune system. It is likely that a combination of viral, host (genetic) and environmental factors contributes to this variation.

Clinical manifestations

The sequelae of untreated HIV infection can be broadly considered in five categories:

- Opportunistic infections, that is, infections that would not normally cause disease in an immunocompetent host, for example, *P. jiroveci* pneumonia and cytomegalovirus (CMV)
- Infections that can occur in immunocompetent patients but tend to occur more frequently, more severely and

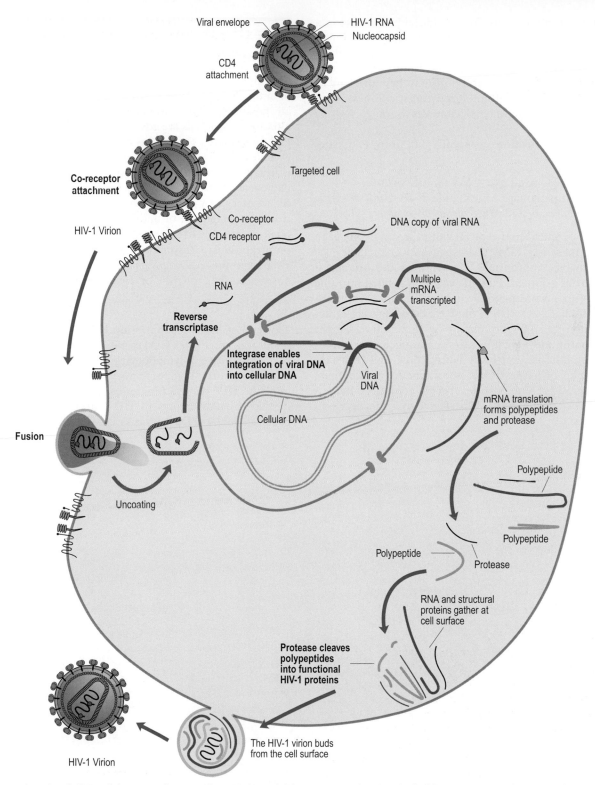

Fig. 41.2 Lifecycle of HIV and the sites of action of currently available antiretroviral agents (in bold).

often atypically in the context of underlying HIV infection, for example, *Salmonella*, herpes simplex and *Mycobacterium tuberculosis*
- Malignancies, particularly those that occur rarely in the immunocompetent population, for example, Kaposi's sarcoma and non-Hodgkin's lymphoma

- Direct manifestations of HIV infection *per se*, for example, HIV encephalopathy, HIV myelopathy and HIV enteropathy
- Consequences of chronic immune activation including premature cardiovascular disease, neurocognitive dysfunction, bone mineral density loss.

In addition, approximately 70% of individuals develop a flu-like illness at seroconversion. This primary HIV infection (PHI) is characterised by fever, arthralgia, pharyngitis, rash and lymphadenopathy. Rarely, the degree of associated CD4 count depletion may be sufficient to result in development of an opportunistic illness such as oropharyngeal/oesophageal candidiasis or *P. jiroveci* pneumonia.

Opportunistic infections generally fall into two categories:

- DNA viruses, for example, CMV and JC virus
- Intracellular pathogens, for example, *P. jiroveci*, *Toxoplasma gondii* and *Mycobacterium avium*.

Although the clinical course of HIV disease varies with each individual, there is a fairly consistent and predictable pattern that enables appropriate interventions and preventive measures to be adopted. Patients can be classified into one of three groups according to their clinical status: asymptomatic, symptomatic or AIDS. Symptomatic disease is characterised by non-specific symptomatology such as fevers, night sweats, lethargy and weight loss, or by complications including oral candidiasis, oral hairy leucoplakia, and recurrent herpes simplex or herpes zoster infections. AIDS is defined by the diagnosis of one or more specific conditions including *P. jiroveci* pneumonia, *M. tuberculosis* infection and CMV disease.

Investigations and monitoring

Current and previous infections

The initial diagnosis of HIV infection is made by the detection of antibodies against HIV. With improved technology, it is usually possible to detect antibodies within 3–4 weeks of infection, although individuals are advised that a 'window period' of up to 3 months after exposure is required before infection can be excluded. After confirmation of HIV infection, the patient is usually tested for prior exposure to a number of potential pathogens, including syphilis, hepatitis A, B and C, CMV, varicella zoster (VZV), and *T. gondii*. This can enable subsequent treatment (in the case of undiagnosed syphilis), vaccination (if no prior exposure to hepatitis A, B, or VZV), prevention (if no prior exposure to *Toxoplasma* and CMV), prophylaxis (if previous exposure to *Toxoplasma*) and can aid subsequent diagnosis (according to CMV or *Toxoplasma* status).

CD4 count

The level of immunosuppression is most easily estimated by monitoring a patient's CD4 count. This measures the number of CD4-positive T-lymphocytes in a sample of peripheral blood. The normal range can vary between 500 and 1500 cells/mm³. As HIV disease progresses, the number of cells falls. Particular complications of HIV infection usually begin to occur at similar CD4 counts (Fig. 41.3) which can assist in

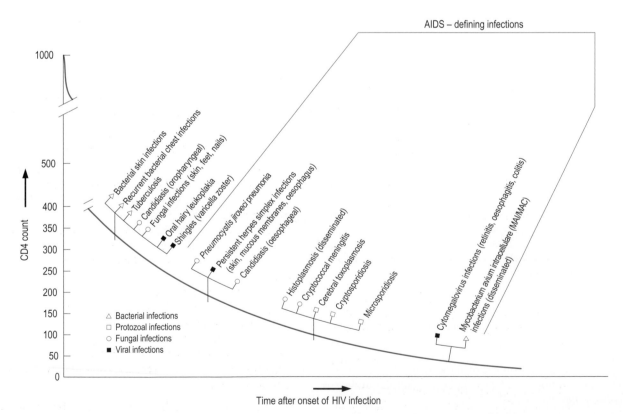

Fig. 41.3 Opportunistic complications of HIV infection and the CD4 count ranges at which they commonly occur.

differential diagnoses and enable the use of prophylactic therapies. For example, patients with a CD4 count of less than 200 cells/mm³ should always be offered prophylaxis against *P. jiroveci* pneumonia. Similarly, both patient and clinician are likely to use the CD4 count as the major indicator of when to consider starting antiretroviral therapy.

Viral load

The measurement of plasma HIV RNA (viral load) estimates the amount of circulating virus in the blood. This has been proven to correlate with prognosis, with a high viral load predicting faster disease progression (Mellors et al., 1997). Conversely, a reduction in viral load after commencement of antiviral therapy is associated with clinical benefit. This measure, in combination with the CD4 count, allows patients and clinicians to make informed decisions regarding when to start and when to change antiviral therapies, enabling the more effective use of such agents. There are on-line calculators utilising viral load and CD4 count to model risk of disease progression or death based on large cohort studies.

Resistance testing

Due to the implications of transmitted (primary) resistance, it is recommended that all patients have a genotypic HIV resistance test performed soon after diagnosis; this will ensure that appropriate initial therapy is selected. Further resistance tests should be performed at any subsequent virological failure to direct therapy choice.

Tropism testing

Viruses may enter the cell using the CCR5 co-receptor, the CXCR4 co-receptor or both co-receptors. Those which just use one co-receptor are known as CCR5-tropic or CXCR4-tropic viruses; those which can use both receptor types are called dual-tropic. Where a mixture of virus populations is present, the term mixed-tropic is used. Different methods of determining tropism are currently under evaluation. The tests must be performed in real time as viral tropism changes as the disease progresses. If CCR5 inhibitors are to be used, it is essential to determine that the virus is CCR5-tropic, that is, that there is no significant use of the CXCR4 receptor.

Drug treatment

The drug treatment of HIV disease can be classified as antiretroviral therapy, the management of opportunistic infections or malignancies, the management of 'non-HIV-related' co-morbidities, and symptom control. For the first decade of the epidemic, most of the available drugs and therapeutic strategies were aimed at treating or preventing opportunistic complications and alleviating HIV-related symptoms. Whilst these are still important, there has been a shift in emphasis towards treatment aimed at reducing the HIV viral load,

restoring immune function and reducing the potential consequences of co-morbidities.

Due to the speed at which new antiretroviral agents are being developed, comprehensive data on drug interactions, side effects, etc., are often lacking. Thus, the ability to apply general pharmacological and pharmacokinetic principles, together with common sense, is required.

The treatment of many of the opportunistic complications of HIV comprises an induction phase of high-dose therapy, followed by maintenance and/or secondary prophylaxis using lower doses. This is due to the high rate of relapse or progression after a first episode of diseases such as *P. jiroveci* pneumonia, cerebral toxoplasmosis (toxoplasmic encephalitis), systemic cryptococcosis and CMV retinitis. Where a cost-effective agent with an acceptable risk/benefit ratio exists, primary prophylaxis may be offered to individuals who are deemed to be at high risk of developing a particular opportunistic infection, for example, *P. jiroveci* pneumonia prophylaxis. Discontinuation of prophylaxis, both primary and secondary, is now usually possible in individuals who demonstrate immunological restoration on Highly Active Antiretroviral Therapy (HAART).

Paradoxically, this immunological restoration may result in apparent clinical deterioration with opportunistic infections during the first few weeks after initiation of HAART. This is known as immune reconstitution inflammatory syndrome (IRIS).

The goals of therapy in HIV-positive individuals are to:

- improve the quality and duration of life;
- prevent deterioration of immune function and/or restore immune status;
- treat and/or prevent opportunistic infections;
- relieve symptoms.

Antiretroviral therapy

Antiretroviral therapy is currently one of the fastest evolving areas of medicine. The specific details of treatment will therefore continue to change as new drugs emerge, although it is likely that the following general principles will remain:

- A combination of three antiretroviral agents, selected on the basis of treatment history and resistance tests, should usually be prescribed to increase efficacy and reduce the development of drug-resistant virus
- Wherever possible, a regimen should contain at least one drug that penetrates the central nervous system and confers protection against HIV-related encephalopathy/ dementia
- Treatment strategies should be adopted that sequence drug combinations, being mindful of potential cross-resistance and future therapy options
- Given the crucial importance of a high level of adherence to these therapies, the regimen adopted for a particular individual should, wherever possible, be tailored to suit the daily lifestyle.

Many organisations, such as the British HIV Association (BHIVA), the European AIDS Clinical Society (EACS) and the International AIDS Society (IAS), produce regularly updated guidelines on the use of antiretroviral therapy, for example, Gazzard et al. (2008). These guidelines include the most up-to-date considerations of:

- when to start therapy;
- what to start with;
- how to monitor, including use of therapeutic drug monitoring and resistance testing;
- when to switch therapy;
- what therapy to switch to;
- treating individuals who have been highly exposed to multiple agents;
- managing individuals with significant co-morbidities, for example, tuberculosis or hepatitis B/C.

Most studies evaluating triple combinations of antiretrovirals have been designed with so-called surrogate marker endpoints, measuring the effect on laboratory parameters such as CD4 count and HIV viral load. These trials are generally smaller and shorter in duration than clinical endpoint studies that are powered to measure the impact on survival and disease progression. The first large clinical endpoint trial that demonstrated the superiority of a triple combination over dual therapy was undertaken by Hammer et al. (1997). Following the results of this trial, the standard approach, where treatment is indicated, has been to use a combination of at least three agents. The reduction in morbidity and mortality associated with HAART has been confirmed in routine clinical practice, as well as in other trials (e.g. Palella et al., 1998; Smit et al., 2006). Subsequent clinical trials have largely been for licensing purposes and/or have served to refine therapeutic choices rather than to change the paradigm of treatment. The concept of intermittent rather than continuous therapy was evaluated in the SMART study but shown to be linked with an increased risk of co-morbidities not previously thought to be associated with HIV (such as cardiovascular disease, hepatic and renal failure) as well as HIV disease progression (El-Sadr et al., 2006). The use of protease inhibitor (PI) 'monotherapy' compared to conventional triple therapy has been evaluated in a number of small studies, for example, Arribas et al. (2009), and is being investigated in longer-term strategic studies. A large international study of early versus deferred treatment, to attempt to address the question of when to initiate treatment, is ongoing.

When to start therapy

Current UK guidelines recommend starting antiretrovirals when the CD4 count drops below 350 cells/mm³. Therapy should be considered at a higher CD4 count in specific situations, for example, in the presence of an AIDS-defining illness or HIV-related morbidity.

Choosing and monitoring therapy

The majority of individuals are currently commenced on a combination of two nucleoside/nucleotide reverse transcriptase inhibitors (NRTIs) and a non-nucleoside reverse

transcriptase inhibitor (NNRTI) or two NRTIs and a boosted PI. The term 'boosted PI' refers to a combination of one PI combined with a low dose (usually 100–200 mg once or twice daily) of ritonavir, another PI. The ritonavir does not directly add to the antiretroviral activity of the regimen; it is used purely as a pharmacokinetic enhancer of the other PI, by increasing the maximum plasma concentration, C_{max}, due to inhibition of cytochrome P450 enzymes in the gut wall and/or extending the half-life, $t_{1/2}$, by inhibition of hepatic cytochrome P450 enzymes. Triple NRTI therapy is no longer recommended, as it is associated with unacceptable rates of virological failure. Alternative strategies, such as NRTI-sparing regimens and boosted PI monotherapy, are currently only routinely recommended in a research setting. More recently, integrase inhibitors have been approved for initial therapy and may be used as an alternative to NNRTIs or PIs.

The aim of initial therapy is to achieve viral load suppression in the plasma to levels below the detection limits of available assays (40 or 50 copies/mL). Such virological suppression is almost invariably accompanied by an elevation in CD4 count and clinical evidence of immune reconstitution. Whilst sustained suppression over many years is usually possible, viral rebound may occur and is often accompanied by the development of resistance to one or more agents in the combination. Upon confirmed virological failure, a resistance test is performed which will help to identify to which agents the virus may have adapted and the extent to which any such resistance mutations may confer cross-resistance to other available drugs. A second-line regimen is then constructed, wherever possible utilising a new class of drug to which the individual has not previously been exposed. Upon virological failure of subsequent regimens, the therapeutic options available become increasingly complex, but with the availability of more agents targeting different parts of the virus life cycle, virological suppression is still usually possible and should remain the goal of treatment.

Many of the antiretrovirals, particularly the PIs and NNRTIs, exhibit a wide range of interactions, especially with other drugs that are metabolised by the cytochrome P450 enzyme system, including prescribed, 'over-the-counter', herbal and recreational drugs. HAART failure (detectable viral load and drug resistance) has been documented following co-administration of hepatic enzyme inducers, including non-prescribed agents such as St John's Wort. Conversely, serious and even fatal toxicities due to enzyme inhibition by the PIs continue to be reported. These include Cushing's syndrome following concomitant use of fluticasone or budesonide inhaler or nasal spray with a PI. This highlights the necessity of taking a comprehensive drug history prior to starting or switching HAART and ensuring patients and prescribers are aware of the need to check the interaction potential of new medicines. General prescribing guidelines for antiretrovirals are presented in Box 41.1 whilst details of common side effects and interactions of the currently available agents are summarised in Tables 41.1 to 41.5.

The routine use of therapeutic drug monitoring is not recommended but blood levels of PIs and NNRTIs should be measured in selected patients, for example, during pregnancy, where there is liver impairment and where there are concerns regarding potentially interacting drugs (Gazzard et al., 2008).

- The Summary of Product Characteristics, current British National Formulary (BNF) and national guidelines should be consulted when managing the treatment of an HIV-positive patient.
- Adverse events should be reported. With greater exposure and long-term use, it is likely that more adverse events will be recognised. Some of these may be class effects associated with particular groups of antiretrovirals and should therefore be monitored even in new agents within a class. Examples include dyslipidaemia and diabetes mellitus with protease inhibitors, mitochondrial myopathy and lipoatrophy with NRTIs, rash with NNRTIs.
- There are limited data on the safety of many antiretroviral drugs when taken during pregnancy, or their long-term effects on babies/children. Updated safety information from the Antiretroviral Pregnancy Register is published twice yearly. Efavirenz has been shown to be teratogenic in animal studies, but comparable data are not available for the other antiretrovirals. Caution should therefore be exercised with all agents. Treatment of women who are planning conception or who are pregnant must be discussed with the relevant experts. All pregnant women who are treated with antiretrovirals should be reported prospectively to the Antiretroviral Pregnancy Register.

HIV mutates readily and resistance to some antiretrovirals, particularly reverse transcriptase inhibitors and integrase inhibitors, develops rapidly in the face of suboptimal treatment, for example, monotherapy or subtherapeutic blood levels. A high level of adherence to treatment is crucial to the sustained, successful outcome of antiretroviral regimens and has been the subject of much research. For example, in one study of people taking their first regimen containing nelfinavir, it was found that at least 95% adherence was required to achieve a sustained response in the majority (78%) of patients. The chances of treatment success declined as the level of adherence dropped, such that 80% of patients whose adherence was below 80% experienced virological failure. Virological success was also found to correlate with a better clinical outcome in terms of fewer hospitalisations, opportunistic infections and deaths (Paterson et al., 2000). Such clinical trial data have also been supported by clinical experience in the UK and elsewhere, although it has yet to be established if the level of adherence required is the same for all regimens and every patient. In view of this, patients should be advised to take HAART as close as possible to the same time every day and certainly within 1 hour of the agreed time each day. If they forget a dose, it should be taken as soon as they remember and then return to the original schedule.

There has been significant progress over recent years in reducing some of the physical burden of therapy, through the development of combination tablets and the use of strategies such as ritonavir boosting to reduce dietary restrictions and dosing frequency. Adherence aids such as pill boxes, medication record cards and alarms (e.g. on mobile phone) can also help to support adherence. However, practical issues are not the only barriers to adherence and the individual's health beliefs and motivation, particularly around HIV and antiretroviral therapy, should also be addressed before treatment is commenced, as these are likely to have a significant impact on outcome (Horne et al., 2004). Although there is little evidence to demonstrate what the optimal interventions to improve adherence are, multidisciplinary and multiagency approaches appear to be most useful (Poppa et al., 2003).

Treatment interruptions

For many reasons, including toxicity, cost and adherence, patients and clinicians have been interested in considering 'drug holidays' or treatment interruptions. However, this strategy is no longer recommended in routine practice (El-Sadr et al., 2006). It is now recognised that there are dangers associated with this approach because of CD4 decline, disease progression, mortality related to co-morbidities, for example, cardiovascular disease, and viral load rebound associated with increased transmission risk and a seroconversion-like syndrome. Further, as different anti-HIV medications have different half-lives, there may be a risk of functional monotherapy, particularly with NNRTIs, and the development of resistance if combinations are stopped abruptly in an unplanned fashion.

Post-exposure prophylaxis

Post-exposure prophylaxis (PEP) involves the use of antiretroviral drugs to prevent infection with HIV after possible exposure, which may be recommended after occupational injuries (DH, 2008) or sexual exposure (Fisher et al., 2006). Whilst PEP is a largely unproven and unlicensed indication for the drugs used, it is supported by animal model data and case–control studies. Where recommended in guidelines, PEP is usually commenced as a 3–5-day starter regimen of two NRTIs and a boosted PI, followed by an ongoing course for a total of 4-week post-exposure. It is believed this will reduce the likelihood of infection by at least 80%, although toxicity issues are not insignificant. Therefore, the decision to prescribe or take PEP must reflect a careful risk/benefit evaluation. Studies of pre-exposure prophylaxis (PREP), using one or two antiretrovirals (orally or topically) before potential exposure to HIV, have so far yielded mixed results, but may offer additional options to reduce transmission.

Nucleoside and nucleotide analogue reverse transcriptase inhibitors

NRTIs are phosphorylated intracellularly and then inhibit the viral reverse transcriptase enzyme by acting as a false substrate. Nucleotide analogues only require two intracellular phosphorylations, whereas activation of nucleoside analogues is a three-stage process. The NRTIs licensed in the UK are:

Abacavir (Ziagen®)
Didanosine (ddI, Videx®)
Emtricitabine (FTC, Emtriva®)
Lamivudine (3TC, Epivir®)
Stavudine (d4T, Zerit®)
Tenofovir (Viread®)
Zidovudine (AZT, Retrovir®)

Table 41.1 General prescribing points for nucleoside/nucleotide analogue reverse transcriptase inhibitors (NRTIs)

Drug, names, manufacturer	Dose and formulation	Administration	Major/common side effects	Significant drug interactions and important pharmacokinetic information
Atripla® (efavirenz + emtricitabine + tenofovir) Bristol Myers Squibb/ Gilead	One tablet od	Tablet contains efavirenz 600 mg, emtricitabine 200 mg + tenofovir 300 mg	See entries for individual drugs	See entries for individual drugs
Abacavir (ABC) Ziagen® ViiV	300 mg bd 600 mg od 300 mg tablets 20 mg/mL oral solution	Can be taken with or without food	Usually well tolerated – Rash, headache, nausea and vomiting, diarrhoea, reduced appetite are most common side effects – Should only be prescribed if HLA B*5701 negative to reduce risk of hypersensitivity (5% incidence in unscreened populations): see BNF/SPC for full details. *Patient must NEVER be rechallenged if abacavir withdrawn due to suspected hypersensitivity.* Discuss with HIV team if reaction suspected. Counsel patient – Lactic acidosis (see BNF for more details) – May increase risk of cardiovascular disease	• Metabolism of methadone may be altered • Rifampicin, phenytoin, phenobarbitone may decrease abacavir levels – unclear significance in clinical practice • Concomitant treatment with abacavir and pegylated interferon + ribavirin associated with an increase in the risk of non-response to anti-HCV therapy – avoid ABC in someone receiving HCV treatment
Combivir® (CBV) (zidovudine + lamivudine) ViiV	One tablet bd	Tablet contains 300 mg zidovudine + 150 mg lamivudine	See entries for individual drugs	See entries for individual drugs
Didanosine (ddI) Videx® Bristol Myers Squibb	If >60 kg, 400 mg od (with tenofovir = 250 mg od) If <60 kg, 250 mg od (with tenofovir = 200 mg od) 400, 250, 200 and 125 mg e-c capsules 25 mg 'buffered' tablets (minimum two tablets/dose) Suspension (named patient)	– Must be taken on an empty stomach (although no food restrictions when taken with tenofovir) – Buffered tablets must be chewed, crushed or dispersed before taking – May be taken with clear apple juice to improve tolerability	– Nausea, bloating, diarrhoea (all may be reduced with e-c formulation) – Dry mouth – Pancreatitis (incidence<1%) (caution in patients with 'high' alcohol intake or history of pancreatitis) – Liver failure rare but reported. Monitor LFTs – Peripheral neuropathy (incidence <10%) – Hyperuricaemia – Lactic acidosis (see BNF for more details) – Shown to increase risk of cardiovascular disease	• Reduce dose in renal impairment (consult product literature) • Tenofovir, ribavirin, ganciclovir and valganciclovir may increase ddI levels ⇒ potential ↑ risk of toxicity • Caution when taking ddI tablets together with drugs adsorbed by antacids. No interaction with ddI capsules • Caution with drugs associated with pancreatitis
Emtricitabine (FTC) Emtriva® Gilead	200 mg od 200 mg capsules 10 mg/mL oral solution	Can be taken with or without food	– Headache most common – Also nausea, diarrhoea, dizziness; harmless skin discoloration – especially in darker skins – Lactic acidosis (see BNF for more details)	• No clinically significant interactions noted so far • Reduce dose in renal impairment (consult product literature) • Has anti-HBV activity
Kivexa® (abacavir + lamivudine) ViiV	One tablet od	Tablet contains 600 mg abacavir + 300 mg lamivudine	See entries under individual drugs (NB: Patients who have had a hypersensitivity reaction to ABC must NEVER be rechallenged with ABACAVIR, KIVEXA or TRIZIVIR)	See entries under individual drugs

Drug	Dose	Administration	Side effects	Notes
Lamivudine (3TC) Epivir® ViiV	150 mg bd 300 mg od 150 and 300 mg tablets Oral solution (10 mg/mL)	Can be taken with or without food	Generally well tolerated – GI disturbances, headache, anaemia and neutropenia have been reported but not common – Lactic acidosis (see BNF for more details) – Recurrent hepatitis can occur in chronic hepatitis B carriers on discontinuation of 3TC	• Reduce dose in renal impairment (consult product literature) • Increased risk of neutropenia with high-dose co-trimoxazole and ganciclovir, valganciclovir or foscarnet • Has anti-HBV activity
Stavudine (D4T) Zerit® Bristol Myers Squibb	If >60 kg, 40 mg bd If <60 kg, 30 mg bd 20, 30 and 40 mg capsules Oral solution (1 mg/mL)	Can be taken with or without food	– Peripheral neuropathy (following discontinuation symptoms may worsen before improvement noted) – Pancreatitis (rare) – Lactic acidosis (see BNF for more details) – Associated with increased risk of lipoatrophy/lipodystrophy syndrome	• Caution with drugs associated with peripheral neuropathy (e.g. didanosine, vincristine, thalidomide, isoniazid)
Tenofovir (TDF) Viread® Gilead	300 mg od Tenofovir disoproxil 245 mg tablet (equivalent to Tenofovir disoproxil fumarate 300 mg)	Can be taken with or without food Can be dispersed in water	– Diarrhoea, nausea and vomiting, flatulence and headache most common (incidence>10%) – Renal impairment and hypophosphataemia reported – monitor serum creatinine and phosphate	• Reduce dose in renal impairment (consult product literature) • Mostly eliminated unchanged in the urine – possible interactions with nephrotoxic drugs or drugs that are excreted renally (e.g. ganciclovir, cidofovir, probenecid) – monitor closely • Has anti-HBV activity
Trizivir® (abacavir + lamivudine + zidovudine) ViiV	One tablet bd	Tablet contains abacavir 300 mg, lamivudine 150 mg and zidovudine 300 mg	See entries under individual drugs (NB: Patients who have had a hypersensitivity reaction to ABC must NEVER be rechallenged with ABACAVIR, KIVEXA or TRIZIVIR.)	• See entries under individual drugs
Truvada® (tenofovir + emtricitabine) Gilead	One tablet od	Tablet contains emtricitabine 200 mg + tenofovir 300 mg Can be dispersed in water	See entries under individual drugs	• See entries under individual drugs
Zidovudine (AZT) Retrovir® ViiV	Usual dose 250 mg bd (300 mg bd in Combivir and Trizivir) 100, 250 mg capsules 50 mg/5 ml syrup iv infusion	Can be taken with or without food (take with/after food to improve GI tolerance)	– Nausea, vomiting, headache, fatigue and muscle pain more common in first few weeks and usually wear off – Haematological toxicities (e.g. neutropenia, anaemia) may develop after ~6 weeks – Myopathy may be associated with long-term therapy (>12 months) – Lactic acidosis (see BNF for more details) – Associated with increased risk of lipoatrophy/ lipodystrophy syndrome	• Clarithromycin can ↓ AZT absorption • Rifampicin may decrease AZT levels – unclear significance in clinical practice • Phenytoin levels may be altered • Increased risk of toxicity with ribavirin, probenecid and myelotoxic drugs (e.g. ganciclovir/valganciclovir and high-dose co-trimoxazole)

od, once daily; bd, twice daily; e-c, enteric coated; iv, intravenous; GI, gastro-intestinal; BNF, British National Formulary; LFTs, liver function tests; HCV, hepatitis C virus; HBV, hepatitis B virus.

Table 41.2 General prescribing points for non-nucleoside reverse transcriptase inhibitors (NNRTIs)

Drug, names, manufacturer	Dose and formulation	Administration	Major/common side effects	Significant drug interactions and important pharmacokinetic information
Efavirenz (EFV) Sustiva® Bristol Myers Squibb	600 mg od (usually at night) – Increase to 800 mg od with rifampicin – Dose of oral solution: 720 mg od (24 ml) due to altered bio-availability 600 mg tablets 200 mg capsules 30 mg/mL oral solution	Can be taken with or without food. Manufacturer recommends taking on an empty stomach to improve tolerability Taken at night to minimise sedative effect, but can be taken during the day if preferred	– CNS disturbances (from sedation/feeling 'stoned'/dizzy and impaired concentration to vivid dreams, mood swings and hallucinations) – Caution in patients with previous or current psychiatric illness – Rash (in about 18% of adults) mostly in first 2 weeks, usually mild; severe rash rare – Raised LFTs – more common if hepatitis B or C co-infected – Hyperlipidaemia – monitor – Avoid in early pregnancy if possible – animal studies show teratogenic effects; effective contraception should be used	• Caution on stopping EFV-containing regimen due to long half-life • Metabolised by cytochrome P450 hepatic enzymes – caution with other drugs which affect these enzymes • Avoid clarithromycin, St John's Wort, ergotamines, caution with anticonvulsants • Mixed inhibitor and inducer of CYP450 enzymes – caution with other drugs metabolised by these enzymes; use alternatives wherever possible. Perform TDM on potentially affected drugs where indicated (e.g. phenytoin) • *Increases levels of midazolam* – avoid or start with low doses and titrate and monitor carefully; do not use in outpatients, caution in day case attenders (*NB*: Manufacturer advises avoid.) • May get altered levels of methadone, erectile dysfunction agents sildenafil (Viagra®), tadalafil (Cialis®), vardenafil (Levitra®) and warfarin (monitor INR) among others
Nevirapine (NVP) Viramune® Boehringer-Ingelheim	200 mg od for first 14 days, then 200 mg bd. 400 mg od unlicensed dose. 200 mg tablets 50 mg/5 ml oral suspension	Can be taken with or without food. If dosing interrupted for >7 days, NVP must be restarted at lead-in dose (200 mg od for 2 weeks)	– Rash (in about 20%; most common in first 6 weeks); severe rash rare but monitor closely – Raised LFTs/hepatitis (check every 2 weeks for first 2 months) – Caution on restarting NVP if previously discontinued due to rash or hepatitis/↑LFTs – See BNF for more details – Also nausea, headache, sedation, fatigue – Should not be started in women with CD4 >250 cells/mm³ or men with CD4 >400 cells/mm³: greater risk of rash-associated hepatic events	• *Caution on stopping NVP-containing regimen due to long half-life* • Metabolised by cytochrome P450 hepatic enzymes – caution with other drugs which may affect these enzymes • *Avoid St John's Wort, rifampicin, caution with anticonvulsants* • Inducer of cytochrome P450 – caution with other drugs metabolised by these enzymes; use alternatives wherever possible. Perform TDM on potentially affected drugs where indicated • *May get altered levels of methadone and warfarin (monitor INR)* • May decrease levels of erectile dysfunction agents sildenafil (Viagra®), tadalafil (Cialis®), vardenafil (Levitra®)
Etravirine (TMC-125) Intelence® Janssen	200 mg bd 400 mg od unlicensed dose 100 mg tablets	Take with food to improve bioavailability. Can be dispersed in water.	– Rash (in >10%) – severe rash (inc Steven-Johnson syndrome) reported but rare – Nausea – Diarrhoea, abdominal pain – Headache, pyrexia, fatigue	• *Caution on stopping etravirine-containing regimen due to long half-life* • Metabolised by cytochrome P450 hepatic enzymes – caution with other drugs which may affect these enzymes • *Avoid St John's wort, carbamazepine, clarithromycin, rifampicin* • Mixed inhibitor and inducer of cytochrome P450 enzymes – caution with other drugs metabolised by these enzymes; use alternatives wherever possible. Perform TDM on potentially affected drugs where indicated • *May get altered levels of methadone and warfarin (monitor INR)* • May get decreased levels of erectile dysfunction agents sildenafil (Viagra®), tadalafil (Cialis®), vardenafil (Levitra®)

od, once daily; bd, twice daily; BNF, British National Formulary; LFTs, liver function tests; TDM, therapeutic drug monitoring; INR, international normalised ratio.

Table 41.3 General prescribing points for protease inhibitors

Drug, names, manufacturer	Dose and formulation	Administration	Major/common side effects	Significant drug interactions and important pharmacokinetic information
Atazanavir (ATV) Reyataz® Bristol Myers Squibb	300 mg (with 100 mg ritonavir) od 400 mg (with 100 mg ritonavir) od with enzyme inducers or interacting meds 300, 200, 150 mg capsules	Take with or after food to enhance bioavailability	Most common: – Nausea, diarrhoea, headache, rash, jaundice Also – Hyperbilirubinaemia (may need dose ↓ or stop if ≥ Grade 3 or 4) – Raised LFTs – more common in Hepatitis B or C co-infection – Does not appear to ↑ lipids – ECG changes – Other protease inhibitor 'class side effects', for example, lipodystrophy syndrome: body shape changes (see BNF for more details)	• Metabolised by cytochrome P450 hepatic enzymes – caution with other drugs which may affect these enzymes – *rifampicin contraindicated, avoid St John's Wort* • Inhibits cytochrome P450 enzymes. Caution with other drugs metabolised by these enzymes as may get ↑ in levels. *Do NOT co-administer with simvastatin, ergotamines, antiarrhythmics* • *Increases levels of midazolam* – avoid or start with low dose and titrate and monitor carefully; do not use in outpatients, caution in day case attenders (NB: Manufacturer advises avoid.) • May increase levels of corticosteroids, including inhaled/intranasal steroids (avoid fluticasone and budesonide) • May require dose alteration of warfarin (monitor INR), methadone, bupropion (Zyban®) • *H₂ antagonists and proton pump inhibitors significantly decrease atazanavir levels* – discuss with specialist HIV team before co-prescribing. Avoid antacids within 2 h of ATV dose • Caution with erectile dysfunct on agents sildenafil (Viagra®), tadalafil (Cialis®) and vardenafil (Levitra®) – reduce initial dose (e.g. maximum dose sildenafil 25 mg in 48 h) • *If boosted, see ritonavir for full list of potential interactions*
Darunavir (TMC-114) Prezista® Janssen	600 mg bd (with ritonavir 100 mg bd) 800 mg od (with ritonavir 100 mg od) 400, 600 mg tablets	Take with food to improve bioavailability	Most common: – Nausea, vomiting diarrhoea, constipation, abdo pain – Headache, rash – Hyperlipidaemia Also – Raised LFTs. – Caution in sulphonamide allergy – Other protease inhibitor 'class side effects', for example, lipodystrophy syndrome: metabolic/body shape changes (see BNF for more details)	• Metabolised by cytochrome P450 hepatic enzymes – caution with other drugs which may affect these enzymes – *rifampicin contraindicated, avoid St John's Wort* • Inhibits cytochrome P450 enzymes. Caution with other drugs metabolised by these enzymes as may get ↑ in levels. *Do NOT co-administer with ergotamines, antiarrhythmics* • *Increases levels of midazolam* – avoid or start with low dose and titrate and monitor carefully; do not use in outpatients, caution in day case attenders (NB: Manufacturer advises avoid.) • May increase levels of corticosteroids, including inhaled/intranasal steroids (avoid fluticasone and budesonide) • May require dose alteration of warfarin (monitor INR), methadone, bupropion (Zyban®) • *Caution with statins (including pravastatin)* – start with lowest dose and titrate according to response. *Simvastatin CONTRAINDICATED* • Caution with erectile dysfunction agents sildenafil (Viagra®), tadalafil (Cialis®) and vardenafil (Levitra®) – reduce initial dose (e.g. maximum dose sildenafil 25 mg in 48 h) • *See ritonavir for full list of potential interactions*

Continued

Table 41.3 General prescribing points for protease inhibitors—cont'd

Drug, names, manufacturer	Dose and formulation	Administration	Major/common side effects	Significant drug interactions and important pharmacokinetic information
Fosamprenavir (FAPV) Telzir® ViiV	700 mg bd (with 100 mg bd ritonavir) unlicensed doses: – 1400 mg od (with 200 mg od ritonavir) – 1400 mg bd (unboosted) 700 mg tablets 50 mg/mL oral solution	Can be taken with or without food	Most common: – Nausea and vomiting, diarrhoea – Rash – Fatigue Also – Raised LFTs – Hyperlipidaemia – Other protease inhibitor 'class side effects', for example, lipodystrophy syndrome: metabolic/lipid/body shape changes (see BNF for more details)	• Metabolised by cytochrome P450 hepatic enzymes – caution with other drugs which may affect these enzymes – *rifampicin contraindicated, avoid St John's Wort, carbamazepine* • Inhibits cytochrome P450 enzymes. Caution with other drugs metabolised by these enzymes as may get ↑ in levels. *Do NOT co-administer with simvastatin, ergotamines, antiarrhythmics* • *Increases levels of midazolam – avoid or start with low dose and titrate and monitor carefully; do not use in outpatients, caution in day case attenders.* (NB: Manufacturer advises avoid.) • May increase levels of corticosteroids, including inhaled/intranasal steroids (*avoid fluticasone and budesonide*) • May require dose alteration of warfarin (monitor INR), methadone, bupropion (Zyban®) • Caution with erectile dysfunction agents sildenafil (Viagra®), vardenafil (Levitra®) and tadalafil (Cialis®) – reduce initial dose (e.g. maximum dose sildenafil 25 mg in 48h) • *If boosted, see ritonavir for full list of potential interactions.*
Indinavir (IDV) Crixivan® Merck Sharp and Dohme	800 mg every 8 h With ritonavir: 800 mg (with 100 mg ritonavir) bd or 400 mg (with 400 mg ritonavir) bd ↓ dose in hepatic insufficiency 200 and 400 mg capsules	Best on an empty stomach >1 h before food or >2 h after meals May take with light, low fat (<5 g fat) snacks. No food restrictions if with ritonavir. Store with desiccant. Drink >1.5 L water per day (even if taking with ritonavir)	– Nephrolithiasis – Hyperbilirubinaemia – Increases in AST and ALT – Rash, dry skin, pruritus, hair loss – Ingrown toenails – Taste perversion – Haemolytic anaemia – Other protease inhibitor 'class side effects', that is lipodystrophy syndrome: metabolic/lipid/body shape changes (see BNF for more details)	• Metabolised by cytochrome P450 hepatic enzymes – caution with other drugs which may affect these enzymes – *rifampicin contraindicated, avoid St John's Wort, carbamazepine. Indinavir increased by ketoconazole and itraconazole* • Inhibits cytochrome P450 enzymes. Caution with other drugs metabolised by these enzymes as may get – in levels. *Do NOT co-administer with simvastatin, ergotamines, antiarrhythmics* • *Increases levels of midazolam – avoid or start with low dose and titrate and monitor carefully; do not use in outpatients, caution in day case attenders* (NB: Manufacturer advises avoid.) • May increase levels of corticosteroids, including inhaled/intranasal steroids (*avoid fluticasone and budesonide*) • *May require dose alteration of warfarin (monitor INR), methadone, bupropion (Zyban®)* • Administer indinavir and didanosine tablets at least 1 h apart (ok to take with e-c caps) • Caution with erectile dysfunction agents sildenafil (Viagra®), vardenafil (Levitra®) and tadalafil (Cialis®) – reduce initial dose (maximum dose sildenafil 25 mg in 48h) • *If boosted, see ritonavir for full list of potential interactions*

Drug	Dose	Administration	Side effects	Interactions/cautions
Kaletra® (LPV/r) (lopinavir + ritonavir) Abbott	2 tablets bd; 5 ml bd (=400/100 mg bd); 4 tablets od (not recommended if >3 protease inhibitor resistance mutations present) Tablets: 200 mg lopinavir with 50 mg ritonavir; 100 mg lopinavir with 25 mg ritonavir; 400/100 mg lopinavir/ritonavir in 5 ml oral solution	Tablets: No food restrictions. Liquid: Take with or after food — Oral solution has high alcohol and propylene glycol content. Caution with disulfiram or metronidazole. Tablets: store at room temperature. Store liquid in refrigerator (stable at <25 °C for 6 weeks)	Most common: – Diarrhoea, nausea, vomiting, headache, rash, dyslipidaemias – Raised LFTs (esp. AST and ALT and GGT. More common if hepatitis B or C co-infected – Other protease inhibitor 'class side effects', that is, lipodystrophy syndrome: metabolic/lipid/body shape changes (see BNF for more details)	• Metabolised by cytochrome P450 hepatic enzymes – caution with other drugs which may affect these enzymes – rifampicin contraindicated, avoid St John's Wort, carbamazepine • Inhibits cytochrome P450 enzymes. Caution with other drugs metabolised by these enzymes as may get ↑ in levels. Do NOT co-administer with simvastatin, ergotamines, antiarrhythmics • Increases levels of midazolam – avoid or start with low dose and titrate and monitor carefully; do not use n outpatients, caution in day case attenders (NB: Manufacturer advises avoid.) • May increase levels of corticosteroids, including inhaled/intranasal steroids (avoid fluticasone and budescnide) • May require dose alteration of warfarin (monitor INR), methadone, bupropion (Zyban®) • Caution with erectile dysfunction agents sildenafil (Viagra®), tadalafil (Cialis®) and vardenafil (Levitra®) – reduce initial dose (e.g. maximum dose sildenafil 25 mg in 48 h) • See ritonavir for full list of potential interactions
Nelfinavir (NFV) Viracept® Roche	1250 mg bd; 750 mg tds; 250 mg tablets	Take with or after food to increase bio availability (up to 2 h after full meal, or with small meal/snack)	Most common: – Diarrhoea and flatulence, nausea. Also – Hyperglycaemia/diabetes – Other protease inhibitor 'class side effects', that is, lipodystrophy syndrome: metabolic/lipid/body shape changes (see BNF for more details)	• Metabolised by cytochrome P450 hepatic enzymes – caution with other drugs which may affect these enzymes – rifampicin contraindicated, avoid St John's Wort, carbamazepine • Inhibits CYP450 enzymes. Caution with other drugs metabolised by these enzymes as may get ↑ in levels. Do NOT co-administer with simvastatin, ergotamines, antiarrhythmics • increases levels of midazolam – avoid or start with low dose and titrate and monitor carefully; do not use in outpatients, caution in day case attenders (NB: Manufacturer advises avoid.) • May increase levels of corticosteroids, including inhaled/intranasal steroids (avoid fluticasone and budesonide) • May require dose alteration of warfarin (monitor INR), methadone, bupropion (Zyban) • Caution with erectile dysfunction agents sildenafil (Viagra), vardenafil (Levitra) and tadalafil (Cialis) – reduce initial dose (max dose sildenafil 25 mg in 48 h)
Ritonavir (RTV) Norv r® Abbott	Usually used to 'boost' other protease inhibitors at doses of 130–200 mg od-bd; 600 mg bd (antiretroviral dose); 100 mg tablets; 400 mg/5 ml oral solution	Do not administer liquid formulation with disulfiram or metronidazole due to high alcohol content (tablets ok with metronidazole). Take with or after food if possible (to reduce GI intolerance). Tablets and liquid stored at room temperature.	– Asthenia, – Nausea, vomiting, – Diarrhoea, abdominal pain, – Anorexia, – Taste perversion, – Circumoral and peripheral paraesthesiae – Other protease inhibitor 'class side effects', that is, lipodystrophy syndrome: metabolic/lipid/body shape changes (see BNF for more details)	• Metabolised by cytochrome P450 hepatic enzymes – caution with other drugs which may affect these enzymes – rifampicin contraindicated, avoid St John's Wort, carbamazepine • Extremely potent inhibitor of cytochrome P450 enzymes. Caution with other drugs metabolised by these enzymes as may get ↑ in levels. Do NOT co-administer with ergotamines, antiarrhythmics, pethidine, piroxicam, amphetamines (inc. ecstasy). Caution with diazepam, antifungals (e.g. ketoconazole), clarithromycin, and carbamazepine • Increases levels of midazolam – avoid or start with low dose and titrate and monitor carefully; do not use in outpatients or day case attenders (NB: Manufacturer advises avoid.) • Caution with statins – start with lowest dose and titrate according to response. Simvastatin CONTRAINDICATED.

Continued

Table 41.3 General prescribing points for protease inhibitors—cont'd

Drug, names, manufacturer	Dose and formulation	Administration	Major/common side effects	Significant drug interactions and important pharmacokinetic information
				• May increase levels of corticosteroids, including inhaled/intranasal steroids (avoid fluticasone and budesonide) • May require dose alteration of warfarin (monitor INR), methadone, bupropion (Zyban®) • Caution with erectile dysfunction agents sildenafil (Viagra), tadalafil (Cialis) and vardenafil (Levitra) – reduce initial dose (e.g. maximum dose sildenafil 25mg in 48h) • See BNF/data sheet for full list of contraindications and caution drugs before prescribing
Saquinavir (SQV) Invirase® Roche	1000mg (with 100mg ritonavir) bd Unlicensed doses: – 400mg (with 400mg ritonavir) bd – 1600–2000mg od (with 100mg ritonavir od) 200mg capsules, 500mg tablets	Take with or after food (up to 2h after a full meal)	– Diarrhoea – Nausea – Abdominal discomfort/wind – Raised LFTs – Prolonged QT interval – Other protease inhibitor 'class side effects', that is, lipodystrophy syndrome: metabolic/lipid/body shape changes (see BNF for more details)	• Metabolised by cytochrome P450 hepatic enzymes – caution with other drugs which may affect these enzymes – rifampicin contraindicated, avoid St John's Wort, carbamazepine. Co-administration of clarithromycin, ketoconazole, ranitidine or cimetidine may increase levels of saquinavir • Inhibits cytochrome P450 enzymes. Caution with other drugs metabolised by these enzymes as may get ↑ in levels. Do NOT co-administer with simvastatin, ergotamines, antiarrhythmics • Increases levels of midazolam – avoid or start with low dose and titrate and monitor carefully; do not use in outpatients, caution in day case attenders • May increase levels of corticosteroids, including inhaled/intranasal steroids (avoid fluticasone and budesonide) • May require dose alteration of warfarin (monitor INR), methadone, bupropion (Zyban®) • Caution with erectile dysfunction agents sildenafil (Viagra®), tadalafil (Cialis®) and vardenafil (Levitra) – reduce initial dose (e.g. max dose sildenafil 25mg in 48h) • If boosted, see ritonavir for full list of potential interactions
Tipranavir (TPV) Aptivus® Boehringer Ingelheim	500mg bd: co-administer with 200mg bd ritonavir 250mg capsules	Take with or after food to improve GI tolerance Store in refrigerator (once opened, container may be stored below 30 °C for 60 days)	– Diarrhoea – Nausea, vomiting – Fatigue – Headache – Elevated LFTs – Other protease inhibitor 'class side effects', that is, lipodystrophy syndrome: metabolic/lipid/body shape changes (see BNF for more details)	• Metabolised by cytochrome P450 hepatic enzymes – caution with other drugs which may affect these enzymes – rifampicin contraindicated, avoid St John's Wort, carbamazepine • Inhibits cytochrome P450 enzymes. Caution with other drugs metabolised by these enzymes as may get ↑ in levels. Do NOT co-administer with simvastatin, ergotamines, antiarrhythmics • Increases levels of midazolam – avoid or start with low dose and titrate and monitor carefully; do not use in outpatients, caution in day case attenders (NB: Manufacturer advises avoid.) • May increase levels of corticosteroids, including inhaled/intranasal steroids (avoid fluticasone and budesonide) • May require dose alteration of warfarin (monitor INR), methadone, bupropion (Zyban®) • Caution with erectile dysfunction agents sildenafil (Viagra®), tadalafil (Cialis®) and vardenafil (Levitra®) – reduce initial dose (e.g. maximum dose sildenafil 25mg in 48h) • See ritonavir for full list of potential interactions

od, once daily; bd, twice daily; e-c, enteric coated; GI, gastro-intestinal; BNF, British National Formulary; LFTs, liver function tests; INR, International normalised ratio; AST, Aspartate transaminase; ALT, alanine transaminase; GGT, γ glutanyl transferase.

Table 41.4 General prescribing points for Integrase Inhibitors

Drug, names, manufacturer	Dose and formulation	Administration	Major/common side effects	Significant drug interactions and important pharmacokinetic information
Raltegravir Isentress® Merck Sharp and Dohme	400 mg bd 400 mg tablets	Can be taken with or without food	– Nausea, headache – Dizziness, vertigo – Abdominal pain, flatulence, constipation – Pruritus, arthralgia, fatigue – Raised creatine kinase – Myopathy and rhabdomyolysis reported but rare	• *Metabolised by glucuronidation* – caution with potent inducers of this pathway, for example, rifampicin. (No effect on cytochrome P450 enzymes) • Levels increased by proton pump inhibitors – clinical significance uncertain • Levels decreased by ritonavir, tipranavir, efavirenz, St John's Wort, nevirapine, no need for dose adjustment

bd, twice daily.

In addition, there are a number of combination formulations of NRTIs that may be used to reduce pill burden:

Abacavir + lamivudine (Kivexa®)
Tenofovir + emtricitabine (Truvada®)
Zidovudine + lamivudine (Combivir®)
Zidovudine + lamivudine plus abacavir (Trizivir®)

There is also one formulation combining two NRTIs with an NNRTI:
Tenofovir + emtricitabine + efavirenz (Atripla®)

Other triple and quadruple mixed class co-formulations are in development.

Most antiretroviral regimens will include two NRTIs, together with a PI and/or an NNRTI. In the UK, the most commonly prescribed NRTI combination as first-line therapy is tenofovir with emtricitabine (either as the combination formulation Truvada® or, with efavirenz, as Atripla®) which has the benefits of once daily administration and an improved toxicity profile compared to older therapies. A number of combinations should be avoided. These include: zidovudine and stavudine (intracellular competition resulting in antagonism); stavudine and didanosine (unacceptable toxicity); tenofovir and didanosine (unacceptable rates of virological failure and potential for CD4 decline).

Non-nucleoside reverse transcriptase inhibitors

NNRTIs inhibit the reverse transcriptase enzyme by binding to its active site. They do not require prior phosphorylation and can act on cell-free virions as well as infected cells. The NNRTIs available include:

Efavirenz (Sustiva®)
Nevirapine (Viramune®)
Etravirine (Intelence®)

Resistance to NNRTIs occurs rapidly in incompletely suppressive regimens and it is therefore essential that they are prescribed with at least two NRTIs or a combination of NRTIs and PIs. Cross-resistance between nevirapine and efavirenz, which are currently used as first-line NNRTIs, is high. The first of the second-generation NNRTIs, etravirine, is active against some viruses resistant to these agents. Rilpivirine (expected to be licensed in 2011) also has a different resistance profile, but is likely to be used as an alternative first-line NNRTI.

The NNRTIs have much longer plasma half-lives than PIs and NRTIs, so when stopping an NNRTI-containing combination, consideration should be given to either continuing the other agents for a period after cessation of the NNRTI or switching to a boosted PI prior to regimen discontinuation.

Protease inhibitors

PIs bind to the active site of the HIV-1 protease enzyme, preventing the maturation of the newly produced virions so that they remain non-infectious. The following PIs are currently available:

Atazanavir (Reyataz®)
Darunavir (Prezista®)
Fosamprenavir (Telzir®)
Indinavir (Crixivan®)
Lopinavir co-formulated with ritonavir (Kaletra®)
Nelfinavir (Viracept®)
Ritonavir (Norvir®)
Saquinavir (Invirase®)
Tipranavir (Aptivus®)

The use of ritonavir-boosted PIs has superseded use of single PIs, due to better pharmacokinetic profiles, superior efficacy data and reduced likelihood of resistance development. Newer second-generation PIs such as tipranavir and darunavir are effective against many viruses resistant to the earlier PIs. Darunavir is used in first-line PI therapy as a once-daily boosted agent (800 mg with 100 mg of ritonavir); for patients with significant PI resistance a higher dose of 600 mg twice daily, each with ritonavir 100 mg, is used.

Table 41.5 General prescribing points for entry inhibitors

Drug, names, manufacturer, mode of action	Dose and formulation	Administration	Major/common side effects	Significant drug interactions and important pharmacokinetic information
Enfuvirtide (T-20) Fuzeon® Roche Fusion Inhibitor	90 mg bd Ideally every 12 h, but dosing interval of 8–16 h allowed (i.e. 4 h flexibility for each dose) 90 mg/mL powder and solvent for solution for s/c injection Each vial contains 108 mg enfuvirtide, 1 ml of reconstituted solution contains 90 mg enfuvirtide	Single use vials, reconstitute with 1.1 ml water for injection (may take up to 45 min to dissolve powder, DO NOT shake vial) Once reconstituted can be stored in fridge for 24 h (i.e. can make up more than 1 dose at once)	– Injection site reactions very common (pain/discomfort, erythema, nodules/cysts) but not usually requiring discontinuation – Other common side effects; insomnia, headache, lymphadenopathy, eosinophilia – Increased rate of bacterial infections (especially pneumonia) reported – Hypersensitivity reactions requiring discontinuation reported, but rare	• No clinically significant pharmacokinetic interactions expected
Maraviroc Celsentri® ViiV CCR5 Antagonist	Dose varies with co-administered medication: 300 mg bd if not with significant enzyme inhibitors/inducers 150 mg bd with significant enzyme inhibitors (e.g. protease inhibitors) 600 mg bd with significant enzyme inducers (e.g. NNRTIs, rifampicin) 150, 300 mg tablets	Can be taken with or without food. Must only be prescribed for patient with recently confirmed CCR5 tropic virus (i.e. not CXCR4 or dual/mixed tropic virus)	– Nausea most common – Vomiting, abdominal pain, constipation, bloating – Dizziness, paraesthesia, somnolence – Rash – Asthenia – Insomnia – Raised LFTs – Dose limiting adverse reaction in clinical trials, postural hypotension	• Metabolised by cytochrome P450 hepatic enzymes, caution with other drugs which may affect these enzymes as dose will need to be adjusted. Do not co-administer with St John's Wort • Does not inhibit or induce any cytochrome P450 enzymes • See product literature for detailed information on dosing • Adjust dose in renal impairment if co-administered with an enzyme inhibitor (see product literature) • Contraindicated in patients with peanut or soya allergy (contains soya lecithin)

bd, twice daily.

An alternative booster to ritonavir, cobicistat, is currently in development and is likely to be co-formulated with PIs as well as elvitegravir (see below).

Entry inhibitors

There are currently two types of entry inhibitors (fusion inhibitors and CCR5 inhibitors) with one agent available in each class. Fusion inhibitors block the structural rearrangement of HIV-1 gp41 and thus stop the fusion of the viral cell membrane with the target cell membrane, preventing viral RNA from entering the cell. CCR5 inhibitors selectively bind to the human chemokine receptor CCR5, preventing CCR5-tropic HIV-1 from entering cells.

Enfuvirtide (T-20, Fuzeon®), a fusion inhibitor, is administered subcutaneously and is largely used in heavily treatment experienced patients. The main side effect is injection site reactions. However, following the licensing of new agents from different antiretroviral classes, enfuvirtide is now rarely used.

Maraviroc (Celsentri®), a CCR5 inhibitor, is indicated for use in patients with only CCR5-tropic virus, which is determined by a tropism test just prior to commencing treatment. It is usually used in patients with resistance to one or more other antiretroviral classes.

Integrase inhibitors

Integrase inhibitors bind to the integrase enzyme, thus blocking the integration of viral DNA into host DNA. There is currently one licensed agent, raltegravir (Isentress). Whilst this was initially used in patients with resistant virus, it is increasingly being used either in first-line regimens or where tolerability issues arise with initial therapy. Other agents in development include elvitegravir and dolutegravir. Elvitegravir requires boosting and is being developed as a co-formulation with cobicistat.

Toxicity of antiretroviral therapies

As more antiretroviral agents have become available and the number of patient-years of exposure to them has increased, our understanding of their various toxicities has grown significantly.

Whilst there are many individual drug toxicities (see Tables 41.1–41.5), there are also a number of class-specific or therapy-related toxicities (Carr and Cooper, 2000).

Mitochondrial toxicity. Mitochondrial toxicity is increasingly recognised in patients with prolonged exposure to nucleoside analogue antiretrovirals, particularly stavudine, didanosine and, to a lesser extent, zidovudine, and is thought to explain such side effects as peripheral neuropathy, myopathy, pancreatitis and lactic acidosis. If these problems should arise, management is to switch the likely causative agent, if possible (McComsey and Lonergan, 2004).

Rash and hepatitis. These are both recognised side effects of the NNRTI class, although the incidence and severity appear greatest with nevirapine, particularly in patients with a higher CD4 count (>250 cells/mm³ for women and >400 cells/mm³ for men). Management is either close observation (in mild-to-moderate cases) or withdrawal of the causative agent (in severe cases). An abacavir hypersensitivity reaction is well characterised and historically occurs in approximately 6–8% of individuals who receive abacavir. It typically presents in the first 6 weeks of therapy as a progressive illness with fevers, rash and flu-like symptoms. Fatalities have been reported where the drug has subsequently been reintroduced in patients with a prior history of hypersensitivity reaction. Management has traditionally been to withdraw the agent and never reintroduce. However, the use of newer pharmacogenomic techniques, for example, HLA B*5701 testing, and subsequent prescription of abacavir only to those who are B*5701 negative have dramatically reduced the incidence of hypersensitivity reaction (Mallal et al., 2008).

Lipodystrophy. Lipodystrophy has been well reported in individuals on HAART. This is characterised by one or both of lipoatrophy (fat loss, particularly from the face, upper limbs and buttocks) and lipohypertrophy (abnormal fat deposition, particularly affecting the abdomen and neck). Whilst these body shape changes are associated with drug therapy, predominantly stavudine and zidovudine for lipoatrophy and possibly PIs for lipohypertrophy, it is likely that host and disease factors also play a role in aetiology (Carr, 2003; Lichtenstein, 2005). Management at present is to avoid or switch away from the causative agent(s) and/or to use cosmetic approaches (fillers or liposuction). Since the decline in use of the older NRTIs, the incidence of lipodystrophy has decreased dramatically.

Metabolic disturbances. Hypercholesterolaemia and hypertriglyceridaemia, in particular, are frequently seen in patients receiving HAART. Again, the aetiology of these toxicities is likely to represent a combination of drug and host factors. However, they are particularly associated with PIs, although the incidence appears lower with atazanavir. Whilst it is likely that this hyperlipidaemia contributes to an increased cardiovascular disease risk, this needs to be considered in the context of traditional risk factors, for example, smoking, which may be present in this patient group. Management is to reduce all modifiable risk factors and either switch away from the likely causative agent to one more metabolically favourable or consider adjunctive lipid-lowering therapy, taking into consideration potential drug–drug interactions (Schambelan et al., 2002).

Renal impairment and, rarely, Fanconi's syndrome have been reported with tenofovir. Creatinine clearance should be calculated and proteinuria quantified prior to starting therapy with this agent and should be monitored regularly.

Cardiovascular disease. Cohort studies have suggested an increased risk of cardiovascular disease with some PIs (Kaletra® and indinavir) and with the NRTI, abacavir (Sabin et al., 2008; Worm et al., 2010). This risk is independent of the effect on lipids and the mechanism has yet to be determined. As with lipid disturbances, the decision to start or continue these agents needs to be considered as part of a holistic approach to cardiovascular risk.

Opportunistic infections and malignancies

Detailed information on treatment guidelines can be obtained by consulting the relevant national guidelines, for example, British HIV Association guidelines for the management of opportunistic infections (Nelson et al., 2010), tuberculosis (Pozniak et al., 2010), malignancies (Bower et al., 2008). Dosing schedules for the most commonly used drugs used to treat opportunistic infections are summarised in Table 41.6.

Fungal infections

P. jiroveci pneumonia. This remains one of the most common causes of morbidity and mortality in HIV-positive individuals. Classically, patients present with an insidious onset of a non-productive cough, shortness of breath on exertion and an inability to take a deep breath. Fever, anorexia and weight loss are common accompanying symptoms. Patients are usually markedly immunosuppressed, with CD4 counts less than 200 cells/mm^3. Diagnosis is supported by the presence of exercise-induced oxygen desaturation and the typical chest radiographic appearance of bilateral interstitial shadowing, though in mild cases, the chest X-ray may be normal. *P. jiroveci* cannot be cultured in vitro, so the diagnosis is confirmed by demonstration of the organism by immunofluorescence or silver staining, or by nucleic acid amplification techniques (NAAT), of samples obtained by bronchoalveolar lavage. Sputum induction, by nebulisation of hypertonic sodium chloride, is not recommended for obtaining samples unless the procedure is being performed in the treatment centre sufficiently regularly to enable staff to maintain competence, as diagnostic sensitivity of the test is significantly affected by technique.

Treatment is instigated in patients with a proven diagnosis, or empirically where there is a suspicion prior to confirmation. Adequate samples may be obtained to make a diagnosis up to 7–10 days after starting treatment. Oxygen is essential for patients with compromised respiratory function. First-line therapy is high-dose co-trimoxazole for 21 days: oral for mild cases (1920 mg three times daily), and intravenous for moderate-to-severe disease (120 mg/kg/day in divided doses for 3 days, then 90 mg/kg/day for 18 days). Nausea and vomiting commonly occur and may be best managed pre-emptively by administration of a prophylactic antiemetic.

In cases of co-trimoxazole intolerance, several alternative therapies are available. For mild *P. jiroveci* pneumonia, a combination of oral trimethoprim (10–15 mg/kg/day in two divided doses) with dapsone (100 mg daily) may be effective. For moderate-to-severe disease, a combination of clindamycin (intravenous or oral) and primaquine is often used. Intravenous pentamidine is another alternative, though its use may be associated with more significant adverse reactions. Pentamidine should also be given in nebulised form (600 mg) via a suitable nebuliser, for example, Respirgard II, for the first 3 days, to ensure prompt attainment of adequate lung tissue levels. Oral atovaquone suspension can be used for mild-to-moderate *P. jiroveci* pneumonia but must be taken with food, particularly fatty food, to be effective. Glucose-6-phosphate dehydrogenase (G6PD) levels should be checked prior to (or as soon as possible after starting) treatment with co-trimoxazole, dapsone or primaquine.

For cases of moderate-to-severe *P. jiroveci* pneumonia (PaO$_2$ < 9.3 kPa or SpO$_2$ < 92%), adjunctive corticosteroid therapy is recommended, for example, prednisolone 75 mg daily for 5 days, 50 mg for 5 days, and then 25 mg for 5 days. Ventilatory support should be considered for patients in whom the underlying prognosis is good, for example, those presenting for the first time with *P. jiroveci* pneumonia, those without severe co-existing medical complications and those with remaining effective antiretroviral options.

It has been clearly demonstrated that prophylactic therapy reduces both the incidence and severity of *P. jiroveci* pneumonia in patients with either prior disease or those at risk of a first episode, and that this intervention significantly improves survival. Primary prophylaxis is recommended for those individuals with a previous AIDS-defining illness, markedly symptomatic disease (including oral candidiasis), a CD4 count < 200 cells/mm^3 or CD4 percentage <14%. Prophylaxis can be discontinued when CD4 is sustained above 200 cells/mm^3 for over 3 months on HAART.

Co-trimoxazole is the gold standard and also confers protection against toxoplasmosis and some other bacterial infections. Commonly used regimens with proven efficacy are 960 mg daily or three times a week or 480 mg daily. The incidence of adverse reactions to co-trimoxazole in HIV-positive individuals is higher than in the general population, although many patients who are intolerant of high-dose treatment do not experience problems at prophylactic doses. In cases of intolerance, several alternative approaches may be adopted. Desensitisation may be attempted or other agents may be used. Dapsone 100 mg daily, with or without pyrimethamine, according to *Toxoplasma* status, is effective but does not offer such broad protection against bacterial infections. Nebulised pentamidine at a dose of 300 mg every month via an appropriate nebuliser (with prior nebulised or inhaled β$_2$-agonist to prevent bronchospasm) can also be used but does not protect against extra-pulmonary *P. jiroveci* pneumonia.

Oropharyngeal candidiasis. Candidiasis is a frequent manifestation of HIV infection and may occur early in the disease. Clinically, it is usually characterised by white plaques on the oral mucosa, but may present as erythematous patches or as angular cheilitis. If swallowing is difficult (dysphagia) or painful (odynophagia), oesophageal involvement may be suspected.

First-line therapy for oral candidiasis is a systemic agent, usually fluconazole (50 mg daily for 7 days). An alternative is itraconazole (200 mg once daily); the solution has higher bioavailability than the capsule formulation and does not require an acid pH for absorption. Topical therapies are available where there is a clinical decision to avoid systemic antifungals (e.g. in patients with hepatic failure). They are as effective as oral azoles for oropharyngeal disease, but time to yeast clearance is longer and relapse rate is higher.

In cases of oesophageal candida, which is an AIDS-defining illness, systemic therapy is necessary using higher doses of the above agents for a longer duration, for example, fluconazole 100 mg once daily for 2 weeks. Continuous azole therapy or frequent courses of these drugs predispose to the development

Table 41.6 Selected drugs to treat opportunistic infections in HIV disease

Drug	Indication	Dosage: route, frequency, duration	Common or significant side effects include:	Significant interactions	Monitoring	Comments
Aciclovir	Herpes simplex Herpes zoster Prophylaxis/suppression of herpes infections	5–10mg/kg i.v. three times daily for 5–10 days, 200–400mg p.o. five times daily for 5–10 days, 10mg/kg i.v. three times daily for 5–10 days, 800mg p.o. five times daily for 7 days. 200–400mg p.o. twice daily	Nausea, vomiting, abdominal pain, diarrhoea, skin rash, abnormal LFTs extravasation (i.v.), renal impairment (i.v.). Confusion and other CNS effects (i.v.). Rapid increases in blood urea and creatinine levels related to peak plasma levels and the state of hydration of the patient	Ciclosporin, mycophenolate mofetil, tacrolimus, probenecid, lithium, theophyline, nephrotoxic drugs	Renal function (with i.v.)	Higher dose and longer duration for herpes encephalitis or varicella zoster. Patients on HAART with CD4 >300cells/mm³ may be treated as for immunocompetent. Intravenous infusion diluted to 0.5% (w/v) and infused over at least 1h (reduces likelihood of renal toxicity)
Amphotericin 1. Sodium deoxycholate (Fungizone®) 2 Liposomal (AmBisome®) 3. Lipid complex (Abelcet®)	Cryptococcal meningitis and other severe fungal infections	Test dose of 1 mg i.v. (over 10–30min, depending on product), followed by once daily i.v.: 1. 0.25–1.0mg/kg (increased over 3–5 days as tolerated) 2. 1–3.0mg/kg (increased over 2–3 days) 3. 5mg/kg. Duration: 2–6 weeks (total induction period at least 6 weeks)	Fever, chills, nausea and vomiting, headache, anorexia, weight loss, malaise, myalgia, thrombophlebitis, epigastric pain, diarrhoea, renal impairment; hypokalaemia, hypomagnesaemia, anaemia hypotension, vasodilatation, flushing, liver function tests abnorma, hyperbilirubinaemia, alkaline phosphatase increased	Nephrotoxic drugs, antineoplastics, corticosteroids	Renal function, FBC, U+Es	Test dose required before first infusion with any parenteral amphotericin. All i.v. preparations administered in 5% glucose. Pre-and post-hydration with 0.9% sodium chloride may decrease nephrotoxicity. Liposomal and lipid complex formulations generally better tolerated
Atovaquone Suspension	Treatment of mild–moderate PCP Prophylaxis of PCP[a] Treatment of toxoplasmosis[a]	750mg p.o. twice daily with food for 3 weeks 1.5g p.o. twice daily for at least 6 weeks	Nausea, rash, diarrhoea, vomiting, headache, insomnia, fever, increased LFTs, decreased sodium, anaemia, neutropenia. Hyponatraemia, hypersensitivity reactions including angioedema, bronchospasm and throat tightness	Indinavir, metoclopramide, rifampicin, rifabutin, tetracycline	LFTs, U+Es, FBC	Absorption improved by taking with food (especially high fat food); reduced by diarrhoea
Azithromycin	Atypical Mycobacterium infections, toxoplasmosis and PCP (adjunctive therapy or part of combination regimen) MAC prophylaxis	500mg oral daily for MAI treatment or PCP prophylaxis; 1250mg oral once weekly for MAI prophylaxis[b], 1250mg daily for toxoplasmosis treatment[b]	Nausea, vomiting, abdominal discomfort, anorexia, dyspepsia, flatulence, diarrhoea, constipation, raised LFTs. (rare: ototoxicity)	Antacids, theophylline, coumarins, ciclosporin artemether/lumefantrine, ergot derivatives, digoxin, bromocriptine, cabergoline, reboxetine, oestrogens	LFTs, hearing (if on long-term or high-dose therapy)	Less significant drug interactions than with the other macrolides For patients allergic to soya or peanut: risk of hypersensitivity reactions with some formulations and brands

Continued

Table 41.6 Selected drugs to treat opportunistic infections in HIV disease

Drug	Indication	Dosage: route, frequency, duration	Common or significant side effects include:	Significant interactions	Monitoring	Comments
Cidofovir	Cytomegalovirus retinitis	5mg/kg weekly for two doses, then every 2 weeks thereafter	Renal impairment, neutropenia, ocular hypotony, iritis/uveitis, nausea, vomiting, alopecia, rash, asthenia, fever, chills, headache	Other nephrotoxic drugs, agents that are contraindicated with probenecid, tenofovir	Renal function (including urine protein) neutrophils	Must be co-administered with probenecid and intravenous fluids (see SPC/BNF for specific regimen). Caution with handling (potential carcinogen). Avoid if on tenofovir
Clindamycin	Treatment of PCP Toxoplasmosis treatment Toxoplasmosis maintenance	600mg i.v./p.o. four times daily for 3 weeks 600mg i.v./p.o. four times daily for at least 6 weeks 1.2g p.o. daily in 3–4 divided doses	Diarrhoea, abdominal discomfort, oesophagitis, nausea, vomiting, rash, abnormal LFTs, thrombophlebitis (i.v.). Rarely pseudomembranous colitis, blood dyscrasias	Non-depolarising muscle relaxants, suxamethonium, oestrogens, pyrido-stigmine, neostigmine, erythromycin	LFTs, renal function, FBC, diarrhoea	Taken with primaquine for PCP. Taken with pyrimethamine for toxoplasmosis. Higher doses may be used if previous failure of co-trimoxazole (for PCP) or sulfadiazine (for toxoplasmosis)[b]
Co-trimoxazole (trimethoprim + sulpha-methoxazole)	Treatment of PCP Prophylaxis of PCP	Moderate–severe: 120mg/kg i.v in 2–4 divided doses for 3 days, then 90mg/kg for 18 days; mild: 1920mg p.o. three times daily for 3 weeks. Prophylaxis: 480 or 960mg p.o. daily or 960mg three times per week (960mg daily if on rifampicin)	Nausea, diarrhoea, headache, rash, hyperkalaemia, vomiting. (rare: drug fever, blood dyscrasias, serious skin reactions, e.g. Stevens-Johnson syndrome)	Amiodarone, oestrogens pyrimethamine, rifampicin, ciclosporin, lamivudine phenytoin, azathioprine, mercaptopurine, metho-trexate, sulphonylureas, warfarin	FBC, renal function, LFTs rash	For infusion, dilute each 480mg with 125ml of glucose 5% or sodium chloride 0.9% and infuse over 1.5–3h. If fluid restricted, 480mg in 75ml of glucose 5%. Caution in G6PD deficiency
Dapsone	Prophylaxis of PCP Treatment of PCP[a]	100mg p.o. daily (with trimethoprim 10–15mg/kg/ day in divided doses for 3 weeks for PCP treatment)	Anorexia, nausea, vomiting, rash. (rare: blood dyscrasias including methaemoglobinaemia; dapsone syndrome)	Rifamycins, probenecid, oestrogens, antacids	FBC, LFTs	Caution in G6PD deficiency
Famciclovir	Treatment of herpes zoster. Treatment of genital herpes	Doses for immunocompromised patients: zoster use 500mg three times daily for 10 days; genital herpes all episodes use 500mg twice daily for 7 days, for suppression 500mg twice daily	Headache, nausea, diarrhoea, vomiting, abdominal pain, constipation, increased tendency to sweat, pruritus	Probenecid	Renal function	Patients on HAART with CD4 >300 cells/mm³ may be treated as for immunocompetent
Fluconazole	Oesophageal candidiasis Oropharyngeal candidiasis Cryptococcal meningitis treatment Cryptococcal meningitis prophylaxis	100mg p.o. daily for 2 weeks 50mg p.o. daily for 7–14 days 400mg i.v./p.o. daily for ≥8 weeks 200mg p.o. daily	Headache, rash, abdominal pain, diarrhoea, flatulence, nausea, abnormal LFTs, hepatotoxicity	Coumarins, midazolam, sulphonylureas, rifabutin, rifampicin, phenytoin, tacrolimus, ciclosporin, theophylline, zidovudine, terfenadine	Renal function LFTs	Higher doses have been used for treatment and prophylaxis of candida and cryptococcus infections (depending on clinical response and antifungal sensitivities) i.v. route only necessary if patient nil by mouth.

Flucytosine	Cryptococcal meningitis treatment	100mg/kg daily p.o./i.v. in four divided doses for 2 weeks (with i.v. amphotericin)	Nausea, vomiting, diarrhoea, rash (rare: blood dyscrasias, hepatotoxicity)	Renal function FBC, LFTs	Cytarabine	Oral formulation is no longer licensed in the UK but can be imported on named-patient basis
Foscarnet	Cytomegalovirus retinitis treatment Cytomegalovirus retinitis maintenance	180mg/kg/day i.v. in 2–3 divided doses (adjust according to renal function) over 2h for 3 weeks 60, 120mg/kg i.v. once daily over 2h for 5–7 days each week	Renal impairment, alterations in serum calcium, potassium, magnesium and other minerals, headache, rash, convulsions, thrombophlebitis, genital ulceration, anaemia, nausea, vomiting, diarrhoea, paraesthesia	Renal function, LFTs, serum magnesium, potassium, calcium and phosphate, FBC, U+Es	Nephrotoxic drugs, drugs that inhibit renal tubular secretion (e.g. probenecid), i.v. pentamidine. When diuretics are indicated, thiazides are recommended	Good hydration, prompt correction of electrolyte abnormalities and dose adjustment for renal function vital. Wash genital area after micturition to reduce risk of ulceration. Give centrally to prevent phlebitis. If infusion related side effects reduce rate. Adjust maintenance dose for disease state, drug tolerability and renal function
Ganciclovir	Cytomegalovirus induction treatment Cytomegalovirus retinitis maintenance	5mg/kg i.v. twice daily for 3 weeks, 5mg/kg i.v. once every day or 6mg/kg once daily for 5 days each week	Blood dyscrasias, anorexia, renal impairment, abnormal LFTs, central nervous system effects, fatigue, nausea, vomiting, flatulence, abdominal pain, dysphagia, dysgeusia, dyspepsia, constipation, ear pain, injection site reactions, eye disorders and skin disorders	FBC renal function, LFTs	Zidovudine, didanosine, impenem-cilastatin, probenecid, mycophenolate mofetil, nephrotoxic drugs, bone marrow suppressive agents	Give over 1h preferably via central venous access Caution with handling. Special dosage instructions for patients with renal impairment: Women of child bearing potential must be advised to use effective contraception during treatment. Men must be advised to practise barrier contraception during treatment, and for at least 90 days thereafter
Peginterferon alfa	Hepatitis C (in combination with ribavirin) Chronic hepatitis B	See product literature for dose and duration (varies by brand, genotype and initial response) weekly s.c. injection	Severe CNS and psychiatric effects, anorexia, nausea, influenza-like symptoms, lethargy, depression, ocular side effects, rash, myelosuppression, hypertriglyceridaemia	Lipids, renal function, LFTs, TFTs, U+Es, FBC, blood glucose	Theophylline	Longer duration of treatment in HIV-coinfected patients. Should be managed jointly by HIV and hepatology specialists
Pentamidine isetionate	PCP treatment Mild PCP treatment PCP prophylaxis	4mg/kg i.v. once daily for 3 weeks (+600mg nebulised for first 3 days) 600mg nebulised daily for 3 weeks 300mg nebulised every 4 weeks	Intravenous: renal impairment, postural hypotension, leucopenia, hypo/hyperglycaemia, pancreatitis, electrolyte disturbances, nausea, vomiting. Nebulised: cough, bronchospasm	Renal function, blood glucose, blood pressure, U+Es	Nephrotoxic drugs, foscarnet, drugs that prolong QT interval (e.g. quinolones, erythromycin)	Infuse over 1h with patient supine. Caution with handling. Pretreat with bronchodilator if nebulised and use special nebuliser
Primaquine	PCP treatment	15–30mg p.o. daily for 3 weeks	Nausea, vomiting, anorexia, abdominal pain (rare: methaemoglobinaemia, haemolytic anaemia)	FBC	Bone marrow suppressive drugs, artemether/lumefantrine	Avoid in G6PD deficiency

Continued

Table 41.6 Selected drugs to treat opportunistic infections in HIV disease

Drug	Indication	Dosage: route, frequency, duration	Common or significant side effects include:	Significant interactions	Monitoring	Comments
Pyrimethamine	Toxoplasmosis treatment Toxoplasmosis maintenance	100mg on day 1, then 50mg p.o. once daily for at least 6 weeks. Different in SPC 25mg p.o. once daily	Anaemia, leucopenia, thrombocytopenia, rash	Bone marrow suppressive drugs, anti-malarials, methotrexate, antacids, lorazepam, kaolin, highly protein-bound drugs (e.g. coumarins)	FBC	Combined with sulfadiazine or clindamycin. Higher dose can be used if previous treatment failure. Recommend folinic acid 15mg od to reduce bone marrow suppression
Ribavirin	Hepatitis C treatment	Dose depends on product (Copegus or Rebetol), weight and hepatitis C genotype, see SPCs for specific details	Anaemia, neutropenia, thrombocytopenia. For other side effects reported in combination with peginterferon alfa, see earlier entry	Stavudine, zidovudine, didanosine, abacavir	FBC, LFTs, renal function	Given with peginterferon alfa. Colony stimulating factor support may counteract haematological side effects without requiring dose reduction. Teratogenic
Rifabutin	MAI prophylaxis MAI treatment	300, 450mg p.o. once daily with other drugs (consult SPC for specific details) 150mg 3 times a week with Kaletra[b]	Abnormal LFTs, nausea, vomiting, bone marrow suppression, arthralgia, myalgia, jaundice (rare: uveitis, risk increased with concomitant administration of drugs that increase rifabutin levels)	Coumarins, aripiprazole, atovaquone, dapsone, efavirenz, erythromycin, clarithromycin, protease inhibitors, sirolimus, oral hypoglycaemics, azole and triazole antifungals, disopyramide, quinidine, carbamazepine, oestrogens, progestogens	LFTs, renal function	Combine with at least one other drug for MAI treatment. TDM of both agents may be useful when given with Kaletra
Sulfadiazine	Toxoplasmosis treatment[a] Toxoplasmosis maintenance[a]	1–1.5 g i.v./p.o. four times daily for at least 6 weeks. 2 g p.o. daily in divided doses	Nausea, vomiting, rash, bone marrow suppression, crystalluria (and see under co-tri moxazole)	Bone marrow suppressive drugs, ciclosporin, oestrogens, coumarins, methenamine	Renal function, LFTs, FBC	Use with pyrimethamine. Prevent crystalluria by ensuring good fluid input/output. Alkalinising urine with sodium bicarbonate may help if crystals formed
Valaciclovir	Herpes zoster treatment Herpes simplex treatment	1g p.o. three times daily for 7 days. 500mg p.o. twice daily for 5–10 days (initial) or 5 days (recurrent) episodes	Mild headache and nausea (more serious events reported in transplant patients on 8g/day long term)	Ciclosporin mycophenolate mofetil tacrolimus probenecid	Renal function	Interactions more likely to be significant if renal impairment
Valganciclovir	CMV retinitis	Induction treatment: 900mg twice a day with food for 3 weeks. Maintenance: 900mg once daily with food	See ganciclovir, similar potential side effects (except those associated with intravenous administration, e.g. injection site reactions)	As for ganciclovir	FBC, renal function, LFTs	

FBC, full blood count; U+Es, urea and electrolyte levels; LFTs, liver function tests; TFTs, thyroid function tests; MAI, Mycobacterium avium intracellulare; G6PD, glucose-6-phosphate dehydrogenase; PCP, Pneumocystis jiroveci pneumonia; CMV, cytomegalovirus; p.o., oral; i.v., intravenous; s.c., subcutaneous; SPC, Summary of product characteristics; BNF, British National Formulary; w/v, weight/volume; TDM, therapeutic drug monitoring; MAC, Mycobacterium avium complex.
[a]Unlicensed treatment indication in UK.
[b]Unlicensed dose in UK.

of azole resistance. In such instances, an alternative azole or an echinocandin may be used, or occasionally higher than usual doses of the original agent, for example, fluconazole 400 mg daily. In intractable cases, intravenous amphotericin may be required. With the use of HAART, such complications are rarely seen.

Cryptococcus neoformans. This causes a disseminated infection, usually with meningeal involvement, in individuals with HIV infection. Patients present with fever and headaches, often without the characteristic symptoms of meningism such as photophobia and neck stiffness. Diagnosis is normally made on the basis of CSF analysis, though serum cryptococcal antigen and blood cultures may also be indicative.

For patients who are moderately or severely unwell, intravenous amphotericin B deoxycholate (0.7–1 mg/kg/day) or a lipid complex/liposomal formulation, with or without flucytosine (100 mg/kg/day in divided doses, oral or intravenous) is the first-line therapy. The place of flucytosine in therapy remains uncertain, with the only clear benefit seen in patients not on HAART, in whom it speeds the rate of CSF sterilisation and reduces the relapse rate. However, it has not been shown to reduce mortality and can be associated with additional toxicity. Conventional amphotericin is associated with high rates of nephrotoxicity, leading in some cases to acute renal failure and death, although strategies can be employed to minimise adverse effects. However, despite the higher cost, the liposomal form (AmBisome®, 4 mg/kg/day) is now usually the agent of choice due to its more favourable toxicity profile. Many UK hospitals now only stock one intravenous amphotericin product, due to reports of errors following confusion between different formulations because doses, reconstitution procedures and administration vary. The usual duration of amphotericin (± flucytosine) treatment is 2 weeks, after which high-dose fluconazole (400 mg daily orally) should be continued for further 10 weeks. Subsequent maintenance therapy with fluconazole 200 mg daily has been shown to be effective in reducing the incidence of relapse and should be continued for life, or until immune function is restored (for example, CD4 > 100 cells/mm³ in the presence of an undetectable viral load for at least 3 months). In milder cases fluconazole may be given for the entire duration of treatment. Itraconazole (400 mg/day) has been used but is less effective than fluconazole and should be used only if other agents are contraindicated.

Protozoal infections

Toxoplasmosis. *T. gondii* is a frequent cause of central nervous system disease in patients with AIDS. Individuals may present with headaches, fever, confusion, seizures or focal neurological symptoms and signs. Diagnosis is usually based on the appearance of ring-enhancing lesion(s) on computed tomography (CT scan). Definitive diagnosis is based on brain biopsy, which is rarely performed, but is generally made presumptively after response to therapy.

First-line treatment is sulphadiazine and pyrimethamine, with folinic acid to prevent myelosuppression, for 6 weeks, followed by maintenance therapy with lower doses of the same agents until CD4 count is consistently maintained above 200 cells/mm³. The preferred alternative is clindamycin and pyrimethamine with folinic acid, with limited data for atovaquone, co-trimoxazole, clarithromycin and doxycycline. Adjunctive therapy with corticosteroids or anticonvulsants may be used in cases of severe oedema or seizures, respectively.

Cryptosporidiosis. *Cryptosporidium parvum* is a ubiquitous organism and a common cause of diarrhoea in immunocompetent individuals. In patients who are immunocompromised, persistent infection may occur characterised by abdominal pain, weight loss and severe diarrhoea. Diagnosis is generally based on stool analysis.

Although many agents have been investigated for the treatment of cryptosporidiosis, the majority of results have been disappointing. Nitazoxanide is possibly the most promising agent, but failed to demonstrate superiority over placebo in severely immunocompromised patients. The optimal treatment for cryptosporidiosis (and indeed the majority of chronic opportunistic infections) is to increase immunological function with HAART. The mainstay of management in patients who are not able or willing to take HAART remains symptomatic control with nutritional supplementation, adequate hydration and antidiarrhoeal agents.

Bacterial infections

Bacterial infections are common in the context of HIV infection. Recurrent bacterial pneumonia, particularly *Streptococcus pneumoniae*, and diarrhoeal illnesses associated with *Salmonella, Shigella* or *Campylobacter* are particularly common. In general, these are treated the same as in immunocompetent individuals, although recurrent infections and/or septicaemia occur more frequently.

Mycobacteria. In HIV-positive individuals, *M. tuberculosis* (TB) is characterised by increased likelihood of reactivation of latent disease; more rapid progression to clinical disease following acquisition; more frequent extrapulmonary manifestations of tuberculosis; and more rapid progression of HIV disease (if the individual is not receiving HAART). Overall, there is no increase in infectivity of tuberculosis compared with HIV-negative patients.

Definitive diagnosis is reliant on culture of the organism from biological specimens but may be complicated by atypical clinical features and reduced response to tuberculin testing; it is often necessary to initiate treatment empirically.

Treatment for pulmonary and extrapulmonary tuberculosis should follow conventional guidelines for immunocompetent individuals. Meningitis is an unusual but significant complication of tuberculosis. Treatment for all forms of CNS tuberculosis should consist of four drugs (isoniazid, rifampicin, pyrazinamide, ethambutol) for 2 months followed by two drugs (isoniazid, rifampicin) for at least 10 months. Adjunctive corticosteroids (either dexamethasone or prednisolone) should be given to all patients with tuberculous meningitis, regardless of disease severity (Thwaites et al., 2009).

The use of primary and secondary prophylaxis remains controversial but may be appropriate in high-incidence groups. The increased incidence of multidrug-resistant tuberculosis (MDRTB) and the emergence of extremely drug-resistant disease (XDRTB) is a cause for concern and raises many infection control issues. It also highlights the need for antibiotic therapy driven by bacteriological sensitivities.

Managing tuberculosis and HIV co-infection is further complicated by drug–drug interactions between anti-tuberculous and antiretroviral agents, overlapping toxicities and the risk of development of immune reconstitution disease (see later). This is a complex area and treatment should be guided by clinicians with the relevant specialist expertise (Pozniak et al., 2010). One of the most frequent concerns is when to initiate therapy for HIV in an individual receiving TB treatment. This decision is based upon the risk of developing other opportunistic infections in the medium term. HAART is usually started after 2 weeks of tuberculosis treatment in those with severe immunosuppression (CD4 <100 cells/mm³), after 2 months if the CD4 is between 100 and 200 cells/mm³, and on completion of tuberculosis treatment or at 6 months if the CD4 is greater than 200 cells/mm³.

M. avium intracellulare (MAI) or *M. avium* complex (MAC) infection was historically a frequent manifestation of late-stage HIV disease, but is rarely seen now that HAART is widely used. Patients with disseminated infection classically present with fevers, weight loss, diarrhoea and hepatosplenomegaly. Diagnosis is sometimes made presumptively but is usually based on culture of the organism(s). *In vitro* sensitivities may not be good predictors of response to therapy. Therapy may need to be tailored to account for drug interactions with concomitant antiretrovirals, but usually includes azithromycin and ethambutol (ideally with rifabutin). Alternative agents include the quinolones and amikacin. Corticosteroids may be useful for symptomatic control. Although rifabutin, clarithromycin and azithromycin have all been demonstrated to be effective agents for primary prophylaxis against MAI, their cost–benefit remains controversial and use is not widespread in the UK. The strongest indications are for those patients with CD4 <50 cells/mm³ who decline HAART, or who experience HAART failure (without further effective options) or who are receiving chemotherapy.

Viral infections

Cytomegalovirus. CMV is a herpes virus that is acquired by approximately 50% of the general population and over 90% of homosexual men. Like other herpes viruses, once infection has occurred, the virus remains dormant thereafter, but in individuals with advanced immunosuppression, reactivation may occur and cause disease. In the context of HIV infection, the most common sites of disease are the retina and gastro-intestinal tract, though neurological involvement and pneumonitis are well reported.

Diagnosis of CMV retinitis is based on clinical appearance; it may be detected in asymptomatic individuals but usually presents with symptoms of blurred vision, visual field defects or 'floaters'. Untreated CMV retinitis progresses rapidly to blindness and treatment substantially reduces the morbidity associated with this condition. Although previously lifelong treatment had been recommended, where immunological restoration occurs discontinuation may be possible. Conventional therapeutic approaches are based upon an initial induction period of high-dose therapy for 2–3 weeks, until the retinitis is quiescent, followed by lower dose maintenance treatment, with reinduction if disease progression occurs.

The most commonly used agent for induction therapy in the UK is ganciclovir, which can be given intravenously or orally, as the pro-drug valganciclovir. It is usually administered (5 mg/kg) via a central line over 1 h and should be handled as a cytotoxic agent. Valganciclovir is well absorbed and a dose of 900 mg twice daily has been shown to be as effective as intravenous ganciclovir for induction therapy. Significant side effects encountered with these agents include neutropenia, which may require colony-stimulating factor support, and thrombocytopenia. Maintenance treatment may also be given either intravenously (6 mg/kg on 5 days a week) or orally (valganciclovir 900 mg once daily).

Intravenous maintenance therapy requires the insertion of a permanent indwelling catheter and is therefore usually used only when oral administration is not possible. Intravitreal administration of ganciclovir is possible, but rarely used, as this does not confer any systemic protection.

An alternative agent to ganciclovir is foscarnet. It has a less favourable toxicity profile and is thus usually reserved for cases of therapeutic failure with ganciclovir. Its main adverse effects are electrolyte abnormalities, nephrotoxicity that requires dose adjustment or cessation of therapy, and ulceration, particularly of the genitals, which may be prevented by assiduous attention to personal hygiene after micturition. No effective oral formulation is currently available.

Cidofovir requires less frequent administration: two doses at weekly intervals for induction and fortnightly for maintenance, though intravenous administration is again required and nephrotoxicity and other metabolic disturbances are well recognised. A strict regimen of intravenous hydration and oral probenecid (2 g given 3 h prior to infusion and 1 g 2 and 8 h post-cidofovir) must be followed. The risk of nephrotoxicity is increased if cidofovir is co-administered with agents such as tenofovir that are excreted via the same renal tubular anion transporter.

CMV disease of the gastro-intestinal tract usually affects the oesophagus or colon, causing dysphagia and abdominal pain with diarrhoea, respectively. Diagnosis is based upon histological analysis of biopsy specimens. Treatment is as for CMV retinitis induction therapy; maintenance therapy is not usually given unless relapses occur. Neurological disease may present in a variety of ways, is difficult to diagnose and frequently carries a poor prognosis, even with treatment. The optimal agent, dosage and duration of therapy remain undetermined.

Impact of HAART on opportunistic infections

The widespread use of HAART has had a dramatic effect on the incidence, prognosis and clinical aspects of opportunistic infections.

Decreased incidence of opportunistic infections. HAART has resulted in a major reduction in the vast majority of opportunistic infections and a consequent reduction in mortality rates and requirement for hospital admissions.

Withdrawal of prophylaxis. The rise in CD4 count associated with HAART has led to an improvement in functional immunity. Clinical trials have suggested that the withdrawal of both primary and secondary prophylaxis against *P. jiroveci* pneumonia is safe, and similar results are thought to be likely for cryptococcosis, toxoplasmosis, MAI and CMV. Most would consider withdrawing prophylaxis in individuals on successful HAART if the CD4 count is consistently greater than 200 cells/mm^3 (*P. jiroveci* pneumonia, toxoplasmosis, cryptococcosis) or 100 cells/mm^3 (MAI and CMV).

Successful treatment of opportunistic infections. Some previously difficult to treat infections, notably cryptosporidiosis and microsporidiosis, appear to resolve with significant CD4 count improvements associated with HAART. However, in up to 30% of individuals, initiation of HAART can be associated with a clinical deterioration known as immune reconstitution inflammatory syndrome or IRIS. This typically occurs in the first 2–6 weeks after starting HAART and presents as fevers and localised symptoms pertaining to a recently treated or previously undiagnosed opportunistic pathogen. It is most frequently seen with mycobacteria (lymphadenitis with both *M. tuberculosis* and MAI) and CMV (vitritis, iritis and retinal oedema), but has been reported for most infections. Diagnosis is difficult as the signs and symptoms mimic those of resistant disease, non-adherence and co-morbidity. No management strategy is proven but corticosteroids, NSAIDs and immunomodulatory therapies (IL-2 and GM-CSF) have all been used.

Cancers

Although there are a number of malignancies associated with HIV infection, the most common are Kaposi's sarcoma and lymphoma.

Kaposi's sarcoma. This is the most common malignancy in people with HIV infection and may be triggered by infection with human herpes virus 8 (HHV-8). The majority of lesions affect the skin and appear as raised purple papules. These may be single or multiple and in severe cases may result in oedema, ulceration and infection. Visceral involvement is not uncommon but rarely causes clinically significant disease. In some cases, no therapeutic intervention is necessary and cosmetic camouflage may be sufficient. Indeed, treatment of HIV with antiretroviral therapy usually results in improvement, and in most cases, complete resolution, of Kaposi's sarcoma. When individual lesions are troublesome, local radiotherapy or intralesional vinblastine can be beneficial. Alitretinoin gel (0.1%) (9-*cis*-retinoic acid) is a topical, self-administered therapy approved for the treatment of KS in the USA but not licensed in Europe. In cases of widespread cutaneous disease or significant visceral involvement, systemic chemotherapy is used, though this is often withheld until the potential benefits of HAART have been established. The liposomal anthracyclines and taxanes are now the mainstay of systemic chemotherapy for Kaposi's sarcoma (Bower et al., 2008).

Lymphomas. The most common lymphomas in patients with HIV infection are high-grade B-cell (non-Hodgkin's) types. Primary central nervous system lymphomas, which are extremely rare in the general population, are more common in individuals with HIV infection but tend to occur only in those with severe immunosuppression. Diagnosis of lymphoma is usually based upon histological confirmation from biopsy specimens. This may not be possible for primary central nervous system disease. The advent of HAART has dramatically reduced the incidence of all lymphomas. However, whilst it has similarly improved the outcome for most cases, this is unfortunately not true for primary central nervous system lymphomas. Lymphoma of the central nervous system is associated with an extremely poor outcome, and in many cases, even palliative radiotherapy or corticosteroids confer little benefit.

The optimal therapy for HIV-associated lymphomas has yet to be determined, but the management plan should either be supervised by, or have input from, an oncologist with relevant specialist experience. The outcome for patients with relatively preserved immune function or those receiving HAART is comparable to that in the general population. However, many individuals are unable to tolerate treatment without dose modification. Drug interactions between antiretrovirals (particularly PIs) and chemotherapeutic agents need to be considered to minimise the risk of treatment-limiting toxicities, whilst the proactive use of colony-stimulating factors may enable optimal dosing.

Cervical intraepithelial neoplasia and anal intraepithelial neoplasia. These are both associated with human papillomavirus infection, are more common in individuals with HIV infection and may progress to cervical cancer and anal cancer, respectively. It is currently believed that HAART reduces the progression of cervical intraepithelial neoplasia (CIN) but this does not appear to be true of anal intraepithelial neoplasia (AIN), and there are concerns that the incidence of this malignancy may increase with improvements in HIV survival.

The optimal management is a combination of early diagnosis, surgery, chemotherapy and/or radiotherapy. It is possible that screening by smear tests and early treatment, for example, with imiquimod, may reduce the need for such aggressive treatment approaches.

Neurological manifestations

Neurological symptoms may be due to opportunistic infections, tumours or the primary neurological effects of HIV.

HIV encephalopathy or AIDS dementia complex (ADC) is believed to result from direct infection of the central nervous system with HIV itself. Individuals who may otherwise be physically well can be debilitated by profound cognitive dysfunction and amnesia. Although psychometric test results are usually suggestive of the underlying aetiology, it is wise to rule out any other cause with brain scanning and CSF analysis.

The incidence of ADC has reduced dramatically with the use of HAART, and similarly, the use of HAART has been anecdotally associated with an improvement in outcome in many cases. Whilst it is known that the central nervous system penetration of some antiretroviral agents is better than others, the beneficial effects on ADC do not appear to be limited to those agents which penetrate well. Nonetheless, many clinicians would choose to include at least one agent with good penetration of the central nervous system in most HAART regimens, particularly in individuals with cognitive impairment. More recently, there have been increasing reports of more subtle cognitive impairment in patients with HIV receiving effective HAART therapy. The role of varying neuropenetrative agents in either the aetiology or the management of such patients is currently under investigation.

Progressive multifocal leucoencephalopathy (PML) is caused by JC virus and may, at presentation, appear similar to a cerebrovascular accident but will have characteristic white matter lesions on an MRI scan, with or without the presence of JC virus in the CSF. In many cases, the introduction of HAART prevents progression of disease, but it is unlikely to reverse the functional deficit at presentation. The role of adjunctive cidofovir in treatment remains controversial.

Hepatitis B co-infection

There are a number of ways in which HIV can impact on hepatitis B (HBV) infection:

- Hepatitis B vaccination is less successful
- Hepatitis B is less likely to be cleared and hence more likely to become chronic
- Hepatitis B infection is likely to be associated with higher hepatitis B DNA levels
- Progression to cirrhosis is more rapid
- Hepatocellular carcinoma is more common.

Although many individuals with HIV will have hepatitis B serological markers suggestive of previous infection, only 6–10% in most series have active hepatitis B infection.

Management requires an understanding of both viruses and is facilitated by the availability of drugs with dual HIV and hepatitis B activity (Brook et al., 2010). The HAART regimen should include two agents with anti-hepatitis B activity, usually tenofovir with either emtricitabine or lamivudine. If HIV develops resistance to these agents, they can still be continued for their anti-hepatitis B activity.

Hepatitis C co-infection

HIV also impacts on hepatitis C infection in a number of ways:

- Hepatitis C is less likely to be cleared spontaneously
- Higher levels of hepatitis C RNA are seen
- Hepatitis C progresses to cirrhosis more rapidly
- Hepatocellular carcinoma occurs more frequently
- Response to hepatitis C therapy is poor.

In the UK, approximately 5–10% of individuals are co-infected with hepatitis C; there are increasing reports of acute hepatitis C infection in gay men with HIV. In Eastern Europe, where the predominant route of HIV transmission is needle sharing, co-infection rates of over 50% are reported.

The management of hepatitis C/HIV co-infection is complicated (Brook et al., 2010). If treatment for hepatitis C is needed for someone on HAART, the antiretrovirals used must be compatible with hepatitis C therapy (pegylated α interferon and ribavirin). Didanosine, abacavir, stavudine and zidovudine should be avoided. It is commonplace to treat individuals with co-infection for a longer duration, for example, 48 weeks rather than 24 weeks for individuals with genotype 2 and 3 hepatitis C, and possibly 72 weeks for genotypes 1 and 4 – dependent upon early virological responses. Side effects of hepatitis C therapy tend to be more frequent and severe in the co-infected population. The proactive use of the colony-stimulating factors erythropoietin and G-CSF may enable optimal dosing of hepatitis C therapy and thereby improve outcome. The management of HCV is likely to be revolutionised by the availability of increasing numbers of Directly Acting Antivirals (DAAs) of which a large number are currently in development. The optimal way to use these and the potential drug-drug interactions with antiretrovirals have yet to be fully elucidated.

Women with HIV

In addition to the general points covered elsewhere in this chapter, specific issues for women with HIV include:

- Cervical screening should be carried out at least annually, to check for gynaecological manifestations of HIV
- Drug toxicity may manifest in different ways or occur with different frequencies, for example, nevirapine hypersensitivity reaction occurs at a lower CD4 count in women whilst lipodystrophy syndrome may also present differently, with breast hypertrophy commonly seen.

Pregnancy and contraception impact on the medicines prescribed for women of childbearing potential. The factors that need to be taken into account (where appropriate) may include:

- Interactions between many antiretrovirals and oral and injectable contraceptive agents (see Table 41.7). There are no interactions with the levonorgestrel-releasing intrauterine system, Mirena. (*Note*: barrier methods should also be recommended in addition to hormonal contraception, to prevent transmission of HIV and other sexually transmitted infections)
- Potential teratogenicity of the drugs prescribed
- Possible increased toxicity of the drugs prescribed to both mother and child
- The use of antiretroviral agents and other strategies to reduce vertical (mother-to-child) transmission of HIV.

The use of combination antiretroviral therapy, with or without caesarean section, with zidovudine as PEP to the neonate, together with a non-breast feeding strategy has reduced vertical transmission rates from 35% to less than 1% where HIV status is known and where antiretroviral therapies are widely available.

Table 41.7 Interactions between antiretroviral (ARVs) and contraceptive agents

	Combined oral contraceptive pill (COC)	Progesterone-only pill (POP)	Depot contraception-Depomedroxyprogesterone acetate (DMPA)	Implanon® Evra®
NNRTIs				
Efavirenz	C	C	A	C
Etravirine	A	A	B	B
Nevirapine	C	C	A	C
PIs				
Atazanavir/ritonavir	A Use COC with **at least** 30 µcg ethinyloestradiol. The increase in progestin exposure may lead to related side effects.	C	C	A
Atazanavir (unboosted)	A Use COC with **maximum** 30 µcg ethinyl estradiol	C	D	C
Darunavir/ritonavir	C	C	B	C
Foamprenavir/ritonavir	C	C	D	C
Indinavir (unboosted)	A	A	B	A
Lopinavir/ritonavir	C	C	B	C
Nelfinavir	C	C	A	C
Saquinavir/ritonavir	C	C	B	C
Tipranavir/ritonavir	C	C	B	C
Integrase inhibitors				
Raltegravir	A	A	A	A
CCR5 Antagonist				
Maraviroc	A	A	A	A
Entry inhibitors				
Enfuvirtide	A	A	A	A

A, combination can be used safely; B, no formal studies, but no clinically significant interactions expected; C, additional barrier contraceptive must be used or alternative method; D, avoid combination.

Nonetheless, questions remain regarding the optimal therapies to use, the risk of transmission of resistant virus to the neonate and the risk of toxicity from antiretroviral agents administered during pregnancy, particularly in the first trimester. Ideally, all HIV-positive women should be counselled regarding these issues before they become pregnant, so they can make informed decisions regarding both therapy and timing of pregnancy.

Guidelines are available that set out the management of HIV infection in pregnant women and the prevention of mother-to-child transmission (de Ruiter et al., 2008). In general, intervention reflects a risk/benefit evaluation between the efficacy of reducing transmission and the potential harmful effects to the mother and fetus. Where HAART is clinically indicated for the mother herself, this should utilise a regimen of optimal efficacy with a favourable safety profile. Where therapy

is initiated to reduce transmission, this is usually a HAART regimen but could be zidovudine monotherapy if the viral load is low (consistently <10,000 copies/mL). In the latter situation, the time of therapy initiation is guided by the viral load (Read et al., 2010):

if <10,000 copies/mL – start by 26 weeks;
if >10,000 copies/mL – start by 20 weeks;
if >32,000 copies/mL – start without delay.

Adjunctive caesarean section is recommended where monotherapy is used or there is a detectable viral load prior to delivery, but may not be essential if the mother is on fully suppressive HAART. Breastfeeding should be avoided and antiretroviral therapy is usually administered to the newborn for 4 weeks after birth. In the developing world, different strategies may be adopted. For example, single-dose nevirapine monotherapy is effective in reducing transmission but may be associated with the development of resistance, and exclusive breast feeding, with or without antiretrovirals for the baby, may be recommended where water safety is poor.

Ethnicity

It is now recognised that ethnicity as well as gender can affect drug handling and response to treatment. This is due, in part, to epidemiological differences in gene expression. For example, reduced activity of cytochrome P450 2B6, one of the key enzymes involved in the metabolism of NNRTIs, appears to be more common amongst Africans than Caucasians. These drugs, therefore, have a significantly longer plasma half-life in those affected, which may impact on efficacy, toxicity and treatment interruptions. The prevalence of the HLA*B5701 gene, associated with abacavir hypersensitivity, also varies in different ethnic groups, though the clinical implications of this have yet to be fully researched.

As pharmacogenomics becomes more widely incorporated into clinical trials and routine patient care, it is hoped that a greater understanding will be gained of differences in response to treatment, enabling treatment strategies to be individualised and optimised.

Case studies

Case 41.1

Ms A is a 21-year-old UK-born pharmacy student who presented to her primary care doctor with a rash, swollen glands and flu-like illness. A presumptive diagnosis of swine flu was made. She was given a course of oseltamivir (Tamiflu®) and her symptoms largely resolved over the following 2 weeks. Two months later, her male partner attended his dentist for a routine check up and was found to have oral candidiasis. He had no obvious predisposing factors and his dentist thus suggested that he have an HIV test, which was positive. As a result of this, Ms A was advised to have a test and was subsequently found to be HIV positive too, with a CD4 count of 420 cells/mm³ and a plasma HIV RNA (viral load) of 610,000 copies/mL.

One year after her diagnosis, Ms A has had two consecutive CD4 counts below 350 cells/mm³ (the latest being 310) and a viral load of 50,000–95,000 copies/mL. She is advised to start antiretroviral therapy and plans to do this in a few weeks as soon as she has finished her final exams. She currently takes no medication and uses condoms for contraception/sexually transmitted infection prevention. You are part of the multidisciplinary team which will recommend the regimen to be offered/prescribed.

Questions

1. What is the most likely diagnosis for the illness Ms A initially presented with to her primary care doctor?
2. What baseline investigation results would you need to inform your choice of antiretroviral therapy?
3. What would you do if there was a need to start therapy urgently and these results were not available?
4. Assuming all results were normal, which antiretroviral therapy regimen would you suggest and why?
5. What are the main counselling points to discuss with Ms A when she starts antiretroviral therapy?

Answers

1. The most likely diagnosis is PHI, also known as seroconversion syndrome. Approximately 70% of people newly infected with HIV develop PHI symptoms, typically a flu-like illness, with fever, arthralgia, pharyngitis, rash and lymphadenopathy.

2. The most important HIV-specific investigation which must be performed prior to starting treatment is an HIV resistance test (usually a genotype). Failure to do this can result in premature treatment failure and rapid development of multiple class drug resistance. The presence of HIV resistance mutations is likely to affect the choice of regimen.

   Some clinicians would also perform tropism testing at this point, that is, immediately prior to starting therapy, but it would be unlikely to affect treatment choice at this stage, and hence antiretroviral therapy can be started before the result is available, which may be 6 weeks. The rationale for carrying out a tropism test now, even though a CCR5 inhibitor is not generally used first line, is that antiretroviral agents may subsequently need to be changed when the viral load is undetectable, due to toxicity or intolerance. In addition, the Trofile® test can only be reliably performed on samples with a viral load >1000 copies/mL. However, different tropism tests, which can be carried out on samples with low/undetectable viral load, are now available.

   HLA B*5701 testing might also be done at this stage. If negative, there is an extremely low probability of developing a hypersensitivity reaction on exposure to abacavir, should this drug be considered either at this stage or if treatment needs to be switched in future.

   Routine baseline blood tests (U&Es, eGFR, LFTs, etc.) should also be done to assist antiretroviral therapy choice and monitor for subsequent adverse effects. Some clinicians would also perform a urine protein creatinine ratio (UPCR) before starting a tenofovir-containing regimen.

   While CD4 count is a useful indicator of when to start treatment, and both CD4 and viral load are invaluable in monitoring antiretroviral therapy success, they do not usually influence the choice of agents.

3. Genotypic resistance test results usually take about 3 weeks to be reported, so if therapy needs to be started sooner (as in someone newly diagnosed with a CD4 count <200 cells/mm³), then a regimen must be selected that has at least one drug with a high genetic barrier to resistance and to which primary resistance is unlikely to be present. In this case, a ritonavir-boosted PI, such as darunavir 800 mg daily or atazanavir 300 mg daily, with ritonavir 100 mg daily, would usually be combined with two nucleoside/nucleotide reverse transcriptase inhibitors (e.g. Truvada® or Kivexa® 1 tablet daily). Non-nucleosides (NNRTIs) and integrase inhibitors should be avoided in this situation because they have a low genetic barrier to resistance, that is, the presence of a single resistance mutation is sufficient to render them ineffective.

4. If there was no baseline resistance and other blood results were within normal limits, a typical initial regimen would be two NRTIs and an NNRTI, such as Kivexa® (abacavir and lamivudine) and efavirenz or tenofovir, emtricitabine and efavirenz. The latter is available as a combination tablet (Atripla®, 1 tablet daily) which is widely prescribed as a first antiretroviral therapy combination. Although the UK licensed indication is currently only for adults whose viral load has been maintained at <50 copies/mL for >3 months on antiretroviral therapy (e.g. on the same drugs, but

taken as Truvada®, or tenofovir and emtricitabine, plus efavirenz), it is common practice to initiate therapy with Atripla.

5. Medication counselling should include:

- What the medication is and how to take it, as well as any specific storage conditions (eg tenofovir-containing preparations contain a desiccant)
- Potential side effects and how to prevent them, what to do and who to contact about them including out of hours. Check the Summary of Product Characteristics (www.medicines.org.uk) for the specific side effects of the drugs chosen. Generally, patients should be counselled on common/very common or serious potential effects which they may notice or those which will be monitored
- Relevant drug interactions, including with prescribed medicines, herbal and over-the-counter (OTC) preparations, recreational drugs and alcohol
- What to do if a dose is missed, administered late or the patient vomits soon after taking a dose
- The rationale for, and importance of, a high level of adherence for successful treatment, outlining services that are available to support her, such as provision of adherence aids.

Case 41.2

In 1995, Mr B, a 47-year-old man, presented with *P. jiroveci* pneumonia. He had a CD4 count of 123 cells/mm³, and plasma HIV RNA was unknown, as viral load testing was not routinely available in clinics at the time. He made a good response to treatment with high-dose co-trimoxazole and was subsequently commenced on dual combination therapy with zidovudine and zalcitabine (ddC, an NRTI, no longer marketed). He remained on this regimen for 18 months, until HIV RNA testing became available and he was found to have a viral load of 13,000 copies/mL and CD4 242 cells/mm³. His full antiretroviral therapy history, with reasons for switching, is detailed as follows (Table 41.8).

In September 2009 (now aged 62), his viral load remained <40 copies/mL, with CD4 670 cells/mm³. However, his creatinine clearance (calculated using Cockcroft-Gault equation) was 41 mL/min and urine protein:creatinine ratio was significantly raised, at 86 mg/mmol (normal <30 mg/mmol). Both were normal when last monitored 4 months previously. On questioning, he revealed that he had been taking regular ibuprofen (400 mg three

times a day) for the past month, following a wrist fracture, as well as bendroflumethiazide 2.5 mg daily and tamsulosin 400 μcg daily, both of which he has been taking for more than 2 years.

Question

1. What are the possible drug-related causes of his renal dysfunction and what alterations, if any, to his drug therapy would you recommend?

Two weeks after stopping the ibuprofen, Mr B's creatinine clearance is now 52 mL/min and he is prescribed Atripla® 1 tablet daily. His repeat urine protein:creatinine ratio, 1 week after stopping ibuprofen was 42 mg/mmol (improving), with normal urine albumin:creatinine ratio. His serum phosphate was low and fractional excretion of phosphate was 35% (normal < 25%). Although his renal function was improving, it was decided to recommend changing his antiretroviral therapy to boosted darunavir (PI monotherapy), darunavir 800 mg daily and ritonavir 100 mg daily.

2. What information should Mr B be given about the proposed change of regimen?

Answer

1. Tenofovir use has been associated with renal dysfunction, the first sign of which may be a raised UPCR, although there are other causes. Mr B has a raised UPCR and reduced creatinine clearance, suggesting moderate renal dysfunction, which may be tenofovir related. However, regular concomitant NSAIDs and bendroflumethiazide may increase the risk of renal dysfunction. It is possible that the addition of regular ibuprofen has precipitated the renal dysfunction. Therefore, he would be advised to change to an alternative analgesic, if one is still required, starting with regular paracetamol.

Atripla is not recommended for patients with creatinine clearance <50 mL/min, as the doses of emtricitabine and tenofovir need to be adjusted. For creatinine clearance 30–49 mL/min, a dose of 200 mg emtricitabine and 300 mg tenofovir disoproxil fumarate (245 mg tenofovir disoproxil) every 48 h is required. The efavirenz dose remains 600 mg daily. However, Mr B's renal function must be closely monitored, for example, twice a week, to ensure that the doses are adjusted promptly to reflect any

---

Table 41.8 Mr B's ARV treatment history (Case 41.2)

Start date	Drug name, dose and frequency	Stop date	Viral load and CD4 at switch	Reason for changing
Nov 1995	Zidovudine 200 mg tds Zalcitabine 750 μgrams tds	May 1997	VL 13000 CD4 242	Virological failure
May 1997	Stavudine 40 mg bd Didanosine 200 mg bd Indinavir 800 mg tds	Apr 1999	VL <200 (lower limit of detection at that time) CD4 412	Renal stones (indinavir)
Apr 1999	Stavudine 40 mg bd Didanosine 200 mg bd Efavirenz 600 mg od	Jan 2002	VL <50 (lower limit of detection at that time) CD4 503 (stavudine and didanosine)	Lactic acidosis
Jan 2002	Tenofovir df 300 mg od Lamivudine 300 mg od Efavirenz 600 mg od	Mar 2008	VL <40 CD4 633	Simplification (Reduction in number of tablets)
Mar 2008	Atripla 1 tablet od			

change. This is to avoid over- or underdosing, and the associated risks of toxicity and antiretroviral therapy failure.

If the renal dysfunction continued or worsened, despite stopping the ibuprofen and dose adjusting his antiretroviral therapy, the choice of diuretic could be reviewed. If the problem still persists, then a change of antiretroviral therapy might be warranted.

2. Although the use of ritonavir-boosted darunavir monotherapy (darunavir/ritonavir) is an unlicensed indication, there are data from clinical trials, for example, Arribas et al. (2010), to support this approach. Mr B should be informed of this. Other discussion points should include:

- How to take the new regimen: two darunavir 400 mg tablets, plus one ritonavir 100 mg tablet, taken together once daily, at the same time each day (±1 h), with or after food
- How to switch from Atripla® to the new regimen. Atripla® is taken on an empty stomach, usually at night, to reduce CNS side effects and he may wish to take his new antiretroviral therapy at a different time. If he does this, he should ensure the interval between the last dose of Atripla® and the first dose of darunavir/ritonavir is no longer than 25 h
- Storage conditions: Atripla® is supplied with a desiccant; darunavir and ritonavir tablets do not have any special storage requirements.

Case 41.3

Mr C is a 58-year-old homosexual man who was diagnosed HIV positive 25 years previously but has never had any AIDS-defining illnesses. He received 16 months of zidovudine monotherapy during 1993–1994 as part of a study but subsequently remained off therapy until 1996 when, following a fall in his CD4 count to 240 cells/mm³, he was commenced on stavudine, lamivudine and indinavir. His response was excellent, with a rise in his CD4 count to 520 cells/mm³ and a viral load below detection (<50 copies/mL), but in 1999, the indinavir was changed to Kaletra®, following an admission to hospital with indinavir-induced nephrolithiasis. In 2003, when his viral load was still undetectable, the stavudine was switched to abacavir because of marked facial and peripheral lipoatrophy. The facial wasting was successfully treated with a course of polylactic acid (New-Fill®) injections, and there has been a small, gradual natural recovery of subcutaneous limb fat. He has been on pravastatin 40 mg once daily and fenofibrate 160 mg once daily since 2000, when he also stopped smoking.

At his annual health review, his most recent surrogate markers remained excellent, with a CD4 count of 1100 cells/mm³ and a viral load of <40 copies/mL. However, his fasting lipids were total cholesterol 5.9 mmol/L, LDL cholesterol 4.5 mmol/L, HDL 1.0 mmol/L, triglycerides 3.3 mmol/L. His calculated creatinine clearance (Cockcroft and Gault equation) was 45 mL/min (it was >50 mL/min when last checked 4 months ago), he had a fasting glucose of 9 mmol/L and had a raised blood pressure (BP 140/95 mmHg confirmed on two separate occasions). His 10-year cardiovascular risk was calculated to be 21.5%.

Questions

1. What are the limitations of using this cardiovascular risk calculator in this situation? Is the calculated risk likely to be an over- or under-estimate and why?
2. Mr C is concerned about the implications of his annual health review results. What information and advice should he be given?
3. What changes to his drug therapy might you recommend?

Answers

1. The main limitation of using any cardiovascular risk calculator is that the population data underpinning it come from individuals whose HIV status was not recorded. HIV infection itself is thought likely to increase the risk of cardiovascular disease, but there is currently insufficient evidence of the extent of additional risk to be able to quantify this in any of the established cardiovascular disease risk calculations. In addition, some antiretrovirals, for example, abacavir, didanosine and Kaletra have been shown to be associated with an increased risk of cardiovascular disease. This is also not factored into any of the existing cardiovascular risk calculators. In addition, Mr C is already on lipid-lowering therapy, so his untreated lipid markers would be expected to be more abnormal. The calculated 10-year risk of 21.5% is therefore likely to be an underestimate.

2. Mr C should be given general lifestyle advice to follow a healthy balanced diet and take aerobic exercise at least three times a week. Specific lipid-lowering dietary advice could be given. It would be useful to establish if Mr C has changed his lifestyle in the last 4–6 months, for example, change in adherence to lipid-lowering therapy, change in diet, restarted smoking, taking any new medication, including non-prescription and herbal medicines. Any relevant cardiovascular risk factors should then be discussed/addressed. The possibility that two of his antiretrovirals may also be contributing to his cardiovascular risk should also be explained.

3. Given Mr C's high cardiovascular risk, a change of antiretroviral therapy should be considered. The risk associated with Kaletra® use appears to be cumulative, that is, related to length of time on treatment, whereas the data on the nature of the risk associated with abacavir are less clear. However, it would be appropriate to explore the options for changing his antiretroviral therapy. Currently, there are no data on the presence or absence of cardiovascular risk associated with the other two commonly used boosted PIs, atazanavir and darunavir. In the absence of any HIV resistance test results dating from soon after he stopped the zidovudine monotherapy, it should be presumed that some NRTI mutations may be 'archived'. Caution should therefore be exercised before prescribing combinations with a low genetic barrier to resistance, for example, those containing NNRTIs or integrase inhibitors, without PIs.

Assuming Mr C's adherence to his lipid-lowering agents had been good, a change of therapy could be indicated, for example, pravastatin to atorvastatin. It would be reasonable to start with 20 mg atorvastatin, increasing to 40 mg if necessary and tolerated. However, if his antiretroviral therapy is going to be changed, it may be helpful to plan the changes in a stepwise fashion, so that the impact of each adjustment can be assessed. In this case, the lipid-lowering therapy alterations should be effected after the change of antiretroviral therapy. A change to simvastatin would be contraindicated if he remains on a PI.

Case 41.4

Ms D is a 50-year-old social worker who was referred to the hospital accident and emergency department by her primary care doctor following a 4-week history of worsening respiratory symptoms, despite treatment with amoxicillin, followed by clarithromycin. She has lost 3 kg in the last 2 months, has had a non-productive cough for 6 weeks and gets breathless climbing the stairs at home. Pulse oximetry showed desaturation to 91% on exercise and her arterial blood gas sample had a PaO₂ of 8.1 kPa. Chest X-ray showed bilateral interstitial infiltrates. Her past medical history includes irritable bowel syndrome (diagnosed

5 years ago), recurrent vaginal candidiasis for the past 7 years and allergic rhinitis for which she uses fluticasone nasal spray. She is divorced and has a 10-year-old son. She works in an inner city area and has no history of foreign travel outside mainland Europe. The hospital has recently introduced routine (opt out) HIV testing for all acute medical admissions, as a result of which Ms D was found to be HIV positive, with a CD4 count of 47 cells/mm³.

Questions

1. What are the most likely HIV-related differential diagnoses for her respiratory symptoms?
2. How should her respiratory symptoms be managed?
3. When should she start antiretroviral therapy?
4. What drug interactions would you need to consider when managing Ms D both in the first few weeks and also in the longer term?

Answers

1. The history, signs and symptoms (gradual onset, failure to respond to treatment for community acquired pneumonia, weight loss, non-productive cough, breathlessness on exertion, oxygen desaturation, low PaO$_2$ and chest X-ray appearance) are all suggestive of *P. jiroveci* pneumonia. However, some of them could also be consistent with TB which she may have been exposed to as a result of the nature and location of her job. TB would need to be excluded. As Ms D has a significant degree of immunesuppression, the possibility of more than one pathogen/diagnosis must always be considered.
2. Until TB has been excluded, Ms D should be nursed in a negative pressure room. A bronchoscopy should ideally be performed to assist diagnosis. She should be started on treatment for *P. jiroveci* pneumonia immediately with high-dose co-trimoxazole and systemic corticosteroid (see text and Table 41.8 for doses and administration details). Following induction treatment (usually 3 weeks' duration), she should receive secondary prophylaxis until her CD4 count on fully suppressive antiretroviral therapy is maintained above 200 cells/mm³.

   If she responds well to *P. jiroveci* pneumonia treatment and bronchial washings are negative for acid-fast bacilli, then it would be reasonable for her to be managed expectantly with regard to the possibility of TB, that is, not kept in isolation and not started on TB treatment unless relevant symptoms persist or worsen, or new ones develop.

   If TB treatment were required, the standard four-drug (rifampicin, isoniazid, pyrazinamide, ethambutol) 2-month induction regimen, followed by 4 months of rifampicin and isoniazid, plus pyridoxine would be recommended.
3. With a CD4 count of 47 cells/mm³, treatment with antiretroviral therapy would be recommended as soon as possible. Depending on how well she tolerated and responded to the *P. jiroveci* pneumonia treatment, and whether or not TB treatment was also needed, antiretroviral therapy would usually be started within 2–4 weeks of diagnosis. For more information, refer to British HIV Association guidelines for management of opportunistic infections (Nelson et al., 2010) and TB/HIV co-infection (Pozniak et al., 2010).
4. If Ms D did require TB treatment, the hepatic enzyme induction effect of rifampicin would need to be considered. For example, the dose of co-trimoxazole for *P. jiroveci* pneumonia prophylaxis should be a minimum of 960 mg once daily when co-administered with rifampicin.

   The choice and dose of antiretroviral therapy would also be affected if treatment was started after the HIV genotypic resistance test result was known; if no resistance had been found, then efavirenz-containing antiretroviral therapy would be possible. If co-administered with rifampicin, the efavirenz dose should be increased to 800 mg once daily. This would ideally be followed by TDM 2 weeks later, with further dose adjustment if necessary. Although the utility of antiretroviral therapy TDM remains controversial, this is a situation where it is commonly used.

   If PI-based antiretroviral therapy were initiated, either because of the presence of resistance mutations or whilst awaiting the HIV resistance test result, then TB therapy (if required) would need to be altered. Rifabutin (150–300 mg three times a week) would be used instead of rifampicin. PIs also interact with intranasal and inhaled fluticasone and budesonide, resulting in systemic absorption of these steroids, due to inhibition of cytochrome 450 3 A4 in the gut wall and the liver. Beclometasone nasal spray would be a suitable alternative preparation for Ms D's allergic rhinitis.

Acknowledgements

The authors would like to acknowledge the contribution of Claire Richardson for assistance in updating Tables 41.2–41.5, of David Annandale for assistance in updating Table 41.6 and Laura Baber for permission to use Table 41.7.

References

Arribas, J.R., Delgado, R., Arranz, A., et al., 2009. Lopinavir-ritonavir monotherapy versus lopinavir-ritonavir and 2 nucleosides for maintenance therapy of HIV: 96-week analysis. J. AIDS 51, 147–152.

Arribas, J.R., Horban, A., Gerstoft, J., et al., 2010. The MONET trial: darunavir/ritonavir with or without nucleoside analogues, for patients with HIV RNA below 50 copies/ml. AIDS. 24, 223–230.

Bower, M., Collins, S., Cottrill, C., on behalf of the AIDS Malignancy Subcommittee, et al., 2008. British HIV Association guidelines for HIV-associated malignancies 2008. HIV Med. 9, 336–388. Available at http://www.bhiva.org/documents/Guidelines/Malignancy/080627MaligFinal.pdf. Accessed Nov. 2010.

Brook, G., Main, J., Nelson, M., et al., 2010. British HIV Association guidelines for the management of coinfection with HIV-1 and hepatitis B or C virus 2010. HIV Med. 11, 1–30. Available at http://www.bhiva.org/documents/Guidelines/HepBC/2010/hiv_781.pdf. Accessed Nov. 2010.

Carr, A., 2003. HIV lipodystrophy: risk factors, pathogenesis, diagnosis and management. AIDS 17 (Suppl. 1), S141–S148.

Carr, A., Cooper, D.A., 2000. Adverse effects of antiretroviral therapy. Lancet 356, 1423–1430.

de Ruiter, A., Mercey, D., Anderson, J., et al., 2008. British HIV Association and Children's HIV Association guidelines for the management of HIV infection in pregnant women 2008. HIV Med. 9, 452–502. Available at http://www.bhiva.org/documents/Guidelines/Pregnancy/2008/PregnancyPub.pdf. Accessed Nov. 2010.

Department of Health, 2008. HIV post-exposure prophylaxis: guidance from the UK Chief Medical Officers' Expert Advisory Group on AIDS. Department of Health, London. Available at http://www.dh.gov.uk/ab/EAGA/index.htm. Accessed Nov. 2010.

El-Sadr, W.M., Lundgren, J.D., Neaton, J.D., et al., 2006. CD4+ count-guided interruption of antiretroviral treatment. N. Engl. J. Med. 355, 2283–2296.

Fisher, M., Benn, P., Evans, B., et al., 2006. UK guideline for the use of post-exposure prophylaxis for HIV following sexual exposure. Int. J. STD AIDS 17, 81–92.

Gazzard, B., on behalf of the BHIVA Treatment Guidelines Writing Group, 2008. British HIV Association guidelines for the treatment of HIV-1-infected adults with antiretroviral therapy. HIV Med. 9, 563–608. Available at http://onlinelibrary.wiley.com/doi/10.1111/j.1468–1293.2008.00636.x/full. Accessed Nov. 2010.

Hammer, S.M., Squires, K.E., Hughes, M.D., et al., 1997. A controlled trial of two nucleoside analogues plus indinavir in persons with human immunodeficiency virus infection and CD4 cell counts of 200 per cubic millimeter or less. N. Engl. J. Med. 337, 725–733.

Horne, R., Buick, D., Fisher, M., et al., 2004. Doubts about necessity and concerns about adverse effects: identifying the types of beliefs that are associated with non-adherence to HAART. Int. J. STD AIDS 15, 38–44.

Lichtenstein, K.A., 2005. Redefining lipodystrophy syndrome: risks and impact on clinical decision making. J. AIDS 39, 395–400.

Mallal, S., Phillips, E., Carosi, G., et al., 2008. HLA-B*5701 screening for hypersensitivity to abacavir. N. Engl. J. Med. 358, 568–579.

McComsey, G., Lonergan, J.T., 2004. Mitochondrial dysfunction: patient monitoring and toxicity management. J. AIDS 37, S30–S35.

Mellors, J.W., Munoz, A., Giorgi, J.V., et al., 1997. Plasma viral load and CD4 lymphocytes as prognostic markers of HIV-1 infection. Ann. Intern. Med. 126, 946–954.

Nelson, M., Dockrell, D., Edwards, S., on behalf of the BHIVA Guidelines Subcommittee, 2010. British HIV Association guidelines for the treatment of opportunistic infection in HIV-positive individuals 2010. British HIV Association, London. Available at http://www.bhiva.org/PublishedandApproved.aspx.

Paterson, D.L., Swindells, S., Mohr, J., et al., 2000. Adherence to protease inhibitor therapy and outcome in patients with HIV infection. Ann. Intern. Med. 133, 21–30.

Palella Jr., F.J., Delaney, K.M., Moorman, A.C. 1998. Declining morbidity and mortality among patients with advanced human immunodeficiency virus infection. N. Engl. J. Med. 338, 853–860.

Poppa, A., Davidson, O., Deutsch, J., et al., 2003. British HIV Association (BHIVA)/British Association for Sexual Health & HIV (BASHH) guidelines on provision of adherence support to individuals receiving antiretroviral therapy. British HIV Association. Available online at www.bhiva.org. Accessed Nov. 2010.

Pozniak, A.L., Collins, S., Coyne, C.M., on behalf of BHIVA Guidelines Writing Committee, et al., 2010. British HIV Association guidelines for the treatment of TB/HIV co-infection 2010. Available at http://www.bhiva.org/PublishedandApproved.aspx.

Read, P., Khan, P., Mandalia, S., et al., 2010. When Should HAART Be Initiated in Pregnancy to Achieve an Undetectable Viral Load? 17th Conference on Retroviruses and Opportunistic Infections, February 2010. Poster 896. Available at www.retroconference.org/2010/PDFs/896.pdf. Accessed Nov. 2010.

Sabin, C.A., Worm, S.W., Weber, R., et al., 2008. Use of nucleoside reverse transcriptase inhibitors and risk of myocardial infarction in HIV-infected patients enrolled in the D:A:D study: a multi-cohort collaboration. Lancet 371, 1417–1426.

Schambelan, M., Benson, C.A., Carr, A., et al., 2002. Management of metabolic complications associated with antiretroviral therapy for HIV-1 infection: recommendations of an International AIDS Society-USA Panel. J. AIDS 31, 257–275.

Smit, C., Geskus, R., Walker, S., et al., 2006. Effective therapy has altered the spectrum of cause-specific mortality following HIV seroconversion. AIDS 20, 741–749.

Thwaites, G., Fisher, M., Hemingway, C., et al., 2009. British Infection Society guidelines for the diagnosis and treatment of tuberculosis of the central nervous system in adults and children. J. Infect. 59, 167–187.

Worm, S.W., Sabin, C., Weber, R., et al., 2010. Risk of myocardial infarction in patients with HIV infection exposed to specific individual antiretroviral drugs from the 3 major drug classes: the data collection on adverse events of anti HIV drugs (D:A:D) study. J. Infect. Dis. 201, 318–330.

Further reading

Bhagani, S., Sweny, P., Brook, G., 2006. Guidelines for kidney transplantation in patients with HIV disease. HIV Med. 7, 133–139. doi:10.1111/j.1468–1293.2006.00367.x. Available at http://onlinelibrary.wiley.com/doi/10.1111/j.1468–1293.2006.00367.x/full. Accessed Nov. 2010.

British HIV Association, British Association of Sexual Health and HIV, British Infection Society, 2008. UK national guidelines for HIV testing. Available at www.bhiva.org/HIVTesting2008.aspx. Accessed Nov. 2010.

Department of Health, 2005. HIV Infected Health Care Workers: Guidance on Management and Patient Notification. Department of Health, London. Available at http://www.clinical-virology.org/pdfs/DH_4116416.pdf. Accessed Nov. 2010.

Geretti, A.M., on behalf of the BHIVA Immunization Writing Committee, 2008. British HIV Association Guidelines for immunization of HIV-infected adults 2008. HIV Med. 9, 795–848. Available at http://onlinelibrary.wiley.com/doi/10.1111/j.1468–1293.2008.00637.x/full. Accessed Nov. 2010.

Gupta, S.K., Eustace, J.A., Winston, J.A., et al., 2005. Guidelines for the management of chronic kidney disease in HIV-infected patients: recommendations of the HIV Medicine Association of the Infectious Diseases Society of America. Clin. Infect. Dis. 40, 1559–1585.

O'Grady, J., Taylor, C., Brook, G., et al., 2005. Guidelines for liver transplantation in patients with HIV infection. British HIV Association A. HIV Med. 6 (Suppl. 2) 149–153. Available at http://onlinelibrary.wiley.com/doi/10.1111/j.1468–1293.2005.00303.x/pdf. Accessed Nov. 2010.

Useful websites

British Association for Sexual Health and HIV:
www.bashh.org

British HIV Association:
www.bhiva.org

Clinical Care Options (US-based website focusing on HIV, hepatitis and oncology):
www.clinicaloptions.com

European AIDS Clinical Society Guidelines:
www.europeanaidsclinicalsociety.org/guidelines.asp

HIV i-Base (UK-based community provider of wide range of HIV-related information, including drug/treatment updates, conference reports and daily news items):
i-base.info/home/

Johns Hopkins University HIV Guide:
   www.hopkins-aids.edu
Medscape (US-based medical website with HIV specialty home page):
   www.medscape.com
NAM (UK-based community provider of wide range of HIV-related information, including drug/treatment updates, conference reports and daily news items):
   www.aidsmap.com
Toronto General Hospital Immunodeficiency Clinic:
   www.hivclinic.ca/main/home.html

United States National HIV Guidelines (antiretroviral treatment, management of opportunistic infections, co-infections and post-exposure prophylaxis):
   www.aidsinfo.nih.gov/guidelines/
University of California San Francisco HIV Educational Resource:
   www.hivinsite.ucsf.edu
University of Liverpool HIV Pharmacology Group (includes drug interaction charts):
   www.hiv-druginteractions.org

42 Fungal infections

M. Narayanan

Key points

- Fluconazole, a triazole, is considered to be standard therapy for oropharyngeal, oesophageal and vaginal candidiasis.
- Itraconazole and terbinafine are efficacious, non-toxic alternatives to griseofulvin when systemic treatment of dermatophytosis is required.
- Fungi can cause overwhelming deep-seated or systemic infections in immunocompromised hosts that are refractory to antifungal treatment alone.
- Incidence of non-Aspergillus mould infections has increased in transplant recipients over the past decade, and these can be lethal.
- Most therapy for deep-seated fungal infection in the immunocompromised host is empirical due to the difficulties in reaching a rapid, accurate diagnosis of systemic fungal infection.
- Lipid-complexed formulations of amphotericin offer a less toxic alternative to conventional amphotericin in the treatment of systemic fungal infection.
- Voriconazole, a triazole, appears to be an effective alternative to amphotericin in the treatment of invasive aspergillosis.
- Caspofungin is an alternative agent to amphotericin for invasive aspergillosis and may have a role to play in the empirical treatment of febrile neutropenic patients.

Fungi are ubiquitous microorganisms that differ from bacteria in their cellular structure, and this makes them naturally resistant to antibacterial agents (Table 42.1). Fungi are broadly divided into yeasts and moulds. Yeasts are typically round or oval shaped microscopically, grow flat round colonies on culture plates and reproduce by forming buds from their cells. Moulds (e.g. *Aspergillus*, *Mucor*) appear as a collection or mass (mycelium) of individual tubular structures called hyphae that grow by branching and longitudinal extension. They appear as a fuzzy growth on appropriate conducive medium (e.g. *Penicillium* colonies on stale bread or Sabourauds agar). The most commonly seen yeast, *Candida*, occasionally produces pseudohyphae.

There are hundreds of species of fungi found in the environment, but only the important human fungal pathogens and their treatment will be discussed in this chapter. The fungi of medical importance can be divided into four groups (Table 42.2).

Some fungi like *Histoplasma capsulatum*, *Coccidioides immitis*, *Blastomyces dermatitidis* are known as dimorphic fungi (Table 42.2) because they are found in the infected host in yeast form at 35–37 °C temperature but grow as moulds, *in vitro*, at room temperatures (22 °C incubation).

Fungi mainly reproduce by forming spores through mitosis giving rise to two daughter cells. They are known by names given to this imperfect state (asexual reproduction), but the same fungus, for example, *Scedosporium apiospermum* (asexual form) is also known as *Pseudoallescheria boydii* (sexual form). However, for all practical purposes, only the oldest and best-established name for the fungi is used in diagnostic laboratories.

Fungal spore are spread by air, water and direct contact with infected source. Humans usually become infected by inhalation of airborne spores or by inoculation into traumatised skin and mucous membrane.

Laboratory diagnosis

Microscopical examination and culture of fungi is the mainstay of laboratory diagnosis. Appropriate staining of histological sections of affected tissue is helpful in making a

Table 42.1 Important characteristics of a fungal cell	
Fungi	Bacteria
Eukaryotes	Prokaryotes, eubacteria
Cell and cytoplasm	Cell and cytoplasm
Nucleus with multiple chromosomes enclosed in a nuclear membrane	No nucleus or nuclear membrane, has single chromosome
Contains endoplasmic reticulum, golgi apparatus, mitochondria and ribosomes	Other structures absent except ribosomes
Cytoplasmic membrane	Cytoplasmic membrane
Contains phospholipids and sterols	Contains phospholipids and no sterols
Cell wall	Cell wall
Contains chitins, mannans,+/- cellulose	Contains peptidoglycan, lipids and proteins

Table 42.2 Classification of fungi of medical importance

Group	Examples	Infections caused
Yeast	*Candida* spp.	Oral and vaginal thrush
		Deep seated: candidaemia, empyema
	Cryptococcus neoformans	Meningitis
	Saccharomyces cervesiae	Rare systemic infection in immunocompromised host
	Malassezia furfur	
Yeast-like	*Geotrichium candidium*	
	Trichosporon beigelii	
Dimorphic fungi	*Blastomyces dermatitidis*	For first three: deep systemic organ involvement, more commonly in the immunocompromised host
	Coccidioides immitis	Deep subcutaneous infection following trauma
	Histoplasma capsulatum	
	Paracoccidioides brasiliensis	
	Sporothrix schenckii	
Moulds		
1. Hyaline		
a. Zygomyces	*Rhizopus*	Infections in neutropenic patients and those with diabetic ketoacidosis
	Mucor	
	Absidia	
b. Hyalohyphomycosis	*Aspergillus fumigatus* and other *Aspergillus* spp.	Systemic infection: invasive pulmonary or central nervous system involvement
	Fusarium	Fusarium keratitis
	Scedosporium apiospermum	Deep infection in immunocompromised host, for example, transplant patients
2. Dermatophytes	*Trichophyton* spp.	For all three: various skin (ringworm) hair and nail infections
	Microsporum spp.	
	Epidermophyton	
3. Dematiaceous	*Alternaria* spp.	Deep tissue infection with granulomas
	Cladophialora spp.	Chromomycosis, mycetomas

diagnosis when culture growth may or may not be positive. Yeast colonies and moulds are characteristic in their appearance on culture plates and can be preliminarily identified by their shape, colour and temperatures at which they grow. For the genus and species identification of yeasts, microscopic examination and biochemical tests are necessary. Moulds are identified by their morphology and the nature of sporulation on agar medium.

Antifungal sensitivity testing for yeast is done by determining the minimum inhibitory concentration (MIC) of the antifungal agent in the E test® strip method which has now replaced the measurement of 'inhibition zone' by disc testing. E-test® strips are also available for determining sensitivity of antifungal agents against moulds. Molecular diagnosis utilising polymerase chain reaction (PCR) is not available for use in routine practice. Serological diagnosis to look for antibodies in patient's blood is of use only in *Coccidioides* infection. Enzyme-linked immunosorbent assay (ELISA) methods to look for galactomannan antigen in deep *Aspergillus* infection are available but not fully evaluated. A positive test needs to be interpreted in conjunction with other findings. Antigen detection is useful in disseminated *Histoplasmosis* and *Cryptococcosis*.

Fungal infection

It is important to distinguish harmless colonisation with fungi and significant infection, as only the latter would benefit from antifungal treatment.

More often, fungi are a cause of superficial infections of the skin and mucous membranes.

In some susceptible hosts whose immune system is heavily compromised, deep-seated infections involving organs like lungs and brain can manifest as 'difficult to cure' infections, for example, pulmonary aspergillosis or cryptococcal meningitis.

Antifungal agents

Topical and systemic antifungal agents are available to treat mucocutaneous candidiasis, various forms of tinea (ringworm) and other dermatophytosis, onychomycosis and deep-seated systemic infections (e.g. candidaemia, mucor mycoses, fungal endocarditis, osteomyelitis). Some infective conditions and their treatment are dealt with in the sections that follow. The side effects of a range of antifungal agents are set out in Table 42.3.

Table 42.3 Side effects of antifungal agents

Drug	Side effects
Griseofulvin	Mild: headache, gastro-intestinal side effects. Hypersensitivity reactions such as skin rashes, including photosensitivity Moderate: exacerbation of acute intermittent porphyria; rarely, precipitation of systemic lupus erythematosus. Contraindicated in both acute porphyria, systemic lupus erythematosus, pregnancy and severe liver disease
Terbinafine	Usually mild: nausea, abdominal pain; allergic skin reactions; loss and disturbance of sense of taste. Not recommended in patients with liver disease
Amphotericin	Immediate reactions (during infusion) include headache, pyrexia, rigors, nausea, vomiting, hypotension; occasionally, there can be severe thrombophlebitis after the infusion Nephrotoxicity and hypokalaemia Anaemia due to reduced erythropoiesis Peripheral neuropathy (rare) Cardiac failure (exacerbated by hypokalaemia due to nephrotoxicity) Immunomodulation (the drug can both enhance and inhibit some immunological functions)
Flucytosine	Mild: gastro-intestinal side effects (nausea, vomiting). Occasional skin rashes Moderate: myelosuppression (dose related), hepatotoxicity
Fluconazole	Mild: nausea, vomiting and occasional skin rashes; occasionally, elevated liver enzymes (reversible) Moderate or severe: rarely, hepatotoxicity and severe cutaneous reactions, especially in AIDS patients
Itraconazole	Mild: nausea and abdominal pain; occasional skin rashes Moderate or severe: rarely, hepatotoxicity
Voriconazole	Similar to fluconazole and itraconazole Mild: reversible visual disturbances occur in about 30% patients
Caspofungin	Mild: gastro-intestinal side effects; occasional skin rashes

Superficial infection

Candida infections

Epidemiology

Candida is a normal commensal of the human gastro-intestinal tract and skin. Loss of skin and mucosal integrity or use of broad-spectrum antibiotics which alter normal bacterial flora allow overgrowth of endogenous *Candida*. There are more than 100 species of *Candida*, but only a few are important as common human pathogens.

Thrush is candidal infection of the mucous membrane. It can manifest as oral infection, for example, oral thrush in various patient groups, vulvo vaginal thrush in females, balanitis in the uncircumcised man or intertrigo infection in moist skin surfaces in close proximity, for example, groin area. Patients with diabetes and steroid users, whether inhaled or oral, are also prone to infections. Dysphagia due to candidal oesophagitis presents in patients with AIDS and cancer.

Clinical presentation

Oral thrush typically presents as a sore mouth with white curd like patches on the tongue or oral mucosa which can bleed on scraping. Females with vaginal thrush present with itching and a creamy vaginal discharge. Skin infection in babies can present as pustular body rash or nappy rash in the moist perianal area. Candida folliculitis may present in unkempt, bearded men. Nail infection with *Candida* (onychomycosis), or subcutaneous tissue involvement under the nail (paronychia) is seen in people whose occupation involves prolonged hand immersion in water.

In severe oesophageal candidiasis, ulceration or formation of pseudomembranes and, rarely, perforation of lower third of the oesophagus may occur.

Candida can be a cause of hospital-acquired infection in patients as it is found in the hospital environment on inanimate objects or on skin of health care workers.

Treatment

Oral and vaginal candidiasis may be treated by either topical or systemic antifungal agents. The drugs currently available for topical use fall into two groups: the polyenes, of which only amphotericin and nystatin are used clinically, and the imidazoles such as econazole, clotrimazole, miconazole and fenticonazole. These agents are essentially identical in their antifungal activity and the only reasons to choose between them are price and differing preparations. The two systemic agents are both triazoles (fluconazole and itraconazole) and can be given by mouth. Skin infections may also be treated topically, but nail infections are unlikely to respond to a topical antifungal agent alone and require systemic treatment. Oesophagitis will invariably require systemic treatment.

Topical treatment. The polyenes are broad-spectrum antifungal agents that are virtually insoluble in water and which are not absorbed from the gastro-intestinal tract or from skin or mucous membranes. Both nystatin and amphotericin (but particularly nystatin) are available in a wide range of formulations including pessaries, creams, gels, tablets, pastilles, etc. The choice of formulation clearly depends on the site of infection and patient preference.

Systemic treatment. Three triazole agents: fluconazole, itraconazole and voriconazole are available for systemic treatment of oral and vulvo vaginal candidiasis (VVC). A good source of advice on treatment is that from the Infectious Diseases Society of America (Pappas et al., 2009):

Vulvo vaginal candidiasis

- Several topical antifungal agents provide effective therapy; no agent is clearly superior
- A single 150-mg dose of fluconazole is recommended for the treatment of uncomplicated cases
- For recurring vulvo vaginal candidiasis, 10–14 days of induction therapy with a topical or oral azole, followed by fluconazole at a dosage of 150 mg once per week for 6 months, is recommended
- Complicated vulvo vaginal candidiasis requires topical therapy for 7 days or multiple doses of fluconazole (150 mg every 72 h for 3 doses). Recurrent infections with non-albicans *Candida*, for example, *C. glabrata,* may be more difficult to treat.

Candida balanitis

- Candida balanitis can be treated with topical polyenes or imidazoles, or with systemic fluconazole in the same dose as for vaginal infection.

It is sometimes stated that when treating a woman with vaginal candidiasis, the male partner should be treated simultaneously to prevent reinfection. Although there is no evidence to support this approach, it may be considered in women who suffer from repeated vaginal candidiasis.

Guidance on the treatment of topical and systemic therapy (Pappas et al., 2009) are also available for treatment of mild, moderate and severe oropharyngeal and oesophageal candidiasis and suppressive therapy for patients with HIV infection.

Dermatophytosis

Epidemiology

Dermatophytosis, or tinea, is a condition caused by three genera of dermatophyte fungi: *Trichophyton*, *Epidermophyton* and *Microsporum*. Unlike *Candida*, these are moulds which have a predilection for keratinised tissue such as skin, nail and hair. These fungi are very widely distributed throughout the world and may be acquired from the soil (anthrophilic, e.g. *Trichophyton rubrum*), from animals (zoophilic) or from humans (geophilic) infected with the fungus.

Some species are prevalent throughout the world, for example, *Microsporum canis,* while some are area specific, for example, *Trichophyton mentagrophyte* in Europe and New Zealand.

Clinical presentation

The classical clinical presentation of dermatophyte infection of the skin is ringworm (tinea), a circular, inflamed lesion with a raised edge and associated skin scaling. However, presentation is influenced by the site of infection, for example, tinea pedis (athlete's foot) between the toes, tinea cruris on the body, and by the actual species of fungus causing the infection. In general, less severe lesions are produced by human fungal strains, while those acquired from animals can produce quite intense inflammatory reactions.

Dermatophytosis of the nail results in thickened, discoloured nails, while in the scalp, infection presents with itching, skin scaling and inflammation, and patchy hair loss (alopecia).

Rarely, deep dermatophytosis may be seen in immunocompromised patients with involvement of subcutaneous tissue (granuloma).

Diagnosis

The diagnosis of dermatophyte infection is confirmed by collecting appropriate specimens such as material from infected nails and skin. The fungi can be seen microscopically and specimens may also be cultured, but antifungal susceptibility testing is not required.

Treatment

Small or medium areas of skin infection can be treated with topical therapy, but nail, hair and widespread skin infection should be systemically treated with oral antifungal agents.

The most commonly used topical agents are the imidazoles, of which a wide variety is available, including clotrimazole, ecoazole, miconazole, sulconazole and tioconazole. There is little to choose between these agents, all of which are usually applied two or three times daily, continuing for up to 2 weeks after the lesions have healed. Side effects are uncommon and usually consist of mild skin irritation. Other topical agents include amorolfine, terbinafine and tolnaftate.

The main oral antifungals used for dermatophytosis are terbinafine, itraconazole and fluconazole. Griseofulvin is an alternative treatment for tinea capitis.

Terbinafine. Terbinafine was the first member of a new class of antifungal agents, the allylamines, which became available for systemic use. These agents act by inhibition of the fungal enzyme squalene epoxidase, an enzyme involved in the synthesis of ergosterol, an essential component of the fungal cytoplasmic membrane. Although terbinafine has a very broad antifungal spectrum in the laboratory, its *in vivo* efficacy does not correspond to its *in vitro* activity, and it is used only for the treatment of dermatophyte infection.

Terbinafine is the treatment of choice for tinea infections at 250 mg/day for 2–4 weeks, 250 mg/day for 6 weeks for fingernail infection and 12 weeks for toenail infection.

About 70% of an oral dose of terbinafine is absorbed, and the drug appears in high concentrations in the skin. The half-life is about 16–17 h, and therefore the drug can be given once per day. Terbinafine is metabolised in the liver and the metabolites are excreted in the urine so that hepatic or renal dysfunction will prolong the elimination half-life.

Table 42.4 Conditions predisposing to systemic or deep-seated fungal infection

Infection	Predisposing conditions
Systemic candidiasis	Neutropenia from any cause (disease or treatment) Use of broad-spectrum antibiotics which eliminate the normal body flora Indwelling intravenous cannulae, especially when used for total parenteral nutrition Haematological malignancy and HSCT Solid organ transplantation AIDS (particularly associated with severe mucocutaneous infection) Intravenous drug abuse Cardiac surgery and heart valve replacement, leading to *Candida* endocarditis Gastro-intestinal tract surgery Oesophagectomy leak leading to pleural space infection (empyema)
Aspergillosis	Neutropenia from any cause, especially if severe and prolonged Acute leukaemia Solid organ transplantation (mainly lungs) Chronic granulomatous disease of childhood (defect in neutrophil function) Pre-existing lung disease (usually leads to aspergillomas; fungus balls form in the lung rather than invasive or disseminated infection)
Cryptococcosis	AIDS Systemic therapy with corticosteroids Renal transplantation Hodgkin's disease and other lymphomas Sarcoidosis Collagen vascular diseases
Zygomycosis	Diabetic hyperglycaemic ketoacidosis (leading to rhinocerebral infection) Severe, prolonged neutropenia Burns (leading to cutaneous infection)

HSCT, hematopoietic stem cell transplantation.

Itraconazole is the second preferred agent at 200 mg/day for 1–2 weeks and longer, with repeated courses for finger and toenail involvement.

Griseofulvin. The first orally administered treatment for dermatophytosis was griseofulvin, which has now been available for over 40 years. Griseofulvin is active only against dermatophyte fungi and is inactive against all other fungi and bacteria. In order to exert its antifungal effect, it must be incorporated into keratinous tissue, where levels are much greater than serum levels, and therefore it has no effect if used topically.

The usual adult dose is 10–20 mg/kg/day for 6 weeks for treatment of larger lesions in tinea corporis.

Griseofulvin is well absorbed and absorption is enhanced if taken with a high-fat meal. In children, it may be given with milk. A 1000-mg dose produces a peak serum level of about 1–2 mg/L after 4 h, with a half-life of at least 9 h. An ultra-fine preparation of griseofulvin exists which is almost totally absorbed and permits the use of lower doses (typically 330–660 mg daily). This preparation is not available in the UK. Elimination is mainly through the liver and inactive metabolites are excreted in the urine. Less than 1% of a dose is excreted in urine in the active form, but some active drug is excreted in the faeces.

The duration of treatment with griseofulvin is dependent entirely on clinical response. Skin or hair infection usually requires 4–12 weeks' therapy, but nail infections respond much more slowly; 6 months' treatment is often required for fingernails, a year or more for toenail infections. Unfortunately, the rate of treatment failure or relapse in nail infection is high, and may reach up to 60%. Hence, terbinafine and itraconazole may be preferred agents.

Pityriasis versicolor

This is a common superficial skin infection caused by a yeast-like fungus, *Malassezia furfur*. The organism is a member of the normal skin flora and lives only on the skin because it has a growth requirement for medium-chain fatty acids present in sebum.

Clinical presentation

The condition usually appears as patches scattered over the trunk, neck and shoulders. These patches produce scales and may be pigmented in light-skinned individuals, appearing light brown in colour. In dark-skinned patients, the lesions may lose pigment and appear lighter than normal skin.

In some patients, Malassezia yeast is also associated with dandruff and seborrhoeic dermatitis, although the exact role of the yeast in causing this condition remains uncertain. In AIDS patients, seborrhoeic dermatitis may be quite extensive and sudden in onset.

Malassezia folliculitis can appear as greasy papules or pustules on the trunk or face of an HIV-infected individual.

Diagnosis

The diagnosis is made by microscopy of scrapings from the lesion. The specimen is examined for the presence of yeast cells and short hyphae. Culture is not usually required for diagnosis and, since it requires special culture media, is not routinely attempted.

Treatment

Pityriasis versicolor is treated with topical terbinafine cream or a topical imidazole cream such as clotrimazole, econazole or miconazole. Cheaper topical alternatives are 2% selenium sulphide lotion or 20% sodium thiosulphate applied daily for 10–14 days. Relapses are common and treatment may need to be repeated. In severe cases, oral itraconazole (200 mg once daily for 7 days) may be given. Treatment of seborrhoeic dermatitis and folliculitis is undertaken with topical azole creams and 1% hydrocortisone. This condition can also often relapse.

Ear infection

Fungi sometimes infect the external auditory canal, causing otitis externa, the most common causative organisms being various species of *Aspergillus* (such as *A. niger* and *A. fumigatus*) and *Candida albicans* and other *Candida* species. A variety of other fungi found in the environment can also cause this condition. The use of topical antibacterial agents in the ear may predispose to local fungal infection.

Clinical presentation

Fungal infection of the ear usually presents as pain and itching in the auditory canal, sometimes with a reduction in hearing due to blockage of the canal. There may be an associated discharge from the ear. Clinical examination shows a swollen red canal, and the fungal mycelium is sometimes visible as an amorphous white or grey mass.

Diagnosis

The diagnosis of a fungal infection of the external canal can be made by microscopy and culture of material obtained from the ear.

Treatment

Aural toilet with removal of obstructing debris is very important in the management of fungal infections of the external auditory canal. A topical antifungal agent such as nystatin or amphotericin, or an imidazole can also be applied.

Infections with saprophytic fungi

Some saprophytic fungi (normally harmless human commensals) can cause significant infections. An example of such an infection in a host with a normal immune system is fusarium keratitis in contact lens wearers. *Penicillium marneffei* can cause skin infection and disseminated fatal infection in HIV-infected patients in South East Asia. *Scedosporium* pulmonary infections are seen in lung transplant recipients.

A large retrospective data from the USA revealed that the three most common non-Aspergillus moulds causing invasive fungal infection among patients receiving haemopoietic stem cell transplants (HSCT) were *Fusarium*, *Scedospermium* and *Zygomycetes*.

Deep-seated fungal infections

Most deep-seated or systemic fungal infections seen in the UK are the result of some breakdown in the normal body defences, which may be due to disease or medical treatment. Fungi that cause superficial infections can also cause deep-seated infection in immunocompromised patients with leukaemia and lymphoma and those in the post-transplant period of immunosuppression. There are, however, a group of fungi, often referred to rather misleadingly as the pathogenic fungi, which are able to cause systemic infection in a previously healthy person. These infections, which are usually due to dimorphic fungi, include diseases such as histoplasmosis, blastomycosis and coccidioidomycosis. They are rare in the UK but rather more common in the USA and other parts of the world.

Fungal infections in the compromised host

Common mycoses

Epidemiology and predisposing factors

There are a large number of conditions which may predispose the individual to systemic or deep-seated fungal infection. These are summarised in Table 42.4. A breach in the body's mechanical barriers may predispose to fungal infection. For example, fungal infection of the urinary tract occurs most commonly in catheterised patients who have received broad-spectrum antibiotics, while total parenteral nutrition (TPN) is strongly associated with fungaemia, sometimes with unusual fungi such as *Malassezia furfur*. This is due to the use of TPN infusions containing lipids, which are a growth requirement of this organism. Most cases of systemic fungal infection, however, are associated with a defect in the patient's immune system, and the nature of the organisms encountered is often related to the nature of the immunosuppression. Neutropenia, for example, is usually associated with *Candida* species, *Aspergillus* and mucormycosis, while defects of cell-mediated immunity, for example HIV infection, are strongly associated with infection by *Cryptococcus neoformans*. Prolonged diabetic ketoacidosis is a risk factor for developing rhinocerebral zygomycosis where mortality can be as high as 100% if there is significant underlying disease.

Many different fungi have been described as causing systemic fungal infection, but the most common organisms encountered and the conditions they cause are listed in Table 42.5. Of these, *Candida* and *Aspergillus* are by far the most common in the UK.

Table 42.5 Common causes of systemic and deep-seated fungal infection in the UK

Condition/organism	Common clinical presentations
Candidiasis (*Candida albicans, C. glabrata, C. krusei, C. tropicalis,* other *Candida* species)	Fungaemia Colonisation of intravenous cannulae Pneumonia Meningitis Bone and joint infections Endocarditis Endophthalmitis Peritonitis in chronic ambulatory peritoneal dialysis
Aspergillosis (*Aspergillus fumigatus, A. flavus,* other *Aspergillus* species)	Invasive pulmonary aspergillosis Disseminated aspergillosis Aspergilloma Endocarditis
Cryptococcosis (*Cryptococcus neoformans*)	Meningitis Pneumonia Cutaneous infection
Zygomycosis (various species of the genera *Rhizopus, Mucor, Absidia*)	Rhinocerebral infection Pulmonary mucormycosis Surgical wound and burns infection
Malassezia furfur	Cutaneous infection (especially in burns patients) Fungaemia associated with total parenteral nutrition

Clinical presentation

Symptoms can be non-specific like low-grade fever, night sweats, weight loss, cough, chest pain and septic shock in extreme cases (Table 42.6).

Diagnosis

Organ-specific radiological findings backed by laboratory tests, as discussed earlier in this chapter, are the mainstay of diagnosis.

Treatment

Compared to the vast array of antibacterial agents available to treat bacterial infections, there are very few systemic antifungal agents available and these comprise four major categories: the polyenes (conventional and lipid formulations of Amphotericin B), the triazoles (fluconazole, itraconazole, voriconazole and posaconazole), the echinocandins (caspofungin, anidulafungin and micafungin) and flucytosine. To provide optimal therapy to the patient, it is necessary to understand the profile, properties and toxicity of these agents. Table 42.7 details the antifungal spectrum of activity against common fungi.

Antifungal prophylaxis is commonly used to prevent invasive fungal infections in the 'at risk' group of patients.

Amphotericin B

Amphotericin, a member of the polyene group, is obtained from various species of *Streptomyces*. Chemically, it is a large carbon ring of 37 carbon atoms closed by a lactone bond. One

Table 42.6 Clinical presentation of systemic fungal infection

Condition	Clinical presentation
Fungaemia (the presence of fungi in the bloodstream), usually due to *Candida* species	Fever, low blood pressure and sometimes other features of septic shock, especially in neutropenic patients Relatively low-grade fungaemias such as those associated with colonised intravenous cannulae often present only with fever Disseminated infection to multiple organ systems is quite common with *Candida* species, leading to central nervous system disease, endocarditis, endophthalmitis, skin infections, renal disease, bone and joint infection
Pneumonia, most frequently due to *Aspergillus* species	Fever, chest pain and cough which may be non-productive. May progress rapidly, especially with *Aspergillus* infection, to severe respiratory distress, necrosis of the lung and pulmonary haemorrhage Formation of fungal balls in pre-existing lung cavities with or without invasion
Meningitis and other central nervous system infection	*Candida* infection may present as a typical meningitis, although it is often more insidious. Aspergillosis is associated with headache, confusion and focal neurological signs due to the presence of brain infarcts. Cryptococcosis most frequently presents as a chronic, insidious meningitis with headache and alteration in mental state
Mucormycosis	Angioinvasive. The most common presentation of mucormycosis is rhinocerebral infection. Initially an infection of the sinuses, it then spreads locally to the palate, orbit and eventually into the brain, leading to encephalitis Pulmonary disease can present as fungal balls radiologically with symptoms of haemoptysis

Table 42.7 Antifungal spectrum of activity against common fungi (adapted from Dodds Ashley et al., 2006)

Organism	AmB[a]	Flu	Itr	Vor	Pos	Anidulafungin	Caspofungin	Micafungin	Flucytosine
Aspergillus species	+	−	+	+	+	+	+	+	−
A. flavus	±	−	+	+	+	+	+	+	−
A. fumigatus	+	−	+	+	+	+	+	+	−
A. niger	+	−	±	+	+	+	+	+	−
A. terreus	−	−	+	+	+	+	+	+	−
Candida species	+	+	+	+	+	+	+	+	+
C. albicans	+	+	+	+	+	+	+	+	+
C. glabrata	+	±	±	+	+	+	+	+	+
C. krusei	+	−	±	+	+	+	+	+	±
C. lusitaniae	−	+	+	+	+	+	+	+	±
C. parapsilosis	+	+	+	+	+	±	±	±	+
C. tropicalis	+	+	+	+	+	+	+	+	+
Cryptococcus neoformans	+	+	+	+	+	−	−	−	+
Coccidioides species	+	+	+	+	+	±[b]	±[b]	±[b]	−
Blastomyces	+	+	+	+	+	±[b]	±[b]	±[b]	−
Histoplasma species	+	+	+	+	+	±[b]	±[b]	±[b]	−
Fusarium species	±	−	−	+	+	−	−	−	−
Scedosprium apiospermum	±	−	±	+	+	−	−	−	−
Scedosporium prolificans	−	−	−	±	±	−	−	−	−
Zygomycetes	±	−	−	−	+	−	−	−	−

Note: Plus signs (+) indicate that the antifungal agent has activity against the organism specified. Minus signs (−) indicate that the antifungal agent does not have activity against the organism specified. Plus-minus signs (±) indicate agent has variable activity against the organism specified. AmB, amphotericin B; Flu, fluconazole; Itr, itraconazole; Pos, posaconazole; Vor, voriconazole.
[a]Includes lipid formulations.
[b]*In vitro* data show that the echinocandins (specifically, micafungin) may have variable activity against the dimorphic fungi, depending on whether they are in the mycelial or yeast-like form.

side of the molecule contains seven carbon- to-carbon double bonds (polyene) and the other side contains seven hydroxyl groups. It dissolves in organic polar solvents but forms a colloidal suspension of micelles in water which is rendered stable by the addition of the surfactant sodium deoxycholate.

Mode of action. Amphotericin B binds to the ergosterol in fungal cell membrane affecting its integrity by forming pores and therefore cell death. Nystatin, the other polyene, is only used topically because of toxicity associated with its systemic use.

Spectrum of activity. Amphotericin is active against a vast majority of fungi and this is the same for all formulations. Development of resistance is uncommon, although primary resistance has been identified for *Aspergillus terreus*, *Scedosporium* spp., *Trichosporon* spp. and *Candida lusitaniae*.

Pharmacodynamically, the ratio of the peak serum concentration to the MIC is important for its efficacy.

Amphotericin B deoxycholate (ABD). Released in 1950, colloidal in nature, amphotericin B deoxycholate is highly protein bound (99%) and insoluble in water. It penetrates poorly into cerebrospinal fluid. Initial elimination of the drug occurs with a half-life of 24–48 h, but this is followed by very slow elimination (half-life about 14 days). As a consequence, it may take 10 weeks for the drug to disappear from the circulation.

Amphotericin B deoxycholate is given by slow IV infusion in 5% dextrose with a dose range of 0.3–1 mg/kg increased to 1.5 mg/kg for serious invasive infections. The duration of treatment can vary from 1 to 2 weeks to longer, depending on the severity of the infection and the organ system involved.

Adverse effects. Nephrotoxicity is the most serious side effect of amphotericin. Renal failure should be monitored regularly at least every other day, and if the serum creatinine exceeds 250 μmol/L, the drug should be discontinued until the creatinine level falls below this limit. Hypokalaemia is also a problem and may be severe, necessitating replacement therapy.

Azotaemia may be seen in patients after the first few infusions of amphotericin B deoxycholate. Chills, fever and tachypnoea may occur but can be avoided by addition of hydrocortisone 25–50 mg to the infusion solution.

The manufacturer recommends that before commencing treatment, a 1 mg test dose should be given in 50 ml of 5% dextrose over a 1- to 2-h period and the patient monitored for fever, rigors and hypotension. True allergic reactions are rare.

Amphotericin B lipid formulations

The advantage of delivering amphotericin encapsulated in liposomes or as a complex with lipid molecules is that a higher unit dose can be given and there is reduction in toxic effects. Three such preparations are currently available: liposomal amphotericin B (AmBisome®), amphotericin B lipid complex (Abelcept®) and amphotericin B colloidal dispersion (Amphocil®).

Liposomal amphotericin B. In liposomal amphotericin B (AmBisome®), the drug is contained in small vesicles each consisting of a phospholipid bilayer enclosing an aqueous environment. This permits the delivery of higher doses (3 mg/kg is recommended, but doses up to 10 mg/kg have been used in some centres) compared to conventional amphotericin, with very little of the immediate toxicity which is such a problem with the conventional formulation. Higher peak serum concentrations are obtained with the liposomal formulation compared to equivalent doses of the conventional drug, although it is not certain if this is clinically relevant. Liposomal amphotericin is concentrated mainly in the liver and spleen, where it is taken up by cells of the reticuloendothelial system. Concentrations in the lung and kidneys are much lower, which may or may not be clinically important.

There is reduced nephrotoxicity with this formulation, and some of the renal dysfunction which has been described in clinical trials of liposomal amphotericin may have been due to concomitant drugs. Three randomised, comparative clinical trials of liposomal amphotericin versus conventional amphotericin B have shown reduced toxicity due to the liposomal preparation, and there is additional evidence for this from open studies. It is this comparative lack of toxicity which accounts for much of the popularity of this agent, despite its expense. These studies also indicate that this agent performs as well as the conventional preparation in febrile neutropenic patients.

Amphotericin B lipid complex and amphotericin B colloidal dispersion. Amphotericin B lipid complex (Abelcet®) is not a liposomal formulation, but consists of large sheets of amphotericin combined with phospholipids. This formulation gives lower peak serum levels compared to the conventional drug because it is rapidly taken up by tissue macrophages, while concentrations in the lungs and the liver are much higher. Patients seem to experience more immediate side effects than with liposomal amphotericin. There is less clinical trial evidence for the use of this agent compared to the liposomal preparation. Amphotericin B colloidal dispersion (Amphocil®) is a formulation consisting of tiny discs of amphotericin and cholesterylsulphate. Like the lipid complex, it too produces low peak serum levels but high liver concentrations compared to the conventional drug. There is less clinical experience with this preparation than with the liposomal preparation, and it appears to have a higher incidence of certain adverse reactions than conventional amphotericin.

Choosing a lipid preparation. Unfortunately, there are limited comparative trial data between the different lipid formulations. At present, the greatest clinical experience is with liposomal amphotericin B and by reason of this and the reduced incidence of side effects, it is the preferred agent of the three in many centres in the UK. In an ideal world, all patients requiring amphotericin would receive the conventional preparation initially, being changed to a lipid formulation only if they fail to respond to or cannot tolerate the side effects of the conventional form. However, the incidence of side effects and the difficulty in administration of conventional amphotericin have in practice led to its replacement in most centres with a lipid formulation.

Flucytosine

Amphotericin B and griseofulvin were the only systemic antifungal agents available until the early 1970s, when flucytosine became available for patient use.

Mode of action. Flucytosine (5-fluorocytosine) is a synthetic fluorinated nucleotide analogue. The mode of action is twofold. Following uptake by the cell, which is dependent on the presence of cytosine permease, flucytosine is deaminated to 5-fluorouracil by cytosine deaminase. This in turn is incorporated into fungal RNA in place of uracil, leading to impairment of protein synthesis. Further metabolism of 5-fluorouracil leads to a metabolite that inhibits the enzyme thymidylate synthetase, leading to inhibition of DNA synthesis. Mammalian cells have absent or weak cytosine deaminase activity which accounts for the selective toxicity of flucytosine.

For all practical purposes, flucytosine is only active against yeasts and yeast-like fungi. Inherent resistance occurs in approximately 10% of clinical isolates of *Candida* species, and acquired resistance develops rapidly if the drug is used alone.

There are several resistance mechanisms, some of which result from a single-step mutation giving a high frequency of acquired resistance in organisms exposed to the drug. For this reason, flucytosine should always be given in combination with another agent such as amphotericin, with which it is synergistic.

Pharmacokinetics. Flucytosine is highly soluble in water and over 90% of an oral dose is absorbed from the gastro-intestinal tract. Virtually all the absorbed dose is excreted unchanged in the urine by glomerular filtration. The elimination half-life is about 4 h, but this is greatly prolonged in renal failure and dosage modification is required in patients with renal dysfunction. The degree of protein binding is very low and flucytosine penetrates well into all tissues, including the aqueous humour of the eye, where about 10% of the serum level is achieved, and the CSF, where about 80% of the serum level is achieved.

Administrations. Flucytosine is given orally or by short intravenous infusion. The dose administered by either route in patients with normal renal function is 100–200 mg/kg/day in four divided doses. This must be reduced in renal failure, but the degree of reduction depends on the degree of renal impairment and it is obligatory to monitor the serum levels of flucytosine. Unfortunately, flucytosine assay is now rarely carried out routinely in UK laboratories. Flucytosine is usually given in conjunction with amphotericin which will probably cause some degree of renal dysfunction, so requiring modification of the flucytosine dose. To avoid dose-related marrow toxicity, the peak serum level, obtained at 1 h after an intravenous dose or 2 h after an oral dose, should be maintained in the range 70–80 mg/L and should not be allowed to exceed 100 mg/L.

Side effects. Some of the side effects of flucytosine are given in Table 42.3. The most important toxic effect is a dose-related myelosuppression with neutropenia and thrombocytopenia. This is usually reversible and can be avoided by monitoring serum levels of flucytosine and adjusting the dose accordingly. Hepatotoxicity is also probably a result of high serum levels, and liver function tests should be performed regularly. The drug is teratogenic in some animals and is not recommended in pregnant women for relatively trivial infections such as a fungal urinary tract infection. In cases of a life-threatening fungal infection, which is very rare in pregnancy, the potential benefits of flucytosine must be weighed against the possible risks.

Imidazoles

The imidazoles clotrimazole, econazole, fenticonazole, sulconazole and tioconazole are now principally used for the local treatment of vaginal candidiasis and for dermatophyte infections. Ketoconazole, which first became available in 1979, can be administered for systemic use, but even this agent has been superseded by the triazoles.

Triazoles

Three triazoles are licensed in the UK: fluconazole, itraconazole and voriconazole. They differ substantially from one another in their pharmacokinetic and antifungal activity (Table 42.8). Their main side effects are listed in Table 42.3.

The basic chemical structure of the triazoles is the azole ring, a five-membered ring containing three nitrogen atoms. Their principal mode of action involves one of the nitrogen atoms of the azole ring binding to fungal cytochrome P450 enzymes. This inhibits the demethylation of lansterol and leads to a reduced concentration of ergosterol necessary for a normal fungal cytoplasmic membrane. The propensity, in man, to also inhibit the metabolism of drugs by cytochrome P450 results in a considerable number of drug interactions.

Fluconazole

Clinical use. Fluconazole is available both orally and parenterally and is used only in the treatment and prophylaxis of infections due to yeasts and yeast-like fungi. It is not used for the treatment of infections due to moulds. It is highly effective in the treatment of *Cryptococcus* infection, but the first-line treatment of cryptococcosis of the central nervous system is the combination of amphotericin B plus flucytosine for CNS infection due to this organism. This may be followed by fluconazole, which in HIV-infected patients will be required life long as suppressive treatment to prevent relapse. In immunocompetent hosts, fluconazole may be used as the primary treatment for disease not involving the CNS, such as pulmonary infection.

In patients with candidaemia due to colonised intravenous cannulae, the most important treatment is removal of the infected cannula, but it is common practice to give a short course of antifungal therapy to prevent disseminated infection elsewhere. Although not proven in randomised clinical trials, changing potentially infected central-line catheters in candidaemia patients is probably the most important part of therapy.

In non-neutropenic patients, studies have shown fluconazole and caspofungin to be as efficacious as, and less toxic than, conventional amphotericin B. In such patients, where the infecting organism and its susceptibility to fluconazole are known, it would be reasonable to commence treatment with fluconazole; caspofungin is a potential alternative. In neutropenic patients, and in patients infected with fluconazole-resistant organisms, amphotericin continues to be the treatment of choice. Fluconazole has also been successfully used as prophylaxis against *Candida* infections in neutropenic patients and patients with AIDS, but this in turn has been associated with an increasing incidence of systemic infections with fluconazole-resistant strains.

Resistance. Some units that use fluconazole extensively have noted an increase in the isolation of yeasts resistant to the drug, with the prevalence of resistance related to the extent of use of fluconazole. Resistance in *Candida* species is mainly seen in patients who are given long-term prophylactic fluconazole. This selects out those *Candida* species such as *C. krusei* and *C. glabrata* that are inherently less susceptible to fluconazole. Resistance in *C. albicans*, the most common species infecting humans, is seen mainly in AIDS patients, partly due to the extensive use of fluconazole in treating severe oral and pharyngeal candidiasis in such patients and partly due to the very large numbers of yeasts in the oropharynx of AIDS patients with candidiasis, which increases the chance of resistance due to spontaneous mutation.

Table 42.8 Comparative pharmacokinetics of antifungal agents (adapted from Dodds Ashley et al., 2006)

Pharmacokinetic parameter	Antifungal agent											
	AmB	ABCD	ABLC	LAB	Flu	Itr[a]	Vor	Pos	Anidulafungin	Caspofungin	Micafungin	Flucytosine
Oral bioavailability (%)	<5	<5	<5	<5	95	50	96	ND	<5	<5	<5	80
Food effect	NA	NA	NA	NA	NE	ES	ES	Food	NA	NA	NA	NE
Distribution												
Total C_{max} μcg/mL	0.5–2	4	131	0.1	0.7	11	4.6	7.8	0.83	0.27	0.24	80
AUC, mg × h/L	17	43	14	555	400	29.2	20.3	8.9	99[b]	119	158[b]	62
Protein binding (%)	>95	>95	>95	>95	10	99.8	58	99	84	97	99	4
CSF penetration (%)	0–4	<5	<5	<5	>60	<10	60	NR	<5	<5	<5	75
Vitreal penetration (%)	0–38[c,d]	0–38[c,d]	0–38[c,d]	0–38[c,d]	28–75[c,d]	10[c]	38[c]	26[c,d]	0[d]	0[c]	<1[d]	49[d]
Urine penetration (%)[e]	3–20	<5	<5	4.5	90	1–10	<2	<2	<2	<2	<2	90
Metabolism	Minor Hep	Unk	Unk	Unk	Minor Hep	Hep	Hep	Hep	None	Hep	Hep	Minor intestinal
Elimination	Faeces	Unk	Unk	Unk	Urine	Hep	Renal	Faeces	Faeces	Urine	Faeces	Renal
Half-life (h)	50	30	173	100–153	31	24	6	25	26	30	15	3–6

Note: ABCD, amphotericin B colloidal dispersion; ABLC, amphotericin B lipid complex; AmB amphotericin B; AUC, area under the concentration curve; C_{max}, peak drug concentration; ES, empty stomach; Flu, fluconazole; Hep, hepatic; Itr, itraconazole; LAB, liposomal amphotericin B; NA, not applicable; ND, no data; NE, no effect; Pos, posaconazole; Unk, unknown; Vor, voriconazole.
[a]Data are for oral solution.
[b]For doses of 100 mg/day.
[c]Human.
[d]Animal.
[e]Percentage of active drug or metabolites.

Itraconazole

Itraconazole is available for both oral and intravenous use. The drug was originally available in capsules, but a newer liquid formulation gives better absorption and pharmacokinetic profile than the original capsule preparation, leading to significantly greater bioavailability and higher serum levels. Systemic bioavailability of itraconazole oral solution is around 55% optimised under fasting conditions. Itraconazole is extensively metabolised by the liver, predominantly by the CYP 3A4 isoenzyme system and is known to undergo enterohepatic circulation. This is a broad-spectrum antifungal which is effective against yeasts, dermatophytes, the 'pathogenic' fungi and some filamentous fungi, such as *Aspergillus.*

Clinical use. In deep-seated infection, itraconazole is used to treat infections due to the 'pathogenic' fungi, but there is less published evidence of its use in the treatment of systemic candidiasis and it cannot be recommended for this purpose (Maertens and Boogaerts, 2005). However, it may be useful in patients who are infected with strains resistant to fluconazole, some of which may remain sensitive to itraconazole, and in patients who are for some reason unable to tolerate fluconazole. It has also been used to treat cryptococcosis, despite its poor penetration of cerebrospinal fluid, and in that condition, it is an alternative to fluconazole for patients who cannot take the latter drug. However, one study comparing fluconazole and itraconazole as maintenance treatment for cryptococcosis was discontinued due to the high rate of relapse in the itraconazole arm.

There is now considerable evidence to support the use of itraconazole as a prophylactic agent in immunocompromised patients. It has been shown to be effective in reducing the incidence of systemic fungal infection compared to placebo and to be more effective than fluconazole, although this is due to a greater reduction in infections due to filamentous fungi, including *Aspergillus.*

Voriconazole

Voriconazole is available for both oral and intravenous administration. It has advantages over itraconazole in that its absorption from the gastro-intestinal tract is significantly better and is not affected by reductions in gastric acidity due to disease or concomitant medication. Its spectrum of activity is similar to that of itraconazole, but it is more active against *Fusarium* species, a mould which causes superficial infection of the nails and cornea, and occasionally systemic infection in immunocompromised patients.

Pharmacokinetics. Voriconazole given orally is rapidly and almost fully absorbed (oral bioavailability > 90%) with a maximum serum concentration being achieved in about 2 h after administration under fasting conditions. It is extensively distributed into tissue and penetrates well into the CSF and into vitreous and aqueous humour. It is cleared by hepatic cytochrome P450 metabolism and is involved in many clinically relevant drug–drug interactions. Therapeutic drug monitoring may be indicated in some clinical settings.

Clinical use. The main clinical indication for the use of voriconazole is aspergillosis. Studies have shown improved efficacy compared to conventional amphotericin B in systemic *Aspergillus* infection. The largest randomised control trial demonstrates that voriconazole is superior to amphotericin B deoxycholate as primary therapy of Aspergillosis (Walsh et al., 2008). One particular indication is cerebral aspergillosis. Although rare, this carries a high mortality rate (90% or higher), and one study has shown this to be reduced by voriconazole, presumably due to its better penetration into the central nervous system. In addition to aspergillosis, voriconazole is also licensed for the treatment of *Fusarium* infection and for the management of patients infected with strains of *Candida* resistant to fluconazole. It has been shown to be as efficacious as amphotericin B followed by fluconazole in the treatment of candidaemia in patients who were not neutropenic, but it is not licensed for this indication.

Administration. For invasive pulmonary aspergillosis, a loading dose of 6 mg/kg IV every 12 h for 2 doses was given followed by 4 mg/kg every 12 h and converted to oral therapy 200 mg every 12 h depending on clinical review to decide duration of treatment.

Side effects. Voriconazole has a side-effect profile similar to that of other triazoles. Two adverse effects associated with voriconazole are visual disturbance (appearance of bright lights, colour changes or wavy lines) in 45% of patients and cutaneous phototoxicity (rash) in 8% patients. Both side effects are reversible after discontinuation of therapy.

Posaconazole

Posaconazole is the latest triazole to be licensed in the UK. Like itraconazole, it is absorbed slowly, is a highly protein bound (>98%) and reaches a steady state after a period of 7–10 days. Optimal absorption is achieved when taken with a high fatty meal.

Clinical use. Posaconazole is used 200 mg three times daily for prophylaxis of invasive fungal infection during neutropenia or moderate to severe graft versus host disease (GVHD).

Caspofungin

Caspofungin was the first of the echinocandins to become available for routine use, and others, such as micafungin and anidulafungin, have only recently become available. These agents interfere with the production of the fungal cell wall by inhibiting the synthesis of an important component, 1,3-ß-D-glucan. This is a target which does not exist in mammalian cells, providing selective toxicity against fungi. Caspofungin has a significant advantage over the triazoles in that it does not inhibit the cytochrome P450 system and therefore is not associated with such a wide range of drug interactions

Susceptible fungi. The drug has a rather unusual spectrum of activity. It is active against most species of *Candida*, although some are less susceptible than others, but *Cryptococcus* is resistant. The commonly encountered species of *Aspergillus* are susceptible, but the drug is inactive against the dermatophytes and activity against other fungi is variable.

Clinical use. Caspofungin is only available for administration via the intravenous route and does not penetrate into the cerebrospinal fluid. Due to its spectrum of activity, caspofungin is indicated only for candidiasis and aspergillosis. A comparative study showed caspofungin to be as efficacious as conventional amphotericin B in invasive candidiasis. It has been shown to be effective in patients with aspergillosis who failed to respond to, or who could not tolerate, other antifungal agents. Finally, caspofungin was also shown to be as effective as liposomal amphotericin B in the empirical treatment of fungal infection in neutropenic patients and had a lower incidence of unwanted effects (Walsh et al., 2004). In the UK, the drug is licensed for this indication.

Choice of treatment

A recent development has been the use of combinations of antifungal agents to improve on the results of single agents. At the present time, there is little firm evidence to support the use of such combinations. Amphotericin B plus flucytosine in the treatment of cryptococcosis is the only combination where evidence exists of increased efficacy over either agent alone. However, faced with a seriously ill patient not responding to single agents, it is not surprising that many clinicians attempt the use of a combination of antifungals, even though the evidence is that the results are no better than monotherapy.

Practice points regarding the drug toxicity in systemic antifungal agents are detailed in Table 42.9.

Table 42.9 Practice points

Drug toxicity in systemic antifungal agents	
Infusion-related side effects	• Particularly with conventional amphotericin B • Lipid-based preparations also show these, but to a lesser extent
Nephrotoxicity	• Particularly with conventional amphotericin B • Results in renal dysfunction • Cessation of treatment may be required • Drug-level monitoring is not helpful in prevention • Potassium loss and hypokalaemia are a serious complication • Renal toxicity may be potentiated by concomitant nephrotoxic agents
Hepatotoxicity	• Associated with the azole antifungals • Was particularly severe with ketoconazole • The newer triazoles may also cause serious liver damage
Bone marrow suppression	• Associated with flucytosine • Dose-related problem, so drug-level monitoring may help to prevent it • Tends to preclude the use of flucytosine in patients whose marrow is already damaged (e.g. in haematological malignancy or following bone marrow transplant)
Drug interactions	• Associated particularly with the azoles • Due to their mode of action in inhibiting the cytochrome P450 system • A wide range of drugs may be affected, some with serious interactions
Difficulties in drug administration	
Drug precipitation	• Amphotericin B will precipitate out if given in electrolyte-containing infusions • This may also happen in 5% dextrose due to acidity resulting from the manufacturing process
Need for a test dose	• Required for all amphotericin B preparations
Long infusion times and/or large infusion volumes	• A particular problem with conventional amphotericin • Long infusion times mean reduced access to intravenous cannulae for other purposes • Large infusion volumes may be undesirable in patients with renal or cardiac dysfunction
Variable absorption when taken by mouth	• A known problem with itraconazole • Absorption is reduced in the presence of raised gastric pH (e.g. following the use of antacids or drugs such as omeprazole) • Absorption is increased in the presence of food or if taken with a cola drink • Subtherapeutic levels may occur due to poor absorption • Therapeutic drug monitoring is recommended to avoid low levels

Continued

Table 42.9 Practice points—cont'd

Resistance to antifungal agents	
Amphotericin B	• Usually seen as a very broad-spectrum antifungal, but inherent resistance is seen in several clinically significant species: *Aspergillus terreus* *Candida lusitaniae* *Scedosporium apiospermum* • Acquired resistance developing during treatment is very uncommon • Lipid preparations have identical *in vitro* antifungal activity to the conventional form
Flucytosine	• Acquired resistance during treatment is very common in *Candida* species • Monotherapy promotes the rapid development of resistance • Combination therapy with amphotericin will reduce the possibility of acquired resistance developing during treatment
Fluconazole	• Some species of *Candida* are inherently resistant or less susceptible to fluconazole: *C. krusei* *C. glabrata* • Long-term use of fluconazole may result in increased infections with these more resistant strains • Long-term use may also result in reduced susceptibility in strains of *C. albicans*

Case studies

Case 42.1

A 27-year-old woman visits her primary care doctor complaining that her toenails have become distorted and discoloured. Since it looks unattractive, she would like it corrected before her summer beach holiday. The primary care doctor makes the clinical diagnosis of tinea unguium (dermatophytosis of the nail) which is confirmed by laboratory culture of nail scrapings. The doctor knows that this condition is unlikely to respond to topical treatment and therefore consults the British National Formulary for a systemic agent. He finds that griseofulvin, terbinafine and itraconazole are all available for this condition. However, the situation is complicated by the fact that his patient tells him that she is trying to get pregnant and does not want to take anything which might harm a baby. At this point, the doctor seeks specialist advice.

Question

What is the most appropriate (and safe) treatment in this patient?

Answer

This is a difficult issue. Griseofulvin is contraindicated, due to its known teratogenicity in animals. In addition, this drug decreases the effectiveness of oral contraceptives, so it would not be appropriate to give it along with an oral contraceptive agent to prevent pregnancy during use. It is also recommended that oral contraception be continued for at least a month after discontinuing griseofulvin. Therefore, in this patient, it is not an appropriate choice.

The position of itraconazole is a little different. Like griseofulvin, it has the U.S. Food & Drugs Administration (FDA) category C (studies show fetal harm in animals, but evidence in human beings is lacking), but there is at least one report of almost 200 women given itraconazole in the first trimester of pregnancy without evidence of fetal harm. In the current state of knowledge, however, it would be difficult to recommend itraconazole to this patient.

Terbinafine carries FDA category B (no evidence in animal studies of fetal harm, but studies proving safety in pregnant women are not available). Therefore, it could be given to the patient if the benefit outweighs the risk, but since this is not a serious condition, this approach would be difficult to justify.

After some discussion, the patient decided that she wanted the condition treated more than she wanted to become pregnant, so she opted to take a course of terbinafine but return to using her oral contraception until the treatment course was complete.

Case 42.2

A 56-year-old diabetic male with carcinoma of the oesophagus undergoes sub-total oesophagectomy. He spends the early post-operative period on surgical ITU and is sent to the surgical ward for further management. On day 6, post-op, he begins to show signs of sepsis for which antibiotics are commenced. However, 48 h later, he has difficulty in breathing, takes a turn for the worse and is transferred to ITU. Imaging the chest revealed a leak from the oesophagectomy site and fluid collection in the pleural space. Gram stain of aspirated pleural fluid revealed budding yeast cells and sputum culture taken 2 days previously has grown *Aspergillus*.

Question

How should this patient's infection be managed?

Answer

The immediate management of this patient would involve drainage of pleural fluid through an intercostal drain and systemic antifungal therapy. The source is very likely to be oral thrush as the patient is diabetic and the candida has travelled from the mouth/oropharynx through the leak in the oesophagectomy wound into the pleural space. Fluconazole at 400 mg twice daily should be commenced awaiting full culture identification of the yeast and antifungal sensitivities. Urgent review is indicated for surgical intervention to close the leak. The duration of antifungal agent would be normally be 14–21 days.

Re-collection of yeasts in inadequately treated spaces can be a problem. It may be useful to add a second antifungal agent to fluconazole. The presence of *Aspergillus* in sputum may be an environmental contamination; therefore, a second specimen will be needed to confirm.

Aspergillus is not sensitive to fluconazole, in which case amphotericin B or voriconazole may be indicated.

Case 42.3

A 18-year-old boy with acute myeloblastic leukaemia sustained 20% accidental burns injury on face, upper body and right arm at a family barbecue. He had recently left hospital after successful antibiotic treatment for a febrile neutropenic episode post-chemotherapy.

Two weeks after admission to ITU for management of burns, he undergoes a septic episode with septic shock. A blood culture taken through a central line shows Gram-negative bacilli. He is commenced on broad-spectrum antibiotics. His peripheral blood count is 3×10^9/L and he has a markedly raised C-reactive protein (CRP). The patient has suffered a moderate degree of renal failure. Two days later, another blood culture is taken through an arterial line and shows yeast cells on Gram stain. Intravenous fluconazole is added to his treatment. Culture growth from the central line blood culture reveals *Pseudomonas aeruginosa* and *Candida albicans*. The arterial blood culture grows *Candida krusei*. Antifungal sensitivities are awaited.

Question

How should the patient be managed?

Answer

Treatment of infections in burns patients can be challenging as the loss in skin integrity increases the risk of being colonised with various endogenous and hospital-acquired bacteria and fungi. Patients with haematological malignancies and chemotherapy treatment are more vulnerable to opportunistic infections, and this case has an additional co-morbidity on top.

Ideally, antibiotics should be avoided in a patient who has an invasive fungal infection as it is believed that killing the bacterial flora helps fungi thrive in the absence of commensal competition. In this case, the patient has concomitant Gram-negative sepsis and lacks a strong bodily defence system because of his underlying disease condition.

Candida krusei is known to be resistant to fluconazole. It is difficult to treat intravenous catheter and other line infections with systemic antibiotics and antifugals alone. It is imperative that these lines are taken out, and treatment given through temporary peripheral lines for at least 48 h before a new central line is inserted. New lines are very likely to get colonised with the same microorganisms if inserted too early. Both *Candida albicans* and *Candida krusei* can be treated with a lipid formulation of amphotericin (use of non-lipid conventional formulations of amphotericin should be avoided as the patient has a moderate degree of renal failure and his present condition could deteriorate).

The duration of treatment can be decided based on daily clinical follow-up that includes imaging and echo cardiograms for up to 2 weeks to look for seeding of *Candida* in other organs. Choice of antifungals can be reviewed after antifungal sensitivity is made available and amphotericin can be switched to caspofungin if necessary.

References

Dodds Ashley, E.S., Lewis, R., Lewis, S.J., et al., 2006. Pharmacology of systemic antifungal agents. Clin. Infect. Dis. 43, S28–S39.

Maertens, J., Boogaerts, M., 2005. The place for itraconazole in treatment. J. Antimicrob. Chemother. 56, i33–i38.

Pappas, P.G., Kauffman, C.A., Andes, D., et al., 2009. Clinical practice guidelines for the management of candidiasis: 2009 update by the Infectious Diseases Society of America. Clin. Infect. Dis. 48, 503–553.

Walsh, T.J., Teppler, H., Donowitz, G.R., et al., 2004. Caspofungin versus liposomal amphotericin B for empirical antifungal therapy in patients with persistent fever and neutropenia. N. Engl. J. Med. 351, 1391–1402.

Walsh, T.J., Anaissie, E.J., Denning, D.W., et al., 2008. Treatment of aspergillosis: clinical practice guidelines of the Infectious Diseases Society of America. Clin. Infect. Dis. 46, 327–360.

Further reading

Bennett, J.E., 2010. Introduction to mycoses. In: Mandell, G.L., Bennett, J.E., Dolin, R. (Eds.), Principles and Practice of Infectious Diseases, seventh ed. Elsevier, Philadelphia, pp. 3221–3240.

Hay, R.J., 2010. Dermatophytosis and other superficial mycoses. In: Mandell, G.L., Bennett, J.E., Dolin, R. (Eds.), Principles and Practice of Infectious Diseases, seventh ed. Elsevier, Philadelphia, pp. 3345–3355.

Pfaller, M.A., Pappas, P.G., Wingard, J.R., 2006. Invasive fungal pathogens: current epidemiological trends. Clin. Infect. Dis. 43, S3–14.

Rex, J.H., Stevens, D.A., Systemic antifungal agents. In: Mandell, G.L., Bennett, J.E., Dolin, R. (Eds.), Principles and Practice of Infectious Diseases, seventh ed. Elsevier, Philadelphia, pp. 549–563.

Winn, W., Allen, S., Janda, W., et al., 2006. Mycology. In: Koneman's Colour Atlas and Textbook of Diagnostic Microbiology, sixth ed. Lippincott Williams and Wilkins, Philadelphia, pp. 1153–1232.

Thyroid and parathyroid disorders 43

M.D. Page

Key points

- When diagnosing thyroid conditions, the possibility of drug-induced disease should always be considered.
- The treatment of hypothyroidism requires lifelong thyroxine therapy and monitoring.
- Thyroxine replacement therapy should be introduced cautiously in the elderly, particularly those with cardiac disease.
- Thyroxine replacement therapy can be given weekly in patients who forget their daily doses or who are unable to self-medicate.
- Thyrotoxicosis can be treated with thionamide therapy, radioiodine or surgery. The choice will largely be determined by the age of the patient, the cause of the thyrotoxicosis, the severity of the condition, co-morbidity and patient preference.
- Patients treated with thionamide therapy require careful counselling about the symptoms and management of agranulocytosis and should be given written guidance.
- Surgery for hyperparathyroidism is only required in a minority of patients.
- Hypoparathyroidism can occur after thyroid surgery. It is managed with vitamin D analogues and requires lifelong monitoring.

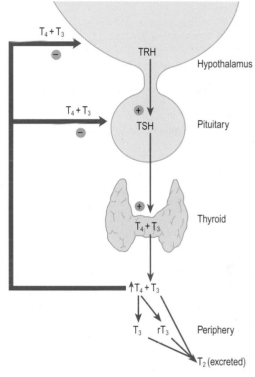

Fig. 43.1 Control of thyroid hormone secretion.

Thyroid physiology

The thyroid gland consists of two lobes and is situated in the lower neck. The gland synthesises, stores and releases two major metabolically active hormones: Tetra-iodothyronine (Thyroxine, T_4) and tri-iodothyronine (T_3). Regulation of hormone synthesis is by variable secretion of the glycoprotein hormone TSH from the anterior pituitary. In turn, TSH is regulated by hypothalamic secretion of the tripeptide thyrotrophin-releasing hormone (TRH) (Fig. 43.1). Low circulating levels of thyroid hormones initiate the release of TSH and probably also TRH. Rising levels of TSH promote increased iodide trapping by the gland and a subsequent increase in thyroid hormone synthesis. The increase in circulating hormone levels feeds back on the pituitary and hypothalamus, shutting off TRH, TSH and further hormone synthesis.

Both T_4 and T_3 are produced within the follicular cells in the thyroid. The stages in synthesis are shown in Fig. 43.2. In summary:

- Thyroglobulin and thyroid peroxidase (TPO) are synthesised by follicular cells.
- Hydrogen peroxide (H_2O_2) is synthesised at the luminal membrane.
- Dietary inorganic iodide is trapped from the circulation and transported to the follicular lumen where it is oxidised by H_2O_2.
- Iodine is then transferred onto the tyrosine residues in thyroglobulin by iodinase enzymes forming mono-iodotyrosine (MIT) and di-iodotyrosine (DIT).
- Subsequently, the formation of T_4 occurs as a result of the coupling of two DIT residues and of T_3 by coupling a DIT and an MIT residue. The hormones are then stored within the gland until their release into the circulation.
- Finally, thyroglobulin is resorbed into the follicular cell, hydrolysed and its amino acids and remaining iodine re-used.

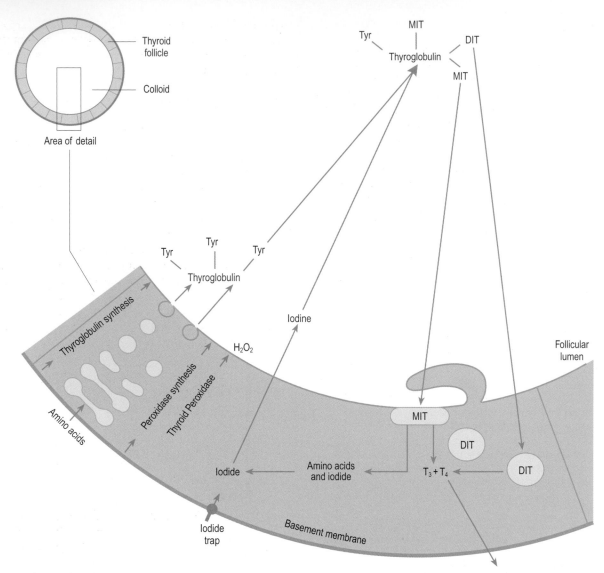

Fig. 43.2 Synthesis of thyroid hormones.

The ratio of T_4:T_3 secreted by the thyroid gland is approximately 10:1. Consequently, the gland secretes approximately 80–100 μcg of T_4 and 10 μcg of T_3 per day. However, only 10% of circulating T_3 is derived from direct thyroidal secretion, the remaining 90% being produced by peripheral conversion from T_4. T_4 can therefore be considered a prohormone that is converted in the peripheral tissues (liver, kidney and brain) either to the active hormone T_3 or to the biologically inactive reverse T_3 (rT_3). In the circulation, the hormones exist in both the active free and inactive protein-bound forms. T_4 is 99.98% bound, with only 0.02% circulating free. T_3 is slightly less protein bound (99.8%), resulting in a considerably higher circulating free fraction (0.2%). Details of protein binding are shown in Table 43.1.

The hormones are metabolised in the periphery (kidney, liver and heart) by deiodination. T_4 and T_3 are also eliminated by biliary secretion of their glucuronide and sulphate conjugates (15–20%). The half-life of T_4 in plasma is about 6–7 days and that of T_3 24–36 h in euthyroid adults. The apparent volume of distribution for T_4 is about 10 L and for T_3 about 40 L.

Table 43.1 Plasma protein binding of thyroid hormones

Carrier protein	Plasma concentration	Proportion of T_4 and T_3 bound (%)
Thyroid-binding globulin (TBG)	15 mg/L	75
Transthyretin (formerly thyroid-binding prealbumin)	250 mg/L	10
Albumin	40 g/L	15

Hypothyroidism

Hypothyroidism is the clinical state resulting from decreased production of thyroid hormones or very rarely from tissue resistance.

Epidemiology

Accurate assessment of the prevalence and incidence of hypothyroidism is difficult due to variation in definitions and population samples. The prevalence of previously undiagnosed, spontaneous, overt hypothyroidism has been estimated to be between 2 and 4 per 1000 of the total population worldwide. However, if all cases of previously diagnosed hypothyroidism and the effects of previous thyroid surgery and radioiodine treatment are included, this prevalence rises to approximately 10 per 1000. In the UK, primary hypothyroidism is common with a prevalence of 14/1000 women (but <1/1000 men). Despite these data, population screening for autoimmune hypothyroidism is thought to be probably not cost-effective unless incorporated into a screening programme for other conditions. Although the disease may occur at any age, most patients present between 30 and 60 years of age.

Aetiology

Primary hypothyroidism accounts for more than 95% of adult cases. It is usually due to a failure of the thyroid gland itself as a result of autoimmune destruction, or the effects of treatment of thyrotoxicosis. Hypothyroidism may be drug induced. Amiodarone and lithium cause hypothyroidism in around 10% of patients treated (see later). Secondary disease is due to hypopituitarism, and tertiary disease due to failure of the hypothalamus. Peripheral hypothyroidism is due to tissue insensitivity to the action of thyroid hormones. A more extensive classification is shown in Box 43.1.

Iodides may produce hypothyroidism in patients who are particularly sensitive to their ability to block the active transport pump of the thyroid gland. Iodine absorption from topical iodine-containing antiseptics has been shown to cause hypothyroidism in neonates. This is potentially very dangerous at a critical time of neurological development in the newborn infant. Transient hypothyroidism may be seen in 25% of iodine-exposed infants.

Clinical manifestations

Hypothyroidism can affect multiple body systems, but symptoms are mainly non specific and gradual in onset (Box 43.2). Symptoms are frequently vague especially in the early stages. It is common for symptoms to be incorrectly attributed by patients and their relatives to increasing age. The reverse is also common in that patients who have read about, or have friends/family with, hypothyroidism will assume that it is responsible for symptoms of fatigue and weight gain. Thus, hypothyroidism is often confused with simple obesity and depression. Thyroid function tests give accurate diagnosis in all cases.

The most useful clinical signs are myotonic (slow-relaxing) tendon reflexes, bradycardia, hair loss and cool, dry skin. Effusions may occur into pericardial, pleural, peritoneal or joint spaces. Mild anaemia of a macrocytic type is quite common and responds to thyroxine replacement. Pernicious anaemia is a frequent concomitant finding in hypothyroidism. Other, organ-specific autoimmune diseases such as Addison's disease may be associated.

Myxoedema coma

Myxoedema coma is a rare but potentially fatal complication of severe, untreated hypothyroidism. Coma can be precipitated by hypothermia, stress, infection, trauma and certain

---

Box 43.1 Classification of hypothyroidism

Primary hypothyroidism
Congenital hypothyroidism
    Agenesis
    Inherited enzyme defects
Immune
    Hashimoto's thyroiditis
    Spontaneous hypothyroidism in Graves' disease
    Postpartum hypothyroidism
Iatrogenic
    Postoperative hypothyroidism
    Hypothyroidism after radioactive iodine
    External neck irradiation
    Drugs – antithyroid thionamides, amiodarone, lithium, elemental iodide
Iodine deficiency
Subacute (viral)

Secondary/tertiary hypothyroidism
Hypopituitarism – any cause
Hypothalamic disease

Peripheral hypothyroidism
Insensitivity to thyroid hormones

Box 43.2 Signs and symptoms of hypothyroidism

Skin and appendages	Dry, cool, flaking, thickened skin Reduced sweating Yellowish complexion. Puffy facies and eyes Sparse, coarse, dry hair Brittle nails
Neuromuscular system	Slow speech Poor memory and reduced cognitive function Somnolence Carpal tunnel syndrome Psychiatric disturbance Hearing loss Depression Muscle pain and weakness Delayed deep tendon reflexes
Metabolic abnormalities	Raised total and LDL cholesterol Macrocytic anaemia
Gastro-intestinal	Weight gain with decreased appetite Abdominal distension and ascites Constipation
Cardiovascular	Reduced cardiac output Bradycardia Cardiac enlargement

drugs, notably β-blockers and respiratory depressants, including anaesthetic agents, narcotics, phenothiazines and hypnotics. The condition is a medical emergency and should be treated rapidly and aggressively.

The term 'myxoedema' used to be synonymous with hypothyroidism. It is now reserved for advanced disease in which there is swelling of the skin and subcutaneous tissues.

Investigations

The laboratory investigation of hypothyroidism is extremely simple. Usually clinical assessment, combined with a single estimation of thyroid hormones and TSH, is sufficient to make the diagnosis. In primary disease, the levels of free T_4 and T_3 are low and the TSH level rises markedly. Some laboratories offer only TSH as a first-line test of thyroid function though this can result in delayed diagnosis of secondary or tertiary hypothyroidism, which should be suspected on the basis of a low free T_4 along with low TSH levels.

Elevation of the TSH level occurs early in the course of thyroid failure and may be present before overt clinical manifestations appear. It is important to appreciate that hypothyroidism is not one disease but a spectrum. Early hypothyroidism may be asymptomatic or the symptoms less obvious and non-specific, but a normal TSH with normal free T4 effectively excludes the diagnosis.

A chest radiograph may detect the presence of effusions, and an electrocardiogram (ECG) is useful, especially in patients with angina or coronary heart disease, in whom replacement therapy needs to be introduced gradually.

Testing thyroid function

As indicated earlier (and later in the section on thyrotoxicosis), a clinical assessment and measurement of free T_4 and TSH are usually all that are necessary to arrive at an accurate diagnosis of thyroid state. All modern TSH assays now employ double antibody immunometric techniques, which are robust and highly reliable. Moreover, these assays are now so sensitive that they are able to identify thyrotoxic patients with TSH levels below the normal euthyroid range. Commercial free T_4 and free T_3 assays, however, are all indirect methods and are subject to interference from drugs and other disease states. As such, both T_3 and T_4 can be decreased as a non-specific consequence of systemic illness ('sick euthyroid' syndrome) and depression along with a host of drugs (Surks and Sievert, 1995), which can interfere with thyroid hormone metabolism and free hormone assays (Table 43.2). Such patients require specialist assessment and collaboration with the local laboratory to rule out confounding disease and pituitary failure.

Treatment

The aims of treatment with thyroxine are to ensure that patients receive a dose that will restore well-being and that usually returns the TSH level to the lower end of the normal range (Vanderpump et al., 1996). All patients with symptomatic

Table 43.2 Drug effects on thyroid function

	Clinical/biochemical effects
Decrease TSH secretion	
Dopamine Glucocorticoids Octreotide	Hypothyroidism (rarely clinically important)
Alter thyroid hormone secretion	
Iodide (amiodarone, contrast agents)	Both hyper- and hypothyroidism
Lithium	Hypothyroidism
Decrease T_4 absorption	
Colestyramine/colestipol Aluminium hydroxide Ferrous sulphate Calcium carbonate Multivitamins Sevelamer Protein pump inhibitors Sucralfate	Increased thyroxine dose requirement
Alter T_4 and T_3 metabolism Increased hepatic metabolism	
Phenobarbital Phenytoin Rifampicin Carbamazepine	Low T_4 and T_3 levels Normal or increased TSH
Reduce conversion of T_4 to T_3 B-blockers Propylthiouracil Amiodarone Glucocorticoids	Lower T_3 levels Normal or increased TSH
Reduce T_4 and T_3 binding Furosemide Salicylates and NSAIDs Heparin	Increased measured free T_4 in some assays
Increase thyroglobulin levels Oestrogen and tamoxifen Opiates and methadone	Increased total T_4
Others Cytokines – interferon and interleukin 2	Thyroiditis. Can produce hypothyroidism and thyrotoxicosis

hypothyroidism require replacement therapy. T_4 is usually the treatment of choice except in myxoedema coma where T_3 may be used in the first instance. Before commencing T_4 replacement, the diagnosis of glucocorticoid deficiency must be excluded to prevent precipitation of a hypoadrenal crisis. If in doubt, hydrocortisone replacement should be given concomitantly until cortisol deficiency is excluded.

The initial dose of T_4 will depend on the patient's age, severity and duration of disease and the coexistence of cardiac disease. In young, healthy patients with disease of short duration, T_4 may be commenced in a dose of 50–100 μcg daily. As the drug has a long half-life, it should be given once daily. The most convenient time is usually in the morning. After 6 weeks on the same dose (not a shorter interval as TSH takes this time to stabilise after a dose change), thyroid function tests should be checked. The TSH concentration is the best indicator of the thyroid state, and this should be used for further dosage adjustment. A raised TSH concentration indicates inadequate treatment, poor adherence or both. The majority of patients will be controlled with doses of 100–200 µcg daily, with few patients requiring more than 200 µcg. In adults, the median dose required to suppress TSH to normal is 125 µcg daily. In the majority of patients, once the appropriate dose has been established, it remains constant. During pregnancy, an increase in the dose of thyroxine by 25–50% is needed to maintain normal TSH levels.

Exacerbation of myocardial ischaemia, infarction and sudden death are all well-recognised complications of T_4 replacement therapy. Patients with coronary heart disease may be unable to tolerate full replacement doses because of palpitations, angina or heart failure. Elderly patients may have undiagnosed ischemic heart disease. In these two groups of patients, treatment should therefore be started with 25 µcg daily and increased slowly by 25 µcg every 4–6 weeks. During this time, the patient's clinical progress should be carefully monitored. In some patients, T_4 may be better tolerated if a β-blocker such as propranolol is given concomitantly. Some authorities recommend starting with 5 µcg of T_3, the rationale being that if adverse effects occur, these can be alleviated more rapidly with a dose reduction due to the shorter half-life of T_3.

It is important to avoid both under- and overtreatment. Hypothyroidism is very rarely life threatening, but adverse effects may result from prolonged overtreatment (which is indicated by a TSH level suppressed below the normal range). Though T_4 exerts an effect on many organs and tissues, it is the effect on bone and the heart that give the greatest cause for concern. There is evidence that bone density is reduced in patients taking excessive T_4 replacement therapy (Faber and Galloe, 1994; Uzzan et al., 1996), and that atrial fibrillation is more common if TSH is suppressed (Sawin et al., 1994). In order to minimise the risk of development of these complications, the dose of T_4 should be carefully tailored to the needs of each individual patient. Some patients will have undetectable serum TSH levels while taking thyroxine and may complain of recurrent fatigue if the dose is reduced to permit the TSH to rise. In these patients, it may be permissible to leave the dose unchanged if levels of free T_4 and T_3 are normal, after a discussion of the relative risks and benefits with the patient (Vanderpump et al., 1996).

Patient care

Hypothyroidism requires lifelong treatment with T_4. Patients on long-term drug therapy are recognised to have a low adherence with their medication regimen. Treatment with T_4 is often terminated because patients feel well and think that treatment is no longer required. Patients should understand the effects of drug holidays on their health and thyroid function tests and should know that a normal TSH indicates adequate dosage. Written advice should be provided and monitoring of dosage should continue annually. There are a series of excellent patient information leaflets available on the British Thyroid Association website at www.british-thyroid-association.org.

Despite adequate counselling, some patients persistently forget to take their tablets reliably, leading to variable thyroid state and wildly fluctuating test results. Other patients lack capacity to self-medicate reliably. There is evidence to show that weekly dosing with T_4 is a safe and acceptable way to manage this type of patient, in whom family members or community staff can supervise treatment (Grebe et al., 1997; Rangan et al., 2007). There are no guidelines yet published, but in practice, patients are normally started on 500–700 µcg T_4 weekly. Dose changes are made in exactly the same way by assessing TSH levels after 6 weeks of stable dosing.

Rarely, patients are seen in whom TSH levels fluctuate or remain elevated despite high doses of thyroxine and in whom adherence seems to be very good. There are a number of possible causes for this, including malabsorption of thyroxine which can be due to coeliac or inflammatory bowel disease or a number of commonly prescribed drugs (Table 43.2). Such patients will need a careful sequential assessment by an endocrine service (Morris, 2009).

Prevention

At present, nothing can be done to prevent autoimmune thyroid failure from developing; however, much can be done to ensure early detection and treatment. Careful follow-up of patients who have undergone radioiodine treatment, subtotal thyroidectomy or completed a course of treatment for thyrotoxicosis is essential along with monitoring of those prescribed amiodarone and lithium. An increase in TSH with normal concentrations of T_3 and T_4 will indicate the onset of hypothyroidism before the patient becomes symptomatic. Box 43.3 shows the prevalence of hypothyroidism after treatment for thyrotoxicosis.

Box 43.3 Prevalence of thyroid disturbance after treatment for thyrotoxicosis

Thyroidectomy
6–75% develop hypothyroidism over their lifetime, dependent on the amount of remnant tissue.
Risk highest during first year after surgery

Antithyroid drugs (>6 month course)
43% relapse with thyrotoxicosis in the first year
13–21% relapse with thyrotoxicosis in the next 4 years

131I therapy
24–90% develop hypothyroidism over their lifetime, depending on dose given

Hyperthyroidism/thyrotoxicosis

Hyperthyroidism is defined as the production by the thyroid gland of excessive amounts of thyroid hormones. Thyrotoxicosis refers to the clinical syndrome associated with prolonged exposure to elevated levels of thyroid hormone. This distinction is important when evaluating thyroid function tests (Table 43.3).

Epidemiology

Hyperthyroidism is a common condition. It has been estimated that there are 4.7/1000 women with active disease. When previously treated cases were included, the population prevalence rose to 20/1000 in women. As for hypothyroidism, it is much less common in men who have a lifetime prevalence of around 2/1000 (Tunbridge et al., 1977).

Aetiology

Hyperthyroidism is a disorder of various aetiologies. In clinical terms, thyrotoxicosis is the result of persistently elevated levels of thyroid hormones.

Graves' disease

Graves' disease is the commonest cause of thyrotoxicosis. It is an autoimmune condition and results from production of an abnormal IgG immunoglobulin which is able to occupy the TSH receptor on the thyroid follicular cell. Here, it mimics the effect of TSH, causing cell division and stimulating thyroid hormone secretion. These stimulatory imunoglobulins are known as thyroid receptor antibodies (TRABs). Very rarely, the TRABs are inhibitory to the TSH receptor, resulting in hypothyroidism.

Ninety per cent of patients with Graves' disease are young women often with a family history of the condition. In addition to the effects of thyrotoxicosis, around 30% of patients develop additional features including a congestive ophthalmopathy which is thought to result from antibody-mediated inflammation of orbital contents. Pretibial myxoedema, gynaecomastia and thyroid acropachy are rare manifestations.

In pregnancy, the maternal TRABs can pass across the placenta to the fetus resulting in transient neonatal thyrotoxicosis.

Nodular disease

Toxic multinodular goitre is also common but more often affects older women in whom an euthyroid nodular goitre may have been present for many years. Individual nodules become autonomous, producing T_3 and/or T_4. Clinically, the thyrotoxicosis is generally less severe and more gradual in onset. Often, only T_3 levels are elevated, though the TSH will be suppressed in all cases. Thyrotoxicosis may also be caused by single autonomous thyroid adenomas. These are benign well-differentiated tumours that secrete excessive amounts of thyroid hormones.

Table 43.3 Aetiology of hyperthyroidism

	Condition	Frequency	Clinical features	I^{131} uptake
Thyrotoxicosis (increased hormone synthesis)				
	Graves' disease	70%	Antibody mediated (TRABs) 90% are young women Diffuse goitre Ophthalmopathy (30%) Pretibial myxoedema Acropachy Transmissible to neonate	Increased
	Multinodular goitre	20%	Benign autonomous nodules Often secrete T_3 Older women Always relapse after withdrawal of thionamides	Increased
	Toxic single adenoma	5%		Increased
	Iodine induced	<1%	Increased urine iodine	Variable
	HCG induced	Rare	Molar pregnancy or choriocarcinoma	Increased
	TSH dependent	Rare	Pituitary tumour	Increased
Thyroiditis (thyroid destruction and leakage of stored thyroid hormones)				
	Acute	2%	Probably viral Neck pain – often severe	Absent
	Silent	2%	Viral Autoimmune	Absent
	Amiodarone induced	<1%	Increased urine iodine	Absent

TRABs, thyroid receptor antibodies.

Thyroiditis

If the thyroid is inflamed by viral or rapid autoimmune attack, the resulting follicular cell death will result in the release of pre-formed thyroid hormones. This usually presents as a painful mildly enlarged and tender thyroid. There is a brief period of hyperthyroidism before thyroid hormone levels fall to subnormal. Most often, this period of hyperthyroidism does not lead to clinically apparent thyrotoxicosis and in any event is brief, but it is common for these patients to be prescribed thionamides which compound the ensuing hypothyroidism. It is therefore necessary to be aware of these conditions. Neck pain with disturbed TFTs should prompt referral for specialist assessment which will usually include a request for an iodine uptake scan. Iodine uptake is absent in hyperthyroidism associated with thyroiditis.

Clinical manifestations

Thyrotoxicosis is characterised by increases in metabolic rate and activity of many systems due to excessive circulating quantities of thyroid hormones. There is a wide spectrum of clinical disturbances. The signs and symptoms reflect increased adrenergic activity, especially in the cardiovascular and neurological systems (Box 43.4). Not all manifestations will be seen in every patient. Additional clinical features will depend on the underlying cause of the thyrotoxicosis (Table 43.3).

The clinical features of thyrotoxicosis in the elderly may not be so obvious. Signs and symptoms of cardiovascular disturbance tend to predominate, atrial fibrillation is frequent and the patient may develop congestive cardiac failure.

Box 43.4	Signs and symptoms of thyrotoxicosis
Skin and appendages	Warm, moist skin Thinning or loss of hair Increased sweating Heat intolerance
Nervous system	Insomnia Irritability, nervousness Lid retraction – staring eyes Symptoms of an anxiety state Psychosis
Musculoskeletal	Fine motor tremor Proximal muscle weakness Rapid deep tendon reflexes Osteoporosis
Gastro-intestinal	Weight loss despite increased appetite Thirst Diarrhoea
Cardiovascular	Palpitations, tachycardia Shortness of breath on exertion Atrial fibrillation Congestive cardiac failure Worsening angina

Unexplained heart failure after middle age should always arouse suspicion of thyrotoxicosis.

The extrathyroidal manifestations of Graves' disease deserve separate mention. Most frequent is ophthalmopathy due to inflammation and expansion of the contents of the orbit. The eye is pushed forward (proposed) such that white sclera appears between the iris and the lower lid. Congestive changes develop including peri-orbital oedema, conjunctival swelling and redness. The extraocular muscles are swollen and become tethered leading to failure of movement of the globe of the eye and thus diplopia. Severe disease causes pressure in the orbit, which can compress the optic nerve leading to blindness. The cutaneous features of Graves' disease include thickening of the pretibial skin (myxoedema), onycholysis (separation of the nail from the nail bed) and acropachy (similar to finger clubbing).

Investigations

In those with suspected thyrotoxicosis, it is good practice to document the diagnosis with two sets of thyroid function tests. If the diagnosis is in doubt, treatment should be withheld because unless severe, thyrotoxicosis can usually be safely observed whilst awaiting the results of investigations. Plasma free T_4 (and/or T_3) levels are elevated. The TSH level is suppressed to subnormal levels in all causes of thyrotoxicosis, except the exceptionally rare cases of TSH secreting pituitary adenomas.

In the overwhelming majority of patients, the combination of the clinical findings and simple investigations is sufficient to make a firm diagnosis. Radioactive iodine uptake scans will differentiate those patients with thyroiditis. Measurement of TRABs will identify Graves' disease patients. If the diagnosis is still equivocal, the clinical findings should be reassessed and particular attention paid to the patient's drug history. There are a number of drugs that may modify the clinical features or interfere with the tests.

Treatment

A number of factors need to be considered when choosing the most appropriate form of therapy for an individual patient (Table 43.4). There are usually a number of therapeutic options available, and the patient should be involved in the deciding on treatment. The decision may also be influenced by physician preference, which in turn can depend on the facilities available. Three forms of therapy are available, including anti-thyroid drugs, surgery and radioactive iodine. There is no general agreement as to the specific indications for each form of therapy, and none of them is ideal, all being associated with both short- and long-term sequelae. Neither surgery nor radioactive iodine should be given until the patient has been rendered euthyroid due to the risk of inducing a thyroid crisis.

In children, surgery may be difficult and the complication rate is higher. Also, radioiodine has been avoided due to concern about the potential development of thyroid malignancy, though there are no data which suggest this to be a

Table 43.4 Treatments available for thyrotoxicosis

	Adverse effects (%)	Contraindications	Cautions
Thionamides Carbimazole Propylthiouracil	Rash/arthropathy (5%) Agranulocytosis (0.3%) Hepatitis (rare)	Previous severe allergy Cross reactivity in 10%	Pregnancy – PTU preferred. Do not use block/replace regimens
Radioiodine	Hypothyroidism requiring lifelong T_4	Pregnancy	Ensure euthyroid first Ophthalmopathy may deteriorate
Surgery	Hospital stay Neck scar Surgical/anaesthetic risk 10–75% require T_4		Ensure euthyroid first Ophthalmopathy may deteriorate

problem. In pregnancy, radioiodine is not used due to the likelihood of producing a hypothyroid neonate. Thyroid surgery during pregnancy should be deferred until the second trimester if possible and most patients can be controlled with drugs. Thionamide doses should be kept as low as possible, especially in the last 2 months of pregnancy, as excessive treatment may produce goitre in the fetus. Aplasia cutis is said to occur after carbimazole therapy, so propylthiouracil (PTU) is usually used in pregnancy. Pregnant patients with thyrotoxicosis should be under the care of a specialist endocrine unit.

Immediate treatment of thyrotoxicosis

Patients need to have their symptoms addressed and their thyrotoxicosis controlled. β-Blockers in standard antihypertensive doses are effective within a matter of hours and should be offered to all non-asthmatics with severe thyrotoxicosis. Carbimazole (40 mg once a day) or PTU (150 mg twice daily) will render most patients euthyroid within 6 weeks. Adjunctive treatment of cardiac disease and anxiety/sleeplessness may be required.

Graves' disease

A proportion (40–50%) of patients with Graves' disease will achieve a long-lasting remission after a period of euthyroidism on thionamides. The optimal duration of anti-thyroid treatment is unknown and remains a controversial issue (Maugendre et al., 1999), but in most units, the length of the treatment course has fallen to between 6 and 12 months. It is not appropriate to discuss complex treatment decisions with a thyrotoxic patient, so most are well into this period when discussions of their options occur. Remission of Graves' disease is much less likely in those with very large goitres, those who require high-dose thionamide treatment to maintain euthyroidism, those with high TRAB titres and patients who have relapsed once after a course of drug treatment. Such patients should therefore be rendered euthyroid and then have a discussion about either surgical or radioiodine thyroid ablation.

Nodular thyroid disease

As the nodules function autonomously and thyrotoxicosis will always recur when thionamides are stopped, there is no value in attempting to achieve a remission of nodular thyroid disease using prolonged medical treatment. Patients should be rendered euthyroid with drugs and then have a discussion about ablative therapy.

Anti-thyroid drugs

The thionamides, PTU, thiamazole (methimazole) and its precursor carbimazole are equally effective pharmacological therapies for thyrotoxicosis. In the UK, carbimazole is usually used. These drugs prevent thyroid hormone synthesis by inhibiting the oxidative binding of iodide and its coupling to tyrosine residues. PTU, but not carbimazole, inhibits the peripheral deiodination of T_4 to T_3. Thionamides may also have an immunosuppressive action.

Adverse effects. The most common adverse effect of anti-thyroid treatment is rash and arthropathy (5%) and less commonly agranulocytosis, hepatitis, aplastic anaemia and lupus-like syndromes (Table 43.5). Overall, serious effects such as these occur in approximately 0.3% of patients treated. These side effects usually occur during the first 6 weeks of treatment, but this is not invariable. Cross-sensitivity between carbimazole and PTU is around 10%, and the patient can often be safely changed to the alternative agent if an adverse event occurs.

Regular monitoring of white cell counts has been advocated, but is not warranted. Agranulocytosis is a rare event, and even if it does occur, it happens rapidly such that routine monitoring of white cell counts may miss it. At the time of prescription, all patients should be counselled about the possible implication of sore throat, mouth ulcers and pyrexia, and instructed to seek an urgent (within hours) full blood count. This verbal information should be backed up by written advice which should specify where the patient should go for the blood test. An abnormal white cell count should prompt urgent admission under a specialist endocrine team.

Table 43.5 Adverse effects of thionamides

	Adverse effect	Comments
Skin	Pruritic, maculopapular rash	Most common in first 6 weeks May disappear spontaneously with continued treatment Can be treated with an antihistamine Change to alternative agent Occurs in 5% of patients
	Urticarial rash with systemic symptoms, that is fever, arthralgia	Discontinue drug Alternative treatment required
Haematological	Agranulocytosis	Most common in first 6 weeks Incidence increases with age Discontinue drug Reversible Consider alternative treatment Occurs in 0.3% of patients
	Leucopoenia	Transient Continue treatment Does not predispose to agranulocytosis
Other	Hepatitis Vasculitis Hypoprothrombinaemia Aplastic anaemia Thrombocytopenia	Rare Discontinue drug

Treatment regimen

Carbimazole is usually given initially at a dose up to 40–60 mg daily, depending on the severity of the condition. It can be given as a single daily dose in multiples of 20 mg tablets to aid adherence. Although the plasma half-life is short (4–6 h), the biological effect lasts longer (up to 40 h). T_4 concentrations are checked at 6-week intervals until the patient is clinically euthyroid and the T_4 and T_3 levels are normalised. (TSH remains suppressed for at least 4 weeks after resolution of significant thyrotoxicosis, so TSH levels are unhelpful in the early stages of treatment.)

At this point, a decision is made about ongoing treatment. It is simplest to continue a high dose of carbimazole to suppress endogenous thyroid hormone production and to give a standard replacement dose of thyroxine to maintain euthyroidism, the 'block and replacement' regimen. This combination results in a steadier thyroid state, reduces the need for blood monitoring and requires fewer hospital attendances. Since adverse drug effects are allergic and not dose related, it is no more risky than tailored dose regimens.

Pregnancy is a specific situation, however, in which tailored dose PTU should be used. Both the immunoglobulins which cause Graves' disease and thionamide drugs cross the placenta and will affect the fetal thyroid, but maternal thyroxine is not able to reach the fetus. Thus, the lowest possible dose of PTU (preferred to carbimazole in pregnancy) should be used and the fetus closely monitored for heart rate and growth. Breast-feeding is considered to be safe when mothers are taking thionamides.

Patient counselling

Patients should be advised of the importance of regular clinic attendance. This is necessary to monitor both therapeutic outcome and the development of adverse effects. The development of skin rashes, mouth ulcers or a sore throat should be reported by the patient, immediately investigated and a full blood count performed (see Box 43.5). It may be dangerous to treat these symptoms with over-the-counter medication before carrying out further investigations.

It is important for the patient to understand the difference between specific anti-thyroid therapy and symptomatic treatment. The patient should also be advised about the timing of doses to aid adherence. Following completion of a course of treatment, the patient should understand relapse may occur, and medical help should be sought if the initial symptoms recur.

Thyroid ablative therapy

Thyroid ablation is required for all patients with toxic multinodular goitres, those who have relapsed or are likely to relapse after drug therapy for Graves' disease and those who are allergic to thionamides. Thyroid ablation can be achieved by radioiodine or surgery.

Radioactive iodine. Radioiodine therapy is extremely easy to administer by mouth and is very effective for a large majority of patients. It is contraindicated in pregnancy and breastfeeding and is usually avoided in children. It is known to make ophthalmopathy worse in some patients with Graves' disease, but giving prednisolone 0.5 mg/kg for 3 weeks and commencing thyroxine replacement early (3 weeks after radioiodine) can mitigate this. Despite public concern in relation to radioactivity, accumulated experience over more than 60 years has not demonstrated any discernible risk of genetic, leukaemic or lymphoma risk (Vanderpump et al., 1996).

Box 43.5 Counselling points for patients on anti-thyroid drugs

1. Carbimazole can be given as a single daily dose.
2. Identify anticipated duration of treatment.
3. Explain block and replacement regimens.
4. Explain use of adjuvant therapy, for example, β-blockers.
5. Encourage reporting of skin rashes, sore throat or mouth ulcers. Provide written guidance.
6. Ensure the patient understands the need for regular review.
7. Outline management of relapse.

The commonest complication is the development of hypothyroidism. Doses sufficient to cause thyrotoxicosis to remit will result in virtually 100% of patients given radioiodine for Graves' disease becoming hypothyroid and around 50% of those treated for multinodular disease. Patients should be counselled to expect to require lifelong thyroxine treatment after radioiodine therapy.

Anti-thyroid drugs must be withdrawn before radioiodine is given and should not be restarted for at least 3 days afterwards (otherwise, the isotope will not be trapped by the thyroid). The author conventionally recommends they be stopped 7 days before radioiodine. Since the ablative effect of radioiodine usually commences within 2–3 months, many patients with mild or moderate disease will not need to restart their drug treatments, though close patient monitoring is required. Patients with severe thyrotoxicosis should restart their anti-thyroid drugs on day 3. Treatment is then withdrawn periodically to assess the effects of the radioiodine.

The patient receiving radioiodine treatment is effectively radioactive for 6 weeks without ill effect. Since the patients are not at risk from this radioactivity, it seems inherently unlikely that the public faces any risk at all to health. Nevertheless, there are regulations governing exposure to radiation, which must be followed. After a standard 555-MBq dose, a patient must for 14 days avoid close continuous contact (2 m) with other persons for periods of more than 1 h, undertake to be careful in disposing of urine, and must not work. For 24 days, they must avoid close contact with children and pregnant women. In practice, it is these regulations and the concerns they engender in the patient that result in a proportion of patients preferring a surgical approach.

Surgery

Surgery is required for those patients with very large goitres, patients who cannot be persuaded of the safety of radioiodine and those who have reacted adversely to both thionamides in pregnancy. The hyperthyroid patient to be treated surgically should first be rendered biochemically euthyroid whenever possible, but occasionally surgery needs to be performed as a semi-urgent procedure. This may require urgent patient preparation with a combination of anti-thyroid drugs and β-blockers, and iodide given as Lugols solution. Iodide exerts a (usually) transient inhibitory effect on the ability of the gland to trap iodide, and it may also reduce the vascularity of the gland. In doses of 800–1200 mg/day, lithium is an effective anti-thyroid drug for patients who have reacted to thionamides. Lithium levels should be monitored to minimise toxicity. β-Blockers should be introduced and the dose titrated to reduce the pulse rate to below 80 beats/min. They are usually continued for 1 week postoperatively. It is imperative that treatment is given right up to the time of operation and the operation deferred if the pulse rate is not adequately controlled. Inadequate pre-treatment can result in the occurrence of thyroid crisis.

Complications of surgery include the generic ones of anaesthetic risk, bleeding, thromboembolic disease and infection. Specific risks of thyroid surgery include damage to recurrent laryngeal nerves (which may be particularly important to actors, singers and teachers) and hypoparathyroidism as a result of interference of the blood supply to the parathyroids or their inadvertent removal during surgery. If this occurs, tetany will begin within 48 h of the operation, and treatment should be initiated with intravenous calcium gluconate. All patients who have undergone partial thyroidectomy should have serum calcium estimation 3 months after operation since the development of hypoparathyroidism can be delayed. Later complications of thyroidectomy include hypothyroidism and recurrent thyrotoxicosis.

Treatment of complications

Ophthalmopathy

In most patients with Graves' disease, no specific treatment is required for the eyes. The commonest complaint is of 'grittiness', which can be treated with hypromellose eye drops or gel. If lid retraction is severe, inadequate lid closure can result in early morning soreness. This can be alleviated by the short-term use of 5% guanethidine eye drops instilled each night and morning. The eyes should be monitored for any signs of infection, and treated appropriately.

Fortunately, severe eye involvement occurs in less than 2% of patients with Graves' disease. Progressive ophthalmopathy producing severe complications from proptosis, diplopia or visual failure should be treated with high-dose steroid therapy (prednisolone, 60 mg daily) until symptoms resolve. Failure to respond is an indication for orbital irradiation or surgical decompression, but such patients should be under the care of a highly specialised ophthalmic surgeon.

Treatment of localised myxoedema

Myxoedema is usually localised to small areas and is asymptomatic. More extensive disease causes difficulty in walking and considerable discomfort. Probably the most effective therapy is the nightly topical application of steroid creams, such as betamethasone, under occlusive polythene dressings.

Thyroid crisis

This condition can develop in any patient with significant untreated thyrotoxicosis but is most common in those with severe Graves' disease. It is precipitated in such patients by infection, injury, trauma, anesthetics, surgery and radioiodine. There is rapidly progressive tachycardia, muscle weakness (including cardiomyopathy) hyperthermia, sweating and vomiting compounding hypotension with ensuing circulatory collapse. In addition, patients are extremely anxious and often psychotic. It should be managed as a medical emergency in a high-care area. In addition to supportive measures, specific anti-thyroid therapy is required along with drugs, which inhibit deiodination of T_4 to T_3. PTU (inhibits deiodinase) is given orally (or via NG tube) in high dose along with Lugols iodine. Glucocorticoids should be given i.v. as they also inhibit deiodinase. Effective β-blockade is required by i.v. infusion (propranolol preferred as it also inhibits deiodinase).

Drugs and the thyroid

From the previous pages, it will be evident that many commonly used drugs can affect the thyroid. This section draws together the most frequently encountered problems. In clinical practice, drug effects and interactions produce thyrotoxicosis, hypothyroidism or disturb thyroid function tests. It is worth specifically noting amiodarone, which contains large quantities of iodide which is released into the circulation during drug metabolism. The effects of amiodarone on the thyroid are extensive and complex.

Drugs and thyrotoxicosis

Table 43.2 indicates drug treatments associated with thyrotoxicosis. Amiodarone-induced thyrotoxicosis (AIT) is caused by two entirely different mechanisms. Type 1 AIT is similar to iodide-induced thyrotoxicosis and results from activation of nodular disease or of latent Graves' disease in patients with thyroid autoimmunity. In this condition, the thyroid is actively synthesising hormone and treatment is with thionamides. Type 2 AIT has features similar to thyroiditis with leakage of pre-formed thyroid hormone, low uptake of radio-label on scanning and is treated with glucocorticoids. AIT is an extremely challenging condition to manage for multiple reasons. These include difficulty in discrimination between type 1 and type 2 disease, each of which have different treatments, and the facts that most patients are taking amiodarone for serious cardiac dysrhythmias and amiodarone has a very long tissue half-life. These patients should be under the care of a specialist endocrinology team.

A recent observation has been the increased frequency of Graves' disease in patients undergoing bone marrow transplantation, after administration of alemtuzumab (CAMPATH, a monoclonal antibody to CD52 cells), or alpha-interferon for multiple sclerosis and during Highly Active Anti-Retroviral Treatment (HAART) of HIV infection. It is thought that these cases all have immunological reconstitution as an underlying factor in their aetiology (Weetman, 2009).

Drugs and hypothyroidism

Amiodarone is frequently associated with the development of hypothyroidism, particularly in those patients with positive TPO antibodies, indicative of latent Hashimoto's disease. Such patients seem particularly sensitive to the high levels of iodine liberated by drug metabolism, and it is thought that hypothyroidism occurs because of a failure of the patient's thyroid to escape from the suppressive effect of iodine on thyroxine synthesis (the Wolff–Chaikoff effect). If amiodarone can be withdrawn, hypothyroidism will resolve over a period of months. More often, however, amiodarone is continued and thyroxine treatment is required.

Lithium inhibits T_4 and T_3 release from the thyroid (making it a useful adjunctive treatment for thyrotoxicosis in patients who react to thionamides) and causes a goitre in 40% of patients and hypothyroidism in 20%, again more commonly in those with positive TPO antibodies. Like amiodarone, lithium is usually continued and these patients are treated with thyroxine. Drug-related interference with absorption of thyroxine is one of the causes of hypothyroidism in patients treated with thyroxine. Table 43.2 indicates the agents which may be implicated.

Calcium and parathyroid hormone

Physiology

Most individuals possess four parathyroid glands situated posterior to the upper and lower lobes of the thyroid. These glands secrete parathyroid hormone (PTH). Calcium is approximately 50% ionically bound to albumin, and it is the unbound ionised plasma calcium levels which regulate the secretion of PTH, increased calcium concentration suppressing secretion and low levels stimulating it. PTH is an 84-amino acid straight-chain polypeptide which acts on hormone-specific receptors on target tissue cells. PTH acts on the renal tubular transport of calcium and phosphate and also stimulates the renal synthesis of 1,25-dihydroxycolecalciferol.

PTH and vitamin D act to maintain plasma calcium levels within the normal range. PTH increases distal tubular reabsorption of calcium and decreases proximal and distal tubular reabsorption of phosphate. The effects of PTH on bone are complex. The two major cell types in bone are osteoblasts and osteoclasts. Osteoblasts are responsible for the synthesis of extracellular bone matrix and priming of its subsequent mineralisation. Osteoclasts decalcify and digest the protein matrix of bone, liberating calcium. PTH stimulates osteoclast-mediated bone resorption but, in addition, has an anabolic effect on bone, with an increase in osteoblast number and function.

Hypoparathyroidism/hypocalcaemia

Hypoparathyroidism is the clinical state which may arise either from failure of the parathyroid glands to secrete PTH or from failure of its action at the tissue level.

Aetiology

Hypoparathyroidism most commonly occurs as a result of surgery for thyroid disease or after neck exploration and resection of adenoma causing hyperparathyroidism. In experienced hands, the incidence of permanent hypoparathyroidism is less than 1% for all thyroid and parathyroid surgery. Other causes include autoimmune parathyroid destruction either as an isolated idiopathic disorder or as part of a multiple endocrine deficiency characterised by hyposecretion of several endocrine glands. Transient hypoparathyroidism with symptomatic hypocalcaemia can occur in neonates. The condition pseudohypoparathyroidism occurs in patients with defects of the PTH receptor such that though PTH levels are normal (or raised), calcium is low. Increasingly, reports are identifying acute symptomatic hypocalcaemia and hypomagnesaemia complicating the use of omeprazole and other protein pump inhibitors. These patients are severely magnesium depleted and have an acquired hypoparathyroidism which is reversible on stopping the offending drug (Cundy and Dissanayake, 2008).

Clinical manifestations

Most of the clinical features of hypoparathyroidism are due to hypocalcaemia. The decrease in ionised plasma calcium levels leads to increased neuromuscular excitability. The major signs and symptoms are shown in Box 43.6.

Investigations

Hypocalcaemia associated with undetectable or low plasma PTH levels is consistent with hypoparathyroidism. Total plasma calcium levels should always be corrected for any abnormality in the plasma albumin concentration using the following equation.

$$\text{Corrected calcium} = \text{measured calcium} + \{0.02 \times (40 - \text{plasma albumin})\}$$

Hyperphosphataemia is often present. It should be noted that there are many other causes of hypocalcaemia (Box 43.7). Pseudohypoparathyroidism is easily distinguished as it is associated with excessive PTH secretion and reduced target organ responsiveness. Drugs that may produce hypocalcaemia include calcitonin, plicamycin (formerly mithramycin), phosphate, bisphosphonates, phenytoin, phenobarbital, colestyramine, cisplatin, 5-FU and high-dose i.v. citrate or lactate.

Treatment

Severe, acute hypocalcaemia with tetany should be treated with intravenous calcium gluconate. Initially, 10 mL of 10% calcium gluconate is given by slow intravenous injection,

---

Box 43.6 Signs and symptoms of hypocalcaemia
Numbness and tingling in the extremities and around the mouth
Muscle spasm (tetany)
Epilepsy
Irritability
Cataracts (prolonged hypocalcaemia)
Chvostek's sign (facial spasm on tapping the 7th cranial nerve)
Trousseau's sign (spasm of hand when blood pressure cuff inflated above systolic pressure)

Box 43.7 Causes of hypocalcaemia
Hypoparathyroidism
Pseudohypoparathyroidism
Vitamin D deficiency/malabsorption/insensitivity
Acute and chronic renal failure
Chronic alcoholism
Hypomagnesaemia
Drug induced (protein pump inhibitors)
Acute pancreatitis

preferably with ECG monitoring. If the patient can swallow, oral therapy should then be commenced. If further parenteral therapy is required, 20 mL of 10% injection should be added to each 500 mL of intravenous fluid and given over 6 h. The plasma magnesium level should always be measured in patients with hypocalcaemia, and if low, magnesium therapy instituted.

For chronic treatment, PTH therapy is not currently a practical option as the hormone has to be administered parenterally, and the current high cost is prohibitive. Maintenance treatment for hypoparathyroidism is easily achieved with a vitamin D preparation to increase intestinal calcium absorption, often in conjunction with calcium supplementation. Details of the preparations available are given in Table 43.6. Ergocalciferol (vitamin D_2) is difficult to use and is not recommended. It has a long pharmacological and biological half-life, takes 4–8 weeks to restore normocalcaemia and its effects can persist for up to 4 months following withdrawal. In contrast, calcitriol and its synthetic analogue alfacalcidol are much easier to use. Alfacalcidol restores normocalcaemia within 1 week and its effects only persist for 1 week following withdrawal, permitting greater flexibility in dosage manipulation. The usual daily dose is 0.5–2 μcg. Patients need close monitoring initially until stable normocalcaemia is achieved and thereafter at a minimum of 6-month intervals indefinitely.

Hyperparathyroidism

Hyperparathyroidism occurs when there is increased production of PTH by the parathyroid gland. Primary hyperparathyroidism causes hypercalcaemia. Secondary hyperparathyroidism reflects a physiological response to hypocalcaemia or hyperphosphataemia.

Epidemiology

Recent studies in the USA and Europe indicate an incidence rate for primary hyperparathyroidism of 25 cases per 100,000 of the population per year. The incidence is two to three times higher in women than in men, and the disease most commonly presents between the third and fifth decades.

Aetiology

Primary hyperparathyroidism is due to the development of either single parathyroid adenomas or rarely (<5%) hyperplasia of all four glands. It may occur as part of the dominantly inherited multiple endocrine neoplasia (MEN) syndromes.

There are several conditions associated with secondary hyperparathyroidism, including chronic renal failure and vitamin D deficiency. Chronic renal failure is the commonest cause. In the early stages of the disease, a rise in the plasma phosphate concentration causes stimulation of PTH release and, in more advanced renal impairment, reduced 1 α-hydroxylation of vitamin D results in reduced intestinal calcium absorption, hypocalcaemia and further stimulation

Table 43.6 Vitamin D preparations

Drug	Preparations	Activity
Ergocalciferol (calciferol, vitamin D₂)	Calciferol injection 7.5 mg (300,000 units/mL) Calciferol tablets 250 µcg (10,000 units) and 1.25 mg (50,000 units) Calcium and ergocalciferol tablets (2.4 mmol of calcium + 400 units of ergocalciferol)	Requires renal and hepatic activation
Colecalciferol (vitamin D₃)	A range of preparations containing calcium (500–600 mg) and colecalciferol (200–440 units)	Requires renal and hepatic activation
Alfacalcidol (1 α-hydroxycolecalciferol)	Alfacalcidol capsules, 250 ng, 500 ng and 1 µcg Alfacalcidol injection, 2 µcg/mL	Requires hepatic activation
Calcitriol (1,25-dihydroxycholecalciferol)	Calcitriol capsules, 250 ng and 500 ng Calcitriol injection, 1 µcg/mL	Active
Dihydrotachysterol	Dihydrotachysterol oral solution, 250 mg/ml	Requires hepatic activation

of the parathyroid glands. Tertiary hyperparathyroidism occurs in a minority of patients with end-stage renal failure when hyperplastic parathyroid glands become autonomous and secrete PTH in levels that raise calcium levels above normal.

Clinical manifestations

The clinical features of primary hyperparathyroidism are shown in Box 43.8. These are related to the effects of hypercalcaemia itself, plus the effects of mobilisation of calcium from the skeleton and excretion in the urine. With increasingly early recognition of the biochemical abnormalities of primary hyperparathyroidism largely due to automated measurement of plasma calcium, most patients are identified at an early stage with mild or asymptomatic disease. The classical presenting features of bone disease and renal stones are now relatively uncommon. Although radiological evidence of bone disease is now rare in these patients, measurement of bone mineral content by densitometry (DEXA) scanning usually indicates that bone loss is accelerated and the risk of osteoporotic fractures later in life is increased.

Box 43.8 Signs and symptoms in hyperparathyroidism

Anorexia, weight loss
Polydipsia, polyuria
Mental changes: poor concentration and memory
Fatigue
Nausea, dyspepsia and vomiting
Constipation
Hypertension
Renal stones
Conjunctival and corneal 'calcium' deposits
Bone pain and deformity
Pathological fractures

Investigations

Hypercalcaemia is the primary biochemical abnormality in primary hyperparathyroidism. Phosphate levels are often decreased and PTH levels are either inappropriately normal in the face of hypercalcaemia or elevated. In a patient with borderline elevation of calcium and a normal or only marginally elevated PTH, the benign condition familial hypocalciuric hypercalcaemia (FHH) must be excluded. Urine calcium excretion is increased in primary hyperparathyroidism and low in FHH.

There are many other causes of hypercalcaemia, including malignancy (including myeloma), drugs (thiazides, excess vitamin D), thyrotoxicosis, immobilisation and sarcoidosis. In all these situations, PTH levels are undetectable as the normal parathyroid glands appropriately switch off production of PTH in the face of hypercalcaemia. The most common cause of symptomatic hypercalcaemia in clinical practice is that associated with malignancy and this diagnosis must always be excluded.

Localisation of parathyroid tumours is only required in those listed for neck exploration. Most parathyroid surgeons request a neck ultrasound prior to performing a neck exploration. Isotope scanning, CT, MRI and selective venous sampling are reserved for those patients (around 1% in experienced hands) in whom the adenoma cannot be located at the first operation.

Treatment

Surgical removal of the adenoma or removal of all hyperplastic tissue is the only curative treatment for primary hyperparathyroidism; however, the natural history of hyperparathyroidism is not fully documented. Some studies have indicated that over 50% of untreated patients with primary hyperparathyroidism show no deterioration over 5 years, but the longer-term effects on renal function and bone mass remain unknown. In practice, many patients are observed and their specific problems separately addressed. Thus, patients receive bisphosphonates for osteoporosis, anti-hypertensives, acid-lowering therapy and laxatives.

The main indications for surgical treatment are persistent hypercalcaemia > 2.85 mmol/L, symptomatic hypercalcaemia, renal impairment, renal stones and progression of osteoporosis. Postoperatively, temporary hypocalcaemia (hungry bones) is common. In patients with bone disease, treatment with alfacalcidol and calcium supplements should be started on the day before the operation. Approximately 10% of surgically treated patients develop permanent hyperparathyroidism.

Treatment of hypercalcaemia

Severe hypercalcaemia is a common medical emergency. It must be corrected whilst investigation continues to identify the cause. Table 43.7 shows the treatments available. In practice, rehydration and parenteral bisphosphonates, for example, pamidronate 60 mg in 250 mL normal saline over 30 min, will normalise calcium over 72 h in most patients.

Table 43.7 Treatment of hypercalcaemia

Mechanism	Treatment
Increase urinary calcium excretion	Normal saline plus loop diuretic
Reduce bone resorption	Bisphosphonates Calcitonin Gallium, mithramycin
Reduce gastro-intestinal absorption	Glucocorticoids in calcitriol dependent (vitamin D excess, sarcoid and some lymphoma patients)
Chelation Dialysis	Intravenous EDTA or phosphate

Case studies

Case 43.1

Mrs HP is a 49-year-old professional singer with Graves' disease. She was initially treated with carbimazole but developed a severe generalised rash, which necessitated withdrawal of the drug. A similar rash occurred within 2 weeks of starting PTU. She is overtly thyrotoxic with a blood pressure of 160/50 mmHg, a pulse of 110 beats/min and a large thyroid gland with a vascular bruit. Laboratory results show an elevated free T_4 and an undetectable TSH.

Questions

1. What are the options for treatment and what factors would you discuss with her that could influence her choice of treatment modality?

2. Mrs HP elects to have an ablative dose of radioactive iodine. What adjunctive therapy would you now consider?

Answers

1. This lady has experienced true allergic reactions to both available thionamide drugs and remains thyrotoxic. She should be counselled that thyroid ablation is required and that the treatment options include an ablative dose of radioactive iodine or thyroidectomy. It is necessary to consider features which would make surgery preferable. These would include concern about malignancy, features of local compression including difficulty swallowing or respiratory stridor, a large goitre causing cosmetic embarrassment or inability to receive radioiodine treatment (pregnancy, childhood). Radioactive iodine is more often an appropriate choice of treatment in patients who have either failed to achieve a remission with, or who have reacted adversely to, thionamides. It is known to be an entirely safe form of treatment though restrictions are placed on a patient for up to 1 month after the dose to reduce the public's exposure to radioactivity. Specific to this lady is her profession as a singer. She should be warned that surgery can rarely damage the recurrent laryngeal nerve leading to permanent hoarseness. This complication of surgery is often an important factor in choice of treatment for those who use their voice in their work (singers, actors, teachers, etc.).

2. To reduce the risk of inducing a thyroid crisis, attempts to render Mrs HP euthyroid before the dose of radioiodine should be made. If not asthmatic, she should be commenced on full doses of β-blockers. Propranolol-modified release is particularly useful as a once daily regimen will assist adherence and propranolol, unlike many other β-blockers, inhibits peripheral conversion of T_4 to T_3. Lithium should be commenced at 800 mg daily and will effectively reduce thyroid hormone secretion. Lithium has the useful added benefit of enhancing thyroidal retention of radioiodine and improving its efficacy in control of thyrotoxicosis in patients with large goitres.

Case 43.2

Mrs MG is a 66-year-old woman. She has a history of depression over many years and has recently been complaining of increased tiredness, lethargy and weight gain. Thyroid function tests have shown a TSH elevated at 12 mU/L (normal range, 0.3–5 U/L), but her free T4 is normal at 12.7 pmol/L (normal range, 10.5–25 pmol/L). Her TPO antibodies are positive at a dilution of 1:1600.

Questions

1. What is Mrs MG's thyroid state?
2. Should T_4 therapy be instituted, and if so, how should it be monitored?
3. What warnings should she receive about treatment?

Answers

1. Mrs MG has autoimmune thyroid disease and compensated hypothyroidism. The T_4 is being maintained in the normal range by virtue of increased TSH drive to the thyroid. Left alone, the disturbance is likely to get worse.

2. The British Thyroid Association has recommended that thyroxine treatment should be offered to patients with positive TPO antibodies whose TSH is above 10 mU/L and those whose TSH is between 5 and 10 who have symptoms which are compatible with hypothyroidism. Thyroxine should be commenced at 50 μcg daily and the dose adjusted along conventional lines by measurement of TSH at least 6 weeks after each dose change.

3. It is common for the non-specific symptoms of hypothyroidism to be mimicked by other conditions, notably depression. Mrs MG should be counselled that thyroxine treatment, though appropriate, may not reverse her symptoms and that if she remains symptomatic when her TSH has been normalised, alternative explanations for her symptoms will need to be considered.

Case 43.3

Mr DE is a 21-year-old man who has been treated for autoimmune hypothyroidism over 5 years. He is now prescribed thyroxine at 350 μcg daily, but his TSH has remained elevated varying between 24.4 and 68.2 mU/L. He also has alopecia areata which has had a very severe effect on his self-confidence and he has been seeing a private trichologist for advice.

Question

What are the possible causes of failure to satisfactorily treat his hypothyroidism?

Answer

The commonest cause of failure to suppress TSH is patient non-adherence with treatment. This is especially likely in a young patient with an irregular lifestyle and the elderly who are forgetful. Very few patients require as much as 350 μcg daily for an adequate replacement dose.

If assessment of the patient suggests that adherence is good, consideration must be given to malabsorption of thyroxine. This can be associated with inflammatory bowel disease or coeliac disease. A host of commonly prescribed drugs and medicines available over the counter may reduce thyroxine absorption. Amongst others, these include ferrous sulphate, some antacids and multivitamin preparations. In this patient, there may be other agents recommended by the trichologist which could affect thyroxine absorption.

Case 43.4

Mr JJ is 55 years old. Six years previously, he had a myocardial infarct complicated by ventricular tachycardia. He had an implantable defibrillator placed and has been taking amiodarone 200 mg daily. He is complaining of increasing exertional dyspnoea and weight loss. His free T_4 is returned at 99.1 pmol/L (normal range, 10.5–25 pmol/L) with a fully suppressed TSH confirming thyrotoxicosis.

Questions

1. How does amiodarone cause thyrotoxicosis?
2. What investigations should be considered?
3. How should he be managed?

Answers

1. Amiodarone-induced thyrotoxicosis (AIT) has two distinct causes. Type 1 AIT results from activation of latent autoimmune disease (Graves' disease) or nodular thyrotoxicosis, and is believed to be mediated by the high levels of iodine liberated through metabolism of the drug. Type 2 AIT is due to thyroiditis and results from release of pre-formed hormone. It is good practice to check a patient for thyroid autoantibodies and nodular disease prior to commencing amiodarone as patients with these markers are more likely to develop AIT.

2. It can be difficult to distinguish between type 1 and type 2 AIT. Patients should be referred urgently to a specialist endocrine unit. Thyroid autoantibodies should be requested along with an ultrasound of the thyroid, which will confirm nodular disease and will often show characteristic features of thyroiditis.
3. Type 1 AIT responds to thionamides. Type 2 AIT is treated with glucocorticoids. Amiodarone should be discontinued whenever possible, but since most patients have serious underlying coronary disease, this must only be done in conjunction with the patient's cardiologist. In practice, many patients are treated with both agents whilst awaiting the results of investigation and cardiology advice. For Type 2 AIT, if amiodarone can be discontinued, the thyroiditis usually resolves over a period of weeks. Otherwise, hypothyroidism will usually ensue and can be managed with thyroxine. For Type 1 AIT, if amiodarone cannot be stopped, thyroid ablation is required after control is achieved with thionamides. Since radioiodine uptake is characteristically low in patients receiving amiodarone, surgical removal may be necessary.

Case 43.5

Mrs BK is aged 76. During a routine assessment by her primary care doctor, her calcium is found to be 2.74 mmol/L (normal range, 2.25–2.60 mmol/L), her PTH is normal at 5.3 pmol/L (normal range, 1.5–6.5) and she has no symptoms. She has been taking weekly alendronate for osteoporosis over the past 4 years since sustaining a wrist fracture. Repeat DEXA scans have shown improved bone mineral density on this treatment. Review of her record discloses that her calcium was 2.67 at the time of her fracture, but at the time of her hysterectomy, when she was 45, her calcium was measured at 2.26 mmol/L.

Questions

1. Does she have primary hyperparathyroidism? Does she require any additional tests?
2. How should she be treated? What are the indications for neck exploration in primary hyperparathyroidism?

Answers

1. Yes, she has primary hyperparathyroidism. An elevated calcium with an inappropriately elevated PTH points to this diagnosis. If her parathyroid glands were normal, the PTH level would be undetectable in the face of the hypercalcaemia. It is very common for marginal hypercalcaemia to go unrecognised for many years in hyperparathyroidism. In the absence of the previous evidence of normocalcaemia from many years earlier, demonstration of an elevated urine calcium excretion would be required to provide reassurance that she does not have the inherited condition familial hypocalciuric hypercalcaemia (a benign and lifelong marginal elevation of calcium resulting from reduced sensitivity of the calcium sensing receptor in parathyroid cells). Since it is known that she once was normocalcaemic, no additional biochemical investigation is required though a renal scan should be arranged to rule out nephrocalcinosis.
2. Mrs BK can be reassured that no additional treatment is required at present. She should receive advice that her condition requires monitoring by annual calcium measurements and repeat DEXA scans to demonstrate continued response to alendronate. Absolute indications for neck exploration would include the presence of renal stone disease, progressive osteoporosis despite treatment, hypercalcaemic symptoms and calcium above 3.0 mmol/L. Relative indications include young age at diagnosis, a rising calcium over

2.8, osteoporosis or osteopaenia. A majority of patients with hyperparathyroidism can be satisfactorily treated medically.

Case 43.6

Ms JH is 22 years old when she is admitted to hospital after a grand mal convulsion. She is found to have a serum calcium of 1.15 mmol/L (normal range, 2.25–2.60) and an undetectable PTH. She has been very well with no recent symptoms of paraesthesiae or tetany, and has no other biochemical abnormalities.

Questions

1. What is the likely cause of her hypocalcaemia? Does she require any other tests?
2. How should she be treated?
3. What monitoring does she require?

Answers

1. She has hypoparathyroidism which is most likely to be autoimmune. Hypoparathyroidism can be associated with neck surgery, neck malignancy and infiltrative disease. Very rarely, it is due to embryonic failure of development of branchial arches, is congenital and is associated with severe immunological failure. The absence of any previous history in a fit young woman makes other causes of hypoparathyroidism exceedingly unlikely. The absence of symptoms of hypocalcaemia indicates that her calcium has been low for a long time and supports a relatively slowly progressive pathology. Rapid falls to this level (e.g. after neck surgery) are invariably associated with hypocalcaemic symptoms. It is very likely that her magnesium level will also be low, and this should be tested as it may also require treatment in the short-term.

2. The emergency treatment of hypocalcaemia is by regular i.v. infusions of 10% calcium gluconate with magnesium sulphate by slow i.v. infusion in patients with significant hypomagnesaemia. Ms JH will then need oral vitamin D analogues plus calcium supplements to maintain her calcium in the normal range. 1-alpha cholecalciferol is an effective and convenient preparation and the dose required ranges from 0.5 to 2 μcg daily.

3. Once her calcium has been normalised, she will need biochemical monitoring at a minimum of 6-month intervals. She should never be discharged as in some patients the calcium can drift above the normal range. If this is not identified, renal stone disease and renal failure can develop.

References

Cundy, T., Dissanayake, A., 2008. Severe hypomagnesaemia in long-term users of proton-pump inhibitors. Clin. Endocrinol. (Oxf.) 69, 338–341.

Faber, J., Galloe, M., 1994. Changes in bone mass during prolonged treatment subclinical hyperthyroidism due to L-thyroxine treatment: a meta analysis. Eur. J. Endocrinol. 130, 350–356.

Grebe, S.K., Cooke, R.R., Ford, H.C., et al., 1997. Treatment of hypothyroidism with once weekly thyroxine. J. Clin. Endocrinol. Metab. 82, 870–875.

Maugendre, D., Gatel, A., Campion, L., et al., 1999. Antithyroid drugs and Graves' disease: prospective randomised assessment of long-term treatment. Clin. Endocrinol. (Oxf.) 50, 127–132.

Morris, J.C., 2009. How do you approach the problem of TSH elevation in a patient on high-dose thyroid hormone replacement? Clin. Endocrinol. (Oxf.) 70, 671–673.

Rangan, S., Tahrani, A., Macleod, A., Moulik, P., 2007. Once weekly thyroxine treatment as a strategy to treat non-compliance. Postgrad. Med. J. 83, e3. Available at http://www.ncbi.nlm.nih.gov/pmc/articles/PMC2600132/pdf/e3.pdf.

Sawin, C.T., Geller, A., Wolf, P.A., et al., 1994. Low serum thyrotropin concentrations as a risk factor for atrial fibrillation in older persons. N. Engl. J. Med. 331, 1249–1252.

Surks, M.I., Sievert, R., 1995. Drugs and thyroid function. N. Engl. J. Med. 333, 1688–1694.

Tunbridge, W.M., Evered, D.C., Hall, R., et al., 1977. The spectrum of thyroid disease in a community: the Wickham survey. Clin. Endocrinol. (Oxf.) 7, 481–493.

Uzzan, B., Campos, J., Cicherat, M., et al., 1996. Effects on bone mass of long-term treatment with thyroid hormones: a meta-analysis. J. Clin. Endocrinol. Metab. 81, 4278–4289.

Vanderpump, M.P.J., Alquist, J.A.O., Franklyn, J.A., et al., 1996. Consensus statement for good practice and audit measures in the management of hypo and hyperthyroidism. Br. Med. J. 313, 539–544.

Weetman, A., 2009. Immune reconstitution syndrome and the thyroid. Clin. Endocrinol. Metab. 23, 693–702.

Further reading

Beckerman, P., Silver, J., 1999. Vitamin D and the parathyroid. Am. J. Med. Sci. 317, 363–369.

Brown, A.J., 1998. Vitamin D analogues. Am. J. Kidney Dis. 32 (2 Suppl. 2), S25–S39.

Hanna, F.W.F., Lazarus, J.H., Scanlon, M.F., 1999. Controversial aspects of thyroid disease. Br. Med. J. 319, 894–899.

Lourwood, D.L., 1998. The pharmacology and therapeutic utility of bisphosphonates. Pharmacotherapy 18, 779–789.

Newman, C.M., Price, A., Davies, D.W., et al., 1998. Amiodarone and thyroid: a practical guide to the management of thyroid dysfunction induced by amiodarone therapy. Heart 79, 121–127.

Woeber, K., 2000. Update on the management of hyperthyroidism and hypothyroidism. Arch. Intern. Med. 160, 1067–1071.

Diabetes mellitus 44

Elizabeth A. Hackett and Stephen N. J. Jackson

Key points

- Diabetes is a chronic, incurable condition with an estimated 2.6 million individuals diagnosed in the UK, equivalent to over 4% of the population. An estimated 2.3 million have type 2 disease, 0.3 million type 1 disease and another 500,000 are probably undiagnosed.
- Up to 15% of hospital in-patients will have diabetes.
- The cost of treating diabetes and its related complications, around £9 billion, equates to 10% of the total NHS budget.
- Effective control of diabetes (glycaemic levels, blood pressure, dyslipidaemia) reduces the risk of developing long-term complications and saves both lives and money.
- Abdominal fat is metabolically different from subcutaneous fat and is implicated in the development of insulin resistance and type 2 diabetes.
- Extreme hyperglycaemia and hypoglycaemia may lead to diabetic emergencies, both of which carry mortality risks.
- There is a wide variety of insulins and delivery devices available, allowing regimens to be tailored to individual need.
- Dietary modifications and oral medicines may maintain adequate glycaemic control in type 2 diabetes, but in time many patients will eventually require insulin.
- People with diabetes require education and support to enable them to effectively manage their disease, diet and lifestyle.

Box 44.1 Aetiological classification of diabetes mellitus

Type 1 (β-cell destruction, usually leading to absolute insulin deficiency)
Autoimmune
Idiopathic

Type 2 (may range from predominantly insulin with relative insulin deficiency to a predominantly secretory defect with or without insulin resistance)

Other specific types
Genetic defects of β-cell function
Genetic defects in insulin action
Diseases of the exocrine pancreas
Endocrinopathies
Drug or chemical induced, for example, nicotinic acid, glucocorticoids, high-dose thiazides, pentamidine, interferon-α
Infections
Uncommon forms of immune-mediated diabetes
Other genetic syndromes sometimes associated with diabetes
Gestational diabetes

Diabetes mellitus is the most common of the endocrine disorders. It is a chronic condition, characterised by hyperglycaemia and due to impaired insulin secretion with or without insulin resistance. Diabetes mellitus may be classified according to aetiology, by far the most common types being type 1 and type 2 diabetes (Box 44.1). More than 2.6 million people in the UK have diabetes, and by the year 2025, this number is estimated to rise to 4 million.

Type 1 diabetes is a disease characterised by the destruction of the insulin-producing pancreatic β-cells, the development of which is either autoimmune T-cell mediated destruction (type 1A) or idiopathic (type 1B). In over 90% of cases, β-cell destruction is associated with autoimmune disease. Type 1 diabetes usually develops in the young (below the age of 30), although it can develop at any age and is usually associated with a faster onset of symptoms leading to dependency on extrinsic insulin for survival.

Type 2 diabetes is more common above the age of 40, with a peak age of onset in developed countries between 60 and 70 years, although it is being increasingly seen in younger people and even children. The prevalence of type 2 diabetes varies widely in different populations, being six times more common in those of South Asian origin compared with those of Northern European origin. It is caused by a relative insulin deficiency and insulin resistance. Symptoms are generally slower in onset and less marked than those of type 1. Type 2 diabetes may be an incidental finding, particularly when patients present with complications associated with the disease, for example, heart disease. Type 2 disease often progresses to the extent whereby extrinsic insulin is required to maintain blood glucose levels. The differences between type 1 and type 2 diabetes are highlighted in Table 44.1. It is sometimes difficult to distinguish clinically between type 1 and type 2 diabetes. The important thing to be aware of is that it is predominantly the degree of metabolic abnormality that is the key determinant of the form of treatment.

Two other varieties of non-typical diabetes that may be seen are latent autoimmune diabetes in adults (LADA) and maturity-onset diabetes of the young (MODY). LADA occurs in younger, leaner individuals who appear to have type 2 diabetes as they do not become ketotic and may manage without insulin for a time. Antiglutamic acid decarboxylase (GAD) antibodies may be present and the individual usually

685

Table 44.1 Differences between type 1 and type 2 diabetes

Type 1 diabetes	Type 2 diabetes
β-cell destruction	No β-cell destruction
Islet cell antibodies present	No islet cell antibodies present
Strong genetic link	Very strong genetic link
Age of onset usually below 30	Age of onset usually above 40
Faster onset of symptoms	Slower onset of symptoms
Insulin must be administered	Diet control and oral hypoglycaemic agents often sufficient control
Patients usually not overweight	Patients usually overweight
Extreme hyperglycaemia causes diabetic ketoacidosis	Extreme hyperglycaemia causes hyperosmolar hyperglycaemic state

progresses to insulin more rapidly than those with other varieties of type 2 diabetes. MODY was noted over 30 years ago and described a subset of type 2 diabetes of young onset, often with a positive family history. Genetic studies have now identified this to be a monogenic autosomal dominant form of diabetes. MODY related to the glucokinase gene typically causes a resetting of the glucose level with a 'mild' nonprogressive hyperglycaemia in which diet treatment is usually sufficient. Other types of MODY are related to mutations in the hepatocyte nuclear factor genes and usually develop during adolescence or the early 20s. Pharmacological treatment is required, but sulphonylureas are extremely effective and insulin can usually be avoided.

Epidemiology

The incidence of type 1 diabetes is increasing worldwide, for unknown reasons. It is speculated that environmental changes may be causing modification to the diabetes-associated alleles. Also, since the introduction of insulin in the 1930s, an increasing number of people with type 1 diabetes have had children. There are major ethnic and geographical differences in the prevalence and incidence of type 1 diabetes. Figures are highest in Caucasians (especially Scandinavians), while the disorder is rare in Japan and the Pacific area. In northern Europe, the prevalence is approximately 0.3% in those under 30 years of age. Type 1 diabetes may present at any age, but there is a sharp increase around the time of puberty and a decline thereafter. Approximately 50–60% of patients with type 1 will present before 20 years of age.

Type 2 diabetes is much more common than type 1, accounting for 90% of people with diabetes. It usually occurs in those over the age of 40 years. Estimates in the UK suggest that type 2 diabetes currently affects approximately 2.3 million people, and up to another 500,000 are thought to be undiagnosed. The incidence of type 2 rises with age and with increasing obesity. As with type 1, there are major ethnic and geographical variations. In general, in non-obese populations, the prevalence is 1–3%. In the more obese societies, there is a sharp increase in prevalence with estimates of 6–8% in the USA, increasing to values as high as 50% in the Pima Indians of Arizona. Diabetes is six times more common among Asian immigrants in the UK than in the indigenous population. World studies of immigrants have suggested that the chances of developing type 2 are between two and 20 times higher in well-fed populations than in lean populations of the same race.

Aetiology

Both genetic and environmental factors are relevant in the development of type 1 diabetes, but the exact relationship between the two is still unknown. There is a strong immunological component to type 1 and a clear association with many organ-specific autoimmune diseases. Circulating islet cell antibodies (ICAs) are present in more than 70% of those with type 1 at the time of diagnosis. Family studies have shown that the appearance of ICAs often precedes the onset of clinical diabetes by as much as 3 years. Type 1 has been widely believed to be a disease of clinically rapid onset, but the development is related to a slow process of progressive immunological damage. However, it is not currently possible to use screening methods to reliably identify patients who will develop diabetes in the future. The final event that precipitates clinical diabetes may be caused by sudden stress such as an infection when the mass of β-cells in the pancreas falls below 5–10%.

Studies have been carried out in which patients with newly diagnosed type 1 were treated with immunosuppressive therapies such as ciclosporin, azathioprine, prednisolone and antithymocyte globulin. When started soon after diagnosis, these therapies showed transient improvements in clinical measures and increased the rate of remissions in which insulin was not required. However, their use is limited in an otherwise healthy and young population due to potential toxicity and the risks associated with immune suppression.

Studies have investigated the use of anti-CD3 monoclonal antibodies. When newly diagnosed type 1 patients are treated with short courses of anti-CD3 monoclonal antibodies, smaller insulin doses are required. This relates to better preservation of β-cell function.

Type 2 diabetes also has a strong genetic predisposition. Identical twins have a concordance rate approaching 100%, suggesting the relative importance of inheritance over environment. If a parent has type 2, the risk of a child eventually developing type 2 is 5–10% compared with 1–2% for type 1. Type 2 diabetes occurs because of the progressive development of insulin resistance and β-cell dysfunction, the latter leading to an inability of the pancreas to produce enough insulin to overcome the insulin resistance. About 85% of people with type 2 diabetes are obese. This highlights the clear association between type 2 and obesity, with obesity causing insulin resistance. In particular, central obesity, where adipose tissue is deposited intra-abdominally rather than subcutaneously, is associated with the highest risk. Body mass index (BMI) has been used as an indicator for predicting type 2 risk; however, it does not take fat distribution into account, so waist circumference measurements are now being increasingly used.

Pathophysiology

The islets of Langerhans form the endocrine component of the pancreas, constituting 1% of the total pancreatic mass. Insulin is synthesised in the pancreatic β-cells, initially as a polypeptide precursor, preproinsulin. The latter is rapidly converted in the pancreas to proinsulin. This forms equal amounts of insulin and C-peptide through removal of four amino acid residues. Insulin consists of 51 amino acids in two chains (the A chain contains 21 amino acids and B chain contains 30), connected by two disulphide bridges. In the islets, insulin and C-peptide (and some proinsulin) are packaged into granules. Insulin associates spontaneously into a hexamer containing two zinc ions and one calcium ion.

Glucose is the major stimulant to insulin release. The response is triggered both by the intake of nutrients and the release of gastro-intestinal peptide hormones. Following an intravenous injection of glucose, there is a biphasic insulin response. There is an initial rapid response in the first 2 min, followed after 5–10 min by a second response which is smaller but sustained over 1 h. The initial response represents the release of stored insulin and the second phase reflects discharge of newly synthesised insulin. Glucose is unique; other agents, including sulphonylureas, do not result in insulin biosynthesis, only release. Once released from the pancreas, insulin enters the portal circulation. The liver rapidly degrades it and only 50% reaches the peripheral circulation. In the basal state, insulin secretion is at a rate of approximately 1 unit/h. The intake of food results in a prompt five- to tenfold increase. Total daily secretion is approximately 40 units.

Insulin circulates free as a monomer, has a half-life of 3–5 min and is primarily metabolised by the liver and kidneys. In the kidneys, insulin is filtered by the glomeruli and reabsorbed by the tubules and degraded. In both renal and hepatic disease, there is a decrease in the rate of insulin clearance, which may necessitate dosage reduction for those using exogenous insulin. Peripheral tissues such as muscle and fat also degrade insulin, but this is of minor quantitative significance.

The interaction of insulin with the receptor on the cell surface sets off a chain of messengers within the cell. This opens up transport processes for glucose, amino acids and electrolytes.

In type 1 diabetes, there is an acute deficiency of insulin that leads to unrestrained hepatic glycogenolysis and gluconeogenesis with a consequent increase in hepatic glucose output. Also, glucose uptake is decreased in insulin-sensitive tissues such as adipose tissue and muscle; hence, hyperglycaemia ensues. Either as a result of the metabolic disturbance itself or secondary to infection or other acute illness, there is increased secretion of the counter-regulatory hormones glucagon, cortisol, catecholamine and growth hormone. All of these will further increase hepatic glucose production.

In type 2 diabetes, the process is usually less acute, since insulin production decreases over a sustained period of time. Hyperinsulinaemia is able to maintain glucose levels for a period of time, but eventually β-cell function deteriorates and hyperglycaemia ensues. If this cycle is not interrupted, type 2 diabetes develops. Impaired glucose tolerance (IGT), impaired fasting glucose or hyperinsulinaemia may be detected before overt diabetes develops, and if so, a strict diet and exercise regimen leading to weight loss and improved insulin sensitivity may delay or even prevent the onset of diabetes. At the time of diagnosis, those with type 2 diabetes may have already lost about 50% of their β-cell function. Irrespective of treatment, β-cell function continues to decline with time, often leading to the need for regular insulin therapy.

Type 2 diabetes is also associated with the metabolic syndrome (or syndrome X), although the real relevance of this 'syndrome' continues to be debated in the literature (Khan et al., 2005). The metabolic syndrome is a group of risk factors commonly found in those with type 2 diabetes, including insulin resistance, glucose intolerance (type 2 diabetes or IGT), hyperinsulinaemia, hypertension, dyslipidaemia, central obesity, atherosclerosis and increased levels of procoagulant factors, for example, plasminogen activator inhibitor-1 and fibrinogen.

Pathophysiology of insulin resistance

Abdominal fat, found in abundance in the majority of those with type 2 diabetes, is metabolically different from subcutaneous fat and can cause 'lipotoxicity'. Abdominal fat is resistant to the antilipolytic effects of insulin, resulting in the release of excessive amounts of free fatty acids, which in turn lead to insulin resistance in the liver and muscle. The effect is an increase in gluconeogenesis in the liver and an inhibition of insulin-mediated glucose uptake in the muscle. Both these result in increased levels of circulating glucose. Further, excess fat itself may contribute to insulin resistance because when adipocytes become too large they are unable to store additional fat, resulting in fat storage in the muscles, liver and pancreas, causing insulin resistance in these organs.

Excess intra-cavity adipose tissue causes the oversecretion of some cytokines (adipokines or adipocytokines) associated with inflammation, endothelial dysfunction and thrombosis. Examples of such adipokines include plasminogen activator inhibitor-1 (which is prothrombotic), tumour necrosis factor-α and interleukin-6 (which are proinflammatory) and resistin (which causes insulin resistance). The atherosclerosis associated with insulin resistance is due to hypercoagulability, impaired fibrinolysis and the toxic combination of endothelial damage (caused by chronic, subclinical inflammation), oxidative stress and hyperglycaemia. Excess adipose tissue is also thought to cause undersecretion of a beneficial adipokine called adiponectin. Adiponectin suppresses the attachment of monocytes to endothelial cells, thereby protecting against vascular damage. People with type 2 diabetes have lower levels of adiponectin than those without diabetes and weight reduction increases adiponectin levels.

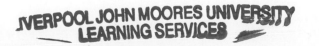

Clinical manifestations

The symptoms of both type 1 and type 2 diabetes are similar, but they usually vary in intensity. Those associated with type 1 diabetes are more severe and faster in onset. The symptoms are related to the osmotic effects of glucose and the abnormalities of energy partitioning. Common symptoms include polyuria (increased urine production, particularly noticeable at night) and polydipsia (increased thirst). These are a consequence of osmotic diuresis secondary to hyperglycaemia. These symptoms are frequently accompanied by fatigue due to an inability to utilise glucose and marked weight loss because of the breakdown of body protein and fat as an alternative energy source to glucose. Blurred vision caused by a change in lens refraction may also occur and patients should be advised that as glucose levels are normalised, vision normally improves and new spectacles should be avoided for the first 3 months of effective treatment of the hyperglycaemia. Patients may also experience a higher infection rate, especially Candida, and urinary tract infections due to increased urinary glucose levels.

Type 1 diabetes

The metabolic abnormality at presentation of an individual with type 1 diabetes is often profound. The symptoms mentioned earlier are usually extreme and of recent (days or weeks) onset. In a significant proportion, the presenting symptoms are those of diabetic ketoacidosis, nausea, vomiting, dehydration, shortness of breath secondary to an attempt by the respiratory system to neutralise the metabolic acidosis caused by the ketones and, in extreme cases, coma.

Type 2 diabetes

Many patients with type 2 diabetes have an insidious onset of hyperglycaemia, with few or no classic symptoms. This is particularly true in obese individuals, whose diabetes may be detected only after glycosuria or hyperglycaemia is found serendipitously. Some patients are unaware of the disease even with marked classic symptoms as they begin so gradually and over such a long period of time. Recurring infections, for example, urinary tract, chest, soft tissue, are common because sustained hyperglycaemia can result in severe impairment of phagocyte function, and raised glucose levels provide a growth medium for bacteria.

Generalised pruritus and symptoms of vaginitis, which may be due to candidal infection, are frequently the initial complaints of women with type 2 diabetes. Patients often present when the complications of sustained hyperglycaemia have already developed, for example, cardiovascular disease or renal disease. Retinopathy may be detected on routine ophthalmological examination. Alternatively, a combination of neuropathy, peripheral vascular disease (PVD) and infection may manifest as foot ulceration or gangrene. In some cases, patients present with hyperosmolar hyperglycaemic state (HHS) where glucose levels in excess of 35 mmol/L are found and excessive dehydration has occurred. Occasionally, patients with type 2 diabetes present with diabetic ketoacidosis, especially in severe infection or in those of African/Caribbean descent.

Diagnosis

In June 2000, the UK formally adopted the World Health Organization criteria for diagnosing diabetes mellitus that was initially published in 1999. It has since been updated and the diagnostic criteria have been reiterated (World Health Organization, 2006).

1. Diabetes symptoms (i.e. polyuria, polydipsia and unexplained weight loss) plus:
   - a fasting serum glucose concentration ≥7.0 mmol/L
   - or serum glucose concentration ≥11.1 mmol/L 2 h after 75 g anhydrous glucose in an oral glucose tolerance test (see later).
2. With no symptoms, diagnosis should not be based on a single glucose determination but requires confirmatory serum venous determination. At least one additional glucose test result, on another day with the value in the diabetic range, is essential, either fasting or from the 2-h post-glucose load. If the fasting value is not diagnostic, the 2-h value should be used.

Current recommendations are that the diagnosis is confirmed by a glucose measurement performed in an accredited laboratory on a venous serum sample. A diagnosis should never be made on the basis of glycosuria or a stick reading of a finger prick blood glucose alone, although such tests are being examined for screening purposes. Glycated haemoglobin (HbA$_{1c}$) is also not currently recommended for diagnostic purposes, although this is currently being considered.

Glucose tolerance test

The patient should not be taking any drugs which interfere with glucose handling. A normal diet with at least 150 g of carbohydrate per day should be consumed for the 3 days before the test, but the patient should be fasted from 8 pm (except for water) on the day before the test. The test should commence at around 9 am with a venous serum glucose test, followed by the administration of 75 g of glucose by mouth over a 5-min period. This is often given in the form of 394 mL of Lucozade® original. The second venous serum glucose sample is then taken 2 h after the drink. The patient should be seated and is not permitted to smoke, eat or drink anything other than water until the test is complete. As there is a risk of later-onset hypoglycaemia in some individuals, it is advisable to suggest that the patient has something to eat immediately upon completion of the test, especially if he/she is planning to drive.

Diabetic emergencies

Hypoglycaemia and extreme hyperglycaemia, causing diabetic ketoacidosis or hyperosmolar hyperglycaemic state, constitute the three acute emergencies associated with diabetes.

Hypoglycaemia

Hypoglycaemia can occur both with insulin treatment and in those taking some oral agents, especially the longer-acting sulphonylureas, for example, chlorpropamide and glibenclamide. Definitions of hypoglycaemia vary, and in particular, there is no WHO definition. However, symptoms caused by the release of counter-regulatory hormones predominantly adrenaline (epinephrine), noradrenaline (norepinephrine) and glucagon tend to occur when the venous serum glucose drops below 3.0 mmol/L in healthy individuals. These symptoms described in Box 44.2 are a normal physiological response to hypoglycaemia and should alert the person to consume carbohydrates. Individuals may not respond appropriately to hypoglycaemia of this degree for several reasons, termed hypoglycaemia unawareness. First, the relevance of the symptoms has not been explained to them. This is an educational failing. It is imperative, therefore, that people with diabetes who are prescribed medication which is known to cause hypoglycaemia should be educated about the autonomic symptoms so that they may take action to avoid further decline of serum glucose. Second, the symptoms simply may not occur because of autonomic neuropathy. One of the commonest complications of diabetes is neuropathy, and when this includes the autonomic nervous system, there are no reliable symptoms to warn the individual that they are hypoglycaemic. A similar situation may occur as a consequence of drugs which suppress autonomic symptoms, such as β-blockers. Third, the patient may have recurrent hypoglycaemia. In those individuals who suffer frequent hypoglycaemic episodes, the autonomic symptoms may cease to occur. There is some evidence that the symptoms can be regained if, for a period of a few weeks, the serum glucose level can be maintained out of the hypoglycaemic range. Finally, the individual may be hypoglycaemia unaware because of alcohol intoxication.

If the serum glucose is allowed to drop to around 2 mmol/L, there are acute changes in cerebral function which lead initially to confusion. This is followed by coma, seizures and death if the glucose drops below about 0.5 mmol/L. Any cerebral malfunction is termed neuroglycopaenia.

Causes of hypoglycaemia

The most common causes of hypoglycaemia are either a decrease in carbohydrate consumption, excess carbohydrate utilisation from unexpected exercise or increase in circulating insulin (Table 44.2).

Nocturnal hypoglycaemia

Sometimes, hypoglycaemia occurs throughout the night. Symptoms may include restlessness, although this may not be identified unless observed by another person. When nocturnal hypoglycaemia occurs, the person often wakes feeling unrested, unwell or with a headache. Contrary to what might be expected, morning blood glucose readings may be high because

---

Box 44.2	Symptoms of hypoglycaemia

Autonomic
Sweating
Trembling
Tachycardia
Palpitations
Pallor

Neuroglycopaenic
Faintness
Loss of concentration
Drowsiness
Visual disturbances
Abnormal behaviour (agitation, aggressiveness)
Confusion
Coma

Other
Hunger
Headache
Perioral tingling/numbness

Table 44.2 Causes of hypoglycaemia

Cause	Comment
Missed meals or delays in eating	Reduced carbohydrate intake, therefore reduction in glucose levels
Not eating the usual amount of carbohydrates	Reduced carbohydrate intake, therefore reduction in glucose levels
Increased doses of insulin	Increased uptake of glucose into cells and increased storage of glucose as glycogen
Increased doses of oral insulin secretagogues	Increased levels of insulin therefore increased uptake of glucose into cells and increased storage of glucose as glycogen
Introduction of other blood glucose-lowering agents to oral insulin secretagogues	Enhanced hypoglycaemic effects
Increase in exercise	Increased uptake of glucose into cells
Excessive alcohol consumption	Impaired gluconeogenesis
Liver disease	Impaired gluconeogenesis and glycogenolysis

a sustained hypoglycaemic episode leads counter-regulatory hormones to raise blood glucose levels. This could present a confusing picture as the obvious solution to a raised blood glucose level in the morning would be to increase the evening/night-time dose of insulin. However, in the case of nocturnal hypoglycaemia, this would make the problem worse. If nocturnal hypoglycaemia is suspected, then blood glucose should be measured at night, for example, 2.00–3.00 am. If confirmed, the patient should either have a snack before bedtime, reduce the evening/night-time dose of insulin, alter the timing of administration of the evening dose of intermediate- or long-acting insulin in order to delay the peak of bioavailability or change the intermediate-acting insulin to a peakless analogue as appropriate. It is important to discuss nocturnal hypoglycaemia with patients as there is often a fear of dying from unrecognised hypoglycaemia in sleep. This fear is unfounded because of the protection from hypoglycaemia severe enough to cause death afforded by the counter-regulatory hormones. This occurs even in those individuals with autonomic neuropathy.

Treatment of hypoglycaemia

If the patient is able to swallow safely without the risk of aspiration, then glucose should be taken orally. However, if unable to swallow or if there is a risk of aspiration because, for example, of a decreased level of consciousness, parenteral treatment should be given, either intravenous glucose or intramuscular glucagon.

The most effective oral treatments are pure sources of glucose, for example, five glucose tablets or glucose drinks such as 150 mL of Lucozade®. In an emergency, hot drinks should be avoided as they might burn and drinks containing milk are not suitable as the fat in milk slows down sugar absorption. Blood glucose levels should be measured about 10–15 min after treating hypoglycaemia. If below 3.5 mmol/L, more glucose should be consumed. If above 3.5 mmol/L and the next meal will be over 1 h, then a long-acting carbohydrate is also required, for example, bread or biscuits. However, if the person is taking an α-glucosidase inhibitor such as acarbose, then monosaccharide carbohydrates must be given because disaccharides and polysaccharides will not be absorbed due to inhibition of the enzymes cleaving carbohydrate into absorbable monosaccharide units.

Should parenteral treatment be required, 25 g of intravenous glucose or 1 mg of intramuscular glucagon is recommended. Glucagon takes approximately 15–20 min to work, but if the person has liver disease (cirrhosis) or is malnourished, then glucagon may not work because glucagon acts by mobilising glucose stores from the liver. In such cases, intravenous glucose must be given. A number of serious extravasation injuries, some necessitating amputation of the affected limb, have been caused by 50% glucose. As a consequence, many hospitals now use 20% glucose.

Diabetic ketoacidosis

Diabetic ketoacidosis is serious, and in developed countries, it has a mortality rate of 5–10%. It occurs because absence of insulin causes extreme hyperglycaemia. At the same time, the normal restraining effect of insulin on lipolysis is removed. Non-esterified fatty acids are released into the circulation and taken up by the liver, which produces acetyl coenzyme A (acetyl CoA). The capacity of the tricarboxylic acid cycle to metabolise acetyl CoA is rapidly exceeded. Ketone bodies, acetoacetate and hydroxybutyrate are formed in increased amounts and released into the circulation. Further, osmotic diuresis, caused by hyperglycaemia, lowers serum volume, causing dizziness and weakness due to postural hypotension. Weakness is increased by potassium loss, caused by urinary excretion and vomiting due to stimulation of the vomiting centre by ketones, and catabolism of muscle protein. When insulin deficiency is severe and of acute onset, all of these symptoms are accelerated. Ketoacidosis exacerbates the dehydration and hyperosmolarity by producing anorexia, nausea and vomiting. As serum osmolarity rises, impaired consciousness ensues with coma developing in approximately 10% of cases. Metabolic acidosis causes stimulation of the medullary respiratory centre, giving rise to Kussmaul respiration (deep and rapid breathing) in an attempt to correct the acidosis. The patient's breath may have the fruity odour of acetone (ketones) commonly described as smelling like pear drops or nail varnish remover.

Precipitating factors for diabetic ketoacidosis in type 1 disease are usually omission of insulin dose, acute infection, trauma or myocardial infarction. Although diabetic ketoacidosis is normally associated with type 1 diabetes, it may rarely occur in people with type 2.

Diagnosis of diabetic ketoacidosis

Diagnosis requires demonstration of hyperglycaemia and metabolic acidosis with the presence of ketones. The biochemical diagnosis of ketoacidosis is usually made at the bedside and confirmed in the laboratory. Urinalysis will show marked glycosuria and ketonuria. A blood glucose test strip usually shows a blood glucose level of more than 22 mmol/L. Formal laboratory measurement of glucose, urea, creatinine, electrolytes and venous bicarbonate should be carried out. Two potentially misleading laboratory results are the white blood cell count and serum sodium. The former will always be raised but correlates with the ketone body level and is not therefore a guide to infection. The serum sodium level will often be low due to the osmotic effect of glucose draining water from the cells and diluting the sodium. The sodium concentration will also be spuriously low if there is marked dyslipidaemia.

Treatment of diabetic ketoacidosis

Treatment comprises fluid volume expansion (initially with 0.9% sodium chloride), correction of hyperglycaemia and the presence of ketones (by infusion of insulin), prevention of hypokalaemia, and identification and treatment of any associated infection. Once the patient is better, they should be reviewed by the diabetes team in order to discuss how to avoid future episodes of diabetic ketoacidosis.

Hyperosmolar hyperglycaemic state

HHS is associated with type 2 disease and has a higher mortality rate (15%) than diabetic ketoacidosis. HHS usually occurs in middle-aged or elderly people, about 25% of whom have previously undiagnosed type 2 diabetes.

In HHS, unlike diabetic ketoacidosis, there is no significant ketone production and therefore no severe acidosis. Hyperglycaemia occurs gradually over a sustained period of time, leading to dehydration due to osmotic diuresis which, if severe, results in hyperosmolarity. Hyperosmolarity may increase blood viscosity and the risk of thromboembolism. Factors precipitating HHS are infection, myocardial infarction, poor adherence with medication regimens or medicines which cause diuresis or impair glucose tolerance, for example, glucocorticoids.

Diagnosis of HHS

The diagnostic features of HHS are hyperglycaemia (often in the region of 55 mmol/L, which is generally much higher than for diabetic ketoacidosis), dehydration and hyperosmolarity. There may be a mild metabolic acidosis but without marked ketone production. Conscious levels on presentation range from slight confusion to coma. In some cases, seizures occur. Serum sodium and potassium levels are usually normal, but creatinine is high. The average fluid deficit is 10 L, so circulatory collapse is common.

Treatment of HHS

Treatment requires fluid replacement to stabilise blood pressure and improve circulation and urine output. Sodium chloride 0.9% or 0.45% (if serum sodium is greater than 150 mmol/L) is given and monitoring of blood pressure and cardiovascular status undertaken. Potassium may be added if required. Insulin treatment is started via intravenous infusion but is not aggressive, since fluid replacement also lowers serum glucose levels. Prophylaxis or treatment for thromboembolism may also be required.

Long-term diabetic complications

Diabetes and its long-term complications cost the NHS substantial amounts of money – approximately 10% of the total budget (£173 million/week).

Although all long-term complications may occur in each type of diabetes, the spectrum of incidence is different. Many patients with type 2 diabetes have had their disease a long time before the diagnosis, by which time many have developed diabetic complications (Figs. 44.1 and 44.2). However, diabetic complications can be limited and sometimes prevented altogether if good management occurs from an early stage. Hyperglycaemia and hypertension are the two major modifiable risk factors that influence the development of diabetic complications.

Patients with diabetes should undergo regular review of their disease management for early signs of associated complications and review of these risk factors and their management. Diabetic complications are frequently divided into macrovascular and microvascular complications. Macrovascular complications arise from damage to large blood vessels and microvascular complications occur from damage to smaller vessels. The general aetiology of macro- and microvascular

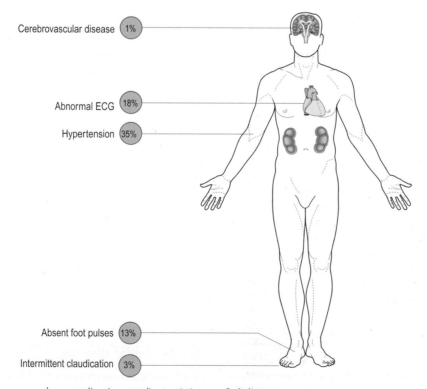

Cerebrovascular disease 1%

Abnormal ECG 18%

Hypertension 35%

Absent foot pulses 13%

Intermittent claudication 3%

Fig. 44.1 Incidence of macrovascular complications at diagnosis in type 2 diabetes.

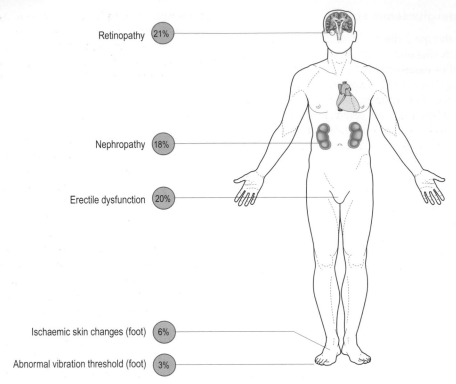

Retinopathy (21%)

Nephropathy (18%)

Erectile dysfunction (20%)

Ischaemic skin changes (foot) (6%)

Abnormal vibration threshold (foot) (3%)

Fig. 44.2 Incidence of microvascular complications at diagnosis in type 2 diabetes.

complications is the same and results from atherosclerosis of the vessels, which may lead to occlusion. The main aims of treatment are, first, to prevent the immediate symptoms associated with diabetes, for example, polyuria, polydipsia, etc., and second, to prevent development, or slow the progression of the long-term disease complications.

Macrovascular disease

The risk of macrovascular complications, including cardiovascular disease (coronary heart disease and stroke) and PVD, is 2–4 times higher for people with diabetes.

Cardiovascular disease

The most common cause of death in people with type 2 diabetes is cardiovascular disease which accounts for an estimated 80% of deaths in this patient group. The risk of a person with diabetes having a myocardial infarction (MI) is the same as someone without diabetes having a second myocardial infarction. The risk of cardiovascular disease is increased further if nephropathy is present. Other cardiovascular disease risk factors are the same as in the non-diabetic population and include smoking, hypertension and dyslipidaemia. However, these risk factors are enhanced in the presence of diabetes, and therefore smokers are encouraged to stop, and individuals with hypertension and lipid disorders are actively reviewed and treated. Silent myocardial infarction (infarction with no symptoms) is more common in those with diabetes and may be due to cardiac autonomic neuropathy. Cerebrovascular disease is also more commonly associated with diabetes, and

patients have a greater mortality and morbidity compared to the general population.

Hypertension. Hypertension is twice as common amongst the diabetic population compared to the general population. It affects over 80% of those with type 2 diabetes. The treatment target ranges for people with diabetes are generally lower than for people without diabetes, as hypertension is associated with the development of macro- and microvascular complications. For people with type 2 diabetes, hypertension is a feature of the metabolic syndrome and is associated with insulin resistance. For those with type 1 disease, it is closely associated with renal disease.

Peripheral vascular disease

PVD affects the blood vessels outside the heart. In people with diabetes, it often affects the arteries of the legs and may give rise to intermittent claudication, a cramping pain experienced on walking, due to reversible muscle ischaemia secondary to atherosclerosis. The iliac vessels can be affected, causing buttock pain and also erectile dysfunction. If PVD is present, the risk of cardiovascular disease increases. About 20% of people with PVD die from myocardial infarction within 2 years of symptom onset.

PVD is also responsible for much of the morbidity associated with diabetic foot problems.

Microvascular disease

Microvascular complications include retinopathy, nephropathy and neuropathy.

Retinopathy

Diabetic retinopathy is the leading cause of blindness in people under the age of 60 in industrialised countries. Twenty years from the onset of diabetes, over 90% of people with type 1, and over 60% of people with type 2, will have diabetic retinopathy. The main problem with diagnosing retinopathy is that it is symptomless until the disease is far advanced. Therefore, if regular screening is not undertaken, diagnosis may not be made early enough for successful treatment intervention. Tight glycaemic control has been shown to prevent and delay the progression of retinopathy in patients with type 1 disease. Likewise, for patients with type 2 diabetes, both tight glycaemic control and tight blood pressure control reduce the risk of developing retinopathy. When retinopathy is detected early, sight may be saved by laser photocoagulation. In advanced cases, surgery may be required.

Pregnancy may worsen moderate-to-severe retinopathy, particularly if there is poor or sudden improvement in glycaemic control. However, tight glycaemic control during pregnancy reduces the long-term risks of retinopathy.

Nephropathy

In diabetic renal disease, the kidneys become enlarged and the glomerular filtration rate (GFR) initially increases. However, if the nephropathy progresses, the GFR starts to decline. Serum creatinine used alone to estimate renal function has limitations. The GFR can be estimated (eGFR). The most popular method is the modified Modification of Diet in Renal Disease (MDRD) formula, which requires serum creatinine, age, sex and ethnicity:

$$eGFR = 175 \times [\text{plasma creatinine } (\mu mol/L) \times 0.011312]^{1.154} \times$$
$$[\text{age in years}]^{0.203} \times [1.212 \text{ if black}] \times [0.742 \text{ if female}]$$

$$eGFR = \text{glomerular filtration rate} (mL/\min \text{ per } 1.73 m^2)$$

The presence of nephropathy is indicated by the detection of microalbuminuria (small amounts of albumin present in urine). If higher amounts of albumin are detected, this is termed proteinuria (or macroalbuminuria) and signifies more severe renal damage. Microalbuminuria is defined as an albumin:creatinine ratio (ACR) greater or equal to 2.5 mg/mmol (men) and 3.5 mg/mmol (women). Proteinuria may be defined as an albumin:creatinine ratio greater than 30 mg/mmol or albumin concentration greater than 200 mg/L. Proteinuria may progress to end-stage renal disease and require dialysis. Albumin in the urine increases the risk of cardiovascular disease, with microalbuminuria associated with 2–4 times the risk, proteinuria with nine times the risk and end-stage renal disease increasing risk by 50 times.

Tight control of both glycaemic levels and blood pressure reduces the risk of developing nephropathy. Angiotensin-converting enzyme (ACE) inhibitors and/or angiotensin receptor blockers (ARBs) are the treatments of choice, since both have been demonstrated to provide renal protective effects additional to their antihypertensive effects. ACE inhibitors and ARBs have been shown to delay the progression to proteinuria in patients with microalbuminuria. Although not proven for all individual drugs in these classes, it is considered to be a class effect. However, these drugs should be used with care if there is a risk of renovascular disease.

Peripheral neuropathy

Peripheral neuropathy is the progressive loss of peripheral nerve fibres resulting in nerve dysfunction. Diabetic neuropathies can lead to a wide variety of sensory, motor and autonomic symptoms. The most common is the symmetrical distal sensory type, which is particularly evident in the feet and may slowly progress to a complete loss of feeling. It is most prevalent in elderly patients with type 2 diabetes but may be found with any type of diabetes, at any age beyond childhood. Painful diabetic neuropathy is another manifestation of sensory neuropathy; it can be extremely disabling and may cause considerable morbidity. Guidance on the treatment of painful neuropathy is available (National Institute for Health and Clinical Excellence, 2010). Diabetic proximal motor neuropathy is rapid in onset and involves weakness and wasting, principally of the thigh muscles. Muscle pain is common and may require opiate analgesia. Distal motor neuropathy can lead to symptoms of impaired fine co-ordination of the hands and/or foot slapping.

Autonomic neuropathy may affect any part of the sympathetic or parasympathetic nervous systems. The most common manifestation is diabetic impotence. Bladder dysfunction usually manifests as loss of bladder tone with a large increase in volume. Diabetic diarrhoea is uncommon, but can be troublesome as it tends to occur at night. Gastroparesis may cause vomiting and delayed gastro-intestinal transit and variable food absorption, causing difficulty in the insulin-treated patient. Postural hypotension due to autonomic neuropathy is uncommon but can be severe and disabling. Disorders of the efferent and afferent nerves controlling cardiac and respiratory function are more common, but rarely symptomatic. Autonomic neuropathy may also cause dry skin and lack of sweating, both of which may contribute to diabetic foot problems.

Macro- and microvascular disease combined

Diabetic foot problems

Infected diabetic foot ulcers account for the largest number of diabetes-related hospital bed-days and are the most common non-trauma cause of amputations. The rate of lower-limb amputation in people with diabetes is 15 times higher than in the general population. The lifetime risk of a person with diabetes developing a foot ulcer is around 15%. Diabetic foot ulcers are a costly problem and are associated with considerable morbidity. Foot problems often develop as a result of a combination of specific problems associated with having diabetes, that is sensory and autonomic neuropathy, PVD and hyperglycaemia. Poor foot care and poorly controlled diabetes are also contributory factors. Development of foot ulcers may be partly preventable by patient education. People with diabetes learn that their feet are particularly vulnerable, and if problems arise, they must seek immediate professional advice.

There are three main types of foot ulcers: neuropathic, ischaemic and neuroischaemic. Neuropathic ulcers occur when peripheral neuropathy causes loss of pain sensation. The ulcers can be deep but are usually painless and are caused by trauma to the foot which is not noticed until after significant damage has occurred. Ischaemic ulcers result from PVD and poor blood supply causing a reduction in available nutrients and oxygen required for healing. Ischaemic ulcers are painful and usually occur on the distal ends of the toes. Most ulcers have elements of both neuropathy and ischaemia and are termed neuroischaemic.

Diabetic foot ulcers are prone to infection, the most common pathogens being staphylococci and streptococci. Wounds with an ischaemic component are commonly infected with anaerobic organisms.

Charcot arthropathy. This is an uncommon foot complication caused by severe neuropathy. It results in chronic, progressive destruction of joints with marked inflammation. Reduced bone density leads to bone fractures, altered foot shape and gross deformity. Owing to the deformity which occurs, excess pressure over protruding bone frequently leads to ulceration unless footwear is extensively modified.

Treatment

Treatment for people with diabetes includes advice on nutrition, physical activity, weight loss and smoking cessation if appropriate. Drug therapy is prescribed where necessary.

Structured education programmes

It is now considered standard care to offer people with diabetes education to help them manage their diabetes themselves on a day-to-day basis. This should be offered in a structured way and based upon theories of adult learning. Group education is now invariably offered as it offers economic advantages over one-to-one education as well as peer support. Examples of such programmes include DAFNE (Dose Adjustment For Normal Eating) in type 1 diabetes and DESMOND (Diabetes Education for Self Management in the Ongoing and Newly Diagnosed) in type 2 diabetes.

Diet

Dietary control is the mainstay of treatment for type 2 diabetes and plays an integral part in the management of type 1. Dietary recommendations have undergone extensive review in recent years and considerable changes have been made. Generally speaking, healthy eating advice for people with diabetes is the same as for the general population. Some of the general dietary advice that patients should be given is shown in Box 44.3.

Box 44.3 General dietary advice for people with diabetes

- Eat regular meals based on starchy foods such as bread, pasta, potatoes, rice and cereals. Whenever possible, choose high-fibre varieties of these foods, for example, wholemeal bread and wholemeal cereals which have a lower glycaemic index.
- Try to cut down on fat, particularly saturated (animal) fats. Monounsaturated fats such as olive oil are preferred. Use less butter, margarine, cheese and eat fewer fatty meals. Choose low-fat dairy foods, for example, skimmed milk and low-fat yoghurt. Grill, steam or oven bake instead of frying or cooking with oil or other fats.
- Try to eat at least five portions of fruit and vegetables every day. This provides vitamins and fibre as well as helping to balance the overall diet.
- Cut down on sugar and sugary foods. Sugar can still be used as an ingredient in foods and baking as part of a healthy diet. Use sugar-free, low-sugar or diet squashes and fizzy drinks, as sugary drinks cause blood glucose levels to rise quickly.
- Use less salt as high intake can raise blood pressure. Food can be flavoured with herbs and spices instead of salt.
- Drink alcohol in moderation. Two units/day for a woman and three for a man. A small glass of wine or half a pint of normal strength beer is one unit. Never drink on an empty stomach as alcohol can exacerbate hypoglycaemia.

Carbohydrates and sweeteners

The blood glucose level is closely affected by carbohydrate intake. Previous guidance for people with diabetes recommended eating about the same amount of carbohydrate at approximately the same time each day and generally advised restriction of carbohydrates. As a consequence of this advice, a number of people tended to eat more fat. Current guidance for carbohydrate consumption still emphasises the importance of total carbohydrate intake, but it focuses on selecting carbohydrates with a lower glycaemic index, that is carbohydrates which give sustained release of sugars over time, as opposed to carbohydrates with a high glycaemic index that give high peaks in blood glucose concentration. Examples of carbohydrates with a low glycaemic index include beans, pulses and starchy foods like wholemeal pasta and wholegrain bread. Total carbohydrate consumption should not exceed 45–60% of energy intake, with monounsaturated fat and carbohydrate combined making up 60–70% of energy intake.

Sucrose or 'sugar' may be included in the diet, according to the new guidance, but sucrose should account for no more than 10% of total energy and should be spaced throughout the day, rather than being consumed all in one go. Sugar alcohols, for example, sorbitol, maltitol and xylitol, often used as sugar substitutes in diabetic foods, are expensive and may cause diarrhoea. They are therefore considered to confer little advantage over sucrose. Non-nutritive or intense sweeteners such as aspartame, saccharin, acesulphame K, cyclamate and sucralose may be useful, especially for those who are overweight.

Alcohol. Alcohol contains carbohydrates and, if consumed in excess, may cause hyperglycaemia. However, more dangerously, it is also associated with later-onset (up to 16 h post-alcohol) hypoglycaemia and hypoglycaemia unawareness.

Alcohol must be restricted to the same maximum weekly quantities as for the general population, that is, 14 units (women) and 21 units (men), with 1–2 alcohol-free days per week. In these quantities, alcohol has cardioprotective effects.

Fats

Since obesity is a major problem in type 2 diabetes and fats contain more than twice the energy content per unit mass than either carbohydrate or protein, consumption of fats should be limited. Monounsaturated fats have a lower atherogenic potential and are therefore recommended as the main source of dietary fat. Intake of fat should be less than 35% of total energy consumption, with saturated and trans-unsaturated fats accounting for less than 10% of energy intake and mono-unsaturated fats providing 10–20%.

Examples of monounsaturated fats are olive oil and rapeseed (also known as canola) oil. Saturated fats are chiefly of animal origin, for example, beef, pork, lamb, whole milk products with some found in plants, for example, cocoa butter, coconut oil and palm oil. Trans-unsaturated fats are found in hydrogenated vegetable oils and hard margarines. N-6 polyunsaturated fats such as cornflower, sunflower, safflower, soyabean oil and seed oils should account for less than 10% of energy intake, and n-3 polyunsaturated fats (fish oils) should be eaten as fish, rather than fish oil supplements, once or twice a week.

Protein

For adults without nephropathy, protein intake is recommended as less than 1 g/kg of body weight, equivalent to about 10–20% of total energy intake. For those with nephropathy, protein intake may need to be further restricted, but this requires expert dietetic advice and supervision.

Fibre

There is no quantitative dietary recommendation for fibre intake. Dietary fibre has useful properties in that it is physically bulky, and it delays the digestion and absorption of complex carbohydrates, thereby minimising hyperglycaemia. For the average person with type 2 diabetes, 15 g of soluble fibre from fruit, vegetables or pulses is likely to produce a 10% improvement in fasting blood glucose, glycated haemoglobin and low-density lipoprotein cholesterol (LDL-C). Insoluble fibre from cereals, wholemeal bread, rice and pasta has no direct effect on glycaemia or dyslipidaemia, but it has an overall benefit on gastro-intestinal health and may help in weight loss by promoting satiety.

Salt

Sodium chloride should be limited to a maximum of 6 g/day. A reduction in salt intake from 12 to 6 g/day has been shown to produce a reduction in systolic blood pressure of 5 mmHg and a reduction of 2–3 mmHg in diastolic pressure.

Obesity management in type 2 diabetes

Obesity management is a very important issue in type 2 diabetes owing to the insulin resistance which occurs as a consequence of excess adipose tissue. Whilst any loss of weight in those who are overweight or obese is of benefit in diabetes in that it is associated with an improvement in dyslipidaemia, hypertension and glycaemic control, bariatric surgery can lead to profound improvements. Recent studies have shown that laparoscopic banding can induce remission of type 2 diabetes in 48% of individuals and Roux-en-y bypass procedures can induce remission in 84%. More importantly, bariatric surgery is associated with a 92% relative risk reduction in diabetes-specific mortality and consequently should be offered to those with diabetes who have a BMI of 35 kg/m^2 or higher (National Institute for Health and Clinical Excellence, 2006). For those with a BMI of 28 kg/m^2 or greater, it is recommended that the pancreatic and gastric lipase inhibitor, orlistat, be considered as the modest weight reduction which can be achieved with this agent yields benefits in diabetes control.

Insulin therapy in type 1 diabetes

All patients with type 1 diabetes require treatment with insulin in order to survive. Exogenous insulin is used to mimic the normal physiological pattern of insulin secretion as closely as possible for each individual patient. However, a balance is required between tight glycaemic control and hypoglycaemia risk. If the risk of hypoglycaemia is high, then it may be necessary to aim for less tight glycaemic control. There is a wide variety of insulin preparations available which differ in species of origin, onset of action, time to peak effect and duration of action (Table 44.3).

Species of origin

Until the 1980s, insulin was obtained and purified from the pancreas of pigs and cows. Human sequence insulins have subsequently been developed using recombinant DNA technology and are now the most common insulins in use. Many of the animal-derived products have been withdrawn, but some animal insulins continue to be available. Porcine insulin only differs from human insulin in one amino acid at the end of the B chain (position B30). Human insulin may be produced semi-synthetically by enzymatic modification of porcine insulin (emp). However, most human insulin is manufactured using genetic engineering and recombinant DNA technology. This is done by inserting either synthetic genes for the insulin A chain and B chain, or the proinsulin gene, or a proinsulin-like precursor into *Escherichia coli* (crb, prb) or yeast cells (pyr). The cells are fermented, resulting in large amounts of the recombinant protein, which is then converted into insulin and purified. More recently, human insulin analogues have been developed through genetic and protein engineering, to produce insulin molecules with differing pharmacokinetic properties.

It is now standard practice to commence all patients requiring insulin on human insulin. In those who have been changed from animal to human insulin, there has been concern that

Table 44.3 Insulin preparations

Preparation	Origin	Onset (h)	Peak (h)	Duration (h)
Soluble insulin				
Human Actrapid (pyr)	H	0.5	2–5	8
Humulin S (prb)	H	0.5	1–3	5–7
Hypurin Bovine Neutral	B	0.5/1	2–5	6–8
Apidra (insulin glulisine)	H	0.25	1	3–4
Humalog (insulin lispro)	H	0.25	1–1.5	2–5
Novorapid (insulin aspart)	H	0.25	1–3	3–5
Hypurin Porcine Neutral	P	0.5/1	2–5	6–8
Insuman Rapid (crb)	H	0.5	1–3	7–9
Biphasic insulin				
Humulin M3 (prb)	H	0.5	1–8.5	14–15
NovoMix 30	H	0.25	1–4	Up to 24 h
Humalog Mix 25	H	0.25	1–2	22
Humalog Mix 50	H	0.25	1–2	22
Hypurin Porcine 30/70	P	0.5	4–12	24
Insuman Comb 15 (prb)	H	0.5	2–4	12–20
Insuman Comb 25 (prb)	H	0.5	2–4	12–19
Insuman Comb 50 (prb)	H	0.5	1–4	12–16
Isophane insulin				
Hypurin Porcine Isophane	P	2	6–12	24
Insuman Basal (crb)	H	1	3–4	12–20
Human Insulatard (pyr)	H	2	4–12	24
Humulin I (prb)	H	0.5	2–8	18–20
Hypurin Bovine Isophane	B	2	6–12	24
Insulin zinc suspension (mixed)				
Hypurin Bovine Lente	B	2	8–12	30
Protamine zinc				
Hypurin Bovine PZI	B	4	10–20	36
Long-acting analogues				
Lantus (insulin glargine)	H	2–4	No peak	20–24
Levemir (insulin detemir)	H	2–4	6–14	16–20

Insulin preparations classified as being of human (H), beef (B) or pork (P) origin; prb, proinsulin recombinant bacteria; crb, chain recombinant bacteria; pyr, precursor yeast recombinant.

human insulin may be associated with an increased risk of hypoglycaemic unawareness, although current evidence suggests that this is unlikely if the switch is done appropriately. Human insulin may be more potent dose for dose than animal insulin due to the formation of antibodies. Conventionally, doses are reduced by 25% or more when changing from animal to either human or analogue insulin.

Insulin preparations

The onset of action, peak effect and duration of action are determined by the insulin type and by the physical and chemical form of the insulin.

Fast-acting insulins. Conventional fast-acting insulins are soluble insulins (also known as neutral insulins). After subcutaneous injection, soluble insulin appears in the circulation within 10 min. The concentration rises to a peak after about 2 h and then declines over a further 4–8 h. This absorption curve can be contrasted with the physiological insulin concentration curve, where peak concentrations are reached 30–40 min after a meal and decline rapidly to 10–20% of peak levels after about 2 h.

The fast-acting recombinant insulin analogues (insulin lispro, insulin aspart and insulin glulisine) are more rapidly absorbed than the non-analogue soluble insulins and have a shorter duration of action. The analogues therefore offer more flexibility. They are more convenient for some patients as they can be given immediately before a meal rather than the 30 min before recommended for human soluble insulin. Another benefit is a reduced risk of hypoglycaemia because of the shorter duration of action. These pharmacokinetic differences arise as the short-acting analogues remain as monomers (single units) unlike regular soluble human insulins which self-associate into a hexameric (6-unit) form. Hexamers need to dissociate into dimers and monomers to be readily absorbed from subcutaneous tissue, which causes delayed absorption.

Intermediate-acting insulins. Conventional intermediate-acting insulins are insoluble, cloudy suspensions of insulin complexed with either protamine (also known as isophane or NPH insulin) or zinc (lente insulin).

Over time, insulin dissociates from the protamine, which gives the preparation its extended activity. The onset of action is usually 1–2 h with the peak effect being seen at 4–8 h. There is considerable inter-patient variation in the duration of action, but it usually requires twice-daily administration to adequately cover a 24-h period. Protamine insulin and soluble insulin do not interact when mixed together. Therefore, ready-mixed (biphasic) preparations are available containing both isophane and soluble insulin.

Long-acting insulins. More recently, long-acting insulin analogues such as insulin glargine and insulin detemir have been developed using recombinant DNA technology. They both have a duration of action of about 24 h, a more predictable, flat profile of action with no pronounced peaks and less inter- and intra-subject dosing variability.

Insulin glargine differs from human insulin as two arginine molecules have been added to the B chain at the C-terminal end. This alters the isoelectric point from pH 5.4 to 6.7. Also, the neutral amino acid glycine replaces the asparagine residue at position A21. The changes mean that insulin glargine remains soluble at a slightly acidic pH. The product is buffered at a pH of 4. Once it is injected into subcutaneous tissue, it forms a microprecipitate in the more neutral surrounding pH. This allows slow absorption from the injection site.

Insulin detemir has a long duration of action and is formulated at neutral pH. It differs from human insulin by omission of the amino acid threonine at position B30 and the attachment of a fatty acid chain (myristic acid) to lysine at position B29. The modification allows the insulin molecule to reversibly bind to albumin, via the fatty acid chain, following absorption from subcutaneous injection. This reduces the amount of free, active insulin detemir (bound insulin is inactive). The long duration of action is produced by dissociation of the insulin molecule from albumin.

Insulin delivery

All the currently licensed insulin products are available only by injection. An inhaled insulin product available for a short period of time is no longer obtainable. The subcutaneous route is routinely used for maintenance therapy, as opposed to the intravenous route which is sometimes used in hospital. Insulin can be injected subcutaneously into the outer aspect of the thigh, abdominal wall, buttocks or upper arm. However, injecting into the arm is incredibly difficult and is therefore not usually a site of choice. The main advantages associated with subcutaneous injection are accessibility, which allows most patients to administer their own insulin. However, this route cannot be regarded as physiological as it delivers insulin to the systemic rather than portal circulation.

A small number of patients still use disposable plastic syringes with insulin from a vial as their means of insulin administration, although the vast majority now use pen injection devices. Insulin pens may either be refillable or disposable. Although not in themselves improving diabetic control, they are popular amongst users since they are compact and more convenient as they remove the need to draw up insulin from a vial.

Intravenous insulin delivery should be used in the management of ketoacidosis and hyperosmolar states. The intravenous route is also preferable for diabetic patients due to have major surgery and who may be 'nil by mouth' after surgery. The short half-life of insulin (3–5 min) means that changes in infusion rate have a rapid effect on insulin action and glycaemic control. Intravenous insulin is commonly delivered as either a continuous insulin infusion at a variable rate or an infusion made with a fixed amount of insulin, with glucose and potassium in the same bag. The former is also commonly referred to as a 'sliding scale' insulin regimen, in which the rate of infusion is adjusted according to frequent blood glucose readings, usually hourly. It is administered with a co-infusion of glucose (with potassium, unless patient is hyperkalaemic). The latter type of insulin infusion is known as GKI (glucose, potassium, insulin), GIK or the Alberti regimen. Intravenous insulin regimens are not routinely recommended for patients who are eating and drinking.

Insulin regimens

Standard insulin regimens for managing type 1 disease vary between two to five injections daily. They must be tailored to the individual patient and will depend on lifestyle, willingness to achieve the best control and ability to cope with both injecting insulin and subsequent monitoring of blood glucose. The chosen insulin regimen is negotiated between patient and health care professional and may change throughout life according to priorities and patient preference. Starting doses of insulin and the ratio of short- to intermediate-acting insulin are very variable. In patients who are very active, such as manual workers and those who exercise regularly, the starting dose should be kept low to reduce the risk of significant hypoglycaemia.

Mealtime plus basal regimens. The best control for type 1 diabetes may be attained using a mealtime plus basal regimen, also referred to as a basal-bolus regimen. This mimics normal physiological insulin release more closely than other regimens. A mealtime plus basal regimen requires mealtime injections of insulin with a fast-acting preparation, preferably with an analogue, plus one or two injections of a basal (intermediate- or long-acting) insulin. This may require up to five injections a day. As a general rule, with this regimen, the soluble insulin injections given before each meal usually comprise 40–60% of the total daily dosage. Some individuals may benefit from exogenous insulin delivery via a continuous subcutaneous insulin infusion administered via a pump worn on their person. The pump can be programmed to give a different basal rate of infusion at different times of day, and boluses are then provided by the pump at mealtimes. There are specific indications for pump therapy (National Institute for Health and Clinical Excellence, 2008).

These regimens offer the most flexibility of dosing and eating habits, and often better blood glucose control. A number of patients have been taught to count mealtime carbohydrates and calculate their own insulin dose on the basis of the preprandial blood glucose concentration, which allows greater scope for 'normal eating'. An example is the DAFNE (dose adjusted for normal eating) programme (DAFNE Study Group, 2002), in which patients are required to attend structured, group education on five consecutive days.

The disadvantage of mealtime plus basal regimens is that they require multiple injections, unless a pump is *in situ*, and require regular blood glucose monitoring and the ability of the patient to match insulin doses according to carbohydrate intake, exercise levels and prevailing glucose levels. For some people, this is either too difficult or unsuitable.

Twice-daily regimens. The mealtime plus basal regimen may be too hard for some, for example, school-age children, to manage. In this type of situation, a twice-daily regimen may be more suitable. The simplest and most effective twice-daily regimens use premixed insulin, comprising a short- or rapid-acting plus an intermediate-acting insulin. Regular human insulin mixes and analogue mixes are available. The regular human insulin mixes should be given 30 min before breakfast and 30 min before the evening meal, whereas analogue mixes may be given immediately before these meals. The longer-acting component of the insulin mix given at breakfast time must span the lunchtime meal and the evening dose must bridge the night time. Twice-daily regimens using intermediate- or long-acting insulins alone are not sufficient for maintenance control of type 1 diabetes. Occasionally, they are used in newly diagnosed patients who are not acutely ill, adding the short-acting preparation if and when indicated by self-monitoring.

Adjusting the insulin dose

The information on which insulin dosage adjustment is based should be derived from blood glucose self-monitoring and the incidence and timing of hypoglycaemia. On twice-daily fast- and intermediate-acting insulin regimens, the soluble insulin may be considered as acting up to the next meal or to bedtime, while the extended-acting insulins act up to the next injection. The glucose concentration at the end of the period can be taken as a measure of the appropriateness of the relevant dose.

Adjustments to a dose of insulin should depend on the degree of insulin resistance present. In order to determine a suitable adjustment dose, the effect of other dosage adjustments in the same patient should be taken into consideration, as should the total insulin dose. For example, a 2-unit dose increase in someone taking 6 units of insulin would be a 33% dosage increase; however, a 2-unit dose increase in someone taking 60 units of insulin would be proportionately much less and make less impact.

Storage of insulin

Insulin formulations are stable if kept out of light, and they are not subject to freezing or extremes of heat. Loss of potency of 5–10% occurs in vials kept at high ambient room temperatures for 2–3 months. Insulin should therefore be stored in a domestic refrigerator except for the vial(s), cartridge(s) or pens in current use which, depending on the individual preparation, may be stable for 4–6 weeks (see manufacturers' recommendations). When pen injector devices are in use, they should never be stored in a refrigerator as there have been reports of devices 'seizing up' when stored in the cold. Also, the injecting of cold or refrigerated insulin is undesirable because it is more painful and the insulin absorption profile is altered.

Adverse effects of insulin

Hypoglycaemia is a common physiological complication of insulin therapy and is often a source of great anxiety to patients and carers. The symptoms (see Box 44.2) may occur at different blood glucose levels in different individuals.

Thickening of subcutaneous tissues can occur at injection sites because of recurrent injection in the same area, known as lipohypertrophy. As well as looking unsightly, it can result in impaired and erratic insulin absorption, leading to poor glycaemic control. The solution is to rotate injection sites. Bruising is usually a sign of superficial injections. Localised skin reactions occasionally occur but resolve even with continued use of the same insulin preparation.

Systemic allergic reactions rarely occur with the current universal use of highly purified insulins. Though not usually species specific, it is worthwhile trying insulin of a different species if allergy occurs. Also, some patients may experience allergy to the excipients within the insulin product or to the needle used for administration. If this is suspected, it is helpful to seek the advice of an immunologist and try an insulin product with different excipients.

Management of type 2 diabetes

About 80% of patients with type 2 diabetes are overweight at diagnosis, and this is known to cause insulin resistance. This means that higher doses of medication may be required to control blood glucose levels. Advice on weight loss through increased physical exercise and calorie restriction, in addition to education about general healthy eating, is required. Targets for weight should be to maintain a normal BMI of between 20 and 25 kg/m² or a waist circumference of less than 88 cm in women and 102 cm in men, which lowers the risk of developing insulin resistance. In those who are already overweight or obese, however, an achievable target of 10–15% body weight loss should be discussed as, if achieved, this will have significant benefits in overall diabetes control.

Some people are able to normalise their glycaemic control by weight loss and attention to diet (diet controlled). Nevertheless, such individuals still invariably have diabetes and are at risk of developing diabetic complications. Hyperglycaemia may still occur, especially in times of stress or if dietary control is lost, and consequently they should be monitored regularly.

For over 75% of people with type 2 diabetes, dietary measures and exercise alone do not produce adequate glycaemic control and oral hypoglycaemic therapy is required. Within

3 years of diagnosis, a large majority of patients will require oral drug therapy. In the UK, there are six classes of oral agents currently available: a biguanide (metformin), sulphonylureas (glibenclamide, gliclazide, glimepiride, glipizide, tolbutamide), meglitinides (repaglinide and nateglinide), a thiazolidinedione (pioglitazone), an α-glucosidase inhibitor (acarbose) and the dipeptidyl peptidase-4 inhibitors (saxagliptin, sitagliptin and vildagliptin).

Acarbose has been poorly tolerated in trials, with only 39% of those receiving the drug still taking it after 3 years. The main reason for non-adherence appears to be flatulence. Acarbose is rarely prescribed in the UK but is popular in other countries such as Germany. Metformin remains the cornerstone of oral treatment for type 2 diabetes. The sulphonylureas and meglitinides are known as insulin secretagogues, since they both enhance secretion of insulin from the pancreatic β-cells. The relatively recent introduction of the dipeptidyl peptidase inhibitors (DPP-4 inhibitors) has been welcomed and is a useful new class of drug, particularly for those in whom weight is a problem, since they do not cause weight gain like many of the other drug treatments. Likewise, the incretin mimetics, another new class of injectable drugs, are often helpful for the obese population since they are associated with weight reduction.

In type 2 diabetes, the progressive decline in β-cell function with time and increasing insulin resistance means people with this disease show a progressive loss of glycaemic control and usually require two or three drugs to maintain control before ultimately requiring insulin.

The factors used to select a particular treatment include the patient's clinical characteristics, such as their degree of hyperglycaemia, weight and renal function (Fig. 44.3). In acutely ill people with significant hyperglycaemia, insulin therapy may well be required, albeit transiently because acute illness leads to an increase in stress hormones, all of which are anti-insulin.

Biguanides

Metformin is the only biguanide available in the UK. The mechanism of action of biguanides is still not completely understood. However, the principal mode of action is via potentiation of insulin action at an unknown intracellular locus, resulting in decreased hepatic glucose production by both gluconeogenesis and glycogenolysis. Metformin also stimulates tissue uptake of glucose, particularly in muscle, and is thought to reduce gastro-intestinal absorption of carbohydrate. The action of metformin does not involve stimulation of pancreatic insulin secretion and therefore it is still a beneficial agent when β-cell function has declined. Another advantage of metformin over insulin secretagogues, and sulphonylureas, in particular, is that it does not cause hypoglycaemia and is not associated with weight gain. Metformin has a short duration of action, with a half-life of between 1.3 and 4.5 h, and does not bind to serum proteins. It is not metabolised and is totally renally eliminated.

It has been shown that diabetes-related death was reduced by 42% in overweight subjects who took metformin for 10 years, compared to those who took conventional therapies such as a sulphonylurea or insulin. Myocardial infarction was also reduced by 39% over the 10-year follow-up period. Consequently, metformin has become the first-line therapy for glycaemic control when oral agents are indicated especially in overweight and obese patients.

Adverse effects. The most common adverse effects of metformin, affecting about a third of patients, result from gastro-intestinal disturbances including anorexia, nausea, abdominal discomfort and diarrhoea. In some patients, diarrhoea can be extreme and can preclude metformin use. However, the gastro-intestinal side effects are usually transient and can be minimised by starting with a low dose, increasing the dose slowly and administering the drug with or after food. A suggested regimen is to start with 500 mg daily for 1 week, then 500 mg twice daily for 1 week, increasing the dosage at weekly intervals until the desired glycaemic response is achieved or intolerance occurs. The maximum licensed dose is 3 g/day, but doses of more than 2 g/day often cause intolerance. If the initial dose of 500 mg daily causes side effects, then some prescribers reduce the starting dose to 250 mg daily for a week. This may be difficult for some patients as the 500 mg strength tablets are not scored and are not easy to halve.

Two modified-release metformin preparations are now available and permit once-daily dosing. Clinical evidence suggests that these formulations cause fewer problems with gastro-intestinal side effects. The maximum licensed dose of the modified-release preparations (2 g daily) differs from the standard preparation.

The two previously available biguanides, phenformin and buformin, were withdrawn due to deaths associated with lactic acidosis. Lactic acidosis is a rare complication with metformin, with an estimated incidence of five cases per 100,000 patient-years. However, it is potentially life threatening. Patients at most risk are those with renal insufficiency in whom the drug accumulates, individuals with co-existing conditions where lactate accumulates, and those who are unable to metabolise lactate. In practice, metformin should not be prescribed for patients who have renal impairment (eGFR <45 mL/min/1.73 m^2) and should be stopped in anyone with an eGFR <30 mL/min/1.73 m^2. Metformin should also be stopped in severe liver disease, uncontrolled cardiac failure or severe pulmonary insufficiency. It should be withdrawn in patients with severe intercurrent illness, for example, acute myocardial infarction or septicaemia, or those undergoing major surgery or requiring investigation using radiographic contrast media and should only be restarted once renal function has been evaluated and determined as within acceptable limits.

Role of metformin. Metformin is useful in obese patients with diabetes as it does not cause weight gain. If there are no contraindications, it can be used in conjunction with diet as second-line therapy in patients not adequately controlled on diet alone. As it has a different mode of action to the sulphonylureas, meglitinides, thiazolidinediones, α-glucosidase inhibitors and DPP-4 inhibitors, it can be valuable when prescribed in combination.

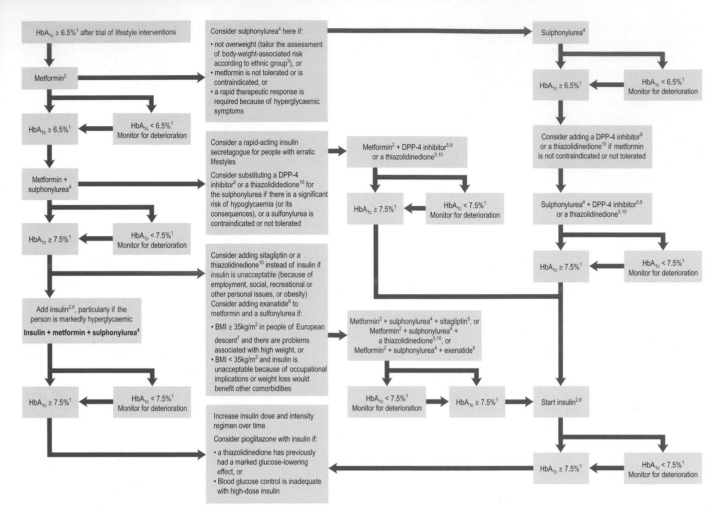

Fig. 44.3 Algorithm for the treatment of glycaemic control in type 2 diabetes. (1) or individually agreed target, (2) with active dose titration (3) see the NICE clinical guideline on obesity (www.nice.org.uk/CG43), (4) offer once-daily sulphonylurea if adherence is a problem, (5) only continue DPP-4 inhibitor or thiazolidinedione if reduction in HbA$_{1c}$ of at least 0.5 percentage points in 6 months, (6) only continue exenatide if reduction in HbA$_{1c}$ of at least 1 percentage point and weight loss of at least 3% of initial body weight in 6 months, (7) with adjustment for other ethnic groups, (8) continue with metformin and sulfylurea (and acarbose if used), but only continue other drugs that are licensed for use with insulin. Review the use of sulphonylurea if hypoglycaemia occurs, (9) DPP-4 inhibitor refers to saxagliptin, sitagliptin or vidagliptin, (10) thiazolidinedione refers to ploglitazone.

Sulphonylureas

Mode of action. The major action of this class of drug relies on the ability of the pancreas to secrete insulin and hence requires functioning β-cells to exert a beneficial effect. Sulphonylureas lower blood sugar by increasing pancreatic β-cell sensitivity to glucose, allowing more insulin to be released from storage granules for a given glucose load. Sulphonylurea therapy is also associated with increased tissue sensitivity to insulin, resulting in improved insulin action. Studies also suggest that sulphonylureas may promote an increased systemic bioavailability of insulin due to reduced hepatic extraction of the insulin secreted from the pancreas.

Pharmacokinetics. The pharmacokinetic parameters of oral hypoglycaemic agents are shown in Table 44.4. Chlorpropamide is the slowest and longest acting agent, but it is now very rarely used. Although glibenclamide has been shown to

have a short elimination half-life, it has a prolonged biological effect, which may be explained by slower distribution and the existence of a deep compartment, possibly the islet cells. All sulphonylureas are metabolised by the liver to some degree and some may have active metabolites.

Choice of drug. There are many factors which influence the choice of sulphonylurea. These may relate to the drug itself, the patient or the prescriber. There are few well-controlled long-term clinical comparisons between sulphonylureas. It would appear that, when dosage is individualised and governed by the effect on fasting blood glucose, there is little or no difference in clinical efficacy between different agents. In general, if a patient is not well controlled on the maximum dosage of one sulphonylurea, it is not worthwhile changing to another one.

Adverse effects. The frequency of adverse effects from sulphonylureas is low. They are usually mild and reversible on

Table 44.4 Pharmacokinetic properties of oral hypoglycaemic agents

Drug	Main route of elimination	Elimination half-life (h)	Duration of action (h)	Daily dose range	Doses per day
Sulphonylureas					
First generation					
Tolbutamide	Hepatic	4–24	6–10	0.5–2 g	1–3
Chlorpropamide	Hepatic (80%) Renal (20%)	24–48	24–72	100–500 mg	1
Second generation					
Glibenclamide	Hepatic (40%) Biliary (60%)	2–4	16–24	2.5–15 mg	1–2
Glipizide	Hepatic	2–4	6–24	2.5–40 mg	1–3
Gliclazide	Hepatic	10–12	10–24	40–320 mg	1–2
Glimepiride	Renal (60%) Biliary (40%)	5–8	12–24	1–6 mg	1
Biguanides					
Metformin	Renal	1–5	5–8	1–3 g	2–3
Meglitinides					
Repaglinide	Hepatic	1	4–6	1–16 mg	3 (with each main meal)
Nateglinide	Hepatic	1	3–4	180–540 mg	3 (with each main meal)
Thiazolidinediones					
Pioglitazone	Hepatic	5–6	16–24	15–30 mg	1
Dipeptidyl pepidase-4 inhibitors					
Sitagliptin	Renal	10–12	12–24	100 mg	1
Vildagliptin	Renal	3	10–12	50 mg	1–2
Saxagliptin	Renal and hepatic	2–3	At least 24 h	5 mg	1
Incretin mimetics					
Exenatide	Renal	2–3	Data not available	5–10 mcg	2
Liraglutide	No main organ identified	13	Data not available	0.6–1.8 mg	1

drug withdrawal (Table 44.5). The most common adverse effect is hypoglycaemia, which may be profound and long lasting. Hypoglycaemia due to sulphonylureas is often misdiagnosed, particularly in the elderly. The major risk factors for the development of hypoglycaemia include use of a long-acting agent, increasing age, renal or hepatic dysfunction and inadequate carbohydrate intake. The major side effect is, however, weight gain.

Other adverse effects are rare; blood dyscrasias occur in 0.1% of patients and rashes in up to 3%. Chlorpropamide can produce troublesome flushing after ingestion of alcohol, and about 5% of patients develop hyponatraemia due to its effect on increasing renal sensitivity to antidiuretic hormone (ADH). Most patients are asymptomatic with this problem, but occasionally severe hyponatraemia is observed. However, as mentioned earlier, this agent is no longer used in routine practice.

Sulphonylurea dosage. The dosage should be individualised for each patient. The lowest possible dose required to attain the desired levels of blood glucose, without producing hypoglycaemia, should be used. Treatment should start with a low dose and be increased if necessary approximately every 2 weeks. For many agents, the maximum effect is seen if the dose is taken half an hour before a meal, rather than with or after food. The number of daily doses required will depend on the agent used and the total daily dose. For several drugs, it becomes necessary to administer the drug two or three times daily when the dose is increased.

A modified-release preparation of gliclazide is available. A dose of 30 mg of the modified-release product is equivalent to 80 mg of the standard-release preparation.

Drug interactions. Several drugs can interfere with the efficacy of sulphonylureas by influencing either their pharmacokinetics or pharmacodynamics, or both. Despite much literature about displacement interactions with sulphonylureas, the clinical significance is doubtful. Many reported cases involve first-generation agents, which have a different protein-binding site from the second-generation agents, which bind in a non-ionic fashion and are not readily displaced. Ingestion of alcohol can cause hypoglycaemia in itself and can also prolong the hypoglycaemic effect of sulphonylureas.

Table 44.5 Adverse effects of sulphonylureas

Adverse effect	Comments
Gastro-intestinal	Affects approximately 2% Most commonly nausea and vomiting Dose related Advise patient to take with or after food
Dermatological	Affects 1–3% Usually occur within the first 2–6 weeks Most commonly: generalised photosensitivity, pruritus, maculopapular rash May require discontinuation of drug Cross-sensitivity between sulphonylureas is common Rare cases of severe allergic reactions, for example, erythema multiforme Stevens–Johnson syndrome
Haematological	Rare cases of fatal agranulocytosis or pancytopenia Other haematological effects usually reversible on discontinuing drug Some reports of reversible haemolytic anaemia
Hepatic	Mild, reversible elevation of liver function tests Cholestatic jaundice Usually a hypersensitivity reaction associated with fever, rash and eosinophilia
Cardiovascular	Possible excess of cardiovascular mortality in patients treated with tolbutamide (not proven)
Hypothyroidism	Association not proven May be rare cases
Alcohol flush	Rarely seen with sulphonylureas other than chlorpropamide Change to another agent
Syndrome of inappropriate antidiuretic hormone (SIADH)	Chlorpropamide and, to a lesser extent, tolbutamide enhance the effect of ADH on the kidney Results in hyponatraemia Risk factors are increasing age, congestive cardiac failure and diuretic therapy
Hypoglycaemia	The most common adverse effect and may be severe and prolonged Highest incidence with chlorpropamide and glibenclamide All sulphonylureas and meglitinides have been implicated Risk factors include increasing age, impaired renal or hepatic function, reduced food intake, weight loss Decrease dose, change to a shorter-acting agent or discontinue sulphonylurea therapy

Meglitinides

The meglitinides are insulin-releasing agents (insulin secretagogues), also called 'post-prandial glucose regulators'. They are characterised by a more rapid onset and shorter duration of action than sulphonylureas. Their site of action is pharmacologically distinct from that of the sulphonylureas. Repaglinide, a benzoic acid derivative, was the first member of the class. It is licensed for use as a single agent when diet control, weight reduction and exercise have failed to regulate glucose levels, or in combination with metformin. Nateglinide was introduced later and is a derivative of the amino acid d-phenylalanine. Nateglinide is only licensed for combination therapy with metformin when metformin alone is inadequate.

Mode of action. Like the sulphonylureas, the meglitinides stimulate first-phase insulin secretion by inhibiting ATP-sensitive potassium channels in the membrane of the pancreatic β-cells. This causes depolarisation and gating of the calcium channels (which are voltage sensitive), increasing the intracellular concentration of calcium and stimulating insulin release. The release of insulin only occurs in the presence of glucose. As glucose levels drop, less insulin is secreted. Conversely, if carbohydrates are consumed and glucose levels rise, insulin secretion is enhanced.

Pharmacokinetics. The pharmacokinetic properties of the meglitinides confer a rapid onset and a short duration of action. The individual parameters are shown in Table 44.4. The meglitinides are extensively metabolised in the liver, repaglinide by oxidative biotransformation and direct conjugation with glucuronic acid. The cytochrome P450 enzymes CYP2C8 and CYP3A4 have been shown *in vitro* to be involved its metabolism. Nateglinide is metabolised predominantly by cytochrome P450 enzyme CYP2C9 and to a lesser extent by CYP3A4. Repaglinide has no active metabolites, but nateglinide has partially active metabolites, one-third to one-sixth the potency of the parent compound. The meglitinides should be taken immediately before main meals, although the time can vary up to 30 min before a meal. The pharmacokinetic profile of meglitinides offers some advantages in patients with poor renal function or irregular eating habits.

Adverse effects. The meglitinides may cause a range of side effects, most commonly hypoglycaemia, visual disturbances, abdominal pain, diarrhoea, constipation, nausea and vomiting. More rarely, hypersensitivity reactions can occur as well as elevation of liver enzymes. The meglitinides may also cause weight gain.

Dosage. The recommended starting dose for repaglinide is 500 μcg before or with each meal, increasing as necessary (depending on blood glucose measurements) every 1–2 weeks to a maximum single dose of 4 mg and a maximum daily dose of 16 mg. When patients are transferred from other therapies, the recommended starting dose is 1 mg preprandially. The recommended starting dose of nateglinide is 60 mg three times a day before meals, which may be subsequently increased to 120 mg three times a day. The maximum single dose is 180 mg, which may be given with the three main meals of the day.

Drug interactions. Drugs which induce or inhibit the cytochrome P450 enzymes CYP2C8 and CYP3A4 interact with repaglinide. Examples of drugs which enhance or prolong the hypoglycaemic effect include gemfibrozil, clarithromycin, ketoconazole, itraconazole, trimethoprim, other hypoglycaemic drugs, monoamine oxidase inhibitors, non-selective β-blockers, ACE inhibitors, salicylates, NSAIDs, octreotide, alcohol and anabolic steroids. Drugs which induce cytochrome P450 enzymes may also interact, for example, rifampicin and phenytoin, and may decrease repaglinide serum levels. Drugs that inhibit CYP2C9 may interact with nateglinide. Drugs that may enhance or prolong the hypoglycaemic effect include ACE inhibitors, gemfibrozil and fluconazole. The hypoglycaemic effects of nateglinide may be reduced by diuretics, corticosteroids and β-blockers.

Role of meglitinides. The meglitinides are an effective hypoglycaemic therapy in type 2 diabetes. They may be most beneficial in patients who experience problems with post-prandial glucose elevation and as single therapy in patients who eat at unpredictable times or have a tendency to miss meals. However, no outcome studies have been undertaken, and so their long-term use has not been proven to be more effective than the less expensive sulphonylureas. Therefore, their exact place in therapy is currently unclear.

Thiazolidinediones

Research into the action of the thiazolidinediones, also known as glitazones, has led to greater understanding of the development of type 2 diabetes. Only one glitazone, pioglitazone, is currently available following the removal of rosiglitazone from the UK market in 2010. Pioglitazone has been shown to have a significant benefit on macrovascular morbidity and mortality, demonstrating the benefit of a glucose-lowering agent on macrovascular disease (Dormandy et al., 2005).

Mode of action. The glitazones act as agonists of the nuclear peroxisome proliferator-activated receptor-γ (PPAR-γ). PPAR-γ is mostly expressed in adipose tissue but is also found in pancreatic β-cells, vascular endothelium and macrophages. It is also expressed weakly in those tissues that express predominantly PPAR-α, for example, skeletal muscle, liver and heart. The thiazolidinediones lower fasting and post-prandial glucose levels in addition to lowering free fatty acid and insulin concentrations. They enhance insulin sensitivity and promote glucose uptake and utilisation in peripheral tissues. They also suppress gluconeogenesis in the liver and, by increasing insulin sensitivity in adipose tissue, suppress free fatty acid concentrations. In addition, patients with IGT have shown increased insulin secretory responses. However, they do not have a direct effect on insulin secretion. The indirect effects of glitazones on adipose tissue are due to alterations in the regulation of gene expression. Various adipokines (adiponectin, tumour necrosis factor-α, resistin and 11β-hydroxysteroid dehydrogenase 1) are regulated by PPAR-γ agonists in animal studies. Other effects of glitazones on the vasculature include antiatherogenic effects thought to be caused by a reduction in the inflammatory response, decrease in vasoconstriction and an increase in plaque stability.

Pharmacokinetics. Pioglitazone is metabolised extensively in the liver to both active and inactive metabolites (see Table 44.4).

Adverse effects. Pioglitazone has been associated with weight gain and oedema, particularly in patients with hypertension and congestive cardiac failure. Since the thiazolidinediones can lead to a worsening of heart failure that may be fatal, pioglitazone should not be used in patients with a previous history of or pre-existing heart failure. Combination therapy with insulin and thiazolidinediones has been found to result in a higher incidence of oedema. There is also an increased risk of bone fracture with pioglitazone, and it should be used with caution in post-menopausal women. Anaemia occurs in about 1% of patients and is seen as a small decrease in the haemoglobin concentration during the first 4–12 weeks of therapy. However, it is suggested this decrease is due to dilutional effects caused by an increase in serum volume. Pioglitazone caused weight gain of around 3.5 kg during clinical trials. Some patients also experience headache, abdominal pain, myalgia and upper respiratory infection. Pioglitazone may also elevate liver transaminases.

Rosiglitazone was withdrawn from the UK market because use was associated with an increased risk of cardiovascular disorders, including heart attacks and heart failure. Another thiazolidinedione, troglitazone, was withdrawn from the UK market in 1997 because of liver failure linked to a toxic metabolite of troglitazone.

Dosage. Pioglitazone is started at a dose of 15 mg or 30 mg and may be increased to 45 mg once daily. In combination with metformin or a sulphonylurea, the current dose can be continued. Administration of pioglitazone may be either with or without food. Dosage adjustment is not necessary in patients with mild or moderate renal impairment or in the elderly. However, neither agent should be used in patients with severe renal impairment or in those with hepatic impairment.

Drug interactions. Pioglitazone is metabolised by cytochrome P450 CYP3A4. Therefore, drugs which induce or inhibit this enzyme interact with pioglitazone. Ketoconazole, itraconazole, erythromycin and fluconazole increase serum concentrations, while rifampicin and phenytoin decrease serum levels of pioglitazone.

Role of thiazolidinediones. Thiazolidinediones improve glycaemic control in patients, especially in those with insulin resistance, by reducing HbA_{1c} levels up to 1.5% compared to sulphonylurea or metformin alone.

Glitazones should be used as third-line therapy after life style modification and the use of metformin or a sulphonylurea as monotherapy. However, if glycaemic control remains poor, pioglitazone can be used either with metformin if treatment with a sulphonylurea is unsuitable, with a sulphonylurea if treatment with metformin is unsuitable, or with metformin and a sulphonylurea if insulin is unsuitable (National Institute for Health and Clinical Excellence, 2009). Treatment should only be continued if, after 6 months of treatment, the HbA_{1c} has reduced by 0.5% of its starting value.

Monotherapy with a thiazolidinedione may be a valuable treatment option for patients who are known to be insulin resistant. Triple therapy can be an alternative to transferring a patient to insulin, but the modest reduction in HbA_{1c} usually means that many patients will eventually require insulin. It is important to be aware that owing to their mode of action involving changes in gene transcription, thiazolidinediones take up to 3 months to have their maximum effect on glycaemic control.

α-glucosidase inhibitors

Acarbose reduces carbohydrate digestion by interfering with gastro-intestinal glucosidase activity. Although overall carbohydrate absorption is not significantly altered, the post-prandial hyperglycaemic peaks are markedly reduced. Acarbose is minimally absorbed in unchanged form from the gastro-intestinal tract.

Adverse effects. The most common adverse effect of acarbose is abdominal discomfort associated with flatulence and diarrhoea. These symptoms usually improve with continued treatment but can be minimised by starting with a low dose and titrating slowly.

Systemic adverse effects are rare but high doses have been associated with idiosyncratic elevations of serum hepatic transaminase levels. Patients titrated to the maximum dose of 200 mg three times daily should be closely monitored, preferably at monthly intervals for the first 6 months. If elevated transaminase levels are observed, reduction in dose or withdrawal of therapy should be considered.

Role of acarbose. Acarbose is a therapeutic option in type 2 patients inadequately controlled by diet alone, or by diet and other oral hypoglycaemic agents. However, the gastro-intestinal side effects do limit the use of acarbose in clinical practice.

Dipeptidyl peptidase-4 inhibitors

The DPP-4 inhibitors are a new class of drugs that work on the incretin system. They are also commonly referred to as the 'gliptins'.

Mode of action. DPP-4 inhibitors block the normal inactivation of incretins (glucagon like peptide-1 [GLP-1] and glucose-dependent insulinotropic peptide [GIP]). Incretins play a role in increasing endogenous insulin in response to a high glucose load, that is, post-prandially. They also reduce the amount of glucose produced by the liver when glucose levels are sufficiently high. By blocking DPP-4, these drugs prolong incretin activity and inhibit glucagon release. This in turn causes a decrease in blood glucose and an increase in insulin secretion.

Pharmacokinetics. DPP-4 inhibitors are predominantly renally excreted. However, there is also a degree of hepatic metabolism involved in the elimination process, which varies with each drug. Sitagliptin is mainly excreted as unchanged drug in the urine, with a small metabolic contribution from the liver via the cytochrome P450 system. The kidney is thought to be mainly responsible for metabolic hydrolysis of vildagliptin to an inactive compound. Although saxagliptin is mainly eliminated renally, some hepatic biotransformation does occur via the cytochrome P450 system (CYP3A4/5), which results in a metabolite with half the potency of the parent compound. The pharmacokinetic parameters of the DPP-4 inhibitors are detailed in Table 44.4.

Adverse effects. All three DPP-4 inhibitors have been linked to gastro-intestinal side effects and upper respiratory tract infection. DPP-4 inhibitors do not cause hypoglycaemia, but they have the potential to cause hypoglycaemia when prescribed with other agents that can produce this effect. Vildagliptin has been associated with rare reports of liver dysfunction. Therefore, it is recommended liver function tests are performed prior to starting treatment, at 3-monthly intervals for the first year and then periodically thereafter.

Drug interactions. DPP-4 inhibitors have a low potential for interaction with other medicines. However, as both sitagliptin and saxagliptin are metabolised by cytochrome P450 3A4/5 (and CYP2C8 for sitagliptin), they have the potential to interact with potent inducers or inhibitors of these enzyme. In practice, few drugs have been formally assessed. Therefore, general advice is to monitor blood glucose levels carefully if one of these drugs is co-prescribed with sitagliptin or saxagliptin.

Role of dipeptidyl peptidase-4 inhibitors. DPP-4 inhibitors are licensed for use as dual therapy with metformin, a sulphonylurea or a thiazolidinedione. Sitagliptin is also licensed as both mono- and triple therapy with metformin and a sulphonlyurea or a thiazolidinedione. Similar to the thiazolidinediones, it is recommended that a DPP-4 inhibitor is used as third-line therapy typically in those who still do not have adequate control or cannot tolerate treatment with metformin and/or a sulphonylurea. DPP-4 inhibitors are also useful if further weight gain is likely. However, if insulin resistance is a key factor, then treating with a thiazolidinedione may be a better choice.

Incretin mimetics

The incretin mimetics, as the name suggests, mimic the effects of incretins. The two currently licensed in the UK, exenatide and liraglutide, are only available as subcutaneously injectable products. Incretin mimetics have both been demonstrated to cause weight loss, which is a particularly beneficial effect in many patients with type 2 diabetes.

Mode of action. The incretin mimetics bind to and activate the glucagon-like peptide-1 (GLP-1) receptor, hence increasing insulin secretion, suppressing glucagon secretion, increasing satiety and slowing gastric emptying. All of these effects help to lower blood glucose levels.

Pharmacokinetics. Incretin mimetics have a longer duration of action than endogenous GLP-1. Exenatide is eliminated primarily by renal clearance. However, the specific organ responsible for liraglutide elimination has not been identified. Table 44.4 details additional pharmacokinetic parameters of the incretin mimetics.

Adverse effects. Both incretin mimetics have been associated with nausea, and other gastro-intestinal disturbances. However, once therapy has been established, the incidence of these side effects decreases. Acute pancreatitis has also been rarely reported. For this reason, both patients and their carers should be advised of the signs and symptoms of this complication and advised to stop taking the drug and seek medical attention immediately if they occur. Since the incretin mimetics cause glucose-dependent insulin release, hypoglycaemia is uncommon and in most cases can be attributed to other agents taken concurrently

Drug interactions. The potential for drug interactions with the incretin mimetics is low. However, as they can cause a delay in gastric emptying, they may influence the absorption of other medicines administered at the same time. For this reason, it is advised that any narrow therapeutic index drugs taken concomitantly are monitored carefully. Also, if other oral medicines are being taken where the threshold concentration is important (e.g. antibiotics), it is advised that these should be taken at least 1 h before exenatide. This may be assumed for liraglutide, although this is not specifically stated in the summary of product characteristics.

Role of incretin mimetics. It is recommended that exenatide be added to metformin and a sulphonylurea as third-line therapy (as an alternative to insulin, thiazolidinediones or DPP-4 inhibitors) for patients who have either a BMI of ≥35 kg/m², are of European decent (adjustments to this threshold may be made for other ethnic groups at greater risk of cardiac disease) and have other medical problems associated with increased body weight. Alternatively, exenatide may be used in patients with a BMI <35 kg/m² who are not able to take insulin, for example, for occupational reasons, or who have other conditions that would benefit from weight loss. Treatment should only be continued if there has been an HbA_{1c} reduction of at least 1% and a weight loss of at least 3% from starting treatment, over a 6-month period.

Insulin therapy in type 2 diabetes

The younger age of onset of type 2 diabetes and tighter glycaemic targets mean that the majority of patients with type 2 diabetes progress to insulin therapy, since recent evidence confirms that long-term glycaemic improvement reduces the risk of both microvascular (Holman et al., 2008) and macrovascular (Turnbull et al., 2009) complications.

It is currently common practice to introduce insulin to an oral medication schedule, although if hypoglycaemia becomes a problem, then the oral medications may be reduced or stopped. A number of different insulin regimens for use in patients with type 2 diabetes are available, the most common of which include once-daily basal insulin, twice-daily biphasic (pre-mixed) insulin, or prandial insulin, using a rapid/short-acting insulin with meals. Until recently, there have not been any trial data to determine which insulin regimen is most effective in controlling blood glucose levels and minimising hypoglycaemia in patients with type 2 diabetes. However, recent work suggests that patients who have basal insulin or prandial insulin added to their oral therapy have better HbA_{1c} control than those who receive biphasic insulin. In addition, the basal insulin regimen is associated with fewer hypoglycaemic episodes and less weight gain than the other two regimens (Holman et al., 2009). Basal insulin should be titrated to achieve normal fasting glucose levels, and the patient may be taught this self-titration protocol (Davies et al., 2005).

In a lean patient (BMI <25 kg/m²), significant insulin deficiency is more likely and therefore from the outset of insulin treatment either a basal-bolus or twice-daily regimen may be preferred.

In type 2 patients who require temporary insulin during intercurrent illness, a soluble preparation such as Humulin S or Human Actrapid can be given two or three times daily with a small dose of isophane insulin at bedtime to control blood glucose quickly and eliminate symptoms. The dose is selected initially according to the patient's previous insulin requirements, if any, and adjusted according to four times daily blood glucose measurements.

Treating hypertension

The co-existence of hypertension and diabetes dramatically increases the risk of microvascular and macrovascular complications. Most important is the increased risk of cardiovascular disease. Tight control of blood pressure may be a more effective method of preventing complications in patients with type 2 diabetes than tight glycaemic control. It is recommended that, for patients with type 2 diabetes, the target blood pressure should be <140/80 mmHg, or for those with pre-existing kidney, eye or cerebrovascular damage the target should be reduced to <130/80 (National Institute for Health and Clinical Excellence, 2009). First-line blood-pressure-lowering therapy should be a once-daily, generically prescribed angiotensin-converting enzyme (ACE) inhibitor. Exceptions to this are people of African-Caribbean descent, in whom first-line therapy should be an ACE inhibitor plus either a diuretic or a generic calcium-channel blocker.

In young patients with type 1 diabetes, the blood pressure target is <135/80 mmHg. However, if there is abnormal albumin excretion (renal disease) or two features of the metabolic syndrome are present, then the blood pressure target should be lowered to 130/80 mmHg with maximal doses of either an ACE inhibitor or ARB as first-line therapy.

Treating obesity

Obesity is a significant risk factor in the development of type 2 diabetes. Evidence suggests that for each kilogram increase in body weight, the risk of diabetes increases by 4.5%. It is estimated that almost one-fifth of the population has a BMI of over $30\,kg/m^2$ and is therefore obese.

Treatment of obesity may require modification of lifestyle (diet and exercise regimens) to reduce calorie intake and increase calorie utilisation, pharmacological intervention and/or surgery. Currently orlistat, a lipase inhibitor, is the only drug available on prescription for the treating of obesity. Orlistat can also be purchased in community pharmacies as a branded over-the-counter product. Both sibutramine and rimonabant were withdrawn because of unwanted side effects.

Orlistat is licensed for use with a 'mildly hypocalorific diet' to treat obese people (BMI $>30\,kg/m^2$) or overweight patients with a BMI $>28\,kg/m^2$ and associated risk factors. It should be discontinued after 12 weeks if a 5% weight reduction since the start of treatment has not been achieved. Orlistat increases the amount of faecal fat excretion but is associated with a number of gastro-intestinal side effects such as oily leakage from the rectum, flatulence, faecal urgency and incontinence. A greater reduction in the incidence of type 2 diabetes has been observed in patients treated with both orlistat and lifestyle modification (Torgerson et al., 2004).

Over recent years, the use of bariatric surgery has increased in popularity, which is another treatment option for those who are seriously struggling with their weight with a BMI over 35–$40\,kg/m^2$, who have other conditions caused by being overweight such as diabetes.

Patient care

Patient education

Patient involvement is paramount for the successful care of diabetes. This is highlighted in the national service standards for diabetes (Department of Health, 2002) which state that all patients, and carers, where appropriate, will be encouraged to develop a partnership with their clinicians to enable them to manage their diabetes and maintain a healthy lifestyle, often through shared care plans. Structured education for patients with type 2 diabetes is important and should be offered to every patient and/or their carer around the time of diagnosis. It is considered to be an integral part of diabetes care (National Institute for Health and Clinical Excellence, 2009).

Education will depend upon the individual patient and the availability of local resources. Individual tuition is preferable in the early stages after diagnosis and is usually delivered by a diabetes specialist nurse. The educational aspect of care is a gradual and ongoing process. At a later stage, group education can be effective and many patients appreciate and find support in meeting others who have the same disease. Many such programmes are multidisciplinary and involve doctors, nurses, dieticians, pharmacists and chiropodists. It is essential to involve the patient's family and carers in the educational process. Patients can also obtain support and information from specialist organisations such as Diabetes UK (available at www.diabetes.org.uk/home.htm).

Patients require education and information about many subjects, ranging from general lifestyle advice through to knowledge about the medicines they are prescribed (Box 44.4).

Advice about the use of over-the-counter medications, diet, foot care products and diabetic food products is frequently requested.

Annual review

People with diabetes should attend their hospital clinic or primary care practice (if this service is offered locally) for an annual review to screen for diabetic complications. Monitoring and optimising glycaemic control are also undertaken although this should be done on a more regular basis, as should review of patients with known complications. The annual review is increasingly taking place in primary care, with referral to secondary care if required. The typical assessments undertaken at an annual review are described in Box 44.5.

Box 44.4 Patient education in diabetes

1. The disease
   Signs and symptoms
2. Hyperglycaemia
   Signs, symptoms and treatments
3. Hypoglycaemia
   Signs, symptoms and treatments
4. Exercise
   Benefits and effect on blood glucose control
5. Diet
6. Insulin therapy
   Injection technique
   Types of insulin
   Onset and peak actions
   Storage
   Stability
7. Urine testing
   Glucose
   Ketones
8. Home blood glucose testing
   Technique
   Interpretation
9. Oral hypoglycaemic agents
   Mode of action
   Dosing
   Need for multiple therapies
10. Foot care
11. Management during illness
12. Cardiovascular risk factors
    Smoking
    Hypertension
    Obesity
    Hyperlipidaemia
13. Regular medical and ophthalmological examinations

Box 44.5 Annual review for diabetes

Routine assessment
Capillary blood glucose level
Weight, body mass index and waist circumference
Blood pressure
Urinalysis for glucose, protein and ketones
Foot assessment

Laboratory investigations
Fasting lipid profile
HbA$_{1c}$
U&E, creatinine
Liver function tests
Urine specimen for albumin:creatinine ratio (ACR)

Referral, if appropriate
Retinopathy screening (should be done annually)
Dietician
Podiatry
Exercise programme
Smoking cessation programme

Box 44.6 Common therapeutic problems in diabetes

- Achieving normoglycaemia or HbA$_{1c}$ targets
- Achieving an acceptable balance between improving glycaemic control and minimising episodes of hypoglycaemia
- Achieving adequate control in type 2 diabetes with diet alone, especially in patients who are overweight
- Drug-related weight gain, notably with insulin and sulphonylureas
- Achieving blood pressure targets in patients with co-existing hypertension
- Ensuring adherence as drug regimens become complex, requiring multiple drug therapies
- Making insulin therapy acceptable to patients with type 2 diabetes, inadequately controlled with oral therapies

---

Glycaemic management targets

The theoretical ideal for all patients with diabetes is to achieve normoglycaemia. As this is not always possible, the aim is to achieve the best possible control compatible with an acceptable lifestyle for the patient. In some patients, this may mean only symptomatic control, in others this may be tight control. In making this decision, the following factors should be considered: the patient's age, motivation, intelligence, understanding, likely adherence, co-existing diseases, ability to recognise hypoglycaemia, duration of their diabetes and the presence/absence/severity of diabetic complications.

Targets for pre-meal blood glucose of between 4 and 7 mmol/L and post-meal values of <10 mmol/L may be set for most patients, provided there is no significant hypoglycaemia risk. An optimal HbA$_{1c}$ target of 6.5% for most of those with type 2 diabetes has been suggested (National Institute for Health and Clinical Excellence, 2009). However, it is recommended that targets should be individualised and that for some a higher target would be more appropriate especially if there is a risk of hypoglycaemia at the lower target. For those with type 1 diabetes, the recommended target is less than 7.5% (National Institute for Health and Clinical Excellence, 2004).

The diabetes treatment goals in older people may be different and more conservative than in younger adults. For example, some elderly patients may have poor vision and limited manual dexterity, which may or may not be linked to a degree of cognitive impairment. Others may have multiple pathology and take a number of other medications. Therefore, the goals of therapy need to be both individual and realistic. In some people, they will involve only the optimisation of body weight, control of symptoms and avoidance of hypoglycaemia which has an increased risk of severe brain damage and may occur without the usual warning signs in the elderly. In others, reasonably tight control may be appropriate. There

is, therefore, a difficult balance between the use of aggressive treatment with its associated risk of hypoglycaemia and the benefits of reducing complications to maintain an acceptable quality of life. Box 44.6 sets out some of the common therapeutic problems in diabetes.

Monitoring glycaemic control

Clinic monitoring

There are several ways in which glycaemic control can be monitored in primary and secondary care. Estimates of average control are often useful. Glycation of minor haemoglobin components occurs in the blood, with the extent depending on both the amount of glucose present and the duration of exposure of the haemoglobin to glucose. Estimates of glycated haemoglobin (HbA$_{1c}$) provide an index of average diabetes control over the preceding 2–3 months, that is, the lifespan of a red blood cell. HbA$_{1c}$ can be measured at any time, the patient does not need to be fasted, and levels are not normally affected by acute changes in therapy, diet or exercise. However, they may be lower in those with reduced red cell lifespan, for example, pregnancy or advanced renal failure. Serum fructosamine represents the glycation of all serum proteins and gives information about control over the preceding 3 weeks. As albumin is the major serum protein, hypoalbuminaemia may affect fructosamine levels. However, HbA$_{1c}$ is the preferred marker for average glycaemic control.

Home monitoring

Type 1 diabetes. All patients treated with insulin should be offered home blood glucose monitoring (HBGM). Capillary blood is applied to a reagent strip which has been impregnated with enzymes, for example, glucose oxidase. Some home blood glucose monitoring methods require visual comparison of colour changes which correspond to various blood glucose concentrations. More commonly, meters may be used to give readings and are more convenient for people who are colour blind or who have poor eyesight. Home blood glucose monitoring enables patients and carers to make a direct assessment of the effect of changes in medicines, dietary habits, exercise and patterns of illness. It has the additional benefit that it can detect hypoglycaemia and, unlike urine testing in which glycosuria may only be detected some time after changes in blood glucose have occurred, it enables more accurate calculations of insulin doses.

Patients with type 1, who are by definition ketosis prone, should also know how and when to test their urine for ketones. This test need not be carried out as part of routine monitoring but is essential at times of intercurrent illness, especially when the blood glucose is ≥17 mmol/L.

Type 2 diabetes. Many people with type 2 diabetes are treated with diet alone or with oral hypoglycaemic agents, and unless they have problems with hypoglycaemia, urine glucose monitoring should be adequate. This is a simple non-invasive test that can detect hyperglycaemia but not hypoglycaemia. Home blood glucose monitoring is used by some patients with type 2, particularly if control is poor, if they are undergoing medication dose titration, if they are being treated with insulin or if they are prone to hypoglycaemia. It is also recommended that blood glucose monitoring be undertaken before driving and at times of intercurrent illness, when blood glucose levels may be particularly erratic.

Regardless of whether individuals with type 1 or type 2 diabetes are using home blood glucose monitoring or urine testing, it is important they are educated about what to do with the results; otherwise, there is little point in testing.

Case studies

Case 44.1

Mrs TM is a 36-year-old married lady who has type 1 diabetes. She undertook a home pregnancy test because she was feeling particularly nauseated in the mornings and her period was late. The test was positive confirming that she was pregnant. However, at 8 weeks, she experienced vaginal bleeding and abdominal pain. She attended the Accident & Emergency department, where a miscarriage was confirmed. Upon questioning, it was discovered that she had been taking folic acid 400 μcg daily for the previous 6 months but had not received any pre-conception diabetes care. Her most recent HbA$_{1c}$ was 7.3% (56 mmol/mol). Her regular medications are ramipril 10 mg daily, simvastatin 40 mg daily, insulin glargine at night and insulin aspart three times daily with meals.

Questions

1. Why should women of childbearing age be offered advice about pregnancy?
2. What blood glucose targets should Mrs TM have been advised to aim for before and after conceiving?
3. Was she taking appropriate dietary supplements prior to conception?
4. What advice should she be given with respect to her regular medication?

Answers

1. Mrs TM should have been offered preconception advice prior to becoming pregnant because glucose control needs to be optimal to reduce the risks of miscarriage, congenital malformation, stillbirth and neonatal death associated with diabetes in early pregnancy. Preconception advice should also include information for the patient on how diabetes affects pregnancy and how pregnancy affects diabetes, what dietary supplements to take and advice on diabetes-related medicines that are unsafe to take during pregnancy.
2. Mrs TM should aim for an HbA$_{1c}$ target of below 6.1% (43 mmol/mol) before conceiving. During pregnancy, she should aim for fasting blood glucose levels of 3.5–5.9 mmol/L and 1-h postprandial levels of below 7.8 mmol/L.
3. Mrs TM was taking the appropriate dietary supplement; however, the recommended dose for women with diabetes is 5 mg daily, rather than 400 μcg daily. The 5-mg strength tablets are available on prescription.
4. Mrs TM should have been advised to stop her ramipril and simvastatin since both have been associated with an increased risk of birth defects.

Case 44.2

Mr LG is a 47-year-old man with type 2 diabetes. He has recently had basal insulin (insulin detemir) added into his other diabetes medicines: metformin modified release 1 g twice a day and gliclazide 80 mg twice a day. He complains of waking with a headache and feeling 'groggy' and unrested in the morning. His recent blood glucose readings have generally been very good although his before breakfast readings are 10–13 mmol/L. He is worried because he is feeling worse since he started insulin, even though his blood glucose levels are much improved. He has made an appointment with his primary care doctor. His primary care doctor suspects nocturnal hypoglycaemia may be causing his recent symptoms.

Questions

1. What is nocturnal hypoglycaemia?
2. Why might nocturnal hypoglycaemia cause raised blood glucose levels in the mornings?
3. How can the diagnosis of nocturnal hypoglycaemia be confirmed?
4. How should it be treated?

Answers

1. Nocturnal hypoglycaemia is a low blood glucose reading that occurs during the night. Definitions vary but it is generally accepted that a reading of less than 3.5 mmol/L is 'hypoglycaemia'. The normal symptoms of hypoglycaemia may be missed if the patient does not wake. However, signs noticed (often by partners) might include restlessness, sweating and nightmares. Symptoms experienced by the patient in the mornings commonly include headache, lethargy and raised blood glucose levels.
2. Nocturnal hypoglycaemia may be caused by a rebound rise in blood glucose levels due to the 'somogyi effect'. This is the effect of the counter-regulatory hormones, glucagon, cortisol, adrenaline (epinephrine) and growth hormone, which all increase glucose in response to low levels.

3. Commonly, nocturnal hypoglycaemia can be confirmed by undertaking a blood glucose reading in the early hours of the morning, that is, between 2 and 4 am. This may require the patient to set their alarm to be woken at this time.
4. Nocturnal hypoglycaemia once confirmed may be treated by either having a bed-time snack, or by reducing the dose of night-time insulin. In the case of Mr LG, stopping his sulphonylurea may also help resolve the problem. Care must be taken when interpreting raised blood glucose levels in the morning, since the obvious intervention would be to increase the dose of night-time insulin. However when nocturnal hypoglycaemia is the cause, increasing the insulin dose would only make the problem worse and more dangerous for the patient.

Case 44.3

Mr PT is a 69-year-old man with longstanding type 2 diabetes. He has recently noticed that his right shoe has been rubbing his foot, which he finds confusing since he has been wearing these shoes for 6 months with no problems. His whole left foot now looks red and swollen and when Mr PT inspected it closely, he noticed that there was a weeping sore. However, his foot is not painful, so he does not feel too concerned.

Questions

1. What is the most likely reason that Mr PT did not feel any pain associated with the sore?
2. Why might Mr PT's shoe suddenly have started to rub his foot?
3. Should he be more concerned?

Answers

1. Mr PT has probably developed sensory neuropathy in his feet. This usually begins with the loss of the sensation of vibration and then may progressively lead onto the loss of sensation altogether.
2. The shape of the feet of people with diabetes has been observed to change over time. This may be due to the development of neuropathy which can weaken muscles causing alterations to the shape of the arch of the foot and toes. In this case, we know that Mr PT has sensory neuropathy since he is unable to feel the pain of the weeping sore. It is likely that Mr PT may also have motor neuropathy.
3. Mr PT should be concerned because his lack of sensation does not indicate that the foot injury is not serious. He is at risk of developing an infected ulcer and needs prompt treatment to prevent the problem from becoming severe. If he does not seek treatment, he may even risk losing his foot through amputation.

Case 44.4

Miss IL is a 17-year-old teenager with recently diagnosed type 1 diabetes. She has been admitted to hospital with diabetic ketoacidosis (DKA), which was precipitated by a diarrhoea and vomiting bug. As she was vomiting she was not eating, and hence she temporarily stopped injecting her insulin.

She is normally well controlled on a basal bolus insulin regimen comprising insulin glargine (Lantus) at night and insulin glulisine (Apidra) three times daily with meals.

Questions

1. Why was it a mistake for Miss IL not to inject her insulin whilst she was not feeling well enough to eat?
2. What advice should patients on insulin be given regarding glucose management when they are feeling unwell and not able to eat normally?
3. What are the initial management priorities for patients admitted with diabetic ketoacidosis?
4. What is the correct way for subcutaneous insulin to be re-introduced after a patient has been on a continuous intravenous insulin infusion?

Answers

1. This is a common misunderstanding amongst patients and sometimes even health care professionals. When a person is unwell, their basal insulin requirements can often increase, despite not eating. This is because of the stress involved and the increase in the production of counter-regulatory hormones which increase glucose levels.
2. Patients should be counselled on what are commonly referred to as 'sick day rules' and should be given contact numbers for advice if they are unclear or struggling with management. Generally patients need to increase the frequency of glucose monitoring to 4-hourly or more and test urine for ketones on a regular basis. Carbohydrate intake should be maintained as much as possible using sugary drinks or fruit juice, soups, jelly or snack foods if they are having difficulty in eating. Fluid intake is important and patients should be advised to have a glass of water every hour, aiming for 3 L in 24 h. If the blood glucose level is less than 12 mmol/L and ketone result is negative-small, patients should continue their normal insulin dose. If the blood glucose level is between 12 and 18 mmol/L and the ketone result is negative-small, the patient should re-test within 4 h or at the next meal and add 4 extra units of insulin to doses of up to 20 units and 8 extra units to doses greater than 20 units. If the blood glucose level is more than 18 mmol/L and ketones are moderate or large, patients should take 50% extra insulin. If blood glucose is more than 20 mmol/L and ketones are moderate or large, the dose of insulin should be doubled. If the patient is vomiting and blood glucose levels are over 16 mmol/L, then medical help should be sought, especially if there is no improvement after the second test or the next insulin injection.
3. Intravenous sodium chloride 0.9% should be started as soon as possible. A fixed rate intravenous insulin infusion should then be started. Current recommendations are to begin at a rate of 0.1 units/kg. Regular hourly monitoring of blood glucose and ketones should be undertaken and 2-hourly monitoring of serum potassium for the first 6 h.
4. When the patient is biochemically stable, they may be converted back to subcutaneous insulin. The current national guidelines from the Joint British Societies Inpatient Care Group (2010) recommend that long-acting subcutaneous insulin analogues are continued throughout treatment of diabetic ketoacidosis in order to prevent rebound hyperglycaemia when the intravenous infusion is stopped. Therefore, Miss IL's glargine should have been continued. Her rapid-acting insulin (Apidra®) should be re-introduced at the next meal and the intravenous insulin infusion should be stopped 30 min afterwards.

References

DAFNE Study Group, 2002. Training in flexible, intensive insulin management to enable dietary freedom in people with type 1 diabetes: dose adjustment for normal eating (DAFNE) randomised controlled trial. Br. Med. J. 325, 746–749.

Davies, M., Storms, F., Shutler, S., et al., 2005. Improvement of glycaemic control in subjects with poorly controlled type 2 diabetes. Diabetes Care 28, 1282–1288.

Department of Health, 2002. National Service Framework for Diabetes: Standards. Department of Health, London.

Dormandy, J.A., Charbonnel, B., Eckland, D.J.A., et al., 2005. Secondary prevention of macrovascular events in patients with type 2 diabetes in the PROactive Study (PROspective pioglitAzone Clinical Trial In macroVascular Events): a randomised controlled trial. Lancet 366, 1279–1289.

Holman, R., Paul, S., Bethel, M., et al., 2008. 10-year follow-up of intensive glucose control in type 2 diabetes. N. Engl. J. Med. 359, 1577–89.

Holman, R., Farmer, A., Davies, M., et al., 2009. Three-year efficacy of complex insulin regimens in type 2 diabetes. N. Engl. J. Med. 361, 1736–47.

Joint British Societies Inpatient Care Group, 2010. The Management of Diabetic Ketoacidosis in Adults. NHS Diabetes. Available at: http://www.diabetes.nhs.uk/.

Khan, R., Buse, J., Ferrannini, E., et al., 2005. The metabolic syndrome: time for a critical appraisal. Joint statement from the American Diabetes Association and the European Association for the Study of Diabetes. Diab. Care 28, 2289–2304.

National Institute for Health and Clinical Excellence, 2004. Type 1 Diabetes: Diagnosis and Management of Type 1 Diabetes in Children, Young People and Adults. Clinical Guideline 15. NICE, London. Available at: http://www.nice.org.uk/nicemedia/pdf/CG015NICEguideline.pdf.

National Institute for Health and Clinical Excellence, 2006. Obesity: Guidance on the Prevention, Identification, Assessment and Management of Overweight and Obesity in Adults and Children. Clinical Guideline 43. NICE, London. Available at: http://www.nice.org.uk/nicemedia/pdf/CG43NICEGuideline.pdf.

National Institute for Health and Clinical Excellence, 2008. Continuous Subcutaneous Insulin Infusion for the Treatment of Diabetes Mellitus. Technology Appraisal 57. NICE, London. Available at: http://www.nice.org.uk/nicemedia/live/12014/41300/41300.pdf.

National Institute for Health and Clinical Excellence, 2009. Type 2 Diabetes: The Management of Type 2 Diabetes. Clinical Guideline 87. NICE, London. Available at: http://guidance.nice.org.uk/CG87/NICEGuidance/pdf/English.

National Institute for Health and Clinical Excellence, 2010. Neuropathic Pain: The Pharmacological Management of Neuropathic Pain in Adults in Non-Specialist Settings. Clinical Guideline 96. NICE, London. Available at: http://www.nice.org.uk/nicemedia/live/12948/47949/47949.pdf.

Torgerson, J.S., Hauptman, J., Boldrin, M.N., et al., 2004. XENical in the Prevention of Diabetes in Obese Subjects (XENDOS) Study. Diabetes Care 27, 155–161.

Turnbull, F., Abraira, C., Anderson, R., et al., 2009. Intensive glucose control and macrovascular outcomes in type 2 diabetes. Diabetologia 52, 2288–98.

World Health Organization, 2006. Definition and Diagnosis of Diabetes Mellitus and Intermediate Hyperglycemia: Report of a WHO/IDF Consultation. Available at: www.who.int/diabetes/publications/en.

Further reading

Aldhahi, W., Hamdy, O., 2003. Adipokines, inflammation, and the endothelium in diabetes. Curr. Diab. Rep. 3, 293–298.

Diabetes UK in partnership with NHS diabetes, 2009. Putting Feet First. Available at: http://www.diabetes.org.uk/Documents/Reports/Putting_Feet_First_010709.pdf.

Fowler, D., Rayman, G., 2010. Safe and Effective Use of Insulin in Hospitalised Patients. Available at: http://www.diabetes.nhs.uk/.

Gerstein, H.C., Miller, M.E., Byington, R.P., et al., 2008. Action to Control Cardiovascular Risk in Diabetes (ACCORD) Study Group, Effects of intensive glucose lowering in type 2 diabetes. N. Engl. J. Med. 358, 2545–2559.

Joint British Societies Inpatient Care Group, 2010. The Hospital Management of Hypoglycaemia in Adults with Diabetes. NHS Diabetes. Available at: http://www.diabetes.nhs.uk/.

Joint British Societies Inpatient Care Group, 2010. The Management of Diabetic Ketoacidosis in Adults. NHS Diabetes. Available at: http://www.diabetes.nhs.uk/.

Lipsky, B.A., Berendt, A.R., Gunner Deery, H., et al., 2004. Infectious Disease Society of America (IDSA) guidelines – diagnosis and treatment of diabetic foot infections. Clin. Infect. Dis. 39, 885–910.

National Institute for Health and Clinical Excellence, 2010. Liraglutide for the Treatment of Type 2 Diabetes Mellitus. NICE, London. Available at: http://www.nice.org.uk/nicemedia/live/13248/51259/51259.pdf.

Patel, A., MacMahon, S., Chalmers, J., et al., 2008. Action in Diabetes and Vascular Disease: Preterax and Diamicron Modified Release Controlled Evaluation (ADVANCE) Collaborative Group. Intensive blood glucose control and vascular outcomes in patients with type 2 diabetes. N. Engl. J. Med. 358, 2560–2572.

Royal Pharmaceutical Society and National Pharmacy Association, 2010. Integrating Community Pharmacy into the Care of People with Diabetes – A Practical Resource. Royal Pharmaceutical Society and National Pharmacy Association. Available at: http://www.npa.co.uk/Documents/Docstore/NPA-Publications/Integrating_community_pharmacy_into_the_care_of_people_with_diabetes.pdf.

Menstrual cycle disorders 45

K. Marshall and S. Calvert

Key points

- Girls can begin experiencing menstrual disorders once ovulatory cycles are established.
- Up to 95% of women experience changes premenstrually, but severe premenstrual syndrome is more common in the 30–40 year age group.
- The aetiology of premenstrual syndrome is multifactorial, the symptomatology complex and treatment options diverse.
- It has been estimated that 50–80% of women of child-bearing age will suffer from dysmenorrhoea at some time.
- Treatment options vary according to the type of dysmenorrhoea (primary or secondary) but include non-steroidal anti-inflammatory drugs, combined oral contraceptive pills, and progestogen-only preparations.
- Menorrhagia (excessive menstrual blood loss) affects up to 30% of menstruating women. The management of the condition depends upon the cause and can be either surgical or medical.
- Endometriosis (the presence of extrauterine endometrial tissue) can give rise to an array of symptoms including subfertility. Treatment may be designed to improve fertility and manage symptoms. Medical and surgical treatments are available.

Once a girl reaches puberty, various physiological events occur, leading to the onset of menstruation, or the menarche. The average age of the menarche has decreased to around 12.5 years and a halt in this trend towards earlier menarche is not evident. This decline has been attributed to an improvement in nutrition and overall health. Body weight is linked to menarchal age and it is possible that as body fat increases so does serum leptin (hormone which influences calorie intake) which in turn may increase the pulsatile release of gonadotrophin-releasing hormone (GnRH).

Menstruation is an event that occurs relatively late in puberty and 95% of girls reach the menarche between the ages of 11 and 15 years. One UK study has shown that one girl in eight begins to menstruate whilst still at primary school. Even before the first ovulatory cycle has taken place, childhood ovarian activity will have gradually increased the production of oestrogen, leading to the development of the secondary sexual characteristics. These events are probably initiated by the central nervous system (CNS) which ultimately triggers the necessary gonadal changes that will eventually lead to the establishment of the menstrual cycle. It may take up to 2 years

for the hypothalamic–pituitary–gonadal axis to mature and for regular ovulation to take place. In girls who only start to menstruate when they are older, it may take even longer. This should be considered when taking a patient's medical history.

Menstruation itself occurs as a result of cyclic hormonal variations (Fig. 45.1). During the first half or follicular phase of the menstrual cycle, the endometrium thickens under the influence of increasing levels of oestrogen (most notably estradiol, which at the peak of its preovulatory surge reaches around 2000 pmol/L) secreted from the developing ovarian follicles. Once the serum oestrogen level has surpassed a critical point it triggers, by positive feedback, the anterior pituitary to release, about 24 h later, a surge of luteinising hormone (LH; up to 50 iu/L) and after 30–36 h, ovulation follows.

After ovulation, which occurs around day 14 of a 28-day menstrual cycle, and as the luteal phase progresses, the endometrium begins to respond to increasing levels of progesterone. Both progesterone and oestrogen are secreted from the corpus luteum which is formed from the remains of the ovarian follicle after ovulation. The lifespan of the corpus luteum is remarkably constant and lasts between 12 and 14 days; hence, the length of the second half or the luteal phase of the menstrual cycle is between 12 and 14 days. Between days 18 and 22 of a 28-day cycle, both sex steroids peak, with levels of progesterone reaching around 30 nmol/L. As progesterone has a thermogenic effect upon the hypothalamus, basal body temperature

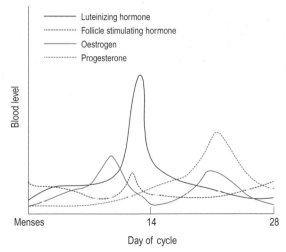

Fig. 45.1 The hormonal events that occur during the menstrual cycle in women.

711

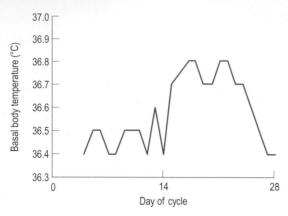

Fig. 45.2 Typical temperature chart from a 28-day ovulatory menstrual cycle.

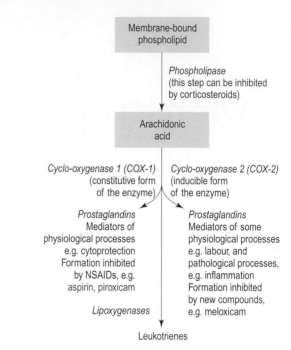

Fig. 45.3 Eicosanoid biosynthesis and inhibition.

increases by about 1 °C in the second half of an ovulatory cycle (Fig. 45.2). Most ovulatory cycles range from 21 to 34 days.

These synchronised changes mean that about a week after ovulation, the endometrium is prepared for implantation, providing fertilisation has taken place. If conception does not occur, then luteolysis begins and steroid levels fall. This means that the endometrium cannot be maintained, there is a loss of stromal fluid, leucocyte infiltration begins and there is intraglandular extravasation of blood. Finally, endometrial blood flow is reduced and this leads to necrosis and sloughing, that is menstruation. Initially, the blood vessels that remain intact after sloughing are sealed by fibrin and platelet plugs; subsequent haemostasis is probably achieved as a result of vasoconstriction of the remaining basal arteries. Nitric oxide may be involved in the initiation and maintenance of menstrual bleeding by promoting vasodilation and inhibiting platelet aggregation. The myometrium is the muscular layers of the uterus that contract spontaneously throughout the menstrual cycle, the frequency of these contractions being influenced by the hormonal milieu. The myometrium is also more active during menstruation. The average blood loss per period is between 30 and 40 mL.

There is evidence which suggests a physiological and pathological role for the local hormones, known as prostaglandins, in the process of menstruation. Prostaglandins are 20-carbon oxygenated, polyunsaturated bioactive lipids, which are cyclo-oxygenase-derived products of arachidonic acid. Indeed, both the myometrium and the endometrium are capable of synthesising and responding to prostaglandins. A potential role for another family of autocoids, the leukotrienes, in the regulation of uterine function remains uncertain, although it is known that leukotrienes can also be synthesised from arachidonic acid by lipoxygenase enzymes (Fig. 45.3).

Disorders associated with menstruation are a major medical and social problem for women which also impact upon their families.

Premenstrual syndrome (PMS)

PMS encompasses both mood changes and physical symptoms. Symptoms may start up to 14 days before menstruation, although more usually they begin just a few days before and disappear at the onset of, or shortly after, menstruation. However, for some women, the beginning of menstruation may not signal the complete resolution of symptoms. Numerous studies have demonstrated that this condition can cause substantial impairment of normal daily activity, including reduced occupational activity and significant levels of work absenteeism. Severity varies from cycle to cycle and may be influenced by other life factors such as stress and tiredness. The most severe form of PMS may be referred to as premenstrual dysphoric disorder (PMDD) as defined by the Modified Diagnostic and Statistical Manual of Mental Disorders appendix IV, or DSM-IV (American Psychiatric Association, 2000) and for which the criteria are set out in Box 45.1. Other bodies (American College of Obstetricians and Gynecologists, 2000) have published diagnostic criteria for PMS (Box 45.2). There is considerable overlap between PMS and PMDD.

Epidemiology

Up to 95% of menstruating women experience some changes premenstrually. Clinically relevant PMS occurs in about 15–20% of these women and PMDD has an estimated incidence of 3–8%. It has been estimated that PMS may account for over 17 million disability-adjusted life years (DALYS) in the European Union. PMS affects young and older women alike and does not appear to be influenced by parity. Severe PMS is more common in the 30–40 year age range, and married women with young children commonly seek help. Certain events may be linked with the onset of PMS, including childbirth, cessation of oral contraceptive use (incidence of reported PMS is lower in pill users), sterilisation, hysterectomy or even increasing age.

Box 45.1 Summary of DSM-IV diagnostic criteria for premenstrual dysphoric disorder (PMDD)

One-year duration of symptoms which are present for the majority of cycles (occur luteal/remit follicular)

Five of the following symptoms (with at least one of these*) must occur during the week before menses and remit within days of menses.
- Irritability*
- Depressed mood or hopelessness*
- Affective lability* (sudden mood swings)
- Tension or anxiety*
- Decreased interest in activities
- Change in sleep patterns
- Difficulty concentrating
- Feeling out of control or overwhelmed
- Lack of energy
- Other physical symptoms, for example, breast tenderness, bloating
- Change in appetite, for example, food cravings

Seriously interferes with work, social activities, relationships

Not an exacerbation of another disorder

Confirmed by prospective daily ratings during at least two consecutive symptomatic cycles

---

Box 45.2 Diagnostic criteria for premenstrual syndrome (PMS)

Patient reports ≥1 of the following affective and somatic symptoms during the 5 days before menses in each of three prior menstrual cycles:

Affective	Somatic
Depression	Breast tenderness
Angry outbursts	Abdominal bloating
Irritability	Headache
Anxiety	Swelling of extremities
Confusion	
Social withdrawal	

Symptoms relieved within 4 days of menses onset without recurrence until at least cycle day 13

Symptoms present in absence of any pharmacological therapy, hormone ingestion, or drug or alcohol abuse

Symptoms occur reproducibly during two cycles of prospective recording

Patient suffers from identifiable dysfunction in social or economic performance

---

PMS may be exacerbated by other stresses, typically those associated with family life. Women with a body mass index over 30 are more likely to suffer from PMS. There is also some evidence that crimes, accidents, examination failure, absenteeism and marital disturbances may be more common premenstrually.

Aetiology

PMS is not seen before puberty, during pregnancy or in post-menopausal women, and therefore, the ovarian hormones have been implicated. The mineralocorticoids, prolactin, androgens, prostaglandins, endorphins, nutritional factors (e.g. pyridoxine, calcium and essential fatty acids) and hypoglycaemia may be involved. In addition, changes in CNS function have been implicated as cerebral blood flow in the temporal lobes is decreased premenstrually in PMS sufferers, and noradrenergic cyclicity is disrupted. As symptoms vary so much from cycle to cycle, and from individual to individual, it is likely that different aetiological factors apply to different women, all of which may be affected by extenuating emotional circumstances. There is some evidence that predisposition to PMDD may be familial.

Hormones

The cyclicity of PMS suggests an ovarian involvement. This is substantiated by the fact that it is still experienced after hysterectomy if the ovaries are left intact and that it disappears during pregnancy and after the menopause. One theory attributes PMS to luteal phase progesterone deficiency leading to a progesterone/estradiol imbalance, but there is no direct clinical evidence to support this in terms of serum progesterone levels. However, the problem could lie at the cellular level, that is, a paucity of functional steroid receptors leading to differential sensitivity to hormones. Alternatively, it could be a central control defect, as ovarian suppression by GnRH analogues can alleviate symptoms in some women; however, the use of these drugs is generally not recommended because of their unwanted effects associated with production of a hypo-oestrogenic state.

The central actions of the sex steroids or their neuroactive metabolites are important. Research into the complex relationship between the steroids and the CNS is ongoing, and progressing with the advent of new tools such as the progesterone receptor modulators. Estradiol increases neuronal excitability possibly via increasing the activity of glutamate (an important excitatory neurotransmitter). Progesterone, and its metabolites, can bind to the γ-aminobutyric acid A (GABA$_A$) receptor, and this interaction would induce an effect similar to that evoked by benzodiazepines. The mineralocorticoid, aldosterone, may be associated with the increase in fluid retention as serum levels of this hormone are elevated in the luteal phase. However, no significant difference in blood levels of this mineralocorticoid has been found between PMS sufferers and non-sufferers. In contrast, one study has found that baseline levels of cortisol were elevated during the luteal phase in PMS sufferers.

Prolactin is secreted from the decidual cells at the end of the luteal phase of the menstrual cycle as well as from the anterior pituitary. This hormone has a direct effect upon breast tissue and hence may be associated with breast tenderness. Prolactin is also associated with stress and has an indirect relationship with dopamine metabolism and release in the CNS. It promotes sodium, potassium and water retention.

However, there are no consistent differences in hormone blood levels of prolactin between PMS sufferers and non-sufferers. Again, the differences could lie at the receptor level. Local hormones such as the prostaglandins may also be implicated in the aetiology of PMS as synthesis of these autocoids can be affected by the sex hormones as well as substrate availability. Prostaglandin imbalance is implicated in PMS as increased synthesis of certain prostaglandins, for example, PGE_2, have antidiuretic and central sedative effects as well as promoting capillary permeability and vasodilation. Deficiencies of others, for example, PGE_1, which can attenuate some of the actions of prolactin, may also contribute to the syndrome.

Vitamins and minerals

Pyridoxine phosphate is a co-factor in a number of enzyme reactions, particularly those leading to production of dopamine and serotonin (5-hydroxytryptamine). It has been suggested that disturbances of the oestrogen/progesterone balance could cause a relative deficiency of pyridoxine, and supplementation with this vitamin appears to ease the depression sometimes associated with the oral contraceptive pill. Decreased dopamine levels would tend to increase serum prolactin, and decreased serotonin levels could be a factor in emotional disturbances, particularly depression. There is some evidence that premenstrual mood changes are linked to cycle-related alterations in serotonergic activity within the CNS and, therefore, serotonin may be important in the pathogenesis of PMS. There are also data to suggest that a variety of nutrients may play a role in the aetiology of PMS, specifically calcium and vitamin D. Further hydroxylation of 25-hydroxyvitamin D_3 ($25(OH)D_3$) takes place in target tissues which include the breast and the endometrium. In the Nurses' Health Study II (NHSII), high total vitamin D intake lowered risk of PMS by almost a third (Bertone-Johnson et al., 2005). Oestrogen influences calcium metabolism by affecting intestinal absorption, and parathyroid gene expression and secretion, so triggering fluctuations throughout the menstrual cycle. Disruption of calcium homeostasis has been associated with affective disorders.

Essential fatty acids

Essential fatty acids, such as γ-linolenic (or gamolenic acid/ GLA), provide a substrate for prostaglandin synthesis. γ-Linolenic is converted into dihomo-γ-linolenic acid, which forms the starting point for the synthesis of prostaglandins of the 1 series (e.g. PGE_1). It has been suggested that women with PMS are abnormally sensitive to normal levels of prolactin and that PGE_1 is able to attenuate the biological effects of this hormone. Hence, if there is a γ-linolenic deficiency, then there is less substrate for PGE_1 synthesis. Therefore, the effect of prolactin with respect to breast tenderness, fluid retention and mood disturbances may be exaggerated. Numerous other dietary factors may also be involved, including excess saturated fats and cholesterol, moderate-to-high alcohol consumption, zinc and magnesium deficiencies, diabetes, ageing and viral infections, all of which hinder the conversion of cis-linolenic acid to γ-linolenic. Pyridoxine, ascorbic acid and niacin also increase conversion of γ-linolenic to PGE_1, while there is some evidence to suggest that linolenic acid metabolite levels are reduced in women with PMS.

Psychological factors

PMS may not be wholly explicable in pathophysiological terms, but it should not be regarded as a psychosomatic disorder as there is no simple relationship between its existence, severity and personality. It is not strictly confined to particular types of women, although there is no doubt that PMS interacts with many aspects of life, especially difficult or stressful times. The latter has been termed the 'vulnerability factor' which, although not a function of the menstrual cycle, can affect the way a woman reacts.

Symptoms

Symptoms occur 1–14 days before menstruation begins and disappear at the onset or shortly after menstruation begins. For the rest of the cycle, the woman feels well. Symptoms are cyclical, although they may not be experienced every cycle, and can be either physical and/or psychological (see Boxes 45.1. and 45.2 for symptomatology). The lives of the 5% or so of women who are severely affected may be completely disrupted in the second half of the menstrual cycle. The symptoms of PMS tend to decrease as a woman gets closer to the menopause as her ovulatory cycles become less frequent.

Management

The first step in the management of PMS is recognition of the problem and realisation that many other women also suffer. Keeping a menstrual diary is useful and will establish any link between symptoms and menstruation, and this will provide a cornerstone for diagnosis. After a few months, it will allow the patient to make predictions and help her deal with changes when they arrive. The effectiveness of medical intervention depends upon which symptoms are being experienced, underlining the importance of a menstrual diary and experimentation. In terms of treatment, self-help and perseverance will be required in the management of PMS. The wide variety of symptoms may require exploring a number of treatment options before optimal relief can be achieved.

Non-pharmacological strategies

Maintenance of good general health is important, especially with respect to diet and possible deficiencies. Dietary modifications that may be helpful include restricting caffeine and alcohol intake. Smoking can also exacerbate symptoms. Exercise may help, as may learning simple relaxation techniques. If fluid retention is a problem, then reducing fluid and salt intake may be of value. Increasing the intake of natural diuretics such as prunes, figs, celery, cucumber, parsley and foods high in potassium such as bananas, oranges, dried fruits, nuts, soya beans and tomatoes may all be useful. Hypoglycaemia may also be involved in premenstrual tiredness, so eating small protein-rich meals more frequently may help.

Results from clinical trials involving pyridoxine (vitamin B_6) have shown conflicting results. However, some women do respond to pyridoxine and show improvement, particularly with respect to mood change, breast discomfort and headache. A typical dosage regimen would be 50 mg twice daily after meals or 100 mg after breakfast. The dose should not exceed 100 mg a day. Gastric upset and headaches have been reported at doses greater than 200 mg. High doses over long periods have also been associated with peripheral neuropathies. Pyridoxine should be commenced 3 days before symptom onset and continued for 2 days after menstruation has started.

Calcium supplementation has shown some activity in reducing emotional, behavioural and physical symptoms. Likewise, there is limited evidence that supplementation with γ-linolenic acid, found in evening primrose oil, gives relief from physical symptoms, especially breast tenderness.

Pharmacological management

Progestogens. Synthetic progestogens, in preparations such as Cyclogest® and Duphaston®, have been used in the past. However, because of the lack of convincing trial evidence and the risk of side effects, the use of progestogens is no longer recommended. Possible side effects include weight gain, nausea, breast discomfort, breakthrough bleeding and changes in cycle length. Problems arise because some synthetic progestogens, especially 19-nor compounds such as norethisterone and levonorgestrel, also display some affinity for glucocorticoid, mineralocorticoid and androgen receptors. The specificity of these synthetic agents is influenced by the substituents present on the steroid nucleus, particularly at C13. For example, the third-generation progestogens that have an ethyl group at C13 (gestodene, desogestrel and norgestimate) have the least androgenic activity of all the 19-nor compounds but are still orally active.

Combined oral contraceptives (COC). Some women are helped by the COC pill because it prevents ovulation from taking place. However, the use of exogenous oestrogen may be contraindicated because it can increase the risk of venous thromboembolism. This occurs because oestrogen decreases blood levels of the potent natural anticoagulant antithrombin III and at the same time increases serum levels of some clotting factors. Women with other risk factors for thromboembolic disease should also avoid this form of therapy. The incidence of venous thromboembolism in healthy, nonpregnant women who are not taking an oral contraceptive is about five to ten cases per 100,000 women per year. For those using COCs containing second-generation progestogens, for example, levonorgestrel, this incidence is about 15 per 100,000 women per year of use. Some studies have reported a greater risk of venous thromboembolism in women using preparations containing the third-generation progestogens desogestrel and gestodene. The incidence in these women is about 25 per 100,000 women per year of use. However, it should be noted that the absolute risk of venous thromboembolism in women

using COCs containing these third-generation progestogens remains very small and well below the venous thromboembolism risk associated with pregnancy.

It is thought that use of third-generation progestogens is associated with increased resistance to the anticoagulant action of activated protein C. Oral contraceptive treatment diminishes the efficacy with which activated protein C down regulates *in vitro* thrombin formation. This is known as activated protein C resistance and is more pronounced in women using the COC pills containing desogestrel than in women using those containing levonorgestrel. However, it has also been recognised that women who do react to third-generation progestogens with venous thromboembolism may be revealing a latent thrombophilia. There are several conditions, congenital or acquired, that can cause thrombophilic alterations. A genetic factor known as factor V Leiden mutation is the most common inherited cause of thrombophilia, and this mutation results in resistance to the effects of activated protein C. Carriers of this mutation have more than a 30-fold increase in risk of thrombotic complications during oral contraceptive use, although this has been disputed (Farmer et al., 2000) because no increase in risk of venous thromboembolism was found with the third-generation progestogens. In conclusion, if there is a history of thromboembolic disease at a young age in the immediate family, then disturbances of the coagulation system must be ruled out.

The combination of ethinylestradiol with drospirenone is also available as an oral contraceptive and appears to be useful in the management of PMS. Drospirenone is a derivative of spironolactone, with affinity for progesterone receptors, but it also acts as a mineralocorticoid antagonist. This progestogen, therefore, alleviates some of the salt-retaining effects of the ethinylestradiol.

Bromocriptine. Bromocriptine stimulates central dopamine receptors and thus inhibits the release of prolactin. It may be useful for breast tenderness and occasionally has beneficial effects upon fluid retention and mood changes. It should be used in small doses, for example, 1–1.25 mg at bedtime with food, to avoid the side effects of nausea and faintness due to hypotension. The dose can be slowly increased to 2.5 mg twice a day if required. It is advised that ergot-derived dopamine receptor agonists, such as bromocriptine, have been associated with pulmonary, retroperitoneal and pericardial fibrotic reactions (Anon, 2002). Excessive daytime sleepiness and sudden onset of sleep can also occur with dopaminergic drugs.

Danazol. Danazol is a synthetic steroid derived from ethisterone. It is weakly androgenic and has been described as an attenuated androgen. Danazol interacts with androgen receptors, but it also has some affinity for the progesterone receptor. It inhibits the pulsatile release of gonadotrophins from the anterior pituitary and so abolishes cyclical ovarian activity, leading to amenorrhoea in the majority of women and a subsequent fall in serum oestrogen levels. However, because of the high incidence of side effects, it tends to be used as a last resort for relief of severe mastalgia and mood changes. These side effects relate to the androgenicity of the compound and include nausea, giddiness, muscular pain, weight gain, acne and virilisation. These can be minimised by using low doses of 200 mg a day.

Gonadotrophin-releasing hormone analogues. GnRH analogues, sometimes referred to as gonadorelin analogues, are useful for managing the physical symptoms, but are less effective with respect to emotional symptoms. These agents inhibit the hypothalamic–pituitary–gonadal axis. However, they can only be used for short periods of time, no more than 6 months, because they induce a hypo-oestrogenic state, and therefore bone loss becomes significant after 6 months' treatment. Should a patient respond well to GnRH analogues for PMS following hysterectomy, because of underlying pelvic pathology, bilateral oophorectomy may also be of benefit.

Prostaglandin synthesis inhibitors. Improvements in tension, irritability, depression, headache and general aches and pains can be seen in some women who take prostaglandin synthesis inhibitors. Most of the information available centres upon the use of mefenamic acid at doses of 250 mg three times a day 12 days before a period is due, increasing to 500 mg three times a day 9 days before the period and continuing until the third day of menstruation. Other inhibitors of prostaglandin synthesis are likely to be just as effective and may be associated with fewer side effects. Some experimental evidence, however, suggests that, in addition to being a cyclo-oxygenase inhibitor, mefenamic acid also has activity as an antagonist at prostaglandin E receptors, and therefore this may be useful if heavy menstrual bleeding is also a problem. For optimum effectiveness, this form of therapy should be started 24 h before the onset of symptoms. However, this starting point may be difficult to predict for women with irregular cycles.

Antidepressants. The selective serotonin reuptake inhibitors (SSRIs) are becoming more popular in the treatment of PMS-related depression because they are effective and well tolerated (Brown et al., 2009). Several randomised controlled trials using fluoxetine, sertraline, citalopram, fluvoxamine or paroxetine concluded that SSRIs are an effective first-line therapy for severe PMS and the side effects at low doses are generally acceptable. Two studies also found that not only do SSRIs improve behavioural symptoms, but some improvement in physical symptoms was also noted. Common side effects experienced include headache, nervousness, drowsiness and fatigue, sexual dysfunction and gastro-intestinal disturbances. Other agents such as tricyclic antidepressants and anxiolytics such as buspirone have been used. However, they appear to improve fewer PMS symptoms than the SSRIs.

St John's Wort has been used to reduce the severity of PMS, but the available evidence is limited.

Dysmenorrhoea

Dysmenorrhoea is usually subdivided into primary and secondary dysmenorrhoea. The former may also be referred to as spasmodic dysmenorrhoea, which is a uterine problem and is predominantly a complaint of young women. Secondary dysmenorrhoea is so called because it occurs secondary to some underlying pelvic pathology such as endometriosis or pelvic inflammatory disease (PID).

Epidemiology

The estimates vary but epidemiological studies suggest that between 50% and 80% of women will suffer from dysmenorrhoea at some time during their reproductive life, and up to 15% of these women will be seriously debilitated by the condition, with social and economic consequences. In the USA, it has been estimated that dysmenorrhoea accounts for the loss of 600 million working hours which equates to >2 billion dollars. Women in Western countries now have fewer pregnancies and this may be a contributory factor in the increasing prevalence of dysmenorrhoea.

Primary dysmenorrhoea

Aetiology and symptoms

The incidence of primary dysmenorrhoea peaks in women in their late teens and early 20s, the pain coinciding with establishment of ovulatory cycles. A typical sufferer will usually complain of lower abdominal pain (cramping), which may radiate down into the thighs, and backache. Some women also suffer gastro-intestinal symptoms (nausea, vomiting, diarrhoea), headaches and faintness. Symptoms are intense on the first day of menses but rarely continue beyond day 1 or 2 of the cycle. Factors that appear to increase the severity include young age at menarche, extended duration of menstrual flow (pain can be most severe when the flow is lighter), smoking and parity (the prevalence and severity of dysmenorrhoea is decreased in parous women). Other factors such as weight, length of menstrual cycle or frequency of physical exercise do not influence the condition.

In terms of aetiology, studies carried out in the 1950s and 1960s first drew attention to the possible role of the prostaglandins. This was followed by many *in vivo* studies which showed that women suffering from primary dysmenorrhoea do have greater concentrations of prostaglandins, predominantly $PGF_{2\alpha}$, and to some extent PGE_2, in their menstrual fluid compared with matched control subjects. Such a prostaglandin imbalance would favour increased myometrial contractility. The effects of the prostaglandins on human myometrium are now well documented, and increased biosynthesis of prostaglandins may also account for the gastro-intestinal problems encountered by some sufferers. A role for the prostaglandins is substantiated by the fact that women whose diet contains more omega-3 fatty acids tend to suffer less. When eicosapentaenoic acid (EPA) is the substrate for prostaglandin biosynthesis, prostaglandins of the three series are produced (e.g. PGE_3 and TXA_3). Such local hormones are less potent stimulators of the myometrium and less effective vasoconstrictors. Other potential mediators are the endothelins, vasoactive peptides produced in the endometrium that may play a role in the local regulation of prostaglandin synthesis, and vasopressin, a posterior pituitary hormone that stimulates uterine activity and decreases uterine blood flow. The smaller branches of the uterine arteries are very sensitive to the vasoconstrictor actions of these mediators, and it is these resistance vessels that are important in the control of uterine blood flow. The interrelationship between blood flow and myometrial activity is summarised in Fig. 45.4.

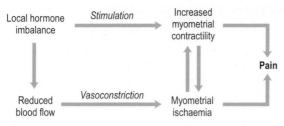

Fig. 45.4 The interactive role of myometrial stimulants and vasoconstrictive agents in the pathway leading to pain in dysmenorrhoea.

Measurements of intrauterine pressure and myometrial activity have been made for research purposes, but there are no simple objective measurements for dysmenorrhoea.

Secondary dysmenorrhoea

Aetiology and symptoms

Secondary dysmenorrhoea tends to afflict women in their 30s and 40s, and usually occurs as a consequence of some other pelvic pathology such as endometriosis or pelvic inflammation. In terms of symptoms, it differs from primary dysmenorrhoea in that the pain may actually start before menstruation begins, continue for the duration of menses and be associated with abdominal bloating, backache and a general feeling of 'heaviness' in the pelvic area. The intra-uterine contraceptive device may also exacerbate menstrual pain, since it causes localised inflammation that triggers the release of prostaglandins. The prostaglandins may also be implicated in the chain of events that lead to pain associated with secondary dysmenorrhoea. For example, if the cause is endometriosis, in which endometrial tissue is found out-side the uterine cavity, then this extrauterine tissue can also synthesise prostaglandins, which may in turn disrupt normal uterine function.

Treatment

In terms of analgesia, the most rational choice would be a non-steroidal anti-inflammatory drug (NSAID) (Zahradnik et al., 2010), as these compounds decrease prostaglandin bio-synthesis by inhibiting cyclo-oxygenase. Differences in anti-inflammatory activity between different NSAIDs are small. However, there is considerable variation in individual patient tolerance and response, and a lack of response to one particular agent does not mean that a patient would not respond to a different NSAID.

Mefenamic acid is frequently used to manage pain due to dysmenorrhoea. As previously stated, this compound not only inhibits prostaglandin production but also appears to possess some prostaglandin E receptor blocking activity which may serve to augment its effect. However, these prepa-rations are not suitable for all women and some, about 30% of women, will not respond. There is substantive evidence (Marjoribanks et al., 2010) that NSAIDs are effective in the treatment of dysmenorrhoea and are more effective than par-acetamol. However, there is insufficient evidence regarding the comparative efficacy of individual agents in terms of superi-ority of analgesia or side-effect profile.

The lack of an effect with an NSAID may be explained by pathway diversion, since the arachidonic acid that was to be converted to a prostaglandin via the action of cyclo-oxygenase can be utilised by an alternative biosynthetic route, leading to increased formation of leukotrienes. Alternatively, the second cyclo-oxygenase enzyme (COX-2), which is generally induced under pathological conditions, may be involved. Many of the currently available NSAIDs are relatively poor inhibitors of COX-2, and if some of the prostaglandins in these uterine disorders are produced via the action of this form of cyclo-oxygenase, then it is not surprising that the NSAIDs are not 100% effective. Celecoxib and etoricoxib have been shown to be effective, although none is currently licensed for use in dysmenorrhoea.

A small study has investigated the use of the leukotriene receptor antagonist montelukast (Singulair®) in the treatment of dysmenorrhoea (Fujiwara et al., 2010). The results suggest blockade of leukotriene receptors alleviate pain and reduce NSAID usage, and this appears to be most effective in women without endometriosis.

It has been estimated that approximately 50% of primary dysmenorrhoea sufferers will gain relief from taking the oral contraceptive pill, although, as this is a condition afflicting young girls, there may be attitudinal problems to the use of these products either in the patient or her parents. The oral contraceptive pill inhibits ovulation and thereby prevents increased luteal phase prostaglandin synthesis and so decreases uterine contractility. However, not all women are suitable can-didates for COC use because of the potential problems asso-ciated with exogenous oestrogen. Contraindications include high blood pressure, obesity and a significant personal or family history of venous thromboembolism. Progestogenic preparations (e.g. dydrogesterone 10 mg twice daily from day 5 to 25 of cycle, norethisterone 5 mg three times daily from day 5 to 24 of the cycle) or progestogen-only pills may be use-ful if they inhibit ovulation. For pain relief, there appears to be no significant difference between the various formulations. Antispasmodics such as hyoscine butylbromide and propan-theline bromide have a very limited role in the treatment of dysmenorrhoea, not least because of their poor oral bioavail-ability. Related compounds such as atropine also have negligi-ble effects upon the human uterus. A summary of the treatment options for dysmenorrhoea is presented in Table 45.1. Future therapy may involve use of vasopressin antagonists. Clinical trials have shown these compounds to be effective and well tolerated and they do not affect bleeding patterns.

For secondary dysmenorrhoea, the best treatment lies in finding the underlying cause and then taking an appropri-ate therapeutic route. For example, if some form of PID is diagnosed that can be attributed to a causative organism, then antimicrobial therapy is appropriate. PID is most com-monly caused by the presence of a sexually transmitted infec-tion. The most frequent causative organisms are *Chlamydia trachomatis* and *Neisseria gonorrhoeae*. In addition, any pro-cedure that may compromise the mucus barrier of the cer-vix, for example, insertion of an intrauterine device, may also

Table 45.1 Summary of treatment options for dysmenorrhoea

Drug	Side effects
NSAIDs	Gastric irritation, which can be minimised by taking with or after food or selecting an agent with less gastrotoxicity, for example, ibuprofen. Hypersensitivity reactions, particularly bronchospasm. Headache, dizziness, vertigo, hearing problems (e.g. tinnitus) and haematuria. NSAIDs may adversely affect renal function and provoke acute renal failure
Combined oral contraceptives	Many side effects are dose related and so the development of the ultra-low-dose preparations (i.e. those containing 20 μcg ethinylestradiol) is beneficial. An alternative to the oral preparations is the low-dose transdermal combined contraceptive which releases 20 μcg ethinylestradiol and 150 μcg of norelgestromin (active metabolite of the third-generation progestogen, norgestimate). The most serious potential adverse effect is the increased risk of thromboembolism due to a decrease in circulating levels of antithrombin III while increasing serum levels of some clotting factors. This risk increases with age and smoking. Analysis of current data suggests that the risk of breast cancer is not increased for most women who use the combined oral contraceptive for the major portion of their reproductive years. Use of the combined oral contraceptive also conveys several health benefits besides being an effective contraceptive. The progestogenic side effects are discussed as follows
Progestogen-only preparations	Use of these agents may cause menstrual disturbances, for example, breakthrough bleeding. Other adverse effects relate to the selectivity of the synthetic hormone, for example, norethisterone is a first-generation progestogen and has some affinity for steroid receptors other than progesterone and so possesses androgenic, oestrogenic and antioestrogenic activity. The third-generation progestogens (gestodene, norgestimate and desogestrel) have the least androgenic activity. This should be advantageous as it is the androgenicity of the compounds that correlates with the decrease in high-density lipoproteins

increase the risk of contracting PID. Treatment of endometriosis will often reduce symptoms of dysmenorrhoea. Surgical treatment for secondary dysmenorrhoea such as hysterectomy is also possible for those women who do not want to become pregnant.

Non-pharmacological management options have recently been reviewed and include high-frequency transcutaneous nerve stimulation (TENS) and acupuncture (Proctor et al., 2002). Both of these therapies showed some potential benefit. There is limited evidence to support the use of uterine nerve ablation and presacral neurectomy, to interrupt the sensory nerve fibres near the cervix blocking the pain pathway. Dietary therapies such as vitamin and mineral supplementation have also been investigated. One study identified that vitamin B₁ 100 mg daily may be effective in relieving pain (Proctor et al., 2002). Magnesium supplementation also shows promising results. Unfortunately, evidence is still lacking to support use of other herbal and dietary therapies, for example, omega-3 fatty acids. Some Chinese herbal medicines have shown interesting results but trial quality is poor.

Menorrhagia

Blood loss is considered to be excessive if it exceeds 80 mL per period, although both women themselves and clinicians find it difficult to objectively quantify blood loss. In practice, it is defined by the woman's subjective assessment of blood loss. Any change in menstruation, whether real or perceived, may be disturbing with respect to social, occupational or sexual activities and can lead to other problems including depression and concern about an undiagnosed problem such as cancer. Physically excessive blood loss will precipitate iron deficiency anaemia (haemoglobin <12 g/dL) which, if left undiagnosed and untreated, will compound the problems outlined earlier.

If a patient has any intermenstrual or postcoital bleeding, then referral to a gynaecologist for endometrial biopsy is essential to exclude intrauterine pathology. Up-to-date cervical cytology is also required. It should also be noted that hormonal contraceptives may cause some irregular spotting or breakthrough bleeding, but this is generally a tolerance effect. Non-oral methods, particularly implants, depots and intrauterine systems decrease bleeding with continued use (see later). WHO recommends a 90-day reference period for reporting vaginal bleeding.

Epidemiology

In the UK, about 30% of women complain of heavy menstrual bleeding, and about 1 in 20 women aged 25–44 years consult their primary care doctor about this problem. Historically, once referred to a gynaecologist, 60% of women could expect to have a hysterectomy within 5 years. Recent changes in the management of women with menorrhagia and new treatment options, particularly endometrial ablations and the levonorgestrel intrauterine contraceptive devices (LNG-IUS), have significantly reduced hysterectomy rates for menorrhagia to a third of the number 10 years ago.

Aetiology and investigation

The aetiology of menorrhagia can be divided into three categories: underlying pelvic pathology, systemic disease and dysfunctional uterine bleeding (Box 45.3). The typical symptoms suggestive of underlying pelvic pathology are presented in Box 45.4. Pelvic pathologies associated with menorrhagia

Box 45.3 Causes of menorrhagia (percentage frequency)

Dysfunctional uterine bleeding (60%), that is cause is unknown

Other gynaecological causes (30%):
- Uterine or ovarian tumours
- Endometriosis
- Pelvic inflammatory disease
- Intrauterine contraceptive devices
- Early pregnancy complications

Endocrine and haematological causes (<5%)
- Thyroid disorders, for example hypothyroidism
- Platelet problems and clotting abnormalities

Box 45.4 Symptoms suggestive of underlying pelvic pathology

Irregular bleeding

Sudden change in blood loss

Intermenstrual bleeding

Postcoital bleeding

Dyspareunia

Pelvic pain

Premenstrual pain

include myomas (fibroids, common benign tumours of the myometrium), endometriosis, adenomyosis (penetration of endometrial tissue into the myometrium), endometrial polyps, polycystic ovarian disease and endometrial carcinoma. Although endometrial cancer is more typically seen in postmenopausal women, approximately 50% of those patients diagnosed with it premenopausally will have associated menorrhagia. Systemic diseases from which menorrhagia may stem include hypothyroidism, disorders involving the coagulation system such as elevated endometrial levels of plasminogen activator and systemic lupus erythematosus. Very few women fall into this group. About 60% of menorrhagia sufferers have no underlying systemic or pelvic pathology and have ovulatory cycles. These patients are said to have dysfunctional uterine bleeding and local uterine mechanisms appear to be important in the control of menstrual blood loss. Occasionally, cycles may be anovulatory, with heavy blood loss because the endometrium has become hyperplastic under the influence of oestrogen. In addition, use of an intrauterine contraceptive device may also increase menstrual blood loss.

Prostaglandins appear to play a role in the aforementioned local mechanisms and have been implicated in menorrhagia. Studies have suggested an association between the type and quantity of endometrial prostaglandin synthesis and the degree of menstrual blood loss. In the mid-1970s, it was discovered that women with heavy periods had raised endometrial levels of $PGF_2\alpha$ and PGE_2 and that blood loss could be reduced by the use of drugs inhibiting

prostaglandin formation. More studies suggested that, in menorrhagic women, there is a shift towards increased biosynthesis of PGE_2, which is known to dilate uterine vasculature and/or increase the number of membrane receptors for this prostanoid. The availability of arachidonic acid, a substrate for prostaglandin synthesis, is also greater in women with menorrhagia. Levels of the vasodilators or their metabolites, PGI_2 and nitric oxide (NO), are also increased in the menstrual blood collected from women with excessive blood loss. It has been suggested that menorrhagia is an angiogenesis-related disease associated with changes in the pattern of vascular fragility involving the upregulation of various vascular endothelial growth factors.

Excessive menstrual blood loss is the most common cause of iron deficiency anaemia in women of reproductive age. In an otherwise healthy, well-nourished woman, it has been estimated that menstrual blood loss would have to exceed 120 mL to precipitate iron deficiency anaemia. Objective measurement of menstrual blood loss is difficult, so measurement of full blood count (including red blood cell indices and serum ferritin levels), and in particular, haemoglobin concentration, gives some indication of blood loss. Thyroid function should also be assessed. If fibroids are suspected, then pelvic ultrasound may be required. Endometrial biopsy is needed if there is an associated irregularity of menstruation or if intermenstrual or postcoital bleeding is present. In the case of regular menses, however, investigation of the uterine cavity would usually only be required in women over the age of 35 years or if medical treatment fails to alleviate symptoms. Young women presenting with dysfunctional uterine bleeding may have underlying coagulopathies such as von Willebrand's disease or Christmas disease, which should be excluded.

Treatment

The management of menorrhagia depends upon the cause of the condition and a woman's desire to conceive. Treatment can be either surgical or medical (Table 45.2). The effectiveness of drug therapy is obviously influenced by the accuracy of the diagnosis. Drug treatment is also influenced by a woman's contraceptive needs; for example, COCs can reduce menstrual blood loss by up to 50%, but in women over 35 years of age who smoke, this form of therapy would need careful consideration. Low-dose luteal phase progestogens are no longer recommended for treatment of heavy but regular periods as they increase menstrual blood loss in this situation. However, they may be of value in women with an irregular cycle. Long-term, long-acting progestogens, however, may render a woman amenorrhoeic. Other hormonally based therapies include the GnRH analogues, although their propensity to induce a hypo-oestrogenic state with long-term use may be problematic (a 6-month course would reduce trabecular bone density by 5–6%). Danazol can reduce menstrual blood loss but its use is generally prohibited by its side-effect profile. However, in 2009, a local vaginal treatment of 200 mg a day was investigated in 55 women (Luisi et al., 2009). Results showed danazol to be effective in reducing blood loss and few

Table 45.2 Summary of drug treatment options for menorrhagia

Drug	Comments
Combined oral contraceptive	See Table 45.1. These preparations are taken for 21 days with a 7-day pill-free (or placebo) period to allow for a withdrawal bleed
Progestogen-only preparations	See Table 45.1. Compounds such as norethisterone can be used, for example, 5 mg three times daily or 10 mg twice daily for the latter half of the cycle. Ten days of therapy should be sufficient from day 15 of the cycle in ovulatory cycles. However, if the cycles are anovulatory, then a minimum of 12 days' therapy is more appropriate. Progestogens for 12 days are also required to prevent endometrial hyperplasia in peri- and postmenopausal women taking oestrogen. When progestogens such as norethisterone are used, the dosage required is higher than that used in the combined oral contraceptive pill, and the adverse effects associated with the synthetic progestogens, particularly the 19-nortestosterone derivatives, may be more pronounced
Intrauterine progestogen-only contraceptive	The levonorgestrel-releasing intrauterine device (LNG-IUS) typically releases 20 μcg of levonorgestrel/24 h. Unlike non-medicated IUCDs, which may increase menstrual blood loss, this device appears to reduce it, as a result of the local endometrial actions of the progestogen. The device also offers contraceptive cover without many of the side effects associated with the non-medicated IUCDs. Progestogen-related side effects should be minimised because of the low dose of levonorgestrel employed. Initially, bleeding patterns may be disrupted, but menstrual blood loss should become lighter within three menstrual cycles
Danazol	Danazol suppress the pituitary–ovarian axis. Side effects include amenorrhoea, hot flushes, sweating, changes in libido, vaginitis and emotional lability. Danazol also causes androgenic side effects such as acne, oily skin and hair, hirsutism, oedema, weight gain, voice deepening and decreasing breast size. Danazol has to be taken daily
GnRH analogues (gonadorelin)	After an initial period of stimulation, these agents suppress the pituitary–ovarian axis. As result of inducing a hypo-oestrogenic state, these compounds should only be used for 6 months because they may decrease trabecular bone density
NSAIDs	These agents only need to be taken for the first 3–4 days of menses
Tranexamic acid	This drug appears well tolerated, but can produce dose-related gastro-intestinal disturbances. Patients who may be predisposed to thrombosis are at risk if given antifibrinolytic therapy. This compound is usually only taken for the first 3 days of menses

IUCDs, intrauterine contraceptive devices; GnRH, gonadotrophin-releasing hormone.

adverse effects were reported. A trial of ormeloxifene, a selective estrogen receptor modulator (similar to raloxifene), 60 mg twice weekly has been used successfully to reduce blood loss with relatively few side effects (Kriplani et al., 2009).

Prostaglandins have been implicated in the aetiology of several forms of menorrhagia. Therefore, NSAIDs may be of use in some patients, especially if there is pain associated with menstruation. The NSAIDs appear to be most effective in women with the heaviest blood loss, for example, mefenamic acid 500 mg three times daily from day 1 until heavy flow ceases.

Women with menorrhagia have greater endometrial fibrinolytic activity, hence the use of antifibrinolytic drugs, which are plasminogen activator inhibitors. Tranexamic acid became available for purchase over the counter in UK pharmacies in 2010 as Cyklo-F®. This can be sold to women aged 18–45 years old with a history of regular heavy menstrual bleeding over several consecutive menstrual cycles. Tranexamic acid reduces menstrual blood loss by up to 50% (Lethaby et al., 2000), the recommended dose being 1 g three times daily starting on the first day of menses for up to 4 days. Agents such as tranexamic acid carry a risk of unwanted thrombogenesis, but this does not appear to be translated into practice as increased numbers of deep vein thromboses. This class of drugs decreases menstrual blood loss better than NSAIDs and oral luteal phase progestogen (Lethaby et al., 2005). However, tranexamic acid should be stopped if it has produced no benefit after three cycles.

The levonorgestrel intrauterine contraceptive devices (also known as intrauterine systems or LNG-IUS) can be left in place for up to 5 years following insertion. They reduce menstrual blood loss by up to 90% after 12 months of use. The levonorgestrel-releasing intrauterine system provides relief from dysmenorrhoea, effective contraception and long-term control of menorrhagia. A study showed that the levonorgestrel-releasing intrauterine device was the most cost-effective treatment followed by ablation surgery (Clegg et al., 2007). In addition, other slow-release progestogenic devices such as nesterone implants and vaginal rings also reduce menstrual blood loss and promote amenorrhoea.

Hysterectomy has been the traditional surgical treatment for menorrhagia, with either an abdominal or vaginal approach used (Marjoribanks et al., 2006). Newer alternatives to hysterectomy include endometrial ablation, which can be done by electrosurgical, laser, microwave or thermal techniques. Endometrial ablation is less invasive than hysterectomy, but recurrence of menorrhagia can occur and amenorrhoea cannot be guaranteed. There is evidence that pretreatment with a single dose of a GnRH agonist before the ablation procedure gives a better result. These preparations cause an initial stimulation of gonadotrophin release which then suppresses the hypothalamic–pituitary axis, producing a hypo-oestrogenic state. If circulating levels of oestrogen are low, then endometrial growth will not be stimulated; thus, it will be thinner, making the surgical endometrial destruction more effective. With GnRH pretreatment, modern techniques such as microwave ablation have achieved amenorrhoea rates of about 50% and patient satisfaction rates of 90%.

Endometriosis

Endometriosis is a condition in which endometrial tissue is found outside the uterus. These so-called ectopic endometrial foci have been found outside the reproductive tract in the gastro-intestinal tract, the urinary tract and even the lungs.

Aetiology

Aetiology remains unclear, although retrograde menstruation, when shed endometrial cells migrate up through the fallopian tubes, would appear to be involved. This may occur because abnormalities in uterine innervation cause disruption in the usual patterns of myometrial contractility with consequent loss of the usual fundocervical polarity. Endometriosis is found in women in whom the normal route for the menstrual flow is disrupted, such as when there is some genital tract abnormality. Women who have frequent and heavier periods also seem to be more likely to suffer from endometriosis. Familial predisposition may also be a factor and several gene polymorphisms have been identified.

Studies suggest that endometrium from endometriosis sufferers tends to be more invasive. This may reflect either biological or genetic differences in the peritoneal milieu and may be explained by the upregulation of certain types of metalloproteinase responsible for the degradation of basement membrane. Endometrial tissue from women with endometriosis has aromatase activity which can be stimulated by PGE_2. Therefore, ostensibly the endometriotic lesions have their own oestrogen supply as aromatase converts androgenic precursors into oestrogen and oestrogen stimulates biosynthesis of PGE_2; thus, the cycle is self-perpetuating. *In vitro* studies have shown that eutopic and ectopic endometrial explants have different lipidomic profiles in terms of their prostaglandin release and the myometrium from endometriosis suffers is more acontractile during menses. Pilot studies in the USA using aromatase inhibitors, such as anastrozole and letrozole, are ongoing.

Epidemiology

Endometriosis was previously considered to be a disease affecting women in their 30s onwards, but increasing use of laparoscopy has revealed that it can occur at any time throughout a woman's reproductive life. The condition is dependent upon oestrogen stimulation, and as such, it does not occur before the menarche or after the menopause. The exact incidence of the disease is unknown, but it is believed to be about 10% in the general female population of reproductive age. One study has found a positive correlation between a menarche before 13 years and increased risk of developing endometriosis.

Symptoms

Although not all women with endometriosis are symptomatic, the pelvis is the most commonly affected site. Consequently, most of the symptoms of endometriosis relate to this region. Symptoms take the form of dysmenorrhoea and pelvic pain. However, the severity of the pain does not necessarily reflect the extent of the disease because women with severe pain may have few lesions, and vice versa. Dyspareunia often with postcoital discomfort is also common. There may also be menstrual irregularities.

The link between endometriosis and infertility is recognised, but the mechanisms involved have not been established. If the ovaries or fallopian tubes themselves are directly affected by the endometriotic lesions, then fertility may be compromised by purely mechanical means. However, the situation is less clear when the endometriosis does not cause any anatomical distortions. In this case, some of the postulated causes of infertility associated with endometriosis include ovulation disorders such as luteinised unruptured follicle syndrome, anovulation, premature ovulation; hyperprolactinaemia; and changes in the peritoneal environment such as extrauterine endometrial material which, like normal endometrium, is subject to control by the ovarian steroids and like its uterine counterpart is also capable of producing prostaglandins. Prostaglandin levels, along with macrophage concentrations, are raised in the peritoneal fluid of women with endometriotic explants, and these may alter tubular and uterine motility within the abdomen.

Outside the reproductive tract, endometrial deposits can be found along the urinary and gastro-intestinal tracts. If the former is involved, then the patient may suffer from cyclical haematuria, dysuria or even ureteric obstruction. If there is gastro-intestinal tract involvement, then symptoms could include dyschezia, cyclical tenesmus and rectal bleeding or even obstruction. Very occasionally, the lesions are found at more distant sites such as the lungs, where they could cause cyclical haemoptysis. A reduction in bone mass in women with endometriosis has also been reported.

Treatment

The aims of treatment in endometriosis are to relieve symptoms and improve fertility if pregnancy is desired. Treatment can be either surgical or medical. Surgery is increasingly performed laparoscopically and can be employed to restore normal pelvic anatomy, divide adhesions or ablate endometriotic tissue using either laser treatment or electrodiathermy. Medical treatment utilises the fact that endometriotic tissue is oestrogen dependent, and any drug therapy that will oppose the effects of oestrogen should, among other things, inhibit the growth of the endometriotic tissue. Hence, the choices of drug treatment are as follows.

- GnRH analogues such as buserelin, goserelin, leuprorelin and nafarelin. These initially stimulate the hypothalamic–pituitary–ovarian axis but thereafter induce a hypo-oestrogenic state by paradoxically inhibiting follicle-stimulating hormone (FSH) and LH release.
- Low-dose COC (20–30 μcg of ethinylestradiol) monophasic preparations have been found to be as effective as GnRH analogues, and they may slow down disease progression in young women and preserve future fertility.
- Compounds with androgenic activity such as danazol also inhibit pituitary gonadotrophin release by interfering with the negative feedback and cause atrophy of endometrial tissue.
- Progestogens such as dydrogesterone, medroxyprogesterone acetate and norethisterone initially cause decidualisation of the endometrial tissue followed by glandular atrophy.

None of the aforementioned drug therapies are free from side effects. Use of the GnRH analogues may evoke menopausal symptoms such as hot flushes, decreased libido, vaginal dryness (topical vaginal lubricants may be helpful), mood changes and headache. The problems associated with the hypo-oestrogenic state limit the long-term use of GnRH analogues. Although lipoprotein levels are not affected adversely, bone mass is, and this loss of bone density may not be entirely reversible after cessation of therapy. Various 'add-back' hormone replacement therapies have been successfully used to minimise bone demineralisation, for example, low-dose oestrogen/progestogen combinations used continuously. Such regimens protect against osteoporosis and other hypo-oestrogenic side effects without apparently affecting clinical efficacy. Pain associated with endometriosis was relieved similarly by gosarelin and a low-dose oral contraceptive (Prentice et al., 1999). However, side-effect profiles differed, for example, hot flushes and vaginal dryness with the former agent and headache and weight gain with the latter.

The androgenic compounds, because of their very nature, are associated with hirsutism, weight gain and acne. Side effects associated with synthetic progestogens relate again to androgenicity, although dydrogesterone is free from virilisation. However, using a levonorgestrel-releasing intrauterine device ensures the low dose of levonorgestrel is delivered locally and the more direct pelvic distribution may be useful in the management of endometriosis. Recent results suggest this device causes the downregulation of endometrial cell proliferation and increased apoptotic activity. Longer-term studies, over 5 years, need to be undertaken to determine how long this effect is maintained and also effectiveness on symptoms such as dyspareunia and dyschezia.

Researchers have also found that certain dietary changes may be beneficial and reduce symptoms. A decreased intake of glycaemic carbohydrates such as sugar, rice and potatoes in addition to reducing/eliminating caffeine and increasing the intake of omega-3 oils such as flax seed oil may also be helpful. In addition, one study found that women with endometriosis tended to have a lower body mass index than those without the condition.

Total pelvic clearance, including the removal of the ovaries, is practical in women who have completed their family. This tends to be a last resort treatment but it is usually effective. However, surgery may be difficult if multiple lesions are present. There is no evidence that hormonal suppression improves surgical outcome.

Neither surgical nor medical management is effective in all cases. Studies suggest that pain associated with endometriosis responds well to both surgical and medical treatment, but symptoms of recurrence occur in about 50% of patients within 5 years of stopping treatment. Fertility may be increased by the use of surgery to remove endometriotic foci causing anatomical distortion. The same benefit is not associated with medical treatment.

Case studies

Case 45.1

A 13-year-old girl is brought to her primary care doctor by her mother. She has been struggling with long, heavy periods for 6 months and as a result is missing time at school.

Questions

1. What non-hormonal treatment options would be considered?
2. What other treatments might be an option?

Answers

1. In young girls, it is worthwhile trying non-hormonal treatment options first as they will tend to have a lower side-effect profile than hormonal treatment. Tranexamic acid at a dose of 1 g three times a day should be taken while bleeding. This is a very simple and effective option with few side effects and a reported 50% reduction in menstrual blood loss. Another option would be to try a non-steroidal preparation such as mefanamic acid (500 mg three times daily from first day of bleeding until period ends), especially if associated dysmenorrhoea is a significant problem. Tranexamic acid and an NSAID can be taken together if required.
2. Cyclical norethisterone (5 mg three times daily from day 5 to day 25 of cycle) can be helpful if the periods are irregular, but it is not recommended for heavy regular periods. Progestogenic side effects such as nausea and bloating can limit use. The COC pill can be very effective at relieving menorrhagia and dysmenorrhoea, provided that there are no contraindications. Sometimes, parents can raise concerns about the use of a contraceptive agent, some parents perhaps believing that it may promote promiscuity.

Case 45.2

A 33-year-old woman has been diagnosed with endometriosis having presented with severe dysmenorrhoea. She has visited the gynaecology clinic to discuss treatment options but is very concerned about her fertility. She does not wish to conceive at the present time but would certainly plan to try for a baby in the next couple of years.

Questions

1. What effect does endometriosis and its treatment have on fertility?
2. What treatment options could be considered?

Answers

1. Severe endometriosis with significant distortion of the pelvic anatomy can cause tubal blockage and hence cause tubal factor infertility. Most patients will have much less severe endometriosis which, although not causing any anatomical abnormality, is associated with a reduction in fertility. Such couples tend to take longer to conceive perhaps because the endometrial deposits create an unfavourable milieu for the egg and sperm. Surgical treatment such as diathermy or laser destruction or excision of endometriotic deposits may improve fertility, although such surgery can be complicated. Medical treatments are not associated with an improvement in fertility rates as many treatment options are contraceptive in themselves and should not be used if women wish to try to conceive. In this situation, symptom control with analgesia may be the best option.
2. As this patient is not wishing to conceive, a trial of medical therapy should be considered. Surgery for endometriosis is a highly skilled procedure which has a significant risk of complications. Medical treatment options include GnRH analogues, the COC pill or a prolonged course of progestogens such as medroxyprogesterone acetate. All have different side effects and contraindications but are all equally effective at reducing symptoms of endometriosis. Currently, the most popular option is a 6-month course of a GnRH analogue which is generally well tolerated. Vasomotor symptoms can be treated with add-back hormone replacement therapy with a continuous combined preparation or tibolone. Treatment is limited to a 6-month course because of the bone loss associated with the

GnRH-induced hypo-oestrogenism. The COC pill can be taken in a conventional way, but anecdotal experience supports tricycling, that is, taking 3 packets back to back and only having a withdrawal bleed after the third packet. Clearly, the usual contraindications to taking a COC pill apply. Progestogens are often poorly tolerated with side effects such as bloating and nausea.

Case 45.3

A 33-year-old with very heavy and prolonged periods presents to her primary care doctor requesting hysterectomy. Her mother had a hysterectomy at age 38 and this patient feels that it is her only option.

Questions

1. What treatment options would you offer this patient before considering hysterectomy?
2. What investigations are necessary?

Answers

1. Before considering treatment, the patient should have a pelvic examination, primarily to exclude large fibroids which are unlikely to respond to medical therapy. Current advice is to recommend a levonorgestrel-releasing intrauterine device as first line for heavy menstrual bleeding (NICE, 2007). If the patient declines this, other options would include tranexamic acid and/or a non-steroidal NSAID such as mefenamic acid taken at the onset of the period. The COC pill could be considered if not contraindicated. Cyclical norethisterone may be of benefit if the menstrual cycle is irregular. Hysterectomy should be reserved as the last option and if medical therapy fails. Consideration should be given to an endometrial ablative procedure before resorting to major surgery.
2. If pelvic examination is normal, the only investigation recommended for this lady is a full blood count to exclude anaemia. If examination suggests the possibility of a pelvic mass, an ultrasound scan should be organised. Further endometrium investigation, by hysteroscopy or endometrial biopsy, in women under 45 with heavy menstrual bleeding and no intermenstrual bleeding, is not indicated unless medical treatment options fail.

References

American College of Obstetricians and Gynecologists, 2000. Premenstrual Syndrome. ACOG Practice Bulletin No 15, ACOG, Washington, DC.

American Psychiatric Association, 2000. Diagnostic and Statistical Manual of Mental Disorders. American Psychiatric Publishing Inc., Arlington, VA.

Anon, 2002. Fibrotic reactions with pergolide and other ergot-derived dopamine receptor agonists. Curr. Probl. Pharmacovigilance 23, 3.

Bertone-Johnson, E.R., Hankinson, S.E., Bendich, A., et al., 2005. Calcium and vitamin D intake and risk of incident premenstrual syndrome. Arch. Intern. Med. 165, 1246–1252.

Brown, J., O'Brien, P.M.S., Majoribanks, J., et al., 2009. Selective serotonin reuptake inhibitors for premenstrual syndrome. Cochrane Database Syst. Rev. 2 Art No. CD001396 DOI: 10.1002/14651858. CD001396.pub2.

Clegg, J.P., Guest, J.F., Hurskainen, R., 2007. Cost-utility of levonorgestrel intrauterine system compared with hysterectomy and second generation endometrial ablative techniques in managing patients with menorrhagia in the UK. Curr. Med. Res. Opin. 23, 1637–1648.

Farmer, R.D.T., Williams, T.J., Simpson, E.L., et al., 2000. Effect of 1995 pill scare on rates of venous thromboembolism among women taking combined oral contraceptives: analysis of General Practice Research Database. Br. Med. J. 321, 477–479.

Fujiwara, H., Konno, R., Netsu, S., et al., 2010. Efficacy of montelukast, a leukotriene receptor antagonist, for the treatment of dysmenorrhea: a prospective, double blind, randomized, placebo-controlled study. Eur. J. Obst. Gynecol. Reprod. Biol. 148, 195–198.

Kriplani, A., Kulshrestha, V., Agarwal, N., 2009. Efficacy and safety of ormeloxifene in management of menorrhagia: a pilot study. J. Obst. Gynaecol. Res. 35, 746–752.

Lethaby, A., Farquhar, C., Cooke, I., 2000. Antifibrinolytics for heavy menstrual bleeding. Cochrane Database Syst. Rev. 4 Art No. CD000249 DOI: 10.1002/14651858.CD000249.

Lethaby, A., Cooke, I., Rees, M.C., 2005. Progesterone or progestogen-releasing intrauterine systems for heavy menstrual bleeding. Cochrane Database Syst. Rev. 4 Art No. CD002126 DOI: 10.1002/14651858.CD002126.pub2.

Luisi, S., Razzi, S., Lazzeri, L., et al., 2009. Efficacy of vaginal danazol treatment in women with menorrhagia. Fert. Ster. 92, 1351–1354.

Marjoribanks, J., Lethaby, A., Farquhar, C., 2006. Surgery versus medical therapy for heavy menstrual bleeding. Cochrane Database. Syst. Rev. 2 Art No. CD003855 DOI: 10.1002/14651858.CD003855. pub2.

Marjoribanks, J., Proctor, M., Farquhar, C., et al., 2010. Nonsteroidal anti-inflammatory drugs for dysmenorrhoea. Cochrane Database. Syst. Rev. 1 Art No. CD001751 DOI: 10.1002/14651858.CD001751. pub2.

NICE, 2007. Heavy Menstrual Bleeding. Clinical Guideline 44, NICE, London. Available at http://www.nice.org.uk/nicemedia/ live/11002/30401/30401.pdf.

Prentice, A., Deary, A., Goldbeck-Wood, S., et al., 1999. Gonadotrophin-releasing hormone analogues for pain associated with endometriosis. Cochrane Database Syst. Rev. 2 Art No. CD000346. DOI: 10.1002/14651858.CD000346.pub2.

Proctor, M.L., Farquhar, C.M., Stones, W., et al., 2002. Transcutaneous electrical nerve stimulation for primary dysmenorrhoea. Cochrane Database Syst. Rev. 1 Art No. CD002123. DOI: 10.1002/14651858. CD002123.

Zahradnik, H.P., Hanjalic-Beck, A., Groth, K., 2010. Nonsteroidal anti-inflammatory drugs and hormonal contraceptives for pain relief from dysmenorrhea: a review. Contraception 81, 185–196.

Further reading

Bachmann, G., Korner, P., 2009. Bleeding patterns associated with non-hormonal contraceptives: a review of the literature. Contraception 79, 247–258.

Barnhart, K.T., Freeman, E.W., Sondheimer, S.J., 1995. A clinician's guide to the premenstrual syndrome. Med. Clin. North Am. 79, 1457–1472.

Fall, M., Baranowski, A.P., Elneil, S., et al., 2010. EAU guidelines on chronic pelvic pain. Eur. Urol. 57, 35–48.

Halbreich, U., 2010. Women's reproductive related disorders. J. Affect. Disord. 122, 10–13.

Ismail, K.M.K., O'Brien, S., 2005. Premenstrual syndrome. Curr. Obst. Gynaecol. 15, 25–30.

Lesley, D., Acheson, N. (Eds.), 2004. Endometriosis. Royal College of Obstetricians and Gynaecologists, London.

May, K., Octavia-Iacob, A., Sweeney, C., et al., 2009. Heavy Menstrual Bleeding Annual Evidence Update. NHS Evidence – Women's Health. Nuffield Department of Obstetrics and Gynaecology, Oxford.

Oelkers, W., 2004. Drospirenone, a progestogen with antimineralocorticoid properties: a short review. Mol. Cell. Endocrinol. 217, 255–261.

O'Flynn, N., Britten, N., 2000. Menorrhagia in general practice – disease or illness? Soc. Sci. Med. 50, 651–661.

Rapkin, A., 2003. A review of treatment of premenstrual syndrome and premenstrual dysphoric disorder. Psychoneuroendocrinology 28, 39–53.

Royal College of Obstericians & Gynaecologists, 2007. Green-top Guideline No. 48. Management of Premenstrual Syndrome. Available at http://www.rcog.org.uk/files/rcog-corp/ uploaded-files/GT48ManagementPremensturalSyndrome.pdf.

Menopause 46

K. Marshall and S. Calvert

Menopause

The UK, like many countries in the developed world, has an ageing population, life expectancy is increasing and women continue to live longer than men, whilst birth rates are declining. Currently, a woman can expect to live about 35% of her life in a post-menopausal state.

Menopause is signalled by a woman's last menstrual period and is defined as the permanent cessation of menstruation resulting from loss of ovarian follicular activity. The occurrence of the last menstruation can only be diagnosed retrospectively and is usually taken as being final if it is followed by a 12-month bleed-free interval; such women are defined as being post-menopausal. The mean age of menopause in the UK is 51 years, and by the age of 54 years, around 80% of women will be post-menopausal. If menopause occurs before 40 years, it would be classed as a premature menopause. Many women will experience erratic periods before the final cessation due to inadequate ovarian oestrogen secretion; these women are described as being peri-menopausal. This transitional phase usually lasts around 4–5 years. The problems associated with menopause result from oestrogen deprivation. Hormone replacement therapy (HRT) reduces the effects of this deprivation and overcomes the associated symptoms.

Menopause is a natural event in the anatomical, physiological and psychological changes which form the female climacteric. Some women will go from the transition of being pre-menopausal to post-menopausal with no symptoms at all. Many will experience the symptoms associated with oestrogen lack, whether in the peri-menopausal or post-menopausal phase, which include:

- vasomotor symptoms
- localised atrophy of urogenital tissues
- osteoporosis
- psychological problems
- coronary heart disease.

Initially, the symptoms are more likely to include vasomotor symptoms such as hot flushes, night sweats and palpitations, and psychological problems such as mood changes, irritability, sleep disturbance, depression and decreased libido. Many women suffer from vaginal dryness and dyspareunia, which serve to enhance the loss of libido, and this in turn can adversely affect psychological well-being. The urethral mucosa may become atrophied, leading to an increased incidence of urinary tract infections or urinary incontinence. In some women, the urethra may eventually become fibrosed, leading to dysuria, frequency and urgency (urethral syndrome). The long-term consequences of oestrogen deprivation are often symptomless. There is a significant loss of calcium from the bones, which may give rise to frequent fractures, and there is a change in the blood lipid profile, which is associated with a rise in coronary heart disease.

Physiological changes

Ovarian

The approaching menopause is associated with loss of ovarian follicular activity. Human ovaries contain approximately 700,000 follicles at birth, but these cells have a high mortality rate and fewer than 500 of them will be ovulated. This number falls progressively with increasing age so that by the time the woman approaches 50 years of age, the number of follicles has fallen to zero or very few. The rate of follicle loss is highest during the decade between 40 and 50 years of age, possibly

725

due to an increase in the rate of degeneration (atresia) of the earliest follicles. Women over the age of 45 years who are menstruating regularly have been shown to have 10 times as many follicles as those with irregular cycles; those who have not had a period for 12 months have few follicles remaining. Thus, the size of the follicular pool is an important determinant in ovarian function.

Ovarian function includes two major roles: the production of eggs (gametogenesis) and the synthesis and secretion of hormones (hormonogenesis). Both of these functions undergo subtle changes with ageing so that fewer ova are produced and they are less readily fertilised, and the hormone levels become irregular. It is the granulosa cells in the developing follicle that normally secrete estradiol, and lack of this follicular activity results in diminishing oestrogen secretion. The diminution in the number of active follicles is followed by an increase in follicle-stimulating hormone (FSH) secretion from the anterior pituitary gland as the normal feedback mechanisms between ovarian estradiol secretion and the hypothalamus–pituitary axis become disrupted. It may be that there is an age-related decrease in sensitivity to feedback inhibition that exacerbates this increase in FSH levels. In women who are still bleeding, an FSH level exceeding 10–12 iu/L on day 2 or 3 of the bleed is indicative of a diminished ovarian response. A high FSH level (above 30 iu/L) and a low estradiol level (below 100 pmol/L) in the plasma characterise menopause. The low oestrogen level fails to stimulate growth of the uterine endometrium. As endometrial growth has not occurred, there can be no menstruation (shedding of the endometrium) and this signifies that menopause has arrived. Since ova are not being released, the production of progesterone from the ovary also ceases and the levels of luteinising hormone (LH) eventually rise. Thus, peri-menopausal and menopausal women are subjected to an increasing ovarian hormone deficiency, as shown in Table 46.1.

When the ovaries are conserved after hysterectomy they will usually continue to produce some estradiol, but the levels of this hormone will decline up to the age of the natural menopause. Post-menopausally, in all women, androstenedione (secreted from the adrenal cortex) is converted in adipose tissue and muscle (peripheral conversion) to estrone, which becomes the major circulating oestrogen (but estrone is about 10 times less potent than estradiol). The levels of FSH and LH remain elevated for many years if no HRT is given, but these elevated levels have no effect on the ovary since the follicles are atretic.

The cessation of reproductive function in the woman and the declining oestrogen production from the ovary are not the only physiological events associated with menopause. For many years, oestrogen was considered to be associated only with the genitourinary system, but its effects are more wide ranging and the major tissues affected include blood vessels, bones and the brain.

Urogenital system

With the failure in ovarian oestrogen production, the number of uterine endometrial oestrogen receptors occupied falls and endometrial growth is not sustained. Thus, in the post-menopausal woman, the endometrium becomes thin and atrophic. Likewise, in the other target tissues containing oestrogen receptors, the basal layers of the vaginal epithelium are no longer stimulated to maintain the vaginal epithelium and produce natural lubricants from the vaginal glands. The result is vaginal atrophy and a thin, dry vagina may result in dyspareunia. Because the lower urinary tract and the lower genital tract share common embryological origin, deprivation of oestrogen can result in urethral and bladder problems. Often, peri-menopausal and post-menopausal women report an increase in urinary frequency, nocturia and urge incontinence. For some women, these changes may become manifest as long as 10 years after menopause.

Bone

Osteoporosis is defined by WHO as a systemic skeletal disease characterised by low bone mass and microarchitectural deterioration of bone tissue leading to enhanced bone fragility and a consequent increase in fracture risk. In 2006, WHO estimated that it affects 200 million women worldwide. In addition, approximately 30% of women over the age of 50 have one or more vertebral fractures compared with one in five men over the age of 50 who will have an osteoporosis-related fracture in their remaining lifetime. The total number of hip fractures in 1950 was 1.66 million, and by 2050, this figure could reach 6.26 million. Twenty percent of people die within 1 year of a hip fracture (Cooper, 1997). Typical morbidities after a vertebral fracture include:

- back pain
- loss of height
- deformity (kyphosis, protuberant abdomen)
- reduced pulmonary function
- diminished quality of life: loss of self-esteem, distorted body image, dependence on narcotic analgesics, sleep disorder, depression, loss of independence.

To contextualise risk, the remaining lifetime probability in women at menopause of a fracture at any one of these sites exceeds that of breast cancer (~12%). Also, the likelihood of a fracture at any of these sites is 40% or more in developed countries (Kanis et al., 2000), a figure close to the probability of

Table 46.1 Ovarian hormone secretion after the onset of the normal menstrual cycle

	Pre-menopausal (normal cyclic)	Peri-menopausal (irregular cycles)	Post-menopausal (cessation of cycle)
Oestrogens	+++	++	+ → −
Progesterone	+++	+	−
Androgens	+	+	+ → −

coronary heart disease. Risk factors for osteoporosis include low body mass index ($<19\,kg/m^2$), smoking, early menopause, family history of maternal hip fracture, long-term systemic corticosteroid use and conditions affecting bone metabolism, especially those causing prolonged immobility. Osteoporosis is most common in white women. People with osteoporosis are at risk of fragility fractures, occurring as a result of mechanical forces which would not ordinarily cause fracture. The clinically relevant outcome in evaluating treatments for osteoporosis is the incidence of fragility fracture as otherwise this condition is asymptomatic and therefore undiagnosed. The most common sites for these fractures are the hip, vertebrae and wrist. In the UK, the combined cost of hospital and social care for patients with a hip fracture amounts to more than £1.73 billion per year (Torgerson et al., 2001). This is very similar to the annual £1.75 billion health care system costs of coronary heart disease costs. The cost of treating all osteoporotic fractures in post-menopausal women has been predicted to increase to more than £2.1 billion by 2020 (Burge, 2001).

Cardiovascular system

Young adult women are protected against the development of hypertension and its deleterious consequences in the cardiovascular system. Levels of low-density lipoprotein cholesterol (LDL-C) and very-low-density lipoprotein cholesterol (VLDL-C) are decreased by oestrogen, and the levels of high-density lipoprotein cholesterol (HDL-C) are increased, thereby giving some protection against atherosclerosis. HDL-C is known to promote cholesterol efflux from macrophages in the arterial wall, thereby reducing atheromatous plaque and conferring a protective effect against heart disease. However, after menopause, this protection is lost and the incidence of high blood pressure and associated cardiovascular disease increases to levels similar to those found in age-matched men.

Oestrogen has direct beneficial effects in the control of blood pressure, possibly via regulating endothelium-mediated control of arteriolar tone. In women deprived of oestrogen, endothelium-dependent vasodilation is impaired. This dysfunction is largely associated with a reduction in nitric oxide availability. Oestrogen increases nitric oxide availability by stimulating endothelial nitric oxide synthase (eNOS). Oestrogen also stimulates the production of other endothelium-derived relaxing factors such as prostacyclin (prostaglandin I_2). Research suggests that the oestrogen receptor (ER)α is important in mediating the vascular effects of oestrogen. Studies using selective ERα agonists are being undertaken. However, many pathways are stimulated by oestrogen receptor activation and the relative importance of these different pathways varies from tissue to tissue.

Miscellaneous

Thinning of the skin, brittle nails, hair loss and generalised aches and pains are also associated with reduced oestrogen levels (Hall and Phillips, 2005) The skin is the largest

non-reproductive target on which oestrogen acts. Oestrogen receptors, predominantly of the ERβ type, are widely distributed within the skin. Both types of oestrogen receptor (ERα and ERβ) are expressed within the hair follicle and associated structures. Thus, epidermal thinning, declining terminal collagen content, diminished skin moisture, decreased laxity and impaired wound healing (selective ERα ligands are being investigated for their wound-healing properties) have been reported in post-menopausal women.

In addition, women also show increasing body weight associated with ageing. This weight gain tends to increase or begin near menopause. Body fat redistribution to the abdomen also occurs independent of weight gain. This type of centralised abdominal fat distribution is widely recognised as an independent risk factor for cardiovascular disease in women.

Psychological changes

Older age at menarche and younger age at menopause are associated with poorer cognitive functioning during ageing. Recent studies have demonstrated that sex steroids have a multifarious and complex relationship with the central nervous system (Hogervorst et al., 2009). For example, there may be a positive correlation between increasing parity and improved executive functioning in response to oestrogen. This temporal relationship between oestrogen deprivation and response to exogenous oestrogen was clearly exemplified in the memory study arm of the WHI (Coker et al., 2010) and MWS studies (Hogervorst and Bandelow, 2010) at the turn of the twenty-first century.

Depression is twice as common in women as in men and may increase during times of changing hormonal levels such as at menopause. Some aspects of decreased central nervous system function have been related to falling oestrogen levels. Preclinical studies have shown oestrogen to have several positive effects on central nervous system function. Perhaps the most important is promotion of acetylcholine synthesis and increased synaptogenesis in the hippocampus. ERβ is expressed in this area of the brain as well as the entorhinal cortex and thalamus, areas crucially involved in explicit memory. Human neuroimaging studies have also indicated that oestrogen influences regional cerebral blood flow in women.

Management

Hormone replacement therapy

HRT is a complicated clinical issue requiring an in-depth risk/benefit assessment. The vast amount of study data are often conflicting, and careful analysis is required. Many factors need to be reviewed before it is prescribed. One important factor is age, as data have shown that if a woman aged less than 35 has a hysterectomy and a bilateral oophorectomy, her risk of non-fatal myocardial infarction is nearly eight times that of her age-matched counterpart who has retained her ovaries. Age at time of HRT prescription in relation to menopausal age, that is, number of years of oestrogen deprivation before replacement, is also of importance when considering outcomes. Individual differences in hormone metabolism (both endogenous and exogenous) are also likely to be important as several different cytochrome enzymes metabolise oestrogen and may be affected by inherited polymorphisms. Therefore, some women may produce oestrogenic metabolites possessing considerable oestrogenic activity, whilst others produce metabolites which are relatively non-oestrogenic. Body mass index (BMI) also influences response to HRT, with increased plasma estradiol levels observed in women with higher BMIs.

HRT is effective for symptomatic relief of menopausal symptoms, and its use is justified when symptoms adversely affect quality of life. Current advice is that the lowest effective dose for a particular woman should be used for the shortest period of time. Local oestrogen replacement may be used to reverse the symptoms of urogenital atrophy as it appears to be more effective than systemic therapy. There is no evidence to suggest that local oestrogen treatment is associated with significant risks.

Treatment with HRT should be reviewed at least annually, with alternative therapies considered for the management of osteoporosis. In the treatment of menopausal symptoms, the benefits of short-term HRT outweigh the risks in the majority of women, but in healthy women without symptoms, the risks outweigh the benefits.

Contraindications to the use of HRT include undiagnosed vaginal bleeding in post-menopausal women, the presence of an oestrogen-dependent tumour, liver disease (where liver function tests have failed to return to normal), active thrombophlebitis, and active or recent arterial thromboembolic disease, for example, angina or myocardial infarction. A history of deep vein thrombosis and pulmonary embolism requires careful evaluation before the use of oestrogen therapy. Use in patients with Dubin–Johnson and Rotor syndromes may also be contraindicated.

Oestrogen therapy

Since the symptoms and long-term effects of menopause are due to oestrogen deprivation, the mainstay of HRT is oestrogen. This may be administered orally or parenterally but, in either case, the oestrogens used are naturally occurring and include:

* estradiol
* estriol
* estrone
* estropipate
* conjugated equine oestrogen (estrone sulphate 40%, equilin sulphate 60%)
* estradiol valerate.

The use of 'natural' oestrogens reduces the risk of the potentially dangerous oestrogenic effects such as raised blood pressure, alteration in coagulation factors and an undesirable lipid profile, which sometimes occur with the more potent synthetic oestrogens used in the oral contraceptive agents. A 'natural' oestrogen is defined as one that is normally found in the human female and has a physiological effect. Natural oestrogens are less potent (up to 200 times) than synthetic oestrogens. As they are naturally occurring compounds, the plasma half-life of these oestrogens is similar to that of the ovarian-secreted oestrogens and the duration of action is shorter than the synthetic oestrogens, such as ethinylestradiol, used in many formulations of the contraceptive pill. The plasma ratio of estradiol to estrone is normally about 1:1 to 2:1, and the aim of HRT should be to preserve this ratio.

There are four main routes of administration for oestrogens in HRT:

* oral
* transdermal (patches/gels/cream)
* subcutaneous (implants)
* vaginal (creams and medicated rings).

The use of oral oestrogen therapy, while convenient for the patient, does mean that the oestrogen will be subjected to conversion to estrone by the liver and the gut, thereby altering the estradiol:estrone ratio in favour of the less active oestrogen, estrone. The oral preparations have different metabolic effects due to first-pass hepatic metabolism. Smoking stimulates metabolism of oestrogens by cytochrome P450 and decreases plasma oestrogen levels by 40–70% in oral oestrogen users. Smoking has no significant effect on plasma oestrogen levels in users of transdermal preparations. Oral delivery compared to transdermal delivery (Table 46.2) also has different effects on lipid levels (Vrablik et al., 2008). In addition, orally administered oestrogens undergo first-pass hepatic metabolism, which may result in some reduction in anti-thrombin III, a potent inhibitor of coagulation. Implants and patches show smaller changes in coagulation, platelet function or fibrinolysis.

More constant levels of oestrogen result from the use of transdermal patches containing estradiol, and these have the added advantage of a more physiological estradiol:estrone ratio (Delmas et al., 1999). However, the adhesive used in these transdermal patches and the alcohol base can cause skin irritation. The patch is applied to the non-hairy skin of the lower body, and care should be taken to ensure that it is placed away from breast tissue. The patch is changed either once or twice a week, thus providing a constant reservoir of estradiol to provide a controlled release into the circulation. Estradiol is also available in a gel formulation, applied daily to the skin over the area of a template (to ensure correct dosage), but

Table 46.2 Effect of HRT administration route on lipid profile

Oral	Transdermal
↓ Low-density lipoprotein	↓ Low-density lipoprotein
↓ Total cholesterol	↓ Total cholesterol
↑ High-density lipoprotein	↔ High-density lipoprotein
↑ Triglycerides	↓ Triglycerides
↑ Bile cholesterol	↔ Bile cholesterol

this formulation may give erratic absorption. The intranasal preparation, administered as a nasal spray, also avoids hepatic first-pass metabolism.

The oestrogen implant gives a constant level of oestrogen from a few days after insertion for up to 6 months. This formulation maintains the best estradiol:estrone ratio and is a convenient method of administration, requiring repeat implants only every 6 months. However, because the levels of oestrogen are constantly raised, there will be some increase in oestrogen receptor numbers, and this can lead to a recurrence of symptoms of oestrogen deficiency due to the presence of unoccupied oestrogen receptors, even in the presence of normal or even high oestrogen levels. This phenomenon, called tachyphylaxis, results in patients becoming symptomatic and requesting repeat implants earlier and earlier. In such cases, it is unwise to treat with additional oestrogen; the patient should receive counselling and perhaps a change of preparation. The disadvantage of the implant is that, once inserted, it cannot be removed readily and even if it is removed, the oestrogen level will take at least a month to fall. There is also evidence that the uterine endometrium, if present, remains stimulated for some time after removal of the implant.

Both the transdermal and implant preparations avoid the first-pass hepatic effects of oral oestrogens and are less likely to affect liver enzyme systems and clotting factors. Some studies show an increase in the incidence of venous thromboembolism (VTE) in women taking HRT. Therefore, patients who have a history of deep vein thrombosis or pulmonary embolism will need careful guidance, with each woman being considered individually, and the relative risks evaluated. Other risk factors include severe varicose veins, obesity or a family history of deep vein thrombosis (DVT). If HRT is justified in such patients, transdermal preparations are a better alternative than oral preparations.

Vaginal creams containing oestrogen are available but generally fail to produce the reliable plasma levels required to protect against the long-term effects of oestrogen deprivation. They provide short-term relief from menopausal symptoms, in particular, atrophic vaginitis. A vaginal ring which releases estradiol at a controlled rate in physiological levels for up to 3 months is an alternative for women who cannot tolerate transdermal patches.

The dose of oestrogen used in HRT sufficient to preserve bone density is usually higher than that necessary to alleviate vasomotor symptoms. The doses suggested to protect bone density are estradiol 2 mg/day orally, 50 μg/day transdermally and 50 mg every 6 months by implant. If the conjugated equine oestrogens are used, the oral dose should be 0.625 mg/day. The lower doses found in vaginal creams may alleviate the vasomotor symptoms but will not protect against osteoporosis. Current guidelines advise the use of the lowest possible dose of HRT to relieve vasomotor symptoms and recommend alternative treatment to prevent and treat osteoporosis.

Oestrogens should be used alone only in women who have undergone a hysterectomy; if the uterus is present, the endometrium will be stimulated and this increase in endometrial growth may be a precursor to development of a malignant condition. Current practice is to administer progestogens with oestrogen. In the early 1970s, when oestrogen was used alone, HRT received a bad press because in women who had not undergone hysterectomy, there was an increased incidence of endometrial carcinoma. In women who have undergone hysterectomy, oestrogens are usually administered continuously.

Progestogen therapy

The only proven reason for adding a progestogen to oestrogen therapy for HRT in women with an intact uterus is to protect the endometrium from hyperplasia and possible neoplasia. There are many preparations which contain progestogens added to oestrogen for a number of days per month. However, to effectively prevent endometrial hyperplasia, the progestogen must be taken for a minimum of 12 days. The minimum dose of progestogen required to protect against hyperplasia depends on the potency of the compound used.

The progestogens commonly available in HRT preparations are either derivatives of progesterone, such as medroxyprogesterone and dydrogesterone, or 19-nortestosterone substitutes such as norethisterone or levonorgestrel. All these synthetic progestogens are active following oral administration and provide adequate protection of the endometrium against oestrogen stimulation. Some transdermal preparations also incorporate a progestogenic compound in the regimen. As with all semi-synthetic or synthetic hormones, these compounds may act on receptors other than the progesterone receptor, and the long-term consequence of this is not predictable.

Progesterone is the only progestogen to act solely on the progesterone receptor, but it has poor oral bioavailability and so it is difficult to achieve satisfactory plasma concentrations. However, the micronised preparations are better absorbed. Progesterone may also be administered at night in the form of a pessary or suppository, or by injection in the form of a long-lasting subdermal implant. The progestogen in HRT is most commonly administered orally or transdermally and usually one of the synthetic progestogens is used.

Oestrogen and progestogen regimens

The monthly withdrawal bleed is perceived by some postmenopausal patients to be an unacceptable side effect of HRT, and this has resulted in the development of a number of regimens in an effort to minimise this effect (Box 46.1). Formulations have been produced with which bleeding only occurs every 3 months instead of every 4 weeks, or it does not occur at all.

Box 46.1 Regimens of combined oestrogen and progestogen therapy for use in HRT

- Oestrogen 28 days + progestogen 12 or 14 days, then repeat without interval (bleed every 4 weeks)
- Oestrogen 70 days + progestogen 14 days followed by 7 days placebo tablets (bleed every 3 months)
- Oestrogen + progesterone continuously (no bleed)
- Oestrogen continuously + Mirena IUS (bleed variable but levonorgestrel likely to reduce bleed and can provoke amenorrhoea)

The use of the 70-day oestrogen preparation, while being more popular with women because bleeding only occurs every 3 months, needs further evaluation as regards endometrial protection. Bleeding can be avoided altogether if a combination of oestrogen and progestogen is given continuously throughout the treatment (continuous combined HRT). Such a preparation should only be given to women who are at least 12 months post-menopausal and have an atrophied endometrium; otherwise, breakthrough bleeding may occur. Bleeding in the first 6 months (usually just spotting) is not uncommon but bleeding after this time should be investigated, although the incidence of endometrial hyperplasia is low with this continuous regimen. Others recommend a 28-day interval between courses of treatment to allow the endometrium to become atrophic in patients who are changing from the cyclical therapy to the continuous combined therapy. Patients who commence cyclical HRT prior to ceasing menstruation should change to a continuous combined preparation only after the age of 54 (when there is an 80% chance that they will be post- rather than peri-menopausal) to reduce the risk of breakthrough bleeding. An alternative option is to use the levonorgestrol-loaded intrauterine system (IUS or Mirena) in conjunction with oral oestrogen. This option can be particularly useful for women intolerant of progestogenic side effects.

Not all progestogens have the same pharmacological profile and these differences have implications for their usage. Two of the most widely used synthetic progestogens are medroxyprogesterone acetate and norethisterone. These are used as the progestogenic component of an HRT regimen in combination with oestrogen but have been shown to increase the risk of breast cancer in long-term HRT users (Million Women Study Collaborators, 2003; Women's Health Initiative, 2002). Structurally, medroxyprogesterone acetate is more similar to natural progesterone than norethisterone. The metabolism of these two compounds is also different, as medroxyprogesterone acetate is the major progestogenic compound rather than one of its metabolites. In contrast, the metabolites of norethisterone exhibit significant activity in addition to a wide range of non-progestogenic actions. Norethisterone also binds to sex hormone–binding globulin, whereas medroxyprogesterone acetate does not.

The most notable difference in steroid receptor-binding affinity between the two synthetic progestogens and endogenous progesterone is that although all the compounds have affinity for the mineralocorticoid receptor, only the natural compound has antagonist activity. As a consequence, the synthetic compounds may be unable to counteract the sodium-retaining and blood pressure–raising effects of the oestrogens used in HRT. Endogenous progesterone affinity for the glucocorticoid receptor is also different, with medroxyprogesterone acetate a more potent antagonist than norethisterone. This may influence their side-effect profiles and impact on inflammation, immune response, adrenal function and bone metabolism.

Tibolone

Tibolone is a synthetic steroid that has oestrogenic, progestogenic and androgenic effects that alleviate menopausal symptoms without a monthly bleed. The oestrogenic effects are weak and should not promote endometrial hyperplasia, but 10–15% of women on this treatment experience breakthrough bleeding. The drug is given continuously but is not suitable for women within 1 year of menopause or immediately after oestrogen therapy because in such cases breakthrough bleeding is most likely to occur. The evidence suggests that this drug is protective against osteoporosis, but the long-term cardioprotective effects remain unclear as there is some evidence of a lowering of HDL-C. It should also be withdrawn if signs of thromboembolic disease occur. The androgenic action of tibolone tends to increase libido. It has been reported that tibolone does have fewer breast-related adverse effects than oestrogenic or oestrogenic–progestogenic HRT regimens.

Raloxifene

Raloxifene is a non-steroidal benzothiophene that binds to some oestrogen receptors and belongs to a class of drugs referred to as selective oestrogen receptor modulators (SERMs). These compounds act selectively on some oestrogen receptors to increase bone mineral density and antagonise oestrogen-dependent effects on breast and endometrial tissues in post-menopausal women. However, there is a reported increased risk of thromboembolism, particularly in the first 4 months of use. Raloxifene cannot be used to treat vasomotor symptoms in peri-menopausal women. In fact, it is reported to induce hot flushes. It has little or no stimulatory effect on the uterine endometrium and is not associated with uterine bleeding.

In summary, raloxifene is a compound that selectively stimulates one group of oestrogen receptors and may be considered a curative treatment for osteoporosis and a preventive agent in the development of oestrogen-dependent breast tumours.

Clinical monitoring

Before initiating HRT, a detailed patient history and physical examination are essential to eliminate medical disorders and genital malignancy. Bone mineral densitometry can also be helpful to establish a baseline for subsequent measurements. Blood tests should include serum electrolytes and creatinine, liver function tests, haemoglobin, lipids and a full blood count. Urine analysis should also be performed. The history and findings from the physical examination may indicate other tests. The patient should have undergone routine cervical smear examination and, preferably, mammography. In women with an intact uterus, any irregular vaginal bleeding should be investigated to exclude endometrial pathology.

After starting therapy, the woman should be seen within 3 months in the first instance and then at intervals between 6 and 12 months so that symptoms may be assessed and any side effects of therapy can be reported. Blood pressure measurements are undertaken on these routine visits; HRT is usually associated with a fall in blood pressure due to a vasodilator action of oestrogen. Hypertension is not a contraindication to treatment with HRT but does need treatment before starting on oestrogen therapy. Some women may have an elevated blood pressure on oral oestrogen but show no such effect with the non-oral route. Weight gain may occur some months after treatment has been initiated, and the patient should be advised to reduce calorie intake accordingly.

Stopping HRT

Guidelines (see Section 7.3.1 British National Formulary) indicate that there are a number of signs and symptoms which suggest that women should be advised to immediately stop taking HRT and these include:

- sudden severe chest pain
- sudden breathlessness or cough with blood-stained sputum
- unexplained severe pain in calf of one leg
- severe stomach pain
- serious neurological effects
- hepatitis, jaundice, liver enlargement
- blood pressure above systolic 160 mmHg and diastolic 100 mmHg
- detection of a risk factor, for example, prolonged immobility after surgery or leg injury.

Once HRT has been stopped, investigation and treatment should be undertaken as appropriate.

Examples of serious neurological effects include unusual severe, prolonged headache. This is especially important if the headache occurs for the first time or it becomes progressively worse. Marked numbness, especially if it suddenly affects one side or part of the body, is important. Other neurological effects are sudden partial or complete loss of vision or disturbance of hearing or other perceptual disorders. HRT should also be stopped if the following occur: dysphasia, bad fainting attack or collapse, a first unexplained epileptic seizure/weakness and motor disturbances.

Alternatives to HRT

HRT remains the most effective treatment for vasomotor symptoms, resulting in 80–90% reduction in hot flushes. Of the non-hormonal agents, serotonin–norepinephrine reuptake inhibitors (SNRIs) such as venlafaxine and its active metabolite desvenlafaxine appear to be the next most useful treatments; gabapentin may be equally effective, whilst clonidine is only modestly effective in reducing hot flushes. Generally, there is a lack of safety information and trial data regarding alternative therapies. Trials with black cohosh, red clover and soy foods, all of which contain phytoestrogens, have yielded conflicting results and have raised concerns about hepatoxicity (black cohosh) and interactions with anti-coagulants (red clover).

Bisphosphonates such as alendronate, etidronate and risedronate are inhibitors of bone resorption and increase bone mineral density by altering osteoclast activation and function. Bisphosphonates are used with care in women with upper gastro-intestinal problems and their posology is complex. They are contraindicated in patients with hypocalcaemia. Etidronate is also contraindicated in patients with severe renal impairment.

Teriparatide, a recombinant human parathyroid hormone, is licensed to treat osteoporosis in post-menopausal women. It stimulates new formation of bone and may increase resistance to fracture. However, it has several contraindications including hypercalcaemia, severe renal impairment, metabolic bone diseases and unexplained elevations of alkaline phosphatase.

A Cochrane review supports the efficacy of strontium ranelate for the reduction of fractures in post-menopausal osteoporotic women (O'Donnell et al., 2006). The main side effect reported was diarrhoea, but the potential vascular and neurological side effects should be explored further. National guidance (NICE, 2010) details the role of alendronate, etidronate, risedronate, raloxifene and strontium ranelate for the primary prevention of osteoporotic fragility fractures in post-menopausal women.

Advances in bone biology may lead to the design of more elegant therapies to deal with osteoporosis. An example would be denosumab, a human monoclonal antibody which binds to the receptor activator of nuclear factor-$\kappa\beta$ ligand (RANKL), which is responsible for osteoclast differentiation, activation and survival. Denosumab therefore mimics the function of osteoprotegerin limiting bone resorption.

Some small studies have shown that aerobic exercise can improve cardiovascular parameters and reduce menopausal symptoms in addition to reducing BMI.

Treatment with HRT

Vasomotor symptoms

Vasomotor symptoms include hot flushes, headaches, insomnia, giddiness and faintness. They occur in about 70–80% of women and result in physical distress in about 50%, lasting for up to 5 years in around one-quarter of the women. Flushes and sweats, particularly night sweats, indicate vasomotor instability and probably result from unoccupied oestrogen receptors on blood vessels. Oestrogens cause a rapid rise in blood flow through the blood vessels, and lack of oestrogen will render the oestrogen receptors in these vessels supersensitive to any subsequent rise in oestrogen level. During the perimenopause and menopause, oestrogen levels tend to fluctuate and it is suggested that it is these fluctuations that result in vasomotor symptoms. The extreme sensitivity of blood vessel oestrogen receptors tends to mean that a clinical response to vasomotor symptoms is achieved with low doses of oestrogen. There is also likely to be central control via a supra-pituitary mechanism incorporating several chemical pathways involving serotonin, noradrenaline and dopamine. General advice regarding diet, for example, avoiding certain foods and drinks that cause vasodilation such as hot spicy foods and alcohol, may be helpful to some women. There is some evidence that regular exercise, which stimulates the production of hypothalamic β-endorphins, may reduce the risk of hot flushes.

Urogenital tract

These symptoms include:

- vaginal dryness and dyspareunia (painful sexual intercourse)
- vaginal discharge and bleeding
- urinary incontinence, urgency of micturition, recurrent symptoms of cystitis.

Symptoms result from oestrogen deficiency in menopausal woman and may be treated either with systemic HRT preparations or with topical applications of oestrogen incorporated into vaginal creams, pessaries and silicone vaginal rings. Such topical routes of administration do result in some systemic absorption of oestrogen through the vaginal mucosa and since this may be erratic, vasomotor symptoms may ensue. Absorption of oestrogen from these topical applications may also stimulate uterine endometrial development, if present. Consequently, it is recommended that these treatments should not be used for more than 6 months. The dose of oestrogen required to stimulate the oestrogen receptors in the vagina and the lower urethra is about 10 μcg/day, and the efficiency of such low doses has been demonstrated in a number of clinical trials. The effect of oestrogen on vaginal symptoms is more marked than its effect on urinary symptoms, but the incidence of urinary sensory dysfunction may be improved. Menopausal atrophic vaginitis may respond to a short course of a topical vaginal oestrogen preparation used for a few weeks and repeated if necessary. Current guidance is that the minimum effective dose should be used for the shortest duration.

Initial treatment with local oestrogen may result in a reaction to the presence of oestrogen in tissues containing oestrogen receptors, such as the breast and vagina. The longer the time between starting HRT and menopause, the greater these effects. During initial treatment, other effects observed include headache, appetite increase and calf muscle cramps, but these side effects usually resolve without intervention. HRT with small doses of an oestrogen (together with a progestogen in women with an intact uterus) is appropriate for alleviating menopausal symptoms such as vaginal atrophy or vasomotor instability.

Bone

In a woman not treated with HRT, approximately 15% of bone mass is lost within 10 years of menopause, resulting in an increased incidence of fracture, typically of the hip. Such fractures take up at least 10% of orthopaedic beds, and the total cost in terms of morbidity and mortality is high. The effect of oestrogen lack is to increase osteoclastic bone resorption. There is an overall increase in bone turnover, more bone is resorbed than replaced and there is an associated increase in the rate of bone loss which may continue for 5–10 years.

Oestrogens may exert effects on bone through the calcium-regulating hormones such as calcitonin and parathyroid-regulating hormones. Evidence also exists for the effect of oestrogens on the local production of bone growth factors, cytokines, in particular osteoprotegerin, which blocks osteoclastogenesis and prostaglandin E$_2$.

The greatest effect of oestrogen on bone is seen with implants, where an approximately 8% increase in vertebral bone density is seen within 1 year of treatment. Estradiol patches are the next most effective route of administration (Fig. 46.1), while oral therapy only achieves an increase in bone density of about 2% per annum. However, 5 years of oral oestrogen therapy will still achieve a lifetime reduction in femoral neck fracture of as much as 50%.

Oestrogen improves the quality and quantity of bone in the post-menopausal woman. It may be started at any time after menopause, and the benefit will continue for the duration of treatment. Bone loss will continue after treatment ceases, which leads into the difficult area of how long treatment should continue. It was previously recommended that to obtain maximum benefit from treatment with oestrogen, the duration of the course should be at least 10 years. However, studies have identified some potential adverse effects of HRT (Million Women Study Collaborators, 2003; Women's Health Initiative, 2002). Therefore, this recommendation is controversial, particularly in women with an intact uterus, where a combined HRT preparation is required as there is probably a greater risk of adverse outcome. Oestrogen given systemically in the peri-menopausal and post-menopausal period or tibolone given in the post-menopausal period also diminishes post-menopausal osteoporosis, but other drugs are preferred.

Raloxifene is licensed for the prevention and treatment of osteoporosis as an alternative to HRT. Raloxifene reduces bone loss and increases bone density at the spine and hip in post-menopausal women. With its oestrogen antagonist effect on breast and endometrium, raloxifene may prove to be an advance over oestrogen treatment in osteoporosis prevention and treatment in post-menopausal women. It does, however, cause hot flushes which may be unacceptable for some.

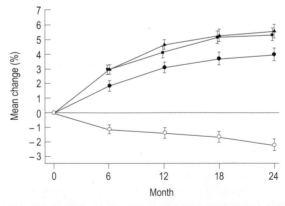

Fig. 46.1 Percentage of change from baseline (mean ± SEM) in lumbar spine bone mineral density in patients receiving placebo (open circles) or transdermal 17β-estradio 50 μcg/day (filled circles), 75 μcg/day (squares) or 100 μcg/day (filled triangles) (from Delmas et al., 1999).

Cardiovascular system

The estimated influence of HRT on the incidence of coronary heart disease, venous thromboembolism and stroke is summarised in Table 46.3.

Coronary heart disease

Women at 45 years are significantly less likely than men to die of coronary heart disease, but by the age of 60 years, the death rate from the disease is similar in both sexes. Oestrogen is probably central to this gender difference as women who experience early loss of endogenous estradiol have an accelerated risk of developing coronary heart disease. Intuitively, it would appear logical that post-menopausal women would gain benefit from receiving exogenous oestrogen. However, there are conflicting views as to whether this is, or is not, the case. A 4-year study of women with coronary heart disease in the USA (Heart and Estrogen-Progestin Replacement Study, HERS) who were also receiving HRT (conjugated equine oestrogen and medroxyprogesterone acetate) demonstrated no significant reduction in stroke (Simon et al., 2001). This was in contrast to the increased risk of myocardial infarction in the first year of starting HRT in the original HERS report (Hulley et al., 1998). The Women's Health Initiative (2002), another US-based study, also reported an increase in coronary events in the first year of receiving HRT.

The relevance of both studies to UK practice has been challenged as both involved use of conjugated equine oestrogen/ medroxyprogesterone acetate regimens. In the UK, natural progesterone is preferred, and this differs from medroxyprogesterone acetate in that it does not attenuate the beneficial effects of oestrogen in reducing the development of coronary artery atherosclerosis and protecting against coronary vasospasm. A study (De Vries et al., 2006) using the UK General Practice Research Database found HRT was associated with a decrease in risk of acute myocardial infarction, and there was no difference between the different oestrogen–progestogen combinations. A recent study found that transdermal but not oral oestrogen replacement therapy significantly reduced atherogenic index of plasma (Vrablik et al., 2008). This occurred by increasing HDL particle size and therefore improving the antiatherogenic properties.

The International Menopause Society consensus statement (2009) states that HRT can be given to women around the age of natural menopause without increasing the risk of coronary heart disease and may even decrease the risk in this age group. HRT is not contraindicated in women with hypertension, and in some cases, HRT may even reduce blood pressure. HRT is contraindicated in women with a history of myocardial infarction, stroke or pulmonary embolism.

Venous thromboembolism

It is known that the oestrogen in the combined oral contraceptive pill contributes to thromboembolic disorders. Whether the same applies to the oestrogen in HRT is unclear as the dose of oestrogen found in HRT is much lower and more physiological than that in the oral contraceptive pill. Analysis of the results from the Women's Health Initiative (2002) has confirmed that there is an increased risk of pulmonary embolism with HRT and the risk is greater with oral HRT than transdermal oestrogen.

Table 46.3 Estimated influence of HRT on incidence of gynaecological cancers, venous thromboembolism, stroke and CHD (MHRA/CHM, 2007)

Risk	Age range (years)	Background incidence per 1000 women in Europe not using HRT		Additional cases per 1000 women using oestrogen only HRT (estimated)		Additional cases per 1000 women using combined (oestrogen-progestogen) HRT (estimated)	
		Over 5 years	Over 10 years	For 5 years' use	For 10 years' use	For 5 years' use	For 10 years' use
Breast cancer	50–59	10	20	2	6	6	24
	60–69	15	30	3	9	9	36
Endometrial cancer	50–59	2	4	4	32	NS	NS
	60–69	3	6	6	48	NS	NS
Ovarian cancer	50–59	2	4	<1	1	<1	1
	60–69	3	6	<1	2	<1	2
Venous thromboembolism	50–59	5		2		7	
	60–69	8		2		10	
	60–69	9		3		3	
Coronary heart disease	70–79	29–44		NS		15	

Note: Where background incidence or additional cases have not been included in the table, this indicates a lack of available data. NS indicates a non-significant difference.

Oral oestrogen, in contrast to the transdermal route, undergoes extensive first-pass metabolism. This increases the production of prothrombotic factors in the liver and is associated with a reduction in fibrinogen and factor VII activation, such as von Willebrand's factor and anti-thrombin, and enhanced fibrinolysis (RCOG, 2004). HRT is also associated with increased resistance to activated protein C.

Whilst oestrogen exposure and age increase the risk of venous thromboembolism, they do not explain the increased risk seen in the first year of HRT use. An underlying thrombophilia, a known risk in hyperoestrogenic situations, is thought to be the additional factor that makes certain women susceptible to venous thromboembolism. Guidelines (RCOG, 2004) to manage the risk of venous thromboembolism have been produced for women starting or continuing HRT (Box 46.2). The selective oestrogen receptor modulators (SERMS) such as raloxifene are considered to carry the same risk of thrombosis as oestrogen-containing HRT.

Overall, minimising cardiovascular risk whilst obtaining the benefits of HRT is influenced by the age of the women treated, their body mass index, cardiovascular health and menopausal history, the timing of initiation of HRT, the formulation of the product used, and polymorphism.

Cancer

Details of the estimated influence of HRT on the incidence of cancer are presented in Table 46.3.

Colorectal cancer

Colorectal cancers tend to occur in women over 50, and several studies have indicated that HRT can reduce the risk by around 35%. The exact mechanism for this protective effect on the colon is unclear, although it has been suggested that oestrogen may decrease the formation of potentially carcinogenic bile acids.

Table 46.4 Properties of progestogens and their link to breast cancer (adapted from Campagnoli et al., 2005)

Progestogen	Action
19-Nortestosterone derivatives, medroxyprogesterone acetate	Oestrogenic activity Influence on 17β-hydroxysteroid dehydrogenase
19-Nortestosterone derivatives, medroxyprogesterone acetate	Metabolic effects, opposing those of oestrogen, on insulin sensitivity. Hepatic effects, opposing those of oestrogen, that is increasing IGF-1 (insulin-like growth factor), decrease in sex hormone-binding globulin
19-Nortestosterone derivatives	Binding to sex hormone-binding globulin with consequent reduction in capacity to bind oestrogen

Ovarian cancer

The risk of ovarian cancer risk is known to be affected by exogenous hormones, with a reduced incidence consistently reported in users of oral contraceptives. The relationship between the hormones used in HRT and ovarian cancer is, however, less clear. Women who use oestrogen plus a progestogen do not appear to be at increased risk of ovarian cancer, perhaps because the progestogenic component has an apoptotic effect on the ovarian epithelium. This has been supported

---

Box 46.2 Summary of guidelines for dealing with the risk of venous thromboembolism (VTE) in women receiving HRT (adapted from RCOG, 2004)

Women starting or continuing HRT
- Women starting or continuing HRT should be counselled with regard to perceived benefits and possible risks for their individual situations, including consideration of alternative therapies.
- All women commencing HRT should be counselled about the risk of VTE, should be aware of the signs and symptoms of VTE and should be able to access medical help rapidly if they suspect that they have developed a thrombus.
- Universal screening of women for thrombophilic defects prior to or continuing the prescription of HRT is inappropriate.
- Prior to commencing HRT, a personal history and a family history assessing the presence of VTE in a first- or second-degree relative should be obtained.
- HRT should be avoided in women with multiple pre-existing risk factors for VTE.

Women with a personal or family history of VTE
- Testing for thrombophilia should be discussed with, and available for, women with a personal or family history of VTE.
- In women with a previous VTE, with or without underlying heritable thrombophilia, oral HRT should be usually avoided in view of the relatively high risk of recurrent VTE.
- In women with a personal history of VTE but with an underlying thrombophilic trait identified through screening, HRT is not recommended in high-risk situations such as anti-thrombin deficiency or with combinations of defects.
- In women over 50 years with a history of VTE within the previous year, a full clinical history and examination with appropriate investigations is warranted for underlying disease.
- If a woman who is on HRT develops VTE, HRT should be discontinued.
- If a woman wants to continue on HRT after VTE, long-term anti-coagulation should be considered.

by studies in small groups of women with a mutation in either the *BRCA1* or *BRCA2* gene (point mutations associated with breast and ovarian cancer) which demonstrated that HRT did not adversely influence the risk of developing ovarian cancer. In contrast, other large HRT trials have suggested a possible increase in risk of ovarian cancer, particularly in women who have had a hysterectomy and are receiving long-term oestrogen-only HRT.

Endometrial cancer

Unopposed oestrogen therapy at least doubles the risk of endometrial cancer, but the addition of a progestogen, either in continuous combined or sequential regimens, reduces this risk. Of the two regimens, continuous combined administration is more effective than sequential therapy in reducing the risk of endometrial hyperplasia.

Breast cancer

Breast cancer is the most common cause of disease and death in middle-aged women, affecting around one in 11 women before the age of 75 in developed countries. Over the past 20 years, there has been a growing body of evidence to suggest that progesterone contributes to the development of breast cancer. Evidence to support this came from trials in which use of combined regimens increased breast cancer risk more than oestrogen alone. This is thought to have occurred because the synthetic progestogens possessed some non-progesterone like effects that potentiated the proliferating action of oestrogen. In the USA, the most commonly used progestogen in HRT was medroxyprogesterone acetate combined with conjugated equine oestrogen and administered orally. In contrast, in central and southern Europe, a wider range of progestogens is used, particularly the 19-nortestosterone derivatives. Studies investigating the use of natural micronised progesterone to improve bioavailability in HRT regimens have demonstrated no increased risk of breast cancer. *In vitro* studies with medroxyprogesterone have found it promotes the reproductive transformation of estrone into estradiol by influencing the activity of 17β-hydroxysteroid dehydrogenase. The properties of the synthetic progestogens are outlined in Table 46.4.

The relationship between different HRT regimens and breast cancer is complex (Table 46.4). There are many potential confounders to be considered when interpreting trial data, for example, time of initiation of therapy, in relation to menopausal status, body mass index, prior hormone use, etc. Chlebowski et al. (2009) reported on the decline in breast cancer in the USA after a reduction in HRT usage following publication of the WHI trial (2002). This prompted a response from the President of the International Menopause Society (Sturdee, 2009) summarised as follows:

- Decline in breast cancer rates started at least 3 years before the WHI study was halted (which led to a dramatic drop in HRT use). This implies that decline in breast cancer rates must be independent of the reduction in HRT use.

- Breast cancer takes years to develop and at least a decade to reach the detectable stage. If HRT use causes breast cancer, then the drop in breast cancer rates would not be seen for some time.
- The drop in breast cancer rates could be due to other factors, for example, changes in screening.

Notwithstanding these arguments, the problem on what to advise women contemplating HRT can be problematic. Current advice recommends that the minimum effective dose of HRT should be used for the shortest duration, but for the treatment of menopausal symptoms the benefits of short-term HRT outweigh the risks in the majority of women, especially in those aged under 60 years (Joint Formulary Committee, 2010).

Psychological symptoms

Psychological symptoms include:

- depression
- mood changes and irritability, which may also be associated with other life changes occurring at this time
- exhaustion
- poor concentration and memory
- panic attacks
- lowered libido, which may be exacerbated by the above symptoms together with dyspareunia linked to lack of oestrogen and falling androgen levels.

The role of HRT in this area has not been clearly defined, although in several studies, surgical menopause has been associated with depression, indicating a correlation with oestrogen lack. Many women experience psychological symptoms around menopause, and although these may be associated with oestrogen deficiency, they may also result from the changes in family life that often occur around this time. Disturbance of sleep pattern and sleep deprivation, associated with menopause, are likely to contribute to the psychological symptoms. Many women find treatment with estradiol restores normal sleep and psychological problems are then reduced. Some of the mood changes will respond to counselling and psychotropic drugs. Treatment with oestrogens at high doses (patches of 100 μcg or implants of 50 mg) has also been shown to improve depression scores. If a progestogen is added into the regimen, then the results are less predictable since progestogen use is related to mood changes, particularly in women who have previously suffered from the pre-menstrual syndrome. Age negatively influences almost all sexual function domains in a significant manner.

HRT improves some aspects of sexual function during menopause, but it does not appear to improve the domains of desire and arousal. The lowered libido experienced during menopause is associated with reduced levels of circulating androgen resulting from ovarian failure. It has been demonstrated that subcutaneous implants of testosterone, 100 mg every 6 months, will increase the libido in a high proportion of patients.

Central nervous system

The relationship between oestrogen and neurodegenerative conditions, in particular, Alzheimer's disease (Mulnard et al., 2000), has received attention in the light of an observation that there is an increased incidence of the disease in older women. The development of plaques of amyloid-β, a protein that disrupts nerve cell connections in the brain, occurs more rapidly in the absence of oestrogen. This effect of amyloid-β production results in the symptoms of short-term memory loss and disorientation which occur in Alzheimer's disease (AD). Further studies are essential to clarify the relationship between HRT and Alzheimer's disease. There is some evidence that heavier women, who have higher free estradiol levels, exhibit better cognitive function in several domains. Such women may also have a greater clinical response when using exogenous oestrogen. It should also be noted that conjugated equine oestrogen is composed primarily of oestrone sulphate and this oestrogen has a much lower affinity for oestrogen receptors than oestradiol. Hence, the findings with respect to exogenous oestrogen and neurological function remain equivocal. The length of oestrogen deprivation before supplementation is also important as early administration of oestrogen for a period of several years may yet be found to be beneficial. Evidence is emerging that the progestogenic component in combined HRT is important and medroxyprogesterone acetate usage has been associated with negative cognitive outcomes. The potential of selective oestrogen receptor modulators (SERMs) as neuroprotectants has been evaluated in a breast cancer prevention trial which compared tamoxifen with raloxifene (Yaffe et al., 2001). Both agents were found to have similar effects on cognition. It is possible that HRT may have a neuroprotective effect under certain circumstances in some women and neuroimaging, for example, PIB (Pittsburgh compound B – a fluorescent agent). PET scanning may reveal effects not detectable using cognitive testing.

Case studies

Case 46.1

A 50-year-old patient has been on cyclical combined hormone replacement therapy for 6 months for troublesome hot flushes. Her periods were irregular before starting HRT. The hot flushes have resolved with this treatment and the withdrawal bleeds are acceptable, but she is struggling with the progestogenic side effects. A friend has told her to ask for the 'no-bleed' HRT as she thought this might suit her better.

Questions

1. What is the problem with considering a no-bleed preparation?
2. What other options could you suggest?

Answers

1. No-bleed preparations include continuous combined HRT and tibolone. If these are used in women before they become truly menopausal (rather than just peri-menopausal), they are associated with significant problems of unscheduled bleeding as the dose of hormone in the preparation is insufficient to override any residual ovarian activity. In women who start on HRT while still peri-menopausal, it can be difficult to know when they are truly menopausal. The recommendation therefore is that women should not take continuous combined HRT or tibolone until they are at least 12 months from their last menstrual period or are 54 years of age (when it is estimated that 80% of women will be post-menopausal).
2. Two options could be considered. Tridestra® could be used. This is a preparation where a 14-day course of combined estradiol valerate and medroxyprogesterone acetate is taken following a 70-day course of estradiol valerate. Seven days of inactive tablets follow during which the patient would be expected to have a withdrawal bleed. This means that the patient only experiences a bleed every 3 months rather than monthly. The other option would be to consider using the levonorgesterel IUS as the progestogen component of HRT together with either an oral or transdermal oestrogen preparation. This has the advantage of very few progestogenic side effects and the possibility that the patient will be rendered amenorrhoeic. If the levonorgesterel IUS is used, it should be replaced after 4 years rather than the usual 5 years when used for contraception or as a treatment for menorrhagia.

Case 46.2

An educated 57-year-old lady has been on oestrogen only HRT (Premarin® 1.25 mg) following a hysterectomy and bilateral oophorectomy for menstrual problems 10 years ago. She has mild, well-controlled hypertension. She has no personal or family history of breast disease, but her mother has osteoporosis. Her primary care doctor has suggested she should stop HRT because of concern about the long-term risks. The patient, however, is not keen, as when she tried to stop it in the past, she felt terrible.

Questions

1. What are the risks and also are there any benefits to her continuing with HRT?
2. How could she be managed?

Answers

1. She has a small increased risk of developing breast cancer, but there does not appear to be an increase in the risk of dying from breast cancer. HRT was started at the time her menopause, that is following a surgical menopause. Therefore, her risk of cardiovascular disease or stroke is not increased and may even be reduced. There may be a very small increase in the risk of venous thromboembolism, but this risk is greatest in the first year after starting HRT. There may be a reduction in the risk of developing colo-rectal cancer with HRT use. Treatment with HRT prevents osteoporosis but is not now recommended in the UK as first-line treatment for bone protection because of the balance of risk and benefit and the efficacy of other treatments such as bisphosphonates. For many women, the greatest benefit is the improved quality of life.
2. The lowest dose of HRT which relieves her menopausal symptoms, such as hot flushes, should be used. It would be sensible to halve the dose to start with and then consider a further slow reduction in dose. The patient's osteoporosis risk should be identified by reviewing diet, exercise, body mass index, etc., and bone densitometry. The risks and benefits should be discussed with the patient, taking into consideration both personal and family history. Once all the risk/benefit issues have been discussed and understood, the patient will then be in a position to make the final decision concerning treatment.

Case 46.3

A 43-year-old lady was started on cyclical HRT at the age of 37 when she was diagnosed with an early menopause after a 15-month period of amenorrhoea. She has no significant menopausal symptoms and regular light withdrawal bleeds. However, she has read that HRT should only be continued for 5 years and thinks she might stop HRT now.

Questions

1. Why should she be advised to continue HRT until the age of 50?
2. What advice would you give her regarding the dose and type of HRT?

Answers

1. Once a woman enters menopause, the fall in oestrogen levels increases the risk of cardiovascular disease and also increases bone loss causing a greater risk of osteoporotic fractures. The earlier the menopause, the greater the risk. Concern about breast cancer rates rising with increased HRT was derived from data in women over the average age of the natural menopause, that is, in their 50s, 60s and 70s. Therefore, it should not be extrapolated to women who have undergone early menopause. Women with an early menopause should be advised that any increase in the breast cancer risk only becomes important once HRT use continues beyond 50. In addition, the benefits of continuing HRT up to the age of 50 in terms of cardiovascular and bone health are significant.

2. Current advice is that the lowest dose of HRT to control menopausal symptoms should be used. This can result in the dose of HRT falling below the bone protective dose, and therefore a risk assessment for osteoporosis should be undertaken. This should include assessing lifestyle (dietary calcium, weight, weight-bearing exercise, etc.) in addition to a bone densitometry scan. This lady may wish to consider treatment with levonorgestrel IUS and oral or transdermal oestrogen as there may be a reduction in breast cancer risk associated with this combination when compared with standard cyclical HRT. This is because of limited systemic progestogen absorption. Cardiovascular well-being should be assessed, for example, family history, body mass index, blood pressure, lipids, aerobic exercise and improved where possible. This is especially important if following discussion of the risks and benefits, the patient still decided to stop HRT.

References

Burge, R.T., 2001. The cost of osteoporotic fractures in the UK. Projections for 2000–2020. J. Med. Econ. 4, 51–62.

Campagnoli, C., Abbà, C., Ambroggio, S., et al., 2005. Pregnancy, progesterone and progestins in relation to breast cancer risk. J. Steroid Biochem. Mol. Biol. 97, 441–450.

Chlebowski, R.T., Kuller, L.H., Prentice, R.L., et al., 2009. Breast cancer after use of estrogen plus progestin in postmenopausal women. N. Engl. J. Med. 360, 573–587.

Coker, L.H., Espeland, M.A., Rapp, S.R., et al., 2010. Postmenopausal hormone therapy and cognitive outcomes: the Women's Health Initiative Memory Study (WHIMS). J. Steroid Biochem. Mol. Biol. 118, 304–310.

Cooper, C., 1997. The crippling consequences of fractures and their impact on quality of life. Am. J. Med. 103 (2A), 12S–17S.

Delmas, P.D., Pornel, B., Felsenberg, D., et al., 1999. A dose-ranging trial of a matrix transdermal 17β-estradiol for the prevention of bone loss in early postmenopausal women. Bone 24, 517–523.

De Vries, C.S., Bromley, S.E., Farmer, R.D.T., 2006. Myocardial infarction risk and hormone replacement: differences between products. Maturitas 53, 343–350.

Hall, G., Phillips, T.J., 2005. Oestrogen and skin: the effects of estrogen, menopause, and hormone replacement therapy on the skin. J. Am. Acad. Dermatol. 53, 555–568.

Hulley, S., Grady, D., Bush, T., et al., 1998. Randomised trial of oestrogen plus progestin for secondary prevention of coronary heart disease in postmenopausal women. J. Am. Med. Assoc. 280, 605–613.

Hogervorst, E., Henderson, V.W., Gibbs, R.B., et al. (Eds.), 2009. Hormones, Cognition and Dementia: State of the Art and Emergent Therapeutic Strategies. Cambridge University Press, Cambridge.

Hogervorst, E., Bandelow, S., 2010. Sex steroids to maintain cognitive function in women after the menopause: a meta-analyses of treatment trials. Maturitas 66, 56–71.

International menopause consensus statement, 2009. Aging, menopause, cardiovascular disease and HRT. Climacteric 12, 368–377.

Joint Formulary Committee, 2010. British National Formulary. BNF BMJ Group and Pharmaceutical Press, London.

Kanis, J.A., Johnell, O., Oden, A., et al., 2000. Long-term risk of osteoporotic fracture in Malmo. Osteoporos. Int. 11, 669–674.

MHRA/CHM, 2007. Drug safety advice. Drug Safety Update 1 (2), 2–6. Available at http://www.mhra.gov.uk/mhra/drugsafetyupdate. Access date 10th August 2010.

Million Women Study Collaborators, 2003. Breast cancer and hormone-replacement therapy in the Million Women Study. Lancet 362, 419–427.

Mulnard, R.A., Cotman, C.W., Kawas, C., et al., 2000. Oestrogen replacement therapy for treatment of mild to moderate Alzheimer disease. J. Am. Med. Assoc. 283, 1007–1015.

National Institute of Health and Clinical Excellence, 2010. Alendronate, Etidronate, Risedronate, Raloxifene and Strontium Ranelate for the Primary Prevention of Osteoporotic Fragility Fractures in Postmenopausal Women (Amended), Technology Appraisal 160. NICE, London. Available at http://www.nice.org.uk/TA160. Access date 10th August 2010.

O'Donnell, S., Cranney, A., Wells, G.A., et al., 2006. Strontium ranelate for preventing and treating postmenopausal osteoporosis. Cochrane Database of Systematic Reviews, Issue 4. Art. No.: CD005326 doi:10.1002/14651858.CD005326.pub3.

Royal College of Obstetricians and Gynaecologists, 2004. Hormone Replacement Therapy and Venous Thromboembolism. Guideline 19, Royal College of Obstetricians and Gynaecologists, London. Available at http://www.rcog.org.uk/files/rcog-corp/uploaded-files/GT19HRTVenousThromboembolism2004.pdf. Access date 10th August 2010.

Simon, J.A., Hsia, J., Cauley, J.A., et al., 2001. Postmenopausal hormone and risk of stroke. Heart and Estrogen-progestin Replacement Study (HERS). Circulation 103, 638–642.

Sturdee, D., 2009. President of the International Menopause Society commenting on 'NEJM Article on Breast Cancer and HRT - Comment by International Menopause Society'. Available at http://www.imsociety.org/pages/comments_and_press_statements/ims_press_statement_04_02_09.php. Access date 10th August 2010.

Torgerson, D., Iglesias, C., Reid, D.M., 2001. The effective management of osteoporosis. In: Barlow, D.H., Francis, R.M., Miles, A. (Eds.), The Economics of Fracture Prevention. Aesculpius Medical Press, London, pp. 111–121.

Vrablik, M., Fait, T., Kovar, J., et al., 2008. Oral but not transdermal estrogen replacement therapy changes the composition of plasma lipoproteins. Metab. Clin. Exp. 57, 1088–1092.

Women's Health Initiative, 2002. Risks and benefits of oestrogen plus progestin in healthy postmenopausal women: principal results from the Women's Health Initiative randomized controlled trial. J. Am. Med. Assoc. 288, 321–333.

Yaffe, K., Krueger, K., Sarkar, S., et al., 2001. Cognitive function in postmenopausal women treated with raloxifene. N. Engl. J. Med. 344, 1207–1213.

Further reading

Brockie, J., 2005. Alternative approaches to the menopause. Rev. Gynaecol. Pract. 5, 1–7.

Dantas, A.P.V., Sandberg, K., 2005. Challenges and opportunities associated with targeting oestrogen receptors in treating hypertension and cardiovascular disease. Drug Discov. Today Ther. Strateg. 2, 245–251.

Dubey, R.K., Imthurn, B., Barton, M., et al., 2005. Vascular consequences of menopause and hormone therapy: importance of timing of treatment and type of estrogen. Cardiovasc. Res. 66, 295–306.

Dunkin, J., Rasgon, N., Wagner-Steh, K., et al., 2005. Reproductive events modify the effects of estrogen replacement therapy on cognition in healthy postmenopausal women. Psychoneuroendocrinology 30, 284–296.

Gallagher, J.C., 2008. Advances in bone biology and new treatments for bone loss. Maturitas 60, 65–69.

Hogervorst, E., Bandelow, S., 2010. Sex steroids to maintain cognitive function after the menopause: a meta-analyses of treatment trials. Maturitas 66, 56–71.

Kanis, J.A., Burlet, N., Cooper, C., et al., 2008. European guidance for the diagnosis and management of osteoporosis in postmenopausal women. Osteoporosis International 19, 399–428. doi:10.1007/s00198–008–0560-z.

Panay, N., Rees, M., 2005. Alternatives to hormone replacement therapy for management of menopausal symptoms. Curr. Obstet. Gynaecol. 15, 259–266.

Sturdee, D.W., 2008. The menopausal hot flush: anything new? Maturitas 60, 42–49.

Drugs in pregnancy and lactation 47

P. Russell, L. Yates, E. Grant and P. Golightly

Key points

Drugs in pregnancy

- Assess risk/benefit ratio for the mother-fetus pair.
- Avoid non-essential drugs.
- Where drug treatment is clinically indicated, select an effective agent with the best safety profile.
- Use the lowest effective dose for the shortest possible time.
- Provide timely and accurate counselling to help avoid unfounded maternal fears about drug safety that may otherwise result in non-adherence with drug therapy or unnecessary pregnancy termination.
- Use the statement 'avoid all drugs in the first trimester where possible' cautiously as drug exposure in the second and third trimesters may still result in fetal harm.
- Remember that the harmful effects of a drug on the fetus may differ depending on the trimester of exposure.

Drugs in lactation

- Avoid unnecessary use of drugs.
- Maternal therapy only rarely constitutes a reason to avoid breastfeeding.
- Assess the risk/benefit ratio for both mother and infant.
- Monitor the infant for unusual signs or symptoms.
- Avoid use of new drugs if there is a therapeutic equivalent for which data on use in lactation are available.

Drugs in pregnancy

The use of both prescription and over-the-counter drugs in pregnancy presents a number of challenges to those asked to provide advice to women either pre-conceptually or during pregnancy. This is in part due to the fact that no two cases are the same, and that each enquiry ideally requires an individual risk assessment that takes into account what is known about the drug and its effects on the developing fetus, as well as the woman's personal medical and family history. It is now well recognised that certain drugs, chemicals and other agents, readily cross the placenta and may act as teratogens, resulting in harm to the unborn child. Robust scientific human data on the effects of many of these drugs, particularly newer preparations, are, however, frequently lacking.

There is now a greater appreciation of the risks of drug use in pregnancy, and it is generally accepted that maternal pharmacotherapy should be avoided or minimised where possible.

Nevertheless, it has been estimated that over 80% of expectant mothers take three or four drugs at some stage of pregnancy (Headley et al., 2004) with a significant number of women taking medication at the time their pregnancy is detected. Indications for drug use range from chronic illnesses such as epilepsy and depression to those commonly associated with pregnancy such as hypertension, urinary tract infections and gastro-intestinal complaints.

Approximately 2–3% of all live births are associated with a congenital anomaly. Although exogenous factors such as drugs may account for only 1–5% of these (affecting <0.2% of all live births), given that drug-associated malformations are largely preventable, they remain an important consideration.

Drugs as teratogens

A teratogen is defined as any agent that results in structural or functional abnormalities in the fetus, or in the child after birth, as a consequence of maternal exposure during pregnancy. Examples of drugs that are known to be human teratogens are shown in Box 47.1. The teratogenic mechanism for most drugs remains unclear, but may be due to the direct effects of the drug on the fetus and/or as a consequence of indirect physiological changes in the mother or fetus. Perhaps the best known, and most widely studied teratogen is thalodimide, a mild sedative

---

Box 47.1 Examples of drugs considered to be human teratogens

ACE inhibitors
Androgens
Carbamazepine
Carbimazole
Cytotoxics (some)
Danazol
Diethylstilboestrol
Ethanol
Lithium
Misoprostol
Penicillamine
Phenytoin
Tetracyclines
Thalidomide
Valproic acid
Vitamin A and derivatives, for example, isotretinoin
Warfarin

that was widely marketed as a remedy for pregnancy-related nausea and vomiting. In 1961, thalidomide was withdrawn from the UK market following numerous reports of severe anatomical birth defects in infants of mothers who took the drug in early pregnancy. Whereas external congenital anomalies such as limb abnormalities, spina bifida and hydrocephalus may be obvious at birth, some defects may take many years to manifest clinically or be identified. Examples of delayed effects of teratogens are the behavioural and intellectual disorders associated with *in utero* alcohol exposure and the development of clear-cell vaginal cancer in young women following maternal intake of diethylstilboestrol, used first in the 1930s for the prevention of miscarriage and preterm delivery (Herbst et al., 1971).

Critical periods in human fetal development

The human gestation period is approximately 40 weeks from the first day of the last menstrual period (38 weeks' post-conception) and is conventionally divided into the first, second and third trimesters, each lasting 3 calendar months. Another method for classifying the stage of pregnancy is according to the stage of fetal development. This is a more useful approach when assessing the potential risks associated with drug use in pregnancy.

Pre-embryonic stage (weeks 0–2 post-conception)

The first two weeks post-conception are regarded as the pre-embryonic stage and describe the period up to implantation of the fertilised ovum. Teratogenic exposure during the pre-embryonic stage is thought to elicit an 'all-or-nothing' response, leading either to death of the embryo or complete recovery and normal development of the fetus. Fetal malformations following drug exposure during this period are therefore thought to be unlikely, except where the half-life of the drug is sufficient to extend exposure into the embryonic stage. A good example of the latter is isotretinoin and related vitamin A derivatives which have half-lives up to a week, and which when used systemically, for example, for the treatment of acne and psoriasis, are recognised teratogens (Nulman et al., 1998).

Embryonic stage (weeks 3-8 post-conception)

Organogenesis occurs predominantly during the embryonic stage and, with the exception of the central nervous system, eyes, teeth, external genitalia and ears, is complete by the end of the 10th week of pregnancy. Exposure to drugs during this critical period therefore represents the greatest risk of major birth defects. For this reason, women are often advised to avoid or minimise all drug use in the first trimester whenever possible. It is important to bear in mind however, that very few drugs are in fact proven teratogens and that exposure in the second and third trimesters may still result in fetal harm.

Fetal stage (weeks 9–38 post-conception)

During the fetal stage, the fetus continues to develop, grow and mature and, importantly, remains susceptible to some drug effects. This is especially true for the central nervous system, which can be damaged by exposure to certain drugs, for example, ethanol, at any stage of pregnancy. The external genitalia also continue to form from the seventh week until term, and consequently, danazol, which has weak androgenic properties, can cause virilisation of a female fetus if given in any trimester after the eighth week of pregnancy when the androgen receptors begin to form (Rosa, 1984).

Further examples include the angiotensin-converting enzyme (ACE) inhibitors, which if given in the second and third trimesters can result in fetal renal dysfunction and subsequent oligohydramnios, that is, reduced amniotic fluid volume (Sedman et al., 1995). The non-steroidal anti-inflammatory drugs (NSAIDs) are another important group of drugs that may cause problems specifically in the third trimester. These drugs inhibit prostaglandin synthesis in a dose-related fashion and, when given late in pregnancy, may result in premature closure of the fetal ductus arteriosus and fetal renal impairment (Koren et al., 2006). NSAIDs should therefore be avoided during the third trimester.

Principles of teratogenesis

In 1959, James Wilson, co-founder of The Teratology Society, proposed several principles of teratogenesis that have since been expanded and modified but remain fundamental in assessing whether a drug or chemical exposure during pregnancy is likely to be associated with reproductive or developmental toxicity. A basic understanding of these factors is essential to both the interpretation of preclinical (animal) reproductive toxicity studies and to enable accurate risk assessment in clinical practice. A subset of Wilson's principles are discussed as follows.

Timing of exposure

The stage of pregnancy at which a drug exposure occurs is key to determining the likelihood, severity or nature of any adverse effect on the fetus. Risk both between and within trimesters may be variable. For example, folic acid antagonists, for example, trimethoprim, are associated with an increased risk of neural tube defects if exposure occurs before neural tube closure (third to fourth week post-conception), but not after this period (Hernandez-Diaz et al., 2001). It has also been suggested that trimethoprim should be avoided after 32 weeks' gestation in view of the theoretical risk of severe jaundice in the neonate as a result of bilirubin displacement from protein binding, although clinical evidence to support this is lacking (Dunn, 1964). Unfortunately, the precise period of teratogenic risk is known for very few substances. One drug for which this period has been established is thalidomide, where exposure between days 20 and 36 post-conception is associated with a high risk of congenital malformation (Lenz, 1988; Newman, 1986).

Drug dose

A threshold dose above which drug-induced malformations are more likely to occur has now been demonstrated for certain teratogenic compounds, although for most a 'safe dose' has not been conclusively determined. The likelihood of a dose relationship underlies the recommendation to use the lowest effective dose in pregnancy. For this reason, more frequent monitoring of drug levels may be recommended for certain drugs during pregnancy.

Species

Teratogenicity of a drug may be species dependent. Interestingly, preclinical thalidomide studies in mice and rats did not result in congenital malformation in the offspring (Breitkreutz and Anderson, 2008; Miller et al., 2009; Vorhees et al., 2001). Birth defects or other adverse reproductive outcomes observed in animal studies cannot therefore be simply extrapolated to the human situation. Further, the drug dose and route of administration used in early animal studies may not be comparable to clinical use in humans.

Genotype and environmental interaction

Not all fetuses exposed to known teratogenic drugs show evidence of having been affected *in utero*. It remains undetermined as to whether this variable susceptibility to teratogenic drugs is a result of genetic differences in the exposed mothers, the fetal genotype, modifying environmental factors or a combination of all three. Malformations are reported to occur in only 20–50% of infants born to mothers exposed to thalidomide during the period of greatest risk for embryopathy, that is, days 20–36 post-fertilisation (Lenz, 1966; Newman, 1985).

Similarly, maternal treatment with systemic isotretinoin during the first trimester results in fetal malformation in only 18–35% of the live born infants, with a further 30% of children exhibiting developmental delay in the absence of physical deformity (Benke, 1984; Braun et al., 1984; Hill, 1984).

Pharmacological effect

Pharmacological effects on the fetus are by far the most common drug effects during pregnancy, and the consequences are often minor and reversible compared to the idiosyncratic effects that can lead to major irreversible anomalies. Pharmacological effects are usually dose related and to some extent predictable. Drugs may adversely affect the fetus via effects on the maternal circulation or they may cross the placenta and exert a direct pharmacological effect on the fetus. Equally, drugs are sometimes administered to pregnant women in order to treat fetal disorders; for example, flecainide has been used to resolve fetal tachycardia.

The neonate can also be adversely affected by maternal drug therapy (see Table 47.1). It is generally only at birth that signs of fetal distress are observed due to *in utero* drug exposure or the effects of abrupt discontinuation of the maternal drug supply. The capacity of the neonate to eliminate drugs is reduced, and this can result in significant accumulation of some drugs, leading to toxicity. Neonatal withdrawal effects may require treatment.

Idiosyncratic drug effects in the fetus and neonate are possible but occur rarely compared with pharmacological effects.

Table 47.1 Examples of drugs with pharmacological effects on the fetus or neonate (adapted from Schaefer et al., 2007)

Drug	Possible adverse pharmacological effect	Notes
ACE inhibitors	Fetal and neonatal hypoxia, hypotension, renal dysfunction, oligohydramnios and intra-uterine growth retardation	Monitor fetus if long-term therapy in the second or third trimester
β-Blockers, for example, atenolol	Neonatal bradycardia, hypotension and hyperglycaemia	Neonatal symptoms are usually mild and improve within 48 h. No long-term effects
Benzodiazepines	'Floppy infant syndrome' Withdrawal reactions	Risk if regular use in third trimester Neonatal observation recommended
Corticosteroid (high dose)	Fetal adrenal suppression	Dependent on dose and treatment interval
NSAID	Premature closure of the ductus arteriosus (affecting fetal circulation) and fetal renal impairment (decreased urine output)	Avoid repeated use after week 28. If unavoidable, fetal circulation monitored regularly
Opioids	Neonatal withdrawal symptoms Respiratory depression	Risk if used long-term Risk if used near term
Phenothiazines	Neonatal withdrawal and transient extrapyramidal symptoms	Observation for at least 48 h. Symptoms may last for several weeks
Tricyclic and SSRI antidepressants	Neonatal withdrawal symptoms	Risk if used long-term and/or near term. Observation for at least 48 h

Maternal pharmacokinetic changes

There are a number of maternal changes which occur during pregnancy and are summarised in Table 47.2.

Absorption

Gastric and intestinal emptying time increases by 30–40% in the second and third trimesters (Pavek et al., 2009) and could be important in delaying absorption and time to onset of action for some drugs (Loebstein et al., 1997). There is also a reduction in gastric acid secretion in the first and second trimesters and an increase in mucus secretion. As a consequence of the increase in gastric pH, the ionisation, and hence absorption, of weak acids and bases can be affected.

Cardiac output and respiratory volume increase during pregnancy leading to hyperventilation and increased pulmonary blood perfusion. These changes cause higher pulmonary absorption of anaesthetics, bronchodilators, pollutants, cigarette smoke and other volatile drugs.

Distribution

The volume of distribution of drugs may be altered because of an increase of up to 50% in blood (plasma) volume and a 30% increase in cardiac output. Renal blood flow increases by up to 50% at the end of the first trimester and uterine blood flow increases and peaks at term (36–42 L/h). There is also a mean increase of 8 L in body water (60% to placenta, fetus and amniotic fluid and 40% to maternal tissues). As a consequence, there may be increased dosage requirements for some drugs to achieve the same therapeutic effect, provided these effects are not offset by other pharmacokinetic changes. Both the total plasma and the free-drug concentrations of phenytoin, carbamazepine and valproic acid decrease during pregnancy, but the free-drug fraction (ratio of free to total plasma concentration) may increase (Pavek et al., 2009).

Table 47.2 Summary of pharmacokinetic changes during pregnancy (adapted from Schaefer et al., 2007)

Absorption	Change during pregnancy
Gastro-intestinal motility	↓
Lung function	↑
Skin blood circulation	↑
Distribution	
Plasma volume	↑
Body water	↑
Plasma protein	↓
Fat deposition	↑
Metabolism	
Liver activity	↑↓
Excretion	
Glomerular filtration	↑

Protein binding

Albumin is the main plasma protein responsible for binding acidic drugs such as phenytoin and salicylates, whilst α_1-acid glycoprotein predominantly binds basic drugs, including β-blockers and opioid analgesics. As pregnancy progresses, the plasma volume increases at a greater rate than the increase in albumin which results in hypoalbuminaemia. In addition, steroid and placental hormones occupy the protein-binding sites. This leads to an increase in the fraction of unbound drug. Clinical effect is related to the concentration of unbound drug, which usually remains unchanged even though the total (bound plus unbound) plasma concentration is decreased. Thus, a fall in the total plasma concentration does not usually require an increase in dose. The α_1-acid glycoprotein concentrations remain the same as those in non-pregnancy.

Phenytoin is bound to albumin and exhibits the effects described earlier, but the situation is further complicated by increased hepatic metabolism that may necessitate a dose increase. Consequently, therapy can only be reliably guided by clinical assessment or measurement of unbound rather than total plasma concentration.

Metabolism

The metabolic activity of cytochrome P450 isoenzymes CYP3A4, CYP2D6, CYP 2A6 and CYP 2C9 and uridine 5′-diphosphate glucuronosyltransferase (UGT) isoenzymes (UGT1a1, UGT1A4 and UGT2B7) is increased during pregnancy. Drugs metabolised by these isoenzymes may therefore require dose adjustment. This may decrease the amount of the drug available for transfer across the placenta and thereby influence fetal exposure. In contrast, the metabolic activity of CYP1A2 and CYP2C19 is decreased during pregnancy and drugs metabolised by these isoenzymes may need dose reduction to minimise toxicity (see Table 47.3).

In general, the effects on individual drugs are inconsistent and difficult to predict, but knowledge of the effect of pregnancy on isoenzymes may inform decisions about possible monitoring and/or dose alterations.

Excretion

Within the first few weeks of pregnancy, the glomerular filtration rate (GFR) increases by approximately 50%. Consequently, those drugs which are excreted primarily unchanged by the kidneys, for example, lithium, digoxin and penicillin, show enhanced elimination and lower steady-state concentrations. The following drugs have shown pregnancy-induced increases of 20–65% on their renal elimination (Anderson, 2005):

- Ampicillin
- Cefuroxime
- Ceftazidime
- Cefazolin
- Pipericillin
- Atenolol

Table 47.3 Summary of pregnancy-induced effects on hepatic metabolism of some drugs (adapted from Anderson, 2005)

Isoenzyme	Drugs/probes	Effect on clearance		
		First trimester	Second trimester	Third trimester
CYP1A2	Caffeine	↓ 33%	↓ 50%	↓ 65%
CYP2A6	Nicotine	ND	↑ 54% (combined data)	
CYP2C9	Phenytoin	No effect	No effect	↑ 20%
CYP2C19	Proguanil	ND	↓ 50%	↓ 50%
CYP2D6	Dextromethorphan[a] Metoprolol	ND	ND	↑ 50%
CYP3A4	Cortisol[a] Nifedipine	ND	ND	↑ Variable[b]
UGT1A4	Lamotrigine monotherapy polytherapy	↑ 200% ↑ 65%	↑ 200% ↑ 65%	↑ 300% ↑ 90%
UGT2B7 (limited data)	Morphine	ND	ND	↑ Variable[b]

ND, not detectable.
[a]Dextromethorphan and cortisol used as probes of CYP2D6 and CYP3A4 activity.
[b]Extent variable depending on the drug studied.

- Sotalol
- Digoxin
- Lithium
- Dalteparin sodium
- Enoxaparin sodium

Fetal-placental transfer

Most drugs diffuse easily across the placenta and thus enter the fetal circulation to some extent. In general, the ratio fetal:maternal drug concentration is less than 1. Drugs differ in the extent to which they bind to fetal and maternal proteins. For example, fetal and newborn plasma proteins appear to bind ampicillin and benzylpenicillin with less affinity and salicylates with greater affinity, than maternal proteins. Maternal albumin gradually decreases during pregnancy and fetal albumin concentrations increase, so different fetal: maternal albumin concentrations occur at different stages of pregnancy. The degree of protein binding of any drug is an important determinant of its movement across the placenta. Drugs which are highly protein bound tend to achieve higher maternal and lower fetal concentrations. Drugs with very large molecular weights such as insulin and heparin have negligible transfer. Lipophilic, un-ionised drugs cross the placenta more easily than polar drugs, and weakly basic drugs may become 'trapped' in the fetal circulation due to the slightly lower pH compared with maternal plasma. Some other factors such as enzymes or drug efflux transporters in the placenta may facilitate or restrict the transfer of a drug to the fetus.

Drug dosing in pregnancy

As a general principle, the dose of a drug given at any stage of pregnancy should be as low as possible to minimise potential toxic effects to the fetus. Drug therapy that is considered essential can be tapered to the lowest effective dose either before conception (ideally) or at the time the pregnancy is diagnosed. Where drug exposure during the third trimester is predicted to have an adverse effect on the neonate postpartum, consideration may be given to slowly reducing the dose towards term to minimise the risks to the baby. Such decisions are, however, not always straightforward. Recommendations to wean an expectant mother off antidepressants and antipsychotics to reduce the likelihood of neonatal withdrawal syndrome (characterised by jitteriness, altered muscle tone, poor feeding and irritability) and, in the case of the SSRIs, avoid the possible increased risk of persistent pulmonary hypertension of the newborn (PPHN) are now being challenged. Not only are there insufficient data to conclusively demonstrate neonatal benefit or an optimal time of weaning, but also the increased risk of psychiatric problems and relapse in the immediate postpartum period needs to be taken into account.

Many physiological changes occur during pregnancy which may affect the way the body handles drugs. Knowledge of these changes can allow some prediction of the impact on pharmacotherapy while remaining aware that there is variability in the extent of these changes during the pregnancy, and high inter-individual variability. The need for changes in dosages is influenced by whether the drug is excreted unchanged by the kidneys or which metabolic isoenzymes are involved in its elimination. Women taking drugs with enhanced clearance and for which a good correlation between plasma levels and therapeutic effect exist, should have their plasma concentrations closely monitored and dose adjusted to reduce the risk of suboptimal therapy, for example, phenytoin, carbamazepine, lithium and digoxin. Similarly, highly protein-bound drugs may require free-drug concentration monitoring. However, there is no clear guidance for adjusting doses during pregnancy, and for most drugs, the concentration of free drug, and therefore the effect of that drug, is unchanged.

Pregnancy itself can cause a temporary worsening or improvement of some diseases and in that way influence drug dosages.

Drug selection in pregnancy

Although there are few, if any, drugs for which safe use in pregnancy can be absolutely assured, only a handful of drugs in current clinical use have been conclusively shown to be teratogenic. In general, drugs that have been used extensively in pregnant women without apparent problems are recommended in preference to new drugs for which there is less experience of use. For example, methyldopa is used rarely to treat hypertension in the non-pregnant state but has historically been preferred in pregnancy because of a long history of safe use (Schaefer et al., 2007). However, older drugs may be less effective in terms of controlling maternal illness and are often associated with an increased side-effect risk profile.

In most cases, the decision as to whether to commence or continue with a medication in pregnancy will depend on the risk–benefit analysis for that specific mother–infant pair. A frequent error made by health professionals is to apply the U.S. Food and Drug Administration (FDA) pregnancy risk categories (A (*no demonstrable risk*), B, C, D and X (*teratogenic agents that are considered to be completely contraindicated in pregnancy*) when considering whether or not to prescribe a drug in pregnancy. It is now widely accepted that these categories are oversimplified and are of little practical help in a clinical setting. The FDA has proposed that the existing categories be replaced with more detailed information sheets containing a summary of the fetal risk and the additional maternal factors that need to be taken into consideration. Importantly, the need for a detailed section discussing the available data including observed human versus animal data, the study design, dose exposure, and reported congenital malformations and/or adverse events has been emphasised (see http://www.fda.gov for up-to-date information).

It is worth noting that standard literature sources often contain unhelpful information such as 'do not use in pregnancy unless the benefits outweigh the risks'. This is understandable from a medico-legal point of view but offers little in terms of risk assessment. The primary literature is frequently inadequate because ethical and legal restraints mean that randomised controlled trials are rarely undertaken in pregnant women. Often, the only information that is available is confined to retrospective studies, voluntary reporting schemes and/or animal studies. The rate of anomalies in retrospective studies and voluntary reporting databases may be erroneously elevated due to preferential reporting of abnormal outcomes. Individual case reports are also difficult to interpret as the denominator of drug exposure is unknown, and an abnormal outcome may be coincidental to the drug exposure. More recently, prospective controlled trials have been utilised where the pregnancy outcomes of a defined cohort of women exposed to the drug are compared with outcomes of a matched control group. Complete follow-up of each pregnancy and post-natal monitoring is an essential feature of this type of investigation.

Pre-conception advice

Drug use during the first trimester, in particular, the embryonic stage, carries the greatest risk of malformation as this is when the fetal organs are being formed. Ideally, all unnecessary drug therapy should be discontinued prior to conception. However, inadvertent drug exposure frequently occurs, as approximately half of all pregnancies are unplanned. It is thus critical to make careful drug choices when prescribing for women of reproductive potential.

Women with chronic illnesses requiring drug treatment should be offered specialist counselling before conception, and the options explored to reduce or change drug therapy to a safer agent. Epilepsy is an example, in which, if continued drug treatment is necessary, attempts are made to stabilise treatment with a single drug at the lowest effective dose. It is also important to note that many pregnant women become less adherent to their drug therapy out of concern about possible harm to their infant. In many cases, such as asthma, inflammatory bowel disease, epilepsy, inadequate treatment of the underlying disease may be more detrimental to the mother–fetus pair than the drugs used to treat the condition. It is thus essential that women of reproductive potential are given clear and accurate information so that unrealistic fears about the risks to their baby do not result in unnecessary pregnancy termination or disease relapse.

All women planning a pregnancy should be offered general advice to minimise the risk of congenital anomalies. This includes avoidance of recreational drugs, 'natural' or herbal remedies, alcohol, smoking, vitamin A products, minimisation of caffeine consumption and beginning daily supplementation with at least 400 μcg of folic acid to reduce the risk of neural tube defects. It is recommended that the daily dose of folic acid be increased to around 4–5 mg daily in women who have epilepsy or who have had a previous child with a neural tube defect. Some infectious diseases may carry important fetal consequences if contracted during pregnancy. For example, rubella infection in the first 20 weeks of pregnancy is associated with an increased risk of miscarriage and a syndrome comprising problems such as deafness, cardiac defects and mental retardation in more than 20% of pregnancies. Women who lack immunity to rubella should be immunised prior to conception.

Post-conception advice

It is important to draw distinction between advice given to women pre-conceptually and that provided to a pregnant woman who has already been exposed to a drug. In the former setting, it may be recommended that an alternative preparation be considered or that a drug treatment be stopped where clinically appropriate. This advice often hinges on the lack of definitive safety data and does not automatically translate to exposure to that drug in pregnancy being an indication for discontinuing the drug, additional fetal monitoring or termination of the pregnancy on the basis of the exposure. Any change to the woman's medication should be based on a careful and individual risk assessment and include a discussion with the woman to provide her with accurate up-to-date evidence-based advice. In many such cases, the woman can be reassured that a normal baby is the most likely outcome, or where appropriate be offered additional prenatal investigation to screen for congenital malformation where the risk to fetus is considered to be significant.

Teratology Information Services and Pregnancy Registries

It is difficult to keep up to date with the published literature. There is an increasing need for summary documents that include and critically appraise all available data, and which enable health care providers to have a balanced and informed discussion with patients regarding the risks and benefits of a certain therapy in pregnancy. This is evidenced by the current debate surrounding the teratogenic potential of various antidepressants with conflicting opinion even amongst experts in the field.

Teratology information services (TISs) have been established in several countries across the world and provide evidence-based, up-to-date information and individual case-based risk assessments. In addition to reviewing published literature on drugs, teratology services also have access to specialist online databases and discussion forums. A number routinely collect pregnancy outcome data on the women about whom they receive an enquiry, to enable surveillance for potential teratogens.

For some new drugs, pregnancy registries have been initiated that record all reported drug exposures and follow up the outcome of the pregnancy. These registries are cumulative and work on the basis that specific anomalies would be identified relatively quickly and that there will eventually be sufficient statistical power to detect the magnitude of any increased risk relative to the general population. These registries may be held by a TIS, or by independent groups with an interest in a defined area. The 2009 A/H1N1 influenza pandemic provided an example of teratology services across the globe responding to the urgent need for safety data by establishing registries on antiviral and pandemic vaccine exposure during the pandemic.

Drugs in lactation

Breast milk is the best form of nutrition for young infants. It provides all the energy and nutrients required for the first 6 months of life. The World Health Organization (WHO, 2001) and the United Nations Children's Fund (UNICEF) recommend exclusive breastfeeding for this period. Benefits of breastfeeding include protection of the infant against gastric, respiratory and urinary tract infections (Kramer and Kakuma, 2002), and reduction in rates of obesity

(Horta et al., 2007), juvenile-onset diabetes (Horta et al., 2007) and atopic disease (Fewtrell, 2004). Adults who were breastfed as infants often have lower blood pressure and lower cholesterol levels (Horta et al., 2007). Maternal benefits include reduced risk of developing pre-menopausal breast cancer and delayed resumption of menstrual cycle. Breastfeeding also strengthens the mother–infant bond.

There are few contraindications to breastfeeding, although maternal HIV infection in developed countries is a notable exception. The percentage of women exclusively breastfeeding their infants after 6 months is often less than 20% (Scott et al., 2006). Reasons for early discontinuation of breastfeeding include return to work, concerns about inadequate lactation or safety of drug use.

Breastfeeding mothers frequently require treatment with prescription medicines or may self-medicate with over-the-counter preparations, nutritional supplements or herbal medicines. It is important for health professionals to understand the principles of safe use of medications during lactation in order to provide appropriate advice.

There are two main goals to consider when formulating advice for nursing mothers. These are to protect the infant from maternal drug-related adverse effects and to allow, whenever possible, necessary maternal medication (Berlin et al., 2009).

Transfer of drugs into breast milk

Most drugs pass into breast milk to some degree although transfer is usually low. The drug 'dose' ingested by the infant via breast milk only rarely causes adverse effects. Examples of adverse effects observed in breastfed infants exposed to medication via breast milk are given in Table 47.4, although not all of these are proven to be directly due to the drug ingested via breast milk.

Table 47.4 Adverse reactions reported in breastfed infants

Atenolol	Bradycardia, cyanosis, hypotension
Ciprofloxacin	Pseudomembranous colitis
Codeine	Death
Dapsone	Haemolytic anaemia
Diazepam	Lethargy, sedation, poor suckling
Doxepin	Sedation and respiratory arrest
Erythromycin	Pyloric stenosis
Fluoxetine	Colic, irritability, sedation
Indometacin	Seizures
Lithium	T-wave abnormalities
Naproxen	Prolonged bleeding, haemorrhage, anaemia
Phenytoin	Methaemoglobinaemia

Almost all drugs enter milk by passive diffusion of un-ionised, unbound drug through the lipid membranes of the alveolar cells of the breast, according to the pH partitioning theory. Several factors influence the rate and extent of passive diffusion. These include maternal plasma level, physiological differences between plasma and milk and the physicochemical properties of the drug. Differences in composition between blood and milk determine which physicochemical characteristics influence diffusion.

Milk differs from blood in that it has a lower pH (7.2 vs. 7.4), less buffering capacity and higher fat content. The following drug parameters affect the extent of transfer into milk:

- pK_a. This is a measure of the fraction of the drug that is ionised at a given pH, for example, physiological pH. Highly ionised drugs tend not to concentrate in milk. For basic drugs, for example, erythromycin, a greater fraction will be ionised at an acidic pH, so the milk compartment will tend to 'trap' weak bases. In contrast, acidic drugs, for example, penicillins, are more ionised at higher pH values and will be 'trapped' in the plasma compartment. Drugs with higher pK_a values generally have higher milk/plasma ratios.
- *Protein binding*. Drugs that are highly bound to plasma proteins, for example, warfarin, are likely to be relatively retained in maternal plasma because there is a lower total protein content in the milk. High protein binding essentially restricts the drug to the plasma compartment as only the free fraction of the drug crosses the biological membrane. Milk concentrations of highly protein-bound drugs are usually low.
- *Lipophilicity*. The alveolar epithelium of the breast is a lipid barrier. Transfer of water-soluble drugs and ions is inhibited by this barrier. CNS active drugs usually have the characteristics required to pass into milk.
- *Molecular weight*. Drugs with low molecular weights (<200) readily pass into milk through small pores in the cell walls of alveolar cells. Drugs with higher molecular weights cross cell membranes by dissolving in the lipid layer which may substantially reduce milk concentrations. Proteins such as heparin or insulin with very large molecular weights of > 6000 are virtually excluded from milk.

The profile of a drug that passes minimally into milk would therefore be an acidic drug that is highly protein bound and has low to moderate lipophilicity, for example, most NSAIDs. In contrast, a weakly basic drug that has low plasma protein binding and is relatively lipophilic will achieve higher concentrations in the milk compartment, for example, sotalol.

In the first few days of life, large gaps exist between the alveolar cells. These permit enhanced passage of drugs into milk. By the end of the first week, these gaps close under the influence of prolactin (Lawrence and Lawrence, 2011). There is greater passage of drugs into colostrum (early milk) than in mature milk as the former contains more protein and less fat. There is also some variation in fat and protein content of milk between the beginning and end of a feed, but these changes have less influence on drug passage than the physicochemical properties of the drug.

Another method by which a drug may enter milk is by a pumping system whereby energy is used to effect transfer into milk. The most important example is iodides which pass into milk in high concentrations (Hale, 2010).

Milk to plasma concentration ratio

Several methods have been proposed to determine the amount of drug transferred to breast milk. The milk to plasma (M/P) ratio is often used as a measure of the extent of drug transfer into breast milk. It is usually obtained from case reports or small clinical studies and may be based on paired concentrations or full area under the concentration–time curve (AUC) analysis. M/P ratios that are based on a pair of milk and plasma samples collected simultaneously may be inaccurate as they assume that the concentrations of drug in milk and plasma are in parallel, which may not be the case. It is better to collect multiple samples of plasma and milk across a dosing interval or until the drug is cleared from both phases after a single dose, for determination of an M/P ratio based on the respective AUCs (M/P_{AUC}). Figure 47.1 demonstrates the markedly different estimates of M/P ratio that can be obtained via both sampling methods. The true M/P ratio may vary significantly during the same episode of breastfeeding.

If human-derived M/P ratios are lacking for a particular drug, it may be possible to predict the extent of transfer using known physicochemical properties, for example, pK_a, and a published predictive model (Atkinson and Begg, 1990; Begg et al., 1992). M/P ratios obtained from animal studies should not be used for clinical decision making, as they may not correlate well with human M/P ratios.

Studies in humans demonstrate that most drugs have an M/P ratio less than 1.0, with the range of reported ratios being from around 0.1 to 5.0. It is often thought that drugs with high M/P ratios (e.g. 5.0) are unsafe because the concentration in milk exceeds that in plasma, while those with low ratios (<1.0) are believed to be safe. This is not always the case as the M/P ratio often fails to correlate with the 'dose' of drug the infant

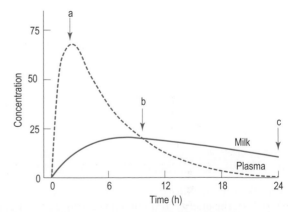

Fig. 47.1 Diagrammatic representation of a drug concentration–time profile in the maternal plasma and milk phases after a single oral dose. The points a, b and c illustrate simultaneous sampling times from both phases. Sampling at 'a' would yield an estimated M/P value of 0.2, at 'b' a value of 1.0, and at 'c' a value of 9.3. All can be misleading. The true M/P ratio calculated by the AUC method is 1.2 when extrapolated to infinity.

ingests via milk. The amount of drug transferred into milk is principally determined by the maternal plasma level. Thus, even where the *M/P* ratio is high, if the maternal plasma level is low, drug transfer is still low. Therefore, the *M/P* ratio must never be used as the sole measure of drug safety in breastfeeding. However, it can be used to estimate the 'dose' ingested via milk, which is a better predictor of safety.

Calculating the infant 'dose' ingested via milk

Infant plasma drug levels are the most accurate indicator of drug exposure, but these are seldom available.

When using quantitative data from milk analyses, the most accurate estimation of the infant 'dose' is from studies in which the milk is collected over a complete dose interval at steady state and the total dose is calculated (Fig. 47.2). Unfortunately, these studies are seldom performed. Therefore, information must be obtained from less than ideal conditions.

If the *M/P* ratio is known from published studies, the likely infant dose (D_{inf}) can be calculated as follows, with some assumptions:

$$D_{inf} = Cp_{mat} \times M/P \times V_{milk}$$

where Cp_{mat} is the average maternal plasma concentration. M/P_{AUC} is used in preference to a ratio based on paired concentrations when available, but this is seldom the case. The volume of milk ingested (V_{milk}) is not known but is generally assumed to be around 150 mL of milk per kilogram of body weight per day. The above equation simplifies if the actual milk concentration data are available:

$$D_{inf} = C_{milk} \times V_{milk}$$

The likely infant plasma drug concentration (Cp_{inf}) can be calculated by:

$$Cp_{inf} = F \times D_{inf} / Cl_{inf}$$

where *F* is oral availability and Cl_{inf} is the infant clearance. Unfortunately, neither *F* nor Cl_{inf} is known accurately for infants, so estimation of the likely steady-state average plasma drug concentration will be very approximate. Weight-adjusted Cl_{inf} values, that is, L/h/kg, are often significantly less than adult values in the early stages of life (Table 47.5).

Given the difficulty in estimating infant plasma drug concentrations, the relative infant dose, for example, compared with a therapeutic infant dose, is often used as a surrogate of exposure. To give some basis for comparison, the likely infant dose from milk can be compared with an infant therapeutic dose. This is reasonable for drugs such as paracetamol that are usually administered to infants but is unsuitable for drugs such as antidepressants that are not. In the absence of a clearly defined range of infant doses, the weight-adjusted maternal dose expressed as a percentage (% dose) is widely used to indicate infant drug exposure.

$$Relative\ infant\ dose\ (RID) = \frac{Dose\ in\ infant\ via\ milk\ [D_{inf}(mg/kg/day)]}{Dose\ in\ mother\ [D_{mat}(mg/kg/day)]} \times 100$$

For the great majority of drugs, this calculation yields infant doses in the order of 0.1–5.0% of the weight-adjusted maternal dose expressed as a percentage (% dose). It is generally thought that relative infant dose values of less than 10% of the maternal dose are probably safe. However, the inherent toxicity of the drug should be taken into account when using this figure.

To calculate the daily infant drug intake via milk, the standard milk intake of 150 mL/kg/day is multiplied by the concentration of the medication in milk:

Estimated daily infant intake = Drug concentration in milk (µcg/L) × 0.15/infant weight (kg)

Some authors use the peak concentration in milk to indicate the maximum infant intake.

Variability

To complicate matters further, there will be significant variability between and within individuals in the values used to estimate infant exposure (i.e. D_{inf}, *F*, Cl_{inf}, where D_{inf} is itself a function of the estimated parameters Cp_{mat}, *M/P*, volume of milk). Some of this variability will change over time due to developing organ function in the maturing baby and part will

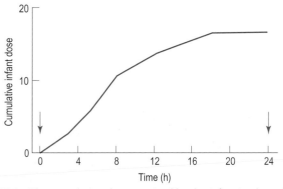

Fig. 47.2 The cumulative dose received by the infant is plotted against time. The arrows represent the maternal dose times. This type of study is undertaken by the mother expressing all the milk, from both breasts, at usual feeding times. An aliquot of milk is taken and assayed for the drug. The volume of milk is measured and the total amount of drug at each time is calculated as the product of concentration and volume. This type of study must be undertaken at steady state.

Table 47.5 Approximate drug clearance by age as percentage of maternal value (Begg, 2000)

24–28 weeks' post-conceptual age	5%
28–34 weeks' post-conceptual age	10%
34–40 weeks' post-conceptual age	33%
40–44 weeks' post-conceptual age	50%
44–68 weeks' post-conceptual age	66%
Over 68 weeks' post-conceptual age	100%

be unexplained variability. In addition to this pharmacokinetic variability, there will be variability in response of the infant to any given concentration of the drug. It is fortunate that most drugs seem to fall readily into safe (RID <10%) based on expected exposure. However, care should be taken when using these values to assess drug safety in lactation, when variability in the estimates of the parameters used may impact on the accuracy of prediction of their safety. This is especially true for those circumstances when initial estimates of these parameters are less precise, for example, in neonates.

Recently, attention has been focused on the possible role of pharmacogenetic factors in affecting the safety of breastfed infants exposed to drugs via milk (Madadi et al., 2009). Sedation (and one death) occurred in infants of mothers with rare genotypes of cytochrome P450 2D6 leading to ultra-rapid metabolism of codeine to morphine. The incidence of these genotypes varies amongst different populations. The overall percentage of Western Europeans with the CYP2D6 ultra-rapid metaboliser phenotype is 5.4% (Ingelman-Sundberg, 2005). Higher percentages have been reported in populations from northeast Africa and the Middle East.

Assessing the risk to the infant

Many factors must be considered when assessing the risk of maternal drug therapy to the breastfeeding infant (Box 47.2).

Inherent toxicity of the drug will be a main factor in determining infant safety. Thus, antineoplastic drugs, radionuclides and iodine containing compounds would be of concern. Multiple maternal therapy with drugs with similar side-effect profiles, for example, psychotropic drugs or anticonvulsants is likely to increase the risk to the infant. Oral bioavailability is an indicator of the drug's ability to reach the systemic circulation after oral administration. Drugs with a low oral bioavailability are either poorly absorbed from the gastro-intestinal tract, broken down in the gut or undergo extensive 'first pass' metabolism in the liver before entering plasma.

The presence of active metabolites, for example, desmethyldiazepam, may prolong infant drug exposure and lead to drug accumulation, especially where drug clearance is low such as in the neonatal period. Similarly, drugs with long half-lives, for example, fluoxetine, may be problematic at this time. Drug clearance by the infant does not reach adult values until 6–7 months (Table 47.5). A premature infant of 30 weeks' gestational age has a drug clearance value of about 10% of the maternal value. It is important to distinguish between gestational age and time after delivery. A 2-week-old infant born at 28 weeks will have a gestational age of 30 weeks.

Box 47.2 Factors affecting infant risk from maternal therapy

Drug adverse reaction profile
Relative infant dose (RID)
Oral bioavailability
Active metabolites
Half-life
Gestational age of the infant
Full maternal drug regimen
Pharmacogenetic factors

The maternal drug regimen can affect infant risk. Single doses or short courses seldom present problems, whereas chronic therapy can be problematic. Topical or inhalation therapy usually results in much lower plasma drug levels and therefore lower passage into milk. Multiple maternal medications increase the risk to the infant.

Reducing risk to the breastfed infant

A number of strategies may be adopted to reduce the risk of drug-related side effects in the breastfed infant. One technique that has been recommended for reducing infant exposure is to give the maternal dose immediately after the infant has been fed with the aim of avoiding feeding at peak milk concentrations. However, this is often impractical, especially where young infants are feeding frequently up to 2 hourly. In addition, accurate data on times of peak levels in milk are often unavailable, and it cannot be assumed that times of peak milk levels mirror those in plasma. This technique should be used selectively, that is, where the drug has a short half-life and where peak and trough levels are predictable, for example, antibiotics, anaesthetics.

Where a single dose of a drug known to be hazardous is given to a breastfeeding mother, for example, a radiopharmaceutical, it will usually be possible to resume breastfeeding after a suitable washout period, calculated as five times the half-life. Where the half-life is very long, the washout period necessary to avoid hazardous exposure to the infant may exceed the period of sustainable lactation.

Breastfeeding mothers should be advised to avoid self-medication. Where drug use is clearly indicated, the lowest effective dose should be used for the shortest possible time. Use of topical therapy such as eye/nasal drops for hay fever would reduce drug exposure in comparison to oral antihistamines.

The maternal regimen should be simplified wherever possible. A review of therapy before delivery will help to reduce risks to the neonate. New drugs are best avoided if a therapeutic equivalent is available for which data on safe use in lactation exists. All infants exposed to drugs via breast milk should be monitored for any untoward effects. Measures to ensure the safety of the breastfed infant are summarised in Box 47.3. Some commonly used drugs thought to be safe to use in mothers of full-term healthy infants are listed in Table 47.6.

Special situations

Neonates and premature infants

Neonates and especially premature infants are at greater risk of developing adverse effects after exposure to drugs via breast milk. Gastric emptying time is significantly prolonged and, in some cases, may alter absorption kinetics. Protein binding is decreased and values for total body water are higher than for adults. Renal function is limited because the kidney is anatomically and functionally immature. The neonate's capacity to conjugate drugs in the liver is often deficient. For example, the half-life of oxazepam (which is subject to glucuronidation) is three to four times longer in neonates than in adults.

Table 47.6 Examples of commonly used drugs thought to be safe for use in breastfeeding mothers of full-term healthy infants[a]

Drug groups	Individual drugs
Antacids	Cetirizine
Bulk laxatives	Clotrimazole
Cephalosporins	Cromoglycate
Inhaled medications, for example, salbutamol	Diclofenac
	Heparin
Penicillins	Ibuprofen
Progestogens	Insulin
Vaccines (except smallpox)	Iron supplements
Vitamins (except high-dose A and D)	Lactulose
	Levothyroxine
	Loratadine
	Nystatin
	Paracetamol
	Warfarin

[a]This table is to be used as a guide only. Expert advice is required when the maternal dose is high, if the infant is premature, has renal or hepatic disease or G6PD deficiency.

Glucose-6-phosphate dehydrogenase deficiency

Infants with glucose-6-phosphate dehydrogenase (G6PD) deficiency are susceptible to adverse effects even when only small amounts of certain drugs are present in milk. G6PD is an enzyme present in erythrocytes that is responsible for maintaining the antioxidant compound glutathione in its active form. Deficiency of this enzyme makes the erythrocyte more susceptible to oxidative stress, resulting in haemolysis. Only small amounts of drug are needed to cause such a reaction. Breastfeeding should be avoided or a safer alternative chosen if the infant has a known or suspected G6PD deficiency and the mother is taking drugs that have been reported to cause oxidative stress (e.g. nitrofurantoin, dapsone).

Allergy

The theoretical possibility exists for an allergic reaction in an infant exposed to a drug in breast milk. Even minimal exposure to the drug could cause an allergic response. However, in practice, such reactions are very rare and only if the infant has already experienced an allergic reaction to a particular drug should maternal use be discouraged or breastfeeding avoided.

Recreational drug use

Accurate details relating to maternal use of recreational drugs may be difficult to obtain. Usage may be chronic or sporadic. The role of the health professional in ensuring the safety of the breastfed infant is important, and the advice should be that substances such as cannabis, LSD and cocaine should be avoided whilst breastfeeding.

Significant amounts of alcohol pass into milk although it is not normally harmful to the infant if the quantity and duration of intake are limited. The occasional consumption of a small alcoholic beverage is acceptable if breastfeeding is avoided for about 2 h after the drink. Chronic or heavy consumers of alcohol should not breastfeed. High intakes of alcohol decrease milk let down and disrupt nursing until maternal levels decrease. Heavy maternal use may cause infant sedation, fluid retention and hormone imbalances in breastfed infants.

Nicotine has been suggested to decrease basal prolactin production although effects may be variable. Ideally, mothers should be encouraged not to smoke whilst breastfeeding. Nicotine and its metabolite, cotinine, are both present in milk. Undertaking smoking cessation with a nicotine patch is a safer option than continued smoking. Whilst transdermal nicotine patches produce a sustained lower nicotine plasma level, nicotine gums produce large variations in peak levels. A 2-3 h washout period is recommended before breastfeeding after maternal use of a nicotine gum.

Caffeine appears in breast milk rapidly after maternal intake. Fussiness, jitteriness and poor sleep patterns have been reported in infants of mothers with very high caffeine intakes equivalent to about 10 or more cups of coffee daily. Preterm and newborn infants metabolise caffeine very slowly and are at increased risk of adverse effects.

Drug effects on lactation

Drugs that affect dopamine activity are the main cause of effects on milk production, mainly mediated by effects on prolactin. Early postpartum use of oestrogens may reduce the volume of milk, but the effect is variable and depends on the dose and the individual response. Progestogen contraceptives are preferred.

Drugs may occasionally be used therapeutically for their effect on lactation. Dopamine agonists such as cabergoline decrease milk production, and this effect may be utilised, for example, after an infant death. Dopamine agonists should not be used routinely for relief of the symptoms of postpartum pain or engorgement which can be managed with simple analgesics or breast support. Dopamine antagonists such as domperidone may be used in cases of inadequate lactation which have not responded to first-line methods such as improved technique or milk expression by hand or pump.

Other drugs may affect lactation as an unwanted side effect, for example, diuretics. When these are used on a long-term basis, infant weight gain should be monitored.

Case studies

Case 47.1

A woman is 6 weeks' pregnant and has been diagnosed with depression that warrants pharmacological intervention. She wishes to recommence venlafaxine, which has been helpful in the past. She is also anxious that the ethanol she consumed around the time of conception may have harmed her baby.

Questions

1. What are the safest antidepressants in the first trimester of pregnancy?
2. Is it reasonable for her to commence venlafaxine?
3. Is there any risk from the ethanol ingestion?

Answers

1. Tricyclic antidepressants (TCAs) have been extensively used in pregnancy and are generally regarded as safe. For this reason, past practice was to recommend that TCAs should be used preferentially for the treatment of depression in pregnancy when considering teratogenic risk to the fetus. TCAs are, however, associated with side effects including risk of maternal cardiotoxicity, particularly in overdose. Further, available data on TCA use in pregnancy do not prove that they are less teratogenic than other antidepressant classes such as SNRIs and SSRIs. An antidepressant other than TCAs may therefore be appropriate for use in pregnancy, and the risks and benefits for each should be considered and ideally discussed with the patient on a case-by-case basis.
2. Experience with the use of venlafaxine and many other antidepressants, for example, moclobemide, in pregnancy is limited. However, in some instances, it may be necessary to use an agent such as venlafaxine. For example, if the mother had a history of severe depression that did not respond to multiple trials of other antidepressants, then venlafaxine may be considered the most appropriate choice of antidepressant for that woman. In this case, any potential risks associated with venlafaxine are likely to be less than those associated with inadequately treated depression.
3. Ethanol is a human teratogen. Fetal alcohol spectrum disorders are characterised by low birth weight, facial dysmorphogenesis and delayed development. A 'safe limit' for alcohol consumption in pregnancy has not been defined, and it is possible that very low amounts of alcohol may produce subtle effects on the fetus. Therefore, the best practice is to avoid all alcohol exposure in pregnancy. In this case, the mother ingested ethanol at the time of conception. She should be reassured that this is regarded as a relatively safe period and is not expected to adversely affect the fetus. However, further ethanol ingestion should be avoided.

Case 47.2

A 30-year-old woman with epilepsy is currently taking valproic acid 1500 mg daily. She wishes to conceive but is concerned about the possibility of birth defects due to valproate exposure in pregnancy. Her seizures have been difficult to control with alternative anticonvulsants.

Questions

1. What are the risks associated with valproate treatment in pregnancy?
2. How can these risks be minimised?

Answers

1. Valproate is a human teratogen, with early first-trimester exposure associated with a 1–2% risk of neural tube defects, as well as other malformations such as orofacial clefts. Valproate has also been associated with neonatal complications such as seizures. It is frequently advised that valproate is avoided in pregnancy and that the valproate dose should be gradually tapered and discontinued prior to conception. However, this is not a realistic option for many women with epilepsy. In fact, seizures may lead to greater problems such as maternal–fetal injury, miscarriage or hypoxia.
2. The patient should be reassured that most pregnancies in women with epilepsy end with a healthy baby without malformations. Concern about the risk of fetal abnormalities may result in reduced adherence, which may have greater maternal–fetal risk than the drug itself. As the patient is not yet pregnant, this is an optimal time for her current drug regime to be reviewed and optimised by a neurologist or health professional with expertise in managing women with epilepsy during pregnancy. There is some evidence to suggest that higher doses/concentrations of valproate are associated with greater risk of malformations. Where valproate remains the drug of choice, the lowest effective dose should be used throughout pregnancy. Monitoring free valproate concentrations may be useful in pregnancy, perhaps with the view to maintaining those concentrations shown to be effective in the non-pregnant stage. However, doses should be adjusted based on clinical need and not concentrations alone. Women with epilepsy should be commenced on high-dose folic acid 4–5 mg daily pre-conceptually. They should also be offered the option of prenatal diagnostic techniques that screen for neural tube defects such as ultrasound and serum α-fetoprotein.

Case 47.3

A 2-day-old full-term infant has excessive shrill crying, is jittery and is feeding poorly. The medical team cannot find any cause for these effects. The mother is worried that they may be due to paroxetine exposure via breast milk and wonders whether St John's wort would be a safer alternative. She has taken paroxetine 20 mg daily throughout pregnancy, and this has been continued after delivery.

You note from a specialist textbook that the likely infant exposure is about 2% of the weight-adjusted maternal dose.

Questions

1. What is the most likely drug-related explanation?
2. Is it safe for the mother to continue to take paroxetine whilst breastfeeding?
3. Is St John's wort a reasonable alternative?

Answers

1. The most likely explanation is a neonatal withdrawal syndrome from SSRI use near term. Symptoms typically occur 12 h–5 days after birth. The adult half-life of paroxetine is about 24 h, but this is much longer in a neonate. There will be a gradual decline in paroxetine plasma levels in the neonate after delivery. Drug exposure in pregnancy is much greater than exposure via milk. There may be some overlap of symptoms resulting from drug transfer into breast milk and from *in utero* exposure – agitation, jitteriness, hypotonia and gastro-intestinal symptoms. However, sedation has only been reported after drug exposure via breast milk. Paroxetine is one of the preferred SSRIs in breastfeeding as the half-life is shorter than most members of the group and the incidence of reported adverse effects is low.
2. The mother should be reassured that the effects are not due to the transfer of excessive amounts of paroxetine into milk. Withdrawal symptoms usually settle after a few days, whereas adverse effects due to the drug via milk will remain with continued exposure. If symptoms persist, further medical advice should be sought.
3. Herbal remedies are often perceived as safe as they are natural. In general, there is a lack of data to support the safe use of herbal remedies in lactation, and their use should be avoided. If a pharmacological treatment is indicated, then a drug for which data in lactation is available, for example, paroxetine should be used.

Case 47.4

A breastfeeding mother returned to see her midwife 4 weeks after delivery of a full-term healthy infant. She is complaining of bilateral nipple pain during and after breastfeeding, a problem that was constant for the past 4 days. She was advised to use miconazole cream 2% to the nipples after each feed. This provided initial relief but symptoms returned after a few days. She was given a course of fluconazole 200 mg daily for 14 days for a presumed candidal infection but expressed concern that the medication might affect the infant.

Questions

1. Is this regimen safe to use in lactation?
2. What other therapeutic measures should be taken?

Answers

1. Topical miconazole is effective in treating superficial candidal infections, but oral therapy with fluconazole is needed when the infection spreads to the milk ducts. Assuming a mean fluconazole milk level of 2.3 mg/L, an infant weight of 4 kg and a milk intake of 150 mL/kg/day:

   The estimated daily infant intake via milk will be 2.3 × 0.15 × 4 = 1.38 mg or 0.345 mg/kg/day.

   This represents 10.35% of the weight-adjusted dose for a 60-kg woman taking 200 mg of fluconazole daily and 5.75% of the paediatric dose of 6 mg/kg/day. The mother may be reassured that the amount of drug reaching the infant via milk is only a small fraction of the dose that would be used to treat an infection in the infant.

2. Candidal infections are easily passed between the mother and the infant, and both should receive treatment. Infants can be treated with nystatin suspension or oral miconazole gel. The latter is not suitable for young infants under 4 months because of the risk of choking on the viscous formulation, and care is still needed with older infants.

Case 47.5

A mother who wishes to give up smoking seeks advice on the safety of nicotine replacement therapy (NRT) whilst breastfeeding. She is currently in the latter stages of pregnancy but does not wish to use these products until after delivery and has not been successful in significantly reducing her smoking without aids.

Questions

1. What effect is smoking likely to have on breastfeeding?
2. Can NRT be used safely whilst breastfeeding?
3. If so, which products are preferred?

Answers

1. Women who smoke during pregnancy are less likely to breastfeed and more likely to wean their infants earlier. Nicotine reduces basal prolactin levels which may lead to a decrease in milk supply. It also causes adrenaline release which may inhibit the release of oxytocin and affect the milk let-down reflex. Tobacco smoke may produce breathing difficulties and other problems in infants. Maternal smoking is a major factor for sudden infant death syndrome (SIDS) and breastfeeding provides significant protection.
2. Ideally, breastfeeding mothers should stop smoking, preferably by using non-pharmacological methods. If this is not possible, most authorities advise that the amount of nicotine passing into milk after use of NRT is very much smaller than that after smoking and less harmful than the second-hand smoke an infant might breathe if the mother continues to smoke. NRT products are devoid of tars, carbon monoxide and respiratory irritants found in cigarettes. Where the infant has breathing difficulties, NRT should be avoided. Other members of the household who smoke should also be encouraged to give up smoking.
3. Breast milk levels of nicotine after use of a 21-mg transdermal patch are roughly equivalent to smoking 17 cigarettes a day. Maternal plasma levels of nicotine after using a nicotine spray are about one-third those of smokers and levels after using a gum are variable but can be similar to those seen after smoking. If possible, nicotine patches should be avoided during breastfeeding because they provide a continuous (but low) passage of nicotine into breast milk. If patches are used, they should be removed at night time to decrease nocturnal exposure. For shorter-acting preparations (e.g. gums, lozenges), it is best to breastfeed immediately before use and allow a 2–3 hour period before resumption of breastfeeding to minimise infant exposure.

Acknowledgements

The contribution of Stephen B. Duffull, Sharon J. Gardiner and David K. Woods to previous versions of this chapter which appeared in earlier editions is gratefully acknowledged.

References

Anderson, G., 2005. Pregnancy-induced changes in pharmacokinetics: a mechanistic-based approach. Clin. Pharmacokinet. 44, 989–1008.

Atkinson, H.C., Begg, J., 1990. Prediction of drug distribution into human milk from physicochemical characteristics. Clin. Pharmacokinet. 18, 151–167.

Begg, E.J., 2000. Clinical Pharmacology Essentials. The Principles Behind the Prescribing Process. Adis International, Auckland.

Begg, E.J., Atkinson, E.J., Duffull, S.B., 1992. Prospective evaluation of a model for the prediction of milk:plasma drug concentrations from physicochemical characteristics. Br. J. Clin. Pharmacol. 33, 501–505.

Benke, P.J., 1984. The isotretinoin teratogen syndrome. J. Am. Med. Assoc. 251, 3267–3269.

Berlin, C.M., Paul, I.M., Vesell, E.S., 2009. Safety issues of maternal drug therapy during breastfeeding. Clin. Pharmacol. Ther. 85, 20–22.

Braun, J.T., Franciosi, R.A., Mastri, A.R., et al., 1984. Isotretinoin dysmorphic syndrome. Lancet 1, 506–507.

Breitkreutz, I., Anderson, K.C., 2008. Thalidomide in multiple myeloma: clinical trials and aspects of drug metabolism and toxicity. Expert Opin. Drug Metab. Toxicol. 4, 973–985.

Dunn, P.M., 1964. The possible relationship between the maternal administration of sulphamethoxypyridazine and hyperbilirubinaemia in the newborn. J. Obstet. Gynaecol. Br. Commonw. 71, 128–131.

Fewtrell, M.S., 2004. The long term benefits of having been breastfed. Curr. Paediatr. 14, 97–103.

Hale, T.W., 2010. Medications and Mothers' Milk, fourteenth ed. Hale Publishing, Amarillo.

Headley, J., Northstone, K., Simmons, H., et al., 2004. Medication use during pregnancy: data from the Avon longitudinal study of parents and children. Eur. J. Clin. Pharmacol. 60, 355–361.

Herbst, A.L., Ulfelder, H., Poskanzer, D.C., 1971. Adenocarcinoma of the vagina. Association of maternal stilbestrol therapy with tumor appearance in young women. N. Engl. J. Med. 15, 878–881.

Hernandez-Diaz, S., Werler, M.M., Walker, A.M., et al., 2001. Neural tube defects in relation to use of folic acid antagonists during pregnancy. Am. J. Epidemiol. 153, 961–968.

Hill, R.M., 1984. Isotretinoin teratogenicity. Lancet 1, 1465.

Horta, B.L., Bahl, R., Martines, J.C., et al., 2007. Evidence on the Long-Term Effects of Breastfeeding. WHO, Geneva.

Ingelman-Sundberg, M., 2005. Genetic polymorphisms of cytochrome P450 2D6 (CYP2D6): clinical consequences, evolutionary aspects and functional diversity. Pharmacogenomics J. 5, 6–13.

Koren, G., Florescu, A., Costei, A.M., et al., 2006. Non-steroidal anti-inflammatory drugs during third trimester and the risk of premature closure of the ductus arteriosus: a meta-analysis. Ann. Pharmacother. 40, 824–829.

Kramer, M.S., Kakuma, R., 2002. Optimal duration of exclusive breastfeeding. Cochrane Database of Systematic Reviews . Issue 1

Art No. CD003517 doi:10.1002/14651858.CD003517. Available at http://www2.cochrane.org/reviews/en/ab003517.html.

Lawrence, R.A., Lawrence, R.M., 2011. Breastfeeding. A Guide for the Medical Profession, seventh ed. Elsevier, Philadelphia.

Lenz, W., 1966. Malformations caused by drugs in pregnancy. Am. J. Dis. Child 112, 99–106.

Lenz, W., 1988. A short history of thalidomide embryopathy. Teratology 38, 203–215.

Loebstein, R., Lalkin, A., Koren, G., 1997. Pharmacokinetic changes during pregnancy and their clinical relevance. Clin. Pharmacokinet. 33, 328–343.

Madadi, P., Ross, C.J., Hayden, M.R., et al., 2009. Pharmacogenetics of neonatal opioid toxicity following maternal use of codeine during breastfeeding: a case control study. Clin. Pharmacol. Ther. 85, 31–35.

Miller, M.T., Ventura, L., Stromland, K., 2009. Thalidomide and misoprostol: ophthalmologic manifestations and associations both expected and unexpected. Birth Defects Res. Part A Clin. Mol. Teratol. 85, 667–676.

Newman, C.G., 1985. Teratogen update: clinical aspects of thalidomide embryopathy: a continuing preoccupation. Teratology 32, 133–144.

Newman, C.G., 1986. The thalidomide syndrome: risks of exposure and spectrum of malformations. Clin. Perinatol. 13, 555–573.

Nulman, I., Berkovitch, M., Klein, J., et al., 1998. Steady-state pharmacokinetics of isotretinoin and its 4-oxo metabolite: implications for fetal safety. J. Clin. Pharmacol. 38, 926–930.

Pavek, P., Ceckova, M., Staud, F., 2009. Variation of drug kinetics in pregnancy. Curr. Drug Metab. 10, 520–529.

Rosa, F.W., 1984. Virilization of the female fetus with maternal danazol exposure. Am. J. Obstet. Gynecol. 149, 99–100.

Schaefer, C., Peters, P., Miller, R.K. (Eds.), 2007. Drugs During Pregnancy and Lactation: Treatment Options and Risk Assessment, second ed. Academic Press, Oxford.

Scott, J.A., Binns, C.W., Oddy, W.H., et al., 2006. Predictors of breastfeeding duration: evidence from a cohort study. Pediatrics 117, e646–e655.

Sedman, A.B., Kershaw, D.B., Bunchman, T.E., 1995. Recognition and management of angiotensin converting enzyme inhibitor fetopathy. Pediatr. Nephrol. 9, 382–385.

Vorhees, C.V., Weisenburger, W.P., Minck, D.R., 2001. Neurobehavioral teratogenic effects of thalidomide in rats. Neurotoxicol. Teratol. 23, 255–264.

World Health Organization 2001 54th World Health Assembly, 2001. Global Strategy for Infant and Young Child Feeding. The Optimal Duration of Exclusive Breastfeeding. WHO, Geneva. Available at http://apps.who.int/gb/archive/pdf_files/WHA54/ea54id4.pdf.

Further reading

Department of Health 2002 Infant feeding, 2000. A Summary Report. DH, London. Available at http://www.dh.gov.uk/en/Publicationsandstatistics/Publications/PublicationsPolicyAndGuidance/DH_4008114.

Department of Health, 2003. Infant Feeding Recommendation. DH, London. Available at http://www.dh.gov.uk/prod_consum_dh/groups/dh_digitalassets/@dh/@en/documents/digitalasset/dh_4096999.pdf.

Hale, T.W., Ilett, K., 2002. Drug Therapy and Breastfeeding: From Theory to Clinical Practice. Parthenon Publishing, New York.

Lee, A., 2006. Adverse Drug Reactions, second ed. Pharmaceutical Press, London.

Schaefer, C., Peters, P.W.J., Miller, R.K. (Eds.) 2007. Drugs During Pregnancy and Lactation. second ed. Elsevier, Amsterdam.

Tomson, G., Sundwall, A., Lunell, N.O., et al., 1979. Transplacental passage and kinetics in the mother and newborn of oxazepam given during labour. Clin. Pharmacol. Ther. 25, 74–81.

Useful websites

UK Teratology Information Service (UKTIS):
www.uktis.org
TOXBASE:
www.toxbase.org
European Network of Teratology Information Services:
http://www.entis-org.com

OTIS (American Organisation of Teratology Information Services):
www.otispregnancy.org
Motherisk (Canadian Teratology information service):
www.motherisk.org.

Prostate disease 48

M. Martinez and M. Satheesh

Key points

Benign prostatic hyperplasia

- Benign prostatic hyperplasia (BPH) is a common condition which increases in prevalence with age.
- A combination of increased adrenergic tone in the prostatic stroma and bladder neck as well as the anatomical effects of an enlarging prostate lead to lower urinary tract symptoms (LUTSs) and bladder outflow obstruction (BOO).
- Surgical treatments such as transurethral resection of the prostate (TURP) are effective, but less invasive procedures such as laser therapy, and less commonly thermotherapy, are used.
- α-Adrenoceptor blocking drugs are effective in reducing symptoms.
- 5α-Reductase inhibitors reduce prostate size, improve symptoms, increase urinary flow rates and reduce the risk of developing complications such as acute urinary retention (AUR) or the need for prostate surgery.

Prostate cancer

- Prostate cancer (PC) typically progresses slowly but is influenced by factors such as tumour grade, stage of the disease, co-morbidities and life expectancy.
- Aetiology is multi-factorial and includes age, race, family history and dietary habit.
- Early detection is difficult because there are no symptoms specific to PC.
- A combination of digital rectal examination (DRE), serum prostate-specific antigen (PSA) and transrectal ultrasonography (TRUS) is used to confirm diagnosis.
- Curative treatments include radical prostatectomy or radiotherapy.
- Treatment depends on the grade and stage of tumour, life expectancy and patient choice.

Prostatitis

- Prostatitis is classified as acute bacterial prostatitis, chronic bacterial prostatitis, chronic prostatitis/chronic pelvic pain syndrome and asymptomatic inflammatory prostatitis.
- There is no absolute diagnostic tool for prostatitis. Diagnosis is based on physical examination and clinical history.
- The pathophysiology of prostatitis is poorly understood and the aetiology is unclear in the majority of patients.
- Prostatitis cases associated with infection or inflammation are treated with antibiotics.
- α-Adrenoceptor antagonists are used for the treatment of chronic prostatitis/chronic pelvic pain syndrome.

Benign prostatic hyperplasia

Epidemiology

Benign prostatic hyperplasia (BPH) is the most common benign tumour in men and is responsible for urinary symptoms in the majority of males over the age of 50 years. Autopsy studies have revealed the histological presence of BPH in 50% of males aged 51–60 years, increasing to 90% in those over 85. By the age of 80 years, virtually all men exhibit one or more of the symptoms associated with BPH.

BPH is seen in all races although the overall size of the prostate varies from race to race.

Pathophysiology

The prostate is a part glandular, part fibromuscular structure about the size of a walnut that surrounds the first part of the male urethra at the base of the bladder (Fig. 48.1). In simple terms, the prostate can be divided into a lobular inner zone encapsulated by an external layer. The inner zone is where benign hypertrophic changes are generally found, whereas most malignant changes originate in the peripheral zone.

Prostatic hypertrophy is directly related to the ageing process and to hormone activity. Within the prostate, testosterone is converted by 5α-reductase to dihydrotestosterone (DHT). DHT is five times more potent than testosterone and is responsible for stimulating growth factors that influence cell division leading to prostatic hyperplasia and enlargement.

Histologically, depending on the predominance of the type of prostatic tissue present, prostatic hypertrophy can be stromal, fibromuscular, muscular, fibroadenomatous or fibromyoadenomatous.

As the prostate enlarges, it can compress the urethra (Fig. 48.2) and this, together with increased adrenergic tone, can lead to bladder outflow obstruction (BOO) and lower urinary tract symptoms (LUTSs). Therefore, the term BPH includes benign prostatic enlargement (BPE), the clinical features associated with urinary obstruction and LUTSs.

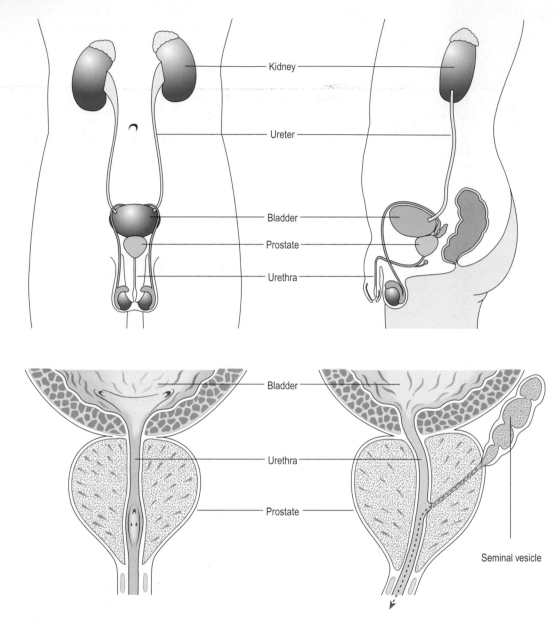

Fig. 48.1 Male urinary system demonstrating the location of the prostate.

Symptoms

Men with BPH can develop bothersome LUTSs that can impact negatively on their quality of life. It is important to emphasise that not all men who experience LUTSs have BPH. LUTSs can have different aetiologies including bladder cancer or stones, urinary tract infection (UTI) or urethral stricture. Furthermore, a histological diagnosis of BPH does not mean the patient will suffer from LUTSs.

LUTSs can be divided into symptoms of failure of urine storage (irritative) and those caused by failure to empty the bladder (obstructive or voiding).

Irritative symptoms

* Frequency
* Nocturia
* Urgency and urge incontinence

Obstructive symptoms

* Poor urinary flow
* Hesitancy in initiation of micturition
* Post-micturition dribble
* Sensation of incomplete emptying
* Occasional acute retention of urine requiring emergency treatment

Examination and investigations

There is a range of investigations and diagnostic tests available for the evaluation of patients with suspected BPH. Some tests are standard during the assessment of all men with LUTSs. Other investigations are optional and are only performed depending on the patient's presentation and the clinician's judgement.

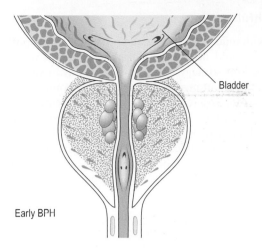

Early BPH

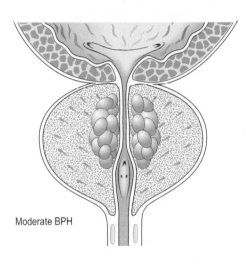

Moderate BPH

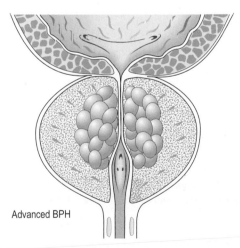

Advanced BPH

Fig. 48.2 Diagrammatic representation of the impact of prostate hyperplasia on the urethra demonstrating overgrowth of cells in the inner zone of the prostate.

History

A focussed medical history of all men with LUTSs should be taken to elucidate the aetiology of their symptoms. As part of the process, LUTSs should be evaluated using a validated

scoring tool such as the international prostate symptom score (IPSS). This can be used to monitor the severity and progression of the disease and assess the impact of therapy on LUTSs.

Physical examination

All patients who present with suspected BPH should undergo a digital rectal examination (DRE) which involves the examiner palpating the prostate with a finger through the rectum wall. A DRE is performed to exclude the presence of prostate cancer (PC) and can also be used to estimate the shape and size of the prostate, although transrectal ultrasonography (TRUS) provides a more accurate measurement of prostate volume.

Urodynamic studies

Simple non-invasive urodynamic studies provide a surrogate measure of BOO. These include maximum flow rate and post-void residual (PVR). Large PVRs of 300 mL, for example, are indicative of bladder dysfunction and predict a poor response to therapy. Definitive proof of BOO requires invasive pressure flow studies.

Imaging

In the past, upper tract imaging involving an ultrasound scan and intravenous urography were used routinely to evaluate LUTSs associated with BPH. These tests are not normally undertaken except in patients with abnormal renal function and LUTSs who should have an ultrasound scan of their kidneys. The following represent the imaging options used for the assessment of men with BPH.

Flexible cystoscopy

Flexible cystoscopy provides an endoscopic image of the bladder for the assessment of prostatic obstruction and informs possible management options. For example, if the prostate has grown and there is intravesical extension, each time the patient tries to void the internal urethral meatus is obstructed. This type of tissue requires surgical removal, whereas simple lateral lobe enlargement may well respond to non-surgical measures.

Prostatic ultrasound scan

Prostatic ultrasound or TRUS uses high-frequency scanners to produce images of the prostate. This imaging is used to obtain an accurate evaluation of the prostate volume and to detect malignant change. TRUS is also used to guide the placement of the needle when obtaining prostatic biopsies.

Other investigations

Other investigations may be carried out to facilitate the diagnostic assessment of patients with LUTSs due to BPH, and these include urinalysis, urine cultures if infection is suspected, and serum creatinine to assess renal function and establish possible upper urinary tract damage. The measurement of serum prostate-specific antigen (PSA) can be considered after counselling the patient, particularly if DRE reveals a nodular or hard prostate.

Treatment

Most men over the age of 50 years exhibit some of the symptoms of BPH. The range of treatment options for the management of BPH includes watchful waiting, medical therapies and surgical interventions. The key issue, therefore, is deciding who should be treated and when.

The British Association of Urological Surgeons has published guidelines for the management of BPH in primary care (Speakman et al., 2004), focussing on when urological referral is required and when non-invasive treatment can be initiated (Fig. 48.3).

Watchful waiting

Men with mild or moderate and not significantly bothersome LUTSs should be offered a trial of watchful waiting. This management strategy does not include any medical or surgical treatment but involves regular active monitoring. In some cases, symptoms remain unchanged for years and no further interventions are necessary since disease progression is minimal. Patients that adopt this modality should be offered education and lifestyle advice (Box 48.1) to manage their urological symptoms together with a review of their medication, particularly diuretics or other medicines known to affect the urinary system.

Therapeutic management

The principal treatment options are α-adrenoceptor blocking drugs, 5α-reductase inhibitors and combination therapy. Phytotherapy is also used in the management of BPH, although the benefits remain unproven.

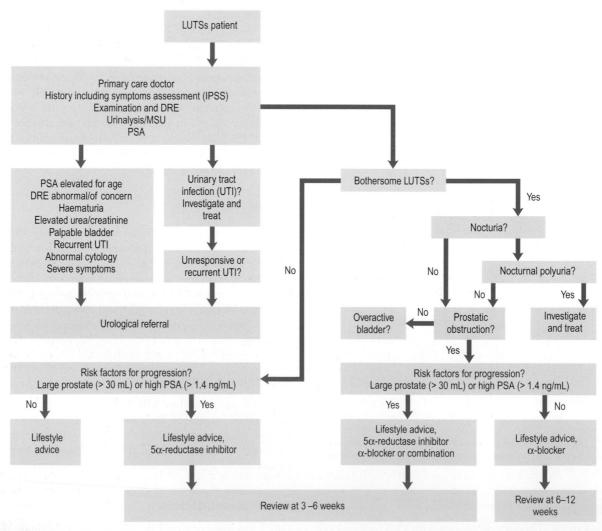

Fig. 48.3 Algorithm for the treatment of lower urinary tract symptoms (LUTSs) in males in primary care (from Speakman et al., 2004) (DRE, digital rectal examination; MSU, mid-stream urine sample; PSA, prostate-specific antigen).

Limit fluid consumption before going out and before going to bed (to reduce urinary frequency and nocturia)
Reduce alcohol and caffeine intake
Schedule toilet visits
Manage constipation
Review medication (including diuretics and other medicines that can affect the urinary system)
Bladder training (encourage patient to go longer between voiding and increase the volume voided)
Use distraction techniques (practice breathing exercises and penile squeezing to control symptoms of irritation)

α-Adrenoceptor blocking drugs

The prostate gland is very responsive to adrenergic stimulation. In fact, prostatic outlet obstruction in BPH is partly due to the hypertrophied bulk of the gland, but it also arises from an increase in adrenergic tone. In the prostate, α_1-receptors predominate and mediate the contraction of the gland's smooth muscle. At least three subtypes of this receptor exist (α_{1A}, α_{1B} and α_{1D}). The α_{1A} is thought to be the dominant receptor in the prostate, although its role clinically has still to be confirmed. This increase in sympathetic tone is potentially reversible by α-adrenoceptor antagonists.

In general, all the agents are considered to produce similar clinical improvements of LUTSs and urinary flow. Benefits can be seen usually within the first few days of therapy and can be maintained in the long-term. α-Adrenoceptor antagonists also have a comparable side-effect profile, which includes postural hypotension, dizziness, fatigue, headache, drowsiness, nasal congestion and ejaculatory dysfunction.

Patients with BPH frequently experience erectile and ejaculatory dysfunction. The treatment of BPH should also aim to improve sexual function. However, the effect of α_1-adrenoceptor antagonists on male sexual function is variable and influenced by the choice of agent and patient characteristics (Van Dijk et al., 2006).

Prazosin. Prazosin was the first α_1-blocker used to relieve the symptoms of BPH but it lacks relative selectivity for α_{1A} receptors and has been associated with many adverse affects such as drowsiness, weakness, headache and postural hypotension (especially after the first dose).

Terazosin. Terazosin was the first in the category to appear in controlled trials aimed at evaluating the efficacy and safety profile of long acting α_1-blockers in the management of BPH. Efficacy is dose dependant and dose titration is necessary, as terazosin can cause postural hypotension. Adverse effects, although generally mild, occur more frequently than with other α_1-adrenoceptor antagonists, resulting in up to a fourfold increase in treatment discontinuation.

Indoramin. Indoramin is readily absorbed from the gastro-intestinal tract and undergoes extensive first-pass hepatic metabolism. Its hypotensive effect may be increased by diuretics and other anti-hypertensive agents. Alcohol has been reported to increase the bioavailability and sedative effects of indoramin.

Doxazosin. Doxazosin has a long half-life of about 22h, which allows for once-daily dosing. When starting treatment, dose titration is recommended to limit postural hypotension. There would appear to be no significant difference in symptom score regardless of whether the standard or controlled-release preparation is used (Kirby et al., 2001).

Tamsulosin. Tamsulosin is a selective inhibitor of the α_{1A}- and α_{1B}-adrenoceptor. It has an elimination half-life of about 13h and is available as a prolonged release formulation that allows once-daily dosing. There is no requirement to titrate the dose upward when initiating treatment. Although the side-effect profile of tamsulosin is similar to other α_1-adrenoceptor antagonists, it is normally well tolerated (O'Leary, 2001). Intraoperative floppy iris syndrome (IFIS) has been reported during cataract surgery in men treated with tamsulosin, as it is highly selective to iris dilator muscle (Chaim et al., 2009). IFIS can lead to complications and poor outcomes during cataract surgery. As a result, it is essential that patients inform their cataract surgeon that they are taking tamsulosin during the pre-operative assessment. It has been recommended to avoid starting treatment and to discontinue treatment with tamsulosin 1–2 weeks before cataract surgery.

Alfuzosin. Alfuzosin displays a higher selectivity for the prostate compared with tamsulosin or doxazosin. It has a half-life of 5h, but it is available as a once-daily formulation. It has a rapid onset of action and good tolerability (MacDonald and Wilt, 2005). It reduces the overall clinical progression of BPH and it appears to have a sustained beneficial effect on quality of life (Roehrborn, 2006). Alfuzosin has the least effect on ejaculatory function. Alfuzosin should not be co-administered with potent inhibitors of cytochrome P450 3A4 such as itraconazole, ketoconazole and ritonavir, since this can lead to a several fold increase to exposure in alfuzosin.

5α-Reductase inhibitors

The primary androgen responsible for the development and progression of BPH is DHT. There are two isoenzymes of 5α-reductase: type 1 is found in most 5α-reductase producing tissues such as the liver, skin and hair; type 2 is predominant in genital tissue, including the prostate. 5α-Reductase inhibitors downregulate prostate growth by blocking the conversion of testosterone to the more potent DHT.

The two agents currently available in this group are finasteride and dutasteride. Both have been shown to reduce prostate volume, to improve symptom scores and flow rates, and reduce the incidence of complications such as acute urinary retention (AUR) and the need for surgical intervention to treat BPH (Roehrborn et al., 2000, 2002). Improvements in LUTSs are normally seen after the first 6 months of treatment and are sustained during continuous treatment (Lam et al., 2003).

Finasteride. Finasteride is a type 2, 5α-reductase inhibitor that can reduce prostate size by about 30%, improve symptom scores and increase urinary flow. Those most likely to benefit are men with a prostate larger than 40mL. Side effects include decreased libido, impotence, reduced ejaculatory volume and, less commonly, gynaecomastia and breast tenderness. Serum concentrations of PSA may be reduced by 50% in the first year of treatment with finasteride, a fact which must be taken into account when attempting to interpret the PSA concentration in men with suspected PC.

Dutasteride. Dutasteride inhibits both type 1 and type 2 isoenzymes of 5α-reductase. Although the clinical significance of this is unclear, this double inhibition can reduce serum dihydotestosterone levels by about 90%. Dutasteride decreases prostate volume by up to 26% and reduces the risk of progression to serious complications of BPH. LUTSs also improve after 6 months of treatment. Dutasteride is well tolerated although side effects which include erectile and ejaculatory dysfunction and breast enlargement occur with similar frequency to finasteride.

Combination therapy

It is well established that α-adrenoceptor antagonists are best for managing acute symptoms but have no impact on reducing the risk of complications such as AUR or progression to prostate surgery. In contrast, 5α-reducatase inhibitors have little impact on short-term acute symptoms but reduce prostate size, improve urinary flow and obstructive symptoms in the long-term. Furthermore, α-adrenoceptor antagonists are effective regardless of prostate volume, whereas the 5α-reductase inhibitors are more suited for the management of LUTSs in men with large prostates. In terms of long-term benefits, continued treatment with 5α-reductase inhibitors decreases the risk of AUR and BPH-related surgery. Therefore, it appears logical to use a combination of an α-adrenoceptor antagonist and a 5α-reductase inhibitor to manage acute symptoms and reduce progression of BPH.

The benefits of using a combination of doxazosin and finasteride compared to monotherapy have been demonstrated in over 3000 men (McConnell et al., 2003). Similarly, the combAT trial (Roehrborn et al., 2010) involved nearly 5000 men with moderate to severe symptoms of BPH and prostate enlargement treated with a combination of dutasteride and tamsulosin. This study demonstrated a significant improvement in BPH symptoms over a 4-year period when compared to either agent used alone. The combination was also found to reduce AUR and progression to BPH-related surgery and, although superior to tamsulosin with respect to these complications, combination therapy was not better than dutasteride. Overall, the adverse events associated with combination therapy were few and treatment was well tolerated.

Combination therapy with an α-adrenoceptor antagonist and a 5α-reductase inhibitor has now been adopted widely into routine practice for the early management of LUTSs and to reduce progression of BPH.

Phytotherapy

A number of plant extracts are reputed to be effective in the management of symptoms of BPH. They include saw palmetto berry (*Serenoa repens*), African plum tree (*Pygeum africanum*), stinging nettle (*Urtica dioica*) and rye grass pollen. Their mechanism of action remains unclear but may exert an anti-inflammatory effect by inhibition of prostanoid formation and perhaps produce some degree of inhibition of 5α-reductase. Most of the data available to support the use of plant extracts derive from poorly designed studies. As evidence to assess efficacy and safety is lacking, phytotherapy remedies are not currently recommended by international guidelines for the management of BPH.

Surgical treatments

Surgical interventions are commonly performed in men with LUTSs caused by BPH that have failed to respond to medical treatment. Surgery is also indicated in patients who develop complications such as intractable or recurrent urinary retention, renal impairment, persistent haematuria, recurrent UTIs or bladder stones.

Transurethral resection of the prostate. Transurethral resection of the prostate (TURP) is a common and effective procedure which achieves a high level of improvement in symptoms and flow rate. It is the preferred surgical intervention in men with a prostate volume between 30 and 80 mL. Sections of prostate are removed using electrical wire loops attached to a tube-like telescope (resectoscope) inserted into the urethra. The tissue removed is collected for histological assessment. There is a small incidence of perioperative mortality associated with TURP along with complications such as bleeding, UTIs and epididymitis. Long-term complications include stress incontinence, urethral and bladder neck strictures and erectile dysfunction.

Open prostatectomy. Open prostatectomy involves the surgical removal of an enlarged prostate. Typically, an incision is made through the lower abdomen although sometimes the incision is between the rectum and the base of the penis. This procedure is now performed infrequently and restricted to very enlarged prostate glands (larger than 100 mL) and those with large bladder stones or bladder diverticula (Stoevelaar and McDonnell, 2001). Open prostatectomy requires a longer hospital stay than transurethral resection and is associated with a higher incidence of bleeding and other complications.

Minimally invasive techniques

Various treatment modalities have been tried as alternatives to TURP to reduce the risks associated with resection. Thermotherapy and laser technology are the most commonly used. Thermotherapy uses techniques such as electrovaporisation and transurethral microwave heat treatment (TUMT), which heats the prostate to cause vaporisation of the tissue. Various types of laser energy can also be used to destroy prostatic tissue mainly by coagulation or vaporisation.

Patient care

Patients generally seek medical help for BPH because of the impact of symptoms on their quality of life. Most men tolerate a high degree of symptoms and impact on daily activities before they seek help. Table 48.1 lists some common

Table 48.1 Common therapeutic problems and proposed management strategies in benign prostatic hyperplasia

Problem	Solution
Patient taking α-blocker still symptomatic after 2 weeks	Patients should be advised that it may take 2–6 weeks before symptomatic treatment relief is seen
Patient taking an α-adrenoceptor blocker complains of cardiovascular adverse effects such as dizziness, syncope, palpitations, tachycardia or angina	These side effects are more likely in elderly patients. They are most common after the first dose and reflect the hypotensive effects of the drugs. They can be reduced by titrating the dose or using more uroselective drugs such as tamsulosin
Sexual dysfunction	Decreased libido or impotence can occur in patients taking finasteride and dutasteride. Abnormal ejaculation can be caused by α-blockers. Tamsulosin in particular can cause a dry climax (retrograde ejaculation). Patients should be forewarned when discussing treatment options
Patient taking finasteride notices breast enlargement	Unilateral or bilateral gynaecomastia is a frequently reported side effect with finasteride and patients need to be counselled accordingly when discussing treatment options
Patient taking finasteride or dutasteride has a sexual partner who is pregnant	Exposure to semen should be avoided as both drugs can cause abnormalities to genitalia in a male fetus. The patient should be advised to use a condom

therapeutic problems in the management of BPH. Patients should receive information about the management options available, the investigations that they need to undergo and possible treatment outcomes and adverse effects. Patients receiving drug therapy should receive specific information about their treatment, including potential benefits, timeline of expected outcomes and possible side effects.

There are two websites which produce particularly useful educational material on prostatic disease: the Men's Health Forum (http://www.menshealthforum.org.uk/) and the Prostate Research Campaign (http://www.prostateuk.org/index.htm).

Prostate cancer

Epidemiology

PC is the second most common cancer in the world and the most common form of cancer in men. Incidence varies from country to country with the highest rates in America, Canada and Scandinavia and the lowest rates in China and other Asian countries (Quinn and Babb, 2002; Gronberg, 2003). In the UK, nearly a quarter of all new male cancer diagnoses are of the prostate. The lifetime risk of PC is 1 in 10 in males in the UK.

The aetiology of PC is multi-factorial. Testosterone and DHT have an important role in the disease as males who undergo castration before puberty do not develop PC. Other factors which can influence the risk of developing PC include the following:

Age. PC is rare before 50 years in Caucasians and before 40 years in Africans, but after this age, the incidence and mortality increase exponentially with every passing decade. Most cases are detected around the age of 70.

Race. Incidence and mortality is high among Caucasians and African Americans and lowest in Chinese males. Environmental factors may play a role in this variation as studies have found an increased incidence in East Asian men who relocate to western countries.

Family history. Presence of PC in a first-degree relative or in multiple family members who need not be first-degree relatives increase risk. Inheritance of a susceptible gene or polymorphism of gene may be responsible for this.

Diet. Although there is no compelling evidence to prove the direct influence of diet, high intake of fat, red meat and dairy produce, typically the main sources of dietary fatty acids in a Western diet, have individually been linked with PC. The low incidence of PC in China and Japan may be due to their use of soya bean products which contain isoflavones and inhibit protein tyrosine kinases responsible for cell proliferation.

Other factors. These include exposure to cadmium (found in cigarette smoke), pesticides, alkaline batteries, radionuclides and heavy metals.

Pathophysiology

The growth and differentiation of cells in the prostate is under androgen control. In the prostate, free testosterone diffuses into the epithelial cells where it is converted to DHT. Various growth factors are present in stromal cells, and the interaction of these with epithelial cells can play a role in cell proliferation and growth. The development of PC is generally a slow, gradual process where cellular structure changes from normal through dysplastic to cancer. High-grade prostatic intra-epithelial neoplasia (HGPIN) represents the precancerous stage of cellular proliferation in prostate cells and can be detected by biopsy. It can predate carcinoma by 10 years or more. There is no link between PC and BPH but they can coexist.

Screening

Population-based screening based on PSA levels is prevalent in the USA, and the annual incidence here has doubled due to this. In the UK, screening is not advocated as the prevailing view is that there is a lack of evidence to support it. Due to the aetiology and nature of PC, most patients will not be symptomatic in their lifetime and screening may increase the risk of overtreatment.

Symptoms

Clinical symptoms of PC are similar to those for BPH, and there are no symptoms which correlate specifically to early PC. As more than 50% of men above the age of 50 years have prostate-related symptoms, it is difficult to detect early PC. Advanced PC typically presents with symptoms of urethral and bladder outlet obstruction, anaemia, weight loss, haematuria or bone pain.

Examination and investigation

Physical examination

A DRE is an important diagnostic tool for PC with an estimated sensitivity of more than 60%. A palpable tumour will have a distinctive texture, but the accuracy of detection may depend on the experience of the clinician. False-positive results can occur in the presence of BPH or cysts.

Imaging

TRUS of the prostate is commonly used to aid the diagnosis of PC. Sensitivity ranges from 48% to 100%. Cancer in the anterior and central region of the prostate can, however, be missed. Computerised tomography, MRI scan of the pelvis and isotope bone scan are also useful to stage PC, but they are not effective as screening methods.

Prostate-specific antigen

Measurement of PSA is an accurate and clinically useful biochemical marker because it is specific to prostate tissue and produced by the columnar epithelial cells in the prostate gland. Unfortunately, PSA is not cancer specific as any damage to the internal architecture of the prostate can result in release. As a consequence, it is not a useful tool for diagnosing cancer on its own, but it is useful in monitoring the effect of treatment or tumour progression in untreated patients. Generally, PSA is high in PC, but it can sometimes be low in high-grade malignancy. The standard assay for PSA measures total prostate-specific antigen (tPSA) and includes all molecular forms. Age-specific ranges are available (Table 48.2) and help make it a better predictor, but this is only a rough guide as variations occur due to racial difference. There is no threshold for PSA below which PC cannot be found.

Table 48.2 Age-specific levels of prostate-specific antigen

Age	Prostate-specific antigen (ng/mL)
40–49	≤2.5
50–59	≤3.5
60–69	≤4.5
>70	≤6.5

Prostate biopsy

This is a definitive method to detect PC. TRUS guided biopsy will help obtain samples from the peripheral and transitional zones of the prostate and other suspicious areas. The peripheral zone of the prostate is the location where the majority of the PC occurs and the most common location for HGPIN. It is difficult to identify PC from trans-urethral resection of the prostate specimens as not much of it occurs in the transitional zone. In the UK, USA and Europe, the most widely accepted histological grading system, which corresponds to biological malignancy, is based on the Gleason scale (Gleason and Mellinger, 1974). Histological examination of biopsy tissue is undertaken to identify cancer cells and these are scored from 1 to 5 depending on the different pattern of glandular tissue (Fig. 48.4). A score of 1 corresponds to well-differentiated cells, while a score of 5 corresponds to poorly differentiated cells. The higher the score, the more aggressive the cancer. The number for the two most common types of cell in the sample are added together to get a Gleason score. The score ranges from 2 to 10. This is an important prognostic factor as it can help predict the future behaviour of the tumour and determine the treatment required.

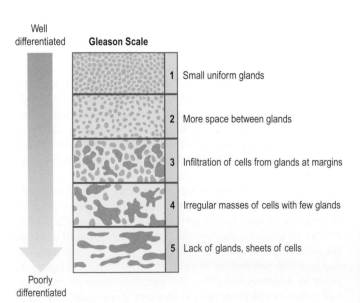

Fig. 48.4 Gleason scale.

Cancer staging

Results from a DRE, biopsy and scan are used to identify the extent of the cancer. The tumour volume, whether there is invasion into or through the capsule, and spread to lymph nodes or bone are all taken into consideration for staging. Staging based on the tumour, node, metastasis (TNM) system is a classification accepted worldwide (Epstein et al., 2005). Based on the TNM classification, PC can be classified into localised disease, locally advanced disease and advanced/metastased disease.

Treatment

The factors that must be considered to aid the treatment decision relate to the tumour and the patient:
Tumour: Staging result, histology, Gleason score and the PSA concentration.
Patient: Age at diagnosis, life expectancy and the presence of co-morbidities such as cardiovascular disease, chronic obstructive pulmonary disease and diabetes (Fig. 48.5).

Localised prostate cancer

Established treatments with curative intent

Active surveillance. It is difficult to distinguish PC which may not cause any problems to that which may grow and spread aggressively. Curative treatment can improve longevity but has side effects which include impotence and incontinence and can affect the quality of life of the individual. Patients on active surveillance are monitored closely by repeated testing of PSA levels, DRE and biopsy with the intention to make a radical intervention to treat if there is disease progression. A 20-year outcome study following conservative management of localised PC found that the annual mortality rates did not support aggressive treatment (Albertsen et al., 2005). Although active surveillance can spare side effects of treatment without compromising survival, regular biopsies used to monitor the disease can also be uncomfortable and carry a risk of infection. The optimal schedule for measuring PSA and repeating biopsies is unclear.

Radical prostatectomy. This is the treatment of choice and the procedure involves the total removal of a prostate, seminal vesicle, distal vasa, ejaculatory ducts and prostatic urethra. In the open procedure, it is performed by the retro pubic or perineal approach based on the surgeon's choice. Laparoscopic prostatectomy, and more recently robotic-assisted laparoscopy, has been developed. The most common complications of prostatectomy are blood loss, post-operative thromboembolism, urinary incontinence, impotence and rectal injury. Systemic review and meta-analysis have shown that the laparoscopic and robotic methods are associated with less blood loss and transfusion, but oncological outcomes, incontinence and erectile dysfunction rates are similar with all three types of prostatectomy.

Radical external-beam radiotherapy. Radiotherapy is used for locally confined disease and more recently for locally advanced disease state as well. In this treatment, high-energy photons produced by a linear accelerator are targeted at the prostate. Sometimes, special particles such as protons and heavy ions are used and have advantages over photons in terms of dose distribution. The side effects of radiotherapy include impotence, genitourinary stricture, rectal bleeding, haematuria and incontinence.

Interstitial brachytherapy. With interstitial brachytherapy radioactive isotope seeds are placed in the prostate under ultrasound or fluoroscopic control. These implants can emit radiation of low energy over several weeks and can be temporary or permanent. This treatment has the potential advantage of less erectile dysfunction than other treatment.

Minimal invasive procedures

The minimal invasive procedures are in the development stage and, although they may be used in some centres, there are no medium- or long-term follow-up data to prove efficacy. The various procedures include:

Cryosurgical ablation of prostate (CSAP). Cryosurgical ablation involves freezing the prostate which results in cell death by protein denaturation, direct rupture of cellular membranes and apoptosis. Freezing is achieved by placing 12–15 cryoneedles into the prostate guided by a transrectal ultrasonograph and using the cryoneedles to create freeze thaw cycles using temperatures of −40 °C.

High-intensity focussed ultrasound (HIFU). In this technique, ultrasound waves from a transducer are focussed on the prostate tissue to cause damage to the cells by mechanical and thermal effects. The malignant tissue is subjected to temperatures above 65 °C and hence is destroyed by coagulative necrosis.

Radio-frequency interstitial tumour ablation (RITA). A needle electrode is placed inside the prostate and radio-frequency waves are delivered through it to heat the tissue up to 100 °C thereby causing necrosis.

Watchful waiting

This approach implies that the patient is observed for symptomatic progression and will only receive palliative treatment when clinical symptoms develop. Since the disease often progresses slowly, watchful waiting is an option for patients with early disease as it maintains their quality of life and avoids complications related to surgery or radiation therapy. On the downside, it is not a curative option, the cancer can metastasise and be a source of pain and reduce life expectancy.

Locally advanced prostate cancer

Hormonal therapy/androgen deprivation therapy

In locally advanced disease involving areas outside the capsule, there is an increased risk of relapse and lymph node metastasis after prostatectomy.

Androgens are produced both in the testes (95%) under the stimulation of luteinising hormone (LH) and luteinising hormone-releasing hormone (LHRH) from the pituitary gland, and in the adrenal glands (5%) under the stimulation of adrenocorticotropic hormone (ACTH). The androgens produced by the adrenal gland are hormone precursors that are enzymatically converted to testosterone and DHT in prostatic and peripheral tissue. Since testosterone is a well-known etiologic factor associated with PC, it follows that testosterone deprivation can be utilised as part of treatment. In practice, this can be achieved by either surgical or medical castration with the response time varying from a few months to years.

Surgical castration. This is further discussed under metastatic disease.

Medical castration. A number of drugs can be used to reduce the levels of testosterone to those achieved by castration.

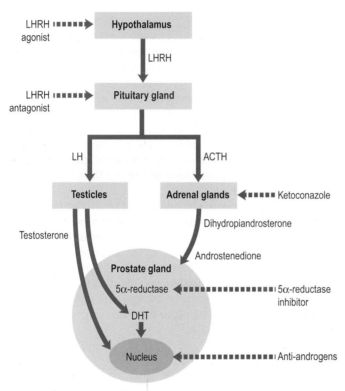

Fig. 48.5 Diagrammatic representation of the site of action of some treatments used in prostate cancer.

LHRH agonists. LHRH is released in the hypothalamus and stimulates the secretion of LH by binding to the LHRH receptors in the pituitary. This LHRH receptor complex is normally broken down by enzymes which lead to the release of lutenising hormone and frees the receptors for further binding with LHRH. LHRH agonists are synthetic analogues that bind to the LHRH receptor and the complex formed is resistant to enzymatic action. Thus, they maintain a continuous presence on the receptor and render the pituitary gland refractory to hypothalamic regulation compared to the pulsatile release in normal individuals. Continuous administration of LHRH agonists exhibits a biphasic response. There is an initial increase in LH, and testosterone release referred to as 'tumour flare up' followed by a fall over the following 1–2 weeks due to the down regulation and decrease in LHRH

release as the receptors are continuously occupied. 'Tumour flare up' is prevented by first initiating treatment with an anti-androgen before the use of LHRH agonist. The anti-androgen is then continued for a further 3–4 weeks. Currently available LHRH analogues include buserelin (nasal spray), goserelin, triptorelin and leuprorelin. Goserelin is administered subcutaneously at monthly or 3 monthly intervals, whereas triptorelin and leuprorelin are administered intramuscularly at monthly or 3 monthly intervals.

In advanced PC, therapy with an LHRH agonist is comparable in efficacy to surgical orchiectomy or diethylstilboestrol but with reduced physical and psychological discomfort of the former or the cardiovascular risks of the latter. There would appear to be little difference between the various formulations of LHRH agonists. UK, U.S. and European guidelines support the use of LHRH agonists as first-line agents in the treatment of advanced PC.

More recently, a novel agonist called histrelin was introduced. This is a 1-year subcutaneous preparation which is surgically implanted.

Anti-androgens. Anti-androgens competitively inhibit the effect of androgens peripherally by competing with testosterone and DHT for binding sites in the prostate. This results in inhibition of cell growth and apoptosis. Based on their chemical structure, the anti-androgens can be further divided into steroidal agents, which include cyproterone acetate, megesterol acetate and medroxyprogesterone, and non-steroidal agents such as nilutamide, flutamide and bicalutamide.

The steroidal agents also possess progestational activity and inhibit leutinising hormone secretion by acting centrally on the pituitary thereby reducing serum testosterone levels. The non-steroidal agents do not possess this additional property. Cyproterone is the most widely used steroidal agent normally administered in two or three daily doses of 100mg despite having a half-life of 30–40h. It can be used to treat the hot flushes associated with LHRH agonists or orchiectomy. Side effects include hepatoxicity, loss of libido and potency, fatigue and depression. Use of medroxy progesterone and megestrol is limited because of less favourable outcomes in clinical trials compared to cyproterone.

Non-steroidal anti-androgens are used in patients who wish to preserve their quality of life as they do not suppress testosterone and hence preserve libido, physical performance and bone mineral density. The disadvantage of nilutamide, flutamide and bicalutamide is a reduced survival when used as monotherapy because of a gradual rise in testosterone. All three agents have side effects of gynaecomastia, gastrointestinal upsets, idiopathic hepato-cellular toxicity and haematuria. Bicalutamide has a better safety and tolerability profile compared to nilutamide and flutamide (Inverson, 2002). Some trials show that non-steroidal anti-androgens used in combination with surgical castration or LHRH agonists bring about complete or total androgen blockade by also reducing the production of androgens from the adrenal glands, which normally accounts for 5% of the body's production, thereby conferring a small survival advantage.

LHRH agonists and the non-steroidal anti-androgen flutamide have been used as neoadjuvant (treatment to reduce tumour size before further surgery or other treatment) or adjuvant (treatment given in addition to primary/initial treatment to reach a treatment goal) with radiotherapy to improve disease-free and overall survival in patients with locally advanced disease.

Metastatic prostate cancer

LHRH agonists

Patients with metastatic cancer of the prostate usually respond to treatment with LHRH agonists and use is as described above for locally advanced disease.

Surgical castration

Surgical castration by bilateral orchiectomy is the treatment of choice for metastatic disease. Advantages include its low cost and morbidity with testosterone levels falling to castration levels within 5–12 h of surgery. The disadvantages include psychological trauma, its irreversible nature and the fact that nearly half experience side effects including loss of libido and potency, hot flushes and bone and muscle loss.

Other palliative treatments

LHRH antagonists. LHRH antagonists, which include abarelix and degarelix, work by competitively binding to LHRH receptors in the pituitary thereby suppressing LH release and creating a rapid and sustained decrease in testosterone levels. They do not cause an initial surge in testosterone levels and hence there is no 'tumour flare up' or need for short-term treatment with anti-androgens unlike the LHRH agonists. Abarelix requires an induction regimen followed by monthly injections and use is associated with anaphylactic reactions. Degarelix is given as a monthly depot injection; the most common side effect is a local reaction at the injection site such as swelling and erythema. Degarelix has a place in high-risk PC where the patient is acutely symptomatic with impending spinal cord compression, ureteric obstruction and urinary retention. Degarelix reduces testosterone, LH and PSA levels faster than LHRH agonists and reduces microsurges of testosterone.

The European Association of Urology (EAU) guidelines on PC recommend the use of LHRH antagonists in patients with metastasis and impending spinal cord compression (Heidenreich et al., 2009).

Bisphosphonates. Skeletal involvement in PC can be disease related or due to androgen depletion therapy. Bisphosphonates are pyrophosphates that inhibit osteoclast activity in bones and hence prevent and treat bone lesions. Pamidronate prevents bone loss but zolendronate not only increases bone mass while on androgen depletion therapy but also reduces skeletal complications in patients with bone metastasis secondary to PC (Saad and Schulman, 2004). Bisphosphonates are also recommended for pain relief when analgesics and palliative radiotherapy to bone have failed. Dental examination needs to be carried out before commencing treatment with a bisphosphonate due to the risk of osteonecrosis of the jaw in those with a history of dental trauma, infection or surgery.

Ketoconazole. This broad-spectrum, imidazole, anti-fungal can be used at a higher dose than is normal for its anti-fungal effect to inhibit the testicular and adrenal cytochrome P-450 enzyme synthesis of sex sterols. It has a rapid onset of action and is usually prescribed at a dose of 400 mg three times daily. As it causes adrenal suppression, hydrocortisone supplementation is necessary. Side effects of ketoconazole include drug-induced toxicity, adrenal suppression and hepatotoxicity.

Dexamethasone. Dexamethasone is used if spinal cord compression is suspected.

Castrate resistant prostate cancer

Androgen deprivation therapy can fail to control disease progression. The reasons for this are unclear but include the clonal selection hypothesis or adaption hypothesis. In the clonal selection hypothesis, the premise is that the basal cells are the stem cells of the prostate and generate secretory epithelial cells. Whilst the secretory epithelial cells undergo apoptosis upon androgen withdrawal, this is not the case with basal or stromal cells. As a consequence, there is selective survival of these androgen independent cells within the tumour. With the adaption hypothesis, there is the assumption that androgen independence may be an intrinsic, but dormant property of some prostate cells that is activated by androgen deprivation. Whatever the explanation, when there is failure of first-line therapy, quality of life can be improved by using single or combination therapy that includes a second-line hormone treatment (oestrogens), corticosteroids, ketoconazole, chemotherapy and bisphosphonates for short-term palliative response.

Oestrogen

Diethylstilboestrol (DES) is a synthetic oestrogen which acts by producing negative feedback on the hypothalamus and anterior pituitary, thereby down regulating the secretion of LHRH and hence the production of testosterone. Diethylstilboestrol is the least expensive of the synthetic oestrogens and causes fewer hot flushes and psychological trauma compared to the surgical option. Side effects include gynecomastia, loss of libido and potency, oedema, nausea and vomiting, and increased risk of thromboembolism. It is usually used in a dose of 1 mg once daily to reduce the risk of cardiovascular side effects as it is associated with increased cardiovascular mortality.

Corticosteroids

Both prednisolone and hydrocortisone are anti-inflammatory and can alter the body's immune response to various stimuli and are used in combination with other treatments.

Chemotherapy

Chemotherapy inhibits cell growth and proliferation; it has a variable response rate and is used as a last resort. In the USA, a regimen using mitoxantrone and prednisolone is approved for use in palliation of advanced PC. In the UK, it is recommended that docetaxel is used within its licensed indication to treat men with hormone refractory metastatic disease. Repeat courses of treatment are not recommended if the disease reoccurs when the planned course is complete.

Chemoprevention

Chemoprevention is defined as the administration of micronutrients, dietary products or drugs to prevent or delay the progression of PC.

Diet

There has been interest in a variety of products and numerous studies have been conducted. Currently in favour are soya-containing foods, green tea, pomegranates and omega-3 fatty acids. Selenium and vitamin E are no longer considered favourable. Similarly, vitamin D and lycopene found in tomatoes are also out of favour due to the lack of positive outcomes.

Drugs

5α-Reductase inhibitors which are currently used in BPH to reduce prostate size due to their inhibitory effect on the production of DHT are thought to have potential for chemoprevention.

Studies with dutasteride have shown it can reduce the risk of PC and improve outcomes in BPH by reducing AUR. On the down side, it appears to increase the risk of cardiac failure and consequently is not routinely used in chemoprevention.

Patient care

Treatment is decided after discussing the various options and side effects with the individual. Urinary and sexual function related problems are common side effects of most treatments in PC and need to be discussed in detail with the patient. Emotional factors like depression may also need to be addressed as they can adversely affect the quality of life of the individual. Some of the common problems associated with PC are listed in Table 48.3. Patients can also be referred to http://www.nhs.uk/prostatecancer for facts, information and details of choices available in the diagnosis and treatment of PC. Information on how to cope with the disease and live with PC together with details of various support organisations are available from http://www.cancerhelp.org.uk, whilst http://www.prostate-link.org.uk describes various patient experiences.

Prostatitis

Epidemiology

The term prostatitis comprises a range of disorders that have been defined and classified (Table 48.4) by the International Prostatitis Collaborative Network (IPCN) into four categories (Krieger et al., 1999).

Prostatitis has been estimated to affect up to 16% of adult men. Unlike BPH and PC, which are more prevalent in older men, prostatitis affects men of all ages.

In most instances (between 90% and 95%), the aetiology of prostatitis is unknown with bacteria isolated in only 5–10% of men presenting with prostatitis.

Table 48.3 Common problems associated with prostate cancer

Problem	Solution
Loss of erectile function after prostatectomy	Phosphodiesterase 5 inhibitors such as sildenafil have shown efficacy in prevention and help improve chance of spontaneous erection. If medication fails or is contraindicated a vacuum device, intraurethral inserts or penile prosthesis may be used
Advanced disease with impending spinal cord compression	Treat with oral dexamethasone and either cyproterone or ketoconazole with external-beam radiotherapy. LHRH agonist treatment is not advisable as the tumour flare up in the initial stage can stimulate tumour growth and exacerbate the condition
Bleeding and coagulation disorder	Prostate cancer can cause disseminated intravascular coagulation as a pathological response to the disease. This is a rare condition where small blood clots are formed in the body, disrupt the normal coagulation process and cause bleeding. This can be further complicated if the patient has co-morbidities which require treatment with anti-coagulants. Prompt treatment of the cancer with hormones and in some cases replacement of blood, platelets and clotting factors may be required
Hot flushes during androgen deprivation therapy	The hypothalamus is the centre for thermoregulation. Orchiectomy and LHRH agonists inhibit some of the peptides involved in thermoregulation. This increases central adrenergic activity and inappropriate stimulation of thermoregulatory centres, causing peripheral body vasodilatation and hot flushes. Low dose cyproterone acetate (100 mg a day) has been used to suppress hot flushes

Table 48.4 International Prostatitis Collaborative Network (IPCN) classification of prostatitis

IPCN classification	Comment
I. Acute bacterial prostatitis	Acute infection of the prostate
II. Chronic bacterial prostatitis	Chronic infection of the prostate
III. Chronic prostatitis/chronic pelvic pain syndrome	No evidence of infection
A. Inflammatory	Leucocytes in prostatic secretions, post prostate massage urine, or semen
B. Non-inflammatory	No evidence of inflammation
IV. Asymptomatic inflammatory prostatitis	Lack of genitourinary symptoms

Pathophysiology

Acute bacterial prostatitis (ABP) is caused by bacterial infection. The most common isolated uropathogen is *Escherichia coli*. Other causative agents include *Proteus* spp., *Klebsiella* spp., *Pseudomonas* spp. and, less commonly, enterococci, *Bacteroides and Staphylococcus* spp. Chronic bacterial prostatitis (CBP) usually involves recurrent bacterial urinary infections caused by the same organism involved in acute bacterial prostatitis. Both syndromes are of infective origin and represent the minority of cases of prostatitis.

In contrast, the aetiology of chronic prostatitis/chronic pelvic pain syndrome is poorly understood. Several possible mechanisms have been proposed including autoimmune disorders, infection, neurogenic inflammation and voiding dysfunction.

Symptoms

In prostatitis, the clinical presentation and symptoms are a strong diagnostic determinant. A validated, nine-point questionnaire, the Chronic Prostatitis Symptom Index (CPSI) quantifies the severity, frequency and location of pain and discomfort. It is also used to assess urinary symptoms and to establish the impact of symptoms on the patient's quality of life.

Patients with acute bacterial prostatitis usually present with symptoms of a UTI which may include dysuria, urinary frequency or urgency, whilst some may present with pain of penile, lower back or perineal origin. Signs and symptoms of systemic infection can be present in some cases and include pyrexia, rigors, malaise and myalgia. Acute bacterial prostatitis can sometimes precipitate AUR due to prostatic inflammation.

In chronic bacterial prostatitis, symptoms of UTI and pain can also be present. Typically, men with chronic bacterial prostatitis remain asymptomatic between infective episodes.

The main feature in chronic prostatitis/chronic pelvic pain syndrome is urological pain (perineum, lower abdomen and back, rectum, penis and testicles). These symptoms are usually present for at least 3 months before a diagnosis can be made. LUTSs and ejaculatory dysfunction can also affect men with chronic prostatitis/chronic pelvic pain syndrome.

Patients with asymptomatic inflammatory prostatitis have no symptoms. The condition is usually diagnosed when patients undergo investigation to assess other genitourinary complaints. For example, prostatitis may be found in biopsies taken from patients investigated for elevated PSA or when leucocytes are found in semen samples from men being investigated for infertility.

Examination and investigations

If acute bacterial prostatitis is suspected, a urine dipstick and culture are performed to reveal the presence of pathogens and leucocytes. Depending on the clinical picture, a blood culture may be indicated to diagnose concomitant bacteraemia. An ultrasound scan of the bladder can be conducted to evaluate the residual volume of urine and problems with voiding and urinary retention.

Chronic bacterial prostatitis is diagnosed in men with a history of recurrent or relapsing UTIs. A positive urine dipstick and culture is a common finding during acute episodes. Microscopy and culture of lower tract urinary secretions (urine and prostatic) between symptomatic periods can be performed and will help identify the prostate as the main focus of infection. Imaging of the urinary tract can be conducted to rule out any structural abnormalities.

Chronic prostatitis/chronic pelvic pain syndrome is a diagnosis of exclusion. Typical disorders which must be excluded include the presence of active urethritis, urogenital cancer, urinary tract disease, functionally significant urethral stricture or neurological disease affecting the bladder (Krieger et al., 1999). The main component of this syndrome is the presence of genitourinary pain. After taking a detailed medical history, the evaluation of symptoms can be done using the Chronic Prostatitis Symptom Index. Other investigations include a DRE, urinalysis, urine culture and cytology, screening for sexually transmitted diseases, urodynamic studies, prostatic TRUS and serum PSA.

Treatment

Acute bacterial prostatitis can present as a serious infection and therapy normally includes empirical treatment with parenteral antibiotics. Commonly used agents include broad-spectrum penicillins, fluoroquinolones or third-generation cephalosporins usually in combination with aminoglycosides. Urine culture and sensitivities will inform the choice of future antibiotic treatment, which is recommended to be continued for 2–4 weeks. General supportive measures such as maintenance of appropriate hydration and pain relief are important. Suprapubic cathetcrisation may be required if AUR is present.

The treatment of chronic bacterial prostatitis involves long courses (at least 4 weeks) of antibiotics. Fluoroquinolones are used as first-choice agents because of good prostatic penetration, their spectrum of anti-bacterial activity and favourable safety profile. If infective episodes are frequent, patients can be offered prophylactic antibiotics for several months with periodic follow-up to monitor progress (McNaughton-Collins et al., 2007).

Since the aetiology of most cases of chronic prostatitis/chronic pelvic pain syndrome is unknown, management often involves empirical treatment. Despite not being considered to have an infective nature, up to 50% of patients with chronic prostatitis/chronic pelvic pain syndrome respond to long courses of fluoroquinolones (Nickel et al., 2001), especially men with symptoms of relatively recent onset (a few weeks). Patients with longstanding symptoms refractory to treatment are less likely to benefit from fluoroquinolones. α-Adrenoceptor antagonists are also used alone or in combination with antibiotics in the management of chronic prostatitis/chronic pelvic pain syndrome. The evidence for efficacy is conflicting but remains an option for patients with persistent symptoms. There are also limited data describing the use of other therapies in chronic prostatitis/chronic pelvic pain syndrome such as fluoxetine, pollen extract, quercertin, finasteride, mepartricin and pelvic electromagnetic therapy.

No treatment is necessary for patients with asymptomatic inflammatory prostatitis since the condition is characterised by the lack of symptoms.

Patient care

Patients need to be made aware that prostatitis is common and affects between 1 and 2 out of every 10 men. The cause is generally poorly understood and it is difficult to diagnose. In chronic cases of prostatitis, symptoms may persist for long periods, although the severity can vary over time. Treatment may involve several therapies. Patients treated with antibiotics must be informed of the importance of completing the prolonged courses necessary to eradicate infection.

The British Prostatitis Support Association has a website (http://www.bps-assoc.org.uk) that offers patients information and support.

Case studies

Case 48.1

A 64-year-old man presents with complaints of poor urinary flow and having to visit the toilet at least twice during the night to pass urine. There is no family history of prostate disease and he is taking no medication.

Question

What investigations are appropriate and how should this patient be managed?

Answer

This patient should be asked to present a frequency volume chart of voided urine and undergo a full clinical examination, including measurement of PSA. The PVR volume of urine within the bladder should be measured after micturition.

If the PSA is within the normal range and the residual volume is less than 100 mL, the patient can be reassured about his condition and a 'watch and wait' policy adopted. If the patient finds this unacceptable, then he should be offered treatment with an α-adrenoceptor antagonist. If he is not hypertensive, a uroselective drug such as tamsulosin can be considered. This should have few systemic side effects and requires no initial titration of dose. If he is hypertensive, a less specific α-blocker may be more appropriate which will serve the dual purpose of an anti-hypertensive agent as well as treating his urinary symptoms. Careful dose titration may be necessary initially to counter any potential postural hypotension. The combination of an α-adrenoceptor antagonist and 5α-reductase inhibitor may be considered the treatment of choice for this patient.

Case 48.2

A 50-year-old man requests treatment from his primary care doctor for a 'bladder infection'. On questioning, he describes symptoms of urinary frequency, urgency and urge incontinence, but fever is absent.

Question

How should this patient be treated?

Answer

The lay person may interpret the symptoms of frequency and urgency as representing a UTI, but in the absence of dysuria this is unlikely. The patient should be referred for a full clinical assessment which should include urodynamic studies, filling and voiding cystometry, an ultrasound scan of the upper urinary tract, measurement of PSA and assessment of renal function. It is likely the patient has an outflow obstruction which has given rise to secondary instability of the detrusor muscle in the bladder, causing involuntary contractions of the bladder and resulting in incontinence. The obstruction may be due either to prostate enlargement or a dysfunctional bladder neck. In either case, treatment with an α-adrenoceptor antagonist is appropriate to reduce the outflow resistance. Should the flow be adequate but symptoms of incontinence persist, then concurrent treatment with an anti-muscarinic drug such as oxybutynin or tolterodine may be necessary to inhibit the cholinergic-mediated contractions of the detrusor.

There is emerging evidence that phosphodiesterase-5 inhibitors may also be useful in the management of LUTSs. It is known there is an abundance of the phosphodiesterase-5 isoenzyme in the prostate, and it is thought this is involved in the regulation of smooth muscle tone. A number of small-scale studies have shown the benefit of agents such as sildenafil and tadalafil, although both are currently licensed only for the treatment of erectile dysfunction. It may be appropriate to prescribe one of these agents for the patient in question.

Case 48.3

A 75-year-old male presents with AUR and a history of nocturia for the past 2–3 months. His medical history includes a heart valve replacement. He denies any haematuria or dysuria and has good flow while passing urine. On DRE, the prostate is found to be hard and nodular on one side and the PSA was 662 ng/mL

Questions

1. What investigations are recommended and how should this patient be managed?
2. What treatment choice is available for this patient?
3. What are the most likely future complications expected in this patient?

Answers

1. Since AUR is painful and can cause renal damage, he needs to be catheterised to relieve his bladder. A hard and nodular prostate on DRE together with elevated PSA suggests PC. The patient needs to have a range of baseline investigations including a TRUS biopsy, MRI of the pelvis and isotope bone scan. Although the DRE is suggestive of PC, the TRUS biopsy helps to grade the cancer using the Gleason scale and helps in making the decision about treatment. The bone scan helps identify bone metastasis which along with the results from MRI is used to stage the cancer based on the TNM score.

   The MRI pelvis revealed an enlarged and irregular prostate with intra-vesicle extension of the medial lobe into the bladder neck. The patient was confirmed to have adenocarcinoma of the prostate with a Gleason score of 8 and with bone metastasis.

2. Surgical castration can bring down the testosterone levels immediately and is relatively inexpensive but may have a psychological impact on the patient in addition to impotence and hot flushes. Medical castration with LHRH analogues would be effective treatment as well. LHRH agonists can be used to treat systemically as it produces response in more than 70% men, but the concern with this group of drugs is the flare up of the disease due to the initial surge in testosterone levels in addition to the other side effects of decreased libido, hot flush and impotence. Flare can precipitate life-threatening symptoms of the disease if the cancer is close to the spinal cord where it may cause spinal cord compression and paralysis. If lymph nodes near the ureter are involved the flare can increase the node size and compress the ureter causing renal impairment. It can also increase bone disease causing severe bone pain. Although initiation of anti-androgens can reduce symptoms of hot flushes associated with flare up to some extent, the preferred option for patients with increased risk of spinal cord compression would be LHRH antagonist as it can reduce testosterone levels much more quickly with no flare up.

   Hormonal treatment was commenced with an LHRH agonist injection together with a 1-month course of cyproterone acetate to protect against tumour flare. His PSA fell from 662 to 130 ng/mL in 5 months and continued to fall to 3.2 ng/mL after 9 months indicating a good response to hormonal treatment. Although the patient wanted to be catheter free, he failed several trials without a catheter and was offered radical radiotherapy and TURP to control local obstructive symptoms.

3. As the disease progresses, the patient can develop hormone resistance and non-hormonal treatment such as chemotherapy with docetaxel and ketoconazole may need to be considered. Osteoporosis is an important potential complication of long-term androgen deprivation therapy and metastatic bone disease and consequently the patient may experience severe bone pain. Palliative radiotherapy to metastatic bone areas and NSAIDs are recommended to control the symptoms initially, but if pain persists use of bisphosphonates may be necessary as they are known to inhibit osteoclast activity and relieve bone pain.

Case 48.4

A 35-year-old man presents with a 3-month history of dysuria, frequency and hesitancy. He also complains of pain in the perineum and discomfort while ejaculating. A DRE reveals the size and shape of his prostate seems to be normal although it is tender on examination.

Question

What are the various conditions that need to be considered and what medication will help confirm the diagnosis?

Answer

A urine dipstick and culture is recommended to rule out UTI. PSA can be measured but is raised in BPH, PC and prostatitis and hence is not a definitive test. The symptoms and physical examination are suggestive of chronic prostatitis. A swab should be taken to rule out chlamydia and other sexually transmitted diseases. Prostatitis needs to be confirmed after ruling out other possibilities like epididymitis, epididymo-orchitis, urethral stricture, renal calculus, PC, bladder and colorectal cancer.

The available evidence suggests a cure or an improvement in symptoms will occur if a quinolone antibiotic is prescribed for 4 weeks. NSAIDs and paracetamol can be used to relieve any associated pain whilst faecal softeners may be required to reduce discomfort and pain when opening bowels.

Case 48.5

A 43-year-old male seeks advice from a community pharmacist regarding his difficulty, over the past 3–4 months, when attempting to start urinating and then urinating for a long time. On questioning, he does not have any other significant medical history and he has no symptoms of a UTI, pain or haematuria.

Questions

1. Is it appropriate to sell over-the-counter tamsulosin to this patient?
2. Does the pharmacist need to maintain a record of the sale?

Answers

1. LUTSs, like hesitancy and weak stream, indicate BPH which is prevalent in one in four men above the age of 40 years. Since it is a very sensitive topic for most males, the patient needs to be consulted in a private area to assess the severity of his symptoms by using the IPSS. This is a sum of seven urinary symptoms which include incomplete emptying, frequency, intermittency, urgency, weak stream, straining and nocturia. If these symptoms severely affect the quality of life and there are no contraindications, a supply of tamsulosin 400 µcg to be taken once daily for 2 weeks initially and then for a further 4 weeks can be made while simultaneously referring the patient to his primary care doctor to confirm diagnosis and to assess his suitability for long-term treatment. If the symptoms do not improve within 14 days or the symptoms worsen, the patient should be asked to discontinue treatment and seek medical advice.

2. Record keeping is necessary to confirm that the doctor has assessed the patient within 6 weeks of initiating treatment and thereby permit further supply. It is important that the patient's consent is obtained to keep this record.

Acknowledgement

Maria Martinez contributed to the sections on benign prostatic hyperplasia and prostatitis whilst Mini Satheesh contributed to the sections on benign prostatic hyperplasia, prostate cancer and the case studies.

References

Albertsen, P.C., Hanley, J.A., Fine, J., 2005. 20-year outcomes following conservative management of clinically localized prostate cancer. J. Am. Med. Assoc. 293, 2095–2101.

Chaim, M., Hatch, W.V., Fischer, H.D., et al., 2009. Association between tamsulosin and serious ophthalmic adverse events in older men following cataract surgery. J. Am. Med. Assoc. 301, 1991–1996.

Epstein, J.I., Allsbrook Jr., W.C., Amin, M.B., ISUP Grading Committee, et al., 2005. The 2005 International Society of Urologic Pathology (ISUP) consensus conference on Gleason grading of prostatic carcinoma. Am. J. Surg. Pathol. 29, 1228–1242.

Gleason, D.F., Mellinger, G.T., 1974. Prediction of prognosis for prostatic adenocarcinoma by combined histological grading and clinical staging. J. Urol. 111, 58–64.

Gronberg, H., 2003. Prostate cancer epidemiology. Lancet 361, 859–864.

Heidenreich, A., Bolla, M., Joniau, S., et al., 2009. Guidelines on prostate cancer. European Association of Urology. Available at http://www.uroweb.org.

Inverson, P., 2002. Antiandrogen monotherapy indications and results. Urology 60 (3 Suppl. 1), 64–71.

Kirby, R.S., Andersen, M., Gratzke, P., et al., 2001. A combined analysis of double blind trials of the efficacy and tolerability of doxazosin-gastro-intestinal therapeutic system, doxazosin standard and placebo in patients with benign prostatic hyperplasia. Br. J. Urol. Int. 87, 192–200.

Krieger, J.N., Nyberg, L., Nickel, J.C., 1999. NIH consensus definition and classification of prostatitis. J. Am. Med. Assoc. 282, 236–237.

Lam, J.S., Romas, N.A., Lowe, F.C., 2003. Long-term treatment with finasteride in men with symptomatic benign prostatic hyperplasia: 10-year follow-up. Urology 61, 354–358.

MacDonald, R., Wilt, T., 2005. Alfuzosin for treatment of lower urinary tract symptoms compatible with benign prostatic hyperplasia: a systematic review of efficacy and adverse effects. Urology 66, 780–788.

McConnell, J.D., Roehrborn, C.G., Bautista, A.M., et al., 2003. The long-term effect of doxazosin, finasteride, and combination therapy on the clinical progression of benign prostatic hyperplasia. N. Engl. J. Med. 349, 2387–2398.

McNaughton-Collins, M., Joyce, G.F., Wise, M., et al., 2007. Prostatitis. In: Litwin, M.S., Saigal, C.S. (Eds.), Urologic Diseases in America. US Department of Health and Human Services, Public Health Service, National Institutes of Health, National Institute of Diabetes and Digestive and Kidney Diseases, US Government Printing Office, Washington, DC. No. 07–5512, pp. 9–41. Available at http://kidney. niddk.nih.gov/statistics/uda/Prostatitis-Chapter01.pdf.

Nickel, J.C., Downey, J., Clark, J., et al, 2001. Predictors of patient response to antibiotic therapy for the chronic prostatitis/chronic pelvic pain syndrome: a prospective multicenter clinical trial. J. Urol. 165, 1539–1544.

O'Leary, M., 2001. Tamsulosin: current clinical experience. Urology 58, 42–48.

Quinn, M., and Babb, P., 2002. International patterns and trends in prostate cancer incidence, survival, prevalence and mortality. Part 1: International comparisons. Br. J. Urol. Int. 90, 162–173.

Roehrborn, C.G. for the ALTESS Study Group, 2006. Alfuzosin 10 mg once daily prevents overall clinical progression of benign prostatic hyperplasia but not acute urinary retention: results of a 2-year placebo-controlled study. Br. J. Urol. Int. 97, 734–741.

Roehrborn, C.G., Bruskewitz, R., Nickel, G.C., et al, 2000. Urinary retention in patients with BPH treated with finasteride or placebo over four years. Eur. Urol. 37, 528–536.

Roehrborn, C.G., Boyle, P.J., Nickel, G.C., et al., on behalf of the ARIA3001, ARIA3002 and ARIA3003 study investigators, 2002. Efficacy and safety of a dual inhibitor or 5-alpha-reductase types 1 and 2 (dutasteride) in men with benign prostatic hyperplasia. Urology 60, 434–441.

Roehrborn, C.G., Siami, P., Barkin, J., et al, 2010. The effects of combination therapy with dutasteride and tamsulosin on clinical outcomes in men with symptomatic benign prostatic hyperplasia: 4-year results from the CombAT study. Eur. Urol. 57, 123–131.

Saad, F., Schulman, C.C., 2004. Role of bisphosphonates in prostate cancer. Eur. Urol. 45, 1–122.

Speakman, M.J., Kirby, R.S., Joyce, A., et al., 2004. Guidelines for the primary care management of male lower urinary tract symptoms. Br. J. Urol. Int. 93, 985–990.

Stoevelaar, H.J., McDonnell, J., 2001. Changing therapeutic regimens in benign prostatic hyperplasia. Pharmacoeconomics 19, 131–153.

Van Dijk, M.M., de la Rosette, J., Michel, M.C., 2006. Effects of α_1-adrenoceptor antagonists on male sexual function. Drugs 66, 287–301.

Further reading

Batista-Miranda, J.E., de la Cruz Diez, M., Bertran, P.A., et al., 2001. Quality of life assessment in patients with benign prostatic hyperplasia. Pharmacoeconomics 19, 1079–1090.

Disantostefano, R.L., Biddle, A.K., Lavelle, J.P., 2006. An evaluation of the economic costs and patient-related consequences of treatments for benign prostatic hyperplasia. Br. J. Urol. Int. 97, 1007–1016.

Kirby, R., Taylor, C. (Eds.), 2005. Your Guide to Prostate Cancer. Hodder Arnold, London.

Luzzi, G., Street, E., Wilson, J., 2008. Clinical Effectiveness Group. United Kingdom National Guideline for the Management of Prostatitis. British Association of Sexual Health and HIV. Available at http://www.bashh.org/documents/1844.

McVary, K.T., 2004. Management of Benign Prostatic Hypertrophy. Humana Press, New Jersey.

Nicholson, T.A., Kirby, M., Miles, A. (Eds.), 2000. The Effective Management of Benign Prostatic Disease and Lower Urinary Tract Symptoms. Aesculapius Medical Press, London.

Sandhu, J.S., Vaughan, E.D., 2005. Combination therapy for the pharmacological management of benign prostatic hyperplasia. Drugs Aging 22, 901–912.

Anaemia 49

C. Acomb and R. Sanderson

Key points

- Anaemia is a common condition which is caused by a number of pathologies and can be subdivided into microcytic, megaloblastic and haemolytic types.
- Iron deficiency is the commonest form of microcytic anaemia worldwide. Once the primary cause has been corrected, ferrous salts are the standard treatment.
- Folate deficiency results in a macrocytic anaemia and is treated with replacement therapy.
- Lack of intrinsic factor prevents absorption of vitamin B_{12} leading to a macrocytic anaemia. Treatment with parenteral B_{12} reverses the blood picture but does not always alleviate the accompanying neuropathy.
- Haemolytic anaemias include the generic disorders of sickle cell anaemia, thalassaemia and glucose-6-phosphate dehydrogenase deficiency. In these diseases, abnormal forms of haemoglobin lead to haemolysis.
- Sideroblastic anaemia is a rare anaemia caused by impaired haem synthesis where the body has adequate iron stores but is unable to incorporate them into haemoglobin.

Anaemia is not one disease, but a condition that results from a number of different pathologies. It can be defined as a reduction from normal of the quantity of haemoglobin in the blood. The World Health Organisation defines anaemia in adults as haemoglobin levels less than 13 g/dL for males and less than 12 g/dL for females. However, there are apparently normal individuals with levels less than this. The low haemoglobin level results in a corresponding decrease in the oxygen-carrying capacity of the blood.

Epidemiology

Anaemia is possibly one of the most common conditions in the world and results in significant morbidity and mortality, particularly in the developing world. Worldwide, over 50% of pregnant women and over 40% of infants are anaemic. In the UK, 14% of women aged 55–64 and 3% of men aged 35–64 have been found to be anaemic.

Aetiology

The low haemoglobin level that defines anaemia results from two different mechanisms:

- Increased haemoglobin loss due to either:
  - haemorrhage (red cell loss) or
  - haemolysis (red cell destruction).
- Reduced haemoglobin synthesis due to either:
  - lack of nutrient or
  - bone marrow failure.

Reduced haemoglobin synthesis leads to either reduced proliferation of precursors or defective maturation of precursors or both (see Table 49.1). It is not unusual to find more than one cause in a single patient.

This chapter will cover some of the more common anaemias that involve drug therapy:

Microcytic anaemias	iron deficiency anaemia
	anaemia of chronic disease
	sideroblastic anaemia
Megaloblastic anaemias	folate deficiency
	vitamin B_{12} deficiency
Haemolytic anaemias	autoimmune haemolytic anaemia
	sickle cell disease
	thalassaemia
	glucose-6-phosphate dehydrogenase deficiency

Table 49.1 Examples of conditions that cause reduced haemoglobin synthesis

Reduced proliferation of precursors	Defective maturation of precursors
Iron deficiency	Vitamin B_{12} deficiency
Anaemia of chronic disease	Folate deficiency
Anaemia of renal failure	Iron deficiency
Aplastic anaemia (primary)	Disorders of
Aplastic anaemia (secondary to drugs, etc.)	– globin synthesis (thalassaemias)
Infiltration of the bone marrow:	– iron metabolism (e.g. sideroblastic)
– leukaemia or lymphoma	Myelodysplastic syndrome
– myelofibrosis	
– metastases	

Normal erythropoiesis

It is thought that white cells, red cells and platelets are all derived from a common cell known as the pluripotent stem cell found in the bone marrow. As these cells mature, they become committed to a specific cell line (Fig. 49.1). The red cells mature through the various stages, during which time they synthesise haemoglobin, DNA and RNA. Reticulocytes are found in the peripheral circulation for 24 h before maturing into erythrocytes. Reticulocytes are released into the peripheral circulation prematurely during times of increased erythropoiesis.

Erythropoietin is a hormone produced by the cells of the renal cortex. The kidney responds to hypoxia and anaemia by increasing the production of erythropoietin. The red cell progenitors BFU-E and CFU-E have receptors on their surface. When erythropoietin binds to these receptors, it promotes differentiation and division, and consequently increased erythropoiesis. Patients with end-stage renal disease fail to produce appropriate amounts of erthropoietin and so develop anaemia. Erythropoietin production is also impaired in other conditions such as rheumatoid arthritis, cancer and sickle cell disease, though the impairment is not as great as in renal disease. Also of interest is the fact that theophylline decreases erythropoietin production, though the clinical relevance of this is uncertain.

Each day approximately 2×10^{11} erythrocytes enter the circulation. Normal erythrocytes survive in the peripheral circulation for about 120 days. Abnormal erythrocytes have a shortened lifespan. At the end of their life, the red cells are destroyed by the cells of the reticuloendothelial system found in the spleen and bone marrow. Iron is removed from the haem component of haemoglobin and transported back to the bone marrow for reuse. The pyrole ring from globin is excreted as conjugated bilirubin by the liver, and the polypeptide portion enters the body's protein pool.

Clinical manifestations

In its mildest form anaemia results in tiredness and lethargy; at its most severe it results in death unless treated. There is some suggestion that even mild anaemia may inhibit physical exercise and result in reduced mental performance. The reduced oxygen-carrying capacity of the blood leads to reduced tissue oxygenation and widespread organ dysfunction (Box 49.1).

A rapid blood loss, for example, haemorrhage, produces shock, with collapse, dyspnoea and tachycardia. Anaemia that develops over a period of time allows the body to partially compensate. As the anaemia becomes worse, more and more signs and symptoms may develop.

Even though in anaemia the amount of haemoglobin is reduced, all the blood that passes through the lungs is fully oxygenated. Increasing the respiratory rate or increasing the FiO_2 (fraction of inspired oxygen) will not improve tissue oxygenation. When the haemoglobin falls below 7 or 8 g/dL, there is almost always a compensatory increase in cardiac output.

Investigations

It is essential to find the cause of the anaemia; there is no place for 'blind' treatment. In most patients, the anaemia is a consequence of a reduced concentration of haemoglobin in each red cell and/or a reduced number of red cells in the peripheral circulation. Blood volumes may be increased in pregnancy and heart failure and haemoglobin concentration appear falsely low. Splenomegaly and signs of heart failure are sure signs of an increased blood volume. A blood transfusion in such a patient would precipitate left ventricular failure.

The most important parameter to assess anaemia is the haemoglobin concentration of the blood. It is also usual to count the number of red cells. In addition the size, shape and colour all contribute to the investigation (Box 49.2). The mean corpuscular volume (MCV) is a useful parameter that helps determine the type of the anaemia. However, care must be

---

Box 49.1 Non-specific signs and symptoms associated with anaemia

Tiredness
Pallor
Fainting
Exertional dyspnoea
Tachycardia
Palpitations
Worsening angina
Worsening cardiac failure
Exacerbation of intermittent claudication

Box 49.2 Anaemia classified by size and colour of red cells

Hypochromic–microcytic
Iron deficiency
Sideroblastic
Anaemia of chronic disease

Normochromic macrocytic
Folate deficiency
Vitamin B$_{12}$ deficiency

Polychromatophilic macrocytic
Haemolysis

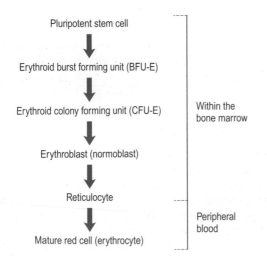

Fig. 49.1 Simplified diagram of some of the stages within erythropoiesis.

taken since the MCV indicates the average size of the cells. If there are two pathologies, where one causes large cells and other causes small cells, the MCV may appear normal or be misleading. Following on from this baseline other investigations may be required. Bone marrow examination by either aspiration or trephine may be needed to make a diagnosis.

Iron deficiency anaemia

Epidemiology

Iron deficiency anaemia is the commonest form of anaemia worldwide and may be present in up to 20% of the world's population. A diet deficient in iron, parasitic infestations, for example, hookworm (causing blood loss), and multiple pregnancies contribute to its high prevalence in underdeveloped countries. Even in Western societies, it has been reported that as many as 20% of menstruating females show a rise in haemoglobin levels on iron therapy.

Aetiology

In Western societies, the commonest cause of iron deficiency is due to blood loss. In women of childbearing age, this is most commonly due to menstrual loss. Amongst adult males, the most likely cause is gastro-intestinal bleeding. Other causes of blood loss associated with iron deficiency anaemia include haemorrhoids, nosebleeds or postpartum haemorrhage. A loss of 100 mL of blood represents the amount of iron normally absorbed from a Western diet over 40 days. The major causes of iron deficiency are listed in Box 49.3.

Pathophysiology

The elimination of iron is not controlled physiologically, so the homeostasis is maintained by controlling iron absorption. Iron is absorbed mainly from the duodenum and jejunum. Absorption itself is inefficient; iron bound to haem (found in red meat) is better absorbed than iron found in green vegetables. The presence of phosphates and phytates in some vegetables leads to the formation of unabsorbable iron complexes, whilst ascorbic acid increases the absorption of iron. In a healthy adult, approximately 10% of the dietary iron intake will be absorbed. Iron is transported around the body bound to a serum protein called transferrin. Normally, this protein is only one-third saturated with iron.

Anaemia may result from a mismatch between the body's iron requirements and iron absorption. The demand for iron varies with age (Table 49.2). Diets deficient in animal protein or ascorbic acid may not provide sufficient available iron to meet

Table 49.2 Typical daily requirements of iron

Infant (0–4 months)	0.5 mg
Adolescent male	1.8 mg
Adolescent female	2.4 mg
Adult male	0.9 mg
Menstruating female	2.0 mg
In pregnancy	3–5 mg
Postmenopausal female	0.9 mg

the demand. Poor nutrition in children in inner cities in the UK frequently leads to anaemia. Milk fortified with iron given to inner city infants up to the age of 18 months has been shown to increase haemoglobin levels and improve developmental performance compared to unmodified cow's milk (Williams et al., 1999). A systematic review showed that iron supplementation in children over seven improved intelligence tests scores in those who were initially anaemic (Sachdev et al., 2005). However, universal iron supplementation may not be appropriate because there is a theoretic increased risk of susceptibility to infectious diseases, although this has only been demonstrated for diarrhoea (Gera and Sachdev, 2002) and malaria in endemic areas (Prentice et al., 2007). Targeting supplementation only to children with anaemia and withholding iron supplementation during malaria treatment is sensible as iron may inhibit treatment, and absorption of oral iron is blocked by the inflammatory response.

Malabsorption of iron has been reported in patients with coeliac disease and in 50% of patients following partial gastrectomy. Tetracyclines, penicillamine and fluoroquinolines bind iron in the gastro-intestinal tract and reduce the absorption of iron from supplements. They probably do not affect the absorption of dietary iron.

During pregnancy, there is an increase in red cell mass but there is also a proportionally bigger increase in plasma volume, which results in a physiological dilutional anaemia. It is thought that the gut increases its ability to absorb iron during pregnancy to meet the additional demands of fetal red cell production. Some of the increased demand is met by the stopping of menstruation. If, however, there is inadequate iron absorption, then anaemia may result.

Clinical manifestations

In addition to the general symptoms of anaemia, various other features may be present (Box 49.4). The colour of the skin is very subjective and often unreliable. Patients at risk of heart failure may present with breathlessness when anaemic. Koilonychia, dysphagia and pica are found only after chronic iron deficiency and are relatively rare.

A full blood count is an essential screening test. The cells of the peripheral blood are microcytic and hypochromic with poikilocytes (often pencil shaped) and occasional target cells

---

Box 49.3 Major causes of iron deficiency anaemia

Inadequate iron absorption
  Dietary deficiency
  Malabsorption
Increased physiological demand
Loss through bleeding

Box 49.4   Features of iron deficiency anaemia

Pale skin and mucous membranes
Painless glossitis
Angular stomatitis
Koilonychia (spoon shaped nails)
Dysphagia (due to pharyngeal web)
Pica (unusual cravings)
Atrophic gastritis

(abnormal thin erythrocytes which when stained show a dark centre and peripheral ring).

The main parameter used to help establish the iron status of the patient is the serum ferritin. The serum ferritin level is low in iron deficiency anaemia and markedly raised in iron overload. It is a good measure of the iron stores in the body. Care needs to be used in interpreting raised ferritin levels as these are sometimes found in cancer, inflammatory conditions and liver disease. Serum iron is a less useful parameter and exhibits diurnal variation, being higher in the morning.

Investigations

The aim of treatment is to correct the anaemia and replenish iron stores. Although the treatment of iron deficiency anaemia is relatively simple, it should not be embarked upon lightly. It is important to resolve the underlying cause as far as possible. Since gastro-intestinal blood loss is the most common cause in men and postmenopausal women, examination of the upper and lower tract is an important investigation. If necessary, this may need to include upper gastro-intestinal tract endoscopy, colonoscopy, barium enema and small bowel biopsy.

Over-the-counter sales of iron should be discouraged except in those patients who have been fully investigated. It is not unknown for patients to be given iron unnecessarily, resulting in iron overload. Also, giving iron therapy to a patient who is continuing to bleed from their gastro-intestinal tract will not help resolve the underlying problem.

Treatment

Prophylaxis of iron deficiency anaemia was widely used in pregnancy (together with folic acid); however, it is now only used for women who have additional risk factors for iron deficiency, for example poor diet. Prophylaxis may also be used in menorrhagia, after partial gastrectomy and in some low birth weight infants, for example, premature twins.

If gastro-intestinal investigation has been performed and any underlying cause treated, all patients should receive iron supplementation to correct their anaemia and replenish stores. Oral iron in the ferrous form is cheap, safe and effective in most patients. Depending on the state of the body's iron stores, it may be necessary to continue treatment for up to 6 months to both correct the anaemia and replenish body stores. The standard treatment is ferrous sulphate 200 mg two to three times a day. It typically takes between 1 and 2 weeks for the haemoglobin level to rise 1 g/dL. An earlier indication

of the patient's response can be seen by looking at the reticulocyte count, which should start to rise 2–3 days after starting effective treatment. Nausea or abdominal pains trouble some patients and this tends to be related to the dose of elemental iron. Giving the iron with food makes it better tolerated but tends to reduce the amount absorbed. Alternative salts of iron are sometimes tried; these tend to have fewer side effects simply because they contain less elemental iron (Table 49.3). Taking fewer ferrous sulphate tablets each day would have the same effect. A change in bowel habit (either constipation or diarrhoea) is sometimes reported, and this is probably not dose related. During the early stages of treatment, the body absorbs oral doses of iron better. Absorption is commonly around 15% of intake for the first 2–3 weeks but falls off to an average of 5% thereafter. It has been shown that for some patients eradication of *Helicobacter pylori* aids recovery from iron deficiency anaemia (Annibale et al., 1999).

There are a number of modified-release oral preparations available. They have no clear therapeutic advantage over ferrous sulphate and are not recommended. Indeed, the modified-release characteristic may cause the oral iron to be carried into the lower gut, which is much poorer at absorbing iron than the duodenum. Modified-release preparations may be more likely to exacerbate diarrhoea in patients with inflammatory bowel disease or diverticulae.

There is a limited place for parenteral iron in iron deficiency anaemia; it should be reserved for patients who fail on oral therapy, usually because of poor adherence or intolerable gastro-intestinal side effects. For most patients when equivalent doses of oral and parenteral iron are used, there is no difference in the rate of at which the haemoglobin level rises. Patients who have lost blood acutely may require blood transfusions. The need for a rapid rise in haemoglobin is not an indication for parenteral iron. Intravenous iron has been shown to have some benefit during the perioperative management of anaemia in selected patients undergoing orthopaedic surgery, but not been observed in other types of surgery (Beris et al., 2008).

There is a risk of anaphylactoid reactions with intravenous iron but the incidence appears to be lower with the newer products than with the older preparations which have now been discontinued. Patients given the newer licensed

Table 49.3   Elemental iron content of common oral preparations

Preparation	Approximate iron content (mg)
Tablets	
Ferrous sulphate 210 mg	68
Ferrous gluconate 300 mg	35
Ferrous fumarate 322 mg	100
Ferrous fumarate 210 mg	68
Oral liquids	
Ferrous fumarate 140 mg in 5 mL	45
Ferrous sulphate 125 mg in 1 mL	25
Sodium feredetate 190 mg in 5 mL	27.5

products, iron dextran (CosmoFer®), iron sucrose (Venofer®), iron III isomaltoside (Monofer®) and ferric carboxymaltose (Ferinject®) should have a test dose, and there should be facilities for cardiopulmonary resuscitation available. The dose for all products is calculated from the body weight and iron deficit. The manufacturer's product information provides details on administration. Some products can be given as a bolus injection (small doses) or by a short intravenous infusion or by a total dose infusion method. There seems to be a higher incidence of adverse reactions with the total dose infusions. Iron dextran may also be given by deep intramuscular injection. Intravenous iron should not be given during acute bacterial infections, since it may stimulate bacterial growth. As intravenous iron significantly reduces the oral absorption of iron, there is no rationale for giving oral iron for several days after administering intravenous iron.

Patient care

It is usual practice to advise patients to take iron products with or after meals as this probably reduces the incidence of nausea. Patients should be told that their faeces may become darker and that this is nothing to worry about. This is important in patients who have had malaena since they may associate their dark stools with the bleed and worry that they are still bleeding from the gastro-intestinal tract. The length of treatment, and adherence should be discussed and an explanation given that iron stores need to be replenished and that this takes time.

Anaemia of chronic disease

Epidemiology

This is the second most common form of anaemia (after iron deficiency). It is associated with a wide variety of inflammatory diseases including arthritis, malignancies, inflammatory bowel disease, HIV and other infections. It is increasingly being referred to as 'anaemia of inflammation'. Related to anaemia of inflammation are the anaemias associated with chronic kidney disease and chronic heart failure.

Aetiology

In anaemia of inflammation, there appears to be impaired response to erythropoietin and the inflammatory cytokines lead to a reduction in the availability of circulating iron. This cytokine-mediated shift of iron from the circulation into reticuloendothelial system leads to iron restricted erythropoiesis, despite normal iron stores. In malignancies, in addition to the anaemia of inflammation, the cytotoxic treatments themselves decrease erythrocyte production through their anti-proliferative effects on the bone marrow. Certain cytotoxic agents, such as platinum-based therapies, are more likely to cause anaemia.

In chronic kidney disease and chronic heart failure, the reduced renal blood flow leads to a decreased production of erythropoietin.

Pathophysiology

During infections, inflammation and cancer, the inflammatory cytokines, in particular interleukin-6 released from macrophages, lead to an increased production of hepcidin. Hepcidin, a peptide produced by hepatocytes, plays a key role in iron availability. The hepcidin causes

- increased uptake of iron by hepatocytes;
- reduced iron absorption;
- reduced release of iron from macrophages.

The reduction of circulating iron is thought to limit this essential nutrient's availability to invading microbes and tumour cells, blocking their proliferation.

In addition, the inflammatory cytokines increase the production of white blood cells which potentially lead to fewer stem cells being available for red cell production.

Clinical manifestations

Patients have the general symptoms of anaemia in addition to their symptoms of the chronic inflammatory condition. The anaemia frequently leads to a reduced quality of life for these patients.

Investigation

Patients have a hypochromic microcytic anaemia similar to iron deficiency anaemia, but the two conditions can be differentiated by reviewing other serum factors (see Table 49.4).

Treatment

Treating the underlying chronic condition is important. Blood transfusions are rarely needed in anaemia of inflammation. Oral iron therapy is not usually indicated despite the apparent reduced iron availability since these patients have a functional iron deficiency rather than an actual iron deficiency; also, the raised hepcidin levels reduce the oral absorption of iron.

A number of patients with chronic renal failure appear to have a functional iron deficiency that responds to intravenous iron. These patients, despite receiving oral iron and erythropoietin analogues, do respond with a rise in haemoglobin when given regular intravenous iron together with an erythropoietin

Table 49.4 Differentiation between iron deficiency anaemia and anaemia of chronic disease

Test	Iron deficiency anaemia	Anaemia of chronic disease
Serum iron	Low	Low
Serum ferritin	Low	Normal or high
Serum transferrin	High	Normal or low
Total iron binding capacity	High	Low

analogue (Silverberg et al., 1996). Intravenous iron in combination with erythropoietin analogues is widely used in chronic kidney disease. The patient's serum ferritin is monitored to check for iron overload. Concerns have been expressed about the possible long-term complications of intravenous iron, for example, atherosclerosis or increased risk of infection (Cavill, 2003). There appears to be a slightly increased risk of infections, but the improvement in anaemia leads to an improved quality of life.

Patients with anaemia-associated inflammatory bowel disease or with rheumatoid arthritis respond to intravenous iron; however, the use of intravenous iron in chronic inflammatory conditions is not generally recommended because of an increased risk of infections and also possible increased risk of acute cardiovascular events. Some small studies have shown intravenous iron to be beneficial in patients with heart failure, but currently this should be reserved for patients with proven iron deficiency and failure on oral iron (Dec, 2009).

Some patients with chronic disorders respond to erythropoietin analogues, none are licensed for use in chronic disease states other than anaemia associated with chronic renal failure or cancer. Elevated endogenous erythropoietin levels in patients with heart failure are associated with adverse outcomes (Felker, 2010). Some clinical trial data show a higher mortality and increased risk of tumour progression in patients with anaemia associated with cancer who have been treated with erythropoietins. It is not recommended that erythropoietin analogues are routinely used in the management of cancer treatment-induced anaemia (NICE, 2008). However, they may be considered, in combination with intravenous iron, for:

- women receiving platinum-based chemotherapy for ovarian cancer who have symptomatic anaemia with a haemoglobin concentration of 8 g/100 mL or lower. The use of erythropoietin analogues does not preclude the use of existing approaches to the management of anaemia, including blood transfusion when necessary;
- patients who cannot be given blood transfusions and who have profound cancer treatment-related anaemia that is likely to have an impact on survival.

Tocilizumab, the interleukin-6 antagonist monoclonal antibody licensed for use in rheumatoid arthritis, has been shown to improve haemoglobin levels (Raj, 2009). It has also been suggested that drugs which downregulate interleukin-6 may have some effect (Altschuler and Kast, 2005). Olanzepine and quetiapine (potent H_1 antagonists) are known to be regulators of interleukin-6 but are not used clinically for this purpose. Furthermore, it is not known what the other effects of modifying interleukin-6 or hepcidin would have on the chronic inflammatory condition.

Patient care

Some patients hearing they have anaemia may be tempted to go and purchase iron or other supplements. Careful explanation will help them make an informed decision.

Sideroblastic anaemias

Epidemiology

Sideroblastic anaemias are a group of conditions that are diagnosed by finding ring sideroblasts in the bone marrow. There are both hereditary and acquired forms. The hereditary forms are rare, whilst some of the acquired forms are relatively common with as many as 30% of alcoholics admitted to hospital having sideroblastic anaemia.

Aetiology

In the majority of hereditary forms, there is an X chromosome-linked pattern of inheritance. Both autosomal dominant and autosomal recessive families have been described. The main defect is a reduced activity of the enzyme 5-aminolevulinate synthase (ALAS) which is involved in haem synthesis.

The acquired forms include idiopathic forms, forms associated with myeloproliferative disorders and forms secondary to the ingestion of drugs (Box 49.5). Regardless of the cause, there is impaired haem synthesis, where the body has adequate iron stores but is unable to incorporate it into haemoglobin.

Pathophysiology

An examination of the bone marrow typically shows a number of erythroblasts that have iron granules surrounding the cell nucleus. These cells are known as ring sideroblasts. In the hereditary forms, there are low levels of ALAS. This mitochondrial enzyme is involved in the first step in the synthesis of haem and requires pyridoxal phosphate as a co-factor. Pyridoxine is a precursor for pyridoxal.

Drugs and toxins

Alcohol can lead to the formation of ring sideroblasts. Ethanol is metabolised to acetaldehyde. It is the acetaldehyde that lowers the levels of ALAS and pyridoxal. Isoniazid is a known cause of sideroblasts. In slow acetylators of

---

Box 49.5 Acquired sideroblastic anaemia

Associated with other disorders
Myelodysplastic syndromes
Myeloid leukaemia
Myeloma
Collagen diseases

Associated with drugs and toxins
Alcohol
Isoniazid
Chloramphenicol
Penicillamine
Pyrazinamide
Cycloserine
Progesterone (single case report)
Copper deficiency (associated with penicillamine, triethylene tetramine and tetrathiomolybdate)

isoniazid, the drug reacts with pyridoxal and the resulting product is then rapidly excreted. Pyridoxine prophylaxis is usually given to all patients on isoniazid. Doses of chloramphenicol over 2 g a day invariably lead to sideroblasts. This is thought to be due to the inhibition of mitochondrial protein synthesis. Sideroblastic anaemia is also associated with copper deficiency which can be caused by an overdose of the chelators: penicillamine, trientine and the experimental tetrathiomolybdate. These are all used in the treatment of Wilson's disease.

Clinical manifestations

The hereditary forms typically develop in infancy or childhood. The anaemia can be severe or mild (haemoglobin typically 4–10 g/dL). There may be splenomegaly, which can lead to mild thrombocytopenia. The idiopathic acquired forms tend to develop insidiously usually in middle age or later. Many patients may be asymptomatic for long periods. In the forms associated with other disorders, the clinical picture tends to be dominated by the underlying diseases.

Investigations

The common finding in all forms is the presence of sideroblasts in the bone marrow. In the hereditary form, the red cells in the peripheral blood are hypochromic and microcytic. Despite this, there are frequently increased iron stores in the bone marrow. The serum iron and ferritin may also be high. In the acquired forms, the peripheral blood has hypochromic cells, which may be either normocytic or macrocytic.

Treatment

In patients with the hereditary forms, large doses of pyridoxine (typically 100–200 mg daily or even up to 400 mg) may reduce the severity of the anaemia. Long-term high-dose pyridoxine has been associated with peripheral neuropathy and so lower maintenance doses are sometimes tried. There have been case reports of patients responding to parenteral pyridoxal-5-phosphate after failing to respond to pyridoxine. Patients with an acquired form occasionally respond to high-dose pyridoxine, and a 2- to 3- month trial may be helpful in symptomatic patients. The response tends to be slow and only partial. Haem arginate (licensed for use in porphyria) has been shown to increase the red cell count and decrease the number of ring sideroblasts in some patients with acquired sideroblastic anaemia, in common with other conditions where an increased turnover of cells in the bone marrow and folate supplements are often necessary.

Although the peripheral blood cells are frequently hypochromic and microcytic, the condition is associated with increased iron stores; therefore, iron supplements should be avoided. The drugs and toxins (Box 49.5) tend to cause a reversible anaemia. Removing the offending agent usually resolves the anaemia.

Iron overload

Inevitably, some patients fail to respond to these treatments and frequent blood transfusions are required. This leads to the complications of iron overload and sensitisation and the risk of blood-borne virus transmission. The chelating agent desferrioxamine is given either by intravenous or by subcutaneous infusion. It binds free iron and iron bound to ferritin. Therapy should be considered when the serum ferritin level reaches 1000 μcg/L. Patients with very high ferritin levels may need daily infusions. Daily subcutaneous infusions using a disposable infusor or small infusion pump are suitable for home use. In the UK, a number of commercial healthcare companies provide a desferioxamine home care service. Published evidence suggests that for an equivalent dose, a longer infusion time results in increased iron excretion. Intravenous infusions can be given whenever the patient comes into hospital for a blood transfusion. Small doses (<200 mg) of vitamin C increase the effectiveness of desferrioxamine probably by facilitating iron release from the reticuloendothelial system. Higher doses of vitamin C are reported to increase the cardiotoxicity of iron overload. Patients with cardiac failure should not be given vitamin C with desferrioxamine. Desferrioxamine should not be given concurrently with prochlorperazine as prolonged unconsciousness may result.

There are two oral agents (desferiprone and deferasirox) licensed for iron overload. Deferiprone unfortunately causes reversible neutropenia in some patients and weekly neutrophil counts are required. It is licensed for patients intolerant of desferrioxamine. Deferasirox has been more recently introduced and comes as a dispersible tablet that needs to be taken at least 30 min before food. It is associated with a high incidence of gastro-intestinal ulcers and renal impairment. Decreased hearing and lens opacities have been reported. Auditory and ophthalmic testing is recommended before the start of treatment and at regular intervals thereafter (every 12 months).

Patient care

Few patients with hereditary or the idiopathic acquired forms have completely reversible anaemia. Patients need to be aware that treatment with pyridoxine may take several months before any signs of improvement are seen. They should be advised not to purchase over-the-counter iron or vitamin supplements, particularly ascorbic acid or pyridoxine, without discussing it with their consultant.

Megaloblastic anaemias

The megaloblastic anaemias are macrocytic anaemias (raised MCV). There is an abnormality in the maturation of haematopoietic cells in the bone marrow. In addition to abnormal red cells, the white cells and platelets may be affected. The two major causes are folate deficiency and vitamin B_{12} deficiency. Pernicious anaemia is a specific autoimmune disease that causes malabsorption of vitamin B_{12} due to a lack of intrinsic factor.

Epidemiology

Folate deficiency anaemia

Much of the world's population has a marginal dietary intake of folate. Body stores are low, and as soon as there is a decrease in dietary intake or there is increased folate demand, deficiency readily occurs.

Vitamin B$_{12}$ deficiency anaemia

Strict vegans (e.g. Hindus) commonly have low vitamin B$_{12}$ levels due to their dietary deficiency though actual anaemia is rarer. All patients who have had a total gastrectomy and up to 15% of those with a partial gastrectomy will develop vitamin B$_{12}$ deficiency anaemia.

Pernicious anaemia

Pernicious anaemia is found most commonly in people of northern European descent. In Britain, the incidence is about 120 per 100,000 being higher in Scotland than in the south of England. Pernicious anaemia is usually a disease of the elderly, the average patient presenting at 60 years of age.

Non-megaloblastic macrocytic anaemia caused by alcohol abuse, hypothyroidism or paroxysmal nocturnal haemoglobinuria will not be discussed in this chapter.

Aetiology

Folate deficiency anaemia

Folate is readily available in a normal diet. Fruit, green vegetables and yeast all contain relatively large amounts of folate. Despite this relative abundance of folate in many foods, dietary deficiency is common, either as the sole cause of the folic acid deficiency anaemia or in conjunction with increased folate utilisation.

Vitamin B$_{12}$ deficiency anaemia

Deficiency occurs from inadequate intake or malabsorption. The only dietary source of vitamin B$_{12}$ (cyanocobalamin) is from food of animal origin. It is present in meat, fish, eggs, cheese and milk. Cooking does not usually destroy vitamin B$_{12}$. Daily requirements are between 1 and 3 µcg. Deficiency arises either from inadequate intake over a prolonged period or more commonly, in the West, from impaired absorption due to lack of intrinsic factor.

Malabsorption occurs if the distal ileum is removed; it may also occur with certain intestinal pathologies, particularly stagnant loop syndrome, tropical sprue and fish tapeworm infestation. Passive absorption does take place in the jejunum, but this is very inefficient and usually accounts for less than 1% of an oral dose.

Pathophysiology

The common biochemical defect in all megaloblastic anaemias is the inhibition of DNA synthesis in maturing cells.

Folate deficiency anaemia

The folate found in food is mainly conjugated to polyglutamic acid. Enzymes found in the gut convert the polyglutamate form to monoglutamate, which is readily absorbed. During absorption, the folate is methylated and reduced to methyltetrahydrofolate monoglutamate. This travels through the plasma and is transported into cells via a carrier specific for the tetrahydrofolate form. Within the cell, the methyl group is removed (in a reaction requiring vitamin B$_{12}$) and the folate is reconverted back to a polyglutamate form (Fig. 49.2). It has been suggested that the polyglutamate form prevents the folate leaking out of cells. The folate eventually acts as a coenzyme involved in a number of reactions including DNA and RNA synthesis. Defective DNA synthesis mainly affects cells with a rapid turnover, for example, gastro-intestinal cells and red blood cells, hence the sore tongue and anaemia seen in folate deficiency. During DNA synthesis, the folate coenzyme is oxidised to the dihydrofolate form, which is inactive and has to be reactivated by the enzyme dihydrofolate reductase. This is the enzyme inhibited by methotrexate and to a lesser extent by trimethoprim and pyrimethamine. Co-trimoxazole has been shown to increase the severity of megaloblastic anaemia.

Vitamin B$_{12}$ deficiency

Absorption of vitamin B$_{12}$ is mainly by an active process. Enzymes in the stomach release vitamin B$_{12}$ from protein complexes. One molecule of vitamin B$_{12}$ then combines with one molecule of a glycoprotein called intrinsic factor. The intrinsic factor protects the vitamin B$_{12}$ from breakdown by microorganisms. There are specific receptors in the distal ileum for the intrinsic factor-vitamin B$_{12}$ complex. The vitamin B$_{12}$ enters the ileal cell and is then transported through the blood attached to transport proteins. Intrinsic factor does not appear in the blood.

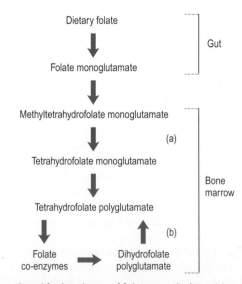

Fig. 49.2 Simplified pathway of folate metabolism: (a) vitamin B$_{12}$ is required as a coenzyme for this reaction: (b) the enzyme dihydrofolate reductase converts inactive dihydrofolate back to the active tetrahydrofolate.

Since intrinsic factor is only produced by the gastric parietal cells, a total gastrectomy always leads to vitamin B$_{12}$ deficiency. Approximately 10–15% of patients who have had a partial gastrectomy also develop deficiency. The onset of anaemia is usually delayed because the body typically has stores of 2–3 mg, which is sufficient for 2–3 years. Vitamin B$_{12}$ is a coenzyme for the removal of a methyl group from methyltetrahydrofolate. Lack of vitamin B$_{12}$ traps the folate as methyltetrahydrofolate and prevents DNA synthesis (Fig. 49.2). The exact mechanism by which vitamin B$_{12}$ deficiency causes neuropathy is not clear but may be due to a defect in the methylation reactions needed for myelin formation.

Pernicious anaemia

Pernicious anaemia is probably autoimmune in origin. Patients typically have a gastric atrophy and no (or virtually no) intrinsic factor secretion. Although not present in all patients, two different antibodies have been found in the serum of some patients with pernicious anaemia.

Clinical manifestations

In addition to the general features of anaemia, megaloblastic anaemia, of which folic acid deficiency and B$_{12}$ deficiency anaemia are the two most common examples, has certain characteristics described in Box 49.6.

Folate deficiency anaemia

Alcoholics and the elderly are particularly prone to nutritional deficiency. Elderly people living alone on tea and toast are typical examples of patients at risk. Many alcoholics develop deficiency due to their poor diet; although some beers contain small amounts of folate, spirits contain none. A number of drugs have been implicated in causing folate deficiency (Box 49.7). Actual megaloblastic anaemia from drug therapy is uncommon, and the exact mechanism(s) has not always been established. Serious malabsorption can occur in tropical sprue and coeliac disease. Reduced absorption is seen in Crohn's disease and following partial gastrectomy or jejunal resection.

There is a physiological increase in folate utilisation during pregnancy. There may be an increased utilisation in various

---

Box 49.6 Features of megaloblastic anaemia

Glossitis (sore, pale, smooth tongue)
Angular stomatitis
Altered bowel habit (diarrhoea or constipation)
Anorexia
Mild jaundice
Insidious onset
Sterility
Bilateral peripheral neuropathy (mainly vitamin B$_{12}$ deficiency)
Melanin skin pigmentation (rare)
Fever (mainly vitamin B$_{12}$ deficiency)

Box 49.7 Drugs implicated in causing folate deficiency

Malabsorption
Phenytoin
Barbiturates
Sulphasalazine
Colestyramine
Oral contraceptives

Impaired metabolism
Methotrexate
Pyrimethamine
Triamterene
Pentamidine
Trimethoprim

---

pathological conditions, in association with inflammation or in a number of chronic haemolytic anaemias, particularly thalassaemia major, sickle cell disease and autoimmune haemolytic anaemia. Chronic folate deficiency probably predisposes patient to thrombosis, depression and neoplasia (Green and Miller, 1999).

Vitamin B$_{12}$ deficiency anaemia

The megaloblastic anaemia caused by vitamin B$_{12}$ deficiency has similar features to folate deficiency (Box 49.6). In addition to the macrocytosis, anisocytosis and poikilocytosis, there is often mild thrombocytopenia. The spleen may be slightly enlarged and there may be a slight fever. Mild jaundice may be present due to the increased breakdown of haemoglobin found in the abnormal red cells. The onset is slow and insidious, so patients often present late or are diagnosed during other investigations. The feature that separates vitamin B$_{12}$ deficiency from the other megaloblastic anaemias is progressive neuropathy. It is symmetrical and affects the legs rather than the arms. Patients notice a tingling in their feet and a loss of vibration sense. Occasionally, patients have muscle weakness, difficulty in walking or experience frequent falls.

Investigations

Folic acid deficiency anaemia

Many patients are symptomless initially, and the diagnosis is made following a full blood count carried out for another reason. The peripheral blood reveals large oval red cells. Anisocytosis and poikilocytosis are common. Some of the neutrophils are hypersegmented, and thrombocytopenia may be present. The red cell folate concentration accurately reflects folate stores and is a more preferable parameter than the serum folate concentration, which is subject to changes in diet and does not correlate as closely with anaemia.

Vitamin B$_{12}$ deficiency anaemia

Following the detection of macrocytes in the full blood count, one of the first investigations will be the determination of the serum vitamin B$_{12}$ level. The serum vitamin B$_{12}$ level is low in mild anaemia and may be very low if there is marked megaloblastic anaemia or neuropathy. If there is no concurrent folate deficiency, the serum folate level tends to be raised whilst the red cell folate level falls, possibly due to a failure of folate polyglutamate synthesis in cells. False positives (low vitamin B_{12} level without true deficiency) may be seen in multiple myeloma, excessive ascorbic acid intake and pregnancy. In contrast, liver disease, lymphoma, autoimmune disease and myeloproliferative disorders may lead to a false-negative result (normal levels in the presence of true deficiency).

The detection of autoantibodies is helpful to distinguish pernicious anaemia from other forms. The presence of intrinsic factor antibodies is virtually diagnostic of pernicious anaemia being rarely found in any other condition. However, it is not a very sensitive test since only half the patients with pernicious anaemia have these antibodies. Gastric parietal cell antibodies are found in 85% of patients with pernicious anaemia (a more sensitive test) but unfortunately also found in up to 10% of people without pernicious anaemia (less specific) (see Table 49.5).

Oral vitamin B_{12} absorption can be measured using the Schilling test though this is now rarely used in practice as most vitamin B_{12} deficiencies are treated in the same way. The test measures the absorption of radiolabelled oral dose of vitamin B_{12}.

Treatment

It is necessary to establish whether the patient with megaloblastic anaemia has vitamin B_{12} deficiency or folic acid deficiency or both. Treatment of vitamin B_{12} deficiency with folic acid may lead to the resolution of the haematological abnormalities but does not correct the neuropathy, which continues to deteriorate. If it is not possible to delay until a definitive diagnosis is made, both folic acid and vitamin B_{12} may be given.

Folate deficiency anaemia

Folate deficiency is usually managed by replacement therapy. The duration of the treatment depends on the cause of the deficiency. Changes in dietary habits or removal of any precipitating factor should also be considered.

The normal daily requirement of folic acid is approximately $100\,\mu cg$ a day; despite this, the usual treatment doses given are 5–15 mg a day. Even in malabsorption states, because of these large doses, sufficient folate is usually absorbed. Therefore, parenteral folic acid treatment is not normally required. Treatment for 4 months will normally be sufficient to ensure that folate deficient red cells are replaced.

Large doses of folic acid can produce a partial haematological response in patients with vitamin B_{12} deficiency. The blood picture appears nearly normal but the neurological damage due to the vitamin B_{12} deficiency continues. Folic acid therapy should not be started until vitamin B_{12} deficiency has been excluded. It has also been suggested that patients on long-term folic acid therapy should have their vitamin B_{12} levels checked at regular intervals (e.g. yearly).

Pregnancy. The folate requirement increases in pregnancy and is higher in twin pregnancies. Folate deficiency regularly occurs in patients with a poor diet who do not take supplements. Prophylaxis with folate (350–500 μcg daily) is now frequently given in pregnancy, often in combination with iron, starting before conception and during the first 12 weeks of pregnancy. It is important that these products with low doses of folate are not used to treat megaloblastic anaemia. Although this low-dose folate should be started before conception to prevent a first occurrence of neural tube defect, higher doses (5 mg daily) are required in women with a history of neural tube defects and again continued until week 12 (DH, 1992).

Vitamin B_{12} deficiency anaemia

The majority of patients with vitamin B_{12} deficiency require lifelong replacement therapy. Occasionally, specific therapy related to the underlying disorder may be all that is necessary, for example, treatment of fish tapeworm.

Since the anaemia has developed slowly, the cardiovascular system does not tolerate blood transfusions very well and is easily overloaded. Transfusions should not normally be given. In severe cases where emergency transfusion is deemed necessary, packed cells may be given slowly whilst blood (mainly plasma) is removed from the other arm. Diuretics may also need to be given, especially if the patient has congestive heart failure and poorly tolerates fluid overload.

For most patients, a definite diagnosis is made before treatment is started. The standard treatment is hydroxocobalamin 1 mg intramuscularly three times a week for 2 weeks then 1 mg every 3 months. Where there is neurological involvement, a slightly higher dose regimen is recommended, 1 mg on alternate days, until no further improvement then 1 mg every 2 months. There is no evidence that larger doses than those recommended provide any additional benefit in neuropathy. In the UK, hydroxocobalamin is the treatment of choice. It is retained in the body longer than cyanocobalamin, and reactions to it are very rare. US texts recommend cyanocobalamin rather than hydroxocobalamin because of the fear that some patients appear to develop antibodies to the vitamin B_{12} transport protein complex in the serum. The haematological response to both is probably identical. A small amount of passive absorption of vitamin B_{12} does take place from the gastro-intestinal tract. High (1 mg) daily oral and sublingual doses of cyanocobalamin are absorbed in sufficient quantities to manage pernicious anaemia. There have been calls for this oral regimen

Table 49.5 Autoantibodies in pernicious anaemia

	Intrinsic factor antibodies	Parietal cell antibodies
Patients *with* pernicious anaemia	Detected in 50% of patients	Detected in 85% of patients
People who do not have pernicious anaemia	Rarely detected	Detected in up to 10%

to replace regular injections as used in other countries. This is potentially cheaper than injections, but this indication is currently unlicensed. It may be worth considering in patients who are unable to have injections. In the UK, cyanocobalamin tablets are not available on the NHS except to treat or prevent vitamin B_{12} deficiency in a patient who is a vegan or who has proven vitamin B_{12} deficiency of dietary origin.

Hypokalaemia develops in some patients during the initial haematological response because potassium is an intracellular ion used in the production of new cells. Potassium supplements may be needed in the elderly and patients receiving diuretics or digoxin. The serum iron level also falls as it is incorporated into haemoglobin. The more severe the anaemia, the more likely it is to see a fall in the serum potassium or iron level.

Not only is it very gratifying to follow the response to treatment, but it is also important to monitor the response to ensure that the patient returns to normal without any attendant problems. There is often a subjective improvement before an objective one. Typically, the patient feels better within 24–48 h, and yet there may be no discernible haematological response. The first haematological change in the peripheral blood is a rise in the reticulocyte count starting around day 3 or 4 and peaking after 7–8 days. The more severe the anaemia, the higher the peak reticulocyte count. The reticulocyte count should remain raised whilst the haematocrit is less than 35%. Failure to remain raised during this time indicates the need for further evaluation. The arrest or slowing down of erythropoiesis may be due to inadequate stores of other essential factors, for example, iron, or may be due to coexisting disease such as hypothyroidism or infection.

The red cells return to normal and the platelet count rises to normal (or even higher) after 7–10 days. The haemoglobin takes much longer to return to normal. It should rise by approximately 2–3 g/dL each fortnight. Neurological damage may be irreversible. Peripheral neuropathy of recent onset often partially improves, but any spinal cord damage is irreversible even with optimum therapy.

Patient care

Folic acid deficiency anaemia

In patients who have a dietary component to their deficiency, appropriate nutritional advice should go alongside their folic acid therapy. If the cause of the deficiency has been eliminated, patients can expect to receive folic acid for approximately 4–6 months. In patients with a continuing requirement, for example, haemolytic anaemia patients can expect lifelong treatment. Those commencing folic acid therapy can anticipate feeling better after a few days but should be informed that their blood count will take much longer to return to normal.

Vitamin B_{12} deficiency anaemia. Patients feel subjectively better very shortly after their first hydroxocobalamin injection. They can be told that their sore tongue will start to improve within 2 days and return to normal after 2–4 weeks. Patients need to be informed that they need regular injections, usually every 3 months. Surprisingly, some patients say that

they feel they are ready for this injection as they approach their appointment time and feel better after their injection.

Haemolytic anaemias

In the haemolytic anaemias, there is a reduced life span of the erythrocytes. Anaemia occurs when the rate of destruction of the erythrocytes exceeds their rate of production. There are a wide range of haemolytic anaemias with both genetic and acquired disorders (Table 49.6). Only autoimmune haemolytic anaemia, sickle cell anaemia, thalassaemia and glucose-6-phosphate dehydrogenase deficiency will be briefly discussed. Haemolytic anaemias account for approximately 5% of all anaemias.

General clinical manifestations

Patients with acute haemolytic anaemia commonly complain of malaise, fever, abdominal pain, dark urine and jaundice. They have haemoglobulinaemia, hyperbilirubinaemia, reticulocytosis and increased urobilinogen levels in the urine. Patients with chronic haemolytic anaemia also usually have splenomegaly. Their anaemia is usually normochromic and normocytic.

General treatment

Many patients with chronic haemolytic anaemia will have an over active bone marrow to compensate for the chronic haemolysis. This increases demand for folate and therefore folic acid supplements are often required, particularly for patients with a poor diet. Patients who require frequent transfusions are at risk of iron overload and require chelation therapy with desferioxamine, desferiprone or deferasirox (as previously discussed under sideroblastic anaemia).

Autoimmune haemolytic anaemia

Epidemiology

This is a range of conditions consisting of warm autoimmune haemolytic anaemia (WAIHA) and cold autoimmune haemolytic anaemia also known as cold agglutinin disease (CAD).

Table 49.6 Some examples of haemolytic anaemias

Genetic disorders of	Examples
Haemoglobin	Sickle cell anaemias
	Thalassaemias
Energy pathways	Glucose-6-phosphate deficiency
Membrane	Hereditary spherocytosis
	Hereditary ovalcytosis
Acquired disorders	
Immune	Autoimmune
	Rh or ABO incompatibility
Non-immune	Infections (parasitic, bacterial)
	Drugs and chemicals
	Hypersplenism

Both forms can be subdivided into idiopathic and acquired forms, and the condition is found in all races. The most common form being idiopathic WAIHA occurring in approximately 40% of all cases with an incidence of between 1 in 4000 and 1 in 80,000. Idiopathic CAD tends to present in middle age.

Aetiology

WAIHA is frequently associated with other diseases with an immunological component, for example, chronic lymphocytic leukaemia, systemic lupus erythematosus and hepatitis B. Acquired CAD is sometimes associated with viral or bacterial infections: cold agglutinins develop in more than 60% of patients following infectious mononucleosis but haemolytic anaemia is rare. A number of drugs have been implicated as leading to immune haemolysis (Box 49.8).

Pathophysiology

The anaemia results from the presence of autoantibodies which agglutinate or lyse the patient's own erythrocytes. In WAIHA, the haemolysis is usually extravascular and mediated by IgG. These antibodies react best at body temperature. CAD is usually mediated by IgM and is capable of fixing complement. The IgM antibody attaches to the erythrocytes and causes them to agglutinate at temperatures below 37°C resulting in impaired blood flow to fingers, toes, nose and ears when exposed to cold.

Clinical manifestations

The symptoms in WAIHA depend on the severity of the haemolysis. In CAD, there is a range in severity of the clinical manifestations from an inconsequential laboratory finding of a benign variety to serious manifestations, such as acute haemolytic crises and Raynaud-type phenomena. A common complaint is painful fingers and toes with purplish discolouration associated with cold exposure. In chronic CAD, the patient is more symptomatic during the colder months.

Investigations

A positive direct Coomb's test indicates the presence of antibodies to red blood cells. Further laboratory serological testing helps determine the exact nature of the reaction.

Box 49.8 Drugs associated with autoimmune haemolytic anaemia

Ciclosporin
Fludarabin
Interferon A
Levodopa
Mefenamic acid
Methyldopa
Penicillin
Quinine
Quinidine

Drug-induced haemolytic anaemia may be difficult to distinguish from other forms of autoimmune haemolytic anaemia, and a clear medication history will help. The antibodies produced may react with the red cells only in the presence of the drug (or one of its metabolites) or may also react without the drug being present.

Treatment

Treatment is dependent on the specific cause (Pruss et al., 2003). In WAIHA, the standard treatment is high-dose corticosteroids. Patients who do not respond can be managed with azathioprine or cyclophosphamide. Blood transfusions are necessary in severe cases, although providing blood free from underlying alloantibodies is difficult. Rituximab, the anti CD-20 monoclonal antibody, has been shown to be beneficial in some patients who fail to respond to the forementioned conventional anti-inflammatory therapy. However, this is an unlicensed indication. (D'Arena et al., 2007) Patients with CAD need to be kept warm with supportive measures as well as treated for any underlying disorder.

Patient care

Patients requiring rituximab will require careful explanation of its unlicensed use and the necessary pretreatment with paracetamol and chlorphenamine.

Sickle cell anaemia

Epidemiology

Sickle cell disease is a hereditary condition. Several different variants of sickle cell disease exist. It is found in a number of ethnic groups, mainly in populations that originate from tropical regions. In the UK, approximately 5000 people, largely from the Afro-Caribbean population, have sickle cell disease.

Aetiology

Patients with sickle cell disease have a different form of haemoglobin. Patients with the most common variant of sickle cell disease have haemoglobin S (Hb S). Normal haemoglobin is usually designated Hb A. Haemoglobin S has valine substituted for glutamic acid as the sixth amino acid in the β-polypeptide compared with normal haemoglobin. Patients with homozygous haemoglobin S develop many problems including anaemia.

Sickle cell trait is where a person is a carrier of the gene (heterozygous for the sickle cell gene). These people are usually asymptomatic. Sickle cell trait provides some protection from malaria and is more common in those ethnic groups originating from geographical areas that are endemic for malaria. The offspring from a father with the trait and a mother with the trait has a one in four chance of having sickle cell disease (Fig. 49.3).

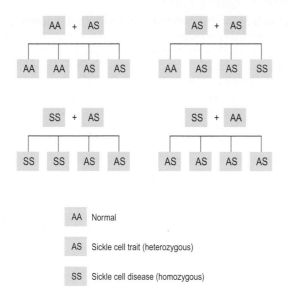

AA	Normal
SS	
AS	Sickle cell trait (heterozygous)
SS	Sickle cell disease (homozygous)

Fig. 49.3 Inheritance patterns in sickle cell trait and sickle cell disease.

Pathophysiology

The membrane of red cells containing haemoglobin S is damaged, which leads to intracellular dehydration. In addition, when the patient's blood is deoxygenated, polymerisation of haemoglobin S occurs, forming a semisolid gel. These two processes lead to the formation of crescent-shaped cells known as sickle cells. Sickle cells are less flexible than normal cells (flexibility allows normal cells to pass through the microcirculation). The inflexibility leads to impaired blood flow through the microcirculation, resulting in local tissue hypoxia. Anaemia results from an increased destruction (haemolysis) of red cells in the spleen. Some red cells in patients with sickle cell disease contain fetal haemoglobin (Hb F). These cells do not become sickle cells.

Clinical manifestations

Patients with severe variants of the disease have chronic anaemia, arthralgia, anorexia, fatigue and splenomegaly. They have crises more frequently than patients with other variants of the disease. A crisis can be precipitated by infection and fever, dehydration, hypoxia or acidosis. A combination of these factors is sometimes present. The clinical manifestation of a crisis can vary with the most common being an infarct crisis. Infarction of the long bones and larger joints or an infarction of a large organ, for example, the liver, lungs or brain, may all occur. Severe pain is a common feature, depending on the site of the infarction. Destructive bone and joint problems are frequently seen.

Investigations

The common form usually presents in the first year of life. From then on, the patients have a chronic haemolytic anaemia interspersed with crises. Abnormal haemoglobin can be detected using electrophoresis. The proportion of haemoglobin S is a useful monitoring parameter. Regular serum ferritin determinations identify the need for desferrioxamine therapy and are used to monitor progress.

Treatment

Patients with sickle cell disease have a high incidence of pneumococcal infections. A number of studies have shown the benefit of prophylactic antibiotics. Penicillin V 250 mg twice a day is usual for adults with erythromycin prescribed for patients allergic to penicillin. Administration of pneumococcal vaccine and *Haemophilus influenzae* vaccine is now common. Folic acid is commonly used because of the high turn over of red cells.

Attempts have been made to increase the proportion of haemoglobin F and reduce the proportion of haemoglobin S in the circulation. Several drugs (Box 49.9) have been shown (some only in animal models) to stimulate fetal haemoglobin production (Charache et al., 1995).

Hydroxycarbamide is effective and may reduce the frequency of crises but is limited by its cytotoxicity. Erythropoietin has been shown to increase haemoglobin F in some animal models, but this has yet to be fully demonstrated in humans. Transfusions and exchange transfusions have also been used to decrease the proportion of haemoglobin S. This is limited by the usual complications of chronic infusions: iron overload, the risk of blood-borne virus transmission and sensitisation.

Sickle cell crises require prompt and effective treatment. Removal of the trigger factor, hydration and effective pain relief are the mainstays of treatment. Appropriate antibiotic therapy should be started at the first signs of infection. Strong opioids are required for pain relief. Traditionally, many patients have been given frequent intramuscular injections of pethidine. Pethidine is not ideal since it is short acting, not very potent and repeated injections lead to the accumulation of metabolites that have been associated with seizures. Morphine is a more logical choice of opioid and has been successfully used in patient-controlled analgesia systems.

Patient care

Patients need to be encouraged to take their prophylactic penicillin and folic acid therapy regularly between crises. During a crisis, some health professionals worry about the patient developing opioid addiction. While this may happen, it is also important to recognise that crises are extremely painful and the patient requires effective analgesia.

Box 49.9 Drugs that may increase fetal haemoglobin production

5-Azacytidine
Cytarabine
Vinblastine
Hydroxycarbamide
Erythropoietin
Short chain fatty acids (butyrates, valproate)

Thalassaemias

Epidemiology

The thalassaemias are a group of inherited autosomal recessive diseases. The β thalassaemias occur mainly in populations from around the Mediterranean, North and West Africa, Middle East and Indian subcontinent. More than 100 β thalassaemia mutations have been identified, and they tend to produce severe anaemia. The α thalassaemias are more common, of which the milder variants do not cause severe anaemia, whilst the severe homozygotes lead to death *in utero* or infancy.

Aetiology

In α thalassaemia, there is either no α chain production (α^0 thalassaemia) or reduced production of a chain (α^+ thalassaemia). Similarly for β thalassaemia. Heterozygotes are usually symptomless, whilst homozygotes are more severely affected, as are compound heterozygotes in which there is a thalassaemia gene and a gene from another haemoglobin variant, for example, haemoglobin S.

Pathophysiology

In β thalassaemias, there is a reduced or absent production of the globin β chain. This leads to a relative excess of α chain which when unpaired become unstable and precipitates in the red cell precursors. There is ineffective erythropoiesis and those mature cells that reach the circulation have a shortened life span.

In α thalassaemias, the pathology is slightly different. The deficiency of α chains leads to an excess of γ or β chains. This time erythropoiesis is less affected, but the haemoglobin produced (haemoglobin Bart's or Haemoglobin H) is unstable when the cells are in the circulation and precipitates as the cells grow older. This leads to a shortened life span with the spleen trapping many of the cells. Haemoglobin Bart's or haemoglobin H is also physiologically useless.

Clinical manifestations

The anaemia causes erythropoietin production to increase and results in expansion of the bone marrow. In severe disease, this causes bone deformity and growth retardation. The spleen is actively involved in removing the abnormal mature cells from the circulation and becomes enlarged.

Investigations

For β thalassaemia, the diagnosis is relatively straightforward: haemolytic anaemia from infancy and racial background. Haemoglobin electrophoresis is used to determine the amounts of abnormal haemoglobin.

Treatment

There is currently no effective treatment. Patients with thalassaemia minor (those who carry the thalassaemia gene, but still make enough normal haemoglobin) usually do not require treatment. Many patients with severe forms are dependent on blood transfusions from an early age. This inevitably leads to iron overload. Desferrioxamine, deferiprone and deferasirox are routinely needed for such patients (see sideroblastic anaemia for additional information). Splenectomy helps some patients, and allogeneic stem cell transplant is used in severe cases. Prevention is actively explored with genetic counselling programmes in Italy and Greece, and antenatal screening in a number of countries.

As in sickle cell disease, much attention is being placed on the idea of switching the bone marrow to the production of fetal haemoglobin rather than the defective adult haemoglobin of β thalassaemia. It is likely that a combination of drugs (hydroxycarbamide and erythropoietin) will provide some clinical improvement.

Patient care

Drug therapy does not currently play a large part in treatment. If hydroxycarbamide becomes standard treatment, pharmacists will become involved in educating the patient particularly with regard to its cytotoxic nature.

Glucose-6-phosphate dehydrogenase deficiency

Epidemiology

Glucose-6-phosphate dehydrogenase (G6PD) deficiency is a recessive hereditary disease and affects approximately 400 million people worldwide. There are more than 300 different forms of G6PD deficiency, only some of which cause anaemia. The most common form of G6PD deficiency is found in 15% of black Americans. It causes anaemia when the individual is exposed to a trigger factor. A more severe form is the Mediterranean variant of G6PD deficiency. Some of these individuals may have chronic haemolytic anaemia even in the apparent absence of exposure to a precipitating factor.

Aetiology

There are a large number of variants of G6PD activity found in different populations and ethnic groups. G6PD is an erythrocyte enzyme that is indirectly involved in the production of reduced glutathione. Glutathione is produced in response to, and protects red cells from, oxidising reagents.

Pathophysiology

G6PD is essential for the production of (NADPH) in erythrocytes. If there is a deficiency in G6PD, this decreases the production of NADPH which is needed to keep glutathione in a reduced form. Reduced glutathione helps erythrocytes deal with oxidative stress. Hence, in G6PD deficiency, if the erythrocytes are exposed to an oxidising agent, the cell membrane becomes damaged, the haemoglobin becomes oxidised and forms what are known as Heinz bodies. Some of the red cells haemolyse and others have their Heinz bodies removed by the spleen to form 'bite cells'.

Clinical manifestation

Clinically, the two most important types of G6PD deficiency occur in the black population and in people originating from the Mediterranean. The black population has a milder form that results in an acute self-limiting haemolytic anaemia following exposure to an oxidising agent, for example, infection, acute illness, broad beans (fava) beans or drugs (Box 49.10). The haemolytic anaemia is self-limiting because the young cells produced by the bone marrow have higher levels of G6PD activity than old cells. Following exposure to the oxidising agent, the old cells are haemolysed but the new cells produced in response are more capable of tolerating the insult until they grow old. In the Mediterranean form of the disorder, the enzyme activity is very low, haemolysis is not usually self-limiting and, indeed, some patients have a chronic haemolytic anaemia despite the absence of an obvious causative factor.

Investigations

The history and the clinical findings steer the diagnosis, which is then confirmed by measuring G6PD activity. Care must be taken during the acute phase since there are increased numbers of young cells with higher levels of activity that may be misleading. The increased numbers of young cells result from the selective destruction of older cells and the increased production of reticulocytes.

Treatment

Prevention of haemolysis by avoiding trigger factors (drugs or food) is important. Vaccination against hepatitis A and hepatitis B may reduce attacks. In cases of acute haemolytic anaemia, the causative oxidising agent should be stopped and general supportive measures adopted. In chronic haemolytic anaemia, most patients become reasonably well adjusted to their anaemia. They need to avoid known precipitating factors to prevent acute episodes occurring on top of their chronic haemolytic anaemia.

There is no specific drug treatment. During acute episodes, the patient should be kept well hydrated to ensure good urine output to prevent haemoglobin damaging the kidney. Blood transfusions may be necessary. Vitamin E (an antioxidant) appears to have little clinical benefit in preventing haemolysis.

Patient care

Since drug therapy does not play a large part in the management of these patients, pharmacists do not often become involved in patient education. Patients can be given a list of drugs to avoid, but since most of these drugs are prescription only medicines, it is important that patients remind health care professionals of their condition.

Case studies

Case 49.1

Mr HA, a 60-year-old single unemployed man, was admitted to hospital for investigation of anaemia. He presented with a 6-month history of lethargy, chest pain, dizziness and falls and a past history of having a gastrectomy 26 years ago. The drug history on admission showed that Mr HA was taking diazepam and GTN spray.

Review of systems revealed no vomiting and no melaena. He complained of some indigestion after meals and reported his appetite was fine if someone else cooked. On examination he was pale, with a blood pressure of 140/80, pulse 90 and haematoglobin level of 2.5 g/dL (normal range: 13.5–18.0 g/dL). A gastroscopy was normal and a biopsy showed no evidence of coeliac disease. A barium enema was normal and faecal occult bloods (FOBs) negative.

Over the first 2 days, he was transfused with 8 units of blood and given furosemide 40 mg with alternate bags. On day 7 he was started on ferrous sulphate 300 mg three times a day, folic acid 5 mg twice daily and ascorbic acid 200 mg three times a day.

Questions

1. What additional questions should Mr HA have been asked at admission?
2. Comment on the use of vitamin C in Mr HA.
3. How long should Mr HA remain on ferrous sulphate?

Answers

1. Although Mr HA's prescribed drugs were documented, it is possible that he was taking purchased medication. On admission, he complained of indigestion over the last 3 months, and on questioning revealed that he was self-medicating with aluminium hydroxide mixture. From a theoretical point of view, antacids may reduce the amount of iron absorbed by increasing the pH of the stomach and by reducing the solubility of ferrous salts. It is unlikely that this contributed significantly to the development of his anaemia, but if he intends to continue using an antacid after discharge, which he should be discouraged from doing, it would be better not to take a dose of the antacid within 1–2 h of his ferrous sulphate. It would also be worth checking to see if he has been self-medicating with a purchased

---

Box 49.10 Common drugs implicated in causing haemolysis in G6PD deficiency

Drugs to be avoided in all variants
Ciprofloxacin (and probably other quinolones)
Dapsone
Methylene blue
Primaquine (reduced dose may be used in milder variants)
Nalidixic acid
Sulphonamides (including co-trimoxazole)

Drugs to be avoided in more severe variants
Aspirin (low dose used under supervision)
Chloramphenicol
Chloroquine (may be acceptable in acute malaria)
Menadione
Probenecid
Quinidine
Quinine (acceptable in acute malaria)

aspirin or ibuprofen-based product, both drugs have been implicated in causing gastro-intestinal blood loss, though in this case his gastroscopy was normal and FOBs negative.

2. Ascorbic acid increases the absorption of iron in some patients, it probably keeps iron in solution either in the ferrous form or by being a soluble chelat with the ferric form. In most patients, this has little clinical benefit. It may be an advantage in Mr HA since he may also benefit from a short course of multivitamins.

3. Mr HA needs to continue iron therapy until he has at least replenished his iron stores. This may take up to 6 months after which time he should be reassessed, taking into account whether he is now having a suitable diet. In practice, since his iron was dangerously low on admission, it may be quite reasonable to leave him on iron for the rest of his life.

Case 49.2

Mr WK, a 46-year-old mechanic, is referred to hospital by his primary care doctor. He gave a history of diarrhoea and vomiting a week ago and now was complaining of headaches and feeling 'lousy'. His doctor had given him metoclopramide and ferrous sulphate. Mr WK did not appear jaundiced although he said he had noticed his urine was unusually dark a few weeks ago. On examination, he was obese with a blood pressure of 120/80 mmHg and had a pulse of 80. Rectal examination revealed black stools. He had a normal gastroscopy with three negative FOBs. His serum biochemistry showed a normal level of alanine transaminase and a slightly raised total bilirubin level. Mr WK's reticulocyte count was 13.5% (normal range: 0.5–1.5%). He was diagnosed with having G6PD deficiency, probably triggered by an infection.

Questions

1. How do you explain Mr WK's dark urine and dark stools?
2. Would Mr WK benefit from any medication following admission?
3. Why is it necessary to repeat his red cell G6PD levels after 2 months?

Answers

1. Mr WK's dark urine was a consequence of his haemolytic anaemia. Bilirubin is a breakdown product of haemoglobin that is transported to the liver and conjugated before being excreted in the bile. Bacteria in the intestine converts this to urobilinogen, most of which is excreted in the stools. Small amounts of urobilinogen are reabsorbed and some of this appears in the urine. Urobilinogen is oxidised to urobilin, which is coloured. During episodes of haemolysis, erythrocytes are destroyed faster than normal, and hence there is an increase in the formation of bilirubin and increased excretion of urobilinogen in the urine. Also during haemolysis, free haemoglobin may be released into the blood. If the haemolysis is severe enough, the normal mechanism for removing haemoglobin from the circulation is overcome and haemoglobin may appear in the urine. Dark stools may indicate melaenia and upper gastro-intestinal bleeding. In Mr WK's case, his gastroscopy was normal and he had three negative FOBs. His dark stools were due to the ferrous sulphate prescribed by the primary care doctor prior to admission.

2. His raised reticulocyte count indicates he is rapidly replacing his lost red cells. Erythropoiesis consumes folate and iron and since his folate is towards the lower end of the reference range, it may be worth giving him a short course of folate supplements.

3. Young red cells tend to have higher levels of enzyme activity than more mature cells. Determining G6PD levels during the acute phase may be misleading since there is a relatively high proportion of young cells. Mr WK's result 2 months later would more accurately represent his normal state.

Case 49.3

Ms PR, a 58-year-old lady, was admitted to the emergency department. She had fallen over and bruised herself but had not broken any bones. On examination, it was noted that she appeared pale with possibly a lemon-yellow tinge to her skin, she was slightly confused and had paraesthesiae of the feet and fingers. She has a past history of heart failure and was taking furosemide and enalapril. She was admitted for investigation and discovered to have a macrocytic anaemia. Pernicious anaemia was suspected. Folate level, vitamin B_{12} levels and Schilling test were carried out before commencing treatment.

Questions

1. What are the features that may lead you to consider a diagnosis of pernicious anaemia?
2. Can Miss PR have a blood transfusion after samples have been taken for folate and vitamin B_{12}?
3. The red cell folate is reported as 150 mg/L (reference range: 160–640 mg/L). Would Ms PR benefit from folate therapy?

Answers

1. Macrocytic anaemia and paraesthesia are typical features, though not diagnostic of pernicious anaemia. Patients may be mildly jaundiced which is often described as lemon-yellow in colour. Interestingly, pernicious anaemia is more common in women than men and is associated with blue eyes and early greying of the hair. Miss PR may have other features of pernicious anaemia which include glossitis, angular stomatitis and altered bowel habit.

2. Patients with pernicious anaemia develop their anaemia over a long period of time and tend not to tolerate increases in blood volume very well. A transfusion may result in fluid overload and precipitate heart failure. Miss PR already has heart failure, so unless she becomes severely compromised by anaemia, a transfusion should not be given. In patients who have such pronounced anaemia that an urgent transfusion is required, an exchange transfusion of a small volume of packed cells may be appropriate.

3. In vitamin B_{12} deficiency folate tends to leak from cells and the red cell folate is often low (serum folate is sometimes raised). Many patients initially require both folate and vitamin B_{12} although folate can usually be stopped after a short course. Folate therapy must never be given to patients who have not been fully investigated for vitamin B_{12} deficiency. If vitamin B_{12}-deficient patients are given large doses of folate without hydroxocobalami, the full blood count may appear to improve but the peripheral neuropathy from the vitamin B_{12} deficiency progresses.

Case 49.4

Mrs GN, a 76-year-old retired factory worker, was seen by her primary care doctor, complaining of tiredness. She had been seen 2 months earlier and started on ferrous sulphate for microcytic anaemia. Initially, she had felt better but the tiredness soon returned. A bone marrow aspiration revealed increased erythropoiesis, iron stores and red cell precursors.

A diagnosis of sideroblastic anaemia was made and it was decided to give her monthly transfusions. She was started on pyridoxine 50 mg three times a day in addition to ferrous sulphate.

Questions

1. What are the potential problems with Mrs GN's treatment?
2. After 3 months there appeared to be little benefit to show from pyridoxine. How might management be improved?

Answers

1. Mrs GN's bone marrow aspiration and serum ferritin level showed that she has high levels of stored iron. Repeated monthly transfusions will also have contributed to further iron accumulation. In sideroblastic anaemia, the bone marrow appears to be inefficient at incorporating the iron into haem. The administration of iron leads to iron overload which may result in damage to the heart, liver and endocrine organs. The ferrous sulphate must be stopped. If iron accumulation remains a problem, desferrioxamine therapy must be tried.
2. Pyridoxine does not always improve the blood picture in patients with sideroblastic anaemia. In sideroblastic anaemia, the dose of pyridoxine required is usually 400 mg daily. So, in the case of Mrs GN, an increase in dose should be tried. In addition, patients with sideroblastic anaemia often do not realise that pyridoxine is not just a simple vitamin but a specific treatment for anaemia. Therefore, counselling the patient may improve adherence.

Case 49.5

Mrs RO, a 70-year-old retired teacher, presented with a history of increased tiredness over the last 6 weeks. She has a past history of a partial gastrectomy 4 years ago. On questioning, her relevant symptoms included 'pins and needles' in her toes and loose bowels. She said that she had never been a good eater but ate red meat twice a week.

Questions

1. Why was it 4 years after her gastrectomy before Mrs RO developed vitamin B_{12} deficiency?
2. How long will it take for Mrs RO to respond to treatment?
3. What therapy will Mrs RO require?

Answers

1. Vitamin B_{12} requires intrinsic factor produced by the stomach for absorption. Patients with a total gastrectomy and some with a partial gastrectomy malabsorb vitamin B_{12}. Most patients have good body stores and even if no new vitamin B_{12} enters the body (e.g. following a total gastrectomy) it will take at least 2 years to deplete the stores.
2. Many patients will feel better within days of starting treatment with hydroxocobalamin and before a change in their haemoglobin concentration can be detected. Mrs RO's blood picture may take a number of weeks to return to normal. However, her 'pins and needles' may be a sign of peripheral neuropathy which can be irreversible and may not respond to the hydroxocobalamin treatment.
3. Mrs RO will require lifelong replacement therapy. The standard treatment for vitamin B_{12} deficiency is hydroxocobalamin 1 mg intramuscularly three times a week for 2 weeks, then 1 mg every 3 months. If neurological involvement is identified, as in the case of Mrs RO, then a slightly higher dose regimen is recommended of 1 mg on alternate days until no further improvement, followed by 1 mg every 2 months thereafter.

References

Altschuler, E.L., Kast, R.E., 2005. Using histamine (H1) antagonists in particular atypical antipsychotics to treat anaemia of chronic disease via interleukin-6 suppression. Med. Hypotheses 65, 65–67.

Annibale, B., Marignani, M., Monarca, B., et al., 1999. Reversal of iron deficiency anaemia after *Helicobacter pylori* eradication in patients with asymptomatic gastritis. Ann. Intern. Med. 131, 668–672.

Beris, I., Munoz, M., Garcia-Erce, J.A., et al., 2008. Perioperative anaemia management: consensus statement on the role of intravenous iron. Br. J. Anaesth. 100, 599–609.

Cavill, I., 2003. Intravenous iron as adjuvant therapy: a two edged sword? Nephrol. Dial. Transplant. 18 (Suppl. 8), viii24–viii28.

Charache, S., Terrin, M.L., Moore, R.D., et al., 1995. Effect of hydroxyurea on the frequency of painful crises in sickle cell anaemia. N. Engl. J. Med. 332, 1317–1322.

D'Arena, G., Califano, C., Annunziata, M., et al., 2007. Rituximab for warm-type idiopathic autoimmune hemolytic anemia: a retrospective study of 11 adult patients. Eur. J. Haematol. 79, 53–58.

Dec, W.G., 2009. Anemia and iron deficiency – new therapeutic targets in heart failure? N. Engl. J. Med. 361, 2475–2477.

DH, 1992. Folic Acid and the Prevention of Neural Tube Defects: Report from an Expert Advisory Group. Department of Health, London.

Felker, M., 2010. Too much, too little, or just right? Untangling endogenous erythropoietin in heart failure. Circulation 121, 191–193.

Gera, T., Sachdev, H.P.S., 2002. Effect of iron supplementation on incidence of infectious illness in children: systematic review.

Br. Med. J. 325, 1142. Available at http://www.bmj.com/content/325/7373/1142.full.pdf.

Green, R., Miller, J.W., 1999. Folate deficiency beyond megaloblastic anaemia: hyperhomocysteinemia and other manifestations of dysfunctional folate status. Semin. Haematol. 36, 47–64.

National Institute for Health and Clinical Excellence, 2008. Epoetin Alfa, Epoetin Beta and Darbepoetin Alfa for Cancer Treatment-Induced Anaemia. Technology Appraisal 142. NICE, London. Available at http://www.nice.org.uk/nicemedia/pdf/TA142Guidance.pdf.

Prentice, A.M., Ghattas, H., Doherty, C., et al., 2007. Iron metabolism and malaria. Food Nutr. Bull. 28 (4 Suppl.), S524–S539.

Pruss, A., Salama, N., Ahrens, A., et al., 2003. Immune hemolysis-serological and clinical aspects. Clin. Exp. Med. 3, 55–64.

Raj, D.S., 2009. Role of interleukin in the anaemia of chronic disease. Semin. Arthritis Rheum. 38, 382–388.

Sachdev, H.P.S., Gera, T., Nestel, P., 2005. Effect of iron supplementation on mental and motor development in children: systematic review of randomised controlled trials. Public Health Nutr. 8, 117–132.

Silverberg, D.S., Blum, M., Peer, G., et al., 1996. Intravenous ferric saccharate as an iron supplement in dialysis patients. Nephron 72, 413–417.

Williams, J., Wolff, A., Daly, A., et al., 1999. Iron supplemented formula milk related to reduction in psychomotor decline in infants from inner city areas: randomised study. Br. Med. J. 318, 693–698.

50 Leukaemia

G. Jackson and G. Jones

Key points

- Leukaemias are uncommon malignancies.
- Acute lymphoblastic leukaemia (ALL) is the most common malignancy in childhood.
- With the exception of ALL, leukaemias are more common in the elderly.
- Age is one of the most important prognostic factors in the treatment of leukaemia. With the exception of neonates, older patients are less likely to be cured than younger patients.
- The treatment of leukaemia is continually improving with the introduction of more focused therapy and improvements in supportive care.
- The use of bone marrow transplantation in the treatment of all forms of leukaemia is increasing. Some of the results are exciting, but the short- and long-term problems of this type of intensive treatment need to be considered.

Table 50.1 Incidence of leukaemia in the UK (Leukaemia and Lymphoma Research, 2010)

	New cases/year	Incidence per 100,000 of the population
CLL	2750	4.58
CML	750	1.5
ALL	650	1.00
AML	1950	3.25

Leukaemias and lymphomas are the commonest forms of haematological malignancy. Although rare, they are of particular interest in that dramatic improvements in the prognosis of patients with these cancers have been achieved through the use of chemotherapy, and cure is now a possibility for many patients.

Many forms of leukaemia exist, but they are all characterised by the production of excessive numbers of abnormal white blood cells. The leukaemias can be broadly divided into four groups:

- acute myeloblastic leukaemia (AML)
- acute lymphoblastic leukaemia (ALL)
- chronic myelocytic leukaemia (CML)
- chronic lymphocytic leukaemia (CLL)

The adjectives 'myeloid' and 'lymphoid' refer to the predominant cell involved, and the suffix-cytic and -blastic to mature and immature cells, respectively. These characteristics can be determined by a combination of cellular appearances, surface antigen expression and cytogenetic features. The international standard for leukaemia classification is the WHO system (Swerdlow et al., 2008).

Epidemiology

Haematological malignancies account for only 5% of all cancers; of these, CLL is the most common form of leukaemia. UK incidence data are presented in Table 50.1. CLL mainly affects an older age group: 90% of patients are over the age of 50 and nearly two-thirds are over 60 years old at diagnosis. It rarely occurs in young people and is twice as common in men as in women. CML is primarily a disease of middle age with the median onset in the 40–50 year old age group, but it can occur in younger people.

Acute leukaemia is rare, with a total annual incidence of approximately 4 per 100,000 population. The more common form of the disease is AML, which accounts for 75% of cases. The incidence of AML rises steadily with age, occurring only rarely in young children. In contrast, ALL is predominantly a childhood disease, with the peak incidence in the 3–5 year age group, and is the most common childhood cancer.

Aetiology

In common with other cancers, the aetiology of leukaemia is not fully understood. Leukaemia is thought to result from a combination of factors that induce genetic mutations which allow mutated cells to proliferate faster than normal cells and/or to fail to die in response to normal apoptotic signals. Epidemiological studies have, however, identified a number of specific risk factors for the development of leukaemia, which are described as follows.

Radiation

The association between the ionising radiation and the development of leukaemia is evident from nuclear disasters such as Hiroshima and more recently Chernobyl. Long-term follow-up of survivors of Nagasaki and Hiroshima has shown an increase in all forms of leukaemia other than CLL. The link is also apparent for patients who received radiotherapy for the treatment of malignant and non-malignant conditions such as Hodgkin's disease or ankylosing spondylitis. The effect of chronic low-level exposure to radiation is less certain.

Exposure to chemicals and cytotoxic drugs

There is a small but definite risk of acute leukaemia occurring in patients successfully treated for other malignancies with cytotoxic and immunosuppressive agents. The combination of chemotherapy, especially alkylating agents such as cyclophosphamide and radiotherapy, presents the highest risk. This has practical implications as an increasing number of patients achieve a 'cure' as a result of combination therapy, while occupational exposure of health professionals to these agents is also an area of concern. Occupational exposures to paint, insecticides and solvents, in particular, the aromatic solvent benzene, have all been associated with the development of leukaemia, but it is difficult to be certain whether such exposures genuinely cause the disease.

Viruses

Human T-cell lymphotrophic virus, an RNA retrovirus endemic in Japan and the West Indies, has been linked to a rare T-cell leukaemia/lymphoma.

Genetic factors

Down's syndrome, constitutional trisomy of chromosome 21, is associated with an increased risk of leukaemia. Disorders that predispose to chromosomal breaks such as Fanconi's anaemia and ataxia telangectasia are also associated with an increased risk of developing acute leukaemia. These alterations may permit the expression of oncogenes, which promote malignant transformation.

Haematological disorders

Many patients with other haematological disorders have a greatly increased risk of developing leukaemia, particularly AML. These disorders include the myelodysplastic syndromes, the non-leukaemic myeloproliferative disorders, aplastic anaemia and paroxysmal nocturnal haemoglobinuria.

Pathophysiology

In leukaemia, the normal process of haemopoiesis is altered (Fig. 50.1). Transformation to malignancy appears to occur in a single cell, usually at the pluripotential stem cell level, but it may occur in a committed stem cell with capacity for more limited differentiation. Accumulation of malignant cells leads to progressive impairment of the normal bone marrow function.

Acute leukaemias

In acute leukaemia, the normal bone marrow is replaced by a malignant clone of immature blast cells derived from the myeloid (in AML) or lymphoid (in ALL) series. More than 20% of the cellular elements of the bone marrow are replaced with blasts. This is usually associated with the appearance of blasts in the peripheral circulation accompanied by worsening pancytopenia as a result of the marrow's reduced ability to produce normal blood cells as the proportion of malignant cells increases. In ALL, the blasts may infiltrate lymph nodes and other tissues such as liver, spleen, testis and the meninges, in particular. In AML, blasts tend to infiltrate skin, gums, liver and spleen.

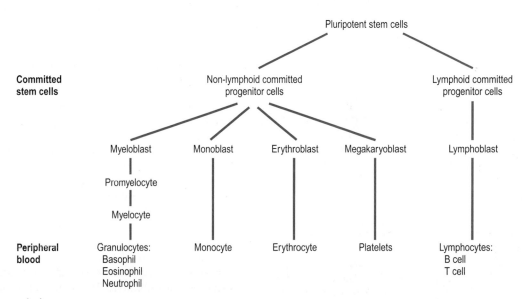

Fig. 50.1 Haemopoiesis.

Classification of acute myeloblastic leukaemia

AML has traditionally been classified on the basis of morphological features of the disease. Subtypes displaying granulocytic, monocytic, erythroid and megakaryocytic differentiation can be demonstrated. Recently, the World Health Organization (WHO) has updated this system (Table 50.2). AML is now classified using a combination of morphological, genetic and immunological cell marker features (surface antigen expression) in an attempt to define disease groups of greater prognostic significance (Swerdlow et al., 2008).

Classification of acute lymphoblastic leukaemia

As with AML, the WHO classification system takes account of morphological, genetic and immunological features. The disease is, however, mainly classified immunologically, based on the presence or absence of B- or T-cell markers (Table 50.3). Each subtype displays different clinical presentations, response to treatment and, ultimately, prognosis, with pre-B having the best prognosis and B-ALL the worst. It is worth noting that B-ALL (Burkitt's type), which is associated with translocations of the myc gene normally located on chromosome 8, seems to be a morphologically and biologically distinct form of leukaemia.

Table 50.2 WHO classification of AML

Subgroup	Examples
AML with recurrent genetic abnormalities	Inversion chromosome 16 (inv 16) t(15;17) t(8;21)
AML with multilineage dysplasia Therapy-related AML	
AML not otherwise classified	AML without maturation AML with granulocytic maturation AML with granulocytic and monocytic differentiation AML with monocytic differentiation AML with erythroid differentiation AML with megakaryocytic differentiation

Table 50.3 Classification of ALL

Pre-B ALL	Possessing the common ALL antigen CD 10
B cell type	B-ALL of Burkitt's type
T cell type	T-ALL
Null	Non-B, non-T and lacking the common ALL antigen CD 10

Chronic leukaemias

In chronic leukaemia, the normal bone marrow is replaced by a malignant clone of maturing haemopoietic cells.

Chronic lymphocytic leukaemia

CLL is characterised by a clonal expansion of morphologically mature lymphocytes of B-cell origin. These cells accumulate in the peripheral blood and give rise to a lymphocytosis that may be very marked. Lymphocytes accumulate in lymph nodes and spread to the liver and spleen, which become enlarged. The bone marrow is progressively infiltrated. Although the malignant lymphocytes appear morphologically normal, they are functionally deficient.

Chronic myelocytic leukaemia

The characteristic feature of CML is the predominance of maturing myeloid cells in blood, bone marrow, liver, spleen and other organs. CML was the first cancer to be associated with a specific chromosomal abnormality: the Philadelphia chromosome translocation (Ph) seen in over 90% of cases. This is a translocation of genetic material between the long arms of chromosome 22 and chromosome 9. This results in the apposition of the BCR gene (chromosome 22) and the ABL gene (chromosome 9). This novel BCR-ABL gene encodes a fusion protein which has tyrosine kinase activity. This genetic event is believed to be crucial in the pathogenesis, or perhaps even to initiate the development, of CML since overactivity of the tyrosine kinase results in the uncontrolled growth characteristic of leukaemic cells (Cilloni and Saglio, 2009).

Clinical manifestations

Acute leukaemia

Most of the clinical manifestations of acute leukaemia are related to bone marrow failure. The disease commonly presents with a short history, and left untreated, it is rapidly fatal. Symptoms of infection, anaemia and bleeding are common and life-threatening presenting problems. Bleeding may be particularly severe in one subtype of AML, acute promyelocytic leukaemia (APL). This condition is associated with a translocation of genetic material between chromosomes 15 and 17, t(15;17). Disseminated intravascular coagulation (DIC) is commonly the presenting feature of this disease. Some patients with AML develop symptoms and signs due to infiltration of major organs by leukaemic cells.

The involvement of other tissues such as spleen, liver, lymph nodes and meninges is more common in ALL than AML. Involvement of the central nervous system (CNS) may give rise to headaches, vomiting and irritable behaviour. CNS disease is rare at presentation, but develops in up to 75% of children with ALL unless specific prophylactic treatment is given. Less commonly, patients present with features of hypermetabolism, hyperuricaemia or generalised aches and pains.

Chronic leukaemia

Chronic myelocytic leukaemia

Patients with CML commonly present with non-specific symptoms, such as malaise, weight loss and night sweats. The main physical sign is an enlarged spleen that may give rise to abdominal discomfort. Hepatomegaly is also detected in approximately 40% of newly diagnosed patients. Neutropenia and thrombocytopenia are uncommon at presentation. Thus, unlike the acute leukaemias, patients with CML rarely present with symptoms of infection or haemorrhage. In up to 30% of cases, patients are asymptomatic and the disease is detected as a result of a routine blood test performed for other reasons.

CML is a triphasic disease. The initial chronic phase may last from several months to 20 years; the median is around 5 years. During this time, treatment can alleviate symptoms and reduce the white blood count (WBC) and spleen size, allowing patients to lead near normal lives. An accelerated phase eventually occurs where the disease becomes more aggressive with progressively worsening symptoms: unexplained fevers, bone pain, anaemia, thrombocytopenia or thrombocytosis. Finally, after a period of weeks or months, a blast crisis occurs, resembling fulminating acute leukaemia. In a small percentage of patients, this occurs abruptly with no prior accelerated phase.

Chronic lymphocytic leukaemia

An increasing number of patients are diagnosed as having CLL by chance, when a full blood count is performed for an unrelated reason. Symptomatic patients often suffer B symptoms: night sweats, unexplained fever and weight loss. At diagnosis, findings may include generalised lymphadenopathy and some enlargement of the liver and spleen. The course of CLL is variable; in some patients, the disease may remain indolent for many years, while others experience a steady deterioration in their health. Survival typically varies from 2 to 20 years depending on the extent of disease. Patients are immunocompromised with a reduction in serum gammaglobulin and are at increased risk of bacterial and viral infections. There is an increased susceptibility to autoimmune disease, particularly immune haemolytic anaemias and thrombocytopenia. With progressive disease, bone marrow failure becomes apparent, resulting in fatigue, infection and bleeding, and the disease becomes less responsive to treatment. Patients with CLL also have an increased risk of developing a more aggressive malignancy such as high-grade non-Hodgkin's lymphoma (known as Richter's transformation) or prolymphocytic leukaemia (PLL).

Investigations

Examinations of peripheral blood and bone marrow are the key laboratory investigations carried out in cases of suspected leukaemia. However, some additional investigations can help in the diagnosis and classification of this group of diseases. Some of the main findings at diagnosis are presented in Table 50.4.

Table 50.4 Findings at diagnosis in leukaemia

	AML	ALL	CML	CLL
WBC	↑ in 60%, may be N or ↓	↑ in 50%, may be N or ↓↓	↑↑ commonly 100×10^9–250×10^9 L^{-1}	Commonly ↑
Differential WBC	Mainly myeloblasts	Mainly lymphoblasts	Granulocytes ↑↑, especially neutrophils, myelocytes, basophils and eosinophils <10% blasts present	>5×10^9 L^{-1} monoclonal lymphocytes
RBC	Severe anaemia	Severe anaemia	Anaemia common	Anaemia in 50% of patients, generally mild
Platelets	↓↓	↓↓	Usually ↑, may be N or ↓	↓ in 20–30%
Bone marrow aspiration and trephine	Predominantly blasts	Predominantly blasts	Hypercellular blasts < 10%	Lymphocytic infiltration
Cytogenetic analysis	Important abnormalities detected	Important abnormalities detected	Presence of Ph chromosome	
Lymphadenopathy	Rare	Common	Rare	Common
Splenomegaly	50%	60%	Usual and severe	Usual and moderate
Other features	DIC, high urate	High urate, CNS involvement	↑ Serum uric acid	Immune paresis

N, normal; ↓, reduced; ↑, increased; WBC, white blood cells; DIC, disseminated intravascular coagulation; Ph, Philadelphia; RBC, red blood cells.

In acute leukaemia, leukaemic blast cells are usually seen on the peripheral blood film. The blasts of ALL and AML are distinguished using morphology, cytochemical stains, cytogenetics and cell surface antigen analysis. In CML, the principal feature is a leucocytosis with WBC usually ranging from $10 \times 10^9 \, L^{-1}$ to $250 \times 10^9 \, L^{-1}$ and comprising the complete spectrum of myeloid cells. In CLL, it is lymphocytes, in particular, which are increased, with clonal lymphocyte counts exceeding $5 \times 10^9 \, L^{-1}$. Non-random chromosome abnormalities are increasingly being identified in patients with leukaemia. The information obtained from cytogenetic analysis of bone marrow or peripheral blood cells can be used to confirm the diagnosis and classification of leukaemia and may provide a guide to the likely response to treatment and prognosis.

Treatment

Although significant progress has been made in the treatment of leukaemia, work continues to further improve prognosis. As leukaemias are rare malignancies, the most important studies are undertaken on a national or international basis. In addition to the specific anti-leukaemia treatment, general supportive therapy is vital to manage both the disease and the complications of therapy.

Acute leukaemia

At the outset, intensive combination chemotherapy is given in the hope of achieving a complete remission (CR). This initial phase of treatment is termed induction or remission induction chemotherapy. A CR can only be achieved by virtual ablation of the bone marrow, followed by recovery of normal haemopoiesis. If two cycles of therapy fail to induce CR, an alternative drug regimen can be used. If this is unsuccessful, it is unlikely that CR will be achieved. The subsequent duration of the first remission is closely linked to survival.

Remission is defined as the absence of all clinical and microscopic signs of leukaemia, less than 5% blast forms in the bone marrow and return of normal cellularity and haemopoietic elements. Despite achieving CR, occult residual disease (also termed minimal residual disease or MRD) will persist, and further intensive therapy is given in an attempt to sustain the remission. This post-remission consolidation therapy may comprise chemotherapy or a combination of chemotherapy and bone marrow transplantation.

Acute lymphoblastic leukaemia

Treatment of ALL in childhood has been one of the success stories of the past 3 decades. Over 80% of children will achieve a remission lasting more than 5 years, and current studies are often focused on trying to identify the 20% of children with poor risk disease and treating them more aggressively (Vrooman and Silverman, 2009). Unfortunately, the results in adults are not so impressive. The combination of vincristine, prednisolone, anthracyclines and asparaginase induces CR in about 90% of children with ALL and 80% of adults, although sadly relapse is far more common in adults (Table 50.5). Other active drugs in the treatment of ALL include methotrexate, 6-mercaptopurine, cyclophosphamide and mitoxantrone.

Table 50.5 Treatment of ALL (adapted from MRC protocol UKALL 12-2005)

	Dose	Route	Regimen
Induction (4 weeks)			
Vincristine	1.5 mg/m²	i.v.	Weekly for 4 weeks
Prednisolone	40 mg/m²	oral	Daily for 4 weeks
L-Asparaginase	6000 u/m²	i.m.	3 × weekly for 3 weeks
Daunorubicin	45 mg/m²	i.v.	Daily for 2 days
Intensification (1 week)			
Vincristine	1.5 mg/m²	i.v.	1 dose
Daunorubicin	45 mg/m²	i.v.	Daily for 2 days
Prednisolone	40 mg/m²	oral	Daily for 5 days
Etoposide	100 mg/m²	i.v.	Daily for 5 days
Cytarabine	100 mg/m²	i.v.	2 × daily for 5 days
Thioguanine	80 mg/m²	oral	Daily for 5 days
CNS prophylaxis (3 weeks)			
Cranial irradiation	24 Gy		
Methotrexate	i.t. weekly for 3 weeks also given during induction and intensification		
Maintenance therapy (2 years)			
Methotrexate	20 mg/m²	oral	Weekly
6-Mercaptopurine	75 mg/m²	oral	Daily
Prednisolone	40 mg/m²	oral	5 days/month
Vincristine	1.5 mg/m²	i.v.	Monthly

i.m., intramuscular; i.v., intravenous; i.t., intrathecal; MRC, Medical Research Council; ALL, acute lymphoblastic leukaemia.

Patients with ALL are at a high risk of developing CNS infiltration. Cytotoxic drugs penetrate poorly into the CNS which thus acts as a sanctuary site for leukaemic cells. For this reason, all patients with ALL receive CNS prophylaxis. Cranial irradiation plus intrathecal methotrexate or high-dose systemic methotrexate can be used.

Maintenance treatment is important to sustain a CR. It is usually milder than induction or consolidation chemotherapy, but is carried on for at least 18 months. Treatment usually consists of weekly methotrexate and daily 6-mercaptopurine with intermittent vincristine and prednisolone.

The treatment of relapsed disease varies with the site of relapse. Isolated CNS or testicular relapse may be successfully treated with radiation and reinduction therapy. Cure can still be achieved for some patients. Bone marrow relapse is much more difficult to cure, especially if it occurs early.

A small proportion of paediatric patients and a larger proportion of adult patients have the Philadelphia chromosome translocation within their ALL blasts. Such patients have a relatively poor prognosis and therefore require more intensive therapy. There is some evidence that drug combinations including imatinib may enhance the response of these leukaemias to therapy.

Acute myeloblastic leukaemia (non-acute promyelocytic leukaemia)

As for ALL, the treatment of AML involves induction and consolidation chemotherapy. In AML therapy, however, the chemotherapy regimens used to achieve remission are much more myelotoxic, and patients require intensive supportive care to survive periods of bone marrow aplasia (Fig. 50.2). The pyrimidine analogue cytarabine has formed

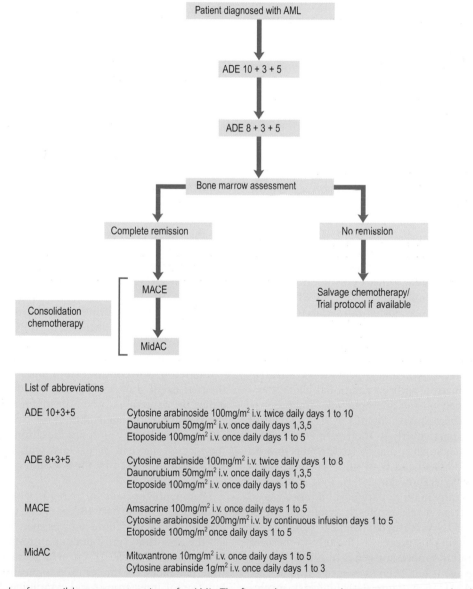

List of abbreviations

ADE 10+3+5	Cytosine arabinoside 100mg/m² i.v. twice daily days 1 to 10 Daunorubium 50mg/m² i.v. once daily days 1,3,5 Etoposide 100mg/m² i.v. once daily days 1 to 5
ADE 8+3+5	Cytosine arabinside 100mg/m² i.v. twice daily days 1 to 8 Daunorubium 50mg/m² i.v. once daily days 1,3,5 Etoposide 100mg/m² i.v. once daily days 1 to 5
MACE	Amsacrine 100mg/m² i.v. once daily days 1 to 5 Cytosine arabinoside 200mg/m² i.v. by continuous infusion days 1 to 5 Etoposide 100mg/m² once daily days 1 to 5
MidAC	Mitoxantrone 10mg/m² i.v. once daily days 1 to 5 Cytosine arabinside 1g/m² i.v. once daily days 1 to 3

Fig. 50.2 One example of a possible treatment regimen for AML. The figure demonstrates that patients are treated with initial induction therapy, then remission is consolidated with at least two courses of chemotherapy. This figure provides a summary only and should not be used as a guide to prescribing or dispensing therapy.

the basis of treatment for AML for 20 years. The addition of daunorubicin and oral thioguanine has achieved a CR rate of 75% in patients under the age of 60 years and about 50% in those over 60 years (Dohner et al., 2010). The precise dose and scheduling of these agents is continually being refined in order to improve the response rates. Despite the numbers of patients who achieve CR following induction therapy, the majority relapse, with only about 25% becoming long-term disease-free survivors (Stone et al., 2004). Thus, in common with ALL, additional post-remission therapy is required. Intensive consolidation chemotherapy with high-dose cytarabine and daunorubicin or amsacrine appears to improve survival rates to approximately 50% after 3 years, with even more encouraging results being obtained in patients under 25 years of age (Dohner et al., 2010; Robak and Wierzbowska, 2009). There is generally no role for maintenance therapy in AML. Similarly, CNS prophylaxis is not routinely indicated though patients thought to be at particularly high risk of CNS disease, such as those with testicular or sinus involvement, should receive prophylactic therapy.

An alternative approach to post-remission therapy is stem cell transplantation. In patients under 40 years of age, allogeneic bone marrow transplantation has resulted in disease-free survival of 45–65% at 5 years post-transplant. These patients are considered cured of their disease. Only about 10% of patients are suitable for allogeneic bone marrow transplants, and there is little evidence to suggest that autologous stem cell transplantation improves the outcome for patients with AML in first CR. It is always worth remembering that AML is most common in the elderly, and intensive intravenous chemotherapy regimens are not always appropriate for this population of patients.

Treatment of AML in relapse is difficult and the prognosis is generally poor. Encouraging results have been seen using a combination of fludarabine, cytosine arabinoside and granulocyte colony-stimulating factor (G-CSF). Novel approaches in AML therapy are often piloted in this group of poor-risk patients. A combination of anti-CD33 antibody, which targets myeloid blasts, with calicheamicin, an anthracycline antibiotic, is a promising and effective approach (Stone et al., 2004), but appears most effective when given in combination with conventional chemotherapy. A newly developed purine analogue, clofarabine, has also been shown to have activity against AML. This drug is a promising agent, particularly in the treatment of older patients, as pilot studies suggest that its toxic effects may be less severe than those associated with other chemotherapy regimens (Robak and Wierzbowska, 2009). 5-Azacytidine is also of interest, especially in older patients and those whose disease has evolved from myelodysplastic syndrome MDS. This agent inhibits DNA methyltransferase resulting in DNA hypomethylation. This process is thought to increase activity of some tumour suppressor genes resulting in antitumour effects. The agent has been shown to slow the rate of progression to AML in patients with high-risk myelodysplastic syndrome and is currently the subject of clinical trials in AML.

Acute Promyelocytic Leukaemia

This subtype of AML deserves special consideration as the treatment is quite different from that of other AML variants. APL is associated with the t(15;17) translocation which involves a genetic translocation of material between chromosomes 15 and 17. The disease is clinically characterised by the presence of disseminated intravascular coagulopathy (DIC) at presentation. Since these patients are so prone to life-threatening haemorrhage at diagnosis, the management of a new case of APL is considered a medical emergency. The leukaemic cells are exquisitely sensitive to all-trans retinoic acid (ATRA), which induces blast maturation and can induce remission when used as a single agent (Sanz et al., 2009; Soignet and Maslak, 2004). Using a combination of ATRA and anthracycline chemotherapy, it is now possible to achieve long-term cure in >80% patients. There are some data to suggest that the ongoing use of ATRA in consolidation and maintenance treatment improves outcome further. A number of studies have been published demonstrating the efficacy of arsenic trioxide (ATO) in treating relapsed or refractory APL. Comparison of ATRA and anthracyclines against ATO and ATRA is now the subject of a large UK study of newly diagnosed patients (AML 17). The latter regimen has the potential advantage of avoiding significant myelosuppression.

Chronic leukaemia

Chronic myelocytic leukaemia

Until recently, the treatment of CML has been essentially palliative, producing modest increases in survival, but with the main aim of keeping patients asymptomatic by normalising the WBC. Hydroxycarbamide was the most widely used drug in the management of CML in chronic phase. Treatment with hydroxycarbamide is initiated at a dose of 1.5–2 g/day and usually brings the WBC under control within 1–2 weeks. The dose can then be reduced to a maintenance dose of 0.5–2 g/day. Withdrawing or reducing the dose abruptly can cause a rebound increase in WBC. The side effects of hydroxycarbamide are generally mild but include rashes and gut disturbances.

Interferon can control symptoms of CML but was also the first agent shown to modify the disease process. It promotes the expression of suppressed normal haemopoiesis at the expense of the malignant clone. Studies have shown that interferon-α therapy prolongs the chronic phase and improves the median survival of patients with CML, and its effects seem to be enhanced by the addition of low-dose cytarabine (Sawyers, 1999).

Therapeutic options for patients with CML have changed dramatically in the past 10 years due to the development of imatinib mesylate. This drug was specifically designed to target the abnormal tyrosine kinase product of the BCR-ABL fusion gene (Fig. 50.3). In a large randomised controlled trial, patients were randomised to receive imatinib or a combination of interferon-α and cytarabine. Many patients were intolerant of the interferon and cytarabine combination and crossed over to receive imatinib after trial commencement.

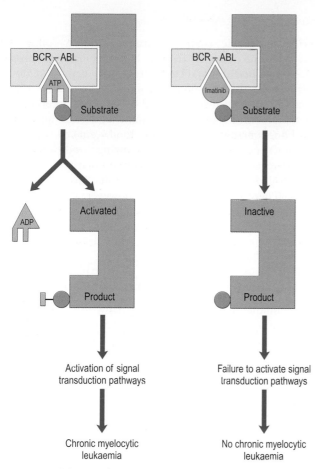

Fig. 50.3 Inhibition of BCR-ABL protein by imatinib. The protein product of the BCR-ABL fusion gene (BCR-ABL protein) acts as a constitutively active tyrosine kinase and uses ATP, bound within a kinase pocket in the molecule, to phosphorylate tyrosine (o) in a variety of substrates. In doing so, ATP (adenosine triphosphate) is reduced to ADP (adenosine diphosphate) which falls out of the kinase pocket to be replaced by further ATP. Imatinib prevents the action of the BCR-ABL protein by blocking ATP entry into the kinase pocket.

Despite this problem, progression-free survival at 1 year was 97% in the imatinib arm and 80% in the interferon and cytarabine arm in an intention-to-treat analysis (O'Brien et al., 2003). The Philadelphia chromosome became undetectable in 68% of imatinib recipients compared to 7% of those in the alternative arm (Hughes et al., 2003). However, more sensitive testing methods, such as real-time polymerase chain reaction (PCR), have now shown that many patients who are Philadelphia chromosome negative still possess very low levels of the abnormal BCR-ABL gene produced by the Philadelphia translocation.

Dasatinib and nilotinib are second-generation tyrosine kinase inhibitors (TKIs) designed to overcome resistance to imatinib caused by mutations in the kinase domain of BCR-ABL. Both agents work well as second-line therapies, producing complete cytogenetic responses in about 50% of patients. The use of dasatinib and nilotinib in newly diagnosed patients is currently being evaluated in ongoing clinical trials. Due to the effectiveness of imatinib therapy and the development of second-generation agents, allogeneic stem cell transplantation is now rarely used to treat CML, but it does represent a potentially curative option for patients with resistant disease.

Transformation of CML into acute leukaemia can be treated in the same manner as *de novo* acute leukaemia, in an effort to achieve a second chronic phase. Treatment is slightly more successful if transformation is lymphoid rather than myeloid. Imatinib, typically at higher doses than are used in chronic phase disease, can also be used to attempt to return patients to chronic phase disease. In general, remissions are rare and the median survival is less than 6 months.

Chronic lymphocytic leukaemia

Currently, there is no cure for CLL. All treatment is, therefore, considered palliative. There is no evidence that early treatment of asymptomatic patients improves outcome. Indications for treatment are:

- rapidly increasing WBC
- increasing or troublesome lymphadenopathy
- systemic symptoms
- marrow failure
- autoimmune complications.

Formerly, the alkylating agent chlorambucil was the most common agent used in the treatment of CLL. Corticosteroids can reduce the lymphocyte count without contributing to myelosuppression and are used to treat autoimmune phenomena such as haemolytic anaemia and immune thrombocytopenia. The use of purine analogues, particularly fludarabine, marked the beginning of an exciting phase in the treatment of CLL. Although CRs were unusual, good responses were seen even in patients whose leukaemia was resistant to alkylating agents. With regard to initial therapy of CLL, fludarabine-treated patients show a higher response rate than patients treated with chlorambucil. However, no survival advantage for the use of fludarabine has been demonstrated (Rai et al., 2000). More recently, a large randomised study comparing fludarabine and cyclophosphamide with and without the anti-CD20 antibody, rituximab, has been published (Hallek et al., 2009). This study demonstrated an overall response rate of 86% and 73%, respectively. The median progression-free survival with rituximab is the best published in a large randomised controlled trial to date, at 40 months. This combination of fludarabine, cyclophosphamide and rituximab has been adopted, in the UK, as the regimen of choice for first-line treatment of CLL as long as patients are considered fit enough. Chlorambucil remains an excellent choice for patients with significant co-morbidities as the treatment is less immunosuppressive.

Splenic complications may necessitate splenectomy or splenic irradiation. Radiotherapy can also be used to control localised painful lymphadenopathy. Combination chemotherapy, such as CHOP (see Chapter 51) used in lymphoma, may be beneficial in advanced disease. Campath-1H is a humanised monoclonal anti-CD52 antibody. CD52 is present on most lymphocytes including malignant lymphocytes in CLL. Binding of this antibody induces both antibody-mediated and complement-mediated T-cell cytotoxicity against malignant B cells. In relapsed patients, the duration of response to Campath-1H is relatively short. However, the agent is currently being studied, both in combination with other drugs and as a possible means of purging the bone marrow of residual cells prior to autologous stem cell harvest and transplantation.

Patients with CLL are very susceptible to infection. Herpes viruses, in particular herpes zoster, can cause significant problems. This susceptibility is increased because many treatments, such as campath-1H and fludarabine, have generalised anti-lymphocyte action and are not absolutely specific for malignant lymphocytes.

Stem cell transplantation

The potential role of stem cell transplantation is increasingly being explored in the management of all types of leukaemia.

The basic principle

This technique provides a means of rescuing the patient from the potentially lethal effects on the bone marrow of ablative therapy given in an attempt to eradicate all traces of disease (Fig. 50.4). The conditioning regimen most commonly used is a combination of high-dose cyclophosphamide and total body irradiation. Other conditioning regimens include high-dose melphalan, etoposide, busulphan or cytarabine.

Following administration of conditioning therapy, 2–3 days elapse to allow its elimination from the body, and then previously harvested stem cells are reinfused peripherally. The stem cells will return to and repopulate the marrow, restoring normal haemopoiesis. Peripheral blood counts recover in 2–4 weeks. Throughout this time, patients require intensive supportive care and the procedure, particularly allogeneic stem cell transplantation, causes significant morbidity and has a mortality rate of 5–30%.

The source of stem cells

During allogeneic stem cell transplantation (allograft), stem cells are obtained from a human leucocyte antigen (HLA)-matched donor. These stem cells can be removed directly from the bone marrow, under general anaesthetic, or harvested from the peripheral blood. Under certain circumstances, in the absence of a matched donor, an autologous bone marrow or peripheral blood stem cell transplant (autograft) can be performed. Following conditioning, the patients receive their own cryopreserved marrow or peripheral blood stem cells, previously harvested from them while in CR. There is a potential risk, however, that stem cells obtained in this way may contain undetected, residual disease. Attempts have been made to purge the bone marrow of disease *in vitro*, but these have generally been unsuccessful.

Peripheral blood stem cell transplantation

This technique for rescuing bone marrow following ablative conditioning therapy is used to restore haemopoiesis (Russell, 1998). Patients receive the haematopoetic growth factor G-CSF, either alone or following an infusion of high-dose chemotherapy such as high-dose cyclophosphamide. Patients receive G-CSF for a period of about 7 days. This stimulates the release of stem cells into the peripheral circulation. Stem cells are then harvested from the peripheral circulation by a process of cell pheresis. The harvested cells can then be reinfused, fresh, into the patient following conditioning therapy or frozen and stored for later use.

Peripheral stem cell transplantation offers some advantages over conventional bone marrow transplant techniques; collection of peripheral stem cells negates the need for general anaesthesia and it has been found that the haemopoietic recovery period following transplantation is shortened by 5–10 days. This technique can also be used to harvest stem cells from allogeneic donors. In this case, G-CSF is used alone to stimulate stem cell release into the peripheral circulation. It is sometimes impossible to harvest enough stem

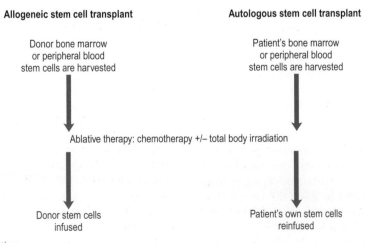

Fig. 50.4 Stem cell transplantation.

cells from patients to allow an autologous transplant to be performed. The commonest reason for this is that the patient has been heavily pretreated with chemotherapy or radiotherapy. A new CXCR4 chemokine antagonist, plerixafor, is now available. This agent is thought to reduce adhesion of stem cells within the bone marrow milieu. It can be given along with G-CSF and allows a proportion of patients who have failed to mobilise stem cells using G-CSF alone to mobilise cells for an autograft.

Complications

Infection is almost inevitable in patients undergoing bone marrow transplantation. Other significant complications of allografts include interstitial pneumonitis and hepatic veno-occlusive disease, but the major life-threatening complication is acute graft-versus-host disease (GVHD). The likelihood of graft-versus-host disease occurring increases with age, and for this reason, myeloblative allografts are largely restricted to patients under 45 years of age. Graft-versus-host disease is caused by T-lymphocytes in the donated marrow reacting to host tissues. The severity of the reaction ranges from a mild maculopapular rash to multisystem organ failure with a high mortality rate. Acute graft-versus-host disease typically occurs within 100 days of the bone marrow transplantation and typically presents with fever, rash, diarrhoea and liver dysfunction. Prophylactic therapy is routinely given with methotrexate or ciclosporin, alone or in combination, for 6–12 months post-transplant. Should acute graft-versus-host disease develop, high-dose methylprednisolone, ciclosporin, antithymocyte globulin and, more recently, anticytokine monoclonal antibodies, for example, anti-TNF (tumour necrosis factor) antibodies, have been used to treat the condition.

Chronic graft-versus-host disease can occur after 3 months following bone marrow transplantation. It is a multisystem disorder associated with chronic hepatitis, severe skin inflammation and profound immunosuppression. Treatment is successful in approximately 50% of patients and consists of immunosuppression with azathioprine and prednisolone together with prophylactic antibiotics. Ciclosporin and thalidomide have also been used successfully in the treatment of chronic steroid-refractory graft-versus-host disease. The main cause of death amongst patients with chronic graft-versus-host disease is infection.

Reduced intensity allografting

Myeloablative allogeneic transplantation, as described earlier, is a very intensive procedure associated with significant morbidity and mortality, hence its restriction to younger patients. Attempts have been made to reduce the intensity of transplant conditioning regimens whilst using increased immunosuppression to facilitate marrow engraftment. Although such an approach reduces the intensity of therapy delivered to any residual tumour, the possible downside of this reduction is offset by an immunological graft-versus-tumour effect and by reduced early post-transplant mortality. This form of

Table 50.6 Indications for allogeneic stem cell transplantation in leukaemia

AML	First remission with the exception of patients with good risk genetic abnormalities: t(15;17), t(8;21) and inversion of chromosome 16
CML	Chronic phase but only if patient fails to respond to first- and second-line tyrosine kinase inhibitors
ALL	First remission in adults Second remission in children
CLL	Not generally appropriate as part of standard therapy but under investigation within several clinical studies

transplant is often offered to older patients who are considered unfit to receive a standard allograft. However, the long-term outcomes of this approach are under continual review. Several trials now suggest that the overall survival after myeloablative and reduced intensity transplants may be similar though the causes of death in the two groups are different. More patients die of disease relapse after reduced intensity transplants, and more die of transplant-related complications in the myeloablative group (Pollack et al., 2009).

The place of stem cell transplantation

The place of stem cell transplantation in the management of a particular form of leukaemia depends very much on the prognosis of patients treated with conventional chemotherapy (Table 50.6). For example, the results of intensive chemotherapy in children with ALL are good, and bone marrow transplantation is generally only considered for children who have relapsed and in whom a second remission can be achieved. However, conventional treatment of adults is less successful, and allogeneic bone marrow transplantation may be offered to adults in first remission.

Patient care

Supportive care

The treatment of CLL and CML is largely carried out on a hospital outpatient basis, with patients taking oral medication at home or attending outpatient clinics on a weekly or monthly basis for injections of chemotherapy. Patients are routinely monitored to follow the progress of disease and to observe treatment-related side effects. Supportive therapy such as blood transfusions can also be given on an outpatient basis. In contrast, the intensity of induction and consolidation regimens used in the management of patients with acute leukaemia renders them severely pancytopenic. Therapy is usually given as a hospital inpatient with patients often remaining in hospital following treatment for 3–4 weeks until their bone marrow recovers sufficiently. This is in contrast to therapy for most solid tumours where, following administration of treatment, patients are often well enough to remain at home until their next cycle of chemotherapy is due.

Advanced leukaemia, bone marrow transplantation and aggressive chemotherapy for acute leukaemia all result in pancytopenia. Red cell transfusions are given to patients to maintain their haemoglobin above 9–10 g/dL. Evidence of bleeding includes petechial haemorrhages in skin and mucous membranes, and patients receiving aggressive treatment must be examined daily for any of the above signs. Platelet concentrates are given to thrombocytopenic patients who have signs of bleeding and are given prophylactically should platelets fall below 10×10^9 L^{-1}. The probability of infection developing rises as the WBC, specifically the neutrophil count, falls. With an absolute neutrophil count of below 0.5×10^9 L^{-1}, patients are at high risk of infection, with the risks being even greater if the period of neutropenia is prolonged.

Chapters 51 and 52 examine many of the non-haematological toxicities which result from the use of cytotoxic drugs, and these are clearly pertinent to haematology patients. The major contributors to morbidity and mortality in patients with leukaemia are relapsed disease and infection.

Infection in the immunocompromised patient

A number of intrinsic and extrinsic factors all contribute to the risk of infection in this vulnerable group of patients (Fig. 50.5).

While cross-infection can occur via staff, other patients or contaminated objects, the main sources of infection in this group of patients are endogenous, arising from commensal gut and skin organisms. The normal host defences to infection are broken down; damage to mucous membranes, particularly in the gastro-intestinal tract, occurs with chemotherapy and radiotherapy, allowing infecting organisms to enter the bloodstream. Most infections in neutropenic patients arise from three main sites: the gastro-intestinal and respiratory tracts, and the skin. Table 50.7 lists the main pathogens responsible for infection in this group of patients.

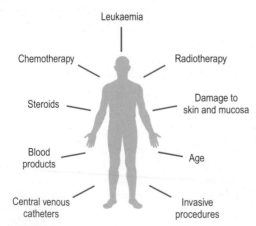

Fig. 50.5 Infection risk in immunocompromised patients.

Table 50.7 Pathogens commonly causing infection in neutropenic patients

Gram-negative bacteria	*Pseudomonas* spp. *Escherichia coli* *Klebsiella* spp. *Enterobacter* spp. *Proteus* spp. *Serratia* spp. *Legionella pneumophilia*
Gram-positive bacteria	*Streptococcus* spp. *Staphylococcus epidermidis* *Staphylococcus aureus*
Anaerobes	*Clostridium difficile* *Clostridium perfringens* *Bacteroides* spp.
Fungi	*Candida* spp. *Aspergillus* spp.
Viruses	Herpes simplex Herpes zoster Cytomegalovirus Hepatitis
Protozoa	*Pneumocystis carinii*

Preventive measures

Oral hygiene. Mouth care is important in all patients receiving chemotherapy but particularly neutropenic patients. Patients are generally asked to use mouthwashes regularly, and prophylactic antifungal therapy may also be given. Although it is important to avoid any sort of trauma to the oral mucosa, teeth should be cleaned regularly using a soft toothbrush. Attention must also be paid to the care of dentures. Patients require careful counselling on mouth care, stressing the importance of oral hygiene.

Prophylactic anti-infectives. In general, prophylactic antibiotics are avoided because of the possible development of resistant organisms, but they may have a place in the management of periods of prolonged myelosuppression following chemotherapy and bone marrow transplantation. Prophylactic antifungal agents are often given and patients undergoing bone marrow transplantation and therapy for ALL require prophylaxis against herpes virus and *Pneumocystis carinii* (Table 50.8).

Gut decontamination. Gut decontamination using a combination of non-absorbable oral antibiotics and antifungal agents reduces the burden of potentially pathogenic organisms in the intestine. One such combination includes neomycin sulphate, colistin sulphate, nystatin and amphotericin. However, opinions are divided over this practice, as gut decontamination can lead to the overgrowth of resistant organisms.

Growth factors. An exciting development in the care of patients with leukaemia has been the production of haemopoietic growth factors using recombinant DNA technology. The first of these, G-CSF, given daily by subcutaneous

Table 50.8 Prophylactic anti-infectives

Gram-negative bacteria	Ciprofloxacin
Candidiasis	Nystatin Fluconazole Itraconazole
Herpes simplex	Aciclovir
Pneumocystis carinii	Co-trimoxazole

injection or intravenous infusion after completion of chemotherapy, stimulates neutrophil production and may reduce the duration of neutropenia by up to 7 days. The cost of these compounds is a major issue and results of studies investigating the effects of G-CSF on morbidity and mortality, following chemotherapy, have been disappointing (Smith et al., 2006). Newer pegylated growth factors have been introduced. These have a longer half-life than standard agents, and thus fewer injections are required. The impact of these agents on morbidity and mortality post-chemotherapy, however, remains controversial.

Aseptic technique. Careful attention should be paid to the care of intravenous cannulae, particularly central venous catheters. The increased incidence of staphylococcal infection in immunocompromised patients can largely be attributed to their use. Invasive procedures, such as venepuncture, must be carried out using strict aseptic technique. Similarly, urinary catheters are a major source of infection and their use should be avoided if at all possible.

Protective isolation. Reverse barrier isolation during periods of neutropenia, nursing in strict sterile environments and high-efficiency particulate air (HEPA) filtration have been used in an attempt to reduce infection rates. This is extremely demanding for staff and patients alike and is generally only appropriate following bone marrow transplantation.

Treatment of infection

Commonly, neutropenic patients show no signs of focal infection; they are unable to form pus. The only clinical manifestations of septicaemia might be general malaise, fever or hypotension. A patient's condition can deteriorate very rapidly, with collapse occurring within hours of the first signs of infection. Treatment should be instigated as soon as infection is suspected. Following a clinically serious febrile episode (temperature: 37.5 °C for more than 1 h or 38 °C or more on a single reading), samples are taken for culture; these may include blood, urine, sputum and stool cultures along with line and throat swabs. Intravenous antibiotics must be started empirically without delay (Sipsas et al., 2005). Standard empirical therapy varies from unit to unit but may involve the combination of an aminoglycoside with an antipseudomonal penicillin such as piperacillin to provide broad-spectrum bactericidal cover. In penicillin-allergic patients, ceftazidime or cefotaxime may be substituted, but local resistance patterns are of paramount importance. Antibiotics with a broad spectrum of activity, such as ciprofloxacin, have been used as single agents.

Vancomycin or teicoplanin are often prescribed if an infected central venous catheter is suspected, to provide additional cover against Gram-positive organisms. Microbiological advice should be sought in cases of methicillin-resistant *Staphylococcus aureus* (MRSA) infection. Metronidazole may be added to the antibiotic regimen to cover anaerobes if the clinical presentation suggests that the source of the infection may be oral, perineal or gut. Anti-infective therapy should subsequently be modified on the basis of cultures, but in the majority of neutropenic patients, a causative organism is never identified.

If the pyrexia persists for more than 4 days in spite of broad-spectrum antibiotics, or if the patient's condition is deteriorating, systemic fungal infection should be suspected. Empirical antifungal therapy for neutropenic patients with antibiotic-resistant fever reduces mortality and is considered a standard of care. A number of broad-spectrum agents are now available for use in this setting, including standard amphotericin, lipid formulation of amphotericin, caspofungin and voriconazole. Intravenous amphotericin is often the first choice to ensure that *Aspergillus* and *Candida* are covered. The main limitation of amphotericin is its toxicity, in particular, nephrotoxicity. Lipid formulation of amphotericin may be appropriate in patients with pre-existing renal impairment or in cases where conventional amphotericin has induced nephrotoxicity. Voriconazole is a useful agent with a similarly broad spectrum of activity. Hepatotoxicity, visual disturbances and prolonged QT interval are the most common side effects of voriconazole. This agent has the advantage of being available as both intravenous and oral preparations, so the conversion from parenteral to oral therapy is straightforward.

Although the antifungal activity of the echinocandin, caspofungin, is more limited than that of amphotericin or voriconazole, it has been shown to be effective for empirical therapy as it has good efficacy against *Candida* and *Aspergillus* spp. It has the advantage of reduced toxicity in comparison with other available agents. The most common side effect is hepatotoxicity. Since this agent has a relatively limited spectrum of activity, it is probably best avoided in the setting of presumed fungal sinus or CNS infection, which are often caused by fungi other than *Aspergillus* or *Candida* spp. Table 50.9 lists some of the common problems encountered in the treatment of the leukaemias.

The following practice points should be used to control infection in immunocompromised patients.

- Measures to prevent infection are important.
- Particular attention should be paid to scrupulous hand washing, mouth care and the use of antifungal, antiviral and antipneumocystis prophylaxis for patients at high risk.
- Preventive measures do not eliminate the risk of infection.
- Treatment of fever in a neutropenic patient is a medical emergency.
- Empirical antifungal therapy should be used to treat neutropenic patients with antibiotic resistant fever, at high risk of fungal infection.

Table 50.9 Common therapeutic problems in the leukaemias

Problem	Cause	Solutions
Mucositis and oral ulceration	Chemotherapeutic agents directly toxic to mucosal epithelium Radiotherapy is directly toxic to the mucosa and also reduces saliva production by salivary glands Vulnerable mucosa is likely to be attacked by infective agents, for example, herpes simplex, *candida*	Regular mouth toilet including the use of antibacterial mouthwash Prophylactic use of antiviral and antifungal agents for patients in whom myelosuppression is likely to be prolonged
Fever in neutropenic patients	Infection predominantly caused by bacteria and/or fungi	Broad-spectrum antibiotics must be commenced as soon as blood cultures have been taken A strategy of planned progressive therapy including use of an antifungal agent in non-responsive fever is appropriate
Graft-versus-host disease (GVHD)	T lymphocytes from the donor react against host tissues	Use a sibling donor if possible Use the donor most closely HLA matched to the patient Consider T-cell depletion of graft (though this may increase the risk of disease relapse) Prophylactic therapy with methotrexate and ciclosporin Treat GVHD with corticosteroids, ciclosporin, anti-thymocyte, globulin, FK 506, anticytokine monoclonal antibodies Irradiate all blood products
Late complications of treatment	Risks of haemopoietic malignancy and non-haemopoietic malignancy are increased post-chemotherapy Late cardiotoxicity secondary to anthracyclines	Aim to tailor therapy to the underlying disease, that is, do not overtreat and do not undertreat Do not exceed maximum cumulative doses of anthracyclines Liposomal anthracyclines may be useful in the future

Case studies

Case 50.1

A 30-year-old woman recently diagnosed with CML attends the haematology clinic to discuss the options for treatment.

Questions

1. Which treatment options are available?
2. Which treatment is likely to be the best choice for this patient?

Answers

1. There are clearly a number of potential treatment options which need to be explored with the patient.
   The various treatment options are:

   - palliative therapy with hydroxycarbamide to control cell counts
   - interferon-α
   - interferon-α and cytosine
   - imatinib
   - allogeneic matched sibling transplant

   - matched unrelated donor (MUD) transplantation if a matched sibling is not available
   - treatment as part of a clinical trial which is likely to involve imatinib in varying doses or in combination with other effective agent.

2. A purely palliative approach is unlikely to be acceptable to a young patient, but hydroxycarbamide can still be used acutely to control high cell counts. There is no doubt that use of interferon-α alone results in cytogenetic remission in a small percentage of patients, and this effect is enhanced by the addition of cytosine. The side effects of interferon-α include flu-like and affective symptoms. The addition of cytosine increases myelosuppression and risk of mucositis. Although these treatments can induce cytogenetic remission, the duration of such responses is unclear and only a minority of patients respond completely. The high risk of side effects and the low chance of complete cytogenetic response to interferon-α, with or without cytosine, are likely to make these therapeutic modalities unattractive to this patient.

   It remains true that allogeneic stem cell transplantation is the only proven curative therapy for patients with CML. The difficulty with this approach is that the mortality rate for transplant recipients remains high. The 1-year mortality rate for a 30-year-old patient transplanted using a sibling donor is approximately 15–20%, and this may rise to 25–30% if a MUD has to be used. The major causes of death in this group are GVHD and infection. In addition to this high risk of mortality in the short-term, there is also a risk of long-term morbidity post-allograft. Chronic graft-versus-host disease can have a significant impact on quality of life for many patients and requires long-term medical follow-up. Ironically, patients with a degree of chronic graft-versus-host disease are at reduced risk of disease relapse since a graft-versus-host response is also associated with a graft-versus-leukaemia effect; some disparity between the immune systems of the transplant donor and recipient is helpful. In addition to these problems, all transplanted patients are at increased risk of a second malignancy developing later in life as a consequence of the conditioning therapy received as part of the transplant and probably also as a consequence of deficiencies within the transplanted immune system.

Given the problems associated with the various therapeutic strategies discussed earlier, it is not surprising that there was great excitement surrounding the development of a targeted tyrosine kinase inhibitor, imatinib. Results with this agent, particularly for patients with newly diagnosed chronic phase disease, are excellent. Complete cytogenetic responses have been seen, although very sensitive quantitative PCR techniques can still detect the abnormal BCR-ABL gene in the vast majority of CML patients in whom the Philadelphia chromosome itself is undetectable. In addition, the drug has been shown to delay progression to accelerated phase disease or blast crisis. It is still not possible, however, to say that imatinib cures patients with CML.

Although no randomised study has been undertaken, it is clear from historical data that, in the short-term, the mortality associated with allogeneic stem cell transplantation far exceeds that associated with imatinib. In addition to these very encouraging data which pertain to the effect of the drug on the disease, the side effects of imatinib are generally mild and patients report this agent far easier to tolerate than interferon-α. The main side effects are rash, cytopenias, fluid retention and abnormalities of liver function tests.

Given the efficacy of imatinib and the fact that the drug is generally very well tolerated, imatinib is regarded as the initial treatment of choice for the vast majority of patients with CML. Ongoing management involves haematological and molecular monitoring of the patient to determine whether they have a good response to imatinib. In the event of a good response, the patient continues to take the drug. If at a later stage the molecular response to the agent begins to diminish, then transplantation is reconsidered. Amongst patients who fail to respond or respond poorly to imatinib, transplantation options are likely to be considered at an earlier stage.

Case 50.2

A patient with AML is currently in first CR and has a fully HLA-matched brother who is medically fit. You have been asked to counsel the potential transplant donor about stem cell collection.

Questions

1. What methods are available for the collection of stem cells for haemopoietic stem cell transplantation?
2. What are the advantages and disadvantages of each of these stem cell collection methods for the transplant donor?
3. What are the advantages and disadvantages of each of these stem cell collection methods for the transplant recipient?

Answers

1. There are two main methods of collection of haemopoietic stem cells from a sibling donor. These are:

   - direct harvesting of cells from the bone marrow in the pelvis;
   - collection of circulating peripheral blood stem cells using an apheresis technique after stimulation of the stem cell compartment using (G-CSF).

2. Direct harvesting of marrow stem cell from the bone marrow is an operative procedure and is performed under general anaesthetic. Clearly, there are risks associated with the use of general anaesthesia, but the risk of death associated with this approach is less than 1 in 10,000 procedures. Marrow harvesting involves a hospital stay, usually for one night post-operatively, but some units also require donors to be admitted the night before surgery. Donors are likely to experience pain around the pelvis, and there is a risk of mechanical back pain in the short to medium term due to pressure applied to the pelvis during repeated needle insertions. This risk is increased in those with a history of back problems prior to the procedure. Indeed, such potential donors may prefer a peripheral blood stem cell harvesting approach. Donors must be warned about bruising and potential infection at the site of their wounds.

   One of the other potential problems associated with marrow harvesting is that it is impossible to select the type of blood cell harvested and a large component of the volume of fluid collected comprises red blood cells. This can lead to a degree of anaemia in the donor who may take several weeks to normalise their haemoglobin. It is usually possible to avoid blood transfusion in this situation as it is unusual for donors to be significantly symptomatic. Nonetheless, donors must be warned that the need for allogeneic blood transfusion is a possibility with this procedure.

   Peripheral blood stem cell harvesting has several advantages over direct marrow harvesting from the iliac crests. The procedure can be undertaken during hospital outpatient visits and does not require the use of a general anaesthetic. As the stem cell-harvesting procedure allows selective collection of mononuclear cells, significant anaemia is very unlikely after this procedure. Clearly, red cells do circulate within the apheresis circuit, and if the circuit clots off and has to be disconnected from the donor, then red cells will be lost. This is unlikely to be of clinical significance unless the donor is a child and hence has a relatively low blood volume.

   Disadvantages of this approach include the need for stimulation of donor haemopoiesis by the G-CSF.

   Marrow stimulation can result in significant pain especially around the shoulders, back and pelvic girdle. Most donors can manage this pain at home with simple analgesia, but very occasionally hospital admission is required for pain control. Very occasionally patients develop splenic pain, and there have been a couple of reports of splenic rupture in normal donors after G-CSF stimulation, but this is very rare. One difficulty with the use of G-CSF is that it has only been in routine use for the past 15 years. This makes it impossible to categorically reassure potential stem cell donors that use of G-CSF in this way is absolutely safe in the long-term. There is, however, currently no evidence that acting as a peripheral blood stem cell donor increases one's risk of leukaemia development later in life. Some potential donors find this element of uncertainty difficult and prefer to undertake a marrow harvest in which the risks, although present, are better quantified.

   The apheresis procedure itself involves the donor lying relatively still with a needle in one or both arms (depending upon the type of apheresis kit used) for approximately 4–5 h. Some collections can be done in one procedure, but some donors will need to be harvested in two procedures, over 2 days.

One prerequisite for peripheral blood stem cell donation is that the potential donor has good enough peripheral veins to allow reliable venous access. If this is not the case and the donor prefers to donate using this method, a temporary central venous line has to be inserted.

Most donors tolerate the apheresis procedure with few problems. One of the most common complications of the procedure is hypocalcaemia which results from calcium binding by the citrate anticoagulant used to prevent clotting within the apheresis circuit. Donors may notice perioral tingling or paraesthesia in other areas and are asked to report this immediately. The problem is easily treated by reducing the concentration of anticoagulant in the circuit and by asking the donor to drink a small amount of milk. If this problem is not picked up early, the consequences can be more severe, with the development of tetany which would require intravenous calcium replacement.

In summary, peripheral blood stem cell donation is generally a less invasive and better-tolerated procedure than direct stem cell harvest from the marrow space. However, the associated procedural risks are more easily quantifiable for the latter procedure.

3. There are some potential advantages, to the transplant recipient, in the use of peripheral blood stem cells as opposed to bone marrow stem cells. Engraftment is quicker, so the recipient spends less time in the neutropenic phase, and hence the risk of infection is reduced. Similarly, there is evidence that duration of hospital stay is reduced when peripheral blood stem cells are used. One potential disadvantage of this approach is that the graft includes a larger dose of T-lymphocytes than a graft of stem cells derived directly from the marrow (approximately a 10-fold increase). There is some evidence that rates of chronic graft-versus-host disease are increased amongst recipients of peripheral blood stem cells, but this observation has not been borne out in all studies. This potential disadvantage of peripheral blood stem cells is negated if a T-cell-depleted approach is used, as is the case for most matched unrelated procedures.

Case 50.3

A 25-year-old woman is admitted with newly diagnosed AML. Once her condition is stabilised, the consultant seeks her consent to start intensive chemotherapy.

Questions

1. How should the consultant ensure the consent process is performed as well as possible?
2. What side effects should the consultant discuss?

Answers

1. It is vital that consent is taken only after very careful discussions. Consent for such intensive chemotherapy usually requires several conversations. The final consent conversation should be done in a quiet private room if possible, and interruptions should be kept to a minimum. The patient should be allowed to have a friend, partner or relative present if they wish, and ideally a clinical nurse specialist should be present too. If possible, the patient should be given some written material on chemotherapy before consent even if it is important the treatment is started promptly. The patient should be given a clear explanation of their potential treatment options and should be informed of any clinical trials that may be available to them. It is vitally important to fully inform patients regarding their condition and its prognosis, and about treatment options and their potential advantages

and disadvantages. Only if the patient has all the necessary information can they decide on the treatment option that is most appropriate/acceptable to their individual circumstances.

2. The consent discussion should include a discussion of all common side effects and less common but severe side effects of treatment. Common side effects of AML chemotherapy would include nausea, vomiting, mucositis, tiredness, malaise, infections, hair loss, bleeding and anaemia. Patients should be warned that they will require transfusions of blood and platelets. They will always need good venous access and usually a Hickman or other long-term in-dwelling central line. They will need to be warned they will have to spend at least 3–4 weeks in hospital. Severe side effects may include infertility and a premature menopause in young women. Options for the prevention and treatment of infertility must be discussed before treatments commences. Anthracyclines can be associated with cardiac problems, infections and bleeding can be life threatening and patients must be warned that they may not respond to therapy or may relapse after treatment. They should also be warned that a cure cannot be guaranteed. There is a risk of treatment-related mortality of around 1–2%. Longer-term risks include a greater lifetime risk of cancers including skin cancer and lung cancer, particularly in smokers.

Case 50.4

A 24-year-old patient with ALL is undergoing chemotherapy and needs intrathecal chemotherapy to prevent relapse in the meninges. Giving drugs by this route is EXTREMELY DANGEROUS. Several patients have died as a result of the inadvertent administration of vinca alkaloids into the CSF.

Question

What steps have been taken nationally to try to prevent the inadvertent intrathecal injection of vincristine and other agents not suitable for intrathecal use?

Answer

In the UK, there are now strict guidelines for administration of intrathecal chemotherapy. It can only be performed in hospital units which have passed a rigorous peer review process. The procedure must be undertaken in a specially designated area. Intravenous drugs must not be given in this area. The intrathecal drugs must only be prescribed by a consultant or specialist registrar who has been trained to prescribe or give intrathecal chemotherapy and whose name appears on a locally held register. Drugs for intrathecal administration must only be prescribed on a specially designated prescription sheet. Once the prescription has arrived in pharmacy, the drugs must be manufactured and checked by pharmacists trained in the manufacture and checking of intrathecal prescriptions. The drugs must be positively labelled 'for intrathecal use only' and must be dispensed by a trained pharmacist. They can only be dispensed once the patient has been given any intravenous drugs that are due that day. The doctor collecting the drugs must sign to confirm that the i.v. drugs, if due, have been given before the drugs are dispensed. The drugs must only be dispensed to a doctor trained and on the register for giving intrathecal drugs. The intrathecal drugs must be transported in a specially designated container, and if they need to be stored, then it must be in a separate, specially designated fridge, that is separate from any intravenous chemotherapy. Once the procedure is under way, the intrathecal drugs must be checked by the registered doctor and by a nurse who has been trained and appears on a register of nurses trained to check intrathecal drugs. The drugs should also be checked by the patient or a patient's representative. Intrathecal drugs must not be given in hospitals not approved for the procedure, in non-designated areas, outside office hours or at the weekend unless there are exceptional circumstances. All staff working on oncology or haematology units should be taught about the rules for giving intrathecal therapy.

In addition, in order to prevent inadvertent vincristine administration into the intrathecal space, hospitals giving intrathecal chemotherapy should follow special rules for labelling vinca alkaloid prescriptions and vinca alkaloids should be made up in a minimum volume of 20 mL in order to prevent intrathecal administration.

Case 50.5

A 37-year-old dental technician presented with acute promyelocytic leukaemia (APL). He had a number of bleeding problems at presentation. He was randomised on an APL trial to be commenced on oral all-trans retinoic acid (ATRA) and arsenic trioxide (ATO).

Questions

1. Why is ATRA used in this circumstance and what are its side effects?
2. Why is ATO used in this circumstance and what are its side effects?

Answers

1. APL is a variant of AML which presents with coagulation defects, low platelet counts and severe bleeding. Patients are at risk of severe haemorrhage at presentation but have a relatively good prognosis with chemotherapy. ATRA can rapidly correct the coagulopathy found at presentation. This agent also increases the likelihood of the patient entering remission, when combined with standard high-dose chemotherapy. It is also used as a maintenance agent and when used with 6-mercaptopurine and methotrexate, it increases the number of patients who remain in long-term remission. The side effects of ATRA include dry eyes and a dry mouth. In addition, ATRA can cause a severe and life-threatening sterile pneumonitis. It is important to recognise this syndrome quickly as it often responds to high-dose dexamethasone and if left untreated leads to respiratory failure and death.

2. ATO has been shown to bring about remission in patients who have APL in association with the 15;17 chromosomal translocation and the PML:RARA genetic abnormality. It is not considered a conventional chemotherapeutic agent and seems to work in a synergistic fashion with ATRA. There is a lot of interest in combining these agents in an attempt to reduce the exposure of these patients to chemotherapy. Side effects include the APL differentiation syndrome, similar to the ATRA differentiation syndrome.

ATO can cause QT interval prolongation and complete atrioventricular block. QT prolongation can lead to a torsade de pointes-type ventricular arrhythmia, which can be fatal. The risk of torsade de pointes is related to the extent of QT prolongation, concomitant administration of QT prolonging drugs, a history of torsade de pointes, pre-existing QT interval prolongation, congestive heart failure, administration of potassium-wasting diuretics or other conditions that result in hypokalemia or hypomagnesemia. Prior to initiating therapy with ATO, a 12-lead ECG should be performed and serum electrolytes (potassium, calcium and magnesium) and creatinine should be assessed; pre-existing electrolyte abnormalities should be corrected and, if possible, drugs that are known to prolong the QT interval should be discontinued. For QTc greater than 500 ms, corrective measures should be completed and the QTc reassessed with serial ECGs prior to considering using ATO.

Case 50.6

A 57-year-old man with a 6-year history of CLL presented with a rising white cell count, worsening lymphadenopathy and hepatosplenomegaly. Treatment was commenced with oral fludarabine 40 mg/m² and oral cyclophosphamide 250 mg/m² daily for 3 days with rituximab given on day 1 (FC-R).

Question

What additional precautions would you advise the physician to take and why?

Answer

Fludarabine, cyclophosphamide and rituximab are a very powerful combination available for the initial treatment of CLL. It has been used as a second-line therapy, although recent data support its use as a first-line therapy. It has been associated with more frequent and deeper remissions which are longer than single-agent therapy. It is a very immunosuppressive combination with activity against both T- and B-cells, and patients treated with this regime are at high risk of developing *Pneumocystis* pneumonia. It is important that patients are given prophylaxis against this severe infection. Herpes virus infections including herpes simplex and herpes zoster are also common, and most patients are given acyclovir prophylaxis.

As patients are immunosuppressed, they are also at risk of developing transfusion related graft-versus-host disease. This is a complication of blood product transfusion, caused by engraftment of lymphocytes from the transfused product, which is frequently fatal. This complication can be prevented by irradiation of blood products prior to transfusion. Rituximab is an antibody-based therapy and can be associated with significant reactions which can occasionally be severe and life threatening (see Chapter 51).

References

Cilloni, D., Saglio, G., 2009. CML: a model for targeted therapy. Balliere's Best Pract. Res. Clin. Haematol. 22, 285–294.

Dohner, H., Estey, E.H., Amadori, S., et al., 2010. Diagnosis and management of acute myeloid leukaemia in adults: recommendations from an international expert panel, on behalf of the European LeukaemiaNet. Blood 115, 453–474.

Hallek, M., Fingerle-Rowson, G., Fink, A.M., et al., 2009. First-line treatment with fludarabine (F), cyclophosphamide (C), and rituximab (R) (FCR) improves overall survival (OS) in previously untreated patients (pts) with advanced chronic lymphocytic leukemia (CLL): results of a randomized phase III trial on behalf of an international group of investigators and the German CLL Study Group. Blood 114, 535.

Hughes, T.P., Kaed, J., Branford, S., et al., 2003. Frequency of major molecular responses to imatinib or interferon-alpha plus cytarabine in newly diagnosed chronic myeloid leukaemia. N. Engl. J. Med. 349, 1423–1432.

Leukaemia and Lymphoma Research, 2010. Disease Facts. Available at: www.beatbloodcancers.org/leukaemia.

O'Brien, S., Guilhot, F., Larson, R.A., et al., 2003. Imatinib compared with interferon and low-dose cytarabine for newly diagnosed chronic-phase chronic myeloid leukaemia. N. Engl. J. Med. 348, 994–1004.

Pollack, S.M., O'Connor Jr., T.P., Hashash, J., et al., 2009. Non-ablative and reduced intensity conditioning for allogeneic hematopoietic stem cell transplantation: a clinical review. Am. J. Clin. Oncol. 32, 618–628.

Rai, K.R., Peterson, B.L., Appelbaum, F.R., et al., 2000. Fludarabine compared with chlorambucil as primary therapy for chronic lymphocytic leukaemia. N. Engl. J. Med. 343, 1750–1757.

Robak, T., Wierzbowska, A., 2009. Current and emerging therapies for acute myeloid leukaemia. Clin. Ther. 31, 2349–2370.

Russell, N.H., 1998. Developments in allogeneic peripheral blood progenitor cell transplantation. Br. J. Haematol. 103, 594–600.

Sanz, M.A., Grimwade, D., Tallman, M.S., et al., 2009. Management of acute promyelocytic leukaemia: recommendations from an expert panel on behalf of European LeukaemiaNet. Blood 113, 1875–1891.

Sawyers, C.L., 1999. Medical progress: chronic myeloid leukaemia. N. Engl. J. Med. 340, 1330–1340.

Sipsas, N.V., Bodey, G.P., Kontoyiannis, D.P., 2005. Perspective for the management of febrile neutropenic patients with cancer in the 21st century. Cancer 103, 1103–1113.

Smith, T.J., Khatcheressian, J., Lyman, G.H., et al., 2006. Update of recommendations for the use of white blood cell growth factors: an evidence-based clinical practice guideline. J. Clin. Oncol. 24, 3187–3205.

Soignet, S., Maslak, P., 2004. Therapy of acute promyelocytic leukaemia. Adv. Pharmacol. 51, 35–58.

Stone, R.M., O'Donnell, M.R., Sekeres, M.A., 2004. Acute myeloid leukaemia. Hematology 2004, 98–117.

Swerdlow, S.H., Campo, E., Harris, N.L., et al., 2008. WHO Classification of Tumours of Haematopoietic and Lymphoid Tissues, fourth ed. IARC Press, Lyon.

Vrooman, L.M., Silverman, L.B., 2009. Childhood ALL: update on prognostic factors. Curr. Opin. Pediatr. 21, 1–8.

Further reading

Hoffbrand, A.V., Pettit, J.E., Moss, P.A.H., 2006. Essential Haematology, fifth ed. Blackwell Publishing, Oxford.

Howard, M.R., Hamilton, P.J., 2007. Haematology: An Illustrated Colour Text, third ed. Churchill Livingstone, Edinburgh.

Negrin, R.S., Blume, K.G., 2005. Allogeneic and autologous hematopoietic stem cell transplantation. In: Kaushansky, K., Lichtman, M.A, Beutler, E., Kipps, T.J., et al. (Eds.), Williams' Hematology. seventh ed. McGraw-Hill Medical Publishing Division, New York.

Provan, D., Gribben, J.G., 2005. Molecular Hematology, second ed. Blackwell Publishing, Oxford.

Lymphomas 51

L. Cameron and C. Loughran

Lymphoma is cancer of the lymphatic system and accounts for approximately 3% of new cases of cancer reported in the UK each year. The primary cancerous cell of origin is the lymphocyte; as a result, there is often considerable overlap between lymphomas and lymphoid leukaemias. Lymphomas are subdivided into two main categories: Hodgkin's lymphoma (HL) and non-Hodgkin's lymphoma (NHL). Both HL and NHL can be further classified based on histology.

The site of malignancy is usually a lymph node. Extranodal disease, most frequently of the stomach, skin, oral cavity and pharynx, small intestine and CNS, can occur and is more common in NHL than HL.

Hodgkin's lymphoma

Hodgkin's disease, now known as HL, was first described by Thomas Hodgkin in 1832. HL accounts for 30% of all lymphomas and has an incidence in the UK of 2.2 per 100,000 for women and 3.3 per 100,000 for men. It is predominantly a disease of young adults, having a peak incidence between the ages of 15 and 35 years.

Aetiology

The cause of HL is unknown, but a number of risk factors have been identified. Epstein–Barr (glandular fever) virus has been identified in 50% of HL cases and is likely to be associated with an increase in risk of developing HL. Certain associations have been identified which suggest a genetic link with HL; for example, same-sex siblings of patients with HL have a 10 times higher risk of developing the disease. Patients with reduced immunity, for example, AIDS or those taking immunosuppressants, may have an increased risk of developing HL.

Pathology

The diagnosis is made by histological examination of an excised lymph node biopsy. The characteristic pathological finding in HL is the identification of a large, abnormal binucleate lymphocyte called a Reed-Sternberg cell. HL as classified by the World Health Organization (WHO) has two distinct entities: classic HL and nodular lymphocyte-predominant Hodgkin's lymphoma (NLPHL). Classic Hodgkin's is further subdivided into four histological types:

- *nodular sclerosis*: this is the most common type in the UK, predominant in young adults and females, and has an excellent prognosis
- *mixed cellularity*: this is second most common type of classic HL and more common in males (70% male)
- *lymphocyte depleted*: this carries a poor prognosis and is more common in HIV-positive individuals
- *lymphocyte rich*: this is a rare type of classic HL

NLPHL accounts for 5% of HL cases and is more common in men.

Signs and symptoms

HL usually presents with painless enlargement of lymph nodes, often in the neck. About 40% of patients will present with fever, night sweats and/or weight loss. These have prognostic significance and are designated B symptoms; others include malaise, itching (25%) or pain at the site of enlarged nodes after drinking alcohol. Bone pain may result from skeletal involvement. Primary involvement of the gut, central nervous system or bone marrow is rare.

If lymph nodes in the chest are involved, patients may present with breathlessness. There is often a disturbance of immune function due to a progressive loss of immunologically competent T-lymphocytes, with patients becoming particularly prone to viral and fungal infections.

Laboratory findings

Laboratory findings include normochromic, normocytic anaemia, a raised erythrocyte sedimentation rate and eosinophilia. One-third of patients have a leucocytosis due to an increase in neutrophils. Advanced disease is associated with lymphopenia (lymphocytes $<0.6 \times 10^9$ L^{-1}). Plasma lactate dehydrogenase (LDH) is raised in 30–40% of patients at diagnosis and has been associated with a poor prognosis.

Investigations and staging

Once the diagnosis has been made on biopsy, further investigations are needed to assess disease activity and the extent of its spread through the lymphoid system or other body sites. This is called staging and is essential for assessing prognosis, with cure rates for localised tumours (stage I or II) being much higher than those for widespread disease (stage IV). The staging of HL is assessed by the Cotswolds modification of the Ann Arbor classification system (Box 51.1). Information about prognostic factors such as mediastinal mass and bulky disease is included in the classification system. The tests required to establish the stage include a complete history, physical examination, FBC, urea and electrolytes (U and Es), chest X-ray and computed tomography (CT). Other useful tests include erythrocyte sedimentation rate (ESR), serum LDH and liver function tests (LFTs). Positron emission tomography (PET) can be used to detect active residual disease.

Management

HL is potentially curable and, in general, sensitive to both chemotherapy and radiotherapy; therefore, the two main goals of treatment are to maximise the likelihood of cure whilst minimising the risk of late toxicity such as infertility. Stage of disease is the biggest factor in treatment choice and outcome. The management of classic HL is determined by the stage of the disease, and this is summarised in Fig. 51.1. Localised NLPHL frequently involves one isolated lymph node and tends to be indolent (slow growing). If there are no risk factors, it can be

Box 51.1 Cotswolds modification of the Ann Arbor classification system for Hodgkin's lymphoma	
Clinical stage	**Defining features**
I	Involvement of a single lymph node region or lymphoid structure
II	Involvement of two or more lymph node regions on the same side of the diaphragm
III	Involvement of lymph node regions or structures on both sides of the diaphragm: III$_1$ – with or without involvement of splenic, hilar, coeliac or portal nodes III$_2$ – with involvement of para-aortic, iliac or mesenteric nodes
IV	Involvement of extranodal site(s) beyond that designated E
Modifying characteristics	A: no symptoms B: fever, drenching sweats, weight loss X: bulky disease >one-third width of the mediastinum >10 cm maximal dimension of nodal mass E: involvement of a single extranodal site, contiguous or proximal to known nodal site CS: clinical stage PS: pathological stage

treated with IFRT alone (30 Gy); all other types are treated as advanced (stage III or IV) classic HL.

In Europe, the treatment of classic HL is determined by whether the disease is staged as early favourable disease, early unfavourable disease, advanced disease or relapsed (see Box 51.2).

Early-stage (favourable) disease

The cure rate for patients with stages I and IIA disease is greater than 90%. Patients with stages I and IIA disease may be cured with radiotherapy alone (wide or extended field irradiation). However, due to radiation-related late effects, cardiac toxicity and secondary malignancy and the incidence of relapse (25–30%), most receive combined modality treatment (chemotherapy and radiotherapy). This usually consists of two to four cycles of ABVD (Adriamycin (doxorubicin), bleomycin, vinblastine, dacarbazine) chemotherapy followed by IFRT of 20–30 Gy (Diehl et al., 2004). The aim of chemotherapy is to destroy subclinical disease outside the field of radiotherapy.

Where disease is confined to above the diaphragm, the mantle field is used (Fig. 51.2). The inverted Y is employed when the disease is confined below the diaphragm. This group of patients have a relapse-free survival rate of 80% at 5–10 years. Patients should be considered for entry into the National Cancer Research Institute (NCRI) 18–30 study or NCRI Lymphoma Groups PET in Hodgkin's Disease Study.

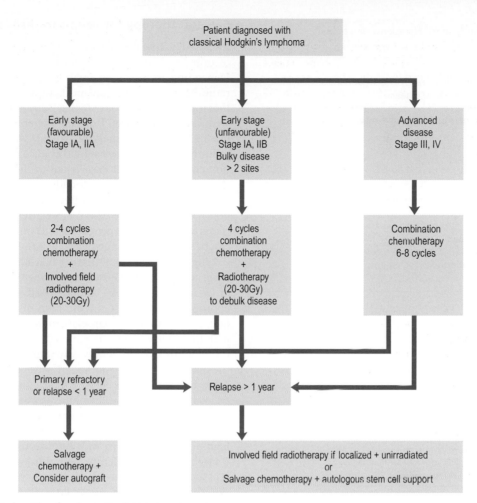

Fig. 51.1 Treatment algorithm for classic Hodgkin's lymphoma.

Early-stage (unfavourable) disease

Patients with stage I or II presenting with bulky disease, B symptoms or with more than two sites of disease are considered to be poor risk if treated with radiotherapy alone. B symptoms are any of the following symptoms: unexplained loss of weight, unexplained fever, drenching night sweats. These patients are treated with four to six cycles of combination chemotherapy, for example, ABVD, and radiotherapy (20–30 Gy) to sites of bulky disease. Patients should be considered for entry into the NCRI 18–30 study.

Advanced disease

Patients with advanced disease (stages III and IV) are treated with combination chemotherapy. The first widely used combination chemotherapy regimen was MOPP (mechlorethamine, vincristine (Oncovin), procarbazine and prednisolone) which produced a response rate of 80% and long-term disease-free survival of approximately 50%. ABVD has replaced MOPP chemotherapy as the regimen of choice as it is as effective but less toxic in terms of fertility, haematological toxicity, and the development of acute leukaemia and myelodysplasia. Six

to eight cycles of ABVD is considered the current standard treatment for advanced disease.

Despite advances in HL, 30–40% of patients progress or relapse and respond poorly to salvage chemotherapy. A number of regimens have been investigated to both increase dose intensity and density of treatment, for example, BEACOPP (bleomycin, etoposide, Adriamycin (doxorubicin), cyclophosphamide, vincristine, procarbazine, prednisolone) and escalated BEACOPP (Table 51.1). In a trial comparing escalated BEACOPP, standard BEACOPP and COPP-ABVD, escalated BEACOPP demonstrated increased overall survival compared with the other two treatment arms but at the cost of significant toxicity (Engert et al., 2009). First-line escalated BEACOPP can only be recommended currently as part of a clinical trial. A study to investigate the role of BEACOPP and PET imaging in patients with advanced HL is under way and will close in 2012 (UK Clinical Research Network Study Portfolio, 2010).

Other options for patients unlikely to tolerate ABVD include ChlVPP (chlorambucil, vinblastine, procarbazine, prednisolone) and CHOP (cyclophosphamide, doxorubicin (hydroxydaonorubicin), vincristine (Oncovin), prednisolone, rituximab.

Box 51.2 Disease staging for Hodgkin's lymphoma (West of Scotland Blood Cancer Network, 2009)

Early stage
European Organisation for Research and Treatment of Cancer (EORTC) risk factors in localised disease

A. Favourable (patients must have all features)
1. Clinical stage 1 or 2
2. Maximum of three nodal areas involved
3. Age less than 50 years of age
4. ESR< 50 mm/h
5. Mediastinal/thoracic mass ratio < 0.33 at D5/6

B. Unfavourable
1. Clinical stage 2 with 4 or more nodal areas involved
2. Age >50 years of age
3. ESR >50 mm/h without B symptoms or >30 mm/h with B symptoms (fever, night sweats, weight loss)
4. Mediastinal/thoracic ratio >0.33 at D5/6ᵃ

Advanced stage
Hasenclever score
1. Age >45 years of age
2. Male gender
3. Serum albumin <40 g/L
4. Hb <10.5 g/dL
5. Stage 4 disease
6. Leucocytosis, that is, WCC >15 × 10^9 L^{-1}
7. Lymphopenia, that is, <0.6 × 10^9 L^{-1} or <8% of total WCC

ᵃMediastinal/thoracic ratio >0.33 at D5/6 – thoracic ratio of maximum transverse mass diameter greater than or equal to one-third (0.33) of the internal transverse thoracic diameter measured at the T5/6 intervertebral disc level.

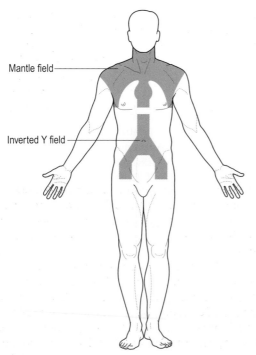

Mantle field

Inverted Y field

Fig. 51.2 The mantle and inverted Y fields commonly employed in the treatment of Hodgkin's lymphoma with radiotherapy (from Souhami and Tobias, 1998, p. 437, with permission from Blackwell Science).

Salvage therapy for relapsed disease

Relapsed disease refers to disease progression after completion of primary treatment which resulted in a complete remission. Depending on previous treatment, options include salvage radiotherapy, salvage chemotherapy or high-dose chemotherapy with autologous stem cell support. In this procedure, stem cells are collected from the patient and returned following high-dose chemotherapy. Patients who relapse after initial radiotherapy alone have a good chance of cure with combination chemotherapy, at least equal to that of patients initially treated with chemotherapy for advanced disease. Occasionally, radiotherapy is used if the disease is localised and previously non-irradiated. Those who relapse after combination chemotherapy have a worse prognosis, although durable remissions can be obtained with further conventional therapy.

Length of remission following first-line chemotherapy influences the success of subsequent salvage therapy and so failure of chemotherapy can be used to classify disease and determine appropriate therapy. If the duration of remission was greater than 12 months (late relapse), then the patient can be re-treated with their initial chemotherapy, salvage regimen or considered for high-dose chemotherapy with autologous transplantation.

Commonly used chemotherapy salvage regimens are listed in Table 51.2. If relapse occurs less than a year after treatment (early relapse), then high-dose chemotherapy with autologous stem cell support should be considered. A patient who has never achieved complete remission (primary refractory disease) should receive high-dose chemotherapy with autologous stem cell support.

High-dose chemotherapy plus autologous stem cell support is associated with a 40–50% 5-year survival rate. However, the significant toxicity of autologous stem cell transplantation means that it should be reserved for patients in whom there is a clear increase in chance of cure. Allogeneic transplant is an option in patients relapsing after autologous transplant (Brusamolino et al., 2009).

New agents

The anti-CD20 antibody rituximab has shown remission in 80% of cases of NLPHL, but due to short follow-up, its use is still considered experimental. Other monoclonal antibodies targeting CD30, which is expressed in the majority of classic HL cases, are being investigated. The most promising of these is a novel immunotoxin conjugate SGN-35 (Younes, 2009).

Panobinostat, a histone deacetylases (HDAC) inhibitor, has been granted orphan drug designation for the treatment of HL.

Gemcitabine has shown activity in relapsed classic HL with response rates up to 79% in a small series of heavily pretreated patients (Ng et al., 2005). Bortezomib and lenalidomide licensed for myeloma are also being investigated in those who have relapsed HL.

Non-Hodgkin's lymphoma

The NHLs are a heterogeneous group of lymphoid malignancies ranging from indolent, slow-growing tumours to aggressive, rapidly fatal disease. Paradoxically, the

Table 51.1 Combination chemotherapy regimens effective in the treatment of Hodgkin's lymphoma

Regimen	Dose and route	Frequency
ABVD (28-day cycle)		
Doxorubicin	25 mg/m^2 i.v.	Days 1 and 15
Bleomycin	10,000 iu/m^2 i.v.	Days 1 and 15
Vinblastine	6 mg/m^2 i.v.	Days 1 and 15
Dacarbazine	375 mg/m^2 i.v.	Days 1 and 15
BEACOPP escalated (21-day cycle)[a]		
Bleomycin	10,000 iu/m^2 i.v.	Day 8
Etoposide	200 mg/m^2 i.v.	Days 1–3
Adriamycin (doxorubicin)	35 mg/m^2 i.v.	Day 1
Cyclophosphamide	1250 mg/m^2 i.v.	Day 1
Vincristine	1.4 mg/m^2 i.v. (max. 2 mg)	Day 8
Procarbazine	100 mg/m^2 orally	Days 1–7
Prednisolone	40 mg/m^2 orally	Days 1–14
BEACOPP standard dose (21-day cycle)[a]		
Bleomycin	10,000 iu/m^2 i.v.	Day 8
Etoposide	100 mg/m^2 i.v.	Days 1–3
Adriamycin (doxorubicin)	25 mg/m^2 i.v.	Day 1
Cyclophosphamide	650 mg/m^2 i.v.	Day 1
Vincristine	1.4 mg/m^2 i.v. (max. 2 mg)	Day 8
Procarbazine	100 mg/m^2 orally	Days 1–7
Prednisolone	40 mg/m^2 orally	Days 1–14
ChlVPP		
Chlorambucil	6 mg/m^2 orally	Days 1–14
Vinblastine	6 mg/m^2 i.v.	Days 1 and 8
Procarbazine	100 mg/m^2 orally	Days 1–14
Prednisolone	40 mg/m^2 orally (max 60 mg)	Days 1–14

[a]Escalated BEACOPP and standard BEACOPP have shown activity in Hodgkin's lymphoma, but their usage is not standard in the UK.

Table 51.2 Salvage chemotherapy regimens effective in the treatment of lymphoma

Regimen	Dose and route	Frequency
DHAP		
Cisplatin	100 mg/m^2 i.v.	Days 1
Cytarabine	2000 mg/m^2 i.v. 12 hourly	Day 2
Dexamethasone	40 mg orally	Days 1–4
ESHAP		
Etoposide	40 mg/m^2 i.v.	Days 1–4
Methylprednisolone	500 mg/m^2 i.v.	Days 1–5
Cytarabine	2000 mg/m^2 i.v.	Day 1
Cisplatin	25 mg/m^2 i.v.	Days 1–4
ICE		
Ifosfamide	5000 mg/m^2 i.v.	Day 2
Carboplatin[a]	AUC 5 i.v.	Day 2
Etoposide	100 mg/m^2 i.v.	Days 1–3
IVE		
Epirubicin	50 mg/m^2 i.v.	Days 1
Etoposide	200 mg/m^2 i.v.	Days 1–3
Ifosfamide	3000 mg/m^2 i.v.	Days 1–3

AUC, area under the curve; GFR, glomerular filtration rate.
[a]Carboplatin dose (mg) = target AUC (mg/mL × min) × (GFR (mL/min) + 25).

more aggressive NHLs are more susceptible to anticancer therapy. The overall incidence of NHL in the UK is 11 per 100,000 per year and accounts for approximately 3% of all cancers in the UK. The disease is rare in subjects under 30 years of age and the incidence steadily increases with increasing age; the median age at presentation is about 60. NHL is slightly more common in men than in women (1.5:1).

Aetiology

The aetiology is unclear although immunosuppression, for example, following organ transplantation, may predispose to the development of lymphoma. Viruses have been implicated in the pathogenesis of NHL; for example, Burkitt's lymphoma is one of the most common neoplasms to develop in HIV-related immunosuppressed patients, human T-lymphotrophic virus type 1 (HTLV-1) is associated with a rare type of T-cell lymphoma, the adult T-cell leukaemia/lymphoma (ATLL) and Epstein–Barr Virus (EBV) is associated with post-transplant lymphoproliferative disorder (PTLD). Exposure to certain chemicals such as pesticides and solvents can increase the risk of developing NHL. There is an increased incidence of gastro-intestinal lymphomas in patients with Crohn's disease.

Signs and symptoms

The most common presentation of NHL is painless lymphadenopathy, frequently in the neck area in the supraclavicular and cervical regions. Spread of disease is haematogenously (via the blood), and so extranodal sites may be involved. Signs and symptoms of infection, anaemia or thrombocytopenia may be present in patients with bone marrow involvement. Hepatosplenomegaly may also be present. Patients may also present with any of the following symptoms: unexplained loss of weight, unexplained fever, drenching night sweats. These symptoms are described as B symptoms and patients without these symptoms are classified as category A. B symptoms are more commonly seen in advanced or aggressive NHL but may be present in all stages and histological subtypes.

Laboratory findings

Laboratory examinations may reveal anaemia, a raised erythrocyte sedimentation rate and a raised serum LDH level. There may be a reduction in circulating immunoglobulins, and a monoclonal paraprotein may be seen in a small number of cases. The immune disruption caused by the disease may also result in an increased susceptibility to viral infection or autoimmune haemolytic anaemia or thrombocytopenia.

Histopathology and classification

There have been many attempts to classify the NHLs into histological categories that have clinical significance. Despite this, many problems and areas of confusion remain. Approximately 85% of NHLs are of B-cell origin, while 15% are of T-cell origin or are unclassifiable.

There are two classification systems in common use. The Working formulation, developed in 1982, divides the lymphomas into low, intermediate and high grade. More recently, the revised European–American lymphoma (REAL) classification system has been developed (Table 51.3) and adopted by the World Health Organization (Box 51.3) to classify the grade of lymphoma. The REAL/WHO classification incorporates some diagnoses not included in the Working formulation and is a list of lymphomas using morphology, immunophenotype, genotype and clinical behaviour. It recognises the three major categories of lymphoid malignancies: B-cell neoplasms, T-cell/natural killer cell neoplasms and HL. However, in practice, the clinical behaviour of lymphomas informs the treatment strategies employed as these are based on the initial classification into indolent (low grade) or aggressive (intermediate and high grade) NHL. A more biologically relevant classification of lymphoma using the REAL/WHO classification and immunological and molecular characteristics increases the diagnostic specificity and improves selection and targeting of therapy.

Diagnosis

Diagnosis is based on a thorough history, physical examination and investigation of a lymph node. A definitive diagnosis of NHL can only be made by biopsy of pathological lymph

Table 51.3 Clinical grade and frequency of lymphomas in the REAL classification

Diagnosis	% of all cases
Indolent lymphomas	
Follicular lymphoma	22
Marginal zone B-cell, mucosa-associated lymphoid tissue	8
Chronic lymphocytic leukaemia/small lymphocytic lymphoma	7
Marginal zone B-cell nodal	2
Lymphoplasmacytic lymphoma	1
Aggressive lymphoma	
Diffuse large B-cell lymphoma	31
Mature (peripheral) T-cell lymphomas	8
Mantle cell lymphoma	7
Mediastinal large B-cell lymphoma	2
Anaplastic large cell lymphoma	2
Very aggressive lymphomas	
Burkitt's lymphoma	2
Precursor T-lymphoblastic	2
Other lymphomas	7

nodes or tumour tissue. An expert histopathologist may need to utilise sophisticated techniques such as immunocytochemistry (e.g. CD20) or genotyping to obtain an accurate subclassification.

Chromosomal abnormalities are of diagnostic importance. Most translocations involve genes associated with either proliferation (e.g. c-MYC) or apoptosis (e.g. BCL-2).

Additional investigations should also be performed to accurately stage the disease and exclude other disease. FBC from peripheral blood and routine biochemistry and uric acid should be performed. Peripheral blood lymphocytosis (increased lymphocytes) with circulating malignant cells is common in low grade and mantle cell lymphomas. A bone marrow aspirate and trephine are required to exclude leukaemia and will detect bone marrow involvement, which is more common than in HL. CT scans of the chest, abdomen and pelvis are required to assess the extent of the disease. The use of PET scans, capable of locating sites not thought to be affected from CT scan images, is increasing. Lumbar punctures should be performed for patients at high risk of CNS involvement, for example, Burkitt's lymphoma. Erythrocyte sedimentation rate, LDH and serum β_2-microglobulin levels may indicate disease activity and can be of prognostic importance.

Staging

Determining the extent of disease in patients with NHL provides prognostic information and is useful in treatment planning. Patients with extensive disease usually require different therapy from those with limited disease. The NHLs can be staged according to the Ann Arbor classification (see Box 51.1). In this system, NHL is defined as stage I, II, III or IV, stage I being disease limited to a single lymph node

Table 51.4 International prognostic index

Factor	Adverse prognosis
Age	≥60 years
Ann Arbor stage	III or IV
Plasma lactate dehydrogenase level	Above normal
Number of extranodal sites of involvement	≥2
Performance status	≥ECOG 2 or equivalent

ECOG, Eastern Co-operative Oncology Group.

it is not curable, patients survive for prolonged periods with minimal symptoms. Aggressive (high-grade) lymphomas result in death within weeks or months if untreated. These lymphomas, however, are very responsive to chemotherapy and up to 50–60% may be cured with combination chemotherapy (Fig. 51.3).

CD20 is essential for cell cycle regulation and cell differentiation. It is expressed on normal B-cells and the majority of malignant B-cell lymphomas. The introduction of rituximab, a monoclonal antibody with specificity for CD20, has changed the way patients with NHL are treated and is now incorporated into most chemotherapy regimens. The mechanism of action of rituximab is not fully understood but is thought to involve complement-mediated lysis of B-cells and antibody-dependent cellular cytotoxicity. Other potential mechanisms include induction of apoptosis and inhibition of cell cycle progression.

Indolent non-Hodgkin's lymphoma

The median age at which patients present with indolent NHLs is 50–60 years, and generally patients have a good performance status. If left untreated, indolent NHL has a comparatively long survival (median: 9 years). Follicular lymphoma is the most common of the indolent lymphomas. For the minority of patients presenting with limited-stage disease (stage I), radiotherapy to the involved field is generally used. However, the majority (80%) of patients present with advanced disease (stages II–IV) where the aim of treatment is to reduce disease bulk and offer symptom relief. Rituximab, cyclophosphamide, vincristine, prednisolone (R-CVP) is used as the first-line treatment for advanced (stage III or IV) follicular lymphoma following the results of a study comparing R-CVP with CVP (cyclophosphamide, vincristine, prednisolone) (Marcus et al., 2005). This approach has been incorporated into national guidance (NICE, 2006). R-CHOP (rituximab, cyclophosphamide, doxorubicin, vincristine, prednisolone) can also be used as first-line treatment for young patients with aggressive disease and is an option in relapsed disease (Table 51.5).

and stage IV being advanced disease, with involvement of extralymphatic sites. The International Prognostic Index (Table 51.4) uses the following factors as predictors of poor prognosis: elevated LDH, stage III or IV disease, greater than 60 years of age, the higher the number of extranodal sites involved and the Eastern Co-operative Oncology Group (ECOG) performance status of two or higher. Other prognostic factors include bulky disease, presence of B symptoms and transformation from low- to high-grade disease. Prognostic indicators are important because they inform the treatment plan to avoid overtreating those with good prognosis and undertreating those with poor prognosis.

Treatment

When designing a treatment plan for an individual patient, various factors must be taken into account. These include the patient's age and general health, the extent or stage of the lymphoma and the particular histological subtype. Indolent (low-grade) lymphoma tends to run a slow course and although

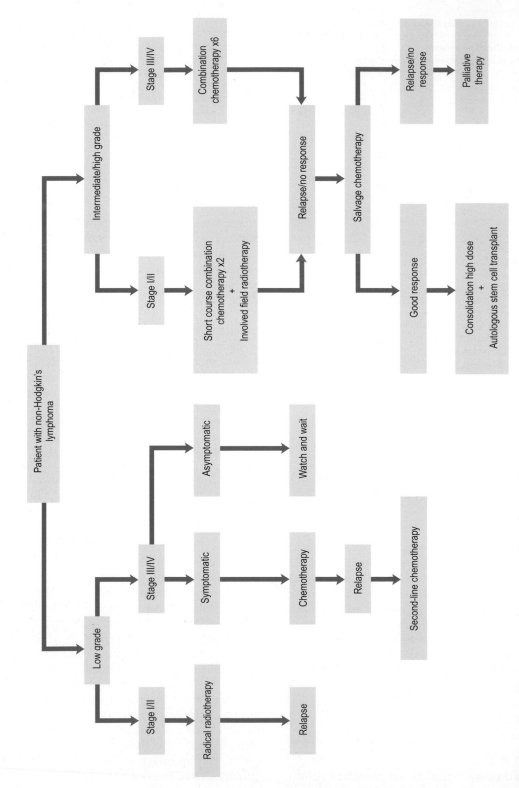

Fig. 51.3 Typical treatment algorithm for non-Hodgkin's lymphoma.

Table 51.5 Chemotherapy regimens effective in the treatment of non-Hodgkin's lymphoma

Drug	Dose and route	Day of administration
R-CHOP (21-day cycle)		
Cyclophosphamide	750 mg/m² i.v.	Day 1
Doxorubicin (hydroxydaunorubicin)	50 mg/m² i.v.	Day 1
Vincristine (Oncovin)	1.4 mg/m² (max 2 mg) i.v.	Day 1
Prednisolone	100 mg orally	Days 1–5
Rituximab	375 mg/m² i.v.	Day 1
R-CVP (21-day cycle)		
Cyclophosphamide	750 mg/m² i.v.	Day 1
Vincristine (Oncovin)	1.4 mg/m² (max 2 mg) i.v.	Day 1
Prednisolone	100 mg orally	Days 1–5
Rituximab	375 mg/m² i.v.	Day 1
FC (28-day cycle)		
Fludarabine	40 mg/m² orally	Days 1–3
Cyclophosphamide	250 mg/m² daily orally	Days 1–3
CHOP (21-day cycle)		
Cyclophosphamide	750 mg/m² i.v.	Day 1
Doxorubicin (hydroxydaunorubicin)	50 mg/m² i.v.	Day 1
Vincristine (Oncovin)	1.4 mg/m² (max 2 mg) i.v.	Day 1
Prednisolone	100 mg orally	Days 1–5

For patients who are asymptomatic at diagnosis, adopting a 'watch and wait' policy with active monitoring and initiating treatment when symptomatic is an option. Patients could be considered for recruitment to clinical trials, there are ongoing studies comparing R-CVP with R-FC (rituximab, fludarabine, cyclosphosphamide) followed by rituximab maintenance and investigating the benefit of bendamustine compared to R-CVP. If patients fail to tolerate the standard treatment options, an oral alkylating agent, for example, chlorambucil, with or without a steroid can be used. Repeated courses may be given.

Relapsed indolent non-Hodgkin's lymphoma

Relapsed patients may be re-treated with rituximab if the time to relapse post-rituximab is greater than 6 months (NICE, 2008). If the time to relapse is less than 6 months, Yttrium-90 labelled ibritumomab tiuxetan (Zevalin®) may be considered. Zevalin® is a new therapeutic development that utilises monoclonal antibodies as tumour-specific vehicles to deliver systemic radiation therapy concurrent with immunotherapy to the targeted tumour. However, for some resistant or relapsing patients, particularly if their condition is too poor to merit further radical chemotherapy, palliation will be appropriate. Radiotherapy may be an option in this situation and this is being evaluated through an ongoing clinical trial.

Aggressive non-Hodgkin's lymphoma

The median age of presentation of aggressive NHL is 60–70 years when 50–60% of patients will present with an advanced stage of the disease. The most common presentation is diffuse large B-cell lymphoma (DLBCL), and therefore the treatment strategies described later refer to this alone. Other aggressive lymphomas, for example, mantle cell, are managed differently. The most important strategy when treating this group of patients is to maintain the dose intensity of chemotherapy and minimise any delay in chemotherapy administration. Treatment is given with curative intent.

The treatment for advanced-stage aggressive NHL is six cycles of the combination of R-CHOP chemotherapy (NICE, 2003). Doxorubicin can cause cardiotoxicity and patients with a reduced cardiac ejection fraction or co-morbidities may not tolerate R-CHOP. The use of gemcitabine (R-GCVP) is currently being investigated for this patient group as part of a clinical trial. The addition of bortezomib to R-CHOP in DLBCL is also being investigated as a clinical trial for patients with high-risk disease.

Relapsed aggressive non-Hodgkin's lymphoma

Combination chemotherapy with R-CHOP probably cures 40–60%. This, therefore, implies that over half of all patients have refractory disease or relapse after first treatment.

In younger patients with aggressive NHL, the aim will be to introduce remission with further chemotherapy, using an alternative, salvage regimen, and then to consolidate remission with high-dose therapy (HDT). HDT is usually supported by mobilised peripheral blood stem cells (PBSCs) and an autologous PBSC transplantation (auto-PBSCT). Lymphoma is the most frequent indication for auto PBSCT in Europe. The European Group for Blood and Marrow Transplantation (EBMT) suggests that the upper age limit for autologous transplantation is 65 years. HDT, with autologous stem cell support, is also used as part of primary treatment for younger patients with indolent lymphoma. Patients who receive HDT after their initial treatment can have progression-free survival rates of around 50% at 5 years.

To induce a remission in patients with aggressive lymphoma and relapsed disease, it may be reasonable to use the same or similar regimen used for front-line chemotherapy. However, in most cases, the regimen chosen introduces new agents that are potentially not cross-resistant with those used in the initial treatment regimen. There are several salvage regimens in use and they generally have response rates of between 40% and 70%. Examples of salvage regimens are ICE (ifosfamide, carboplatin, etoposide), ESHAP (etoposide, methylprednisolone, cytarabine, cisplatin) and DHAP (cisplatin, cytarabine, dexamethasone) (see Table 51.2). Gemcitabine, a pyrimidine analogue, may be of benefit for patients with relapsed or refractory disease after two lines of treatment. Gemcitabine is used in combination with other agents, such as cisplatin and methylprednisolone. Rituximab can also be added to these salvage regimens. PBSCs are usually harvested after the second course of the salvage regimen. Patients then receive a high-dose regimen such as BEAM (carmustine, etoposide, cytarabine, melphalan) (Table 51.6) conditioning prior to stem cell infusion (autograft). Patients should only undergo an autograft if they have demonstrated a response to salvage chemotherapy.

CNS prophylaxis for diffuse large B-cell lymphoma. Approximately 5% of patients with DLBCL develop CNS disease. The optimum approach to CNS prophylaxis is uncertain, and it usually involves a course of intrathecal chemotherapy.

The updated national guidance for the safe administration of intrathecal chemotherapy (DH, 2008) sets out the minimum requirements of a hospital providing an intrathecal chemotherapy service.

Very aggressive lymphoma

Burkitt's lymphoma is a rare form of B-cell NHL which occurs most commonly in children and young adults. The median age of adult patients is 30 years. Untreated, survival is measurable in days or weeks, and it is widely accepted that combination chemotherapy should be urgently commenced. Intensive chemotherapy is necessary, together with CNS prophylaxis, and cure is possible in a high proportion of cases.

Multi-agent chemotherapy regimens including high-dose methotrexate, high-dose cytarabine, etoposide and ifosfamide are used and a schedule such as CODOX-M (cyclophosphamide, vincristine, doxorubicin, high-dose methotrexate)/IVAC (ifosfamide, etoposide, high-dose cytarabine) is common.

There is an on-going debate about the value of adding rituximab to the CODOX-M/IVAC regimen.

Lymphoblastic lymphomas/leukaemia

Lymphoblastic lymphomas comprise about 2% of adult NHLs. Patients are often treated with the same regimens used in acute lymphoblastic leukaemia (ALL). Despite a very high rate of complete responders, long-term survival remains poor. Patients who fail after first-line chemotherapy have a long-term disease-free survival of less than 10%. These cases are subsequently treated as leukaemias (see Chapter 50).

Patient care

The chemotherapy regimens used to treat HL and NHL (see Tables 51.1 and 51.5) are usually administered on a hospital outpatient basis with the patient visiting the clinic regularly for assessment and treatment. The patient is monitored by FBCs carried out before each cycle of chemotherapy and at the 'nadir' between cycles. The nadir is when the blood count is at its lowest point, usually 10–14 days after the first day of chemotherapy. The interval between each cycle of chemotherapy enables normal body cells to recover before the patient receives further treatment. Disease response to treatment is monitored by repeating some of the diagnostic investigations, such as CT, at suitable intervals and the use of PET. If there is little or no response to treatment, a different chemotherapy regimen will be used or a decision made to withdraw from active therapy and provide optimum supportive care.

Counselling and support

Counselling is an essential part of the care of the cancer patient and involves not only the explanation of drug therapy and investigations but also the provision of psychological support for the patient and family. Prior to treatment with chemotherapy, the patient will be counselled by the doctor, chemotherapy nurse and, increasingly, by oncology pharmacists. It is necessary to explain how the chemotherapy is to be given and discuss both potential and inevitable side effects. The probability of successful treatment must be weighed against the prospect of serious and life-threatening adverse effects. Patients must be made aware of the long-term complications of chemotherapy and radiotherapy, such as secondary malignancy.

The support available to the cancer patient, to help cope with both the illness and its treatment, has improved dramatically in recent years. Multidisciplinary teams working within specialised units have become skilled in anticipating the problems of lymphomas and their treatment. In addition, many charities provide care, support and advice such as Macmillan Cancer Support (www.macmillan.org.uk) and the Lymphoma Association (www.lymphoma.org.uk).

Patient-specific treatment modifications

The selection of appropriate therapy must also take into consideration the individual patient. Factors include the patient's age, renal and hepatic function and underlying medical conditions, such as heart disease, diabetes or chronic pulmonary disease. The patient's tolerance of side effects and complications of therapy may then be predicted. The decision is based on an understanding of the pharmacodynamics and pharmacokinetics of the drugs being used as well as the clinical condition of the patient.

Table 51.6 Conditioning chemotherapy for autologous transplantation

Drug	Dose and route	Day of administration
BEAM		
Carmustine	300 mg/m² i.v.	6 days before reinfusion
Etoposide	200 mg/m² i.v.	5–2 days before reinfusion
Cytarabine	200 mg/m² 12 h i.v.	5–2 days before reinfusion
Melphalan	140 mg/m² i.v.	1 day before reinfusion
Reinfusion of stem cells		Day 0
LACE		
Lomustine	200 mg/m² orally	7 days before reinfusion
Etoposide	1000 mg/m² i.v.	7 days before reinfusion
Cytarabine	2000 mg/m²	6–5 days before reinfusion
Cyclophosphamide	1800 mg/m² i.v.	4–2 days before reinfusion
Reinfusion of stem cells		Day 0

Supportive care

During a course of chemotherapy, the patient requires supportive care to minimise the adverse effects of treatment. The common adverse effects of the chemotherapy regimens discussed in this chapter are outlined in Table 51.7. These will occur to varying degrees depending on the combination of drugs and the doses used as well as individual patient factors.

Nausea and vomiting

Nausea and vomiting is the most distressing and most feared adverse effect of chemotherapy. Its effect on the patient should not be underestimated, and its treatment is an important part of supportive care. The severity will depend on the combination of drugs used. For example, oral chlorambucil is generally well tolerated by almost all patients and requires no antiemetic cover. Regimens such as ABVD, which is highly emetic, will make most patients vomit if no antiemetics are given. Aprepitant, an NK1 receptor antagonist, is licensed for cisplatin chemotherapy regimens and may be useful for managing emesis with DHAP, ESHAP, etc. The patient should be counselled on the appropriate use of prescribed antiemetics (see Table 51.7).

Tumour lysis syndrome

The lymphomas are, in general, highly sensitive to chemotherapy. The resulting lysis of cells which occurs following initiation of chemotherapy may lead to hyperuricaemia,

Table 51.7 Adverse effects associated with chemotherapy regimens used in the lymphomas with supportive measures and counselling points

Adverse effect	Cytotoxics implicated	Supportive measures	Counselling points
Bone marrow suppression	Chlorambucil Cyclophosphamide Dacarbazine Etoposide	Blood transfusion Platelet transfusions Mouth care Antibiotic therapy for febrile episodes	Expect tiredness Report bleeding or unusual bruises Importance of good personal hygiene Adhere to mouth care regimen
	Vinblastine	Granulocyte-colony stimulating factor	Avoid people with infections
	Prednisolone	(GCSF)	Monitor temperature Report febrile episodes or signs of infection immediately
Nausea and vomiting Mucositis	Cyclophosphamide Doxorubicin	Antiemetic therapy	Emphasise regular use. A short course is more effective than 'as required' treatment
	Procarbazine Dacarbazine		Take tablets before meals Report episodes of vomiting (especially if taking oral cytotoxics). For dexamethasone, emphasise short course not to be continued to ensure the patient does not receive repeat prescriptions from primary care doctor
	Doxorubicin	Mouth care regimen	Importance of good oral hygiene, instruct how mouthwashes are used, stress importance of regular use
Tumour lysis syndrome	High tumour load sensitive to chemotherapy	Hydration, allopurinol	Stress importance of regular allopurinol until appropriate to stop
		Rasburicase	Drink plenty of fluids
Alopecia	Cyclophosphamide Doxorubicin, etoposide	Provision of wig if wanted	Hair usually regrows on completion of therapy
Impaired gonadal function	Alkylating agents Procarbazine, doxorubicin (to a lesser degree)	Sperm storage	Refer to doctor, depends on regimen, reversible in some cases
Neuropathy	Vincristine	Discontinue use or substitute vinblastine	Report tingling sensations or difficulty with buttons, jaw pain or stiffness
Constipation			Do not self treat but refer to doctor
Cardiomyopathy	Doxorubicin		Report breathlessness, tiredness
Lung fibrosis	Bleomycin		Report breathlessness

hyperkalaemia and hypocalcaemia in patients with bulky disease, and result in urate nephropathy. There is a high incidence of tumour lysis syndrome (TLS) in tumours with high proliferation rates and tumour burden such as Burkitt's lymphoma and T-lymphoblastic lymphoma. The mainstay of TLS prevention is hydration with the patient encouraged to maintain a high fluid intake. Hyperuricaemia is controlled with allopurinol and close monitoring of renal function, serum urate levels and electrolytes. Allopurinol must be commenced before chemotherapy and continued until the tumour load has reduced and serum urate levels are normal. In aggressive forms of NHL, rasburicase, a recombinant urate oxidase, may be indicated as prophylaxis. Allopurinol should not be prescribed concurrently with rasburicase because it will inhibit the production of uric acid, the substrate for rasburicase.

Rasburicase can also be used to treat TLS but will only correct hyperuricaemia. Treatment of TLS should include vigorous hydration and diuresis. Historically alkaline diuresis has been recommended, but overzealous alkalinisation can lead to problems such as metabolic acidosis (Cairo and Bishop, 2004). Hypocalcaemia should be corrected if the patient is symptomatic, but this may increase calcium phosphate deposition. Hyperkalaemia and hyperphosphataemia should be corrected; patients may require haemofiltration or dialysis.

Mucositis

Chemotherapy may cause mucositis, which is inflammation of or damage to the surface of the gastro-intestinal tract. In the mouth, this may lead to painful ulceration, local infection and difficulty in swallowing. Dependent on the severity of mucositis, patients may require analgesia from benzydamine mouthwash to systemic opiates. Disruption of the mucosal barrier will give bacteria and fungi easier systemic access. A mouth care regimen should therefore be instituted with myelosuppressive therapy. This involves good oral hygiene, for example, gentle brushing with a toothbrush to remove plaque or rinsing with saline to remove debris. An antiseptic mouthwash such as chlorhexidine 0.2% should also be used regularly to prevent infection. Palifermin, keratinocyte growth factor (KGF), may have a role in autologous haemopoietic stem cell support.

Bone marrow suppression

Myelosuppression is usually the dose-limiting factor with these regimens, and it is necessary to carry out FBCs before treatment to confirm that recovery has occurred. Each chemotherapy protocol should be referred to so as to ensure appropriate management. Generally, if the platelet count is below 100×10^9 L^{-1} and/or the absolute neutrophil count (ANC) is less than 1×10^9 L^{-1}, the subsequent dose may be reduced or treatment delayed by a week.

Anaemia is treated with blood transfusions and thrombocytopenia with platelet transfusions as necessary. Erythropoietin administration reduces blood transfusion requirements and can improve quality of life. However, the evidence suggesting improvement in patient survival is inconclusive.

Neutropenia is the most life-threatening acute toxicity; the neutropenic patient is at constant risk from infections. Seemingly minor infections such as cold sores can spread rapidly, and infections not seen in the normal population, such as systemic fungal infections, can occur. Supportive measures involve reducing the risks and the aggressive treatment of any infectious episodes. The patient is counselled to avoid contact with people with infection or those who may be carriers. Most infections, however, are from an endogenous source such as the gut or skin. The patient is educated on the importance of good personal hygiene, mouth care, how to monitor body temperature and to report any febrile episodes immediately. Co-trimoxazole 960 mg may be prescribed as prophylaxis against *Pneumocystis* pneumonia in patients receiving chemotherapy for lymphomas, particularly in those receiving a regimen containing fludarabine. Thorough and frequent hand washing helps to prevent the transmission of opportunistic infection to the neutropenic patient.

Febrile neutropenia

A febrile episode in the neutropenic patient is an indication for immediate treatment with broad-spectrum intravenous antibiotics. Susceptibility to infection is likely when the neutrophil count is less than 1×10^9 L^{-1} with increasing risk at levels less than 0.5×10^9 L^{-1} and 0.01×10^9 L^{-1}. Fever, usually defined as a temperature above 38 °C maintained for 1 h or 38.3 °C on one occasion, may be the only sign of infection. The patient should be assessed to determine the site of infection, if possible. Blood cultures from all venous access ports and any other appropriate cultures, for example, midstream urine sample and stool sample, are taken and then antibiotic therapy commenced. Blood cultures are taken prior to starting antibiotics to increase the likelihood of obtaining a positive culture. Infection with Gram-negative bacilli, for example, *Escherichia coli*, *Klebsiella pneumoniae* and *Pseudomonas aeruginosa,* and Gram-positive cocci, for example, coagulase-negative staphylococci, β-haemolytic streptococci, enterococci, and *Staphylococcus aureus* is probable in this situation. First-line therapy should cover these common pathogens. Options include carbapenems, a third-generation cephalosporin or antipseudomonal penicillin with or without an aminoglycoside. If the patient does not respond to this combination within 24–48 h, then second-line therapy, which may include a glycopeptide for Gram-positive cover, is commenced.

Gram-positive infections are becoming more common with the use of indwelling intravenous catheters. If positive microbiological cultures are found, the appropriate antibiotic can be prescribed on the basis of sensitivities; however, if the patient is responding to empiric therapy, the antibiotics should not be changed. Only one-third of suspected infections are ever confirmed, and the pathogen may not be isolated. The febrile episode may not be due to infection; non-infectious causes include blood transfusion and underlying disease.

Growth factor support

Patients with persistent neutropenia or those who have repeated admissions for neutropenic sepsis may be supported with granulocyte-colony-stimulating factor (GCSF). There is evidence that patients with lymphomas receiving a reduced dose of chemotherapy as a consequence of myelosuppression have a worse prognosis when compared with patients who receive full doses. GCSF is indicated as primary prophylaxis, before any episode of febrile neutropenia, for regimens where there is a high (>40%) incidence of febrile neutropenia. GCSF has been investigated as a prophylactic measure to increase the dose intensity of chemotherapy in regimens such as CHOP-14 (cyclophosphamide, hydroxydaunorubicin (doxorubicin), Oncovin (vincristine), prednisolone at 14-day intervals) and BEACOPP-14 (bleomycin, etoposide, Adriamycin (doxorubicin) cyclophosphamide, vincristine, procarbazine, prednisolone at 14-day intervals).

Case studies

Case 51.1

Mr RB is a 50-year-old man receiving a course of fludarabine and cyclophosphamide (see Table 51.5) for mantle cell lymphoma. He has no other medical problems and has normal renal and hepatic function.

Questions

1. What are the key counselling points for the oral chemotherapy drug fludarabine?
2. What antibacterial agent would you expect to see prescribed with fludarabine?
3. What antiemetic regimen would you recommend with the fludarabine and cyclophosphamide?

Answers

1. Immunocompromised patients, for example, those receiving purine analogues, fludarabine, cladribine and pentostatin, are at risk of developing transfusion-associated graft versus host disease (TAGVHD), a rare but usually fatal complication of transfusion.

   Viable T-lymphocytes in donated blood can recognise the recipient as 'foreign', leading to fever, skin rash, hepatitis and bone marrow involvement. Death occurs in 90% of cases, predominantly due to infection.

   γ-Irradiation of cellular blood components is the mainstay of TAGVHD prevention. Patients should be given an appropriate patient information leaflet and an alert card. The risk of TAGVHD is minimised by informing transfusion staff and the patient of their need for irradiated blood products.
2. Mr RB should be prescribed co-trimoxazole prophylactically to prevent *Pneumocystis jiroveci* infection.
3. Chemotherapy drugs are grouped by how likely they are to cause emesis if antiemetics are not given, called emetogenic potential. Antiemetic regimens are then prescribed to prevent the degree of vomiting expected for each group.

   Fludarabine is rarely emetogenic and oral cyclophosphamide is moderately emetogenic. Therefore, the regimen should be classified and treated as moderately emetogenic.

Dexamethasone, granisetron and metoclopramide are frequently employed for moderately emetogenic regimens. Guidelines for antiemetic use in oncology are available (American Society of Clinical Oncology, 2006). As corticosteroids are associated with immunosuppression, some clinicians prefer not to use them for emesis prevention with FC chemotherapy.

Case 51.2

Mrs BC is a 72-year-old widow who has been newly diagnosed with low-grade NHL. She has been seen in the hospital outpatient haematology clinic and has brought a prescription to the pharmacy for chlorambucil 10 mg daily for 14 days. When she hands in her prescription, she expresses concern about the side effects of the tablets. The doctor who saw her had spent a lot of time talking to her about her treatment, but she feels confused with all the information given.

Questions

1. What are the side effects of chlorambucil?
2. How would you counsel this patient?

Answers

1. Chlorambucil, an alkylating agent, is generally well tolerated. The major side effect is bone marrow suppression. Other side effects are uncommon and include nausea and vomiting, rash, mucositis and diarrhoea. Hepatotoxicity and jaundice have been reported. Mrs BC is an elderly patient and is thus more likely to experience toxicity because of deteriorating renal and hepatic function and underlying medical conditions.
2. Mrs BC may be distressed by her diagnosis and may not have been able to absorb all the information she was given in the clinic. She may also be seeking confirmation of information.

   Mrs BC should be counselled to complete the course of tablets as prescribed. She should be told that she will probably feel tired and be more prone to infection because the tablets lower the blood count and resistance to infection. She should be advised to inform the haematologist if she feels unwell. Chlorambucil is unlikely to make her feel nauseous, but if this occurs she should inform the doctor, who will be able to prescribe an antiemetic.

Case 51.3

Mr F is 56 years old and was diagnosed with stage III high-grade NHL (DLBCL) over 10 weeks ago. Since then, he has received three cycles of R-CHOP and has come to the hospital for his nadir blood count. He complains of painful mouth ulcers and a sore throat. On examination, he has mucositis and oropharyngeal candidiasis. He has a white blood cell count (WCC) of 3.2 (normal range: 3.5–11 × 10^9 L^{-1}) with ANC of 0.8 × 10^9 L^{-1}.

Questions

1. How would you treat Mr F's *Candida* infection?
2. How would you counsel this patient?

Answers

1. Mr F has an ANC of 0.8 × 10^9 L^{-1} and is therefore neutropenic (ANC <1.0 × 10^9 L^{-1}). Localised candidal infections can spread rapidly in the immunosuppressed patient, so local therapy with

an antifungal mouthwash will be inadequate therapy. A course of fluconazole, 100 mg daily for at least 7 days, should be prescribed. Therapy should continue for a further 7 days if Mr F is still neutropenic or if the thrush has not completely resolved.

An antibacterial mouthwash, such as chlorhexidine 0.2% 10 mL four times daily, should be used. As Mr F is complaining of pain, an analgesic should be added. Benzydamine mouthwash, a locally acting analgesic, could be prescribed initially. If this does not give adequate pain relief, then systemic analgesics such as dihydrocodeine should be given.

2. Regular mouth care reduces the risk of infection but does not entirely remove it. It is not necessarily a reflection of how well the patient has adhered to his mouth care regimen. Chlorhexidine mouthwash should be used first, held in the mouth as long as possible, ensuring the entire mucosa is covered before spitting out. The mouthwash should be used after meals and at bedtime. He should not eat or drink for at least half an hour after using the mouthwash.

The benzydamine mouthwash should be used before meals as Mr F will probably find eating painful. He should be advised to use a soft toothbrush, to eat soft foods and to avoid hot and spicy dishes. He may be reassured that once his blood count recovers, his mouth ulcers should resolve and that the fluconazole should relieve his sore throat.

Case 51.4

Mr D, 38 years old with advanced HL, is admitted to the haematology ward at the local hospital as an emergency. He had a temperature of 39 °C on the morning of admission, feels generally unwell but has no specific symptoms. It is 12 days since he started his third cycle of ABVD. On admission, he is taking the following medication:

- co-trimoxazole 960 mg twice daily on 3 days a week
- chlorhexidine 0.2% mouthwash 10 mL four times daily

Blood cultures are taken and piperacillin + tazobactam 4.5 g i.v. three times daily and gentamicin 480 mg i.v. once daily are prescribed, to be commenced immediately. Blood biochemistry results are normal; his FBC was Hb 10.8 (normal range: 13.5–18.0 g/dL for men), WCC 2.5 (normal range: 3.5–11 × 10^9 L^{-1}), neutrophil count 0.6 (normal range: 1.5–7.5 × 10^9 L^{-1}) and platelets 150 (normal range 150–400 × 10^9 L^{-1}). Mr D weighs 86 kg and is 186 cm tall.

Questions

1. Comment on the rationale for the antibiotic therapy prescribed.
2. How would you monitor this patient?
3. What would be an appropriate second-line regimen if he remains pyrexial?
4. What modifications would need to be made to subsequent cycles of chemotherapy?

Answers

1. Mr D's FBC is probably at its nadir following his last course of chemotherapy. He is neutropenic and febrile; fever is

often the only sign of infection in neutropenic patients. Immunosuppression is also a feature of HL and contributes to susceptibility to infection. Treatment should commence immediately after cultures have been taken, as infection can be rapidly fatal in these patients. The antibiotics selected should provide broad-spectrum cover and follow local policy as there are institutional variations in predominant pathogens and antimicrobial sensitivities. The organisms responsible for infectious episodes are constantly changing: in the 1970s, Gram-negative infections predominated but now Gram-positive organisms account for 65% of positive cultures. As Gram-negative infections are more rapidly fatal, first-line therapy should be biased towards these infections. Piperacillin, an antipseudomonal penicillin, and gentamicin therefore form an appropriate combination to use in this patient. Piperacillin + tazobactam monotherapy may be sufficient in cases of uncomplicated neutropenic sepsis.

The dose of piperacillin + tazobactam is appropriate. Infection is considered to be severe in these patients as signs and symptoms are often muted. Single daily dose gentamicin is at least as effective as multiple dosing and less nephrotoxic; it is more convenient and cost effective and overcomes deficiencies of the traditional method such as subtherapeutic dosing and inadequate monitoring. The dose is 5–7 mg/kg and has been calculated correctly for Mr D. He has normal renal function, so no dose modifications are necessary.

2. Monitor temperature, pulse and blood pressure and any patient symptoms for signs of improvement or deterioration. Blood biochemistry should be checked daily to detect any deterioration in renal function. Microbiology reports should be checked and antibiotics reviewed if any micro-organisms have been cultured. However, no change should be made to antibiotics if the patient is showing signs of improvement. The administration of gentamicin should be monitored, checking both administration and sampling time for drug levels. The results should be checked and recommendations for dose modification made where appropriate, using a method such as the Hartford monogram.

3. If the patient remains pyrexial 24–48 h after the first-line antibiotics have been commenced, consideration should be given to broadening cover, for example, adding vancomycin if the patient has mucositis or line infection. If blood cultures show growth, found in only 30–40% of neutropenic patients, the choice of antibiotics should be on the basis of sensitivities. It is important to note that febrile episodes lasting several days may involve more than one infecting organism.

The patient's FBC should start to recover from day 14 but may be delayed by this infection. It is unusual for patients on conventional chemotherapy for HL to require more than one change to antibiotic therapy, and clinical improvement is often seen with recovery of neutrophil count. If Mr D is still pyrexial at 96 h, then the likelihood of fungal infection must be considered and an intravenous amphotericin-based product or caspofungin commenced if appropriate. The incidence of fungal infection is increasing in patients with prolonged neutropenia. As Mr D's neutropenia is short lived, he is more likely to have a bacterial infection.

4. A dose reduction for subsequent cycles of chemotherapy may be considered. However, as this patient is being treated with curative intent, it may be more appropriate to give GCSF and maintain the dose intensity.

Acknowledgements

The authors thank Denise Blake and Mary Maclean for permission to use material originally included in their chapter that appeared in the third edition of this book.

References

American Society of Clinical Oncology, 2006. Guideline for antiemetics in oncology: update 2006. J. Clin. Oncol. 24, 2932–2947.

Brusamolino, E., Bacigalupo, A., Barosi, G., 2009. Classical Hodgkin's lymphoma in adults: guidelines of the Italian Society of Hematology, the Italian Society of Experimental Hematology, and the Italian Group for Bone Marrow Transplantation on initial work-up, management, and follow-up. Haematologica 94, 550–565.

Cairo, M.S., Bishop, M., 2004. Tumour lysis syndrome: new therapeutic strategies and classification. Br. J. Haematol. 127, 3–11.

Department of Health, 2008. HSC 2008/001: Updated National Guidance on the Safe Administration of Intrathecal Chemotherapy. Department of Health, London. Available at: http://www.dh.gov.uk/en/Publicationsandstatistics/Lettersandcirculars/Healthservicecirculars/DH_086870.

Diehl, V., Thomas, R.K., Re, D., 2004. Part II: Hodgkin's lymphoma – diagnosis and treatment. Lancet Oncol. 5, 19–26.

Engert, A., Diehl, V., Franklin, J., et al., 2009. Escalated-dose BEACOPP in the treatment of patients with advanced-stage Hodgkin's lymphoma: 10 years of follow up of the GHSG HD9 Study. J. Clin. Oncol. 27, 4548–4554.

Marcus, R., Imrie, K., Belch, A., et al., 2005. CVP chemotherapy plus rituximab compared with CVP as first-line treatment for advanced follicular lymphoma. Blood 105, 1417–1423.

National Institute for Health and Clinical Excellence, 2003. Rituximab for Aggressive Non-Hodgkin's Lymphoma. NICE, London. Available at: http://guidance.nice.org.uk/TA65/Guidance/pdf/English.

National Institute for Health and Clinical Excellence, 2006. Rituximab for the treatment of follicular lymphoma. NICE technology appraisal guidance A 110, NICE, London. Available at http://www.nice.org.uk/nicemedia/pdf/TA110guidance.pdf.

National Institute for Health and Clinical Excellence, 2008. Rituximab for the treatment of relapsed or refractory stage III or IV follicular non-Hodgkin's lymphoma. NICE technology appraisal guidance 137, NICE, London. Available at http://www.nice.org.uk/nicemedia/pdf/TA137guidance.pdf.

Ng, M., Waters, J., Chau, I., et al., 2005. Gemcitabine, cisplatin and methylprednisolone (GEM-P) is an effective salvage regimen in patients with relapsed and refractory lymphoma. Br. J. Cancer 92, 1352–1357.

Souhami, R., Tobias, J. (Eds.), 1998. Cancer and Its Management. Blackwell Science, Oxford.

Younes, A., 2009. Novel treatment strategies for patients with relapsed classical Hodgkin lymphoma. Hematology (American Society Hematology Education Program), 507–519.

UK Clinical Research Network Study Portfolio RATHL, 2010. A Randomized Phase III Trial to Assess Response Adapted Therapy Using FDG-PET Imaging in Patients with Newly Diagnosed Advanced Hodgkin's Lymphoma. Available at http://public.ukcrn.org.uk/search/StudyDetail.aspx?StudyID=4488.

West of Scotland Blood Cancer Network, 2009. Clinical Management Guidelines Hodgkin's Lymphoma Version 3.0. Available at http://www.medednhsl.com/meded/clinicalgpp/pdf/WoSCAN_CMG_Hodgkins_v3_0_August_2009.pdf.

Further reading

Dearden, C., Matutes, E., 2000. Non-Hodgkin's lymphoma. Medicine 28, 71–77.

Evens, A.M., Winter, J.N., Gordon, L.I., et al., 2011. Non-Hodgkin's lymphoma. In: Pazdur, R., Coia, L.R., Hoskins, W.J., et al. (Eds.), Cancer Management: A Multidisciplinary Approach. 13th ed. PRR Melville, New York, Chapter 27. Available at: http://www.cancernetwork.com/cancermanagement-12.

Laport, G.F., Williams, S.F., 1998. The role of high-dose chemotherapy in patients with Hodgkin's disease and non-Hodgkin's lymphoma. Semin. Oncol. 25, 503–517.

Leonard, J.P., Coleman, M. (Eds.), 2006. Hodgkin's and Non-Hodgkin's Lymphoma. Springer-Verlag, New York.

Yahalom, J., Strauss, D., 2011. Hodgkin's lymphoma. In: Pazdur, R., Coia, L.R., Hoskins, W.J., et al. (Eds.), Cancer Management: A Multidisciplinary Approach, 13th ed. PRR Melville, New York, Chapter 26. Available at http://www.cancernetwork.com/cancer-management-12.

Provan, D., Singer, C.R.J., Baglin, T., et al., 2009. Oxford Handbook of Clinical Haematology. third ed. Oxford University Press, Oxford.

52 Solid tumours

N. Wood and A. Lamont

Key points

- Cancer involves a group of relatively normal cells dividing without the controls that usually prevent the cells from growing beyond their usual size, site and nutritional base.
- Cancer is now considered a long-term illness with many subgroups.
- Cancer is a collective term for several diseases each with its own characteristics and natural history according to where it has started. Even for a single site of origin, such as breast cancer, major biological and histological differences can be shown.
- Before treatment, patients must be carefully 'staged' to establish the type and extent of disease.
- Depending on the stage of disease, the aim of treatment may be cure, prolongation of survival or symptom control.
- Cytotoxic chemotherapy is the main treatment for disseminated disease.
- Treatment options depend not only on the 'gold standard' of treatment but also patient factors and preferences.
- Targeted medical therapies are becoming more common, generally have fewer side effects and are given over a longer term than conventional chemotherapy.

The term 'cancer' is used to describe more than 200 different diseases, including those affecting discrete organs (solid tumours) and haematological malignancies (which are not localised in the same way). Whereas some tumours are benign and may be harmless, this chapter will focus on the management of patients with solid malignancies which require some form of treatment. Treatment is generally carried out in specialised cancer centres, cancer units or for some agents, in the patient's home. Therapy may include surgery, radiotherapy, chemotherapy and biological or targeted therapy as single modalities or in combination. Care of the cancer patient demands a broad range of services involving a multidisciplinary team working across the hospital, community and hospice network.

Epidemiology

Cancer is a common disease, and more than one in three people will develop some form of cancer in their lifetime. Although more than a quarter of a million people develop cancer each year in the UK, it is predominantly a disease of the elderly, with 74% of new cases diagnosed in people aged over 60 years. Of all deaths in the UK, one in four is due to cancer. The most common single cause of death (22%) is lung cancer, which is potentially preventable by a reduction in tobacco smoking.

Prostate cancer is now the most common cancer in men (24%) followed by lung (15%) and bowel (14%) cancer. In women, breast cancer is the most common (31%) followed by bowel (12%) then lung (12%). However, there are regional variations. From 1979 to 2008, mortality rates from cancer fell by 20% (Cancer Research UK, 2010).

Aetiology

The causes of cancer may be categorised as either environmental or genetic, although these may be interrelated and the causes of some cancers may be multifactorial.

Environmental factors

Increasingly, lifestyle factors play a large part in the development of many cancers. Cigarette smoking has been identified as the single most important cause of preventable disease and premature death in the UK. The beneficial effect of stopping smoking on the cumulative risk of death from lung cancer reduces with increasing age (Doll et al., 2004). Smoking causes about 90% of lung cancer deaths, and the link between tobacco and cancer was established more than 50 years ago.

The most important lifestyle factor for bowel cancer is diet, while cervical cancer is primarily linked to sexual behaviour through the transmissible agent human papilloma virus (HPV) and secondarily to smoking.

Table 52.1 lists a number of other factors which have been associated with cancer development.

Genetic factors

A number of rare tumours are known to be associated with an inherited predisposition, where an individual is born with a marked susceptibility to cancer. This is due to the inheritance of a single genetic mutation which may be sufficient to greatly increase the risk of one or more types of cancer. Examples include the paediatric malignancies, Wilms' tumour of the kidney and bilateral retinoblastoma, a rare cancer of the eye. Some common cancers such as breast, ovarian and colorectal

Table 52.1 A–K of factors associated with specific cancer sites: An empirical basis for recommending lifestyle changes (Jankowski and Boulton, 2005)

Factor	Associated cancer
Alcohol consumption >3 units a day	Most squamous cancers, especially bladder and oesophagus
Body mass index >25 and certainly >30	All solid cancers
Cigarette smoking at any level (even passive smoking)	Bladder, lung, head and neck, oesophagus and oropharyngeal cancers
Diet, especially one that is high in fat	All solid cancers
Exercising <30 min a day	All solid cancers
Family history of cancer (in at least one first-degree relative and at least three people in two or more generations)	Inherited cancer syndromes, including breast, colorectal, diffuse gastric, ovarian, prostate and uterine cancers
Genital and sexual health (sexually transmitted infections)	Cervical cancer
Health-promoting drugs that may decrease global cancer risks (but need a careful risk/benefit analysis)	Colonic adenomas can be treated with low-dose aspirin but can have serious side effects Hormone replacement therapy linked with breast cancer
Intense sunburn	Melanoma
Job-related factors	Lung cancer (exposure to asbestos and particulates), skin cancer (contact with arsenic)
Known disease associations	Colorectal cancer has predisposing mucosal pathology – adenomas, coeliac disease, ulcerative colitis

cancer may also show a tendency to occur in families, but these represent a small proportion of the overall presentation of common cancers where identifiable risk factors are relevant in only 5–10% of cases, although when the genetic factor is present the cancers tend to have their onset at a younger age (Garber and Offit, 2005).

Screening and prevention

Screening

Screening programmes aim to detect pre-malignant changes or early-stage cancer in asymptomatic individuals in the general population to provide earlier and thus more effective treatment. Any screening test must be simple, reliable, highly specific (to exclude healthy individuals) and highly sensitive (detection: 90–95%). For a screening programme to be effective in reducing morbidity and mortality, there must also be an available, effective, safe and economically viable treatment that can be applied to the abnormalities detected by the screening test. Screening is well established for cancers of the breast, cervix and, more recently, bowel. Population screening for prostate cancer using the prostate-specific antigen (PSA) blood test remains more controversial due to the lack of specificity and sensitivity of the test, and to the limited evidence on the viability and effectiveness of the treatment options in early-stage disease. It is currently not recommended for use in screening programmes in the UK

but is used in the USA. The evidence base for ovarian cancer screening using the blood test CA125 and pelvic ultrasound is evolving through clinical trials.

Prevention

The strong association between cancer risk and lifestyle factors means there is great potential for the primary prevention of cancer through:

- Avoiding tobacco use, especially exposure to cigarette smoke
- Moderate alcohol consumption
- Healthier eating
- Limiting exposure to sunlight and artificial tanning UV exposure
- Encouraging physical exercise
- Maintaining a healthy body weight
- Maintaining adequate protection from asbestos fibres, radon and other occupational and environmental risk factors.

Chemoprevention

Chemoprevention is the prevention of cancer by using medication. The most common example is tamoxifen (pre-menopausal women) or an aromatase inhibitor (post-menopausal women) prescribed daily for 5 years to reduce the risk of developing breast cancer in high-risk women. However, these treatments are not without their side effects, such as menopausal symptoms and increased risk of thromboembolic events. Therefore, the risk-benefit ratio to each patient needs to be carefully assessed.

Another potential future development is the effect of aspirin as a chemopreventive agent for colorectal cancer. Maximal effect requires long-term use of high-dose aspirin that may increase the risk of gastro-intestinal bleeding. Non-steroidal anti-inflammatory drugs (NSAIDs) and selective cyclooxygenase-2 (COX-2) inhibitors may also be candidates for chemoprevention. However, the regular use of these drugs may also cause gastro-intestinal bleeding and increase the risk of cardiovascular events (Herszényi et al., 2008)

Cancer at the cellular level

Cancer arises from the changes in genes that regulate cell growth. For a normal cell to transform into a cancer cell, genetic changes must occur to the genes that regulate cell growth and differentiation. The nature of the genetic change may be a single point change to a DNA nucleotide, or the complete loss/gain of an entire chromosome. However, the most important factor is that a gene which regulates cell growth and/or differentiation must be altered to allow the cell to grow in an uncontrolled manner. Most cancers require a series of genetic mutations in a cell before an invasive tumour results.

Oncogenes

Oncogenes are where the normal gene, called a proto-oncogene, mutates and is then expressed at inappropriately high levels, therefore increasing the function of that gene. Examples of proto-oncogenes are genes that encode growth factors, signal transducers and transcription factors.

Tumour suppressor genes

Tumour suppressor genes are normal genes which have a protective effect against oncogenes, and are also known as 'anti-oncogenes'. The tumour suppressor gene's normal function is usually to control the cell cycle or act as a check point in division. When this function becomes lost due to mutations affecting both copies of the gene in a potentially malignant cell, other genetic mutations have a greater likelihood of progressing to cancer. An example is the *TP53* gene which codes for the suppressor protein product p53.

The p53 protein acts as a regulator of cell growth and proliferation and controls passage from G1 to S phase in cell division (see Fig. 52.1). Agents which damage DNA cause p53 to accumulate. This accumulation of p53 switches off replication in the cell, arresting the cell cycle and allowing time to repair. If repair fails, p53 may trigger cell suicide by apoptosis. Thus, p53 controls and halts the proliferation of abnormal cell growth.

The cancer cell

Cancer cells differ from normal cells in that they function differently. Inherently unstable, they may display different protein or enzyme content and chromosomal abnormalities (such as translocations or deletions) which may be associated with

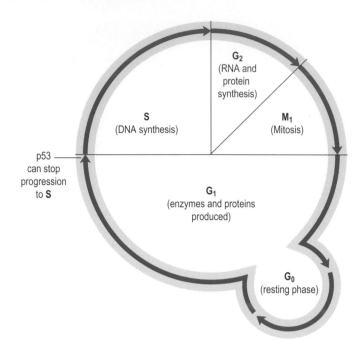

Fig. 52.1 Normal cell cycle.

differences in their susceptibility to chemotherapy or radiotherapy. The changes in internal structure and function lead to changes in their appearance which are visible under light microscopy, for example, larger and more varied appearance of the cell nuclei, and loss of the appearances of specialised cell function such as gland formation. This allows them to be easily detected, particularly when these lead to changes in the way clusters of cells form structures as a group and relate to normal cells in a tissue or organ.

Tumour growth

A solid tumour represents a population of dividing and non-dividing cells. The time it takes for a tumour mass to double is known as the doubling time. The latter will vary depending on the type of tumour but for most solid tumours it is about 2–3 months. In most solid tumours, the growth rate is very rapid initially (exponential growth) and then slows as the tumour increases in size and age, a pattern described as Gompertzian growth (see Fig. 52.2). The growth fraction is the percentage of actively dividing cells in the tumour, and this decreases with increasing tumour size.

This pattern of tumour growth kinetics has implications for chemotherapy treatment. Generally, chemotherapy is most successful when the number of tumour cells is low and the growth fraction high, which is the situation in the very early stages of cancer.

Tumour spread

As a primary tumour grows, it both pushes the normal surrounding cells aside and invades between them into normal tissue. It is this property of invasion that characterises a

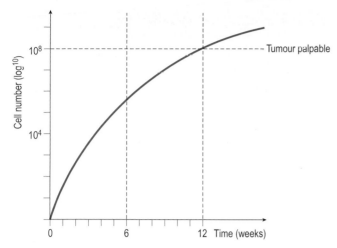

Fig. 52.2 Example of Gompertzian growth of cancer cells.

malignant tumour and leads to distant spread of the disease, since the abnormal cells often infiltrate through the walls of blood vessels and the lymphatic system. Malignant cells are then released from the infiltrating cluster of tumour cells and are transported by the blood or lymphatic fluid to other organs of the body where they can subsequently form secondary cancers or metastases. The pattern of spread tends to be predictable for different tumour types, influenced by the anatomy of the primary site and by differences in the local factors affecting the viability of malignant cells when they become deposited elsewhere. For example, breast cancer usually metastasises to the lymph nodes under the arm, lungs and central nervous system, while prostate cancer tends to metastasise to bone. Generally, when the primary is first detected, the larger the tumour mass the more likely that it has metastasised to other sites.

Patient management

Clinical assessment

Presentation

The clinical features of cancer vary with tumour type. Generally, patients most commonly present with non-specific complaints which include weight loss, unexplained anaemia, malaise, lethargy or pain, or they may have a specific localising symptom such as bleeding from an identifiable site, a non-healing ulcer, a minor symptom such as a cough or hoarseness not resolving in the usual way or the presence of a painful or painless lump. In general, solid tumours are first clinically detectable when there are approximately 10^8–10^9 tumour cells present in a tumour mass in the range of 1–10 g. The patient is usually in the terminal stages of the disease when there are 10^{12} cells present and a tumour burden of around 1 kg. A tumour may be detected by chance during a routine physical examination or by screening or through identification of early symptoms. However, if this does not occur or these symptoms are not present or not recognised, then the disease at presentation is commonly at a stage where there is a high risk that metastatic spread has already occurred at a microscopic level even if that is not clinically detectable.

Before treatment, each patient must undergo a thorough assessment to establish diagnosis, stage of disease and general fitness level. These factors will influence the choice of treatment and give a guide to prognosis.

Diagnosis

An accurate diagnosis is usually made from a tissue sample taken from a suspected primary or secondary tumour, according to the initial clinical investigations. This sampling procedure, biopsy, may be obtained by an open operation, or less invasively by endoscopy. Such samples may be obtained, for example, during bronchoscopy when lung cancer is suspected or, as in the case of a patient presenting with a breast lump, aspiration through a fine needle.

Malignant tumours vary in their sensitivity to chemotherapy. For example, there are two major groups of lung cancer: small-cell and non-small-cell lung cancer. Each of these groups is treated with different combinations of surgery, radiotherapy and chemotherapy drugs. Therefore, precise histopathology is important.

Tumour markers

Tumour markers are usually proteins associated with a malignancy and are clinically useful to:

- Diagnose a specific tumour
- Monitor response to treatment
- Estimate prognosis
- Detect recurrent disease
- Screen a healthy population or a high risk population for the presence of cancer.

They may be detected in a solid tumour, in circulating tumour cells in peripheral blood, in lymph nodes, in bone marrow or in other body fluids. A number of the tumour markers are presented in Table 52.2.

Staging investigations

Since the cancer is often disseminated at the time of presentation, it is vital that patients undergo thorough staging investigations to establish the extent and nature of disease. This will determine the most appropriate treatment offered to the patient. Baseline investigations range from clinical examination, blood tests, liver function tests, diagnostic imaging such as chest and skeletal X-rays, ultrasound, computed tomography (CT), magnetic resonance imaging (MRI) and positron emission tomography (PET), depending on the disease type and likely pattern of spread. Clinical guidelines for staging and management of malignancies of the various body systems have been produced at local and national level in most developed countries, with relatively minor variations according to local custom and practice (e.g. NICE in UK, see http://www.nice.org.uk/ for guidance and NCI in USA, see http://www.cancer.gov/ for guidance).

Table 52.2 Examples of tumour markers used in detection, diagnosis and monitoring

Tumour marker	Indicative cancer
CA125	Ovarian cancer, although non-specific
α-Fetoprotein (AFP) β-Human chorionic gonadotrophin (β-HCG)	Testicular tumour
5-Hydroxyindole acetic acid (5HIAA)	Carcinoid tumours
Thyroglobulin	Thyroid cancer
α-Fetoprotein	Hepatocellular carcinoma
Prostate-specific antigen	Prostate cancer
Human chorionic gonadotropin	Gestational trophoblastic tumours

Box 52.1 Performance status scales

Karnofsky performance index
100 Normal, no complaints, no evidence of disease
90 Able to carry on normal activity, minor signs or symptoms of disease
80 Normal activity with effort, some signs or symptoms of disease
70 Cares for self, unable to carry on normal activity or do active work
60 Requires occasional assistance but is able to care for most of own needs
50 Requires considerable assistance and frequent medical care
40 Disabled, requires special care and assistance
30 Severely disabled, hospitalisation is indicated, although death is not imminent
20 Very sick, hospitalisation necessary, active supportive treatment is necessary
10 Moribund, fatal processes progressing rapidly
WHO performance scale
0. Able to carry out all normal activity without restriction
1. Restricted in physically strenuous activity but ambulatory and able to carry out light work
2. Ambulatory and capable of all self-care but unable to carry out any work; up and about more than 50% of waking hours
3. Capable of only limited self-care; confined to bed more than 50% of waking hours
4. Completely disabled; cannot carry on any self-care; totally confined to bed or chair

Staging classification

Staging is essentially a measure of how far a tumour has progressed in its development at the time of diagnosis, while grading is a measure of how aggressive its behaviour is likely to be in future based on the microscopic appearance of the cells of the tumour. Both measures are relevant to the patient and clinical team in planning the management.

Most tumours are classified according to the TNM (tumour–nodes–metastases) system where T (0–4) indicates the size of the primary tumour, N (0–3) the extent of lymph node involvement and M (0–1) the presence or absence of distant metastases. Each solid tumour site has a specific grading and staging classification such as Dukes staging in colorectal cancer (Cancer Research UK, 2009) and Gleason scoring for grading prostate cancer (Berney, 2007).

Performance status

The patient's general level of fitness (performance status) at the time of diagnosis is often a surprisingly reliable indicator of prognosis independent of disease-related factors, and will help determine if they are likely to withstand intensive chemotherapy; this therefore influences the choice of treatment. A number of physical rating scales have been devised to assess performance status, including the Karnofsky performance index (Karnofsky and Burchenal, 1949) and the World Health Organization (WHO) performance scale (Box 52.1).

Prognostic factors

These are factors that can predict how the disease is likely to behave and determine an outcome in individual patients. For example, Table 52.3 lists prognostic factors in patients with colorectal cancer.

Table 52.3 Prognostic factors in patients with colorectal cancer

Favourable	Unfavourable
Good performance status	Presence of nodal involvement
No penetration of the tumour through the bowel wall	Presence of distant metastases
Absence of nodal involvement	Bowel obstruction and bowel perforation
Absence of distant metastases	

Treatment

Treatment goals

After the diagnosis of cancer has been confirmed and the extent of disease fully investigated, the goals of treatment have to be considered. Depending on stage of disease, the goal can be the following (and may change throughout treatment):

- Cure – Patients are said to be 'cured' of cancer when they are completely disease free and have a normal life expectancy. The smaller the tumour bulk when treatment is given, the greater the potential of achieving cure. A common measure of 'cure' is the 5-year disease-free survival rate
- Prolong survival while maintaining patient quality of life
- Provide palliative care with relief of symptoms such as pain.

Childhood malignancies, choriocarcinoma and testicular tumours in adults are most responsive to chemotherapy and these patients are frequently cured, even with advanced disease. However, for most patients treated with chemotherapy, cure is less likely and treatment will be given to maximise the probability of cure, prolong survival or be purely palliative. The decision is influenced by factors such as the extent of the disease as well as co-existing symptoms and concurrent medical conditions, performance status and, importantly, the patient's wishes. The possibility of medium-to long-term survival justifies aggressive treatment but with palliative therapy it is particularly important that the toxicity of treatment is carefully weighed against the potential benefits.

Treatment guidelines

Consensus on the best approach to managing each particular type of cancer is continually evolving, based on the evidence from clinical research most reliably in the form of randomised controlled trials. National guidelines aim to promote equity for patients and ensure a consistent treatment approach taking account of the boundaries of affordability for the healthcare system. In the absence of clinical consensus, patients should be encouraged to participate in clinical trials.

Treatment methods

Three main options are available for the treatment of patients with solid tumours: surgery, radiotherapy and chemotherapy. Targeted and biological therapies are at present minor modalities, and it is hoped that these will be employed more as their effectiveness improves. Each treatment may play a number of roles, either alone or in combination, depending on the disease, stage and grade.

Role of surgery

Surgery can be curative when solid tumours are confined to one primary anatomical site or region as in localised disease. It can also be used to remove isolated metastatic masses with curative intent in rare circumstances or to deal with anatomical consequences of a tumour as a palliative procedure, such as relief of bowel obstruction by defunctioning colostomy. Surgical techniques may be used to support chemotherapy administration when given by continuous infusion or by the intraperitoneal route. Surgery may also play a role in diagnosis through tissue biopsy or in staging to ascertain the extent of tumour involvement such as in ovarian cancer. In the latter, it may also be used to debulk or reduce the size of the tumour to effect pain relief or to improve the effectiveness of subsequent radiation or chemotherapy. However, with more widespread disease, systemic treatment becomes necessary, with chemotherapy playing a major role

Role of radiotherapy

Radiotherapy can be used to cure cancer, reduce the symptoms of the tumour, reduce the size of the tumour ready for surgery or to prevent re-occurrence of the tumour after surgical removal. It can be used alone or in combination with surgery and/or chemotherapy. A full exposition of the role of radiotherapy is beyond the scope of this chapter, which concentrates on the role of systemic agents. However, the combination of radiotherapy and systemic treatment is becoming increasingly employed as research shows the benefit to disease control and long-term survival, for example, in carcinoma of the uterine cervix (Green et al., 2009).

Systemic therapy

This encompasses cytotoxic chemotherapy, hormonal, biological and targeted therapies, but the term does not usually encompass the modalities of nutritional, complementary, alternative, or other 'holistic' interventions, even if employed within a conventional medical environment.

Cytotoxic chemotherapy

Chemotherapy regimen

Although chemotherapy is sometimes administered as a single agent, it is more usual to combine two or more drugs to achieve additive or synergistic effects. Generally, drugs used in combination should have established efficacy as single agents, different mechanisms of action and differing toxicity profiles to allow their use at optimal doses.

Chemotherapy scheduling

As chemotherapy does not specifically target malignant cells, any actively proliferating normal cell will be at potential risk of damage, in particular the cells of the bone marrow. This causes a fall in the white blood cell count and with many cytotoxic drugs, the white blood count is at its lowest level (nadir) around 10 days after treatment. Recovery generally occurs by day 20 post-treatment, and therefore chemotherapy treatment is usually repeated every 3–4 weeks. With agents such as mitomycin and lomustine, haematological recovery may be delayed for 42–50 days following treatment, in which case the interval between treatment cycles needs to be increased. In most cases, a course of treatment will comprise a maximum of six cycles of chemotherapy, although in some less common cancers such as sarcomas and in paediatrics, the regime may continue with a much longer period of adjuvant or consolidation therapy.

Figure 52.3 demonstrates the tumour cell kill for each cycle of chemotherapy together with the healthy normal cell kill. Chemotherapy works in situations where the healthy normal cells recover faster or more completely from the effects of chemotherapy compared to the tumour cells. This allows the tumour cells to be progressively killed off, whilst not having a detrimental effect on the patient.

Chemotherapy dose

The dose of most chemotherapy agents is calculated using the patient's body surface area (BSA) and is usually given in the form of milligrams per square meter. Body surface area may

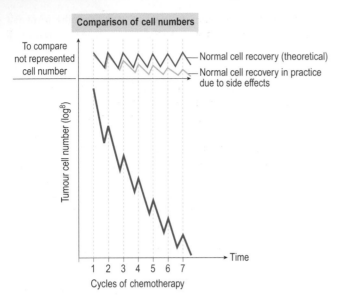

Fig. 52.3 The effect of chemotherapy on tumour mass and healthy cells.

be calculated from the height and weight of the patient using a nomogram and may need to be recalculated for subsequent cycles of chemotherapy if the patient experiences significant weight changes. Table 52.4 gives an example of a chemotherapy regimen used in breast cancer. The reliability of body surface area as a predictor of the effective safe dose is diminished for patients who are either very thin (cachectic) or grossly overweight (morbidly obese) since it does not then reflect a reasonable estimate of lean body mass.

Adjuvant chemotherapy

Adjuvant chemotherapy means literally 'additional treatment' and is usually given after surgery or radiotherapy when all detectable disease has been removed, but where there remains

Table 52.4 Example of a chemotherapy regimen FEC–T (Fluorouracil, epirubicin, cyclophosphamide, docetaxel (Taxotere®)) for breast cancer

Indication	Adjuvant Breast Cancer	
Length of cycle	21 days	
No. of cycles	3 cycles of FEC followed by 3 cycles of Taxotere® (Docetaxel)	
FEC		
Fluorouracil	IVB	500 mg/m² day 1
Epirubicin	IVB	100 mg/m² day 1
Cyclophosphamide	IVB	500 mg/m² day 1
T		
Docetaxel	IVI over 1 h	100 mg/m² day 1

IVB, i.v. bolus; IVI, i.v. infusion.

a statistical risk of relapse due to undetectable disease. Adjuvant therapy is, therefore, used to increase the likelihood of cure. Only patients whose cancers have a high or intermediate risk of recurrence tend to be selected for adjuvant chemotherapy since it is not desirable to expose patients whose disease may already have been cured by surgery or radiotherapy to the toxicity of chemotherapy treatment.

In colorectal cancer, for example, adjuvant chemotherapy provides significant disease-free survival benefit by reducing the recurrence rate and also increases overall survival. This indicates the curative role of chemotherapy in the adjuvant setting (Sargent et al., 2009). Similarly, in breast cancer, adjuvant treatment has been shown to increase recurrence-free survival (Levine and Whelan, 2006), and trials are underway to determine which agents and in what combination further improvements in overall survival will be obtained. A recent trial has shown that three-weekly AC/T (doxorubicin, cyclophosphamide, docetaxel [Taxotere®]) is significantly inferior to CEF (cyclophosphamide, epirubicin, 5-flourouricil) or EC/T (epirubicin, cyclophosphamide, docetaxel [Taxotere®]) in terms of recurrence-free survival (Burnell et al., 2010). This is important, as standard treatment choices should move to the superior regimen.

Neo-adjuvant chemotherapy

In neo-adjuvant chemotherapy, chemotherapy is given before local therapy, often preoperatively, to reduce tumour size and facilitate surgical removal. Neo-adjuvant chemotherapy has been of particular value in cases of breast cancer, non-small-cell lung cancer, advanced head and neck cancer, and bone tumours. In Ewings sarcoma, it allows limb-sparing surgery as an alternative to amputation. It also improves survival with reduced morbidity in osteosarcoma.

Synchronous chemoradiation

In several cancers, chemotherapy alongside radical radiotherapy is now established. Agents such as cisplatin are commonly used as a 'radiosensitiser' in head and neck, oesophageal and cervical cancers. The use of cetuximab in combination with radiotherapy for a certain type of head and neck cancer is also recommended (National Institute for Health and Clinical Excellence, 2008). Although common, the use of the term 'radiosensitiser' in this context is somewhat inaccurate and is distinct from the 'true' radiosensitising drugs such as nimorazole, which interact at a chemical level with very short-lived radiation-induced free radicals, and the effect is better termed 'combined modality therapy'.

Adverse effects of cytotoxic drugs

Most cytotoxic drugs have been developed because of their effect on dividing cells. Consequently and as previously mentioned under chemotherapy scheduling, proliferating normal tissue such as bone marrow is at risk. Myelosuppression is frequently the dose-limiting toxicity with these compounds. Neutropenia and thrombocytopenia place patients at risk of life-threatening infection and bleeding, respectively.

The other acute adverse effects occurring most frequently include nausea and vomiting, mucositis, anorexia and alopecia. Individual drugs will also give rise to specific adverse effects, some of which may not be reversible on stopping treatment. Cardiotoxicity, nephrotoxicity and pulmonary toxicity, which are specific to the chemotherapeutic agent or class, may depend on cumulative drug exposure, the schedule of administration and previous therapy. Long-term side effects include infertility due to suppression of ovarian and testicular function and occasionally the induction of a second malignancy.

Chemotherapy-related toxicity is an important issue. Not only can it result in prolonged hospitalisation and a reduction in patients' quality of life, but also successful treatment can be compromised. A reduction in dose intensity, that is the dose of cytotoxic delivered for unit time, because of dose reductions or treatment delays can result in reduced response rates and survival. Recently, the use of granulocyte-colony-stimulating factors (G-CSF) to prevent dose-limiting toxicity of myelosuppression has started to become standard practice. This is often used in adjuvant treatments where the dose intensity given is paramount, and the goal of treatment is cure.

Chemotherapy-specific adjunctive treatments

Both ifosfamide and cyclophosphamide are metabolised to the inactive acrolein which is responsible for bladder toxicity. The co-administration of mesna, a sulphydryl-containing compound which binds to acrolein, has reduced the incidence of haemorrhagic cystitis associated with intravenous regimens of ifosfamide and high-dose cyclophosphamide.

Calcium leucovorin or folinic acid is a reduced form of folic acid and is in effect an 'antidote' to the cytotoxic methotrexate. Folinic acid is effectively used as a form of 'rescue' when high doses of intravenous methotrexate are used to limit the exposure to methotrexate to a defined period of time.

Targeted therapies

In recent years, there has been an increased understanding of biochemical signalling pathways involved in the growth and progression of tumours. This has allowed the development of therapies targeted specifically at the cell receptors involved. A number of these are described. As they are targeted at tumour cells, they suppress disease without inflicting the non-selective toxic effects of cytotoxic chemotherapy on the patient.

Epidermal growth factor receptor

The epidermal growth factor receptor (EGFR) is a transmembrane protein with an intracellular tyrosine kinase domain. Extracellular binding of the epidermal growth factor receptor induces tyrosine phosphorylation which activates signal cascade pathways. These ultimately lead to cellular proliferation and metastasis. Epidermal growth factor receptor expression is low in normal tissues, and overexpression is associated with a variety of tumours including non-small-cell lung cancer, colon, and head and neck.

Inhibitors of epidermal growth factor receptor (also known as human epidermal growth factor receptor type 1 [HER1]) include:

- Small molecules such as the orally administered erlotinib used in the treatment of non-small-cell lung cancer and imatinib used in the treatment of gastro-intestinal stromal tumours (GIST) which specifically inhibit tyrosine kinase.
- Monoclonal antibodies such as cetuximab which binds to the epidermal growth factor receptor. Cetuximab has demonstrated synergy when given in combination with irinotecan chemotherapy, offering prolonged survival in selected patients with metastatic colorectal cancer.

Vascular endothelial growth factor receptor

Angiogenesis is the formation of new blood vessels on which tumour growth depends. Vascular endothelial growth factor (VEGF) is key in angiogenesis and its overexpression has been associated with increased vasculature, aggressive disease and poor prognosis. The monoclonal antibody bevacizumab inhibits VEGF, thereby reducing new blood vessel growth and interstitial pressure within the tumour, allowing improved chemotherapy access. Studies have demonstrated meaningful survival benefits when bevacizumab is administered in conjunction with chemotherapy in patients with advanced or metastatic colorectal cancer (Hurwitz et al., 2004).

Human epidermal growth factor receptor type 2

Overexpression of human epidermal growth factor receptor 2 (HER2) is associated with a particularly aggressive form of breast cancer (about 20% cases are HER2 positive) linked with a poor prognosis. Trastuzumab, a humanised monoclonal antibody, specifically targets human epidermal growth factor receptor 2 and is only effective in patients with elevated levels. It is used widely in metastatic and early breast cancer (National Institute for Health and Clinical Excellence, 2002, 2006a). The use of trastuzumab in other cancers that express human epidermal growth factor receptor 2 is also under investigation. Trastuzumab has also been licensed for use in human epidermal growth factor receptor 2 positive gastric cancer.

Capecitabine

Although capecitabine does not target a particular receptor, it is mentioned in this section, as it preferentially targets tumour cells.

Capecitabine is a fluoropyrimidine carbamate precursor of 5-fluorouracil (5FU). Given orally, it is converted via enzyme pathways to 5-fluorouracil. As these enzymes are found in higher concentrations in tumour cells, treatment is effectively targeted. Capecitabine has been shown to be at least as effective as intravenous 5-fluorouracil (Twelves et al., 2008), and it is widely used in practice. This is of a particular benefit where the total regimen can then be given orally rather than intravenously.

Management of patients receiving cytotoxic chemotherapy

Prescription verification

Over recent years, there has been considerable effort to improve the quality and safety of chemotherapy services for adult patients (National Chemotherapy Advisory Group, 2009). In particular, the importance of all chemotherapy prescriptions being checked by appropriately trained and competent pharmacists is now recognised. A checklist of key points an authorised pharmacist must undertake to verify any prescription for systemic anti-cancer therapy prior to preparation and release has been determined (British Oncology Pharmacy Association, 2010) and is presented in Box 52.2.

Box 52.2 Standards for chemotherapy prescription verification (British Oncology Pharmacy Association, 2010)

1. Check prescriber's details and signature are present and confirm they are authorised to prescribe SACT
2. Ensure regimen has been through local approval processes, for example, clinical governance and financial approval and/or is included on a list of locally approved regimens
3. On the first cycle, check the regimen is the intended treatment as documented in a treatment plan, in the clinical notes or in the electronic record
4. Check regimen is appropriate for patient's diagnosis, medical history, performance status and chemotherapy history (using the treatment plan, clinical notes or electronic record)
5. Check there are no known drug interactions (including with food) or conflicts with patient allergies and other medication(s)
6. Check that the timing of administration is appropriate, that is the interval since last treatment
7. Check patient demographics (age, height and weight) have been correctly recorded on prescription
8. Check body surface area (BSA) is correctly calculated, taking into account recent weight. Note there should be local agreement for frequency of monitoring and checking patient's weight
9. Check all dose calculations and dose units are correct and have been calculated correctly according to the protocol and any other relevant local guidance, for example, dose rounding/banding
10. Check cumulative dose and maximum individual dose as appropriate
11. Check reason for and consistency of any dose adjustments, for example, reduction(s) or escalations and ensure reason is documented
12. Check method of administration is appropriate
13. Check laboratory values, FBC, U&Es and LFTs are within accepted limits if appropriate
14. Check doses are appropriate with respect to renal and hepatic function and any experienced toxicities
15. Check other essential tests have been undertaken if appropriate
16. Check supportive care is prescribed and it is appropriate for the patient and regimen
17. Sign and date prescription as a record of verification

SAT, Systemic anticancer therapy

Cumulative dosing

The use of doxorubicin is limited by a dose-dependent cardiomyopathy. A number of other factors have been implicated, including treatment schedule, patient age and pre-existing cardiac disease, but dose is the most important. The maximum recommended cumulative dose is 550 or 400 mg/m^2 for patients who have received radiotherapy to the mediastinum. Therefore treatment should be monitored closely to make sure the cumulative dose is not exceeded throughout the patient's lifetime. All other anthracycline antibiotics also have a lifetime cumulative dose limit.

Dose modification or delay

Appropriate investigations must be carried out before each treatment to ensure that patients are fit for chemotherapy. In particular, the patient's haematological, renal and hepatic function should be investigated. For some cytotoxic drugs, it may be necessary to adjust the dose, or even stop treatment, in the presence of renal or hepatic impairment to ensure that delayed excretion or reduced metabolism does not result in excess toxicity. Therefore, the individual summary of product characteristics (SPC) for the chemotherapy agent should be consulted and can be found at http://www.medicines.org.uk.

If the bone marrow does not recover sufficiently between cycles of treatment, then a dose reduction or a delay in treatment may be necessary. In general, patients with a neurophil below 1×10^9/L or a platelet count below 100×10^9/L should not be given myelosuppressive cytotoxics at full doses.

Drug interactions

Prescriptions for cancer chemotherapy are often complex, sometimes involving combinations of both parenteral and oral cytotoxic drugs, intravenous fluids and other supportive therapies. The potential for drug interactions to arise is considerable. However, care is required when assessing the clinical significance of potential drug interactions. A documented interaction does not necessarily imply that drugs should not be used together but can necessitate close monitoring of the patient.

Patient information and counselling

All patients must be provided with information about their treatment, including any anticipated side effects. Patients should be encouraged by health professionals to ask questions about their treatment.

Patients must understand the different medication, the specific role of each medicine and duration of treatment. Duration of treatment is particularly important to prevent highly potent medicines from being inadvertently continued beyond their intended course.

Symptom control

Nausea and vomiting

Chemotherapy-induced nausea and vomiting (CINV) is one of the most frequently experienced side effects encountered by chemotherapy patients and is considered to be the most distressing. In extreme cases, poor symptom control can result in patients refusing further treatment.

In selecting an appropriate anti-emetic regimen, relevant factors include the emetogenic potential of the chemotherapy drugs prescribed, the putative mechanism(s) of inducing emesis, and the likely onset and duration of symptoms. Individual patient characteristics also have to be taken into consideration. For example, predisposing factors which increase a patient's susceptibility to emesis following chemotherapy treatment are:

- Poor control with prior chemotherapy.
- Female sex.
- Younger age <50 years.
- A current or prior history of low chronic alcohol intake.
- History of sickness: pregnancy/travelling/surgery.
- Anxiety.
- Smoking.
- Radiation to gastro-intestinal tract, liver or brain.
- Other medications: various medications can cause nausea and vomiting such as anaesthetic agents, anti-depressants, anti-microbials, anti-fungals, iron, levodopa, carbidopa, NSAIDs.

Differences in the severity of emesis can also occur between patients receiving the same type of chemotherapy and even between treatment cycles in the same patient; however, modern drug treatment can successfully control CINV for the majority of patients.

The 5-hydroxytryptamine type 3 ($5HT_3$) receptor antagonists, which include dolasetron, granisetron, ondansetron, palonosetron and tropisetron, have become the standard management of acute CINV when treating patients with moderately emetogenic chemotherapy regimens. For highly emetogenic chemotherapy regimens such as those including cisplatinum, the use of the NK_1 inhibitor, aprepitant, together with a $5HT_3$ antagonist is becoming the gold standard. These agents are most effective in dealing with acute emesis (less than 24 h duration) when combined with a potent steroid such as dexamethasone.

It is important to achieve optimal control of nausea and vomiting at the outset to avoid subsequent anticipatory symptoms which can prove very difficult to treat.

The route of administration for anti-emetics is an important consideration. With intravenous chemotherapy, it may be simpler to administer all treatments by the intravenous route. Alternatives to the oral route may be useful when vomiting occurs and include the rectal and buccal route.

Pain control

Drug therapy remains the cornerstone of effective pain management but it is often undertreated, thus highlighting the importance of regular patient assessment and appropriate dose or drug treatment changes. For example, patients experiencing intolerable side effects to morphine may be transferred to oxycodone or transdermal fentanyl skin patches. Analgesia should be prescribed both regularly and for breakthrough pain, and stimulant laxatives should be prescribed to prevent constipation. Combinations of analgesics which have synergistic activity, for example, opiates plus NSAIDs, can be highly effective whilst minimising dose-related side effects of each agent.

The route of administration is also important. When patients are unable to manage oral medication, it is important to assess the use of alternative routes such as the rectal, subcutaneous, epidural and transdermal routes.

Bone marrow suppression

Myelosuppression following chemotherapy is common, and for some patients profound. The risk of systemic infection can be reduced by good oral hygiene and mouth care using antiseptic mouthwashes and anti-fungal prophylaxis. Patients must be advised to immediately report symptoms of infection and bruising. Platelet transfusions may be required, but fever or other evidence of infection occurring in a neutropenic patient when the neutrophil count is less than 1.0×10^9/L must be aggressively treated with broad-spectrum intravenous antibiotics to prevent overwhelming infection.

The duration and depth of neutropenia can be dramatically reduced by the administration of G-CSF which stimulate neutrophil production and, in cases of severe neutropenia, effectively rescue the patient. Once the patient's neutrophil count has recovered sufficiently, their use may be safely discontinued. These agents may also be used prophylactically in patients with a high risk of febrile neutropenia before receiving chemotherapy.

Blood transfusions are commonly required by patients at some stage of their treatment due to anaemia. Alternatively, erythropoietin may be useful in some patients receiving chemotherapy to shorten the period of anaemia and improve the patient's quality of life where blood transfusions are not possible.

Extravasation

Extreme care must be taken when administering cytotoxic drugs parenterally because of the dangers of extravasation. Extravasation, which is the accidental leakage of an intravenous drug into the surrounding tissue, can cause pain, erythema and severe local necrosis, resulting in permanent tissue damage. The patient must be asked to immediately report any pain or a stinging sensation at the injection site since the degree of damage is determined by the amount of drug extravasated and the speed at which it is detected. If extravasation is suspected, the administration of further chemotherapy must stop and remedial treatment must commence as soon as possible. The effectiveness of such therapy varies according to the agent extravasated.

Inpatient or outpatient treatment

The majority of patients receive chemotherapy in the outpatient clinic or day-care setting, where cytotoxics are administered mainly by short intravenous infusion at 3- or 4-week intervals. Other treatments include monoclonal antibodies,

Table 52.5 National Cancer Institute common toxicity criteria for anaemia (haemoglobin) (Cancer Therapy Evaluation Program, 1998)

Adverse event, Grade	0	1	2	3	4
Haemoglobin (Hgb)	WNL	<LLN–10.0 g/dL <LLN–100 g/L <LLN–6.2 mmol/L	8.0–<10.0 g/dL 80–<100 g/L 4.9–<6.2 mmol/L	6.5–<8.0 g/dL 65–<80 g/L 4.0–<4.9 mmol/L	<6.5 g/dL <65 g/L <4.0 mmol/L

WNL, within normal limits; LLN, lower limit of normal.

which usually require close monitoring of the patient for several hours in case of anaphylactic reactions. More complex treatments, such as cisplatinum-containing regimens which require prehydration with intravenous fluids, need the patient to attend all day.

Currently, inpatient treatment of chemotherapy only occurs for the small minority of treatments, and this number is declining further as novel ways of administering long infusions are being developed.

Domiciliary treatment

Oral cytotoxic drugs can safely be taken at home so long as the patient is informed and able to monitor side effects. Availability of a 24-h helpline is essential for these patients should they encounter problems whilst on treatment (National Chemotherapy Advisory Group, 2009). In the future, administration of intravenous treatments, such as the monoclonal antibody trastuzumab, may be carried out more frequently in the home setting, particularly when safety permits and where patient preference becomes an influential factor.

Monitoring anti-cancer therapy

As well as desirable outcomes, treatment with chemotherapy may result in a variety of undesirable outcomes; both require careful monitoring.

Toxicity

The toxicity resulting from treatment is routinely assessed following each cycle of chemotherapy, and may result in therapy being modified on subsequent cycles, for example, a dose reduction, a delay in treatment or, in some cases, an alternative treatment. A number of international rating scales are available for rating predictable acute reactions arising from chemotherapy, including that of the National Cancer Institute Common Toxicity Criteria (for an example, see Table 52.5). Standardising the assessment of treatment-related toxicity in this way allows comparison to be made between published reports of clinical trials.

Response to treatment

Throughout treatment, the response to therapy is closely monitored, noting changes in performance status, symptoms and objective measurements of the tumour. This may necessitate repeating some or all of the initial staging investigations. Should the initial treatment prove ineffective, an alternative can then be considered without delay. Assessment of response should be formally documented before proceeding to further therapy.

Definitions of response. These have been standardised by the WHO:

- *Complete response or remission* (CR). Disappearance of all recognisable tumour masses and/or biochemical changes directly related to the tumour and resolution of symptoms determined by two observations at least a month apart.
- *Partial response* (PR). Decrease by 50% or more in all tumour masses, measured by the product of the longest × the widest perpendicular diameters for at least a month.
- *Stable disease* (SD) *or no change* (NC). Changes smaller than those described above for PR or less than for progressive disease for at least a month.
- *Progressive disease* (PD). Occurrence of any new lesion or increase in the longest × widest perpendicular diameters of measurable disease by at least 25%.

Again, this allows comparison of results between different reported studies. An update of the WHO guidelines has been published (Therasse et al., 2000) called RECIST or Response Evaluation Criteria in Solid Tumours. To avoid confusion, it is important to stipulate in trial protocols which system will be used. Although clinical response indicates tumour sensitivity, it may not necessarily predict long-term survival nor does it measure other benefits such as quality of life.

Case studies

Case 52.1

Mrs BH, a 53-year-old post-menopausal mother of two teenage children, has recently completed six cycles of FEC(100)-T (5-fluorouracil, epirubicin, cyclophosphamide, docetaxel) as adjuvant chemotherapy for her node-positive early breast cancer. She tolerated her chemotherapy well and did not require any dose reductions or delays.

Her receptor status at diagnosis was oestrogen receptor positive and progestogen receptor negative (ER+/PR–); she was also HER2 positive.

Her oncologist has recommended that she commences adjuvant treatment with trastuzumab.

Questions

1. What treatment regimen for trastuzumab should be followed?
2. What side effects of trastuzumab should Mrs BH be informed about when giving consent for treatment?
3. What other treatments should be considered for this patient?

Answers

1. Trastuzumab targets the epidermal growth factor receptor (EGFR) and is indicated for the treatment of early breast cancer overexpressing HER2 following surgery, chemotherapy (neo-adjuvant or adjuvant) and radiotherapy if applicable as recommended by National Institute for Health and Clinical Excellence (2006a). The product license for trastuzumab recommends the dosing schedule used in the HERA study (Piccart-Gebhart et al., 2005), that is loading dose of 8 mg/kg body weight, followed by 6 mg/kg body weight 3 weeks later and then 6 mg/kg repeated at three-weekly intervals administered as infusions over approximately 90 min. This is continued for 12 months, stopping sooner if disease reoccurs.

2. The most common side effects experienced by patients are infusion related, such as fever and chills, usually following the first or second treatment. Patients should be closely monitored for at least 6 h after the start of the first infusion and if the treatment has been well tolerated, for 2 h after the start of subsequent infusions. If a reaction occurs, the infusion should be stopped, appropriate symptomatic treatment administered and treatment recommenced at a slower rate only when the symptoms have subsided. Trastuzumab has been associated with cardiotoxicity and patients who have previously received anthracyclines are at increased risk. All patients should have their cardiac function closely monitored at baseline and every 3 months during the period that they are being treated with trastuzumab (National Institute for Health and Clinical Excellence, 2006a). There was an approximate 5% increase in the number of patients with a significant change in cardiac function in the HERA study (Piccart-Gebhart et al., 2005).

3. In view of her receptor status, this patient should be offered hormonal treatment. Depending on the perceived level of risk of recurrence as estimated using a model such as the Nottingham Prognostic Index (Galea et al., 1992), she should be offered either 5 years' treatment with an aromatase inhibitor or planned sequential treatment with tamoxifen switching to an aromatase inhibitor after 2–3 years' therapy. The long-term effect on cardiovascular health (tamoxifen) or bone health (aromatase inhibitors) together with the expected level of benefits should be used to guide choice of treatment. Further information can be found in national guidance for the early management of breast cancer with hormonal treatments (National Institute for Health and Clinical Excellence, 2006a).

Case 52.2

Mr BS, a 67-year-old man with a history of localised prostate cancer, is reviewed by his oncologist. Mr BS was previously treated with radical radiotherapy and more recently several lines of hormonal therapy.

His PSA has risen over the last 6 months and is now 80 ng/mL. It was 0.1 ng/mL on completion of radical radiation therapy. He also complains that his longstanding back pain controlled by low-dose NSAIDs has now become much worse and is out of control.

Questions

1. What is the most likely cause of Mr BS's back pain and raised PSA?
2. What treatment options should be discussed with the patient?

3. Why should he be referred for a dental examination before commencing any further treatment?

Answers

1. The fact that the PSA is markedly raised suggests a recurrence of prostate cancer. Moderate rises in the PSA would have warranted a change in hormonal therapy. The elevated PSA together with the increased back pain suggest metastatic bone disease as a result of distant recurrence of his prostate cancer. This could be confirmed with plain film X-rays or by bone scan. The risk of both local and distant recurrence depends on the stage at presentation.

2. Treatment options for recurrent prostate cancer include second-line hormonal therapy, chemotherapy with or without corticosteroids, and best supportive care. Localised radiotherapy to specific bone lesions could improve his back pain; this would depend on the distribution of treatable lesions identified. The choice of therapy depends on the symptoms, the site of relapse, performance status of the patient and the presence of other co-morbidities. Best supportive care can be provided with radiotherapy, bisphosphonates, steroids and analgesics, and is the only option for patients who are too ill to tolerate further systemic intervention. Tolerability of chemotherapy is of concern, particularly because most patients with prostate cancer are elderly and many have other medical problems. Mr BS has already received more than one line of hormonal therapy; his tumour is unlikely to respond to further hormonal manipulation. An alternative strategy that is available is the use of radioactive isotopes such as Strontium 89 for systemic treatment of multiple bone metastases. The use of chemotherapy in the treatment of hormone-refractory prostate cancer should be considered in patients with a Karnofsky performance status of 60% or greater. Further information on the use of docetaxel for the treatment of hormone-refractory metastatic prostate cancer is available (National Institute for Health and Clinical Excellence, 2006b).

3. Future treatment options for this patient may include use of bisphosphonates to stabilise his bone lesions and reduce his pain. Long-term use of bisphosphonates has been associated with osteonecrosis of the jaw; the risk is exacerbated by poor dental hygiene, concurrent dental procedures, chemotherapy, corticosteroids and malignant disease. Examination and preventive dental treatment should be considered for patients prior to commencing therapy with bisphosphonates in order to avoid any invasive procedures, for instance dental extraction, during bisphosphonate therapy.

Case 52.3

Mr SG, a 46-year-old patient, was diagnosed with Dukes' C colon cancer several months ago. Since then, he has undergone a left hemicolectomy. He is currently receiving capecitabine monotherapy as adjuvant treatment. He telephones the pharmacy department for advice on how to cope with the side effects he is currently experiencing.

Questions

1. What side effects are commonly associated with capecitabine?
2. How do these differ from those associated with intravenous 5-fluorouracil?
3. What advice should he be given?

Answers

1. Side effects most commonly associated with capecitabine treatment are mainly related to the skin and the gastro-intestinal tract.

- Palmar–plantar erythema (hand–foot syndrome) 57%
- Diarrhoea 47%
- Nausea 35%
- Stomatitis 23%
- Vomiting 18%
- Fatigue 16%

2. Although capecitabine is converted enzymatically to 5-fluorouracil, there is a difference in the frequency with which specific side effects are experienced, making it more akin to continuous infusions of 5-flourouracil. Patients receiving intermittent bolus therapy with 5-fluorouracil are more likely to experience the gastro-intestinal side effects, particularly diarrhoea or stomatitis, rather than the cutaneous reactions. Myelosuppression may also infrequently be a problem encountered by these patients.

3. Mr SG should be instructed to contact the emergency telephone number he would have been given with his treatment from the hospital looking after him.

    If detected early, side effects usually improve within 2–3 days. Treatment may be reinstated at the same dose if side effects are moderate, or at a reduced dose if more severe. Symptomatic relief for palmar–plantar erythema may be provided by the use of emollients. There is little evidence to support the use of specific antidotes.

Case 52.4

Mrs PQ, a 59-year-old women, has non-small-cell lung cancer. She has had a course of gemcitabine combined with carboplatin and now requires second-line chemotherapy. The doctor has suggested erlotinib.

Questions

1. What type of treatment is erlotinib and how is it given?
2. What common side effects should Mrs PQ be informed about when she is giving consent for treatment?
3. What other treatments should be considered for this patient?

Answers

1. Erlotinib is an epidermal growth factor receptor/human epidermal growth factor receptor type 1 (EGFR also known as HER1) tyrosine kinase inhibitor. Erlotinib potently inhibits the intracellular phosphorylation of EGFR. Epidermal growth factor receptor is expressed on the cell surface of normal cells and cancer cells. In non-clinical models, inhibition of epidermal growth factor receptor phosphotyrosine results in cell stasis and/or death. It is an oral tablet given once a day until disease progression or unacceptable toxicity.

2. Rash (75%) and diarrhoea (54%) were the most commonly reported adverse drug reactions (ADRs). In general, rash manifests as a mild or moderate erythematous and papulopustular rash, which may occur or worsen in skin areas exposed to the sun. For patients who are exposed to the sun, protective clothing, and/or use of sun screen (with minimum SPF 15, e.g. mineral-containing) may be advisable. The rash generally starts about 8–10 days after starting treatment but usually improves after a few weeks. Diarrhoea is usually mild and

can be controlled with anti-diarrhoeal drugs. Fatigue, nausea and vomiting and sore mouth are also quite common. Some people also develop sore, red eyes (conjunctivitis) or dry eyes.

3. Docetaxel is the other second-line treatment currently available for the treatment of non-small-cell lung cancer.

Case 52.5

Mrs GH is a 64-year-old post-menopausal women with metastatic breast cancer. She has had several cycles of chemotherapy including previous anthracyclines and she had her third cycle of capecitabine 8 days ago. Mrs GH is feeling 'a bit unwell' and her husband thinks she is not at all her usual self, and is, therefore, worried about her.

Questions

1. What side effect may Mrs GH be suffering from?
2. How would you explain to Mrs GH how to take a cycle of capecitabine?
3. What are the possible patient safety concerns regarding oral chemotherapy?

Answers

1. Mrs GH may be suffering from neutropenic sepsis. The signs can be difficult to identify with a small elevation in temperature and a general feeling of not being well. It is important that Mrs GH is prescribed IV antibiotics as soon as possible before she succumbs to the infection. Chemotherapy patients are all at varying degrees of risk for neutropenic sepsis due to the marked decrease in neutrophils in the body due to the chemotherapy. She should also have a blood test to check her neutrophil level, but administration of antibiotics should not wait for these results. Each hospital will have guidelines or a protocol in place to treat neutropenic sepsis in patients receiving chemotherapy.

2. Take the capecitabine dose morning and evening, 12 h apart with a glass of water. Mrs GH should take the capecitabine for 14 days and then stop for 7 days. In addition, it is important to make sure that Mrs GH understands her correct dose.

3. Healthcare workers and their staff must be made aware that the prescribing, dispensing and administering of oral anti-cancer medicines should be carried out and monitored to the same standard as injected therapy. This requires:

- Healthcare organisations to prepare local policies and procedures that describe the safe use of these oral medicines
- Treatment to be initiated by a cancer specialist
- All oral anti-cancer medicines to be prescribed only in the context of a written protocol and treatment plan
- Non-specialists who prescribe or administer on-going oral anti-cancer medication to have ready access to appropriate written protocols and treatment plans
- Staff dispensing oral anti-cancer medicines to be able to confirm that the prescribed dose is appropriate for the patient
- Patients to be fully informed and receive verbal and up-to-date written information about their oral anticancer therapy from the initiating hospital.

Acknowledgment

The authors acknowledge the contribution of J. So and G. Saunders to versions of this chapter which appeared in previous editions.

References

Berney, D.M., 2007. The case for modifying the Gleason grading system. Br. J. Urol. Int. 100, 725–726.

British Oncology Pharmacy Association, 2010. Standards for clinical pharmacy verification of prescriptions for cancer medicines. Available at http://www.bopawebsite.org/tiki-page.php?pageName=Position+Statements.

Burnell, M., Levine, M.N., Chapman, J.A.W., et al., 2010. Cyclophosphamide, epirubicin, and fluorouracil versus dose-dense epirubicin and cyclophosphamide followed by paclitaxel versus doxorubicin and cyclophosphamide followed by paclitaxel in node-positive or high-risk node-negative breast cancer. J. Clin. Oncol. 28, 77–82.

Cancer Research UK, 2009. Dukes stages of bowel cancer. Available at http://www.cancerhelp.org.uk/type/bowel-cancer/treatment/dukes-stages-of-bowel-cancer.

Cancer Research UK, 2010. Cancer in the UK: July 2010 factsheet. Available at http://info.cancerresearchuk.org/prod_consump/groups/cr_common/@nre/@sta/documents/generalcontent/018070.pdf.

Cancer Therapy Evaluation Program, 1998. Common toxicity criteria, Version 2.0. DCTD, NCI, NIH, DHHS. Available at http://ctep.cancer.gov/protocoldevelopment/electronic_applications/docs/ctcv20_4–30–992.pdf.

Doll, R., Peto, R., Boreham, J., et al., 2004. Mortality in relation to smoking: 50 years' observations on male British doctors. Br. Med. J. 328, 1519. Available at http://www.bmj.com/content/328/7455/1519.full.

Galea, M.H., Blamey, R.W., Elston, C.E., et al., 1992. The Nottingham prognostic index in primary breast cancer. Breast Can. Res. Treat. 22, 207–219.

Garber, J.E., Offit, K., 2005. Hereditary cancer predisposition syndromes. J. Clin. Oncol. 23, 276–292.

Green, J.A., Kirwan, J.J., Tierney, J., et al., 2009. Concomitant chemotherapy and radiation therapy for cancer of the uterine cervix (Review). The Cochrane Library Issue 4. Available at http://www.cochranejournalclub.com/chemoradiotherapy-for-cervical-cancer-clinical/pdf/CD002225_standard.pdf.

Herszényi, L., Farinati, F., Miheller, P., et al., 2008. Chemoprevention of colorectal cancer: feasibility in everyday practice? Eur. J. Cancer Prevent. 17, 502–514.

Hurwitz, H., Fehrenbacher, L., Novotny, W., et al., 2004. Bevacizumab plus irinotecan, fluorouracil and leucovorin for metastatic colorectal cancer. New Engl. J. Med. 350, 2335–2342.

Jankowski, J., Boulton, E., 2005. Cancer prevention. Br. Med. J. 331, 618.

Karnofsky, D.A., Burchenal, J.H., 1949. The clinical evaluation of chemotherapeutic agents in cancer. In: MacLeod, C.M. (Ed.), Evaluation of Chemotherapeutic Agents. Columbia University Press, New York.

Levine, M., Whelan, T., 2006. Adjuvant chemotherapy for breast cancer – 30 years later. N. Engl. J. Med. 355, 1920–1922.

National Chemotherapy Advisory Group, 2009. Chemotherapy services in England: ensuring quality and safety. Department of Health, London. Available at http://www.dh.gov.uk/en/Publicationsandstatistics/Publications/DH_104500.

National Institute for Health and Clinical Excellence, 2002. Guidance on the use of trastuzumab for the treatment of advanced breast cancer. NICE, London. Available at http://www.nice.org.uk/nicemedia/pdf/advancedbreastcancerno34PDF.pdf.

National Institute for Health and Clinical Excellence, 2006a. Trastuzumab for the adjuvant treatment of early-stage HER2-positive breast cancer. NICE, London. Available at http://www.nice.org.uk/nicemedia/live/11586/33458/33458.pdf.

National Institute for Health and Clinical Excellence, 2006b. Docetaxel for the treatment of hormone refractory prostate cancer. NICE, London. Available at http://www.nice.org.uk/nicemedia/live/11578/33348/33348.pdf.

National Institute for Health and Clinical Excellence, 2008. Cetuximab for the treatment of locally advance squamous cell cancer of the head and neck. NICE, London. Available at http://www.nice.org.uk/nicemedia/live/12006/40996/40996.pdf.

Piccart-Gebhart, M.J., Procter, M., Leyland-Jones, B., et al., 2005. Trastuzumab after adjuvant chemotherapy in HER2-positive breast cancer (HERA Study). N. Engl. J. Med. 353, 1659–1672.

Sargent, D., Sobrero, A., Grothey, A., et al., 2009. Evidence for cure by adjuvant therapy in colon cancer: observations based on individual patient data from 20,898 patients on 18 randomized trials. J. Clin. Oncol. 27, 872–877.

Therasse, P., Arbuck, S.G., Eisenhauer, E.A., et al., 2000. New guidelines to evaluate the response to treatment in solid tumours. J. Natl. Cancer Inst. 92, 205–216.

Twelves, C., Scheithauer, W., McKendrick, J., et al., 2008. Capecitabine versus 5-FU/LV in stage III colon cancer: updated 5-year efficacy data from X-ACT trial and preliminary analysis of relationship between hand-foot syndrome (HFS) and efficacy. Gastr. Cancers Symp. Abstr. 274. Available at http://www.asco.org/ascov2/Meetings/Abstracts?&vmview=abst_detail_view&confID=53&abstractID=10524.

Further reading

Allwood, M., Wright, P., Stanley, A., 2002. The Cytotoxics Handbook, fourth ed. Radcliffe Medical Press, Oxford.

Department of Health, 2009. Chemotherapy Services in England: Ensuring Quality and Safety. A Report from the National Chemotherapy Advisory Group. Department of Health, London. Available at: http://www.dh.gov.uk/en/Publicationsandstatistics/Publications/PublicationsPolicyAndGuidance/DH_104500.

Devita, V.T., Lawrence, T.S., Rosenberg, S.A., et al., 2008. DeVita, Hellman, and Rosenberg's Cancer – principles and practice of oncology, eighth ed. Lippincott, Williams and Wilkins, Philadelphia.

Smith, I., Chua, S., 2006. ABC of breast diseases. Medical treatment of early breast cancer: adjuvant treatment. Br. Med. J. 332, 34–37.

Useful websites

British Oncology Pharmacy Association, Available at http://www.bopawebsite.org.

Cancer statistics, Available at http://info.cancerresearchuk.org/cancerstats/keyfacts/index.htm.

National Extravasation Information Service website, Available at http://www.extravasation.org.uk.

53 Rheumatoid arthritis and osteoarthritis

D. J. Pang and G. M. Brough

Key points

Rheumatoid arthritis

- Rheumatoid arthritis is the most common inflammatory arthritis affecting 1% of the population.
- It affects 5% of women and 3% of men over 65 years of age.
- The aetiology is unclear.
- Non-pharmacological treatment includes physiotherapy, occupational therapy, education and psychological support.
- On diagnosis of rheumatoid arthritis, early treatment with aggressive disease-modifying anti-rheumatic drugs (DMARDs) should commence to prevent joint destruction.
- Cytokine inhibitors are used in patients who do not respond to DMARD treatment. There are several agents available which target different cytokines in the inflammatory pathway.
- Non-steroidal anti-inflammatory drugs (NSAIDs) may be considered for symptomatic relief and should be co-prescribed with a proton pump inhibitor.
- Steroids are useful for rapid relief of symptoms and in the early stages of DMARD introduction.

Osteoarthritis

- Osteoarthritis is uncommon under the age of 35 years.
- A wide variety of factors are thought to predispose a patient to osteoarthritis including genetic factors, age and mechanical overloading of the joint.
- Lifestyle changes such as maintaining optimal weight and undertaking regular exercise are an essential part of treatment.
- Paracetamol and topical NSAIDs are considered first-line treatments.
- Intra-articular steroids and opioids may be used for severe pain.
- Oral NSAIDs may be useful and should be co-prescribed with a proton pump inhibitor.

Rheumatoid arthritis

Rheumatoid arthritis is one of the most common inflammatory disorders affecting the population worldwide. It is a systemic inflammatory disease which affects not only the joints but a wide range of extra-articular organs. The disease, if not treated early, will lead to progressive joint deformity and increased morbidity and mortality.

Rheumatoid arthritis is a potentially fatal illness, with mortality increased twofold and an average decrease in life expectancy of 7–10 years. Patients with rheumatoid arthritis have an increased prevalence of other serious illnesses. The predominant conditions leading to this increased co-morbidity and mortality include infections, renal impairment, cardiovascular disease and lymphomas. The incidence of lymphoma is twofold higher than expected before taking into account the disease-modifying immunosuppressant drugs used in treating rheumatoid arthritis.

Epidemiology

Approximately 1% of the population worldwide is affected by rheumatoid arthritis, with females being two to three times more commonly affected. The prevalence of rheumatoid arthritis increases with age in both sexes; nearly 5% of women and 3% of men over the age of 65 years are affected by the disease. The peak age of incidence is about 30–50 years in women and slightly older in men. Rheumatoid arthritis also affects young children and its classification and treatment differs slightly from adults.

Aetiology and pathophysiology

The cause of rheumatoid arthritis remains unclear with hormonal, genetic and environmental factors playing a key role. Genetic factors contribute 53–65% of the risk of developing this disease. The HLA-DR4 allele is associated with both the development and severity of rheumatoid arthritis. Cigarette smoking is a strong risk factor for developing rheumatoid arthritis. A study of over 3000 women clearly linked the length of time that people had smoked with rheumatoid arthritis (Karlson et al., 1999). Patients with a smoking history of 25 years or more were increasingly likely to develop seropositive disease with nodules and erosions on radiology.

Pathologically, rheumatoid arthritis is characterised by the infiltration of a variety of inflammatory cells into the joint. The synovial membrane, which is normally acellular, becomes highly vascularised and hypertrophied, creating a so-called pannus formation. There is proliferation of synovial fibroblasts and an increase in the number of inflammatory cells present within the joint. The inflammatory cells involved in rheumatoid arthritis include T-cells (predominantly CD4 helper cells), B-cells, macrophages and plasma cells. Cytokines are released by these cells which cause the synovium to release proteolytic enzymes, resulting in the destruction of bone and cartilage. Key cytokines involved in rheumatoid arthritis include tumour necrosis factor (TNF)-α, interleukin-1, interleukin-6 and granulocyte macrophage colony-stimulating factor (GM-CSF). These play a crucial role in the pro-inflammatory reaction.

Clinical manifestations

There are different patterns of clinical presentation of rheumatoid arthritis. The disease may present as a polyarticular arthritis with a gradual onset, intermittent or migratory joint involvement, or a monoarticular onset. In addition, extra-articular manifestations may be present (Box 53.1). Extra-articular features occur in approximately 75% of seropositive patients and are often associated with a poor prognosis.

Disease onset is usually insidious with the predominant symptoms being pain, stiffness and swelling. Typically, the metacarpophalangeal and proximal interphalangeal joints of the fingers, interphalangeal joints of the thumbs, the wrists, and metatarsophalangeal joints of the toes are affected during the early stages of the disease. Rheumatoid arthritis–associated deformities affecting multiple joints of the hands are shown in Fig. 53.1. Other joints of the upper and lower limbs, such as the elbows, shoulders and knees, are also affected. Morning stiffness may last for 30 min to several hours, and usually reflects the severity of joint inflammation. Up to one-third of patients also suffer from prominent myalgia, fatigue, low-grade fever, weight loss and depression at disease onset.

Rheumatoid arthritis shows a marked variation of clinical expression in individual patients both in the number and pattern of joints affected, disease progression and the rapidity of joint damage. Disease activity may not abate in 10–20% of cases. Remission has been reported in a small proportion of patients but usually is very rare without disease-modifying anti-rheumatic drugs (DMARDs).

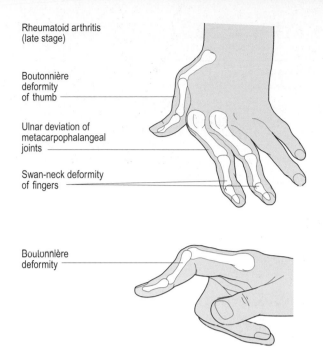

Fig. 53.1 Typical ulnar deviation, swan neck and boutonnière deformities.

Diagnosis

A clinical diagnosis of rheumatoid arthritis is made based on the patient's history, presenting symptoms and clinical findings. Family history is useful, as well as investigations including blood tests, ultrasound for the presence of synovitis and X-rays. The latter is used to demonstrate joint destruction which indicates a late manifestation of the disease.

Emphasis on early diagnosis and treatment is extremely important to prevent disease activity, duration and ultimately joint destruction. The American Rheumatism Association (ARA) criteria (Box 53.2) were principally designed for disease classification in patients with established disease and are not sensitive for patients in the early stages of rheumatoid arthritis (Arnett et al., 1988). The Disease Activity Score

---

Box 53.1 Examples of the extra-articular features of rheumatoid arthritis

Amyloidosis
Carpal tunnel syndrome
Episcleritis
Felty's Syndrome
Fever
Lymphadenopathy
Nodules; may be subcutaneous or within the lungs, eyes or heart
Osteoporosis
Pericarditis
Pleural and pericardial effusions
Scleritis
Vasculitis

Box 53.2 American Rheumatism Association criteria for the diagnosis of rheumatoid arthritis

- Morning stiffness in and around the joints for at least 6 weeks, lasting at least 1 h before maximal improvement
- Swelling of three or more joints for at least 6 weeks
- Swelling of the wrist, metacarpophalangeal or proximal interphalangeal joints for at least 6 weeks
- Symmetric joint swelling for at least 6 weeks
- Hand X-ray changes typical of rheumatoid arthritis that must include erosions or unequivocal bony decalcification around the joints
- Rheumatoid subcutaneous nodules
- Positive rheumatoid factor

The presence of at least 4 of these indicates a diagnosis of rheumatoid arthritis.

Box 53.3 Summary of DAS28 criteria in the assessment of rheumatoid arthritis

DAS28 is a composite formula. Four parameters are used to calculate a disease severity score:

1. Number of swollen joints out of a total of 28 specified joints
2. Number of tender joints out of a total of 28 specified joints
3. Erythrocyte sedimentation rate
4. Patient's interpretation of wellbeing, with 0 being at their best and 100 their worst

Programmed calculators are used to determine the final DAS28. DAS28 does not take into account other features of a patient's disease, such as synovitis and other clinical symptoms.

High disease activity: DAS28 of >5.1
Moderate disease activity: DAS28 of >3.2 to 5.1
Low disease activity: DAS28 of 2.6–3.2
Remission: DAS28 of <2.6

Box 53.4 American College of Rheumatology (ACR 20) response assessment in rheumatoid arthritis

At least 20% improvement in:
Swollen joint count
Tender joint count
and 20% improvement in any three of the following:
Patient assessed global disease activity
Evaluator assessed global disease activity
Patient pain assessment
Functional disability (using a health assessment questionnaire)
Acute phase response (ESR or CRP)
ACR 50 and 70 are determined as above but the relative improvement in response is 50% or 70%, respectively.

CRP, C-reactive protein; ESR, erythrocyte sedimentation rate.

---

using 28 joint counts (DAS28) and American College of Rheumatology (ACR) response are some of the tools used by rheumatologists to assess disease activity and to monitor the patient's response to treatment (see Boxes 53.3 and 53.4).

Investigations

Inflammatory markers, including C-reactive protein (CRP) and erythrocyte sedimentation rate (ESR), are usually but not always elevated in active disease and are useful for monitoring response to treatment. Rheumatoid factor (RF) is an autoantibody directed against the host immunoglobulin and is most commonly found in rheumatoid arthritis. Routinely performed tests only detect immunoglobulin M rheumatoid factor (IgM RF) which is present in 75–80% of patients with rheumatoid arthritis (termed seropositive disease) and 5% of normal subjects. Those patients who do not have a detectable RF are said to be 'seronegative'. RF is not specific to rheumatoid arthritis and is also present in patients with chronic lung and liver disease, other connective tissue diseases, neoplasia, infections (particularly bacterial endocarditis) and cryoglobulinaemia.

Anti-cyclic citrullinated peptide antibodies (anti-CCP antibody) are a more specific test for rheumatoid arthritis with a specificity of 90–96% compared with the specificity of IgM

RF of 85%. They are more useful for the early detection of rheumatoid arthritis in a patient with inflammatory arthritis. The sensitivity of both anti-CCP antibody and IgM RF is approximately 70%.

Antinuclear antibodies (ANA) and extractable nuclear antigens (ENA) are useful for establishing the differential diagnosis, such as other connective tissue diseases presenting or associated with an arthritis. ANA is almost universally positive in systemic lupus erythematosus and only positive in 20% of patients with rheumatoid arthritis.

Other abnormal laboratory tests include an elevated alkaline phosphatase, an elevated platelet count, a decreased serum albumin and a normochromic, normocytic anaemia. White cell count, particularly neutrophils, is elevated in patients with infected joints and is also elevated whilst the patient is on steroids.

Treatment

There are four primary goals in the treatment of rheumatoid arthritis:

- Symptom relief including pain control
- Slowing or prevention of joint damage
- Preserving and improving functional ability
- Achieving and maintaining disease remission

Once the diagnosis has been established, an individualised care plan with treatment goals should be agreed, including monitoring of disease severity using objective measures such as the ACR or DAS28 scores. The ultimate aim is to achieve disease remission, which can be defined by a number of methods including a target DAS28 of less than 2.6, CRP, or a reduction in signs and symptoms of disease activity. If remission cannot be achieved, the aim of therapy is to minimise joint destruction and to preserve function. The longer the period of remission or the best possible reduction in disease activity that can be achieved, the better the long-term outcome.

Patients should have access to a multidisciplinary team to address the pharmacological and non-pharmacological aspects of disease management. Education is extremely important as patients cope better if they understand their condition and have realistic expectations of the benefits and disadvantages of their treatment strategies. Patients may need psychological support and employment counselling to help them adjust to living with their condition. Occupational therapy aims to provide support and aid to allow patients to improve function and limit disability in their activities of daily living. This includes devices to alleviate tasks which may be troublesome for those with restricted manual dexterity, such as twisting lids to open bottles. Physiotherapy involves assessment of function and designing a programme to aid pain relief and rehabilitation. The programme should aim to improve general fitness through regular exercise, and tailor exercises to the individual patient to enhance joint flexibility and muscle strength. Alternative short-term pain relief options may also be explored such as transcutaneous electrical nerve stimulators

(TENS) and hydrotherapy. Surgical interventions, such as synovectomy and arthroplasty, may be useful to relieve pain and restore function.

Drug treatment

The pharmacological management of rheumatoid arthritis is evolving rapidly as more advanced therapies become available. The advent of biological therapies has brought new technologies which target different cytokine pathways involved in the pathogenesis of rheumatoid arthritis and have revolutionised disease management.

There are four main categories of drugs employed in the management of rheumatoid arthritis: non-steroidal anti-inflammatory drugs (NSAIDs) including cyclo-oxygenase (COX)-2 inhibitors, glucocorticoids, DMARDs and biological therapies. Simple analgesia also has a small role to play in basic symptom relief and includes paracetamol, codeine, and paracetamol and opiate combination products. These analgesics do not have any anti-inflammatory effect and will not aid disease modification. The aim of analgesia is to achieve symptom relief and reduce the need for long-term use of NSAIDs, COX-2 inhibitors and glucocorticoids.

Guidance for the treatment of rheumatoid arthritis has been issued and this is summarised in Fig. 53.2.

Non-steroidal anti-inflammatory drugs

The analgesic and anti-inflammatory properties of NSAIDs are used to reduce joint pain and swelling. However, as with simple analgesics, these drugs provide only symptomatic relief to improve joint function, and so should always be used in combination with other agents which modify the disease process.

The COX enzyme converts arachidonic acid into prostaglandins and thromboxanes. These prostanoids have a variety of physiological functions, and are also believed to be responsible for causing pain and swelling in inflammatory conditions. There are two main isoforms of the COX enzyme:

Table 53.1 NSAIDs currently licensed in the UK

Non-selective NSAIDs	COX-2 inhibitors
Aceclofenac	Celecoxib
Acemetacin	Etoricoxib
Azapropazone	
Dexibuprofen	
Dexketoprofen	
Diclofenac	
Etodolac	
Fenbufen	
Fluribprofen	
Ibuprofen	
Indometacin	
Ketoprofen	
Meloxicam	
Nabumetone	
Naproxen	
Piroxicam	
Tenoxicam	
Tiaprofenic acid	

COX-1 produces prostaglandins required for homeostatic functions, such as maintaining the gastric mucosa, support of renal function and platelet function. COX-2 is responsible for the production of inflammatory prostanoids.

NSAIDs vary in their selectivity for the COX-1 and COX-2 isoforms, and are categorised as either non-selective NSAIDs or selective COX-2 inhibitors, otherwise known as the coxibs (Table 53.1). Non-selective NSAIDs generally block both COX-1 and COX-2, whereas the coxibs have higher selectivity for the COX-2 isoform. However, COX-2 selectivity in NSAIDs varies according to the dose of drug given, which is demonstrated by the dose-related toxicity exhibited by some agents such as ibuprofen. The three most commonly used non-selective NSAIDs have differing levels of COX-1 or COX-2 selectivity: diclofenac is COX-2 'preferential', whereas ibuprofen and particularly naproxen preferentially inhibit COX-1. Originally, inhibition of COX-2 was thought to be involved solely with the anti-inflammatory, anti-pyretic and analgesic properties of NSAIDs. However, it is possible that COX-2 inhibition may also impair endothelial health, cause a prothrombotic state and promote cardiovascular disease.

Safety

In 2004, rofecoxib, a selective COX-2 inhibitors, was withdrawn from the worldwide market due to evidence of an increased risk of confirmed serious thrombotic events that included myocardial infarction and stroke, following long-term use. In the following years, similar evidence against the other COX-2 inhibitors and also against some of the non-selective NSAIDs accumulated.

At present, the exact cardiovascular risk for individual selective COX-2 inhibitors and NSAIDs is not known. Evidence from clinical trials of COX-2 inhibitors suggests that about 3 additional thrombotic events per 1000 patients/year may occur in the general population (MHRA, 2006).

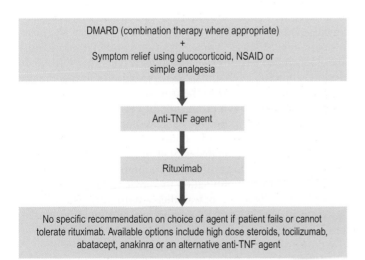

DMARD (combination therapy where appropriate)
+
Symptom relief using glucocorticoid, NSAID or simple analgesia

↓

Anti-TNF agent

↓

Rituximab

↓

No specific recommendation on choice of agent if patient fails or cannot tolerate rituximab. Available options include high dose steroids, tocilizumab, abatacept, anakinra or an alternative anti-TNF agent

Fig. 53.2 Treatment algorithm for rheumatoid arthritis (NCCCC, 2009).

A dose-dependent increase in cardiovascular risk is associated with use of celecoxib, high-dose diclofenac (150 mg/day) and high-dose ibuprofen (2400 mg/day). There does not appear to be an increased risk of myocardial infarction in association with low-dose ibuprofen (≤1200 mg/day). Naproxen is associated with a lower risk of arterial thrombotic events than COX-2 inhibitors. There may be some increased cardiovascular risk in all patients receiving any NSAID, irrespective of their baseline risk or duration of therapy. The key message is that patients should use the lowest effective dose and the shortest duration of treatment necessary to control symptoms to minimise the risk of adverse events.

The most common adverse events of NSAIDs are those that predominantly inhibit COX-1 and cause adverse gastro-intestinal effects. These range from minor symptoms, including dyspepsia, nausea and diarrhoea, to more serious events, such as gastric erosion, bleeding and duodenal and gastric ulceration. Patients are at a higher risk of serious gastro-intestinal complications if they are over 65 years of age, have a previous history of gastro-intestinal ulceration/bleeding or peptic ulcer disease, or are taking concomitant anti-platelet, anti-coagulation or steroid therapy. There are several gastroprotective agents available which may be used to reduce adverse events, including H_2 antagonists, misoprostol and proton pump inhibitors (PPIs). PPIs, such as omeprazole and lansoprazole, have been shown to be particularly effective at preventing gastric and duodenal ulcers with NSAIDs. All patients taking a non-selective NSAID or COX-2 inhibitor should receive concomitant treatment with a PPI to minimise gastro-intestinal adverse effects.

Aspirin inhibits the COX enzyme irreversibly through a different mechanism of action to the NSAIDs. Therefore, there is an increased risk of gastro-intestinal toxicity if aspirin and non-selective NSAIDs are used concomitantly, and the gastro-intestinal advantage of using a selective COX-2 inhibitor is severely reduced. Low-dose aspirin should only be co-prescribed with NSAIDs where absolutely necessary.

All NSAIDs may potentially cause adverse cardio-renal effects such as oedema, hypertension and heart failure. The distribution of COX-1 and COX-2 differs in the kidney, but there is no evidence to suggest differing degrees of isoform inhibition have an impact on the severity of cardio-renal adverse effects. Pharmacokinetic parameters, such as half-life and metabolism, may affect both thrombotic and cardio-renal properties of NSAIDs.

Choice of agent

Evidence suggests that all non-selective NSAIDs and COX-2 inhibitors are of similar efficacy, but vary in their toxicity profiles. However, there is individual patient variability in terms of response to a given NSAID, and so some patients may need to try several agents before reaching an effective and well-tolerated agent. Non-selective NSAIDs or COX-2 inhibitors should be used at the lowest effective dose for the shortest possible period of time. There are no recommendations on which agent to use first-line as all NSAIDs have analgesic effects of similar magnitude. However, as these drugs vary in terms of potential gastro-intestinal, liver and cardio-renal toxicity, it is advised that the choice of drug should take into account the patient's individual risk factors, including age.

Disease-modifying anti-rheumatic drugs

Joint damage is known to occur early in rheumatoid arthritis and is largely irreversible. The need for early intervention with DMARDs as part of an aggressive approach to minimise disease progression has become standard practice and is associated with better patient outcome. Early introduction of DMARDs also results in fewer adverse reactions and withdrawals from therapy (NCCCC, 2009).

The DMARDs that are commonly used for rheumatoid arthritis and have clear evidence of benefit are methotrexate, sulphasalazine, leflunomide and intramuscular gold (O'Dell, 2004). There is less compelling evidence for the use of hydroxychloroquine, D-penicillamine, oral gold, ciclosporin and azathioprine, although these agents do improve symptoms and some objective measures of inflammation. The exact mechanism of action of these drugs is unknown. All DMARDs inhibit the release or reduce the activity of inflammatory cytokines, such as TNF-α, interleukin-1, interleukin-2 and interleukin-6. Activated T-lymphocytes have been implicated in the inflammatory process, and these are inhibited by methotrexate, leflunomide and ciclosporin.

Patients should be made aware that the DMARDs all have a slow onset of action. They must be taken for at least 8 weeks before any clinical effect is apparent, and it may be months before an optimal response is achieved. Whilst early initiation of DMARDs is crucial, it is important to ensure the patient is maintained on therapy to maintain disease suppression. This itself is a challenge, due to the toxicity profiles of the majority of these drugs (see Table 53.2). The majority of the DMARDs require regular blood monitoring. Guidelines are available on the action to take in the event of abnormal blood results (Chakravarty et al., 2008).

Recommendations regarding the use of DMARDs in rheumatoid arthritis are summarised in Box 53.5 (NCCCC, 2009). Patients with a new diagnosis of rheumatoid arthritis should be offered combination DMARD therapy as first-line therapy as soon as possible, ideally within 3 months of the onset of persistent disease symptoms. The combination therapy should include methotrexate and at least one other DMARD, usually sulphasalazine and/or hydroxychloroquine. Evidence suggests that combination therapy appears to be superior in terms of benefits to symptoms, quality of life, remission rates and slowing of joint damage, when compared to monotherapy. Once sustained and satisfactory levels of disease control have been achieved, the doses of drugs should be cautiously reduced to levels that continue to maintain disease control.

In patients where combination therapy is not appropriate, for example where there are contraindications to a drug due to existing co-morbidities, DMARD monotherapy should be started, placing greater emphasis on fast escalation to a clinically effective dose rather than on choice of agent (NCCCC, 2009).

Table 53.2 DMARDs used in the treatment of rheumatoid arthritis

| Name | Dose | Adverse reactions | Monitoring | | Time period to benefit |
			Baseline	Long-term	
Auranofin (oral gold)	3 mg two to three times daily	Rash, oral ulceration, proteinuria, myelosuppression	FBC Urinalysis U&E LFTs	FBC and urinalysis every 4 weeks	4–6 months
Azathioprine	1–3 mg/kg/day	Myelosuppression, hepatic impairment	FBC U&E LFTs TPMT assay	FBC and LFTs weekly for 6 weeks, then every 2 weeks until dose is stable for 6 weeks, then monthly. If maintenance dose is achieved and stable for 6 months consider reducing monitoring to every 3 months U&E every 6 months	6 weeks to 3 months
Ciclosporin	2.5–4 mg/kg/day (in two divided doses)	Hypertension, renal dysfunction, gingival hyperplasia, electrolyte imbalance, hyperlipidaemia	FBC U&E LFTs Fasting lipids CrCl BP	FBC and LFTs monthly until dose and trend stable for 3 months, then every 3 months thereafter U&E every 2 weeks until dose and trend stable for 3 months, then monthly thereafter Periodic lipid check Regular BP check – maintain ≤ 140/90	3 months
D-penicillamine	Usual maintenance 500–750 mg daily	Nausea, anorexia, myelosuppression, rashes, taste disturbances	FBC U&E Urinary protein	FBC and urinalysis every 2 weeks until dose stable for 3 months, then monthly thereafter	3–6 months
Hydroxychloroquine	200–400 mg daily	Ocular toxicity, GI and visual disturbances	FBC U&E LFT Visual acuity	Annual review with optometrist	2–3 months
Leflunomide	10–20 mg daily Loading dose is not commonly used in practice due to GI side effects	Weight loss, hypertension, GI disturbances, myelosuppression	FBC U&E LFTs BP Weight	FBC and LFTs monthly for 6 months, then every 2 months thereafter if stable Monthly bloods should be continued long-term if co-prescribed with another immunosuppressant or potentially hepatotoxic agent Regular BP and weight checks	8–12 weeks, although longer if the loading dose is not given
Methotrexate	7.5–25 mg once weekly	Hepatotoxicity, myelosuppression, pneumonitis, nausea and vomiting	FBC U&E LFTs Chest X-ray	FBC, U&E, LFTs every 2 weeks until MTX dose and monitoring stable for 6 weeks, then monthly thereafter until dose and disease stable for 1 year. Following this, reduction in frequency of monitoring may be considered depending on various patient factors, for example renal impairment	6 weeks to 3 months

Table 53.2 DMARDs used in the treatment of rheumatoid arthritis—cont'd

Name	Dose	Adverse reactions	Monitoring		Time period to benefit
			Baseline	Long-term	
Sodium aurothiomalate (IM gold)	10 mg test dose, then 50 mg weekly until significant response or total dose of 1000 mg has been given	Rash, oral ulceration, proteinuria, myelosuppression	FBC Urinalysis U&E LFTs	FBC and urinalysis every 4 weeks	Usually when 500 mg cumulative dose has been reached
Sulphasalazine	500 mg to 3 g daily	GI disturbances, myelosuppression, hepatotoxicity	FBC U&Es LFTs	FBC and LFTs monthly for first 3 months, then every 3 months thereafter. Reduce frequency after first year if dose and results are stable	3 months

BP, blood pressure; CrCl, creatinine clearance; FBC, full blood count; GI, gastro-intestinal; IM, intramuscular; LFTs, liver function tests; MTX, methotrexate; TPMT assay, thiopurine methyl transferase; U&E, Urea and electrolytes, including creatinine

---

Box 53.5 Key points regarding DMARD therapy (NCCCC, 2009)

Introduce DMARD therapy early (within 3 months ideally)
Use combination DMARDs involving methotrexate and at least one other DMARD
Use monotherapy where combination DMARD therapy is not appropriate, with rapid escalation to therapeutic dose
Withdraw cautiously when disease is stable to doses that maintain disease control

---

There are many factors that influence the choice of DMARD: relative efficacy, severity of disease, convenience, monitoring requirements, patient co-morbidities, cost, time period to benefit, prescriber's experience and success rates with the drug, side effects and patient adherence. Studies have shown that methotrexate has the best benefit to toxicity ratio. Both sulphasalazine and hydroxychloroquine are also favourable in terms of low incidence of serious adverse effects, although hydroxychloroquine alone does not slow radiological damage. Most patients started on a DMARD will not be taking it 3–4 years later because of adverse reactions or lack of efficacy. Despite promising results initially, some patients experience disease reactivation at a later stage and become unresponsive to treatment.

Methotrexate

Methotrexate is recognised as the gold standard DMARD in the management of rheumatoid arthritis. It is given as a once weekly dose and can be given orally or parenterally via the intramuscular or subcutaneous routes. Patients usually begin on oral therapy; parenteral methotrexate may be considered in those who do not respond adequately to the maximum tolerated oral dose, or in those who suffer from gastro-intestinal side effects. Doses used, whether administered by the parenteral or oral route, are similar, although bioavailability is greater with parenteral administration. Methotrexate is primarily excreted unchanged by the kidneys and so elderly patients or those with renal impairment may require lower doses. Methotrexate is a folic acid antagonist and acts by reversibly inhibiting dihydrofolate reductase, the enzyme that reduces folic acid to tetrahydrofolic acid. Concomitant administration of oral folic acid reduces adverse effects of methotrexate and improves continuation of therapy and adherence. Doses used range from 5 mg weekly to 5 mg daily except on the day of methotrexate administration.

Methotrexate is associated with lung, liver and bone marrow toxicities. As a consequence, strict monitoring is advised and alcohol intake should be minimised. Methotrexate pneumonitis is usually seen within the first year of treatment, but can sometimes occur after long-term therapy. Myelosuppression can cause significant falls in blood cell counts. It is more likely to occur in the elderly, patients with renal impairment or patients who are also taking anti-folate drugs. A clinically significant drop in cell count calls for immediate withdrawal of methotrexate, and folinic acid rescue therapy. Patients should be counselled to report any of the following warning symptoms immediately to a healthcare professional: blood disorders, for example sore throat, bruising, mouth ulcers; liver toxicity, for example nausea, vomiting, abdominal discomfort, dark urine; and respiratory effects, for example shortness of breath, persistent dry cough.

Following a number of patient incidents involving methotrexate toxicity, guidance on safe use was issued by the National Patient Safety Agency (Box 53.6). Methotrexate-monitoring booklets are routinely given to patients when therapy is initiated. The booklet contains information to reinforce counselling points such as warning symptoms and drug interactions, and has sections where prescribers can enter in dose details (in number and strength of tablets) and record blood results. Methotrexate tablets are available as 2.5-mg and 10-mg strengths; most pharmacies will dispense the 2.5-mg strength only for non-chemotherapy indications such as rheumatoid arthritis.

All prescriptions must specify a dose
The term 'as directed' should be avoided on prescriptions
The strength of tablets supplied should remain consistent to avoid confusion regarding dose
Issue all patients with a methotrexate monitoring booklet
Counsel patient:

- Strength and number of tablets to take
- Monitoring requirements
- Warning symptoms of methotrexate, for example sore throat, persistent cough, vomiting
- To inform other healthcare professionals that he/she is taking methotrexate

Sulphasalazine

Sulphasalazine has been shown to slow joint erosions and suppress inflammatory activity in rheumatoid arthritis. Blood dyscrasias usually occur within the first 3–6 months of treatment, therefore necessitating close monitoring in the initiation period. Patients should also be counselled to report warning symptoms of unexplained bleeding, bruising, purpura, sore throat, fever or malaise. Enteric-coated tablets are available to minimise gastro-intestinal side effects.

Hydroxychloroquine

Hydroxychloroquine is significantly less effective than other DMARDs and historically was reserved for milder cases of rheumatoid arthritis. It still has a place in therapy, particularly in combination with other DMARDs, as it seems to give some symptomatic relief to patients and is the least toxic of the DMARDs. It has also been used relatively safely in pregnancy. Regular visual assessment for retinopathy is recommended as long-term use of anti-malarial agents has been linked to ocular toxicity.

Leflunomide

Leflunomide has a long half-life of approximately 2 weeks, and consequently a loading dose may be given to achieve therapeutic drug levels more quickly. However, in practice, the loading dose is often omitted due to intolerable gastro-intestinal side effects such as diarrhoea. Leflunomide is associated with hepato- and haemato-toxicity, and should be used with caution if co-prescribed with drugs which also cause these adverse effects. Washout procedures using colestyramine or activated charcoal may be necessary when switching to another DMARD, in the event of a serious adverse effect or before conception in females.

Gold

Gold can be given via intramuscular injection as sodium aurothiomalate, or orally as auranofin. Intramuscular gold is more effective than oral. These drugs can be used over a long period of time provided the patient does not experience side effects such as proteinuria, blood disorders, rashes, gastro-intestinal side effects or bleeding.

Other DMARDs

D-Penicillamine is less commonly used, as side effects such as rashes, taste loss and vomiting, are common. It can be effective in some patients, but doses above 750 mg daily are associated with a high incidence of adverse effects. Azathioprine and ciclosporin can be used in refractory rheumatoid arthritis, but use is limited due to monitoring requirements and high incidence of side effects.

Glucocorticoids

Steroids can be given via the oral, intramuscular or intra-articular routes. They act by inhibiting cytokine release and give rapid relief of symptoms and decrease inflammation. Prednisolone is the most commonly used oral steroid. Intra-articular injections, such as triamcinolone or methylprednisolone, are administered into inflamed joints for local anti-inflammatory action, pain relief and to reduce deformity. The effects of the injection tend to last for approximately 4 weeks and should generally not be repeated more than three times a year into an affected joint. Intramuscular and, less commonly intravenous, injections are used as high-dose pulse therapy to control aggressive disease flares.

Steroids are also used as a bridging therapy and are particularly useful when introducing DMARDs which may take several months to take effect. There are various studies which demonstrate steroids are disease modifying in slowing radiological damage over 2 years. Doses of prednisolone 7.5 mg daily have been suggested to reduce the rate of joint destruction in moderate to severe rheumatoid arthritis of less than 2 years' duration (NCCCC, 2009).

Ideally, steroids should be reserved for short-term use in new-onset rheumatoid arthritis because of their long-term complications and adverse effects. However, because they exert such a potent anti-inflammatory effect, it may be difficult in some patients to withdraw therapy as the disease tends to flare with dose reductions. Gradual reducing regimens should be used with the aim to reach the lowest possible maintenance dose. A reducing rate as slow as 1 mg/month may even be necessary in some patients. Steroids can induce osteoporosis, which is a known complication associated with rheumatoid arthritis itself. Prophylactic therapy, such as calcium and vitamin D supplementation and bisphosphonates, should be considered in patients on steroids at a high dose or for an extended period of time. Gastroprotection may also be necessary in the form of H_2 antagonists or proton pump inhibitors. Other adverse effects associated with steroids are diabetes, increased risk of infection, hypertension and weight gain.

Biological therapies

Over the past decade, there have been significant advances in the treatment of rheumatoid arthritis due to emerging biological therapies. The so-called biologics in rheumatoid arthritis are

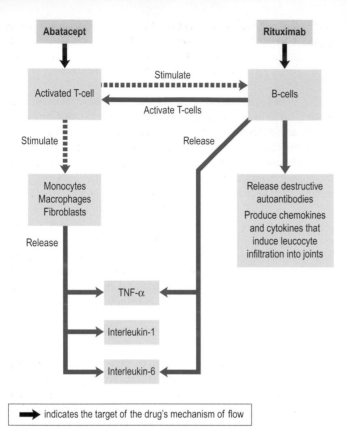

→ indicates the target of the drug's mechanism of flow

Fig. 53.3 Biologic agents and their targets in the inflammatory pathway.

usually well tolerated, with the most common adverse effects being mild infusion reactions, such as headache and urticaria. Anaphylaxis and delayed hypersensitivity reactions have also been rarely reported. As infliximab is a part murine monoclonal antibody, it is thought to carry a higher risk of developing human anti-chimeric antibodies (HACAs). HACAs are associated with an increased frequency of infusion-related reactions and can be minimised by administering with an immunomodulatory therapy.

Adalimumab is a recombinant human monoclonal antibody that binds to and neutralises TNF-α. Etanercept is a human TNF fusion protein that binds to TNF cell surface receptors, thereby inhibiting interaction of TNF-α with its receptors. Certolizumab pegol is a pegylated antibody fragment which binds and neutralises TNF-α and is thought to have a relatively more rapid onset of action. Golimumab is the most recent addition to this family of agents and has the advantage of having a less frequent dosing schedule. (Table 53.3). Optimum clinical benefit is achieved when these drugs are used in combination with methotrexate. However, adalimumab, etanercept and certolizumab pegol can be used alone as monotherapy in patients for whom methotrexate is not appropriate or not tolerated.

Safety

The anti-TNF agents are generally well tolerated, with the main side effects being injection site reactions with the subcutaneous agents, and infusion-related reactions with infliximab.

genetically engineered monoclonal antibodies which selectively target different parts of the inflammatory pathways (Fig. 53.3). Activated T-cells release pro-inflammatory cytokines including TNF-α, interleukin-1 and interleukin-6. Adalimumab, etanercept, golimumab, infliximab and certolizumab pegol target TNF-α, anakinra and tocilizumab target the interleukins, whilst abatacept and rituximab act on T-cells and B-cells, respectively.

In current practice, biologics are used after a patient has failed DMARDs, although there is emerging evidence to suggest they should be used earlier in the disease. Combination DMARD therapy is increasingly advocated and may lead to earlier use of biologics. For example, a patient may now be trialled on two DMARDs, including methotrexate, over a period of 6 months and if the response is inadequate could be eligible for an anti-TNF agent within a year of diagnosis.

Anti-TNF agents

There are five anti-TNF agents available: adalimumab, etanercept, golimumab, infliximab and certolizumab pegol. All inhibit TNF-α which is an inflammatory cytokine found in high concentrations within the joint synovium of rheumatoid arthritis patients.

Infliximab was the first anti-TNF agent licensed for the treatment of rheumatoid arthritis. It is a chimeric human-murine monoclonal antibody that binds with high affinity to TNF-α, thereby neutralising its activity. Infliximab is the only anti-TNF agent which is given by intravenous infusion and must be given concomitantly with methotrexate. It is

Table 53.3 Biologic agents used in the treatment of rheumatoid arthritis and typical dose regimens in adults

Drug	Usual dose	Route
Adalimumab	40 mg every 2 weeks	Subcutaneous
Certolizumab pegol	400 mg at week 0, 2 and 4, then 200 mg every 2 weeks thereafter	Subcutaneous
Etanercept	25 mg twice weekly or 50 mg weekly	Subcutaneous
Golimumab	50 mg monthly	Subcutaneous
Infliximab	3 mg/kg at week 0, 2 and 6, then every 8 weeks thereafter	Intravenous infusion
Rituximab	1 g then 1 g 2 weeks later Max 2 courses/year	Intravenous infusion
Abatacept	750 mg at week 0, 2 and 4, then every 4 weeks thereafter[a]	Intravenous infusion
Anakinra	100 mg daily	Subcutaneous
Tocilizumab	8 mg/kg every 4 weeks	Intravenous infusion

[a]For a patient weighing between 60 and 100 kg; dose modifications are necessary for patients outside this weight range.

There are fewer monitoring requirements compared to the DMARDs and less frequent dosing, making these drugs potentially more appealing. However, the long-term safety of these drugs is being monitored in the UK by the British Society of Rheumatology Biologics Registry. This database collects data on efficacy and safety outcomes of all patients on biologics in a variety of rheumatological conditions including rheumatoid arthritis.

Patients using anti-TNF agents are more susceptible to serious infections such as sepsis, and opportunistic infections. A number of serious infections, including some fatalities, have been reported. Patients should not start anti-TNF therapy in the presence of infection. Those who develop infection whilst receiving treatment should stop and wait until the infection is controlled. The anti-TNF agents have long half-lives and temporary cessation of therapy should be considered prior to and after surgery. Reactivation of hepatitis B and latent tuberculosis has been reported. All patients should be screened for tuberculosis using appropriate tests, such as the tuberculin skin test and a chest X-ray. Active tuberculosis must be treated before an anti-TNF agent is initiated.

Malignancies, including lymphoma, have been reported in studies and post-marketing surveillance of the anti-TNF agents. Caution should be exercised with the use of anti-TNF agents in patients with previous malignancy.

All the anti-TNF agents except etanercept are contraindicated in New York Heart Association (NYHA) grade III/IV heart failure, and all should be used with caution in those with mild heart failure.

Place in therapy

Guidance on the use of adalimumab, etanercept, infliximab (NICE, 2007) and certolizumab pegol (NICE, 2010a) have been published, with the appraisal of golimumab pending. Adalimumab, certolizumab, etanercept or infliximab are recommended as treatment options in adults who meet the following criteria:

- Active rheumatoid arthritis with a DAS28 greater than 5.1 on at least two occasions, 1 month apart.
- Have undergone trials with two DMARDs, including methotrexate, unless contraindicated. A trial of a DMARD is defined as being normally of 6 months, with 2 months at standard dose, unless significant toxicity has limited the dose or duration of treatment.

Patients should be assessed for treatment efficacy using DAS28 every 6 months and continue treatment only if an adequate response is demonstrated 6 months after initiation. An adequate response is currently defined as an improvement in DAS28 of 1.2 points or more.

Changes in eligibility criteria have been suggested (Deighton et al., 2010) which recommend patients should have tried two DMARDs, but those with DAS28 > 3.2 and at least three or more tender joints and three or more swollen joints should be eligible for an anti-TNF agent. Whether NICE will adapt their guidance accordingly is unclear.

Use of the anti-TNF agents above their starting doses as listed in Table 53.3 is not advocated. According to their product licences, doses of adalimumab and infliximab may be escalated according to response, but this does not generally occur in practice.

Generally, the least expensive anti-TNF agent should be used although patient aspects may also affect choice of drug. There are differences between dosing frequencies of the anti-TNF agents, which should be discussed with the patient to ensure drug administration is easily incorporated into their lifestyle, thereby improving adherence. The subcutaneous agents are also available in pen formulations, making it easier for self-administration in patients who have problems with manual dexterity. Patients who are unable to self-administer the subcutaneous anti-TNF agents may choose to receive infliximab as a hospital day case. As infliximab is only licensed to be used in combination with methotrexate, adalimumab, certolizumab and etanercept are favoured in patients where methotrexate cannot be taken.

Rituximab

Rituximab is a chimeric human-murine monoclonal antibody which binds to the C20 antigen on B-lymphocytes to mediate B-cell lysis. It causes depletion of peripheral B-cells which play a role in the pathogenesis of rheumatoid arthritis. Recovery of B-cells appears to occur 6 months after treatment, with some patients showing prolonged B-cell depletion persisting up to 2 years after treatment (Emery et al., 2004).

Rituximab in combination with methotrexate is licensed for the treatment of severe active rheumatoid arthritis in patients who have had an inadequate response or intolerance to other DMARDs including one or more anti-TNF agent. Rituximab is also licensed for non-Hodgkin's lymphoma and chronic lymphocytic leukaemia, both using a different dosing schedule to that of rheumatoid arthritis. A course of rituximab consists of two intravenous infusions administered as a day case in hospital: 1000-mg infusion followed by a second 1000-mg infusion 2 weeks later. The course may be repeated every 6 months depending on patient response. Disease response varies between patients in that some achieve disease remission after one course and do not require re-treatment, whilst others require further repeat infusions every 6–12 months.

Rituximab is generally well tolerated, and the most common adverse effects are infusion-related reactions including fever, changes in blood pressure and rash. Minor infusion-related side effects can be managed by reducing the rate of infusion and giving treatment for relief of symptoms such as paracetamol. The incidence of adverse effects is minimised by pre-medicating with methylprednisolone, paracetamol and an anti-histamine 1 h prior to the infusion. Hypersensitivity reactions and anaphylaxis are rare but serious side effects.

As with the anti-TNF agents, rituximab increases the risk of infections and should not be used in the presence of active or severe infections. Use has been associated with progressive multifocal leukoencephalopathy. It may also exacerbate existing cardiac conditions such as angina pectoris and atrial fibrillation. Patients with a known history of cardiac disease should be closely monitored during treatment administration for changes in blood pressure and pulse. Anti-hypertensives may be omitted 12 h prior to the infusion. HACAs have been reported in some patients after the first course of rituximab. The presence of HACAs may be associated with worsening of infusion or allergic reactions, and possibly failure to deplete B-cells on further treatment.

In practice, rituximab is used in line with its product license, i.e. after failure of, or intolerance to, DMARD therapy including at least one anti-TNF agent. Patients may continue on rituximab therapy with infusions no more frequent than every 6 months, provided they demonstrate an adequate response of a DAS28 improvement of 1.2 points or more (NICE, 2010b).

Abatacept

Abatacept acts by blocking the full activation of T-cells thereby inhibiting the release of inflammatory cytokines. It is licensed for use in combination with methotrexate in the treatment of moderate to severe active rheumatoid arthritis in adults who have had an insufficient response or intolerance to other DMARDs including at least one anti-TNF agent and who cannot receive rituximab because they have a contraindication to rituximab, or when rituximab is withdrawn due to an adverse event (NICE, 2010a).

Anakinra

Anakinra blocks the binding of interleukin-1 to its receptor, thus inhibiting the inflammatory effects of interleukin-1. The evidence of its benefit in rheumatoid arthritis is weak and it is considered modestly effective. There are no trials directly comparing anakinra with other biologic agents; adjusted indirect comparisons suggest that anakinra may be significantly less effective at relieving the clinical signs and symptoms of rheumatoid arthritis than anti-TNF agents in combination with methotrexate. Anakinra is not cost effective in the treatment of rheumatoid arthritis and availability for routine use in the NHS has not been supported (NCCCC, 2009).

Tocilizumab

Tocilizumab acts by binding to interleukin-6 receptors. Interleukin-6 is a pro-inflammatory cytokine produced by a variety of cells including T- and B-cells, and has been implicated in the pathogenesis of rheumatoid arthritis and other inflammatory diseases. Tocilizumab is licensed for use in combination with methotrexate in the treatment of moderate to severe active rheumatoid arthritis in adults who have had an insufficient response or intolerance to other DMARDs including at least one anti-TNF agent. It is given as a monthly intravenous infusion at a dose of 8 mg/kg and requires regular monitoring of liver function tests and full blood count.

Tocilizumab is recommended for the treatment of rheumatoid arthritis in patients who fulfil the following criteria (NICE, 2010c):

- The patient has not responded adequately to one or more anti-TNF agents

and

- The patient cannot receive rituximab due to a contraindication or
- The patient cannot receive rituximab as they have experienced an adverse effect to treatment or
- The patient has not responded adequately to rituximab treatment.

Which biologic?

More biological therapies for the treatment of rheumatoid arthritis, with new mechanisms of action and targets in the inflammatory pathway, are expected to become available in the near future. Cost is a major factor in the use of biologics with many costing in the region of £10,000 per patient per annum. The decision as to which agent to use is further confounded by the absence of clinical trials that directly compare efficacy between the different biologics.

At present, anti-TNF agents remain the first-line biological therapy. Following failure or intolerance to one anti-TNF agent, patients should then be treated with rituximab. However, if patients cannot receive rituximab due to a contraindication, adverse effect, or intolerance to methotrexate, there remains a number of treatment options (see Fig. 53.4).

Rheumatoid arthritis and pregnancy

The management of rheumatoid arthritis during pregnancy is a common challenge, with disease activity improving in approximately 70–80% of patients. Disease activity usually decreases in the first trimester, and this lasts for a number of weeks to months into the postpartum period. Subsequently, 90% of patients will then experience a flare usually during the first 3 months.

Although case control studies of pregnancy outcome demonstrate a slight increase in spontaneous abortion in women with rheumatoid arthritis, most reports have failed to show an increase in fetal morbidity. Medication may potentially increase this risk, for example, steroids may restrict intrauterine growth. Women with active rheumatoid arthritis or other types of inflammatory arthritis may have children with lower birth weights.

None of the available drug treatments for rheumatoid arthritis are absolutely safe in pregnancy. A prescriber must carefully assess the risks and benefits of treatment in consultation with the patient. In patients with active rheumatoid arthritis during pregnancy, prednisolone is recommended at the lowest dose (below 20 mg daily if possible) to control the disease. Sulphasalazine and hydroxychloroquine are considered safe to prescribe by most obstetric physicians. Many of the DMARDs are contraindicated in pregnancy as they are known teratogens, and some require a washout period before conception, such as leflunomide.

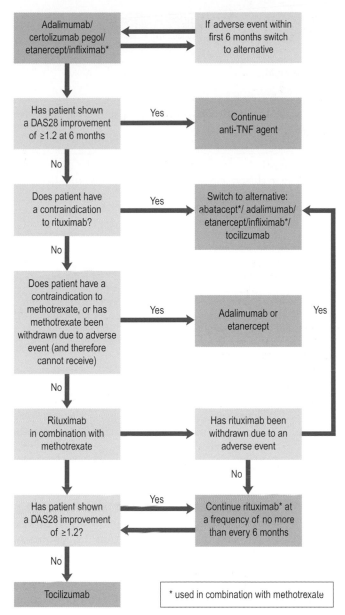

Fig. 53.4 Algorithm following introduction of an anti-TNF agent in the management of rheumatoid arthritis.

Patient care

Patient education and counselling are vital aspects in the management of rheumatoid arthritis. Patients should be encouraged to engage actively in their pharmacological and non-pharmacological treatment, and take responsibility for ensuring their medication regimen is safe and effective. Medicine information sheets are available from the Arthritis Research UK with further information available on their website (http://www.arthritisresearchuk.org/). Monitoring of the potentially toxic DMARDs is essential as non-adherence with the monitoring schedule may have serious consequences. Patients should be reminded of the warning symptoms that must trigger them to contact a healthcare professional. They should also be counselled to inform healthcare professionals of all the medication they are taking before starting a new

medicine, and this includes use of over-the-counter products such as ibuprofen or aspirin.

Shared care agreements between secondary and primary care are often employed for DMARD therapy. This involves a primary care clinician continuing to prescribe and monitor drug treatment which has been initiated by a hospital specialist. Clear guidelines stating responsibilities of both parties, and the action required in the event of toxicity is defined within the document. The main advantage of shared care is that the patient will not be required to attend regular hospital appointments for blood tests and will be managed in primary care.

Some of the common therapeutic problems that are encountered in the management of rheumatoid arthritis are outlined in Table 53.4.

Osteoarthritis

Osteoarthritis is a chronic disease and the most common of all rheumatological disorders. It particularly affects individuals over the age of 65 years and is the major cause of hip and knee replacements in developed countries.

Osteoarthritis was previously thought to be the consequence of ageing, thereby leading to the term degenerative joint disease. However, it is now thought to be the result of a complex interplay of multiple factors including joint integrity, genetic predisposition, local inflammation, mechanical forces and cellular and biochemical processes.

Epidemiology

The prevalence of osteoarthritis increases with age. Generally, osteoarthritis is uncommon under the age of 35 years with 0.1% of people affected between the ages of 25–34 years, but 80% of people affected above the age of 55 years. It occurs in all populations irrespective of race, climate or geographical location. Obesity is the strongest modifiable risk factor and has been shown to particularly affect the knees. Trauma or injury due to diseases, such as rheumatoid arthritis, will predispose a joint to developing osteoarthritis.

A strong genetic component is thought to be present, particularly in women with hand involvement. An inherited defect in type II collagen genes is linked to the development of early-onset polyarticular osteoarthritis.

Aetiology

Osteoarthritis is a complex disease involving bone, cartilage and the synovium. It is generally believed to be an imbalance in erosive and reparative processes. There are a wide variety of factors predisposing an individual to this condition including the following:

- Increasing age
- Gender
- Genetic predisposition
- Congenital abnormality such as Perthes disease of the hip

Table 53.4 Examples of therapeutic problems encountered in the management of rheumatoid arthritis

Problem	Solution
NSAID not providing adequate symptom control	Consider alternative NSAID Review DMARD dose If patient has been on DMARD for a sufficient time period but with no improvement, consider alternative disease-modifying agent, i.e. another DMARD or a biologic agent Consider short-term systemic steroids for rapid relief of symptoms
Patient non-adherent with DMARD monitoring regimen	Education and counselling If patient still unwilling to comply, the safest option would be to consider swapping to DMARDs that require less stringent blood monitoring, for example hydroxychloroquine or sulphasalazine However, relative drug efficacy must also be considered
Nausea and vomiting with methotrexate	Ensure patient is taking folic acid Add anti-emetic therapy Change to parenteral methotrexate
Disease flares when trying to withdraw systemic steroids	Use a slower withdrawal regimen, for example decrease by 1 mg each month If patient cannot be withdrawn completely from steroids, consider reducing to lowest dose possible as maintenance treatment
Side effects of long-term steroids	Aim to use steroids for short-term treatment only Ensure concomitant treatment of PPI, bisphosphonate and calcium and vitamin D preparations are prescribed where appropriate
Patient cannot tolerate stinging at injection site associated with adalimumab or etanercept administration	Consider switching to infliximab

- Obesity
- Previous injury either due to sport or occupation
- Previous disease such as rheumatoid arthritis or gout
- Systemic disorders such as acromegaly
- Neuropathic joint disease such as a Charcot joint

Pathogenesis

The pathogenesis of osteoarthritis has been classified into four stages:

1. Initial repair
2. Early-stage osteoarthritis
3. Intermediate-stage osteoarthritis
4. Late-stage osteoarthritis

Initial repair is characterised by proliferation of chondrocytes synthesising the extracellular matrix of bone. Early-stage osteoarthritis results in degradation of the extracellular matrix as protease enzyme activity exceeds chondrocyte activity. There is net degradation and loss of articular cartilage. Intermediate osteoarthritis is associated with a failure of extracellular matrix synthesis and increased protease activity, further increasing cartilage loss. Finally, late-stage osteoarthritis may result in complete loss of cartilage with joint space narrowing in the most severe of cases. Bone outgrowths (osteophytes) appear at the joint margins, and there is sclerosis of the adjacent bone. Deformity is common at this stage.

Clinical manifestations

Osteoarthritis is traditionally classified by aetiology into idiopathic and secondary forms. Idiopathic can be further divided into localised and generalised depending on the number of joints involved. Localised osteoarthritis most commonly affects the hands, feet, hip, knees and spine, and less commonly the shoulder, temporomandibular, sacroiliac and wrist joints. Pain is increased by movement and loading on the joint, and may radiate beyond the joint itself, as in leg pain associated with spinal disease, and knee pain radiating from the hip. Stiffness in the early morning lasts for less than 30 min, unlike that due to rheumatoid arthritis; it may also occur after periods of rest and throughout the day.

In the hands, the most commonly affected joints are the distal interphalangeal joints or Heberden's nodes, the proximal interphalangeal joints (Bouchard's nodes) and the base of the thumb, the first carpometacarpal joint. Hip pain is particularly felt in the groin. Unlike rheumatoid arthritis, there is no extra-articular disease.

Investigations

Osteoarthritis is primarily diagnosed by its clinical presentation. Confirmation and progression can be achieved by radiography with the presence of joint space narrowing, bone sclerosis, cysts and deformity. There is a lack of conformity between symptoms and radiological findings. On arthroscopy normal cartilage is smooth, white and glistening, while osteoarthritic cartilage is yellowed, irregular and ulcerated. Synovial fluid analysis should be carried out if one suspects infection or crystal arthropathy such as gout or pseudogout. Blood tests usually reveal a normal ESR and CRP.

Treatment

The aims of treatment are pain relief, optimisation of function and minimisation of disease progression. There are three core interventions which should be considered for every person with osteoarthritis where possible:

- Education, advice and access to information
- Strengthening exercises to improve muscle strength and aerobic fitness training
- Weight loss if overweight or obese

Guidelines are available for the management of osteoarthritis (NCCCC, 2008). If the three core interventions are not sufficient, paracetamol and topical NSAIDs can be added in to the treatment regimen. Paracetamol and topical NSAIDs are deemed 'relatively safe pharmaceutical options' compared to other available agents such as oral NSAIDs, opioids and intra-articular steroids. Other interventions which may also be considered include joint arthroplasty, transcutaneous electrical nerve stimulation (TENS), supports and braces, or manual therapy involving manipulation and stretching.

Paracetamol is the first-line drug treatment and should be used alongside core treatment. Regular dosing may be required as 'when required' administration may lead to reduced efficacy.

Topical NSAIDs, capsaicin and rubefacients are widely used for local relief of pain and inflammation. Topical treatments are perceived as self-management, and this has a positive effect on a patient's perception of their disease.

Due to the recent safety concerns with non-selective NSAIDs and COX-2 inhibitors, treatment regimens have moved towards opioids for uncontrolled pain. This should be balanced against adverse effects such as constipation and drowsiness, particularly in the elderly population.

There is a large amount of evidence supporting the efficacy of NSAIDs in reducing pain and stiffness in osteoarthritis. However, there is no strong evidence to suggest a consistent benefit over paracetamol. Non-selective NSAIDs or COX-2 inhibitors may be considered in patients where paracetamol and/or topical NSAIDs do not provide adequate pain relief, based on careful consideration of the patient's risk factors, as discussed earlier in the chapter. This does not include etoricoxib which is associated with a greater risk of causing fluid retention and aggravating hypertension. NSAIDs should be used at the lowest dose for the shortest period of time possible, and patients should also be prescribed a PPI.

Intra-articular steroids may be of benefit in reducing pain and inflammation in joints. Evidence suggests that they provide short-term reduction in pain, although improvement in function is less clear. They should be considered as an adjunct to core treatment for the relief of moderate to severe pain in osteoarthritis.

Hyaluronan is an endogenous molecule found in the synovial fluid. Its key functions are to increase viscosity of synovial fluid and lubrication within the joint. Synthetic intra-articular injections of hyaluronan are thought to provide pain relief and improve joint function, although there is limited evidence to support this. The synthetic hyaluronans are expensive and not currently recommended.

Nutraceuticals is a term which describes food supplements believed to have health benefits. The most widely used of these agents in osteoarthritis are glucosamine and chondroitin. They are available in a multitude of preparations, combinations, strengths and purities and can be purchased over the counter and via the internet. There is, however, little available evidence of efficacy to support their use.

Case studies

Case study 53.1

Mrs JS is a 46-year-old woman who has been referred by her primary care doctor to the rheumatology outpatient clinic in the local hospital. Her presenting complaint is a symmetrical pattern of inflammation in the joints of her hands, knees and shoulders, and severe pain and stiffness which are worse in the morning. She is a gardener and is finding it increasingly difficult to continue her job due to limited joint function. Her investigations and X-rays confirm a diagnosis of severe seropositive rheumatoid arthritis, including a high CRP and ESR. She takes citalopram for depression and has no other remarkable medical or drug history.

Questions

1. What treatment should be introduced for Mrs JS?
2. What key counselling points should be covered regarding her DMARD therapy?

Answers

1. DMARD treatment should be initiated immediately for Mrs JS as she has seropositive disease which is associated with a poorer outcome. She has no other co-morbidities which contraindicate her to any of the DMARDs. Combination treatment should be started with methotrexate and sulphasalazine as she has severe active disease. Folic acid should be also prescribed at 5 mg weekly. Some clinicians may opt for triple combination therapy of methotrexate, sulphasalazine and hydroxychloroquine.

   Her disease activity is impacting on her life and so rapid relief of symptoms is necessary. Methotrexate and sulphasalazine will take between 6 and 12 weeks to take effect. Multiple joints have been affected, and therefore local steroid injections are inappropriate. Oral prednisolone 30 mg daily should be started, with the aim to withdraw steroids after about 3 months.

   Prednisolone will usually alleviate pain and inflammation effectively and so a NSAID should not be required. However, if additional short-term relief is necessary, an as-required regimen with an NSAID, such as ibuprofen 400 mg three times a day or naproxen 500 mg twice a day, may be offered. A PPI should be co-prescribed, for example omeprazole 20 mg daily. Paracetamol may also be taken, and may be substituted for co-codamol if the pain is severe and uncontrolled.

Other non-pharmacological measures should be considered, such as physiotherapy. Counselling and psychological support may be particularly important for Mrs JS. Most patients find it useful to have one key healthcare professional to refer to for advice and if they have any problems – this role is usually managed by a specialist nurse.

Mrs JS is started on methotrexate 7.5 mg weekly and sulphasalazine 500 mg twice a day as her disease-modifying treatments.

2. Mrs JS should be counselled on the following:

- Her dose of methotrexate is 3 × 2.5 mg tablets and this should be taken as a single dose on the same day each week. This dose will be increased over the next few weeks.
- Folic acid is given to minimise adverse effects of methotrexate, and should be taken weekly, but not on the same day as methotrexate.
- Both DMARDs will take several weeks to take full effect.
- She will need regular blood monitoring and she should be counselled about possible adverse effects on the liver and bone marrow.
- Warning symptoms to report to a healthcare professional include any sign of infection, unexplained bleeding, bruising, purpura, sore throat, fever, malaise, dyspnoea, persistent dry cough, mouth ulcers, nausea or vomiting.
- A methotrexate-monitoring booklet should be given to Mrs JS and she should be advised that it must be shown to any healthcare professional before receiving any additional medication or treatment.

Case study 53.2

Mr TP is a 58-year-old man who has been on methotrexate 20 mg weekly for the last 2 years for rheumatoid arthritis. He has found that his symptoms are worsening, and he has been taking more regular NSAIDs and analgesia in the last month for pain relief. He has tried sulphasalazine and leflunomide in the past, but was unable to continue therapy due to gastro-intestinal side effects.

Questions

1. How would you manage Mr TP's worsening disease activity?
2. After discussion with Mr TP and consideration of other co-morbidities, the treatment plan is to add in an anti-TNF agent. What additional information is required to ensure Mr TP meets eligibility criteria for treatment?
3. Mr TP admits that he is needle-phobic and does not like the idea of giving himself weekly or fortnightly injections. What treatment options are available to him?

Answers

1. Mr TP is on DMARD monotherapy, and so an additional agent may be beneficial. However, he has not tolerated sulphasalazine and leflunomide which are regarded as the more effective DMARDs, as well as methotrexate. Hydroxychloroquine could be added in alongside methotrexate, but this is unlikely to provide adequate disease modification.

Another treatment option would be to introduce one of the biological agents. The anti-TNF agents are licensed to be used

after failure of DMARDs, and would be the next logical step in Mr TP's treatment regimen.

2. Patients should demonstrate severe active disease, measured by two DAS28 assessments greater than 5.1, one month apart. A tender joint count and a swollen joint count should be carried out, ESR should be measured, and Mr TP's perception of his disease severity should be scored on a scale from 0 to 100 on a visual analogue scale. These parameters can then be used to calculate a DAS28 using an online calculator.
3. Adalimumab and etanercept are subcutaneous injections which are usually self-administered by patients. In some cases, a district nurse may be organised to administer the injection at the patient's home. For Mr TP, the thought of having such frequent injections is not desirable, and this may affect adherence to the medication regimen.

Infliximab is given as an intravenous infusion in hospital, and he would not have to administer the drug himself. It has a less frequent dosing compared to the other anti-TNF agents, and it should be discussed with Mr TP whether he is happy to have an infusion every 8 weeks.

Case study 53.3

Mr AR is a 68-year-old man who has stable rheumatoid arthritis which is well controlled on his current drug regimen:

Sulphasalazine 1 g twice a day
Hydroxychloroquine 200 mg twice a day
Co-codamol 30/500 2 four times a day as required
Diclofenac 50 mg three times a day
Ramipril 5 mg once a day
Aspirin 75 mg once a day
Atorvastatin 40 mg once a day at night
Atenolol 50 mg once a day
He also has a history of myocardial infarction.

Question

Comment on his drug regimen.

Answer

High-dose diclofenac (150 mg/day) has been associated with an increased cardiovascular risk, and Mr AR has a history of myocardial infarction. As a consequence, his diclofenac should be stopped. In addition, Mr AR is on aspirin 75 mg daily, and so is as at a higher risk of gastro-intestinal adverse events if he is also taking an NSAID. In general, patients should not take NSAIDs concomitantly with low-dose aspirin unless absolutely necessary.

The reason for regular NSAID use should be investigated. The effectiveness of his DMARD regimen should also be considered, as his disease progression may be causing additional pain and inflammation of the joints. The next step in his disease-modifying treatment would be to consider a third DMARD, such as methotrexate. He may also be a candidate for anti-TNF therapy.

Alternative symptomatic relief that could be offered would be local steroid injections or modifications to his simple analgesia regimen, such as regular paracetamol with codeine as required. Some prescribers may consider using low-dose ibuprofen 400 mg three times a day on an as required basis, although the risk versus benefit regarding gastro-intestinal adverse effects should be considered.

References

Arnett, F.C., Edworthy, S.M., Bloch, D.A., et al., 1988. The American Rheumatism Association 1987 revised criteria for the classification of rheumatoid arthritis. Arthritis Rheum. 31, 315–324.

Chakravarty, K., McDonald, H., Pullar, T., et al., on behalf of the British Society for Rheumatology, British Health Professionals in Rheumatology Standards, Guidelines and Audit Working Group in consultation with the British Association of Dermatologists, 2008. BSR/BHPR guideline for disease-modifying anti-rheumatic drug (DMARD) therapy in consultation with the British Association of Dermatologists. Rheumatology. doi:10.1093/rheumatology/kel216b. Available at http://www.rheumatology.org.uk/includes/documents/cm_docs/2009/d/diseasemodifying_antirheumatic_drug_dmard_therapy.pdf.

Deighton, C., Hyrich, K., Ding, T., et al., on behalf of BSR Clinical Affairs Committee & Standards, Audit and Guidelines Working Group and the BHPR, 2010. BSR and BHPR rheumatoid arthritis guidelines on eligibility criteria for the first biological therapy. Rheumatology doi:10.1093/rheumatology/keq006b.

Emery, P., Sheeran, T., Lehane, P.B., et al., 2004. Efficacy and safety of rituximab at 2 years following a single treatment in patients with active rheumatoid arthritis. Arthritis Rheum. 50, (Suppl. 9): S659.

Karlson, E.W., Lew, J.M., Cook, N.R., et al., 1999. A retrospective cohort study of cigarette smoking and risk of rheumatoid arthritis in female health professionals. Arthritis Rheum. 42, 910.

Medicines and Healthcare Products Regulatory Agency, 2006. Cardiovascular safety of NSAIDs and selective COX-2 inhibitors. Current Problems in Pharmacovigilance 31, 7.

National Collaborating Centre for Chronic Conditions, 2008. Osteoarthritis: National Clinical Guideline for Care and Management in Adults. Royal College of Physicians, London. Available at http://www.gserve.nice.org.uk/nicemedia/pdf/CG59NICEguideline.pdf.

National Collaborating Centre for Chronic Conditions, 2009. Rheumatoid Arthritis: National Clinical Guideline for the Management and Treatment in Adults. NICE, London. Available at http://www.nice.org.uk/nicemedia/pdf/CG79NICEGuideline.pdf.

National Institute for Health and Clinical Excellence, 2007. Adalimumab, Etanercept and Infliximab for the Treatment of Rheumatoid Arthritis. Technology Appraisal 130. NICE, London. Available at http://www.nice.org.uk/nicemedia/pdf/TA130guidance.pdf.

National Institute for Health and Clinical Excellence, 2010a. Certolizumab Pegol for the Treatment of Rheumatoid Arthritis. Technology Appraisal 186. NICE, London. Available at http://www.nice.org.uk/nicemedia/live/12808/47544/47544.pdf.

National Institute for Health and Clinical Excellence, 2010b. Adalimumab, etanercept, infliximab, Rituximab and Abatacept for the Treatment of Rheumatoid Arthritis After the Failure of a TNF Inhibitor. Technology Appraisal 195. NICE, London. Available at http://www.nice.org.uk/nicemedia/live/13108/50413/50413.pdf.

National Institute for Health and Clinical Excellence, 2010c. Tocilizumab for the Treatment of Rheumatoid Arthritis. In: Technology Appraisal 198. NICE, London. Available at http://www.nice.org.uk/nicemedia/live/13100/50391/50391.pdf.

O'Dell, J.R., 2004. Therapeutic strategies for rheumatoid arthritis. N. Engl. J. Med. 350, 2591–2602.

Further reading

Firestein, G., Panayi, G.S., Wollheim, F.A. (Eds) 2006. Rheumatoid Arthritis. Oxford University Press, Oxford.

Hochberg, M.C., Silman, A.J., Smolen, J.S., et al., 2008. Rheumatoid Arthritis. Elsevier Health Sciences, London.

Sharma, L., Berenbaum, F. (Eds) 2007. Osteoarthritis. Elsevier Health Sciences, London.

Taylor, P.C., 2007. Rheumatoid Arthritis in Practice. Royal Society of Medicine Press Ltd, London.

Useful websites

American College of Rheumatology. http://www.rheumatology.org.

Arthritis Research UK. http://www.arthritisresearchuk.org/.

British Society of Rheumatology. http://www.rheumatology.org.uk/.

54 Gout and hyperuricaemia

T. Hawkins and A. Cunnington

Key points

- Gout is the most common inflammatory joint disease in men and is strongly age related.
- The prevalence of gout has increased over recent decades.
- It is caused by the deposition of monosodium urate crystals within articular and periarticular tissue.
- The degree of elevation of uric acid levels above the saturation point for urate crystal formation is a major determinant in precipitating an attack.
- Not all people with hyperuricaemia develop gout.
- Gout is normally the result of an interaction between genetic, constitutional and environmental risk factors.
- The aim of long-term therapy is to reduce the serum uric acid level sufficiently so that crystals can no longer form and existing crystals are dissolved.
- Non-pharmacological measures such as lifestyle and dietary modification play an important role in the management of gout.
- Unmanaged recurrent attacks can result in progressive cartilage and bone erosion, deposition of tophi, secondary osteoarthritis and disability.

Introduction

Gout is the most common inflammatory joint disease in men and the most common inflammatory arthritis in older women. It is caused by deposition of monosodium urate crystals in joints and soft tissues following chronic hyperuricaemia. Chronic hyperuricaemia is associated with disorders of purine metabolism due to under excretion or over production of uric acid, the final metabolite of endogenous and dietary purine metabolism. Gout usually presents as a monoarthritis in the first metatarsophalangeal joint (big toe) of the foot and is often referred to as podagra (from the Greek 'seizing the foot'). Subsequent attacks may be polyarticular. Other commonly affected joints include the mid-foot, ankle, knee, wrist and finger joints. Although the attack is extremely painful, it is usually self-limiting resolving spontaneously in 1–2 weeks. Acute attacks are managed with rest, ice and one of the following pharmacological agents: NSAIDs, colchicine or corticosteroids. Some patients may only ever experience one attack, but often a second attack occurs within 6–12 months, with increased risk of subsequent attacks. Patients with recurrent attacks require long-term prophylaxis with drugs that lower the serum urate level. The drug of choice is usually allopurinol, however, a small percentage of patients are unable to tolerate allopurinol and require treatment with an alternative urate-lowering agent such as febuxostat or a uricosuric agent such as benzbromarone, sulphinpyrazone or probenecid. It is essential that pharmacological measures are combined with non-pharmacological measures such as dietary and lifestyle modification to prevent recurrent attacks. Inappropriate management of gout can result in chronic tophaceous gout with polyarticular, destructive low-grade joint inflammation, joint deformity and tophi.

Epidemiology

Gout is one of the oldest recognised diseases and was identified by the Egyptians in 2460 BC. Hippocrates described it as 'arthritis of the rich' due to the association with certain foods and alcohol. Gout affects 1–2% of adults in developed countries, and in recent decades there has been a significant rise in its prevalence and incidence (Zhang et al., 2006). The USA has seen a doubling in the number of cases with the rate of gout increasing to 4.1% in older males. However, unlike the rest of the world, prevalence in the UK appears not to be rising and from 2000 to 2005 remained at 1.4% (Rider and Jordan, 2010). The increasing numbers in many developed countries have been attributed to trends in lifestyle leading to increased risk of gout, for example, obesity, metabolic syndrome, hypertension, alcohol consumption and increased age of the general population. Although the Maori population have a marked genetic predisposition to gout, prior to 1700 they did not experience this inflammatory joint disease. It was changes in diet and lifestyle following European settlement that led to the appearance and increasing prevalence in the country. New Zealand now has probably the highest prevalence in the World with one in eight men affected (Richette and Bardin, 2010). A similar pattern has also been seen in Eastern China, where gout was considered a very rare disease in the 1980s. Changes in diet and lifestyle due to Western influences have seen its prevalence rise to 1.1% in Eastern China in 2008.

In the UK, the presentation of gout in men before the age of 45 years is unusual, but in those over the age of 75 years prevalence is greater than 7% in men and 4% in women (Doherty, 2009; Jordan et al., 2007; Zhang et al., 2006).

Gout is predominantly a disease of men with a male to female ratio of 3.6:1. In women, it tends to develop after menopause when levels of oestrogen, a known uricosuric, fall.

Although environmental factors are clearly implicated in the development of gout, studies have shown that inheritance also plays an important role. In recent years, research into the genetic background of gout has identified several renal urate transporters including URAT-1 and GLUT-9 and the genes that encode them, for example, *SLC22A12* and *SLC2A9*, respectively. Polymorphisms in these genes are associated with increased hyperuricaemia and gout (Dalbeth and Merriman, 2009; Doherty, 2009).

Pathophysiology

Uric acid is mainly a by-product from the breakdown of cellular nucleoproteins and purine nucleotides synthesised *de novo* with about a third coming from the breakdown of dietary purine intake (Fig. 54.1). Uric acid is a weak acid with a pK_a of 5.75, and at the physiological pH of the extra-cellular compartment 98% of uric acid is in the ionised form of urate. This is mainly present as monosodium urate due to the high concentration of sodium in the extra-cellular compartment. Human beings and higher primates lack the enzyme uricase that degrades uric acid to the highly soluble allantoin resulting in higher concentrations of urate close to the level of solubility. Monosodium urate has a solubility limit of 380 μmol/L; when the concentration exceeds 380 μmol/L, there is a risk of precipitation and the formation of monosodium urate crystals.

The production of urate is dependent upon the balance between purine ingestion, *de novo* synthesis in the cells and the actions of xanthine oxidase at the distal end of the purine pathway. Xanthine oxidase is the enzyme that catalyses the oxidation of hypoxanthine, the breakdown product from the catabolism of cellular nucleoproteins and purine nucleotides, to xanthine and xanthine to uric acid.

Gout can be classified as primary or secondary, depending on the presence or absence of an identified cause of hyperuricaemia.

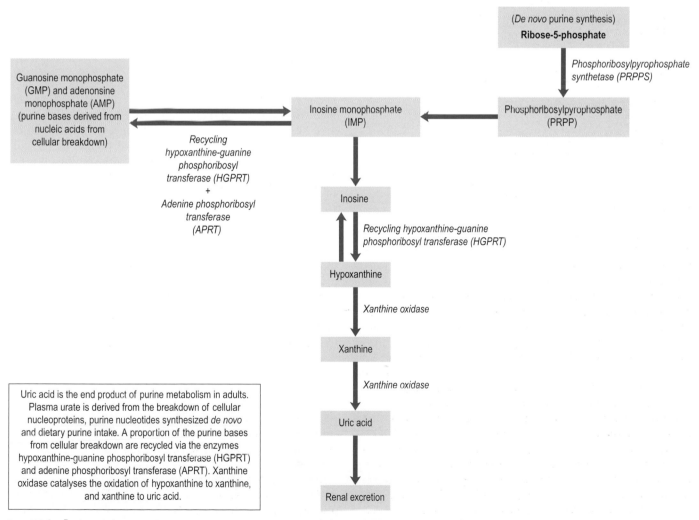

Uric acid is the end product of purine metabolism in adults. Plasma urate is derived from the breakdown of cellular nucleoproteins, purine nucleotides synthesized *de novo* and dietary purine intake. A proportion of the purine bases from cellular breakdown are recycled via the enzymes hypoxanthine-guanine phosphoribosyl transferase (HGPRT) and adenine phosphoribosyl transferase (APRT). Xanthine oxidase catalyses the oxidation of hypoxanthine to xanthine, and xanthine to uric acid.

Fig. 54.1 Purine pathway.

Primary gout is not a consequence of an acquired disorder, but is associated with rare inborn errors of metabolism and isolated renal tubular defects in the fractional clearance of uric acid. A rare group of enzyme defects result in an increased *de novo* purine synthesis such as hypoxanthine-guanine phosphoribosyl transferase deficiency (Lesch-Nyhan syndrome), phosphoribosyl pyrophosphate synthetase super activity, glucose-6 phosphatase deficiency and myogenic hyperuricaemia (Table 54.1).

Secondary gout is the consequence of the use of specific drugs or develops as a consequence of other disorders. Certain diseases are associated with enhanced nucleic acid turnover, for example, myeloproliferative and lymphoproliferative disorders, psoriasis and haemolytic anaemia, and can lead to hyperuricaemia. Renal mechanisms are responsible for the majority of hyperuricaemia in individuals with over production representing less than 10% of patients with gout. The kidney excretes about two-thirds of the uric acid produced daily with the remainder being eliminated via the biliary tract with subsequent conversion to soluble allantoin by colonic bacterial uricase. Approximately 90% of the daily load of urate filtered by the kidneys is re-absorbed. This re-absorption process is mediated by specific anion transporters such as URAT-1 which is located on the apical side of the renal proximal tubular cells and is an important determinant of urate re-absorption (Richette and Bardin, 2010). The URAT-1 transporter is targeted by a number of drugs including benzbromarone, probenecid, losartan and sulphinpyrazone.

Table 54.1 Causes of primary and secondary gout

Primary gout	Secondary gout
Idiopathic	Increased uric acid production
Rare enzyme deficiencies	Lymphoproliferative/
Hypoxanthine-guanine phosphoribosyl transferase deficiency (HPRT)	Myeloproliferative
	Chronic haemolytic anaemias
	Secondary polycythemia
Phosphoribosyl pyrophosphate synthetase super-activity	Severe exfoliative psoriasis
Ribose-5-phosphate	Gaucher's disease
AMP-deaminase deficiency	Cytotoxic drugs
	Glucose-6 phosphate deficiency
	High purine diet overproduction
	Reduced uric acid secretion
	Renal failure
	Hypertension
	Drugs (diuretics, aspirin, ciclosporin)
	Lead nephropathy
	Alcohol
	Down's Syndrome
	Myxoedema
	Beryllium poisoning

Risk factors

Hyperuricaemia is one of the main risk factors for gout and occurs in about 15–20% of the population (Doherty, 2009). Fortunately, only a minority of individuals with increased serum uric acid levels develop gout suggesting the importance of other contributing factors (Box 54.1).

Genetics

Common primary gout in men often shows a strong familial predisposition, although the genetic basis for this is not fully understood. A polymorphism of the *SLC22A12* gene which encodes for URAT-1 has been associated with under excretion of uric acid and hyperuricaemia in German Caucasians (Graessler et al., 2006). While in a Japanese cohort, another mutation of the *SLC22A12* gene has been shown to be protective for the development of gout (Taniguchi et al., 2005).

The recently identified glucose and fructose transporter (GLU9) also acts as a high-capacity urate transporter in the proximal renal tubules (Dalbeth and Merriman, 2009). Polymorphism in the gene which encodes for this transporter (SLC2A9) has been reported to influence serum uric acid levels, and a significant association with self-reported gout has been described (Dalbeth and Merriman, 2009).

Renal disease

Gout is frequently associated with kidney disease, each being a risk factor for the other. Hyperuricaemia is associated with primary kidney disease, but kidney damage may arise secondary to gout as a consequence of the deposition of urate crystals in the interstitium and tubules of the kidney. Historically, gout was associated with significant renal impairment; however, progressive renal failure directly due to gout is now rare and mainly limited to inadequately treated patients with primary purine overproduction associated with purine enzyme defects, rare forms of inherited renal disease, chronic lead intoxication and renal disease as a consequence of uncontrolled disease states associated with gout e.g. hypertension, type 2 diabetes and congestive cardiac failure. Men with gout have a two-fold higher risk of kidney stones than patients without gout (Jordan et al., 2007). The likelihood of stones increases with serum urate concentration, extent of urinary acid secretion and low urine pH.

Box 54.1 Risk factors for gout

Genetics
Renal disease
Co-morbidities, for example, obesity, dyslipidaemia, glucose intolerance, hypertension
Diet
Alcohol consumption
Medication

Co-morbidities

Metabolic syndrome is a multiplex risk factor for atherosclerotic cardiovascular disease that consists of atherogenic dyslipidaemia, raised blood pressure, increased blood glucose, and both prothrombotic and pro-inflammatory states. In the USA, metabolic syndrome is present in 63% of those with gout compared to 25% of those without gout (Choi et al., 2007). Other studies have shown obesity, weight gain and hypertension all to be independent risk factors for the development of gout (Choi et al., 2005).

Diet

Gout has often been associated with a rich lifestyle and excesses in diet. In particular, gout is higher in people who consume large quantities of red meat. There is also an increased risk associated with seafood consumption, but to a lesser extent than with red meat. In contrast, a diet high in purine-rich vegetables does not increase the risk, and the consumption of low-fat dairy products reduces the relative risk of gout with each additional dairy serving. The consumption of soft drinks sweetened with sugar (not diet drinks) has also been linked to an increase in the number of gout cases particularly in USA (Choi and Curham, 2008). The mechanism of action is thought to be an increase in uric acid levels caused by an increase in adenine nucleotide degradation. Vitamin C (ascorbic acid) has been shown to have a modest uricosuric effect (Huang et al., 2005). The consumption of cherries, but no other fruits, has also been shown to decrease uric acid levels.

Alcohol

Increased daily consumption of alcohol is associated with a higher risk of gout. Beer carries the greatest risk, probably due to its high purine content, followed by spirits. However, a moderate consumption of wine is not associated with an increased risk of developing gout (Jordan et al., 2007). The mechanism of action involved is thought to be the metabolism of ethanol to acetyl coenzyme A leading to adenine nucleotide degradation, with resultant increased formation of adenosine monophosphate, a precursor of uric acid. Alcohol also raises lactic acid levels in blood, which inhibits uric acid excretion.

Medication

A number of drugs are associated with increased uric acid levels (Box 54.2). The use of both loop and thiazide diuretics is the most common modifiable risk factor for secondary gout, especially in the elderly. It is thought loop and thiazide diuretics may precipitate an attack via volume depletion and reduced renal tubular secretion of uric acid. Aspirin has a bimodal effect; low doses inhibit uric acid excretion and increase urate levels, while doses greater than 3 g/day are uricosuric.

The prescribing of ciclosporin in organ transplant patients is an independent risk factor for new-onset gout in this group. The proposed mechanism of action is the interaction

---

Box 54.2 Examples of drugs known to raise serum urate levels

Alcohol
Aspirin
Ciclosporin
Cytotoxic chemotherapy
Diuretics (both loops and thiazides)
Ethambutol
Levodopa
Pyrazinamide
Ribavarin and interferon
Teriparatide

---

of ciclosporin with the hOAT10 transporter that mediates urate/glutathione exchange in the kidney (Bahn et al., 2008). Radiotherapy and chemotherapy in patients with neoplastic disorders can cause hyperuricaemia because of increased cell breakdown; to overcome this, prophylactic treatment may be given with allopurinol, commencing 3 days before therapy.

Presentation and diagnosis

An acute attack of gout has a rapid onset, with pain being maximal at 6–24 h of onset and spontaneously resolving within several days or weeks. The first attack usually affects a single joint in the lower limbs in 85–90% of cases, most commonly the first metatarsophalangeal joint (big toe). The next most frequent joints to be affected are the mid-tarsi, ankles, knees and arms. The affected joint is hot, red and swollen with shiny overlying skin. Even the touch of a sheet on the affected joint is too painful for the patient to bear. The patient may also have a fever, leucocytosis, raised erythrocyte sedimentation rate (ESR), and the attack may also be preceded by prodromal symptoms such as anorexia, nausea or change in mood. Following resolution of the attack, there may be pruritis and desquamation of the overlying skin on the affected joint.

Monosodium urate crystals preferentially form in cartilage and fibrous tissues where they are protected from contact with inflammatory mediators. The deposition of crystals may continue for months or years without causing symptoms; it is only when the crystals are shed into the joint space or bursa that inflammatory reaction occurs precipitating an acute attack of gout. The shedding of crystals can be triggered by a number of factors including direct trauma, dehydration, acidosis or rapid weight loss. The acute phase response associated with intercurrent illness or surgery may also precipitate an attack; during this phase, there is increased urinary urate excretion with a lowering of serum uric acid which leads to partial dissolution of monosodium urate crystals and subsequent shedding of crystals into the joint space.

The shed crystals are phagocytosed by monocytes and macrophages, activating the NACHT–LRR–PYD-containing protein-3 (NALP3) inflammasome and triggering the release of interleukin-1β (IL-1β) and other cytokines, a subsequent infiltration of neutrophils and the symptoms of an acute attack (Dalbeth and Haskard, 2005). The NALP3 inflammasome (cryopyrin) is a complex of intracellular proteins that is activated on exposure to microbial elements, such as bacterial RNA and toxins. Activation of NALP3 leads to the release of caspase-1, which is required for cleavage of pro-IL-1β to active IL-1β (Richette and Bardin, 2009). IL-1β has been shown to be critically associated with the inflammatory response induced by monosodium urate crystals (Rider and Jordan, 2010).

A third of patients will have normal uric acid concentrations during an acute attack of gout due to increased urinary urate excretion. The most appropriate time to measure serum urate for monitoring purposes is when the attack has completely resolved. The gold standard for the diagnosis of gout is the demonstration of urate crystals in synovial fluid or in a tophus by polarised light microscopy (Zhang et al., 2006). Crystals may be found in fluid aspirated from non-inflamed joints, even in those joints which have not previously experienced an attack. The crystals are large (10–20 μm) and needle shaped with a strong, intense, characteristic light pattern under polarised light. In contrast, the calcium pyrophosphate dehydrate crystals associated with pseudo-gout are small rhomboid crystals of low intensity. Gout and septic arthritis may co-exist and in order to exclude septic arthritis synovial fluid is sent for Gram staining and culture.

Fig. 54.3 Chronic tophaceous gout.

Course of disease

The course of gout follows a number of stages; initially, the patient may be asymptomatic with a raised serum uric acid level (Fig. 54.2). Some patients may only ever experience one attack, but often a second attack occurs within 6–12 months. Subsequent attacks tend to be of longer duration, affect more than one joint and may spread to the upper limbs. Untreated disease can result in chronic tophaceous gout, with persistent low-grade inflammation in a number of joints resulting in joint damage and deformity. The disease is characterised by the presence of tophi (Fig. 54.3), monosodium urate crystals surrounded by chronic mononuclear and giant-cell reactions. Tophi deposition can occur anywhere in the body, but they are commonly seen on the helix of the ear, within and around the toe or finger joints, on the elbow, around the knees or on the Achilles tendons. The skin overlying the tophi may ulcerate and extrude white, chalky material composed of monosodium urate crystals.

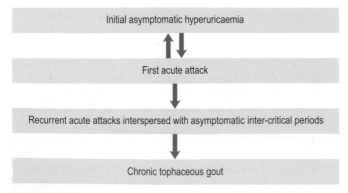

Initial asymptomatic hyperuricaemia

⬆⬇

First acute attack

⬇

Recurrent acute attacks interspersed with asymptomatic inter-critical periods

⬇

Chronic tophaceous gout

Fig. 54.2 Schematic representation of the stages of gout.

Treatment

The management of gout can be split into the rapid resolution of the initial acute attack and long-term measures to prevent future episodes (see Box 54.3).

Gout is often associated with other medical problems including obesity, hypertension, excessive alcohol and the metabolic syndrome of insulin resistance, hyperinsulinaemia, impaired glucose intolerance and hypertriglyceridaemia. This contributes to the increased cardiovascular risk and deterioration of renal function seen in patients with gout. Management is not only directed at alleviating acute attacks and preventing future attacks, but also identifying and treating other co-morbid conditions such as hypertension and hyperlipidaemia. Pharmacological measures should be combined with non-pharmacological measures such as weight loss, changes in diet, increased exercise and reduced alcohol consumption.

Management of an acute attack

Drugs used in the management of an acute attack include NSAIDs, colchicine and corticosteroids. NSAIDs are the recommended first-line agents, but in a number of patients their use is contraindicated and a second-line agent is indicated

Box 54.3 Treatment aims in gout
Rapid alleviation of the acute attack
Prevention of future attacks
Lower serum uric acid levels to below saturation point
Reduce risk of co-morbidities, for example, cardiovascular disease
Lifestyle modification

(Box 54.4). Where the pain is not adequately controlled by treatment, paracetamol and weak opiate analgesics, for example, codeine or dihydrocodeine may be added to the regimen to provide additional relief. Treatment should be continued until the attack is terminated, usually between 1 and 2 weeks. The affected joints should also be rested for 1–2 days and initially treated with ice which has a significant analgesic effect during an acute attack.

A complete medication review should be performed, and ideally medication which is likely to have contributed to the attack discontinued. Where loop and thiazide diuretics are being used for the management of hypertension alone, an alternative anti-hypertensive agent should be considered according to national guidance. Losartan, an angiotensin receptor blocker effective in hypertension, has been shown to have uricosuric properties and is a suitable agent in hypertensive patients with gout (Sica and Schoolwerth, 2002; Takahashi et al., 2003). In patients with heart failure, diuretics are often essential and cannot be discontinued. Certain NSAIDs may be preferable in patients on diuretics with both indometacin and azapropazone (no longer licensed in the UK) demonstrating an increase uric acid secretion. Moreover, the diuretic effect of furosemide appears unaffected by azapropazone and azapropazone's ability to promote uric acid secretion is sustained (Williamson et al., 1984).

Allopurinol should not be commenced during an acute attack as it may prolong or precipitate another attack. However, in patients already established on allopurinol therapy, allopurinol should always be continued during the attack. Aspirin at analgesic doses (600–2400 mg/day) should be avoided as it blocks urate secretion. The continuation or initiation of low-dose aspirin (75–150 mg/day) is recommended in patients with cardiac disease as the benefits outweigh the minimal effect on serum uric acid levels.

Non-steroidal anti-inflammatory drugs

Maximum doses of an NSAID should be commenced rapidly after the onset of an attack and then tapered 24 h after the complete resolution of symptoms. The usual treatment period is 1–2 weeks. NSAIDs act by direct inhibition of cyclo-oxygenase-1 (COX-1) and cyclo-oxygenase-2 (COX-2) via blockade of the cyclo-oxgenase enzyme site. The subsequent inhibition of prostaglandin production reduces inflammation, but also results in additional activities on platelet aggregation, renal homeostasis and gastric mucosal integrity.

Although the NSAIDs differ in chemical structure, they all have similar pharmacological properties in terms of anti-inflammatory and analgesic action, and have similar drug interactions. For a number of years, indometacin was considered the NSAID of choice in gout largely because it was one of the first NSAIDs shown to be effective in the management of gout. However, it has not been shown to be of superior efficacy or safety when compared to other NSAIDs used in the management of acute gout (Jordan et al., 2007).

Azapropazone (1200–1800 mg/day) has been shown to have both anti-inflammatory and uricosuric effects during an acute attack. Unfortunately, use is associated with a higher risk of upper gastro-intestinal side effects when compared to other high-dose NSAIDs (diclofenac, ibuprofen, naproxen, indometacin and ketoprofen), and this significantly restricts its use.

Overall, there is no convincing evidence to promote the use of one NSAID over another in the management of acute gout.

In an effort to reduce the side effects of NSAIDs, and particularly the gastro-intestinal side effects, agents were developed to selectively block COX-2 and have minimal effect on COX-1. COX-2 selective agents are recommended for use in patients who are at high risk of developing gastro-intestinal side effects, but they are not recommended for routine use. It should be noted that the selective benefit of COX-2 inhibitors is lost in patients taking low dose aspirin. The selective COX-2 inhibitor etoricoxib in a daily dose of 120 mg has been shown to give comparable rapid relief of pain in acute gout to indometacin 50 mg three times daily but with fewer side effects (Schumacher et al., 2002). However, a systematic review and meta-analysis of studies involving etoricoxib have demonstrated an increased risk of cardiovascular thromboembolic events (Aldington et al., 2005). Although there are currently no data directly comparing the cardiovascular risk associated with selective and non-selective NSAIDs, it is recommended that the use of COX-2 inhibitors is avoided in patients with established heart disease, cerebrovascular disease or peripheral vascular disease.

NSAIDs should be avoided in patients with heart failure, renal insufficiency and a history of gastric ulceration. Care should also be exercised in elderly patients with multiple pathologies. When prescribing an NSAID, the need for gastric protection should be considered in patients at increased risk of a peptic ulcer, bleed or perforation.

Colchicine

Colchicine is an alkaloid derived from the autumn crocus (colchicum autumnale) and has been reported to have been used in the treatment of gout since the 6th century AD. Colchicine has a slower onset of action than NSAIDs but is recommended in patients where NSAIDs are contraindicated. It should be started as soon as possible after the onset of an attack.

Although the mode of action of colchicine in gout is not fully understood, it is thought to arrest microtubule assembly in neutrophils and inhibit many cellular functions. It suppresses monosodium urate crystal-induced NALP3 inflammasome-driven caspase-1 activation, IL-1β processing and release, and L-selectin expression on neutrophils. Colchicine also blocks the release of a crystal-derived chemotactic factor from neutrophil lysosomes, blocks neutrophil adhesion to endothelium by modulating the distribution of adhesion molecules on the endothelial cells and inhibits monosodium urate crystal-induced production of superoxide anions from neutrophils (Nuki, 2008).

Although widely used, there are few studies that demonstrate the efficacy of colchicine. A single, randomised, controlled trial has compared the benefits of colchicine to placebo in acute gouty flare (Ahern et al., 1987). Patients were given 1 mg of colchicine followed by 500 μcg every 2 h until the attack stopped or they felt too ill to continue taking colchicine. Colchicine was found to be superior to placebo with an absolute reduction of 34% for pain and a 30% reduction in clinical symptoms such as palpation, swelling, redness and pain. The number needed to treat (NNT) with colchicine to reduce pain was 3 and the NNT to reduce clinical symptoms was 2. All participants given colchicine experienced gastro-intestinal side effects such as diarrhoea and/or vomiting. There are no studies comparing colchicine to either NSAIDs or corticosteroids in an acute flare of gout.

The current dose of colchicine licensed for the management of an acute attack of gout is 1 mg initially, followed by 500 μcg every 2–3 h until relief of pain is obtained or vomiting or diarrhoea occurs. A maximum of 6 mg should be given per course and treatment should not be repeated within 3 days. This dosage regimen frequently causes diarrhoea and other toxic side effects, particularly in elderly patients (Morris et al., 2003; Terkeltaub et al., 2008). It is therefore recommended that a dose of 500 μcg given twice or four times a day should be used to reduce toxicity. Intravenous colchicine is no longer licensed in the UK because use has been associated with a number of fatalities (2% mortality rate).

Common side effects associated with colchicine are abdominal cramps, nausea, vomiting, and rarely bone marrow suppression, neuropathy and myopathy. Side effects are more common in patients with hepatic or renal impairment. The dose of colchicine should be reduced in mild to moderate renal impairment, for example creatinine clearance 10–50 mL/min, and it should not be used in patients with severe renal impairment, for example creatinine clearance less than 10 mL/min. Care should also be exercised in patients with chronic heart failure due to colchicine's ability to constrict blood vessels and stimulate central vasomotor centres.

Colchicine is metabolised by CYP3A4 and excreted by p-glycoprotein; toxicity can be caused by drugs that interact with its metabolism and clearance, and this includes macrolides, ciclosporin and protease inhibitors. The absorption of vitamin B$_{12}$ may be impaired by chronic administration of high doses of colchicine.

Corticosteroids

Corticosteroids are usually considered where use of an NSAID or colchicine is contraindicated or in refractory cases. They may be given intravenously, intramuscularly or direct into a joint (intra-articular) when only one or two joints are affected. In patients with a monoarthritis, an intra-articular corticosteroid injection is highly effective in treating an attack.

Intramuscular triamcinolone acetonide 60 mg has been shown to be as safe and effective as indometacin 50 mg three times daily in treating an acute attack of gout with earlier resolution of symptoms in the steroid group (Alloway et al., 1993). Common doses of intra-articular steroids are 80 mg of methylprednisolone acetate for a large joint such as a knee; 40 mg of methylprednisolone acetate or 40 mg of triamcinolone acetonide for a smaller joint such as a wrist or elbow. Oral prednisolone 30 mg daily for 5 days has also been shown to be equally efficacious to indometacin 50 mg three times a day for 2 days or 25 mg three times a day for 3 days plus paracetamol and has fewer adverse events (Man et al., 2007). Oral steroid regimens used in practice include prednisolone 30 mg daily for 1–3 days with subsequent dose tapering over 1–2 weeks. Intramuscular steroid injections (methylprednisolone acetate 80–120 mg) may sometimes be used to prevent the precipitation of a flare on initiation of prophylactic treatment for gout. Corticosteroids may have fewer adverse events than other acute treatments when used short term, particularly in the elderly.

Interleukin-1 inhibitors

IL-1β is critically associated with the inflammatory response induced by monosodium urate crystals (Rider and Jordan, 2010). Anakinra, an IL-1 receptor antagonist, has been shown to reduce the pain of gout and bring about complete resolution by day 3 in the majority of patients after a course of three 100-mg subcutaneous injections (McGonagle et al., 2007; So et al. 2007). Other IL-1 inhibitors, such as rilonacept, are under development.

Management of chronic gout

The presence of hyperuricaemia is not an indication to commence prophylactic therapy. Some patients may only experience a single episode and a change in lifestyle, diet or concurrent medication may be sufficient to prevent further attacks. Patients who suffer one or more acute attacks within 12 months of the first attack should normally be prescribed prophylactic urate-lowering therapy (see Fig. 54.4). There are, however, some groups of patients where prophylactic therapy should be instigated after a single attack. These include individuals with uric acid stones, the presence of tophi at first presentation and young patients with a family history of renal or cardiac disease. The criteria for starting prophylactic therapy for gout is detailed in Box 54.5.

The aim of prophylactic gout treatment is to maintain the serum urate level below the saturation point of monosodium urate (300 μmol/L). If the serum urate is maintained below this level, crystal deposits dissolve and gout is controlled. Prophylactic treatment should not be initiated until an acute attack of gout has completely resolved, usually 2–3 weeks

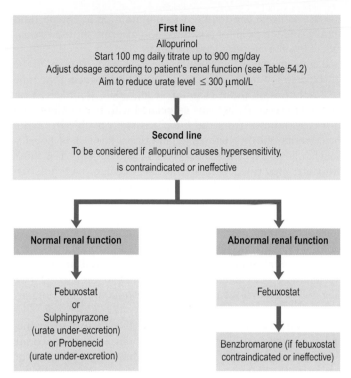

First line
Allopurinol
Start 100 mg daily titrate up to 900 mg/day
Adjust dosage according to patient's renal function (see Table 54.2)
Aim to reduce urate level ≤ 300 μmol/L

↓

Second line
To be considered if allopurinol causes hypersensitivity,
is contraindicated or ineffective

Normal renal function

↓

Febuxostat
or
Sulphinpyrazone
(urate under-excretion)
or Probenecid
(urate under-excretion)

Abnormal renal function

↓

Febuxostat

↓

Benzbromarone (if febuxostat
contraindicated or ineffective)

Fig. 54.4 Management of chronic gout in patients requiring urate-lowering therapy.

Box 54.5 Criteria for starting prophylactic therapy for gout

One or more acute attacks within 12 months of the first attack
Tophi present at the first presentation of an acute attack
Presence of uric acid stones
Need to continue medication associated with raised uric acid levels, for example diuretics
Young patients with a family history of renal or cardiac disease

Box 54.6 Classification of prophylactic agents used to lower serum urate

Uricostatic agents: allopurinol, febuxostat
Uricosuric agents: benzbromarone, probenecid, sulphinpyrazone
Uricolytic agents: rasburicase, polyethylene glycol-uricase

Table 54.2 Recommended dose of allopurinol in patients with diminished renal function

Creatinine clearance (mL/min)	Dose
0	100 mg three times a week
10	100 mg alternate days
20	100 mg daily
40	150 mg daily
60	200 mg daily
>100	300 mg daily

after symptom resolution. Once started, prophylactic treatment should be continued indefinitely even if further acute attacks develop.

Drugs that lower serum uric acid can be classified into three groups according to their pharmacological mode of action (Box 54.6).

Uricostatic agents

Uricostatic agents act on the enzyme xanthine oxidase. Xanthine oxidase catalyses the oxidation of hypoxanthine to xanthine and subsequently xanthine to uric acid (Fig. 54.1). Hypoxanthine comes from the catabolism of cellular nucleoproteins and purine nucleotides. Blocking the action of this enzyme reduces the production of uric acid. Agents in this group include allopurinol and febuxostat.

Allopurinol. Allopurinol is the prophylactic agent of choice in the management of recurrent gout. In order to become pharmacologically active, allopurinol must be metabolised by the liver to oxypurinol. Oxypurinol has a much longer half-life than allopurinol, 14–16 h compared to 2 h. Both allopurinol and oxypurinol are renally excreted, with oxypurinol undergoing re-absorption from the renal tubule. In patients with reduced renal function, the half-life of oxypurinol is increased with the risk of accumulation and toxicity. It is, therefore, essential that a patient's renal function is checked prior to the prescribing of allopurinol and the dose adjusted accordingly (Table 54.2). In patients with normal renal function, the starting dose is 100 mg/day; this is gradually increased in 100-mg increments every 2–3 weeks until the optimal serum urate level (<300 μmol/L) or the maximum dose is reached. The maxi-

mum recommended daily dose in patients with normal renal function is 900 mg/day. A decrease in serum urate will occur within a couple of days of introducing allopurinol therapy with a peak effect at 7–10 days. The dissolution of tophi may take up to 6–12 months with effective therapy.

Approximately 3–5% of patients treated with allopurinol suffer from an adverse reaction. Intolerance usually manifests itself as a hypersensitivity reaction within the first 2 months of treatment. Adverse effects reported with allopurinol therapy include rash, fever, worsening renal failure, hepatotoxicity, vasculitis and even death. Severe toxic effects arise in less than 2% of patients. The risk of toxicity increases with renal impairment, age and concurrent drug therapy such as diuretics.

Prior to the availability of febuxostat, allopurinol desensitisation was attempted in patients with a mild hypersensitivity to allopurinol. This involved starting with a very low dose (50 μcg daily) and gradually increasing the dose over a period of several weeks to 100 mg daily. Desensitisation is now only considered where the reaction has been mild and there is an absence of alternative treatment options.

Azathioprine and mercaptopurine are metabolised by xanthine oxidase, co-administration of allopurinol reduces the metabolism of these two medicines leading to accumulation and toxicity. The dose of azathioprine or mercaptopurine should be reduced to approximately a quarter of the normal dose when co-prescribed with allopurinol. In addition, full blood counts should be performed at regular intervals to identify potential toxicity. High-dose allopurinol (>600 mg/day) increases carbamazepine blood levels by approximately one third; the same effect is not associated with lower doses of allopurinol (<300 mg/day).

Febuxostat. Febuxostat is a more selective and potent inhibitor of xanthine oxidase than allopurinol and has no effect on other enzymes involved in purine or pyrimidine metabolism (Lawrence Edwards, 2009). It is licensed for the treatment of chronic hyperuricaemia in conditions where urate deposition has already occurred including a history, or presence of, tophus and/or gouty arthritis. It is recommended as a second-line agent in patients who are intolerant of allopurinol or for whom allopurinol is contraindicated.

Febuxostat is more effective than fixed-dose allopurinol 300 mg in lowering uric acid concentrations in trials of up to 40 months' duration (Schumacher et al., 2008, 2009). However, a reduction in the incidence of episodes of acute gout has not been demonstrated.

The recommended starting dose for febuxostat is 80 mg once daily. If the serum uric acid is greater than 357 μmol/L, after 2–4 weeks, the dose should be increased to 120 mg once daily. The increased potency and good oral bioavailability of febuxostat leads to rapid decreases in serum uric acid levels permitting the testing of levels 2 weeks after starting therapy or adjusting the dose. No dosage adjustment is necessary in patients with mild or moderate renal impairment; however, there are no current recommendations for use in patients with severe renal impairment, for example creatinine clearance <30 mL/min. In patients with mild hepatic impairment, the dose should not exceed 80 mg daily; the use of febuxostat has not been studied in patients with severe hepatic impairment. Febuxostat should not be given to patients with ischaemic heart disease or congestive heart failure because of cardiovascular side effects. When initiating therapy with febuxostat, gout flare prophylaxis should be prescribed for at least 6 months.

The most common adverse effects include respiratory infection, diarrhoea, headache and liver function abnormalities. It is recommended liver function should be tested in all patients prior to the initiation of therapy and periodically thereafter based on clinical judgement. The use of febuxostat is not recommended in patients concomitantly treated with mercaptopurine or azathioprine and in patients taking theophylline, serum levels of theophylline should be monitored.

Uricosuric agents

Uricosuric agents increase uric acid excretion primarily by inhibiting post-secretory tubular absorption of uric acid from filtered urate in the kidney. They are indicated as second-line agents in those who are urate under-excreters and are dependent on the patient having an adequate level of renal function. These agents should be avoided in patients with urate nephropathy or those who are over producers of uric acid due to the high risk of developing renal stones. Patients receiving a uricosuric agent are required to maintain an adequate fluid intake, and the need for alkalinisation of urine should be considered to prevent urate precipitation

Benzbromarone. Benzbromarone has been shown to be effective in lowering serum urate levels and reducing the time to resolution of tophi (Kumar et al., 2005; Reinders et al. 2009). However, its use was associated with hepatoxicity and it was withdrawn from the UK. It is still possible to obtain benzbromarone on a named patient basis. The risk of hepatotoxicity has been estimated to be 1:17,000 patients. For those who are prescribed benzbromarone, regular liver function tests must be performed during the first 6 months of therapy, and the hepatotoxic risk associated with the medicine should be clearly explained to the patient at the outset.

The dose ranges from 50 to 200 mg daily. It remains active in mild to moderate renal impairment and is indicated where there is a contraindication to other agents used in the management of gout such as allopurinol and febuxostat (see Fig. 54.4). Diarrhoea may be troublesome in approximately 10% of patients.

Sulphinpyrazone. Sulphinpyrazone is effective in reducing the frequency of gout attacks, tophi and plasma urate levels at doses of 200–800 mg/day. It has the same mode of action on the kidney as benzbromarone and probenecid all of which inhibit URAT-1 transporter resulting in reduced urate re-absorption. However, in addition to this, sulphinpyrazone inhibits prostaglandin synthesis resulting in a similar adverse effect profile to NSAIDs, for example gastro-intestinal ulceration, acute renal failure, fluid retention, elevated liver enzymes and blood disorders. The use of sulphinpyrazone is reserved for use in patients with adequate renal function who are underexcretors of uric acid and intolerant or resistant to treatment with allopurinol.

Probenecid. Probenecid monotherapy is less effective than the other agents in this group and generally not recommended. It may have a role as an add-on agent when allopurinol alone is insufficient. Doses of 0.5–2.0 g/day have been used. As with sulphinpyrazone, it is ineffective in renal impairment. Dyspepsia and reflux may be troublesome in some patients, and it can interact with renally excreted anionic drugs. It is no longer marketed in the UK.

Uricolytics

Uricolytic drugs convert uric acid to allantoin through the actions of the enzyme urate oxidase (uricase). Allantoin is more soluble than uric acid and readily excreted by the kidney. Uricolytics are indicated for hyperuricaemia associated with tumour lysis syndrome and are not indicated for other forms of hyperuricaemia.

Rasburicase. Rasburicase, a recombinant form of the enzyme urate oxidase (uricase), is derived from a cDNA code from a modified *Aspergillus flavus* strain expressed in a modified strain of *Saccharomyces cerevisiae*. It is licensed to treat tumour lysis syndrome and is given intravenously at a dose of 0.2 mg/kg in short courses for 5–7 days. Rasburicase has a half-life of approximately 19 h. No dosage adjustment is required in patients with renal or hepatic impairment.

Rasburicase is generally well tolerated, but adverse effects include fever, nausea, vomiting, rash, diarrhoea, headache, allergic reactions and the development of auto-antibodies.

Polyethylene glycol-uricase (PEG-uricase). PEG-uricase is a pegylated, recombinant form of uricase. Pegylation of the molecule reduces the risk of patients developing auto-antibodies and lengthens the half-life of the drug. It is effective in reducing tophi. The use of PEG-uricase has been associated with severe infusion reactions in a small minority of patients; this and its high cost are likely to limit its use. It may have a role in severe, refractory cases or as a short-term treatment to remove tophi prior to the initiation of conventional urate-lowering therapies.

Preventing gout flare

When prophylactic treatment is commenced, there is a risk of precipitating an acute gout attack, or 'mobilisation flare', for approximately 12 months. Mobilisation flares are thought to be caused by the rapid fall in serum urate following the initiation of urate lowering. The risk of precipitating an acute attack can be reduced by delaying the initiation of long-term urate-lowering therapy until the acute attack has completely resolved and prescribing colchicine or an NSAID during the treatment initiation period.

Colchicine

Colchicine is the agent of first choice to prevent the precipitation of a flare when commencing chronic gout treatment. Low doses of colchicine (500 μcg orally twice a day) should be prescribed and continued for at least 6 months. There are no randomised controlled trial data assessing the effectiveness of colchicine as a single agent to prevent recurrent gout, but it has been shown to help reduce mobilisation flares for up to 6 months after starting allopurinol.

NSAIDs

If there are no contraindications to the use of NSAIDs, they may be considered second line to colchicine in patients' intolerant to colchicine. NSAIDs should be continued for a maximum of 6 weeks.

Patient care

It is important to inform patients about the disease, its curable nature, the aims of drug therapy and how to prevent and handle flares. The need for dietary and lifestyle changes should also be stressed. The UK Gout Society website can assist in providing patients with information about the condition and how it should be managed (http://www.ukgoutsociety.org/). In over-weight patients, gradual weight loss should be encouraged, very rapid weight loss should be avoided as it can cause ketosis and result in raised uric acid levels with the likelihood of precipitating an attack. Low purine diets are difficult to

adhere to; a calorie-restricted diet with low carbohydrate (40% of energy), high protein (30% of energy) and unsaturated fat (30% of energy) should be recommended. The importance of avoiding or reducing alcohol consumption should also be emphasised.

Patients at risk of recurrent attacks should be issued with a suitable NSAID to treat the attack as soon as possible. The patient should be clear on what dose to take, when to initiate therapy, how long to take the medication for and any possible side effects to look out for. The patient should also be advised to avoid certain over-the-counter medicines which may exacerbate an attack, for example the use of aspirin as an analgesic.

Those taking long-term prophylactic therapy need to understand the importance of continuing therapy despite being asymptomatic. They should avoid running out of medication, as a short gap in therapy may precipitate an attack. Patients receiving uricosuric agents should be advised to maintain a fluid intake of at least 2 L/day to reduce the risk of uric acid stone formation in the kidneys.

Case studies

Case 54.1

Mr TH is a 50-year-old, slightly over-weight (95 kg) male who presents with an extremely painful big toe. He states that the pain started suddenly in the early hours of the morning and that he cannot even bear to put a sock over his foot. He can think of no recent trauma to his foot. He has no other symptoms and there is no previous significant medical history apart from high blood pressure for which he takes bendroflumethiazide (2.5 mg in the morning). On examination, the toe is red, hot, swollen and extremely painful on palpation. The patient also has an elevated blood pressure of 150 mm/95 mmHg. On questioning about his weekly alcohol intake, he states that he usually does not exceed 21 units/week, but that it was a friend's 50th birthday party recently and he might have had considerably more to drink than usual. Blood results show a slightly raised C-reactive protein, other parameters are normal including renal function; however, his serum urate is slightly raised (390 μmol/L). A diagnosis of acute gout is made.

Questions

1. What initial therapy would you recommend to treat the patient's acute attack of gout?
2. What risk factors could have contributed to the acute attack?
3. Should this patient be placed on therapy to prevent further attacks?
4. What lifestyle and dietary advice would you give to the patient to assist in preventing further attacks?

Answers

1. Initial therapy should be directed at promptly and safely resolving the pain. Drugs used in the management of an acute attack include NSAIDs, colchicine and corticosteroids. NSAIDs are indicated as first-line agents, but there are a number of patients

who cannot take these medicines, and this includes those with renal impairment, heart failure or a history of gastric ulceration. Caution should also be exercised in elderly patients with multiple pathologies as they are prone to develop side effects with NSAIDs, particularly gastric symptoms. Colchicine has a slower-onset action then NSAIDs (6h vs. 2h) and is usually indicated where NSAIDs are contraindicated. When only a single joint is affected, an intra-articular injection directly into the joint may be considered; however, this is often too painful for the patient to bear.

As the patient has no contraindications, it would be appropriate to start an NSAID at maximal dose for 2–3 days and then reduce and continue for a further 7–10 days. There is no evidence to promote the use of one NSAID over another in the management of an acute attack; the main issue is to start therapy as soon as possible at maximal dose provided there are no contraindications. When initiating an NSAID, the need for gastric protection should be considered particularly in those aged over 65 years, previous history of peptic ulcer disease or gastro-intestinal complications and other medicines associated with gastro-intestinal side effects.

COX-2 inhibitors such as etoricoxib selectively block the COX-2 pathway resulting in reduced gastro-intestinal side effects. These agents are recommended for patients with high risk of gastro-intestinal side effects, but they are not recommended for routine use. Etoricoxib has been shown to be as equally effective as indometacin with fewer adverse effects. However, a systematic review and meta-analysis of etoricoxib showed an increased risk of cardiovascular and thromboembolic events associated with its use. It is recommended that COX-2 inhibitors be avoided in patients with established heart disease, cerebrovascular disease or peripheral vascular disease.

Where the patient's pain is not adequately controlled by an NSAID, simple and low-potency opiate analgesia can be added to the regimen. The affected joint should be rested for 1–2 days and the affected area treated with ice.

2. Hyperuricaemia (raised serum uric acid levels) is one of the main risk factors for the development of gout; however, not all patients with a raised serum uric acid level will go on to develop gout. Studies have shown obesity, weight gain and hypertension all to be independent risk factors for the development of gout. Mr TH is slightly over-weight and has a history of hypertension. Measurement of his serum lipid levels should be considered as dyslipidaemia is commonly associated with gout.

Loop and thiazide diuretics are one of the most common modifiable risk factors associated with gout. It is thought they exert their action via volume depletion and the reduced tubular renal secretion of uric acid. In patients with heart failure, diuretics are often essential and cannot be discontinued. Mr TH's bendroflumethiazide is being used for the management of hypertension and a change to an alternate hypertensive agent should be considered. Losartan, an angiotensin receptor blocker, has been shown to have both anti-hypertensive and urate-lowering properties and is suggested as a suitable agent in hypertensive patients with gout.

Alcohol consumption is an important risk factor for the development of gout. The mechanism of action is thought to be due to the metabolism of ethanol to acetyl coenzyme A leading to adenine nucleotide degradation and a subsequent rise in the levels of adenosine monophosphate which is a precursor of uric acid. Beer drinking is associated with the highest risk due to its high purine content. It is recommended that males restrict their alcohol consumption to less than 21 units/week and that both male and female patients have at least 3 alcohol-free days per week. Beer, stout, port and fortified wines should be avoided. Two 125-mL glasses of wine per day are considered acceptable and two pub-sized measures of spirits are considered safer than half a pint of many beers.

3. In uncomplicated gout, specific long-term treatment to reduce plasma uric acid concentration should only be given if a second attack or further attacks of gout occur within 1 year. The need for preventative therapy is not indicated in this patient; he has uncomplicated gout and his bendroflumethiazide can be switched to an alternate anti-hypertensive agent which is not linked to an increase in uric acid levels. For some patients, changes in diet and lifestyle plus the removal of medicines contributing to the attack may be sufficient to prevent further flares. Where prophylactic therapy is indicated, it should only be commenced after complete resolution of the flare.

4. Lifestyle modification can be effective in preventing further attacks. Moderate physical exercise can be beneficial; however, intense muscular exercise should be avoided as it can lead to a rise in uric acid levels. In over-weight patients, gradual weight loss should be encouraged. Rapid weight loss can precipitate ketosis and a subsequent rise in the urate pool. Mr TH should be given appropriate dietary advice. It is the regular consumption of foods containing purines rather than the absolute purine content of a particular food that is important. The UK Gout Society (http://www.ukgoutsociety.org/) provides a fact sheet with dietary recommendations and the purine content of various foods for patients. Ideally, total daily purine intake should not exceed 200mg/day, and foods such as shellfish, offal and sardines should be avoided. Dairy products have been shown to be beneficial in lowering serum uric acid, and even the addition of yoghurt on alternate days has been shown to reduce levels. The consumption of soft drinks sweetened with fructose or sucrose (not diet drinks) should be limited. Cherries whether sweet, tart, juice or fruit have a urate-lowering potential.

As previously discussed, Mr TH should also moderate his alcohol consumption.

Case 54.2

Mr SB, a 45-year-old man, has recently been treated for his second acute attack of gout within 8 months of his first episode. The symptoms have now resolved and his primary care doctor is unsure if Mr SB should be commenced on prophylactic medication. Mr SB has no family history of renal disease, but his father died of a myocardial infarction aged 52. He takes no regular medication and has no other significant previous medical history.

Questions

1. Is it appropriate to initiate prophylactic treatment?
2. What prophylactic treatment would you recommend?

Answers

1. Patients who suffer one or more acute attacks of gout in a year should be commenced on prophylactic therapy. However, prophylactic therapy is recommended for some patients at the first acute attack. These include patients with uric acid stones, tophi and young patients with a family history of renal or cardiac disease. Mr SB is relatively young and there is a family history of cardiac disease. The initiation of prophylactic therapy should therefore be considered.

2. Allopurinol is the first-line choice for prophylactic treatment of hyperuricaemia. Patients with normal renal function should be commenced on 100 mg daily and the dose gradually increased by 100 mg increments at 2–3 week intervals until the serum urate level has been reduced to less than 300 µmol/L. Serum urate levels may be artificially low during an acute attack. The level should be checked following the acute episode and prophylactic therapy, if deemed appropriate, should not be commenced until

after the flare has resolved. Serum urate levels should fall within 2 days and peak at 7–10 days with the introduction of allopurinol and with dose increases.

Renal function should be checked prior to starting allopurinol to ensure that the correct dosage is prescribed based on the patient's creatinine clearance. Reduced renal function increases the half-life of allopurinol's active metabolite, oxypurinol. If the dose is not reduced according to renal function, the patient is at risk of oxypurinol accumulation and toxicity.

Mr SB does not take regular medication, but current medication should always be checked for interactions with allopurinol, for example azathioprine, mercaptopurine, carbamazepine.

As prophylactic treatment is being initiated, Mr SB is at risk of a mobilisation flare for approximately 12 months. Prophylaxis treatment for mobilisation flares should be recommended. First-line choice for the prevention of mobilisation flares is colchicine (500 µcg twice daily for 6 months). For patients who are intolerant to colchicines, NSAIDs offer a second-line choice, provided there are no contraindications to NSAID therapy. NSAIDs should be continued for a maximum of 6 weeks.

Case 54.3

Mrs DM, a 72-year-old woman, was admitted to hospital with dehydration and loss of consciousness, following a fall. On admission, she was taking bendroflumethiazide 2.5 mg each morning, candesartan 8 mg each morning, simvastatin 10 mg at night, paracetamol 1 g four times a day and the week before admission had been started on allopurinol 300 mg once a day for gout. On day 2 of her admission, she developed a rash and fever, her creatinine clearance was 23 mL/min and her ALT 156 international units/L. After investigation, she was diagnosed as having a hypersensitivity reaction to allopurinol. The allopurinol was stopped immediately.

Questions

1. What risk factors does this patient have for developing a hypersensitivity to allopurinol?
2. What prophylaxis treatment option would you recommend for following the allopurinol hypersensitivity reaction?

Answers

1. Severe toxic effects caused by allopurinol occur in less than 2% of patients taking allopurinol; however, the mortality risk is high in this group. The risk of allopurinol toxicity is increased for patients with renal impairment, old age and concomitant drugs. Mrs DM has all of these risk factors. Her renal function may have been impaired prior to admission due to her age, but this

may have been further exacerbated by a period of dehydration caused from extended stasis following a fall. Bendroflumethiazide may have contributed to her fall, dehydration and history of gout. Her blood pressure requires close monitoring to ensure she is not suffering from postural hypotension or that the combination of two anti-hypertensive drugs is not causing her blood pressure to drop too low. Ideally, bendroflumethiazide should be avoided in this patient and if needed an alternate anti-hypertensive prescribed. Mrs DM's starting dose of allopurinol is considerably higher than that which would normally be recommended, the high dose in combination with renal impairment may have caused an accumulation of the active metabolite of allopurinol, oxypurinol, which would have increased the risk of toxicity. Renal function should be checked in all patients prior to commencing allopurinol. For normal renal function, a starting dose of 100 mg once a day is recommended. For abnormal renal function, the product data sheet should be consulted for appropriate dose reduction. Hypersensitivity reactions usually occur up to 2 months following the initiation of allopurinol. Allopurinol should be stopped immediately in patients with symptoms of hypersensitivity reaction.

2. The choice of second-line prophylaxis treatment to replace allopurinol should be based on both renal function and pathophysiology of the disease.

Febuxostat is recommended in mild to moderate renal impairment, but there are no data in severe renal impairment. In patients with mild hepatic impairment, the dose of febuxostat must not exceed 80 mg once a day. Febuxostat is initiated at 80 mg daily but can be increased to 120 mg daily if the serum urate has not decreased adequately after 2–4 weeks of therapy. Febuxostat should not be used in patients with a history of cardiovascular disease.

In normal renal function, sulphinpyrazone or probenecid is indicated in urate under excretors when febuxostat is not appropriate. However, sulphinpyrazone can increase sodium and water retention and may worsen Mrs DM's heart failure. Probenecid is less effective than other uricosuric agents and is generally not used.

Benzbromarone is effective in moderate renal impairment and may be considered if febuxostat is contraindicated or ineffective. Baseline liver function tests must be performed as well as regular monitoring during the first 6 months of therapy. Benzbromarone is only available on a named patient basis, patients must have failed or been intolerant of other therapies and understand that the use of benzbromarone is associated with liver toxicity.

Allopurinol desensitisation should only be considered when all other prophylactic treatments have failed and is not appropriate for patients who have suffered a severe hypersensitivity reaction.

Acknowledgements

The authors thank Professor Philip Conaghan, Centre for Musculoskeletal Disease, Leeds Teaching Hospital NHS, for his invaluable comments regarding the structure and content of this chapter.

References

Ahern, M.J., Reid, C., Gordon, T.P., et al., 1987. Does colchicine work? The results of the first controlled study in acute gout. Aust. N. Z. J. Med. 17, 301–304.

Aldington, S., Shirtcliffe, P., Weatherall, M., et al., 2005. Systematic review and meta-analysis of the risk of major cardiovascular events with etoricoxib therapy. N. Z. Med. J. 118 (1223) U1684.

Alloway, J.A., Moriarty, M.J., Hoogland, Y.T., et al., 1993. Comparison of triamcinolone acetonide with indomethacin in the treatment of acute gouty arthritis. J. Rheumatol. 20, 111–113.

Bahn, A., Hagos, Y., Reuter, S., et al., 2008. Identification of a new urate and high affinity nicotinate transporter, hOAT10 (SLC22A13). J. Biol. Chem. 283, 16332–16341.

Choi, H.K., Curham, G., 2008. Soft drinks, fructose consumption, and the risk of gout in men: prospective cohort study. Br. J. Med. 336, 309–312.

Choi, H.K., Atkinson, K., Karlson, E.W., et al., 2004. Purine rich foods, dairy and protein intake, and the risk of gout in men. N. Engl. J. Med. 350, 1093–1103.

Choi, H.K., Atkinson, K., Karlson, E.W., et al., 2005. Obesity, weight change, hypertension, diuretic use, and risk of gout in men: the health professionals follow-up study. Arch. Int. Med. 165, 742–748.

Choi, H.K., Ford, E.S., Li, C., et al., 2007. Prevalence of metabolic syndrome in patients with gout: the Third National Health and Nutrition Examination Survey. Arthritis Rheum. 57, 109–115.

Dalbeth, N., Haskard, D.O., 2005. Mechanisms of inflammation in gout. Rheumatology 44, 1090–1096.

Dalbeth, N., Merriman, T., 2009. Crystal ball gazing: new therapeutic targets for hyperuricaemia and gout. Rheumatology 48, 222–226.

Doherty, H., 2009. New insights into the epidemiology of gout. Rheumatology 49, 613–614.

Lawrence Edwards, N., 2009. Febuxostat: a new treatment for hyperuricaemia in gout. Rheumatology 48 (Suppl. 2), ii15–ii19.

Graessler, J., Graessler, A., Unger, S., et al., 2006. Association of the human urate transporter 1 with reduced renal uric acid excretion in a German Caucasian population. Arthritis Rheum. 54, 292–300.

Huang, H.Y., Appel, L.J., Choi, M.J., et al., 2005. The effects of vitamin C supplementation on serum concentrations of uric acid: results of a randomized controlled trial. Arthritis Rheum. 52, 1843–1847.

Jordan, K.M., Cameron, S., Snaith, M., et al., on behalf of the British Society for Rheumatology and British Health Professionals in Rheumatology Standards, Guidelines and Adult Working Group (SGAWG), 2007. British Society for Rheumatology and British Health Professionals in Rheumatology guideline for the management of gout. Rheumatology doi:10.1093/rheumatology/kem056b.

Kumar, S., Ng, J., Gow, P., 2005. Benzbromarone therapy in management of refractory gout. N. Z. Med. J. 118 (1217), U1528.

Man, C.Y., Cheung, I., Cameron, I., et al., 2007. Comparison of oral prednisolone/paracetamol and oral indomethacin/paracetamol combination therapy in the treatment of acute gout like arthritis: a double blind randomized, controlled trial. Ann. Emerg. Med. 49, 670–677.

McGonagle, D., Tan, A.L., Shankaranarayana, S., et al., 2007. Management of treatment resistant inflammation of acute or chronic tophaceous gout with anakinra. Ann. Rheum. Dis. 66, 1683–1684.

Morris, I., Varughese, G., Mattingly, P., 2003. Lesson of the week – colchicine in acute gout. Br. Med. J. 327, 1275–1276.

Nuki, G., 2008. Colchicine: its mechanism of action and efficacy in crystal-induced inflammation. Curr. Rheumatol. Rep. 10, 218–227.

Reinders, M.K., Haagsma, C., Jansen, T.L., et al., 2009. A randomised controlled trial on the efficacy and tolerability with dose escalation of allopurinol 300–600mg/day versus benzbromarone 100–200mg/day in patients with gout. Ann. Rheum. Dis. 68, 892–897.

Richette, P., Bardin, T., 2010. Gout. Lancet 375, 318–328.

Rider, T.G., Jordan, K.M., 2010. The modern management of gout. Rheumatology 49, 5–14.

Schumacher, H.R., Boice, J.A., Daikh, D.I., et al., 2002. Randomised double blind trial of etoricoxib and indometacin in treatment of acute gouty arthritis. Br. Med. J. 324, 488–492.

Schumacher, H.R., Becker, M.A., Wortmann, R.L., et al., 2008. Effects of febuxostat versus allopurinol and placebo in reducing serum urate in subjects with hyperuricaemia and gout: a 28-week, phase III, randomized, double blind, parallel-group trial. Arthritis Rheum. 59, 1540–1548.

Schumacher, H.R., Becker, M.A., Lloyd, E., et al., 2009. Febuxostat in the treatment of gout; 5-yr findings of the FOCUS efficacy and safety study. Rheumatology 48, 188–194.

Sica, A.D., Schoolwerth, A.C., 2002. Part 1. Uric acid and losartan. Curr. Opin. Nephrol. Hypertens 11, 475–482.

So, A., De Smedt, T., Revas, S., et al., 2007. A pilot study of IL-1 inhibition by anakinra in acute gout. Arthritis Res. Ther. 9, R28.

Takahashi, S., Moriwaki, Y., Yamamoto, T., et al., 2003. Effects of combination treatment using anti-hyperuriaemic agents with fenofibrate and/or losartan on uric acid metabolism. Arthritis Res. Ther. 72, 671–674.

Taniguchi, A., Urano, W., Yamanaka, M., et al., 2005. A common mutation in an organic anion transporter gene SLC22A12, is a suppressing factor for the development of gout. Arthritis Rheum. 52, 2576–2577.

Terkeltaub, R., Furst, D.E., Bennett, K., et al., 2008. Low dose (1.8mg) vs high dose (4.8mg) oral colchicine regimens in patients with acute gout flare in a large, multicentre, randomized, double-blind, placebo controlled, parallel group study. Arthritis Rheum. 58 (Suppl. 9), 1944.

Williamson, P.J., Ene, M.D., Roberts, C.J., 1984. A study of the potential interactions between azapropazone and frusemide in man. Br. J. Clin. Pharmacol. 18, 619–623.

Zhang, W., Doherty, M., Pascual, E., et al., 2006. EULAR evidence based recommendations for gout. Part I: diagnosis. Report of a task force of the EULAR Standing Committee for International Clinical Studies Including Therapeutics (ESCISIT). Ann. Rheum. Dis. 65, 1301–1311, doi 10.1136/ard.2006.055251.

Further reading

Choi, H.K., Mount, D.B., Reginato, A.M., 2005. Pathogenesis of gout. Ann. Int. Med. 143, 499–516.

National Institute for Health and Clinical Excellence, 2008. Febuxostat for the management of hyperuricaemia in people with gout. Technology Appraisal No. 164, NICE, London. Available from http://www.nice.org.uk/nicemedia/live/12101/42738/42738.pdf.

Zhang, W., Doherty, M., Bardin, T., et al., 2006. EULAR evidence based recommendations for gout. Part II: management. Report of a task force of the EULAR Standing Committee for International Clinical Studies Including Therapeutics (ESCISIT). Ann. Rheum. Dis. 65, 1312–1324, doi 10.1136/ard.2006.055269.

Glaucoma 55

L. C. Titcomb and S. D. Andrew

Key points

- Glaucoma is a large group of disorders with widely differing clinical features.
- Chronic open-angle glaucoma (COAG) is a chronic progressive disease of insidious onset.
- The aim of treatment in COAG is to reduce the intraocular pressure (IOP) to a target pressure, specific to the patient, preventing further damage to the nerve fibres and the development of further visual field defects.
- A wide range of drugs is used to treat COAG. Laser treatment or surgery may be undertaken if the target pressure is not attained with medical therapy.
- COAG is a symptomless disease until well advanced. Concordance with therapy is an important issue.
- Acute primary angle-closure glaucoma (PACG) is a medical emergency that must be treated rapidly to prevent blindness.
- The aim of medical treatment in acute PACG is to reduce the IOP in preparation for laser treatment or surgery.
- A wide range of drugs can provoke an attack of PACG in susceptible individuals.

The term 'glaucoma' does not represent a single pathological entity. It consists of a large group of disorders with widely differing clinical features. It is, therefore, difficult to attempt a single definition of the term. High intraocular pressure (IOP) was previously used as a diagnostic criterion for glaucoma, but more recently, it has been recognised purely as the most important risk factor for the disease. This is because glaucoma can occur even in patients with normal IOP (normal-pressure chronic open-angle glaucoma, COAG). The 'normal' IOP (10–21 mmHg) is a statistical description of the range of IOP in the population and is not applicable to an individual subject. It is thought to increase with age, at the rate of approximately 1 mmHg every decade after the age of 40 years in the Western population. There is a circadian cycle of IOP, with maximum levels often occurring between 8 and 11 a.m. and minimum levels between midnight and 2 a.m. This may affect IOP readings taken in outpatient clinics at different times of the day. The normal diurnal variation is between 3 and 5 mmHg, and this is wider in untreated glaucoma. Although a raised IOP is not the only cause of glaucoma, it is the only parameter that can currently be changed by pharmacological intervention and therefore plays an important part in the evaluation of disease progression.

Current thinking is that once the rate of disease progression has been established, a 'target IOP' can be set. The target IOP is defined as a dynamic, clinical judgement about what level of IOP is considered by the healthcare professional treating the patient to be sufficiently low to minimise or arrest disease progression or onset and avoid disability from sight loss within a person's expected lifetime.

It is, however, extremely difficult to accurately assess in advance the IOP level at which further damage will occur for any one patient. As the correct target IOP is only discovered with hindsight, one limitation is that the chosen target IOP may not be low enough and a patient must get worse before it is realised that the target IOP was inadequate. There is no single safe IOP level for all patients, but in general, the aim is to achieve at least a 25–30% reduction from the initial IOP at which damage occurred. In advanced disease, the aim is to achieve an IOP level below 18 mmHg at all times. This can be used as a good method to set an initial target IOP. However, it is essential that the patient receives regular periodic re-evaluation so that the target IOP can be adjusted according to disease progression and treatment adjusted accordingly.

Epidemiology

The World Health Organisation has estimated that globally there are 12.5 million people blind from glaucoma with the total number affected by this condition at around 66 million. Approximately 13% of UK blindness registrations are ascribed to glaucoma, and around 2% of people older than 40 years have COAG, a figure which rises to almost 10% in people older than 75 years. With changes in population demographics, the number of individuals affected by glaucoma is expected to rise. Based on these estimates, there are around 500,000 people affected by COAG in England and Wales, who receive over a million glaucoma-related outpatient visits in the hospital eye service annually. Once diagnosed, affected individuals require lifelong monitoring for disease control and to detect possible progression of visual damage. Once lost, vision cannot be restored. Disease control with prevention or at least minimisation of ongoing damage is therefore paramount to maintain sight.

The diseases which make up the group known as glaucoma are usually classified according to the manner in which aqueous humour outflow is impaired.

Chronic open-angle glaucoma

COAG, also referred to as chronic simple glaucoma, is associated with a relative obstruction to aqueous outflow through the trabecular meshwork and is a chronic progressive disease of insidious onset, usually affecting both eyes. It is frequently an inherited condition, with approximately 10% of first-degree relatives of COAG sufferers eventually developing the disease. Two conditions similar to COAG are normal-tension glaucoma, where the IOP is not raised on initial screening although signs of damage are present, and ocular hypertension (OHT), elevated IOP in the absence of visual field loss or glaucomatous optic nerve damage. It is estimated that 3–5% of those over 40 years have OHT, around one million people in England. OHT represents a major risk for future development of COAG with visual damage. Lowering IOP has been shown to protect against conversion to COAG.

Primary angle-closure glaucoma

Primary angle-closure glaucoma (PACG), or closed-angle glaucoma, is a condition in which closure of the angle by the peripheral iris results in a reduction in aqueous outflow. It occurs in predisposed eyes and is frequently unilateral. There are ethnic variations as the disease affects approximately 1 in 1000 Caucasian adults over the age of 40 years, about 1 in 100 Asians (especially mongoloids) and Hispanics, and 2–4 per 100 Inuits (Eskimos). It occurs in four times as many females as males.

Secondary glaucomas

Secondary glaucomas can arise for a number of reasons, including inflammation, intraocular tumour, raised episcleral venous pressure, or congenitally due to developmental abnormalities.

Aetiology

The factors that determine the level of IOP are the rate of aqueous humour production and the resistance encountered in the outflow channels. A fine balance between these is necessary to keep the pressure within the eye in the range of 16–21 mmHg.

Production of aqueous humour occurs in the ciliary epithelium by two mechanisms: secretion due to an active metabolic process, independent of the level of IOP, and ultrafiltration influenced by the level of blood pressure in the ciliary capillaries and the level of IOP.

Outflow of aqueous humour occurs by two routes. Approximately 80% of total outflow is through the trabecular meshwork into the canal of Schlemm and into the venous circulation via the aqueous veins. The uveoscleral pathway accounts for the remaining 20% through the ciliary body into the suprachoroidal space, to be drained into the ciliary body, choroid and sclera via the venous circulation.

Pathophysiology

The primary site of damage is thought to be the optic nerve head, rather than any other point along the nerve axon. This most easily explains the progressive loss of visual field. Studies of axoplasmic flow show a vulnerability of the nerves to elevated IOP as they pass through the optic disc.

In COAG, increased resistance within the drainage channels causes the rise in IOP. It is thought that the main route of resistance to aqueous outflow lies in the dense juxtacanalicular trabecular meshwork, or the endothelium lining the inner wall of Schlemm's canal.

In PACG, the rise in IOP is caused by a decreased outflow of aqueous humour, due to closure of the chamber angle by the peripheral iris. It occurs in predisposed eyes, and the predisposing factors can be anatomical or physiological. The anatomical characteristics are lens size, corneal diameter and axial length of the globe. The lens continues to grow throughout life. This brings the anterior surface closer to the cornea. Slackening of the suspensory ligaments increases this movement. Both factors occur very gradually and lead to a progressive shallowing of the anterior chamber. The depth of the anterior chamber and width of the chamber angle are related to corneal diameter, and those eyes predisposed to PACG are observed to have a corneal diameter less than that seen in normal eyes. A short eye, which is frequently also hypermetropic, has a small corneal diameter and a thick and relatively anteriorly located lens.

The physiological precipitating factors of PACG in predisposed eyes are not fully understood. Two theories currently exist. The dilator muscle theory suggests that contraction of the dilator muscle causes a posterior movement, which increases the apposition between the iris and anteriorly located lens and the degree of physiological pupillary block. The simultaneous dilation of the pupil renders the peripheral iris more flaccid, and causes the pressure in the posterior chamber to increase and the iris to bow anteriorly. Eventually, the peripheral iris obstructs the angle and the IOP rises (Fig. 55.1).

The sphincter muscle theory postulates that the sphincter of the pupil precipitates angle closure. The pupillary blocking force of the sphincter is greatest when the diameter of the pupil is about 4 mm.

Clinical manifestations

COAG is typically characterised by the following: an IOP greater than 21 mmHg, an open-angle, glaucomatous cupping and visual field loss. COAG, because of its insidious onset, is usually asymptomatic until it has caused a significant loss of visual field. In some eyes, subtle signs of glaucomatous retinal nerve damage can be detected prior to development of pathological cupping and detectable field loss. The earliest clinically significant field defect is a scotoma, which is an area of depressed vision within the visual field. Patients with COAG frequently show a wider swing in IOP than normal; therefore, a single pressure reading of 21 mmHg or less does not exclude

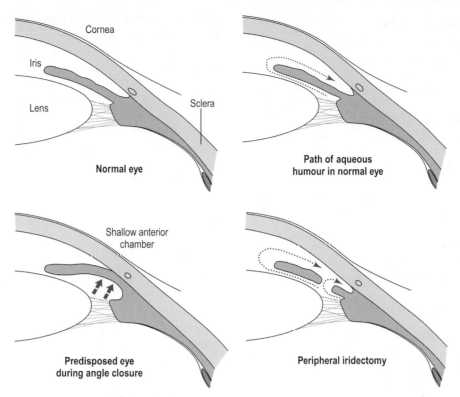

Fig. 55.1 Changes to the eye seen during closed-angle glaucoma.

the diagnosis. It may be necessary to measure IOP at different times of the day, or at periodic intervals.

Acute PACG is due to a sudden closure of the angle and a severe elevation in IOP. The symptoms include rapidly progressive visual impairment, periocular pain and congestion of the eye. In severe cases, nausea and vomiting may occur. The signs include injection of the limbal and conjunctival vessels, giving a 'ciliary flush'. The IOP usually lies between 50 and 80 mmHg and causes corneal oedema with epithelial vesicles. The anterior chamber is shallow and iridocorneal contact can be observed. The pupil is vertically oval and fixed in a semi-dilated position. It is unreactive to light and accommodation. The fellow eye usually has a shallow anterior chamber and a narrow angle. The optic nerve head is oedematous and hyperaemic.

Investigations

IOP may be measured by tonometry, such as indentation tonometry in which a plunger is applied to the cornea and the amount of indentation on the eye reflects the pressure within it. Tonography is a technique used to measure the outflow of aqueous humour from the eye, resulting from indentation of the eye, using a tonometer. Gonioscopy is used to estimate the width of the chamber angle, with the aid of a slit lamp. Perimetry is important for both the diagnosis and management of glaucoma by detecting early scotomata and larger changes in visual field. Other investigations which should be routinely offered to patients include a central corneal thickness measurement (CCT), as this has an effect on the measured IOP and may affect the efficacy of certain drug treatments (Johnson et al., 2008), and fundus examination for optic nerve assessment with dilatation using stereoscopic slit-lamp biomicroscopy. There are also guidelines for the monitoring of these patients and at what intervals their IOP, optic nerve head and visual fields should be checked (National Institute for Health and Clinical Excellence, 2009).

In patients with COAG, cupping of the optic disc becomes progressively apparent and is used in both diagnosis and assessment of the efficacy of treatment. The increased IOP appears to push the optic disc back into an excavation. This is known as glaucomatous cupping.

The colour of the optic disc will be observed to change from a creamy pink colour, due to the rich capillary network seen in the healthy eye, to increased pallor with advancing disease as the optic nerve tissue progressively atrophies.

Treatment

Chronic open-angle glaucomas

The aim of treatment in COAG is to reduce the raised IOP to the target value, preventing further damage to the nerve fibres and the development of further visual field defects to maintain the patient's visual function and quality of life. The key to effective treatment is careful and regular follow-up, including measurement of visual acuity, tonometry, gonioscopy, evaluation of the optic disc, CCT and perimetry, which is of primary importance.

The actual safe level of IOP is unknown, the importance of disc and field assessment being underlined by evidence that IOP does not rise above the 'normal' range in up to 50% of glaucomas (normal-pressure glaucomas). However, in many cases, maximal retardation of the disease process is achieved if the IOP is maintained in the lower teens. The effect on the visual field and the appearance of the optic disc are the only indications that IOP is being controlled at a safe level. A raised IOP without field or disc changes may not require treatment but will need regular review.

The initial treatment of COAG is usually medical. Topical administration is the preferred type of therapy, and there is a wide range of preparations available (Table 55.1). The chosen drug should be administered at its lowest concentration and as infrequently as possible to obtain the desired effect over the whole 24-h period as a high level of diurnal variation in IOP has been shown to be a more important factor in visual field development than the average IOP. A drug with few potential side effects should be chosen, with oral therapy retained as the final option. The prostaglandin analogues latanoprost and travoprost and the prostamide bimatoprost are indicated for first-line use, as are the β-blockers as these produce the greatest fall in IOP (Table 55.2). Carbonic anhydrase inhibitors and sympathomimetics, which result in a smaller fall in IOP, are reserved for patients unresponsive to first-line drugs, in patients in whom the first-line agents are contraindicated or as adjunctive therapy.

In most cases, the initial topical treatment is with a prostaglandin analogue or prostamide. If this is ineffective, another prostaglandin or prostamide may be substituted or a β-blocker used instead. Patients not reaching their target pressure on one first-line agent may be prescribed another concomitantly. Alternatively, a carbonic anhydrase inhibitor or a sympathomimetic may be added to one of the first-line drugs. Guidance on the treatment of people with OHT or suspected COAG has been published (National Institute for Health and Clinical Excellence, 2009). The treatment options (Table 55.3) take into account central corneal thickness and age, although age thresholds are only appropriate where vision is normal (OHT with or without suspected COAG) and the treatment is purely preventative. Pilocarpine is no longer recommended by NICE but is recommended as a second-line agent in European guidelines (European Glaucoma Society, 2008). Oral therapy with carbonic anhydrase inhibitors is usually reserved for use as the final stage of treatment in those complex glaucomas awaiting surgery (Fig. 55.2).

It has been proposed that the improved control of IOP with newer therapies has led to a reduction in surgery for glaucoma (Kenigsberg, 2007). However, some patients still require surgical intervention to reach their target pressure.

The most frequently performed surgical procedures create a fistula to act as a new route for aqueous outflow and the

Table 55.1 Drugs used in the treatment of chronic open-angle glaucoma

Therapeutic category	Primary mechanism
Topical prostaglandins	Increase aqueous outflow
Topical prostamides	Increase aqueous outflow
Topical β-blocking agents	Decrease aqueous formation
Topical miotics	Increase aqueous outflow
Topical adrenergic agonists	Increase aqueous outflow and decrease aqueous formation
Topical carbonic anhydrase inhibitors	Decrease aqueous formation
Oral carbonic anhydrase inhibitors	Decrease aqueous formation

Table 55.2 Comparison of reduction in intraocular pressure (IOP) with a range of ocular hypotensive drugs (adapted from van der Valk et al., 2009)

Drug	Relative IOP change from baseline at trough (%) (95% CI)	Relative IOP change from baseline at peak (%) (95% CI)
Bimatoprost	−28 (−29 to −27)	−33 (−35 to −31)
Travoprost	−29 (−32 to −25)	−31 (−32 to −29)
Latanoprost	−28 (−30 to −26)	−31 (−33 to −29)
Timolol	−26 (−28 to −25)	−27 (−29 to −25)
Betaxolol	−20 (−23 to −17)	−23 (−25 to −22)
Dorzolamide	−17 (−19 to −15)	−22 (−24 to −20)
Brinzolamide	−17 (−19 to −15)	−17 (−19 to −15)
Brimonidine	−18 (−21 to −14)	−25 (−28 to −22)
Placebo	−5 (−9 to −1)	−5 (−10 to 0)

Table 55.3 Treatment of people with ocular hypertension or suspected COAG (National Institute for Health and Clinical Excellence, 2009)

Central corneal thickness	More than 590 μm		555–590 μm		Less than 555 μm		
Untreated IOP (mmHg)	>21 to 25	>25 to 32	>21 to 25	>25 to 32	>21 to 25	>25 to 32	>32
Age (years)	Any	Any	Any	Treat until 60	Treat until 65	Treat until 80	Any
Treatment	No treatment	No treatment	No treatment	β-blocker	Prostaglandin analogue	Prostaglandin analogue	Prostaglandin analogue

most frequently performed surgery of this type, trabeculectomy, appears more effective in controlling IOP than laser trabeculoplasty, in which a series of laser burns is applied to the trabecular meshwork to improve the outflow of aqueous humour. (Rolim de Moura et al., 2007).

Primary angle-closure glaucoma

The medical management of acute PACG is essentially to prepare the eye for surgical treatment. The aim of treatment is to decrease the IOP and associated inflammation. Analgesics and antiemetics are sometimes needed, dependent on symptom severity, to make the patient comfortable. It is usual to treat the unaffected eye prophylactically with miotics (Fig. 55.3).

Paralysis of the iris sphincter usually occurs at an IOP of more than 60 mmHg, due to ischaemia. Therefore, intensive miotic therapy, previously the treatment of choice in many cases of PACG, is usually ineffective and the IOP needs to be lowered by drugs that reduce aqueous humour production rather than by trying to pull the peripheral iris away from the angle with miotics. An intravenous loading dose of mannitol is usually the first drug of choice with intravenous acetazolamide a possible alternative. This is followed by oral treatment, sometimes in combination with corneal indentation, to physically force aqueous humour into the peripheral anterior chamber and artificially open the angle. This should allow the IOP to drop sufficiently to relieve iris ischaemia and allow the sphincter to respond to pilocarpine therapy.

Once the IOP has been reduced medically, the condition is treated surgically, by either surgical peripheral iridectomy or laser iridotomy, to remove an area of the peripheral iris to allow flow of aqueous humour through an alternative pathway (see Fig. 55.1). Filtration surgery is indicated if a large proportion of the angle has been permanently closed by adhesions between the iris and the cornea.

Drug treatment

Ocular prostanoids: prostaglandin analogues and prostamides

The National Institute for Health and Clinical Excellence (2009) guideline does not differentiate between the prostaglandin analogues and the prostamide bimatoprost, but recommends one of this class for the treatment of COAG, certain patients with OHT and certain COAG suspects (see Table 55.4)

The prostaglandin analogues, latanoprost, travoprost and tafluprost, are ester compounds thought to achieve a fall in IOP primarily by increasing the uveoscleral outflow with no significant effect on other parameters of aqueous humour dynamics, while the prostamide bimatoprost is thought to increase outflow through both trabecular and uveoscleral outflow pathways. However, there is still debate about the precise mechanisms of action of this group (Lim et al., 2008; Toris et al., 2008).

All the drugs in this class are licensed for the reduction of elevated IOP in open-angle glaucoma and OHT, and are administered once daily in the evening.

In a meta-analysis, these drugs have been shown to have a greater effect on both peak and trough readings of IOP than timolol, betaxolol, dorzolamide, brinzolamide or brimonidine, producing falls in IOP of 28–29% at trough and 31–33% at peak as shown in Table 55.2 (van der Valk et al., 2009).

Randomised head-to-head evaluations of prostaglandin therapy demonstrate similar efficacy, but differing hyperemia effects with bimatoprost and travoprost causing more hyperaemia than latanoprost (Eyawo et al., 2009; Honrubia et al., 2009). However, these studies were conducted before the introduction of the new formulations of bimatoprost 0.01% and the benzalkonium chloride–free travoprost.

The prostanoids have some interesting local side effects (Table 55.5). Pigmentation of the iris occurs in patients with mixed colour (green-brown or blue-brown) irides after 3–6 months of use and is a result of increased deposition of melanin in the melanocytes. An increase in the length and thickness of the eyelashes and pigmentation of the palpebral skin are also known side effects. Use of these drugs may lead to disruption of the blood–aqueous barrier in patients with aphakia and pseudophakia (no or false lens, respectively) and increase the risk of developing cystoid macular oedema; they should be used with caution in such patients. Reactivation of herpes simplex infection has been reported with bimatoprost, travoprost and latanoprost.

Latanoprost

Latanoprost, which is converted to its active free acid on entering the eye, was the first of the prostanoids to be launched and is the market leader. Like timolol amongst the

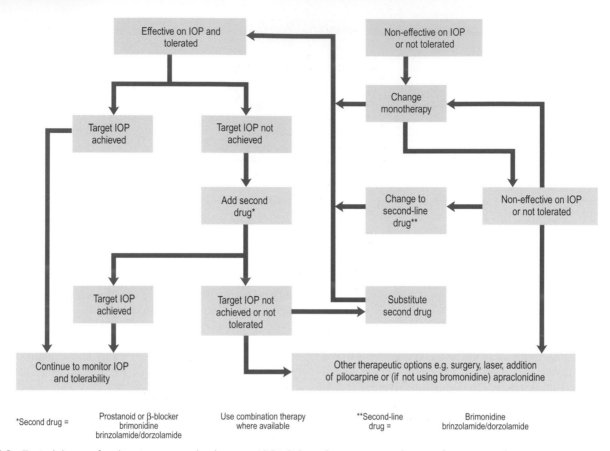

Fig. 55.2 Topical therapy for chronic open-angle glaucoma (COAG) based on recommendations of European Glaucoma Society (2008).

β-blockers, latanoprost is the drug in this class against which new drugs or combinations are assessed. It must be administered in the evening for maximum effect (Stewart et al., 2008). Latanoprost is generally very well tolerated. Serious adverse drug reactions were reported in only 17/3936 (0.43%) patients using latanoprost over a 5-year period (Goldberg et al., 2008), and patient persistence with latanoprost therapy is better than that with all other frequently used monotherapies (Rahman et al., 2009). Latanoprost is not heat stable and requires refrigeration; however, it is stable enough to be stored at room temperature for the 4-week in-use period applied in the UK. The concentration of the preservative benzalkonium chloride in latanoprost eye drops and bimatoprost 0.01% may prevent their use in certain patients. The benzalkonium chloride concentration in these formulations is 0.02%, which is four times that in bimatoprost 0.03% eye drops. The current formulation of travoprost, launched in January 2011, contains polyquaternium-1 rather than benzalkonium chloride.

Travoprost

Like latanoprost, travoprost is an ester pro-drug, converted to its active acid form by corneal hydrolytic enzymes as it is absorbed through the eye. Travoprost acid is a potent full agonist for prostaglandin $F_{2\alpha}$-receptors, producing 100% efficacy, whereas the comparable efficacy for latanoprost is 92%. It is highly selective, with no significant activity at non-prostanoid receptors and low affinity for the other prostanoid receptors responsible for pain, etc. It appears to be generally well tolerated by patients and is relatively free of systemic side effects, although abdominal cramp has been reported.

Patients treated with travoprost show good diurnal fluctuation control, and an ocular hypotensive effect was shown to last for over 3 days. Patients previously treated with β-blockers, α_2-agonists, carbonic anhydrase inhibitors, latanoprost and the dorzolamide-timolol fixed combination respond to travoprost. Administration time is not as important with travoprost as with latanoprost as no statistical difference was noted in the percentage fall in IOP whether travoprost was administered in the morning or in the evening (Stewart et al., 2008). Travoprost is a stable compound throughout a range of temperatures, and the commercially available product does not require refrigeration.

Tafluprost

Tafluprost is the first of the prostanoids available in a preservative-free form. In terms of efficacy and safety, it has been shown to be equivalent to a preserved preparation of tafluprost (Hamacher et al., 2008) and useful in patients allergic to, or intolerant of, benzalkonium chloride.

Tafluprost as adjunctive therapy to timolol results in consistently greater reductions in IOP compared with vehicle in patients with glaucoma or OHT that is inadequately controlled with timolol monotherapy (Egorov and Ropo, 2009).

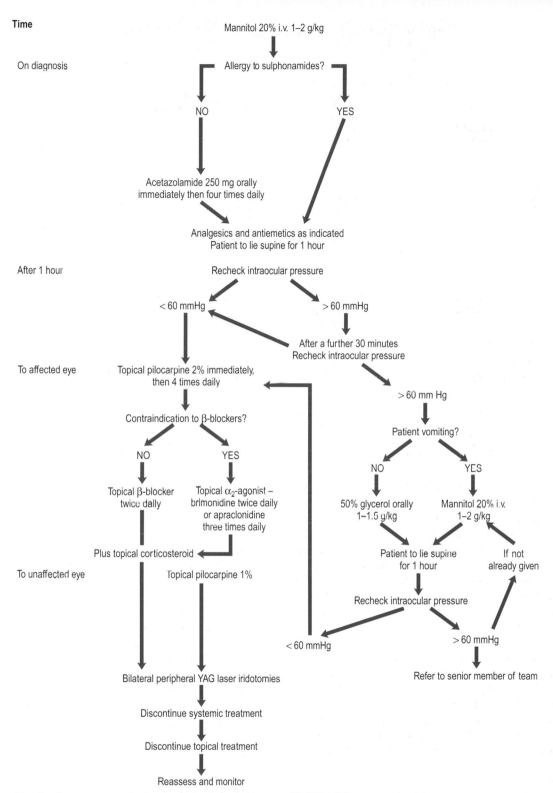

Fig. 55.3 Algorithm for the treatment of primary angle-closure glaucoma (PACG). YAG, yttrium aluminium garnet.

Bimatoprost

Bimatoprost is a fatty acid amide, pharmacologically similar to prostaglandin $F_{2\alpha}$1-ethanolamide (prostamide $F_{2\alpha}$).

Several mechanisms of action have been proposed including activity of bimatoprost or its free acid, 17-phenyl PGF_{2a}, at the prostaglandin $F_{2\alpha}$ receptor, prostamide mimetic activity, and inhibition of PGF synthase which leads to an increase in endogenous $PGF_{2\alpha}$. Although the free acid has been found in human eyes, its presence alone does not explain the 24-h efficacy of bimatoprost or its hypotensive superiority over

Table 55.4 Ocular prostanoids

	Bimatoprost		Latanoprost	Tafluprost	Travoprost
Trade name	Lumigan		Xalatan	Saflutan	Travatan
Pharmacological class	Prostamide		Prostaglandin analogue	Prostaglandin analogue	Prostaglandin analogue
Strength	0.03%	0.01%	0.005%	0.0015%	0.004%
Preservative	Benzalkonium chloride 0.005%	Benzalkonium chloride 0.02%	Benzalkonium chloride 0.02%	None	Polyquaternium-1 0.001%
Storage requirements	≤25 °C	≤25 °C	2–8 °C until opened then ≤25 °C for period of use of 4 weeks	2–8 °C	≤25 °C

latanoprost. The pharmacology of bimatoprost itself is not explained wholly by its interaction with known prostaglandin $F_{2\alpha}$ receptors. It is administered once daily in the evening; more frequent administration may lessen the IOP-lowering effect.

Bimatoprost lowers the IOP to a greater extent than any other topical ocular hypotensive (van der Valk et al., 2009), an effect (see Table 55.2) which is sustained for at least 4 years (Williams et al., 2008). It is superior to latanoprost in terms of response rate, fall in IOP and the percentage of patients reaching their target IOP. In some studies, bimatoprost is reported to be as effective as the fixed combination of latanoprost and timolol. Many patients are non-responsive to latanoprost as they do not achieve a fall in IOP greater than 10%, although a large proportion of patients show a 20% or more fall in IOP with bimatoprost. Patients not reaching their target on latanoprost achieved lower IOPs when switched to bimatoprost (Sonty et al., 2008). Such patients achieve better diurnal control with bimatoprost than with a fixed combination of dorzolamide and timolol (Sharpe et al., 2008).

Generally, bimatoprost causes similar ocular side effects to latanoprost and travoprost, but while all the ocular prostanoids cause subclinical ocular inflammation, bimatoprost and travoprost cause this to a lesser degree than latanoprost. However, bimatoprost causes hyperaemia more frequently than latanoprost, although this is described as mild. This may contribute to the higher discontinuation rate seen with bimatoprost therapy (Rahman et al., 2009). To address this issue, the manufacturers of bimatoprost have introduced a lower strength (0.01%) version containing a higher concentration of benzalkonium chloride to aid penetration of the drug. In a 12-month study, the bimatoprost 0.01% was equivalent to bimatoprost 0.03% in lowering IOP and demonstrated improved tolerability, including less frequent and severe conjunctival hyperemia (Katz et al., 2010).

β-Adrenoceptor antagonists

The exact mechanism of action of β-adrenoceptor antagonists (β-blockers) in lowering IOP has not been fully established but is thought to result from the blockade of ciliary β-receptors, preventing the cyclic AMP-induced rise in aqueous secretion, as they have been shown to reduce aqueous humour formation rather than increase outflow. Although there are both β_1- and β_2-receptors in the eye, the latter predominate and even cardioselective β-blockers are thought to work by blockade of β_2-receptors. Genetic factors have been shown to be important in patients' response to this group of drugs (Nieminen et al., 2007, Sidjanin et al., 2008).

Four drugs are available in the UK for topical administration: betaxolol, carteolol, levobunolol and timolol (Table 55.6). β-Blockers have a number of important properties in addition to β-adrenoceptor blockade. These include intrinsic sympathomimetic activity (ISA), cardioselectivity and membrane-stabilising activity, which are all of importance when considering the side effects seen with these agents (Table 55.7). The property of membrane stabilisation is relevant to the incidence of ocular side effects. The absence of anaesthetic properties reduces the number and severity of foreign body and dryness sensations, anaesthesia of the cornea and dry eye syndrome.

Ocular side effects of topically administered β-blockers are shown in Table 55.8.

It has been suggested that those β-blockers that show ISA are less likely to produce bronchospasm and peripheral vascular side effects. Carteolol is the only commercially available drug that shows ISA. The selectivity of cardioselective β-blockers diminishes with increasing dosage, even within the therapeutic range. Betaxolol is the only commercially available topical β-blocker that demonstrates cardioselectivity.

A degree of bradycardia is commonly seen with all β-blockers, and β-blocker eye drops have been identified as the cause of episodes of orthostatic hypotension and syncope in elderly patients (Müller et al., 2006). The use of topical β-blockers in patients on verapamil, diltiazem, disopyramide, quinidine or amiodarone could potentiate bradycardia and should be avoided. Topical β-blockers are generally avoided in patients with normal-tension glaucoma because the nocturnal fall in arterial pressure causes a potentially dangerous reduction in ocular perfusion.

The precipitation of bronchospasm in susceptible patients can occur with the administration of as little as one drop of timolol. Those β-blockers that show cardioselectivity or

Table 55.5 Side effects of prostanoids

Ocular	Systemic
Asthenopia	Abdominal cramp
Allergic conjunctivitis	Asthenia
Blepharitis	Asthma
Blepharospasm	Bradycardia
Browache	Dizziness
Cataract	Dyspnoea
Conjunctival follicles, papillae	Elevated liver function
Conjunctival hyperaemia	Headache
Cystoid macular oedema	Hirsutism
Corneal erosion	Hypertension
Conjunctival oedema	Hypotension
Deepening of lid sulcus	Infection (primarily URTIs)
Distichiasis	Peripheral oedema
Eye discharge	Skin rash
Eye pain	
Eyelash changes – increased number, length, thickness, pigmentation, misdirection, poliosis	
Eyelid oedema, eyelid retraction	
Eyelid and periocular skin darkening	
Foreign body sensation	
Increase in vellus hair on eyelids	
Increased iris pigmentation	
Iritis	
Lid margin crusting	
Localised skin reactions on the eyelids	
Ocular burning, dryness, irritation pruritus, fatigue	
Photophobia	
Punctate epithelial erosions	
Retinal haemorrhage	
Tearing	
Uveitis	
Visual disturbance	

URTIs, upper respiratory tract infection

Table 55.6 Ophthalmic β-blockers

Drug	Brand name	Strength (%)	Daily dosage frequency
Betaxolol	Betoptic® solution	0.5	2
	Betoptic® suspension[a]	0.25	2
Carteolol	Teoptic®	1	2
		2	2
Levobunolol	Betagan®[a] and generic form	0.5	1–2
Timolol	Timoptol®[a] and generic form	0.25	2
		0.5	2
	Timoptol-LA®	0.25	1
		0.5	1
	Nyogel®	0.1	1
	Cosopt®[a] (with dorzolamide 2%)	0.5	2
	Xalacom® (with latanoprost 0.005%)	0.5	1
	DuoTrav® (with travoprost 0.004%)	0.5	1
	Ganfort® (with bimatoprost 0.03%)	0.5	1
	Combigan® (with brimonidine 0.2%)	0.5	2
	Azarga® (with brinzolamide 1%)	0.5	2

[a]Available in unit dose and multidose forms.

Table 55.7 Pharmacological profile of ophthalmic β-blockers

	β-blocking potency[a]	ISA	Cardioselectivity	Membrane-stabilising activity
Betaxolol	3–10	–	++	+
Carteolol	30	++	–	–
Levobunolol	6	–	–	–
Timolol	5–10	–	–	+

ISA, intrinsic sympathomimetic activity.
[a]Propranolol = 1

ISA are less likely to cause bronchoconstriction, and it has been demonstrated that respiratory function improved in patients whose treatment was changed from timolol to betaxolol or an adrenergic agonist, these same patients having previously been asymptomatic.

All topical β-blockers have been reported to cause bronchospasm; hence, 'at-risk' patients with a tendency to airway disease who require therapy for glaucoma should be treated with

Table 55.8 Ocular and systemic side effects of topical β-blockers

Ocular	Systemic
Allergic blepharoconjunctivitis	*Central nervous system*
Burning and itching	Anxiety
Blurred vision	Depression
Conjunctival hyperaemia	Fatigue
Corneal anaesthesia	Hallucinations
Dryness	Irritability
Foreign body sensation	Sleep disturbances
Macular oedema	*Endocrine*
Nasolacrimal duct obstruction	Hypoglycaemia (insulin induced)
Pain	*Gastro-intestinal*
Punctate keratitis	Nausea
Uveitis	Diarrhoea
	Vascular
	Arrhythmias
	Bradycardia
	Hypotension
	Peripheral vasoconstriction
	Reduced stroke volume
	Respiratory
	Bronchoconstriction
	Dyspnoea

extreme caution. Prescribers are advised that β-blockers, even those with apparent cardioselectivity, should not be used in patients with asthma or a history of obstructive airways disease unless no alternative treatment is available. In such cases, the risk of inducing bronchospasm should be appreciated and appropriate precautions taken. Lacrimal occlusion with intracanalicular plugs has been shown to almost completely prevent the bronchoconstriction caused by topical timolol in asthmatics by inhibiting or decreasing systemic absorption of the medication.

Ocular β-blockers are generally not contraindicated in diabetes, although a cardioselective agent may be preferable. However, they are best avoided in patients who suffer frequent hypoglycaemic attacks as they may mask the signs and symptoms of acute hypoglycaemia.

Systemic side effects of topically administered β-blockers are shown in Table 55.8.

The long-term benefits of β-blockers on visual function preservation have been shown to be less than would be expected. This may be due to adverse effects on the ocular microcirculation whereby the β-blockers interfere with endogenous vasodilation and cause optic nerve head arteriolar vasoconstriction. The various β-blockers demonstrate marked differences in their vasoconstrictive effect, with betaxolol possibly demonstrating the least vasoconstriction.

Betaxolol

In theory, because of its cardioselectivity, betaxolol should have fewer adverse effects on the pulmonary system. It should also have fewer adverse cardiovascular effects because of comparatively lower systemic β-receptor occupancy after ocular administration. Maximum occupancies for β_1 and β_2 receptors after ophthalmic administration were 52% and 88% for carteolol, 62% and 82% for timolol, and 44% and 3% for betaxolol, respectively. The lack of systemic effects of betaxolol compared with timolol has been highlighted by Easton who reported the case of an 85-year-old lady who developed atrial fibrillation on having her β-blocker eye drops changed from timolol to betaxolol (Easton, 2007)

However, betaxolol is less effective than other β-blockers as an ocular hypotensive agent (van der Valk, 2009). On initiation of treatment, the fall in IOP is slower than with other topical β-blockers. The 0.25% suspension is as effective as the 0.5% solution and is better tolerated by the patient (Yalvac et al., 2007). Experimental studies showed the drug reaches the retina after topical administration and displays a voltage-dependent L-type calcium channel-blocking activity, which probably leads to improved retinal perfusion. This effect may explain the significant improvement in visual field performance seen with betaxolol in a comparison study with timolol in open-angle glaucoma. The significant improvement with betaxolol occurred despite the more effective reductions in IOP with timolol.

Carteolol

It has been suggested that because of the ISA of carteolol, attributable to its metabolite 8-hydroxycarteolol found in the plasma, smaller changes are seen in pulmonary and cardiovascular parameters than are seen with the non-cardioselective β-blockers without ISA. Carteolol appears to be neutral in its effect on serum lipid levels, whereas timolol adversely affects high-density lipoprotein cholesterol (HDL-C) and the total cholesterol/HDL-C ratio. Carteolol is generally well tolerated and has been shown to be as effective as timolol at lowering IOP in the majority of patients. It has a greater vasodilator effect on the retinal and choroidal vasculature than timolol and levobunolol but less than that of betaxolol. It is the least lipophilic of the topical β-blockers and consequently is likely to show a lower incidence of central nervous system side effects.

Levobunolol

Levobunolol is the potent L-isomer of bunolol. It is metabolised to dihydrolevobunolol in the eye, prolonging the drug's half-life and making it one of only two topical β-blockers licensed for once-daily use. It is as effective with once-daily dosing as the usual twice-daily regimen. It is not cardioselective, showing greater affinity for the β_2-receptor, and does not possess ISA. It is reported to be as effective as timolol 0.5% and metipranolol 0.6% (now discontinued) in lowering IOP and more effective than betaxolol 0.5%. The incidence of allergic contact dermatitis is greater with levobunolol than timolol (Jappe et al., 2006), and a greater percentage of patients on levobunolol than timolol or betaxolol discontinued the drug due to adverse effects (Rahman et al., 2009). Its effect on tear volume and corneal epithelial barrier function is similar to that produced by timolol, and it has less effect on non-invasive break-up time of the precorneal tear film. This may be attributable to its formulation which includes polyvinyl alcohol. Levobunolol appears to have no effect on the retinal and choroidal vasculature.

Timolol

This non-cardioselective β-blocker without ISA was the first to be introduced, and as such is the agent against which all newer β-blockers were compared. It is effective in the long-term treatment of glaucoma, often in conjunction with other antiglaucoma therapy in terms of IOP lowering. Many patients can be placed on once-a-day therapy provided the IOP is maintained at satisfactory levels. However, the presentation of timolol in a prolonged-release formulation (a polysaccharide-based, gel-forming solution) leads to a prolonged corneal contact time and increased penetration of timolol into the eye. This is the preferred form for once-daily administration. Both timolol eye gels, 0.1% and 0.5%, have been shown to be as effective as the 0.5% solution administered twice daily. The 0.1% gel has the advantage of a much lower drug load, giving rise to plasma levels of timolol 10 times lower than achieved after twice-daily dosage of timolol 0.5% eye drops. The concentration of timolol achieved in the aqueous humour following administration of the 0.1% gel formulation, despite being approximately 40% of that following administration of the 0.5% solution is sufficient to occupy 100% of β_1- and β_2-receptors (Volotinen et al., 2009). Timolol is available in combination products with the carbonic anhydrase inhibitors brinzolamide and dorzolamide, the prostaglandin analogues latanoprost and travaprost, the prostamide bimatoprost and the sympathomimetic brimonidine (see Table 55.6).

Sympathomimetic agents

The original sympathomimetic drug used in the treatment of OHT and open-angle glaucoma, adrenaline (epinephrine) and its lipophilic pro-drug dipivefrine have been discontinued. Adrenaline (epinephrine) is an α- and β-adrenoreceptor agonist. It decreases IOP by reducing aqueous inflow via an α-mediated vasoconstriction in the ciliary body and increased outflow due to a dilation of the aqueous and episcleral veins. Adrenaline (epinephrine) is a mydriatic and therefore its use is contraindicated in PACG and in patients who show a shallow anterior chamber, because of the risk of precipitating angle closure. More selective sympathomimetics apraclonidine and brimonidine are in use today.

Apraclonidine

Apraclonidine (a derivative of clonidine) was the first of the selective adrenergic agonists to be introduced. This drug, which acts predominantly on α_2 but also on α_1-receptors, reduces the rate at which aqueous humour is produced due to ciliary vasoconstriction. Eye drops containing apraclonidine 1% are used to control or prevent postsurgical elevation of IOP following anterior segment laser surgery.

Eye drops containing a 0.5% solution are licensed for the short-term adjunctive treatment of patients on maximally tolerated medical therapy who require additional IOP reduction to delay laser treatment or glaucoma surgery, but the benefit for most patients is less than 1 month. Apraclonidine 0.5% is as effective in lowering IOP as brimonidine 0.2%, but has less effect on blood pressure and heart rate. Although an off-licence use, apraclonidine is sometimes used in children in whom brimonidine is strictly contraindicated (Wright and Freedman, 2009).

Ocular and systemic side effects of α_2-agonists are shown in Table 55.9.

Brimonidine

More α_2-selectivity is seen with brimonidine, which results in miosis rather than mydriasis. Vasoconstriction of microvessels is also not seen. It is thought to increase uveoscleral outflow as well as reducing aqueous production. Brimonidine administered twice daily is almost as effective as timolol twice a day at peak. However, bromonidine is significantly less effective at trough, and some consider it to be more efficacious when administered three times a day, the frequency used in the USA. Brimonidine may be used as monotherapy to lower IOP in patients with open-angle glaucoma or OHT who are intolerant of β-blockers or in whom β-blockers are contraindicated, as there is no effect on pulmonary function

Table 55.9 Ocular and systemic side effects of topical α_2-agonists

Ocular	Systemic
Ocular pruritus	Dry mouth/nose
Discomfort	Headache
Tearing	Asthenia
Hyperaemia	Bradycardia
Conjunctival and lid oedema	Depression
Lid retraction, conjunctival blanching and mydriasis (reported after perioperative use of apraclonidine)	
Miosis (reported with brimonidine)	
Uveitis	

and only minimal cardiovascular effect. It may also be used as an adjunctive therapy in those patients whose IOP is not adequately controlled with a single agent as its IOP-lowering activity has been shown to be additive to that of β-blockers and prostaglandin analogues.

A database containing details of drug use in 956 glaucoma patients over 18 years shows that brimonidine had the highest proportion of discontinuations due to adverse effects (Rahman et al., 2009). It has high allergenicity and may increase the likelihood of allergy to preparations subsequently used.

A formulation of brimonidine, brimonidine-Purite 0.15%, given twice daily, has been shown to be as effective as brimonidine 0.2% twice a day. It has a more favourable safety and tolerability profile, a reduced incidence of allergic conjunctivitis and better patient satisfaction and comfort rating. In a 4-month study, co-administration of latanoprost and brimonidine 0.15% results in a greater fall in IOP than co-administration of latanoprost and brinzolamide or dorzolamide (Bournias and Lai, 2009). This product is not available in the UK.

Brimonidine is contraindicated in patients receiving monoamine oxidase inhibitors or antidepressants which affect noradrenergic transmission, and there is the possibility of brimonidine potentiating or causing an additive effect with CNS depressants. Its use is contraindicated in children in whom it causes drowsiness, ataxia, pallor, irritability, hypotension, bradycardia, miosis and respiratory depression (Lai Becker et al., 2009).

Experimental evidence in animals has demonstrated that brimonidine is a potential neuroprotective agent. However, to date, clinical trials have failed to translate into similar efficacy in humans (Saylor et al., 2009).

Commercially available preparations of sympathomimetic agents are shown in Table 55.10.

Miotics

Miotics act to increase the outflow of aqueous humour by a stimulation of ciliary muscle and an opening of channels in the trabecular meshwork. Miotics are directly acting parasympathomimetic agents that act at muscarinic receptors. The only such drug currently available commercially in the UK is pilocarpine.

Miosis is an unwanted incidental effect and can cause considerable difficulties to patients. Reduced visual acuity, especially in the presence of central lens opacities, spasm of accommodation, accompanied by severe frontal headache (browache) and diminished night vision may cause poor adherence in many patients.

Ocular side effects of pilocarpine are shown in Box 55.1. In eyes with narrow angles, PACG may be precipitated by an aggravation of pupillary block. Systemic side effects are due to parasympathetic stimulation and include anxiety, bradycardia, diarrhoea, nausea, vomiting and sweating (Box 55.2).

The onset of action of pilocarpine is 20 min, but its short duration of action necessitates four times daily dosing. The frequency of instillation of pilocarpine eye drops is a major disadvantage, and advances have been made to reduce the inconvenience of a four-times-daily dosage regimen. A slow-release gel preparation, Pilogel (Table 55.11), has been introduced. A single daily application, administered at bedtime, allows low IOP to be maintained for 24 h, with the patient sleeping through the more troublesome ocular side effects.

Box 55.1 Ocular side effects of topical pilocarpine
Allergic conjunctivitis
Blurred vision
Ciliary/conjunctival injection
Ciliary spasm
Induced myopia
Lens changes (chronic use)
Lid twitching
Pain
Pigment epithelial cells
Poor night vision
Posterior synechiae
Pupillary block
Retinal tear/detachments
Uveitis
Vitreous haemorrhage

Box 55.2 Systemic side effects of topical pilocarpine
Bradycardia
Bronchial spasm
Browache, headache
Diarrhoea
Hypotension
Lacrimation
Nausea and vomiting
Pulmonary oedema
Salivation
Sweating

Table 55.10 Available ocular products containing sympathomimetic agents

Drug	Trade name	Strength	Daily dosage frequency
Apraclonidine	Iopidine®	1%	1 h prior to surgery and on completion
	Iopidine®	0.5%	3
Brimonidine	Alphagan®	0.2%	2

Table 55.11 Commercially available forms of pilocarpine

Drug	Trade name	Strength	Daily dosage frequency
Pilocarpine	Generic presentation	0.5–4%	4
	Minims®	2%	4
	Pilogel®	4%	1

Carbonic anhydrase inhibitors

There are many forms of the enzyme carbonic anhydrase, three of which (CA-I, CA-II and CA-IV) are present in ocular tissues. In the ciliary epithelium, the inhibition of CA-II slows the formation of bicarbonate ions and their secretion into the posterior chamber of the eye. This reduces the sodium transport into the posterior chamber and decreases aqueous humour production, resulting in lower IOP. Inhibition of other forms of the enzyme results in many side effects.

Acetazolamide

This is the only systemic carbonic anhydrase inhibitor available in the UK. Although it is amongst the most potent ocular hypotensive agents available, it has limited use in the long-term management of glaucoma due to poor patient adherence following occurrence of side effects. The systemic side effects are shown in Box 55.3.

Paraesthesia occurs in almost all patients on commencement of therapy but usually disappears on continued therapy. The malaise complex can include fatigue, depression, weight loss and decreased libido.

Acetazolamide is also available in injection form, and given either intramuscularly or, preferably, intravenously. It is useful in the preoperative/emergency treatment of closed-angle glaucoma.

Topical carbonic anhydrase inhibitors

The topical carbonic anhydrase inhibitors dorzolamide and brinzolamide are useful alternatives to acetazolamide in glaucoma management. They are licensed as monotherapy for patients with OHT or open-angle glaucoma resistant to β-blockers or those in whom use of β-blockers is contra-indicated. Dorzolamide is also licensed for the treatment of pseudo-exfoliative glaucoma, and limited clinical data in paediatric patients are available. Both drugs are licensed as adjunctive therapy to β-blockers and brinzolamide to prostaglandin analogues, although there is evidence to suggest that dorzolamide is as efficacious as brinzolamide when added to latanoprost (Nakamura et al., 2009).

Table 55.12 Side effects of topical carbonic anhydrase inhibitors

Ocular	Systemic
Blurred vision	Dry mouth
Burning/stinging	Dyspnoea
Conjunctivitis	Headache
Eyelid pain/discomfort	Nausea
Fatigue	Taste perversion
Itching	
Nasolacrimal duct obstruction	
Ocular discharge	
Tearing	

Dorzolamide is used either alone three times a day or concurrently with a β-blocker or twice daily with a prostaglandin analogue. While the licence for brinzolamide states that the drug can be used twice a day as monotherapy, some patients may respond better to a three times daily dosage. Mean changes in IOP with brinzolamide administered twice daily and three times daily and dorzolamide administered three times daily are equivalent. However, the fall in IOP achieved with these agents is less than that seen with timolol 0.5% twice daily.

Side effects similar to those of systemic sulphonamides may occur and should be watched for. The most common side effects are shown in Table 55.12. Of the two topical carbonic anhydrase inhibitors, brinzolamide appears to cause less burning and stinging on instillation due to the neutral pH (7.5) of the formulation. This is reflected in a much greater discontinuation rate with dorzolamide (31%) than with brinzolamide (14%) (Rahman et al., 2009).

Animal studies suggested that both topical carbonic anhydrase inhibitors may improve ocular blood flow independent of the IOP; however, while this has been well established for dorzolamide in humans, data for brinzolamide are limited. It remains to be established whether this effect can help reduce visual field loss in patients with glaucoma.

Combination products

A large number of patients require more than one medication to achieve target pressure. A need for the patient to use two products concomitantly may lead to confusion, with multiple instillation of one product and non-use of the other. Also, if the second drop is instilled too soon after the first, wash-out of the first product with the second drop, overflow of the precorneal tear film and a dilution of both products may occur. In addition, the patient receives a larger dose of preservative which can irritate the eye and

Box 55.3 Side effects of systemic carbonic anhydrase inhibitors

Acidosis
Diarrhoea
Drowsiness
Elevated uric acid
Hypokalaemia
Nausea/vomiting
Malaise complex
Paraesthesia
Sulphonamide crystalluria
Sulphonamide sensitivity
Transient myopia

is a common reason for non-tolerance of the regimen. The combination of two drugs in one topical ophthalmic preparation may improve adherence and result in a reduction in preservative load. Single rather than multi-drop combinations are recommended to improve adherence and maintain patients' quality of life.

For a combination of two drugs to be an acceptable alternative to the prescriber, the fixed combination must be more effective than either of the components used alone and at least as effective as the drugs administered separately, that is not demonstrate antagonism. In addition, adverse effects of the fixed combination must not be more numerous or more frequently encountered than with the components administered separately. There are six products in which timolol is combined with a second ocular hypotensive agent. They differ slightly in their therapeutic indications.

Fixed combination of timolol and dorzolamide

A combination of timolol 0.5% and dorzolamide 2% (Cosopt®) was the first topical ocular hypotensive combination to be marketed. It is indicated in the treatment of elevated IOP in patients with open-angle glaucoma or pseudoexfoliative glaucoma when topical β-blocker monotherapy is not sufficient. The fixed combination of dorzolamide and timolol is more effective than either timolol or dorzolamide alone, and as effective as its two components administered separately. In a review of its efficacy compared with other ocular hypotensives, an 80% response rate was reported for the fixed combination of dorzolamide and timolol (Yeh et al., 2008). It has also been reported to be a useful agent when used adjunctively with latanoprost, resulting in a further fall in IOP. Although generally well tolerated, the main problem with Cosopt® is burning and stinging on instillation. Although discontinuation of the combination in trials is low, Cosopt® has been found to be the third most frequently discontinued eye product in practice (Rahman et al., 2009).

Fixed combination of timolol and latanoprost

A combination of timolol 0.5% and latanoprost 0.005%, marketed as Xalacom®, was first launched in the UK in 2001, shortly before the launch of travoprost and bimatoprost. Xalacom® is indicated for the reduction of IOP in patients with open-angle glaucoma and OHT who are insufficiently responsive to topical beta-blockers or prostaglandin analogues. It is administered once a day and has been shown to be more effective when administered in the evening than in the morning (Takmaz et al., 2008). It is unclear whether fixed combinations of prostaglandin analogues with timolol are superior to prostaglandin analogues alone.

Fixed combination of timolol and brimonidine

A combination of timolol 0.5% with brimonidine 0.2% is marketed as Combigan® and is indicated for the reduction of IOP in patients with COAG or OHT who are insufficiently responsive to topical beta-blockers.

The fixed combination has been shown to be superior in reducing IOP than either brimonidine or timolol alone and is as safe and effective as concomitant treatment with the individual components. Use of the combination product has been shown to result in a 24% fall in IOP (Papaconstantinou et al., 2009). Use of the brimonidine/timolol combination results in a greater number of side effects than timolol alone has fewer side effects than brimonidine alone (Sherwood et al., 2006) and fewer cases of allergy than brimonidine used alone (Motolko, 2008).

Fixed combination of timolol and travoprost

A fixed combination of travoprost 0.004% and timolol 0.5% (DuoTrav®) has been shown to be more effective than either of its components and is as efficacious as the components administered concomitantly while fewer side effects are reported with the combination product (Gross et al., 2007). The fixed combination of travoprost and timolol is indicated to decrease IOP in patients with open-angle glaucoma or OHT who are insufficiently responsive to topical β-blockers or prostaglandin analogues. Although the Summary of Product Characteristics states that the dose is one drop in the affected eye(s) once daily, in the morning or evening, it has been shown that an evening dose demonstrates better 24-h pressure control (Konstas et al., 2009).

Fixed combination of timolol and bimatoprost

A fixed combination of bimatoprost 0.03% and timolol 0.5% (Ganfort®) is available for the reduction of IOP in patients with open-angle glaucoma or OHT who are insufficiently responsive to topical β-blockers or prostaglandin analogues. The fixed combination has been shown to be more effective than either of its components used alone and as effective as the components used in their usual dosing regimen, that is bimatoprost once daily in the evening and timolol twice daily, used concomitantly. Conjunctival hyperaemia has been reported more frequently by patients on bimatoprost (39%) than the bimatoprost/timolol fixed combination (23%) with the lowest incidence in those receiving timolol (7%) (Brandt et al., 2008).

Fixed combination of timolol and brinzolamide

A fixed combination of brinzolamide 1% and timolol 0.5% (Azarga®) is a recently launched combination topical ocular hypotensive presentation. The combination is indicated to reduce IOP in adult patients with open-angle glaucoma or OHT for whom monotherapy has produced insufficient IOP reduction. It has greater IOP-lowering efficacy than brinzolamide or timolol alone (Kaback et al, 2008). Brinzolamide/timolol administration leads to a 30–33% fall in IOP at trough and 34–35% at peak and is better tolerated than, and preferred to, the dorzolamide/timolol combination, probably because of the neutral pH (7.2) of the suspension (Manni et al., 2009; Mundorf et al., 2008).

Hyperosmotic agents

Hyperosmotic agents are of great value during PACG emergencies due to their speed of action and effectiveness. The most commonly used agents are oral glycerol and intravenous mannitol, although both isosorbide and urea have been used in the past. Hyperosmotic agents act by drawing water out of the eye and therefore lower IOP. The maximal effect of glycerol is seen within 1 h and lasts for about 3 h, while mannitol acts within 30 min with effects lasting for 4–6 h.

Glycerol

Glycerol is given orally, usually as a 50% solution in water, the dose being 1–1.5 g/kg body weight given as a single dose. It is not a strong diuretic but may cause headaches, nausea and vomiting. Although it is metabolised to glucose in the body, it may be given to diabetics who are well controlled. All practitioners should be aware of the difference in dose in mL required for a 50% solution of glycerol formulated as a 50% w/v solution and one formulated as a 50% v/v solution (Table 55.13).

Mannitol

Mannitol is given as a 20% solution in water for intravenous administration. The dose is 1–2 g/kg body weight up to a maximum of 500 mL given over 30–40 min at a rate not exceeding 60 drops/min. It is a strong diuretic and as large volumes are required, it may cause problems due to cardiovascular overload, pulmonary oedema and stroke. Cerebral dehydration leads to headache and the patient may experience chills and chest pain. Mannitol is now generally preferred over acetazolamide as an initial treatment for PACG.

Patient care

Chronic open-angle glaucoma

When the condition is first diagnosed, patients should be told that the disorder cannot be cured but only controlled by the regular use of the prescribed treatment. As patients may not be aware of progression of the disease, the result of non-adherence with treatment should be made clear and the importance of regular attendance at clinics stressed.

The existence of a patient self-help group, the International Glaucoma Association (http://www.glaucoma-association.com), should be brought to the patient's attention. They will be able to put the patient in contact with their nearest support group.

The patient's technique for instillation of eye drops should be checked and corrected if necessary. Emphasis should be on the dose (one drop), the position of instillation, into the temporal side of the lower conjunctival sac, and the importance of punctal occlusion to minimise systemic side effects.

The preferred times for administration of topical medication should be discussed with the patient. Prostaglandins, prostamides and the gel form of pilocarpine are best administered at bedtime; a 12-hourly regimen should be employed for twice-daily drugs; 8-hourly for drugs given three times a day; and as near a 6-hourly regimen as practical for the

Table 55.13 Doses of hyperosmotic agents used in the treatment of POAG

Oral glycerol 50% at 1 g/kg				i.v. Mannitol 20% w/v[a]		
50% w/v solution		50% v/v solution				
Weight (kg)	Dose (mL)	Weight (kg)	Dose (mL)	Weight (kg)	Dose at 1 g/kg (mL)	Dose at 2 g/kg (mL)
40	80	44.5	70	40	200	400
50	100	50.8	80	50	250	500
60	120	57.2	90	60	300	–
		63.5	100	70	350	–
70	140	69.9	110	80	400	–
		76.2	120	90	450	–
80	160	82.6	130	100	500	–
90	180	88.9	140			
		95.3	150			
100	200	101.7	160			
For each additional 5 kg	Add 10 mL	For each additional 6.4 kg	Add 10 mL			

[a]Maximum dose 500 mL.

aqueous formulation of pilocarpine. β-Blockers given once daily should be administered in the morning. The importance of allowing a reasonable interval between drops should be emphasised. Sometimes, the order of instillation of different types of eye drop is important for pharmacological or practical reasons. For example, the instillation of pilocarpine should always precede that of a sympathomimetic to prevent pain in the eye resulting from a strong miosis following a weak mydriasis. The instillation of aqueous eye drops, which remain in the conjunctival sac for a maximum of 10 min, should precede that of viscous eye drops, for example hypromellose eye drops, or suspensions (e.g. dexamethasone 0.1% eye drops) where the contact time is prolonged.

Eye drops containing benzalkonium chloride should not be instilled if soft contact lenses are in situ. The patient should be instructed to remove the lens immediately before instillation and replace it approximately 30 min later.

As there is a hereditary component to COAG, patients should be told to advise first-degree relatives to be screened.

Such people over the age of 40 years are entitled to free eye tests by their optometrist.

Primary angle-closure glaucoma

Patients found to have shallow anterior chambers and narrow angles are normally promptly listed for peripheral iridectomies. However, if the procedure is delayed, they should be advised of the symptoms of an attack of acute PACG and details of the factors that are likely to precipitate an attack so that they can be avoided. They should be advised that there are a number of prescription and non-prescription drugs that they should not take (Lachkar and Bouassida, 2007). When visiting the doctor and purchasing medicines from a pharmacy, the patient should always remember to mention their condition, and the prescriber should ensure that the drug is appropriate for a patient prone to angle closure. Examples of drugs contraindicated in this condition are listed in Table 55.14. Note that the absence of a drug from this list does not imply safety.

Table 55.14 Drugs contraindicated in narrow-angle glaucoma

Therapeutic class		Examples
Antimuscarinics	Topical	Atropine, cyclopentolate, homatropine, tropicamide
	Antispasmodic	Atropine, dicycloverine, hyoscine, propantheline
	Motion sickness	Hyoscine, promethazine, cyclizine
	Bronchodilator	Ipratropium, tiotropium
	Urinary retention	Darifenacin, fesoterodine, flavoxate, oxybutynin, propiverine, solifenacin, tolterodine, trospium
Drugs used in anaesthesia		Glycopyrronium, ketamine, suxamethonium
Antidepressants		Amitriptyline, amoxapine, citalopram, clomipramine, dosulepin, doxepin, duloxetine, fluvoxamine, imipramine, lofepramine, maprotiline, mirtazapine, nortriptyline, paroxetine, phernelzine, reboxetine, sertraline, trazodone, trimipramine, venlafaxine
Antipsychotics		Chlorpromazine, clozapine, flupentixol, fluphenazine, olanzapine, pericyazine, perphenazine, pipotiazine, promazine, risperidone, sulpiride, thioridazine, trifluoperazine, zuclopentixol
Antihistamines		Alimemazine, antazoline, cetirizine, chlorphenamine, clemastine, cyproheptadine, diphenhydramine, hydroxyzine, loratidine, pizotifen
Antiarrhythmics		Disopyramide
Antiepileptics		Carbamazepine, topiramate
Sympathomimetics		Adrenaline, cocaine, dipivefrine, ephedrine, isometheptene, naphazoline, phenylephrine, pseudoephedrine, salbutamol, xylometazoline
Drugs used in the treatment of ADHD		Atomoxetine, dexamfetamine, methylphenidate, ritodrine
Drugs used in the treatment of parkinsonism		Benserazide, carbidopa, entacapone, levodopa, orphenadrine, procyclidine, selegiline, trihexyphenidyl,
Non-steroidal anti-inflammatory drugs		Mefenamic acid
Sulphonamide derived drugs		Acetazolamide, co-trimoxazole, hydrochlorothiazide, sulphasalazine
Miscellaneous		Botulinum toxin, carboprost, paracalcitol, pilocarpine

Following an attack of angle closure and surgical treatment of the disorder, the patient should be told that the drugs previously contraindicated can be safely taken provided that iridectomy/iridotomy remains patent.

Patient adherence

The patient is more likely to comply with the prescribed treatment if the drug or drugs can be administered according to a simple, infrequent dosage regimen and cause no or few, local or systemic side effects.

Thus, a patient treated with a once-daily prostaglandin analogue or prostamide or once- or twice-daily β-blocker would be expected to adhere to the regimen better than someone treated with pilocarpine, with its unfortunate side effects and inconvenient four-times-a-day dosage regimen. Common side effects of topical and systemic medication should be fully discussed with the patient so that the hyperaemia encountered with the prostanoids and the paraesthesia with acetazolamide are not unexpected, leading to premature discontinuation of therapy.

As glaucoma is predominantly a disease of elderly people, physical disability may prevent successful treatment, however conscientious the patient. For example, rheumatoid arthritis may reduce the patient's ability to squeeze the bottle of eye drops, while the tremor of Parkinson's disease can make correct positioning of instillation difficult. Various aids have been introduced to help with correct positioning and squeezing of eye drops, and these should be made available to patients so disabled.

Patients with poor visual acuity can be helped by colour coding of eye drop labels and supplying bottles labelled with large print. Some manufacturers have endeavoured to enhance adherence by including dose-reminder caps and facilitating instillation by supplying aids to open or position the bottle. Other manufacturers have made their eye drop containers easier to squeeze or supply aids to squeeze the bottle. A list of such devices, some of which are available on prescription, others free of charge from manufacturers of drugs used in the treatment of glaucoma is available on the International Glaucoma Association's website (http://www.glaucoma-association.com/).

Where self-medication is impossible, a simple infrequent dosage regimen is more likely to be achieved when a relative, a neighbour or the district nursing service becomes responsible for administration of the medication. In these cases, a drug administered once daily, such as a long-acting timolol preparation or a prostaglandin analogue or bimatoprost, has an obvious advantage over one that should be administered at 12-hourly intervals. If pilocarpine is required and bedtime administration is possible, the prescribing of pilocarpine ophthalmic gel will be more practical than pilocarpine eye drops, the administration of which is totally impractical for anyone other than someone living with the patient.

Common therapeutic problems in glaucoma are listed in Table 55.15.

Table 55.15 Common therapeutic problems in glaucoma

Problem	Comments
Lack of adherence	Treatment perceived to be worse than disease Complex multiple drug regimens Frequency of dosing Inability to differentiate between different types of medication Inability to instil medication
Contraindication to therapy	Pilocarpine in uveitis β-Blockers in asthma, bradycardia, heart block, uncontrolled heart failure Prostaglandin analogues and prostamides in aphakia Wide range of topical and systemic drugs in shallow anterior chamber α_2-agonists in depression Carbonic anhydrase inhibitors in renal failure
Intolerance to drug	Miosis and ciliary spasm with pilocarpine Red eye with prostaglandin analogues, bimatoprost Bronchospasm with β-blockers Paraesthesia with acetazolamide
Use outside licensed indications	Paediatric patients Pregnant women Nursing mothers
Hypersensitivity	To active drug To preservative in multidose formulations

Case studies

Case 55.1

Mrs SJ, a 49-year-old nurse with asthma, visits her optometrist for an annual eye check because her father has glaucoma. Although the optometrist has never detected any problem before, on this occasion he decides to refer her to an ophthalmologist because her IOPs are 27 left eye and 20 mmHg right eye, even though there are no signs of glaucomatous damage.

The ophthalmologist confirms the optometrist's findings and measures this lady's central corneal thickness at 570 μm. In accordance with National Institute for Health and Clinical Excellence (2009) guidelines, she decides to initiate ocular hypotensive therapy in the left eye.

Question

What treatment should the ophthalmologist prescribe?

Answer

It is recommended that patients under 60 years of age with OHT or suspected COAG and a central corneal thickness of between

555 and 590 μm are treated with an ocular hypotensive agent (National Institute for Health and Clinical Excellence, 2009). The recommended therapy is a topical β-blocker which typically reduces IOP by approximately 25%. However, β-blockers are contraindicated in patients with asthma and the ophthalmologist needs to choose an alternative agent with equivalent or better efficacy.

If β-blockers are contraindicated, a prostaglandin analogue could be prescribed.

The ophthalmologist initiates latanoprost eye drops 0.005%, one drop in the left eye at night and arranges to see Mrs SJ again in 3 months to assess her response to therapy.

Case 55.2

Mr FT, a 67-year-old retired bank manager, has COAG in both eyes and a history of herpes simplex infection of the right eye. His IOP has been controlled on timolol eye drops 0.5% twice a day in each eye which he tolerates well. At this appointment, the optometrist working in the hospital's clinic noted an increased IOP in the right eye and deterioration in the visual field in that eye. She feels that Mr FT requires an additional ocular hypotensive agent in his right eye and asks the ophthalmologist in the clinic for an opinion.

Question

What treatments should the ophthalmologist consider for Mr FT?

Answer

Patients with COAG would normally be offered a prostaglandin analogue as first-line treatment, but in Mr. FT's case this therapy is contraindicated because of his history of herpes simplex infection. He is already on a β-blocker, the other group of drugs recommended as first-line therapy, so the ophthalmologist should consider surgical intervention or the addition of a second ocular hypotensive agent. Mr. FT is not at all keen on the idea of surgery and expresses a preference for further medical therapy. Other classes of ocular hypotensives which have an additive effect with timolol are the carbonic anhydrase inhibitors brinzolamide and dorzolamide and the sympathomimetic brimonidine. The ophthalmologist explains to the patient that he can continue to use timolol in both eyes and an additional drop in his right eye or use timolol in his left eye and a combination drop containing timolol and a second agent in his right eye. Mr FT decides on the latter option and leaves with a prescription for timolol eye drops 0.5%, twice daily for his left eye and Azarga® eye drops, twice daily for his right eye together with a date for a review appointment in 2 months.

References

Bournias, T.E., Lai, J., 2009. Brimonidine tartrate 0.15%, dorzolamide hydrochloride 2%, and brinzolamide 1% compared as adjunctive therapy to prostaglandin analogs. Ophthalmology 116, 1719–1724.

Brandt, J.D., Cantor, L.B., Katz, L.J., et al., 2008. Ganfort Investigators Group II 2008 Bimatoprost/timolol fixed combination: a 3-month double-masked, randomized parallel comparison to its individual components in patients with glaucoma or ocular hypertension. J. Glaucoma. 17, 211–216.

Easton, P.J., 2007. A cardiovascular benefit of ophthalmic beta-blockade. Age and Ageing. 36, 351.

Egorov, E., Ropo, A., 2009. Adjunctive use of tafluprost with timolol provides additive effects for reduction of intraocular pressure in patients with glaucoma. Eur. J. Ophthalmol. 19, 214–222.

European Glaucoma Society, 2008. Terminology and Guidelines for Glaucoma, third ed. Editrice Dogma, Savona. Available at http://www.eugs.org/eng/EGS_guidelines.asp.

Eyawo, O., Nachega, J., Lefebvre, P., et al., 2009. Efficacy and safety of prostaglandin analogues in patients with predominantly primary open-angle glaucoma or ocular hypertension: a meta-analysis. Clin. Ophthalmol. 3, 447–456.

Goldberg, I., Li, X.Y., Selaru, P., et al., 2008. A 5-year, randomized, open-label safety study of latanoprost and usual care in patients with open-angle glaucoma or ocular hypertension. Eur. J. Ophthalmol. 18, 408–416.

Gross, R.L., Sullivan, E.K., Wells, D.T., et al., 2007. Pooled results of two randomized clinical trials comparing the efficacy and safety of travoprost 0.004%/timolol 0.5% in fixed combination versus concomitant travoprost 0.004% and timolol 0.5%. Clin. Ophthalmol. 1, 317–322.

Hamacher, T., Airaksinen, J., Saarela, V., et al., 2008. Efficacy and safety levels of preserved and preservative-free tafluprost are equivalent in patients with glaucoma or ocular hypertension: results from a pharmacodynamics analysis. Acta Ophthalmol. (Copenh) 86 (S242), 14–19.

Honrubia, F., García-Sánchez, J., Polo, V., et al., 2009. Conjunctival hyperaemia with the use of latanoprost versus other prostaglandin analogues in patients with ocular hypertension or glaucoma: a meta-analysis of randomised clinical trials. Br. J. Ophthalmol. 93, 316–321.

Jappe, U., Uter, W., Menezes de Pádua, C.A., et al., 2006. Allergic contact dermatitis due to beta-blockers in eye drops: a retrospective analysis of multicentre surveillance data 1993–2004. Acta Derm. Venereol. 86, 509–514.

Johnson, T.V., Toris, C.B., Fan, S., 2008. Effects of central corneal thickness on the efficacy of topical ocular hypotensive medications. J. Glaucoma. 17, 89–99.

Kaback, M., Scoper, S.V., Arzeno, G., et al., 2008. Brinzolamide 1%/timolol 0.5% Study Group. Intraocular pressure-lowering efficacy of brinzolamide 1%/timolol 0.5% fixed combination compared with brinzolamide 1% and timolol 0.5%. Ophthalmology 115, 1728–1734.

Katz, L.J., Cohen, J.S., Batoosingh, A.L., et al., 2010. Twelve-month, randomized, controlled trial of bimatoprost 0.01%, 0.0125%, and 0.03% in patients with glaucoma or ocular hypertension. Am. J. Ophthalmol. 149, 661–671.

Kenigsberg, P.A., 2007. Changes in medical and surgical treatments of glaucoma between 1997 and 2003 in France. Eur. J. Ophthalmol. 17, 521–527.

Konstas, A.G., Tsironi, S., Vakalis, A.N., et al., 2009. Intraocular pressure control over 24 hours using travoprost and timolol fixed combination administered in the morning or evening in primary open-angle and exfoliative glaucoma. Acta Ophthalmol. (Copenh) 87, 71–76.

Lachkar, Y., Bouassida, W., 2007. Drug-induced acute angle closure glaucoma. Curr. Opin. Ophthalmol. 18, 129–133.

Lai Becker, M., Huntington, N., Woolf, A.D., 2009. Brimonidine tartrate poisoning in children: frequency, trends, and use of naloxone as an antidote. Pediatrics 123, e305–e311. Available at http://pediatrics.aappublications.org/cgi/reprint/123/2/e305.pdf.

Lim, K.S., Nau, C.B., O'Byrne, M.M., et al., 2008. Mechanism of action of bimatoprost, latanoprost, and travoprost in healthy subjects. A crossover study. Ophthalmology 115, 790–795.

Manni, G., Denis, P., Chew, P., et al., 2009. The safety and efficacy of brinzolamide 1%/timolol 0.5% fixed combination versus dorzolamide 2%/timolol 0.5% in patients with open-angle glaucoma or ocular hypertension. J. Glaucoma. 18, 293–300.

Motolko, M.A., 2008. Comparison of allergy rates in glaucoma patients receiving brimonidine 0.2% monotherapy versus fixed-combination brimonidine 0.2%-timolol 0.5% therapy. Curr. Med. Res. Opin. 24, 2663–2667.

Müller, M.E., van der Velde, N., Krulder, J.W., et al., 2006. Syncope and falls due to timolol eye drops. Br. Med. J. 332, 960–961.

Mundorf, T.K., Rauchman, S.H., Williams, R.D., et al., 2008. Brinzolamide/Timolol Preference Study Group. A patient preference comparison of Azarga (brinzolamide/timolol fixed combination) vs

Cosopt (dorzolamide/timolol fixed combination) in patients with open-angle glaucoma or ocular hypertension. Clin. Ophthalmol. 2, 623–628.

Nakamura, Y., Ishikawa, S., Nakamura, Y., et al., 2009. 24-hour intraocular pressure in glaucoma patients randomized to receive dorzolamide or brinzolamide in combination with latanoprost. Clin. Ophthalmol. 3, 395–400.

National Institute for Health and Clinical Excellence, 2009. Glaucoma: Diagnosis and Management of Chronic Open Angle Glaucoma and Ocular Hypertension. NICE, London. Available at http://guidance.nice.org.uk/CG85.

Nieminen, T., Lehtimäki, T., Mäenpää, J., et al., 2007. Ophthalmic timolol: plasma concentration and systemic cardiopulmonary effects. Scand. J. Clin. Lab. Invest. 67, 237–245.

Papaconstantinou, D., Georgalas, I., Kourtis, N., et al., 2009. Preliminary results following the use of a fixed combination of timolol-brimonidine in patients with ocular hypertension and primary open-angle glaucoma. Clin. Ophthalmol. 3, 227–230.

Rahman, M.Q., Montgomery, D.M., Lazaridou, M.N., 2009. Surveillance of glaucoma medical therapy in a Glasgow teaching hospital: 26 years' experience. Br. J Ophthalmol. 93, 1572–1575.

Rolim de Moura, C., Paranhos A. Jr, Wormald, R., 2007. Laser trabeculoplasty for open angle glaucoma. Cochrane Database Syst. Rev. 4. Art. No.: CD003919. DOI: 10.1002/14651858.CD003919.pub2.

Saylor, M., McLoon, L.K., Harrison, A.R., et al., 2009. Experimental and clinical evidence for Brimonidine as an optic nerve and retinal neuroprotective agent: an evidence-based review. Arch. Ophthal. 127, 402–406.

Sharpe, E.D., Williams, R.D., Stewart, R.D., et al., 2008. A comparison of dorzolamide/timolol-fixed combination versus bimatoprost in patients with open-angle glaucoma who are poorly controlled on latanoprost. J. Ocul. Pharmacol. Therapeut. 24, 408–413.

Sherwood, M.B., Craven, E.R., Chou, C., et al., 2006. Twice-daily 0.2% brimonidine-0.5% timolol fixed-combination therapy vs monotherapy with timolol or brimonidine in patients with glaucoma or ocular hypertension: a 12-month randomized trial. Arch. Ophthal. 124, 1230–1238.

Sidjanin, D.J., McCarty, C.A., Patchett, R., et al., 2008. Pharmacogenetics of ophthalmic topical beta-blockers. Personal. Med. 5, 377–385.

Sonty, S., Donthamsetti, V., Vangipuram, G., et al., 2008. Long-term IOP lowering with bimatoprost in open-angle glaucoma patients poorly responsive to latanoprost. J. Ocul. Pharmacol. Therapeut. 24, 517–520.

Stewart, W.C., Konstas, A.G., Nelson, L.A., et al., 2008. Meta-analysis of 24-hour intraocular pressure studies evaluating the efficacy of glaucoma medicines. Ophthalmology 115, 1117–1122.

Takmaz, T., A ik, S., Kürkçüolu, P., et al., 2008. Comparison of intraocular pressure lowering effect of once daily morning vs evening dosing of latanoprost/timolol maleate combination. Eur. J. Ophthalmol. 18, 60–65.

Toris, C.B., Gabelt, B.T., Kaufman, P.L., 2008. Update on the mechanism of action of topical prostaglandins for intraocular pressure reduction. Surv. Ophthalmol. 53 (Suppl. 1), S107–S120.

van der Valk, R., Webers, C.A., Lumley, T., et al., 2009. A network meta-analysis combined direct and indirect comparisons between glaucoma drugs to rank effectiveness in lowering intraocular pressure. J. Clin. Epidemiol. 62, 1279–1283.

Volotinen, M., Mäenpää, J., Kautiainen, H., et al., 2009. Ophthalmic timolol in a hydrogel vehicle leads to minor inter-individual variation in timolol concentration in aqueous humor. Eur. J. Pharmaceuti. Sci. 36, 292–296.

Williams, R.D., Cohen, J.S., Gross, R.L., et al., 2008. Bimatoprost Study Group. Long-term efficacy and safety of bimatoprost for intraocular pressure lowering in glaucoma and ocular hypertension: year 4. Br. J. Ophthalmol. 92, 1387–1392.

Wright, T.M., Freedman, S.F., 2009. Exposure to topical apraclonidine in children with glaucoma. J. Glaucoma. 18, 395–398.

Yalvac, I.S., Basci, N.E., Dulger, B., et al., 2007. Penetration of betaxolol HCL ionic suspension 0.25% and betaxolol HCL solution 0.50% into the aqueous humor. Eur. J. Ophthalmol. 17, 368–371.

Yeh, J., Kravitz, D., Francis, B., 2008. Rational use of the fixed combination of dorzolamide – timolol in the management of raised intraocular pressure and glaucoma. Clin. Ophthalmol. 2, 389–399.

Further reading

Costagliola, C., dell'Omo, R., Romano, M.R., et al., 2009. Pharmacotherapy of intraocular pressure: part I. Parasympathomimetic, sympathomimetic and sympatholytics. Exp. Opin. Pharmacother. 10, 2663–2677.

Costagliola, C., dell'Omo, R., Romano, M.R., et al., 2009. Pharmacotherapy of intraocular pressure – part II. Carbonic anhydrase inhibitors, prostaglandin analogues and prostamides. Exp. Opin. Pharmacother. 10, 2859–2870.

Harvey, R., 2009. In the management of acute angle closure glaucoma is intravenous acetazolamide now an outdated treatment? Eye News 15, 44–50.

Martinez, A., Sanchez, M., 2009. Bimatoprost/timolol fixed combination vs latanoprost/timolol fixed combination in open-angle glaucoma patients. Eye (Lond) 23, 810–818.

56 Drug-induced skin disorders

S. Walsh and D. Creamer

Key points

- Drug-induced skin reactions are common, accounting for 30% of all reported adverse drug reactions.
- Diagnosis requires a comprehensive drug history and knowledge of likely causative drugs.
- Treatment involves drug withdrawal and general supportive measures.
- All skin eruptions will cause morbidity but the severe reactions, such as Stevens–Johnson syndrome/toxic epidermal necrolysis, are associated with appreciable mortality.
- Certain individuals are at higher risk of drug eruptions, for example patients with HIV infection.
- Some types of drug reaction can cause systemic as well as skin involvement, affecting the hepatic, haematological and lymphatic systems.

Adverse drug reactions (ADRs) are an inevitable consequence of modern drug therapy. They are an important cause of iatrogenic illness in terms of morbidity and mortality. ADRs can cause serious harm to the patient, as well as carrying medico-legal and economic consequences. Fortunately, only about 2% of all drug-induced skin reactions are severe and very few are fatal. However, all drug-induced skin eruptions can cause morbidity, affect the patient's confidence in the prescriber and future adherence with medication. Therefore, it is important that all drug-associated rashes are carefully evaluated and documented. It is essential that the patient is made aware of his or her sensitivity, as subsequent exposure to the drug may cause a more severe eruption. At population level, both reporting of adverse events via the MHRA 'Yellow card scheme' and post-marketing surveillance of new drugs have a role in identifying patterns of drug eruption.

It is important to remember that the potential of an individual drug to cause a skin eruption is variable. Any drug can potentially cause any reaction pattern in the skin. Some drugs such as ferrous sulphate seldom produce a rash, while others, for example, carbamazepine, penicillin antibiotics and sulphasalazine, are far more likely to precipitate a skin eruption.

Diagnosis

It is often difficult to determine the cause of a drug-induced eruption because:

- Almost any drug can affect the skin
- Unrelated drugs produce similar reactions
- The same drug may produce different reaction patterns in different patients
- Some drug reactions are difficult to distinguish from specific skin diseases such as acne, eczema and psoriasis.

In most cases, diagnosis of a drug-induced skin eruption is based on the history and the temporal association of the onset of the rash to the commencement of the medication. Particular difficulties are presented by the patient taking combined preparations, for example co-tenidone, which contains both a diuretic and a β-blocker. Excipients contained in medication, such as preservatives, stabilisers or colours, may be the culprit rather than the drug itself. Changes in brand of medication may for this reason provoke a skin reaction in someone who appears to have been established on a drug for some time and suddenly develops a rash. Patients may be taking preparations acquired over the counter, or from an alternative practitioner, which they may not immediately volunteer when asked about current medication. If a patient presents with a rash and is currently taking, or has recently finished, medication it is important to:

- Take an accurate drug history, including over-the-counter medicines, herbal and homeopathic preparations and any injections. Record both generic and brand name of medicines.
- Ask if the patient has any history of drug sensitivity.
- Ascertain when the eruption started in relation to drug use (the latency of onset of the eruption).

Definitive diagnosis of a drug-induced dermatosis would require drug re-challenge; however, this is not recommended due to the possibility of provoking a more severe reaction on second exposure (Li Wan Po and Kendall 2001).

Drug-induced skin disorders

In this chapter, drug reactions will be considered under the following headings: drug reactions causing changes to skin function; mild drug-induced skin disorders; severe drug-induced skin disorders.

Drug reactions causing changes to skin function

Some drugs alter the ability of the skin and associated structures (hair and nails) to perform their function normally.

Abnormal photosensitivity

Drugs may induce an excessive sensitivity to sunlight. Ultraviolet wavelengths of sunlight (290–400 nm) are able to interact with certain drugs in the skin to provoke abnormal photosensitivity. An eruption occurring on all uncovered skin implicates exposure to a systemic photosensitising agent, for example, a patient who commences bendroflumethiazide and subsequently develops sunburn on a cloudy day. A localised eruption indicates a reaction to a locally applied topical photosensitiser and subsequent exposure to light. This may be seen in individuals who are sensitive to a component of sunscreens such as benzophenone, a chemical sun block.

Drug-induced photosensitivity can be either phototoxic or photoallergic (Box 56.1). Phototoxic reactions, which are more common, resemble severe sunburn and can progress to blistering. They are dose dependent for both the drug and sunlight, occur within 5–15 h of taking the drug and subside quickly on drug withdrawal. Photoallergic rashes are usually eczematous, but may be lichenoid, urticarial, bullous or purpuric. They are not dose dependent and occur following exposure to normal amounts of sunlight exposure. The onset can be delayed by weeks or months, while recovery is often slow following drug withdrawal. Rarely, a photoallergic state can persist for years after the drug responsible has been discontinued.

Patients receiving known photosensitising drugs should be advised to avoid strong sunlight. They should also be advised to use a broad-spectrum topical sunscreen, providing both UVA protection (indicated by the 'star rating' on the bottle) and UVB cover (indicated by the sun protection factor, SPF).

Pigmentary changes

The skin's colour can be altered by drugs: hyper-pigmentation, hypo-pigmentation and discoloration can all potentially be induced by a variety of medicines (see Fig. 56.1 and Table 56.1). Pigmentary changes can be widespread or localised. The most common examples of localised pigmentation are the facial blue–black pigmentation in individuals on amiodarone or minocyline, and melasma facial pigmentation occurring in some women taking the combined oral contraceptive pill. Generalised pigmentary change induced by drugs is rare, but can occur with chemotherapeutic agents such as bleomycin. This may have the appearance of generalised hyper-melanosis, or may take on a more flagellate appearance with multiple linear areas of hyper-pigmentation.

The mechanism of drug pigmentation is not always known; however, proposed pathogenetic mechanisms are:

(1) Drug or drug metabolite deposition in the dermis and epidermis. An example of this would be agyria, in which systemic absorption of silver from, for example, topical silver sulphadiazine, causes a slate-grey discolouration of the skin.

(2) Enhanced melanin production with or without an increase in the number of active melanocytes. This appears to be the pathogenetic mechanism in melasma and also bleomycin-induced pigmentation (Moncada et al., 2009)

Nail changes

The growth and colour of finger and toenails can be modified by drugs. Abnormalities of texture and architecture of the nail unit can also be drug-induced. Blue discoloration of the nails can result from therapy with mepacrine, while a blue–black pigmentation may accompany treatment with minocycline and certain cytotoxic drugs such as hydroxyurea.

Box 56.1 Drugs causing light-induced eruptions

Topical preparations
Topical non-steroidal anti-inflammatory drugs (NSAIDs)
Components of sunscreen such as para-aminobenzoic acid (PABA), benzophenone

Systemic drugs
Phototoxic reactions
Amiodarone
Nalidixic acid
NSAIDs
Chlorpromazine
Tetracyclines
Photoallergic reactions
Griseofulvin
NSAIDs
Sulphonamides
Sulphonylureas
Thiazide diuretics

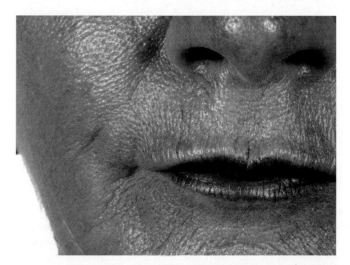

Fig. 56.1 Minocycline pigmentation: this female patient was taking minocycline for 2 years for treatment of rosacea and developed unsightly grey pigmentation round the mouth. This did not respond to stopping the medication.

Table 56.1 Drugs causing skin pigmentation

Drug	Pigmentation
Amiodarone	Blue-Grey
Anticonvulsants	Brown
Antimalarials	Blue-Grey
β-Blockers	Brown
Imatinib	Hypo/Hyperpigmentation
Imipramine	Blue/Grey
Mepacrine	Blue/black
Methyldopa	Brown
Oral contraceptives	Brown spots/patches
Phenothiazines	Brown/Blue-Grey
Psoralens	Brown
Tetracyclines	Blue-Black

Box 56.2 Drugs causing hair disorders

Alopecia
Acetretin
Anticoagulants
Anticonvulsants
Antithyroid drugs
β-Blockers
Cimetidine
Cytotoxic drugs
Gold salts
Interferons
Isotretinoin
Leflunomide
Lithium
Sodium valproate
Statins
Tacrolimus

Hirsutism/hypertrichosis
Acetazolamide
Anabolic steroids
Androgens
Corticosteroids (topical and systemic)
Ciclosporin
Danazol
Minoxidil
Oral contraceptives
Penicillamine
Phenytoin
Tamoxifen
Verapamil

Potassium permanganate solutions will dye nails brown. White nails (leuconychia) can result from treatment with chemotherapy agents, especially, cyclophosphamide, doxorubicin and vincristine. Beau's lines, transverse depression of the nail, represent interruption to the normal growth of the nail matrix, and are caused by systemic infection, metabolic upset, or occasionally by drugs. In the drug-induced form, the most common cause is again chemotherapy agents, similar to those which cause leuconychia.

Onycholysis is characterised by separation of the nail plate from the underlying nail bed. Any cytotoxic agent may induce onycholysis by direct toxicity to the matrix. Photo-onycholysis describes lifting of the nail plate and is caused by the combination of a photosensitising drug, for example minocycline, oxytetracycline and UVA exposure.

Hair changes

Drugs may exert an effect on the hair follicle itself or on the growth cycle of hair. The cycle of hair growth involves anagen (the growth phase of the hair), catagen (the resting phase) and telogen (the shedding phase). Either loss of hair or excessive growth of hair may result.

Loss of hair. Drug-induced alopecia (Box 56.2) may be partial or complete. The temporal relationship between the introduction of the drug and the subsequent loss of hair depends on the part of the hair cycle with which the drug interferes. Cytotoxic drugs interfere with the 'anagen' or growth phase of the hair cycle, and so loss is rapid and complete; it begins shortly after administration of the drug and the effect is dose dependent and fortunately reversible, but a delay of several weeks is common before regrowth begins.

Delayed hair loss following the introduction of a drug is a more insidious process and may not be noticed immediately by the patient. In this scenario, the drug is often interfering with the 'telogen' or shedding part of the hair cycle, moving follicles through this phase more quickly. Hair is shed at a rate that exceeds that at which the follicles can produce new hair, resulting in a thinning effect. Given the length of the hair cycle, this type of hair loss can occur 2–4 months after a drug is initiated. Retinoid therapy, including isotretinoin prescribed for acne, or acitretin for psoriasis, may induce a telogen alopecia.

Androgens promote shrinking of hair follicles and shorten duration of the growth stage of the hair-follicle cycle (anagen stage). Drugs with androgen activity can induce male-pattern baldness, for example exogenously administered testosterone, which may be prescribed for hypogonadism in men and occasionally in post-menopausal women as an adjunct to hormone replacement therapy. Oestrogens are known to prolong the anagen stage and counteract androgenetic alopecia. Oestrogenic stimuli may cause the hair follicle to shift into anagen phase and vice versa. Use of the oestrogen receptor antagonist tamoxifen in women with breast cancer can exacerbate female pattern hair loss. Tamoxifen competes for the oestrogen receptor and produces an environment with relative hyperandrogenism, which may augment the androgen action on follicles.

Excessive hair. Hirsutism is excessive hairiness, especially in women, in the male pattern of hair growth, while hypertrichosis is the growth of hair at sites not normally hairy. Both conditions can be drug induced and in some cases the same drug can produce both patterns of hair growth (see Box 56.2). The capacity of minoxidil to produce hypertrichosis was noted during early trials of this drug as an antihypertensive. It is infrequently used for its originally intended purpose, as it produces profound postural hypotension, but its most noticeable side effect has been exploited as a topical preparation for the treatment of male pattern baldness.

Changes to the skin's immune system and skin malignancy

The skin's innate immune surveillance system detects and repairs UV-induced DNA damage thus limiting the tendency to cutaneous carcinogenesis. Drug-induced immunosuppression places an individual at an increased risk of skin cancer, notably squamous cell and basal cell carcinomas. As well as a reduction in immune surveillance, immunosuppression increases susceptibility to the human papilloma virus, some strains of which may predispose to the development of squamous malignancy. Patients taking drugs such as azathioprine, ciclosporin, tacrolimus, mycophenolate mofetil and chemotherapeutic agents should be counselled about the importance of sun protection to minimise the risk of development of malignant and pre-malignant skin cancers. Certain high-risk patients on immunosuppressant drugs, particularly renal transplant recipients, should undergo formal follow-up with skin monitoring by a dermatologist on a yearly basis.

Mild drug-induced skin disorders

Mild drug reaction patterns in the skin are numerous; some of the more commonly seen morphologies are discussed in this section.

Drug-induced exanthems

A drug-induced exanthem (widespread rash) is the most common type of drug reaction in the skin. Exanthems are characterised by erythema (redness) and may be morbilliform (resembling measles) or maculopapular (a mixture of flat and raised areas) (see Fig. 56.2). Less frequently there may be blisters, which may be small (vesicles) or larger (>5 mm, bullae), and the skin may feel hot, burning or itchy.

The proportion of the body surface area (BSA) involved varies from case to case but when severe, involving more than 90% of the BSA, the presentation is referred to as 'erythroderma', which is discussed later. In theory, any drug is capable of producing a drug-induced exanthem in the skin, but in practice, common causes include antibiotics (e.g. sulphonamides, ampicillin, isoniazid), anticonvulsants (e.g. phenytoin, carbamazepine) and antimalarials (chloroquine).

Most drug-induced exanthems begin within 7 days of commencing a drug, the mechanism being a delayed (type IV) hypersensitivity (Burns et al., 2004). If the drug can be identified, it should be stopped, appropriate symptomatic relief instituted with antihistamines and topical steroids. A clear record of the reaction should be made in the patient's notes.

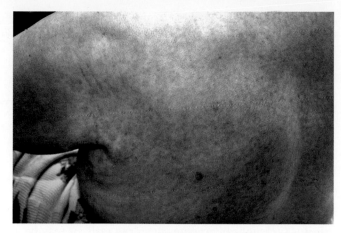

Fig. 56.2 Drug exanthem: maculopapular, itchy eruption appeared 4 days following the introduction of a course of co-amoxiclav for a respiratory tract infection. Note the linear marks indicating excoriation (scratching) on the left posterior shoulder.

Both the patient and his primary care doctor should be made aware of the reaction for the purposes of future avoidance.

An exanthematous reaction commonly occurs following administration of ampicillin (or its derivatives, including amoxicillin) to patients suffering from glandular fever (infectious mononucleosis). It does not usually represent a true penicillin allergy, but a complex interplay between viral factors (infectious mononucleosis being caused by Epstein Barr virus) and drug epitopes (Burns et al., 2004). This reaction to the drug would not be expected to be seen in the same patient in the absence of the virus.

Urticaria and angioedema

Urticaria, also known as hives, describes the appearance of red, itchy weals on the skin (Fig. 56.3). Angioedema is a more serious, related condition in which the patient develops deep soft-tissue swellings, mostly notably on the face. Urticaria and angioedema can be either allergic, a reaction between an antigen and specific mast cell-bound IgE, or non-allergic.

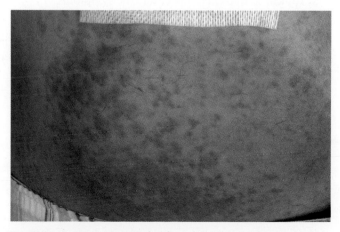

Fig. 56.3 Urticaria: patient developed the classic raised red itchy weals of urticaria following the commencement of ibuprofen for musculoskeletal pain.

Drugs are recognised triggers of urticaria and angioedema (Box 56.3) and can also exacerbate pre-existing urticaria. The most important culprits are the NSAIDs and opiates, both of which lower the threshold for mast cell degranulation. ACE inhibitors and angiotensin receptor blockers (ARBs), for example candesartan, can provoke angioedema in a susceptible individual.

Drug-induced urticaria/angioedema can be a cutaneous manifestation of anaphylaxis, and in this situation, urgent medical attention is needed with administration of adrenaline, antihistamine and intravenous corticosteroid.

Pruritus

Pruritus (itching) can accompany a drug rash, or may be an isolated symptom provoked by a medication. The most common trigger of drug-induced pruritus is the administration of opiate analgesics and their related synthetic derivatives such as tramadol. Opiate-induced pruritus is centrally mediated, rather than by peripheral nerves; therefore, antihistamines do not, in general, ameliorate the itch. This can pose a particular problem in the palliative care setting where opiate analgesics are required regularly.

Fixed drug eruptions

Fixed drug eruption is characterised by one or more inflammatory patches that recur at the same cutaneous or mucosal site(s) each time the patient is exposed to the offending drug (Fig. 56.4). The eruption usually involves the torso, hands, feet, face or genitalia, and is characterised by a deep red, circular, well-demarcated patch. They take between 2 and 24h to develop following drug ingestion. On the first drug exposure, there is usually only one lesion, but subsequent exposure can result in multiple lesions.

The group of drugs with the potential to cause a fixed drug eruption is virtually limitless, but some of the drugs more commonly responsible are listed in Box 56.4.

Once the drug has been stopped, the lesions resolve and may leave an area of post-inflammatory hyperpigmentation. This may be the only physical sign at the time the patient presents. Topical steroids may ameliorate the symptoms.

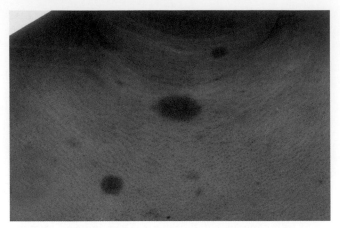

Fig. 56.4 Fixed drug eruption: female patient developed persistent macular inflamed areas on her upper chest wall 2 months after starting a new combined oral contraceptive pill. A fixed drug eruption was suspected and the lesions resolved after stopping the medicine.

Box 56.4 Drugs causing fixed drug eruptions

Ampicillin
Aspirin
Barbiturates
Dapsone
Metronidazole
NSAIDs
Oral contraceptives
Phenytoin
Quinine
Sulphonamides
Tetracyclines

Acneiform eruptions

Acne may be drug-induced or drug-exacerbated. One of the most commonly prescribed drugs to produce an acneiform eruption is corticosteroid, in either topical or oral form. Illicit use of anabolic steroids by athletes can also produce this effect, occasionally in its most severe form, acne fulminans. Other drugs which may worsen or provoke acne include ciclosporin, lithium and progesterone-only oral contraceptives.

A new class of anticancer drug, endothelial growth factor receptor antagonists, for example cetuximab, commonly produce an acneiform eruption. The papules and pustules which occur are more monomorphic than those seen in idiopathic acne. Interestingly, studies have shown that there is a positive correlation between the severity of the acneiform eruption and response of the cancer to the treatment (Saltz et al., 2003; Susman, 2004) Most drug-induced or drug-exacerbated acne can be managed with the same treatments as used in idiopathic acne, such as topical agents, oral tetracycline antibiotics, erythromycin, or in severe cases, oral retinoids. Examples of drugs which may cause an acneiform eruption are given in Box 56.5.

Box 56.3 Drugs causing urticaria/angioedema

Antibiotics (particularly penicillins, and especially when given by the parenteral route)
Barbiturates
ACE inhibitors
Angiotensin receptor blockers
Levamisole
NSAIDs
Opiate analgesics
Phenolphthalein
Quinine
Rifampicin
Sulphonamides
Thiopental
Vancomycin

Box 56.5 Drugs causing acne

Androgens (in women)
Corticosteroids (oral and topical) and ACTH (including inhaled
preparations)
Ciclosporin
EGFR antagonists (cetuximab)
Ethambutol
Haloperidol
Isoniazid
Lithium
Oral contraceptives
Phenobarbital
Phenytoin
Propylthiouracil

EGFR, Epidermal growth factor receptor.

Psoriasiform eruptions

Drugs can either exacerbate psoriasis in predisposed patients or induce psoriasiform rashes in previously unaffected patients (see Box 56.6). The psoriasiform eruptions mimic psoriasis and are characterised by itchy, scaly red patches on the elbows, forearms, knees, legs and scalp. Drugs which have a well-established effect of worsening pre-existing psoriasis include β blockers, lithium, antimalarials and ACE inhibitors.

Lichenoid eruptions

Drug-induced lichenoid eruptions (see Box 56.7) resemble lichen planus, occurring as flat mauve lesions. However, they may be atypical, showing scaling and confluence. The lesions can be seen at any site, but are found mainly on the forearms, neck and on the inner surface of the thighs. The eruption resolves with drug withdrawal, with or without topical steroids, but post-inflammatory hyperpigmentation is often long lasting.

Eczematous eruptions and contact dermatitis

Retinoid drugs (such as isotretinoin, acitretin and alitretinoin) and statins have a drying effect on the skin, and can exacerbate pre-existing eczema or precipitate eczema in a susceptible individual. Irritant contact dermatitis may be seen in preparations with an alcohol base, such as topical antibiotics, or with the application of topical preparations which are inherently irritant such as benzoyl peroxide, tar or dithranol.

Box 56.6 Drugs which exacerbate psoriasis

ACE inhibitors
Antimalarials – chloroquine, mepacrine
Biological therapy targeting tumour necrosis factor alpha (TNF-α)
(occasionally – slightly paradoxical given that such drugs are also
given to *treat* psoriasis)
β-Blockers (most frequently atenolol, oxprenolol and propranolol)
Corticosteroids, for example prednisolone
G-CSF
Lithium
NSAIDs

G-CSF, Granulocyte-colony stimulating factor.

Box 56.7 Drugs causing lichenoid eruptions

Antimalarials – chloroquine, mepacrine
Aspirin
ACE inhibitors
β-Blockers
Calcium channel blockers, for example amlodipine, nifedipine
Carbamazepine
Ethambutol
Gold salts
Imatinib
Interferon-α
Lithium
Methyldopa
NSAIDs
Penicillamine
Phenothiazines
Quinine
Sulphonylureas

Allergic contact dermatitis is a delayed (type IV) hypersensitivity reaction which can develop to any topical preparation, for example eye drops in a sensitised individual. Most commonly, this will be to excipients contained in the preparation, such as preservatives, for example sodium metabisulphite, fragrances or stabilisers, but may be to the drug itself. In all cases of irritant or allergic contact dermatitis, the patient should be counselled to stop the preparation. Patch testing carried out by a dermatologist is a useful way of investigating patients in whom a diagnosis of allergic contact dermatitis is suspected.

Erythema nodosum

Erythema nodosum is an acute inflammatory reaction with painful subcutaneous nodules, usually but not exclusively found on the shins. Erythema nodosum is usually a complication of infection with, for example, streptococcus or tuberculosis, or is a cutaneous manifestation of an inflammatory condition such as sarcoidosis. In its drug-induced form, it may be caused by oral contraceptives, sulphonamide antibiotics, salicylates, penicillins and gold salts.

Severe drug-induced skin disorders

Erythema multiforme (EM), Stevens–Johnson syndrome (SJS) and toxic epidermal necrolysis (TEN) are all idiosyncratic, immunologically mediated severe drug eruptions. For our purposes, these diseases may be considered to be on a spectrum, from the mild and self-limiting at one end (EM) to the fulminating severe at the other (TEN).

Erythema multiforme

EM is an eruption of target-like lesions which are characterised by concentric red and pale rings with, in severe cases, central blistering. EM typically occurs on the limbs rather than the trunk but mucous membrane surfaces, such as the eye, the mouth and the genital tract, may also become involved. A significant proportion of EM cases are caused by infection,

Box 56.8 Drugs causing erythema multiforme

Allopurinol
Antiretrovirals, for example nevirapine
Barbiturates
Carbamazepine
Cimetidine
Dapsone
Gold salts
Isoniazid
Lamotrigine
Leflunomide
Macrolide antibiotics
Mefloquine
NSAIDs
Penicillins
Phenytoin
Rifampicin
Sulphonamides

particularly herpes simplex virus reactivation; however, in some patients, EM is triggered by a drug (see Box 56.8). Drug-induced EM will usually present within 2 weeks of starting a new medication. Once the responsible drug has been stopped, treatment is symptomatic with paracetamol, topical steroids and appropriate topical therapy for the mouth and other involved mucosal surfaces.

Stevens–Johnson syndrome and toxic epidermal necrolysis

Stevens–Johnson syndrome (SJS) and toxic epidermal necrolysis (TEN) are terms used to describe a life-threatening, mucocutaneous drug hypersensitivity syndrome characterised by blistering and epidermal sloughing (Fig. 56.5). In SJS, there is epidermal detachment of <10% BSA, in TEN there is detachment of >30% of the BSA, while cases with 10–30% involvement are labelled SJS/TEN overlap. The systemic problems which accompany widespread epidermal loss such as high losses of heat and fluid, and the heightened risk of infection due to diminished barrier function can cause serious morbidity, similar to extensive burns. TEN carries a mortality rate of approximately 30%, but this can rise to 90% mortality in the presence of co-morbidities. HIV-infected patients and patients with systemic lupus erythematosus (SLE) have an enhanced risk of developing SJS/TEN. Drugs causing SJS/TEN are listed in Box 56.9.

Clinical features. A prodrome of fever, malaise, and upper respiratory tract symptoms may precede the eruption by a few days. Involvement of the mucous membranes of the eyes, mouth, and nose is a prominent early feature. Eye involvement results in blepharitis, haemorrhagic conjunctivitis, mucus secretion, and pseudomembranes. Ophthalmological input is required early if long-term sequelae such as blindness from corneal opacities and synechiae are not to occur. Urethral involvement must also be anticipated and the patient catheterised if strictures are not to complicate the disease course. Mouth involvement causes an erosive and haemorrhagic mucositis. On the skin, dusky red macules 1–3 cm in diameter appear at any site and evolve to become confluent. The skin lesions pass through vesicular and bullous phases before epidermal detachment occurs. Shearing pressure to the skin causes detachment of involved epidermis (positive Nikolsky's sign). In TEN, there is widespread epidermal loss and sloughing of the necrotic epidermis which peels back to leave large areas of exposed dermis. Denuded dermis exudes serum, becomes secondarily infected and readily bleeds. The patient is in severe pain and is usually extremely ill. The visceral manifestations that result from widespread epithelial loss include pneumonia, pancreatitis, thromboembolic disease, renal and hepatic impairment.

The patient with SJS/TEN will require full supportive care, preferably in an intensive care unit. Patients with SJS with less extensive involvement may be managed in a lower-dependency environment, but should be monitored closely

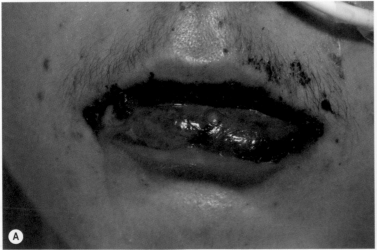
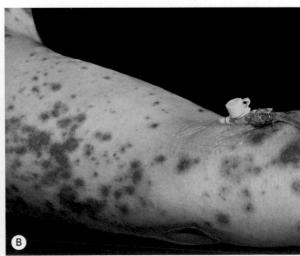

Fig. 56.5 Stevens–Johnson syndrome is a serious, idiosyncratic reaction of the skin and mucous membranes to a drug. It results in blistering and subsequently widespread epidermal loss and can have a high mortality rate.

Box 56.9 Drugs causing Stevens–Johnson syndrome and toxic epidermal necrolysis

Allopurinol
Antiretrovirals, for example nevirapine
Carbamazepine
Co-trimoxazole
Dapsone
Gold salts
Lamotrigine
Leflunomide
NSAIDs, for example meloxicam, diclofenac
Penicillins, for example amoxicillin, ampicillin
Phenobarbitone
Phenolphthalein
Phenylbutazone
Phenytoin
Sulphadiazine
Sulphasalazine
Tetracyclines, for example doxycycline

Box 56.10 Common causes of Drug Reaction with Eosinophilia and Systemic Symptoms (DRESS)

Allopurinol
Antiretrovirals, for example efavirenz
Carbamazepine
Cotrimoxazole
Lamotrigine
Minocycline
Phenobarbitone
Phenytoin
Sulphadiazine
Sulphasalazine
Vancomycin

for signs of progression in the first 48 h of admission. A multidisciplinary approach, including dermatologists, ophthalmologists and intensive care physicians, is critical to a successful outcome. Following drug withdrawal, the management is supportive, including prompt treatment of infection, careful attention to thermoregulation, fluid balance and skin care, and introduction of appropriate eye and lid care. The literature has failed to identify one treatment which definitively improves outcomes, but agents which have been used include systemic steroids, ciclosporin and intravenous immunoglobulin.

Drug Reaction with Eosinophilia and Systemic Symptoms

Drug Reaction with Eosinophilia and Systemic Symptoms (DRESS) is sometimes known as Drug-Induced Hypersensitivity Syndrome (DIHS) and is a distinct, severe and potentially fatal drug-induced skin disorder. The drugs commonly associated with this syndrome are listed in Box 56.10.

Typically, the dermatosis of DRESS is an extensive, inflammatory, maculo-papular exanthem. Other skin signs may also be present including pustules, purpura, blisters, target-like lesions and facial oedema (Fig. 56.6). To meet the diagnostic criteria, there will also be a haematological abnormality, either a raised eosinophil count (>1.5×10^9/L) or the presence of atypical lymphocytes on the blood film. There is prominent systemic involvement in DRESS, most commonly fever, lymph node enlargement and liver function abnormalities. Less typically, there is renal, pulmonary or cardiac involvement.

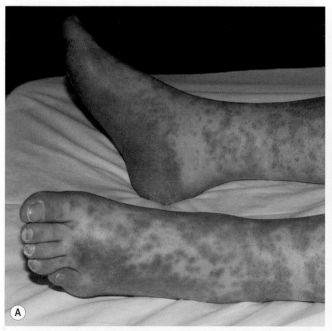
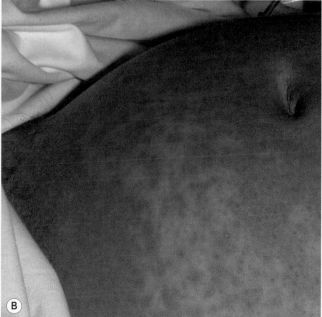

Fig. 56.6 Drug Reaction with Eosinophilia and Systemic Symptoms (DRESS): female patient developed a severe systemic reaction following commencement of phenytoin for seizure prophylaxis after brain surgery. She had an erythematous urticated eruption as seen above accompanied by lymphadenopathy, derangement of liver function, and a circulating eosinophilia.

DRESS is characterised by its long latency of onset with the syndrome usually presenting between 2 and 8 weeks after commencement of the causative drug. This is an important point to note in the medication history, as often the drug responsible may be overlooked if it is considered to have been started 'too long ago'.

DRESS is accompanied by significant morbidity while the mortality has been estimated at 10%. Systemic steroids are usually administered, and may be beneficial, but there are no randomised controlled trials to support use. Management involves stopping the suspected drug, and supportive care dictated by extent of involvement.

Acute Generalised Exanthematous Pustulosis

Acute Generalised Exanthematous Pustulosis (AGEP) describes a reaction pattern to a drug consisting of widespread sterile, monomorphic pustules studding the skin in a generalised fashion. Such patients are generally systemically unwell with a fever and the complications of generalised skin inflammation including excessive heat and fluid loss. The differential diagnosis would include pustular psoriasis. Although the condition is self-limiting, potent topical steroids may accelerate resolution. The drugs which can cause AGEP are summarised in Box 56.11.

Erythroderma and exfoliative dermatitis

Erythroderma is the term used to describe any pattern of drug reaction in the skin where more than 90% of the BSA is involved. This is usually an extension of a severe drug-induced exanthem. The erythrodermic patient often feels shivery and may have lymphadenopathy and fever. The large surface area involved in erythroderma leads to substantial losses of heat and fluid from the body. This puts the patient at risk of electrolyte imbalances, hypothermia, and with the loss of skin barrier function, infection. Admission to hospital is indicated in cases of erythroderma, and management is supportive, with intravenous fluids, warming measures, and treatment of infection. Topical corticosteroids are often prescribed but must be used with caution since significant amounts will be systemically absorbed across the erythrodermic skin. During recovery, the patient will desquamate, referred to as the exfoliative phase. Drugs commonly provoking this pattern of reaction are similar to those which cause a drug-induced exanthem (Box 56.12).

Lupus erythematosus

Syndromes indistinguishable from Lupus erythematosus (LE) may occur following drug administration (see Box 56.13) and can be accompanied by seroconversion to antinuclear antibody (ANA) positivity. Serological clearance of ANA may occur after drug withdrawal, but this may take months or years.

The cutaneous manifestations of drug-induced LE include the characteristic butterfly-shaped rash on the face, photosensitive erythema on dorsal hands and neck, and annular lesions on limbs.

Box 56.12   Drugs causing exanthemous eruptions

Amoxicillin
Ampicillin[a]
Bleomycin
Captopril
Carbamazepine
Chlorpromazine
Co-trimoxazole
Gold salts
Nalidixic acid
NSAIDs
Phenytoin
Penicillamine

[a]Ampicillin rashes do not necessarily indicate penicillin hypersensitivity, but may seen when administered to a patient with glandular fever (see text).

Box 56.11   Drugs causing acute generalised exanthematous pustulosis

Allopurinol
Amoxicillin
Carbamazepine
Cefuroxime
Co-trimoxazole
Doxycycline
Macrolide antibiotics, for example, erythromycin, pristinamycin
Metronidazole
Lamotrigine
Phenytoin
Sulphasalazine
Vancomycin

Box 56.13   Drugs causing lupus erythematosus

Anticonvulsants: phenytoin
β-Blockers
Chlorpromazine
Griseofulvin
Hydralazine
Isoniazid
Lithium
Methyldopa
Oral contraceptives
Penicillamine
Phenytoin
Procainamide
Propylthiouracil
Sulphasalazine
Terbinafine
Biological therapy targeting tumour necrosis factor alpha (TNF-α), for example infliximab

Biological therapy targeting tumour necrosis factor alpha (TNF-α) such as infliximab and etanercept has been found to provoke lupus both in its systemic and limited cutaneous forms.

Vasculitis

Vasculitis is characterised pathologically by inflammation in vessel walls and clinically as palpable purpuric lesions most commonly found on the lower limbs. Cutaneous vasculitis without other organ involvement is the rule, but systemic involvement, such as renal, can occasionally occur. The purpuric areas on the legs may become ulcerated and require specialist dermatology input.

Drugs are the cause of approximately 10% of cutaneous vasculitis cases and should be considered in any patient with small vessel vasculitis (Box 56.14). Withdrawal of the causative drug is often sufficient to resolve the clinical manifestations without the need for treatment with systemic corticosteroids or more powerful immunosuppressants.

Skin necrosis

The term widespread cutaneous necrosis describes extensive skin infarction which often heralds a severe systemic coagulopathy. Widespread cutaneous necrosis can be triggered by a reaction to warfarin, or less commonly to heparin. In warfarin or coumarin skin necrosis, the buttocks and breasts are the most commonly involved sites. Discontinuation of the anticoagulant responsible is essential; however, ongoing management of the coagulopathy is critical and patients need to be assessed by a haematologist.

Box 56.14 Drugs that may cause cutaneous vasculitic reactions

ACE inhibitors
Allopurinol
Amiodarone
Aspirin
Carbamazepine
Carbimazole
Diltiazem
Erythromycin
Furosemide
Gold
Haematopoietic growth factors (G-CSF and GM-CSF)
Hydralazine
Interferons
Methotrexate
Minocycline
NSAIDs
Penicillamine
Propylthiouracil
Sulphasalazine
Sulphonamides
Thiazides
Thrombolytic agents

G-CSF, Granulocyte-colony stimulating factor; GM-CSF, Granulocyte-macrophage colony-stimulating factor.

Patient care

Withdrawal of the likely offending drug should be the first intervention in cases of suspected drug eruption. This should be done in consultation with the prescribing physician, as an alternative drug may be required to control the patient's condition. General methods which will provide symptomatic relief in a mild, limited drug eruption include emollients, soap substitutes and oral antihistamines. A mild topical corticosteroid may also be appropriate. In cases where the eruption is more extensive, or if a mucosal surface is involved, specialist care provided by a dermatologist will be necessary.

Case studies

Case 56.1

A 36-year-old female patient with a long history of chronic idiopathic urticaria attends her local pharmacy for some advice. Her skin disease is usually well controlled with an occasional dose of cetirizine which she buys over the counter. She has recently begun taking ibuprofen for muscular pain associated with her marathon training, but has found to her dismay that her urticaria has become much worse and is flaring on a daily basis.

Questions

1. What is the likely cause of the deterioration in the control of urticaria?
2. What management should be advised?
3. What other group of drugs is likely to produce this effect?

Answers

1. Non-steroidal anti-inflammatory drugs (NSAIDs) are known to increase the frequency of attacks of urticaria in susceptible individuals. It is likely that the self-medicating with ibuprofen has lessened the patient's control of her urticaria.
2. In the first instance, the ibuprofen should be stopped. An alternative such as paracetamol could be advised for the musculoskeletal symptoms. An enquiry should be made as to whether or not any symptoms suggestive of angioedema, such as lip/tongue swelling, or difficulty breathing, have accompanied the urticaria, as this would imply a need for medical attention. In the acute phase, regular administration of an antihistamine such as chlorphenamine should help to relieve rapidly the symptoms. The patient should be warned that the ability of NSAIDs to worsen urticaria is a 'class effect' and that similar symptoms may be produced with drugs such as aspirin, meloxicam and naproxen.
3. Opiate analgesics lower the threshold for mast cell degranulation, which is the most important pathophysiological mechanism in the production of urticaria. Thus, morphine and related products such as codeine should be avoided.

Case 56.2

A 69-year-old male patient with a history of psoriasis attends the pharmacy looking for advice. In the past, his skin disease has always been well controlled with topical preparations. He was recently admitted to hospital with a myocardial infarction and has noticed a marked deterioration in his psoriasis since discharge. During his admission, he was commenced on:

Aspirin 75 mg daily
Simvastatin 20 mg daily
Atenolol 25 mg daily
Enalapril 5 mg daily

Questions

1. What is the likely reason for the exacerbation of his psoriasis?
2. How should this be treated?

Answers

1. The patient's psoriasis could have worsened due to the stress of his recent illness, but it is probably secondary to the introduction of atenolol or enalapril. Both β-blockers and ACE inhibitors have been associated with the worsening of psoriasis.
2. Given the recent myocardial infarct, any interruptions or substitutions to treatment must be made in conjunction with the patient's primary care doctor or cardiologist. The worsening of psoriasis with β-blockers is likely to be a class effect, and therefore substituting a different β-blocker is unlikely to resolve the problem. The treating physician may wish to prescribe an alternative antihypertensive such as a calcium channel blocker. If this does not ameliorate the situation, then the ACE inhibitor may be suspected, and trial stoppage may be considered. An ARB (angiotensin receptor blocker) such as candesartan may be acceptable as an alternative.

Case 56.3

A 37-year-old man presents with swelling of his upper lip. He asks if this could be stress induced as he has had several previous episodes of localised swelling of the face over the last 6–12 months.
He has been taking bendroflumethazide and enalapril for hypertension for the last 3 years, but has not taken any other medications recently.

Questions

1. What condition do his symptoms suggest?
2. Could this be drug-induced?
3. How should the condition be treated?

Answers

1. This pattern of localised swelling of the face is characteristic of angioedema.
2. Angioedema is a known adverse effect of ACE inhibitors with an overall incidence of 0.5–1%. Although this commonly occurs in the first week of treatment, delayed-onset angioedema can occur even after many years of treatment.
3. Since angioedema can be life-threatening, any suspect drug should be stopped. There is a very low incidence of this occurring with an angiotensin II receptor blocker (ARB), and this may be a suitable alternative for this patient. The acute presentation of angioedema is treated with antihistamine and corticosteroids. If the patient presents with respiratory symptoms, subcutaneous epinephrine (adrenaline) is indicated.

Case 56.4

Miss AF is a 15-year-old renal transplant patient who attends the pharmacy 6 weeks following transplant. She is very distressed about the growth of facial hair and the worsening of acne.

Questions

1. What are the possible causes of Miss AF's skin complaints?
2. What other side effects should be enquired about?
3. How might these conditions be treated?

Answers

1. It is likely that Miss AF is receiving transplant immunosuppression that includes ciclosporin and prednisolone. The ciclosporin is most likely to have caused the growth of facial hair. Both the oral corticosteroid and the ciclosporin may have aggravated pre-existing acne or precipitated new-onset acne.
2. Ciclosporin may cause gingival hyperplasia, tremor, paraesthesia and nausea. Corticosteroids can cause increased appetite/weight gain, alterations of mood (euphoria, depression), sleep disturbance, gastritis and numerous other side effects.
3. Hirsutism is a side effect of ciclosporin that many young transplant patients have to cope with, and depilatory creams are commonly used. Tacrolimus is an alternative long-term immunosuppressant which is less likely to cause acne and hirsutism and which may be used in place of ciclosporin.

Case 56.5

An 85-year-old gentleman with rheumatoid arthritis, Mr DC, attends the local pharmacy with a persistent lesion on his left upper cheek, abutting the eyelid (Fig. 56.7), which has recently been bleeding. For the last 18 years, his rheumatoid arthritis has been treated with methotrexate. You know Mr DC is a retired naval officer, and his skin is severely sun damaged. He tells you he has had a number of basal cell carcinomas in the past and is concerned that this may be another.

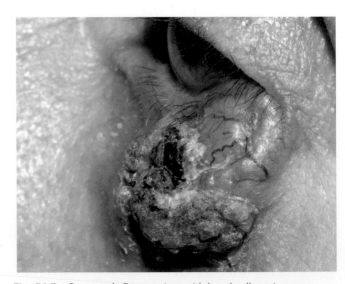

Fig. 56.7 Case study 5 – a patient with basal cell carcinoma.

Questions

1. What is the likely diagnosis?
2. What risk factors does the patient have for this diagnosis?
3. How should he be advised?

Answers

1. This is likely to be another basal cell carcinoma (BCC). Basal cell carcinomas are the most common type of skin cancer in the western world, presenting as pearly papules with a central area of ulceration and creeping telangiectatic vessels at their surface. They usually occur on sun-exposed sites and are related to high cumulative levels of sun exposure.
2. Mr DC has a number of risk factors for developing a basal cell carcinoma:

   - Age: these lesions tend to occur in the older age group, presumably because of their high level of actinic damage accrued over many years. In addition, sunscreen was not as widely used in mid-to-late 20th century as it is today.
   - Immunosuppressed state: Mr. DC has been on an immunosuppressant for 18 years resulting in his tumour surveillance mechanisms being attenuated.
   - Occupation: it is likely that Mr DC will have served in some very sunny climates. A history of active service with the Armed Forces should always prompt health-care professionals to ask about the patient's history of sun exposure.

3. Firstly, the patient should be asked to consult his primary care doctor or dermatologist as the lesion will require treatment. If left unattended, basal cell carcinomas continue to grow and can become locally invasive. Secondly, Mr. DC should be advised of the importance of sun protection, using a high factor (30 or above) sunscreen, with good UVA protection (as indicated by the star rating system on the back of the bottle). A hat provides excellent cover for the scalp and face. The sun should be avoided completely between the hours of midday and 2 pm, when the levels of ultraviolet light are at their highest.

Case 56.6

A 56-year-old man, Mr SW, presents to the pharmacy in an alarmed state. In recent months, he has had several episodes of gout and was recently prescribed allopurinol. He has now taken four doses of the drug. Last night, Mr SW developed an unusual rash on his palms and soles, which this morning has developed blisters. The rash has now extended to involve his arms and legs. He also complains of 'mouth ulcers', a gritty feeling in the eyes, and pain on passing urine. Mr SW is not feverish now, but had a raised temperature overnight.

Questions

1. What is the likely diagnosis?
2. How should Mr SW be managed?

Answers

1. This patient is developing SJS. He has a blistering eruption which commenced peripherally, which is classical for this disorder. Mr SW now has evidence of mucosal site involvement, including the oral mucosa and conjunctivae, with urethral involvement suggested by his history of dysuria. Allopurinol is a common culprit for this condition.
2. Patients with suspected SJS need urgent dermatological assessment and often require inpatient care. The suspected drug should be withheld. Following admission to hospital, a full blood count, urinalysis, blood culture, skin swabs and a chest X-ray should be performed to screen for infection. An ophthalmological opinion should be sought to ensure that no synechiae (scarring) of the eyes forms because this can occasionally arise with the degree of inflammation seen in this patient. Catheterisation is required if urethral mucosal involvement is suspected, to prevent strictures forming due to scarring. Mr SW should not be exposed to allopurinol or related drugs again, as recurrence is likely.

Case 56.7

A 24-year-old female, Ms AM, was commenced on the combined oral contraceptive pill last month. Ms AM is concerned because she has noticed the appearance of raised red nodules on both shins, which are tender to touch, and have been becoming more numerous over the last 3 days. She has never had any such eruption before. There is no recent travel history, and Ms AM has no rashes elsewhere, nor does she have any arthralgia.

Questions

1. What is your diagnosis?
2. What is the likely cause of this eruption and what are the other possible causes?
3. What is the prognosis?

Answers

1. Ms AM has developed erythema nodosum, an inflammatory condition seen on the anterior legs, usually bilaterally. Erythema nodosum is a Latin term meaning 'red lumps', it represents a pathological process in which subcutaneous fat becomes inflamed.
2. The combined oral contraceptive pill is the most likely precipitant in this case. However, a full drug and medical history should be taken as other medicines may cause erythema nodosum, for example antibiotics or NSAIDs. A very common cause of erythema nodosum in young people is streptococcal throat infection. A travel history is important as the same clinical reaction pattern may be brought about by tuberculosis. Finally, a number of other medical problems such as ulcerative colitis and Crohn's disease, or sarcoidosis may also produce erythema nodosum.
3. The patient should see a dermatologist to have the other causes of erythema nodosum excluded. The management of erythema nodosum is supportive, with regular NSAIDs or paracetamol given for pain. The combined oral contraceptive pill should be stopped, and Ms AM switched to a different form of contraception.

Case 56.8

A 17-year-old girl, Miss AW, asks for some advice regarding a widespread itchy rash which has appeared suddenly over the last 24 h. Miss AW visited her primary care doctor 4 days ago complaining of a sore throat and a productive cough. Having auscultated the chest, the primary care doctor suspects a respiratory tract infection and prescribes amoxicillin. Five days later, Miss AW develops a widespread maculopapular rash. She attends the pharmacy for advice, and you suspect the rash to be drug-induced.

Questions

1. What is the cause of the eruption?
2. How should Miss AW be managed?
3. Should Miss AW be advised to avoid penicillin antibiotics in the future?

Answers

1. This is likely to be an amoxicillin-induced drug eruption.
2. The antibiotic should be stopped and the clinical indication for an alternative preparation assessed by the primary care doctor. An antihistamine and a mild/moderate potency topical corticosteroid should provide symptomatic relief. If the patient does not obtain relief with such treatment, if the rash is becoming widespread, or if there are any features of a systemic illness such as fever or enlarged lymph nodes, the patient should see the primary care doctor.
3. The reaction may be provoked by any antibiotic in the penicillin group, so the patient needs to be informed of the need to avoid all such antibiotics in the future.

References

Breathnach, S.M., 2004. Drug eruptions. In: Burns, T., Breathnach, S.M., Cox, N., et al. (Eds.), Rook's Textbook of Dermatology. seventh ed. Blackwell Publishing, Oxford.

Li Wan Po, A., Kendall, M.J., 2001. Causality assessment of adverse effects: when is rechallenge ethically acceptable. Drug Saf. 24, 793–799.

Moncada, B., Sahagun-Sanchez, L.K., Torres-Alvarez, B., et al., 2009. Molecular structure and concentration of melanin in the stratum corneum of patients with melasma. Photodermatol. Photoimmunol. Photomed. 25, 159–160.

Saltz, L., Kies, M., Abbruzzese, J.L., et al., 2003. The presence and intensity of the cetuximab-induced acne-like rash predicts increased survival in studies across multiple malignancies. Proc. Am. Soc. Clin. Oncol. 22, 204 (Suppl; abstract 817).

Susman, E., 2004. Rash correlates with tumour response after cetuximab. Lancet Oncol. 5, 647.

Further reading

Litt, J.Z., 2010. Litt's Drug Eruption Reference Manual Including Drug Interactions, sixteenth ed. Informa Healthcare, London.

Weller, R.P.J.B., Hunter, J.A.A., Savin, J.A., et al., 2008. Clinical Dermatology, fourth ed. Blackwell Publishing, Oxford.

Eczema and psoriasis 57

A. Abdul-Wahab and N. Desai

Key points

- Eczema and psoriasis are common, chronic skin diseases with significant impact on quality of life.
- Emollient therapy is the mainstay of treatment for most types of eczema.
- Active inflammation should be treated with a topical steroid of appropriate potency.
- Eczematous skin is often secondarily infected and appropriate recognition of secondary bacterial and viral infections is mandatory.
- Systemic steroids should be avoided in psoriasis.
- New effective systemic agents are now available, including biologic agents, for which careful patient selection and regular monitoring are important.
- Eczema and psoriasis are inflammatory skin conditions commonly encountered in clinical practice. Although the conditions both manifest as erythematous, pruritic rashes, their morphology, distribution, long-term treatment options and outcomes may differ significantly. Both conditions can be functionally and socially disabling. Patient education, support and guidance with topical treatments are therefore extremely important.

Eczema

The terms 'eczema' and 'dermatitis' may be used interchangeably and describe the same clinical and histological entity. Eczema is an itchy erythematous (red) eruption consisting of ill-defined erythematous patches or papules. The skin surface is usually scaly and as time progresses, constant scratching leads to thickened, 'lichenified' skin.

Pathology and clinical features

Acute eczema is an inflammatory process leading to oedema in the epidermis. The oedema is seen histologically in the epidermis as 'spongiosis'. Oedema manifests as fluid that collects into tiny blisters which may then coalesce. This is seen histologically as intraepidermal vesicles and clinically as pompholyx blisters on thicker palmar and plantar skin, and as excoriated, ruptured crusted vesicles elsewhere. Tightly packed keratinocyte cells in the epidermis usually prevent transepidermal fluid loss and the entry of pathogens. This barrier function of the skin is lost in eczema. A schematic diagram demonstrating the normal skin epidermis and the effects on the barrier function during an acute eczema flare is shown in Fig. 57.1.

In the chronic form of eczema, prolonged rubbing and scratching results in a thickened epidermis and an increase in the upper horny cell layer of keratin, termed hyperkeratosis. Clinically, the skin appears thick, leathery, scaly and 'lichenified' with exaggerated skin markings, like tree bark (Fig. 57.2). Both acute and chronic stages are accompanied by a heavy chronic inflammatory cell infiltration of the dermis and epidermis. The main consequent symptom of these pathological processes is itch. The dictum of 'if it's not itchy, it's not eczema' holds true.

Clinical types

Atopic eczema

Atopic eczema is the commonest skin disorder of childhood, affecting between 10% and 20% of school age children in the UK. The aetiology is a combination of genetic, environmental and immunological factors.

The term 'atopy' describes an exaggerated propensity to form IgE to common allergens. In later life, approximately half of eczema patients will develop associated atopic disorders such as asthma and allergic rhinitis. The molecular pathology in atopic eczema is complex. The epidermal Langerhans cells have high-affinity IgE receptors through which the T-helper cells (T_h2 and T_h1) release cytokines and mediate skin inflammation.

Atopic eczema is diagnosed clinically and the criteria for definition include chronic itchy skin with three or more of the following: a history of flexural involvement of the skin creases, visible flexural involvement, dry skin, other atopic disease or onset within the first 2 years of life. The clinical course and distribution change through puberty and adulthood. In infants, common areas affected are face, neck and nappy area. Through childhood, flexural sites such as folds of the elbows and backs of the knees are classically involved (see Fig. 57.3). Symptoms usually improve with age and approximately 60% have resolution of symptoms by the age of 16.

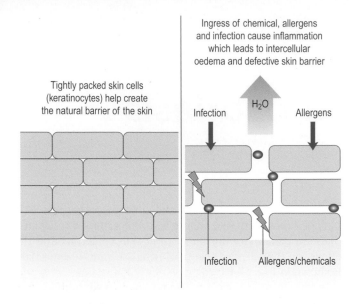

Fig. 57.1 Schematic diagram demonstrating the normal skin epidermis (left) and the effects on the barrier function (right) during an acute eczema flare.

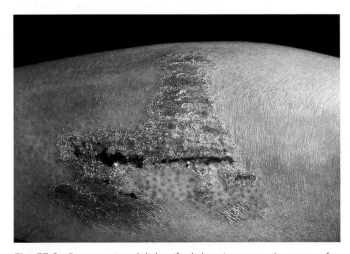

Fig. 57.2 Dry, excoriated, lichenified chronic eczema (courtesy of M. Carr).

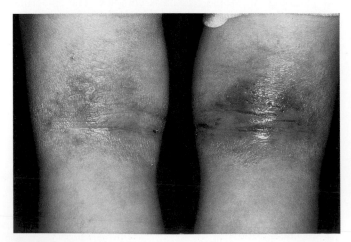

Fig. 57.3 Flexural eczema in childhood (courtesy of M. Carr).

Exacerbating factors

A number of factors can aggravate atopic eczema:

- Extremes of temperature
- Irritants: soap, detergents, shower gels, bubble baths and water
- Stress
- Infection, either bacterial or viral
- Contact allergens
- Food allergens
- Inhaled allergens
- Airborne allergens.

The commonest trigger in the paediatric population is secondary infection, either bacterial or viral. Bacterial colonisation is common on the skin of those with atopic dermatitis and may result in the invasive infection triggering an acute flare. *Staphylococcus aureus* and *Streptococcus* spp. are most often responsible (Fig. 57.4).

Viral infections such as herpes simplex and molluscum contagiosum may also complicate atopic eczema. Eczema herpeticum is caused by the widespread dissemination of herpes simplex virus in eczematous skin and is a dermatological emergency. It requires urgent assessment and treatment with systemic aciclovir.

In some cases of severe atopic eczema, food allergy may be a contributory factor, particularly if a clear temporal relationship is detected by the parents. These cases should be referred to a paediatric allergy specialist, with access to a paediatric dietician, as unsupervised dietary restriction should be avoided in children. Most children tend to grow out of food allergies over time with the exception of nut and shellfish allergies.

Contact dermatitis

Contact dermatitis is classified as either allergic contact dermatitis (ACD) or irritant contact dermatitis (ICD).

Allergic contact dermatitis

ACD is a delayed type IV hypersensitivity reaction that develops in response to an antigen to which the host immune system has been previously sensitised. As a consequence, symptoms rarely develop on first exposure to the stimulus and

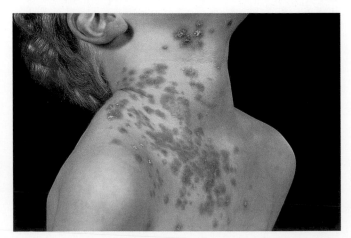

Fig. 57.4 Impetigo complicating atopic eczema (courtesy of M. Carr).

may only manifest months or years later following repeated re-exposure.

Many common compounds can lead to ACD. The most common compounds implicated are:

- Metals, for example nickel and cobalt
- Neomycin, a topical antibiotic found in over-the-counter preparations sold in some countries
- Fragrance ingredients, for example Balsam of Peru
- Rubber compounds
- Hair dyes, for example p-phenylediamine
- Plants, for example poison ivy.

Diagnosis relies heavily on a detailed patient history as well as recognising the pattern and distribution of the eczematous rash. Although the signs are usually localised to the area exposed to the allergen, secondary generalised eczema may develop.

The standard confirmatory investigation is patch testing and is used to differentiate allergic from ICD. This involves application of a standard, with or without a specialised range of compounds, to the patient's back over 72 h. This is followed by examination for a cutaneous reaction at day 2 and day 4. Identification of relevant compounds allows the patient to avoid the substance in the future, and this will hopefully reduce symptoms. Common areas of the body affected by ACD, with corresponding probable sensitisers, are listed in Table 57.1.

Irritant contact dermatitis

This is the most common form of occupational dermatitis and the commonest cause of hand eczema (Fig. 57.5). Unlike ACD, ICD is not immunologically mediated. The mechanism involves disruption of the epidermal permeability barrier and a direct cytotoxic effect depending on the irritant. Patients with pre-existing epidermal barrier dysfunction such as atopic eczema are at higher risk. The occupation of the individual may also be a risk factor, especially those working as builders, hairdressers, gardeners, healthcare workers and chefs. Irritants include detergents, oils, water, inorganic

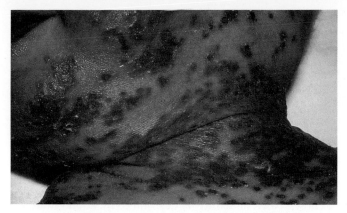

Fig. 57.5 Contact dermatitis to cement in a building worker (courtesy of M. Carr).

acids, alcohols and plastics. Preventative skin care is key and this includes the use of barriers such as emollients or cotton gloves in addition to avoiding suspected irritants.

Seborrhoeic dermatitis

This common disorder is usually confined to areas with high sebum production. The likely aetiological mechanism is overgrowth of the commensal yeast *Malassezia furfur* (Pityosporum ovale). The clinical features are pink-yellow greasy patches with 'bran-like' scale which occur in the sebaceous-rich scalp, nasal folds, medial eyebrow, pre-sternal region and flexural sites. In the first few months of life, it manifests as coherent scaling of the scalp with inflammation and ooze, known as 'cradle cap'. In adults, the symptoms are usually mild with a chronic, relapsing course. Extensive and severe seborrhoeic dermatitis can be seen in patients with underlying HIV infection or Parkinson's disease. Treatment usually includes topical imidazoles.

Discoid eczema

Discoid eczema is also known as 'nummular dermatitis' and is a type of chronic eczema presenting with disseminated coin-shaped eczematous lesions of the extremities. Middle-aged males are most commonly affected.

Stasis eczema

Stasis eczema is also called stasis dermatitis, gravitational dermatitis or varicose eczema. It is a clinical component of chronic venous insufficiency seen in addition to other features which include varicose veins, skin discolouration, peripheral oedema, leg discomfort and non-healing ulcers. Clinical features include scaly eczematous plaques confined to the lower legs. Multiple topical medicines and dressings often lead to a secondary ACD. Management of stasis eczema should address the underlying cause.

Asteatotic eczema

Asteatotic eczema, also called eczema craquele, usually affects the lower legs and appears as dry, cracked skin likened to 'cracked paving'. This is associated with increasing age, low

Table 57.1 Common locations for allergic contact dermatitis and possible sensitisers

Location	Possible sensitising agents
Periorbital	Airborne allergens, nail polish, contact lens solution
Umbilicus	Nickel hypersensitivity to belt/jean button
Neck	Antiseptic in soap, cosmetics
Hairline	PPD in hair dye, hair perming solution
Hands	Latex or rubber accelerators in gloves, nickel, fragrances, protein contact dermatitis in food preparation, irritant contact dermatitis due to water

PPD, p-phenylediamine.

humidity and frequent bathing. Treatment consists of emollients and mildly potent topical steroids.

Treatment

First-line treatment of eczema should include an emollient and soap substitute for washing. Topical steroids are used for anti-inflammatory effect. Systemic treatments for adult atopic eczema include oral prednisolone, ciclosporin and azathioprine. If there is a secondary bacterial infection, then this should be treated with oral antibiotics. The antibiotic(s) should be chosen based on sensitivity determined by wound swab.

Emollients

Emollients, topical hydrating agents consisting of fat or oil to soften the skin, are the mainstay of eczema management. Emollients are effective first-line treatments for all types of eczema, and regular, liberal use will reduce topical steroid requirements. The greasier products have more emollient effect (see Fig. 57.6). They are often underused and the need to educate the patient regarding use of sufficient quantities is vital. Dry skin is aggravated by soap and bath products, and therefore an emollient soap substitute for washing is advisable.

Topical corticosteroids

Topical steroids act as anti-inflammatory agents and are extremely useful and important in managing eczema. In recent years, the public have veered from overuse of topical steroids causing long-lasting side effects, to high levels of anxiety regarding possible side effects concerning their use. This can commonly lead to under treatment in children. Therefore, patient/carer education regarding appropriate topical steroid use is a crucial part of eczema management.

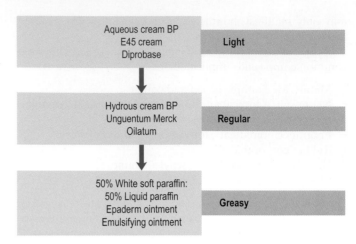

Fig. 57.6 Commonly used emollients used in dry skin conditions (adapted from MeReC, 1998).

Topical steroids are classified into four main groups according to potency: mild, moderately potent, potent and very potent (Table 57.2). The choice of topical steroid is dependent on the site and severity of skin disease. Potent and very potent steroids should be avoided on delicate sites such as the face, genitals and flexures. The periorbital region should be treated with caution due to the thin skin increasing the likelihood of absorption and risk of cataracts or glaucoma. Treatment should be reviewed regularly and tailored accordingly. It is also important to remember that any form of occlusion will increase the absorption of steroid applied.

Side effects are mainly local and include striae (stretch marks), telangiectasia (visible dilated small blood vessels), epidermal thinning, purpura (bruising), acne and perioral dermatitis. Lower frequency side effects include poor wound healing, spread or worsening of untreated infections and hypertrichosis. Hypopigmentation is a temporary side effect of long-term topical steroid use and is frequently

Table 57.2 Comparative potencies of topical corticosteroid preparations

UK Steroid Group	Trade name	Strength	Relative strength compared to hydrocortisone
Hydrocortisone 0.5–2.5%	Hydrocortisone	Mild	1
Fluocinolone acetonide 0.0025%	Synalar 1:10 dilution®		
Betamethasone valerate 0.025%	Betnovate RD®	Moderately potent	2.5× stronger
Clobetasone butyrate 0.05%	Eumovate®		
Fluocinolone acetonide 0.00625%	Synalar 1 in 4 dilution®		
Fludroxycortide 0.0125%	Haelan®		
Betametasone valerate 0.1%	Betnovate®	Potent	10× stronger
Mometasone furoate 0.1%	Elocon®		
Clobetasol propionate 0.05%	Dermovate®	Very potent	50× stronger

exploited in illegal 'skin bleaching' agents. Rarely, adrenal suppression or Cushing's syndrome due to systemic absorption may occur.

Local and systemic side effects are extremely rare with appropriate use and duration of topical steroid treatment. Patients should be advised to spread preparations thinly either once or twice daily. The recommended amount used can be quantified using a fingertip unit (Fig. 57.7). The quantity in this unit is sufficient to cover an area the size of two adult palms. Table 57.3 details the quantities for application to different sites required for twice-daily treatment for 1 week.

Base

Topical corticosteroids are available in ointment (oil based), cream (water based), aqueous or alcoholic solution, gel, foam or shampoo formulation for the scalp. In general, ointment preparations are preferable to creams in eczema management because they are absorbed better and have fewer preservative chemicals. Alcoholic solutions may lead to irritation and should not be applied to acutely inflamed or broken skin.

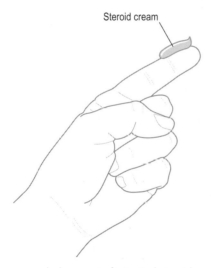

Steroid cream

Fig. 57.7 Recommended amount of a topical steroid corresponding to one fingertip unit.

Table 57.3 Minimum quantity of topical application required for twice daily treatment for 1 week (courtesy of M. Carr).

Age	Whole body	Trunk	Both arms and legs
6 months	35	15	20
4 years	60	20	35
8 years	90	35	50
12 years	120	45	65
Adult (70 kg)	170	60	90

Allergies

Both immediate and delayed hypersensitivity reactions to topical corticosteroids can occur, although not commonly. These can be reactions to either the steroid molecule itself or the vehicle in which it is found. Allergic reactions to one topical steroid may cross-react to others. Therefore, allergy testing is mandatory for such patients. Betamethasone may be less likely to cause allergic reactions than other topical preparations.

Antibiotics and steroid combinations

Combination preparations can be useful in treating mild bacterial infection of eczematous skin. Long-term use should be limited due to the risks of sensitisation and antibiotic resistance. In general, invasive infection is best managed with oral antibiotics.

Calcineurin inhibitors

The past decade saw the introduction of topical calcineurin inhibitors for the treatment of chronic eczema. These non-steroid immunomodulators inhibit calcineurin phosphatase which is important in T-lymphocyte activation. The main side effect is burning or stinging on initial application, but this usually improves after a few days. Although a theoretical risk of increased malignancy exists with these agents, studies have not shown an association between exposure to topical calcineurin inhibitors and increased rates of cutaneous malignancy. Calcineurin inhibitors should not be used on infected skin and are generally not very useful in severely inflamed eczematous skin. Their greatest value appears to be in maintenance therapy.

Tacrolimus ointment (Protopic®) is a calcineurin inhibitor derived from the oral transplant medicine FK506. The 0.1% and 0.03% preparations are indicated in the treatment of moderate to severe atopic dermatitis in adults and children over the age of 2 years. Tacrolimus is now also used in clinical practice as a second-line agent for other steroid responsive dermatoses.

Pimecrolimus 1% cream (Elidel®) is indicated for short-term or intermittent long-term use in mild to moderate atopic dermatitis. Studies have shown that it is effective, well tolerated and has minimal adverse effects in the long-term control of eczema in children aged over 2 years (Langley et al., 2008). Furthermore, this has resulted in the reduced use of topical steroids leading to a lower risk of steroid-induced side effects (Kapp et al., 2002).

Antihistamines

Pruritis is the most distressing feature of eczema. Oral antihistamines have no direct effect on pruritis in eczema; their main effect is sedation. Sedating antihistamines may cause day time drowsiness, and caution should be taken when driving and also if prescribed to school age children.

Topical imidazoles

Ketoconazole as a shampoo or cream is effective in reduction of *Pityosporum ovale* on the skin and is therefore useful in the treatment of seborrhoeic dermatitis. As the disease runs a chronic, relapsing course regular or intermittent use is usually necessary.

Coal tar preparations

Tar creams and ointments can be used in the management of hyperkeratotic, lichenified eczema. These are less cosmetically acceptable than other topical preparations, but coal tar is an effective anti-pruritic.

Bandaging

In children with atopic eczema, occlusion with bandages is useful to prevent scratching and potentiate the action of ointments and creams on the skin. Wet wrapping involves the application of emollients and steroids under a double layer to keep the inner layer moist. Parents can be trained to apply these bandages at home.

Systemic therapies

Systemic steroids

Oral prednisolone can be used as a short-term treatment in the management of severe acute eczema that needs rapid control. Long-term treatment with oral steroids is now rarely used due to the risk of side effects including hypertension and osteoporosis.

Ciclosporin

Ciclosporin is a systemic immunosuppressant that blocks activation of T-lymphocytes. It is effective as a short-term bridging therapy in severe chronic adult eczema and has a rapid onset of action. Intermittent courses at doses of 2.5–5 mg/kg/day are useful, but dose-related renal nephrotoxicity is inevitable and limits treatment duration to a maximum of 8–12 months. Other side effects include hypertension and increased risk of malignancy. A detailed patient history is required to determine if there is a previous history of gynaecologic or prostate malignancy. During treatment with ciclosporin, patients also require close monitoring of renal function and blood pressure.

Azathioprine

Azathioprine is a purine analogue that inhibits DNA synthesis and can be effective as monotherapy in adult eczema. Bone marrow suppression and toxicity are the major concerns. A higher risk of marrow suppression occurs in individuals with low levels of thiopurine methyltransferase (TPMT), and this should be assessed at screening. Patients with borderline TPMT levels require a lower dose of azathioprine. Patients with low levels of TPMT should not be offered this treatment.

Methotrexate

Methotrexate is occasionally used in unresponsive adult atopic eczema, but randomised controlled trials are lacking. A small prospective trial has shown that methotrexate can be effective and well tolerated as a second-line therapy for the treatment of moderate to severe atopic eczema in adults (Weatherhead et al., 2007).

Mycophenolate mofetil

Mycophenolate mofetil is an oral systemic agent that prevents T- and B-cell proliferation, thereby reducing inflammatory cytokine release. This can be used as an alternative in severe adult atopic dermatitis where azathioprine or ciclosporin are contraindicated. Side effects are gastro-intestinal upset, bone marrow suppression and an increased risk of infection.

Phototherapy

Phototherapy can be effective in select cases of atopic dermatitis. Narrow-band UVB is the therapy of choice (Gambichler et al., 2005; Meduri et al., 2007). The potential side effects of all types of phototherapy include burning, premature ageing and a small increased risk of skin cancer. A small proportion of patients have photosensitive eczema, and this should be determined by taking a detailed patient history before prescribing phototherapy treatment. A treatment course requires a patient to attend two or three times a week for at least 6 weeks.

Dietary supplements

Current evidence suggests that probiotics are not an effective treatment for eczema and may carry a small risk of adverse events such as infection and small bowel ischaemia. There is no evidence for use of evening primrose oil. The use of Chinese herbal medications in atopic eczema is under close scrutiny, and conflicting results have been obtained. Liver function should be monitored as hepatitis is a known side effect of some Chinese herbal medicines.

Interactions with drugs used in the treatment of eczema and psoriasis are shown in Table 57.4.

Patient care

It is important to recognise that eczema affects many aspects of a patient's life and has considerable effects on the family. Quality-of-life factors affected include body image, irritability and loss of sleep due to profound itch and limitations to work and hobbies (Fig. 57.8). A multidisciplinary approach is often needed in overcoming these issues, and healthcare workers including primary care doctors, dermatologists, specialist nurses, pharmacists and teachers may be involved. Patients with eczema should aim to lead as normal a life as possible, and school staff and employers can play an important part in achieving this goal.

Patient and parental education is important as treatments are designed to control and manage the disease. Although atopic eczema is likely to improve throughout childhood, expectations of an immediate cure need to be addressed. Advice and support through contact with other patients and their families can be obtained from the National Eczema Society (www.eczema.org). An algorithm for the management of eczema is shown in Fig. 57.9.

Psoriasis

Psoriasis is a chronic inflammatory disorder of the skin and joints. The current prevalence in Europe and North America is estimated to be between 1% and 3%. The usual presentation is with well-demarcated red plaques with an overlying scale.

Table 57.4 Interactions with drugs used in the treatment of eczema and psoriasis (courtesy of M. Carr)

	Interacting drug	Outcome
Methotrexate	Aspirin	Increased plasma concentration and toxicity of methotrexate
	NSAIDs	Increased plasma concentration and toxicity of methotrexate
	Probenecid	Increased plasma concentration and toxicity of methotrexate
	Phenytoin	Increased bone marrow toxicity
	Sulphonamides	Increased toxicity
	Trimethoprim	Increased antifolate effect of methotrexate
Azathioprine	Allopurinol	Enhanced effect and toxicity of azathioprine
	Warfarin	Inhibition of anticoagulant effect
	Cimetidine	Enhanced myelosuppression
	Indometacin	Increased risk of leucopenia
Ciclosporin	NSAIDs	Increased risk of nephrotoxicity
	Aminoglycosides	Increased risk of nephrotoxicity
	Co-trimoxazole	Increased risk of nephrotoxicity
	Ciprofloxacin	Increased risk of nephrotoxicity
	Ketoconazole	Increased plasma concentration of ciclosporin
	Itraconazole	Increased plasma concentration of ciclosporin
	Erythromycin	Increased plasma concentration of ciclosporin
	Oral contraceptives	Increased plasma concentration of ciclosporin
	Calcium channel blockers	Increased plasma concentration of ciclosporin
	Phenytoin	Decreased plasma concentration of ciclosporin
	Carbamazepine	Decreased plasma concentration of ciclosporin
	Rifampicin	Decreased plasma concentration of ciclosporin
Acitretin	Methotrexate	Increased plasma concentration of methotrexate

Aetiology

The aetiology of psoriasis is a combination of genetic and environmental factors. In most cases, there is a genetic predisposition and up to 70% of patients report a family history of psoriasis. Recent advances in genome-wide association

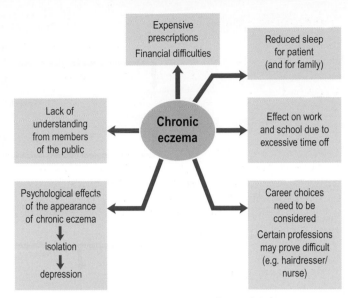

Fig. 57.8 The social and psychological effects of chronic eczema.

studies have led to the identification of at least nine chromosomal psoriasis susceptibility loci. Multiple genes are likely to influence disease susceptibility, severity and clinical subtype. The strongest association is with HLA-CW*06.

Precipitating factors

Non-inherited factors also have a role in triggering psoriasis in predisposed individuals. These are described as follows.

Infections

Bacterial infections have been implicated as triggers for psoriasis. Streptococcal infections, particularly pharyngitis, frequently precede the onset of guttate psoriasis. HIV infection can aggravate psoriasis. The severity of the psoriasis is greater in this patient population.

Drugs

Drugs can exacerbate or induce psoriasis in predisposed individuals. The most common causative agents are lithium, ß-blockers, anti-malarials, non-steroidal anti-inflammatory drugs (NSAIDs), tetracyclines and rapid withdrawal of systemic corticosteroids.

Alcohol and smoking

Excess alcohol consumption may exacerbate established psoriasis. Additionally, psoriasis is associated with high rates of alcoholism due to the psychological stresses of the disease.

Smoking is strongly associated with palmoplantar psoriasis; up to 95% of patients with this variant are smokers at disease onset. Smoking cessation should be actively addressed due to a likely improvement in disease status and associated risk reduction of ischaemic heart disease. It has been suggested that psoriasis,

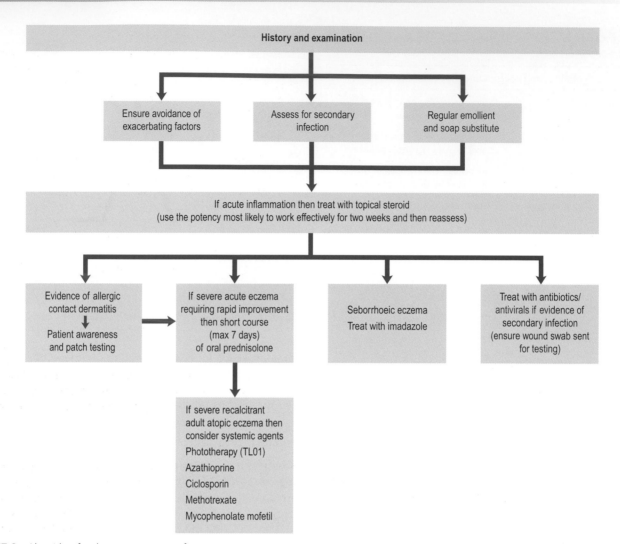

Fig. 57.9 Algorithm for the management of eczema.

particularly if severe, may be an independent risk factor for athero-sclerosis, myocardial infarction and stroke (Mehta et al., 2010).

Emotional stress

Anecdotal observations and frequent patient reports identify stress as an important trigger factor for psoriasis. Clinical evidence has demonstrated that the onset and severity of psoriasis can correlate with prior stress (Kirby et al., 2008). Furthermore, psychological distress and depression can occur as a consequence of psoriasis.

Koebner phenomenon

The Koebner phenomenon refers to psoriatic lesions which occur at sites of injury to the skin, such as a cut, burn, scratch or surgical scar, in patients with psoriasis.

Pathology and clinical features

The clinical features of psoriasis, well-demarcated, erythematous scaly plaques, are explained by the histological features (Fig. 57.10). Common sites affected include the scalp, buttocks, elbows, knees and nails.

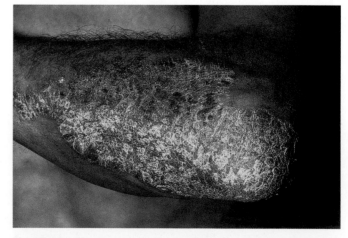

Fig. 57.10 Chronic scaly plaque psoriasis on an elbow (courtesy of M. Carr).

Histologically, the epidermis is thickened (acanthosis), with a thickened upper horny layer (hyperkeratosis) which is reflected by the clinical features of thick, scaly skin. The build of scale is due to increased epidermal turnover. The differentiation of cells through the epidermis terminating in the keratin horny layer normally takes approximately 40 days. Epidermal turnover in psoriatic skin may be as rapid as 7 days. In the dermis, the capillaries are dilated, tortuous and closer to the surface of the skin. This explains Auspitz's sign which is the appearance of pinpoint bleeding after scraping off psoriasis scales.

Inflammatory cells are present in all layers of psoriatic skin; granulocytes are predominant and form microabscesses in the epidermis. Lymphocytes and Langerhans cells are also increased. The presence of lymphocytes in the epidermis led to hypotheses of an immunological cytokine-mediated process causing epidermal hyperproliferation and changes in vascular structure. T-cells, dendritic cells and cytokines such as tumour necrosis factor alpha (TNFα), interleukin (IL)-12 and IL-23 all contribute to its pathogenesis. This is confirmed by the therapeutic effect of drugs that suppress T-lymphocyte function, such as ciclosporin, in psoriasis.

Clinical types

Psoriasis vulgaris

Psoriasis vulgaris, also known as chronic plaque psoriasis, is the most common variant. It can occur at any age but most often begins in young adulthood and has a chronic relapsing course. The typical psoriatic lesion is a red, sharply demarcated plaque with overlying silvery scale. The distribution is usually symmetrical and involves extensor sites such as the elbows and knees. The sacrum, scalp and nails are also commonly affected. The plaques may itch but not usually to the severity of eczematous plaques. Treatment is aimed at management of disease rather than cure.

Guttate psoriasis

Guttate psoriasis is more commonly seen in children and young adults and is characterised by a widespread scaly eruption of small 'teardrop-like' scaly plaques (Fig. 57.11). The presentation is often acute and can appear 10–14 days after a streptococcal upper respiratory tract infection. Topical treatments or UVB phototherapy are usually effective. Spontaneous resolution is common; however, guttate psoriasis may be the first manifestation of psoriasis in predisposed individuals.

Scalp psoriasis

Involvement of the scalp may be the only manifestation of psoriasis in some patients, but may also occur in psoriasis vulgaris. This appears as scaly demarcated plaques extending to the hairline and around the ears. Hair loss is rare.

Psoriatic nail disease

The nails are frequently affected in psoriasis. In a small proportion of patients, the nails are the only area affected. Changes include nail pitting, nail ridging, onycholysis (separation of the nail from the nail bed), hyperkeratosis under the nail and complete nail destruction. These symptoms can be cosmetically disfiguring. Topical treatments are rarely effective for psoriatic nail disease. Systemic treatments such as methotrexate, when prescribed for generalised psoriasis, may also improve nail disease.

Palmoplantar psoriasis

At these sites on the palms and soles, there is sharp demarcation of the involved areas (Fig. 57.12). Palmoplantar psoriasis can take two forms: either inflamed hyperkeratotic fissured skin which can be very painful or sterile pustules on an erythematous base which dry to leave small brown macules (palmoplantar pustulosis). The pustular form is much commoner in smokers.

Flexural psoriasis

Psoriasis can occur at flexural sites such as the axillae, groin, submammary areas and genitalia. Due to friction and moisture within skin folds, lesions differ in appearance from classical psoriasis and tend to be red and glazed rather than scaly. Affected areas tend to be clearly demarcated. Secondary infections,

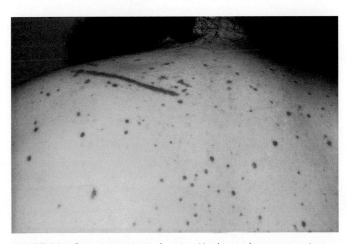

Fig. 57.11 Guttate psoriasis showing Koebner phenomenon in scratch mark (courtesy of M. Carr).

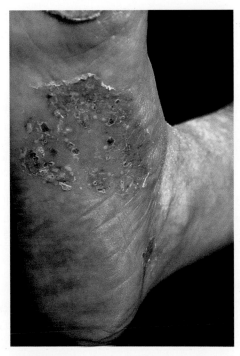

Fig. 57.12 Pustular psoriasis of sole (courtesy of M. Carr).

and general malaise. Pustular psoriasis may be precipitated by the withdrawal of systemic or very potent topical steroid. Therefore, oral steroids are avoided in the management of stable psoriasis.

Psoriatic arthropathy

Approximately 25% of psoriatic patients suffer with an associated arthropathy. There are five patterns of psoriatic arthropathy; monoarthopathy, rheumatoid arthritis-like, osteoarthritis-like, sacroiliitis-like and arthritis mutilans. Rheumatoid factor is negative in these patients. Some treatments effective for skin psoriasis are also effective in psoriatic arthropathy including methotrexate, and biological agents with action against TNFα.

Treatment

Many patients with psoriasis have mild disease and require only emollient therapy to prevent drying and fissuring of the elbows and knees. Other treatment options should take into account the type of psoriasis, patient occupation and lifestyle factors as well as disease severity. This will ensure improved patient compliance and better outcome.

Topical therapy

First-line treatment of mild to moderate psoriasis should include an emollient as well as a topical treatment. Mild to moderate topical steroids are useful for delicate skin sites such as the face and flexures. Dithranol and tar products are effective, but limitations of use include irritation, messy application and potent odour. Topical treatments may be technically difficult to apply to the scalp area; patient education and demonstration is key. Topical vitamin D analogues are well tolerated.

Vitamin D analogues

Vitamin D analogues inhibit keratinocyte differentiation and production. The most commonly prescribed Vitamin D analogue is calcipotriol. This is commonly used within primary care for mild localised psoriasis and is available as a lotion, ointment, cream or scalp treatment. Patients should be advised to avoid use on delicate skin sites such as the face and flexures due to irritation. Hypercalcaemia due to systemic absorption can occur if the maximum weekly dose exceeds 100 g. Efficacy may be enhanced when used in combination with a topical steroid.

Steroids

Topical steroids are cosmetically acceptable and easy to apply. Mild to moderately potent steroids are of greatest value in acutely inflamed psoriasis to reduce inflammation. Reduction of inflammation is important as it then allows other treatments to be introduced that would otherwise irritate acutely inflamed plaques. Topical steroids have a number of limitations. The use of potent steroids on large areas of psoriasis is associated with

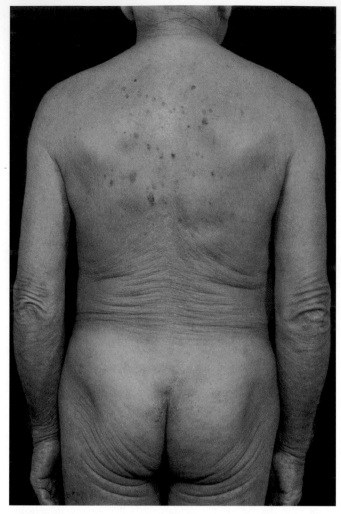

Fig. 57.13 Erythrodermic psoriasis, courtesy of St John's Institute of Dermatology, London.

particularly with *Candida* are common. Potent steroids are not advised at these sites due to the high risk of skin atrophy.

Erythrodermic psoriasis

Erythroderma, or exfoliative dermatitis, is a severe, potentially life-threatening condition in which more than 90% of the body surface is red and scaly (see Fig. 57.13). This can occur as a consequence of either eczema or psoriasis. Skin function is impaired and patients suffer dehydration, electrolyte imbalance, temperature dysregulation and serious secondary infection. These patients need urgent hospital admission, medical supportive therapy and topical treatment. Initially, bland emollients such as white soft paraffin and mild to moderate topical steroids should be used. Underlying conditions, such as psoriasis, can then be treated with appropriate systemic agents.

Generalised pustular psoriasis

This is an acute, unstable form of psoriasis manifesting as widespread sheets of tiny sterile pustules on an erythematous base. The patient is usually systemically unwell with fever risks of local atrophy and systemic absorption. Furthermore, there is a rebound effect on withdrawal. Potent steroids should be reserved for localised disease, such as thicker acral sites, often in combination with salicylic acid if there is hyperkeratosis. In general, very potent steroids should be avoided.

Coal tar

Along with dithranol, coal tar is one of the oldest topical treatments for psoriasis. Coal tar has anti-inflammatory, antibacterial, anti-pruritic and antimitotic effects. A variety of preparations are available including bath preparations, shampoos, creams and ointment. Coal tar concentrations of 1–10% can be used, but use of higher concentrations should occur in a supervised setting. Coal tar in combination with topical steroids can be effective, for example Alphosyl HC®. The efficacy of tar is enhanced when used with UVB light therapy (Goerkerman regimen). The main limitations of tar are irritation of delicate skin sites, odour and temporary staining of skin and clothing. The theoretical risk of carcinogenesis due to polycyclic aromatic hydrocarbons has not been demonstrated in long-term clinical practice.

Dithranol

Dithranol (anthralin in the USA) is a synthetic anthracene derivative which has an anti-proliferative and anti-inflammatory effect on the skin. It is one of the older treatments used for stable, chronic plaque psoriasis. Although effective, practical drawbacks include burning and irritation of normal skin, staining of clothes as well as a strong odour. In current practice, dithranol is most commonly used as a short contact regimen within a dermatology day centre setting. The starting concentration of dithranol is usually 0.5% which can be increased slowly if tolerated up to 3%.

Salicylic acid

This is useful to reduce scale, particularly while treating hyperkeratosis of the palms and soles. It can be mixed with coal tar, steroid or urea.

Topical retinoids

Retinoids are less effective than vitamin D analogues in the treatment of psoriasis. Irritation is a possible side effect to therapy.

Topical treatment of psoriasis at special sites
Scalp

Tar shampoo is effective in mild scalp psoriasis. However, a descaling agent is required as part of therapy for thicker plaques. Coconut oil compounds, peanut oil and greasy emollient with salicylic acid can be used as descaling agents. A topical steroid can then be applied for inflammatory disease. Treatment does require considerable time and commitment from the patient.

Genitals

The genital regions are prone to irritation and mild to moderate topical steroids can be used. In addition, it is also important to inform patients that treatments used on other parts of the body may be too potent and irritant for genital areas.

Nails

Before treatment of psoriasis, fungal infections of the nails should be excluded. Topical treatments often have poor efficacy in psoriasis affecting the nail, and systemic therapy is preferred.

Phototherapy

The majority of psoriatic patients exhibit improvement of symptoms on sunny holidays, with only 10% of patients reporting deterioration in symptoms on sun exposure. Phototherapy has an immunosuppressive effect on skin and has been used in the treatment of psoriasis for over 80 years. Narrow-band UVB (311–313 nm) is preferable to broadband UVB (290–320 nm) due to increased safety and reduced risk of burning.

PUVA

PUVA (psoralens plus UVA light) has a valuable role in the treatment of stable moderate to severe psoriasis. Psoralens are drugs that are activated by long-wave ultraviolet light (320–400 nm), thereby interfering with DNA synthesis and reducing epidermal turnover. The two psoralens available in the UK are 8-MOP (methoxypsoralen) and 5-MOP. These are taken orally 2 h before exposure to UVA light. The eyes are always protected due to the risk of cataracts and patients are given sunglasses to wear for 12 h after treatment. The treatment is usually given twice a week for a 6-week period. Total cumulative dosage is carefully monitored.

The commonest adverse effect is nausea due to ingestion of oral psoralens. The most serious adverse effect is an increased risk of long-term cutaneous malignancy. Those with fair skin types and on past or present immunosuppresion are at greatest risk. Due to these risks, PUVA is usually reserved for patients resistant to UVB therapy.

Systemic therapy

Systemic therapy is indicated in severe widespread psoriasis, intolerant of or rapidly relapsing after topical therapy and phototherapy. Objective measures of disease severity and impact on quality of life are used routinely to assess need for systemic therapy and treatment response and include the Psoriasis Area and Severity Index (PASI) and the Dermatology Quality of Life Index (DLQI). Systemic treatments commonly prescribed in psoriasis include methotrexate, acitretin and ciclosporin. Drug interactions are important and a detailed patient drug history is important. New biologic agents are used in severe disease which is unresponsive to oral immunosuppressant treatment. Common adverse effects and monitoring requirements of systemic treatments of eczema and psoriasis are presented in Table 57.5.

Table 57.5 Common adverse effects and monitoring requirements for systemic treatments of eczema and psoriasis

Therapy	Adverse Effects	Monitoring requirements
Methotrexate	Hepatic fibrosis; myelosuppression; nausea; pulmonary fibrosis; teratogenic (contraindicated in both males and females for 4 weeks before and 3 months after treatment)	FBC U&E LFT Pro-collagen III peptide (P3NP) ±Liver biopsy Chest X-Ray (screening)
Hydroxyurea	Myelosuppression; skin reaction; teratogenic; liver toxicity (narrow therapeutic window)	FBC U&Es LFT
Ciclosporin	Renal nephrotoxicity Hypertension Gingival hypertrophy	FBC U&E LFT Lipid profile Blood pressure Urinalysis
Acitretin	Teratogenic (including up to 2 years post-treatment) Dryness of mucous membranes and skin Hyperostoses, increased serum triglyceride Occasional hepatotoxic reaction	FBC U&E LFT Lipid profile
Fumaric Acid Esters	Gastro-intestinal side effects Flushing Lymphopenia Proteinuria Renal failure	FBC U&E LFT Urinalysis
Azathioprine	Myelosuppression Deranged liver function Gastro-intestinal effects	TPMT pre-treatment FBC/U&E/LFT

U&Es, urea and electrolytes; LFTs, liver function tests; FBC, full blood count; TPMT, thiopurine methyl transferase genetic polymorphism screening.

Methotrexate

Methotrexate is a folic acid antagonist used in moderate to severe psoriasis. In males and females of non-childbearing potential, this tends to be the first-line systemic agent. It is also effective in psoriatic arthropathy. Methotrexate is given as a once weekly oral low dose regimen, with an initial test dose of 5 mg increasing up to 30 mg weekly. Acute toxicity occurs due to the effect of methotrexate on folic acid metabolism of rapidly dividing cells in the bone marrow and gastro-intestinal tract. This can cause myelosuppression or gastro-intestinal bleeding. In such cases, folinic acid rescue can be used to oppose the folate antagonist effect at a dose of 120 mg folinic acid over 12–24 h intravenously or intramuscularly in divided doses, followed by 15 mg/kg orally every 6 h for 48 h. Hepatic fibrosis is the commonest long-term risk and regular monitoring of liver function is necessary. Some patients complain of nausea and other gastro-intestinal side effects as well as lethargy. Folic acid 5 mg taken on the days methotrexate is not prescribed can reduce these adverse effects.

Patient monitoring in methotrexate therapy is detailed in Table 57.5. Liver function tests do not reliably predict hepatic fibrosis; supportive investigations are therefore required. Liver biopsy remains the gold standard. Recently, the measurement of serum pro-collagen three peptide levels has led to a reduction of liver biopsies for detection of hepatic fibrosis in these patients (Chalmers et al., 2005).

Acitretin

Acitretin, a vitamin A derivative that inhibits epidermal proliferation, is effective for disorders of keratinisation including chronic plaque psoriasis. The starting dose is usually 25–30 mg daily for 2–4 weeks increasing to 75 mg daily for short periods and according to clinical response. Mucocutaneous side effects, hair loss and lethargy are common. Acitretin should be avoided in women of childbearing potential because of the teratogenic risk. However, it is a safer option for patients with chronic infection for whom immunosuppression is contraindicated. Patients should be warned that a rebound response is occasionally seen when stopping treatment, and therefore a long-term maintenance dose is usually advised.

Ciclosporin

Ciclosporin is an effective treatment for all variants of psoriasis with a fairly rapid mode of action. The dose is 2–5 mg/kg. Similar to eczema management, continuous ciclosporin treatment for more than 1 year is not advised due to renal nephrotoxicity. Adverse events include hypertension, hypertrichosis, paraesthesia, tremor and increased risk of infections. There is also of an increased risk of skin cancer in conjunction with ciclosporin use in patients who have previously had phototherapy.

Hydroxyurea/hydroxycarbamide

Hydroxyurea/hydroxycarbamide is a drug with similar effects on bone marrow and germ cells to methotrexate but without the hepatotoxic effects. Relapse occurs on stopping treatment.

Fumaric acid esters

Fumaric acid esters have been used since the early 1960s and affect both keratinocytes and T-cell activity. It is licensed in Europe, but not in the UK, for severe, relapsing, chronic, plaque psoriasis. The main side effects are gastro-intestinal upset and flushing.

Biologic therapy

Biologic therapies or 'biologics' are drugs designed to block specific molecular steps important in immune-mediated disease. They have been used successfully in rheumatoid arthritis, inflammatory bowel disease and are now licensed for use in chronic plaque psoriasis. Their use is recommended for patients with severe plaque psoriasis defined as a PASI ≥ 10 and DLQI > 10 who have failed at least two standard systemic agents including methotrexate, ciclosporin and acitretin or one systemic agent and phototherapy (Smith et al., 2009).

TNFα antagonists

TNFα is a pro-inflammatory cytokine that plays a central role in the pathogenesis of psoriasis. The tumour necrosis factor antagonists: infliximab, adalimumab and etanercept all have potent immunosuppressant action and have proven efficacy in severe psoriasis. Serious adverse effects include infection, in particular reactivation of tuberculosis, exacerbation of severe cardiac failure, demyelinating disease and a potential risk of malignancy (solid organ tumours and lymphoma). Careful patient selection and regular monitoring are important.

Etanercept is a genetically engineered receptor fusion protein with affinity for soluble TNFα. The dose is 25 mg twice weekly via subcutaneous injection. Higher doses of 50 mg twice a week are used in psoriatic arthropathy. The most frequent side effects are injection site reactions.

Infliximab is a chimeric monoclonal antibody against TNFα. It is also used in Crohn's disease, ulcerative colitis, ankylosing spondylitis and rheumatoid arthritis. Clinical trials have demonstrated rapid onset and good efficacy in psoriasis.

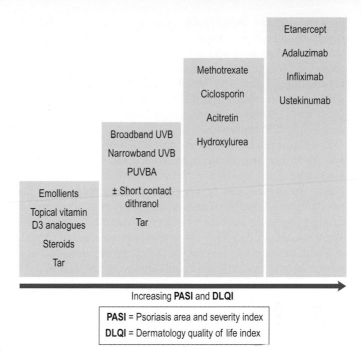

Fig. 57.14 Treatment algorithm for psoriasis.

Infliximab is administered at a dose of 5 mg/kg by intravenous infusion every 8 weeks after a loading dose at weeks 0, 2 and 6. Observation and nursing care on a day unit are therefore required.

Adalimumab is humanised monoclonal antibody against TNFα that is administered in a bolus of 80 mg subcutaneously and then 40 mg on alternate weeks.

Other biologic agents used in psoriasis

Ustekinumab is the newest available biologic agent used in the treatment of psoriasis. It is a fully human monoclonal antibody that prevents IL-12 and IL-23 from binding receptor proteins. A dose of 45 mg (or 90 mg in patients weighing >100 kg) is administered subcutaneously at week 0, 4 then every 12 weeks. In light of the limited patient exposure to this treatment, ustekinumab is reserved for use as a second-line biologic agent where TNF therapy has failed or cannot be used.

Efaluzimab, a T-cell modulator, was withdrawn in 2009 due to an increased risk of progressive multifocal leucoencephalopathy.

A treatment algorithm for psoriasis is shown in Fig. 57.14.

Patient care

Psoriasis is a chronic disease associated with significant psychosocial disability and reduction in quality of life. As well as effects related to depression; impact on body image and sexual relationships should be considered. Coexistent psoriatic arthropathy may have a severe impact on function and lead to significant time away from work or education. Support and understanding of individual patients' needs and lifestyles will improve adherence to treatment. Psoriasis can be associated with alcohol misuse, and a drug and alcohol history should always be sought. Systemic and biologic treatments require regular attendance and blood tests, and therefore patients with poor attendance records may not be suitable for such treatment. Ultimately, responsibility lies with the patient to ensure regular treatment.

The chronicity of this disease may lead to treatment 'fatigue' and frustration with messy topical therapies. There are numerous alternatives and newer formulations are generally less messy. Treatments can be expensive and information on the entitlement to benefits to replace clothing ruined by ointments or washing machines worn out by constant use is available. The Psoriasis Association (www.psoriasis-association.org.uk) provides an excellent service for this, together with practical advice from fellow sufferers about day-to-day problems.

Case studies

Case 57.1

A 3-year-old child with known atopic eczema is seen in clinic with a widespread, excoriated, dry rash (see Fig. 57.15). Her eczema symptoms started at the age of 6 weeks. Her sleep has always been poor due to the marked itch symptoms at night. She has had two recent courses of oral antibiotics for presumed bacterial skin infection. Her normal skin treatment involves hydrocortisone 1% ointment to affected areas twice daily. Her parents are concerned regarding the possible triggers of her eczema flares and are keen to pursue possible allergy testing.

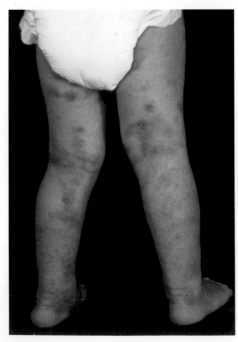

Fig. 57.15 Case study 1 – a young child with moderate/severe atopic eczema courtesy of St John's Institute of Dermatology, London.

Question

What advice could be given to the child's parents?

Answer

Fig. 57.15 shows a young child with moderate/severe atopic eczema. Ill-defined, dry, erythematous patches of eczema are visible. A few of the patches around her ankles appear crusty and eroded. This may represent secondary infection.

Management should include regular topical emollient therapy. The correct quantities should be emphasised. A regular soap substitute should be prescribed.

Wound swabs should always be taken before prescribing an oral antibiotic for presumed infected eczema.

A moderately potent steroid ointment should be administered daily, along with a regular, greasy topical emollient. When a moderately potent or potent topical steroid is prescribed for a child, medical follow-up must be arranged. Regular use of potent steroids is not advised and will lead to local side effects including skin atrophy. If the treatment is ineffective, a short admission to hospital or regular day care should be arranged for further intensive topical treatments or dressings.

Time should be spent explaining to the parents the aetiology of atopic eczema. Although eczema is usually a chronic disease with no 'cure', it should also be explained that approximately 60% of children will have minimal or no symptoms after the age of 16.

Allergy testing is commonly requested by parents, but as most children will grow out of their symptoms as well as food sensitivities, formal testing is not always appropriate. Allergy testing may involve blood tests, including RAST tests, and skin prick tests. These may not be a pleasant experience for a young child. A positive result does not directly correlate with the effect of allergen avoidance on the course of atopic eczema. High street or internet allergy tests have no benefit in atopic eczema.

Case 57.2

A 22-year-old male nurse attends outpatients complaining of dry, painful eczema affecting his hands. He had previously suffered with childhood eczema and asthma. Since starting his new job, his symptoms have developed causing severe pain, fissures, itch and dry skin. His finger pulps are particularly affected. He attended occupational health and was then advised to see a dermatologist.

Question

What is the likely cause of his symptoms and what advice should be given?

Answer

The aetiology of hand dermatitis is often complex and multi-factorial. An atopic predisposition, irritant factors as well as allergic contact type IV hypersensitivity may all play a part. In view of his atopic eczema during childhood, he is at greater risk of irritant and ACD than the general population. The need for this patient to constantly wash his hands with antiseptic hand wash and excessive contact with water is likely to be an exacerbating factor. Alternatives to antiseptic washes include a moisturising soap substitute, for example Dermol 500®.

A potent topical steroid and emollient with a good barrier effect should be prescribed. Tape impregnated with a steroid preparation, for example Haelan® tape may be useful to protect fissured areas on his hands. Patch testing would be the next step to investigate a possible allergic contact component to his symptoms.

Young adults with moderate or severe eczema should be given career guidance to avoid occupations at higher risk of leading to ICD, for instance hairdressing, domestic cleaning or working in a healthcare environment that requires constant hand washing.

Case 57.3

A 28-year-old male management executive with lifelong atopic eczema has attended with worsening severity of his eczema. He has been using emollients and moderately potent topical steroids for many years and feels that these are no longer having an effect. Over the past year, he has required two short courses of oral steroids. His sleep is affected and he cannot afford to take any further time off work.

Question

What are the treatment options for this man?

Answer

This patient needs effective treatment before he becomes erythrodermic. High-dose systemic steroids over a 2-week period may have a rapid effect but are not a long-term option. His topical regime should be explored to ensure adequate quantities of emollient are being used. In addition, his aims, expectations and medical issues should be explored with a view to possible systemic treatment.

If more than a few weeks of treatment are anticipated, ciclosporin is a possible treatment option. Pre-treatment screening should include blood pressure, urinalysis and blood tests including renal function. A short course of ciclosporin treatment no longer than 12 months would alleviate his symptoms, improve his mental well being and give him a break from his chronic skin disease. If longer-term systemic management is anticipated, azathioprine would be an option, but efficacy would only be evident after approximately 8 weeks of treatment.

Case 57.4

A 9-year-old boy with known atopic eczema presented with a vesicular, blistering eruption over his face and trunk (see Fig. 57.16). His mother noticed the blisters 48 h ago and brought him to hospital as he was unwell and feverish. He had been using topical steroids and emollients regularly for his moderate atopic eczema. His sister has recently been suffering with cold sores.

Question

Fig. 57.16 shows the young patient with eczema herpeticum. What advice would you give this patient and his mother?

Answer

Eczema herpeticum, Kaposi's varicelliform eruption, is an important and serious complication that can occur in eczema patients. This is a medical emergency and early treatment with aciclovir may prove lifesaving. This widespread eruption occurs following inoculation of herpes simplex virus to skin damaged by eczema. This then spreads rapidly and can affect the eyes and lungs. It usually

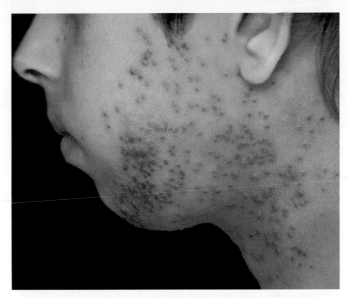

Fig. 57.16 Case study 4 – a young patient with eczema herpeticum courtesy of St John's Institute of Dermatology, London.

manifests in young children with atopic eczema. Typically, the tiny blisters, vesicles, develop in large numbers on eczematous skin and patients are systemically unwell. The blisters or erosions appear 'punched out' and may be pustular. Eye involvement, as suggested in Fig. 57.16, necessitates urgent ophthalmological review as herpes simplex ocular infection can lead to corneal ulceration, stromal keratitis, iritis and permanent visual loss.

Children with atopic eczema and their parents should be educated to recognise the signs and symptoms of eczema herpeticum.

Case 57.5

A 33-year-old electrician presents to clinic with a 5-month history of a mildly itchy eruption occurring around the nasal area and eyebrows (see Fig. 57.17). He describes it as occasionally scaly and is very concerned regarding the cosmetic appearance. On examination, he also has mild scale and erythema affecting the scalp. The dandruff shampoos he usually purchases from his local community pharmacy have been ineffective. The diagnosis is seborrheic dermatitis.

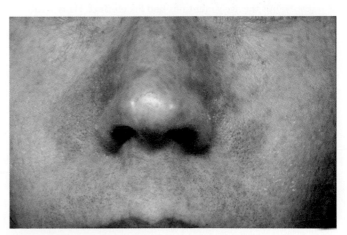

Fig. 57.17 Case study 5 – man with seborrheic dermatitis, courtesy of St John's Institute of Dermatology, London.

Question

What options would you offer for topical treatment?

Answer

Ketoconazole shampoo and ketoconazole 2% cream will reduce the population of *Pityosporum ovale* on the skin which may benefit symptoms. If symptomatic and itchy, a mild topical steroid with antifungal may be an option. In addition, patients should be counselled that seborrheic dermatitis is a common condition which may be chronic and periodic exacerbations may occur.

Case 57.6

A 55-year-old woman presents with a history of longstanding chronic plaque psoriasis. Since the age of 16, she has had numerous topical treatments which have not adequately managed her symptoms. Over the past 18 months, she has noticed swelling and pain over the proximal joints of both hands, which is much worse in the morning. On examination, she has early signs of deformity. NSAIDs have not alleviated her symptoms, and her function at work is now affected.

Question

What management options should be offered for this patient?

Answer

Psoriatic arthopathy affects up to 30% of patients with psoriasis. The resulting pain and functional disability of this arthropathy can be debilitating. However, non-steroidal anti-inflammatory medicines improve symptom control. Other treatment options include methotrexate, ciclosporin and TNFα antagonists. These medicines would also have a beneficial effect on this patient's psoriasis. Both rheumatology and dermatology services are required in the management of such patients.

Case 57.7

A 45-year-old man with psorasis has been complaining of an itchy scaly scalp for the last 8 months. He has seen his primary care doctor who as prescribed a topical steroid preparation (Betacap®), but this treatment has had little effect. He is troubled by thick scale and severe itch at night.

Question

What treatment options could be considered?

Answer

Treatment of scalp psoriasis differs from other forms of psoriasis because of the presence of thick hair. Topical treatments can be difficult and messy to apply. In addition, phototherapy is not usually effective at this site. Almost all topical preparations used to treat psoriasis on the body have equivalent scalp preparations, although the application method varies. Coal tar shampoos are usually suitable first-line treatments for scalp psoriasis. Aqueous and alcoholic scalp preparations will not penetrate thick scale which needs to be softened with emollient preparations first.

Arachis oil, provided the patient is not peanut allergic, or coconut oil are commonly used for this. Salicylic acid and coal tar preparations are often effective, and sometimes these are mixed with a coconut oil base (Sebco®, Cocois®). These preparations should be left on for approximately 1 h and then washed off. Topical steroids may be effective for inflamed skin, but will not penetrate thick scale. Intermittent rather than prolonged use of topical steroids is advised.

Case 57.8

A 45-year-old man has become increasingly disabled with palmoplantar pustular psoriasis. He has had frequent crops of inflamed pustules on the palms and soles which dry up to form crusts and scaling followed by painful fissuring of the skin. This has made his job as a joiner increasingly difficult, and he has had prolonged periods of absences through illness. He has tried emollients, topical steroid applications and steroid combinations but with only temporary relief.

Question

What are the best options for the treatment of this man?

Answer

Firstly, the patient should be advised to use regular emollient therapy. A topical treatment should also be prescribed such as a potent topical steroid in combination with a base such as propylene glycol or salicylic acid. Occlusion with either cotton gloves or cling film can improve skin penetration. However, this condition can be chronic and very disabling for manual workers, and therefore systemic therapy may be advised. In such cases, oral acitretin may be given for long-term use. The patient's fasting lipids and liver function should be monitored. If oral acitretin is contraindicated, hand and foot PUVA can be used. Patients diagnosed with palmoplantar pustulosis should be advised to stop smoking and be provided with appropriate support. This is because palmoplantar pustulosis has been found to improve after cessation of smoking (Michaëlsson et al., 2006).

Case 57.9

A 24-year-old man presents at the clinic with a 10-year history of plaque psoriasis affecting his elbows, knees and sacral area, with a few small plaques elsewhere. He is otherwise fit and well. He regularly plays football and is embarrassed by the appearance of his skin. He has tried Betnovate RD® ointment (0.025%), which smoothed the plaques a little, and calcipotriol ointment, which removed the scale from the plaques but did not clear them.

Question

What treatment could this patient try next?

Answer

As the patient only has a few localised plaques, a treatment course of short contact dithranol creams may be suitable. A starting concentration of 0.5% dithranol is tolerated by most patients. The dithranol strength can then be increased every 5–7 days. The effect can be enhanced by UVB treatment twice weekly at a dermatology department. The usual staining and burning with dithranol is minimised by short contact therapy, and any discolouration fades quickly after the treatment has stopped.

Case 57.10

A 35-year-old male patient with chronic plaque psoriasis has been reviewed. He has severe plaque psoriasis occurring on more than 50% of his body surface area. He has tried topical treatments and has also had UVB and PUVA therapy with little improvement. A course of methotrexate has failed to improve his symptoms and his work and psychological wellbeing are suffering. His PASI score is 25 and DLQI is 13.

Question

What treatment options could now be offered?

Answer

This patient would be considered eligible to receive treatment with any of the licensed biologic agents. Eligibility is based on having severe disease. This is defined as PASI score greater than 10 and a DLQI greater than 10 in addition to being unresponsive/intolerant to standard systemic therapy. Pre-treatment screening for infection including active or latent tuberculosis, congestive cardiac failure, demyelination and malignancy is required.

References

Chalmers, R.J., Kirby, B., Smith, A., et al., 2005. Replacement of routine liver biopsy by procollagen III aminopeptide for monitoring patients with psoriasis receiving long-term methotrexate: a multicentre audit and health economic analysis. Br. J. Dermatol. 152, 444–450.

Gambichler, T., Breuckmann, F., Boms, S., et al., 2005. Narrowband UVB phototherapy in skin conditions beyond psoriasis. J. Am. Acad. Dermatol. 52, 660–670.

Kapp, A., Papp, K., Bingham, A., et al., 2002. Flare reduction in eczema with Elidel (infants) multicenter investigator study group. Long-term management of atopic dermatitis in infants with topical pimecrolimus, a non steroid anti-inflammatory drug. J. Allergy Clin. Immunol. 110, 277–284.

Kirby, B., Richards, H.L., Mason, D.L., et al., 2008. Alcohol consumption and psychological distress in patients with psoriasis. Br. J. Dermatol. 158, 138–140.

Langley, R.G., Eichenfield, L.F., Lucky, A.W., et al., 2008. Sustained efficacy and safety of pimecrolimus cream 1% when used long term (up to 26 weeks) to treat children with atopic dermatitis. Pediatr. Dermatol. 25, 301–307.

Meduri, N.B., Vandergriff, T., Rasmussen, H., et al., 2007. Phototherapy in the management of atopic dermatitis: a systemic review. Photodermatol. Photoimmunol. Photomed. 23, 106–112.

Mehta, N.N., Azfar, R.S., Shin, D.B., et al., 2010. Patients with severe psoriasis are at increased risk of cardiovascular mortality: cohort study using the General Practice Research Database. Eur. Heart J. 3, 1000–1006.

MeReC, 1998. The use of emollients in dry skin conditions. MeReC Bull. 12, 45–48.

Michaëlsson, G., Gustafsson, K., Hagforsen, E., 2006. The psoriasis variant palmoplantar pustulosis can be improved after cessation of smoking. J. Am. Acad. Dermatol. 54(4), 737–738.

Smith, C.H., Anstey, A.V., Barker, J.N., et al., 2009. British Association of Dermatologists' guidelines for biologic interventions for psoriasis. Br. J. Dermatol. 161, 987–1019.

Weatherhead, S.C., Wahie, S., Reynolds, N.J., et al., 2007. An open-label, dose-ranging study of methotrexate for moderate to severe adult atopic eczema. Br. J. Dermatol. 156, 346–351.

Further reading

Ashton, R., Leppard, B., 2004. Differential Diagnosis in Dermatology, third ed. Radcliffe publishing limited, Oxford.

Boyle, R.J., Bath-Hextall, F.J., Leonardi-Bee, J., et al., 2008. Probiotics for treating eczema. Cochrane Database Sys. Rev. 4 Art No. CD006135. DOI: 10.1002/14651858.CD006135.pub2.

Brown, S., Reynolds, N.J., 2006. Atopic and non-atopic eczema. Br. Med. J. 332, 584–588.

Buxton, P., 2003. ABC of Dermatology, fourth ed. BMJ Books, London.

Ghaffar, S.A., Clements, S.E., Griffiths, C.E., 2005. Modern management of psoriasis. Clin. Med. 5, 564–568.

Hui, R.L., Lide, W., Chan, J., et al., 2009. Association between exposure to topical tacrolimus or pimecrolimus and cancers. Ann. Pharmacother. 43, 956–963.

Menter, A., Griffiths, C.E., 2007. Current and future management of psoriasis. Lancet 370, 272–284.

Williams, H.C., (Ed.), 2000. Atopic Dermatitis. Cambridge University Press, Cambridge.

58 Wounds

S. Holloway and K. Harding

Key points

- Acute wound healing should progress through an orderly sequence of events to re-establish tissue integrity.
- A functional blood vessel network is fundamental for wound healing.
- Changes occur in the repaired tissue for up to 2 years with the scar tissue becoming stronger with time.
- A number of intrinsic and extrinsic factors can affect the healing process and include age, diabetes, infection, nutrition, smoking and drugs.
- Wounds are costly to treat and therefore accurate assessment of a patient and his/her wound is important.
- Assessment should be part of an ongoing process with opportunity for regular re-assessment.
- Acute wounds such as surgical incisions heal quickly with minimal complications; chronic wounds such as diabetic foot ulcers, leg ulcers and pressure ulcers take longer to heal.
- The management of patients with diabetic foot ulcers needs to include treatment of their diabetes as well as local wound management and off-loading techniques to reduce foot pressures.
- Venous leg ulcers are the most common cause of ulceration in the population and require the external application of compression bandages/hosiery to aid healing. These ulcers can be complicated by gravitational eczema; therefore, treatment of the surrounding skin is of equal importance.
- The majority of pressure ulcers are preventable. Management of patients requires a multi-disciplinary approach with the use of pressure-reducing/pressure-relieving support surfaces and repositioning as adjunctive measures to ensure appropriate care.

A wound can be thought of as any break in the integrity of the skin (Enoch and Leaper, 2005), although when this is due to minor trauma it might be termed a cut or an abrasion. Such wounds tend to heal fairly quickly by the process of regeneration of tissue and cells and generally do not pose any long-term problems. However, the time it takes for a wound to heal will depend on a number of factors related to the nature of the wound, the individual and environment. Many of these factors will be dealt with at different points throughout this chapter.

Structure of the skin

The skin is made up of the epidermis and dermis below which is the sub-cutis, muscle and bone. Within the epidermis, there are four layers:

- Stratum corneum
- Stratum granulosum
- Stratum spinosum
- Stratum basale.

Within the very thin structure of the epidermis, some of the key cells required for healing are present, in particular keratinocytes, dendritic cells and melanocytes.

The dermis is separated into the papillary and reticular dermis and is thicker than the epidermis. It is joined to the epidermis by structures known as rete ridges or 'pegs'. In uninjured tissue, this arrangement helps the skin to maintain its normal function, something which can be affected when a wound occurs or as an individual's skin changes with age. Like the epidermis, the dermis also contains many of the key cells/structures that are required for the normal healing response to occur; these include:

- Fibroblasts; for the production of collagen
- Endothelial cells; to stimulate blood vessel growth
- Leucocytes; such as lymphocytes, neutrophils and macrophages
- Smooth muscle cells
- Extracellular matrix.

The functions of the skin and factors that affect skin condition are listed in Table 58.1. How these roles link to wounds and wound healing will be explored in more detail later.

Wound healing

In adults, a scar is the normal end product of most injuries, with occasionally excessive scarring, that is hypertrophic or keloid complicating matters. However, wound healing can also be scarless, such as in fetal skin or the oral mucosa

Table 58.1 Functions of the skin and factors affecting skin condition

Functions of the skin	Factors affecting skin condition
Protective covering	Dryness
Moisture retention	Age
Sensation	Environment
Regulation of body temperature	Nutrition
Release of waste	Hydration
Absorption of nutrients, that is Vitamin D	

(Desai, 1997a; Wysocki, 2007). This type of healing presents an interesting concept and may offer some significant developments in the future. There are also many individuals for whom healing is delayed, and includes wounds often referred to as 'chronic' or 'non-healing'. Other terminology is used in clinical practice to describe how wounds heal and includes:

- Primary intention
- Delayed primary closure
- Secondary intention.

Essentially, healing by primary intention (Fig. 58.1) describes where the wound edges are opposed, that is brought together by sutures, staples or glue and wound healing occurs mainly by connective tissue formation. Delayed primary healing is used where there may be a risk of contamination or infection, that is if the patient has undergone emergency abdominal surgery. In this instance, some of the layers of tissue are stitched, and the sutures are placed in readiness for the remainder of the wound to be closed after 48 h when the risk of infection is less. In contrast, secondary healing (Fig. 58.2) describes a situation where the wound is left open to heal by the normal processes. This type of healing is relevant to many of the types of wounds that will be discussed later.

Any injury to the skin will result in a sequence of events aimed at repairing the defect. Figure 58.3 shows the process of wound healing and is divided into four phases:

- Haemostasis
- Inflammation
- Proliferation
- Remodelling or maturation.

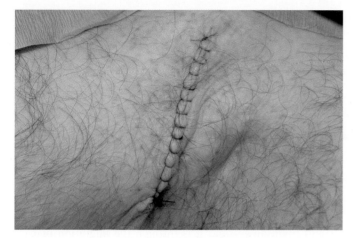

Fig. 58.1 Example of wound healing by primary intention.

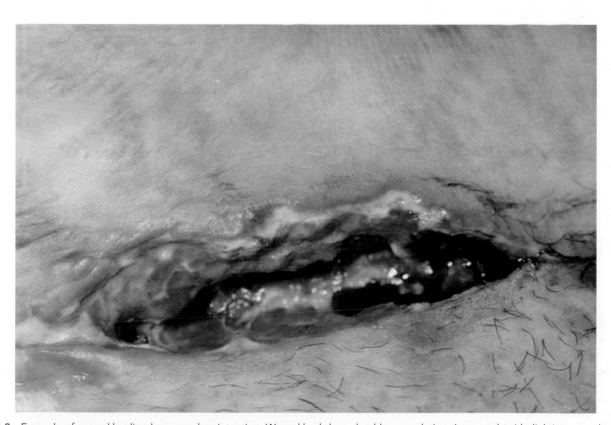

Fig. 58.2 Example of wound healing by secondary intention. Wound bed shows healthy granulation tissue and epithelial tissue can be seen at the wound edges.

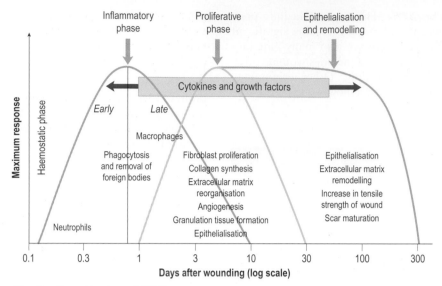

Fig. 58.3 Phases of wound healing (from Enoch et al 2008).

An insult to the tissues causes a number of systemic processes to occur simultaneously. Platelets aggregate and adhere to the sub-endothelium; coagulation factors as well as growth factors are also released. Through changes in the platelet structure and function, thrombin and fibrin are released to aid clot formation and reduce excess blood loss. Once this has occurred, haemostasis is said to have been established. The initial fibrin matrix provides the scaffold for the subsequent structure. This process relies on the individual having a normal clotting response and may be affected by drugs or systemic disease.

Following haemostasis, the inflammatory phase extends from day 0 through to about day 10 in normal healing and involves neutrophils (early inflammation), and macrophages (late inflammation). Neutrophils phagocytose bacteria and kill foreign bodies by producing oxygen metabolites such as hydroxyl radicals, hydrogen peroxide and superoxide ion. In normal healing, the numbers of neutrophils decrease in number over time leading to an increase in the number of macrophages present. The key function of macrophage is to digest bacteria, dead tissue and old neutrophils. There is some evidence to suggest that in wounds which are not healing it may be the inflammatory phase and its related cells that are at fault. The classic signs of inflammation are well reported and include:

- Redness
- Swelling
- Heat
- Pain.

These signs are normal and should not be considered as indicating the presence of infection.

The proliferative phase begins approximately 1 day post-injury and should be resolving by about day 30. There are three main activities that occur during this time and include:

- Granulation tissue formation – requires new blood vessels and formation of collagen
- Contraction of the wound
- Epithelialisation.

The presence of a functional blood vessel network is fundamental for wound healing to progress. Angiogenesis, the formation of blood vessels, is required to supply oxygen to the wound environment and it is through the migration of capillaries through the provisional matrix that the vasculature is re-established. Endothelial cells migrate and proliferate to eventually join the existing blood supply to the injured area. Once this has occurred, granulation tissue can form to begin to repair the defect. The provisional tissue laid down (Fig. 58.2) is made up of fibrin, fibronectin, collagen and glycosaminoglycans. Through the action of fibroblasts, collagen is produced and the continued presence of macrophages ensures the wound is kept 'clean'. Collagen production is essential for healing to progress and in particular Types I, III and IV are required.

In conjunction with the laying down of granulation tissue, the wound edges begin to contract at around day 8, and this process assists wound closure. The key cell involved is the myofibroblast which applies tension to the surrounding matrix to induce contraction. The normal process of contraction should not be confused with contracture, which is an abnormal feature of scarring.

Around the same time, it may also be possible to see signs of epithelialisation occurring (Fig. 58.2). Keratinocytes, the cell associated with this process, are initiated hours after injury; they migrate from the edge of a wound over the provisional matrix laid down or they dissect through it. Hair follicles can act as islands of regenerating epithelium in some areas. The wound bed can be easily damaged during the proliferative phase, with simple things like incorrect dressing choice causing significant damage. Moist wound healing (MWH) principles (Winter, 1962) are encouraged to support the normal physiological process of healing.

The final phase of the healing process is termed remodelling or maturation. During this time, the initial collagen that has been laid down is synthesised by enzymes ultimately leading to a more ordered network that increases in structure and strength over time. However, this repaired area is never as strong as normal tissue and is always at risk of breakdown should circumstances occur. These final changes can take place for up to a year or more after the initial insult.

Factors affecting wound healing

Generally, wound healing should progress as described above; however, a number of factors that affect healing have been identified (Grey and Harding, 2008). A summary of these is provided in Table 58.2, some of which include:

- Age
- Diabetes
- Infection
- Nutrition
- Smoking
- Drugs.

Age

Younger patients appear to have an increased rate of healing, and there are differences in fetal healing that mean the regeneration process is superior with little or no inflammation or scarring (Desai, 1997b). In comparison, wound repair in the elderly is slower (Ashcroft et al., 2002), and management may be more challenging because of concurrent disease processes. This is a particular problem in the proliferative and remodelling phases where tissue appears to be more friable and fragile. The overall effects of age on wound healing appear to be:

- Decreased inflammatory response
- Delayed angiogenesis
- Decreased collagen synthesis and degradation
- Slower epithelialisation.

Diabetes

Diabetes poses many problems for patients with wounds and management is often challenging because of concurrent peripheral neuropathy (PN), peripheral arterial disease (PAD), neuro-ischaemia and infection (Table 58.3).

Infection

Bacterial invasion of wounds is very common. In fact, any break in the skin integrity places the wound at risk of local contamination or infection and if untreated can lead to systemic infection. The spectrum of infection from colonisation through to infection is demonstrated in Fig. 58.4. The difficulty may be in recognising when such circumstances are present. The normal inflammatory signs were discussed earlier, and these should be borne in mind when examining a patient's wound. However, there are additional local signs that may be present in wounds healing by primary or secondary intention (Fig. 58.5) that suggest an infective process; these include:

- Increased pain
- Delayed wound healing
- Wound bleeds easily
- Friable, fragile tissue
- Pocketing/bridging of tissue
- Wound breakdown (dehiscence).

Infection in a wound can often be diagnosed by clinical signs and symptoms alone and unless a systemic infection is suspected, that is the patient complains of flu-like symptoms, can

Table 58.2 Intrinsic and extrinsic factors affecting wound healing

Intrinsic factors systemic local		Extrinsic factors
Age	Blood supply	Nutrition
Uraemia	Changes in oxygen tension	Smoking
Jaundice	Vessel trauma	Radiotherapy
Diabetes	Abnormal scarring	Infection
Anaemia	Haematoma	Drugs
Hormones	Local infection	Iatrogenic influences
Malignant disease		Wound dressings

Table 58.3 Complications of diabetes

Peripheral neuropathy	Causes damage to nerves that leads to a lack of the protective pain sensation, but the blood supply remains good. Very common and can lead to foot deformities and abnormal walking patterns. Neuropathy should be considered in terms of sensory, autonomic and motor changes. The foot is usually warm, numb and dry with palpable foot pulses
Peripheral arterial disease	Often develops as a result of atherosclerosis but develops at a faster rate in diabetic patients. Can affect the large (macro) and small (micro) vessels leading to decreased blood flow to the legs and feet, which can ultimately lead to minor or major amputations. The foot is often cool, clammy with absent or reduced foot pulses
Neuro-ischaemia	A combination of peripheral neuropathy and peripheral arterial disease
Infection	More common in diabetic patients, probably because they have an associated defective immunity. The neutrophil and lymphocyte response is slow (partly due to vascular problems); therefore, the inflammatory and subsequent phases are impaired. Hence, these patients have an increased tendency to develop infections

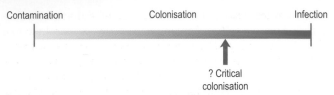

Fig. 58.4 Schematic representation for the outcome of bacterial invasion.

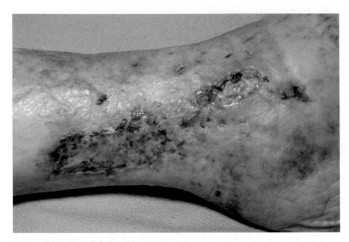

Fig. 58.5 Infection in a granulating wound.

be treated locally with topical antimicrobial dressings rather than oral antibiotics.

In recent years, there has been increased recognition that bacteria have the ability to build up colonies that present a challenge in terms of the management of bacterial load. Known as biofilms, they have the ability to resist removal and have been implicated in delayed healing of a number of wound types. The removal of dead and devitalised tissue from the wound bed seems to have some effect in preventing the growth of biofilms (Wolcott and Rhoads, 2008); however, this method is not suitable for all wounds; hence, other approaches are being sought.

The choice of topical treatment for the management of local wound infection will be dealt with in a later section.

Nutrition

The nutritional requirements for wound healing have been the subject of debate with limited evidence as to the exact dietary components for individual wound types. In general, if the patient has a balanced diet, this should be sufficient for the normal processes to take place. However, a diet that is lacking in vital nutrients can lead to delayed wound healing and wound breakdown. In the extreme, the patient can become malnourished with surgical patients most at risk of protein energy malnutrition (PEM). Box 58.1 outlines the nutritional factors that should be considered in the assessment of individuals, many of which have been incorporated in nutritional risk assessment tools. Individuals at most risk of nutritional deficiencies are those affected by:

- Ill-health in old age
- Cancer
- Chronic neurological disease

Box 58.1 Nutritional assessment and treatment options

General nutritional assessment to include
Current appetite
Food intake
Patient's ability to eat/chew/swallow
Presence of dentures

Specialist nutritional assessment
Anthropometric measurements such as:
Body Mass Index (BMI), % weight loss, haemoglobin, skin fold thickness, grip strength, serum albumin
Gut function
Total energy requirements

Nutrients required for healing
Protein
Zinc
Copper
Iron

Vitamins required for healing
A
B complex
C
E

Treatment options
Modified normal diet: increase high energy/protein foods
Modified normal diet plus nutritional supplementation
Total enteral support
Naso-gastric feeding
Total parenteral nutrition
Percutaneous endoscopic gastrostomy (PEG)

- Chronic inflammatory bowel disease
- Surgery (pre- and post-operatively)
- Stroke
- Acute and chronic pain
- Immuno-deficiency disease such as HIV and AIDS.

Smoking

Smoking is known to be detrimental to health generally, and in addition the effect of nicotine and carbon monoxide on skin and muscles is well documented (Møller et al., 2002). These substances reduce the oxygen levels in the tissues and can lead to the formation of thrombi. A good blood supply and adequate vascularisation is important for normal wound healing. There has been debate about the period of time patients should abstain from smoking to reduce relevant, potential complications. This has been suggested to vary from 4 (Sorensen et al., 2003) to 8 weeks (Møller et al., 2002). However, the role of nicotine replacement interventions in further reducing complications is less clear.

Drugs

There are certain drugs that are suggested to have an effect on the healing process. These include NSAIDs, corticosteroids and immunosuppressive agents (Grey and Harding, 2008),

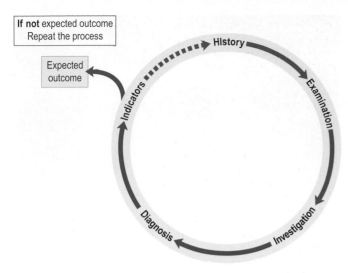

If not expected outcome
Repeat the process

Expected outcome

History

Examination

Investigation

Diagnosis

Indicators

Fig. 58.6 Assessment of a patient with a wound.

which affect the inflammatory response, collagen synthesis and mitosis, respectively. Whilst drugs do not generally cause wounds, there have been recent reports that nicorandil, used for the treatment of angina, may cause peri-anal wounds that resolve on cessation of the medication (Baker et al., 2007).

Wound assessment

Wounds are costly to treat; therefore, it is important to appreciate the various considerations that need to be taken into account when assessing a patient. Assessment should not be viewed as a one-off occurrence but instead should be undertaken as part of an ongoing process with the emphasis on the patient, not just their wound.

A structured approach to the assessment of a patient with a wound is required. The six key elements of the original wound healing matrix are listed here and the key concepts depicted in Fig. 58.6:

- Phase of wound healing
- Aetiology
  - Acute, that is surgical, trauma, burns
  - Chronic, that is leg ulcers, diabetic foot ulcers, pressure ulcers
- Clinical manifestation
  - Size
  - Shape
  - Characteristics, that is exudate, odour, tissue type
- Environment and care
  - Primary care
  - Secondary care
- Healthcare system and resources
- Site of the wound.

Diabetic foot ulcers

Epidemiology

It was estimated that there were 1.4 million people diagnosed as diabetic in 2002 with these figures expected to double by 2010 (Cradock and Shaw, 2002). The cost of treating individuals

with diabetes accounts for at least 9% of the acute health-care costs in the UK. These costs, however, do not take into account the personal cost to the individual, such as a reduction in the ability to work and time they may need to take off work (Waters and Holloway, 2009). Diabetic foot problems are the most common cause for admission, and patients admitted to hospital for in-patient care are often hospitalised for 4–6 weeks, which obviously increases the financial costs considerably.

One of the major risks to patients with diabetic foot disease is that of amputation, which could be minor, that is mid-foot to toe; or major, that is mid-foot and above. National Service Frameworks for diabetes (Department of Health, 2001) have emerged to address this and, in turn, have been built upon (Department of Health, 2007a,b). Of concern is that up to 85% of amputations are preceded by foot ulcers. Therefore, if the incidence of foot ulcers can be reduced, this might lead to a reduction in amputations.

Aetiology

Individuals with diabetes are at risk of a number of systemic complications (see Chapter 44).

The two main causes of foot ulceration in patients with diabetes are:

- Neuropathy
- Ischaemia

PN causes damage to the nerves that leads to a lack of the protective pain sensation and is present in 75% of patients with diabetes. In this group of individuals, the blood supply to the extremities remains good, but the foot becomes insensate and can subsequently become deformed. This leads to an abnormal walking pattern and potentially tissue breakdown from abnormal pressures placed upon the foot. The characteristics of the diabetic foot are set out in Table 58.4. Unfortunately, the early systemic changes associated with the onset of diabetes may be present for up to 12 years before a diagnosis is

Table 58.4 Clinical features of a diabetic foot with neuropathy or arterial disease

Characteristic	Peripheral neuropathy	Peripheral arterial disease
Temperature	Warm	Cool
Foot pulse	Present/'bounding'	Absent/reduced
Pain	Commonly no pain NB Painful diabetic neuropathy is a rare but potential feature	Pain on walking (intermittent claudication) Depends on degree of neuropathy
Site of ulcers	Toes and metatarsal heads	Lateral (outer) border of foot
Callus (hard skin)	Present	Absent

made, by which time damage has already begun to occur and is often irreversible.

PAD usually occurs as a result of atherosclerosis. This often results in a reduction in blood flow to the lower limbs and pain on walking (claudication), pain at rest with possible progression to gangrene and amputation. PAD is common in the elderly and is not just a complication of diabetes, although people who have diabetes are at an increased risk of developing it. Foot ulceration due to PAD is less common, accounting for approximately 5% of cases.

Neuropathy can be related to lack of sensation (sensory neuropathy) and may also cause atrophy and weakness of muscles in the foot (motor neuropathy). In addition, there are effects on the autonomic nervous system which can cause changes in blood flow and sweat secretion (autonomic neuropathy). Each of these elements needs to be considered as each has significant effects on the lower limb in individuals with diabetes.

Clinical signs

The clinical features of a diabetic foot with PN and PAD are summarised in Table 58.4 and their typical presentations shown in Fig. 58.7 and Fig. 58.8, respectively. There are a number of factors that place patients at increased risk of ulceration including foot deformity; ill-fitting footwear; mechanical injury, for example treading on a sharp object; thermal injury, for example heat from a fire, or stepping into a hot bath; and chemical trauma typically caused by an over-the-counter preparation purchased to remove hard skin. National guidelines outline the processes that should be in place to ensure the monitoring of patients deemed at risk (Department of Health, 2001, 2007a,b; National Institute of Health and Clinical Excellence, 2004). One of the key issues

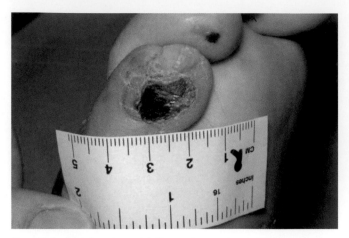

Fig. 58.8 Peripheral arterial disease in a patient with diabetes.

to consider is that the feet of patients with diabetes do not ulcerate spontaneously, instead any one, or combination, of the factors discussed could be to blame.

Diagnosis

It is essential that individuals with diabetes are cared for within a multi-disciplinary framework with the responsibilities for management of the patient clearly defined.

Initial assessment should include a clinical examination of the foot and may also require objective testing, for example an X-ray. The key features of this examination are set out in Table 58.5. In addition, further tests such as a full blood count, examination of urine, alternate imaging methods,

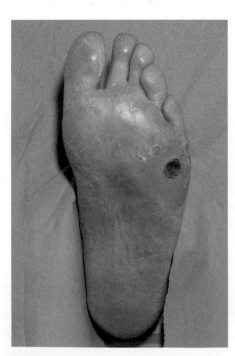

Fig. 58.7 Diabetic foot ulcer caused by peripheral neuropathy.

Table 58.5 Examination of the diabetic foot		
Clinical examination		**Objective test**
Shape and deformities	Toe deformities Foot deformities Callus	X-ray
Sensory function	Vibration Protective sensation	Biothesiometry Semmes–Weinstein filament
Motor function	Wasting Weakness Ankle reflexes	Electrophysiological tests
Autonomic function	Reduced sweating Callus Warmth Appearance of veins on the foot	Quantitative sweat test
Vascular status	Foot pulses Temperature Swelling	Non-invasive Doppler studies, ankle brachial pressure index and/or toe pressure indices

that is magnetic resonance imaging, colour duplex scans and angiograms, may be indicated.

Infection in the diabetic foot is a real risk and a common complication. It has been estimated that 20–50% of diabetic ulcers are infected. The severity of the infection will depend on the nature of the bacteria, but commonly cellulitis and osteomyelitis occur in patients with neuropathic ulcers with gangrene being more associated with PAD. Bacterial cultures from ulcers are usually polymicrobial with both Gram-positive and Gram-negative organisms as well as anaerobic bacteria. There should be concern if any of the following features occur:

- Difficulty walking and/or applying shoes
- Swelling in part or all of the foot
- Redness or other discolouration
- Foot becomes hotter than normal
- Discharge or unusual odour
- Open sores or blisters
- Nausea, vomiting or high temperature
- Difficulty maintaining blood glucose control.

Treatment

Infection

The signs of infection are often delayed or insidious in patients with diabetes. Virtually all diabetic foot infections require antimicrobial therapy, but this alone is rarely sufficient. If soft-tissue infection is superficial, then oral, relatively narrow spectrum antibiotics for 1–2 weeks are indicated (Lipsky and Berendt, 2006); however, if there is cellulitis and spreading infection, parenteral antibiotic therapy may be required for up to 4 weeks. In addition to antibiotics, the patient may require hospitalisation if removal of dead or devitalised tissue is required. An X-ray of the foot may also be advisable if the tissue loss is over the bone, and referral to a vascular or orthopaedic specialist may be necessary for surgery.

Other considerations

Treatment of a diabetic foot ulcer should also include:

- Podiatry
- Skin and wound care
- Provision of footwear to remove/redistribute weight
- Offloading options to include orthoses/custom-made insoles
- Patient education
- Pain relief
- Control of diabetes
- Multidisciplinary team approach.

The range of treatment options will be determined by whether there is neuropathy and/or PAD present, as well as the presence of ulcers and/or infection. The debridement of callus and devitalised tissue is essential as it enables the true dimensions of the ulcer to be established (Edmonds and Foster, 2000). Dressings are important but should not be viewed in isolation to the other essential aspects of treatment listed above. Key

aspects in the choice of dressing for diabetic foot ulcers are how it will perform in a shoe, whether it will withstand pressure and shear forces, how well it will absorb any fluid from the wound and how often the dressing needs to be changed and cost effectiveness.

Prevention of recurrence

Many of the considerations discussed above are also important in terms of preventing a recurrence of ulceration and should be borne in mind when planning the management of individuals with diabetes. Ideally, ulceration should be prevented via intensive screening programmes, although unfortunately this is not always achievable. In addition, the maintenance of tight control over blood glucose and blood pressure is required together with the monitoring of cholesterol and initiation of antiplatelet therapy. Guidelines (National Institute of Health and Clinical Excellence, 2008) recommend the following:

- Blood pressure ≤140/80
- Blood glucose <7 mmol/L or $HbA1_c$ <6.5%
- Total cholesterol <5.0 mmol/L
- Antiplatelet therapy for those with or at risk of cardiovascular disease.

Leg ulcers

Epidemiology

The prevalence of leg ulcers in the Western world is 0.11–0.18% (Briggs and Closs, 2003). There is a preponderance of 2.8:1 female to male ratio, with venous disease being the main cause of ulceration. The risk of leg ulceration increases with age.

The estimated cost in the UK of all leg ulcers is between £200–600 million pounds with the costs of individual ulcer treatment between £557–1366 over a year (Tennvall and Hjelmgren, 2005). Between 60% and 90% of patients are managed in the community.

Aetiology

Leg ulcers can be classified as follows:

- Venous
- Arterial
- Mixed, that is ulcers that have a venous and arterial component
- Diabetic; typically on the foot, rather than the leg
- Autoimmune, for example rheumatoid arthritis.

Venous ulcers

Ulcers of venous origin account for the majority of all leg ulcers. There are a number of reasons why they occur and include failure of the calf muscle pump to work effectively, which leads to pooling of fluid in the lower limb and oedema. This can lead to high pressures in the lower limb on walking, known as venous hypertension. This swelling can lead to poor oxygenation of the tissues and trapping of harmful substances such as growth factors and enzymes. Ultimately, this can lead to tissue breakdown precipitated by simple trauma such as knocking the leg.

The calf muscle pump relies on an adequate level of mobility; therefore, anything that might affect this such as increasing age, obesity and trauma predisposes the individual to a sequence of events if they also have poor venous return.

Risk factors associated with the development of venous ulcers include deep vein thrombosis (DVT), varicose veins, or surgery/trauma to the leg.

Clinical signs

Venous disease. As a result of venous hypertension and leakage of fluid, red blood cells are deposited in the tissues causing discolouration known as haemosiderin. This can often be seen on the lower limb and may be red or brown in colour. Varicose veins may also be visible as will oedema (swelling) and a characteristic change known as lipodermatosclerosis (LDS). Over time, the limb may develop a typical inverted 'champagne bottle' appearance. Venous ulcers are typically shallow and develop in the gaiter area (Fig. 58.9). Patients may also have associated gravitational eczema.

Diagnosis

The key element is the accuracy of the assessment and should include:

• Clinical history
• Clinical investigation
• Assessment of the limb
• Assessment of the ulcer.

Table 58.6 summarises the key aspects of the assessment of an individual with a leg ulcer.

Assessment of ankle brachial pressure index (ABPI). The use of a hand-held Doppler device is used to assess the arterial blood flow. Ideally, this test should be undertaken on any patient presenting with a leg ulcer. Furthermore, it should

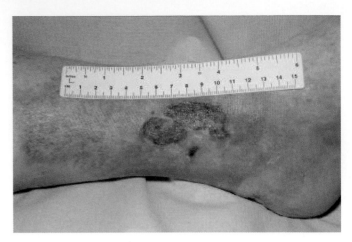

Fig. 58.9 Venous leg ulceration.

be carried out on first presentation as well as at subsequent intervals depending on whether the ulcer is improving or not. Essentially, the ankle brachial pressure index compares the patient's brachial (arm) and ankle systolic pressures:

$$ABPI = \frac{\text{highest ankle systolic pressure}}{\text{highest brachial systolic pressure}}$$

The patient should rest for 20 min before the assessment and the pressures should be measured supine (lying down). Two measurements should be taken from the foot and the highest value used in the calculation.

The ankle brachial pressure index is not a definitive measure of arterial status but merely serves as an indicator of blood flow. Other clinical signs and symptoms also need to be taken into account.

As a general principle, the ankle brachial pressure index or ratio should be ≥ 1.0 in individuals with no arterial disease. However, this should not be relied upon in the presence of diabetes as calcification of arteries can occur and lead to falsely high ABPI readings. In this instance, a Duplex scan would be a more reliable indicator of vascular status. Furthermore, both hypo- and hypertension can affect the readings.

Table 58.6 Factors to be taken into account in the assessment of an individual with a leg ulcer

Clinical history	Clinical investigations	Assessment of both limbs	Assessment of the ulcer
Family history	Blood pressure	Oedema	Year first ulcer occurred
Varicose veins	Ankle brachial pressure index	Site of ulcer	Site of ulcer/previous ulcers
Deep vein thrombosis/pulmonary embolus	Full blood count	Depth of wound	Size of ulcer(s)
Phlebitis		Appearance of wound bed	Number of previous episodes
Surgery or fracture of the leg		Surrounding skin	Time free of ulcers
Heart disease/stroke		Perfusion of feet	Past treatment (successful or not)
		Presence of pulses	Previous/current uses of compression bandaging
Diabetes		Ankle brachial pressure index	
Peripheral arterial disease			
Chest pain/angina			
Smoker			
Rheumatoid arthritis			
Medication			
Allergies			

Treatment

The mainstay of treatment for confirmed venous ulceration is compression bandaging. Known as graduated compression, specific bandage systems are used to apply external pressure to aid venous return. The ABPI must be ≥ 0.8 for this treatment to be used. Although there is much debate about which bandage system is preferable, the choice should be based on an individual patient assessment and may include:

- Short stretch systems
- Multi-layer systems

The aim of most systems is to create pressures of 40 mmHg at the ankle decreasing up to the knee to assist in venous return. In addition to bandaging, the patient should be encouraged to keep mobile, which could be as simple as undertaking ankle exercises to improve blood flow. Leg elevation and rest should also form part of overall management.

Even where arterial disease has been excluded as a complication, the patient should be monitored carefully for signs of compromised blood flow as serious injury such as skin necrosis or in the extreme amputation may be required.

Other treatment options may include antibiotics if systemic infection is suspected or topical antimicrobial dressings for local infection which include iodine- or silver-based products.

Intermittent pneumatic compression, surgery, skin grafting, bioengineered skin and pharmacological treatments such as oxypentifylline have all been suggested as adjuvant therapies to compression therapy (Robson et al., 2006).

General wound care should include cleansing of the ulcerated area with saline or tap water to maintain cleanliness and hygiene as well as debridement of any dead or devitalised tissue. Dressings should be simple and as low adherent as possible as they have to perform well under the bandage system. There is a need to be aware of the potential of contact sensitivity to the dressings, bandages, or skin treatments used.

Gravitational eczema is commonplace in patients with venous disease and is related to the changes caused by venous hypertension. The patient may complain of intense itching, and scratch marks may be visible on examination. It is important to distinguish eczema from contact sensitivity and cellulitis as each of these requires a different treatment. Treatment of eczema will include a combination of a topical corticosteroid such as clobetasone butyrate (Eumovate®) or mometasone furoate (Elocon®) creams and emollients such as Epaderm® or similar mixtures of white soft paraffin and liquid paraffin to manage this inflammatory condition.

Prevention of recurrence

Once a venous ulcer is healed, compression hosiery (in the form of stockings) are required. This hosiery is classed as 1, 2 or 3 depending on the level of pressure applied. Class 3 stockings and tights provide strong support (25–35 mmHg at the ankle) and are the preferred choice to prevent recurrence of venous ulcers. Table 58.7 provides the compression values for hosiery. Ideally, they will need to be worn for life or at least a minimum of 5 years. Unfortunately, recurrence is common often because of the inconvenience associated with the wearing of stockings. Patient education and follow-up is essential. Community leg ulcer clinics have been established in many areas of the UK and have shown to be effective in supporting patients.

Table 58.7 British national formulary compression values for hosiery

Compression class	Level of support	Compression hosiery (British Standard)
Class 1	Light	14-17 mm Hg*
Class 2	Medium'	18-24 mm Hg*
Class 3	Strong	25-35 mm Hg*

*compression provided at the ankle

Arterial ulcers

Arterial ulceration is commonly associated with atherosclerosis and peripheral artery disease, much of which has been discussed previously in relation to diabetic foot disease. Both macro- and micro-disease may be present.

Clinical signs

The classic clinical features of arterial insufficiency are:

- Intermittent claudication/rest pain
- Colour changes, for example pallor
- Muscle atrophy/weakness
- Poor perfusion, for example cool limb
- Loss of skin hair
- Thickening/hardening of the nails
- Ulceration
- Gangrene.

Arterial ulcers often appear 'punched out' (Fig. 58.10) and have a pale wound bed. The significant feature is pain, with many patients reporting pain on walking known as intermittent claudication. As the disease progresses, patients may also report that their pain is worse at rest, particularly when their legs are elevated. This feature affects their ability to sleep, eat and keep mobile which can ultimately mean they are unable to leave the house.

Diagnosis

A simple test known as Buerger's Test (see glossary) is normally used to look for positive signs of disease. If it is possible, a Doppler test should also be undertaken to calculate the patient's ankle brachial pressure index. Typically, an ankle brachial pressure index of 0.6–0.8 indicates a degree of arterial disease, whilst a value ≤0.6 is considered to be indicative of considerable disease. In addition, a colour Duplex scan is usually required to ascertain the extent of the disease. If treatment is required, an angiogram will usually be undertaken to examine the affected vessels.

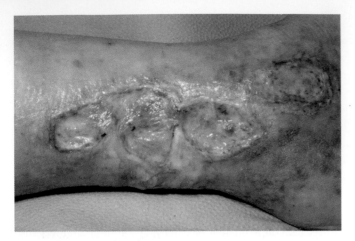

Fig. 58.10 Arterial leg ulceration.

Treatment

An angioplasty may be carried out to improve the blood supply. Where this is not possible, vascular reconstruction may be advised to try and prevent further progression. Treatment will also include pain relief, prevention of infection and nutritional support. In addition, smoking cessation advice may be needed as might pharmaceutical intervention for cholesterol or lipid lowering purposes.

Prevention of recurrence

The main risk for individuals with arterial disease is amputation (minor or major). The patient plays a key role in prevention as many of the predisposing factors are lifestyle issues such as giving up smoking, eating a healthy diet and exercise. It may also be necessary to continue taking medication as discussed previously.

Mixed ulcers

While the term 'mixed ulceration' is used in clinical practice to describe ulcers with an element of venous and arterial disease, technically it is not a diagnosis. Patients present with venous and arterial symptoms, and an ankle brachial pressure index is likely to be between 0.6 and 0.8. Treatment is directed at the symptoms causing most concern, with compression bandaging only used under close supervision. The management options are as discussed previously for venous and arterial ulcers.

Pressure ulcers

Epidemiology

Previously referred to as *bed sores* or *pressure sores*, this wound type is now generally referred to as a pressure ulcer (National Institute of Health and Clinical Excellence, 2005) and defined as:

> *localised injury to the skin and/or underlying tissue usually over a bony prominence, as a result of pressure, or pressure in combination with shear. A number of*

contributing or confounding factors are also associated with pressure ulcers, the significance of these factors is yet to be elucidated.

(European Pressure Ulcer Advisory Panel and National Pressure Ulcer Advisory Panel, 2009)

The prevalence of pressure ulcers across five European countries was 18.1% (Clark et al., 2004). This helps us establish the burden of pressure ulcers perhaps locally, nationally and globally but does not necessarily provide information on the quality of care (European Pressure Ulcer Advisory Panel and National Pressure Ulcer Advisory Panel, 2009). Table 58.8 provides the most recent data on incidence.

Common sites of pressure ulcers

Pressure ulcer damage can occur anywhere on the body, but are most common over bony prominences including:

- Sacrum
- Heels
- Buttock
- Trochanter.

Sacral damage often occurs from the patient slipping down the bed or whilst sitting in a chair with shear forces causing the most damage. Injury to other areas is more likely to be due to direct pressure over a bony prominence. In acutely ill patients, equipment such as nasal cannula can even cause pressure damage to the nose.

Aetiology

As the name implies, this sort of wound is caused by external pressure on the tissues which, if sustained, leads to decreased capillary flow, ischaemia and capillary thrombosis. In turn, fluid escapes from the vasculature into the surrounding tissues causing oedema, accumulation of metabolic waste and cell death.

There are different types of pressure that may be implicated in the onset of damage, and it is both the type and duration of pressure that is of importance. The types of pressure are listed as follows:

- Capillary closing pressure
- Vertical pressure
- Tissue interface pressure
- Shear and friction forces.

Table 58.8 Incidence of pressure ulcers in UK

	Grade distribution	Annual incidence
Grade I	34.9%	140,000
Grade II	41.2%	170,000
Grade III	12.9%	50,000
Grade IV	11.0%	50,000

In addition to pressure, other factors that may influence the development of the damage are:

- Reactive hyperaemia
- Reperfusion injury
- Patient age: extremes of age most at risk
- Nutritional status: extremes of weight most at risk
- Mobility status
- Condition of peripheral circulation
- Continence status.

Clinical signs

Early signs of damage may present as a red area on the skin that remains even after the pressure has been relieved, or damage may present as broken skin or an abrasion. Pressure ulcers are now classified using four categories or stages (rather than grades):

Category/stage I: Non-blanchable redness of intact skin

Intact skin with non-blanchable erythema (in normal tissue if you use light finger pressure on an area it turns white, once the pressure is released it returns to the normal colour very quickly; where damage is present the tissue does not 'blanch', i.e. turn white) of a localised area usually over a bony prominence. Discolouration of the skin, warmth, oedema, hardness or pain may also be present. Darkly pigmented skin may not have visible blanching but may be painful, firm, soft, warmer or cooler as compared to adjacent tissue.

Category/stage II: Partial skin loss or blister

Partial thickness loss of dermis presenting as a shallow open ulcer with a red pink wound bed, without slough. May also present as an intact or open/ruptured serum-filled or serosanguinous filled blister.

Category/stage III: Full thickness skin loss (fat visible)

Full thickness tissue loss. Sub-cutaneous fat may be visible but bone, tendon or muscle is not exposed. Some slough may be present. May include undermining and tunnelling.

Category/stage IV: Full thickness tissue loss (muscle/ bone visible)

Full thickness tissue loss with exposed bone, tendon or muscle. Slough or eschar may be present. Often includes undermining and tunnelling.

Diagnosis

Pressure ulcers are usually diagnosed on clinical appearance and presenting history. Using the classification system outlined above, it is also possible to determine the stage of ulcer.

X-rays of the ulcer may be required, especially if it is over a bony area, to exclude any underlying infection in the bone (osteomyelitis). In addition, blood tests to examine inflammatory markers may also be useful in determining the presence of infection.

If undermining or tunnelling is present, further ultrasound scans may be required to examine the full extent of the wound and to identify any collection of fluid.

Treatment

The care of patients with pressure ulcers will depend on the category/stage of the damage, but there are interventions common to all patients and these include (National Institute of Health and Clinical Excellence, 2003, 2005):

- Appropriate support surface (mattress and seating/ cushions) to redistribute pressure and reduce shear forces
- Repositioning (turning) schedule to meet the needs of the individual
- Wound cleansing with normal saline or potable water
- Debridement of dead or devitalised tissue using an appropriate method
- Dressings that meet the wound characteristics
- Treatment of infection via local or systemic route as appropriate
- Skin care and hygiene, particularly if the patient is incontinent
- Negative pressure wound therapy may be a suitable adjuvant therapy
- Surgical reconstructive intervention in complex cases.

Other therapeutic interventions include electrical stimulation, laser therapy and ultrasound.

Prevention of pressure ulcers

The majority of pressure ulcers are preventable. Prevention strategies should take into account the aetiology of the ulcer and also the risk factors discussed. Important considerations in terms of prevention include:

- Patient repositioning
- Use of equipment
- Skin care
- Nutritional support.

An individual's potential risk of developing damage should be assessed with a view to identifying those that are vulnerable. Once an individual is deemed to be at risk of skin breakdown, the aim should be to improve tissue tolerance which can be achieved using the elements described above.

Principles of wound management

There are a number of principles to wound management including:

- Knowledge of wound healing physiology
- Assessment of the patient
- Assessment of the wound/ulcer
- Assessment of the tissue type
- Recognition of factors affecting healing
- Knowledge of dressings available
- Availability of resources.

The health care professional needs to be clear about the aim of management, and the expected outcome before the most appropriate treatment can be selected. Table 58.9 outlines the main considerations to be taken into account. Whilst wound healing is often viewed as the eventual outcome in some instances this may not be feasible; therefore, alternative aims should be identified to demonstrate success.

Assessment of the tissue type should include examination of the following:

- Dead, devitalised tissue, that is slough, necrosis
- Infected tissue
- Granulating, that is pink
- Epithelial tissue, that is pink, silvery tissue at the edges of a wound.

Once this information has been established, then the choice of local treatment should be more apparent. The selection of a dressing will depend on:

- Treatment objective
- Stage of healing
- Tissue type
- Site and size of the wound
- Frequency of the dressing change
- Comfort/cosmetic appearance
- Where/by whom the dressing is to be changed
- If the dressing is available.

Table 58.9 Criteria to consider in choosing appropriate wound management

Aim	Criteria
Protect from	Drying out
	Infection
	Further damage
Debride using	Autolytic methods
	Mechanically
	Sharp/Surgical
	Larvae
Control	Bleeding
	Exudate
	Pain
	Odour

Box 58.2 lists the main types of dressings available. Dressings alone will not heal a wound, and other aspects of care may need to be taken into account including:

- Compression bandages for patients with venous ulcers
- Pressure relieving equipment for individuals with or at risk of pressure ulcers
- Footwear and off-loading devices for patients with diabetic foot disease

---

Box 58.2   Wound management products

Basic wound contact dressings, that is knitted viscose/polymer dressings
Low adherent dressings – indicated for clean granulating wounds with a light amount of exudate. NB Dressing may stick so be cautious of trauma on removal
  Absorbent dressings – are also low adherent and suitable for mild and moderate (but not viscous) exudate

Advanced wound dressings
Hydrogel – generally donates liquid to aid autolytic debridement of sloughy, necrotic wounds. Available in amorphous or sheet form depending on the size and shape of the wound. Choice will depend on the amount of exudate present.
  Vapour permeable films and membranes – also allow the passage of water vapour and oxygen but remain impermeable to water and bacteria. They allow viewing of the wound and are flexible and conform to awkward wound shapes. Mainly suitable for partial thickness wounds and formulated with and without an absorbent pad for exudate management. Use would be avoided in infected and highly exuding wounds.
  Soft polymer – often with added silicone. Designed to be non-adherent and are useful if the skin/wound is fragile and where further damage is to be avoided. They can be used on wounds that have light to moderate exudate but may require a secondary absorbent dressing if large amounts of exudate are present.
  Hydrocolloids – semi-permeable to water vapour and oxygen, and gel in the presence of exudate. Promote autolytic debridement and are also useful on granulating wounds as they can be left in place for a number of days. Generally, these dressings are indicated for moderate to heavy exudate, careful monitoring for maceration of the wound edges and surrounding skin would be important.
  Foam – suitable for most types of wounds but requires a moist wound interface. Can absorb various levels of exudate with some having better fluid handling capacity than others. Presented in adhesive and non-adhesive forms, the choice of which is often based on the integrity of the patient's surrounding skin.
  Alginate – usually fibrous dressings, made from seaweed, some have haemostatic properties. Require moisture so are not suitable for dry wounds. They are suitable for exuding wounds and can aid autolytic debridement. Available as packing material (ropes) or flat sheets, the choice of which depends on the size and shape of the wound. May require a secondary dressing to hold in place.
  Capillary action – contraindicated in bleeding wounds but useful for exuding wounds, particularly when slough is present. Absorbent core absorbs and contains the exudate which minimises the risk of maceration. A secondary dressing is also required.
  Odour absorbent – utilise activated charcoal to absorb odour from wounds. Some require a suitable primary contact layer whilst others are layered and provide a non-adherent wound contact interface. The cause of the odour should always be established as underlying infection may require additional treatment.

Continued

Box 58.2 Wound management products—cont'd

Antimicrobial – used to treat local rather than spreading or systemic infection. Can be used to reduce the levels of bacteria in the wound. The amount of exudate should be a consideration when choosing an antimicrobial dressing.

Honey – medical honey is anti-inflammatory as well as antimicrobial and can aid with debridement of the wound and combating odour. Caution should be exercised in diabetic patients and its use should be avoided if a patient is allergic to bees/bee stings.

Iodine – available as povidone-iodine or cadexomer-iodine, preparations are useful in clinically infected wounds. Iodine is effective against a wide range of bacteria, but its effect can be diluted if large amounts of exudate are present. Cadexomer-iodine is effective at debriding wounds. Iodine can cause sensitivity and systemic absorption can occur especially from large wounds or prolonged use.

Silver – used when infection is suspected. Available in different presentations and can be used on all wound types that have clinical signs of infection and where exudate is present. Skin discoloration can occur and systemic absorption can occur therefore use is contraindicated in pregnancy and neonates.

Specialised dressings

Protease-modulating matrix – acts on the proteolytic enzymes in chronic wounds and re-establishes normal enzymatic activity. Can be used on non-healing wounds that do not seem to be progressing.

Silicone keloid dressings – used to reduce hypertrophic and keloid scarring, therefore are not appropriate for open wounds. A staged approach to application is advised with increasing wear time being indicated. Dressings can be washed and re-used.

Adjunct dressings and appliances

Surgical absorbents – useful as secondary layer over a primary wound contact layer. Absorb exudate but allow leakage of exudate ('strike-through'). Can adhere to the wound bed and fibres may be shed, therefore should be used cautiously.

Wound drainage pouches – use when other exudate absorbing dressings are not sufficient to manage the fluid levels; wound drainage bags may be useful as a means to containing the leakage.

Complex adjunct therapies

Topical negative pressure – useful for acute and chronic cavity wounds and shallower wounds healing by secondary intention; topical negative pressure or vacuum-assisted closure aims to stimulate angiogenesis, remove excess exudate, reduce the bacterial burden and stimulate the production of granulation tissue.

Sterile larvae (maggots) – useful for debridement of sloughy wounds. Once applied they can remain *in situ* for 3 days before replacing. Now available contained within a net bag to simplify application.

Growth factors – Becalpermin (Regranex®) licensed for full thickness, diabetic neuropathic foot ulcers.

Bandages

Compression (multi-layer) – provide compression for treatment of venous ulcers. Correct application of bandage is essential as the incorrect application technique can be hazardous. A Doppler assessment to establish the patient's ankle brachial pressure index (ABPI) is essential prior to application. Systems include high compression, short stretch and multi-layer (4 layer and 2 layer). Choice is often dependent on patient preference.

Compression hosiery – prevents recurrence of venous ulcers. Ankle brachial pressure index should be established prior to application. Class III is preferred.

Compression garments – for management of lymphoedema. Used in conjunction with intermittent pneumatic compression systems.

Skin care

Skin barriers that protect the peri-wound area are important as wound exudate contains enzymes that can cause damage to tissues. Simple silicone-based creams or petroleum-based ointments can be useful in providing a protective layer for fragile skin.

- Topical negative pressure for cavity wounds healing by secondary intention.
- Nutritional supplementation
- Drugs to influence healing
- Surgical interventions.

Case studies

Case 58.1

A 64-year-old diabetic man has an ulcer on the sole of his foot. He cannot recall how he sustained the injury and the wound is not painful. The patient feels otherwise well (Fig. 58.11).

Questions

1. What is the most likely cause of the ulceration?
2. What are the key concerns in ensuring appropriate management?
3. What are the options for assessment and treatment?

Answers

1. From the position and the appearance, this is likely to be a neuropathic diabetic foot ulcer as these commonly present on the plantar (sole) aspect of the foot. They are usually painless and can leak large amounts of exudate if they are deep. Note the signs of macerated tissue around the edges of the wound.

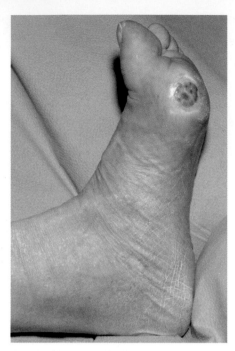

Fig. 58.11 Case 58.1

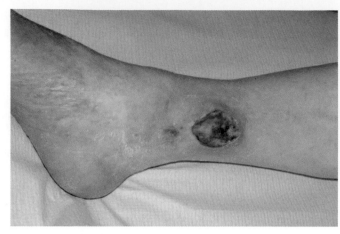

Fig. 58.12 Case 58.2

2. The most common complication of this sort of ulcer is infection. Local infection of the wound bed can quickly lead to spread of infection (cellulitis) in patients with diabetes as they have a slower immune response and do not mount a defence mechanism quickly. In addition, an assessment of the patient's glucose control should be undertaken as poor glucose management can exacerbate complications. Finally, a review of the patient's footwear should be considered as the patient may require further off-loading techniques to assist wound healing.

3. Assessment of the foot should be undertaken to establish the extent of the neuropathy. Vascular assessment is also required to examine the blood flow to the limb. Local wound assessment should include a description of the tissue present, the size of the wound (to include depth) and the amount of exudate as this will determine not only the topical dressing to be applied but also whether further investigations are required.

   As the ulcer has some depth, the wound will need packing gently with a dressing that has good fluid handling capacity. A secondary dressing will be needed to secure the contact layer, and the footwear should be suitable enough to accommodate the dressing without causing further pressure.

Case 58.2

A 71-year-old lady has ulceration on the gaiter area of her lower leg (Fig. 58.12).

Questions

1. What is the likely cause and how would this be established?
2. What treatment does the patient require?
3. What advice would be required in the short and long-term?

Answers

1. The ulcer is typical of a venous ulcer, caused by venous hypertension which damages the veins and causes leakage of cells and fluid ultimately leading to tissue breakdown often caused by minor trauma. A medical history should be taken to establish likely predisposing factors; the limb should be assessed for colour, oedema and the presence of pain. The ulcer is likely to be shallow, with irregular edges and surrounding skin may demonstrate changes associated with venous disease such as haemosiderin, LDS or gravitational eczema.

2. Local treatment will include a non-adherent dressing if the wound bed is clean and granulating. Surrounding skin will require emollients for hydration and/or topical steroids if eczema is present. The most important treatment will be the application of graduated compression using a multi-layer bandage system.

3. The patient should be encouraged to take gentle exercise (sufficient to ensure ankle flexion) and also elevate the leg when sitting. The patient must continue to wear the compression bandages (day and night) until healed unless pain, discomfort or skin colour changes occur, in which case they should seek medical attention. In the long-term, the patient should be assessed for compression hosiery which should be continued for at least 5 years post-healing to prevent recurrence.

Case 58.3

A 59-year-old spinally injured, wheelchair-bound patient has a pressure ulcer extending into the underlying tissues (Fig. 58.13).

Questions

1. What is the likely stage/category of the ulcer?
2. What are the factors that have led to the development of the ulcer?
3. What are the key concerns in selecting the most appropriate product (s) to manage (a) the ulcer (b) the patient?

Answers

1. This is likely to be a Stage/Category III ulcer as on further examination no bone can be felt at the base of the wound (bleeding noted in the image is due to probing of the ulcer and is also due to the presence of local infection in the tissues).

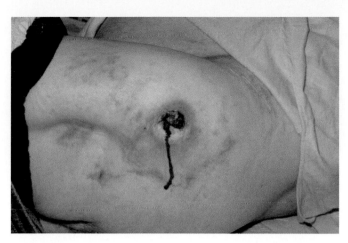

Fig. 58.13 Case 58.3

2. The patient has sustained a spinal injury and as a consequence their mobility will be limited, and they will not sense the need to change position regularly as they have lost the sensory clues to undertake this. The ulcer has probably been caused by direct pressure over a bony prominence which has led to the compression of tissue and vessels leading to damage.

(a) An assessment of the ulcer should be undertaken to include the size of the ulcer, presence of undermining or tunnelling, the type of tissue in the wound bed (to include presence of bone) and the amount of exudate. A cavity wound such as this should be packed gently and secured with a non-adhesive type dressing as skin stripping may occur on dressing removal otherwise. An antimicrobial dressing could be used.

(b) The patient's wheelchair and cushion should be assessed to determine whether they are suitable. The patient should also be asked about how often they relieve the pressure when sitting and be reminded that ideally this should be every 15 min. The patient should be encouraged to remain off the affected area until it has healed and the use of an appropriate mattress should be discussed. Other aspects such as skin care (to include the peri-wound area), skin hygiene and nutrition should also be reviewed.

References

Ashcroft, G.S., Mills, S.J., Ashworth, J.J., 2002. Ageing and wound healing. Biogerontology 3, 337–345.

Baker, R.P., Al-Kubati, W., Atuf, M., et al., 2007. Nicorandil-induced severe perianal ulceration. Techn. Coloproctol. 11, 343–345.

Briggs, M., Closs, S.J., 2003. The prevalence of leg ulceration: a review of the literature. EWMA J. 3(2), 14–20.

Clark, M., Defloor, T., Bours, G., 2004. A pilot study of the prevalence of pressure ulcers in European hospitals. In: Clark, M., (ed.), Ulcers Pressure: Recent Advances in Tissue Viability. Quay Books, Salisbury, pp. 8–22.

Cradock, S., Shaw, K., 2002. The diabetes national standards framework. Setting the standard. Pract. Diab. Int. 19, 3.

Department of Health, 2001. National Service Framework for Diabetes: Standards. DH, London.

Department of Health, 2007a. Working Together for Better Diabetes Care. DH, London.

Department of Health, 2007b. The Way Ahead: The Local Challenge Improving Diabetes Services. DH, London.

Desai, H., 1997a. Ageing and wounds part 1: fetal and post-natal healing. J. Wound Care 6, 192–196.

Desai, H., 1997b. Ageing and wounds part 2: healing in old age. J. Wound Care 6, 237–239.

Edmonds, M., Foster, A., The Ulcerated Foot. 2000. Managing the Diabetic Foot. Blackwell Science, London.

Enoch, S., Grey, J.E., Harding, K.G., 2008. Recent advances and emerging treatments. In: Grey, J.E., Harding, K.G., ABC of Wound Healing. BMJ Books, Blackwell Publishing. Oxford.

Enoch, S., Leaper, D.J., 2005. Basic science of wound healing. Surgery 23, 37–42.

European Pressure Ulcer Advisory Panel (EPUAP) and National Pressure Ulcer Advisory Panel (NPUAP), 2009. Prevention and Treatment of Pressure Ulcers: Quick Reference Guide. NPUAP, Washington DC.

Grey, J.E., Harding, K.G., 2008. ABC of Wound Healing. BMJ Books, Blackwell Publishing, Oxford.

Lipsky, B.A., Berendt, A.R., 2006. Infection of the foot in persons with diabetes: epidemiology, pathophysiology, microbiology, clinical presentation and approach to therapy. In: Boulton, J.M., Cavanagh, P.R., Rayman, G. (Eds.), The Foot in Diabetes, fourth ed. John Wiley, Chichester, pp. 159–168.

Møller, A., Villebro, N., Pedersen, T., et al., 2002. Effect of preoperative smoking interventions on postoperative complications: a randomised clinical trial. Lancet 359, 114–117.

National Institute of Health and Clinical Excellence, 2003. Pressure ulcer prevention: pressure ulcer risk assessment and prevention, including the use of pressure-relieving devices (beds, mattresses and overlays) for the prevention of pressure ulcers in primary and secondary care. NICE, London. Available at http://www.nice.org.uk/nicemedia/pdf/CG7_PRD_NICEguideline.pdf.

National Institute of Health and Clinical Excellence, 2004. Type 2 diabetes: prevention and management of foot problems. NICE, London. Available at http://www.nice.org.uk/CG010NICEguideline.

National Institute of Health and Clinical Excellence, 2005. Pressure ulcers – prevention and treatment. NICE, London. Available at http://www.nice.org.uk/nicemedia/pdf/CG029publicinfo.pdf.

National Institute of Health and Clinical Excellence, 2008. Type 2 diabetes: national clinical guideline for management in primary care (update). NICE, London. Available at http://www.nice.org.uk/nicemedia/linve/11983/40803/40803.pdf.

Robson, M.C., Cooper, D.M., Aslam, R., et al., 2006. Guidelines for the treatment of venous leg ulcers. Wound Repair Regen. 14, 649–662.

Sorensen, L.T., Karlsmark, T., Gottrup, F., 2003. Abstinence from smoking reduces incisional wound infection: a randomized controlled trial. Ann. Surg. 238, 1–5.

Tennvall, G.R., Hjelmgren, J., 2005. Annual cost of treatment for venous leg ulcers in Sweden and the United Kingdom. Wound Repair Regen. 13, 13–18.

Waters, N., Holloway, S.L., 2009. Personal perceptions of the impact of diabetic foot disease on employment. Diab. Foot 12, 119–131.

Winter, G.D., 1962. Formation of the scab and the rate of epithelialization of superficial wounds in the skin of the young domestic pig. Nature 193, 293–294.

Wolcott, R.D., Rhoads, D.D., 2008. A study of biofilm-based wound management in subjects with critical limb ischaemia. J. Wound Care 17, 145–155.

Wysocki, A.B., 2007. Anatomy and physiology of the skin and soft tissue. In: Bryant, R.A., Nix, D.P. (Eds.), Acute and Chronic Wounds: Current Management. Mosby, St Louis, pp. 39–55.

SECTION 4

APPENDICES

Medical abbreviations

25 OHD	25-hydroxy vitamin D		**AHA**	autoimmune haemolytic anaemia
5-ASA	5-aminosalicylic acid		**AHD**	autoimmune haemolytic disease
5-HIAA	5-hydroxyindolacetic acid		**AIDS**	acquired immune deficiency syndrome
5-HT	5-hydroxytryptamine (serotonin)		**AIP**	asymptomatic inflammatory prostatitis
A & O	alert and oriented		**AIT**	amiodarone induced thyrotoxicosis
A & P	anterior and posterior		**AK**	above knee
	auscultation and percussion		**ALA**	aminolaevulinic acid
A & W	alive and well		**ALD**	alcoholic liver disease
A&E	accident and emergency		**ALF**	acute liver failure
AAA	abdominal aortic aneurysm		**ALG**	antilymphocyte globulin
	acute anxiety attack		**ALL**	acute lymphocytic leukaemia
AAAAA	aphasia, agnosia, apraxia, agraphia and alexia		**ALP**	alkaline phosphatise
Ab	antibody		**ALT**	alanine transaminase
ABCD	amphotericin B colloidal dispersion			argon laser trabeculopasty
ABD	amphotericin B deoxycholate		**AMA**	against medical advice
abd.	abdomen (abdominal)		**AMI**	acute myocardial infarction
	abduction		**AML**	acute myeloid leukaemia
ABE	acute bacterial endocarditis		**AMP**	adenosine monophosphate
ABG	arterial blood gases		**ANA**	antinuclear antibody
ABMT	autologous bone marrow transplant		**ANC**	absolute neutrophil count
ABP	acute bacterial prostatitis		**ANF**	antinuclear factor
ABVD	adriamycin (doxorubicin), bleomycin,		**ANP**	atrial natriuretic peptide
	vinblastine, dacarbazine		**Anti-HbAb**	anti-hepatitis B antibody
ACAT	acylcholesterol acyltransferase		**AOB**	alcohol on breath
ACBS	aortocoronary bypass surgery		**AP**	alkaline phosphatase
ACD	allergic contact dermatitis			angina pectoris
ACE	angiotensin-converting enzyme			antepartum
Acid phos.	acid phosphatase			anterior pituitary
ACR	albumin:creatinine ratio			anteroposterior
ACT	activated clotting time			aortic pressure
AD	Alzheimer's disease			apical pulse
ADC	AIDS dementia complex			appendectomy
ADH	antidiuretic hormone			artificial pneumothorax
ADL	activities of daily living		**APB**	atrial premature beat
ADP	adenosine diphosphate		**APC**	activated protein C
ADR	adverse drug reaction			atrial premature contraction
ADT	androgen deprivation therapy		**APD**	action potential duration
ADU	acute duodenal ulcer		**APKD**	adult polycystic kidney disease
AED	antiepileptic drug		**APP**	amyloid precursor protein
AF	atrial fibrillation		**APSAC**	anisoylated plasminogen streptokinase
AFB	acid-fast bacillus			activated complex
AFP	a-fetoprotein		**APTT**	activated partial thromboplastin time
AGEP	acute generalised exanthematous pustulosis		**AR**	aortic regurgitation
AGL	acute granulocytic leukaemia			apical/radial (pulse)
AGN	acute glomerulonephritis		**ARB**	angiotensin receptor blocker

ARDS	adult respiratory distress syndrome		Bx.	biopsy
ARF	acute renal failure		C	complement
AS	aortic stenosis		C & P	cystoscopy and pyelogram
	arteriosclerosis		C & S	culture and sensitivity
A–S attack	Adams–Stokes attack		c/o	complains of
ASB	asymptomatic bacteriuria		$C_1, C_2, ...$	cervical vertebrae 1, 2, ...
ASCA	anti-*Saccharomycs cerevisiae* antibodies		CA	cancer
ASD	atrial septal defect			carcinoma
ASLO titre	antistreptolysin-O titre			cardiac arrest
AST	aspartate transaminase			coronary artery
ATG	antithymocyte globulin		Ca	carcinoma
ATN	acute tubular necrosis		CABG	coronary artery bypass graft
AUC	area under the curve		CAD	coronary artery disease
AUR	acute urinary retention		CAH	chronic active hepatitis
AV	aortic valve		CAP	community acquired pneumonia
	atrioventricular		CAPD	continuous ambulatory peritoneal dialysis
A-V	arteriovenous		CAT	computed axial tomography
AVNRT	atrioventricular nodal re-entry tachycardia		CAVH	continuous arteriovenous haemofiltration
AVR	aortic valve replacement		CBA	cost–benefit analysis
	augmented V lead, right arm (ECG)		CBP	chronic bacterial prostatitis
AVRT	atrioventricular re-entry tachycardia		CBT	cognitive behaviour therapy
AVS	arteriovenous shunt		CC	chief complaint
AXR	abdominal X-ray			current complaint
B Bx.	breast biopsy		CCF	congestive cardiac failure
BACUP	British Association of Cancer United Patients		CCU	coronary care unit
BBB	bundle branch block		CEA	cost-effectiveness analysis
BBBB	bilateral bundle branch block (ECG)		CF	cardiac failure
BCAA	branched-chain amino acid			complement fixation
BCC	basal cell carcinoma			cystic fibrosis
BCG	bacille Calmette–Guérin		CFT	complement fixation test
BDA	British Diabetic Association		CGL	chronic granulocytic leukaemia
BE	base excess		CGN	chronic glomerulonephritis
BEACOPP	bleomycin, etoposide, adriamycin (doxorubicin), cyclophosphomide, Oncovin (vincristine), procarbazine, prednisolone		CHB	complete heart block
			CHD	coronary heart disease
			CHF	congestive heart failure
BEAM	carmustine, etoposide, cytarabine, melphalan		CHM	Commision on Human Medicines
BG	blood glucose		CHO	carbohydrate
BHS	beta haemolytic streptococci		CHOP	cyclophosphamide, hydroxydaunorubicin (doxorubicin), Oncovin (vincristine), prednisolone
BIA	bioelectrical impedance analysis			
BJ protein	Bence-Jones protein		CHOP-R	cyclophosphamide, hydroxydaunorubicin (doxorubicin), Oncovin (vincristine), prednisolone, rituximab
BKA	below knee amputation			
BM	bowel movement			
BMI	body mass index			
BMT	bone marrow transplant		CI	cardiac index
BNO	bowels not open			cerebral infarction
BOR	bowels open regularly		CINV	chemotherapy-induced nausea and vomiting
BP	bypass, blood pressure		CIVA	centralized intravenous additive
BPA	British Paediatric Association		CK	creatine kinase (same as CPK)
BPD	bronchopulmonary dysplasia		CKD	chronic kidney disease
BPE	benign prostatic enlargement		CL	clubbing
BPH	benign prostatic hyperplasia		ClCr	creatinine clearance
BS	blood sugar		CLD	chronic liver disease
	bowel sounds			chronic lung disease
	breath sounds		CLL	chronic lymphocytic leukaemia
			CMA	cost minimization analysis
BSA	body surface area		CML	chronic myelocytic leukaemia
BW	body water		CMV	cytomegalovirus
	body weight		CNS	central nervous system

CNS	coagulase negative staphylococci		CV	cardiovascular
CO	cardiac output			central venous
CoA	co-enzyme A			cerebrovascular
COAD	chronic obstructive airways disease			contingent valuation
COC	combined oral contraceptive		CVA	cerebrovascular accident (stroke)
COD	cause of death			costovertebral angle
COG	closed angle glaucoma		CVD	cardiovascular disease
COLD	chronic obstructive lung disease		CVP	central venous pressure
COP	capillary osmotic pressure		CVVH	continuous venovenous haemofiltration
COPD	chronic obstructive pulmonary disease		Cx	cervical, cervix
COX	cyclo-oxygenase		CXR	chest X-ray
CP	cor pulmonale		d	dead
	creatine phosphate			deceased
CP	chronic prostatitis		D & C	dilation and curettage
CPA	cardiopulmonary arrest		D & V	diarrhoea and vomiting
	cerebellar pontine angle		D/C	discontinue
CPAP	continuous positive airway pressure		D/S	dextrose and saline
CPD	continuous peritoneal dialysis		D5W	dextrose 5%
CPK	creatine phosphokinase		DADs	delayed after depolarisation
CPN	chronic pyelonephritis		DAFNE	(insulin) dose adjustment for normal eating
CPPS	chronic pelvic pain syndrome		DBP	diastolic blood pressure
CPPV	continuous positive pressure ventilation		DDx.	differential diagnosis
CPR	cardiopulmonary resuscitation		DES	diethylstilboestrol
CPSI	chronic prostatitis symptom index		DEXA	dual energy X-ray absorptiometry
CPZ	chlorpromazine		DH	drug history
CR	cardiorespiratory		DIC	disseminated intravascular coagulation
	clot retraction		DILD	drug-induced liver disease
	colon resection		DILI	drug-induced liver injury
	complete remission		DIP	drug-induced parkinsonism
	conditional reflex		DIT	di-iodotyrosine
	crown-rump		DKA	diabetic ketoacidosis
CRD	chronic renal disease		DLBCL	diffuse large B cell lymphoma
CRF	chronic renal failure		DLE	discoid lupus erythematosus
	corticotrophin-releasing factor			disseminated lupus erythematosus
CRP	C-reactive protein		DM	diabetes mellitus
CSAP	cryosurgical ablation of prostate			diastolic murmur
CSF	cerebrospinal fluid		DMARDS	disease-modifying antirheumatic drugs
CSH	chronic subdural haematoma		DNA	did not attend (outpatients)
CSM	carotid sinus massage		DOA	dead on arrival
	cerebrospinal meningitis		DOB	date of birth
CSP	carotid sinus pressure		DOD	date of death
CSR	Cheyne–Stokes respiration		DOE	dyspnoea on exertion
	correct sedimentation rate		DOTS	Directly Observed Treatment Short course TB programme
CSS	carotid sinus stimulation		DRE	digital rectal examination
	central sterile supply		DROP	dyslipidaemia, insulin resistance, obesity and high blood pressure
CSU	catheter specimen of urine			
CT	circulation time		DSM	*Diagnostic and Statistical Manual of Mental Disorders*
	clotting time			
	computer tomography		DTI	direct thrombus imaging
	Coombs' test		DTP	diphtheria, tetanus, pertussis (vaccine)
	coronary thrombosis		DTs	delirium tremens
cTnI	cardiac troponin I		DU	diagnosis undetermined
cTnT	cardiac troponin T			duodenal ulcer
CTZ	chemoreceptor trigger zone		DUB	dysfunctional uterine bleeding
CUA	cost–utility analysis		DUE	drug use evaluation
CUG	cystourethrogram			

DVT	deep vein thrombosis	**FRC**	functional reserve capacity
Dx.	diagnosis		functional residual capacity
DXT	deep X-ray therapy	**FSH**	follicle-stimulating hormone
E/I	expiration–inspiration ratio	**FSNGN**	focal segmental necrotising glomerulonephritis
EADs	early after depolarisations	**FT4**	free thyroxine
EBV	Epstein–Barr virus	**FTI**	free thyroxine index
ECBV	effective circulating blood volume	**FUO**	fever of unknown origin
ECF	extracellular fluid	**FVC**	forced vital capacity
ECFV	extracellular fluid volume	**Fx.**	fracture
ECG	electrocardiogram	**G6PD**	glucose-6-phosphate dehydrogenase
ECHO	echocardiogram	**GA**	general anaesthesia
	echoencephalogram		general appearance
ECMO	extracorporeal membrane oxygenation	**GABA**	g-aminobutyric acid
ECT	electroconvulsive therapy	**GABAA**	g-aminobutyric acid A
EDD	expected date of delivery	**GAD**	glutamic acid decarboxylase
EDV	end-diastolic volume	**GAD**	generalised anxiety disorder
EEG	electroencephalogram	**Gamma-GT**	g-glutamyl transferase
EENT	eyes, ears, nose and throat	**GB**	gallbladder
EGFR	epidermal growth factor receptor		Guillain–Barré (syndrome)
ELBW	extremely low birth weight	**GBM**	glomerular basement membrane
ELISA	enzyme-linked immunosorbent assay	**GBS**	Glasgow-Blatchford score
EM	ejection murmur	**G-CSF**	granulocyte-colony stimulating factor
EM	erythema multiforme	**GDM**	gastro-intestinal diabetes mellitus
EMG	electromyogram	**GF**	glomerular filtration
EN	erythema nodosum		gluten-free
ENT	ears, nose and throat	**GFR**	glomerular filtration rate
EP	ectopic pregnancy	**GGT**	g-glutamyl transpeptidase (transferase)
ER	(o)estrogen receptor	**GI**	gastro-intestinal
ERCP	endoscopic retrograde cholangiopancreatography	**GIK**	glucose, insulin and potassium
ERP	effective refractory period	**GLA**	g-linolenic acid
ESBL	extended spectrum beta lactamase	**GM seizure**	grand mal seizure
ESHAP	etoposide, methylprednisolone, cytarabine, cisplatin	**GM-CSF**	granulocyte macrophage colony stimulating factor
ESM	ejection systolic murmur	**GN**	glomerulonephritis
ESN	educationally subnormal	**GNDC**	Gram-negative diplococci
ESP	end-systolic pressure	**GnRH**	gonadotrophin-releasing hormone
ESR	erythrocyte sedimentation rate	**GORD**	gastro-oesophageal reflux disease
ESRF	end-stage renal failure	**grav.**	gravid (pregnant)
ET	endotracheal tube	**GRE**	glycopeptide-resistant enterococci
ETT	exercise tolerance test	**GS**	general surgery
FAS	fetal alcohol syndrome		genital system
FB	finger breadths	**GTN**	glyceryl trinitrate
FBS	fasting blood sugar	**GTT**	glucose tolerance test
FCE	finished consultant episode	**GU**	gastric ulcer
FeNa	fractional excretion of sodium		genitourinary
FEV	forced expiratory volume		gonococcal urethritis
FEV1	forced expiratory volume in 1 second	**GUS**	genitourinary system
FFA	free fatty acids	**GVHD**	graft-versus-host disease
FFP	fresh frozen plasma	**H & L**	heart and lungs
FH	familial hypercholesterolaemia	**h/o**	history of
	family history	**HAA**	hepatitis-associated antigen
FHH	familial hypocalciuric hypercalcaemia	**HACAs**	human anti-chimeric antibodies
FMD	fludarabine, mitoxantrone, dexametasone	**HAP**	hospital-acquired pneumonia
FOB	faecal occult blood	**HAS**	human albumin solution
FP	frozen plasma	**HAV**	hepatitis A virus
		HB	heart block

Hb (Hgb)	haemoglobin
HbA$_1$	glycated haemoglobin
HbA$_{1c}$	glycated haemoglobin
HbA$_2$	haemoglobin found in b-thalassaemia carriers
HBAg	hepatitis B antigen
HBD	hydroxybutyrate dehydrogenase
HBDH	hydroxybutyrate dehydrogenase
HBGM	home blood glucose monitoring
HbS	sickle haemoglobin in sickle cell disease
HBsAG	hepatitis B surface antigen
HBV	hepatitis B virus
HCAI	healthcare-associated infections
Hct. (hct.)	haematocrit
HCV	hepatitis C virus
HDL	high-density lipoprotein
HDL-C	high-density lipoprotein cholesterol
HDT	high-dose therapy
HER1	human epidermal growth factor receptor type 1
HER2	human epidermal growth factor receptor type 2
HF	heart failure
HHV	human herpes virus
Hib	*Haemophilus influenzae* type b
HIE	hypoxic-ischaemic encephalopathy
HIFU	high intensity focussed ultrasound
HIT	heparin induced thrombocytopaenia
HIV	human immunodeficiency virus
HLA	human lymphocyte antibody
HMD	hyaline membrane disease
HMMA	4-hydroxy-3-methoxymandelic acid
hMPV	human metapneumovirus
HO	house officer
HONK	hyperosmolar non-ketotic hyperglycaemia
HPEN	home parenteral and enteral nutrition
HPI	history of present illness
HPN	home parenteral nutrition
HPRT	hypoxanthine-guanine phosphoribosyl transferase deficiency
HPV	human papilloma virus
HR	heart rate
HRS	hepatorenal syndrome
HRT	hormone replacement therapy
HS	half strength
	Hartmann's solution
	heart sounds
HSA	human serum albumin
HSCT	hematopoietic stem cell transplantation
HSV	herpes simplex virus
HT, HTN	hypertension
HUS	haemolytic uraemic syndrome
HVA	homovanillic acid
HVD	hypertensive vascular disease
Hx.	history
i.v.	intravenous
IADHS	inappropriate antidiuretic hormone syndrome
IBC	iron binding capacity
IBD	inflammatory bowel disease
IBS	irritable bowel syndrome

IC	intercostal
	intracerebral
	intracranial
ICA	islet cell antibody
ICD	*International Classification of Diseases*
ICD	implantable cardioverter-defibrillator
ICD	impulse control disorder
ICE	ifosfamide, carboplatin, etoposide
ICF	intracellular fluid
ICH	intracerebral haemorrhage
ICM	intracostal margin
ICS	intercostal space
ICS	inhaled cortocosteroids
ICU	intensive care unit
ID	intradermal
IDDM	insulin-dependent diabetes mellitus
IDL	intermediate-density lipoprotein
IDL-C	intermediate-density lipoprotein cholesterol
IDP	intradialytic parenteral nutrition
IEP	immunoelectrophoresis
IFRT	involved field radiotherapy
Ig	immunoglobulin
iGAS	invasive group A streptococcal infection
IGT	impaired glucose tolerance
IHC	immunohistochemistry
IHD	ischaemic heart disease
IHR	intrinsic heart rate
IMI	inferior myocardial infarction
IMP	impression
Inf. MI	inferior myocardial infarction
INR	international normalized ratio
IOP	intraocular pressure
IPCN	International Prostatitis Collaborative Network
IPF	idiopathic pulmonary fibrosis
IPI	International Prognostic Index
IPP	intermittent positive-pressure inflation with oxygen
IPPB	intermittent positive-pressure breathing
IPPV	intermittent positive-pressure ventilation
IRDS	idiopathic respiratory distress syndrome
ISA	intrinsic sympathomimetic activity
ISDN	isosorbide dinitrate
ISI	International Sensitivity Index
ISMN	isosorbide mononitrate
IT	intrathecal(ly)
ITT	insulin tolerance test
IUCD	intrauterine contraceptive device
IUD	intrauterine death
	intrauterine device
IVD	intervertebral disc
IVH	intraventricular haemorrhage
IVP	intravenous push
	intravenous pyelography
IVSD	interventricular septal defect
IVU	intravenous urography
J	jaundice
JVD	jugular venous distension
JVP	jugular venous pressure

KA	ketoacidosis
KCCT	kaolin-cephalin clotting time
KLS	kidney, liver, spleen
KS	Kaposi's sarcoma
KUB	kidneys, ureters, bladder
L	left
	lower
	lumber
L & A	light and accommodation
L & U	lower and upper
L & W	living and well
L$_1$, L$_2$, …	lumbar vertebrae 1, 2, …
LA	left arm
	left atrium
	local anaesthesia
LABA	long-acting β_2-adrenoceptor agonist
LAD	left anterior descending
LADA	latent autoimmune diabetes in adults
LAMA	long acting antimuscarinic
LBBB	left bundle branch block
LBM	lean body mass
LBW	low birth weight
LCAT	lecithin-cholesterol acyltransferase
LCT	long-chain triglyceride
LD, LDH	lactate dehydrogenase
LDL	low-density lipoprotein
LDL-C	low-density lipoprotein cholesterol
LDS	lipodermatosclerosis
LE	lupus erythematosus
LFT	liver function test
LH	luteinizing hormone
LHRH	luteinizing hormone-releasing hormone
LIF	left iliac fossa
LK	left kidney
LKKS	liver, kidneys, spleen
LKS	liver, kidney, spleen
LL	left leg
	left lower
	lower lobe
LLL	left lower lobe
	left lower lid
LLQ	left lower quadrant
LMN	lower motor neurone
LMP	last menstrual period
LMWH	low molecular weight heparin
LN	lymph node
LNG-IUS	levonorgestrel intrauterine system
LNMP	last normal menstrual period
LOM	limitation of movement
LP	lumbar puncture
Lp(a)	lipoprotein a
LPA	left pulmonary artery
LS	left side
	liver and spleen
	lumbosacral
	lymphosarcoma
LSD	lysergic acid diethylamide
LSK	liver, spleen, kidneys

LSM	late systolic murmur
LT	leukotriene
LTBI	latent tuberculosis infection
LTC	long-term care
LTOT	long-term oxygen therapy
LUL	left upper lobe
LUQ	left upper quadrant
LV	left ventricle
LVDP	left ventricular diastolic pressure
LVE	left ventricular enlargement
LVEDP	left ventricular end-diastolic pressure
LVEDV	left ventricular end-diastolic volume
LVET	left ventricular ejection time
LVF	left ventricular failure
LVH	left ventricular hypertrophy
LVP	left ventricular pressure
M	male
	married
	metre
	mother
	molar
	murmur
M:P	milk-to-plasma ratio
MABP	mean arterial blood pressure
MAC	*Mycobacterium avium* complex
MAI	*Mycobacterium avium-intracellulare*
MALT	mucosal-associated lymphoid tissue
MAMC	mid-arm muscle circumference
MAO-A	monoamine oxidase A
MAO-B	monoamine oxidase B
MAOI	monoamine oxidase inhibitor
MAP	mean arterial pressure
MARS	molecular adsorbent recycling system
MBC	minimum bactericidal concentration
MBP	mean blood pressure
MCH	mean corpuscular cell haemoglobin
MCHC	mean corpuscular cell haemoglobin concentration
MCP	metacarpophalangeal (joint)
MCT	medium-chain triglycerides
MCV	mean corpuscular cell volume
MD	mitral disease
	muscular dystrophy
MDI	metered-dose inhaler
MDM	mid-diastolic murmur
MDMA	methylene dioxymethamphetamine, ecstasy
MDRD	modification of diet in renal disease formula for GFR estimation
MDRST	multidrug-resistant *S. enterica* serovar typhi
MDRTB	multidrug-resistant tuberculosis
MDR-TB	multidrug-resistant tuberculosis
MDS	myelodydsplastic syndrome
MEN	multiple endocrine neoplasia
met.	metastatic (metastasis)
MGN	membranous glomerulonephritis
MH	medical history
	menstrual history
MHPG	methoxyhydroxyphenylglyccrol

MHRA	Medicines and Healthcare products Regulatory Agency
MI	myocardial infarction
	mitral incompetence
MIC	minimum inhibitory concentration
MID	multi-infarct dementia
MIRU	mycobacterial interspersed repetitive unit typing
MIT	monoiodotyrosine
ML	middle lobe
	midline
MMR	measles, mumps, rubella
MMSE	mini mental state examination
MODY	maturity-onset diabetes of the young
MOPP	mustine, Oncovin (vincristine), procarbazine, prednisolone
MOTT	mycobacteria other than tuberculosis
MPJ	metacarpophalangeal joint
MR	mitral regurgitation
MRA	magnetic resonance angiography
MRD	minimal residual disease
MRDM	malnutrition-related diabetes mellitus
MRI	magnetic resonance imaging
MRSA	methicillin-resistant *Staphylococcus aureus*
MS	mitral stenosis
	multiple sclerosis
	musculoskeletal
MSL	midsternal line
MSSA	methicillin-sensitive *Staphylococcus aureus*
MSU	midstream urine specimen
MTB	*Mycobacterium tuberculosis*
MTI	minimum time interval
MTP	metatarsophalangeal
MUD	matched unrelated donor
MV	minute volume
	mitral valve
MVP	mitral valve prolapse
MVPP	mustine, vinblastine, procarbazine, prednisolone
MVR	mitral valve replacement
MWH	moist wound healing
N	normal
N & T	nose and throat
N & V	nausea and vomiting
NAAT	nucleic acid amplification techniques
NAD	no appreciable disease
	normal axis deviation
	nothing abnormal detected
NADPH	nicotinamide adenine dinucleotide phosphate hydrogen
NAFLD	non-alcoholic fatty liver disease
NAG	narrow angle glaucoma
NAI	neuraminidase inhibitor
NAPQI	*N*-acetyl-*p*-benzoquinoneimine
NARI	noradrenergic reuptake inhibitor
NARTI	nucleoside analogue reverse transcriptase inhibitor
NASH	non-alcoholic steatohepatitis

NaSSA	noradrenergic and specifc serotonergic antidepressant
NBM	nil by mouth
NEC	necrotizing enterocolitis
NG	nasogastric
NHL	non-Hodgkin's lymphoma
NIDDM	non-insulin-dependent diabetes mellitus
NKHA	non-ketotic hyperosmolar acidosis
NLPHL	nodular lymphocyte-predominant Hodgkin's lymphoma
NMR	nuclear magnetic resonance
NMS	neuroleptic malignant syndrome
NNRTI	non-nucleoside reverse transcriptase inhibitor
NOF	neck of femur
NS	nephrotic syndrome
	nervous system
	normal saline
	no specimen
NSAID	non-steroidal anti-inflammatory drug
NSFTD	normal spontaneous full-term delivery
NSR	normal sinus rhythm
NSTEMI	non-ST-elevated myocardial infarction
NSU	non-specific urethritis
NT	nasotracheal (tube)
NTS	nucleus tractus solitarius
NVD	nausea, vomiting, diarrhoea
O	oedema
O & A	observation and assessment
O & E	observation and examination
O/A	on admission
O/E	on examination
OA	osteoarthritis
OAD	obstructive airway disease
OAG	open angle glaucoma
OB	occult blood
OCD	obsessive compulsive disorder
OD	overdose
OGTT	oral glucose tolerance test
OH	occupational history
OHT	ocular hypertension
OI	opportunistic infection
OKGA	ornithine salt of a-ketoglutaric acid
OLT	orthoptic liver transplantation
OPA	outpatient appointment
OPD	outpatient department
OSAHS	obstructive sleep apnoea hypopnoea syndrome
OT	occupational therapy
P & A	percussion and auscultation
P & V	pyloroplasty and vagotomy
PA	pernicious anaemia
	pulmonary artery
PACG	primary angle-closure glaucoma
PaCO$_2$	arterial carbon dioxide tension
PAD	peripheral arterial disease
PAF	platelet-activating factor
PAH	pulmonary artery hypertension
pANCA	perinuclear antineutrophil cytoplasmic antibodies

PaO$_2$	arterial oxygen tension
PAPS	primary antiphospholipid syndrome
PAS	P-aminosalicylic acid
	pulmonary artery stenosis
PAT	paroxysmal atrial tachycardia
PAWP	pulmonary artery wedge pressure
PB	premature beats
PBC	primary biliary cirrhosis
PBI	protein-bound iodine
PBSCT	peripheral blood stem cell transplantion
PC	prostate cancer
PCA	patient-controlled analgesia
PCAS	patient-controlled analgesia system
PCI	percutaneous coronary intervention
PCO$_2$	partial pressure of carbon dioxide
PCR	polymerase chain reaction
PCS	portocaval shunt
PCV	packed cell volume
PD	peritoneal dialysis
PDA	patent ductus arteriosus
PE	physical examination
	pleural effusion
	pulmonary embolism
PEARLA	pupils equal and react to light and accommodation
PEF	peak expiratory flow
PEFR	peak expiratory flow rate
PEG	percutaneous endoscopic gastrostomy
PEJ	percutaneous endoscopic jejunostomy
PEM	prescription event monitoring
PEM	protein energy malnutrition
PEP	post exposure prophylaxis
PERLA	pupils equal, react to light and accommodation
PERRLA	pupils equal, round, react to light and accommodation
PET	position emission tomography
PF	peak flow
PF4	platelet factor 4
PFR	peak flow rate
PFT	pulmonary function test
PG	prostaglandin
P-gp	P-glycoprotein
PH	past history
	patient history
	personal history
	prostatic hypertrophy
	pulmonary hypertension
PHI	primary HIV infection
PI	present illness
	protease inhibitor
PICC	peripherally inserted central catheter
PID	pelvic inflammatory disease
PIN	prostatic intra-epithelial neoplasia
PIP	proximal interphalangeal joint
PIVD	protruded intervertebral disc
PJB	premature junctional beat
PJC	premature junctional contraction
PJP	*Pneumocystis jiroveci* pneumonia
PKU	phenylketonuria

PL	product licence
PLL	prolymphocytic leukaemia
PMDD	premenstrual dysphoric disorder
PMH	past medical history
PMI	past medical illness
PMN	polymorphonucleocyte
PMS	premenstrual syndrome
	postmenopausal syndrome
PMT	premenstrual tension
PMV	prolapsed mitral valve
PN	percussion note
	peripheral nerve
	peripheral neuropathy
PND	paroxysmal nocturnal dyspnoea
	postnasal drip
PO$_2$	partial pressure of oxygen
POAG	primary open-angle glaucoma
POMR	problem-oriented medical record
PONV	postoperative nausea and vomiting
PPAR-g	proliferative-activated receptor-g
PPD	purified protein derivative
PPH	postpartum haemorrhage
PPI	proton pump inhibitor
PPNG	penicillinase-producing *Neisseria gonorrhocae*
PPV	positive-pressure ventilation
PR	per rectum
	progestogen receptor
PRCA	pure red cell aplasia
PREP	pre-exposure prophylaxis
PROM	premature rupture of membranes
PS	pulmonary stenosis
	pyloric stenosis
PSA	prostate-specific antigen
PSG	presystolic gallop
PSGN	poststreptococcal glomerulonephritis
PSVT	paroxysmal supraventricular tachycardia
PT	parathyroid
	paroxysmal tachycardia
	physical therapy
	physical training
	posterior tibial (pulse)
	prothrombin time
PTC	percutaneous cholangiogram
PTH	parathyroid hormone
PTLD	post-transplant lymphoproliferative disorder
PTSD	post traumatic stress disorder
PTT	partial thromboplastin time
PTTK	partial thromboplastin time kaolin
PTU	propylthiouracil
PU	pass urine
	per urethra
	peptic ulcer
PUD	peptic ulcer disease
	pulmonary disease
PUO	pyrexia (fever) of unknown origin
PUVA	psoralen and ultraviolet A radiation
PV	vaginal examination (per vagina)
PVB	premature ventricular beat

PVC	premature ventricular contraction
PVD	peripheral vascular disease
PVP	pulmonary venous pressure
PVR	post-void residual
PVT	paroxysmal ventricular tachycardia
Px.	past history
	prognosis
QALY	quality-adjusted life-year
R	respiration
RA	renal artery
	rheumatoid arthritis
	right arm
	right atrial (atrium)
RAST	radio-allergosorbent test
RBBB	right bundle branch block
RBC	red blood cell
	red blood (cell) count
RBS	random blood sugar
R-CVP	rituximab, cyclophosphamide, vincristine, prednisolone
RDS	respiratory distress syndrome
REMS	rapid eye movement sleep
Re-PUVA	PUVA treatment with retinoids
RF	renal failure
	rheumatic fever
	rheumatoid factor
RFT	respiratory function tests
Rh factor	rhesus factor
RHF	right heart failure
RHL	right hepatic lobe
rhuEPO	recombinant human erythropoietin
rhuGM-CSF	recombinant human granulocyte-macrophage colony-stimulating factor
RIF	right iliac fossa
RIMA	reversible inhibitor of monoamine oxidase type A
RITA	radiofrequency interstitial tumour ablation
RK	right kidney
RL	right leg
	right lung
RLC	residual lung capacity
RLD	related living donor
RLL	right lower lobe (lung)
RLQ	right lower quadrant (abdomen)
RP	radial pulse
RPGN	rapidly progressive glomerulonephritis
RPI	resting pressure index
RQ	respiratory quotient
RR	respiratory rate
RR & E	round, regular and equal (pupils)
RRT	renal replacement therapy
RS	respiratory system
RSF	rheumatoid serum factor
RSV	respiratory syncytial virus
RTA	road traffic accident
rt-PA	recombinant plasminogen activator
RUL	right upper lobe
RUQ	right upper quadrant
RV	residual volume
	right ventricle
RVH	right ventricular hypertrophy
RVOT	right ventricular outflow tract
SA	sinoatrial (node)
	Stokes–Adams (attacks)
	surface area
SAH	subarachnoid haemorrhage
SARS	severe acute respiratory syndrome
SARS CoV	severe acute respiratory syndrome-associated coronovirus
SB	seen by
	shortness of breath
SBE	subacute bacterial endocarditis
	shortness of breath on exertion
SBO	small bowel obstruction
SBP	spontaneous bacterial peritonitis
sCT	spiral computed tomography
SCU	see SCUF
SCUF	slow continuous ultrafiltration
SDD	selective decontamination of the digestive tract
SEM	systolic ejection murmur
SERM	selective estrogen receptor modulator
SGOT	serum glutamate-oxaloacetate transaminase
SGPT	serum glutamate-pyruvate transaminase
SH	social history
SIADH	syndrome of inappropriate antidiuretic hormone
SIDS	sudden infant death syndrome
SJS	Stevens–Johnson syndrome
SLE	systemic lupus erythematosus
SmPC	summary of product characteristics
SNRI	serotonin-noradrenaline reuptake inhibitor
SOA	swelling of ankle(s)
SOAP	subjective, objective, assessment, plan
SOB	short of breath
SOBOE	short of breath on exertion
SP	systolic pressure
SPA	suprapubic aspiration
SPC	Summary of Product Characteristics
SR	sinus rhythm
	sustained release
SS	serotonin syndrome
SSI	surgical site infection
SSRI	selective serotonin reuptake inhibitor
ST	sinus tachycardia
stat.	immediately (Latin: statim)
STD	sexually transmitted disease
STS	sodium tetradecyl sulphate
STS	serological tests for syphilis
SV	stroke volume
SVI	stroke volume index
SVT	supraventricular tachycardia
SWS	slow-wave sleep
Sx.	symptoms
T	temperature
T & C	type and cross-match

T & X	type and cross-match	TUMT	transurethral microwave heat treatment
T₃	tri-iodothyronine	TUR	transurethral resection
T₄	thyroxine	TURB	transurethral resection of the bladder
TAGvHD	transfusion-assisted graft-versus-host disease	TURP	transurethral resection of the prostate
TB	tuberculosis	TV	tidal volume
TBA	to be administered	TVN	tissue viability nurse
	to be arranged	TWOC	trial without catheter
TBG	thyroid-binding globulin	Tx.	transfusion
TBI	total body irradiation		treatment
TBM	tuberculous meningitis	U & E	urea and electrolytes
TBW	total body weight	UBIC	unsaturated iron-binding capacity
TC	total capacity	UC	ulcerative colitis
	total cholesterol	UFH	unfractionated heparin
	tricarboxylic acid cycle	UPCR	urine protein creatinine ratio
TCA	tricyclic antidepressant	URTI	upper respiratory tract infection
TDM	therapeutic drug monitoring	US	ultrasound
TEN	toxic epidermal necrolysis (Lyell's syndrome)	UTI	urinary tract infection
TENS	transcutaneous electrical nerve stimulation	UVA	ultraviolet A
TF	tissue factor	UVB	ultraviolet B
TFTs	thyroid function tests	V/Q	ventilation-perfusion ratio
TGF	tubuloglomerular feedback	VaD	vascular dementia
TGs	triglycerides	VC	vital capacity
TH	thyroid hormone (thyroxine)		vulvovaginal candidiasis
THA	tetrahydroaminoacridine	VD	venereal disease
THC	tetrahydrocannabinol	VDRL	Venereal Disease Research Laboratory (test for syphilis)
TIA	transient ischaemic attack	VEGF	vascular endothelial growth factor
TIBC	total iron-binding capacity	VF	ventricular fibrillation
TIMP	tissue inhibitor of metalloproteinases	VHD	valvular heart disease
TIPSS	transjugular intrahepatic portosystemic shunting	VKA	vitamin K antagonist
TKI	tyrosine kinase inhibitor	VLBW	very low birth weight
TLC	total lung capacity	VLDL	very low-density lipoprotein
	tender loving care	VMA	vanillyl mandelic acid
TLCO	transfer factor of the lung for carbon monoxide	VNTR	variable number of tandem repeats typing
TLS	tumour lysis syndrome	VP	venous pressure
TNF	tumour necrosis factor	VPC	ventricular premature contraction
TNF-α	tumour necrosis factor alpha	VS	vital signs
TNM	tumour node metastasis	VT	ventricular tachycardia
TP & P	time, place and person	VTE	venous thromboembolism
t-PA	tissue plasminogen factor	VTEC	verotoxin-producing E. coli
TPMT	thiopurine methyl transferase	VUR	vesicoureteric reflux
TPMT	thiopurine methyltransferase testing	VVC	vulvo vaginal candidiasis
TPN	total parenteral nutrition	WBC	white blood cell
TPR	temperature, pulse, respiration		white blood count
tPSA	total prostate specific antigen	WCC	white cell count
TRABs	thyroid receptor antibodies	WHO	World Health Organization
TRH	thyrotrophin-releasing hormone	WPW	Wolff–Parkinson–White (syndrome)
TRUS	transrectal ultrasonography	WR	Wassermann reaction
TSF	triceps skinfold thickness	WTA	willingness to accept
TSH	thyroid-stimulating hormone	WTP	willingness to pay
TTA	transtracheal aspiration	XDR-TB	extensively drug resistant tuberculosis
TTO	to take out (to take home)	ZE	Zollinger–Ellison (syndrome)
TUIP	transurethral incision of the prostate	ZIG	zoster immune globulin
		ZPP	zinc protoporphyrin

Glossary

Acanthosis nigricans Diffuse velvety acanthosis with grey, brown or black pigmentation, chiefly in axilla and other body folds, occurring in an adult form, often associated with an internal carcinoma and in a benign, nevoid form, more or less generalised.

Achlohydria Absence of hydrochloric acid from maximally stimulated gastric secretion.

Acral Pertaining to or affecting a limb or other extremity.

Acropachy Clubbing of the fingers and toes with distal periosteal bone changes and swelling of the overlying soft tissues.

Addisonian crisis The symptoms that accompany an acute onset or worsening of Addison's disease, including fatigue, nausea and vomiting, loss of weight, hypotension, fever and collapse.

Adenomyosis Penetration of an endometrial tissue into the myometrium.

Agenesis Absence of an organ.

Agyria Congenital malformation or absence of the convolutions of the cerebral cortex.

Alloimmunity Immunity to an alloantigen.

Alport syndrome Hereditary disease of the kidneys that primarily affects men. Heterogeneous group of conditions may manifest including glomerulonephritis, hematuria, proteinuria, hypertension, nephrotic syndrome, end-stage renal disease, and variably accompanied by sensorineural deafness, coloured urine, swelling, cough, poor vision. Eventually, kidney dialysis or transplant may be necessary.

Amphipathic Molecules containing groups with characteristically different properties, for example both hydrophilic and hydrophobic properties.

Amphoteric Having opposite characters, that is capable of acting as an acid and a base.

Anoxaemia Reduction of blood oxygen content below physiological levels.

Anthropometry The science which deals with the measurement of the size, weight and proportions of the human body.

Aphakia No lens.

Aplasia cutis Localised failure of development of skin.

Apnoea Cessation of breathing.

Apoptosis Programmed destruction of cells; mechanism that keeps cell numbers in check by eliminating senescent cells or those without useful cell function.

Arachnoiditis Inflammation of the arachnoidea, a delicate membrane inter-posed between the dura mater and the pia mater.

Ataxia telangectasia Hereditary disorder with severe progressive cerebellar ataxia, associated with oculocutaneous telangectasia, sinopulmonary disease with frequent respiratory infections and abnormal eye movements.

Atelectasis Incomplete expansion of a lung.

Atretic Without an opening; characterised by atresia.

Auspitz's sign Removal of a yellow-white, sharply demarcated plaque of psoriasis, results in pinpoint hemorrhage.

Azoospermia Absence of spermatozoa in the semen, or failure of formation of spermatozoa.

Bacteriuria The presence of bacteria in the urine.

Barrett's oesophagus A precancerous condition in which normal cells lining the oesophagus are replaced with abnormal cells that may develop into an adenocarcinoma.

Beau's lines Transverse depression of the nail that represents interruption to the normal growth of the nail matrix.

BK virus A human polyomavirus that causes widespread infection in childhood and remains latent in the host; believed to cause hemorrhagic cystitis and nephritis in immunocompromised patients.

Bronchiectasis Characterised by dilation of the small bronchi and bronchioles, associated with the presence of chronic pulmonary sepsis. It presents as a chronic cough, often with the production of large amounts of purulent, foul-smelling sputum, and may eventually lead to repeated episodes of pneumonia and respiratory failure.

Bronchoalveolar lavage A procedure performed during bronchoscopy in which the bronchial tree is literally washed (lavaged) with a small volume of sterile saline. The saline is then collected and sent for microbiological or cytological examination.

Bronchoscopy The procedure in which a flexible fibreoptic endoscope is inserted into the bronchial tree to allow direct visualization of the bronchi and, if required, the collection of specimens for microbiology or histology.

Brugada syndrome A genetic disease characterised by an abnormal electrocardiogram and an increased risk of sudden cardiac death. More prevalent in those from South East Asia.

Bruxism Tooth grinding.

Budd–Chiari syndrome Symptomatic obstruction or occlusion of the hepatic veins, usually of unknown origin but probably caused by neoplasms, strictures, liver disease, trauma, systemic infections or haematological disorders.

Buerger's test Two part test to assess adequacy of the arterial supply to the leg.

Cachectic A profound and marked state of general ill health and malnutrition.

Cardiogenic emboli Emboli originating from the heart; caused by abnormal function of the heart.

Carpal tunnel syndrome A complex of symptoms resulting from compression of the median nerve in the carpal tunnel, with pain and burning or tingling paraesthesias in the fingers and hand, sometimes extending to the elbow.

Catamenia Term used to designate age at onset of menses.

Cataract An opacity of the crystalline lens of the eye.

Cavitation Formation of cavities. For example, in the lungs when the liquefied centre of a tuberculous lesion drains (usually into a bronchus).

Charcot's arthropathy A destructive arthropathy (disease of any joint) with impaired pain perception or position sense.

Cholelithiasis The presence or formation of gallstones.

Chondrocyte A mature cartilage cell embedded in a lacuna (a small pit or hollow cavity) within the cartilage matrix.

Christmas disease Haemophilia B.

Churg–Strauss syndrome Allergic granulomatosis.

Chvostek's sign Spasm of the facial muscles elicited by tapping the facial nerve in the region of the parotid gland, seen in tetany.

Coarctation of the aorta A localised malformation characterised by deformity of the aortic media, causing narrowing, usually severe, of the lumen of the vessel.

Cognitive Pertaining to cognition; that operation of the mind by which we become aware of objects of thought or perception; it includes all aspects of perceiving, thinking and remembering.

Corneal arcus Crescentic deposition of lipids in the cornea.

Cor pulmonale Persistent lung damage, eventually leads to increased blood pressure in the pulmonary arteries (pulmonary hypertension), which in turn leads to stress on the right ventricle, right ventricular hypertrophy and heart failure. This process is known as cor pulmonale.

Cryptogenic Obscure, doubtful or unascertainable origin.

Cytotoxin A toxin or antibody that has a specific toxic action upon cells of special organs.

Denudation Removal of the epithelial covering from any surface.

Diarthrodial joint A joint characterised by mobility in a rotary direction.

Dimorphic Occurring in two distinct forms.

Disseminated intravascular coagulation (DIC) In this condition vigorous activation of the clotting cascade causes widespread intravascular deposition of fibrin and consumption of clotting factors and platelets. There are numerous potential triggers for this process, including severe sepsis, burns, massive transfusion and placental abruption.

Diverticulosis The presence of circumscribed pouches or sacs of variable size called diverticula that occur normally or are created by herniation of the lining mucous membrane through a defect in the muscular coat of a tubular organ such as the gastro-intestinal tract.

Ductopenia Absence/shortage of ducts; typically absence of interlobular bile ducts.

Dubin–Johnson syndrome Familial chronic form of non-haemolytic jaundice due to a defect in the excretion of conjugated bilirubin and other organic anions.

Dupuytren's contracture Shortening, thickening and fibrosis of the palmar fascia, producing a flexion deformity of a finger. The term also applies to a flexion deformity of a toe.

Dyschezia Difficult or painful evacuation of faeces from the rectum.

Dyskinesia Impairment of the power of voluntary movement, resulting in fragmentary or incomplete movements.

Dyspareunia Difficult or painful intercourse.

Dyspnoea Difficult or laboured breathing.

Dystonia Disordered tonicity of muscle.

Dysuria Painful or difficult urination.

Eclampsia Convulsions and coma occurring in a pregnant or puerperal woman, associated with hypertension, oedema and/or proteinuria.

Electrodiathermy Heating of the body tissues due to their resistance to the passage of an electric current.

Elliptocytosis A hereditary disorder in which the majority of erythrocytes are elliptical in shape, and characterised by varying degrees of increased red cell destruction and anaemia.

Emphysema A state in which the alveoli of the lung become dilated, possibly with destruction of the alveolar walls, leading to large empty air spaces which are useless for gas exchange. It is often seen accompanying chronic bronchitis but may be due to inherited disorders such as a_1-antitrypsin deficiency.

Encephalopathy Any degenerative disease of the brain.

Endophthalmitis Inflammation involving the ocular cavities and their adjacent structures.

Enterostomy The formation of a permanent opening into the intestine through the abdominal wall.

Enterotoxin A toxin arising in the intestine.

Episcleritis Inflammation of the loose connective tissue forming the external surface of the sclera.

Epstein–Barr virus A herpes virus originally isolated from Burkitt lymphomas and believed to be the aetiological agent in infectious mono-nucleosis or closely related to it.

Euthymic Normal state of thymus.

Exanthema Widespread rash usually occurring in children caused by toxins, drugs, micro-organisms or autoimmune disease.

Faecal Occult blood in the stools. Called 'occult' because it is partly digested and therefore no longer red in colour. Usually detected by means of a chemical test.

Fanconi's anaemia A rare hereditary disorder, transmitted in a recessive manner and having a poor prognosis, characterised by pancytopenia, hypoplasia of the bone marrow, and patchy brown discoloration of the skin due to the deposition of melanin, and associated with multiple congenital anomalies of the musculoskeletal and genitourinary systems.

Fastidious organism Organism which will only grow with specialist culture media or under certain physiological conditions.

Feculent Having dregs or a sediment.

Felty's syndrome Combination of chronic rheumatoid arthritis, splenomegaly, leucopenia, pigmented spots on the skin of the lower extremities.

Fibroadenoma Benign tumour that is made of glandular and fibrous tissue and typically occurs in breast tissue.

Fibromuscular Composed of fibrous and muscular tissue.

Fistula An abnormal passage or communication, usually between two internal organs or from an internal organ to the surface of the body.

Foreign body giant cells Giant cells resembling Langhan's giant cells, having clusters of nuclei scattered in an irregular pattern throughout the cytoplasm, characteristic of granulomatous inflammation due to invasion of the tissue by a foreign body.

Gastroschisis Congenital fissure of the abdominal wall not involving the site of insertion of the umbilical cord, and usually accompanied by protrusion of the small and part of the large intestine.

Gaucher's disease Group of hereditary disorders of glucocerebroside metabolism characterised by accumulation of glucocerebroside in the spleen, liver, lungs, bone marrow, and sometimes the brain leading to splenomegaly, hepatomegaly, erosion of the cortices of the long bones and pelvis, and CNS impairment.

Glasgow-Blatchford score Screening tool to assess likelihood that a patient with an acute upper gastro-intestinal bleed will require medical intervention.

Glomerulonephritis Nephritis characterised by inflammation of the capillary loops in the glomeruli of the kidney.

Glossitis Inflammation of the tongue.

Goerkerman regimen Combination of coal tar and UVB light to bombard the skin with anti-psoriasis treatment.

Gonioscopy Estimate of the width of the eye chamber angle, measured using a slit-lamp.

Goodpasture's disease Autoimmune disease characterised by glomerulonephritis and hemorrhaging from the lung.

Granuloma A tumour-like mass or nodule of granulation tissue, with actively growing fibroblasts and capillary buds; it is due to a chronic inflammatory process associated with infectious disease or with invasion by a foreign body.

Guillain–Barré syndrome Acute febrile polyneuritis.

Haematuria Blood in the urine.

Haem(at)opoiesis The formation and development of blood cells.

Harris Benedict equation Equation first developed in 1919 to predict basal energy expenditure.

Hasenclever score Prognostic score for Hodgkins disease.

Haustral Pertaining to the haustra of the colon, denoting sacculations in the wall of the colon produced by adaptation of its length.

Heberden's nodes Gelatinous cysts or bony outgrowths on the dorsal aspects of the distal interphalangeal joints.

Heinz bodies Inclusion bodies in red blood cells resulting from oxidative injury to and precipitation of haemoglobin, seen in the presence of certain abnormal haemoglobins and erythrocytes with enzyme deficiencies.

Henoch–Schönlein purpura An acute or chronic vasculitis primarily affecting skin, joints and the gastro-intestinal and renal systems.

Hepatorenal syndrome Development of renal failure secondary to liver disease.

Hirschsprung's disease Congenital megacolon.

Horner's syndrome Sinking in of the eyeball, ptosis of the upper eyelid, slight elevation of the lower lid, constriction of the pupil, narrowing of the palpebral fissure, anhidrosis and flushing of the affected side of the face; caused by paralysis of the cervical sympathetic nerves.

Horton's syndrome Migrainous neuralgia; also called paroxysmal nocturnal cephalalgia.

Huntington's chorea A rare hereditary disease characterised by chronic progressive chorea and mental deterioration terminating in dementia. The age of onset is variable but usually occurs in the fourth decade of life.

Hyaline membrane A layer of eosinophilic hyaline material lining the alveoli, alveolar ducts and bronchioles, found at autopsy in infants who have died of respiratory distress syndrome of the newborn.

Hypermelanosis Excessive deposition of melanin.

Hypersplenism A condition characterised by exaggeration of the inhibitory or destructive functions of the spleen, resulting in deficiency of the peripheral blood elements, singly or in combination, hypercellularity of the bone marrow, and usually splenomegaly.

Hypertrichosis Growth of hair at sites not normally hairy.

Hypophonic Reduced volume of speech.

Hypovolaemia Abnormally reduced volume of circulating fluid in the body/plasma.

Ileus Obstruction or lack of smooth muscle tone in the intestines.

Immunoblastic Pertaining to or involving the stem cells (immunoblasts) of lymphoid tissue.

Index case The first detected case in a particular series that prompts investigation into other patients.

Interstitial nephritis Inflammation of the renal interstitial tissue resulting from arterial, arteriolar, glomerular or tubular disease which destroys individual nephrons.

Intussusception The prolapse of one part of the intestine into the lumen of an immediately adjoining part.

Jod–Basedow syndrome Thyrotoxicosis produced in a patient with goitre, when given a bolus of iodine.

Kayser–Fleischer ring A grey-green to red-gold pigmented ring at the outer margin of the cornea, seen in progressive lenticular degeneration and pseudosclerosis.

Koebner phenomenon Induction of new psoriasis skin lesions following local trauma or injury to the skin.

Koilonychia Dystrophy of the fingernails, in which they are thin and concave, with edges raised.

Kussmaul's respiration Air hunger.

Kwashiorkor Insufficient protein provision.

Kyphosis Abnormally increased convex curvature of the spinal column.

Labyrinthitis Inflammation of the labyrinth; otitis interna.

Lacunar syndrome Small infarct or small cavity in brain tissue that develops after the necrotic tissue of a deep infarct is resorbed.

Laminectomy Excision of the posterior arch of a vertebra.

Laparoscopy Examination of the interior of the abdomen by means of a laparoscope.

Lesch–Nyhan syndrome Rare disorder of purine metabolism due to deficiency of the enzyme hypoxanthine-guanine phosphoribosyl-transferase and characterised by physical and mental retardation, self-mutilation of fingers and lips by biting, choreoathetosis, spastic cerebral palsy and impaired renal function.

Leucocytosis Total white cell count in excess of $11 \times 10^9 \, L^{-1}$.

Leuconychia White nails.

Lichenoid Resembling the skin lesions designated as 'lichen' – the name applied to many different kinds of papular skin.

Liddle's Syndrome Autosomal dominant disorder in which the kidneys excrete potassium but retain too much sodium and water, leading to high blood pressure diseases in which the lesions are typically small, firm papules that are usually set very close together.

Lipaemia retinalis Retinal deposition of lipid.

Lipohypertrophy Thickening of subcutaneous tissues at injection sites because of recurrent injection in the same area.

Livedo reticularis A peripheral vascular condition characterised by a reddish blue netlike mottling of the skin and extremities.

Lyme disease A multisystem tick-borne disorder caused by the spirochaete *Borrelia burgdorferi*. Clinical manifestation includes an erythematous macule followed by systemic disorders such as arthralgias, myalgias and headache followed by neurological manifestations, cardiac involvement and a migratory polyarthritis.

Lymphadenopathy Disease of the lymph nodes.

Lymphoblastic Pertaining to a lymphoblast.

Maculopapular An eruption consisting of both macules (areas distinguishable by colour from their surroundings, e.g. spots) and papules (small circumscribed, superficial, solid elevations of the skin).

Malleolus medialis The rounded protruberance on the medial surface of the ankle joint.

Malrotation Abnormal or pathological rotation.

Marasmus Insufficient energy provision.

Melaena The passage of dark stools stained with blood pigments or with altered blood.

Menorrhagia Excessive and prolonged uterine bleeding occurring at the regular intervals of menstruation.

Microalbuminuria Small amounts of albumin present in the urine.

Miliary Literally, resembling small round millet seeds. Miliary tuberculosis is so called because the chest radiograph usually shows miliary speckling.

Morbilliform Resembling the eruption of measles.

Mucositis Inflammation of a mucous membrane.

Mycosis fungoides A rare, chronic, malignant, lymphoreticular neoplasm of the skin and, in the late stages, the lymph nodes and viscera, marked by the development of firm, reddish, painful tumours that ulcerate.

Myelofibrosis Replacement of the bone marrow by fibrous tissue occurring in association with a myeloproliferative disorder or secondary to another disorder.

Myoclonus Shock like contractions of a group of muscles.

Myoglobulinuria Presence of myoglobin in the urine.

Myomas Fibroids, common benign tumours of the myometrium.

Myometrium The muscular layers of the uterus that contract spontaneously throughout the menstrual cycle.

Myopathy Unexplained muscle soreness or weakness.

Myositis Inflammation of a voluntary muscle.

Necrobiosis lipoidica A dermatosis usually occurring in diabetics characterised by necrobiosis (swelling and distortion of collagen bundles in the dermis) of the elastic and connective tissue of the skin, with degenerated collagen occurring in irregular patches, especially in the upper dermis.

Nephrolithiasis Formation of uric acid calculi in the kidneys.

Nikolsky's sign Easy separation of the outer portion of the epidermis from the basal layer on exertion of firm sliding pressure by the finger or thumb.

Nocturia Waking at night to pass urine.

Nystagmus Involuntary rapid movement of the eyeball, which may be horizontal, vertical, rotatory or mixed.

Obligate intracellular pathogen An organism that cannot be cultured using artificial media since it requires living cells for growth.

Oligohydramnios Presence of less than 300ml of amniotic fluid at term.

Oliguria Diminished urine output.

Onycholysis Separation of the nail from its bed.

Oophorectomy Removal of an ovary or ovaries.

Ophthalmopathy Any disease of the eye.

Opsonization The rendering of bacteria and other cells subject to phagocytosis.

Orchiectomy Excision of one or both testis(es).

Orosomucoid a_1-acid glycoprotein, a glycoprotein occurring in blood plasma.

Orthopnoea Difficult breathing except in an upright position.

Orthoptic Correcting obliquity of one or more visual axis.

Osler's nodes Small, raised, swollen tender areas, about the size of a pea and often bluish in colour but sometimes pink or red, occurring most commonly in the pads of the fingers or toes, in the palm or the soles of the feet.

Osteomalacia Reduced mineralization.

Osteophyte A bony or osseous outgrowth.

Pallidotomy A stereotaxic surgical technique for producing lesions in the globus pallidus or extirpation of it by other means.

Palmar striae Yellow raised streaks across the palms of the hands.

Pancytopenia Deficiency of all cell elements of the blood.

Panmyelopathy A pathological condition of all the elements of the bone marrow.

Paroxysmal nocturnal dyspnoea Difficult or laboured breathing at night that recurs in paroxysms.

Pericarditis Inflammation of the fibrous sac (pericardium) that surrounds the heart and the roots of the great vessels.

Petechial Characterised by pinpoint, non-raised, round, purplish red spots caused by intradermal or submucous haemorrhage.

Phaeochromocytoma A tumour of chromaffin tissue of the adrenal medulla or sympathetic paraganglia. The cardinal symptom that represents the increased secretion of adrenaline and noradrenaline is hypertension, which may be persistent or intermittent.

Phagocytosis The engulfing of micro-organisms, cells and foreign particles by phagocytes.

Phlebitis Inflammation of a vein.

Pica A craving for unnatural articles of food.

Pneumaturia Passage of urine charged with air.

Polycythaemia rubra vera A myeloproliferative disorder in which the abnormal bone marrow overproduces red blood cells (white cells and platelets may also be raised).

Polymorphic Occurring in several or many forms.

Polyp A protruding growth from a mucous membrane.

Pompholyx A skin eruption on the sides of the fingers, toes, palms or soles, consisting of discrete round intraepidermal vesicles 1 or 2 mm in diameter, accompanied by intense itching and occurring in repeated self-limited attacks lasting 1 or 2 weeks.

Porphyria Any of a group of disturbances of porphyrin metabolism, characterised by marked increase in formation and excretion of porphyrins or their precursors.

Pretibial myxoedema Localised myxoedema associated with preceding hyperthyroidism and exopthalmus, occurring typically on the anterior (pretibial) surface of the legs where mucin deposits as plaques and papules.

Priapism Persistent, abnormal erection of the penis, usually without sexual desire, and accompanied by pain and discomfort.

Prinzmetal's angina A variant of angina pectoris in which the attacks occur during rest.

Proptosis A forward displacement or bulging, especially of the eye.

Pseudophakia False lens.

Pyruvate kinase deficiency A deficiency in the glycolytic (metabolic) pathway of red blood cells that results in haemolysis.

Pyuria Presence of pus in the urine.

Raeder's syndrome A syndrome consisting of the Horner syndrome but without loss of sweating on the affected side of the face.

Reed–Sternberg cells Giant histiocytic cells, typically multinucleate, most often binucleate; the nuclei are enclosed in abundant amphophilic cytoplasm and contain prominent nucleoli.

Retinopathy Any non-inflammatory disease of the retina.

Retroperitoneal fibrosis Deposition of fibrous tissue in the retroperitoneal space, producing vague abdominal discomfort, and often causing blockage of the ureters with resultant hydronephrosis and impaired renal function.

Retrosternal Situated or occurring behind the sternum.

Reiter's syndrome Triad of nongonococcal urethritis, conjunctivitis, and arthritis frequently with mucocutaneos lesions.

Reye's syndrome An acute and often fatal childhood syndrome of encephalopathy and fatty degeneration of the liver, marked by rapid development of brain swelling and hepatomegaly and by disturbed consciousness and seizures.

Rhabdomyolysis Dissolution of muscle associated with excretion of myoglobin in the urine.

Rockall score Scoring system to identify patients at risk of adverse outcome following acute upper gastro-intestinal bleed.

Roth's spots Round or oval white spots sometimes seen in the retina early in the course of subacute bacterial endocarditis.

Rotor's syndrome Chronic familial non-haemolytic jaundice differing from Dubin–Johnson syndrome in the lack of liver pigmentation.

Sarcoidosis A chronic, progressive, generalised granulomatous reticulosis of unknown aetiology, involving almost any organ or tissue.

Schofield equation An equation to predict basal metabolic rate; may be used to estimate the total calorie intake required to maintain current body weight.

Sclerotherapy The injection of sclerosing solutions in the treatment of haemorrhoids or varicose veins.

Scotoma An area of depressed vision within the visual field, surrounded by an area of less depressed or of normal vision.

Sézary syndrome Generalised exfoliative erythroderma produced by cutaneous infiltration of reticular lymphocytes and associated with intense pruritus, alopecia, oedema, hyperkeratosis, pigment and nail changes.

Shy–Drager syndrome Orthostatic hypotension, urinary and rectal incontinence, anhidrosis, atrophy of the iris, external ophthalmoplegia, rigidity, tremor, loss of associated movements, impotence, atonic bladder, generalised weakness, fasciculations, and neuropathic muscle wasting.

Sickle cell anaemia A hereditary haemolytic anaemia occurring almost exclusively in black people, characterised by arthralgia, acute attacks of abdominal pain, ulcerations of the lower extremities and with sickle-shaped erythrocytes in the blood.

Sjögren's syndrome A symptom complex of unknown aetiology, usually occurring in middle-aged or older women, in which keratoconjunctivitis is associated with pharyngitis sicca, enlargement of the parotid glands, chronic polyarthritis and xerostomia.

Sloughing material Soft, gel-like material often found in ulcer bases. Composed of tissue exudate and cellular debris.

Spherocytosis The presence of spherocytes (thick, almost spherical, red blood cells) characterised by abnormal fragility of erythrocytes, jaundice and splenomegaly.

Splinter haemorrhages Linear haemorrhages beneath the nail.

Steatosis Fatty degeneration.

Stenosis Narrowing or stricture of a duct or canal.

Stevens–Johnson syndrome A severe form of erythema multiforme in which the lesions may involve the oral and anogenital mucous membranes in association with constitutional symptoms, including malaise, prostration, headache, fever, arthralgia and conjunctivitis.

Stromal keratitis Immune-mediated nonsuppurative stromal inflammation with an intact epithelium usually linked to a causative disorder such as Epstein Barr virus, herpes zoster and simplex, mumps, measles, Lyme disease, tuberculosis.

Subchondral Beneath a cartilage.

Subluxation An incomplete or partial dislocation.

Supranuclear palsy Pseudobulbar paralysis.

Sweet's syndrome Acute febrile neutrophillic dermatosis.

Sympathetic ileus Failure of gastro-intestinal motility secondary to acute non-gastro-intestinal illness, for example hyaline membrane disease or septicaemia.

Tamponade Surgical use of the tampon; also pathological compression of a part, as compression of the heart by pericardial fluid.

Telangiectasia Prominent surface blood vessels.

Tendon xanthomas Yellow papules or nodules or lipids deposited in tendons.

Tenesmus Straining, especially ineffectual and painful straining at stool or in urination.

Tenosynovitis Inflammation of a tendon sheath.

Thalassaemia A heterogeneous group of hereditary haemolytic anaemias that have in common a decreased rate of synthesis of one or more haemoglobin polypeptide chains and are classified according to the chain involved (a, b, g). The homozygous form (thalassaemia major) is incompatible with life. The heterozygous form (thalassaemia minor) may be asymptomatic or marked by mild anaemia.

Thrombocytopenia Decrease in the number of blood platelets.

Thrombocytosis Increased number of platelets in blood.

Thrombophilia A tendency to the occurrence of thrombosis.

Thromboplastin Phospholipid-protein extract of tissue that promotes the activation of factor X by factor VIII.

Tonometry Measurement of intraocular pressure.

Tophi Deposits of monosodium urate crystals, typically in subcutaneous and periarticular areas.

Trephine Biopsy examination of an intact core of tissue (e.g. liver, bone marrow) obtained through a wide-bore needle.

Tropical sprue A malabsorption syndrome occurring in the tropics and subtropics. Protein malnutrition is usually precipitated by the malabsorption, and anaemia due to folic acid deficiency is particularly common.

Trousseau's sign Spasmodic contractions of muscles provoked by pressure upon the nerves which go to them; seen in tetany.

Tuberoeruptive xanthomas Groups of flat or yellowish raised nodules on the skin over joints, especially the elbows and knees.

Tuberous sclerosis Congenital familial disease characterised by tumours on the surfaces of the lateral ventricles and sclerotic patches on the surface of the brain and marked clinically by progressive mental deterioration and epileptic convulsions.

Tubular cast A cast formed from gelled protein precipitated in the renal tubules and moulded to the tubular lumen; pieces of these casts break off and are washed out with the urine.

Uraemic frost Crystalline area deposited on the skin.

Urethral Pertaining to the urethra, the membranous canal conveying urine from the bladder to the exterior of the body.

Variant angina *See* Prinzmetal's angina.

Volvulus Intestinal obstruction due to a knotting and twisting of the bowel.

Von Willebrand's disease A lack of or a defective plasma protein (von Willebrand factor) necessary for the adhesion of platelets to vascular elements when a blood vessel is damaged.

Wernicke–Korsakoff syndrome The co-existence of Wernicke's disease (acute onset of mental confusion, nystagmus, ophthalmoplegia and gait ataxia, due to thiamine deficiency) with Korsakoff's syndrome (a gross disturbance in recent memory, sometimes compensated for by confabulation).

West's syndrome A form of myoclonus epilepsy with onset in infancy or early childhood and characterised by seizures involving the muscles of the neck, trunk and limbs, with nodding of the head and flexion and abduction of the arms. Mental retardation is common.

Wilson's disease Characterised by progressive accumulation of copper within body tissues, particularly erythrocytes, kidney, liver and brain, and associated with liver and lenticular degeneration.

Xanthelasma Yellow plaques or nodules of lipids deposited on eyelids.

Xenotransplantation Transplantation of tissue from another species.

Xerosis Dry skin.

Index

Note: Page numbers followed by *b* indicate boxes, *f* indicate figures, and *t* indicate tables.

A

abacavir
  HIV infection, 628*t*
  pharmacogenetics, 66
abarelix, 763
abatacept, 842
ABCB1 gene, 56–57
abciximab
  arterial thromboembolism, 386
  ST elevation myocardial infarction, 324
ABC transporters, 56–57
abdominal pain in liver disease, 242
ABL gene, 788, 793
absence attacks, 491
absorption (of drugs), 35
  drug interactions, 52
  in the elderly, 150
  in neonates, 124
  in pregnancy, 742
  in renal replacement therapy, 267
ABVD (adriamycin, bleomycin, vinblastine, dacarbazine), Hodgkin's lymphoma, 804, 805, 807*t*
acanthosis, 900–901
acarbose
  adverse effects, 704
  diabetes mellitus, 699, 704
accelerated hypertension, 296–297, 299*t*
accountability, 16–17
acebutolol
  arrhythmias, 370
  coronary heart disease, 318*t*
ACE inhibitors *see* angiotensin converting enzyme (ACE) inhibitors
acenocoumarol, 381
acetazolamide
  epilepsy, 497
  glaucoma, 865, 873
acetylcholine
  affective disorders, 466
  anxiety, 456
acetylcholinesterase inhibitors
  and dementia, 153
  and diarrhoea, 215*t*
acetylcysteine
  hepatotoxicity antidote, 231
  paracetamol overdose, 232
aciclovir
  meningitis, 592
  opportunistic infections in HIV, 639*t*
  postherpetic neuralgia, 529
acid-base balance, 83, 260
acidosis
  in acute kidney injury, 264

in chronic kidney disease, 287
  metabolic, 83
acid suppression, peptic ulcer disease, 169–170, 173
acipimox, 407
acitretin
  drug interactions, 899*t*
  eczema, 904*t*
  psoriasis, 904, 904*t*
acneiform eruptions, drug-induced, 884, 885*b*, 890
acquired immune deficiency syndrome (AIDS), 621
  see also HIV infection
acrolein, 825
activated charcoal, paracetamol overdose, 232
activated partial thromboplastin time (APTT), 92–93, 379
activated protein C, 715
acupuncture, 527
  dysmenorrhoea, 718
  pregnancy-associated nausea and vomiting, 541
acute coronary syndrome (ACS), 320–329
  causes, 320–321
  classification, 322*f*
  definition, 320–321
  diagnostic criteria, 321
  mortality rates, 321
acute generalised exanthematous pustulosis (AGEP), 888, 888*b*
acute kidney injury (AKI), 255–271
  case studies, 269*b*
  causes, 255–259, 256*f*
  classification, 255–259, 255*t*
  clinical evaluation, 260, 261*f*
  clinical manifestations, 259–260
  course, 260–262
  definition, 255, 256*f*
  diagnosis, 260, 261*f*
  incidence, 255
  intra-renal, 257–259, 257*t*
    definition, 255*t*
    vs. pre-renal, 259, 259*t*
  management, 262–263
    drug therapy and renal auto-regulation, 263
    early preventative and supportive strategies, 262–263
  mortality rates, 261
  non-dialysis treatment, 263–265
    acidosis, 264
    hyperkalaemia, 264
    hyperphosphataemia, 264
    hypocalcaemia, 264
    infection, 264
    nutrition, 265
    uraemia and intravascular volume overload, 263–264
    uraemic gastro-intestinal erosions, 264–265
  parenteral nutrition in, 110–111
  post-renal, 259
    course and prognosis, 261

definition, 255*t*
  pre-renal, 256–257, 256*f*
    course and prognosis, 260–262
    definition, 255*t*
    vs. intra-renal, 259, 259*t*
  prognosis, 260–262
  renal replacement therapy *see* renal replacement therapy
  RIFLE criteria, 255, 256*f*
  staging, 256*f*
  with volume depletion, 259, 259*t*
  with volume overload, 259*t*, 260
  vs. chronic kidney disease, 272
acute liver failure (ALF), 250
  in acute liver disease, 238
  characteristics of types of, 223*t*
  drug-induced, 222, 222*f*
acute lymphoblastic leukaemia (ALL), 133, 786
  case studies, 800
  classification, 788, 788*t*
  clinical manifestations, 788
  epidemiology, 786
  pathophysiology, 787
  treatment, 790–791, 790*t*, 812
acute myeloblastic leukaemia (AML), 786
  case studies, 799, 800
  classification, 788, 788*t*
  clinical manifestations, 788
  epidemiology, 786
  pathophysiology, 787
  treatment, 791–792, 791*f*
acute peritoneal dialysis, 266–267, 267*f*, 267*t*
acute promyelocytic leukaemia (APL), 788, 792, 801
acute renal failure (ARF) *see* acute kidney injury (AKI)
acute tubular necrosis (ATN), 257–258, 257*t*, 260–261
adalimumab
  guidance on the use of, 841
  inflammatory bowel disease, 199, 200, 200*t*, 201–202, 203*t*
  psoriasis, 905
  rheumatoid arthritis, 840
Addison's disease, 80
adefovir, hepatitis B, 251
adenosine
  adverse effects, 367*t*
  arrhythmias, 371–372
adenosine triphosphate (ATP), 371–372
adenoviruses, 214, 573
adherence/non-adherence, 5, 24
  antiretrovirals, 627
  children, 141–142
  costs of, 121–122
  elderly, 158
  glaucoma treatment, 877–878
  intentional, 24

likelihood of, 5–6
tuberculosis treatment, 617
unintentional, 24
adipokines, 687
adiponectin, 687
adolescents
  adverse drug reactions, 65
  definition, 132
adrenaline
  chronic heart failure, 343
  neonates, 124
adrenergic receptors *see* α-adrenoceptors;
    α$_1$-adrenoceptors; α$_2$-adrenoceptors;
    β-adrenoceptors
adrenocorticotropic hormone (ACTH), 761–762
adriamycin *see* doxorubicin
adsorption, 52
adult polycystic kidney disease (APKD), 275
adult T-cell leukaemia/lymphoma (ATLL), 807
adverse drug events (ADEs), 63
adverse drug reactions (ADRs), 62–75
  affecting the liver *see* drug-induced liver disease
      (DILD)
  assessing the safety of drugs, 63
  benefits of pharmaceutical care, 4
  in breastfed infants, 745*t*
  case studies, 73, 74
  in children, 144
  classification, 63–64
    DoTS system, 64, 65*t*
    Rawlins-Thompson classification, 63–64, 64*t*
  cost of, 4
  definitions, 63
  in the elderly, 158
  epidemiology, 68
  factors affecting susceptibility to, 64–67
    age, 65
    co-morbidities and concomitant medicine
      use, 65
    erythrocyte glucose 6-phosphate
      dehydrogenase (G6PD) deficiency, 66
    ethnicity, 66
    gender, 65
    pharmacogenetics, 66
    porphyrias, 67
  formulation issues, 67–68
  immunological reactions, 67, 67*t*
  pharmacovigilance and epidemiological
     detection methods, 68–71
    case-control studies, 70–71
    cohort studies, 70
    published case reports, 70
    spontaneous reporting, 68–69, 69*t*
    Yellow Card Scheme, 69–70
  rates of, 4
  risk management of, 120–121
  roles of health professionals, 71–74
    explaining risks to patients, 72–74
    identifying and assessing ADRs, 71
    monitoring therapy, 72
    presenting ADRs, 71–72
  skin *see* skin disorders, drug-induced
  time-dependent, 64
  topical drugs, 136
advertising of medicines, 27
affective disorders, 465–478
  aetiology, 466
    biochemical factors, 466
    endocrine factors, 466
    environmental factors, 466
    genetic causes, 466
    physical illness and side effects of
      medication, 466, 467*b*
  case studies, 476*b*

classification, 465
clinical manifestations, 467
common therapeutic problems in management
    of, 475*t*
epidemiology, 465–466
investigations, 467–468
patient care, 474–478
rating scales, 468
severity, 467
treatment, 469–474, 475*t*
affective reactions of benzodiazepines, 459
age
  adverse drug reactions, 65
  and chronic kidney disease, 272
  and dyslipidaemia, 396
  and fibrinolysis, 324
  and hormone replacement therapy, 727–728
  and prostate cancer, 759
  risk for drug-induced liver disease, 223
  and surgical site infection, 599
  and total cholesterol, 390
  and venous thromboembolism, 377
  and wound healing, 913
  see also geriatrics
agomelatine, depression, 472
agonists, 57
agoraphobia, 456
agranulocytosis, 89*t*, 676
AIDA, 30, 30*t*
AIDS *see* acquired immune deficiency syndrome
    (AIDS)
AIDS dementia complex, 645–646
airflow limitation, chronic obstructive pulmonary
    disease, 433, 434*b*
airflow obstruction, chronic obstructive
    pulmonary disease, 435, 435*t*
airflow optimisation, bronchitis/chronic
    obstructive pulmonary disease, 549
airway remodelling, 433
akathisia, 481
alanine transaminase (ALT), 85
  in liver disease, 244
  liver function tests, 86
albumin, 53
  in the elderly, 150
  extracellular fluid osmolality, 77
  in liver disease, 244
  liver function tests, 84–85
  pregnancy, 742, 743
  and serum calcium, 81
albumin creatinine ratio (ACR), 277–278
alcohol
  children and, 134
  diabetes mellitus, 694–695
  distribution in the elderly, 150
  and drug metabolism, 54
  and dyslipidaemia, 395
  effect on lipoprotein levels, 394*t*
  and folate deficiency anaemia, 777
  gout, 851
  hepatotoxicity, 224
  and liver disease, 240–241
  in oral preparations, 139
  and psoriasis, 899–900
  sideroblastic anaemia, 774–775
  transfer into breast milk, 749
aldosterone, 273
  effects of, 341–342
  premenstrual syndrome, 713
aldosterone antagonists
  chronic heart failure, 336, 339*t*, 341–342
  hypertension, 304*b*
alendronate
  adverse effects, 154

alternatives to HRT, 731
  osteoporosis, 154
alfacalcidol, 287
  hypoparathyroidism/hypocalcaemia, 680, 681*t*
  osteoporosis, 154
Alfalfa, 59
alfuzosin, benign prostatic hyperplasia, 757
alimemazine, 285
aliphatics, schizophrenia, 483*t*
aliskiren, hypertension, 301
alitretinoin, Kaposi's sarcoma, 645
alkaemia, 82
alkaline phosphatase
  in liver disease, 244
  liver function tests, 84, 85–86
alkalosis, 81, 83
allantoin, 856
allergic contact dermatitis, 894–895, 895*t*
allergic rhinitis *see* hay fever
allergy, drug, 749
  see also adverse drug reactions (ADRs)
allopurinol
  drug interactions, 61, 198
  gout, 853, 855–856
  interstitial nephritis, 258–259
  tumour lysis syndrome, 813–814
all-trans retinoic acid (ATRA), acute
    promyelocytic leukaemia, 792
alopecia
  chemotherapy-induced, 813*t*
  drug-induced, 882, 882*b*
α$_1$-acid glycoprotein, 53, 150
α-adrenoceptor blockers
  benign prostatic hyperplasia, 757, 758
  and diarrhoea, 215*t*
  hypertension, 301, 303*t*
    in diabetes, 305
    indications/contraindications, 307*t*
α-adrenoceptors, age-related changes, 151
α$_1$-adrenoceptors, age-related changes, 151
α$_2$-adrenoceptors, age-related changes, 151
α-agonists, 57
α-antagonists, 57
α$_1$-antitrypsin
  deficiency, 241
  liver disease, 244
α$_1$-blockers
  hypertension in chronic kidney disease, 284–285
  urinary incontinence, 156–157
α-glucosidase inhibitors, diabetes mellitus, 704
5α-reductase, urinary incontinence, 157
5α-reductase inhibitors
  benign prostatic hyperplasia, 757–758
  prostate cancer, 764
α-synuclein, 508
α thalassaemias, 782
Alport syndrome, 277
alprazolam
  anxiety disorders, 459
  profile, 458*t*
alteplase
  ST elevation myocardial infarction, 323*t*, 324
  stroke, 153
  venous thromboembolism, 385
alternative medicines *see* complementary and
    alternative medicines
aluminium hydroxide, hyperphosphataemia, 287
alveolitis, 433
Alzheimer's disease, 152–153, 736
amantadine
  influenza, 546
  Parkinson's disease, 513
American College of Rheumatology (ACR)
    response, 833–834

American Rheumatism Association (ARA) criteria, 833–834, 833*b*
American Society of Anaesthesiology (ASA) classification of physical status, 598*t*
amfebutamone *see* bupropion
amfetamines, 58
amikacin
  hypomagnesaemia, 82
  mycobacteria, 644
  tuberculosis, 616*t*
amiloride
  ascites, 247*t*
  hyperkalaemia, 80
amino acids
  essential, 98
  parenteral nutrition, 98–99
  stability, 107
amino acid solutions, electrolyte-free, 265
aminoglycosides
  acute pyelonephritis, 568
  acute tubular necrosis, 257*t*
  cystic fibrosis, 556*t*
  drug distribution in children, 137
  elimination in children, 138
  hypocalcaemia, 82
  meningitis, 587–588
  in neonates
    infections, 127
    monitoring in, 129
  pneumonia, 554*t*
5-aminolaevulinate synthase, 774
5-aminolaevulinic acid (ALA), 67
aminophylline, 39, 47
  asthma, 418*t*, 422
  chronic obstructive pulmonary disease, 439
  intravenous, 422, 422*t*
Aminoplasmal®, 98, 99*t*
4-aminopyridine, 152
aminosalicylates
  formulations, 197–198, 197*t*
  inflammatory bowel disease, 193, 196–198, 196*f*, 197*t*, 203*t*
aminotransferases, liver disease, 244
Aminoven®, 98, 99*t*
amiodarone
  adverse effects, 367*t*, 370–371
  arrhythmias, 359, 363, 365, 370–371
  dosage, 370
  hypothyroidism, 671, 679
  pharmacokinetics, 368*t*, 370
  thyrotoxicosis, 679
amisulpride, schizophrenia, 483*t*
amitriptyline
  anxiety disorders, 461
  depression, 470
  pain, 526
  sedative properties, 470
amlodipine
  chronic heart failure, 343–344
  clinical trials, 302
  studies, 299–300
ammonia, 83
  hepatic encephalopathy, 248
  liver function tests, 86
amoebiasis, 580
amoxicillin
  bacteriuria of pregnancy, 570
  bronchitis/chronic obstructive pulmonary disease, 549–550
  cholera, 579–580
  gastro-intestinal infections, 579
  Helicobacter pylori eradication, 171, 172
  hepatotoxicity, 234
  meningitis, 587–588, 591

otitis media, 548
pneumonia, 551
urinary tract infections, 568*t*
amphotericin
  acute tubular necrosis, 257*t*
  candidiasis, 657
  fungal ear infections, 659
  infection in neutropenia, 797
  opportunistic infections in HIV, 639*t*
  oropharyngeal candidiasis, 638–643
amphotericin B
  cryptococcus neoformans, 643
  fungal infections in compromised host, 660–662
  and hypomagnesaemia, 82
  lipid formulations *see* amphotericin B lipid formulations
  meningitis, 591–592
  mode of action, 661
  pharmacokinetics, 664*t*
  spectrum of activity, 661–662
amphotericin B deoxycholate (ABD), 662
amphotericin B lipid formulations, 662
  amphotericin B lipid colloidal, 662, 664*t*
  amphotericin B lipid complex, 662, 664*t*
  choosing, 662
  liposomal amphotericin B, 662, 664*t*
ampicillin
  cholera, 579–580
  gastro-intestinal infections, 579
  meningitis, 587–588, 589*t*, 591
amsacrine, acute myeloblastic leukaemia, 791–792
amylase, liver function tests, 86
amyloid, 152–153
amyloid-β, 736
amyloid precursor protein (APP), 152–153
anabolic steroids, 884
anaemia, 769–785
  aetiology, 769–771
  case studies, 783*b*
  of chronic disease, 773–774, 773*t*
  in chronic kidney disease, 278, 286–287
  classification, 770*b*
  clinical manifestations, 770, 770*b*
  definition, 769
  epidemiology, 769
  haemolytic *see* haemolytic anaemias
  in inflammatory bowel disease, 191, 204
  investigations, 770–771
  iron deficiency *see* iron deficiency anaemia
  macrocytic, 93
  megaloblastic *see* megaloblastic anaemias
  microcytic, 769*t*, 784
  sideroblastic *see* sideroblastic anaemia
  treatment, 814
anaesthetic agents
  acute tubular necrosis, 257*t*
  local, 524–525
  pain, 525*t*
anakinra
  gout, 854
  rheumatoid arthritis, 842
analgesia
  epidural, 524
  solid tumours, 827
  stimulation-produced, 527
analgesic drugs, 520–525
  agonist-antagonists, 523
  non-opioid, 520–521, 525
  partial agonists, 523
  strong opioids, 520, 522–523
  weak opioids, 520, 521–522
analgesic ladder, 520, 520*f*
anal intraepithelial neoplasia (AIN), 645
Ananas comosus, 59

androgen deprivation therapy, prostate cancer, 761–763
androgens
  effect on lipoprotein levels, 394*t*
  hair changes, 882
androstenedione, 726
Angelica, 59
angina
  atherosclerosis, 313–314
  Prinzmetal's, 317–318, 319
  stable, 315–317
    characteristics, 315
    symptom relief and prevention, 317–320
      beta-blockers, 317–318, 318*t*
      calcium channel blockers, 318–319
      ivabradine, 320
      nicorandil, 319
      nitrates, 319, 320*t*
      ranolazine, 320
    treatment, 315, 316*f*
      ACE inhibitors, 317
      antithrombotic drugs, 315–317
      statins, 317
  unstable, 313–314, 320, 327
angioedema, drug-induced, 883–884, 884*b*, 890
angiogenesis, 912
angioplasty, arterial leg ulcers, 920
angiotensin converting enzyme (ACE), 273
angiotensin converting enzyme (ACE) inhibitors
  acute kidney injury, 262, 262*f*
  adverse reactions, 66, 74, 339–340, 347–348
  arrhythmias, 365
  chronic heart failure, 336, 338–341, 340*t*, 344, 350
  clinical trials, 302
  contraindications, 341
  coronary heart disease, 317
  diabetic nephropathy, 693
  diarrhoea, 215*t*
  disease interactions, 348*t*
  drug interactions, 348*t*
  effect on lipoprotein levels, 394*t*
  hyperkalaemia, 80
  hypertension, 156, 301, 302–304, 303*t*, 304*b*
    in chronic kidney disease, 283–284
    in diabetes, 305, 705
    indications/contraindications, 307*t*
    in pregnancy, 306
    in renal disease, 305
  intolerance, 339–340
  pre-renal acute kidney injury, 256–257
  as pro-drugs, 348
  self-monitoring, 345*t*
  ST elevation myocardial infarction, 326
  teratogenicity, 740, 741*t*
angiotensin I, 273
angiotensin II, 262, 273
  escape phenomenon, 284
angiotensinogen, 273
angiotensin receptor blockers (ARBs)
  acute kidney injury, 262, 262*f*
  adverse reactions, 347–348
  chronic heart failure, 336, 340*t*, 341, 344
  diabetic nephropathy, 693
  diarrhoea, 215*t*
  drug interactions, 348*t*
  hypertension, 156, 301, 302–304, 303*t*
    in chronic kidney disease, 283–284
    in diabetes, 705
    indications/contraindications, 307*t*
    in pregnancy, 306
  pre-renal acute kidney injury, 256–257
Anglo Scandinavian Cardiac Outcomes Trial (ASCOT) study, 299–300, 302, 306

anidulafungin, 664*t*

anion exchange resins, pruritus in liver disease, 245

anisocytosis, 89*t*

ankle brachial pressure index (ABPI), 918

Ann Arbor classification system, Cotswolds modification of, 804, 804*b*

anorexia, 242

antacids

  absorption, 52

  diarrhoea, 215*t*

  gastro-oesophageal reflux disease, 173–174

  peptic ulcer disease, 178

antagonists, 57

anthracyclines

  acute lymphoblastic leukaemia, 790

  acute promyelocytic leukaemia, 792

  Kaposi's sarcoma, 645

  nausea and vomiting, 540

anti-androgens, prostate cancer, 762–763

antiarrhythmic drugs, 366–373

  class I, 366–368, 367*t*

  class IA, 368–369

  class IB, 369

  class IC, 369

  class II, 367*t*, 369–370

  class III, 367*t*, 370–371

  class IV, 367*t*, 371

  electrophysiological effects of, 366*t*

  pharmacokinetics, 368*t*

antibiotics

  bronchitis, 549–550

  chronic obstructive pulmonary disease, 438–439, 549–550

  cystic fibrosis, 555–556

  diarrhoea, 214, 215*t*, 217–218

  elimination, 56

  gastro-intestinal infections, 573–574, 578–581

  hepatic encephalopathy, 248

  infection in neutropenia, 797

  inflammatory bowel disease, 186, 193, 202, 203*t*

  interstitial nephritis, 258–259

  intrathecal and intraventricular administration, 593, 593*t*

  neonates

    infections, 127

    monitoring in, 129

    necrotizing enterocolitis, 128

    respiratory distress syndrome, 130

  otitis media, 548

  pain, 525*t*

  pneumonia, 553–554

  prophylaxis

    leukaemia, 796, 797*t*

    surgical site infection *see* surgical site infection, prevention/antibiotic prophylaxis

    urinary tract infections, 570

  prostatitis, 765, 766

  quinolone *see* quinolone antibiotics

  renal transplantation, 292

  resistance, 567

    urinary tract infections, 566

  sore throat, 547

  urinary tract infections, 568*t*

anti-CD33 antibody, 792

anti-CD3 monoclonal antibodies, 686

anticholinergic agents

  absorption, 52

  adverse effects, 151

  antiemesis, 538

  asthma, 415

  constipation, 210

  Parkinson's disease, 514

  schizophrenia, 485

anticholinesterases, 152

anticoagulants, 246

  metabolism, 55, 55*t*

  monitoring, 91–95

    activated partial thromboplastin time (APTT), 92–93

    D-dimers, 93

    folate, 93–95

    international normalised ratio (INR), 92

    iron, 93

    iron binding, 93

    one stage prothrombin time, 91

    transferrin, 93

    vitamin B_{12}, 93–95

    xanthochromia, 93

  non-ST elevation myocardial infarction, 327–329

  ST elevation myocardial infarction, 324, 326

  stroke, 153, 154

  venous thromboembolism, 381–384

anticonvulsants *see* antiepileptic agents

anti-cyclic citrullinated peptide antibodies, 834

anti-cytokine monoclonal antibodies, 795

antidepressants

  adverse effects, 469

  anxiety disorders, 460–461

  choice of, 472

  dependence, 469

  depression, 469

  diarrhoea, 215*t*

  drug-induced parkinsonism, 509–510

  hepatitis C, 251–252

  insomnia, 450

  pain, 525–526, 525*t*

  premenstrual syndrome, 716

  ST elevation myocardial infarction, 326

  withdrawal, 469

  see also tricyclic antidepressants

antidiabetic agents, 215*t*

antidiarrhoeals, 202

antidiuretic hormone (ADH), 76, 273

  and blood pressure, 296

  extracellular fluid osmolality, 78

  oesophageal varices, 250

  secretion, 78

antidopaminergics, 538

antidotes, 231

antiemetics, 215*t*, 536–539

antiepileptic agents

  action, 497, 497*f*

  adverse reactions, 66

  altering drug regimens, 494

  development, 497

  diarrhoea, 215*t*

  dose changes, 494–495

  drug interactions, 499*t*

  follow-up, 496

  initiation of therapy, 494

  long-term, 493

  maintenance dosage, 494, 498*t*

  mania, 474

  metabolism, 54

  monitoring, 496–497

  neonates, monitoring in, 129

  neuropathic pain, 530

  newer, 495*t*, 503–506

  pain, 525*t*, 526

  pharmacokinetics, 498*t*

  profiles, 497–503

  starting dosage, 498*t*

  withdrawal, 494, 496

antifibrinolytic drugs, menorrhagia, 720

antifungals, 655

  administration difficulties, 666*t*

  adverse effects, 656*t*

  diarrhoea, 215*t*

  infection in neutropenia, 797

  pharmacokinetics, 664*t*

  resistance, 666*t*

  spectrum of activity, 661*t*

  toxicity, 666*t*

antiglutamic acid decarboxylase (GAD) antibodies, 685–686

antihistamines

  absorption, 52

  antiemesis, 536–538, 541

  eczema, 897

  insomnia, 448*t*, 450

  pain, 526

  pruritus

    in chronic kidney disease, 285

    in liver disease, 245

Anti-hypertensive and Lipid Lowering treatment to prevent Heart Attack Trial (ALLHAT), 300, 302

antihypertensives, 155

  adverse effects, 308

  classes, 299–304

  clinical trial evidence, 302

  drug selection, 302

  and dyslipidaemia, 395

  hepatotoxicity, 228

  hypertension in chronic kidney disease, 283

  recommendations for drugs sequencing, 302–304

anti-IgE monoclonal antibodies, asthma, 419

anti-inflammatories, asthma, 418–419

anti-ischaemic drugs, non-ST elevation myocardial infarction, 329

antilymphocyte globulin (ALG), 291

antimalarials

  diarrhoea, 215*t*

  psoriasis, 899

antimicrobial catheters, 569

antimicrobials

  diarrhoea, 217–218

  hepatotoxicity, 228

  inappropriate prescribing of, 15

  meningitis, 587–593

  pharmacokinetics, 587–593

  urinary tract infections, 566

  see also antibiotics; antifungals; antivirals

antimotility agents, 217

antimuscarinic drugs

  asthma, 11*t*

  urinary incontinence, 157

anti-neutrophil cytoplasmic antibodies (ANCA), 258

antinuclear antibodies (ANA)

  lupus erythematosus, 888

  rheumatoid arthritis, 834

antioncogenes, 820

antioxidants

  and coronary heart disease, 315

  and dyslipidaemia, 400–401

antiplatelet therapy

  non-ST elevation myocardial infarction, 327–329

  ST elevation myocardial infarction, 322, 324, 326

  stroke, 153

antiproteinase imbalance, 433

antiprotozoal agents, 215*t*

antipsychotic drugs

  adverse effects, 486–488

  anxiety disorders, 461

  depot formulations, 485, 485*t*

  diarrhoea, 215*t*

  individual response, 481

  interactions, 475*t*, 485

  long-acting formulations, 484–485

  mania, 473

  mode of action, 480–481

antipsychotic drugs *(Continued)*
  neuroleptic equivalence, 484, 484*t*
  side effects, 481–482
  therapeutic drug monitoring, 485–486
antiretroviral therapy
  adherence/non-adherence, 627
  choosing and monitoring, 626–627, 627*b*
  highly active *see* highly active antiretroviral
     therapy (HAART)
  in HIV infection, 625–637
  post-exposure prophylaxis, 627
  starting, 626
  studies, 626
  toxicity of, 637
  treatment interruptions, 627
antispasmodics
  dysmenorrhoea, 717
  pain, 525*t*
antithrombin III deficiency, 377
antithrombotic drugs
  coronary heart disease, 315–317
  non-ST elevation myocardial infarction,
    327
antithymocyte globulin (ATG), 291, 795
anti-thyroid drugs, 676
  adverse effects, 676
  counselling, 677, 677*b*
  regimens, 677
anti-TNF agents
  adverse effects, 841
  place in therapy, 841
  psoriasis, 905
  rheumatoid arthritis, 840–841
  safety, 840–841
antivirals
  diarrhoea, 215*t*
  see also antiretroviral therapy
anxiety disorders, 454–464
  aetiology, 456
  case studies, 462*b*
  in chronic heart failure, 337*t*
  clinical manifestations, 456
  and coronary heart disease risk, 313
  definitions, 454–455
  differential diagnosis, 457
  epidemiology, 454–455
  investigations, 457
  neurotransmitters, 456
  pathophysiology, 455–456
  ST elevation myocardial infarction, 326
  symptoms, 454–455, 454*f*
  treatment, 457–463
    antidepressants, 460–461
    benzodiazepines, 457–460, 458*t*, 460*b*
    pharmacotherapy, 457–463, 462*t*
    psychotherapy, 457
  types of, 454–455, 455*t*
anxiolytics
  anxiety *see* anxiety disorders, treatment
  pain, 526
aorta, coarctation of the, 297
aplasia, 89*t*
apnoea, neonates, 128
apolipoprotein C-II deficiency, familial, 393
apomorphine, Parkinson's disease, 514
apo-proteins (apo), 390
appendicectomy, 186
apraclonidine, glaucoma, 871, 872*t*
Aptivus©, 631*t*
aqueous humour, 862
arachidonic acid, menorrhagia, 719
arachidonic acid pathway, 164, 164*f*
arachnoid mater, 584–585
arachnoid villi, 584–585

area postrema, 535–536
area under the concentration time curve (AUC),
  35, 35*f*
area-under-the-curve (AUC), 54–55
aripiprazole, schizophrenia, 483*t*
aromatase inhibitors, chemoprevention, 819
arousal systems, 455–456, 456*f*
arrhythmias, 354–375
  abnormal impulse formation, 356–358
    abnormal automaticity, 356–357, 357*f*
    triggered activity, 357–358, 357*f*
  abnormal impulse propagation, re-entry, 358,
    358*f*
  cardiac action potential, 354–355, 355*f*
  case studies, 374*b*
  in chronic heart failure, 337*t*
  clinical problems, 358
  common therapeutic problems, 373*t*
  diagnosis, 358–359
  drug therapy, 366–373
  management, 358–359
  mechanisms, 356–358
  normal cardiac conduction, 355–356, 356*f*
  normal cardiac electrophysiology, 354–356
  patient care, 373–374
  refractoriness, 355
  during ST elevation myocardial infarction, 325
  Vaughan-Williams classification, 366–373
  see also specific types
arsenic salts, 203*t*
arsenic trioxide (ATO), 792
arterial blood gases, 83
arterial leg ulcers, 919–920, 920*f*
  clinical signs, 919
  diagnosis, 919
  prevention of recurrence, 920
  treatment, 920
arterial thromboembolism (ATE), 385–388
  aetiology, 385
  patient care, 387–388
  treatment and prevention, 385–386
    aspirin, 385–386
    clopidogrel, 386
    dipyridamole, 386
    glycoprotein IIb/IIIa inhibitors, 386
    prasugrel, 386
arthritis, 155
  see also osteoarthritis; rheumatoid arthritis
arthropathies
  psoriatic, 902
  in ulcerative colitis, 190
artificial sweeteners, 139
ascites
  in liver disease, 243, 246–248
  management, 246–248, 246*b*, 247*t*
    diuretics, 246–247
    paracentesis, 247
    transjugular intrahepatic portosystemic
     shunting, 247, 247*f*
  refractory, 247
  spontaneous bacterial peritonitis, 247–248
aseptic technique, 797
Asian ginseng, 59
AS METTHOD, 5–6, 6*b*
asparaginase, 790
aspartame, 139
aspartate transaminase (AST), 85
  in liver disease, 244
  liver function tests, 86
aspergillosis, 658*t*, 660*t*, 667
Aspergillus sp., 659
aspiration pneumonia, 555
aspirin
  adverse effects, 65, 386

arterial thromboembolism, 385–386
  chemoprevention, 820
  coronary heart disease, 11*t*, 12*t*, 315–316
  and dementia, 153
  drug-induced asthma, 412–413
  drug interactions, 836
  gout, 851, 853
  hepatotoxicity, 223, 226
  hypertension, 306
  interactions, 59
  in liver disease, 246
  non-ST elevation myocardial infarction,
    327–328
  peptic ulcer bleeding, 165
  pharmacokinetics, 385–386
  ST elevation myocardial infarction, 322, 324
  stroke, 153, 362, 363
Assign risk calculator, 397–398
asteatotic eczema, 895–896
asthma, 412–430
  acute severe, 414, 420–422, 421*f*
  aetiology, 412–413
  case studies, 428*b*
  in children, 133
  chronic, 415–422
  clinical manifestations, 413–414
  definition, 412
  drug interactions, 11*t*
  epidemiology, 412
  extrinsic, 413
  inhalation devices, 423–427, 424*t*
    breath-actuated metered dose inhalers, 426,
     426*f*
    for children, 425*t*
    dry powder inhalers, 426, 426*f*
    metered dose aerosol inhalers, 424–425
    metered dose inhaler with a spacer extension,
     425–426
    nebulisers, 426–427
  intrinsic, 413
  investigations, 414–415
  ladder of knowledge, 422, 423*b*
  pathophysiology, 413
  patient care, 422–429, 423*b*
  patient knowledge/education, 423
  refractory/difficult to treat, 414
  self-management programs, 427–429
  treatment, 415–422
    acute severe asthma, 420–422
    chronic asthma, 415–422
    preventer medication, 418–420
    reliever medication, 415–418
  triggers, 412–413, 413*t*
astroviruses, 214
atazanavir, 631*t*
atenolol, 318*t*
  arrhythmias, 370
  clinical trials, 302
  hypertension, 309
    in chronic kidney disease, 284
    in pregnancy, 306
  stable angina, 317–318
  studies, 299–300
atherosclerosis
  coronary heart disease, 313–314, 314*f*
  plaques, 313–314
athlete's foot, 657
atonic colon, 212–213
atonic seizures, 491
atopic eczema, 893–894, 906, 906*f*, 907, 907*f*
atorvastatin
  adverse reactions, 73
  dyslipidaemia, 402
  metabolism, 55, 404

atovaquone
    opportunistic infections in HIV, 639t
    Pneumocystis jiroveci pneumonia, 638
atracurium, 126
atrial fibrillation, 334, 362–364
    case studies, 374
    classification, 362
    emergency management, 363
    long-term management, 363
    rhythm control, 363–364
    stroke risk, 362–363, 362f, 374
    treatment, 336
    ventricular rate control, 363
atrial flutter, 359, 360f
atrial natriuretic peptide (ANP), 296
atrioventricular node, 356–357
atrioventricular re-entry tachycardia (AVRT),
        360, 361f
Atripla©, 628t
atropine
    arrhythmias, 365–366
    diarrhoea, 217
    dysmenorrhoea, 717
    in the elderly, 152
auranofin, 836, 837t, 839
Australian National Blood Pressure Study Group,
        302
auto-antibodies, 244
autoimmune haemolytic anaemia, 779–780,
        780b
autoimmune hepatitis (AIH), 241, 252
automated peritoneal dialysis (APD), 292
autonomy, 17, 17b
autosomal dominant polycystic kidney disease, 277
average costs, 117
AV nodal re-entry tachycardia (AVNRT), 360, 361f
5-azacytidine, 792
azapropazone, gout, 853
azathioprine
    adverse effects, 198
    autoimmune hepatitis, 252
    drug interactions, 198, 899t
    eczema, 898, 904t
    graft-versus-host disease, 795
    inflammatory bowel disease, 198, 200–201, 203t
    interactions, 61
    interstitial nephritis, 258–259
    metabolism, 55t
    psoriasis, 904t
    renal transplantation, 289t, 291
    rheumatoid arthritis, 836, 837t
azithromycin
    gastro-intestinal infections, 578, 579, 580
    Legionnaire's disease, 552
    mycobacteria, 644
    opportunistic infections in HIV, 639t
    tuberculosis, 616t
azole ring, 663
azotaemia, 662
aztreonam, pneumonia, 554t

B

Bacillus cereus, 214
    gastro-intestinal infections, 574t, 576t
    investigations, 577
    treatment, 578
back pain, 530, 533
baclofen, 527
bacterial infections
    in atopic eczema, 894
    in HIV infection, 643–644
    and psoriasis, 899
    wounds, 913–914, 914f

bacterial meningitis, 593t
    aetiology, 585
    diagnosis, 586–587
    drug treatment, 587–593, 588t
    epidemiology, 585
    presentation, 586
bacteriuria
    asymptomatic, 561
    of pregnancy, 569–570
    significant, 561
    treatment, 566
Baker's cyst, 378
balanitis, candida, 657
balloon tamponade, oesophageal varices, 249–250
balsalazide, inflammatory bowel disease, 196, 203t
bandaging, eczema, 898
barbiturates, 54
bariatric surgery, 706
baroreceptor reflex, 296
Barrett's oesophagus, 173, 175
basal cell carcinoma, 890, 890f
basiliximab, renal transplantation, 291
basophilia, 89t
basophils, 90
BCG vaccine, 608, 617
BCR gene, 788, 793
BEACOPP (bleomycin, etoposide, adriamycin,
        cyclophosphamide, vincristine,
        procarbazine, prednisolone), Hodgkin's
        lymphoma, 805, 807t
BEAM (carmustine, etoposide, cytarabine,
        melphalan), non-Hodgkin's lymphoma,
        811–812
Beau's lines, 881–882
Beck Depression Inventory, 468
beclometasone inhaler, 11t, 12t, 419, 419t
behaviour
    medicines-taking, 5
    pharmaceutical consultation, 6, 6b
benchmarking, prescribing influences, 29
bendroflumethiazide
    chronic heart failure, 337, 339t
    clinical trials, 302
    hypertension, 300
    photosensitivity, 881
beneficence, 18
benefits, communicating, 23–24
benign prostatic hyperplasia (BPH), 753–759
    case study, 767
    common therapeutic problems, 759t
    epidemiology, 753
    examination, 754–756
    investigations, 754–756
    pathophysiology, 753
    patient care, 758–759
    symptoms, 754
    treatment, 756–758, 759t
benperidol, schizophrenia, 483t
benserazide, Parkinson's disease, 511
benzamides, schizophrenia, 483t
benzbromarone, gout, 856
benzodiazepines
    abuse, 460
    adverse effects, 450–451, 459–460, 460b
    anxiety disorders, 457–460
        choice of, 459
        role in treating, 459
    dependence, 459–460
    drug interactions, 451, 460
    effect on neonates, 124
    in the elderly, 152
    insomnia, 448–449, 448t
    mechanism of action, 449, 458–459
    pain, 526

pharmacokinetics, 448–449, 457–458
    in pregnancy and lactation, 460
    profile of selected, 458t
    teratogenicity, 741t
    withdrawal, 460, 460b
benzyl alcohol, 141
benzylpenicillin
    meningitis, 589, 589t
    pneumonia, 551
β-adrenoceptor agonists
    asthma, 415–417
    long-acting, 415–417
    short-acting, 415
β-adrenoceptor antagonists *see* β-blockers
β-adrenoceptors, 151
β₂-agonists, 57
    adverse reactions, 420b
    asthma, 11t, 418, 420, 422
    chronic obstructive pulmonary disease, 437
    drug interactions, 423t
β-blockers
    adverse effects, 317, 318, 349, 367t, 370,
        868–869, 870t
    anxiety disorders, 462
    arrhythmias, 325, 359, 361, 363, 365, 369–370
    cardioselective, 299
    chronic heart failure, 336, 340t, 341
    clinical trials, 302
    coronary heart disease, 11t
    diarrhoea, 215t
    disease interactions, 348t
    drug-induced asthma, 412–413
    drug interactions, 348t
    dyslipidaemia, 395
    effect on lipoprotein levels, 394t
    effect on neonates, 124
    glaucoma, 868–871, 869t
    hypertension, 155–156, 299–300, 302–304,
        303t, 304b
        in chronic kidney disease, 284
        in diabetes, 305
        in the elderly, 304
        indications/contraindications, 307t
        in pregnancy, 306
    interactions, 57
    lipid solubility, 370
    non-ST elevation myocardial infarction, 329
    pharmacokinetics, 318t
    properties, 318t
    psoriasis, 899
    self-monitoring, 345t
    stable angina, 317–318, 318t
    ST elevation myocardial infarction, 326
    teratogenicity, 741t
    thyrotoxicosis, 676
betahistine, antiemesis, 541
β-lactams
    allergy, 604–605, 605t
    resistance, 566
    urinary tract infections, 566, 568
betamethasone, 124, 126
β thalassaemias, 782
betaxolol, 318t
    adverse effects, 868
    glaucoma, 868, 869t, 870
bevacizumab, solid tumours, 825
bicalutamide, prostate cancer, 762
bicarbonate, 83
    acidosis, 264
    extracellular fluid osmolality, 77
Bifidobacteria, 186
biguanides
    adverse effects, 699
    diabetes mellitus, 699, 701t

bilateral renal artery stenosis, 262, 262*f*
bile acid binding agents
    adverse effects, 406–407
    drug interactions, 406*t*
    dyslipidaemia, 403*t*, 405–407
biliary excretion, 56
biliary fistula, 105*t*
bilirubin
    conjugated, 85
    in liver disease, 244
    liver function tests, 84, 85
    unconjugated, 85
bimatoprost
    adverse effects, 868
    glaucoma, 864, 865, 867–868, 868*t*, 874
    and timolol, 874
bioavailability, 35
biochemical tests, 76–84, 77*t*
    arterial blood gases, 83
    bicarbonate and acid-base, 83
    calcium, 81–82
    creatinine, 82–83
    drug-induced liver disease, 228
    glucose, 77*t*, 84
    glycated haemoglobin, 84
    liver disease, 244
    magnesium, 82
    phosphate, 82
    potassium, 79–81
    sodium and water balance, 76–79, 77*f*, 77*t*
    urea, 77*t*, 83
    uric acid, 84
    see also laboratory data
biofilms, 914
biological agents
    choice of, 842
    contraindications, 201
    inflammatory bowel disease, 193, 199–202,
        200*t*, 203*t*
    psoriasis, 905
    rheumatoid arthritis, 839–840, 840*f*, 840*t*
biopsy urease test, *Helicobacter pylori*, 167–168
bipolar disorder
    case studies, 476, 477
    clinical features, 467, 467*b*
    definition, 465
    incidence, 465–466
    management, 468
bisacodyl, constipation, 157, 211, 212
bismuth chelate
    adverse reactions, 178
    peptic ulcer disease, 178
bismuth salts, inflammatory bowel disease, 203*t*
bismuth subsalicylate, diarrhoea, 217
bisoprolol, 318*t*
    chronic heart failure, 340*t*
    stable angina, 317–318
bisphosphonates
    absorption, 52
    alternatives to HRT, 731
    diarrhoea, 215*t*
    hypercalcaemia, 81
    hypocalcaemia, 82
    osteoporosis, 154
    pain, 525*t*
    prostate cancer, 763
bivalirudin
    non-ST elevation myocardial infarction,
        328–329
    ST elevation myocardial infarction, 324
    venous thromboembolism, 380
black cohosh, 731
bladder, menopausal changes, 726
bleomycin, Hodgkin's lymphoma, 804, 805, 807*t*

blood
    cultures, gastro-intestinal infections, 577
    glucose during ST elevation myocardial
        infarction, 325
    pH, 83
blood pressure
    high *see* hypertension
    home/ambulatory measurements, 297
    low *see* hypotension
    measurement, 295
    normal values, 295
    regulation, 296
Blood Pressure Lowering Treatment Trialists
        Collaboration, 302
blue bloater, 434
boceprevir, hepatitis C, 252
body mass index (BMI)
    and dyslipidaemia, 396
    parenteral nutrition, 97*t*
body surface area, 138
body weight
    and dyslipidaemia, 399–400
    and hormone replacement therapy, 727–728
bone marrow
    leukaemia, 788
    sideroblastic anaemia, 775
    suppression, chemotherapy, 813*t*, 814, 827
    transplantation, 792
bone(s)
    disease in chronic kidney disease, 279–280,
        279*f*
    menopausal changes, 726–727, 732
    metastatic pain, 529, 531*t*
    tuberculosis, 614
    in ulcerative colitis, 190
Borage, 59
Borago officinalis, 59
bortezomib, Hodgkin's lymphoma, 806
botulinum toxin, 527
botulism, 576
bowel cancer, 818
Braak hypothesis, 508
bradycardia, 365–366
    AV block, 365
    first degree, 365
    management, 365
    second degree, 365
    sinus, 365
    third degree, 365
bradykinesia, 508
bradykinin
    and blood pressure, 296
    hypertension, 301
bran, constipation, 212
breast cancer
    adjuvant chemotherapy, 824
    case study, 830
    and hormone replacement therapy, 734*t*, 735
breastfeeding *see* lactation/breastfeeding
breast milk
    benefits of, 745
    transfer of drugs into, 745–751
    see also lactation/breastfeeding
breath-actuated metered dose inhalers, 426,
        426*f*
breathlessness *see* dyspnoea
bretylium
    adverse effects, 367*t*
    arrhythmias, 370
    pharmacokinetics, 368*t*
brimonidine
    contraindications, 872
    glaucoma, 871–872, 872*t*, 874
    and timolol, 874

brinzolamide
    glaucoma, 873, 874
    and timolol, 874
British Hypertension Society (BHS), 297
British National Formulary (BNF), 18
Bromelain, 59
bromocriptine
    parkinsonism, 153
    premenstrual syndrome, 715
bronchiectasis, 433
bronchiolitis, 432, 433, 550
bronchitis
    acute, 549–550
    chronic, 431, 549
    in chronic obstructive pulmonary disease, 434
    clinical features, 549
    definition, 549
    diagnosis, 549
    lung function tests, 435
    treatment, 549–550
bronchoconstriction, 412–413
bronchodilators
    asthma, 415–418, 418*t*
    chronic obstructive pulmonary disease, 436–438,
        439
    comparison, 417*t*
    dosage, 418*t*
    high-dose, 437
    inhaled, 415–417
    long-acting, 437
    oral, 417–418
    short-acting β-adrenoceptor agonists, 415, 437
bronchopneumonia, 551
bronchopulmonary dysplasia (BPD), 126–127
bronchospasm, 868–870
buccal route of administration
    children, 139
    drug absorption in children, 136–137
    neonates, 124
Budd-Chiari syndrome (BCS), 227, 241
budesonide
    asthma, 417
    autoimmune hepatitis, 252
    inflammatory bowel disease, 195, 203*t*
Buerger's Test, 919
bulimia, 535
bumetanide, chronic heart failure, 338, 339*t*
bundle of His, 356, 366, 366*t*
bupivacaine
    local anaesthesia, 524
    postherpetic neuralgia, 529
buprenorphine, 523
bupropion, smoking cessation, 436, 441–442
Burkholderia cepacia complex, 555, 556
Burkitt's lymphoma, 807, 812
burn pain, 531–533
buserelin, prostate cancer, 762
buspirone, anxiety disorders, 461
butyrophenones, 483*t*, 538

C

cabergoline, Parkinson's disease, 512
caeruloplasmin, 244
Caesarian section, antimicrobial prophylaxis, 603
caffeine
    neonates, 130
        apnoea, 128
        transfer into breast milk, 749
calamine lotion, 246
calcineurin inhibitors
    eczema, 897
    renal transplantation, 290
    topical, 897

calcipotriol, psoriasis, 902
calcitonin
    and hypocalcaemia, 82
    osteoporosis, 155
calcitriol, 279, 287
    hypoparathyroidism/hypocalcaemia, 680,
        681t
    osteoporosis, 154
calcium, 81–82
    in acute kidney injury, 265
    osteoporosis, 154
    and parathyroid hormone, 679–684
    premenstrual syndrome, 714, 715
    supplements, 81, 264
    see also hypercalcaemia; hypocalcaemia
calcium acetate, hyperphosphataemia, 287
calcium antagonists see calcium channel blockers
calcium carbonate, hyperphosphataemia, 287
calcium channel blockers
    arrhythmias, 363
    clinical trials, 302
    effect on lipoprotein levels, 394t
    hypertension, 156, 283, 301, 303t, 304, 304b
        in chronic kidney disease, 283
        in diabetes, 305
        in the elderly, 304
        indications/contraindications, 307t
        in pregnancy, 306
    metabolism, 55
    stable angina, 318–319
calcium gluconate, hyperkalaemia, 81, 264
calcium leucovorin, 825
calcium phosphate precipitation, 106, 106t
calf muscle pump, 917–918
Calgary Cambridge framework, 21, 21f
calicheamicin, acute myeloblastic leukaemia, 792
campath-1H, chronic lymphocytic leukaemia,
        793–794
Campylobacter, 214, 217, 573
    gastro-intestinal infections, 574t, 576t
    transmission, 573
    treatment, 578, 581t
cancer
    cells, 820, 821f
    in children, 133
    in HIV, 623, 637–651
    and hormone replacement therapy, 733t,
        734–735
    pain, 528–529
        adjuvant drugs and treatments, 528
        case study, 532
        opioid use, 528
        specific syndromes, 528–529
    parenteral nutrition in, 111
    venous thromboembolism, 377
    see also tumours; solid. specific cancers
candesartan, chronic heart failure, 340t, 350
Candida sp.
    ear infections, 659
    fungal meningitis, 585
candidiasis, 656–657, 660t
    balanitis, 657
    clinical presentation, 656
    ear infections, 659
    epidemiology, 656
    neonates, 127, 127t
    oesophageal
        presentation, 656
        treatment, 656–657
    oral
        presentation, 656
        treatment, 656–657
    oropharyngeal, 638–643
    skin, 656–657

systemic, 658t
    treatment, 656–657, 663
    vaginal, 657
        presentation, 656
        treatment, 656–657
cannabinoids
    antiemesis, 539
    pain, 527
capecitabine, 825
capreomycin, tuberculosis, 616t
capsaicin, osteoarthritis, 845
capsicum, 59
captopril
    chronic heart failure, 340t
    clinical trials, 302
Captopril Prevention Project (CAPPP), 302
carbamazepine
    absorption, 42
    adverse effects, 66, 498, 500t
    distribution, 42
    drug interactions, 499t
    elimination, 42
    epilepsy, 498
    mania, 474
    metabolism, 53, 54, 55t
    pharmacokinetics, 42–43, 45t, 498, 498t
    plasma concentration-response relationship, 42
    postherpetic neuralgia, 529
    practical implications, 42–43
    rectal administration, 140
    trigeminal neuralgia, 529
carbapenems
    cystic fibrosis, 556t
    gastro-intestinal infections, 579
carbidopa, Parkinson's disease, 511
carbimazole
    hyperthyroidism, 675–676, 677
    thyrotoxicosis, 676
carbohydrates, diabetes mellitus, 694–695
carbonic acid-bicarbonate buffer system, 83
carbonic anhydrase inhibitors
    adverse effects, 873b, 873t
    glaucoma, 864, 873, 873b, 873t
    topical, 873
carboplatin
    and hypomagnesaemia, 82
    nausea and vomiting, 540
    non-Hodgkin's lymphoma, 811–812
cardiac action potential, 354–355, 355f
cardiac arrhythmias see arrhythmias
cardiac glycosides
    chronic heart failure, 342t
    self-monitoring, 345t
cardiac markers, 77t, 87
    creatine kinase, 87
    lactate dehydrogenase, 87
    troponins, 87
cardiac output, 334
cardiomyopathy, chemotherapy-induced, 813t
cardiovascular disease, 312
    antiretroviral toxicity, 637
    and chronic kidney disease, 275
    COX-2 inhibitors risk, 835, 836
    in diabetes mellitus, 692
    hypertension risk for, 295, 298
    and lipid profile, 389–390
cardiovascular system, menopausal changes, 727,
        733–734
carmustine, non-Hodgkin's lymphoma, 811–812
carteolol, 318t
    adverse effects, 868
    glaucoma, 868, 869t, 870
carvedilol, 318t, 340t
case-control studies, 70–71

case reports, 70
caspofungin
    adverse effects, 797
    clinical use, 666
    fungal infections in compromised host, 663,
        665–666
    infection in neutropenia, 797
    pharmacokinetics, 664t
    susceptible fungi, 666
castration
    medical, 762–763
    surgical, 762, 763
catechol-O-methyl transferase (COMT), 512
catechol-O-methyl transferase (COMT) inhibitors,
        Parkinson's disease, 512–513
Cates plot, 72, 73f
catheter ablation, arrhythmias, 364
catheter-associated urinary tract infections, 569
catheters, antimicrobial, 569
CCR5 inhibitors, 637
CD20, 809
CD4 count in HIV infection, 624–625
cefaclor, 223t
cefalexin
    bacteriuria of pregnancy, 570
    otitis media, 548
    urinary tract infections, 568t
cefixime
    hepatotoxicity, 223t
    otitis media, 548
cefotaxime
    infection in neutropenia, 797
    meningitis, 587–588, 589, 589t, 590, 591
    neonates
        infections, 127
        respiratory distress syndrome, 130
    spontaneous bacterial peritonitis, 247–248
ceftazidime
    acute pyelonephritis, 568
    infection in neutropenia, 797
    meningitis, 587–588
    neonatal infections, 127
    pneumonia, 554t
    urinary tract infections, 569t
ceftriaxone
    gastro-intestinal infections, 579
    meningitis, 588–589, 589t, 590, 591
cefuroxime
    acute pyelonephritis, 568
    urinary tract infections, 569t
celecoxib, 62
celiprolol, 318t
Celsentri©, 636t
central corneal thickness (CCT), 863
centralised intravenous additive services (CIVAS), 141
central nervous system (CNS)
    in leukaemia, 788, 791
    and the menopause, 736–737
central venous pressure (CVP), 260
cephalin, 92
cephalosporins
    acute pyelonephritis, 568
    bronchitis/chronic obstructive pulmonary
        disease, 549–550
    cystic fibrosis, 556t
    epiglottitis, 548
    gastro-intestinal infections, 573–574, 579
    interstitial nephritis, 258–259
    meningitis, 587–588, 589–590
    neonates
        infections, 127
        respiratory distress syndrome, 130
    pneumonia, 554t
    sore throat, 547

cephalosporins *(Continued)*
  spontaneous bacterial peritonitis, 247–248
  surgical site infection prophylaxis, 601
  urinary tract infections, 567
cerebrospinal fluid (CSF), 584–585, 586, 587
cerivastatin, dyslipidaemia, 402
certolizumab pegol
  guidance on the use of, 841
  inflammatory bowel disease, 199, 200*t*, 202, 203*t*
  rheumatoid arthritis, 840
cervical cancer, 818
cervical intraepithelial neoplasia (CIN), 645
cetirizine, pruritus in liver disease, 245, 245*t*
cetuximab
  adverse reactions, 884
  solid tumours, 825
CHADS$_2$ score, 362, 362*f*
CHA2DS2-VASc, 362–363
chamomile, 59, 61
channelopathies, 354, 364–365
Chan Su, 59
Charcot arthropathy, 694
chelation, 52
chemical exposure, leukaemia risk, 787
chemoreceptor trigger zone (CTZ), 535–536
chemotherapy, 823–825
  adjuvant, 824
  adverse effects, 813, 813*t*, 824–825
  chemotherapy-specific adjunctive treatments, 825
  neo-adjuvant, 824
  patient management, 826–830
    cumulative dosing, 826
    domiciliary treatment, 828
    dose modification or delay, 826
    drug interactions, 826
    inpatient/outpatient treatment, 827–828
    monitoring anti-cancer therapy, 828–830
    patient information and counselling, 826
    prescription verification, 826, 826*b*
    symptom control, 826–827
  prostate cancer, 763–764
  regimen, 823–825, 824*t*
    dose, 823–824
    scheduling, 823
  response to treatment, 828–830
  synchronous chemoradiation, 824
  toxicity, 828
chemotherapy-induced nausea and vomiting, 540, 540*b*, 540*t*, 813, 813*t*
chest pain, coronary heart disease, 315
chest radiography
  chronic obstructive pulmonary disease, 435
  tuberculosis, 612
child health clinics, 135
children, 132–148
  adherence, 141–142
  adverse drug reactions, 65, 144
  bacteriuria in, 566
  biochemical ranges, 143*t*
  case studies, 146–147
  concordance, 141–142
  consent, 17
  constipation, 212
  counselling, 141–142
  definition, 132
  dehydration, 214–215, 216–217
  demography, 132–134
    alcohol use, 134
    asthma, 133
    cancer, 133
    congenital anomalies, 132–133
    drug use, 134

eczema, 133
    hay fever, 133
    infections, 133–134
    mental health disorders, 134
    nutrition and exercise, 134
    smoking, 134
  drug absorption, 135–137
  drug distribution, 137
  drug excretion, 138
  drug metabolism, 137–138
  drug therapy in, 138–141
    buccal route, 139
    choice of preparation, 139–141
    dosage, 138–139, 138*t*
    dose regimen selection, 141, 142*t*
    intranasal route, 140
    nasogastric and gastronomy administration, 140
    oral route, 139–140
    parenteral route, 140–141, 140*t*
    pulmonary route, 141
    rectal route, 140
  estimate glomerular filtration rate, 274
  fluid requirements, 140, 140*t*
  gastroenteritis, 214
  hepatotoxicity risk, 232
  insomnia, 451
  licensing of medicines, 145–146
  medication errors, 144–145
  medicines in schools, 142–143
  meningitis, 588–590, 588*t*
  mental health disorders, 134
  monitoring parameters, 143–144, 143*t*
  normal, 134–135
  parenteral nutrition, 112–115
    formulation and stability issues, 112–113
    heparin, 113
    nutritional requirements, 112, 112*t*
    route of administration, 113–115
  service frameworks, 146–148
  stages of development, 136*f*
  tuberculosis, 614
  urinary tract infection prophylaxis, 570–572
  urinary tract infections, 562, 563, 568
Chinese ginseng, 59
Chlamydia pneumoniae, 313
Chlamydia trachomatis, 563, 717–718
chloral hydrate, 140
chlorambucil
  chronic lymphocytic leukaemia, 793
  Hodgkin's lymphoma, 805, 807*t*
chloramphenicol
  adverse reactions, 65
  gastro-intestinal infections, 579
  meningitis, 588, 589, 589*t*, 590
  sideroblastic anaemia, 774–775
chlordiazepoxide, 458*t*
chloride, extracellular fluid osmolality, 77
chlorphenamine
  pruritus
    in chronic kidney disease, 285
    in liver disease, 245, 245*t*
chlorpromazine
  drug-induced parkinsonism, 509–510
  hepatotoxicity, 223, 223*t*
  schizophrenia, 483*t*
chlortalidone
  clinical trials, 302
  hypertension, 155
ChlVPP (chlorambucil, vinblastine, procarbazine, prednisolone), Hodgkin's lymphoma, 805, 807*t*
cholecalciferol, 279
cholera, 579–580

cholestasis
  aetiology, 225–226
  clinical presentation, 228
  drugs associated with, 226*t*
  pathophysiology, 226–227
cholesterol
  and coronary heart disease, 313–315
  high-density lipoprotein *see* high-density lipoprotein cholesterol (HDL-C)
  intermediate-density lipoprotein cholesterol *see* intermediate-density lipoprotein cholesterol (IDL-C)
  low-density lipoprotein *see* low-density lipoprotein cholesterol (LDL-C)
  total *see* total cholesterol (TC)
  very low-density lipoprotein *see* very low-density lipoprotein cholesterol (VLDL-C)
cholesterol absorption inhibitors, dyslipidaemia, 407
cholesterol ester transfer protein (CETP) inhibitors, dyslipidaemia, 407–410
choline acetyltransferase, 151
cholinergic system, age-related changes, 152
cholinesterase inhibitors
  adverse effects, 152
  dementia, 152
  Parkinson's disease, 516
chondrodysplasia punctata, 381
CHOP (cyclophosphamide, doxorubicin, vincristine, prednisolone, rituximab), Hodgkin's lymphoma, 805
chronic heart failure (CHF), 333–353
  aetiology, 334
  case studies, 350*b*
  classification, 333, 333*t*
  clinical manifestations, 335, 335*t*
  epidemiology, 333–334
  investigations, 335–336, 336*t*
  pathophysiology, 334–335
  patient care, 344–352
  patient education and self-monitoring, 344–345, 345*t*
  symptoms, 333, 334
  treatment, 336–344
    guidelines, 344
    monitoring effectiveness of, 345–346, 346*t*
    monitoring safety of, 346–352
    potential problems, 346–348, 349, 350–352
chronic kidney disease (CKD), 272–294
  anaemia, 278–279
  bone disease, 279–280
  case studies, 292*b*
  causes of, 275–277
  classification, 273*t*
  clinical manifestations, 277–281, 277*f*
  common therapeutic problems in, 288*t*
  diagnosis, 281–282
  and dyslipidaemia, 395
  electrolyte disturbances, 280–281
  fluid overload, 278
  haematuria, 278
  hypertension, 278
  implementation of regular dialysis, 292–293
  incidence, 272
  investigations, 281–282
  monitoring, 281–282
  muscle function, 280
  neurological changes, 280
  nocturia, 278
  polyuria, 278
  prognosis, 282–283
  proteinuria, 278
  renal function measurement, 273–275

chronic kidney disease (CKD) *(Continued)*
  renal transplantation, 288–292
  renin-angiotensin-aldosterone system, 272–273, 273*f*
  significance of, 275
  treatment, 283–288
  uraemia, 278
  urinary tract features, 277–278
  vs. acute kidney injury, 272
chronic lymphocytic leukaemia (CLL), 786
  case study, 801
  clinical manifestations, 789
  epidemiology, 786
  pathophysiology, 788
  supportive care, 795–796
  treatment, 793–794
chronic myelocytic leukaemia (CML), 786
  case study, 798
  clinical manifestations, 789
  epidemiology, 786
  pathophysiology, 788
  supportive care, 795–796
  treatment, 792–793
chronic obstructive pulmonary disease (COPD), 431–445
  acute exacerbations, 439, 549–550
  aetiology, 432–433
  case studies, 443*b*, 558–559
  clinical features, 434–435, 549
  clinical manifestations, 434–435
  definition, 431
  diagnosis, 434, 549
  epidemiology, 431, 431*t*
  inflammation, 433
  investigations, 435, 436*t*
  oxidative stress, 433
  pathology, 431–432
    central airways, 431
    lung parenchyma, 432
    peripheral airways, 432
    pulmonary vasculature, 432
  pathophysiology, 433–434
  patient care, 440–445
  proteinase and antiproteinase imbalance, 433
  risk factors, 432*t*
  stable, 436–439
  systemic effects, 434
  treatment, 436–440, 549–550
    acute exacerbations of COPD, 439
    of hypoxia and cor pulmonale, 439–440
    stable COPD, 436–439
Chronic Prostatitis Symptom Index (CPSI), 765
chylomicron remnants, 390
chylomicrons, 390
ciclesonide, asthma, 419*t*
ciclosporin
  adverse effects, 199, 290
  distribution, 44
  drug interactions, 290, 290*b*, 899*t*
  dyslipidaemia, 396
  eczema, 898, 904*t*
  effect on lipoprotein levels, 394*t*
  elimination, 44
  gout, 851
  graft-versus-host disease, 795
  and hypomagnesaemia, 82
  inflammatory bowel disease, 198–199, 203*t*
  metabolism, 54, 54*t*, 55
  pharmacokinetics, 44–49, 45*t*
  plasma concentration-response relationship, 44
  practical implications, 44
  psoriasis, 904*t*, 905
  renal transplantation, 289*t*, 290
  rheumatoid arthritis, 836, 837*t*

cidofovir
  cytomegalovirus, 644
  opportunistic infections in HIV, 639*t*
cigarette smoking
  affect on wound healing, 914
  and cancer risk, 818
  cessation, 436, 440–442
  in children, 134
  and chronic obstructive pulmonary disease, 432
  and coronary heart disease, 315, 330
  and drug metabolism, 54
  and dyslipidaemia, 396
  and inflammatory bowel disease, 186, 204
  and psoriasis, 899–900
  and rheumatoid arthritis, 832
  and surgical site infection, 599
cilazapril, chronic heart failure, 340*t*
ciliary dysfunction, chronic obstructive pulmonary disease, 433
cimetidine
  distribution, 150
  drug interactions, 177
  peptic ulcer disease, 177
cinnarizine, drug-induced parkinsonism, 509–510
ciprofloxacin
  acute pyelonephritis, 568
  bacteriuria of pregnancy, 570
  bronchitis/chronic obstructive pulmonary disease, 550
  cystic fibrosis, 556
  diarrhoea, 217
  gastro-intestinal infections, 578–579
  hepatotoxicity, 223*t*
  meningitis, 589*t*, 591
  metabolism, 55
  pneumonia, 554*t*
  tuberculosis, 616*t*
  urinary tract infections, 568*t*, 569*t*
cirrhosis, 238–239, 239*f*, 240
  alcoholic, 240–241
  drug-induced, 226*t*
cisplatin
  and hypocalcaemia, 82
  and hypomagnesaemia, 82
  nausea and vomiting, 540
  non-Hodgkin's lymphoma, 811–812
citalopram, depression, 471
civil wrongs, 16
clarithromycin
  bronchitis/chronic obstructive pulmonary disease, 549–550
  drug interactions, 176
  gastro-intestinal infections, 578
  Helicobacter pylori eradication, 171, 172
  interactions, 59
  straws, 139
  tuberculosis, 616*t*
clearance (CL), 34
  capacity limited, 36
  increasing, 36–37
clindamycin
  gastro-intestinal infections, 573–574
  opportunistic infections in HIV, 639*t*
  Pneumocystis jiroveci pneumonia, 638
  pneumonia, 554*t*
  toxoplasmosis, 643
clinical governance, 19, 20*b*
clinical negligence, 16
clinical pharmacy, 2–13
  definition, 3*t*
  development of, 2–3
  functions and knowledge, 7–12
  patient details, 7–8

pharmaceutical care *see* pharmaceutical care
pharmaceutical consultation *see* pharmaceutical consultation
  quality assurance, 12–13
clinical trials
  drug safety, 63
  pre-marketing, 63
clobazam, epilepsy, 498–500
clofarabine, acute myeloblastic leukaemia, 792
clofazimine, tuberculosis, 616*t*
clomethiazole
  distribution, 150
  metabolism, 150
clomipramine
  anxiety disorders, 461
  depression, 470
clonazepam
  adverse effects, 500*t*
  anxiety disorders, 459
  epilepsy, 500
  neonatal seizures, 128–129
  pain, 526
  pharmacokinetics, 498*t*
  profile, 458*t*
clonidine
  alternatives to HRT, 731
  hypertension in chronic kidney disease, 285
  pain, 527
clopidogrel
  arterial thromboembolism, 386
  coronary heart disease, 11*t*, 12*t*, 316
  metabolism, 55, 55*t*
  non-ST elevation myocardial infarction, 327–328, 329
  peptic ulcer disease, 169
  ST elevation myocardial infarction, 322, 324
  stroke, 153
Clostridium botulinum, 527, 574*t*
Clostridium difficile, 214, 216, 264, 265, 575, 578
  gastro-intestinal infections, 574*t*, 576*t*
  investigation, 577
  surgical site infection, 601, 606
  treatment, 580, 581*t*
Clostridium perfringens, 214
  gastro-intestinal infections, 574*t*, 576*t*
  treatment, 578
clotting abnormalities
  in liver disease, 246, 246*f*
  management, 246
cloxacillin, 225–226
clozapine
  mode of action, 481
  monitoring therapy, 72
  Parkinson's disease, 516
  and refractory illness, 482
  schizophrenia, 482, 483*t*
cluster headaches, 531
coagulation, 92*f*
  disorders, 231
  tests, 91
  in liver disease, 244
coal tar preparations
  eczema, 898
  psoriasis, 903
co-amoxiclav
  acute pyelonephritis, 568
  bacteriuria of pregnancy, 570
  bronchitis/chronic obstructive pulmonary disease, 549–550
  hepatotoxicity, 223, 234
  otitis media, 548
  pneumonia, 554*t*
  spontaneous bacterial peritonitis, 247–248
  urinary tract infections, 568*t*, 569*t*

cobalamins, 93
co-beneldopa, 511
co-careldopa intestinal gel, 511
Coccidioides immitis, 585
Cockcroft Gault formula, 37, 83, 144, 274, 274*f*
codeine
    absorption, 52
    analgesia, 522, 523*t*
    diarrhoea, 217
codeine diphenoxylate, inflammatory bowel
        disease, 202
CODOX-M (cyclophosphamide, vincristine,
        doxorubicin, methotrexate),
        non-Hodgkin's lymphoma, 812
cognitive behavioural therapy (CBT)
    anxiety disorders, 457
    depression, 472
    obsessive-compulsive disorder, 457
    post-traumatic stress disorder, 457
cognitive biases influencing prescribing, 28, 28*t*
cognitive function, in geriatrics, 151
cognitive impairment, benzodiazepines, 459
cohort studies, 70
colchicine, gout, 852–854, 857
cold agglutinin disease (CAD), 779–780
cold autoimmune haemolytic anaemia, 779–780
colds, 545
colecalciferol, hypoparathyroidism/hypocalcaemia,
        681*t*
colesevelam
    drug interactions, 406*t*
    dyslipidaemia, 405, 406
colestipol
    drug interactions, 406*t*
    dyslipidaemia, 405, 406
    patient counselling, 407
    pruritus in liver disease, 245
colestyramine
    absorption, 52
    drug interactions, 406*t*
    dyslipidaemia, 405, 406
    inflammatory bowel disease, 202, 203*t*
    patient counselling, 407
    pruritus in liver disease, 245, 245*t*
colitis, 188
    chronic, 188
    clinical features, 188–189
    diversion, 188
    pseudomembranous, 188, 202
    ulcerative *see* ulcerative colitis
collagen, 912
colloid dressings, leg ulcers, 156
colloid replacement, ascites, 247
colorectal cancer
    adjuvant chemotherapy, 824
    case study, 829
    and hormone replacement therapy, 734
colostomy, electrolyte content of, 105*t*
combined oral contraceptives (COCs)
    drug interactions, 176
    and dyslipidaemia, 396
    dysmenorrhoea, 717, 718*t*
    endometriosis, 722
    and hypertension, 306, 308
    interactions, 60
    menorrhagia, 719–720, 720*t*
    metabolism, 54*t*
    premenstrual syndrome, 715
    venous thromboembolism risk, 733
Combivir©, 628*t*
Commission on Human Medicines (CHM), 145
community-acquired pneumonia, 550–552
    case study, 558
    causative organisms, 550–551, 551*t*

clinical features, 551
    diagnosis, 551
    prevention, 552
    treatment, 553*t*
        empiric, 552
        targeted, 551–552
competence, 19–20
competency frameworks, 19–20, 20*t*
complementary and alternative medicines
    antiemesis, 539
    interactions, 50
complex partial seizures, 491–492
complex regional pain syndrome, 530, 532
compression bandaging, 919
compression hosiery, 919
computed tomography (CT)
    chronic kidney disease, 282
    liver disease, 244
concordance, children, 141–142
confidentiality, 17
    breach of, 16
confusion in the elderly, 152, 152*b*
congenital anomalies, 132–133, 277
conjunctivitis, 191
Conn's syndrome, 297
consent, 17, 17*b*
    Gillick competence, 17
constipation, 209–214
    aetiology, 209–210
    case studies, 219*b*
    causes of, 210, 211*t*
    chemotherapy-induced, 813*t*
    in chronic kidney disease, 285
    common therapeutic problems, 218*t*
    definition, 209
    diagnostic algorithm, 212*f*
    differential diagnosis, 210
    in the elderly, 151, 157, 209
    general management, 210–214
        drug treatment, 211–214
        non-drug treatment, 210–211
    incidence, 209
    opioid-induced, 524
contact dermatitis, 894–895
    allergic, 894–895, 895*t*
    drug-induced, 885
    irritant, 895, 895*f*
contingent valuation, 117–118
continuous ambulatory peritoneal dialysis
        (CAPD), 292
continuous arterio-venous haemofiltration
        (CAVH), 266
continuous positive airway pressure (CPAP)
    neonates
        apnoea, 128
        bronchopulmonary dysplasia, 126
        respiratory distress syndrome, 125–126
continuous venovenous haemofiltration (CVVH),
        266
contraception
    combined oral *see* combined oral contraceptives
        (COCs)
    HIV infection and, 646
Control Hypertension and Hypotension
        Immediately Poststroke Study
        (CHHIPPS), 305–306
controlled drugs, 16
copper
    adult daily reference range, 102*t*
    deficiency, 101–102, 774–775
    excess *see* Wilson's disease
co-proxamol, 522
corneal microdeposits, amiodarone, 371
coronary angiography, coronary heart disease, 315

coronary artery disease (CAD) *see* coronary heart
        disease (CHD)
coronary heart disease (CHD), 312–332
    acute coronary syndrome *see* acute coronary
        syndrome (ACS)
    aetiology, 313–314
    case studies, 331*b*
    and chronic heart failure, 334
    clinical syndromes, 315–320
    common therapeutic problems, 330*t*
    definition, 312
    drug interactions, 11*t*
    drugs for, 11*t*
    epidemiology, 312–313
    and hormone replacement therapy, 733, 733*t*
    and hypertension, 295
    modification of risk factors, 314–315, 314*t*
    patient care, 330
    prevalence, 313
    risk factors, 313, 313*b*, 391–392
    stable angina *see* angina, stable
coronary steal, 319
cor pulmonale, 434, 439–440
corpus luteum, 711–712
corticosteroids
    adverse reactions, 420*b*
        acneiform, 884
        in children, 144
    antiemesis, 539
    asthma, 418–419, 419*t*, 420*b*, 422
    autoimmune hepatitis, 252
    bacterial meningitis, 592–593
    bronchopulmonary dysplasia, 126–127
    cancer pain, 528
    chronic lymphocytic leukaemia, 793
    chronic obstructive pulmonary disease, 438,
        439
    drug interactions, 423*t*
    dyslipidaemia, 396
    eczema, 896–897, 896*t*, 898
    effect on neonates, 124, 126
    gout, 852–853, 854
    hepatotoxicity management, 231
    inflammatory bowel disease, 193–195, 194*b*,
        203*t*
    inhaled, 11*t*, 418–419, 419*t*, 420*b*
    metabolism, 54*t*
    mycobacteria, 644
    neonates, 126–127
    osteoarthritis, 845
    pain, 525*t*
    Pneumocystis jiroveci pneumonia, 638
    prostate cancer, 763
    renal transplantation, 289*t*, 290, 291
    teratogenicity, 741*t*
    topical
        adverse effects, 896–897
        allergies, 897
        base, 897
        combined with antibiotics, 897
        eczema, 896–897, 896*t*
        psoriasis, 902–903
        tuberculosis, 643
cortisol, affective disorders, 466
Corynebacterium diphtheriae, 546
cost-benefit analysis (CBA), 117–118
cost-effectiveness analysis (CEA), 118
cost-minimisation analysis (CMA), 118
cost(s)
    of adverse drug reactions, 4
    average, 117
    categorisation of, 117
    fixed, 117
    incremental, 117

marginal, 117
opportunity, 117
prescribing, 116
variable, 117
cost-utility analysis (CUA), 118–119
co-trimoxazole
opportunistic infections in HIV, 639t
Pneumocystis jiroveci pneumonia, 638
urinary tract infections, 567–568
Cotswolds modification of Ann Arbor
classification system, 804, 804b
Counahan-Barratt equation, 144
counselling
anti-thyroid drugs, 677, 677b
bile acid binding agents, 407
chemotherapy, 826
children, 141–142
drug-induced liver disease, 233–234
lymphomas, 812
rheumatoid arthritis, 834–835, 843
statins, 405
tuberculosis, 618–619
COX-1, 521
inhibition, 165
rheumatoid arthritis, 835
COX-2, 521
inhibitors
chemoprevention, 820
choice of agent, 836
coronary heart disease, 316–317
in liver disease, 246
osteoarthritis, 845
peptic ulcer disease, 165, 173
rheumatoid arthritis, 835
safety, 835
rheumatoid arthritis, 835
selective drugs, 521
COX (cyclo-oxygenase)
COX-1 *see* COX-1
COX-2 *see* COX-2
inhibition, 164
rheumatoid arthritis, 835
Coxsackie viruses, 585
cranberry juice, 58, 570
C-reactive protein (CRP), 91, 314
creatine kinase (CK), 74, 87, 87t
creatinine, 82–83
acute kidney injury, 255, 259, 260, 265
children, 144
chronic kidney disease, 274
creatinine clearance, 274, 274f
estimation of, 37
Crixivan©, 631t
Crohn's disease
case studies, 205, 206
clinical features, 188–189
colitis, 188–189
definition, 185
diet and, 185, 186
drug treatment
aminosalicylates, 196
antibiotics, 202
biologic agents, 199, 200–201
budesonide, 195
colestyramine, 202
thalidomide, 202
epidemiology, 185
fish oils, 202
gastroduodenal and oral disease, 189
genetic factors, 186
infection, 186
location and distribution, 187–188, 187f, 187t
lymphomas in, 807
nutritional therapy, 192

perianal disease, 189
small bowel, ileocaecal and terminal ileal
disease, 188
smoking, 186
stricturing, 189, 189f
surgical treatment, 204
vs. ulcerative colitis, 189t
Crohn's Disease Activity Index (CDAI), 192
cromones, asthma, 419
Crown report, 15
cruciferous vegetables, 58
cryopyrin, 851–852
cryosurgical ablation of prostate (CSAP), 761
cryptococcal meningitis, 593t
in HIV patients, 592
treatment, 591–592
cryptococcosis, 658t, 660t, 663
Cryptococcus neoformans, 591
fungal meningitis, 585
HIV infection, 643
cryptosporidiosis, 573, 643
Cryptosporidium, 214
gastro-intestinal infections, 576t
treatment, 580, 581t
crystalloids, acute kidney injury, 263
cultures
blood, 577
sputum, 551, 553
stool, 216, 577
urine, 565–566
Cumberlage report, 15
CURE study, 327
cyanocobalamin, 776, 778–779
cyclic adenosine monophosphate (cAMP), 151
cyclizine, antiemesis, 285
cyclo-oxygenase *see* COX (cyclo-oxygenase)
cyclophosphamide
acute lymphoblastic leukaemia, 790
chronic lymphocytic leukaemia, 793
Hodgkin's lymphoma, 805, 807t
metabolism, 825
nausea and vomiting, 540
non-Hodgkin's lymphoma, 809, 811, 812
cycloserine, tuberculosis, 616t
CYP450 enzymes
and adverse drug reactions, 66
benzodiazepines, 457–458
classification, 53
CYP1A2, 54t, 55
CYP2C9, 54t, 55, 66
CYP2C19, 54t, 55, 66, 176
CYP2D6 (debrisoquine hydroxylase), 53, 54t, 66
CYP2E1, 54t
CYP3A, 53, 54–55, 176
CYP3A4, 54t, 55, 56–57, 58
CYP3A5, 66
drug interactions, 53
enzyme inhibition, 54–55
identification, 55–56
pharmacogenetics, 66
in pregnancy, 742, 743t
proton pump inhibitors metabolism, 176
statin metabolism, 404
cyproterone, prostate cancer, 762
cystic fibrosis (CF), 138, 555–556
case study, 559
clinical features, 555
infecting organisms, 555
treatment, 555–556
cystitis, 561, 563, 566
cytarabine
acute myeloblastic leukaemia, 791–792
chronic myelocytic leukaemia, 792–793
non-Hodgkin's lymphoma, 811–812

cytochrome P450 enzymes *see* CYP450
enzymes
cytokine inhibitors, 215t
cytomegalovirus (CMV)
of the gastro-intestinal tract, 644
in HIV infection, 644
neonates, 127
retinitis, 644
cytosine arabinoside, acute myeloblastic
leukaemia, 792
cytotoxic agents
acute tubular necrosis, 257t
adverse effects, 824–825
and diarrhoea, 215t
leukaemia risk, 787
therapeutic index, 138–139
see also chemotherapy
cytotoxin-associated gene A (CagA), 164
cytotoxins, gastro-intestinal infections, 575

D

dabigatran
stroke, 154
venous thromboembolism, 382–384
dacarbazine, Hodgkin's lymphoma, 804, 807t
daclizumab, renal transplantation, 291
danaparoid, venous thromboembolism, 380
danazol
adverse effects, 722
endometriosis, 722
menorrhagia, 719–720, 720t
premenstrual syndrome, 715
dandruff, 658
Danshen, 59
dantrolene, pain, 527
dantron, constipation, 212
dapsone
opportunistic infections in HIV, 639t
Pneumocystis jiroveci pneumonia, 638
daptomycin, meningitis, 589t, 590
darbepoetin alfa, 286
darifenacin, urinary incontinence, 157
darunavir, HIV infection, 631t, 635
darusentan, hypertension, 301
dasatinib, chronic myelocytic leukaemia, 793
DASH (Dietary Approaches to Stop
Hypertension) diet, 298
DaTSCAN, Parkinson's disease, 510
daunorubicin, acute myeloblastic leukaemia,
791–792
D-dimers, 88t, 93
debrisoquine hydroxylase (CYP2D6), 53, 66
decision analysis, 119–120, 119t, 120t
deep vein thrombosis (DVT), 376, 377–378
diagnosis, 93
in hormone replacement therapy, 729
investigations, 378
deferasirox
iron overload, 775
thalassaemias, 782
deferiprone
iron overload, 775
thalassaemias, 782
degarelix, prostate cancer, 763
dehydration
and diarrhoea, 214–216
treatment/rehydration, 216–217, 216t
delayed afterdepolarisations, 357–358, 357f
demeclocycline, hypernatraemia, 79
dementia, 152–153
with Lewy bodies, 152
in Parkinson's disease, 516
see also Alzheimer's disease

denosumab, 731
depression
  adverse effects of benzodiazepines, 459
  biochemical factors, 466
  case studies, 476, 477
  clinical features, 467
  and coronary heart disease risk, 313
  definition, 465
  genetic, 466
  incidence, 465–466
  management, 468
  menopause, 727, 735
  in Parkinson's disease, 509
  ST elevation myocardial infarction, 326
  treatment, 469–473
    drugs, 469–472
    non-drug, 472–473
dermatitis. *see also specific types*
Dermatology Quality of Life Index (DQLI), 903
dermatophytosis, 657–658
  clinical presentation, 657
  diagnosis, 657
  epidemiology, 657
  treatment, 657–658
dermis, 910
desferrioxamine
  hepatotoxicity antidote, 231
  iron overload, 775
  thalassaemias, 782
desmethyl-diazepam, 150
desmopressin
  absorption in children, 137
  intranasal administration, 140
desvenlafaxine, 731
detrusor instability, 156–157
developmental model, schizophrenia, 480
dexamethasone
  antiemesis, 539, 540, 542
  bacterial meningitis, 592–593
  cancer pain, 528
  non-Hodgkin's lymphoma, 811–812
  prostate cancer, 763
  tuberculosis, 643
dexamethasone suppression test, 466
dextromoramide, 522
dextropropoxyphene, 522
DHAP (cisplatin, cytarabine, dexamethasone),
    non-Hodgkin's lymphoma, 811–812
diabetes mellitus, 685–710
  aetiology, 686–687
  affect on wound healing, 913, 913t
  annual review, 706, 707b
  antipsychotics, 486
  β-blockers in, 317
  case studies, 708b
  causing chronic kidney disease, 276
  classification, 685b
  clinical manifestations, 688
  common therapeutic problems, 707b
  and coronary heart disease risk, 313
  diabetic emergencies, 688–691
  diagnosis, 688
  dyslipidaemia, 394–395, 405
  epidemiology, 686
  foot problems, 693–694 (*see also* diabetic foot
    ulcers)
  glycaemic management targets, 707
  hypertension in, 305, 307
  latent autoimmune diabetes in adults (LADA),
    685–686
  long-term complications, 691–694
    macro- and microvascular disease combined,
      693–694
    macrovascular disease, 691f, 692

microvascular disease, 692–693, 692f
  maturity-onset diabetes of the young (MODY),
    685–686
  monitoring glycaemic control
    in the clinic, 707
    at home, 707–709
  myocardial infarction, 325
  parenteral nutrition in, 111
  pathophysiology, 687
    of insulin resistance, 687
  patient care, 706–709, 706b
  surgical site infection, 599
  treatment, 694–706
    diet, 694–695
    hypertension, 705
    insulin therapy, 695–698
    obesity, 706
    structured education programs, 694
    type 1, 695–698
    type 2, 698–705
  type 1, 394
    aetiology, 686
    definition, 685, 685b
    incidence, 686
    insulin therapy, 695–698
    monitoring glycaemic control, 707–708
    symptoms, 688
    vs. type 2, 686t
  type 2, 394–395
    aetiology, 686–687
    definition, 685, 685b
    incidence, 686
    insulin therapy, 705
    management, 698–705
    monitoring glycaemic control, 708–709
    obesity management, 695
    symptoms, 688
    vs. type 1, 686t
diabetic foot ulcers, 915–917
  aetiology, 915–916, 915t
  case study, 923
  clinical signs, 916, 916f
  diagnosis, 916–917, 916t
  epidemiology, 915
  prevention of recurrence, 917
  treatment, 917
diabetic ketoacidosis, 690
  diagnosis, 690
  treatment, 690
diabetic nephropathy, 276
diabetic peripheral polyneuropathy, 529, 531–532
Diagnostic and Statistical Manual of Mental
    Disorders *see* DSM IV
diamorphine
  absorption, 52
    in children, 137
  analgesia, 523t
  cancer pain, 528
  effect on neonates, 125
  intranasal administration, 140
diarrhoea, 209, 214–220
  aetiology, 214
  case studies, 219b
  common therapeutic problems, 218t
  definition, 214
  electrolyte content of, 105t
  gastro-intestinal infections, 578
  incidence, 214
  investigations, 216
  medicines causing, 215t
  proton pump inhibitors adverse effects, 176
  signs and symptoms, 214–216
  traveller's, 214, 579
  treatment, 216–220

dehydration, 216–217, 216t
  drug treatment, 217–220
  general measures, 216
diastolic dysfunction, 334
diazepam
  anxiety disorders, 459
  distribution in the elderly, 150
  epilepsy, 500
  neonates, 124
    seizures, 128–129
  pain, 526
  pharmacokinetics, 498t
  profile, 458t
  rectal administration, 140
dibenoxazepine tricyclics, schizophrenia, 483t
diclofenac
  hepatotoxicity, 223t
  inflammatory bowel disease, 186
dicloxacillin, 225–226
didanosine, HIV infection, 628t, 635
diet
  affect on wound healing, 914
  and cancer risk, 818
  diabetes mellitus control, 694–695, 694b
  and dyslipidaemia, 400–401
  and endometriosis, 722
  and gout, 851
  and inflammatory bowel disease, 185–186
  and iron deficiency anaemia, 771
  modification in chronic kidney disease, 285, 286
  and prostate cancer, 759, 764
  vasomotor symptoms, menopause, 731–732
dietary supplements, eczema, 898
diethylene glycol poisoning, 67
diethylstilboestrol (DES), prostate cancer, 763
diffuse large B-cell lymphoma (DLBCL), 811,
    812
digitalis, 62
digitoxin, chronic heart failure, 342t
digoxin
  absorption, 38, 52
  action and uses, 37, 342, 372
  adverse reactions, 65, 342, 349, 372–373
  arrhythmias, 359, 363, 372–373
  bioavailability in children, 135
  chronic heart failure, 336, 342, 342t, 344
  disease interactions, 348t, 372t
  distribution, 38
    in the elderly, 150
  drug interactions, 38, 348t, 372t
  in the elderly, 150, 152
  elimination, 38
  and hypomagnesaemia, 82
  pharmacokinetics, 37–38, 45t, 46, 368t, 372
  plasma concentration-response relationship,
    37
  practical implications, 38
dihydrocodeine, 522, 523t
dihydropyridines
  adverse effects, 301, 349
  hypertension, 301, 303t
    in chronic kidney disease, 283
  stable angina, 319
dihydrotachysterol, hypoparathyroidism/
    hypocalcaemia, 681t
dihydrotestosterone (DHT), 753
  prostate cancer, 759
  urinary incontinence, 157
di-iodotyrosine (DIT), 669
dilator muscle theory, 862
diloxanide, diarrhoea, 218
diltiazem
  adverse effects, 73, 156, 349
  arrhythmias, 325, 359

coronary heart disease, 11t, 12t
hypertension, 156, 301
  in chronic kidney disease, 283
interactions, 59
pharmacokinetics, 368t
stable angina, 319
dimercapto succinic acid (DMSA) scan, 282
dipeptidyl peptidase (DPP-4) inhibitors, 699
  adverse effects, 704
  diabetes mellitus, 701t, 704
  drug interactions, 704
  mode of action, 704
  pharmacokinetics, 704
Dipeptiven®, 98
diphenoxylate, diarrhoea, 217
diphenylbutylpiperidines, schizophrenia, 483t
dipipanone, analgesia, 522
dipsticks, urinary tract infection, 564
dipyridamole
  arterial thromboembolism, 386
  stroke, 153
directly observed therapy (DOT), tuberculosis, 617–618
disability in Parkinson's disease, 515
discoid eczema, 895
discounting, 119
Disease Activity Score using 28 joint counts (DAS28), 833–834
disease-modifying anti-rheumatic drugs (DMARDs)
  choice of, 838
  combination therapy, 836
  key points, 838b
  monotherapy, 836
  onset of action, 836
  rheumatoid arthritis, 836–839, 837t
disinhibition, benzodiazepines, 459
disopyramide
  adverse effects, 367t
  arrhythmias, 368–369
  distribution, 53
  pharmacokinetics, 368t
distribution (of drugs)
  in children, 137
  drug interactions, 53
  in the elderly, 150
  in neonates, 124–125
  in pregnancy, 742–743
  in renal replacement therapy, 268
  volume see volume of distribution (V_d)
dithranol, psoriasis, 902, 903
diuretics
  adverse effects, 346–347
  ascites, 246–247, 247t
  chronic heart failure, 336, 337–338, 339t
  disease interactions, 348t
  drug interactions, 348t, 475t
  and dyslipidaemia, 395
  hypertension, 300–301, 303t, 307t
    in chronic kidney disease, 284
    in pregnancy, 306
  loop see loop diuretics
  neonatal heart failure, 127
  patient education, 344
  self-monitoring, 345t
  thiazide see thiazide diuretics
dobutamine, chronic heart failure, 342t, 343
docetaxel, prostate cancer, 763–764
docusate sodium, constipation, 157, 214
dofetilide, adverse effects, 367t
domperidone, antiemesis, 538, 541, 542
donepezil
  and dementia, 152, 153
  hepatotoxicity, 223t

Dong Quai, 59
dopamine
  in acute kidney injury, 263
  affective disorders, 466
  chronic heart failure, 342t, 343
  premenstrual syndrome, 714
dopamine agonists
  Parkinson's disease, 512
  side effects, 512
dopamine receptors, 481
dopaminergic agents, 215t
dopexamine, chronic heart failure, 342t
dorzolamide
  glaucoma, 873, 874
  and timolol, 874
dosulepin, depression, 470
DoTS system, 64, 65t
doxapram
  chronic obstructive pulmonary disease, 439
  neonatal apnoea, 128
doxazosin
  benign prostatic hyperplasia, 757, 758
  clinical trials, 302
  hypertension, 301
doxepin, depression, 470
doxorubicin
  Hodgkin's lymphoma, 804, 805, 807t
  non-Hodgkin's lymphoma, 809, 811, 812
  solid tumours, 826
doxycycline
  cholera, 579–580
  interactions, 60
D-penicillamine, rheumatoid arthritis, 836, 837t, 839
dressings, wound, 922, 922b
dronedarone, arrhythmias, 363
drospirenone, 715
drug abuse
  benzodiazepines, 459–460
  in children, 134
drug-associated nausea and vomiting, 541
drug-induced hypersensitivity syndrome (DIHS), 887–888, 887f
drug-induced liver disease (DILD), 222–237
  aetiology, 224–226
  antidotes, 231
  case studies, 235b
  cholestatic, 224–225
  clinical manifestations, 227–228
  cytotoxic, 224–225
  dose-related, 225t
  enzyme elevation, 222–223, 223t
  epidemiology, 222–223, 222f
  idiosyncratic, 224–225, 225t, 229
  incidence, 222
  intrinsic, 224–225, 225t
  investigations, 228
  pathophysiology, 226–227
  patient care, 232–236
  patient counselling, 233–234
  pruritus, 231
  risk factors, 223–224
    age, 223, 224t
    concurrent diseases, 224, 224t
    enzyme induction, 224, 224t
    gender, 223, 224t
    genetics, 224, 224t
    polypharmacy, 224, 224t
    pre-existing liver disease, 223, 224t
    pregnancy, 224, 224t
  risk minimisation, 234–236, 234b
  treatment, 228–232
    diagnosis, 228–229, 230b
    long-term, 231
    management, 231–232

    rechallenge, 231
    supportive, 231
    withdrawal, 229–231
drug interactions, 50–61
  case studies, 11t, 59, 60, 61
  definition, 50
  drug-disease, 8
  drug-drug, 8–9
  drug-food, 58
  drug-herb, 58–59
  drug-patient, 8
  epidemiology, 51
  high risk drugs, 51b
  mechanisms, 51–59
  pharmacodynamic interactions, 57–58
    additive or synergistic interactions, 57, 57t
    antagonistic interactions, 57
    drug or neurotransmitter uptake interactions, 58
    serotonin syndrome, 57–58
  pharmacokinetic interactions, 51–57
    absorption, 52
    drug distribution, 53
    drug metabolism, 53–56
    elimination, 56–57
  safety measures, 50
  susceptible patients, 51
  therapeutic benefits of, 50
  see also specific drugs
drug reaction with eosinophilia and systemic symptoms (DRESS), 887–888, 887f
drug(s)
  adherence see adherence/non-adherence
  administration, 9, 9t, 10–12
  advertising, 27
  affect on wound healing, 914–915
  communicating risks/benefits of, 23–24
  controlled, 16
  dosage, 9
  and dyslipidaemia, 395–396
  economic evaluation of, 120
  establishing the need for, 7–8, 10
  evaluating effectiveness, 10–12
  and gout, 851
  hepatotoxicity, 242
  history, 8, 8b
  and inflammatory bowel disease, 186
  monitoring, 10, 12, 72
    in the elderly, 158
    in neonates, 129
  patient advice/education, 10, 12
  prescribing see prescribing (of drugs)
  provision, 9–10
  and psoriasis, 899
  reconciliation, 4, 24
  regimens, 9
  safety, 63
  selection, 8–9, 10
drug transport proteins, 52, 56–57
drug use process (DUP), 2, 3t, 5
dry powder inhalers (DPIs), 426, 426f
DSM IV
  affective disorders, 468
  premenstrual dysphoric disorder, 713b
  schizophrenia, 479
dual energy, 99–100, 100b
duloxetine
  anxiety disorders, 461
  depression, 472
  pain, 526
duodenal ulcer, 162, 163f, 164, 165, 174f
Duodopa®, 511
Dupuytren's contracture, 242
dura mater, 584–585

dutasteride, benign prostatic hyperplasia, 758
dyes in oral preparations, 139
dysentery, 214, 217, 218, 575
dyslipidaemia, 389–411
  aetiology, 392–396
    primary dyslipidaemia, 392–393
    secondary dyslipidaemia, 393–396
  case studies, 408b
  epidemiology, 389–390
  lipid-lowering therapy, 401–410
    bile acid binding agents, 405–407, 406t
    cholesterol absorption inhibitors, 407
    cholesterol ester transfer protein (CETP)
      inhibitors, 407–410
    fibrates, 405
    fish oils, 407
    nicotinic acid and derivatives, 407
    soluble fibre, 407
    statins, 402–405
  lipid transport, 390–392
  lipoprotein metabolism, 390–392
  risk assessment, 396–399
    primary prevention, 396–399
    secondary prevention, 399
  treatment, 399–401
    drugs, 401
    lifestyle, 399–401, 400b
    lipid profile, 399
dysmenorrhoea, 716–718
  aetiology, 716–717
  epidemiology, 716
  pain management, 531
  primary, 716–717
  secondary, 717
  symptoms, 716–717
  treatment, 717–718, 718t
dyspareunia, 732
dyspepsia, 162–163, 165
  antacids, 178
  decision algorithm, 167f
  drugs causing, 166b
  gastro-oesophageal reflux disease, 173
  patient education, 178–179
  symptom subgroups, 166b
dyspnoea
  in asthma, 414
  in chronic heart failure, 337t
  in the elderly, 156
dystonia, 481

E

ear infection, fungal, 659
early afterdepolarisations, 357, 357f
echocardiography, chronic heart failure, 335–336
echoviruses, 585
ecological model, schizophrenia, 480
eczema, 893–898
  asteatotic, 895–896
  atopic, 893–894, 894f, 906, 906f, 907, 907f
  case studies, 906, 906f, 907, 907f
  in children, 133
  clinical features, 893, 894f
  discoid, 895
  drug-induced, 885
  gravitational, 919
  pathology, 893
  patient care, 898
  stasis, 895
  treatment, 896–898, 900f
    antihistamines, 897
    bandaging, 898
    calcineurin inhibitors, 897
    coal tar preparations, 898

dietary supplements, 898
  drug interactions, 899t
  emollients, 896
  phototherapy, 898
  systemic therapies, 898, 904t
  topical corticosteroids, 896–897
  topical imidazoles, 897
  types, 893–896
eczema herpeticum, 894, 907, 907f
efaluzimab, psoriasis, 905
efavirenz
  hepatotoxicity, 223t
  HIV infection, 628t, 630t
eicosapentaenoic acid (EPA), dysmenorrhoea, 716
elderly people see geriatrics
electrocardiography
  normal, 355–356, 356f
  stable angina, 315
electroconvulsive therapy (ECT), depression,
  472–473
electroencephalography (EEG), epilepsy, 492
electrolytes, 77t
  acute kidney disease, 260
  acute kidney injury, 265
  cholera, 579–580
  chronic kidney disease, 280–281, 280t
  content of gastro-intestinal secretions, 105t
  gastro-intestinal infections, 578
  parenteral nutrition, 103
elimination half-life, 35
elimination (of drugs), 34–35
  in children, 138
  clearance, 34
  drug interactions, 56–57
  first-order, 34, 34f
  in neonates, 125
  total body, 34
elimination rate constant (k_e), 34, 46
emesis see nausea and vomiting
EMLA, 136, 156
emollient laxatives, 214
emollients, eczema, 896, 896f
emotional arousal system, 455
emphysema, 432
  in chronic obstructive pulmonary disease,
    434–435
  lung function tests, 435
emtricitabine
  hepatitis B in HIV, 646
  HIV infection, 628t, 635
Emtriva©, 628t
enalapril
  chronic heart failure, 340t
  clinical trials, 302
encephalopathy
  hepatic, 248, 249t
  HIV, 645–646
  hypertensive, 296–297
ENCORE, 5–6, 6b
endocrine/autonomic arousal system, 455
endocrine factors, affective disorders, 466
endometrial ablation, menorrhagia, 721
endometrial cancer, 718–719, 735
endometriosis, 721–723
  aetiology, 721
  case study, 723
  epidemiology, 721
  symptoms, 721
  treatment, 721–723
endorphins, 519–520
endoscopic band ligation, oesophageal varices, 250
endoscopy
  inflammatory bowel disease, 191
  peptic ulcer disease, 166, 168–169

endothelins, dysmenorrhoea, 716
endotracheal intubation, neonates, 125–126
end-stage renal failure, 275
  causes of, 275
  clinical manifestations, 277
  renal transplantation, 288
energy
  dual, 99–100, 100b
  parenteral nutrition, 99–101, 100b
enfuvirtide, HIV infection, 636t, 637
enoximone, chronic heart failure, 342t
entacapone, Parkinson's disease, 513
Entamoeba, 214, 576t
entecavir, hepatitis B, 251
enteric fever, 575–576
  investigations, 577
  treatment, 579–581, 581t
enteric microflora, 186
Enterobacter sp., 591
  surgical site infection, 599–600
  urinary tract infections, 562
enterohepatic shunt, 56
enterotoxin, 214, 575
enteroviruses, 585
entry inhibitors, HIV infection, 636t, 637
environmental factors
  affective disorders, 466
  inflammatory bowel disease, 185–186
  solid tumours, 818, 819t
enzyme(s)
  induction, 54, 54t
    risk for drug-induced liver disease, 224
  inhibition, 54–55, 55b, 55t
  liver function tests, 85
eosinophilia, drug-induced, 887–888, 887f
eosinophils, 90
epidermal growth factor receptor (EGFR), 825
epidermis, 910
Epidermophyton, 657
epidural analgesia, 524
epidural local anaesthetics, 525
epiglottitis, acute, 547–548
epilepsy, 489–506
  aetiology, 490
  case studies, 504b
  chronic, 496
  clinical manifestations, 491–492
  common therapeutic problems in, 504t
  cryptogenic, 490
  diagnosis, 492
  epidemiology, 489–490
  evidence for clinical use of newer drugs,
    503–506
  febrile convulsions, 493
  incidence, 490
  intractable, 496, 501
  mortality, 490
  pathophysiology, 490–491
  prevalence, 490
  prognosis, 490
  seizures see seizures
  severe myoclonic epilepsy of infancy, 503
  status epilepticus, 493
  treatment, 492–503, 492b
    general principles of, 493–496
    long-term, 493
    monitoring, 496–497
    during seizures, 493
epinephrine see adrenaline
episcleritis, 191
Epivir©, 628t
eplerenone
  chronic heart failure, 339t, 341–342
  ST elevation myocardial infarction, 326

epoetins, 286
Epstein-Barr virus (EBV)
    and lymphomas, 807
    pharyngitis (sore throat), 546
eptifibatide, arterial thromboembolism, 386
ergocalciferol, 681t
erlotinib, solid tumours, 825
erythema multiforme, drug-induced, 885–886, 886b
erythema nodosum, 190–191
    drug-induced, 885, 891
erythrocyte glucose-6-phosphatase dehydrogenase
        (G6PD) deficiency see glucose-6-
        phosphatase dehydrogenase (G6PD)
        deficiency
erythrocyte sedimentation rate (ESR), 88t, 91
erythroderma, 883
    drug-induced, 888, 888b
erythrodermic psoriasis, 902, 902f
erythromycin
    adverse reactions, 65
    cholera, 579–580
    cystic fibrosis, 555–556
    diarrhoea, 217
    gastro-intestinal infections, 578
    hepatotoxicity, 223, 231
    Legionnaire's disease, 554
    metabolism, 53
    otitis media, 548
    pneumonia, 551
erythropoiesis, 88
    normal, 770, 770f
erythropoietin, 88, 770
    in sickle cell anaemia, 781
erythropoietin analogues, 774
Escherichia coli, 127
    antibiotic resistance, 567
    diarrhoea, 214, 217–218
    gastro-intestinal infections, 574–575, 574t, 576t
    transmission, 573
    treatment, 578, 579
    urinary tract infections, 562
    verotoxin-producing, 133–134, 575, 576t
escitalopram
    depression, 471, 472
    drug interactions, 176
ESHAP (etoposide, methylprednisolone,
        cytarabine, cisplatin), non-Hodgkin's
        lymphoma, 811–812
eslicarbazepine acetate, epilepsy, 501
esmolol
    arrhythmias, 370
    coronary heart disease, 318t
esomeprazole
    drug interactions, 176
    formulations available, 175t
    intravenous, 175
    peptic ulcer disease, 173t, 175, 175t
essential fatty acids, 714
estradiol
    dose, 729
    hormone replacement therapy, 728–729
    menopause, 726, 732
    premenstrual syndrome, 713
estrone, 726
etanercept
    guidance on the use of, 841
    psoriasis, 905
    rheumatoid arthritis, 840
ethambutol
    adverse effects, 616, 616t
    mycobacteria, 644
    tuberculosis, 612, 613, 613t, 614, 643
ethanol see alcohol
ethics, prescribing (of drugs), 17–18

autonomy, 17, 17b
beneficence, 18
justice and veracity, 18
non-maleficence, 17–18
ethinylestradiol, 715
ethionamide, tuberculosis, 616t
ethnicity/race
    and adverse drug reactions, 66
    and chronic kidney disease, 272
    and coronary heart disease, 313
    and dyslipidaemia, 396
    and HIV infection, 648–651
    and hypertension, 296, 304–306, 307
    and inflammatory bowel disease, 186–187
    and prostate cancer, 759
ethosuximide
    adverse effects, 500t
    drug interactions, 499t
    epilepsy, 501
    pharmacokinetics, 498t
etidronate
    adverse effects, 154
    alternatives to HRT, 731
    osteoporosis, 154
etoposide
    Hodgkin's lymphoma, 805
    non-Hodgkin's lymphoma, 811–812
etoricoxib, gout, 853
etravine, HIV infection, 630t, 635
EUROPA study, 317
evening primrose oil, 59
exanthems, drug-induced, 883, 883f, 888b
excitation-contraction coupling, 354
excretion (of drugs)
    in pregnancy, 742–743
    in renal replacement therapy, 268
    see also elimination (of drugs)
exenatide, 704–705
exercise
    children, 134
    and coronary heart disease, 330
    and dyslipidaemia, 401
exfoliative dermatitis, drug-induced, 888
extended-spectrum β-lactamase (ESBL)-producing
        bacteria, 566
extensively drug-resistant tuberculosis (XDR-TB),
        608, 609
extracellular fluid (ECF), 76
    osmolality, 77, 78
    potassium, 79
    volume, 78, 137, 137t
extracorporeal membrane oxygenation (ECMO), 126
extractable nuclear antigens (ENA), rheumatoid
        arthritis, 834
extravasation, 827
eye contact, 22
eye drops administration, 875–876
eye movement desensitisation and reprocessing
        (EMDR), 457
eyes
    in chronic kidney disease, 278
    in ulcerative colitis, 191
ezetimibe, dyslipidaemia, 403t, 407

F

factor VIII, 91
factor V Leiden
    thrombophilia, 715
    venous thromboembolism, 377
faecal softeners, 214
famciclovir, opportunistic infections in HIV, 639t
familial apolipoprotein C-II deficiency, 393
familial combined hyperlipidaemia, 393

familial hypercholesterolaemia, 392–393, 399b
familial lipoprotein lipase deficiency, 393
familial type III hyperlipoproteinaemia, 393
famotidine, peptic ulcer disease, 177
fats, 695
fatty acids, 100–101
fatty liver disease, non-alcoholic, 241
febrile convulsions, 493
febrile neutropenia, 814
febuxostat, gout, 856
felbamate
    adverse effects, 501
    epilepsy, 501
felodipine
    chronic heart failure, 343–344
    interactions, 58
    metabolism, 55
fenofibrate, dyslipidaemia, 393–394, 405
fenoldopam, acute kidney injury, 263
fentanyl
    absorption in children, 136–137
    analgesia, 522, 523t
    intranasal administration, 140
    patches, 136
ferritin, 88t
    anticoagulant therapy monitoring, 93
    in liver disease, 244
ferrous sulphate, 772
fetal cell transplantation, Parkinson's disease,
        514–515
feverfew, 59, 61
fibrates
    adverse effects, 405
    drug interactions, 406t
    dyslipidaemia, 403t, 405
fibre intake, 210–211
    in diabetes mellitus, 695
fibrin, 91
fibrinogen, 91, 314
fibrinogen gamma 10034T, venous
        thromboembolism, 377
fibrinolytic agents
    adverse effects, 324
    categories, 324
    contraindications, 324–325, 325b
    ST elevation myocardial infarction, 322, 323,
        323t, 324–325
    venous thromboembolism, 384–385
fibroids, 719
Fibroscan, 244
fibrosis
    liver, 227
    pulmonary, 371, 433, 813t
finasteride
    benign prostatic hyperplasia, 757–758
    urinary incontinence, 157
finger clubbing, 242
fish, dyslipidaemia, 400
fish oils
    dyslipidaemia, 400, 407
    inflammatory bowel disease, 202, 203t
fixed costs, 117
fixed drug eruptions, 884, 884b, 884f
flecainide
    adverse effects, 367t
    arrhythmias, 359, 361, 365
    pharmacokinetics, 368t
flexible cystoscopy, benign prostatic hyperplasia, 755
flexural psoriasis, 901–902
flu see influenza
flucloxacillin
    cystic fibrosis, 555–556
    hepatotoxicity, 223, 224, 225–226
    neonates, respiratory distress syndrome, 130

fluconazole
  absorption, 52
  candidiasis, 656–657
  clinical use, 663
  cryptococcus neoformans, 643
  fungal infections in compromised host, 663
  meningitis, 592
  opportunistic infections in HIV, 639t
  oropharyngeal candidiasis, 638–643
  pharmacokinetics, 664t
  resistance, 663
flucytosine
  administrations, 663
  adverse effects, 663
  cryptococcus neoformans, 643
  fungal infections in compromised host, 662–663
  meningitis, 591–592
  mode of action, 662–663
  opportunistic infections in HIV, 639t
  pharmacokinetics, 663, 664t
fludarabine
  acute myeloblastic leukaemia, 792
  chronic lymphocytic leukaemia, 793
fluid balance in acute kidney disease, 260
fluid intake, constipation, 210–211
fluid overload, 263–264
  children, 140
  in chronic kidney disease, 278
fluid replacement
  in acute kidney injury, 263
  cholera, 579–580
  gastro-intestinal infections, 578
  hyperosmolar hyperglycaemic state, 691
  oesophageal varices, 249
fluid requirements, factors affecting, 98t
fluid retention in chronic kidney disease, 286
flumazenil, 459
fluoroquinolones
  gastro-intestinal infections, 573–574, 578–579
  Legionnaire's disease, 552
  prostatitis, 766
  urinary tract infections, 566, 569
5-fluorouracil (5FU), 825
fluoxetine
  depression, 469, 471
  interactions, 58, 60
flupentixol, schizophrenia, 483t
fluphenazine
  drug-induced parkinsonism, 509–510
  schizophrenia, 483t
flutamide, prostate cancer, 762–763
fluticasone, asthma, 419t
fluvastatin
  dyslipidaemia, 402
  metabolism, 55, 404
fluvoxamine, depression, 471
focal atrial tachycardia, 359
focal segmental necrotising glomerulonephritis
    (FSNGN), 258
focal seizures, 491–492
foetal development, 740
foetal-placental transfer, 743
folate deficiency anaemia
  aetiology, 776
  clinical manifestations, 777
  drugs implicated in, 777b
  epidemiology, 776
  investigations, 777
  pathophysiology, 776
  patient care, 779
  treatment, 778
folic acid/folates, 88t
  anticoagulant therapy monitoring, 93–95
  deficiency in chronic kidney disease, 286

pre-conceptual, 744
  in sickle cell anaemia, 781
  supplementation during pregnancy, 133
folinic acid, 825
  toxoplasmosis, 643
follicle-stimulating hormone (FSH), 726
follicular lymphoma, 809
folliculitis
  candida, 656
  Malassezia, 658, 659
fondaparinux
  non-ST elevation myocardial infarction, 328–329
  ST elevation myocardial infarction, 324
  venous thromboembolism, 380
food(s)
  adding medicines to, 139
  allergy, 894
  poisoning, 214, 573, 577, 578
  see also diet; nutrition
foot problems in diabetes mellitus, 693–694
  see also diabetic foot ulcers
forced expiratory volume (FEV)
  asthma, 414
  chronic obstructive pulmonary disease, 435
forced vital capacity (FVC)
  asthma, 414
  chronic obstructive pulmonary disease, 435
formoterol, asthma, 417, 418t
formularies, 29
formulation choice, 32
fosamprenavir, HIV infection, 631t
foscarnet
  cytomegalovirus, 644
  opportunistic infections in HIV, 639t
fosfomycin, urinary tract infections, 567–568
fosinopril, chronic heart failure, 340t, 341
FP-CIT SPECT, Parkinson's disease, 510
fractional excretion of sodium (FENa), 259
fractures, osteoporotic, 726–727
Framingham risk charts, 396–397
Fraser guidance, 17
free fatty acids, 248
frontotemporal dementia, 152
fumaric acid esters
  eczema, 904t
  psoriasis, 904t, 905
fungaemia, 660t
fungal infections, 654–668
  case studies, 667b
  classification, 655t
  in the compromised host, 659–668
    choice of treatment, 666–668
    clinical presentation, 660, 660t
    diagnosis, 660
    epidemiology, 659–668
    predisposing factors, 659–668
    treatment, 660
  deep-seated, 659, 660t
  in HIV, 638
  laboratory diagnosis, 654–655
  superficial, 656–659
fungal meningitis, 660t
  aetiology, 585
  diagnosis, 586–587
  epidemiology, 585
  presentation, 586
fungi, 654
  characteristics, 654t
  classification, 655t
  definition, 654
  reproduction, 654
furazolidine, cholera, 579–580
furosemide
  acute kidney injury, 263

adverse reactions, 64
ascites, 247, 247t
chronic heart failure, 338, 339t, 351
distribution in the elderly, 150
elimination in children, 138
gout, 853
hypercalcaemia, 81
and hypocalcaemia, 82
and hypomagnesaemia, 82
interstitial nephritis, 258–259
neonates
  bronchopulmonary dysplasia, 127
  heart failure, 131
fusarium keratitis, 659
fusion inhibitors, 637
Fuzeon©, 636t

G

GABA see γ-aminobutyric acid (GABA)
gabapentin, 495t, 496
  adverse effects, 500t
  alternatives to HRT, 731
  epilepsy, 501
  pharmacokinetics, 44, 498t
  plasma concentration-response relationship, 44
  postherpetic neuralgia, 529
galantamine, dementia, 152, 153
gallstones, 191
gametogenesis, 726
γ-aminobutyric acid$_A$ (GABA$_A$) receptors, 449,
    449f, 458–459, 458f
γ-aminobutyric acid (GABA)
  anxiety disorders, 456, 458–459, 458f
  hepatic encephalopathy, 248
γ-glutamyl transpeptidase
  in liver disease, 244
  liver function tests, 86
ganciclovir
  cytomegalovirus, 644
  opportunistic infections in HIV, 639t
garlic, 59, 61
gas exchange abnormalities, 434
gastric acidity, 575
gastric acid secretion, 164
gastric juice, electrolyte content of, 105t
gastric lavage, paracetamol overdose, 232
gastric ulcers, 165, 170f
gastric varices, 249–250
gastrin, 164
gastroenteritis, 214
  causes of, 576t
  clinical presentation, 575
  definition, 573
  investigations, 576
  transmission, 573
gastro-intestinal erosions, uraemic, 264–265
gastro-intestinal infections, 573–583
  aetiology, 573–574
  case studies, 582b
  causes, 574t
  clinical manifestations, 575–576
  epidemiology, 573–574
  investigations, 576–577, 577f
  pathophysiology, 574–575
  patient care, 581–583
  transmission, 573
  treatment, 578–581
    problems with, 581t
gastro-intestinal motility
  effect of drugs on, 52, 210
  mechanisms of, 210
gastro-intestinal secretions, electrolyte content
    of, 105t

gastro-intestinal tract, 209–210, 210f
cytomegalovirus, 644
effect of NSAIDs on, 836
haemorrhage/bleeding, 94
in the elderly, 157
pH, 52
potassium loss from, 80
symptoms in chronic kidney disease, 285
ulceration (see also duodenal ulcer; gastric ulcers; peptic ulcer disease)
in the elderly, 157
gastro-oesophageal reflux disease (GORD), 162
antacids, 178
symptoms, 174b
treatment, 173–175, 174f
gastrostomy administration of drugs, 140
gate control theory of pain, 519, 519f
gatifloxacin, gastro-intestinal infections, 579
gemcitabine
Hodgkin's lymphoma, 806
non-Hodgkin's lymphoma, 811–812
gender
adverse drug reactions, 65
chronic kidney disease, 272
constipation, 209
coronary heart disease, 313
dyslipidaemia, 396
risk for drug-induced liver disease, 223
generalised anxiety disorder (GAD), 454–455, 455t
antidepressants, 460, 461
pregabalin, 461
recommended drug treatments, 462t
generalised seizures, 491
genetic liver disorders, 241–242
genetic model, schizophrenia, 480
genetics
affective disorders, 466
causing chronic kidney disease, 277
gout, 850
inflammatory bowel disease, 186–187
leukaemia risk, 787
Parkinson's disease, 507–508
prostate cancer, 759
rheumatoid arthritis, 832
risk for drug-induced liver disease, 224
solid tumours, 818–819
genitals, psoriasis, 903
gentamicin
acute pyelonephritis, 568
adverse effects, 39
clinical use, 39
distribution, 39
dosage
changing, 39
initial, 39
once daily, 39–40, 40f
elimination, 39
and hypomagnesaemia, 82
meningitis, 589t, 593t
neonates, 125
respiratory distress syndrome, 130
pharmacokinetics, 39–40, 45t
renal clearance in children, 138t
therapeutic range, 39
urinary tract infections, 569t
geriatrics, 149–160
adverse drug reactions, 65, 459
case studies, 159b
common clinical disorders, 152–157
arthritis, 155
cardiac failure, 156
constipation, 157, 209, 212
dementia, 152–153
gastro-intestinal ulceration and bleeding, 157

hypertension, 155–156
leg ulcers, 156
myocardial infarction, 156
osteoporosis, 154–155
parkinsonism, 153
stroke, 153–154
urinary incontinence, 156–157
dehydration, 216–217
epilepsy in, 490
and folate deficiency anaemia, 777
hypertension, 304–305, 309
insomnia, 451
pharmacodynamics, 150–152
age-related changes in specific receptors/target sites, 151–152
reduced homeostatic reserve, 151
pharmacokinetics, 149–150
principles and goals of drug therapy, 157–158
sleep patterns, 447
urinary tract infections, 562, 563
Giardia, 214, 218, 580
Giardia lamblia, 576t
Gilbert syndrome, 242
Gillick competence, 17
ginger, antiemesis, 539, 541
Ginkgo, 59
ginseng, 59, 61
Glamin®, 98, 99t
Glasgow-Blatchford score, 166
glaucoma, 861–879
aetiology, 862
case studies, 877b
chronic open-angle
clinical manifestations, 862–863
epidemiology, 861, 862
pathophysiology, 862
patient care, 875–876
treatment, 863–865, 866f
clinical manifestations, 862–863
common therapeutic problems, 877t
epidemiology, 861–862
chronic open-angle glaucoma, 862
primary angle-closure glaucoma, 862
secondary glaucomas, 862
investigations, 863
pathophysiology, 862
patient adherence, 877–878
patient care, 875–878
chronic open-angle glaucoma, 875–876
primary angle-closure glaucoma, 876–877
primary angle-closure
clinical manifestations, 863
drugs contraindicated in, 876t
epidemiology, 862
pathophysiology, 862, 863f
patient care, 876–877
treatment, 865, 867f
secondary, 862
treatment, 863–865
β-blockers, 868–871, 869t, 870t
carbonic anhydrase inhibitors, 873, 873b, 873t
chronic open-angle glaucomas, 863–865, 864t, 865t
combination products, 873–874
hyperosmotic agents, 875, 875t
miotics, 872, 872b, 872t
ocular prostanoids, 865–868, 868t, 869t
primary angle-closure glaucoma, 865
sympathomimetic agents, 871–872, 871t, 872t
Gleason scale, 760, 760f
glibenclamide, diabetes mellitus, 700
gliptins see dipeptidyl peptidase (DPP-4) inhibitors
glitazones see thiazolidinediones

global introspection, 69
Global Registry of Acute Coronary Events (GRACE), 321
glomerular filtration rate (GFR), 82, 83, 268
in children, 138
in chronic kidney disease, 272
in diabetes mellitus, 693
estimate (eGFR), 37, 274, 274f
graphical plots of, 282
in pregnancy, 742
glomerulonephritis, 258
chronic, 276
focal segmental necrotising, 258
rapidly progressive, 258
GLU9, 850
glucagon, 690
glucocorticoids
effect on lipoprotein levels, 394t
meningeal tuberculosis, 614
rheumatoid arthritis, 839
glucosamine, 74
glucose, 77t
in acute kidney injury, 265
extracellular fluid osmolality, 77
hyperkalaemia, 264
hypoglycaemia, 690
insulin release, 687
oral rehydration solutions, 216–217
parenteral nutrition, 100, 100t
serum, 84
glucose-6-phosphatase dehydrogenase (G6PD) deficiency, 782–785
adverse drug reactions, 66
aetiology, 782
in breastfed infants, 749
clinical manifestation, 783, 783b
epidemiology, 782
investigations, 783
pathophysiology, 782
patient care, 783–785
treatment, 783
glucose tolerance test, 688
L-glutamine, 98
glycaemic control, diabetes, 707–709
glycated haemoglobin, 84
glycerol, 139, 875
glyceryl trinitrate (GTN)
chronic heart failure, 340t, 343
coronary heart disease, 11t, 12t
stable angina, 319, 320t
ST elevation myocardial infarction, 321
glycogen storage disease, 241
glycopeptides, surgical site infection prophylaxis, 604
glycoprotein IIb/IIIa receptor antagonists
arterial thromboembolism, 386
non-ST elevation myocardial infarction, 327, 329, 329f
ST elevation myocardial infarction, 324
Glycyrrhizin glabra, 59
GnRH analogues see gonadotrophin-releasing hormone (GnRH) analogues
goitre, toxic multinodular, 674, 676
gold, rheumatoid arthritis, 836, 837t, 839
golimumab, rheumatoid arthritis, 840
gonadotrophin-releasing hormone (GnRH) analogues
adverse effects, 722
endometriosis, 722
menorrhagia, 719–720, 720t, 721
premenstrual syndrome, 716
gonioscopy, glaucoma, 863
Goodpasture's disease, 258
goserelin, prostate cancer, 762

gout, 848–860
  case studies, 857b
  course of disease, 852, 852f
  definition, 848
  diagnosis, 851–852
  epidemiology, 848–849
  pathophysiology, 849–850, 850b, 850t
  patient care, 857–859
  presentation, 851–852
  preventing flare, 857
  primary, 850, 850t
  risk factors, 850–851
  secondary, 850, 850t
  tophi, 852, 852f
  treatment, 852–857, 852b
    acute gout, 852–854, 853b
    chronic gout, 854–857, 855b, 855f, 855t
governance see clinical governance
graduated compression, 919
graft-versus-host disease (GVHD), 795
grand mal seizures, 491
granisetron, antiemesis, 540
granulation tissue, 912
granulocyte colony-stimulating factor (G-CSF)
  acute myeloblastic leukaemia, 792
  lymphomas, 815
granulomatous hepatitis, 226t, 227
grapefruit juice, 50, 55, 58
Graves' disease, 674
  case study, 682
  extrathyroidal manifestations, 675
  ophthalmopathy, 678
  treatment, 676
gravitational dermatitis, 895
gravitational eczema, 919
Griess test, 564
griseofulvin, dermatophytosis, 658
growth factors
  hepatitis C, 251–252
  leukaemia, 796–797
  lymphomas, 815–816
growth hormone antagonists, 215t
gut decontamination, 796
guttate psoriasis, 901, 901f
gynaecomastia, 243

H

HAART see highly active antiretroviral therapy
    (HAART)
haem arginate, sideroblastic anaemia, 775
haematological disorders, 787
haematology data, 88–90, 88t
  D-dimers, 88t
  descriptive terms, 89t
  erythrocyte sedimentation rate (ESR), 88t
  ferritin, 88t
  haemoglobin, 88t, 90
  iron, 88t
  mean cell haemoglobin concentration (MCHC),
      88t, 89–90
  mean cell haemoglobin (MCH), 88t, 89
  mean cell volume (MCV), 88t, 89
  packed cell volume (PCV), 88t, 89
  paediatric, 143t
  platelets (thrombocytes), 88t, 90
  red blood cell count, 88–89, 88t
  red cell folate, 88t
  reticulocytes, 88t, 89
  serum B$_{12}$, 88t
  total iron binding capacity (TIBC), 88t
  transferrin, 88t
  white blood cell count, 88t, 90, 90f
haematuria in chronic kidney disease, 277–278

haemochromatosis, 241, 242
haemodiafiltration, 266
haemodialysis, 265–266, 266f, 267t, 292
haemofiltration, 266, 267t
  continuous arterio-venous, 266
  continuous venovenous, 266
  slow continuous ultrafiltration, 266
haemoglobin, 88t, 90, 94
  concentration, 770–771
  glycated, 84
  low see anaemia
haemoglobin S, 780, 781
haemolytic anaemias, 769t, 779–785, 779t
  autoimmune, 779–780, 780b
  case study, 784
  clinical manifestations, 779
  treatment, 779
haemolytic uraemic syndrome (HUS), 133–134,
    575, 578
Haemophilus influenzae
  bronchitis, 549
  chronic obstructive pulmonary disease,
      438–439
  cystic fibrosis, 555
  otitis media, 548
  pneumonia, 552
  type b (Hib), 585, 588, 589
    chemoprophylaxis, 590–591, 590b, 591b
    epiglottitis, 547
    treatment, 590
haemopoiesis, 787, 787f
haemorrhage
  heparin-induced, 379
  torrential venous, 243
  warfarin-induced, 381, 384t
haemorrhagic disease of the newborn, 128
haemorrhagic stroke, aspirin-induced, 386
haemosiderin, 918
hair
  drug-induced changes, 882–883, 882b
  excessive, 882–883
  loss of, 882
haloperidol
  mania, 473
  schizophrenia, 483t
halothane hepatotoxicity, 223, 224, 234
Hamilton Depression Rating Scale, 468
Harris Benedict equation, 99
Harvey-Bradshaw Index (HBI), 192
hawthorn, 59
hay fever, 133
headache, 530–531
  see also migraine
head circumference, 135
Health and Social Care Act (2001), 16
healthcare-associated infections (HCAIs), 596
  see also surgical site infection
health professionals, roles in adverse drug
      reactions, 71–74
heart
  normal cardiac conduction, 355–356, 356f
  sinus rhythm, 354
  sounds, 335
  see also entries beginning cardiac
heart block, 365
heart failure
  chronic see chronic heart failure (CHF)
  in the elderly, 156
  neonates, 127, 131
  parenteral nutrition in, 111
  with preserved ventricular ejection fraction
      (HFPEF), 334
  during ST elevation myocardial infarction, 325
height, children, 135

Heinz bodies, 782
Helicobacter pylori, 162b
  and coronary heart disease risk, 313
  detection, 166–168
  in the elderly, 157
  epidemiology, 163, 163f
  eradication, 166, 171–172
  pathogenesis, 163–164
Henderson-Hasselbalch equation, 83, 83f
heparin
  adverse effects, 379
  atrial fibrillation, 363
  hepatotoxicity, 223t
  low molecular weight see low molecular weight
      heparin (LMWH)
  non-ST elevation myocardial infarction, 327,
      328–329
  parenteral nutrition in children, 113
  ST elevation myocardial infarction, 324
  stroke, 153
  unfractionated see unfractionated heparin
  venous thromboembolism, 379–380, 387
heparinoids, venous thromboembolism, 380
hepatic clearance, 150
hepatic encephalopathy, 248, 249t
hepatic microsomal enzyme inducers, 396
hepatitis
  acute, 226t, 227
  antiretroviral toxicity, 637
  autoimmune, 241, 252
  chronic
    active, 226t, 227
    biochemical tests, 244
    granulomatous, 226t, 227
hepatitis A virus (HAV), 239, 244
hepatitis Be antigen (HBeAg), 240, 251
hepatitis Bs antigen (HBsAg), 251
hepatitis B virus (HBV), 239–240
  acute liver failure, 250
  in HIV, 646
  laboratory investigation, 244
  liver biopsy, 244
  management, 251
  vaccine in neonates, 130
hepatitis C virus (HCV), 239, 240
  in HIV, 646
  laboratory investigation, 244
  liver biopsy, 244
  management, 251–252
  sustained virologic response, 251–252
hepatitis D virus (HDV), 239, 240
hepatitis E virus (HEV), 239, 240
hepatocellular carcinoma, 240
hepatocellular jaundice, 242–243
hepatocytes, 238
hepatomegaly, 242
hepatorenal syndrome, 246–248, 257t
hepatotoxicity see drug-induced liver disease
      (DILD)
hepcidin, 93
herbal medicines, 58–59
  hepatotoxicity, 230b
  interactions, 50
hereditary haemochromatosis (HH), 241
herpes zoster infection, 529
high-density lipoprotein cholesterol (HDL-C),
      389, 390
  and cardiovascular disease, 389
  lipid profile, 399
  menopause, 727
  metabolism, 390
  optimal, 389t
  reverse cholesterol transport pathway,
      390–391

high-grade prostatic intra-epithelial neoplasia (HGPIN), 759
high-intensity focused ultrasound (HIFU), 761
highly active antiretroviral therapy (HAART)
  AIDS dementia complex, 646
  failure, 626
  HIV infection, 625
  impact on opportunistic infections, 645
Hippocratic Oath, 17–18
hirsutism, drug-induced, 882–883, 882b
hirudins, venous thromboembolism, 380
histamine H₁ antagonists see antihistamines
histamine H₂ antagonists
  absorption, 52
  adverse reactions, 177
  drug interactions, 177–178
  peptic ulcer disease, 169–170, 172, 173, 177–178
Histoplasma capsulatum, 585
HIV infection, 621–653
  breastfeeding in, 745
  case studies, 648b
  CD4 count, 624–625
  clinical manifestations, 622–624
  drug treatment, 625–651
    antiretroviral therapy, 625–637
    opportunistic infections and malignancies, 637–651
  epidemiology, 621
  and ethnicity, 648–651
  hepatitis B co-infection, 646
  hepatitis C co-infection, 646
  investigations and monitoring, 624–625
  lifecycle, 623f
  lymphomas in, 807
  neurological manifestations, 645–646
  pathogenesis, 621–622, 622f, 623f
  pharmacogenetics, 66
  primary, 624
  resistance testing, 625
  transmission to neonates, 127
  tropism testing, 625
  tuberculosis in, 609, 612, 615
  viral load, 625
  virus structure, 622f
  in women, 646–648
HIV-protease inhibitors, 54
HLA-*B570, 66
HLA-B*1502, 66
HLA-*B5701, 66
HMG-CoA, 402
Hodgkin's lymphoma, 803–806
  aetiology, 803
  case study, 816
  investigations and staging, 804, 806b
  laboratory findings, 804
  management, 804–805
    advanced disease, 805, 807t
    early-stage (favourable) disease, 804
    early-stage (unfavourable) disease, 805
  new agents, 806
  pathology, 803
  salvage therapy for relapsed disease, 806, 807t
  signs and symptoms, 804
  types, 803
homeostatic reserve, reduced in geriatrics, 151
HOPE study, 317, 326
hormonal analogues, 525t
hormone replacement therapy (HRT), 727–731
  alternatives to, 731
  case studies, 736, 737
  clinical monitoring, 730–731
  and coronary heart disease, 315
  effects, 725
  and hypertension, 306

menopause, 727–731
  bone, 732
  cancer, 734–735
  cardiovascular system, 733
  central nervous system, 736–737
  psychological symptoms, 735
  urogenital tract, 732
  vasomotor symptoms, 731–732
oestrogen see oestrogen therapy
oestrogen and progestogen regimens, 729–730, 729b
osteoporosis, 154–155
prescribing, 727–728
progestogen therapy, 729–730
prostate cancer, 761–763
raloxifene, 730
stopping, 731
tibolone, 730
hormonogenesis, 726
horse chestnut, 59, 61
hospital-acquired (nosocomial) pneumonia, 552–555
  causative organisms, 552–553, 553b
  clinical features, 553
  diagnosis, 553
  prevention, 554–555
  treatment, 553–554, 554t
hot flushes, 731–732, 736
house dust mite, 412–413
human epidermal growth factor receptor type 1 (HER1), 825
human epidermal growth factor receptor type 2 (HER2), 825
human growth hormone, 203t
human metapneumovirus (hMPV), 545
human T-lymphotrophic virus type 1 (HTLV-1), 807
hyaline membrane disease see respiratory distress syndrome (RDS)
hyaluronan, osteoarthritis, 845
hydralazine
  chronic heart failure, 336, 340t, 343, 344
  hypertension, 301
    in chronic kidney disease, 285
    in pregnancy, 306
hydrazine, 224
hydrochlorothiazide
  clinical trials, 302
  and hypomagnesaemia, 82
hydrocortisone
  asthma, 422
  inflammatory bowel disease, 193, 195, 203t
  prostate cancer, 763
hydrocortisone sodium succinate, inflammatory bowel disease, 195
hydrogen ions, 281
hydrogen peroxide, 669
hydromorphone
  analgesia, 522, 523t
  cancer pain, 528
hydroxocobalamin, 778–779
hydroxycarbamide
  chronic myelocytic leukaemia, 792
  psoriasis, 905
  in sickle cell anaemia, 781
hydroxychloroquine, rheumatoid arthritis, 836, 837t, 839
5-hydroxytryptamine (5HT) see serotonin
hydroxyurea
  eczema, 904t
  nail changes, 881–882
  psoriasis, 904t, 905
25-hydroxy vitamin D (25-OHD), 82
hydroxyzine
  anxiety disorders, 461

pruritus in liver disease, 245, 245t
hyoscine butylbromide, dysmenorrhoea, 717
hyoscine hydrobromide
  antiemesis, 538, 541
  patches, 136
hyperaldosteronism, 297
Hyperamine®, 99t
hyperammonaemia, 86
hyperbilirubinaemia
  in neonates, 125
  unconjugated, 85
hypercalcaemia, 81
  causes of, 681
  effect on digoxin pharmacokinetics, 38
  treatment, 682–684, 682t
hypercholesterolaemia, 313–314
  antiretroviral toxicity, 637
  familial, 392–393, 399b
hyperemesis gravidarum, 541
hypergammaglobulinaemia, 88
hyperglycaemic hyperosmolar non-ketotic coma, 94
hyperkalaemia, 80–81, 81b, 261
  in acute kidney injury, 264
  in chronic kidney disease, 281, 281f, 286
  treatment, 264
hyperkeratosis, 893, 900–901
hyperlipidaemia, familial combined, 393
hyperlipoproteinaemia, familial type III, 393
hypermagnesaemia, 82
hypernatraemia, 78–79, 79b, 280t
hyperosmolar hyperglycaemic state (HHS), 691
  diagnosis, 691
  treatment, 691
hyperosmotic agents, glaucoma, 875, 875t
hyperparathyroidism, 81, 280, 680–684
  aetiology, 680–681
  case study, 683
  in chronic kidney disease, 287–288
  clinical manifestations, 681, 681b
  epidemiology, 680
  investigations, 681
  treatment, 681–682
hyperphosphataemia, 82, 264, 279–280, 287, 680
hyperpigmentation
  drug-induced, 881
  in liver disease, 242
hyperresponsiveness, asthma, 412–413
hypersensitivity reactions to drugs, 67, 67t
  see also adverse drug reactions (ADRs)
hypertension, 295–311
  blood pressure regulation, 296
  case studies, 307b
  causes of, 296b
  causing chronic kidney disease, 276
  and chronic heart failure, 334
  in chronic kidney disease, 278
  clinical presentation, 296–297
  complications, 295b
  in diabetes mellitus, 692, 705
  in the elderly, 155–156
  epidemiology, 296, 296b
  essential, 296
  genetic factors, 296
  malignant (accelerated), 296–297, 299t
  management, 297–298
    assessment, 297–298
    contributing factors, 297
    determination of cardiovascular risk, 298
    diagnosis, 297
    evidence of end-organ damage, 297–298
    home/ambulatory blood pressure measurements, 297
    secondary causes, 297

hypertension *(Continued)*
  menopause, 727
  ocular, 862, 864
  risk for cardiovascular disease, 295
  salt-sensitive, 278
  treatment, 155–156, 298–309
    ancillary drugs, 306–309
    antihypertensives *see* antihypertensives
    in chronic kidney disease, 283–285
    drugs, 283–285, 283, 298–299 *see also*
      antihypertensives)
    non-pharmacological approaches, 298
    special patient groups, 304–306
    target blood pressures, 298–299, 299*t*
    thresholds, 298, 299*t*
  white coat, 297
Hypertension in the Very Elderly Trial
  (HYVET), 305
Hypertension Optimal Treatment (HOT) study, 298
hypertensive encephalopathy, 296–297
hyperthyroidism, 674–678
  aetiology, 674–675, 674*t*
  amiodarone-induced, 371
  and chronic heart failure, 334
  clinical manifestations, 675
  effect on digoxin pharmacokinetics, 38
  epidemiology, 674
  investigations, 675
  nodular disease, 674, 676
  treatment, 675–678
  treatment of complications, 678
  see also thyrotoxicosis
hypertrichosis, drug-induced, 882–883, 882*b*
hypertriglyceridaemia, 391–392, 637
hyperuricaemia, 848–860
  definition, 848
  pathophysiology, 850
  prevalence, 850
  risk factors, 850
hypnotic drugs
  adverse effects, 450–451
    over sedation and hangover effects, 450–451
    rebound insomnia, 450
    tolerance and dependence, 450
  choice of, 451–452
  drug interactions, 451
  duration and timing of administration, 452
  insomnia, 447–448
  rate of elimination, 451–452
hypoalbuminaemia, 84, 85, 244
hypocalcaemia, 82, 264, 279–280, 279*f*, 679–680
  aetiology, 679–680
  case study, 684
  clinical manifestations, 680, 680*b*
  investigations, 680, 680*b*
  treatment, 680
hypochromia, 89*t*
hypoglycaemia, 689–690
  causes of, 689, 689*t*
  nocturnal, 689–690
  symptoms of, 689, 689*b*
  treatment, 690
hypogonadism, 243
hypokalaemia, 80, 80*b*
  diuretic-induced, 347
  effect on digoxin pharmacokinetics, 38
  in vitamin B_{12} deficiency anaemia, 779
hypomagnesaemia, 38, 82
hyponatraemia, 79, 79*b*, 280*t*
  diuretic-induced, 347
hypoparathyroidism, 679–680
  aetiology, 679–680
  case study, 684
  clinical manifestations, 680, 680*b*

investigations, 680, 680*b*
  treatment, 680
hypoperfusion, acute tubular necrosis, 257*t*
hypophosphataemia, 82
hypopigmentation, drug-induced, 881
hypotension, 257
  ACE inhibitor-induced, 339
  in the elderly, 151
hypothalamic-pituitary-adrenal (HPA) axis,
  466
hypothalamic-pituitary-thyroid (HPT) axis, 466
hypothyroidism, 670–673
  aetiology, 671
  amiodarone-induced, 371
  case studies, 682, 683
  classification, 671*b*
  clinical manifestations, 671–672
  drug-induced, 671, 679
  and dyslipidaemia, 395
  effect on digoxin pharmacokinetics, 38
  epidemiology, 671
  investigations, 672
  patient care, 673
  prevention, 673
  signs and symptoms, 671*b*
  treatment, 672–673
hypovolaemia, 256–257, 260
hypoxaemia, 439–440
hypoxia, 38
hypoxic-ischaemic encephalopathy (HIE), 129
hysterectomy, 721

I

ibandronate, osteoporosis, 154
ibuprofen
  leg ulcers, 156
  neonates, 126, 130
  patent ductus arteriosus, 130
ICD 10
  affective disorders, 468, 468*b*
  bipolar disorder, 467, 467*b*
  schizophrenia, 479
ICE (ifosfamide, carboplatin, etoposide),
    non-Hodgkin's lymphoma, 811–812
ifosfamide
  metabolism, 825
  non-Hodgkin's lymphoma, 811–812
ileostomy, 105*t*
imatinib
  chronic myelocytic leukaemia, 792–793
  metabolism, 54
  solid tumours, 825
imidazoles
  candidiasis, 656–657
  dermatophytosis, 657
  eczema, 897
  fungal ear infections, 659
  fungal infections in compromised host, 663
  pityriasis versicolor, 659
  topical, 897
imipenem, meningitis, 589*t*
imipramine
  adverse effects, 470
  anxiety disorders, 461
  depression, 470
  metabolism, 470
  toxicity, 470
immune disorders
  hepatic, 241
  renal, 258
immune reconstitution inflammatory syndrome
    (IRIS), 625
immune system

and gastro-intestinal infections, 575
  skin, 883
immunisations
  childhood, 133, 135
  chronic obstructive pulmonary disease, 438–439
immunocompromised patients
  infections in, 796–801, 796*t*
  meningitis treatment in, 591
  respiratory infection in, 556–559, 557*t*
  tuberculosis in, 615
immunoglobulins, 88, 244
immunological adverse drug reactions, 67, 67*t*
immunosuppressants
  acute tubular necrosis, 257*t*
  asthma, 419
  and diarrhoea, 215*t*
  inflammatory bowel disease, 193, 198–199,
    200*b*, 203*t*
  liver transplantation, 250–251
  monitoring, 199
  renal transplantation, 289–292, 289*t*
impulse control disorders (ICDs), 512
inappropriate sinus tachycardia, 359
incentives, prescribing, 29
incontinence, urinary *see* urinary incontinence
incremental cost, 117
incretin mimetics
  adverse effects, 705
  diabetes mellitus, 701*t*, 704–705
  drug interactions, 705
  mode of action, 705
  pharmacokinetics, 705
incretins, 704
indapamide, hypertension, 155, 305
independent prescribing, non-medical, 16
indinavir, HIV infection, 631*t*
indometacin
  adverse reactions, 67
  elimination, 56
  gout, 853
  neonates, 126, 130
  respiratory distress syndrome, 130
indoramin, benign prostatic hyperplasia, 757
infants
  definition, 132
  meningitis, 586, 587–588, 588*t*
  premature, drug transfer into breast milk, 748
  urinary tract infections, 561, 563
infection(s)
  in acute kidney injury, 264
  affect on wound healing, 913–914, 914*f*
  in children, 133–134
  and coronary heart disease risk, 313
  diabetic foot, 917
  diarrhoea, 214
  in HIV, 622–623
  in inflammatory bowel disease, 186, 204
  in leukaemia
    in immunocompromised patients, 796–801, 796*t*
    prevention, 796–797
    treatment, 797–801
  neonates, 127, 127*t*
  viral *see* viruses/viral infections; *specific viruses*
infective meningitis *see* meningitis, infective
inflammatory bowel disease (IBD), 185–208
  aetiology, 185–187
    environmental, 185–186
    genetic, 186–187
  case studies, 205*b*
  clinical manifestation, 188–191
  disease location, 187–188
  epidemiology, 185
  future treatments, 202
  investigations, 191–192

clinical assessment tools, 192
endoscopy, 191
laboratory findings, 191–192
radiology, 191
stool tests, 192
pathophysiology, 187–188
patient care, 204–207
surgical treatment, 204
treatment, 192–204
drug treatment, 192–204, 193*t*, 194*b*, 194*f*, 195*f*, 203*t*
nutritional therapy, 192
see also Crohn's disease; ulcerative colitis
inflammatory renal disease, 258
infliximab
case study, 205
contraindications, 201
guidance on the use of, 841
inflammatory bowel disease, 199, 200–201, 200*t*, 203*t*
psoriasis, 905
rheumatoid arthritis, 840
influenza, 545–546, 551
informed patients, 27
infusion pumps, parenteral nutrition, 104
inhalation absorption (of drugs), 137, 141
inhalation devices, 423–427, 424*t*, 442, 442*t*
inotropes
in acute kidney injury, 263
chronic heart failure, 342*t*, 343
insomnia, 446–453
aetiology, 447
case studies, 452*b*
clinical manifestations, 447
definitions, 446
differential diagnosis, 447
epidemiology, 446
investigations, 447
pathophysiology, 446–447
patient care, 451–452
rebound, 450
sleep systems, 446–447
treatment, 447–450, 448*t*
benzodiazepines, 448–449
hypnotic drugs, 447–448
melatonin, 450
non-drug, 447
zaleplon, 450
zolpidem, 449–450
zopiclone, 449
types of, 451
insulin
circulation, 687
deficiency *see* diabetes mellitus
hyperkalaemia, 264
release, 687
resistance, 687
synthesis, 687
insulin therapy, 695–698
administration routes, 137
adverse effects, 698
delivery, 697
dose adjustment, 698
preparations, 696–697, 696*t*
fast-acting insulins, 696–697
intermediate-acting insulins, 697
long-acting insulins, 697
regimens, 697–698
mealtime plus basal, 697–698
twice-daily, 698
type 2 diabetes, 705
species of origin, 695–696
storage of insulin, 698
in type 2 diabetes, 705

integrase inhibitors, HIV infection, 637
Intelence©, 630*t*
intensive care, 146
interferon therapy
chronic myelocytic leukaemia, 792–793
hepatitis B, 251
hepatitis C, 251–252
interleukin-1 inhibitors, gout, 854
intermediate-density lipoprotein cholesterol (IDL-C), 390
International Classification of Diseases *see* ICD 10
International Glaucoma Association, 875
international normalised ratio (INR), 92
in liver disease, 244
target in venous thromboembolism, 382*t*
International Prognostic Index, non-Hodgkin's lymphoma, 808–809, 809*t*
International Prostatitis Collaborative Network (IPCN) classification of prostatitis, 765*t*
international sensitivity index (ISI), 92
interpersonal skills, 21
interstitial brachytherapy, 761
interstitial fluid, 76
interstitial nephritis, 258–259
intestinal motility, 575
intracellular fluid (ICF), 76, 77
intractable epilepsy, 496, 501
intradialytic parenteral nutrition (IDPN), 110–111
intramuscular route of administration
drug absorption in children, 136
neonates, 124, 129
intranasal route of administration
children, 140
drug absorption in children, 137
intraocular pressure (IOP)
glaucoma, 861, 864*t*
high, 861
level of, 862
measurement, 863
normal, 861
target, 861
intraosseous route of administration, 136
intravascular fluid overload, 263–264
intravascular monitoring in acute kidney disease, 260
intravenous urography (IVU), chronic kidney disease, 282
Invirase©, 631*t*
iodine/iodide, 669
hyperthyroidism, 678
hypothyroidism, 671
IONA study, 319
ipratropium bromide
adverse reactions, 420*b*
asthma, 418*t*, 422
irinotecan, metabolism, 54
iron, 88*t*
adult daily reference range, 102*t*
anticoagulant therapy monitoring, 93
binding, 93
hepatotoxicity, 231
overload, 775
typical daily requirements, 771*t*
iron deficiency anaemia, 93, 771–773
aetiology, 771
in chronic kidney disease, 286
clinical manifestations, 771–772, 772*b*
epidemiology, 771
following bleeding peptic ulcer, 179
in inflammatory bowel disease, 204
investigations, 772
major causes, 771*b*
menorrhagia, 719
pathophysiology, 771
patient care, 773

treatment, 772–773
vs. anaemia of chronic disease, 773*t*
irritant contact dermatitis, 895, 895*f*
ischaemic heart disease *see* coronary heart disease (CHD)
ischaemic leg ulcers, 156
ischaemic nephropathy, 276
Isentress©, 631*t*
islet cell antibodies (ICAs), 686
isoniazid
adverse effects, 615, 616*t*
hepatotoxicity, 222–223, 223*t*, 224
sideroblastic anaemia, 774–775
tuberculosis, 612, 613, 613*t*, 614, 615, 617, 643
isoprenaline
arrhythmias, 365–366
chronic heart failure, 342*t*
isosorbide dinitrate
chronic heart failure, 340*t*, 343
stable angina, 319, 320*t*
isosorbide mononitrate
chronic heart failure, 340*t*, 343
stable angina, 320*t*
isotretinoin, 394*t*
ispaghula husk, constipation, 211, 212
itching *see* pruritus
itraconazole
absorption, 52
candidiasis, 656–657
clinical use, 665
dermatophytosis, 658
fungal infections in compromised host, 665
meningitis, 592
oropharyngeal candidiasis, 638
pharmacokinetics, 664*t*
pityriasis versicolor, 659
ivabradine
arrhythmias, 359
stable angina, 320

J

jaundice
common causes of, 243*f*
hepatocellular, 242–243
in liver disease, 242–243, 243*f*
jejunostomy, 105*t*
Joint British Societies (JBS2), 396, 397*f*, 398*f*
joints
tuberculosis, 614
in ulcerative colitis, 190
jugular venous pressure (JVP), 335
junctional re-entry tachycardia, 360–361, 361*f*
justice and veracity, 18

K

Kaletra©, 631*t*
kanamycin, tuberculosis, 616*t*
kaolin
activated partial thromboplastin time, 92
diarrhoea, 217
kaolin-cephalin clotting time (KCCT), 379, 380
Kaposi's sarcoma, 621, 645
keratinocytes, 912
Kernig's sign, 586
ketamine, 526
ketoconazole
absorption, 52
eczema, 897
fungal infections in compromised host, 663
prostate cancer, 763
shampoo, 897
ketones, 690

kidney(s)
  acute injury/failure *see* acute kidney injury (AKI)
  auto-regulation, 263
  biopsy, 282
  blood flow changes, 56
  drug elimination, 56
  extrinsic renal tract obstruction, 277
  function
    assessment, 281
    assessment in children, 144
    measurement of, 273–275
  potassium loss from, 80
  renal perfusion optimisation, 263
  renal tubule *see* renal tubule
  stones, 276
  transplantation *see* renal transplantation.
  see also entries beginning renal
kininase, hypertension, 301
Kivexa©, 628*t*
Klebsiella sp., 562
Koebner phenomenon, 900, 901*f*
Kupffer cells, 238
kwashiorkor, 96

L

labetalol, 318*t*
  clinical trials, 305–306
  hypertension in pregnancy, 306
  metabolism in the elderly, 150
laboratory data, 76–95
  biochemical data, 76–84
  blood tests, 91
  cardiac markers, 77*t*, 87
  case studies, 94, 95
  haematology data, 88–90
  immunoglobulins, 88
  liver function tests, 77*t*, 84–86
  monitoring anticoagulant therapy, 91–95
  tumour markers, 87–88
labyrinthitis, 541
lacosamide, 495*t*
  adverse effects, 500*t*
  epilepsy, 501
  pharmacokinetics, 44
  plasma concentration-response relationship, 44
lactate dehydrogenase, 87
lactation/breastfeeding
  benzodiazepines in, 460
  drug effects on, 749–751
  drugs in, 745–751
    adverse reactions in infants, 745*t*
    calculating infant dose ingested via milk, 747
    case studies, 750, 751
    milk to plasma concentration ratio, 746–747
    reducing risk, to infant, 748
    risk assessment, to infant, 748
    special situations, 748–749
    transfer into breast milk, 745–751
    variability, 747–748
lactic acid bacteria, 218
lactic acidosis, 699
Lactobacilli, 186
lactulose
  constipation, 213–214
  hepatic encephalopathy, 248, 249*t*
lamivudine
  hepatitis B, 251
    in HIV, 646
  HIV infection, 628*t*
lamotrigine, 495, 495*t*, 496
  adverse effects, 66, 500*t*, 501
  drug interactions, 499*t*
  epilepsy, 501

mania, 474
  pharmacokinetics, 44, 498*t*
  plasma concentration-response relationship, 44
lansoprazole
  adverse effects, 176
  coronary heart disease, 11*t*, 12*t*
  drug interactions, 176
  formulations available, 175*t*
  interactions, 61
  peptic ulcer disease, 173*t*, 175*t*
lanthanum, hyperphosphataemia, 287
laser therapy, benign prostatic hyperplasia, 758
latanoprost
  adverse effects, 865–866
  glaucoma, 864, 865–866, 868*t*, 874
  and timolol, 874
latent autoimmune diabetes in adults (LADA),
    685–686
law of Tort, 16
laxatives
  bulk-forming agents, 212
  classification, 211
  constipation in chronic kidney disease, 285
  faecal softeners/emollient, 214
  hepatic encephalopathy, 248
  and hypomagnesaemia, 82
  osmotic, 213–214
  stimulant, 212–213
lecithin, 152
leflunomide, rheumatoid arthritis, 836, 837*t*, 839
left ventricular systolic dysfunction (LVSD)
  causes of, 334
  ejection fraction, 334
  treatment, 337*t*
Legionnaire's disease, 550–551, 552, 554
leg ulcers, 917–920
  aetiology, 917
  arterial, 919–920, 920*f*
    clinical signs, 919
    diagnosis, 919
    prevention of recurrence, 920
    treatment, 920
  case study, 924
  in the elderly, 156
  epidemiology, 917
  mixed, 920
  venous, 917–919, 918*f*
    clinical signs, 918
    diagnosis, 918, 918*t*
    prevention of recurrence, 919
    treatment, 919
lenalidomide, Hodgkin's lymphoma, 806
lepirudin, venous thromboembolism, 380
leucocyte esterase test, 564
leucocytosis, 89*t*
leuconychia, 881–882
leucopenia, 89*t*
leukaemia, 133, 786–802
  acute lymphoblastic *see* acute lymphoblastic
    leukaemia (ALL)
  acute myeloblastic *see* acute myeloblastic
    leukaemia (AML)
  acute promyelocytic, 788, 792, 801
  aetiology, 786–787
  case studies, 798*b*
  chronic lymphocytic *see* chronic lymphocytic
    leukaemia (CLL)
  chronic myelocytic *see* chronic myelocytic
    leukaemia (CML)
  clinical manifestations, 788–789
  common therapeutic problems in, 798*t*
  epidemiology, 786
  investigations, 789–790
  pathophysiology, 787–788

  patient care, 795–801
  treatment, 790–795
leukapheresis, 202
leukonychia, 242
leukotriene receptor antagonists
  adverse reactions, 420*b*
  asthma, 419
leukotrienes, menstrual cycle, 712
leuprorelin, prostate cancer, 762
levetiracetam
  adverse effects, 500*t*
  epilepsy, 501
  pharmacokinetics, 44
  plasma concentration-response relationship, 44
levobunolol, glaucoma, 868, 869*t*, 870–871
levodopa
  co-careldopa intestinal gel, 511
  controlled-release, 511
  immediate-release, 511
  long-term levodopa syndrome, 511
  parkinsonism, 153
  Parkinson's disease, 510, 511, 512, 516
  preparations, 511
levofloxacin, bronchitis/chronic obstructive
    pulmonary disease, 550
levomepromazine
  antiemesis, 538
  cancer pain, 528
  pain, 528
  schizophrenia, 483*t*
levonorgestrel intrauterine contraceptive devices
    (LNG-IUS), menorrhagia, 720, 720*t*
Lewy bodies, 507–508
libido and the menopause, 735
licensing of medicines for children, 145–146
  licensing process, 145
  recent legislation, 145–146
  unlicensed and off-label medicines, 145
lichenoid eruptions, drug-induced, 885, 885*b*
lidocaine
  adverse effects, 367*t*
  arrhythmias, 369
  distribution, 53
    in the elderly, 150
  inflammatory bowel disease, 203*t*
  local anaesthesia, 524
  neonatal seizures, 128–129
  pharmacokinetics, 368*t*
linezolid
  interactions, 58
  meningitis, 589*t*, 590
  pneumonia, 554*t*
lipid clearance monitoring, 101
lipid destabilisation, parenteral nutrition, 106–107,
    107*t*
lipid emulsions, 100*t*, 101*f*
lipid-lowering therapy, 401–410, 402*t*, 403*t*
  bile acid binding agents, 405–407, 406*t*
  cholesterol absorption inhibitors, 407
  cholesterol ester transfer protein (CETP)
    inhibitors, 407–410
  fibrates, 405
  fish oils, 407
  hypertension, 306–309
  nicotinic acid and derivatives, 407
  soluble fibre, 407
  statins, 402–405
  ST elevation myocardial infarction, 325–326
lipid profile
  disorders adversely affecting, 394*b*
  dyslipidaemia, 399
  effect of HRT administration route on, 728*t*
  in liver disease, 244
  optimal, 389*t*

lipid transport, 390–392
lipodermatosclerosis (LDS), 918
lipodystrophy, antiretroviral toxicity, 637
lipophilicity, drug transfer into breast milk, 746
lipoprotein(a), 393
lipoprotein lipase, 390, 393
lipoprotein(s)
  effects of drugs on, 394t
  high-density lipoprotein cholesterol see high-
    density lipoprotein cholesterol (HDL-C)
  intermediate-density lipoprotein see
    intermediate-density lipoprotein
    cholesterol (IDL-C)
  low-density lipoprotein cholesterol see low-
    density lipoprotein cholesterol (LDL-C)
  metabolism, 390–392, 391f
  very low-density lipoprotein cholesterol see
    very low-density lipoprotein cholesterol
    (VLDL-C)
liquid paraffin, 214
liquorice, 59
liraglutide, 704–705
lisinopril
  chronic heart failure, 340t, 351
  clinical trials, 302, 305–306
Listeria monocytogenes, 585, 588, 591, 593t
lithium
  absorption, 474
  bioavailability, 474
  depression, 472
  discontinuation, 474
  distribution, 40
  dose-dependent effects, 40
  dose-independent effects, 40
  elimination, 40–41
  and hypercalcaemia, 81
  hypernatraemia, 79
  hyperthyroidism, 678, 679
  interactions, 475t
  mania, 473–474
  pharmacokinetics, 40–41, 45t, 47
  practical implications, 41
  and psoriasis, 899
  serum levels, 474
liver
  adverse effects of drugs on see drug-induced
    liver disease (DILD)
  biopsy, 228, 244
  bloody supply, 238
  drug metabolism, 53
  fibrosis, 227, 240–241
  functions, 238, 238f
  necrosis, 225, 226, 226t, 227
  transplantation, 250–251
  see also entries beginning hepatic
liver disease, 238–254
  acute, 238
  acute liver failure (ALF), 238
  case studies, 252b
  causes of, 239–242
    alcohol, 240–241
    drugs, 242
    immune disorders, 241
    metabolic and genetic disorders, 241–242
    non-alcohol-related fatty liver disease, 241
    vascular abnormalities, 241
    viral infections, 239–240
  chronic, 238–239
  disease specific therapies, 251–254 (see also
    specific diseases
  drug-induced see drug-induced liver disease
    (DILD)
  investigations, 244
  parenteral nutrition in, 110

patient care, 244–251
  acute liver failure, 250
  ascites, 246–248, 246b, 247t
  clotting abnormalities, 246, 246f
  hepatic encephalopathy, 248, 248b, 248t, 249t
  liver transplantation, 250–251
  oesophageal varices, 248–250, 249f
  pruritus, 244–246
  risk for drug-induced liver disease, 223
  signs of, 242, 242t
  symptoms of, 242
  tuberculosis in, 615
liver enzymes elevation, drug-induced, 222–223, 223t
liver function tests (LFTs), 77t, 84–86, 244
  albumin, 84–85
  alkaline phosphatase, 85–86
  ammonia, 86
  amylase, 86
  bilirubin, 85
  drug-induced liver disease, 228
  enzymes, 85
  γ-glutamyl transpeptidase, 86
  in hepatotoxicity, 233–234, 233t
  transaminases, 86
Liverpool Care Pathway (LCP), 528
loading dose, 32
local anaesthetics, 524–525
local guidelines, 29
lofepramine, depression, 470
lomustine, 823
long-term levodopa syndrome, 511
loop diuretics
  acute kidney injury, 263
  chronic heart failure, 338, 339t, 343, 344
  dyslipidaemia, 395
  gout, 851
  hypertension, 300, 304b
    in chronic kidney disease, 284
  hypokalaemia, 80
loperamide, diarrhoea, 217
lopinavir, HIV infection, 631t
loratidine
  pruritus
    in chronic kidney disease, 285
    in liver disease, 245
lorazepam
  anxiety disorders, 459
  profile, 458t
losartan
  chronic heart failure, 340t
  gout, 853
Losartan For Endpoint reduction in hypertension
  (LIFE) study, 299–300, 302
lovastatin
  dyslipidaemia, 402
  metabolism, 404
low birth weight (LBW), 124
low-density lipoprotein cholesterol (LDL-C), 389,
  390
  and cardiovascular disease, 389
  lipid profile, 399
  menopause, 727
  metabolism, 390
  optimal, 389t
low molecular weight heparin (LMWH)
  adverse effects, 379
  non-ST elevation myocardial infarction, 327
  venous thromboembolism, 379, 380
lumbar puncture, 586
lung function tests, chronic obstructive pulmonary
  disease, 435
lung(s)
  hyperinflation, 433
  mesothelioma, 529

parenchyma, 432
vasculature, 432
see also entries beginning pulmonary
lupus anticoagulant, venous thromboembolism,
  377
lupus erythematosus, drug-induced, 888–889, 888b
luteinising hormone (LH), 761–762
  menopause, 726
  menstrual cycle, 711
luteinising hormone-releasing hormone (LHRH),
  761–762
luteinising hormone-releasing hormone (LHRH)
  agonists, prostate cancer, 762, 763
luteinising hormone-releasing hormone (LHRH)
  antagonists, prostate cancer, 763
lymecycline, 60
lymph nodes, tuberculosis of peripheral, 614
lymphoblastic lymphomas/leukaemia, 812
lymphocytes, 90
lymphomas, 803–817
  Burkitt's, 807, 812
  case studies, 815b
  diffuse large B-cell, 811, 812
  follicular, 809
  in HIV infection, 645
  Hodgkin's see Hodgkin's lymphoma
  mantle cell, 815
  non-Hodgkin's see non-Hodgkin's lymphoma
  patient care, 812–816
    counselling and support, 812
    patient-specific treatment modifications, 812
    supportive care, 813–816

M

macroalbuminuria see proteinuria
macrogols, constipation, 211, 213–214
macrophages, wound healing, 912
Madopar®, 511
magnesium, 82
  acute kidney injury, 265
  dysmenorrhoea, 718
  hypermagnesaemia, 82
  hypomagnesaemia, 82
  infusions, arrhythmias, 325
magnesium salts, constipation, 213
magnesium sulphate, asthma, 422
magnetic resonance angiography (MRA), chronic
  kidney disease, 282
magnetic resonance imaging (MRI)
  chronic kidney disease, 282
  deep vein thrombosis, 378
  epilepsy, 492
  liver disease, 244
Maillard reaction, 107
malabsorption, 52
Malassezia furfur, 658, 659, 660t, 895
malignancy see cancer
malignant hypertension, 296–297, 299t
malnutrition, 96
  incidence, 96
  nutrition screening, 96
Malnutrition Advisory Group of the British
  Association of Parental and Enteral
  Nutrition (BAPEN), 96
mania
  clinical features, 467
  definition, 465
  treatment, 473–474
mannitol
  acute kidney injury, 263
  glaucoma, 865, 875
mantle cell lymphoma, 815
Mantoux test, 611

marasmus, 96
maraviroc, HIV infection, 636t, 637
marginal costs, 117
marketing authorisation (MA), 145
maturity-onset diabetes of the young (MODY),
    685–686
mean cell haemoglobin concentration (MCHC),
    88t, 89–90
mean cell haemoglobin (MCH), 88t, 89
mean cell volume (MCV), 88t, 89
mean corpuscular volume (MCV), 770–771
mechanical ventilation, neonates, 125–126
mechlorethamine, Hodgkin's lymphoma, 805
Medicago sativa, 59
Medical Dictionary for Regulatory Affairs
    (MedDRA), 70
medication-related problems (MRPs), 3–4, 4b
medication review, 25–26, 25t
medicines *see* drug(s)
Medicines and Health care Products Regulatory
    Authority (MHRA), 69–70, 71, 145
Medicines and Human Use (Prescribing;
    Miscellaneous Amendments) Order
    (2006), 16
Medicines for Children Research Network
    (MCRN), 146
medicines management, definition, 3t
medicines-taking behaviour, 5
medicines use review (MUR), 5
Mediterranean diet, 400
medroxyprogesterone acetate, 730
mefenamic acid
    dysmenorrhoea, 717
    premenstrual syndrome, 716
megaloblastic anaemias, 769t, 775–777
    aetiology, 776
    clinical manifestations, 777–779, 777b
    epidemiology, 776
    investigations, 777–778
    pathophysiology, 776–777
    patient care, 779
    treatment, 778–779
meglitinides
    adverse effects, 703
    diabetes mellitus, 699, 701t, 702–703
    dosage, 703
    drug interactions, 703
    mode of action, 702
    pharmacokinetics, 702–703
melatonin, insomnia, 448t, 450
melphalan, non-Hodgkin's lymphoma, 811–812
Melt® technology, 139
memantine, dementia, 153
menadiol sodium phosphate, coagulation
    disorders, 231
menarche, 711
meningeal tuberculosis, 614
meningitis, infective, 584–595
    aetiology, 585
    bacterial *see* bacterial meningitis
    case studies, 594b
    clinical manifestations, 586
    diagnosis, 586–587
    drug treatment, 587–593, 588t, 589t
    epidemiology, 585
    fungal *see* fungal meningitis
    in HIV infection, 643
    meningococcal *see* meningococcal meningitis;
        Neisseria meningitidis
    neonates, 127t
    pathophysiology, 586
    patient care, 593–595
    pneumococcal *see* pneumococcal meningitis;
        Streptococcus pneumoniae

prevention of person-to-person transmission,
    594–595
    shunt-associated, 591, 592t
    tuberculous *see* tuberculous meningitis
    viral *see* viral meningitis
meningitis C vaccination, 135
meningococcal meningitis, 590–591, 590b, 591b
    see also Neisseria meningitidis
menopause, 725–738
    case studies, 736b
    definition, 725
    management, 727–731
    physiological changes, 725–727
        bone, 726–727
        cardiovascular system, 727
        miscellaneous, 727
        ovarian, 725–726
        urogenital system, 726
    psychological changes, 727
    treatment, 731–737
    vasomotor symptoms, 731–732
    see also hormone replacement therapy (HRT)
menorrhagia, 718–721
    aetiology, 718–719
    case studies, 722, 723
    causes of, 719b
    epidemiology, 718
    investigation, 718–719
    treatment, 719–721, 720t
menstrual cycle
    body temperature, 711–712, 712f
    disorders, 711–724
    hormonal events in, 711–712, 711f
menstruation, 711
Mental Capacity Act (2005), 17, 17b
mental health disorders, 134
menthol, pruritus in liver disease, 245t, 246
mepacrine, 881–882
mepacrine hydrochloride, 580
mercapto acetyl tri-glycerine (MAG3), 282
mercaptopurine
    adverse effects, 198
    drug interactions, 198
    inflammatory bowel disease, 198, 203t
6-mercaptopurine
    acute lymphoblastic leukaemia, 790, 791
    inflammatory bowel disease, 198
meropenem
    meningitis, 589t, 591
    pneumonia, 554t
    urinary tract infections, 569t
mesalazine
    formulations, 197, 198
    inflammatory bowel disease, 196–197, 196f,
        198, 203t
mesothelioma of the lung, 529
metabolic acidosis, 83
metabolic alkalosis, 83
metabolic disorders
    antiretroviral toxicity, 637
    causing chronic kidney disease, 276
metabolic liver diseases, 241–242
metabolic syndrome, 687, 851
metabolism (of drugs)
    in children, 137–138
    drug interactions, 53–56
        predicting, 55–56
    in the elderly, 150
    in neonates, 125
    in pregnancy, 742, 743t
    in renal replacement therapy, 268
metastatic bone pain, 529
metered dose aerosol inhalers (MDIs), 424–425,
    424f

breath-actuated, 426, 426f
    with a spacer extension, 425–426, 425f, 426f
metformin
    adverse effects, 699
    diabetes mellitus, 699
methadone
    analgesia, 522, 523t
    cancer pain, 528
methionine, 231
methotrexate
    acute lymphoblastic leukaemia, 790, 791
    adverse reactions, 64, 198, 420b, 838
    drug interactions, 176, 899t
    eczema, 898, 904t
    graft-versus-host disease, 795
    inflammatory bowel disease, 198, 203t
    interactions, 198
    non-Hodgkin's lymphoma, 812
    pharmacokinetics, 838
    psoriasis, 904, 904t
    rheumatoid arthritis, 836, 837t, 838
    safety, 838, 839b
    toxicity, 56
methylcellulose, constipation, 212
methyldopa
    hypertension, 301
        in chronic kidney disease, 285
        in pregnancy, 306
methylprednisolone
    acute lymphoblastic leukaemia, 791
    graft-versus-host disease, 795
    inflammatory bowel disease, 193, 195
    non-Hodgkin's lymphoma, 811–812
    postherpetic neuralgia, 529
    renal transplantation, 291
    rheumatoid arthritis, 839
methylprednisolone acetate, gout, 854
meticillin-resistant *Staphylococcus aureus*
    (MRSA), 127, 599–600, 605
metipranolol, glaucoma, 869t
metoclopramide
    absorption, 52
    adverse reactions, 65
    antiemesis, 285, 538, 539, 541, 542
metolazone
    acute kidney injury, 263
    chronic heart failure, 338, 339t
    hypertension in chronic kidney disease, 284
metoprolol, 318t
    arrhythmias, 370
    chronic heart failure, 340t
    hypertension in chronic kidney disease, 284
    stable angina, 317–318
metronidazole
    amoebiasis, 580
    diarrhoea, 218
    gastro-intestinal infections, 580
    Helicobacter pylori eradication, 171, 172
    hepatic encephalopathy, 248, 249t
    infection in neutropenia, 797
    inflammatory bowel disease, 202, 203t
    necrotizing enterocolitis, 128
    neonates, 128
mexiletine
    adverse effects, 367t
    arrhythmias, 369
    pharmacokinetics, 368t
mianserin, depression, 472
micafungin, 664t
Michaelis-Menten model, 41
microalbuminuria, 693
microbial contamination, parenteral nutrition, 107
microcytic anaemias, 769t, 784
microflora, 575

micronutrients, 101–103, 102*b*
microscopic polyangiitis, 258
microscopy, urinary tract infections, 564–565
Microsporum, 657
midazolam
    absorption in children, 136–137
    intranasal administration, 140
    neonates, 128–129
    seizures, 128–129
midstream urine sample (MSU), 563–564
migraine, 531, 541
miliary tuberculosis, 608–609, 614
milk to plasma concentration ratio, 746–747, 746*f*
milrinone, chronic heart failure, 342*t*
mineralocorticoids
    deficiency, 80
    excess, 80
minerals
    dysmenorrhoea, 718
    premenstrual syndrome, 714
mini tablets, 139
minocycline
    interactions, 60
    nail changes, 881–882
    pigmentation, 881*f*
minoxidil
    hair changes, 882–883
    hypertension, 301
    hypertension in chronic kidney disease, 285
miosis, 872
miotics
    adverse effects, 872*b*
    glaucoma, 865, 872, 872*b*, 872*t*
mirtazapine
    anxiety disorders, 461
    depression, 472
misoprostol, peptic ulcer disease, 173, 173*t*
mithramycin, hypocalcaemia, 82
mitochondrial toxicity of antiretrovirals, 637
mitomycin, 823
mitoxantrone
    acute lymphoblastic leukaemia, 790
    prostate cancer, 763–764
MMR vaccine, 63, 133, 186
moclobemide
    anxiety disorders, 461
    depression, 471
Modification of Diet in Renal Disease (MDRD)
        study equation, 37, 83, 274, 693
molecular weight, drug transfer into breast milk,
        746
mometasone, asthma, 419*t*
monoamine oxidase inhibitors (MAOIs)
    affective disorders, 466
    anxiety disorders, 461
    depression, 470–471
    effects, 471
    interactions, 50, 58, 470–471, 475*t*
    reversible, 470–471
    traditional, 470–471
monoamine oxidase type B, 513
monoamine oxidase type B inhibitors, Parkinson's
        disease, 513
monobactams, cystic fibrosis, 556*t*
monoclonal antibodies
    renal transplantation, 290, 291
    tuberculosis, 201
monocytes, 90
mono-iodotyrosine (MIT), 669
monosodium urate, 84, 849, 851
monounsaturated fats, 695
montelukast
    asthma, 419
    dysmenorrhoea, 717

MOPP (mechlorethamine, vincristine,
        procarbazine, prednisolone), Hodgkin's
        lymphoma, 805
Moraxella catarrhalis, 438–439, 549
morphine
    analgesia, 522, 523*t*
    cancer pain, 528
    diarrhoea, 217
    neonates, 126
motion sickness, 541
moulds, 654–655, 655*t*
moxifloxacin
    bronchitis/chronic obstructive pulmonary
        disease, 550
    meningitis, 590
    metabolism, 55
    pneumonia, 552
moxonidine, hypertension, 301
MPTP (1-methyl-4-phenyl-1,2,3,6-
        tetrahydropyridine), 507
MRSA *see* meticillin-resistant *Staphylococcus
        aureus* (MRSA)
mucolytics, chronic obstructive pulmonary
        disease, 438
mucormycosis, 660*t*
mucositis, chemotherapy-induced, 813*t*, 814
mucus hypersecretion, 433
multidrug-resistant tuberculosis (MDR-TB), 608,
        609
murine-human chimeric antibodies, 327
muromonab, renal transplantation, 289*t*
muscle relaxants, 525*t*, 526–527
muscles in chronic kidney disease, 280
MUST (Malnutrition Universal Screening Tool),
        96
mycobacteria, 643–644
Mycobacterium africanum, 608
Mycobacterium avium intracellulare (MAI), 644
Mycobacterium bovis, 608
Mycobacterium leprae, 608
Mycobacterium paratuberculosis, 186
Mycobacterium tuberculosis, 608, 612, 643, 644
mycophenolate
    autoimmune hepatitis, 252
    inflammatory bowel disease, 198, 199
mycophenolate mofetil (MMF)
    eczema, 898
    renal transplantation, 289*t*, 290, 291
Mycoplasma pneumoniae, 552
myocardial infarction
    acute, 320
    in diabetes mellitus, 692
    in the elderly, 156
    and hypertension, 295
    non-ST-elevation, 320, 321
        classification, 322*f*
        high-risk patients, 328*t*
        prognosis, 321
        treatment, 326–329
    risk, 313
    silent, 692
    ST-elevation
        classification, 322*f*
        complications, 325
        prevention of further infarction, 325–326
        prognosis, 321
        treatment, 321–326
myocardial ischaemia, 312
myoclonic seizures, 491
myocytes, 354
myofascial pain, 530
myopathy, statin-associated, 87, 404
myxoedema, 678
myxoedema coma, 671–672

N

N-acetyl-*p*-benzoquinoneimine (NABQI), 232,
        520–521
nadolol, 318*t*
nails
    candida infection, 656
    dermatophytosis, 657
    drug-induced changes, 881–882
    fungal infections, 667
    in liver disease, 242
    psoriasis, 901, 903
Na/K-ATPase pumps, 79, 80
nalidixic acid, diarrhoea, 217
nalmefene, pruritus in liver disease, 245
naloxone
    pruritus in liver disease, 245
    respiratory depression in neonates, 125
NALP3 inflammasome, 851–852
naltrexone, pruritus in liver disease, 245, 245*t*
naproxen
    in chronic heart failure, 351
    hepatotoxicity, 223*t*
naringenin, 58
naringin, 58
nasogastric route of administration, 140
natalizumab, inflammatory bowel disease, 200–201
nateglinide
    diabetes mellitus, 702
    dosage, 703
    pharmacokinetics, 702–703
National Cancer Institute Common Toxicity
        Criteria, 828, 828*t*
National Congenital Anomaly System (NCAS), 132
national guidelines, 29
National Institute for Health and Clinical
        Excellence guidelines *see* NICE
        guidelines
National Prescribing Centre competency
        framework, 19–20, 20*t*
National Service Frameworks (NSFs)
    influence on prescribing, 27
    paediatric, 146–148
natriuretic peptide hormone, 78
nausea and vomiting, 535–544
    case studies, 542*b*
    causes, 536, 536*t*
    central causes, 536, 536*t*
    chemotherapy-induced, 540, 540*b*, 540*t*, 813,
        813*t*, 826–827
    chronic kidney disease, 285
    common therapeutic problems, 537*t*
    drug-associated, 541
    epidemiology, 535
    labyrinthitis, 541
    migraine, 541
    motion sickness, 541
    opioid-induced, 523
    palliative care-associated, 542, 542*b*
    pathophysiology, 535–536, 537*f*
    patient management, 536
    peripheral causes, 536
    post-operative, 539
    pregnancy-associated, 540–541
nebivolol, 318*t*, 340*t*
nebulisers, 426–427
neck pain, 530
necrosis, liver, 225, 226, 226*t*, 227
necrotizing enterocolitis
    adverse drug effects, 139
    neonates, 127–128, 127*t*
nedocromil sodium
    adverse reactions, 420*b*
    asthma, 419

...am, analgesia, 525
...sseria gonorrhoeae, 563, 717–718
...eisseria meningitidis, 585, 588, 589
nelfinavir, HIV infection, 631t
neomycin
  absorption, 52
  hepatic encephalopathy, 249t
neonates, 124–131
  adverse drug reactions, 65
  bacterial meningitis, 585
  case studies, 130, 131
  definition, 132
  drug absorption, 124
  drug distribution, 124–125
  drug elimination, 125
  drug metabolism, 125
  drug transfer into breast milk, 748
  major clinical disorders, 125–129
    apnoea, 128
    bronchopulmonary dysplasia, 126–127
    haemorrhagic disease of the newborn, 128
    infection, 127, 127t
    necrotizing enterocolitis, 127–128
    patent ductus arteriosus, 126
    respiratory distress syndrome, 125–126
    seizures, 128–129
  meningitis, 587–588, 588t, 593t
  premature, 124, 132
  principles and goals of therapy, 129–131
    avoiding harm, 129
    patient and parent care, 130–131
    rapid growth, 129
    therapeutic drug monitoring, 129
    time-scale of clinical changes, 129–130
  terminology, 125t
  theophylline metabolism, 38
  urinary tract infections, 561, 563
nephropathy, diabetic, 693
nephrotic syndrome, 395
nephrotoxins, 262–263, 268–270
neural tube defects, 133
neuraminidase inhibitors (NAIs), influenza, 546
neurokinin-1 (NK₁) receptor antagonists,
    antiemesis, 538–539
neuroleptic malignant syndrome (NMS), 486–488
neuroleptics see antipsychotic drugs
neurological changes in chronic kidney disease,
    280, 287
neurological manifestations of HIV, 645–646
neuroma, 530
neurones, 490–491
neuropathic pain, 529–530, 531t
  in cancer, 528
  case study, 531–532
  causes of, 529t
  specific syndromes, 529–530
neuropathy, 530
  chemotherapy-induced, 813t
  diabetic peripheral, 529
neuroprotective agents, stroke, 153
neurotransmitters, 490–491
  affective disorders, 466
  anxiety, 456
  and pain, 519–520
neutropenia, 89t
  febrile, 814
  fungal, 659
  lymphomas, 814
  prevention of infection in, 797
  treatment of infection in, 797
neutrophilia, 89t
neutrophils, 90, 912
nevirapine
  hepatotoxicity, 223t

HIV infection, 630t
New York Heart Association (NYHA)
    classification, 333, 333t
niacin, hepatotoxicity, 223t
NICE guidelines
  hypertension management, 297
  influence on prescribing, 27
  prescribing strategies, 29
nicorandil, stable angina, 319
nicotinamide adenine dinucleotide phosphate
    (NADPH), 782
nicotine
  inflammatory bowel disease, 203t
  transfer into breast milk, 749
nicotine replacement therapy (NRT), 436, 440–441,
    441t
nicotinic acid
  adverse effects, 407
  dyslipidaemia, 393–394, 403t, 407
nifedipine, 150
night sweats, 731–732
nilotinib, chronic myelocytic leukaemia, 793
nilutamide, prostate cancer, 762
nitazoxanide
  cryptosporidiosis, 643
  gastro-intestinal infections, 580
nitrates
  chronic heart failure, 336, 340t, 343, 344
  commonly used, 320t
  coronary heart disease, 11t, 12t
  drug interactions, 348t
  metabolism in the elderly, 150
  non-ST elevation myocardial infarction, 329
  patient education, 344–345
  preparations, 319
  self-monitoring, 345t
  stable angina, 319, 320t
  ST elevation myocardial infarction, 326
  tolerance, 319
nitric oxide, 319
  and blood pressure, 296
  menorrhagia, 719
  neonates, 126
nitric oxide-releasing NSAIDs, 165
nitrite test, 564
nitrofurantoin
  bacteriuria of pregnancy, 570
  hepatotoxicity, 223
  urinary tract infections, 566, 568, 568t
nitrogen balance, 99
nitroprusside, chronic heart failure, 340t
nizatidine, peptic ulcer disease, 177
N-methyl-D-aspartate (NMDA) antagonists,
    dementia, 152
nociceptors, 519
nocturia, 277–278
nocturnal hypoglycaemia, 689–690
non-adherence see adherence/non-adherence
non-alcoholic fatty liver disease (NAFLD), 241
non-alcoholic steatohepatitis (NASH), 241
non-Hodgkin's lymphoma, 806–812
  aetiology, 807
  case studies, 815
  diagnosis, 808
  histopathology and classification, 808
  laboratory findings, 808
  signs and symptoms, 808
  staging, 808–809
  treatment, 809–812, 810f, 811t
    aggressive non-Hodgkin's lymphoma, 811
    indolent non-Hodgkin's lymphoma, 809–811
    lymphoblastic lymphoma/leukaemia, 812
    relapsed aggressive non-Hodgkin's
        lymphoma, 811–812

relapsed indolent non-Hodgkin's lymphoma,
    811
  very aggressive non-Hodgkin's lymphoma,
    812
non-maleficence, 17–18
non-medical prescribing, 15–16
non-nucleoside reverse transcriptase inhibitors
    (NNRTIs), HIV infection, 626, 630t,
    635
non-peptide synthetics, 327
non-steroidal anti-inflammatory drugs (NSAIDs)
  acute tubular necrosis, 257t
  adverse reactions, 62, 836, 883–884
  analgesia, 521, 527
  chemoprevention, 820
  choice of agent, 836
  chronic heart failure, 350, 351
  clinical considerations, 521
  currently licensed (UK), 835t
  diarrhoea, 215t
  drug-induced asthma, 412–413
  drug interactions, 836
  dysmenorrhoea, 717, 718t
  elimination, 56
  gout, 852–853, 857
  guidance on use of, 521
  hepatotoxicity, 224, 228
  inflammatory bowel disease, 186
  interstitial nephritis, 258–259
  liver disease, 246
  menorrhagia, 720, 720t
  mode of action, 521
  nitric oxide-releasing, 165
  osteoarthritis, 845
  peptic ulceration, 162b
    epidemiology, 163
    pathogenesis, 164–165, 164f
    prophylaxis, 172–173
    risk factors, 164b
    treatment, 172
  pre-renal acute kidney injury, 256–257
  and psoriasis, 899
  rheumatoid arthritis, 835–836
  safety, 835–836
  teratogenicity, 740, 741t
non-verbal communication, 21–22
noradrenaline
  in acute kidney injury, 263
  affective disorders, 466
  chronic heart failure, 343
  drug interactions, 58
  water balance, 76
norepinephrine see noradrenaline
norethisterone, 730
norfloxacin
  hepatotoxicity, 223t
  metabolism, 55
  spontaneous bacterial peritonitis, 247–248
noroviruses, 214, 573
nortriptyline
  depression, 470
  drug-induced parkinsonism, 509–510
Norvir©, 631t
NO TEARS medication review, 26, 26t
nuclear factor of activated T-cells (NFAT), 290
nuclear medicine investigations, chronic kidney
    disease, 282
nucleoside/nucleotide reverse transcriptase
    inhibitors (NRTIs), HIV infection, 626,
    627–635, 628t
nucleus tractus solitarus (NTS), 535
nummular dermatitis, 895
nurses prescribing drugs, 16
nutraceuticals, osteoarthritis, 845

nutrition
    in acute kidney injury, 265
    affect on wound healing, 914, 914b
    children, 134
    screening, 96
nutritional therapy, inflammatory bowel disease, 192
nutrition support teams, 97
nystatin
    candidiasis, 657
    fungal ear infections, 659

O

obesity
    childhood, 134
    in diabetes mellitus, 695, 698, 706
    and dyslipidaemia, 395
    and hypertension, 298, 307, 308
    osteoarthritis risk, 843
obsessive-compulsive disorder (OCD), 454–455,
        455b, 455t, 457
    antidepressants, 460, 461
    benzodiazepines, 459
    case study, 462
    recommended drug treatments, 462t
occupational therapy, rheumatoid arthritis,
        834–835
octreotide, oesophageal varices, 250, 250t
ocular hypertension (OHT), 862, 864
ocular prostanoids, 868t
    adverse effects, 869t
    glaucoma, 865–868
oedema
    in chronic kidney disease, 286
    epidermal see eczema
    peripheral, 243, 246
oesophageal candidiasis
    presentation, 656
    treatment, 656–657
oesophageal ulceration, 162
oesophageal varices, 248–250, 249f
    drug treatment, 250, 250t
    endoscopic management, 249–250
    prevention of rebleeding, 250
    transjugular intrahepatic portosystemic
        shunting, 250
oesophagitis, 173–174, 175
oestradiol, 394t
oestrogen(s)
    blood pressure control, 727
    bone loss, 732
    diminishing, 726
    dyslipidaemia, 396
    effect on lipoprotein levels, 394t
    hair changes, 882
    menstrual cycle, 711
    osteoporosis, 154–155
    venous thromboembolism, 377
oestrogen therapy
    administration, 728
        effect on lipid profile, 728t
    dose, 729
    implants, 729
    menopause, 728–729, 732
    natural oestrogens, 728
    oral, 728t
    with progestogen, 729–730, 729b
    prostate cancer, 763
    transdermal patches, 728–729
    vaginal creams, 729
off-label medicines, 18, 19b
    for children, 145
ofloxacin, tuberculosis, 616t
olanzapine, schizophrenia, 483t, 484

oliguria, 255, 259, 260–261
olsalazine, inflammatory bowel disease, 196, 203t
omalizumab, asthma, 419
omega-3 fatty acids, 400
    dyslipidaemia, 407
    dysmenorrhoea, 716
    inflammatory bowel disease, 202, 203t
omeprazole
    absorption, 52
    drug interactions, 176
    formulations available, 175t
    Helicobacter pylori eradication, 172
    interstitial nephritis, 258–259
    intravenous, 175
    peptic ulcer disease, 173t, 175, 175t
oncogenes, 820
ondansetron, antiemesis, 285, 540
on-off phenomenon, 511
ONTARGET study, 305
onycholysis, 882
onychomycosis, 656
ophthalmic route of administration, 136
ophthalmopathy, hyperthyroidism, 678
opioid antagonists, pruritus in liver disease, 245
opioid receptors, 519–520
opioids
    absorption, 52
    addiction, 524
    adverse effects, 523–524, 883–884
    cancer pain, 528
    clinical considerations, 523
    constipation, 210
    dependence, 524
    effect on neonates, 124, 125
    epidural, 524
    relative potencies of, 523t
    smooth muscle spasm, 524
    special delivery techniques, 524
    strong, 522–523
    teratogenicity, 741t
    tolerance, 524
    weak, 521–522
opportunistic infections
    in HIV, 622, 624, 624f, 637–651, 639t
    impact of HAART on, 645
opportunity cost, 117
optometrists, prescribing drugs, 16
oral candidiasis
    presentation, 656
    treatment, 656–657
oral contraceptives see combined oral
        contraceptives (COCs)
oral hygiene
    in immunocompromised patients, 796
    mucositis, 814
oral rehydration solutions, 216–217, 216t
oral route of administration, 135, 139–140
oral syringes, 139
Organisation for Economic Co-operation and
        Development (OECD), 116
orlistat
    absorption, 52
    obesity in diabetes, 706
ormeloxifene, menorrhagia, 719–720
oropharyngeal candidiasis, 638–643
orthodox sleep, 446
orthostatic circulatory responses, in geriatrics, 151
oseltamivir, influenza, 546
osmosin, 67
osmotic laxatives, 213–214
osteoarthritis, 843–846
    aetiology, 843–844
    clinical manifestations, 844
    epidemiology, 843

investigations, 844–845
    pain management, 530
    pathogenesis, 844
    treatment, 845–846
osteodystrophy, renal, 279–280, 279f, 287–288
osteomalacia, 94
osteomyelitis, neonatal, 127t
osteoporosis, 154–155, 204
    definition, 726
    fractures, 726–727
    heparin-induced, 379–380
    menopause, 726, 732
    prevention, 154
    risk factors, 726–727
    treatment, 154–155
otitis externa, 659
otitis media, 548
ovarian cancer, 734–735
ovaries
    menopausal changes, 725–726
    premenstrual syndrome, 713
overactive bladder syndrome, 157
overflow incontinence, 156
overweight children, 134
ovulation, 711–712
oxazepam, 458t
oxcarbamazepine, 495, 496
    adverse effects, 66, 500t
    epilepsy, 501–502
oxidative stress, chronic obstructive pulmonary
        disease, 433
oxiracetam, dementia, 152
oxprenolol
    anxiety disorders, 462
    coronary heart disease, 318t
oxybutynin, urinary incontinence, 157
oxycodone
    analgesia, 522
    cancer pain, 528
oxygen therapy
    asthma, 422
    bronchiolitis, 550
    chronic obstructive pulmonary disease, 439–440,
        442–445, 443t
    continuous long-term, 439–440, 442
    intermittent (short burst), 439
    neonates
        bronchopulmonary dysplasia, 126, 127
        respiratory distress syndrome, 125–126
oxypurinol, gout, 855
oxytetracycline, 60

P

p53 protein, 820
pacemaker activity, 356–357, 357f
pacemaker potential, 354–355
packaging and labelling of drugs, 158
packed cell volume (PCV), 88t, 89
PaCO₂ (partial pressure of carbon dioxide), 83
paediatrics see children
pain, 519–534
    acute, 519, 520
    adjuvant medication, 525–527, 525t
    aetiology, 519–520
    assessment, 520
    cancer see cancer, pain
    case studies, 531b
    definition, 519
    management, 520 (see also analgesia)
    neuroanatomy of pain transmission, 519
    neuropathic see neuropathic pain
    neurophysiology, 519–520
    neurotransmitters and, 519–520

(Continued)

sistent, 519, 520
ostoperative, 527
ST elevation myocardial infarction, 321–322
treatment of pain syndromes, 527–533
Paling palette, 72
paliperidone, schizophrenia, 483*t*
palivizumab, bronchiolitis, 550
palliative care
  associated nausea and vomiting, 542, 542*b*
  parenteral nutrition in, 111
palmar erythema, 242
palmoplantar psoriasis, 901, 908
palonosetron, antiemesis, 540
p-aminosalicylate (PAS), tuberculosis, 612, 616*t*
Panax ginseng, 59
pancreatic cancer, 528–529
pancreatic fistula, 105*t*
pancreatitis
  parenteral nutrition in, 111
  serum amylase, 86
pancuronium, 126
pancytopenia, 89*t*, 796
panic attacks, 456
panic disorder, 454–455, 455*b*, 455*t*
  antidepressants, 461
  benzodiazepines, 459
  recommended drug treatments, 462*t*
panobinostat, Hodgkin's lymphoma, 806
pantoprazole
  drug interactions, 176
  formulations available, 175*t*
  intravenous, 175
  peptic ulcer disease, 173*t*, 175, 175*t*
PaO₂ (partial pressure of oxygen), 83
paracentesis, ascites, 247
paracetamol
  absorption, 52
  analgesia, 520–521, 527
  dose, 521
  metabolism, 54*t*, 137–138, 520–521, 521*f*
  neonates, 124
  osteoarthritis, 845
  overdose/toxicity, 232, 235
    acute liver failure, 250
    biochemical tests, 244
    hepatotoxicity, 222, 224, 225, 231, 232, 232*f*,
      233, 235
paradoxical effects of benzodiazepines, 459
paradoxical sleep, 446–447
paraldehyde
  neonates, 124
    seizures, 128–129
  rectal administration, 140
parasites
  diarrhoea, 214, 216
  gastro-intestinal infections, 577
parathyroid gland disorders, 669–684
parathyroid hormone peptides, osteoporosis, 155
parathyroid hormone (PTH), 81, 82, 279–280
  calcium and, 679–684
parenteral administration of drugs
  children, 140–141
    dead space, 141
    displacement volume, 141
    excipients, 141
    fluid overload, 140
    intravenous access, 140
    lack of suitable paediatric formulations, 140–141
    rates of infusion, 141
  in urinary tract infections, 569*t*
parenteral nutrition, 96–115
  administration, 103–105
    central route, 104

cyclic infusions, 105
    infusion control, 104
    licensed ready-to-use products, 105
    peripherally inserted central catheters, 104
    peripheral route, 103–104, 103*b*
    routes of, 103–104
    standardised formulations, 104–105
  amino acids, 98–99, 99*t*
  body mass index, 97*t*
  in cancer and palliative care, 111
  in cardiac failure, 111
  case study, 113*b*, 114*t*
  children, 112–115
    formulation and stability issues, 112–113
    heparin, 113
    nutritional requirements, 112, 112*t*
    route of administration, 113–115
  complications, 109–110, 109*b*
    line occlusion, 110
    line sepsis, 109
    refeeding syndrome, 110, 110*t*
  in diabetes mellitus, 111
  electrolytes, 103
  energy, 99–101
    dual energy, 99–100, 100*b*
    glucose, 100, 100*t*
    lipid emulsions, 100–101, 100*t*, 101*f*
  indications for, 96–97
  initial assessment, 108
  intradialytic, 110–111
  in liver disease, 110
  long term, 111
  malnutrition *see* malnutrition
  micronutrients, 101–103
    factors affecting requirements of, 102*b*
    trace elements, 102, 102*t*
    vitamins, 102–103, 103*t*
  monitoring, 108–109
  nutrition screening, 96
  nutrition support teams, 97
  osmolarity of formulations, 104
  in pancreatitis, 111
  pharmaceutical issues, 105–108
    chemical stability, 107
    drug stability, 108
    filtration, 108
    light protection, 108
    microbial contamination, 107
    physical stability, 106–107
    shelf-life and temperature control, 107–108
  regimen components, 97–103
  in renal failure, 110–111
  in respiratory disease, 111
  in sepsis and injury, 111
  in short bowel syndrome, 111
  water volume, 97–103
paricalcitol, 287
parkinsonism, 153
  differential diagnosis, 509, 509*t*
  drug-induced, 509–510
  epidemiology, 507
parkinson-like side-effects, antipsychotic drugs, 481
Parkinson's disease, 507–518
  aetiology, 507–508
  case studies, 516*b*
  clinical features, 508–509
  differential diagnosis, 509–510
  epidemiology, 507
  investigations, 510
  motor features, 508
  non-motor features, 509
  pathophysiology, 508
  patient care, 515–518
  treatment, 510–515

Parkinson's Disease Society, 515
paronychia, 656
paroxetine, depression, 471
paroxysmal nocturnal dyspnoea (PND), 156
partial dopamine agonists, schizophrenia, 483*t*
partial pressure of carbon dioxide (PaCO₂), 83
partial pressure of oxygen (PaO₂), 83
partial seizures, 491–492
patent ductus arteriosus (PDA), 126, 130
patient-controlled analgesia (PCA), 524
patient education
  chemotherapy, 826
  chronic heart failure, 344–345, 345*t*
  diabetes mellitus, 694, 706, 706*b*
  peptic ulcer disease, 178–179
  rheumatoid arthritis, 834–835, 843
patient information leaflets (PILs), 24, 27, 72
peak and trough levels, 36
peak expiratory flow (PEF), 414
pegylated interferon alfa
  hepatitis C in HIV, 646
  opportunistic infections in HIV, 639*t*
pegylated interferon alfa-2a
  hepatitis B, 251
  hepatitis C, 251–252
pelvic inflammatory disease (PID), 717–718
pemoline, hepatotoxicity, 234
penicillamine, Wilson's disease, 252
penicillin G, neonatal infections, 127
penicillin(s)
  acute pyelonephritis, 568
  allergy, 604, 606
  elimination in children, 138
  hepatotoxicity, 225–226
  infection in neutropenia, 797
  interstitial nephritis, 258–259
  meningitis, 588
  neonates, respiratory distress syndrome, 130
  otitis media, 548
  resistance, 589–590
  sore throat, 547
  therapeutic index, 139
penicillin V, sickle cell anaemia, 781
Penicillium marneffei, 659
pentamidine
  and hypomagnesaemia, 82
  opportunistic infections in HIV, 639*t*
  Pneumocystis jiroveci pneumonia, 638
pentazocine, analgesia, 523
peptic ulcer disease, 162–184
  bleeding, 165, 168–169
  case studies, 180*b*
  clinical manifestations, 165
  common therapeutic problems, 179*t*
  definition, 162
  duodenal ulcer, 162, 163*f*, 164, 165, 174*f*
  in the elderly, 157
  epidemiology, 163
  gastric ulcer, 165, 170*f*
  Helicobacter pylori, 162*b*
    detection, 166–168
    epidemiology, 163, 163*f*
    eradication, 166, 171–172
    pathogenesis, 163–164
  investigations, 166–168
    endoscopy, 166
    Helicobacter pylori detection, 166–168
    radiology, 166–168
  NSAID-associated, 162*b*
    epidemiology, 163
    pathogenesis, 164–165, 164*f*
    prophylaxis, 172–173, 173*t*
    risk factors, 164*b*
    treatment, 172

pathogenesis, 163–165
patient assessment, 165–166
patient care, 178–183
presentation, 162–163
pyloric stenosis, 169
treatment, 168–175
complications, 168–169
gastro-oesophageal reflux disease, 173–175, 174b, 174f
Helicobacter pylori, 171–172
Helicobacter pylori negative ulcers, 173
NSAID-associated ulcers, 172
NSAID-negative ulcers, 173
stress ulcers, 169–170
ulcer-healing drugs, 175–178, 175t, 176t
uncomplicated disease, 170–172
Zollinger-Ellison syndrome, 169
percutaneous coronary intervention (PCI), 315, 323–324, 327
performance status scales, 822, 822b
pericardial tuberculosis, 614
pericyazine, schizophrenia, 483t
perimetry, glaucoma, 863
perindopril
chronic heart failure, 340t
clinical trials, 302
hypertension, 155, 305
stable angina, 317
peripheral arterial disease (PAD), 915t, 916, 916f
peripheral blood stem cell transplantation, 794–795
peripherally inserted central catheters (PICCs), 104
peripheral nerve injury, 530
peripheral neuropathy, 693, 915–916, 915t, 916f
peripheral oedema, 243, 246
peripheral vascular disease (PVD), 692
peristalsis, 210
peritoneal dialysis
acute, 266–267, 267f, 267t
in chronic kidney disease, 292
complications of, 292
peritonitis, 292
pernicious anaemia
case study, 784
epidemiology, 776
investigations, 778
pathophysiology, 777
peroxisome proliferator-activated receptor (PPAR) agonists, 314, 703
perphenazine, schizophrenia, 483t
persistent pulmonary hypertension, 126
pethidine
absorption, 52
analgesia, 522, 523t
effect on neonates, 125
petit mal seizures, 491
P-glycoprotein, 52, 56–57, 58
inducers, 56–57, 57t
inhibitors, 56–57, 57t
phaeochromocytoma, 297
phantom limb pain, 530
pharmaceutical care, 3–4
benefits of, 4
case study, 10b, 11t, 12t
definition, 3, 3t
delivery, 3
medication-related problems, 3–4
classification, 4b
process, 5t
pharmaceutical consultation, 4–6, 21–23, 21f
behaviours, 6, 7b
building relationships, 21–22
closing the session, 23
competency framework, 20t
explanation and planning, 22–23

gathering information, 22
initiating the session, 22
medicines-taking behaviour, 5
mnemonics, 5–6, 6b
physical examination, 22
postconsultation questions, 7b
process, 5–6, 5t, 6t
providing structure, 22
pharmaceutical industry, influence on prescribing, 28
pharmacodynamics
drug interactions, 57–58
in the elderly, 150–152
pharmacoeconomics, 116–122
application, 122b
choice of comparator, 117
decision analysis, 119–120, 119t, 120t
discounting, 119
economic evaluations, 117–119
cost benefit analysis, 117–118
cost-effectiveness analysis, 118
cost-utility analysis, 118–119
of medicines, 120
incentives and disincentives, 122
medication non-adherents, 121–122
risk management of unwanted drug effects, 120–121
terminology, 117
pharmacogenetics, adverse drug reactions, 66
pharmacokinetics, 32–49
absorption *see* absorption (of drugs)
basic concepts, 33–37
case studies, 45b
in children, 135–138
clinical applications, 37–49
distribution *see* distribution (of drugs)
dosage
adjustment, 36–37
alterations, 32
regimens, 35–36
drug concentration data, 36
drug interactions, 51–57
in the elderly, 149–150
elimination *see* elimination (of drugs)
excretion *see* excretion (of drugs)
formulation choice, 32
general applications, 32
loading dose, 32
metabolism *see* metabolism (of drugs)
peak and trough levels, 36
in pregnancy, 742
therapeutic drug monitoring, 33
time to maximal response, 32, 32f
volume of distribution, 33–34
pharmacovigilance, 68–71
case-control studies, 70–71
cohort studies, 70
published case reports, 70
spontaneous reporting, 68–69, 69t
Yellow Card Scheme, 69–70
pharyngitis (sore throat), 546–547
case studies, 558
causative organisms, 546
clinical features, 546–547
diagnosis, 547
treatment, 547
phenelzine
anxiety disorders, 461
depression, 471
phenobarbital
adverse effects, 500t
in children, 144
bioavailability, 135
distribution, 43

drug interactions, 499t
elimination, 43
epilepsy, 502
hypocalcaemia, 82
neonates, 125
monitoring in, 129
seizures, 128–129
pharmacokinetics, 43, 45t, 498t
plasma concentration-response relationship, 43
practical application, 43
phenothiazines
absorption, 52
antiemesis, 538
schizophrenia, 483t
teratogenicity, 741t
phenytoin
adverse effects, 66, 67–68, 500t, 502
distribution, 41, 53
drug interactions, 499t
elimination, 41
epilepsy, 502
hypernatraemia, 79
hypocalcaemia, 82
interactions, 60
metabolism, 54, 55, 55t
nasogastric administration, 140
neonatal seizures, 128–129
pharmacokinetics, 41–42, 45t, 48, 498t
plasma concentration-response relationship, 41
practical implications, 41–42
pregnancy, 742
Philadelphia chromosome translocation, 791, 792–793
phlebitis, 103
phobias, 454–455, 455t, 457
phosphate, 82
in acute kidney injury, 265
hyperphosphataemia, 82
hypophosphataemia, 82
phosphate-binding agents, hyperphosphataemia, 287
phosphate enemas
constipation, 157, 213
hypocalcaemia, 82
phosphodiesterase inhibitors, chronic heart failure, 342t, 343
photoallergic reactions, 881
photosensitivity
amiodarone-induced, 371
antipsychotics, 486
drug-induced, 881, 881b
phototherapy
eczema, 898
psoriasis, 903
phototoxic reactions, 881
physical examination, 22
physical status classification, 598t
physiotherapy
chronic obstructive pulmonary disease, 439
rheumatoid arthritis, 834–835
phytomenadione
clotting abnormalities, 246
coagulation disorders, 231
see also vitamin K
phytotherapy, benign prostatic hyperplasia, 758
pia mater, 584–585
pilocarpine
adverse effects, 872, 872b
commercially available forms, 872t
glaucoma, 872, 872b, 872t
Pilogel, 872
pimecrolimus, eczema, 897
pimozide, schizophrenia, 483t
pindolol, 318t
pink puffer, 434–435

pioglitazone
  adverse effects, 703
  diabetes mellitus, 703
  dosage, 703
  drug interactions, 703–704
  pharmacokinetics, 703
piperacillin
  infection in neutropenia, 797
  urinary tract infections, 569t
piperazine, schizophrenia, 483t
piperidines, schizophrenia, 483t
pipotiazine, schizophrenia, 483t
piracetam, dementia, 152
pityriasis versicolor, 658–659
  clinical presentation, 658
  diagnosis, 659
  treatment, 659
pivmecillinam, urinary tract infections, 567–568
pK$_a$, 746
placenta, 124
plant sterols, 400
plaque psoriasis, 901, 908, 909
plasma concentration-response relationship see
  specific drugs
plasma proteins, 53
plasminogen activator inhibitors, menorrhagia,
  720
platelet-activating factor (PAF), asthma, 413
platelets (thrombocytes), 88t, 90, 91, 770
pluripotent stem cells, 770
pneumococcal infections
  conjugate vaccines, 548
  pneumonia, 551
  resistance to penicillin, 551–552
  in sickle cell anaemia, 781
pneumococcal meningitis, 585, 588, 589
  treatment, 589–590
  see also Streptococcus pneumoniae
Pneumocystis jiroveci pneumonia (PCP), 638, 621
pneumonia, 550–555
  aspiration, 555
  community-acquired see community-acquired
    pneumonia
  fungal infections, 660t
  hospital-acquired (nosocomial) see hospital-
    acquired (nosocomial) pneumonia
  pneumococcal lobar, 551
poikilocytosis, 89t
poisons, acute tubular necrosis, 257t
pollen, 412–413
polyangiitis, microscopic, 258
polyclonal antibodies, renal transplantation, 291–292
polycystic kidney disease, 297
polyenes, candidiasis, 656–657
polyethylene glycol-uricase (PEG uricase), gout, 857
polymorphonucleocytes see neutrophils
polymyxins, cystic fibrosis, 556t
polypharmacy
  risk for drug-induced liver disease, 224
  schizophrenia, 482–484
polysorbates, 141
polyunsaturated fatty acids, 100–101
polyuria, chronic kidney disease, 277–278
porphyrias, 67
portal hypertension, liver disease, 243
portal tract, 238, 239f
posaconazole
  clinical use, 665
  fungal infections in compromised host, 665
  meningitis, 592
  pharmacokinetics, 664t
postamputation pain, 530
post-conception advice, 744–745
post-exposure prophylaxis, antiretroviral therapy, 627

postherpetic neuralgia, 529
post-operative nausea and vomiting, 539
post-operative pain, 527
post-transplant lymphoproliferative disorder
  (PTLD), 807
post-traumatic stress disorder (PTSD), 454–455,
  455b, 455t, 457
  antidepressants, 460, 461
  benzodiazepines, 459
  case study, 463
  recommended drug treatments, 462t
postural control, in geriatrics, 151
postural hypotension, antipsychotics, 486
postural instability, Parkinson's disease, 508
potassium, 79–81
  acute kidney injury, 265
  chronic kidney disease, 281
  hyperaldosteronism, 297
  hyperkalaemia, 264
  intracellular fluid osmolality, 77
  normal daily dietary intake, 80
  restriction in chronic kidney disease, 286
  secretion, 79
  total body, 79
  urinary tract infections, 566
  see also hyperkalaemia; hypokalaemia
potassium permanganate, nail changes, 881–882
potassium salts, 345t
potassium sparing diuretics
  and hyperkalaemia, 80
  hypertension in chronic kidney disease, 284
practical skills, 21
practolol, 62
pramipexole
  adverse effects, 512
  Parkinson's disease, 512
pramiracetam, dementia, 152
prasugrel
  arterial thromboembolism, 386
  non-ST elevation myocardial infarction, 327–328
  ST elevation myocardial infarction, 324
pravastatin
  dyslipidaemia, 402
  metabolism, 404
prazosin
  benign prostatic hyperplasia, 757
  hypertension, 301
precipitation, parenteral nutrition, 106
pre-conception advice, 744
prednisolone
  acute lymphoblastic leukaemia, 790
  autoimmune hepatitis, 252
  eczema, 898
  effect on neonates, 124
  gout, 854
  graft-versus-host disease, 795
  Hodgkin's lymphoma, 805, 807t
  inflammatory bowel disease, 193–194, 195, 203t
  meningeal tuberculosis, 614
  non-Hodgkin's lymphoma, 809, 811
  prostate cancer, 763–764
  renal transplantation, 291
  rheumatoid arthritis, 839
  tuberculosis, 643
prednisone, autoimmune hepatitis, 252
pre-eclampsia, 306
pregabalin
  adverse effects, 502
  anxiety disorders, 461
  pharmacokinetics, 44
  plasma concentration-response relationship, 44
  postherpetic neuralgia, 529
pregnancy
  bacteriuria in, 566, 569–570

diabetic retinopathy in, 693
drugs in, 739–745
  anti-thyroid drugs, 677
  benzodiazepines, 460
  case studies, 750
  dosing, 743–744
  foetal development periods, 740
  foetal-placental transfer, 743
  maternal pharmacokinetic changes, 742,
    742t
  pharmacological effect, 741
  post-conception advice, 744–745
  pre-conception advice, 744
  principles of, 740–741
  selection, 744
  teratogenicity, 739–745, 739b
  teratology information services, 745
  embryonic stage, 740
  foetal stage, 740
  and folate deficiency anaemia, 777, 778
  HIV infection and, 646, 647
  hypertension in, 306, 309
  and inflammatory bowel disease, 204
  nausea and vomiting in, 540–541
  pre-embryonic stage, 740
  rheumatoid arthritis in, 842
  risk for drug-induced liver disease, 224
  tuberculosis in, 614
pregnancy registries, 745
premature infants, drug transfer into breast milk,
  748
premenstrual dysphoric disorder (PMDD), 712,
  713b
premenstrual syndrome (PMS), 712–716
  aetiology, 713–714
  diagnosis, 713b
  epidemiology, 712–713
  essential fatty acids, 714
  hormones, 713–714
  management, 714–716
  psychological factors, 714
  symptoms, 714
  vitamins and generals, 714
prescribing (of drugs), 9–10, 14–31
  adherence see adherence/non-adherence
  communicating risks/benefits of treatment,
    23–24
  consultation see pharmaceutical consultation
  costs of, 116
  factors influencing, 26–28
    cognitive factors, 28, 28t
    colleagues, 28
    health care policy, 27
    patients, 26–27
    pharmaceutical industry, 28
  inappropriate or irrational, 15
  legal framework, 15–20
    accountability, 16–17
    clinical governance, 19, 20b
    competence and competency frameworks,
      19–20, 20t
    ethical framework, 17–18
      autonomy, 17, 17b
      beneficence, 18
      justice and veracity, 18
      non-maleficence, 17–18
    evolution of non-medical prescribing, 15–16
      non-medical independent prescribing, 16
      supplementary prescribing, 16, 16b
    off-label and unlicensed prescribing, 18, 19b
    prescribing between primary and secondary
      care, 18–19
    professional frameworks, 18
  medication review, 25–26, 25t

process, 21–24
rational and effective, 14–15, 15f
  definition, 14–15
  inappropriate or irrational, 15
repeat, 25
strategies to influence, 29–30
  managerial approaches, 29
  support and education, 30
pressure ulcers, 920–921
aetiology, 920–921
case study, 924
clinical signs, 921
common sites of, 920
definition, 920
diagnosis, 921
epidemiology, 920, 920t
prevention, 921
treatment, 921
Prezista©, 631t
prilocaine, 136
primaquine, opportunistic infections in HIV, 639t
primary antiphospholipid syndrome (PAPS), 377
primary biliary cirrhosis (PBC), 241
hyperpigmentation, 242
management, 252
primary sclerosing cholangitis (PSC), 241, 252
Primene®, 98, 99t
primidone
epilepsy, 502
pharmacokinetics, 43, 45t, 498t
Prinzmetal's angina, 317–318, 319
probenecid
elimination, 56
gout, 856
probiotics
diarrhoea, 218
inflammatory bowel disease, 186, 203t
procainamide
adverse effects, 367t
arrhythmias, 369
pharmacokinetics, 368t
procarbazine, Hodgkin's lymphoma, 805, 807t
prochlorperazine
antiemesis, 285, 538, 541
drug-induced parkinsonism, 509–510
proctitis
treatment, 193, 199, 204
ulcerative colitis, 190
product licence (PL), 145
PROFESS study, 305
progesterone
deficiency, 713
menstrual cycle, 711–712
premenstrual syndrome, 713
progestins, 394t
progestogens
dyslipidaemia, 396
endometriosis, 722
menopause, 729–730
menorrhagia, 719–720
premenstrual syndrome, 715
progressive multifocal leucoencephalopathy
  (PML), 646
PROGRESS study, 305
prolactin, premenstrual syndrome, 713–714
promazine, schizophrenia, 483t
promethazine, antiemesis, 541
propafenone
adverse effects, 367t
arrhythmias, 363
pharmacokinetics, 368t
propantheline bromide, dysmenorrhoea, 717
propiverine, urinary incontinence, 157
propranolol, 318t

absorption, 52
anxiety disorders, 462
arrhythmias, 370
distribution, 53
in the elderly, 150, 151
metabolism, 150
oesophageal varices, 250
propylene glycol
adverse reactions, 141
in oral preparations, 139
propylthiouracil (PTU)
hyperthyroidism, 675–676, 677
thyrotoxicosis, 676
prostaglandin analogues, glaucoma, 865–868
prostaglandins, 56
dysmenorrhoea, 716
kidney perfusion, 256–257
menorrhagia, 719, 720
menstrual cycle, 712
premenstrual syndrome, 713–714
prostaglandin synthesis inhibitors
drug-induced asthma, 412–413
premenstrual syndrome, 716
prostamides, glaucoma, 864, 865–868
prostanoids, ocular, 865–868, 868t, 869t
prostate cancer, 759–764
case studies, 766–767, 829
chemoprevention, 764
common problems associated with, 764t
epidemiology, 759
examination, 760
investigation, 760–761
pathophysiology, 759
patient care, 764
screening, 760
staging, 761
symptoms, 760
treatment, 761–764
  castrate resistant prostate cancer, 763 764
  localised prostate cancer, 761
  locally advanced prostate cancer, 761–763
  metastatic prostate cancer, 763
prostatectomy
open, 758
radical, 761
prostate disease, 753–768
case studies, 766b
see also specific diseases
prostate gland
anatomy, 753, 754f
biopsy, 760
transurethral resection, 758
prostate-specific antigen (PSA), 88
age-specific levels, 760t
prostate cancer, 760
prostatitis, 764–767
acute bacterial, 765
asymptomatic inflammatory, 765
chronic bacterial, 765, 766
chronic prostatitis/chronic pelvic pain
  syndrome, 765, 766
classification of, 765t
definition, 764
epidemiology, 764
examination, 765
investigations, 765
pathophysiology, 765
patient care, 766–767
symptoms, 765
treatment, 765–766
prosthetic implants, 597
protease inhibitors
effect on lipoprotein levels, 394t
HIV infection, 626, 631t, 635

protective isolation, neutropenia, 797
protein
in diabetes mellitus, 695
extracellular fluid osmolality, 77
proteinase imbalance, 433
protein binding, 137
drug transfer into breast milk, 746
in pregnancy, 742
protein C
activated, 715
deficiency, 376–377
protein S deficiency, 377
proteinuria
in chronic kidney disease, 277–278
in diabetes mellitus, 693
Proteus sp, 562
prothianamide, tuberculosis, 616t
prothrombin 20210 mutation, 377
prothrombin time (PT), 84, 91, 244
proton pump inhibitors
absorption, 52
adverse reactions, 176
available formulations of, 175, 175t
clinical use, 177
drug interactions, 176–177
gastro-oesophageal reflux disease, 173–174
Helicobacter pylori eradication, 171
interstitial nephritis, 258–259
peptic ulcer disease, 169–170, 172–173,
  175–177
pharmacokinetics, 175, 176
protozoa
gastro-intestinal infections, 574t
in HIV infection, 643
pruritus
in chronic kidney disease, 285
drug-induced, 884
drug-induced liver disease, 231
in liver disease, 242, 244–246, 245t
management, 244–246
treatment, 231
pseudohypoparathyroidism, 680
pseudomembranous colitis, 188, 202, 216
Pseudomonas aeruginosa, 591
cystic fibrosis, 555–556, 556t
gentamicin, 39
urinary tract infections, 562
psoralens plus UVA light (PUVA), psoriasis, 903
psoriasis, 898–909
aetiology, 899–900
case studies, 908, 909
clinical features, 900–901, 900f
clinical types, 901–902
drug-induced, 885, 885b, 889–890
pathology, 900–901
patient care, 905–909
precipitating factors, 899–900
treatment, 902–905
  biologic therapy, 905
  drug interactions, 899t
  phototherapy, 903
  psoriasis at special fights, 903
  systemic therapy, 903–905, 904t
  topical retinoids, 903
  topical therapy, 902–903
Psoriasis Area and Severity Index (PASI), 903
psoriasis vulgaris, 901
psoriatic arthropathy, 902
psychological changes, menopause, 727, 735
psychomotor impairment, benzodiazepines, 459
psychosis, Parkinson's disease, 516
psychotherapy, anxiety disorders, 457
puberty, 711
pulmonary arteriography, 378

pulmonary embolism (PE), 378
  acute submassive, 378
  diagnosis, 93
  investigations, 378
  maternal death, 376
pulmonary fibrosis, 433
  amiodarone-induced, 371
  chemotherapy-induced, 813*t*
pulmonary hypertension, 434
pulmonary rehabilitation, chronic obstructive
        pulmonary disease, 440
pure red cell aplasia (PRCA), 286
purine analogues, chronic lymphocytic leukaemia, 793
purines, 84
Purkinje fibres, 356, 366, 366*t*
pustular psoriasis, 901*f*, 902, 908
PUVA (psoralens plus UVA light), psoriasis, 903
pyelonephritis
  acute, 258, 561, 568–569
  chronic, 277, 561
pyloric stenosis, 169
pyoderma gangrenosum, 191
pyrazinamide
  adverse effects, 615–616, 616*t*
  tuberculosis, 612, 613, 613*t*, 614, 643
pyridoxine
  premenstrual syndrome, 715
  sideroblastic anaemia, 775
  Wilson's disease, 252
pyrimethamine
  opportunistic infections in HIV, 639*t*
  Pneumocystis jiroveci pneumonia, 638
  toxoplasmosis, 643
pyroxidine phosphate, premenstrual syndrome, 714

Q

QRISK2, 398–399
QT prolongation
  antipsychotics, 486
  drug interactions, 50
quality-adjusted life-years (QALYs), 118–119
quality of life, elderly, 157
quetiapine
  Parkinson's disease, 516
  schizophrenia, 483*t*
quinapril, chronic heart failure, 340*t*
quinidine
  adverse effects, 367*t*
  arrhythmias, 368
  pharmacokinetics, 368*t*
quinolone antibiotics
  absorption, 52
  acute pyelonephritis, 568
  cystic fibrosis, 556*t*
  interstitial nephritis, 258–259
  Legionnaire's disease, 552
  mycobacteria, 644
  urinary tract infections, 567, 568

R

rabeprazole
  drug interactions, 176
  formulations available, 175*t*
  peptic ulcer disease, 175*t*
race *see* ethnicity/race
radiation, leukaemia risk, 786–787
radiocontrast media, acute tubular necrosis, 257*t*
radio-frequency interstitial tumour ablation
      (RITA), 761
radioiodine, 675–676, 677–678
radiology
  drug-induced liver disease, 228

inflammatory bowel disease, 191
peptic ulcer disease, 166.
see also specific modalities
radiotherapy
  alongside chemotherapy, 824
  Hodgkin's lymphoma, 804, 806*f*
  prostate cancer, 761
  solid tumours, 823
raloxifene
  alternative to HRT, 730, 732
  osteoporosis, 155
raltegravir, HIV infection, 631*t*, 637
ramipril
  chronic heart failure, 340*t*
  coronary heart disease, 11*t*, 12*t*
  hypertension, 305
  stable angina, 317
ranitidine, peptic ulcer disease, 169–170, 173*t*, 177
ranolazine, stable angina, 320
rapid eye movement (REM) sleep, 446–447
rapidly progressive glomerulonephritis (RPGN),
    258
rapport, 22
rasagiline, Parkinson's disease, 513
rasburicase
  gout, 856–857
  tumour lysis syndrome, 813–814
rash, antiretroviral toxicity, 637
Rawlins-Thompson classification, 63–64, 64*t*
R-CHOP (rituximab, cyclophosphamide,
    doxorubicin, vincristine, prednisolone),
    non-Hodgkin's lymphoma, 809, 811
R-CVP (rituximab, cyclophosphamide, vincristine,
    prednisolone), non-Hodgkin's
    lymphoma, 809, 811
reactive oxygen species (ROS), coronary heart
    disease, 314
REAL (revised European-American lymphoma)
    classification, 808, 808*t*, 809*b*
reasoning skills, 21
rebound insomnia, 450
reboxetine, depression, 472
record keeping, 158
recreational drug use, and breastfeeding, 749
rectal route of administration
  children, 136, 140
  in inflammatory bowel disease, 193
  neonates, 124
red blood cell count, 88–89, 88*t*
red blood cells, 770
red cell folate, 88*t*
red clover, 59, 731
re-entry, 358, 358*f*
refeeding syndrome, 110, 110*t*
refractoriness, 355
regurgitation, 535
rehydration, 216–217, 216*t*
relationships, building, 21–22
renal artery stenosis
  bilateral, 262, 262*f*
  in hypertension, 297
renal clearance in the elderly, 150
renal disease
  gout, 850
  hypertension in, 305
  tuberculosis in, 614
renal osteodystrophy, 279–280, 279*f*, 287–288
renal perfusion optimisation, 263
renal replacement therapy, 265–270
  acute peritoneal dialysis, 266–267, 267*f*
  approximate clearances of, 267*t*
  characteristics of the ideal drug, 269*b*
  in chronic kidney disease, 292–293
  common adverse effects, 269*f*

convection, 265
diffusion, 265
drug dosage in, 267, 267*t*
factors affecting drug use, 267–270
  absorption, 267
  distribution, 268
  excretion, 268
  metabolism, 268
  nephrotoxicity, 268–270
forms of, 265–267
haemodiafiltration, 266
haemodialysis, 265–266, 266*f*
haemofiltration, 266
primary diagnosis, 276*t*
ultrafiltration, 265
vs. transplantation, 288
renal tract obstruction, 277
renal transplantation, 288–292
  acute tubular necrosis, 257*t*
  donors, 288–289
  end stage renal failure, 288
  immunosuppressants, 289–292, 289*t*
  other precautions, 292
  vs. renal replacement therapy, 288
renal tubule, active excretion, 56
renin, 273
renin-angiotensin-aldosterone antagonists,
    hypertension, 301
renin-angiotensin-aldosterone system, 76
  ascites, 243
  in chronic kidney disease, 272–273
  and hypertension, 296
  kidney perfusion, 256–257
repaglinide
  diabetes mellitus, 702
  dosage, 703
  pharmacokinetics, 702–703
repeat prescriptions, 25
reserpine, affective disorders, 466
residual volume (RV), 435
respiratory depression
  in neonates, 125
  opioid-induced, 523
respiratory disease, parenteral nutrition in, 111
respiratory distress syndrome (RDS)
  case study, 130
  in neonates, 125–126
respiratory failure, acute, 435
respiratory infections, 545–560
  case studies, 558*b*
  common therapeutic problems, 557*t*
  in the immunocompromised, 556–559, 557*t*
  lower respiratory tract, 549–556
  upper respiratory tract, 545–549
respiratory syncytial virus (RSV), 134, 550
retching, 535
reteplase
  ST elevation myocardial infarction, 323*t*, 324
  venous thromboembolism, 385
reticulocytes, 88*t*, 89
retinitis, cytomegalovirus, 644
retinoid drugs
  adverse effects, 885
  topical, psoriasis, 903
retinopathy, diabetic, 693
Retrovir©, 628*t*
reverse cholesterol transport pathway, 390–391
reverse transcriptase, 621–622, 622*f*
revised European-American lymphoma (REAL)
    classification, 808, 808*t*, 809*b*
Reyataz©, 631*t*
Reye's syndrome, 144, 223
rhabdomyolysis, 87, 87*t*, 257*t*
rheumatoid arthritis, 832–843

aetiology, 832–833
case studies, 845, 846
clinical manifestations, 833, 833b, 833f
diagnosis, 833–834, 833b, 834b
epidemiology, 832
investigations, 834
pain management, 530
pathophysiology, 832–833
patient care, 843
therapeutic problems in management of, 844t
treatment, 834–843
abatacept, 842
anakinra, 842
anti-TNF agents, 840–841
biological therapies, 839–840, 840t
disease-modifying anti-rheumatic drugs, 836–839, 837t, 838b, 839b
drugs, 835
non-steroidal anti-inflammatory drugs, 835–836, 835t
in pregnancy, 842
rituximab, 841–842
tocilizumab, 842
rheumatoid factor (RF), 834
ribavirin
bronchiolitis, 550
hepatitis C, 251–252, 646
HIV, 639t, 646
opportunistic infections, 639t
ribonucleic acid (RNA), 89
rifabutin
mycobacteria, 644
opportunistic infections in HIV, 639t
tuberculosis, 616t
rifampicin
adverse effects, 615, 616t
gastro-intestinal infections, 580
hepatotoxicity, 223t, 226
Legionnaire's disease, 552
meningitis, 589t, 590, 591
metabolism, 54
pruritus in liver disease, 245
tuberculosis, 612, 613, 613t, 614, 617, 643
rifaximin
gastro-intestinal infections, 579
hepatic encephalopathy, 248, 249t
RIFLE criteria, 255, 256f
rilpivirine, HIV infection, 635
ringworm, 657
risedronate
adverse effects, 154
alternatives to HRT, 731
osteoporosis, 154
risk management of unwanted drug effects, 120–121
risks, communicating, 23–24, 72–74, 73f
risperidone, schizophrenia, 483t, 485
ritonavir
HIV infection, 626, 631t, 635
metabolism, 55
rituximab
adverse effects, 841
autoimmune haemolytic anaemia, 780
chronic lymphocytic leukaemia, 793
Hodgkin's lymphoma, 805, 806
indications/contraindications, 841–842
non-Hodgkin's lymphoma, 809, 811–812
rheumatoid arthritis, 841–842
rivaroxaban, venous thromboembolism, 384
rivastigmine
dementia, 152
Parkinson's disease, 516
Rockall risk scoring system, 166
rofecoxib

adverse reactions, 62
safety, 835
ropinirole
adverse effects, 512
Parkinson's disease, 512
rosiglitazone, 703
Rosser-Kind matrix, 118
rosuvastatin
dyslipidaemia, 402
metabolism, 404
rotaviruses, 214, 573
vaccine, 218–220
rubefacients, osteoarthritis, 845
rufinamide, epilepsy, 502
rumination, 535

S

Saccharomyces, 218
St John's wort, 50
depression, 473
and drug metabolism, 54
interactions, 59, 61, 475t
salbutamol inhaler
asthma, 415, 418, 418t, 422
coronary heart disease, 11t, 12t
hyperkalaemia, 264
salicylates
adverse reactions, 144
elimination, 56
salicylic acid, psoriasis, 903
saliva, electrolyte content of, 105t
salmeterol, asthma, 418t
Salmonella
diarrhoea, 214, 217–218
gastro-intestinal infections, 573, 574–575, 574t, 576t
transmission, 573
treatment, 578–579, 581t
salt intake
in diabetes mellitus, 695
and dyslipidaemia, 401
salt reduction
ascites in liver disease, 246
hypertension, 298
saprophytic fungi, 659
saquinavir, HIV infection, 631t
Saving Lives programme, 554
saxagliptin, 704
scalp psoriasis, 901, 903, 908
scarlet fever, 546–547
scars, 910–911
Scedospermium, 659
schizophrenia, 479–488
acute psychotic illness, 479–480
case studies, 487b
causes of, 480
chronic, 480
classification, 479
diagnosis, 479–480
drug treatment, 480–488
adverse effects, 486–488
anticholinergic drugs, 485
antipsychotics, 480–481, 483t, 484–485, 486–488
augmentation strategies and polytherapy, 484
clozapine and refractory illness, 482
neuroleptic equivalence, 484
non-acting formulations, 484–485
polypharmacy, 482–484
rationale, 481
selection and dose, 481–482
therapeutic drug monitoring, 485–486
symptoms, 479–480

Schofield equation, 99, 99t
schools, medicines in, 142–143
policies and guidance, 143
responsibility for, medicines, 143
special schools, 143
Schwartz equation, 144
scleritis, 191
sclerosing cholangitis, 191
Scottish Intercollegiate Guideline Network see SIGN
seborrhoeic dermatitis, 658, 659, 895
case study, 907, 907f
secondarily generalised seizures, 492
sedation
antipsychotics, 486
opioid-induced, 523
seizures
febrile convulsions, 493
generalised, 491, 494t
absence attacks (petit mal), 491
atonic seizures, 491
myoclonic seizures, 491
tonic clonic (grand mal) convulsions, 491
incidence, 490
neonates, 128–129
partial/focal, 491–492, 494t
complex partial seizures, 491–492
secondarily generalised seizures, 492
simple partial seizures, 491
treatment during, 493
selective decontamination of the digestive tract (SDD), 554–555
selective oestrogen receptor modulators (SERMs), 730, 736
selective serotonin reuptake inhibitors (SSRIs)
antiemesis, 538, 540
anxiety disorders, 461
depression, 469, 471, 472
hepatotoxicity, 223t
interactions, 58, 475t
pain, 526
premenstrual syndrome, 716
teratogenicity, 741t
selegiline, Parkinson's disease, 513
selenium, 102t
selenium sulphide lotion, pityriasis versicolor, 659
self-monitoring, chronic heart failure, 344–345, 345t
senna, constipation, 157, 212
sensory ataxia, 95
sepsis
acute tubular necrosis, 257t
parenteral nutrition, 109, 111
septicaemia, neonates, 127t
serological markers, drug-induced liver disease, 228
serotonin
affective disorders, 466
nausea and vomiting, 538
premenstrual syndrome, 714
serotonin-dopamine antagonists, schizophrenia, 483t
serotonin-noradrenaline reuptake inhibitors (SNRIs), 472, 731
serotonin syndrome (SS), 57–58, 60
Serratia sp., 562
sertindole, schizophrenia, 483t
sertraline
depression, 471, 472
effect on lipoprotein levels, 394t
serum, 76
sevelamer, hyperphosphataemia, 287
severe acute respiratory syndrome (SARS), 555
severe myoclonic epilepsy of infancy (SMEI), 503
sexual characteristics, liver disease, 243

sexual dysfunction
  antipsychotics, 486
  and the menopause, 735
SGN-35, Hodgkin's lymphoma, 806
Shankapushpi, 59
Shigella, 214, 217
  gastro-intestinal infections, 574–575, 574*t*, 576*t*
  transmission, 573
  treatment, 579, 581*t*
short bowel syndrome, 111
shunt-associated meningitis, 591, 592*t*
sickle cell anaemia, 780–781
  aetiology, 780
  clinical manifestations, 781
  epidemiology, 780
  inheritance patterns, 781*f*
  investigations, 781
  pathophysiology, 781
  patient care, 781
  treatment, 781
sickle cells, 781
sickle cell trait, 780, 781*f*
sideroblastic anaemia, 774–775
  acquired, 774, 774*b*, 775
  aetiology, 774
  case study, 784
  clinical manifestations, 775
  drugs and toxins, 774–775
  epidemiology, 774
  hereditary, 774, 775
  investigations, 775
  iron overload, 775
  pathophysiology, 774–775
  patient care, 775
  treatment, 775
SIGN, prescribing strategies, 29
sildenafil
  metabolism, 55, 55*t*
  neonates, bronchopulmonary dysplasia, 127
silent ischaemia, 315
simple partial seizures, 491
simvastatin
  adverse reactions, 73
  coronary heart disease, 11*t*, 12*t*
  dyslipidaemia, 402, 403*t*
  interactions, 59
  metabolism, 55, 404
  over-the-counter sale, 405
Sinemet®, 511
sinusitis, 548–549
sinus node, 356–357
sinus rhythm, 354
sirolimus
  adverse effects, 291
  renal transplantation, 289*t*, 291
sitagliptin, 704
skeletal muscle relaxants, 525*t*, 526–527
skin
  in liver disease, 242
  menopausal changes, 727
  necrosis, drug-induced, 889
  neonates, 124
  pigmentary changes, 881, 881*f*, 882*t*
  structure, 910
  in ulcerative colitis, 190–191
  warfarin-induced reactions, 381
skin cancer
  case study, 890, 890*f*
  drug-induced, 883
skin disorders, drug-induced, 880–892
  case studies, 889*b*
  causing skin function changes, 881–883
  diagnosis, 880
  mild, 883–885

patient care, 889–892
severe, 885–889
skip lesions, 187–188
SLC2A9, 850
SLC22A12 gene, 850
sleep
  hygiene, 447, 447*b*
  problems and the menopause, 735
  systems, 446–447, 446*f*, 456*f*
sleep apnoea syndrome, 435
sleep attacks, 512
slow continuous ultrafiltration (SCU), 266
small round structured virus (SRSV), 214
small-vessel vasculitis (SVV), 258
smoking *see* cigarette smoking
social phobia, 454–455, 455*t*
  antidepressants, 461
  case study, 463
  recommended drug treatments, 462*t*
sodium
  in acute kidney injury, 265
  balance, 76–79
  in chronic kidney disease, 280, 280*t*
  depletion, 78
  distribution, 78
  excess, 78
  extracellular fluid
    osmolality, 77
    volume, 78
  oral rehydration solutions, 216–217
  restriction in chronic kidney disease, 286
  see also hypernatraemia; hyponatraemia
sodium aurothiomalate, rheumatoid arthritis, 836, 837*t*, 839
sodium bicarbonate, acidosis, 264
sodium channel blockade, 368*t*
sodium citrate
  enemas, constipation, 213
  urinary tract infections, 566
sodium cromoglicate
  adverse reactions, 420*b*
  asthma, 419
  inflammatory bowel disease, 203*t*
sodium nitroprusside
  chronic heart failure, 343
  hypertension, 301
sodium thiosulphate, pityriasis versicolor, 659
sodium valproate
  adverse effects, 500*t*, 502–503
    in children, 144
  drug-induced parkinsonism, 509–510
  drug interactions, 499*t*
  epilepsy, 502–503
  hepatotoxicity, 223, 223*t*, 226, 233
  metabolism, 55*t*
  neonatal seizures, 128–129
  pharmacokinetics, 498*t*
solifenacin, urinary incontinence, 157
soluble fibre, dyslipidaemia, 407
somatostatin, oesophageal varices, 250
sorbitol, 139
sore throat *see* pharyngitis (sore throat)
sotalol
  adverse reactions, 65
  arrhythmias, 359, 361, 363, 370
  pharmacokinetics, 318*t*
sphincter muscle theory, 862
spider naevi, 242
spina bifida, 133
spiral computed tomography, pulmonary embolism, 378
spirometry
  asthma, 414–415
  chronic obstructive pulmonary disease, 435

spironolactone
  adverse reactions, 74, 243
  ascites, 246, 247, 247*t*
  chronic heart failure, 339*t*, 341–342
  drug interactions, 348*t*
  hyperkalaemia, 80
  hypertension, 285, 300–301
  neonatal bronchopulmonary dysplasia, 127
splenomegaly, 242
spontaneous bacterial peritonitis (SBP), 247–248
spontaneous reporting, 68–69
  causality assessment, 69, 69*t*
  signal detection, 68–69
sputum tests/cultures
  pneumonia, 551, 553
  tuberculosis, 611
standard gamble method, 118
stanol esters, 400
staphylococcal infections
  coagulase-negative, 127
  pneumonia, 552
  urinary tract infections, 562
Staphylococcus aureus
  bacterial meningitis, 585
  chronic obstructive pulmonary disease, 438–439
  cystic fibrosis, 555
  diarrhoea, 214
  gastro-intestinal infections, 574*t*, 576*t*
  investigations, 577
  meticillin-resistant *see* meticillin-resistant *Staphylococcus aureus* (MRSA)
  neonates, 127
  surgical site infection, 599–600
  transmission, 573
  treatment, 578
stasis eczema, 895
statins
  adverse effects, 73, 87, 404, 885
  coronary heart disease, 11*t*, 317
  drug interactions, 404*t*
  dyslipidaemia, 402–405
  hepatotoxicity, 223*t*
  hypertension in chronic kidney disease, 285
  non-ST elevation myocardial infarction, 329
  over-the-counter sale, 405
  patient counselling, 405
  pleiotropic properties, 404–405
  stable angina, 317
  ST elevation myocardial infarction, 325
status epilepticus, 493
stavudine, HIV infection, 628*t*, 635
steatohepatitis, 226–227, 241
steatosis
  aetiology, 225
  clinical presentation, 227
  drugs associated with, 226*t*
  pathophysiology, 226–227
stellate cells, 238
stem cell transplantation, 794*f*
  acute myeloblastic leukaemia, 792
  basic principle, 794
  complications, 795
  leukaemia, 794–795
  Parkinson's disease, 514–515
  peripheral blood, 794–795
  place of, 795
  reduced intensity allografting, 795
  source of stem cells, 794
STEPS, 14–15
sterculia, constipation, 212
steroids *see* corticosteroids
steroid-sparing agents, asthma, 419
Stevens-Johnson syndrome, 66

clinical features, 886–887, 886*f*
drug-induced, 886–887, 886*f*, 887*b*, 891
stimulant laxatives, 212–213
stimulation-produced analgesia, 527
stiripentol, epilepsy, 503
stool antigen tests, *Helicobacter pylori*, 166–167
stool examination/tests
    diarrhoea, 216
    gastro-intestinal infections, 577
    inflammatory bowel disease, 192
streptococcal infections
    group B β-haemolytic, 127
    sore throat, 546–547
Streptococcus pneumoniae, 585, 588, 589, 593*t*
    bronchitis, 549
    chronic obstructive pulmonary disease, 438–439
    otitis media, 548
Streptococcus pyogenes, 546
streptokinase
    adverse effects, 324, 385
    leg ulcers, 156
    ST elevation myocardial infarction, 323*t*, 324
    venous thromboembolism, 384–385
streptomycin
    adverse reactions, 65
    tuberculosis, 612, 613*t*, 614, 616*t*
stress
    and anxiety, 456
    and inflammatory bowel disease, 186
    and peptic ulcers, 169–170
    and psoriasis, 900
stress incontinence, 156–157
stroke, 153–154
    and fibrinolytics, 324
    haemorrhagic *see* haemorrhagic stroke
    and hormone replacement therapy, 733*t*
    hypertension in, 295, 305–306, 309
    primary prevention, 154
    risk from atrial fibrillation, 362–363, 362*f*, 374
    secondary prevention, 153–154
    treatment, 153
strontium ranelate
    alternatives to HRT, 731
    osteoporosis, 154
Study of Cognition and Prognosis in the Elderly
        (SCOPE), 304
subarachnoid haemorrhage, 93
subarachnoid space, 584–585
subcutaneous jet injection systems, 136
substance P, 538–539
substantia nigra, 508
subthalamic nucleus, 514
sucralfate
    adverse reactions, 178
    drug interactions, 178
    peptic ulcer disease, 169–170, 178
sulfadiazine
    opportunistic infections in HIV, 639*t*
    toxoplasmosis, 643
sulfapyridine, inflammatory bowel disease, 196
sulfasalazine
    inflammatory bowel disease, 196, 203*t*
    rheumatoid arthritis, 836, 837*t*, 839
sulphanilamide, 67
sulphinpyrazone, gout, 856
sulphonamides
    bioavailability in children, 135
    hepatotoxicity, 223*t*
sulphonylureas
    adverse effects, 700–701, 702*t*
    choice of, 700
    diabetes mellitus, 699, 700–701, 701*t*
    dosage, 701
    drug interactions, 701

mode of action, 700
    pharmacokinetics, 700
sulpiride, schizophrenia, 483*t*
supplementary prescribing, 16, 16*b*
supraventricular tachycardias, 359–364
    atrial fibrillation *see* atrial fibrillation
    atrial flutter, 359, 360*f*
    case study, 374
    focal atrial tachycardia, 359
    inappropriate sinus tachycardia, 359
    junctional re-entry tachycardia, 360–361, 361*f*
surfactant deficiency, 125, 126
surgery
    benign prostatic hyperplasia, 758
    duration of, 597
    hyperthyroidism, 678
    infection after *see* surgical site infection
    Parkinson's disease, 514–515, 514*t*
    solid tumours, 823
    venous thromboembolism, 377
surgical site infection, 596–607
    case studies, 605*b*
    definition, 596, 597*t*
    epidemiology, 596
    pathogenesis, 599–600, 600*f*, 600*t*
    prevention/antibiotic prophylaxis, 600–606
        β-lactam allergy, 604–605, 605*t*
        cephalosporin-free, 603*t*
        choice of antimicrobial, 601–605
        common micro-organisms, 602*t*
        local, 605–606
        number needed to treat, 601*t*
        recommendations, 601*t*
        repeat doses, 604, 605*t*
        susceptibility of common pathogens, 602*t*
        timing and duration, 602–603, 603*f*
        topical, 605–606
    risk factors, 597–599, 598*t*, 599*f*, 599*t*
    surveillance, 596–597
sustained virologic response (SVR), hepatitis
        C virus, 251–252
Sustiva©, 630*t*
Swedish Trial in Old Patients with hypertension-2
        (STOP-2), 304
sweeteners, diabetes mellitus, 694–695
Sweet's syndrome, 191
sympathomimetics
    chronic heart failure, 342*t*
    glaucoma, 864, 871–872, 871*t*, 872*t*
    interactions, 58
syndrome of inappropriate secretion of
        antidiuretic hormone (SIADH), 78, 79
syndrome X, 687
Synthamin®, 98, 99*t*
systemic lupus erythematosus (SLE), 258, 377

T

tacrolimus
    autoimmune hepatitis, 252
    drug interactions, 176
    effect on lipoprotein levels, 394*t*
    hypomagnesaemia, 82
    inflammatory bowel disease, 199
    metabolism, 54
    renal transplantation, 289*t*, 290
    topical, eczema, 897
tafluprost, glaucoma, 865, 866, 868*t*
tamoxifen
    chemoprevention, 819
    hair changes, 882
    and hypercalcaemia, 81
tamsulosin, benign prostatic hyperplasia, 757
tardive dyskinesia, 481, 482

taxanes, Kaposi's sarcoma, 645
tazobactam, urinary tract infections, 569*t*
teicoplanin
    infection in neutropenia, 797
    surgical site infection prophylaxis, 604
telaprevir, hepatitis C, 252
telbivudine, hepatitis B, 251
telmisartan
    clinical trials, 305
    hypertension, 305
Telzir©, 631*t*
temazepam, 458*t*
temocillin, pneumonia, 554*t*
tenecteplase
    ST elevation myocardial infarction, 323*t*, 324
    venous thromboembolism, 385
tenofovir
    hepatitis B, 251, 646
    HIV infection, 628*t*, 635
TENS *see* transcutaneous electrical nerve
        stimulation (TENS)
teratogenicity, 739–745
    drug dose, 740–741
    example drugs, 739*b*
    genotype and environmental interaction, 741
    principles, 740–741
    species, 741
    timing of exposure, 740
teratology information services (TIS), 745
terazosin
    benign prostatic hyperplasia, 757
    hypertension, 301
terbinafine
    dermatophytosis, 657–658
    pityriasis versicolor, 659
terbutaline, asthma, 415, 418, 418*t*
teriparatide
    alternatives to HRT, 731
    osteoporosis, 155
terlipressin, oesophageal varices, 250, 250*t*
testosterone
    effect on lipoprotein levels, 394*t*
    hair changes, 882
    prostate cancer, 759, 761–762
    urinary incontinence, 157
tetracyclines
    absorption, 52
    adverse reactions, 144
    bronchitis/chronic obstructive pulmonary
        disease, 549–550
    cholera, 579–580
    Helicobacter pylori eradication, 172
    hepatotoxicity, 225, 226
    interactions, 60
    and psoriasis, 899
tetra-iodothyronine *see* thyroxine (T₄)
thalassaemias, 782
thalidomide, 62, 739–740
    graft-versus-host disease, 795
    inflammatory bowel disease, 202, 203*t*
T-helper cells, 622
theophylline
    adverse reactions, 420*b*
    asthma, 417, 418*t*
    chronic obstructive pulmonary disease, 437–438
    distribution, 38
    dosage in children, 137*t*
    drug interactions, 423*t*
    elimination, 38
    metabolism, 55
    pharmacokinetics, 38–39, 45*t*, 47, 419*t*
    plasma concentration-response relationship, 38
    practical implications, 39
    product formulation, 39

therapeutic drug monitoring (TDM)
    antiepileptic drugs, 496–497
    practical pharmacokinetics, 33
therapeutic index, 138–139
therapeutic range, 37
thermoregulation, in geriatrics, 151
thermotherapy, benign prostatic hyperplasia, 758
thiacetazone, tuberculosis, 616*t*
thiazide diuretics
    in acute kidney injury, 263
    chronic heart failure, 337, 339*t*
    clinical trials, 302
    and dyslipidaemia, 395
    effect on lipoprotein levels, 394*t*
    and gout, 851
    and hypercalcaemia, 81
    hypertension, 155, 300, 304, 304*b*
        in diabetes, 305
        in the elderly, 304
        in renal disease, 284, 305
    and hypokalaemia, 80
    neonatal heart failure, 127
thiazolidinediones
    adverse effects, 703
    diabetes mellitus, 701*t*, 703–704
    dosage, 703
    drug interactions, 703–704
    mode of action, 703
    pharmacokinetics, 703
thiobenzodiazepines, schizophrenia, 483*t*
thioguanines
    acute myeloblastic leukaemia, 791–792
    drug interactions, 198
    inflammatory bowel disease, 198
thiols, 319
thionamide
    adverse effects, 677*t*
    hyperthyroidism, 675–676
thiopental, 150
thiopurine methyl transferase (TPMT), 198, 898
thioxanthines, schizophrenia, 483*t*
thirst, 76
throat, sore *see* pharyngitis (sore throat)
thrombin, 91
thrombocytes *see* platelets (thrombocytes)
thrombocytopenia
    definition, 89*t*
    heparin-induced, 379
thromboembolism
    arterial *see* arterial thromboembolism (ATE)
    in inflammatory bowel disease, 191
    venous *see* venous thromboembolism (VTE)
thrombolytic agents
    myocardial infarction, 156
    stroke, 153
thrombophilia, 715
thromboplastin, 91
thrombosis, 376–388
    arterial thromboembolism *see* arterial
        thromboembolism (ATE)
    case studies, 387*b*
    definition, 376
    venous thromboembolism *see* venous
        thromboembolism (VTE)
thrush, 656
    see also candidiasis
thyroglobulin, 669
thyroid ablative therapy, 677–678
thyroid crisis, 678
thyroid gland
    disorders, 669–684 (*see also specific disorders*)
        case studies, 682*b*
    drugs and the, 672*t*, 679
    function testing, 672, 675

hormones, 669
    control, 669*f*
    metabolism, 670
    plasma protein binding, 670*t*
    secretion, 670
    synthesis, 670*f*
    physiology, 669–670
thyroiditis, 674*t*, 675
thyroid peroxidase (TPO), 669
thyroid receptor antibodies (TRABs), 674
thyroid stimulating hormone (TSH), 669
    hypothyroidism, 672
    thyroid function testing, 672
thyrotoxicosis
    aetiology, 674–675, 674*t*
    amiodarone-induced, 371
    case study, 683
    clinical features, 675, 675*b*
    drugs and, 679
    epidemiology, 674
    investigations, 675
    treatment, 675–678, 676*t*
thyrotrophin-releasing hormone (TRH), 669
thyroxine (T$_4$), 669, 670
    hypothyroidism, 672
    replacement therapy, 672–673, 677
    thyroid function testing, 672
tiagabine
    adverse effects, 500*t*
    epilepsy, 495*t*, 496, 503
    pharmacokinetics, 44
    plasma concentration-response relationship, 44
tibolone, 730
ticarcillin, cystic fibrosis, 556*t*
time trade-off method, 118
timolol, 318*t*
    adverse effects, 868–869
    and bimatoprost, 874
    and brimonidine, 874
    and brinzolamide, 874
    and dorzolamide, 874
    glaucoma, 866, 868, 869*t*, 871, 874
    and latanoprost, 874
    and travoprost, 874
tinea, 657
tinea cruris, 657
tinea pedis, 657
tinea unguium, 667
tinidazole
    amoebiasis, 580
    gastro-intestinal infections, 580
tiotropium, chronic obstructive pulmonary
    disease, 437
tipranavir, HIV infection, 631*t*, 635
tirofiban, arterial thromboembolism, 386
tissue factor (TF), 91
tissue plasminogen activator, stroke, 153
tizanidine, pain, 527
TNM classification
    prostate cancer, 761
    solid tumours, 822
tobacco use *see* cigarette smoking
tobramycin, hypomagnesaemia, 82
tocilizumab
    anaemia of chronic disease, 774
    rheumatoid arthritis, 842
tolcapone
    hepatotoxicity, 234
    Parkinson's disease, 513
tolterodine, urinary incontinence, 157
tonic clonic convulsions, 491
tonography, glaucoma, 863
tonometry, glaucoma, 863
topical preparations

absorption in children, 136
in inflammatory bowel disease, 193
pruritus in liver disease, 246.
see also specific drugs
topiramate, 495*t*, 496
    adverse effects, 500*t*, 503
    drug interactions, 499*t*
    epilepsy, 503
    pharmacokinetics, 44
    plasma concentration-response relationship, 44
torasemide, chronic heart failure, 338, 339*t*
torrential venous haemorrhage, 243
torsade de pointes, 50, 57, 370
    gender risk, 65
total cholesterol (TC), 389
    and age, 390
    and cardiovascular disease, 389–390
    optimal, 389*t*
total iron binding capacity (TIBC), 88*t*, 93
tourniquets, 603
toxic epidermal necrolysis (TEN), 66
    clinical features, 886–887
    drug-induced, 886–887, 887*b*
toxic multinodular goitre, 674, 676
toxins, gastro-intestinal infections, 575
toxoplasmosis, HIV infection, 643
trace elements, 102, 102*t*, 106
tracheal route of administration, 124
tramadol, analgesia, 523, 523*t*
trandolapril, chronic heart failure, 340*t*
tranexamic acid, menorrhagia, 720, 720*t*
transaminases
    liver function tests, 84, 86
    see also alanine transaminase (ALT); aspartate
        transaminase (AST)
transcutaneous electrical nerve stimulation (TENS)
    analgesia, 527
    dysmenorrhoea, 718
    osteoarthritis, 845
    rheumatoid arthritis, 834–835
trans fats, 400
transferrin, 88*t*, 93
transient insomnia, 451
transjugular intrahepatic portosystemic shunting
    (TIPS)
    ascites, 247, 247*f*
    oesophageal varices, 250
transmitter abnormality model, schizophrenia, 480
transurethral resection of the prostate (TURP),
    758
tranylcypromine, depression, 471
Traub and Johnson equation, 144
traveller's diarrhoea, 214, 579
travoprost
    glaucoma, 864, 865, 866, 868*t*, 874
    and timolol, 874
trazodone, depression, 472
Tredaptive©, 407
tremor, Parkinson's disease, 508
triamcinolone, rheumatoid arthritis, 839
triamcinolone acetonide, gout, 854
triamterene, hyperkalaemia, 80
triazoles, fungal infections in compromised host, 663
Trichophyton, 657
tricyclic antidepressants
    absorption, 52
    affective disorders, 466
    anxiety disorders, 461
    depression, 469, 470
    distribution, 53
    interactions, 475*t*
    neuropathic pain, 530
    pain, 525–526
    Parkinson's disease, 514

postherpetic neuralgia, 529
teratogenicity, 741*t*
trientine, Wilson's disease, 252
trifluoperazine, schizophrenia, 483*t*
Trifolium pratense, 59
trigeminal neuralgia, 529
triglycerides, 389*t*, 391–392
tri-iodothyronine (T₃), 669, 670
  hypothyroidism, 672
  replacement therapy, 672
  thyroid function testing, 672
trimethoprim
  bacteriuria of pregnancy, 570
  cholera, 579–580
  diarrhoea, 217
  gastro-intestinal infections, 579
  Pneumocystis jiroveci pneumonia, 638
  urinary tract infections, 566, 567, 568, 568*t*, 569
trimipramine, depression, 470
triptan drugs, migraine, 531
triptorelin, prostate cancer, 762
Trizivir©, 628*t*
troglitazone, 234, 703
tropism testing, HIV infection, 625
troponins, 87, 321
Truelove and Witts criteria, 192, 192*t*
Truvada©, 628*t*
tuberculin testing, 611–612
tuberculosis, 201, 608–620
  aetiology, 608
  awareness of, 610–611
  bacterial characteristics, 612–613
  BCG vaccine, 608, 617
  bone and joint, 614
  case studies, 559, 618*b*
  chemoprophylaxis, 617
  clinical aspects, 608–609
  definition, 608
  diagnosis, 610–612
    in people with HIV, 612
  directly observed therapy, 617–618
  drug-resistant, 608, 609, 615
  epidemiology, 609–610, 610*t*
  in HIV infection, 609, 612, 643–644
  incubation period, 609
  investigations, 611–612
  latent, 609
  meningeal, 614
  miliary (disseminated), 608–609, 614
  patient care, 617–619
  pericardial, 614
  of peripheral lymph nodes, 614
  public health action, 612
  pulmonary (respiratory), 609, 613
  risk groups, 609
  symptoms, 610–611
  transmission, 609
  treatment, 612–616
    adverse reactions, 615–616, 616*t*
    dosage, 613*t*
    drugs, 612
    monitoring, 615
    regimens, 613–614
    in special circumstances, 614–615
  urinary tract, 562
tuberculous meningitis, 591–592
  diagnosis, 586–587
  presentation, 586
tubuloglomerular feedback (TGF), 263
tumour lysis syndrome, 813–814, 813*t*
tumour markers, 87–88, 821, 822*t*
tumour necrosis factor alpha (TNF-α), 199
tumour necrosis factor alpha (TNF-α) antagonists
  see anti-TNF agents

tumours, solid, 818–831
  aetiology, 818–819
  case studies, 828*b*
  cellular level, 820–821, 820*f*, 821*f*
  clinical assessment, 821–822
  diagnosis, 821
  drug-induced hepatic, 227, 228
  epidemiology, 818
  growth, 820, 821*f*
  performance status, 822, 822*b*
  presentation, 821
  prevention, 819–820
  prognostic factors, 822, 822*t*
  screening, 819
  spread, 820–821
  staging classification, 822
  staging investigations, 821
  targeted therapies, 825
  treatment, 822–823
    chemotherapy *see* chemotherapy
    goals, 822–823
    guidelines, 823
    methods, 823
    radiotherapy, 823
    surgery, 823
  tumour markers, 821, 822*t*
tumour suppressor genes, 820
turmeric, 59
tyramine, 471
  interactions, 58

U

ubiquitin-proteasome system, 507–508
UK Prospective Diabetes Study Group, 299
ulcerative colitis
  acute severe disease, 190
  case studies, 205, 206, 207
  clinical features, 189–191
  definition, 185
  drug treatment
    aminosalicylates, 196
    biologic agents, 199, 200, 201
  epidemiology, 185
  eyes, 191
  fish oils, 202
  genetic factors, 186
  hepatobiliary, 191
  and infection, 186
  joints and bones, 190
  location and distribution, 187*f*, 187*t*, 188
  moderately active disease, 190
  and primary sclerosing cholangitis, 241
  proctitis, 190
  remission, 192
  skin, 190–191
  and smoking, 186
  surgical treatment, 204
  toxic dilatation, 190
  vs. Crohn's disease, 189*t*
ultrasonography
  chronic kidney disease, 282
  deep vein thrombosis, 378
  liver disease, 244
  prostate cancer, 760
  prostatic, 755, 760
unfractioned heparin
  adverse effects, 379
  venous thromboembolism, 379, 380, 380*b*
unipolar disorder, 465
unlicensed medicines for children, 145
unlicensed prescribing, 18, 19*b*
uraemia, 259, 261
  in chronic kidney disease, 278

  dietary modification, 285
  and intravascular volume overload, 263–264
uraemic gastro-intestinal erosions, 264–265
URAT-1 transporter, 850
urea, 77*t*, 83
  in acute kidney injury, 265
  in chronic kidney disease, 274–275
  extracellular fluid osmolality, 77
  liver function tests, 86
urea breath tests, *Helicobacter pylori*, 166–167
ureidopenicillins, cystic fibrosis, 556*t*
urethra, menopausal changes, 726
urethral syndrome, 561, 568, 725
uric acid, 84, 849
uricase, 849
uricolytic agents, 856–857
uricostatic agents, 855–856
uricosuric agents, 856
urinary incontinence, 156–157
urinary pH changes, 56
urinary tract
  abnormalities, 563
  in chronic kidney disease, 277–278
  diseases *see* urinary tract diseases
  infections *see* urinary tract infections (UTIs)
  tuberculosis, 562
urinary tract diseases
  causing chronic kidney disease, 276–277
  chronic pyelonephritis, 277
  extrinsic renal tract obstruction, 277
  reflux disease, 276
  renal stone disease, 276
urinary tract infections (UTIs), 561–572
  in adults, 562, 563
  aetiology, 562
  in babies and infants, 561, 563
  in benign prostatic hyperplasia, 754
  case studies, 570*b*
  in children, 562, 563
  clinical manifestations, 563
  common management problems, 567*t*
  in the elderly, 562, 563
  epidemiology, 561–562
  fungal, 659
  investigations, 563–566
    culture, 565–566
    dipsticks, 564
    microscopy, 564–565
  pathogenesis, 562–563
  prevention and prophylaxis, 570–572
  relapsing, 569
  risk factors, 562
  treatment, 566–570
    acute pyelonephritis, 568–569
    antimicrobial chemotherapy, 566
    bacteriuria of pregnancy, 569–570
    catheter-associated infections, 569
    in children, 568
    duration of, 568
    non-specific treatments, 566
    relapsing UTI, 569
    uncomplicated lower UTI, 567–568
    uncomplicated, 567–568
urine
  culture, 565–566
  midstream sample, 563–564
  testing in chronic kidney disease, 281
urobilinogen, 85
urodynamic studies, benign prostatic hyperplasia, 755
urogenital system
  menopausal changes, 726, 732
  see also urinary tract
urokinase, venous thromboembolism, 385

ursodeoxycholic acid (UDCA)
primary biliary cirrhosis, 252
primary sclerosing cholangitis, 252
pruritus in liver disease, 245, 245*t*
urticaria, drug-induced, 883–884, 883*f*, 884*b*, 889
ustekinumab, psoriasis, 905
uveitis, 191

V

vac A, 164
vaccination *see* immunisations
vaccines, diarrhoea, 215*t*
vaginal candidiasis, 657
presentation, 656
treatment, 656–657
vaginal dryness, 732
valaciclovir, opportunistic infections in HIV, 639*t*
valganciclovir
cytomegalovirus, 644
opportunistic infections in HIV, 639*t*
valproate
distribution, 43
effect on lipoprotein levels, 394*t*
elimination, 43
pharmacokinetics, 43–44, 45*t*
plasma concentration-response relationship, 43
practical implications, 43–44
valproate semisodium, mania, 473
valsartan
chronic heart failure, 340*t*
clinical trials, 302
VALUE study, 302
Vamin®, 98, 99*t*
Vaminolact®, 98, 99*t*
vancomycin
gastro-intestinal infections, 580
infection in neutropenia, 797
meningitis, 589–590, 589*t*, 593, 593*t*
neonates, 125
monitoring in, 129
respiratory distress syndrome, 130
surgical site infection prophylaxis, 604
varenicline
adverse reactions, 74
smoking cessation, 436, 442
variable costs, 117
variceal band ligation, 249–250
variceal bleed, 243
varicose eczema, 895
varicose veins, 918
vascular abnormalities, hepatic, 241
drug-induced, 226*t*, 227
vascular dementia (VaD), 152, 153
vascular endothelial growth factor (VEGF), 825
vasculitis
drug-induced, 889, 889*b*
small-vessel, 258
vasodilators
centrally acting, 303*t*, 307*t*
chronic heart failure, 340*t*
direct-acting, 303*t*, 307*t*
hypertension, 303*t*, 307*t*
in chronic kidney disease, 285
ST elevation myocardial infarction, 324
vasomotor symptoms, menopause, 731–732
vasopressin *see* antidiuretic hormone (ADH)
Vaughan-Williams classification, 366–373
venlafaxine
alternatives to HRT, 731
anxiety disorders, 461
depression, 472
pain, 526

venography, deep vein thrombosis, 378
veno-occlusive disease, 228
venous congestion, 335
venous hypertension, 917–918
venous leg ulcers, 917–919, 918*f*
clinical signs, 918
diagnosis, 918, 918*t*
in the elderly, 156
prevention of recurrence, 919
treatment, 919
venous thromboembolism (VTE), 376–385
aetiology, 376–377
case studies, 387
clinical manifestations, 377–378
diagnosis, 93
epidemiology, 376
hormone replacement therapy, 729, 733–734, 733*t*, 734*b*
investigations, 378
oral contraceptives risk, 715
patient care, 385
recommended target international normalised ratios, 382*t*
treatment, 378–385
fibrinolytic drugs, 384–385
fondaparinux, 380
heparinoids, 380
heparins, 379–380, 380*b*
hirudins, 380
oral anticoagulants, 381–384
prophylaxis, 379
ventilation-perfusion scanning, pulmonary embolism, 378
ventricular fibrillation, 321, 364–365
ventricular tachyarrhythmias, 364–365
emergency management, 365
ongoing management, 365
ventricular tachycardia, 364
complicating structural heart disease, 364
normal heart, 364
verapamil
adverse effects, 156, 301, 349, 367*t*
arrhythmias, 359, 361, 371
hypertension, 156, 301
in chronic kidney disease, 283
pharmacokinetics, 150, 368*t*, 371
stable angina, 319
verbal rating scales, 520
verotoxin-producing *Escherichia coli* (VTEC), 133–134
verotoxins, gastro-intestinal infections, 575
very low birth weight (VLBW), 124
very low-density lipoprotein cholesterol (VLDL-C), 390
menopause, 727
metabolism, 390
Vibrio sp., 214
gastro-intestinal infections, 574*t*, 576*t*
treatment, 578
Videx©, 628*t*
vigabatrin
adverse effects, 500*t*, 503
epilepsy, 495*t*, 496, 503
pharmacokinetics, 44, 498*t*
plasma concentration-response relationship, 44
vildagliptin, 704
vinblastine
Hodgkin's lymphoma, 804, 805, 807*t*
Kaposi's sarcoma, 645
vincristine
acute lymphoblastic leukaemia, 790, 791
Hodgkin's lymphoma, 805
non-Hodgkin's lymphoma, 809, 811, 812
Viracept©, 631*t*

viral hepatitis, 239
biochemical tests, 244
see also specific viruses
viral load, HIV infection, 625
viral meningitis
aetiology, 585
diagnosis, 586–587
epidemiology, 585
presentation, 586
treatment, 592
Viramune©, 630*t*
Viread©, 628*t*
viruses/viral infections
in atopic eczema, 894
diarrhoea, 214
gastro-intestinal infections, 573, 574*t*, 576*t*, 578
in HIV infection, 644
leukaemia risk, 787
liver disease, 239–240
and lymphomas, 807
treatment, 578
visceral muscle function, in geriatrics, 151
visual aids
adverse drug reactions, 72, 73*f*
communicating benefits/risks of treatment, 24
visual analogue scales, 118, 520
vital capacity (VC), 435
vital signs, paediatric, 143*t*
vitamin A, 107
vitamin B_{12}
anticoagulant therapy monitoring, 93–95
serum, 88*t*
vitamin B_{12} deficiency anaemia
aetiology, 776
case study, 785
clinical manifestations, 777
epidemiology, 776
investigations, 777–778
pathophysiology, 776–777
patient care, 779
treatment, 778–779
vitamin C
with iron, 775
stability, 107
vitamin D, 81
deficiency, 82, 94, 279
in chronic kidney disease, 287–288
hypoparathyroidism/hypocalcaemia, 680, 681*t*
osteoporosis, 154
and parenteral nutrition, 102–103
premenstrual syndrome, 714
vitamin D analogues, psoriasis, 902
vitamin E, 107
vitamin K, 246
vitamin K-dependent bleeding *see* haemorrhagic disease of the newborn
vitamin K epoxide reductase (VKOR), 66
vitamin(s)
adult reference range, 103*t*
dysmenorrhoea, 718
fat-soluble, 102
parenteral nutrition, 102–103
and premenstrual syndrome, 714
stability, 107
water-soluble, 102.
see also specific vitamins
volume of distribution (V_d), 33–34, 33*f*
vomiting *see* nausea and vomiting
vomiting centre, 535, 536
vomiting reflex, 536

von Willebrand factor, 91
voriconazole
    absorption, 52
    administration, 665
    adverse effects, 665
    candidiasis, 657
    clinical use, 665
    fungal infections in compromised host, 665
    infection in neutropenia, 797
    meningitis, 592
    pharmacokinetics, 664t, 665
vulnerability model, schizophrenia, 480

W

waist measurement, dyslipidaemia, 399–400
warfarin
    absorption, 52
    action, 381
    adverse effects, 66, 74, 381
    atrial fibrillation, 363
    distribution, 53
        in the elderly, 150
    drug interactions, 177, 383t
    effects, 381
    in the elderly, 152
    interactions, 58, 59, 61, 74
    management of bleeding, 384t
    metabolism, 66, 381
    stroke, 154
    stroke prevention in atrial fibrillation, 362,
        363
    suggested induction schedule, 384t
    venous thromboembolism, 381–382, 384t,
        387
warm autoimmune haemolytic anaemia
        (WAIHA), 779–780
water
    balance, 76–79, 77f, 77t
    depletion, 77–78, 94
    excess, 78
    and extracellular fluid osmolality, 78
    parenteral nutrition, 97–98
    total body water, 137, 137t

Wegener's granulomatosis, 258
weight, children, 134–135
weight gain
    antipsychotics, 486
    menopause, 727
weight loss
    ascites in liver disease, 246
    in diabetes mellitus, 698
    in liver disease, 242
white blood cell count, 88t, 90, 90f
    basophils, 90
    eosinophils, 90
    lymphocytes, 90
    monocytes, 90
    neutrophils, 90
white blood cells, 770
white coat hypertension, 297
WHO see World Health Organization (WHO)
widespread cutaneous necrosis, 889
willingness to accept, 117–118
willingness to pay, 117–118
Wilson's disease, 241, 252–254
Wolff-Chaikoff effect, 679
Wolff-Parkinson-White pattern, 360, 361f
women
    adverse drug reactions, 65
    HIV infection, 646–648
    see also gender
Working formulation, non-Hodgkin's lymphoma,
        808
World Health Organization (WHO)
    adverse drug reactions definition, 63
    causality categories for adverse drug reactions,
        69, 69t
    make medicines child size programme, 146
wounds, 910–925
    assessment, 915, 915f
    case studies, 923b
    healing, 910–915, 911f
        factors affecting, 913–915, 913t
        moist, 912
        phases of, 911, 912, 912f
        by primary intention, 911, 911f
        by secondary intention, 911, 911f

management principles, 921–925, 922b
    skin structure, 910, 910t
    see also surgical site infection
WWHAM, 5–6, 6b

X

xanthine oxidase, 61, 84, 849, 855
xanthochromia, 93

Y

yeasts, 654–655, 655t
Yellow Card Scheme, 69–70, 71
Yerks Dodson curve, 454f
Yersinia, 214

Z

zafirlukast, asthma, 419
zaleplon, insomnia, 448t, 450
zanamivir, influenza, 546
Zerit©, 628t
Zevalin®, non-Hodgkin's lymphoma, 811
Ziagen©, 628t
zidovudine, HIV infection, 628t, 635
zinc
    acute kidney injury, 265
    adult daily reference range, 102t
    deficiency, 101–102
    diarrhoea, 218
    Wilson's disease, 252
ziprasidone, schizophrenia, 483t
Zollinger-Ellison syndrome, 163, 169
zolpidem, insomnia, 448t, 449–450
zonisamide, 495t
    adverse effects, 500t, 503
    drug interactions, 499t
    epilepsy, 503
    pharmacokinetics, 498t
zopiclone, insomnia, 448t, 449
zotepine, schizophrenia, 483t
zuclopenthixol, schizophrenia, 483t
zygomycosis, 658t, 660t